Organ of the International Association of Gero

AF887558

Gerontology

International Journal of Experimental, Clinical and Behavioural Gerontology

Founded 1957 by F. Verzàr as 'Gerontologia',
merged 1975 with 'Gerontologia Clinica',
founded 1959 by E. Woodford-Williams and A.N. Exton-Smith

KARGER

Appears bimonthly:
1 volume per year
(6 issues)

Gerontology

Guidelines for Authors

Gerontology publishes manuscripts on all aspects of experimental, clinical, and behavioural science research into the aging process. It accepts particularly high-quality, original research papers in all disciplines of gerontological research.

Gerontology welcomes those submissions which represent a conceptual advance or an original approach to the understanding of the molecular or behavioural basis of aging. From the clinical angle we would like papers of general interest submitted concerning the aetiology, pathogenesis, prevention and treatment of diseases or abnormalities of the elderly. Papers in the fields of neuroscience, cardiology, infectious disease and immunology, cancer, and epidemiology, to name just a few subjects of interest, will find a place in *Gerontology*, as will those reflecting current developments in the behavioural sciences.
In the section 'Reviews', themes of general interest including nutrition, longevity, psychology, demography, socioeconomic problems in old age such as health-care financing, benefits and risks of physical exercise, and normal and abnormal aging are welcome.

Studies on drugs, e.g. double-blind trials, are already covered by most of the other gerontology journals and are therefore *not considered* for publication in *Gerontology.*
Experimental papers dealing with *mechanisms of developmental phenomena* and which are not related to changes due to old age are not of interest for *Gerontology*.
Authors should indicate whether they wish their article to be considered for the Experimental, Clinical or Behavioural Science section. Manuscripts may be submitted in the following categories:

Review Articles
Original Research Papers/Experimental Section
Original Research Papers/Clinical Section
Original Research Papers/Behavioural Science Section
Debate
Short Communications
Letters to the Editor
Book Reviews
Announcements

Submission

Only original papers written in English are considered and should be sent to:

Prof. Dr. W. Meier-Ruge
Institut für Pathologie der Universität Basel
Gerontologische Forschung
Schönbeinstrasse 40
CH–4003 Basel (Switzerland)

Manuscripts from North America should be sent to:

Donald K. Ingram, PhD
National Institute on Aging
National Institutes on Health
Gerontology Research Center
5600 Nathan Shock Drive
Baltimore, MD 21224 (USA)

Tel. (410) 558 8180
Fax (410) 558 8323
E-Mail doni@vax.grc.nia.nih.gov

Only manuscripts that conform with the Guidelines for Authors will be considered.

Manuscripts should be submitted in triplicate (with three sets of illustrations of which one is an original), typewritten double-spaced on one side of the paper, with a wide margin.

***A statement signed by all authors* saying that they agree with the publication of the paper should accompany the manuscript.**

Original Research Papers must describe new research results, not published or under consideration in another journal. Note: **A maximum of *six authors* is allowed.** All papers should be arranged with an Introduction, Methods, Results and Discussion. An exception is made for Reviews and Debate articles. Abbreviations should be explained and limited to a minimum. All terms abbreviated in the text, abstract and in the figures must, on the first occasion, be given in full, followed by the abbreviation (e.g. electrocardiogram (ECG)). Any papers dealing, partly or wholly, with basic science should include a few lines of description to any concept which may not be well known to some readers who are primarily practising clinicians.

Critical Reviews are either invited by the Editors, or may be submitted for consideration. Invited reviews, if accepted, are not subject to page charges.

The *Debate* Section publishes arguments, critical statements and theoretical papers reflecting the authors' views on mechanisms of the aging process at all levels of biological and medical organization and clinical matters of general interest and controversy.

The *Short Communications* Section is reserved mainly for case reports. Short Communications may be limited to two printed pages.

Letters addressed to the Editor are encouraged if they directly concern articles previously published in this journal and clinical subjects related to the matters discussed. The editor reserves the right to submit copies of such letters to the authors of the articles concerned prior to publication in order to permit them to respond in the same issue of the journal. But letters on general scientific or medical subjects in gerontology are also welcome. Letters to the Editor should be no longer than one printed page.

Disk submission

Do not send a disk before the paper is accepted for publication. The accepted manuscript must match the file on disk exactly. For details, refer to 'Disk Submission' or www.karger.com/journals/disksub.htm. Copy-editing will be executed from the disk version of your manuscript.

Conditions

All manuscripts are subject to editorial review. Manuscripts are received with the explicit understanding that they are not under simultaneous consideration by any other publication or have not already been published. Submission of an article for publication implies the transfer of the copyright from the author to the publisher upon acceptance. Accepted papers become the permanent property of *Gerontology* and may not be reproduced by any means, in whole or in part, without the written consent of the publisher. It is the author's responsibility to obtain permission to reproduce illustrations, tables, etc. from other publications.

Arrangement

Title page: The first page of each paper should indicate the title without any abbreviations, the authors' names, and the institute where the work was conducted. **A short title** for use as running head is also required. The title should adequately describe in the fewest possible words the content of the paper. Avoid abbreviations or jargon.

Full address: The exact postal address complete with postal code must be given at the bottom of the title page. Please also supply phone and fax numbers, as well as your e-mail address.

Key words: For indexing purposes, a list of 3–7 key words (no abbreviations) in English is needed.

Each *Abstract* should be structured as follows:

Background: What prompted the study?
Objective: What is the purpose of the study?
Methods: How was the study carried out?
Results: What are the most important findings?
Conclusion: What is the most important conclusion?

The abstract should not exceed 350 words, and any abbreviations must be explained.

Small type: Paragraphs which can or must be set in smaller type (case histories, test methods, etc.) should be indicated with a 'p' (petit) in the left-hand margin.

Footnotes: Avoid footnotes. When essential, they are numbered consecutively and typed at the foot of the appropriate page.

Tables and illustrations: Tables and illustrations (both numbered in Arabic numerals) should be prepared on separate sheets. Tables require a heading and figure legends should be supplied on a separate sheet. For the reproduction of illustrations, only good drawings and original photographs will be accepted; negatives or photocopies cannot be used. Due to technical reasons, figures with a screen background should not be submitted. When possible, group several illustrations on one block for reproduction (max. size 181 × 223 mm) or provide crop marks. On the back of each illustration, indicate its number, the author's name, and 'top' with a soft pencil.

KARGER

Fax +41 61 306 12 34
E-Mail karger@karger.ch

The Guidelines for Authors are available at:
www.karger.com/journals/ger/ger_gl.htm

Color illustrations: Up to 6 color illustrations per page can be integrated within the text at the reduced price of CHF 660.– / USD 545.00 per page. Color illustrations are reproduced at the author's expense.

References: Identify references in the text with Arabic numerals [in square brackets]. Material submitted for publication but not yet accepted should be noted as 'unpublished data' and not be included in the reference list. The list of references should include only those publications cited in the text. Do not alphabetize; number references in the order in which they are first mentioned in the text. The surnames of the authors followed by initials should be given. There should be no punctuation other than a comma to separate the authors. Cite all authors, 'et al.' is not sufficient. Abbreviate journal names according to the Index Medicus system. (Also see International Committee of Medical Journal Editors: Uniform requirements for manuscripts submitted to biomedical journals. N Engl J Med 1997;336:309–315.)

Examples
(a) Papers published in periodicals: Sun J, Koto H, Chung KF: Interaction of ozone and allergen challenges on bronchial responsiveness and inflammation in sensitised guinea pigs. Int Arch Allergy Immunol 1997;112:191–195.
(b) Monographs: Matthews DE, Farewell VT: Using and Understanding Medical Statistics, ed 3, revised. Basel, Karger, 1996.
(c) Edited books: Parren PWHI, Burton DR: Antibodies against HIV-1 from phage display libraries: Mapping of an immune response and progress towards antiviral immunotherapy; in Capra JD (ed): Antibody Engineering. Chem Immunol. Basel, Karger, 1997, vol 65, pp 18–56.

Page charges
There are no page charges for papers of up to 4 printed pages (i.e., 12 typewritten pages at 33 lines per page, 65 strokes per line, including tables, illustrations and references). Each additional complete or partial page is charged to the author at CHF 275.– / USD 196.00.

Galley proofs
Unless indicated otherwise, galley proofs are sent to the first-named author and should be returned with the least possible delay. Alterations made in galley proofs, other than the correction of printer's errors, are charged to the author. No page proofs are supplied.

Reprints
Order forms and a price list are sent with the galley proofs. Orders submitted after the issue is printed are subject to considerably higher prices.

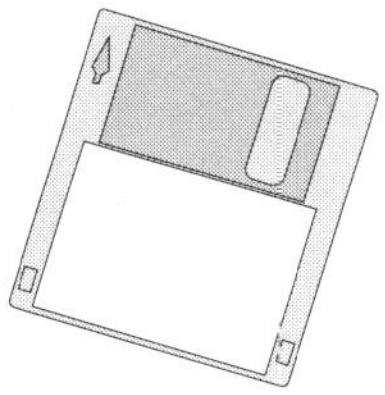

Disk Submission

A **comprehensive version** of these guidelines for the **submission of manuscripts and illustrations on disk** can be accessed online under **www.karger.com/journals/disksub.htm** or requested as a leaflet from the editorial department.

Please follow the general rules on style and arrangement in the **'Guidelines for Authors'** of the journal. Submit a **double-spaced printout** of your manuscript matching the file on disk exactly.

Technical Information
Store only data pertinent to this manuscript. Include your fonts (screen and printer fonts for Macintosh).
For a **text only** manuscript, use a 3.5-inch disk. For **text and illustrations,** use 3.5 or 5.25 Magneto Optical Disc; CD-ROM (DOS or hybrid); iomage Zip/DOS (100 MB), or 44 MB, 88 MB or 200 MB SyQuest. Compress extensive data using ZIP format.

Data Description
Label your disk with the **title of the journal or book** for which it is submitted; a **short version** of the paper's title; your **name,** postal and e-mail address, fax and phone number; **hard and software** used, including the version; and the **complete list of the file names.** File names consist of eight characters before the dot identifying the file and three characters after the dot identifying the application.

Text and Format
The **preferred word-processing package is MS-Word.** Other commonly used PC text programs and ASCII formats are accepted.
Update your data when you revise subsequent to the reviewer's or editor's decision and mark revisions clearly. Manuscripts accepted for publication are subject to **copy editing:** changes and/or questions will be marked in the manuscript, which will be returned to you with your disk and the galley proofs for checking.
Enter your text continuously flush left. Do not use any layout functions. Do not split words at the end of a line. **Do not use indentations.** Use a blank line before and a hard return at the end of paragraphs.
Arrange headings flush left. Insert only **one space after punctuation marks.** Insert Greek letters, mathematical symbols etc. with your word-processing program. Use **boldface and italics** as well as sub- and superscript where appropriate.
Tables are part of the text and should be placed at the end of the text file. Separate the individual parts of a table by lines. Use the tabulator instead of spaces. Format operation data on one line in the same column. **Legends to illustrations are part of the text** and should also be listed at the end of the text file.

Illustrations
Store illustrations as separate files: do not integrate them in your text. Export **line drawings/vector graphics** as TIF, EPS or WMF format. Use Photoshop for processing and retouching **scanned halftone images.** Save the original scan and the processed version. Export **black and white or color images** as TIF or EPS format in their anticipated size in print.
For detailed information on how to submit illustration data on disk please consult the leaflet or **www.karger.com/journals/disksub.htm.**

KI 98 DISK

KARGER

Fax + 41 61 306 12 34
E-Mail karger@karger.ch
www.karger.com

The Journal Home Page is available at:
www.karger.com/journals/ger

General Information

Gerontology

Publication data: 'Gerontology' is published 6 times a year. Volume 47 with 6 issues appears in 2001.

Subscription rates: Subscriptions run for a full calendar year. Prices are given per volume.
Personal subscription:
Subscription + postage and handling
CHF 386.– + CHF 27.40 Europe
CHF 386.– + CHF 40.80 Overseas
USD 297.00 + USD 27.40
+ online subscription per volume:
CHF 39.– / USD 30.00
(Must be in the name of, billed to, and paid by an individual. Order must be marked 'personal subscription'.)
Institutional subscription:
Subscription + postage and handling
CHF 772.– + CHF 34.20 Europe
CHF 772.– + CHF 51.– Overseas
USD 594.00 + USD 34.20
+ online subscription per volume:
CHF 58.– / USD 45.00
Airmail postage: CHF 36.–, USD 30.00. (Extra per volume.)
Discount subscription prices:
Int. Ass. of Gerontology; British Geriatric Society; Gerontological Soc.; American Geriatric Society.

Advertising: Correspondence and rate requests should be addressed to the Publisher.

Microforms: Please direct all enquiries and orders to:
University Microfilms Inc.
300 North Zeeb Road, P.O. Box 1346
Ann Arbor, MI 48106-1346 (USA)

Subscription orders: Orders can be placed at agencies, bookstores, directly with the Publisher
S. Karger AG, P.O. Box
CH–4009 Basel (Switzerland)
or with any of the following distributors:
Deutschland: S. Karger GmbH, Postfach
D–79095 Freiburg
France: Librairie Luginbühl
36, bd de Latour-Maubourg, F–75007 Paris
Great Britain, Ireland: S. Karger Publishers
58 Grove Hill Road
Tunbridge Wells, Kent TN1 1SP, UK
USA: S. Karger Publishers, Inc.
26 West Avon Road, P.O. Box 529
Farmington, CT 06085, USA
India, Bangladesh, Sri Lanka:
Panther Publishers Private Ltd.
39, 6th Cross
Wilson Gardens
Bangalore 560 027, India
Japan: Katakura Libri, Inc.
2F, Marushima Bldg, 4-6-17, Yushima,
Bunkyo-ku, Tokyo 113-0034, Japan

Change of address: Both old and new address should be sent to the subscription source.

Single issues and back volumes: Information can be obtained through the Publisher.

Bibliographic indices: This journal is regularly listed in bibliographic services, including *Current Contents®*.

Copying: This journal has been registered with the Copyright Clearance Center (CCC), as indicated by the code appearing on the first page of each article.
For readers in the US, this code signals consent for copying of articles for personal or internal use, or for the personal or internal use of specific clients, provided that the stated fee is paid per copy directly to
Copyright Clearance Center, Inc.
222 Rosewood Drive
Danvers, MA 01923 (USA)
A copy of the first page of the article must accompany payment. Consent does not extend to copying for general distribution, for promotion, for creating new works, or for resale. In these cases, specific written permission must be obtained from the copyright owner,
S. Karger AG
P.O. Box
CH–4009 Basel (Switzerland).

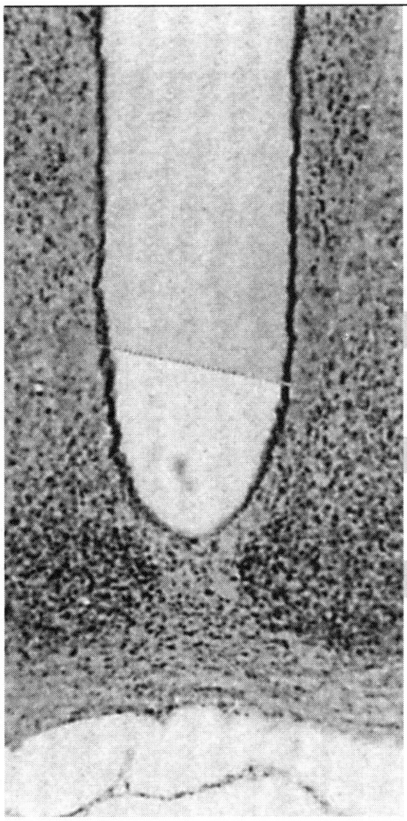

Gerontology

Abstracts

17th World Congress of Gerontology
Vancouver, Canada, July 1–6, 2001

Editors
Gloria M. Gutman, PhD
Andrew V. Wister, PhD
Norman Samaroo, Dip.Gero

KARGER

Basel · Freiburg · Paris · London · New York ·
New Delhi · Bangkok · Singapore · Tokyo · Sydney

ABSTRACTS

Abstracts are arranged numerically by session number

AUTHOR INDEX

Numbers refer to sessions not pages.

ABSTRACT REVIEWERS

Maureen Gorman, PhD
Gloria M. Gutman, PhD
Samuel J. Gutman, MD,
Sandra Hirst, PhD
Belinda McIntosh, BSN
Carol McWilliam, PhD
Carl Taillon, MD
Andrew Wister, PhD

S. Karger
Medical and Scientific Publishers
Basel · Freiburg · Paris · London
New York · New Delhi · Bangkok
Singapore · Tokyo · Sydney

Drug Dosage
The authors and the publisher have exerted every effort to ensure that drug selection and dosage set forth in this text are in accord with current recommendations and practice at the time of publication. However, in view of ongoing research, changes in government regulations, and the constant flow of information relating to drug therapy and drug reactions, the reader is urged to check the package insert for each drug for any change in indications and dosage and for added warnings and precautions. This is particularly important when the recommended agent is a new and/or infrequently employed drug.

P.O. Box, CH–4009 Basel (Switzerland)
ISBN 3–8055–7293–X

Printed in Canada on acid-free paper
by Mitchell Press Limited.

KARGER

Fax + 41 61 306 12 34
E-Mail karger@karger.ch
www.karger.com

SESSION 3

[1] The 80+ Studies: Lund, Reykjavik and Fredericton Longitudinal Studies on Aging

T. Svensson (Gerontology Research Center, Lund, Sweden), J.E. Jónsson (University Hospital, Reykjavik, Iceland), W.L. Randall (Gerontology Program, St. Thomas University, Fredericton, NB, Canada)

The 80+ Studies is the overhead title for the three projects: Lund 80+, Sweden, Reykjavik 80+, Iceland, and Fredericton 80+, Canada. The projects are all longitudinal, use sequential design, are multisdisciplinary, and use the same core protocols concerning some 450 variables. The fact that the study is conducted in three countries with exactly the same set-up gives the unique possibility for researching the cultural influences on aging in advanced age. The study was initiated in Lund in 1988, was expanded to Reykjavik in 1993 and to Fredericton in 1998. The projects study the aging process from age 80 and on. The first cohort to be included at the different sites, in Lund born 1908, in Reykjavik born 1913 and in Fredericton born 1918, are examined once every year until all subjects have died. New cohorts are included and examined every five years i.e. there are now 3 cohorts in Lund, 2 in Reykjavik and 1 in Fredericton under study. The design allows for the study of both aging and cohort effects, and as the cohorts coincide in the three sites cross-cultural differences and similarities can be studied as to their effects on the aging process. The protocols include medical, psychological and social aspects of aging using questionnaires, tests, medical examinations, EKG's and blood samples. The design and methods will be presented and discussed as well as some cross-cultural comparisons.

[2] Images of Aging in India

V. Burholt (Centre for Social Policy Research and Development, Institute of Medical and Social Care Research, University of Wales, Bangor, United Kingdom), G. C. Wenger (Centre for Social Policy Research and Development, Institute of Medical and Social Care Research, University of Wales, Bangor, United Kingdom)

This photographic display presents images of aging in rural and urban areas of Gujarat, India. The intention is to allow the audience to make a comparison between representations of ageing in India and the roles and perceptions of aging associated with their own country. The tradition in India is to live in multi-generation households. Sons remain at home, while daughters marry and move in with and are considered members of their husband's family. Photographs present older people living in multi-generation households ranging in size, with one older person living in a household containing fourteen members. It is possible to compare the differences in the wealth of households, especially with regard to the difference that migration makes to the household income. One picture shows a women who is financially better off than people in other villages and those in her own village who did not have children living abroad. In the context of the multi-generation household, older people continue to contribute to the domestic routine for as long as they are able. Pictures depict grandparental contributions, food preparation and other domestic chores. Very few older people have any pension rights. In addition to domestic contributions many older people continue to work as retirement is not an option, except for the minority whose children are wealthy enough to support them. The pictures show a continuum of affluence, from those working as part of a family business (laundry), to a widow collecting garbage.

[3] Life's Shipwrecks: Images of Old Age in Brazil (1890-1920)

Groisman, Daniel (Instituto of Social Medicine, University of State of Rio de Janeiro - IMS/UERJ, Rio de Janeiro, Brazil)

Purpose: The focus of our presentation is to analize representations, texts and images of old age that were published in brazilian newspapers from 1890 to 1920. This is part of a greater research focusing on the establishment of institutions for the old in Rio de Janeiro at the and of XIX century and beginning of XX. Method: The idea of a history of old age starts from the premise that the ways in which different age groups are distributed and interpreted by society vary according to period and culture. The survey was made through the analysis of primary sources: documents of the period, newspapers, and others. Results: The advent of this new mode of institution in Brazil - a home for old folks - caused intense social mobilization by focusing on the debate on the need to lend assistance to a new group of socially excluded citizens: the elderly. This was particularly evident in a series of newspaper articles published at the period. Conclusion: Analizing this news, we can understand some of the way that old age was viewed at the time. There was a tendency to create negative and positives stereotypes and exacerbate the drama of the elderly, in order to justify the assistance for this people.

[4] The Aging of the Population in China: Basic Countermeasures

Zhang Wenfan (China National Committee on Aging, Beijing, China)

The paper will discuss the development trend of the aging of population in China and the reasons for the population. Further, the author discusses the implications of the aging of population to the economic and social development of China. Lastly, the author discusses the policies options and recommendations to the aging of population in China.

[5] The Aging of the Population in China: National Policy

Zhang Yaqun (Gerontological Society of China, Beijing, China)

This paper will discuss the current status and the future development of the aging of population in China and its characteristics as well. Based on the discussion of the aging development, the author would further discuss on the possible policies to the aging of population and the elderly in China.

[6] Coping with Population Aging in China: A National Strategy

Xiong Bijun (Institute of Gerontology Studies, Chinese Academy of Social Sciences)

China's elderly population aged 60 and over is growing faster than the world, it will pose considerable challenge to public policies, especially in supporting the aged. Population aging in China starts under conditions of a less developed economy; that is, to solve the contradiction between the process of aging and economic development is a major problem to be coped with in meeting aging challenge. Aging rapidly in China will raise the dependency ratio of the aged and lead increasing expenditures for the aged. The basic measures to solve these problems in China are as follow: to establish a social support system, to keep the function of family in supporting the elderly, to encourage the social participation of the elderly and to improve the community-base social services for the elderly.

[7] Marital Status and Households of the Aged in Eastern Europe: A Cross-National Comparison.

T. Koropeckyj-Cox (Sociology Department, University of Florida, USA), E.M. Agree (Population and Family Health, Johns Hopkins School of Public Health, Baltimore, USA), N. Botev (Population Activities Unit, U.N. Economic Commission for Europe, Geneva, Switzerland).

The economic and political transitions in Eastern Europe are taking place within a uniquely challenging demographic environment. Historical patterns of low fertility, war casualties, and stagnant life expectancies in Eastern Europe are reflected in aging populations with highly imbalanced gender ratios and a preponderance of unmarried women in old age. This paper presents a cross-national comparison of the living arrangements of older men and women in six European countries (Bulgaria, Czech Republic, Estonia, Latvia, Lithuania, and Romania). Using data from census microdata samples (prepared by the U.N. E.C.E.) from an early point in the current transitions, we provide (1) a comparative portrait of the marital status, gender, and age distributions of older adults in these countries; and (2) an examination of the relative household well-being (e.g, income, dwelling size, household amenities) of older men and women. We also use multinomial logit models to examine the relationship between marital status, living arrangements, and relative well-being among older persons. The findings highlight the contrast between the living arrangements and well-being of men and women at older ages. Older men at every age are significantly more likely than women to be married and living with a spouse and other relatives. Institutionalization is relatively rare. Large proportions of unmarried women live alone, particularly in the Czech Republic. The relative household well-being of elders and its relation to gender and marital status varies widely among the countries. We discuss the results in terms of their implications for the vulnerability of elders in the context of transition.

[8] Demography of Old Age in the Czech Republic and in its Districts

Z. Kalvach[1-st medical faculty, Charles University, Prague, Czech Republic]

The Czech Republic is expected to rank among the countries with the highest percentage of the elderly in 21st century. Analysis of mortality survival parameters[life expectancy, death probability] for age 0, 65, 75, 65-80 in the Czech Republic since 1899 and in its 76 districts in 5-year periods since 1981. We present rectangularization of survival curves in the 20th century with unusual stagnancy in 1960-1990. Frequency analysis shows long time trends related to ecological changes in industrial areas after 1989. Death probability for the age 65-80[1-[log q80log q65]] seems to be a rather interesting gerontological parameter for longitudinal assessment of demographical trends.

[9] In Recognition of Population aging

Cai Yongqing, (Taiyuan, Shanxi, P.R. China)

Now, the academic circles of the elderly hold that there are two aspects for the problem of the population aging. One is the special demands of the elderly themselves. The other one is a series of social problems which are caused by the constant increase of the aged population. By the investigation, we found that there is another problem, that is, the relationship between the elderly and the society. The above-mentioned study adopts the method of combination of the social investigation and empirical summary, and the achievements of modern gerontology study. The study shows that the existence of the relationship between the elderly and the society is a reality, and it is necessary to solve the problem. It lays stress on the important significance that the elderly blends into the society and takes part in the social development. Conclusion: We must completely recognize the problem of population aging, put the relationship between the elderly and the society in our study and solve the problem of population aging.

[10] China's Family Planning and Population Problems in Relation to Aging

Pu-de Qin (Shanxi Academy of Social Sciences Taiyuan Shanxi china)

China has won great achievements in carrying out the family planning policies which have brought about some negative effects in the meanwhile. That's approaching of population aging. At present, China has to face tremendous pressure and a series of problems. Firstly, lipsidedown-pyramid family structure is changing from 4-2-1 structure into 8-4-2 and quite a few of empty-nest families have come into being. Secondly, problems of providing for the elderly have arisen as a series of problems, such as systems and styles of family-support for the aged. Thirdly, Medical care problems, include medical resources, health care costs and so on. Fourth, the aged reemployment. Fifth, the aged psychological problems. Sixth, community service for the aged and so on. All these problems should get researched as soon as possible and get counter measures to be put forward.

[11] The Aging Population in China: Synthetic Evaluation

Zhou Li-Ping (Population and Development Research Institute, Zhejiang University, Hangzhou, 310028, China) Liu Wen-Han (Zhejiang University of Technology, Hangzhou, 310032, China)

Abstract: China stepped into the aged society at the end of the 20th century. One of the social problems that aging of population leads to is the aging health. The Chinese government is paying more attention to how to improve the aging population health efficiently. Healthy Aging means that the aging population has high quality of life while their life periods prolong. Its purpose is to prolong the aging healthy life period, to make more elderly people have more time to participate in the society's economic activities, and to decrease the negative impacts which aging of population brings about. From the perspectives of sociological, medical and population economics, in this paper, the synthesis evaluation indexes which measuring health quality of the aging population have been putting forward. The contents of the system such as: The physical indexes of the aging include medicine evaluation, ADL, IADL and the states of body health self-evaluation. The psychological indexes of the aging include the status of affection, psychology and cognitive function. The social well-being indexes of the aging include social intercourse, social participation and contribution to the society. By using synthetic evaluation theories, this paper analyzes the status concerning the physical, mental and social well-being of the aging population, and synthetic evaluate the health quality of the aging population in China.

[12] Mortality of the Oldest Old in an Industrial City in Southeast Brazil.

Leticia Marín-León & Marilisa B.A. Barros (State University of Campinas, Campinas, Brazil)

The increasing importance of the oldest old led us to describe the profile of their mortality. Death information from the National Mortality Information System and population data from the State Demographic Office were used to calculate mortality rates from 1980 to 1999. The oldest age group informed by this institution is 75 years and more, thus we could not use the internationally accepted definition of 80 years and more. The socioeconomic differences of the mortality were explored through ecological approach. The mortality rate was studied in 4 homogeneous areas, constructed through the mean of the salary and educational level of the chief of the family in each district of the census. In the study period, the proportional mortality of the oldest old increased, mainly in women, whereas it decreased in the 0-4 group. The trend of the mortality rate indicates a stable risk (around 110 deaths/1.000 men) and showed a small increase in women. Although the leading causes of death did not change, the relative importance of the circulatory diseases diminished and the respiratory diseases augmented. The principal single causes of death in the period 97-99 were pneumonia and acute myocardial infarct, with excess mortality of the male population (1233 versus 966/100000 for pneumonia). Nearly 25% die at home. Although the mortality rate in the poorest area is higher than in the richest, there is no clear trend in the intermediate areas. Further research is needed to analyse inequalities. Public policies should be directed to prevent respiratory infections.

[13] Causes of Death in a Population of Centenarians

L.E. Garcez-Leme; C.R. Carelli; M..M.Amatuzzi.(Hospital das Clínicas da Faculdade de Medicina da Universidade de São Paulo, Brasil)

OBJECTIVE: To study the causes of death in centenarians in São Paulo City, Brazil, METHODS: The authors studied all the death declarations of 1996, finding 76 death declarations of the population over 100 years. RESULTS: This group of centenarians represents 0.1% of the whole number of deaths in São Paulo in 1996 (78.243), with 17 men (22,4%) and 59 women (77.6%). Of these, 47.4% died in his own home, 43% died in hospital and 9.2% in other locations. Distribution of the deaths during the year was regular without preference for any month or season the main causes were related with pneumonia and cardiovascular problems Results are the following: Pneumonia 26.32%; Acute coronary disease 15.8%; Stroke 17.1%; Heart failure 7.9%; Lung diseases other than pneumonia 6.6%; Cancer 6.6%; Malnutrition 5.3%; Infections 5.3%; Arrhythmia 2.7%; Dementia 2.7% and Miscellaneous 7.9%. The results reinforce the necessity of prevention of respiratory infection in this very old population.

[14] The Relation of the Aging Population to Causes of Deaths

Y. Ooe, T. Furukawa, T. Nagakura, H. Kusuoka (Clinical Research Institute, Osaka National Hospital, Osaka, Japan)

Purpose: The number of aged death is increasing to major causes in Japan. And the number of the living elderly is increasing similarly. Whether the aging of population effects on deaths by causes is very important to understand this situation. We investigated the effect on the major causes of death in Japan. Methods: Japanese vital statistics of deaths by causes and age, between 1950 and 1999, were analyzed. The death ratios by causes were compared to the living population at the same age. Malignant neoplasm, heart disease, cerebrovascular disease, pneumonia, tuberculosis, diabetes mellitus, liver disease, accidents and suicide were investigated as major causes of death. Results: According to the vital statistics of Japan, the peak of total deaths by age was shifted to older consistently in this period. And the peak value increased. This was the common trend to the major causes. The increase of death ratios by age was observed in malignant neoplasm, heart disease, cerebrovascular disease, pneumonia and diabetes mellitus. On the other hand, the ratio was decreasing in accidents, suicide, liver disease and tuberculosis. Conclusion: There were two groups of causes. In one group, although the ratio decreased, the number of death increased simply corresponding to the increase of elders. And in the other group, the ratio and the number of death increased.

[15] Longevity in Saint-Petersburg.

L.Lenskaya, (St.Petersburg City Geriatric Centre, Russia)

For all developed countries the propotion of long-living persons in total population is increasing. Modern medical and social aspects of longevity have been studied in Saint-Petersburg. Study was carried out during 1996-1999. Demographic characteristics of longevity in Saint-Petersburg from 1979-1998 have been analyzed. Special groups of centenarians have been selected. In this group some peculiarity nave been marked: absence of oncological pathologies, "disappearing" of some chronic diseases.

[16] Centenarian's History and Historical Background.

K. Kitagawa (Komazawa University, Tokyo, Japan),H. Inagaki, Y. Gondo, Y. Masui (Tokyo Metropolitan Institute of Gerontology, Tokyo, Japan), N. Hirose, Y. Arai, M. Takayama, Y. Ebihara, K. Yamamura, S. Nakazawa (Keio University, Tokyo, Japan), K. Yamashita, H. Shimomura, K. Nishikawa, Y. Lau (Keio Junior college of Nursing, Tokyo, Japan).

Purpose Recently, various researches are performed from the standpoint of clinical psychology, cognitive psychology, development psychology, and healthy psychology to man's growth, development, and aging in psychology. Moreover, the subject of various age groups is used in general in these researches. However, the research by which a history and a historical background of the subject group are examined is very few. This research aimed to examine an educational system, the starting work situation, and the history, and to clarify a history and a historical background of the subject group a dynamic population and educational years. Method The subject is a centinalian of the Tokyo living. Data was Japanese Government, was government and municipal offices, and examined an educational system, a starting work situation, and a historical background by using the publication of Tokyo at the centinalian's dynamic of population and educational years. Result and conclusion The starting work situation was clarified at a survival rate of the centinalian and educational years. In addition, it was clarified that there was a peculiar social, cultural life event to the centinalian who had resided in Tokyo. In a word, examining a history and a historical background of the subject group is thought whether data becomes in the interpretation and become a help of the analysis though is necessary a further examination.

[17] Frailty is a Risk Factor for Mortality in Mexican Elderly People

J.C. García, J.L. Torres, L.M. Gutiérrez-Robledo, S. Villa. (Geriatrics Clinic, National Institute of Medical Sciences and Nutrition, Mexico City)

PURPOSE. Evaluate a short candidate measure of frailty in prediction of death. METHOD. Retrospective cohort from 1994 to 1999 in a Mexican tertiary care center. We used the brief clinical instrument to classify frailty published by Rockwood. The outcome was established from the charts in July 2000. We made survival analysis and proportional hazard model with Cox regression for demographic, functional and morbidity variables. RESULTS. There were 874(37.2%) male and 1477(62.8%) female patients. 1631 (69.4%) were evaluated in the inpatient setting and the rest in the ambulatory unit. Mean age was 76.17 years. In group 1 (not frailty) there were 1022 (43.5%) patients (median survival 59.91 months); in group 2, with only urinary incontinence: 480(20.4%) patients (median survival 75 months, OR .749 IC 95% .596-.991); in group 2 with mild cognitive impairment or two or more dependencies in activities of daily living (ADL) 567(24.1%) patients (median survival 25.98 months, OR 1.94 IC 95% 1.579-2.393); and in group 3 with severe cognitive impairment and three or more dependencies in ADL 282(12%) patients (median survival 14.76 months, OR 3.013 CI 95% 2.285-3.972). In the proportional hazard models the frailty scale continued being significant after adjusting for demographic and basal medical status ($p<0.0001$ Exp B 1.35 IC 95% 1.279-1.427), together with being older than 75 years and being in the inpatient unit. CONCLUSION. Higher levels of frailty are related with mortality in the Mexican elderly population.

[18] Vitality 90+ - A Multidisciplinary Population Study of Nonagenarians

M Jylhä, O. Jolanki, S. Goebler, A. Hervonen (School of Public Health, University of Tampere)

Vitality 90+ is a multidisciplinary prospective population study of people aged 90 or over in the city of Tampere, Finland. The study describes life conditions, ways of life, and heterogeneity of this most rapidly growing age group; examines physical and psychological functioning and their predictors, analyses life stories and personal accounts of the oldest generation alive; and searches for predictors and pathways for successful longevity. The study includes the whole population aged 90 + in Tampere (ca 800 persons, depending on exact date, both community-dwelling and institutionalized. Data sets include repeated mailed surveys with the home-dwelling population, interviews with informal caregivers, measured functional performance and cognitive status, genetic material, history of disease and use of care, and tape-recorded oral life stories and narrative interviews. Institutionalization and mortality are followed in registers. Approximately one third on people aged 90+ live in nursing homes or other institutions. A vast majority of them suffer from dementia diseases. Diagnoses of cardiovascular disease and other chronic disease are frequent also among the home-dwelling people. However, at least 20% of them have no difficulty in mobility and in ca 30% self-rated health is good. In longitudinal follow-up, both mobility problems and self-rated health predicted mortality. In biographic interviews, nonagenarians talk about health as an important, but problematic part of their identity. In this study that includes the whole population aged 90+, we could not find any "survival of the fittest" -effect. In contrast, nonagenarians are a very heterogeneous group with a rather high lifetime prevalence of chronic disease. Indicators that are known to predict mortality in younger age groups, such functional status and self-rated health that, were significant predictors also in nonagenarians.

[19] Freedom and Security: Swiss Guidelines for the use of restraints in the care of elderly

Ch. Chappuis, F. Huber, P. Schwed, A. Wettstein (Swiss Geriatrics Society), M. Gaillard, H. Haske Pelsoeczy, D. Inglin, R. Schmitt-Mannhart, M.C. Thierstein (Swiss Association on Gerontology)

Some years ago, a court in Switzerland sentenced the staff of a hospital to be responsible for a fall of a 91 year old confused lady, who sustained a hip fracture, because they didn't use restraints. The publication of this sentence has upset professionals in geriatric wards and nursing homes. The fear of a major draw back by decades in the management of the confused elderly was substantial. A group of specialists from the Swiss Society on Gerontology and the Swiss Geriatrics Society decided to create guidelines with the intention, to give the institutionalized elderly as much freeedom as possible but also appropriate security. After a long period of discussions, the guidelines were published in 1999 and met considerable attention. The guidelines put on record the need of special structures for care concerning facilities and caregivers. In addition, the decisions have to be reflected in the process of care: Individualized decisions, evaluation by an interdisciplinary team, documentation of the restrictions measures in written form, respectation of the will of the patient and his familiy and mutual information of all involved parties, use of restraints for a limited time only, periodical evaluation of the decisions.

[20] Boomers! Their future is our future: It had better be better than THEY expect!

Jeanne E. Bader[California State University, Long Beach, USA]

The purpose of this poster is to encourage collegial discussion of Boomer aging and its implications for people of ALL ages. Historical review, the research literature and my current research strongly suggest that Boomers will age differently from their parents and grandparents — but that they could age so much better than that if they and we get answers to certain questions and make data-based decisions today. IAG participants are urged to come discuss Boomer aging in their countries and to use this poster presentation as a venue for sharing the results of their own future-oriented research.

[21] Predictors of mortality among nonagenarians: The Danish 1905-cohort survey

Hanne Nybo, Hans Chr. Pedersen, David Gaist, Kjeld Andersen, Bernard Jeune, James Waupel, Kaare Christensen (Epidemiology, Institute of Public Health, University of Southern Denmark-Odense University, Denmark _

PURPOSE: To examine whether well-known risk factors such as smoking, alcohol consumption, BMI, physical and cognitive abilities and health have the same impact on the very old as on younger elderly. This is mainly unresolved as few data are available on predictors of mortality among nonagenarians. METHODS: All Danes born in 1905, irrespective of physical and mental status, were in 1998 invited to participate in a multidimensional survey. Vital status on the cohort was drawn from the Danish Civil Registration System covering all inhabitants in Denmark, yielding a minimum of 15 months follow-up for the 2249 participants. RESULTS: A total of 579 persons died during the follow-up period. Unadjusted Cox Proportional Hazards models showed that smoking, number of diseases, education, and marital status did not influence mortality and the higher the BMI and the weekly intake of alcohol the lower the mortality. Furthermore, difficulty in managing activities of daily living, low performance on the physical and cognitive tests, and low self-rated health were associated with an increase in mortality. However, after controlling for all included variables the association between alcohol consumption, handgrip (males only), chair stand, self-rated health (males only), and mortality became non-significant. CONCLUSION: Among nonagenarians, predictors of mortality such as smoking, obesity, number of diseases, civil status, and education have lost their importance. However, a high disability level, poor physical and cognitive function, and self rated health are strong predictors of mortality, which shows that mortality among nonagenarians is not a stochastic process.

[22] The effect of cohort- and person-specific socioeconomic conditions in childhood on socioeconomic differences in mortality

Ingemar Kåreholt (Aging Research Center, Stockholm, Sweden)

PURPOSE: To examine the effect of person- and cohort-specific socioeconomic conditions in childhood on socioeconomic differences in mortality among adults. Adult socioeconomic conditions are measured as social class from occupation. METHOD: Hazard regressions are used to analyze mortality in a random sample of the Swedish population aged 23 to 99 years (n = 4,201) for the period 1968 to 1994 (29 years). RESULTS: Class differences in mortality (between blue- and white-collar workers) are large in cohorts experiencing harsh socioeconomic circumstances in childhood, and smaller in cohorts with better circumstances in childhood. A similar difference is found for person-specific socioeconomic conditions in childhood, measured as father's social class. Among persons with poor person-specific socioeconomic conditions in childhood, class differences in mortality were larger than among persons with good person-specific socioeconomic conditions in childhood. Among persons with both good person- and cohort-specific socioeconomic conditions in childhood, there were nearly no class differences in mortality. CONCLUSIONS: The results in this paper show that socioeconomic conditions in childhood are important for the development of class differences in mortality among adults. The mortality differences between adult blue- and white-collar workers depend at least a partly on differences in childhood conditions. The results demonstrate the importance of childhood conditions for individual life expectancy.

[23] Health Among the Oldest Old: the Umea 90+ study

Gustavsson J, von Heideken P, Kallin K, Nygren B, Lundman B*, Norberg A*, Gustafson Y (Department of Community Medicine and Rehabilitation, Geriatric Medicine, *Department of Nursing, Umeå University, Umeå, Sweden)*

PURPOSE: To examine health and living circumstances among the oldest old. METHOD: A population based study was performed in the municipality of Umeå, where all persons born before 1906 (n=86) and in 1910 (n=115) were asked to participate. The data collection concisted of structured interviews and assessments in the person´s home. Data was also collected from medical charts, relatives and caregivers. Information about previous and current diseases, medications, vision, hearing and Body Mass Index (BMI, l/m2) was collected. Nutritional status was examined with Minimal Nutritional Assessment (MNA), cognition was tested with Minimal Mental State Examination (MMSE) and prevalence of depression was screened with the Geriatric Depression Scale-15 (GDS-15). RESULTS: One hundred sixtyfive persons (82%) agreed to participate while 25 (12%) refused and 11 persons (6%) died before inclusion. Seventy-nine percent were women, 81% were widows/widowers and 94% lived alone. Almost half of the subjects had impaired vision and/or hearing. Only 2% were not on drug treatment and 78% took more than three medications daily. According to MNA, 61% were at risk of or suffered from malnutrition. MMSE was performed in 132 cases (80%), and 55cored <24 but only 25 0f the total sample had a dementia diagnosis. Signs of mild or moderate depression according to GDS was found in 37% of those (n=105) who were possible to assess. CONCLUSION: Malnutrition, polypharmacy, underdiagnoses of dementia and depression seem to be major health issues among the oldest old.

[24] Optimization of methods of biological age assessment

V. Kroutko, T. Smirnova, V. Dontsov, A. Mamay (National Gerontology Center, Moscow, Russia)

PURPOSE: The analysis of efficiency of the standard technique of biological age (BA) assessment for particular group of patients and optimization of this technique was the purpose of research. METHODS: 195 essentially healthy people (159 women and 36 men) in the age of 20 - 74 years who addressed the aging prevention center in 1995-1999 were inspected. The set of biological age biomarkers (BAB) and the conditions of examination corresponded to the "Kiev test" of BA definition[Voitenko V.P, Tokhar A.V, Polyuhov A.I, 1984], based on the model of multiple linear regression. The set of utilized statistical methods included correlation, dispersion and regression analysis, analysis of variants, t-test, chi-square test and factor analysis. The factor of a multiple determination between BA, defined by the set of biomarkers, and calendar age was adopted as BA definition quality criterion. RESULTS: The quality of BA definition by equations of the "Kiev test" as in its full version including 13 biomarkers, and in reduced version (4 biomarkers) for the ours inspected population has appeared worse as compared with the base Kiev population, for which one these equations were obtained, in 1.5 times for the women and in 2.5 times for the men. The analysis of age dynamics of biomarkers has revealed for some of them reliable non-linear, and in a number of cases even nonmonotone nature. The nonlinear regression has allowed to construct new formulas for BA definition (full and reduced for both sex) with quality of approximation superior to the "Kiev test". CONCLUSION: the efficiency of methods of BA estimation (mathematical models and sets of biomarkers) can be unequal for different populations. The optimization of methods of BA definition requires reference to non-linear nature of age dynamics of BA biomarkers.

[25] Refugees and Aging

Juma Mohammed Omar

The purpose of this study is to let the world know- Who is a refugee and why this program of refugee and Aging is being presented. A refugee is a person who owing to a well founded fear of being persecuted for reasons of religion,nationality,membership of a particular social group or political opinion is outside the country of his nationality and unable to or owing to fear is unwilling to avail himself of the protection of that Country. The method used to carryout this study was by observation,questionaire and interview to the refugee in the camps. The result of the study shows that,the elderly especially reach the places of asylum in a weakened state,hungry,sick or traumatized by events that took place violently in their lives leading to disruption of lives,property or family ties. Harsh climatic conditions is another leading factor that affect the old during the enmasse journeys,many sucumb to death due to diseases. Women either old or young,during this exodus they fell prey to rebels,soldiers or host country citizens who rape them or sexually abuse them this leads to high numbers of loss of lives through Aids. To conclude,it's alot loss to countries to loose lives of loved ones due to this enmass movement of peoples. The study come with posible ammendment which could reduce loss of lives-especally the old in this countries. The international and regional emmergency response capacities in both govermental and NGO's should be strengthened to prevent crises that uproot masses of people. Humanitarians should be prepared to cross borders to help people in their country of origin rather than wait untill a crisis has created enmass movement. International solidarity especially the UNHCR in the context of the refugees issue is of a material support.

[26] Bulgarian Association on Aging (BAA)

I.C. Petrov (Specialized University Hospital of Endocrinology, Nephrology and Gerontology "Academician Ivan Pentchev", Medical University of Sofia, Bulgaria)

The Bulgarian Association on Aging , was founded in 1994 by a group of gerontologists and volunteers connected with the former Sofia Centre of Gerontology and Geriatrics (1963-1972). According to its by-laws, adopted in 1996, BAA is a non-profit association of a wide circle of professionals, researchers, voluntary workers and public figures, who are interested in the wide range of problems related with aging, old age and elderly, and who work with older people, with a conviction and clear desire to assist in improving their health, well-being and quality of life. BAA carries out research in gerontology and geriatrics; it organizes and encourages educational, teaching, diagnostic, therapeutic and consultative activities as well as rehabilitation, social work, charity, publicity, creative work. BAA assists in: improving the health, vitality, longevity, social and psychological well-being, family solidarity, and quality of life of senior citizens, including the stimulation of their independent and active way of living; building of humane and positive attitude towards the elderly people, for respect and warmth, and for their esteem, in an atmosphere which would simultaneously spare and encourage them; developing a consent of our membership for attaining the well-being of all citizens of all ages in this country. BAA members are involved in the practical work with the Health Groups of elderly volunteers within a program of regular physical and social activity throughout the country as well as with peoples with dementia and their families. BAA has now consulting and methodical activities, organizes courses, carries out research in the field of mental health, rural elderly, social gerontology, etc.

[27] The Thai Society of Gerontology and Geriatric Medicine

The Thai Society of Gerontology and Geriatric Medicine, Thailand

The purpose of this presentation is to introduce the Thai Society of Gerontology and Geriatric Medicine with a brief history of this organization, the current number of members, the on going special projects, dates and location of the next national and regional congress. Lt.Dr.Siriphan Sasat The Thai Society of Gerontology and Geriatric Medicine Thailand

[28] The Gerontology and Geriatrics Society of the Ukraine

V.V.Bezrukov (Institute of Gerontology, Kiev, Ukraine

The Gerontology and Geriatrics Society of Ukraine was organized as a Ukrainian branch of the USSR Society founded in Kiev in 1963. Before the fall of the USSR, the USSR Society had convened its five congresses, two of them in Kiev. In 1972, according to the IAG decision, the 9th International Congress of Gerontology (President: Prof. D.F. Chebotarev) was held in Kiev. The Ukrainian Society held its three national congresses: 1st - in 1988 (Dniepropetrovsk), 2nd - in 1994 (Kiev)and 3rd - in 2000 (Kiev). The Society has greatly benefited owing to participation in its activity of the well- known scientists: N.N. Gorev (1900-1992), V.V. Frolkis (1924-1999), D.F. Chebotarev, N.B. Mankovsky, V.V. Bezrukov, G.M. Butenko, O.V. Korkushko and oth. The last (3rd) congress was attended by more than 500 participants. There were 27 scientific sessions and 3 symposia. Currently, the Society lists 200 members. It has regional branches in Kharkov, Odessa, Dniepropetrovsk, Lvov, etc. Working actively in the field of aging is also the Institute of Biology (Kharkov) and the Institute for Eye Diseases and Replacement Therapy (Odessa). The Society issues the "Problems of Ageing and Gerontology" journal since 1990. Affiliated with the Institute of Gerontology are: the Geriatric Rehabilitation Center, the Parkinson's Disease Treatment Center, the Center for Osteoporosis, the Alzheimer Patients Association, the Center "Health of the Elderly". The Society maintains relations with gerontological societies worldwide. The following meetings will take place in 2001: "Osteoporosis: Epidemiology, Diagnosis, Treatment and Prevention" (May, Kharkov); "Accelerated Aging and its Prevention" (October, Odessa). The next national gerontological congress is planned for 2005.

[29] The French Society of Gerontology and Geriatrics

Bernard FORETTE, Alain FRANCO, Robert MOULIAS (French Society of Gerontology and Geriatrics)

The French Society on Geriatrics and Gerontology was one of the twelve founders of the International Association of Gerontology, after the First

International Congress of Gerontology held in Liege (Belgium) in July 1950. A national, multidisciplinary, scientific and educational association, the FSGG has over 3000 members, and gathers 14 regional societies, 6 specialized societies and two Academic Colleges. The FSGG publishes four journals and awards two prizes every year for researchers in the field of aging. For over 30 years, the SFGG has been organizing successful national and international conferences: - Biannual regular national meetings - National meetings on specific issues such as Gerontopsychiatry, Nutrition, Elder abuse, Quality of care, Biology of aging, Dementia, Ethics... - The first and fourth international French speaking congresses of gerontology were held in Paris (1982) and Strasbourg (1994). In Strasbourg, the SFGG gathered 2,500 delegates from French speaking countries all over the world. - Since 1997, the SFGG organizes transatlantic (bilingual) meetings in Paris. These meetings have international participants from many countries and they are acknowledged for CME by the American Medical Association. The SFGG is proud to bid for hosting the XIXth World Congress in Paris in 2009. Paris is not only an attractive city, it is also one of the most accessible, best situated and the most convenient locations in the world to organize efficiently a large international congress in its new conference center. The experience of organizing national and international meetings will ensure a well organized and managed World Congress.

[30] Finnish Gerontological Society (Societas Gerontologica Fennica)

Timo Strandberg, Kaisu Pitkälä, Helsinki University Central Hospital Helsinki, Finland

Societas Gerontologica Fennica (SGF) was founded in 1948 with the aim of promoting scientific research in the field of gerontology. The Society's first president was professor Oswald Renkonen, and the first secretary professor Eeva Jalavisto who later played a central role in SGF, gerontological research and geriatrics in Finland. She published numerous articles about the status and care of elderly in the community. For the remarkable achievements of Eeva Jalavisto, SGF has arranged several symposia named after her and founded the Eeva Jalavisto Prize for notable gerontological research in Finland. The aim of SGF is to promote research and cooperation in the scientific field of gerontotogy through: * Arranging scientific symposiums, educational meetings and congresses * Promoting gerontological research by contributing grants and scholarships * Discussing scientific issues of gerontology in its meetings * Promoting publications in gerontology The Society had also an impact on the origination of geriatrics in Finland by starting a geriatric outpatient clinic in Helsinki in 1952. The yearbook of SGF, called Geron, was published from 1949 to 1985. Thereafter, the Society's proceedings have been actively published in different formats, most lately also on the Internet since 1997 (www.gernet.sci.fi) SGF has been active in the international cooperation, especially Nordic collaboration with the Nordisk Gerontologisk F'rening. Nordic Gerontological Congresses have been arranged in Finland in 1977, 1986 and 1996. SGF has also representatives in the International Association of Gerontology (IAG) and its European Region. In 1998, SGF arranged the congress of the IAG, European Region, Clinical Section. SGF is now also affiliated with EUGMS. Presently Societas Gerontologica Fennica has about 300 members (geriatricians, gerontologists in different fields, and geriatric nurses). The current president of SGF is Timo Strandberg, (e-mail: timo.strandberg@hus.fi), past president Heikki Takkunen and secretary Otto Lindberg.

[31] Czech Society of Gerontology and Geriatrics, Czech Medical Association: Its History and Future

J. Poehnal (Bata Hospital, Zlin and Department of Geriatrics, Institute for Postgraduate Medical Education, Prague, Czech Republic), E. Topinkova (Department of Geriatrics, 1st Medical Faculty, Charles University and Institute for Postgraduate Medical Education, Prague, Czech Republic)

History of professional interest in old age medicine in Czech lands goes back to 1843 when first lectures were held at Medical Faculty, Charles University, Prague by Prof. Hammerník. But it was only in 1958 when Gerontological Section of Czech Society of Internal Medicine, Czech Medical Association was established and, later on in 1962 renamed as Czech Society of Gerontology. Since then membership grew up to 500 members physicians, nurses, social workers and other health care professionals working in the field of gerontology and geriatrics. Growing interest in clinical issues resulted in re-naming as Czech Society of Gerontology and Geriatrics (CGGS) in 1993. From the very beginning main tasks of CGGS were: to promote education in the field of geriatrics and gerontology, to improve clinical practice and care for elderly, to support research, international co-operation and networking, and to influence health and social policy by serving as consulting body for Ministry of Health, Welfare and regional authorities. These tasks are being fulfilled through year-long scientific and educational activities as well as publications (journal Geriatria published together with Slovak Society of Gerontology and Geriatrics, position statements and Gerontologicke aktuality). An overview of current and future activities and contacts are given.

[32] British Geriatrics Society: Improving Knowledge, Standards and Delivery of Care

Richard Lynham (British Geriatrics Society, Majory Warren House 31 St John's Square, London)

The Societys poster relates to its present objectives and work to improve knowledge, standards and delivery of care. This reflects the vision of its founding members in 1947:; for the relief of suffering amongst the aged and infirm1;. The poster describes the operation of the Society, including the: craft committees and special interest groups; Newsletter and scientific journal, Age and Ageing; Compendium of guidelines; website (www.bgs.org.uk); and six-monthly national scientific and regional meetings. The poster relates this to its external work, advising government agencies and other organisations, campaigning publicly for better services for older people, and encouraging multi-professional development and research. The Society has enjoyed a long association with the IAG and is proud to participate in the 2001 World Congress in Vancouver.

[33] Swiss Society of Gerontology

Astrid Stuckelberger, Daniel Inglin (Swiss Society of Gerontology)

Swiss Society of Gerontology (SSG) Astrid Stuckelberger (president) and Daniel Inglin (vice-president) Proportionally to its ageing population, the Swiss Society of Gerontology counts one of the largest national societies by number of members. The SSG includes not only researchers in the universities and medical doctors in geriatrics but a significant number of members from health professionals to specialized professionals doing practical work for or with older people. The objective of the SSG is to forge and encourage interdisciplinary work between and within the scientists and the practitioners as well as advocate and propose sound policies on ageing. For example, in order to implement a long lasting interaction and to help particularly the transfer between research, daily practical work and sound policy building, the Swiss Society of Gerontology has created working groups constituted by experts focusing on specific themes. Ad hoc task force groups meet regularly for a limited period of time and aim at tackling specific issues in order to improve the conditions of ageing and the elderly in Switzerland. The SSG reaches not only the practice, but also contributes to the foundation of new structures and to policy implementation. Three examples will illustrate the different current fields where new facts from science meet the know-how and finds consensus in concrete outcomes such as guidelines: 1) promoting results from the Swiss Research Program on Ageing, 2) work on a consensus building with and for the churches, 3) thematic task forces: age and violence, freedom and security, offers of Post-grade education in Gerontology, freedom and security of the elderly patient, end of life care in pensions, euthanasia-related issues A quarterly newsletter is issued reporting concise scientific information relevant to its member as well as more general information on publications, meetings and conferences related to ageing. A Congress is organized every year scientific and practically oriented meetings alternating between the national congress and more regional meetings. The committee members all represent a specific field in gerontology and geriatrics as well as a linguistic representation of Switzerland. The SSG is involved in international activities by its privileged position and implication in the work with International organisations and the United Nations in Geneva (ie UNECE and the Geneva International Network on Ageing)

[34] The Work of the Hong Kong Association of Gerontology

Edward M F Leung (Hong Kong Association of Gerontology, Hong Kong)

The Hong Kong Association of Gerontology was established in 1986 with the objectives of establish links with gerontology organizations outside Hong Kong to promote mutual understanding and co-operation, promote concern on elderly services, promote development of elderly services to improve quality of life among elderly people, promote development of research in gerontology, promote training and education in gerontology In the past 15 years the Hong Kong Association of Gerontology has organized over 150 seminars and workshop. Hong Kong has been the host of 5th Asia/Oceania Regional Congress of Gerontology in 1995 which attracted over 1100 participants. The Association also publish the Hong Kong Journal of Gerontology which is a peer reviewed journal twice a year and has attracted subscription from all over the world The Association also organize Annual Congress of Gerontology which was attended by over 200 people each year Since November 2000 the Association has established the Hong Kong Institute of Gerontology which offer training for both local an

[35] What is AGECO? Asociacion Gerontologica Costarricense

Francisco Carrillo Castro (Asociacion Gerontológica Costarricense)

Purpose: The general understanding of AGECO, its objectives, strategies, services, programs and activities are oriented towards participation, development, and growth of older people. Method: The method used is description. Results: These programs and services follow strategic lines directed to the target population and the community. They are divided as follows: Consulting The objective is to try to eliminate stereotypes about aging, support programs and strengthen different activities to prevent, promote and educate people on health. The following are some of the main activities in this area: Women and Aging workshops, Specialized technical Advising for Homecare, Inter-institutional training (elderly care centers), Workshop on Jubilation Educational material production, Communitarian Promotion. The Asociación Gerontológica perceives family and community as the media to develop physical and social skills of older people. Some of the areas are: A. Clubs in Communities: The main objective is to offer older people the possibility to improve their interests and knowledge by sharing with others. B. Specialized Clubs: The reason for this is to stimulate social interchange and development of physical, mental, artistic and social capacities. (i.e. Theatre, Literature and Music) C. Physical Activity Clubs: This kind of club gives elderly time to get away of their isolation and loneliness by providing physical activities and improving their physical condition. (i.e. Yoga, Gymnastics, Hydro kinesis) D. Older People Volunteering: The purpose of this area is to motivate people to use their skills, experience and talent for others. Communication AGECO promotes educational and informative messages about the aging process to people through mass media. Some of the activities in this area are: Bulletin La Voz de AGECO (Published every two months), La Edad de Oro Column (Published every week in the most important written media of Costa Rica, newspaper La Nación), La Voz de AGECO, Radio Program (This is a weekly program in one of the highest rating stations, Radio Fides), Antaño y este Año, Radio Program (This is weekly, and it is in the main cultural station in Costa Rica, Radio Nacional), Institutional Relations. The Asociación Gerontológica is related to different national and international associations in order to share experiences and knowledge. Services: In order to look for independent life, the institution supplies auxiliary equipment for low class older people. Equipment such as orthopedic beds, wheelchairs, air mattresses and bath chairs can be rented for a low price. Conclusion: All these areas combined are the reason why AGECO exists: To find the solutions for elderly, and have them enjoy a deserving old age according to their conditions as human beings not only in their personal aspect but also in the familial and social one.

[36] The Australian Association of Gerontology - Celebrating 40 years

Barbara Squires (President), Anna Howe (Immediate Past President, on behalf of the Australian Association of Gerontology)

This Australian Association of Gerontology celebrates its 40th anniversary in 2001 and this poster present an account of the development and activities of the Association in 8 panels: (1) the emblem of the Australian Association of gerontology, (2) its mission to expand knowledge of ageing, (3) the provision of education through Annual Conferences, 4) the promotion of research and scholarships through the RM Gibson Visiting Fellowship and Scientific Research Fund, (5) the dissemination of information through the Australasian Journal on Ageing (6) a profile of the membership and leadership awards (7) the history of the AAG and (8) the future of the AAG as a member of the IAG and especially in the Asia-Oceania Region.

[37] Gerontological Society of the Russian Academy of Sciences

V.N. Anisimov (Department of Carcinogenesis and Oncogerontology, N.N. Petrov Research Institute of Oncology, Saint Petersburg, Russia)

Gerontological Society of the Russian Academy of Sciences (RAS) has been established in March 1994 at the All-Russian constituent conference "Medical and Social Aspects of Gerontology and Geriatrics" held in Saint Petersburg. Since 1997 The Gerontological Society is a member of I.A.G. The Society is a voluntary public scientific organisation of citizens working in the field of gerontology and related sciences. Main objectives of the Society are: facilitating the research development in the sphere of the Russian gerontological science and related fields of physiology and biology and integrating the research results with practice; establishing and maintaining contacts with scientific gerontological organisations of the CIS and other countries and with international non-governmental scientific organisations; holding meetings of researchers with the purpose to exchange scientific information, discuss problems arising in the process of scientific investigations; assisting the Society members in increasing their professional skills and conducting research, inventions and rationalisation proposals; exerting research and methodological assistance in educating the bases of the modern gerontology at high and secondary school, establishing relations with the Russian scientific societies working in the related fields of research; participating in the work of international scientific associations; popularising and spreading knowledge and recent research and technical achievements in the sphere of the Society's activity. By July 1, 2001, the Gerontological Society has comprised 36 regional branches in Moscow, Saint Petersburg, Archangel, Astrakhan, Barnaul, Ekaterinburg, Ivanovo, Khabarovsk, Kursk, Minsk, Nizhny Novgorod, Novokuznetsk, Novosibirsk, Obninsk, Perm, Petrozavodsk, Pushchino, Rostov, Ryazan, Samara, Saratov, Sochi, Stavropol, Tchelyabinsk, Tchita, Tomsk, Tver, Tyumen, Ufa, Ulan-Ude, Ulyanovsk, Vladivostok, Volgograd, Voronezh and Yaroslavl, Yoshkar-Ola. The Society includes over 1500 specialists from more than 40 regions of Russia. Since 1996, the Society published an information bulletin "Herald of the Gerontological Society of the Russian Academy of Sciences". By July 1, 2001, 38 issues of the Herald have been published. Since 1997, the Gerontological Society has published a yearbook "Advances in Gerontology". The Gerontological Society maintains close contact with international organisations engaged in gerontology: the UN Programme on Ageing, I.A.G. and European Region thereof, IABG, etc. Gerontological Society has organised or co-organised over 40 scientific conferences and symposia including ten international ones. Among them there are such significant events as the International Symposium

"Gerontological Aspects of Peptide Regulation of Functions" (Saint Petersburg, 1996), annual conferences "Elderly Patient. Quality of Life" (Moscow, 1996-2000), 2nd European Congress on Biogerontology (Saint Petersburg, 2000). The 1st Russian Congress of Gerontology and Geriatrics was held in 1999 in Samara. 6th European Congress on Clinical Gerontology will held in Moscow (2002). In 1995 there was instituted the Gerontological Society award to the young scientists of Russia for the best work in gerontology. Since then 9 researchers have won the award.

[38] Canadian Association on Gerontology / Association Canadienne de Gérontologie

Pierre Soucie, Linda O'Rourke (Canadian Association on Gerontology, Ottawa, Ontario, Canada)

The Canadian Association on Gerontology (CAG) is a national, multidisciplinary scientific and educational association established to provide leadership in matters related to the aging population. The CAG seeks to improve the lives of older Canadians through the creation and dissemination of knowledge in gerontological policy, practice, research and education. A registered Canadian charity, the CAG was founded on October 15, 1971 and is a member of the International Association of Gerontology. Our membership is a dynamic mix of people interested in the field of gerontology including health care professionals, researchers, academics, administrators, government representatives, national organizational executives, students, and seniors.

[39] Maltese Association of Gerontology and Geriatrics (MAGG)

Joseph Troisi (Institute of Gerontology, University of Malta, Msida, MALTA)

The Maltese Association of Gerontology and Geriatrics was set upon the 12th February 1998. It aims at promoting professional and educational advancement of gerontologists and geriatricians. It seeks to foster the professional education and training of those working in the multi-disciplinary field of ageing. MAGG places great emphasis on research-based mutual education by and of its members. It also stresses the importance of promoting the total well-being of the elderly human person. The Association also acts as a representative r forum of the professional interests of persons working in the field of ageing both locally and internationally. On the 17th December 1999, MAGG was accepted as a member of IAG. It is affiliated with a number of European organisations and associations in the Mediterranean region. It enjoys enjoys a consultative status with the Parliamentary Secretariat for the Care of the Elderly, Government of Malta. Membership is open to professionals engaged in a wide range of areas in the field of ageing. MAGG members also offer their services and expertise to various p private and public organisations engaged in the field of ageing.The Association conducts bi-monthly meetings and lectures for its members on various topics of ageing. Some of these lectures are also open to the general public. Once a year MAGG conducts a one day national seminar which is very well attended by members and others working in the field of ageing. MAGG publishes a bi-monthly newsletter which serves as a link for its members locally and abroad. Every month, the Association members publish feature articles on different aspects of ageing in one of the leading Sunday newspapers. It also runs a one hour informative radio programme on the national station. This is very popular and heavily subscribed to. MAGG is planning an international conference for the Mediterranean region to be held in November 2002. It has its own webpage: http://soc.um.edu.mt/magg

[40] Sociedad Paraguaya de Gerontologia Y Geriatria

E. de Mestral (National Faculty of Medicine, Asunción Δ Paraguay, Past-president of the Paraguayan society of geriatrics)

Founded in 1973

[41] Scoiedad Argentina de Gerontologia Y Geraitria

I. Fainstein (Buenos Aires, Argentina)

The Argentine Society of Gerontology and Geriatrics (SAGG), a pioneer in Latin America, was founded in 1951. Nowadays we have more than 1.500 members. SAGG follows the IAG's objectives and mission statement. Regular sessions are held monthly with the attendance of guest professionals from other societies. Presentations include papers, round tables, invited lectures, and symposia.

[42] German Society of Gerontology and Geriatrics - DGGG

W. Oswald (President of the DGGG)

The poster of the German Society of Gerontology and Geriatrics (DGGG) will be a presentation in five parts. Part 1 will report the origins and the history of the DGGG as well as its actual situation and current trends of development. A survey of the structure of the members and an overview of recent and congresses will be given. Part 2-5 will introduce the four sub-societies or sections of the DGGG. Those arelSection I: Society for the Biology of AgeinglSection II: Society for Geriatric MedicinelSection III: Society for Social and Behavioral Gerontology. Section IV: Society for Social Gerontology and Health Care Services for the Elderly. Each section will present a short portrait of itself which is structured as pro-posed by the Organizing Committee of the Vancouver Congress. That means, that each of the texts will inform about the area of gerontology it deals with: its members and their professions resp. working fields, the topics and contents of meetings, conferences and research projects, aspects of future works.

[43] The British Society of Gerontology

Kate Davidson (Secretary, British Society of Gerontology, UK)

The British Society of Gerontology aims to promote the understanding of human ageing and later life through research and communication. It seeks to foster the application of this knowledge to the improvement of the quality of life in old age. The BSG was established in 1971 to provide a multidisciplinary forum for researchers and other interested members in the field of ageing. Until 1979 it was known as the British Society of Social and Behavioural Gerontology. BSG's main activities are concerned with promoting the exchange of ideas and information. An important element is the programme of meetings, which as well as providing venues for informal discussion and formal presentations, create opportunities for members to publish and disseminate their work. The Society is also increasing its activity in the promotion of research. The Society has actively fostered journal and book publications. With the Centre for Policy on Ageing, it jointly sponsored the first academic journal in British social gerontology, Ageing and Society, and it also publishes a quarterly journal Generations Review. Published six times a year by Cambridge University Press (CUP). Each issue of this premier international journal in social gerontology contains four or five main articles, a progress report or review article, abstracts of significant papers, and about a dozen book reviews. The Society was elected as a member of the International Association of Gerontology (IAG) in 1987 and is affiliated to many other organisations in the UK and abroad.

[44] The Belgian Society of Gerontology and Geriatrics

J.P.Baeyens (Secretary General - Flemish) Michielsen (President) J.Peteremans (Secretary General - French)

The Belgian Society of Gerontology and Geraitrics was founded by Prof. Brull in 1950. Belgium has 10 million inhabitants, flemish, french and german speaking. The Capital is Brussels, the Capital of the European Union too. There are at this moment 300 active members, geriatricians, medicals, (research) nurses, physiotherapists, occupational therapists, psychologists, sociologists, economists, etc. All of them have an university degree. Every Year we have three meetings: one in the winter at Oostende (1200 parcticipants), one in may in Brussels (200 participants), and one in the automs in Liège (500 participants). Every year the proceedings are published. Four times a year a news bulletin is published: G-News. A website is in construction. In Belgium nearby every General Hospital has a Department of Geriatric medicine, headed by an internsit with special competence in geriatric medicine. This compentence can be obtained by a one year training after the recognition as a specialist in Internal Medicine, in a recognized geriatric training center. Every University has a Professor of Geriatric Medicine. Studens have courses in Geriatric Medicine in their curriculum. In september 2002 (22-25-09-2002) the BSGG organises an International Froncophone Congress, only in the french language. Information is available on teh website: http://www.gerontologie2002.com

SESSION 5

Rethinking Intergenerational Relations and Family Care

Ariela Lowenstein (Center for Research and Study of Aging, Faculty of Welfare and Health Studies, The University of Haifa, Haifa, Israel) and Vern L. Bengtson (Andrus Gerontology Center, University of Southern California, Los Angeles, USA), Roseann Giarrusso (Andrus Gerontology Center University of Southern California LA, USA) Du Feng (Department of Human Development and Family Studies Texas Tech University, Lubbock, TX, USA and Vern L. Bengtson Andrus Gerontology Center, University of Southern California LA, CA). Longitudinal Predictors of Change in the Intergenerational Stake Phenomenon over Twenty Years P. Ron (School of Social Work, Faculty of Social Welfare and Health Studies, Haifa University, Israel). Masculine Sex-Role Orientation and Mental Health of Offspring Caring for an Elderly Parent. Chris Phillipson (Applied Social Studies and Social Gerontology, Keele University, Keele, UK). Globalization and intergenerational ties: new solidarities and relationships in the 21st Century Hiroko Akiyama, Hidehiro Sugisawa and Jersey Liang (University of Tokyo, Tokyo Metropolitan Institute of Gerontology, Japan and University of Michigan, USA), Living Arrangements and Intergenerational Support of Japanese Elderly: A Longitudinal Study Over 12 Years

ISSUE: The importance of intergenerational relations and family care is presented within an international perspective and debated. This symposium seeks to make the links between theory and substantive research in intergenerational family relationships. STRUCTURE: The moderator will briefly introduce the session. Five papers address the explicit role of intergenerational relations, within an international perspective, and their impact on family care in different cultural domains. The co-convener will conduct an open discussion first asking for panelist comments and then audience comments. CONTENT: Theoretical aspects and empirical data of intergenerational relations are presented and addressed in five areas: family care and social support, grandparenthood, impact of globalization, living arrangements and gender. Discussion will focus on the nature and value of explicit theorizing in intergenerational family relationships. ANTICIPATED OUTCOME: A greater appreciation of the value of explicit theorizing in intergenerational family relationships. mailto: ariela@research.haifa.ac.il

Globalization and intergenerational ties: new solidarities and relationships in the 21st Century

Chris Phillipson (Centre for Social Gerontology, Keele University, Stoke-on-Trent, England)

Abstract: This paper will explore the new context shaping the production and maintenance of intergenerational ties. In particular, it traces the impact of globalization on care relations, specifically those expressed in intergenerational forms. The argument developed is that globalization is leading to new types of transnational families and communities. Families, it is argued, are in a process of change, reflecting pressures of migration on the one hand, and new forms of global governance on the other hand. Growing old within a global community is resulting in hybrid forms of generational ties within the various global networks and flows. The central question addressed by the paper is: to what extent is globalization creating new forms of care relations, whilst at the same time undermining existing forms of support? A variety of data sets will be drawn upon from a range of studies, to answer this research question. The paper will argue that an increasing number of families are facing the task of managing generational ties at a transnational rather than a national level. This is creating a major challenge for social policy responses to ageing issues. Increasingly, these will need to take account of global pressures and issues, whilst being rooted in national responses and national institutions. The tension between the local and the global, in the framing of social policy, will be explored in the concluding section of the paper.

Living Arrangement and Intergenerational Support of Japanese Elderly: A Longitudinal Study Over 12 Years

Hiroko Akiyama (University of Tokyo and Institute for Social Research University of Michigan), Hidehiro Sugisawa (Tokyo Metropolitan Institute of Gerontology, Japan) and Jersey Liang (Institute for Social Research, University of Michigan)

Living arrangement of Japanese elderly has been increasingly diversified. In the traditional Japanese society, older persons lived with their eldest son's family. During the past 50 years, the proportion of older persons living in such traditional household constantly declined. In 2000, the majority of the older Japanese opt non-traditional living arrangements such as living with spouse, daughter or non-kin. A large number of them live alone. This study addresses three questions: (1) how does loss of resources such as limited income, declined health and loss of spouse, affect the choice of living arrangements? (2) How is intergenerational support provided in various living arrangements? And (3) how do living arrangement and intergenerational support affect well being of Japanese elderly? The data are derived from a longitudinal national survey of the well being of Japanese elderly. A probability sample of 912 older Japanese completed 5 waves of face-to-face interview survey conducted every third year from 1987 to 1999. Analysis results indicate that multiple resource losses are likely to lead to changes in living arrangements of older persons. Regardless, living arrangements, intergenerational support is quite strong and affects the subjective well being of older persons. Daughters are more likely to provide support to elderly parents who live alone in urban areas. Like many Western societies, they are becoming the primary source of support for elderly mothers. Findings will be discussed in broader cultural context.

Longitudinal Predictors of Change in the Intergenerational Stake Phenomenon over Twenty Years

Roseann Giarrusso (Andrus Gerontology Center, University of Southern California, Los Angeles, CA, USA 90089-0191], Du Feng [Department of Human Development and Family Studies, Texas Tech University, Lubbock, TX, USA 79409-1162], and Vern L. Bengtson [Andrus Gerontology Center, University of Southern California, Los Angeles)

PURPOSE: The intergenerational stake phenomenon refers to the generational bias that is evidenced when parents' and children's evaluations of their joint relationship are compared. Parents tend to view the relationship in a more favorable light than their children thereby resulting in a divergence in parent and child reports of affection. The purpose of this study is to examine four possible theoretical explanations for this generational bias: social psychological theories; theories of developmental aging; stress models; and status inheritance models. METHOD: Data on 483 adult child-parent dyads from the 1971 and 1991 waves of the USC Longitudinal Study of Generations are used to investigate longitudinal predictors of change in the size of the difference between parents' and children's ratings of affection (i.e, the intergenerational stake) across 20 years. Analyses are conducted separately for each of four parent-child gender configurations: father-son;

father-daughter; mother-son; and mother-daughter. RESULTS: The results reveal support for social psychological theories of interpersonal attraction for all gender dyad types: the strongest predictor of an increase in the gap between parents' and children's reports of mutual affection from 1971 to 1991 is an increase in the gap between parents' and children's perceptions of attitudinal similarity over the same time period. Limited support is also found for the other three theories, but only for certain parent-child gender configurations. CONCLUSION: It is concluded that research on intergenerational relations should include dyadic level data in order to get a more accurate appraisal of change in adult child-parent relationships across the life course.

Masculine Sex-Role Orientation and Mental Health of Offspring Caring for an Elderly Parent

P. Ron (School of Social Work, Faculty of Social Welfare and Health Studies, Haifa University, Israel)

The study explored coping processes of offspring of old parents based on the Pearlin and Schooler's stress model (1981), focusing on the differences between sons and daughters caring for an old parent, relating to sex-role orientation. The research hypotheses test the relations between characteristics of the caregiving role and mental health of the offspring; between caregivers burden and their mental health; the relations between their self esteem and mental health and between sex role orientation and their mental health. The study was conducted among 345 of the Israel Electricity Company's workers who responded to mail questionnaires - 211 and 224 women. The findings indicate correlations between all the components of the model and accordingly all hypotheses had been confirmed. Among the demographic characteristics, which impact on mental distress were age, family status, origin and socio-economic status. Among the characteristics connected to the caregiving role, it was found that the kind of assistance given, the diversification's and the independence ability are the most important factors related to mental health of the offspring. Regarding the mediators variables in the model: family support and the manly sex role orientation, they functioned as moderating the intensity of the stress experiences. The main contribution of the research is by understanding the meaning of the influence of the manly sex role orientation to the mental health of the caregivers.

SESSION 6

New approaches in the care of outpatients with cognitive disorders

R. Moulias (Hôpital Charles Foix 94200 IVRY - FRANCE) F. Forette (Hôpital Broca, Paris, FRANCE) J.P. Baeyens (Ostende, BELGIUM) L. Bartorelli (Roma, ITALY) M. Selmes-Antoine, Chairperson Foundation Alzheimer Espana (SPAIN) J. Selmes-Van-Den-Bril, Vice Chairman Alzheimer Europe (SPAIN)

Issue. Progress in home care and progress in early diagnosis enlarged number of dements cared in community. Structure. Four points will ve emphasized : • Early diagnosis at predemential stage : why and how (F. Forette, Paris) • Gerontological expertise centers : a key role for outpatient care of elderly with cognitive disorders (J.P. Baeyens, Ostende) • Home care : conditions for a better quality of life for patient and family caregiver (L. Bartorelli, Roma) • Educational intervention for the principal caregivers of patients with alzheimer's disease (M. Selmes and J. Van Den Bril, Madrid) Content. Non recognition of dementia is the main factor for a delayed diagnosis. A panel of criteria may lead to early diagnosis, at predemential stage. Follow up of mild cognitive impairment may lead to an earlier diagnosis leading to new strategies. Among the trails for prevention, some positive outcomes will be shown. The outpatient must get advice from geriatrician (he is over 75 or 80 y.o.), neuropsychologist, and if needed from neurologist, psychiatrist, orthophonist, etc.. and needs medico-technical facilities (as brain C.T. or M.R.I.) in expert centers. The expert center has to precise diagnosis, to start therapy, to inform patient and family, to educate them, to prepare the project of care with community actors and G.P. A study of 33 expertise centers in 15 E.U countries, has lead to specific guidelines and recommendations. Demented patient cannot live alone, or only in case of a mild form. The care project foresee care, helps, social life, respite for caregiver, funding issues, legal issues, crisis and complications, decision making procedures, activities for the patient and for the caregiver : a life project. >From familial and volunteer unformal helps to well organized sectors or networks, an infinity of answers has been proposed in Europe The main lacks were : qualified staff, respite solutions, funding for helps, education and training of staff and family. The familial caregiver must be perfectly informed about the disease of her (his) patient : nature, evolution, symptoms, risks, care, behavioural positive or negative symptomes, how to understand them, how to avoid them, attitude in front of them, complications and of crisis symptoms. She (he) must acquire education and practical skills about helps and care. She (he) must be aware about her own risks (excess work, stress, depression, and age associated diseases). Alzheimer associations have developped education and training for caregiver, volunteers help networks, informations for family, We will describe a 4 years follow up (ALOIS programme) in Madrid experience. Conclusions Home care could be largely improved by : - better information of general population and of health professionals - earlier diagnosis - skilled expertise for care project - progress in home care and home help facilities and better qualification for staff - education and training of familial caregivers

Early diagnosis at predemential stage : why and how

F. Forette (Hôpital Broca, Paris, FRANCE)

Even in developped countries, dementia diagnosis is delayed. Late diagnosis implies many years with suffering and poor quality of life for the patient and his (her) familial caregiver. Evidence based arguments for early diagnosis or better diagnosis at a predemential stage are numerous. In some forms of dementia early anticholinesterase therapy may improve for months or years the patient and so slow down the course of the disease (Lewy bodies disease, Alzheimer, mixed dementia). In some other forms of dementia treatments may improve (normal pressure hydrocephaly) or slow (vascular dementia), (carential encephalopathy) the evolution. In all dementia early diagnosis allows prevention of crisis, education of caregiver, foreseeing of complications, symptomatic treatment for behavioral disorders and so on. For numerous pists for prevention of Alzheimer disease, human therapeutical trials are in course. Tomorrow they will be effective only if started up at a predemential stage.

Educational intervention for principal caregivers of patients with Alzheimer's disease: A 4-year follow up

J. Selmes Van Den BriL, Vice Chairman Alzheimer Europe M. Selmes Antoine, Foundation Alzheimer Espana (SPAIN)

In the cognitive disorders of the elderly the main carer is the familial one: spouse, husband, daughter, daughter in law, grand daughter. So whatever will be the home care and helps given to the patient only the familial caregiver is always present. This fact implies practical issues. The familial carer must be perfectly informed Δ as much she (he) can understand Δ about the disease of her (his) patient : nature, evolution, symptoms, risks, care. This familial caregiver must receive precise information on behavioural positive or negative symptoms, how to understand them, how to avoid them, attitude in front of them. The familial caregiver must acquire education and practical skills about helps: she (he) may have to help his patient to stand up, to wash, to toilet, to eat, to go out, to get up after a fall ... The familial caregiver must be aware of the different complications and of crisis symptoms (both for patient and for herself or himself). Familial caregiver must be aware about her own risks (excess work, stress, depression, and age associated diseases). Alzheimer family associations have widely developed through European Union education and training for caregiver, volunteers help networks, informations for family, etc

Gerontological expertise centers : a key role for outpatient care of elderly with cognitive disorders

J.P. Baeyens, Oostende (BELGIQUE)

Diagnosis and care projects for dementia syndromes in the elderly need a multidisciplinary team. The outpatient must find a geriatrician (he is over 75 or 80 y.o.), a neuropsychologist, he must get if needed advices of neurologist, psychiatrist, rehabilitation specialist, orthophonist, ophtalmologist and have soon access to medico-technical facilities (as brain C.T. or M.R.I.) The role of this expertise is not only of precising an accurate diagnosis in security and starting appropriate therapy without hospitalisation. The expert centre has to inform patient and family, to educate them, toprepare the project of care with community actors and G.P. , to find respite solutions, to foresee - and avoid - crisis and complications. In a study of 33 expertise centres in 15 E.U. (and associated)countries, the running of these centres was studied. Specific guidelines and recommendations were prepared. One Gerontological expertise centre seems to be necessary for 300-500.000 inhabitants inside a hospital with complete geriatric facilities (day hospital, consultation acute care, geriatric rehabilitation, and also long term care). The expert centre must work in narrow link with community care structures

Home care : Conditions for a better quality of life for patient and family caregiver.

L. Bartorelli, S. Eugenio Hospital, Roma (ITALY)

For elderly patients with cognitive disorders, the best place for them to live is in their own home where they can maintain for longer their vital space, their memories, their identity. However, beyond a very mild form of initial dementia, they cannot live alone. There is a large variety of local solutions in the different regions, but all lead to a similar global assistance model based on data evidence. The family caregiver is the key person and coordinator for all or any of the care systems available for the patient - whether those systems be sectorial, or an organized network, or home care services, or free-lance personnel, or volunteers. The care project is prepared only after an accurate medical, psychological and social diagnosis and a careful analysis of the local expertise working together with the G.P. and family caregiver. The care project foresees not only care and assistance but also activities and social life for patients and caregivers, respite for caregivers, decision making procedures, tutelage (representation of the the patient), funding issues : a life project. There are various local adaptations in addressing these issues but the main aspects are 1) a well-trained and qualified staff, 2) education, and respite solutions for the caregivers, 3) funding for assistants. Cooperation between community care and local expertise seems one of the best ways to improve home-care for the demented elderly, assuring a personalized approach as well as dignity of life both for the patient and for the family.

SESSION 7

Clinical applications of CTA and virtual endoscopy in older aneurysm and dissection

Ou Shan xing Vicer Director/MD(Department of Radiology, Liu Hua Qiao Hospital,Guang Zhou,CN),Liu Zhen an Director/MD (Department of Gerontology, Liu Hua Qiao Hospital,Guang Zhou,CN)

PURPOSE:To assess the three-dimensional CT angiography (3D-CTA) and CT virtual endoscopy (CT-VE) for noninvasive imaging in older aneurysms and dissections. METHODS: The study group comprised 50 subjects (40 males and 10 females , mean age of 70 years) was divided into 3 groups. The classification of dissections: DeBakey type I 21 cases, DeBakey type II 5 cases, DeBakey type IIIa 10 cases, IIIb 4 cases ,and aneurysms 10 cases were performed. Images obtained by CTA and CT-VE were analyzed for Between the sizes and types US and MRI in control, then the multilinear regression models were analyzed to the data. RESULTS: The mean size of the aortic diameter involved in part was about 4.8cm (range 3.5-7.0cm).The sizes of the aneurysm and dissection in men were showed significant difference with increasing hypertension, smoking, and age ($p < 0.01$) and positive relative($r=0.90$)in degree of extension. CTVE provided precise information for the relationship between the vascular lesions and the aortic orifices. CONCLUSION: CTA and CTVE enable visualisation of lesions from an infinite number of viewing angles for imaging in older aneurysms and dissection and is useful for treatment planning and follow-up.

Crystallographic picture of blood serum at atherosclerotic defeat of blood vessels.

V.N. Shabalin, S.N. Shatochina (Russian Research Institute of Gerontology, Moscow, Russia)

Purpose: to study age features of crystalline patterns in blood serum of the man at atherosclerotic defeat of blood vessels. Methods. In reference conditions the dehydration of a drop of blood serum arranged between subject and cover glasses was conducted. With a stereomicroscope Leica MZ12 in ordinary light, polarized light, and phase-contrast microscopy the crystalline patterns in a dehydrated blood serum were studied. Blood serum of 478 patients in the age of 65 - 85 years with a different expressiveness of an atherosclerotic defeat of vessels is studied. The monitoring group - 120 healthy people in the age of 25- 45 years. Results. Established, that the exuberant contents of endogenic cholesterol in blood formed the laminated structures in crystallographic picture of blood serum (fig. 1). These patterns are detected in serum of a blood 453 patients of elderly age. They had the vast areas, differed by the expressed polymorphism and permanently were determined at repeated researches. The similar patterns were detected and in young age (for 27 of 120 patients). However they were sparse, did not find out at repeated researches, and had the narrow areas. The most significant fact was the bundles of anisotropic patterns (crystals of calcium salts) with the laminated structures (fig. 2). These bundles were detected for 237 elderly patients having rough atherosclerotic changes in blood vessels with calcification of a vascular wall. The anisotropic inclusions in laminated structures were detected for 5 patients of monitoring group having clinical and laboratory signs of early atherosclerosis. conclusion. The presence in crystallographic picture of dehydrated blood serum the laminated structures having anisotropic inclusions, indicat to severe atherosclerotic defeat of blood vessels.

Effect of DHEA Administration on Vascular Properties in Elderly Healthy Men: A Placebo Controlled Study

O Hanon, X Girerd #, AS Rigaud*, G Franconi#, S Legrain≠, V Faucounau°, EE Baulieu&, F Forette*. * Hôpital Broca, Paris, France # Hôpital Broussais, Paris, France ≠ Hôpital Bichat, Paris, France ° Fondation Nationale de Gérontologie France & INSERM U448 and College de France*

Recent prospective studies have suggested a favorable effect of Dehydroepiandrosterone (DHEA) on cardiovascular morbidity, but direct effect on the arterial system is not known. Objectives : To study the vascular effects of the DHEA of structural and functional vascular parameters in healthy elderly subjects, in a randomized, double-blind, placebo controlled prospective study. Methods : Sixty men (73+/-2 years), considered healthy, were randomized to receive DHEA (50 mg/d) or placebo. Arterial parameters (wall thickness, internal diameter, distensibility) were evaluated for the common carotid and the radial arteries using high resolution echo-tracking devices (NIUS-02(r) and Wall Track System(r)). Arterial stiffness was evaluated by carotid-femoral pulse wave velocity (PWV) measurements. All measurements were performed at inclusion and after one year of treatment. Results : On the whole population blood pressure remained stable but a significant increase in PWV was observed (14.9 to 16.3 m/sec). At the level of the radial artery, significant changes in distensibility (5.1 to 4.2 kPa-1.10-3) and wall thickness (251 to 266 µm) occurred. No modification was observed for the vascular parameters of the carotid artery. No significant interaction was observed between DHEA administration and vascular modifications in a two way ANOVA. Conclusion : These results indicate that, in elderly healthy men, changes in structural and functional properties are observed after a one year follow-up. DHEA administration had no direct effect on the vascular modifications related to aging process.

SESSION 8

Anthropological study of aging among older women in a small Brazilian town

Uchôa, Elizabeth (Centro de Pesquisas René Rachou da Fundação Oswaldo Cruz na Faculdade de Medicina da Universidade Federal de Minas Gerais) Firmo, Josélia. O.A. (Centro de Pesquisas René Rachou da Fundação Oswaldo Cruz) Lima e Costa, Maria Fernanda F(Centro de Pesquisas René Rachou da Fundação Oswaldo Cruz e Faculdade de Medicina da Universidade Federal de Minas Gerais)

Purpose: To study the everyday living conditions of older women living in a small Brazilian town (Bambuí), in order to understand the main problems and strategies used to face up these conditions, and to identify the factors that mediate their quality of life, positively or negatively. Method: Two methods of sampling collection were adopted in a complementary way: 1) ethnographic study: individual interviews with 20 key-informants and 2) reconstruction of life histories of 30 elderly women (>65 years). The qualitative analyses of the data was performed in two steps. After transcription the interviews were entered into a computer, coded and indexed using the computer program Qualittat. Recurrent information categories were identified and their contents analyzed in order to investigate possible interactions among these categories. Results: The analyses of the interviews with key informants and life histories allowed the identification of common problems of older women living in this community (appearance of chronic diseases, impoverishment, loss of autonomy and social isolation). However, there is a remarkable difference between the discourses of key informants on the living condition of older women and their own life histories. The former tended to emphasize the losses and limitations associated with aging and to provide a negative image of aging in Bambui. Conclusion: The analysis of life histories show that losses and limitations do exist, but the actual impact of such problems seem to be mediated by a compensation process of redefinition and adaptations, with make aging much more positive.

Centering The Margins: Taking Account of Lesbians' Experience With Aging

Karen Gallagher (Victoria Lesbian Seniors Care Society, Victoria, BC, Canada)

In the past, gerontology (and other) researchers, caregivers, policy makers and practitioners often have, at best, passively omitted, and at worst, actively discriminated against aging lesbians and gay men. Basing models of gerontology and other policy and practice on heterosexist norms of labour force participation, old age benefits, and the degree of societal embeddedness of familial and community relationships has exposed the homosexual elderly to inadequate gerontological care, alienation from support networks, and the possibility of physical and emotional abuse. Based on interviews with aging lesbians, and the author's experiences with grassroots and non-governmental lesbian/gay organizations, this paper highlights some of the problems for lesbians and gay men within the gerontology system(s). In particular, it focuses on the implications for the lesbian and gay elderly of coping with the loss of autonomy when autonomy has often meant survival, of chosen families when those families are societally shunned, and of sexuality when that sexuality, in all its dimensions, is ignored or considered dysfunctional. Finally, this paper addresses possibilities in gerontological research, policy and practice for greater inclusivity. This paper also highlights a community development project, within the older lesbian community, in a smaller Canadian city.

Mapping Ethnographic Narratives of Canadian Elderly Muslim Women

Parin Dossa (Department of Sociology, Simon Fraser University, Burnaby)

Over the last two decades, global cultural flows together with resurgence of "ethnicity" have led to critical reformulation of disciplinary paradigms. Within anthropology, there has been a modest attempt to disengage from an exclusive western vantage point towards dialogue with other narratives of modernity originating from other historical situations and religious traditions. In this emerging theoretical crossroads, mapping ethnographic narratives of elderly Muslim women in metropolis Vancouver is informative. On the one hand, documenting the multiple contexts of their lives illuminates the process of reformulation of a religious and cultural tradition in a new more secular terrain; on the other hand, examining the intervention strategies of these women in the context of the political economy of social services suggest an alternative narrative of modernity. In this paper, I explore these themes to show the political and social agency of Muslim elderly women. In conclusion, I will comment on the theoretical and methodological implications of this focus for the study of elderly immigrant women.

Middle-aged women: from being invisible to indispensable, 4 research projects on their participation

Christel Geerts, Els Messelis(Free University Brussels, Brussels, Belgium)

About one fifth of all the women in Flanders is between 50 and 65 years. But this group is under-represented in all areas of our social and political life. *We'll present the results of four studies concerning various parameters of the social and political (local) participation of middle-aged women.1. an analysis of 47 women holding a political office (on local level);2. an analysis of 93 female board members of associations for senior citizens or communal senior advisory councils. 3. an analysis of the procedures of 1089 local associations for senior citizens and communal senior advisory boards4. an analysis of 238 female board members of local meso-organisationsOur results point out an under-representation of these women. This low degree of participation has been thoroughly investigated, and the solutions put forward by the respondents have been analysed.The socio-demographic profile of these women has been compared with the profile of Flemish women in general. In the evaluation of their commitment several parameters were taken into account: duration, selection, procedures, intensity, reason and motivation. Their personal appreciation of their participation and their perception of the specific skills of female board members has also been investigated.

Older Women's Lives and Voices: Lessons from participatory research

Joe Cook, Lorna Warren (University of Sheffield UK) and Tony Maltby (University of Birmingham UK)

PURPOSE To investigate and explore 'life story' and autobiographical methods as a research method of understanding older women's lives and to provide a structured platform for their 'quiet voices'. The research is part of the 'Growing Older' programme funded by the UK Economic and Social Research Council. METHOD Eleven small discussion groups with pre-established groups of older women drawn so as to reflect the ethnic mix of Sheffield. The discussions have allowed and developed a range of themes which will be used as a basis of individual interviews during the second phase started January 2001. The whole research process is being professionally filmed as one method of dissemination of the findings and as a training aid for community groups. RESULTS The paper reports the preliminary results but considers important methodological issues of our chosen method. Among the issues that will be presented are four themes 1. Working at community level 2. Benefits and limitations using discussion group format 3. The advantages and limitations of using a participatory research approach and 4. the filming of the process. CONCLUSION The broad conclusions are that despite the ageist barriers to older women exercising social agency when given appropriate platforms to voice their concerns the women are capable and ready to make valuable contributions to the policy making process at local level. This may have important consequences for the planning and implementation of services to local communities.

Social Inequality and Depression in Older Women: Social Policy as Risk or Relief

Alisoun Milne, Lecturer in Social Gerontology (Tizard Centre, University of Kent, Canterbury)

This paper is a review of evidence from the UK. It explores two relationships; that between social inequality and depression in old age and that between social inequality and social policy. Its aim is to elucidate the role of social policy in creating and perpetuating theinequalities, which are associated with the development of old age depression and to explore its potential to address these inequalities. Older women are particularly vulnerable to the psychological effects of life long and age-related inequalities; the majority sufferers of depression in later life are women. Older women are also the group most acutely affected by those social policies, which impact upon the incomes, quality of life and health care of older people. The role of such policies in replicating inequality and in perpetuating - or even deepening - the psychological vulnerability of older women, is identified as a key component in the development of late life depression. Of particular note are pension policy and community care. More recently, social policies, which acknowledge the role of social inequalities in damaging physical and mental health (Acheson, 1998) are being developed. Whilst this is a positive step, the current focus largely ignores the role of inequalities for the mental health of older people, and does nothing to acknowledge that social policy itself has a wide ranging and cumulative impact on the psychological well-being of older women (Milne & Williams, 2000). Ways in which policy could address inequality include alleviating poverty and extending citizenship rights.

SESSION 9

Aging as a Chaos-Driven Process

M. Soloviev (N. N. Petrov Research Institute of Oncology, St. Petersburg, Russia)

PURPOSE: Life span can be significantly changed by simple interventions (e.g. by changing the activity of few genes). It may mean the organism is a metastable system and hence one may hypothesize the gene regulation system (the end point of the most aging-related changes) can be driven by the laws of chaos. METHOD: A computer model of gene regulation was created. The model genes had two states (active and inactive). The connections between genes and associated switching rules were distributed randomly. It was shown (Kauffman, 1993) that such models could be used to research general properties of real systems. The reaction of the model to short-term change of activity of few genes (model of biochemical fluctuations) was studied. RESULTS: The model shows chaotic behavior at many initial conditions. It can be in stable state (changing gene activity regularly) and returns to this state after fluctuations. In the same time there are fluctuations that can switch it in other stable state. It was found that the model forgets its initial state exponentially. CONCLUSION: Short-term changes of activity of few genes may lead to long-term deviations in cell state. Accumulation of the deviated cells leads to aging. It means that even small biochemical instability (necessary for biological control, development and evolution) may cause aging. The exponential forgetting of initial state allows us to correlate the exponent (alpha) in Hompertz's equation with Lyapunov's time (1/alpha) describing such forgetting in chaotic systems. The organism has not forget its initial (healthy) state for a period enough for guaranteed reproduction. It is corresponded with the fact that Lyapunov's time is approximately equal to average age of reproduction in fruit flies, mice, and primitive humans.

Aging versus Reliability: Stochastic Modulations of the Genetic Melodies

V. K. Koltover (Institute of Problems of Chemical Physics, RAS, Russia)

The goal of this study was to understand why, despite complexity of mechanisms, aging is governed by the relatively simple quantitative laws. The concept, that all molecular biological constructions perform their functions with the genetically limited reliability, served as the methodology of this study (Blumenfeld & Koltover, 1972; Koltover, 1997). The universal laws of aging, such as Gompertzian growth of mortality and correlation of longevity with the species- specific resting metabolism, are easily and naturally explained on this basis. For the advanced ages, the theory predicts that the mortality rate can display a plateau or accelerate its run depending upon genotype and phenotype variability of the populations. The random malfunctions of mitochondrial respiratory chains are of the first importance since they produce toxic superoxide radicals. Mitochondria become intensive generators of superoxide radicals after transient anoxia/ischemia conditions. This loss of control for the electron flow is caused by increase in the membrane lipid fluidity (Nohl, Stolze, Koltover, 1993). The reliability of mtSOD defence is also limited. Analysing the stochastic dynamics of appearance and disappearance of superoxide radicals by a reliability "Birth and Death" model, we estimated that approximately 2 radicals from every 100,000 penetrate the mtSOD-defence system. The slipping radicals initiate the chemical reactions of oxidative damages to DNA and other cellular components. Since all defence systems, including DNA-repair enzymes, operate with the limited reliability, stochastic damages accumulate up to the threshold dysfunction level, resulting in apoptosis. To compensate the apoptotic cell loss, cell division is initiated. However, replicative capacity of human diploid cells is also limited owing to the gradual loss of telomeres. Thus, the limited reliability of the mitochondrial enzyme machinery along with the telomere marginotomy causes the loss of functionally competent cells. We estimated that the longevity of human brain could reach 250 years, should the reliability of mtSOD-defence be absolutely perfect. Some low-molecular antioxidants, among them butylated hydroxytoluene (BHT) can increase life-span of laboratory animals (Harman, 1956). In situ, however, the low-molecular "antioxidants" seem to operate not by the direct antioxidant pattern but in an indirect manner (Koltover, 1983). For instance, BHT improves the supply of heart tissue with oxygen through the nitric-oxide/endocrine mechanism, thereby decreasing the free-radical malfunctions in the mitochondrial electron-transport chains (Frolkis, Gorban and Koltover, 1990; Koltover, 1995). Thus, the concept of the limited reliability of biological systems pieces together the free-radical theory of aging and the theory of telomere marginotomy in the unified pattern which is consistent with the data of modern biogerontology.

Global ageing is a consequence of global evolution

H.V.Tereshina (Research Institute of Gerontology, Moscow, Russia)

A new conception of global evolution is developed that is based on the theory of an elementary open chemical system by A.P. Rudenko. It clears up the nature of the main force that moves the process of structural building from molecules to multicellular organisms and populations. The living being is regarded as a self organizing catalytical system (CS). The evolution of living beings starts and proceeds in the thermo stable conditions which occurs to be necessary for the organization and step by step improvementof CSs specialized on one or another source of energy (ES). There exists coevolution of ES and CS which it serves. In this collaboration the ES plays the leading role that realizes not only in the increase of the single CS's complexity but in the behavior of the whole multitude of homogenous CSs. The earth which is considered to be a global open chemical system evolves to the cycling of the processes of synthesis and utilization of monomers and polymers. Mammals and a man belong to the species that utilize polymers. Thus the coevolution of

Homo sapiens and global cyclization appears to be. The ES, its intensiveness and availability, defines the level of the stationary phase and quantity of CS (individuals) of population that interacts with it. This factor makes deaths an inevitable event. The limit of CS's possibilities to gain the energy out of the ES results in the number of offsprings and longevity. The period from birth to death of an individual that species demonstrate while being in the stationary phase is there true longevity. The duration of a specie's existence divides into three periods including growth, stationary phase and degradation. On the first stage number of births prevails over deaths. On the second stage they are equal. Nowadays the global balance between the synthesis and utilization of biopolymers is near to achieve. We are facing the second stage of the mankind's existence, its stationary phase when the number of middle-aged persons increases. Only now we can get to know the real longevity of a human being.

On the nature of aging

Imre Semsei (Molecular Biology Research Laboratory, 3rd Department of Medicine, University of Debrecen, Debrecen, Hungary

The aim of this lecture is to indicate that aging may be multifactorial and the process of senescence may be determined by the information level of the organization. This level itself changes during senescence (including the information level of the genom that also alters by time because of, e.g, its fluid character). According to this approach the aging process is determined by the sum effects of internal (e.g. genom) and external (material, energy, information) factors, although there are some elements that bear more importance than others. Subsequently, the maximal life-span is probably determined by the principle of the weakest element of the chain. Because of the high complexity of the human body where different information systems superpose each other, the cooperation of the elements (counter-effects, regulation) have the same determining importance as the information level of the unit parts (cells) have. The further aim of this paper is to show that the roots of certain diseases (e.g. cancer, autoimmunity) could firmly be linked to the aging process itself. This interpretation offers two ways of influencing the process of senescence. It could be influenced by maintaining the information level of the organism via optimization or by changing this level. All the factors that help to prevent the decrease of the information level of the organism could act against aging and certain diseases, and vice versa: the factors which deteriorate the state of the information system could contribute to the acceleration of the aging process. (MAD 117: 93-108, 2000)

Telomerase and MYC protein in blocking of terminal differentiation. Influence only on replicative senescence.

A. Khalyavkin (Russian Academy of Sciences, Institute of Biochemical Physics, Moscow, Russia)

Current evidence support a point that a somatic stem-like cell is an unrestricted source of a whole tissue renewal in norm. The gradual loss of the division potential in fibroblasts and other cells in vitro (replicative senescence) is a consequence of cellular maturation and terminal differentiation but not of the true senescence of cells. The limitless proliferative capacity, which somatic stem-like cells are thought to possess, is clearly revealed by the constitutive expression of protooncogenes which encode the nuclear immortalizers of MYC type (Schwab &Bishop, 1988). The important function of these proteins is the blocking of cell differentiation (Coppola & Cole, 1986; Dmitrovsky et al, 1986; Prochownik & Kukowska, 1986). The decade after, there are the same results, obtained by means of telomerase constitutive expression (Bodnar et al, 1998; Vaziri & Benchimol, 1998) and the same plausible explanation of it via differentiation blocking (Sharma et al, 1995; Kruk et al, 1996; Zhang et al, 1996). Perhaps this effect is related with the fact that telomerase can activate of c-myc expression (Wang et al, 2000). These and some other findings are compatible with the point that anti-aging processes can, in principle, successfully counteract cellular deterioration and show the essential futility of attempting to search the primary causes of normal aging by purely cytological methods. Some researchers agree with the view that the aging is more a function of breakdown in control mechanisms of the whole organism than of intrinsic changes in individual cells. Even age-related changes of non-dividing long-living neurons, not connected with their differentiation, may be a consequence of senescence and not its primary cause. Why, in this case, does an organism age? The answer might be found by taking into account the influence of external factors on the control efficiency of an organism's self-maintenance.

SESSION 11

Adjuvant transdermal nicotine for treatment-resistant agitation in dementia.

R. Rosin (Geropsychiatry Division, Highline Community Hospital Specialty Center, Tukwila, USA), M.D. Levine (Swedish Medical Center, Seattle, USA)

Purpose: To evaluate whether the addition of transdermal nicotine would ameliorate symptoms of agitation in patients with severe Alzheimer's disease who had had poor responses to traditional medical therapies. Method: Four consecutive patients admitted to our geropsychiatric unit with treatment-resistant agitation had transdermal nicotine added to their pharmacologic regimens. Results: All four patients were markedly improved soon after implementation of the nicotine patch. Consensus opinion among staff was that verbal aggression, physical combativeness, and insomnia were markedly reduced. Patients were discharged to long-term care facilities with transdermal nicotine a part of their new medical regimens. Conclusion: Transdermal nicotine deserves evaluation in a pilot clinical trial to see if it may be useful as adjuvant therapy in demented, agitated patients.

Biventricular Pacing in End-stage Heart Failure

S Utahayasenan,J.K.Dave, A. G. Kocheril (University of Illinois College of Medicine, Urbana-Champaign, US)

PURPOSE Biventricular pacing has emerged as a promising treatment modality for geriatric patients with end-stage congestive heart failure. Typically patients requiring biventricular pacing have New York heart association (NYHA) class IV symptoms and have failed optimal medical treatment. METHODS A 75 year old man with history of coronary artery disease, left ventricular dysfunction, and atrial fibrillation requiring AV node ablation and pacemaker therapy, was evaluated for persistent NYHA class IV symptoms. His medication included optimum doses of warfarin, lisinopril, atenolol, furosemide and digoxin. Examination was remarkable for pulse 61 per minute, BP 120/60mm of Hg, JVD 7cm of water above the sternal angle , bibasilar crackles, and 1+pedal edema. The patient underwent biventircular pacing. A new lead was introduced into a branch of the coronary sinus through left subclavian vein and connected via a Y adapter to the existing right ventricular lead and pulse generator. This procedure was expected to improve his cardiac output, by synchronizing right and left ventricular contraction. RESULTS Within two weeks, the patient reported improvement in dyspnea and fatigue. ON examination, his lungs were clear and he had no pedal edema. He could now walk 2 to 3 blocks and his lasix requirement decreased. Furthermore, he had an improved overall sense of well being. CONCLUSION Preliminary studies show that biventricular pacing is beneficial in advanced congestive heart failure patients. Whether patients with atrial fibrillation would benefit from biventricular pacing is not clear. In this patient with atrial fibrillation, functional class improved from NYHA class IV to NYHA class II after biventricular pacing. When patients are on maximum medical treatment for congestive heart failure, biventricular pacing offers an additional therapeutic option.

Double blind trial on the efficacy and adverse drug reaction of Huperzine in treatment of age-associated memory impairment in 662 cases

Ma Yong-Xing, Lu Pei-Fang, Gu Yue-Di (Department of Aging, Antiaging and Cognitive Function, Shanghai Institute of Gerontology and Geriatrics, Huadong Hospital,Shanghai,China)

Objective: To observe the efficacy and adverse drug reaction of Huperzine in treatment of Age-Associated Memory Impairment (AAMI). Huperzine, a new alkaloid extracted from Huperzia Serrata (Thumb) Trev, is a potent anticholinesterase with minimal toxicity, and may improve the learning and retrieval function of rats. Its facilitation actions were due to an effect on the central cholinergic system. Methods: Double blind trials were performed in 662 cases of AAMI in the aged and preaged with MQ<100 (WMS). The dosage of Huperzine and placebo were all 2 capsules or tablets (0.05mg/cap or tab) Bid for 2 months. The effects were evaluated with MQ(WMS). Results: The mean value of MQ(WMS) before and after treatment were 84.83±13.53 and 97.35±16.58 (P<0.001) in 355 cases treated with Huperzine and 87.8±16.1 and 91.8±16.9 (P<0.001)in 307 cases in the placebo group respectively. A significant difference of mean value of MQ increment between Huperzine 12.47±10.20 and placebo 3.89±8.15 (P<0.001) were observed. The total effective rate of the Huperzine and placebo were 62.82% and 36.81% respectively (P<0.001). No significant adverse drug reactions were observed. We consider that the clinical effect of Huperzine is mainly related to its anticholinesterase action. Conclusions: Huperzine is effective and safe to improve memory and cognitive function in the elderly.

Interactions between herbal and prescribed drug therapy in patients with dementia

J. Dergal, J. Gold, D. Laxer (Baycrest Centre for Geriatric Care, Toronto, Canada), K. Lanctôt (HOPE Research Centre at Sunnybrook & Women's College Health Sciences Centre, Baycrest Centre for Geriatric Care, University of Toronto, Toronto, Canada), P. Rochon (Baycrest Centre for Geriatric Care, University of Toronto, Toronto, Canada)

Purpose: To document herbal medicine use and identify potential drug interactions between herbal medicines and conventional drug therapies in older adults with dementia. Method: We interviewed all patients (or caregivers, as appropriate) attending an outpatient memory disorder clinic between July 4 and August 8, 2000. We documented herbal medicine and conventional drug therapy (i.e. prescribed or over- the-counter) use. To identify potential drug interactions, we reviewed each patient's herbal medicine and conventional drug therapy use, and compared this to interactions reported in the literature. Results: Of the 199 patients attending the clinic, 193 (97%) agreed to be interviewed. Of these 193, 109 (56.5%) were female and 84 (43.5%) were male. Mean age was 73 (SD + 12) years. A total of 59 (30.6%) patients had at some time used herbal medicines, and 31 (16%) were currently using herbal medicines. Of current herbal medicine users, 16 (51.6%) were using more than one herbal medicine. Forty-four herbal medicines were identified as being used by patients. Ginkgo biloba was most frequently used, by 20 (10.4%) of patients. Glucosamine sulfate, Garlic, and Ginseng were also frequently used. Of the 31 herbal medicine users, 10 (33%) were found to be at risk for an adverse drug event due to an interaction between their conventional drug therapy and an herbal medicine. A potential interaction between Ginkgo biloba and acetylsalicylic acid was encountered most frequently. Conclusion: Older people with dementia are frequent users of herbal medicines. Many are at risk for experiencing drug interactions that could lead to preventable adverse drug events.

Medication use patterns among cognitively intact and cognitively impaired community-dwelling older people in Hong Kong

CHAN FHW, LUK JKH, CHIU PKC, PAU MML

BACKGROUND : Whilst some drugs have been reported to be beneficial to cognitive impairment, inappropriate drug use are often causes of delirium. Overseas studies suggested cognitively impaired older people averaged fewer prescribed or over-the counter (OTC) medications per person. However, similar pharmaco-epidemiological studies have not been performed in Hong Kong. PURPOSE : The purpose of the study was to compare the medication use patterns among cognitively intact and cognitively impaired community-dwelling older people in the use of prescription drugs, OTC drugs, health food and Chinese Medicine; and to determine the common indications for these four categories of medications. METHOD : A face-to-face questionnaire survey was performed among older people at nine community centres. The Abbreviated Mental Test (AMT) was used to differentiate between the cognitively intact and cognitively impaired. RESULTS : 385 older people participated in the study, of which 251 (65.2%) were female. The mean age was 74.3 years (SD=+7.8). 38 (9.87%) subjects were classified as cognitively impaired. The cognitively impaired were significantly older, more likely to be female, less educated, single, more dependent in activities of daily living and more likely to be hospitalized in the past 12 months. There was no significant difference between the cognitively imapired and cognitively intact in the use of prescription drugs, OTC drugs,health food and Chinese Medicine. Among the prescription drugs, the most commonly used drugs were those for cardiovascular system (71.2%), gastro-intestinal system(28.8%), endocrine system (26.4%) and analgesia (22.2%). Common indications for OTC drugs included pain relief (47.1%), general improvement of functional state (25.0%), enhancement of immune system (17.3%) and nutritional supplement (16.3%) As for health food, the most common indications were nutrional supplement (69.6%), general improvement of functional state (68.8%) and sleep disturbance (19.2%). Up to a quarter of the subjects were using Chinese Medicine, of whom 46.9% were using them for their immune system and 38.5% for general improvement of functional state. CONCLUSION : Cognitively impaired older people were not taking fewer medications in Hong Kong. A large proportion of community-dwelling older people were consuming non-prescription drugs. With increasing popularity of alternative medicine, physicians should be reminded to enquire any use of OTC drugs, health food, as well as Chinese medicine in order to minimize drug-drug interactions and adverse drug reactions.

Passive 70° Head-Up Tilt Test: An Useful Procedure in the Diagnosis of Unexplained Syncope in the Elderly.

J.D. Soares, (Autonomic Nervous System and Arrhythmia Laboratory - Alfenas University), Minas Gerais, Brazil. A.C. Lopes, (Titularof Internal Medicine - Universidade Federal de São Paulo). P.J.F. Tucci, (Professor of Cardiovascular and Respiratory Physiology - Universidade Federal de São Paulo).

The objective was to determine the usefulness of Head-Up Tilt to induce vasodepressive and cardio-inhibitory syncope in the elderly and to study the effects of different pharmacologic agents and their therapeutic implications. It was studied 34 patients, mean age: 66 +/- 6.0, who had had at least one episode of undetermined syncope, comparatively to 10 normal controls, mean age: 65 +/- 5.6 Δ(p>0.01 Δ T-Student) Both groups were studied with prolonged and passive 70° Head-Up Tilt Test. Pharmacologic and therapeutic tests were performed with etilephrine-oral, dose of 30 to 125 mg a day, during 3 days period; atropine intravenously dose of 0.04 mg/Kg body weight in bolus during 1 minute. The beta blocker, propranolol Δ intravenously, dose of 0.02 mg/Kg in 2 minutes; and transdermal scopolamine, as parasympathetic drug. Among the abnormal group 16 patients had an abnormal response to the Tilt Test, none among the normal controls showed abnormal Tilt Test. The alpha-adrenergic agonist: etilephrine was able to prevent syncope in 11 among 14 patients. The beta-blocker propranolol, was efficient to prevent syncope in 7 out of 14 patients. The authors conclude that the 70° Head-Up Tilt Test is useful for the diagnosis of syncope of undetermined origin in the elderly. The peripheral vasodilation during the test is secondary to the withdrawal of alpha-sympathetic stimulation, and this is the main etiopathogenic mechanism responsible for vaso-vagal syncope. The alpha-adrenergic agonist, etilephrine, effectively prevent the autonomic syncope episodes in acute context. The beta-blocker propranolol was efficient in acute context to prevent syncope in 7 out of 14 patients of the following types: cardio-inhibitory and vasodepressive types, in one year period of follow-up. Seven patients received long-term drug treatment with oral propranolol, selected on the basis of acute drug testing during Tilt. None of these 7 patients had syncopal recurrences or death during the follow-up or any side effects. Among the 11 patients who received chronically etilephrine in the same above dosage, none had syncopal recurrences or death but 5 patients presented cardiac arrhythmias during Holter/24 hs. In a chronic context the beta-blocker was superior to the alpha adrenergic agonist etilephrine considering side effects, in this context this agent, etilephrine, must be better evaluated.

Study on the effect of Choline Piracetam to treat age-associated memory impairment by double blind trial method

Lu Pei-Fang, Ma Yong-Xing, Xie Su-Zhen (Department of Aging, Antiaging and Cognitive Function, Shanghai Institute of Gerontology and Geriatrics, Department of Geriatrics of Huadong Hospital, Shanghai,China)

Objective: To Observe the effect of Choline Piracetam to treat age-associated memory impairment (AAMI) Methods: Double blind trials were performed in 436 cases of AAMI in the aged and pre-aged with MQ<100(WMS). The dosage of Choline Piracetam and placebo were all 2 capsules(0.4g/cap) tid for 2 months. The effect were evaluated with MQ(WMS) and light reaction time. Results: The mean value of MQ(WMS) before and after treatment were 83.50±15.04 and 94.69±16.54(P<0.001) in 218 cases treated with Choline Piracetam and 81.05 ±13.78 and 86.67±16.05 (P<0.001) in 218 cases in placebo group respectively. Significant difference of mean value of WMS increment between Choline Piracetam 11.19±12.13 and placebo 5.55±8.78 (P<0.001) were observed. The total effective rate of the Choline Piracetam and placebo were 57.80% and 33.03% respectively (P<0.01). No significant side effects were observed. Significant decrement of simple and choose light (Red and Green) reaction time were observed between treatment and placebo group. Conclusions: Choline Piracetam may increase MQ, decrease light reaction time. It is effective to improve memory function in the elderly.

SESSION 12

The Aging Immune System: Implications for Immunization

Rita B. Effros (UCLA School of Medicine, Los Angeles, USA) Telemere/Telomerase dynamics in T cells: impact on immunological memory. K.C.P. Hirokawa (Tokoyo Medical and Dental University, Tokoyo, Japan) Effectiveness of intra-nasal immunization of influenza virus with cholera toxin B in old mice. Carlos Franceschi (Italy) Abstract not yet available Beatrix Grubeck-Loebenstein (University of Innsbruck, Austria)An imblance between Th1 and Th2 cytokines may be responsible for lack of antibody production following influenza vaccination in old age. Janet E. McElhaney (Eastern Virginia Medical School, Norfolk, USA) Influence of vaccination is less effective for stimulating a granzyme B response in older adults. Stefan Gravenstein (Eastern Virginia Medical School, Norfolk, USA) Influenza in seniors: biologic implications of clinical presentations.

Issue:Influenza is a serious illness in older adults and vaccine efficacy is limited. Structure: This translational research symposium will present data from vaccine studies in both in animal models and humans and will include a discussion of the biological implications of clinical influenza in older adults. Content: 1. Longitudinal analysis in cell culture of antigen-specific CD8+ memory T cells over time, showed that the robust telomerase activity induced in response to the first and second antigenic stimulations, was not sustained during subsequent antigenic exposures. Once telomerase became uninducible, the antigen-specific memory cells continued to undergo antigen-specific proliferation and telomere shortening until they reached the end-stage of replicative senescence. Although cytotoxic function was maintained, cytokine profiles were altered in senescent T cells. 2. Intranasal immunization of influenza vaccine with cholera toxin B (CTB)gives rise to significant production of IgG antibody in serum and IgA antibody in nasal wash, which was markedly increased in 3 month old and moderately increased in 18 month old mice. Mice at 18 months of age are more susceptible to infection with influenza virus than 3-month old mice; older mice died with a 10-fold lower dose of virus. However, 18-month old mice exposed to a lower dose of virus can survive and obtain strong immunity to the same virus. 3. Decreased diversity of T cell subsets due to the appearance of large expanded clones was accompanied by increased numbers of CD45RO+ and of CD45RA+CD11a++ CD28- T cells. These changes were more pronounced in old non-responders than in responders. T cells from old non-responders also produced interferon gamma, but only little IL-5 following in vitro stimulation with PHA or influenza antigen. While interferon gamma was predomoninantly produced by CD45RO+ T cells in the young control group, CD45RA+CD28- T cells became a main source of interferon gamma in older responders and non-responders. 4. Granzyme B, one of the mediators of CTL activity, is lower in older adults who develop influenza illness. An ex-vivo assay of granzyme B levels in influenza-stimulated PBMC showed >2-fold higher levels of granzyme B in young compared to older adults; CTL frequencies increased by a similar proportion in the two age groups following vaccination. 5. The age-associated increase in the duration of symptoms of influenza can be independently attenuated by anticedent vaccination and zanamivir treatment. The quality of vaccine match affects acute presentation; better match appears to have a greater likelihood but shorter duration of elevated temperature. The duration of influenza incubation appears to be prolonged and speed of seroconversion accelerated in vaccinated compared to unvaccinated institutionalized elderly. Conclusion/ Anticipated Outcomes: Vaccines intended to protect older adults from influenza must take into account dysregulated and reduced immune responses. This will require customizing vaccine formulations and innoculation strategies as well as considering the use of anti-viral therapies to optimize protection against influenza in older adults.

An imbalance between Th1 and Th2 cytokines may be responsible for lack of antibody production following influenza vaccination in old age

Thomas L. Lung, Maria Saurwein-Teissl, Esther Asch, Walter Parson, Imrich Blasko, Dietmar Schönitzer, Emanuelle Trannoy1 and Beatrix Grubeck-Loebenstein (Institute for Biomedical Aging Research of the Austrian Academy of Sciences Innsbruck, Austria); 1Aventis-Pasteur) (Marcy l'Etoile, France)

PURPOSE: Influenza vaccination is frequently not accompanied by the production of specific antibodies in elderly persons. It was the aim of this study to analyse the nature of the underlying molecular and cellular defects. METHOD: We characterized T cell subsets and their clonal composition as well as their in vitro responsiveness to PHA and influenza antigen in young (<35 years) and old healthy (>60 years) volunteers. The old age group consisted of two subgroups, (a) "responders", persons who did and (b) "non-responders", persons who did not produce specific antibodies following influenza vaccination. RESULTS: Old age was in general associated with typical changes in the T cell repertoire. Decreased diversity due to the appearance of large expanded clones was accompanied by increased numbers of CD45RO+ and of CD45RA+ CD11a++CD28- T cells. These changes were more pronounced in old non-responders than in responders. T cells from old non-responders also produced IFN , but only little IL-5 following in vitro stimulation with PHA or influenza antigen. In contrast, stimulated T cells from young persons and to a certain extent from aged responders produced both cytokines in vitro. While IFN was predominantly produced by CD45RO+ T cells in the young control group, CD45RA+CD28- T cells had become a main source of IFN in the old responder as well as in the non-responder group. CONCLUSIONS: These results suggest that loss of type-2 cytokine production with a relative overproduction of IFN by CD28- T cells may to be a cause of insufficient antibody production following influenza vaccination in the elderly.

Effectiveness of intranasal immunization of influenza virus with cholera toxin B in old mice.

Hirokawa K.C.P, Utsuyama M.C.P. and Tamura S.C.Q. (CP Department of Pathology and Immunology, Tokyo Medical & Dental University Graduate School and 2 Department of Pathology, National Institute of Health)

Intranasal immunization of influenza vaccine with cholera toxin B (CTB) gave rise to a significant production of IgG antibody in serum and IgA antibody in nasal wash, markedly in 3 months old and moderately in 18 months old mice. On the contrary, intraperitoneal injection of influenza virus with CTB induced high level of IgG antibody production in serum in both 3 months and 18 months old mice, but not IgA antibody production in nasal wash. Since the nasal mucosa is the most common route of respiratory infection of influenza virus, nasal immunization of vaccine appears to be more effective than systemic route such as peritoneal immunization. Mice at 18 months of age are more susceptible to infection of influenza virus than 3 months old mice; i.e, older mice died of infection of influenza virus at 10 fold less dose of virus. Old mice at 18 months of age exposed to a low dose of virus can survive and obtain strong immunity to the same virus. Namely, these mice become resistant to the 2nd infection with a high dose of influenza virus. These data suggest that vaccination appears to be useful to protect the elderly people from various kinds of infection. One thing to be kept in mind is that vaccination performed in very old people may not work due to depressed immune functions. Thus, vaccination should be started at latest in middle aged people, still having enough capacity to respond to infectious agents. Or one should use some methods to enhance or stimulate the depressed immune capacity of the elderly people at the time of vaccination.

Influenza in Seniors: Biologic Implications of Clinical Presentations.

Gravenstein S. (Glennan Center for Geriatrics and Gerontology, Eastern Virginia Medical School, Norfolk, VA, USA) McElhaney J. Deng Y. (1Glennan Center for Geriatrics and Gerontology, Eastern Virginia Medical School, Norfolk, VA, USA) Drinka P. (2Wisconsin Veterans Home, King, WI, USA;) Ambrozaitis A, Radziusauskiene D.(Department of Infectious Diseases, Vilnius Univeristy, Vilnius, Lithuania.)

Background. Influenza morbidity and mortality increases with age. The clinical presentation and mortality are differentially affected by age, prior vaccination and treatments. How can the presentation be predicted based on the immunesenescent biology? Methods. Clinical data from several studies including prospective surveillance and placebo, rimantadine or zanamivir for primary influenza prevention in nursing home settings and pooled analyses from phase III zanamivir treatment studies on ambulatory adult volunteers are presented for a combined post-hoc analysis of the clinical presentation of influenza. Over 1000 elderly and 1000 young volunteers were enrolled in described studies. Results. There is an age-associated increase in duration of symptoms that can be independently attenuated by antecedent vaccination and zanamivir treatment. The quality of vaccine match affects acute presentation; better match appears to have a greater likelihood but shorter duration of elevated temperature. The duration of influenza incubation appears to be prolonged and speed of seroconversion accelerated in vaccinated compared to unvaccinated institutionalized elderly. Conclusions. Clinical presentation of influenza can be dramatically influenced by vaccination and antiviral treatment or prophylaxis. None of these techniques is 100% effective in influenza prevention, but they offer complementary and potentially synergistic mechanisms that affect presentation and can improve outcomes of natural influenza infection.

Influenza vaccination is less effective for stimulating a granzyme B response in older adults

Janet E. McElhaney, Caroline R. Letter and Stefan Gravenstein Eastern Virginia Medical School School, Virginia (Norfolk, USA)

PURPOSE: To determine age-related differences in the number of virus-specific precursor CTL (pCTL) and Grz B levels after influenza vaccination. METHOD: We measured the number of pCTL by ELISPOT and Grz B levels in lysates of peripheral blood mononuclear cells (PBMC) stimulated with live virus (A/H3N2; A/Sydney, A/Nanchang and A/Shangdong) under ex vivo conditions. RESULTS: Prior to influenza vaccination, healthy young and older adults had similar levels of Grz B. At 4 weeks post-vaccination, the Grz B levels in PBMC from young adults were significantly higher than in the older adults (young, 6.36 U/mg protein; older, 2.78 U/mg; $p=0.0002$). Young adults had a higher proportion of pCTL compared to older adults ($p<0.05$) but the two groups had a similar increase in the number of pCTL in response to vaccination (pre to post; young, 0.45% to 0.50%; older, 0.36% to 0.44% of PBMC). When the level of Grz B was calculated based on the number of pCTL, the young adults were found to have a 4-fold rise in Grz B per pCTL while the older adults showed only a 2-fold rise in response to influenza vaccination. Granzyme B and pCTL frequency were lower for the older influenza strains at baseline and after vaccination. CONCLUSIONS: We conclude that killed virus vaccines are more effective in young compared to older adults for re-stimulating a previously primed response to influenza but only weakly stimulate proliferation of virus-specific pCTL. These results provide insight in to the mechanism of reduced influenza vaccine efficacy in older adults.

Telomere/telomerase dynamics in T cells: impact on immunological memory

Rita B. Effros, Mirabelle Dagarag, Hector F. Valenzuela and Carolyn Spaulding UCLA School of Medicine, California (Los Angeles, USA)

PURPOSE: To identify changes in the aged immune system age that might impact attempts at vaccine-mediated prophylaxis in the elderly. METHOD: The effect of aging was examined at the cellular level, using an in vitro model of human T cell replicative senescence. Human T cells from healthy individuals were stimulated repeatedly with an allogeneic tumor cell line until they reached senescence. Similar experiments were performed using CD8+ T cells from HIV-infected donors stimulated with HIV antigens. The T cells were followed for function, phenotype, cytokine profile, population doublings, telomere length and ability to activate telomerase. RESULTS: Human T cells that are aged in cell culture have many characterstics resembling expanded CD8+ memory T cells populations in the elderly and in younger persons infected with HIV (e.g,short telomeres, poor proliferation, absence of CD28 expression, apoptosis resistance). Longitudinal analysis in cell culture of the same population of antigen-specific memory T cells over time showed that the robust telomerase activity induced in response to the first and second antigenic stimulations was not sustained during subsequent antigenic exposures. Once telomerase became uninducible, the antigen-specific memory cells nevertheless continued to undergo antigen-specific proliferation and telomere shortening until they reach the end stage of replicative senecence. Although cytotoxic function was maintained, cytokine profiles were altered in senescent T cells. CONCLUSIONS: Repeatedly stimulated antigen-specific memory T cells leads to phenotypic, genetic and functional alterations. These observations, combined with our earlier demonstration of age-associated antigen-presentation defects in a murine model of influenza, suggest that vaccines intended to protect the elderly from such viral infections as HIV and influenza require customizing both the immunogen formulation and inoculation strategies to accommodate the unique characteristics of the aged immune system.

SESSION 13

Narrative Matters 1: Perspectives on Stories and Aging

Gary Kenyon (Programme in Gerontology, St. Thomas University, Fredericton, Canada) The Stories We Are: Expanding our Understanding of Time and Wisdom. Jay Gubrium (Department of Sociology, University of Florida, Gainesville, USA) The Practical Mediations of Storytelling. Ruth Ray (Department of English and

Institute of Gerontology, Wayne State University, Detroit, USA) Repeating Ourselves: The Developmental Importance of Oft-Told Tales. Sharon R. Kaufman (Institute for Health and Aging, University of California, San Francisco, USA) Narrative and the Culture of Death in the United States. Riitta-Liisa Heikkinen (The Finnish Centre for Interdisciplinary Gerontology, University of Jyvaskyla, Jyvaskyla, Finland) Aging _ Experience in a Narrative Context: A Ten-Year Follow Up.

The narrative perspective has spread throughout the social sciences and the humanities, even entering into professional applications across the human services, from care and counseling to mediation and advocacy. This is the first of two symposia entitled, "Narrative Matters", to reflect both the substance and the popularity of this perspective. This first session emphasizes the conceptual facets of narrativity. Participants consider, from their varied perspectives, what it means either analytically or methodologically to proceed by considering the storied features of their respective enterprises. In the first paper in the session, Kenyon explores the philosophical foundations of "narrative gerontology", with a particular emphasis on the implications that a storied perspective has for our understanding of time and wisdom. The second paper by Gubrium, drawing from narrative material gathered in a variety of social settings, discusses the ways in which a lifestory belongs, paradoxically, as much to the social context as it does to the individual storyteller. This theme is further elaborated in the third paper by Ray which deals with the developmental influences that the sociocultural dimension of storytelling exerts on our personal stories over time. Ray's findings are based on research carried out with writing groups in senior citizen centers. The fourth paper by Kaufman explores the rapidly expanding narrative interest in the context of death with dignity. By presenting a case study, this paper, as with the previous two contributions, examines narratives at both a subjective or personal level, and at the sociocultural or meta-narrative level. The paper considers the unique insight that a narrative perspective brings to this area of inquiry, in contrast to the dominant medical "story" of death and dying. The session concludes with a paper by Heikkinen in which the results of a longitudinal narrative study in Finland are presented. The theme of this paper is aging as it is experienced and accessed by language in the form of narratives. Further, the discussion in this paper returns to the topics of temporality, discussed in the first paper, as well as considering the issue of embodiment. One conclusion of this study is that narratives provide a particularly effective lens with which to understand the inner life of older persons. The anticipated outcome of Narrative Matters 1 is the further development of a conceptual framework and a language that facilitates the understanding and employment of stories in theory and research in the field of aging. Building on this analysis, the second symposium emphasizes the central role that stories play in various practice contexts. The overall goal of the two symposia is to critically orient to and to appreciate the place of narrative in the practice as well as the representation of lives.

Aging - Experience in a Narrative Context: A Ten-Year Follow Up

Riitta-Liisa Heikkinen (The Finnish Centre for Interdisciplinary Gerontology, University of Jyvaskyla, Jyvaskyla, Finland)

In 1990 we studied 262 persons aged 80 in Jyvaskyla, central Finland. As well as epidemiological data, tape recorded narratives on the aging experience were collected from a sample of 20 participants. A five-year follow-up was carried out with seventeen remaining participants. A 10-year follow-up was carried out in 2000, with ten participants, now aged 90. The findings of this study are considered in light of the themes of aging, bodiliness and temporality. In terms of results, the narratives at age 80 revealed no special feeling of old age itself. At age 85 most narrators said they had crossed the line into old age. These new stories were narratives about change and decline. At age 90, "nothing is the same as before". The sense of "abandonment" was also reflected in the narrators' mood. Their losses exceeded what they could achieve and caused a sense of uncertainty. However, there was also some strength and will-power left, some hope for the future. One of the conclusions of this study is that language provides a means with which to express thoughts and to access the world of experience. Narrativity is a type of discourse with which temporal existence is transformed into linguistic form. This is what our 10-year follow-up highlights: The temporal existence of the human individual. The aging body is also a temporary sketch in existence. Its key characteristic is variability. The narrative served as a means of giving voice to one's bodily experience and inner life.

Narrative and the Culture of Death in the United States

Sharon R. Kaufman (Institute for Health and Aging, University of California, San Francisco, USA)

This paper explores uses of narrative in the context of "death with dignity," a dominant American preoccupation over the last decade. It considers narrative as operating at two levels: first, as storytelling, especially subjective accounts of illness, treatment, hospital technologies and practices; and second, as cultural knowledge or societal meta-narratives, that operate as background assumptions through which individual stories are lived, constructed, and told. Its goal is to explore the limits of the "death with dignity" idea through multiple uses of narrative. The paper presents one case study, drawn from an ethnographic investigation of how death and dying are approached and understood by health professionals, patients, and families in the United States, in order to consider advanced age and common dying trajectories in the American hospital. It will illustrate ways in which medicine is producing a discourse on senescence, in which members of industrial societies form understandings about scientific progress, approach decline, frailty, and finitude, and value a range of dying practices. The impact of that discourse on both understanding and dealing with the end of life is almost entirely unexplored in the field of gerontology. Narrative analysis of one example of hospital death shows how that discourse is constituted and emphasizes how the particular actions and concerns of individual players are informed and constrained by larger sociocultural effects.

Repeating Ourselves: The Developmental Importance of Oft-Told Tales

Ruth Ray (Department of English and Institute of Gerontology, Wayne State University, Detroit, USA)

Narrative approaches to adult development require that we study, not only how an individual's life story changes over time, but the sociocultural influences that promote or impede that change. Through several years of qualitative research on lifestory writing groups in senior citizen centers, I have found that repeated stories — those which are told to the same group multiple times and which would appear to be "set pieces" resistant to change — actually serve as prompts for reflection and reinterpretation. Repetition and recursiveness in talk and writing is typically interpreted by peers as a call for attention and, in many cases, narrative intervention.

The Practical Mediations of Storytelling

Jay F. Gubrium (Department of Sociology, University of Florida, Gainesville, USA)

Storytelling doesn't exist in a social vacuum. It takes place in time and in particular locations, among a variety of others who have agendas of their own about what is narratively relevant. In other words, in practice, local "going concerns" mediate the contents and presentation of narrative accounts. Drawing from narrative material gathered in a variety of social settings, this presentation will consider and illustrate how the local conditions of narration are taken into consideration in storytelling in later life. The theme will be that the characterization, employment, and moral contours of accounts are as much features of social settings as they are personal constructions.

The Stories We Are: Expanding our Understanding of Time

and Wisdom

Gary Kenyon (Programme in Gerontology, St. Thomas University, Fredericton, Canada)

The life as story metaphor gives rise to important implications for our understanding of human development and aging. This paper explores the ontological character of storytelling and storylistening. That is, human beings do not only tell stories periodically as one form of human activity, they "are" stories. This means that the stories we "live" are not only cognitive in nature, they contain emotions and they influence action. Moreover, lives as stories are composed of both facticity, which refers to the narrative setting in which we exist at any point along the lifespan, and a sense of possibility, the ability to restory our lives. These two insights have crucial implications for the ways in which we understand such basic concepts as time and wisdom. The paper discusses the distinction between clock-time and storytime for the purpose of indicating the diverse and creative ways that we can interpret and experience time from a narrative perspective. As to wisdom, the paper considers how a narrative perspective moves us away from specialized and exclusive interpretations of this phenomenon and towards "ordinary wisdom" that may be an integral aspect of our lives as stories.

SESSION 14

Progress in Understanding and Treating Late-life Insomnia

Maurice M Ohayon, MD (Sleep Disorders Center, School of Medicine, Stanford University, Stanford, CA 94305, USA). Prevalence of Insomnia Related to Age in the General Population. Célyne Bastien, (School of Psychology, Université Laval, Bureau 1644, Ste-Foy, Québec G1K 7P4, Canada) Chronic insomnia: sleep EEG power spectra of elderly people using benzodiazepines and drug-free individuals. Colin Shapiro, MD (Department of Psychiatry, The Toronto Hospital, 399 Bathurst Street, Toronto, Ontario M5T 2S8, Canada). Insomnia as a cause and consequence of psychiatric illness: relevance to assessment and treatment Kevin Morgan, (Gerontology Research Unit, Loughborough University, Leicestershire L11 3TU, UK) Psychological treatment in the management of chronic insomnia in primary care: clinical and cost effectiveness Joanne Thompson (Institute of General Practice and Primary Care, University of Sheffield, Sheffield S5 7AU, UK) Factors predicting insomnia treatment outcomes in primary care settings: implications for assessment.

ISSUE Experienced by up to 1 in 3 older people, insomnia represents both a major influence on health and wellbeing in later life, and a significant challenge for health care services throughout the world. Combining clinical and research experience in epidemiology, sleep research, health services research and health economics, this interdisciplinary symposium will present recently completed research findings addressing the prevalence, nature and treatment of late-life insomnia. Overall, the symposium will provide an authoritative, evidence-based overview of current approaches to assessment, diagnosis, treatment, and service delivery. STRUCTURE Following a brief introduction, the symposium will include 5 individual oral presentations, with time for questions allowed after each. Printed summary information will be available from the symposium convenor. CONTENT The first presentation (Ohayon) considers the prevalence and natural history of insomnia, before exploring in greater detail the relationship between ageing and sleep disturbances. Moving from population to laboratory-based research, the second presentation (Bastien) examines the sleeping EEG profiles of those older people who do, and do not, report insomnia symptoms (comparing, in the insomnia group, those taking benzodiazepines, and those drug free). Clinical assessment and innovations in drug management are then specifically considered in the third presentation (Shapiro), while recent results from a controlled evaluation of psychological treatment and treatment costs are then presented (Morgan/Thompson). CONCLUSION/ANTICIPATED OUTCOMES Older people with insomnia can now benefit from a range of effective, evidence-based treatments. Epidemiology and laboratory sleep studies are essential in guiding the clinical assessments which should precede and accompany the efficient deployment of treatment options. Service delivery models, appropriate for national healthcare systems, should continue to be developed.

Chronic Insomnia: Sleep EEG Power Spectra of Elderly People Using Benzodiazepines and Drug-Free Individuals

Célyne H. Bastien, Mélanie LeBlanc (Université Laval, Montréal, Québec, Canada), Julie Carrier (Université de Montréal, Québec, Canada) & Charles M. Morin (Université Laval, Montréal, Québec, Canada)

PURPOSE It is estimated that approximately 10% of older individuals use benzodiazepines (BZDs) chronically as sleep inducers. Although the short-term effects of BZDs on the sleep EEG are well documented (in terms of Sleep Stages, Power Spectral Analysis, etc.) no data exists on the impact of long-term use. METHOD All night sleep EEGs were collected from 3 groups of older volunteers (aged 55+): those suffering from chronic insomnia, but who were drug-free (INS; N=20); those suffering from chronic insomnia and chronically using BZDs (BZD; N=20); and self defined good sleepers not using benzodiazepines (GS; N=20). EEG power spectra were then analysed and compared in the three groups. RESULTS There were no significant differences between INS and GS groups. However, when compared with the INS and GS groups, there was significantly higher EEG fast frequency activity in BZD group. More micro-arousals were also present within the BZD group when compared with INS and GS groups. CONCLUSION Cortical activity appears to be higher in chronic users of BZDs, with long-term use still affecting the EEG. More micro-arousals and increased activity in fast frequency EEG bands in chronic BZD users might reflect poorer sleep quality. Spectral analysis appears to be an efficient tool to quantify chronic BZD use in older people with insomnia.

Factors Predicting Insomnia Treatment Outcomes in Primary Care Settings: Implications for Assessment

Joanne Thompson (Institute of General Practice and Primary Care, University of Sheffield, Sheffield S5 7AU, UK)

PURPOSE While cognitive/behavioural (CBT) treatments have been successful in managing insomnia in clinical trials, not all patients with insomnia are prepared to engage in 'talking therapies' and, among those who do, treatment effects vary. Relatively little research, however, has attempted to identify factors predictive of engagement or response variations following CBT for insomnia. Within an optimal 'mixed-economy' of insomnia management (including educational, psychological, and pharmacological approaches) identifying such factors could help to direct appropriate treatment options, and provide a clinical response to insomnia that is flexible, practical, and lastingly effective. This presentation examines demographic and psychological factors related to: i) the preparedness of patients offered CBT in a clinical trial to engage in treatment; and ii) the expressed satisfaction of those patients who completed CBT treatment. METHOD In the context of a clinical trial a random series of general practice patients (all of whom were chronic benzodiazepine users) were offered a package of psychological therapies for insomnia over 6 sessions (including health education, sleep hygiene, stimulus control procedures, relaxation and cognitive approaches). Treatment was delivered by primary care counsellors supervised by a clinical psychologist. It was made clear at the outset that patients were free to exit from the programme at any time. RESULTS A total of 109 patients attended for psychological treatment (mean age 63.0 years; range 31-89). Of these, 76 patients (70%) completed the full therapy package, with 33 patients exiting early (i.e. before completion). Completion/non-completion was unrelated to age (mean age 63.08y and 63.03y respectively; $t = -0.017$; NS), and showed no significant association with gender ($X2 = 1.2$, $df = 1$; NS). Among completers patient satisfaction ratings were highly positive, with 88% of patients reported the sleep clinic as being quite or extremely helpful. The majority of the remainder were neutral. There were too few patients unsatisfied with the clinic to conduct age/gender statistical analyses. Treatment outcomes were related to health status and health attitudes. CONCLUSION Older age is not a barrier to the delivery of psychological treatments for chronic insomnia.

Insomnia as a Cause and Consequence of Psychiatric Illness: Relevance to Assessment and Treatment

Colin Shapiro, MBBCh (Department of Psychiatry, The Toronto Hospital, 399 Bathurst Street, Toronto, Ontario M5T 2S8, Canada).

PURPOSE Insomnia is commonly encountered in clinical psychiatric practice where it is frequently secondary to underlying emotional and psychiatric disorders. Less recognised, however, are psychological disturbances which originate from, or are exacerbated by, primary sleep disturbances. This presentation examines insomnia as both a consequence and a cause of mental ill health, and considers in particular appropriate assessment strategies and recent innovations in pharmacological treatment. METHOD The information for this presentation has been derived from three sources: i) a review of the clinical and scientific literature; ii) ongoing and recently completed laboratory sleep studies; and iii) clinical case studies. RESULTS Cause/effect relationships between insomnia and a variety of psychiatric disorders can be usefully explored and discriminated using appropriate clinical assessments. Such assessments provide an important guide to effective and efficient pharmacological treatment. CONCLUSION Insomnia represents a major public health issue with direct implications for quality of life, occupational and social performance, and mental health. Pharmacological treatment strategies must be matched to individual patient need.

Prevalence of Insomnia Related to Age in the General Population

Maurice M. Ohayon, M.D, D.Sc, Sleep Disorders Research Center, School of Medicine, Stanford University, Stanford, CA, USA

PURPOSE: Insomnia is a widespread sleep problem in industrialized countries. About 20% of the population suffers of mild to severe insomnia symptoms. Most of epidemiological studies found the prevalence of insomnia symptoms dramatically increases with age and is twice more frequent in women than in men. This increase in elderly people is often presented as part of the aging process namely because of changes in biological sleep patterns. METHOD: Over 24,000 subjects aged between 15 to 100 years and representative of the general population of six European countries (France, the United Kingdom, Germany, Italy, Portugal, Spain) were interviewed by telephone using the Sleep-EVAL system, a computer software designed to assess sleep and mental disorders in the general population. The overall participation rate was 81%. RESULTS: Insomnia symptoms increased with age in all these countries being 12.2% in the young adults (<25 y.o.) and reaching 22.8% in subjects aged 65 years or older. However, this association needs to be temperate with other factors that can better account for the relationship than age itself. Among important contributing factors, there is the presence of physical diseases, mental illnesses, and level of occupation. The prevalence of DSM-IV insomnia disorder diagnoses also increased with age. However, the increase was in two steps: before 45 years, the prevalence was 4.8% and among subjects 45 years or older the prevalence was 7.6% with no significant increase beyond this age. CONCLUSION: Insomnia needs to be assessed using different levels in order to understand its evolution over age.

Psychological Treatment in the Management of Chronic Insomnia in Primary Care: Clinical and Cost Effectiveness

Kevin Morgan (Gerontology Research Unit, Loughborough University, Leicestershire LE11 3TU, UK), Simon Dixon (Sheffield Health Economics Group, University of Sheffield, Sheffield S1 4DA, UK) Nigel Mathers, Joanne Thompson (Institute of General Practice and Primary Care, University of Sheffield, Sheffield S5 7AU, UK), Maureen Tomeny (Department of Clinical Psychology, Central Nottinghamshire Healthcare Trust, Mansfield NG18 4HH, UK)

PURPOSE While the clinical trials evidence shows that chronic insomnia can be effectively treated with appropriate psychological therapies, such treatments are rarely deployed in primary care settings - where most complaints of insomnia are made. This study was designed to evaluate the practicality, cost and clinical effectiveness of a primary care 'sleep clinic' providing short-term cognitive/behavioural treatment in the management of chronic insomnia in primary care settings. METHOD Patients presenting, or recalled, for repeat hypnotic prescriptions in 23 Sheffield general practices were invited to participate in either the clinic (50%) or control (50%) conditions of the study. Clinic patients were offered a package of psychological therapies for insomnia over 6 sessions (including health education, sleep hygiene, stimulus control procedures, relaxation and cognitive approaches). Treatment was delivered by primary care counsellors supervised by a clinical psychologist. Controls were assessed, but received no additional treatment. Outcomes included sleep quality, drug use, and patient ratings of service satisfaction. Detailed economic analyses of treatment costs and National Health Service insomnia care in the UK were conducted alongside the trial. RESULTS A total of 101 and 109 patients participated in the control and clinic groups respectively (total = 210; mean age = 65 years). The sleep clinic was associated with improved sleep quality, reduced hypnotic use, positive ratings of patient satisfaction, and high take-up by general practices. Economic analyses indicated substantial hidden costs associated with hypnotic drug usage. CONCLUSION The primary care sleep clinic model described here can offer a high quality, low risk response to chronic insomnia in general practice settings.

SESSION 15

Changing parameters of ageing in the UK: Evidence for the existence of the Third Age

Martin Hyde. (Department of Social Science and Medicine Imperial College of Science, Technology and Medicine St Dunstan's Rd London W6 UK) David Blane (Department of Social Science and Medicine Imperial College of Science, Technology and Medicine St Dunstan's Rd London W6 UK) Paul Higgs (Department of Psychiatry and Behavioural Sciences University College London Wolfson Building Riding House St London W1N 8AA UK) Dick Wiggins (Department of Sociology City University Northampton Square London EC1 UK)

Purpose: This paper presents findings that demonstrate the existence of a section of the older population in Britain participating in the 'Third Age'. We argue that the Third Age is not a set of personality traits but a social and cultural space created by increased affluence and falling morbidity Method A postal survey of a representative sample of the UK population aged 65-75 years was conducted to investigate the influences on Quality of Life in early old age. The sample was generated from a previously studied population [n = 286]. A response rate of 92 per cent was attained. The questionnaire measured Quality of Life, Social Capital, Social Networks and Consumption behaviour. Contextual data collected via the questionnaire was analysed in conjunction with lifecourse data already held on the respondents using Transitional Data Analysis . Results Our data demonstrate the diversity of experiences and lifestyles in old age. Combining data collected across factors such as Social Networks, Pension adequacy, Quality of Life and the lifecourse we map out the pathways and contextual influences that characterise the Third. Conclusion We conclude that older people in the UK can no longer be viewed as a homogenous category of the population. Whilst it is important to recognise the continued existence of a disadvantaged section of the older population it is neither sociologically nor empirically justified to generalise from them to the whole age group. Increasingly we are seeing the emergence of the reality of a 'Third Age' for many older people.

Influence of wartime deprivation in childhood on health in older age

David Gordon (School for Policy Studies, University of Bristol, Bristol, UK) Liz Lloyd (School for Policy Studies, university of Bristol, Bristol, UK)

The long-term effects of deprivation in childhood on health in older age has been the subject of a range of research, and theoretical explanations have included biological and social dimensions. The risk factors associated with childhood deprivation takes on particular poignancy when associated with violence, conflict and war. The 1999 Jersey Health Survey has produced data from 2000 questionnaire returns (response rate over 60%) which was a wide-ranging investigation into the health of the adult population. Measures of health using Euroqol and self-reported indicators, such as diet and use of health services, were analysed together with responses on socio-economic, lifestyle, environmental and social capital factors. This provided the first opportunity to analyse the health of older people in Jersey and to take into account their experiences of extreme hardship and deprivation during the period of Nazi occupation (1940 - 45). At times during this period the population was reduced to near starvation levels. The population of Jersey has, since the war, included high levels of migration and we have been able to compare the health of middle-aged and older people in currently similar socio-economic circumstances whose childhood and youth experiences were radically difference. The study provides an opportunity to further analyse the complex inter-relationship of socio-economic circumstances and physical and mental health across the life course.

One or Many The Contemporary Composition of the Urban Elderly Population of Canada

Susan Lucas (University of Connecticut, Storrs, USA)

The purpose of this research is to examine the composition of the contemporary urban elderly population of Canada. The breakdown of strict age scheduling associated with the modern lifecourse and population aging have increased the heterogeneity of the urban elderly population. It is argued that the increased heterogeneity of the urban elderly population is reflected in the fracturing of the traditional family status factor and the consequent identification of several old-age family status dimensions. An orthogonally rotated principal components analysis (PCA) using 1991 census tract data for all census metropolitan areas is used to investigate the fracturing of the traditional family status factor and to identify the resultant old-age family status dimensions. In order to account for the variation caused by other changes in the structure of the family status dimension, all family status factors are initially derived. The non old-age family status factors are then excluded from any further analysis. The dimensions derived by the PCA include an old female widow, a young elderly/ mature family and an all elderly widows factor. Based on the results of the analysis it is possible to conclude that the traditional family status factor has fractured and that the urban elderly population of Canada is characterized by the existence of highly differentiated subgroups. These old-age factors and the subgroups of the elderly population they describe are differentiated principally by marital status (the difference between being married or widowed), advanced age (the population aged 85 and over) and being female.

Trends in Later Life, Austria 1971-1998

J. Hörl (Institute of Sociology, Vienna University, Austria)

This paper analyses changes in important areas of late life in Austria. In 1971, 1979, 1987 and 1998 personal interviews were conducted with about 30,000 private households. These interviews were part of the Austrian microcensus sample survey carried out by the governmental statistical office. About three dozen questions were included to investigate details of life styles and social problems of people 60 years and over. Results suggest that the social situation of the elderly has been changing in a positive way in the course of the last quarter of the past century. More people than ever in any age group over sixty now feel healthy and are able to perform activities of daily life without difficulty. At the same time, more elderly are involved in close intergenerational family ties than ever before in the 20th century. In comparison to other developed countries in Austria there is still a relatively frequent incidence of intergenerational living arrangements, especially in smaller rural communities. Of course, for demographic reasons the strong family orientation of today’s elderly will be weakened. Around 2016, approximately, a greater proportion of women (and men) who never had a child will enter young-old age. One consequence will probably be an increase in one-person-households and maybe a greater reliance on non-family institutions, as well as services of all kinds. Such developments should prove even more substantial in the rural areas where the decline in birth rates has been more significant than in the cities and where social services are still relatively sparse.

SESSION 16

Educating the public on Aging through Publications, and Public Relations

Tuvia Mendelson () (Director, Publications & Public Relations, JDC-ESHEL, The Association for the Planning and Development of Services for the Aged in Israel, Jerusalem, Israel)

The purpose of the presentation is to show the importance of producing various publications as educational means of the elderly themselves as well as their relatives and the general public. The press & the electronic media do not respond to the growing need of elderly people, their relatives and caregivers for high-quality, professional & reliable information about the various aspects of aging. The elderly, in many cases, are exposed either to their lack of knowledge about their rights, as well as about the most trivial things related to their age - or to manipulative and inaccurate information. JDC- Eshel has developed hundreds of programs for the elderly, and has established a training center for professionals and paraprofessionals. However in the last few years it became apparent that written and audiovisual educational material is also required. These publications are the best means to spread & provide theoretic and practical information, guide the elderly and their families about the services available, promote good health, improve quality of life, strengthen the elderly self image and change public attitudes. Examples available

Education for older adults who did not benefit from higher education

Martina Winkelmann (Technical University, Berlin, Germany)

Society's developing requests make it necessary for individuals to develop themselves further, which should be supported by pedagogic offers. People who did not attend any post-high school educational institutions or programs have problems participating in workshops for older people. These are mostly targeted for specifically educated senior citizens, and both highlight and increase the differences in the level of education amongst older people. In my study answers to the following questions are acquired by biographical interviews with older adults who are between the ages of 55 and 70 years: To what extent do older people recognize and acknowledge their own educational improvements and in which areas does this happen? When are educational opportunities rejected? In which sectors are learning requirements and support appreciated? First findings lead one to assume that particularly in the sectors of family, health, travel, culture and volunteerism, further education is appreciated. New technologies and information media sectors yield ambivalence in that they are partly rejected, and partly accepted as a new challenge. Many retired people lose social contacts, which used to help them participate in society. Family is not always suitable as a substitute for links to the changing environment, so a gap remains. This gap can be used by pedagogues. Old structures and techniques should be refined to reach older adults without specialized education, since this kind of older person must be addressed in a way that applies to their needs. I will present in brief the results of my research in July.

Further education at an advanced age

Marianne Burbaum (Institut für Kulturanthropologie und Europäische Ethnologie, Johann Wolfgang Goethe Universität Frankfurt, Germany)

The willingness to undertake further education is still limited in Germany. Furthermore only 1/3 of the participants in institutional further education are male. Up to now there are no firm findings available as to why men, contrary to women, show so little interest. Interviews and field research show basically three reasons: -Men are exhausted after a long working life -During their working lives men have participated in enough further education activities -In old age men no longer want to assume a "pupil" role The first reason should lose its significance after a regeneration phase. The second does not apply to those over 65 today. This education has only been in demand to a greater extent for about 10 years. Many of today´s senior citizens were already too old at that time for investment measures. The last-named reason cannot be refuted. Institutional further education calls for subordination. Women tend to accept this role easier due to their generally lower positions in their former jobs. On the other hand men suffer a loss of identity. Case examples prove that they regard criticism as condescension. They are also better at passing on experience and knowledge rather than working on academic topics. Presenting oneself in a „pupil" role usually leads to loss of identity. The personal identity is not the same as the one they had before. In their new environment they do not receive the social recognition which they expect. Identifying with one´s profession is a fundamental factor in the forming of an identity. Being a pupil suggests dependence. Men, who were used to social recognition, want to continue to retain it.

Lifewide learning and elderly in third and fourth age

Kurt Wissendorf Moller (Danish Institute of GerontoEducation (DIGE)).

The paper will present an educational model containing sociological factors active in learning, whether you are in formal or informal learning situations. The model is a result of studies of educational practice and literature in Danish and international educational environments. It's a point, that the longer you live the more your experiences, gathered through your life, will influence the learning process and the outcome of the efforts of learning. Sociological factors of economics, lifestyle and worklife are active elements to be considered in planning and educational processes and products.

The Role of Older Adult Educational Programmes in Class Dynamics in Old Age

Marvin Formosa (Institute Of Gerontology, University Of Malta, Malta)

Despite the fact that older persons do not form part of the productive sector of society, class formation and action are a fundamental attribute of later life. Older persons, similar to their younger peers, are involved in an incessant struggle to maintain or improve their position in the hierarchal social space. An exploratory study found that all older persons, but especially those of middle-class position, experienced a decrease in their objective and subjective class position with the advent of mandatory retirement. Consequently, they resorted to various social strategies to combat such an incidence and consolidate their previously held class position. Field research was conducted in a University of the Third Age in Malta (U3A). Data collection was administered through 'data combination', employing non-participant observation, a mail questionnaire, and elite interviews. The data elicited was consequently analysed through Pierre Bourdieu's (and Passeron, 1977; 1984) critical insights on educational practice and distinction. The study found that membership was especially sought by older persons endowed with a higher than average volume of 'cultural capital', who used to work in professional/managerial occupations and who perceived themselves as 'educated', as a conscious and unconscious strategy to distinguish themselves vis-à-vis their elder peers. The study concluded that U3A was characterised by a liberal ideological ideology, whose membership is largely deployed by middle-class older persons to for garnering honour and prestige, for enacting and displaying one's interpretation of oneself, against the play of downward class mobility resulting from structural and interaction factors.

SESSION 17

Social Networks and the Changing Reality

T.C. Antonucci and H. Akiyama (University of Michigan, Ann Arbor, Michigan, USA) and K. Ajrouch [Eastern Michigan University, Ypsilanti, Michigan, USA) Socioeconomic Status, Social Relations and Health. T.G. van Tilburg, M.I. Broese van Groenou, and C.P.M. Knipscheer (Dept. of Sociology and Social Gerontology, Vrije Universiteit, Amsterdam, The Netherlands) Does Socioeconomic Inequality in Network Size and Support Decrease Over Generations? I. Chi (Dept of Social Work and Social Administration, University of Hong Kong, Hong Kong) and James E. Lubben, (School of Social Welfare, UCLA, California, USA) Health Quality of Life among Chinese Elders in Hong Kong: The Impact of Social Support Networks. H. Litwin (Paul Baerwald School of Social Work, The Hebrew University of Jerusalem, Israel) Correlates of Social Network Type among Elderly Israeli Jews: Continuity and Change. G.C. Wenger and V. Burholt (Centre for Social Policy Research and Development, University of Wales, Bangor, United Kingdom) Predicting Social Change and Informal Care Dynamics in the United Kingdom.

ISSUES. The social network is the sum of one's meaningful interpersonal ties. It is a potential provider of emotional and practical support, as well as a possible source of stress. The social network serves as the human milieu within which people develop and in which they exchange goods and services. The well-being of older people, in particular, is influenced by the structure and the nature of their social networks. This symposium considers the changing nature of the social networks of older persons and examines the impact of such changes on their well-being. STRUCTURE. The symposium draws upon network analyses in different settings to underscore the changes that have occurred in the social networks of older people. In addition, through the different presentations, it presents the major modes of network analysis that have emerged in gerontology in the recent decades. These include unique social network inventories, typologies and analytic strategies developed by the presenters. These means are employed to trace the changing reality of social networks. CONTENT. Antonucci and Akiyama utilize two regionally representative samples from the United States and Japan to consider the impact of social relations on the association between socioeconomic status and health of older people. Trends in which older people with lower levels of education in the United States have smaller networks, feel they receive less support and are less satisfied with the support they receive are viewed vis a vis the elderly of Japan. Van Tilburg, Broese van Groenou and Knipscheer examine the relative impact of childhood and present socioeconomic status on network size and support in old age among older Dutch persons. Their results suggest that socioeconomic inequality in network size may disappear among future generations of older adults, but inequality in emotional support may persist. Chi and Lubben explore social network patterns among the Chinese elderly in Hong Kong and the impact of social support on their health quality of life. They found that network scores correlated with respondents' somatic health, functional health and depression, even after controlling for sociodemographic characteristics. Litwin maps the network dynamics of a national probability sample of elderly Israeli Jews, and identifies the sociodemographic correlates of network formation. The current aged cohort in Israel reflects a high proportion of robust network types, but data also show that advanced old age maintains a strong association with attenuated network structure. Finally, drawing on a longitudinal study in Wales, Wenger and Burholt consider the impact of network changes on informal care in the early decades of the 21st century. Given the growth of independent and private restricted social network types, they predict the emergence of new types of supportive relationships based on affinity rather than consanguinity. ANTICIPATED OUTCOMES. The symposium will provide a unique overview of the major methodological approaches to social network analysis in contemporary gerontology, and a comparative review of the latest findings concerning the interpersonal social milieu of older persons in selected countries in Europe, Asia, North America and the Middle East

Correlates of Social Network Type among Elderly Israeli Jews: Continuity and Change

H. Litwin (Paul Baerwald School of Social Work, The Hebrew University of Jerusalem, Israel)

The social networks of older people tend to change as individuals age. Networks may also vary according to the changing characteristics of their focal elders. The purpose of this analysis was to map the network dynamics of a national probability sample of elderly Israeli Jews, and to identify the correlates of network formation. The study is based upon secondary analysis of data from a 1997 survey by the Israeli Central Bureau of Statistics among people age 60 and over (n=2079). Five network types were derived through the use of K-means cluster analysis: diverse, friends, neighbors, family and restricted. All had a familial base but differed according to other composition factors. Analysis revealed that respondents in diverse networks were more likely to be men with higher incomes, higher education and little disability. Those in the friends network were similar but younger. The neighbor network type was comprised most frequently by lower income women. Respondents in the family network were more likely to have lower incomes and less education, and greater disability despite their younger age. Those in the restricted network were likely to have lower incomes, less education, and greater disability, and were likely to be older as well. In conclusion, the current aged cohort in Israel seems to reflect a greater proportion of older people who have robust network types, due to higher incomes and better health. However, the data also show that advanced old age maintains a strong association with attenuated network structure.

Does Socioeconomic Inequality in Network Size and Support Decrease Over Generations?

T.G. van Tilburg, M.I. Broese van Groenou, C.P.M. Knipscheer (Dept. of Sociology and Social Gerontology, Vrije Universiteit, Amsterdam, The Netherlands)

Previous research revealed that socioeconomic deprived older persons have relatively small personal networks and receive small amounts of support. These network differences in old age may partly be explained by socioeconomic deprivation early in life, reflecting few structural opportunities and personal resources to develop personal relationships during life. However, due to upward socioeconomic mobility during the life course one may recuperate from early social deprivation. The present study examines the relative impact of childhood and present socioeconomic status on network size and support in old age. Since socioeconomic status varies largely by age, specific attention is devoted to differences between birth cohorts. Data are from a survey conducted in 1992 in the Netherlands among 2400 married older adults born between 1903 and 1937. Childhood and current socioeconomic status are indicated respectively by the father's and the respondent's highest educational and occupational level and prestige. Preliminary results indicate that both childhood and current socioeconomic status are positively related to network size, yet only in the oldest birth cohorts and not in the youngest cohorts. Present socioeconomic status is in all birth cohorts positively related to emotional support received, but not to instrumental support received. Effects of childhood status are small or absent. The results suggest that socioeconomic inequality in network size may disappear among future generations of older adults, where inequality in emotional support may persist, reflecting cultural differences in communication and expression of emotions.

Health Quality of Life among Chinese Elders in Hong Kong: The Impact of Social Support Networks

I. Chi (Dept of Social Work and Social Administration, University of Hong Kong, Hong Kong), James E. Lubben, (School of Social Welfare, UCLA, USA)

Hong Kong is mainly a Chinese society, with 98% of its residents comprised of ethnic Chinese. This study examines social network patterns among the Chinese elderly in Hong Kong and the impact of social support on their health quality of life. The analysis is based upon a random sample of persons aged 60 and over (n=334). The Lubben Social Network Scale (LSNS) was administered to measure respondents' social support networks. A score of 20 or less on the scale indicated insufficient network support. Results indicate that a majority of respondents reside with children. Male elders tend more frequently to live with a spouse only or to live alone. Educational attainment positively correlates with living apart from children. Eleven percent of the sample respondents were found to have insufficient support networks and were classified as socially isolated. LSNS scores correlated with respondents' somatic health, functional health and depression, even after controlling for sociodemographic characteristics. It seems that processes of urbanization and modernization in Chinese society in Hong Kong over the past two decades have reduced support functions of families in the care for their older members. Compared to previous eras, there are currently fewer elders residing with children. The problem of social isolation among a minority of elders persists in Hong Kong, and may be increasing. Similar trends are being found in industrialized cities in Asia.

Predicting Social Change and Informal Care Dynamics in the United Kingdom.

G.C. Wenger, V. Burholt (Centre for Social Policy Research and Development, University of Wales, Bangor, United Kingdom)

The Bangor Longitudinal Study of Ageing (BLSA) represents 20 years (1979-1999) of continuous study of the social ageing process in six communities in rural North Wales, UK. Both quantitative and qualitative data were recorded at four yearly intervals regarding the experiences and situations of a cohort of older people, aged 65 or older in 1979 (N=534). One of the outcomes of the study was the identification of a support network typology. On the basis of observations from the BLSA in combination with the impact of four areas of social change, this paper speculates about possible outcomes for informal care in the early decades of the 21st century. Consideration is given to the effects of changes in job security, increasing geographical mobility and family dispersal, divorce and the changed status of women and the emergence of the four generation family as the norm. The quantitative data indicate that in the course of twenty years, people aged 85 and over have become more independent. Three times as many respondents had private restricted networks in 1999 compared with 1979. It is suggested that in the twenty-first century, family care will be less common than it has been in the past. Older people will be more independent and self-directed. New types of supportive relationships based on affinity rather than consanguinity will emerge. There will be an expansion of technological solutions to dependency, but formal services will still be needed to take care of a substantial minority of people in old age.

Socioeconomic Status, Social Relations and Health

T.C. Antonucci, H. Akiyama (University of Michigan, Ann Arbor, Michigan) and K. Ajrouch (Eastern Michigan University, Ypsilanti, Michigan, USA)

It has long been recognized that socioeconomic status (SES) significantly affects health. Further, we know that people of lower SES accumulate an array of disadvantages such as poor nutrition and poor health care, which negatively affects their health. It has also been documented that social relations affect health. In this paper we examine the social relations-SES association among older people in the United States and Japan and if social relations influence the SES-health association. We utilized two regionally representative samples from the United States and Japan to examine these issues. Given recent research recommending that, especially among older people, SES is best measured by education, we examine educational differences in support network (size), receipt of support, and satisfaction with support among older people in the United States and Japan. The US data indicates that there are consistent educational differences. Older people with lower levels of education have smaller networks, feel they receive less support and are less satisfied with the support they do receive. These differences are relatively consistent for both men and women. We examine whether the same pattern of relationships is replicated among older Japanese people and if they are the same for Japanese men and women.Finally, we explore the degree to which positive social relations, even among people of lower levels of education, influence the association between SES and health. In our discussion we consider the implications of these findings for improving the health of older people.

SESSION 18

An Investigation of the Prevalence of Resistive behaviours in Residential Care Facilities [Nursing Homes]

Sandra Cody [Centre for Ageing Studies, Adelaide, Australia]
Author: James Grealy [C&G Education and Research Pty. Limited]

This reports the results of a WorkCover Corp. SA funded investigation into the prevalence of resident resistance to care in residential care facilities. Methodology: The project evaluated documented care practices for fifty-six cognitively impaired nursing home residents. This was correlated with facility and staff data (40 staff), and five days of behavioural incident reporting [690 observations]. A functional definition of resistive behaviours was employed using a 4-point rating scale of resistiveness, ranging from 0, no resistiveness to 3, severe resistiveness. Data was collected from three Commonwealth funded residential care facilities (purposive sample). The results: The three residential care facilities identified 62% of the entire resident population (n=179) to be resistive to care for a period of greater than two weeks. Staff observations of the resident sample (n=56) over a five-day period revealed that 63% of all staff care interventions were met with resistiveness. Only 52.2% of the sample had a diagnosis of dementia. 20% of residents had a recorded psychiatric history. Behavioural histories indicated that 84.8% of the resident sample had two or three other behaviours such as wandering, aggression, being verbally disruptive, or displaying sexual disinhibition. 84.7% of the resident sample were medicated with either or both benzodiazipines and anti-psychotics. The resistive behaviour occurred most frequently during the most intimate contact with the resident. Aggressive behaviours directed toward staff during care delivery constituted only 2.8% of all behavioural episodes. Conclusion: The research has revealed the extensive nature of this behaviour and a high prevalence within this setting.

Behavioural Disturbances in Patients With Dementia Living in Nursing Homes

Gil P, Sánchez-Guevara A, Garnica A, Fariñas F.(Geriatrics Service. Hospital Clinico San Carlos. Madrid. Spain.) and ENERA Study (Pfizer).

AIMS: To know the frequency and main behavioural disturbances in patients with Alzheimer Disease (AD) or Vascular Dementia living in nursing-homes. METHODS: 1791 patients that fulfilled DSM-IV criteria of dementia were included. NINCDS- ADRDA criteria were used for AD and NINCDS-AIREN criteria for Vascular Dementia. Cognitive assessment (MMSE, Pfeiffer, ADAS-COG), functional assessment (BLESSED, KATZ) and behavioural assessment (Neuropsychiatry Inventory, NPI) were carried out in every patient. Develop stage was graded with respect to FAST (Functional Assessment Stages). The following data were included: age, period of disease progression, related diseases, drugs, nutritional assessment, biochemical measurements and neuroimagine techniques. Data base: SPSS, Statistical measurement of common tendency and dispersion, and quantity comparative data t-Student (Confidence interval 95%). RESULTS: n: 1971(mean age 84.1+/- 7, women 75.4%). Dementia type: Alzheimer disease 57%, Vascular dementia: 27.3%. NPI: 21.5 +/- 2.1. Behavioural disturbances night-time behaviours 60%. Anxiety 51.5%. Depression: 31%.Wandering: 28%. Irritability:27.4%. NPI Night Time Depression Wandering A D 27.3 61.3 26.1 40.4 V D 20.5 56.8 30.4 19.3 CONCLUSIONS: 1. Behavioural disturbances are very frequent in elderly living in nursing homes.2 Night time behaviours are the most frequent behavioural disturbances.3 Wandering and Night time behaviours are more frequent in AD than in Vascular Dementia.

Contextual factors associated to the emission of aggressive behaviors among elderly persons suffering from dementia.

G. Primeau, J. Vézina, P. Landreville, J. Aubert, C. Brochu, S. Imbeault, E. Matteau, C. Laplante (School of Psychology, University Laval, Quebec, Canada)

In long-term care institutions, aggressive behaviors (AB) are emitted daily by 24% to 65% of the demented elderly people and have a major impact on their quality of life as well as on the burden experienced by staff members. Although certain biological and psychiatric hypotheses have been proposed to explain the presence of AB, some studies also emphasize the impact of environmental factors. The purpose of the present study is to systematically analyze certain environmental conditions associated to verbal and physical AB. The methodology involved the non-participant, direct observation of 15 patients displaying AB over a period of 12 hours each. A handheld computer permitted the real time coding of the occurrence of AB as well as the recording of the location and the activity performed by the participants. In this study, 216 episodes were found, of which 135 AB were verbal. In 68% of the cases, AB were aimed at the staff members. They occurred principally during the activities of daily living (56%), in the bedroom of the participants (55%). The AB took place primarily between 9:00 and 11:00 AM (40%) and also between 5:00 and 07:00 PM. (30%). These results emphasize the fact that, among the people experiencing extensive cognitive impairment, various environmental factors associated to particular locations and circumstances contribute to the presence of AB.

How do Care Outcomes & Service Patterns Relate to Behavioural Problems Part II: Health Services.

K. Paddock, J. Kozak, & E. Sayre (Sisters of Charity of Ottawa Health Service, Ottawa, Canada).

Behaviour problems are a worrisome issue for those who give professional care to elderly patients. The potential for injury and the distress it causes may hinder staff from giving adequate care to those with behaviour problems. To evaluate the relationship between behaviour problems and health service patterns, a study was undertaken which included 4,414 patients aged 65 and older in Ontario Complex Continuing Care Hospitals. Information regarding behaviour problems and special services or treatments was obtained from the Minimum Data Set (MDS) 2.0. A behaviour problem scale (BPS) was created to represent the level of challenge associated with the patient's behaviour, and logistic regression analyses were utilized to determine if behavioural problems were related to receipt of health services. The range of services included treatments for depression, incontinence, mobility impairments, and communication problems. Restraints, pharmacological treatments, and psychological therapies were also included in the analysis. Preliminary findings indicate that having a higher level of behaviour problems is significantly related to poorer health service patterns. For example, someone with a high BPS score is over 5 times more likely to not be treated for a depression and almost 1.5 times more likely to receive no corrective action for a communication or sensory problem than is someone without behaviour problems. Clinical situations in which services may be appropriately withheld will be discussed in relation to study results. Findings from this study highlight the need to carefully monitor health service patterns for this at-risk population.

SESSION 20

[1] Effects of Family Participation in Caring of the Hospitalized Elderly Patients

T.Arnantapunpong(The Thai Red Cross Nursing College, Rama IV Rd. ,Patumwan,Bangkok 10330 Thailand.) P.Intarasombat and P.Putwatana (Ramathibodi school of nursing, Faculty of medicine, Mahidol university,Rama VI Rd. bangkok10400 Thailand)

The purpose of this quasi-experimental research was to test the effects of family participation in caring of hospitalized elderly patients on patients'recovery and family satisfaction with nursing care. The purposive samples consisted of sixty pairs of relatives and female elderly patients who admitted in to general medical wards in the department of Medicine of King Chulalongkorn Memorial Hospital. The first 15 patients were assigned into the experimental group and the other 15 patients who were assigned into the control group, and then this pattern was rotated. Subjects in both groups received routine nursing care, but the subjects in experimental group received care from family participation in addition. For each patient, functional status and mental status were evaluated before and after the experimental period by using Katz's index of independence in ADL and Folstein's mini-mental state examination respectively. Family satisfaction was measured by the modified La Monica's patient satisfaction scale. The results of the study revealed significant statistical difference ($p<.05$) between the experimental and the control groups in mental status but no significant statistical difference ($p>.05$) in functional status which consisted of ADL, complication and duration of hospitalization. For the family satisfaction, there was significant statistical difference ($p<.01$) between the experimental and the control groups. The findings not only support Orem's self care theory which explains that the dependent care agent can learn and apply knowledge enables to promote well being to the patients but also support Orem's theory of nursing system which explains that the appropriate designed nursing care model using family participation and interpersonal relationship can bring more satisfaction with nursing care.

[2] Examination of family burden degree of old age person care in Japan

A Hattori, K Nakahara, S Matsusita, H Orimo (Division of Internal Medicine, Tokyo Metropolitan Geriatric Hospital, Tokyo, Japan)

PURPOSE: A cross sectional survey was done in order to quantify the background factors that exhaust family caregivers in Japan. METHOD: The study employed a self-recording questionnaire form which included the Pines' burnout scale. RESULTS: Seventy-three caregivers in the house filled in the questionnaire when old age persons (average age 82.7 years old) were sick and entered Tokyo Metropolitan Geriatric Hospital. They reported the difficulty of care for elderly patients in the home and the degree of the difficulty correlated well with their burnout score ($r=-0.517$, $p<0.001$). The caregivers' burnout score did not correlate so well with the level of their patients' basic activities of daily living ($r=-0.307$, $p<0.05$). The older the caregivers, the higher caregivers' burnout score. The worse the health status of caregivers, the heavier were their burnout scores ($p<0.01$). Among the factors for the care of elderly person with dementia, the aid at midnight, the need for observation at any time, and the care refusal all increased the burnout score. On multiple regression analysis using the background factors for the burnout score as explanatory variables, aid for toilet use, aid at midnight, and health status of care person were significant independent contributing factors ($r2=0.40$, $p<0.0001$) CONCLUSION: It became clear that the caregivers in the home were almost burnt out owing to the aid they need to give for the elderly persons' BADL, the mental status of elderly patients, and health status of caregivers.

[3] Geriatric Patients: Privations and Needs of Familiar Support

I. Ferreira; L. Cassimiro; I. Suzuki; L.E.G.Garcez Leme; M.M. Amatuzzi.(Geriatric Unit/Orthopedic Institute University of São Paulo-School of Medicine/São Paulo/Brazil

Objective: 1) Characterize the social profile of the geriatric patients admitted to E.R. in the Orthopedics and Traumatology Institute of the Hospital das Clinicas in the Medicine University of São Paulo. 2) Obtain a better comprehension of the patients familiar psycho- social-economical situation. 3) Identify the privations and needs presented by patients and their families. Method: Retrospective research through 119 psychological and social patients reports, attended by Social and Psychological Services while interned patients in this Institute, from January 1999 to June 2000. Variables demographics, psychosocial and familiar structure had been analyzed. Results: A significant number of admissions, 82.5%, are by trauma. Of those admissions, 66.4% are female with 51.9% older than 80 years old. 33.6% are male with 25% older than 80 years old. In analyzing family infrastructures 52.5% of men and 50.63% of women have unsatisfactory and precarious support and deficient home care. Even with a lack of familiar support, 67.86% of men and 80.7% of women tend to chose a close relative as a caretaker. Conclusion: Family support for a significant number of patients can become deficient because of the limitations of familiar infrastructure and the absence of a community safety net and governmental support.

[4] Towards Empowerment: Reconceptualizing Family Support Groups

Deborah O'Connor , RSW (University of British Columbia, Vancouver, C anada)

Purpose: Family support groups have been recognized as an important and viable means for responding to the needs of family caregivers. How these groups work however is not well understand. The purpose of this qualitative exploratory study was to explore the impact of attending a family support group on the caregiving experience from the perspective of the family member. Method: Personal, semi-structured interviews took place with eleven family members who had participated in at least one family support group. Data was analyzed for themes using a constant comparative categorizing strategy. Results: This analysis suggests that attending a family support group impacts the caregiving experience in four important ways: helping the family member to construct a self-identity as a 'caregiver'; promoting a sense of personal competence; fostering the use of formal support groups; and creating a community context within which to experience the caregiving role. Cumulatively, these have the potential to contribute to a sense of empowerment for the family member by helping him or her to reposition the caregiving experience as more than just a personal issue. This however is conditional upon the approach taken by the group leader. Conclusion: From a political perspective there are implications associated with this reconceptualization of family support groups. This research suggests that the family support group experience can help to make visible to family members what it is they are doing, and help them to understand that their private difficulties are shared by many in similar circumstances. Reframing their experiences as a more public, collective experience assists family members to recognize the societal contributions they are making providing care to their family member. Expectations related to formal support may become more explicit as family members begin to recognize and appreciate their own rights. The potential for family support groups to assist family members in developing a collective voice emerges.

[5] Care of Aging Parents and Friends

C. Westley, W. Forch, K. Fletcher (University of Virginia Health System; Charlottesville, VA USA)

Seventy-two percent of paid and unpaid caregivers of the elderly are family members. Even with help from paid and unpaid caregivers, more than 1/3 of this population has unmet needs. Many times the role of caregiver is thrust on unprepared family and negatively impacts their physical, mental, and emotional health. The number of people age 70 and older is expected to increase substantially over the next several decades compounding problems for both patients as well as informal caregivers. To address this growing problem we collaborated with both in-house and community partners to assess needs for as well as develop and provide programs and services to assist caregivers. This has been accomplished through a "Caregiver Helpline" providing information and support on the telephone; "Foundation for Caregiving" courses teaching essential, hand-on caregiver skills; a resource guide; support groups; a library with videos, books and other resources; and a lunchtime lecture series for audiences consisting of hospital and university staff as well as the general public. These services have allowed us to reach and positively impact families and others who balance caregiving with their many other responsibilities.

[6] Cohort effect of the impact of loss of spouse in Japan

Chieko Kawaai (Tokyo Metropolitan Institute of Gerontology, Tokyo, Japan)

Purpose:During the last decade, there have been various social changes in Japan, such as the bubble economy burst, and the changes of family structure. The purpose of this study is to examine the changes of the impact of spouse's deaths. Method: We conducted the survey within approximately one year of the bereavement and analyzed the data on the 460 middle aged and elderly widowed who experienced the bereavement in 1984, cohort C1, and in 2000, cohort C2. To investigate the impact of the bereavement, we examined the psychosomatic response, grief response, loneliness and the level of the inconvenience of daily life. Further, we conducted the retrospective assessment of marital satisfaction Results: ANOVA demonstrated significant main effect of cohort on loneliness, where C1 showed the higher score. Although the main effect of cohort was not significant on psychosomatic response and the daily life inconvenience, interaction effect was observed in female in C2 showing the higher score than those in C1. The main effect of cohort was not observed on grief response, however interaction effect of cohort and marital assessment was observed. Among the widowed that had good relationships with their spouses before the bereavement, C2 showed higher grief response than C1. Conclusion: Therefore various social changes in Japan have been making the widowed lonelier. And in such environment, it is more difficult for some widowed to adjust to the bereavement, especially for female and those who had good relationships with their spouses.

[7] The relationships among social support and self-care of patients with colostomy

C.W. Kao(National defense medical center, Taipei, Taiwan, R.O.C.)

This is a descriptive study. The main purpose of the study is to investigate the relationship between social support and self-care. Data were collected by visiting and interviewing the patients during pre-discharge. The sample consisted of 61 colostomy patients from five hospitals. To analyze data was by using canonical correlation. One statistically significant canonical correlation was found : 0.901($p<0.001$). Social support explained 81.1% of variance of the self-care. In conclusion, the results of the study showed that self-care was related to social support.

[8] Care Recipient and Caregiver Functioning as Correlates of Reactions to Caregiving

C. M. de Frias, H. A. Tuokko (Department of Psychology, University of Victoria, Victoria, BC, Canada), T. Rosenberg (Capital Health Region, Victoria, BC, Canada)

There is a need to better understand the relations between health status and various caregiver and care recipient characteristics when seeking ways to support caregivers of older adults. Information was available on mental health, physical health, daily functioning, and pain status of 177 consecutive persons (Mage = 81 years) referred to various programs within a comprehensive set of geriatric care services. Similar information was collected on their caregivers (n=133; Mage = 65 years). In addition, caregiver depression using the CES-D and caregiver reactions as assessed by the Caregiver Reaction Assessment (CRA) instrument were also examined. The CRA measures the family members' reactions to caring for an older adult along five dimensions: Impact on Schedule, Caregiver Esteem, Lack of Family Support, Impact on Health, and Impact on Finances. An examination of the psychometric properties of the CRA revealed moderate to high internal consistency among the five domains. Several relations were found between caregiver functioning and caregiver reactions with fewer relations observed between care recipient functioning and caregiver reactions, after controlling for age and gender of the caregiver. The strongest correlates of caregiver reactions included the mental health and depression status of the caregiver. Only one aspect of care recipient functioning (mental health) was related to caregiver reactions (caregiver esteem). In a broad geriatric sample, responses on the CRA were most closely related to other indicators of caregiver functioning, whereas, care recipient characteristics were generally unrelated to caregiver reactions to caring for persons with health impairments.

[9] New ideas for older persons' caretaking - Research on older persons' mutual aid organization for caretaking

Zhu Jiming , Ni Bo (Shanghai Research Center on Aging, Shanghai, China)

It has been over twenty years since Shanghai entered an aging society at the end of the 1970's. Shanghai is confronted with a severe situation of an aging population. Aging, especially the aging of the old-old will definitely result in their deteriorating health. There is a strong need for attendance and caretaking for older persons, but on the other hand, families are reduced to nuclear families. Limited income and fewer family members make it impossible for older persons and their families alone to shoulder the responsibility and bear the financial and spiritual pressure. It is not realistic for the government to solve all the problems involved in the caretaking of older persons. How to take care of older persons has stood out as a social problem that afflicts many families. Establishing a mutual aid organization for older persons is a tentative approach to the aging problem in Shanghai. In the August of 1998, scholars and experts from municipal welfare, finance and labor organizations and bureaus joined together and set up a research team on Older Persons' Mutual Aid Organization in Shanghai. There are two ways: one is taking part in the mutual funds, paying the membership dues for caretaking; the other is taking part in the saving up service hours, the members themselves or their family member should receive some adequate training in caretaking, and use their skill to take care of other older persons, their service hours are kept track of in their personal account. The Older Persons' Mutual Aid Organization assumes taking good care of the old as its mission. The organization will perfect its service and make it a networking system in Shanghai.

[10] The remarriage mode of the aged in China should reform

Ye Nazi (One of the directors of Old Age Institute of China)

Today China is entering the aged society. The number of the aged greater than 60 years old has already reached 120 million, and it is 10 percent of all population in China. There is a special phenomenon in the aged society. It is a problem of remarriage of the aged in China. The physiological conditions, psychological conditions, social conditions and the goal of the aged remarriage are different from those of the young or the middle-aged, and the ethical relationships of the aged are complex in China. According to existing [marriage] law in China, it is low in successful rate or consolidate rate for the aged remarriage. Therefore, in fact, the right of remarriage for the aged has been deprived in China. For this issue it is difficult for remarriage of the aged, there have to have a solution for the way of the aged remarriage in China. In other word, the existing [marriage law] in China has to reform. It should be allowed to remarriage in "cohabiting in terms of law" for the aged in China. That is to say, it should transform from existing single marriage mode to dualistic marriage mode that is also allowed to remarriage in "cohabiting in terms of law" in the same time in China.

[11] The Caring and Being Cared Process in the Family the Aged and His/Her Care

Angela Maria Alvarez e Lucia HisakoTakase Gonçalves [Universidade Federal de Santa Catarina (UFSC) in Florianopolis-Brazil]

PURPOSE: To understand the process and its multivariated dimensions of family care to the sick and /or frail aged living in a family environment. METHOD: The adopted method was one of qualitative research-grounded theory, and the theoretical foundation was one of symbolic interactionism. Families were visited and inquired, in the Province of Florianópolis (State capital of Santa Catarina the south region of Brazil) using a theoretical sampling. The researched families lived in neighborhoods where a public Family Health Program (PSF) is being implemented. RESULTS: Two main phenomena were identified in observing the aged and their caregiver relationship: a)-being cared for in a family context shows the experience of a dependent condition, of care given within the home, and everyday survival, and b) assuming the role of a family member caregiver, with the three living experiences of having to care and being responsible for caring activities; reflecting on the implications of being a caregiver (the complexity of care, the need for one s own care, and the expectation of counting with help from the other members), and looking for the support of care activities (support from the whole family, the community, and institutional social and health resources). CONCLUSION: The public Family Health Program does not contemplate the care and caring process developed by the families for their sick and/or frail aged as it refers to assistance to the aged family, nor does it offer the specific family care to both aged members and their caregivers.

[12] Quality of Life and Health of Caregivers and Non-Caregivers Who Are 65 Years or Older

Anita M. Hubley (The University of British Columbia, Vancouver, Canada) Dawn Hemingway (University of Northern British Columbia, Prince George, Canada) Alex C. Michalos (University of Northern British Columbia, Prince George, Canada) Bruno D. Zumbo (The University of British Columbia, Vancouver, Canada)

The purpose of this study was to compare the quality of life of caregivers and non-caregivers age 65 or older. This sample was taken from a large quality of life survey of 875 individuals age 55 or older living in communities in northern British Columbia, Canada (Michalos, Hubley, Zumbo, and Hemingway, in press). We restricted our sample to (a) individuals 65 years or older because we were particularly interested in seniors, and (b) married individuals because preliminary analyses indicated that marital status was a potentially confounding variable in the caregiver/non-caregiver comparisons. Thus, our sample consisted of 242 respondents ranging in age from 65 to 88 years, with an average age of 72 years. Of these respondents, 49% were females and 26% were caregivers. The specific variables examined were self-reported health, social support, age identity, satisfaction with various life domains, life satisfaction, overall quality of life, and happiness. The caregivers and non-caregivers were, essentially, indistinguishable in terms of these variables. Seniors, whether they were caregivers or not, reported positive levels of quality of life and health status. Caregivers and non-caregivers, however, did differ in terms of: (a) their satisfaction with their romantic relationships with caregivers being less satisfied, and (b) the age they felt mentally with caregivers feeling slightly older mentally than non-caregivers. Thus, caregiver status alone does not appear to result in a significant reduction in many of the dimensions of quality of life in older adults.

[13] A survey on stress and needs of carers of frail community-dwelling elderly

S L Hui, L W Chu, W Hu, W Mok, N Chan, T Ngan, C Liu, W Tsui, (Division of Geriatric Medicine, Department of Medicine, The University of Hong Kong, Pokfulam, HKSAR)

PURPOSE: Population ageing is a global problem. In Chinese tradition, caring for sick and frail elderly is an obligation or perceived family role. However, care-giving is not an easy task for informal carers. In order to help the family carers to look after their frail elders at home and community as long as possible, it is important to know their stress and needs. METHODS: Principle carers of community-dwelling elderly in-patients or out-patients attending the geriatric unit were identified. A structured questionnaire on medical, cognitive and social function of the patient and stress level of the carer was administered. Knowledge and specific needs were assessed. Factors affecting carer stress was analyzed by logistic regression. Relationship between carer stress level was compared to the patient's age using unpaired t-test. RESULTS: 83 carers were interviewed (mean age 52.3±1.8, 64.2% female). 29.1% of them were elderly spouses, 59.5% of the carers were the children and children's spouses. Over 77% of the participants had stressful feeling. 28.4% felt severe stress. The patient's age, self care ability, presence of dementia and behavioural disturbance were determinants of carer stress. 40.7% of carers were in need of help but 75.6% of the interviewees had not received any community social service. Caring had a negative impact on health in 49.4%. Medical knowledge was generally inadequate in carers. CONCLUSION: Stress and lack of social support is common among carers of geriatric patients. Care-giving had adverse health and social consequences on our carers. An improved community network is needed.

[14] The Caregiver Support Centre: An Innovative Response to Caregivers' Needs

Pam Orzeck (CLSC Rene-Cassin/Institute of Social Gerontology of Quebec, Montreal, Canada)

Purpose: To present the unique services and programs of the Caregiver Support Centre offering respite, support, advocacy, education, outreach and prevention for caregivers. The Caregiver Support Centre of the CLSC René-Cassin/Institute of Social Gerontology of Quebec is an innovative multi-faceted service program for caregivers developed at the heart of the community. The Caregiver Support Centre has four components related to caregiving issues: *Direct services to caregivers and seniors in the population *Outreach services to the community *Research and the transfer of knowledge *Teaching/training Each of these four components will be explored within the presentation METHOD: The CLSC René-Cassin/ISGQ is a public health and social service establishment and is affiliated with three universities - University of Montreal, McGill University and University of Quebec at Montreal. The CLSC is integrated into its local community where 27% of the population is 65 years of age or older. This characteristic compelled the establishment to develop, over the course of many years, "cutting edge services" and conduct research in gerontology to respond to the evolving needs of this population. The Caregiver Support Centre has recently published a book on its history and evolution, along with caregiver testimonials, and a section written by three prominent Quebec researchers. Conclusion:The Caregiver Support Centre is a dynamic centre with alternative and innovative responses to caregivers' needs. The centre offers cutting edge services and is involved with various applied research projects. We look forward to presenting our program Thank you very much, Pam Orzeck, MSW

[15] Caring in Later Life: The Needs and Roles of Older Carers

Alisoun Milne, Lecturer in Social Gerontology, (Tizard Centre, University of Kent, Canterbury)

Despite the fact that many vulnerable adults are supported by older carers (ONS, 1998), little is known specifically about this group. This poster will present the key findings of a scoping study exploring the specific nature, characteristics, roles and needs of older carers. The study - commissioned by 'Help the Aged' - interrogated research and policy literature and conducted some secondary analysis of the General Household Survey 1996 relating to family carers. The findings suggest that: over a quarter of all UK carers are elderly, many are spouses, many provide intensive caring over long periods of time and most receive little or no support. Many older carers worry about not being able to continue caring due to their own health problems. Carers under particular strain are those caring for someone with a cognitive impairment and those caring for a relative with a learning disability. The needs and circumstances of minority groups of older carers were also explored; these included carers from ethnic populations, gay carers and former carers. Of particular note are the difficulties faced by carers who's relative has been admitted to a care home. In addition to reviewing what is known, the study also identified research and policy goals. The needs of former carers and a review of services for older carers from ethnic minority populations were identified as research tasks. The study concluded that policy has a clear role in encouraging services to be available to carers at an early stage and alleviating poverty amongst older carers.

[16] Relationships Between the Uses of Welfare Services and Family Caregivers for Elderly

T.Ono(Okayama prefectural University,Soja,Japan) M.Onishi(Ehime University,Shigenobu,Japan) A.Tanaka(Hiroshima University,Hirosshima,Japan)

Purpose: This study was to elucidate the relationships between the uses of welfare service and caregivers of domiciliary care of frail and red-ridden elderly persons. Method: All subjects were persons who used home care nursing services. 41 of the voluntary caregivers agreed to a semi-structured interview in their homes. Result: 1)Welfare services are utilized home help services, care-instrument supplies, bath services, day services, and short-stay services in order of frequency. 2) Almost all caregivers said they felt some physical and mental burden. 3) The elderly with family relations preferred home care. As such, wife/daughter/ husband caregivers felt that they were fulfilling a need for their loved one. 4)Elderly persons were put into nursing homes for short-stay or elderly day services. During these periods home caregivers could relax and rid themselves of stress. Conclusion: Caregivers' use of welfare services resulted in a decrease of burden and stress. In case of extended home care good family relationships and love.

[17] Differences Between Family Support Networks for Elderly Dementia Patients in Two Ethnic Groups

S.M.A.Santos, P. Dalgalarrondo (Postgraduate Program in Gerontology at the State University of Campinas UNICAMP, Campinas/SP Brazil)

We know the importance of family support networks to provide both quality care for elderly dementia patients and quality of life for their caregivers. OBJECTIVE: In this study we present part of our experience with Brazilian families and families of Japanese immigrants or descendants living in Campinas and surroundings. We aim at verifying differences between family support networks in these two ethnic groups and their influence on both the quality of care provided and the caregiver s quality of life. METHOD: We employed a qualitative methodology in which ethnography was a form of describing and understanding the culturally mediated relationship between family support networks and quality of life of elderly and caregivers. Data collection was made at subjects homes, after previous agreement and scheduling, through techniques of participant observation and semi-structured interview. RESULTS: In a graphic representation we show different kinds of family support networks found in these ethnic groups, giving special emphasis to the process of joint construction of networks and to the analysis of the influence of family support networks on caregiving activities. CONCLUSIONS: We identify significant differences between family support networks in the two ethnic groups. We discuss the assessment that primary family caregivers make about the family support they have and how much it interferes in their quality of life.

[18] Interaction of generations in aging society

Dong Zhiying (Scientific Research Bureau, Chinese Academy of Social Sciences)

In the preceding 50 years of new century, it will be faced with the challenge of the summit phase of aging in China. We hope that resources and wealth will be shared in generations without dividing age. These resources and wealth run in order between generations. We create the quietly harmonious atmosphere of society, which everybody can share in common social fruits. The elderly is integrated in the world on an equal basis especially. We shall realize a sustainable development for population aging and society. This is an important problem that we must study. In accordance with the theory of society attribute, there is an exchange for mankind between obligation and right, duty and interest in the interdependent modern world. We have studied instances for generations in aging society, which include economy interaction and culture interaction, whether competition and cooperation, or enterprising and dependency, we all are to reconcile our thinking between youth and the elderly. It must be pointed out that there is a transition from the traditional filial duty ethics civilization to the just ethics civilization in the modern society. We should show not only support for the elderly, but also respect and love to old people, which is a virtue from eastern tradition. Moreover, we insist a personality, which has self-determination, self-respect and self-help consciousness among the elderly. We advocate an equal consciousness between generations, such as social position, participating in society, consumption and education, and so on.

[19] Intergenerational Perspectives: Older persons Through the Eyes of the Younger Generations

Trang Thomas, (RMIT University, Melbourne, Australia)

Our age-separated society has produced myths and misinformation about old age, and a lack of knowledge about older persons has been found common among younger generations. This study explores the attitudes of Australian adolescents towards older people as a function of their relationship with grandparents. Over 200 school students (aged approximately 13 or 14 years) participated in a single session questionnaire study. Both quantitative and qualitative data were collected: information relating to the frequency of adolescent-grandparent contact, propinquity of grandparents' residences to adolescents, and types of relationships between adolescents and their grandparents (e.g, emotional, financial or information support, reciprocal shared common interest, sense of obligations and duties). Typologies of adolescent-grandparent interaction were constructed from the subjects' descriptions of their visits with their grandparents. These variables were then examined in relation to adolescents' attitudes towards older people in general. The results indicate that adolescents' attitudes towards the elderly are more favourable when they have a close relationship with their grandparents, especially maternal. Finally, the paper discusses intergenerational issues in the multicultural context and implications for social policies.

[20] Geographical Distance and Frequency of Contacts between Elderly Parents and Children in Japan

W. Koyano (Seigakuin University, Saitama, Japan), M. Nishimura, T. Ishibashi (Dia Foundation for Research on Ageing Societies, Tokyo, Japan), Y. Yamada (Keio University, Tokyo, Japan)

The traditional living arrangement of Japanese seniors was co-residence with the eldest son. During a 40-year period from 1960, however, the frequency of co-residence drastically decreased, and a new style of intergenerational solidarity has been emerging. In this study, in order to explicate the intergenerational relationships in todays Japan, geographical distance and frequency of contacts between seniors and their adult children were observed. The survey was carried out in 1998 with a nationally representative sample of seniors aged 65 years and over, and 2,311 persons were successfully interviewed (the response rate was 77.0%). The respondents ranged in age from 65 to 100 years, with an average of 72.1 years; 45.1% were men, and the remaining 54.9% were women. The respondents were asked to name all their children, and to indicate geographical distance from and the frequency of contacts with each of the children. 58.1% of the respondents had coresident child(ren); 38.4% had child(ren) not co-residing but living within 30 minutes of transportation time; 73.6% had child(ren), either co-resident or not, living within 30 minutes of distance. Among the children named (n=5,947), 26.8

[21] Intergenerational conflict: Distinctions between inequality, dissatisfaction and protest orientation

A-L. Ellwood, C.A. Konnert (University of Calgary, Calgary, Canada)

Tension between age groups regarding support for programs that benefit the elderly is an issue that has been much discussed but little researched. In this study, group relative deprivation theory was used to examine claims of increasing intergenerational tension and protest among young Canadians. One hundred and forty (45 male, 95 female) undergraduate students completed a questionnaire assessing attitudes toward three groups: the Younger, Baby Boom, and Older generations. Measures of perceived inequality between groups, dissatisfaction/resentfulness, emotional closeness, and strength of group identification were used to predict support for programs that benefit the elderly, attitudes toward the elderly and protest orientation. Results indicated that although participants reported perceptions of inequality and feelings of dissatisfaction, these thoughts and feelings were not associated with support for programs for the elderly or with protest orientation. Perceived inequality and feelings of dissatisfaction were, however, related to negative group attitudes. Higher levels of perceived inequality, dissatisfaction, and willingness to protest were reported toward the Baby Boom generation than toward the Older generation. Given these results, it is suggested that there is little evidence that young Canadians are wanting to protest against any inequality they perceive between themselves and the elderly. Future research should attempt to clarify whether the greater levels of hostility directed toward the Baby Boom generation will hold as the Baby Boom generation ages and becomes part of the Older generation. This issue has considerable implications for policy planning and development.

[22] Children's attitudes towards old age

*Davidovic S,Trailov D,Stevic M, Erdeljan N, and Davidovic M. (*Children's Hospital, University of Belgrade, Yugoslavia *KBC Zvezdara, Center for Geriatric Medicine, Belgrade , Yugoslavia)*

The connection that promotes the healthy ageing the best is the one that concerns children.It provides the first two factors for longevity to those that do not poses those two factors in the first place: optimism and activity. Ee have studied the attitudes about old age of four population groups: *school children (n=99, age range 7-16, with mean age of 10 years) *adolescent (n=107 ,age range 16-18,with mean age of 17 years) *nurses (n=56, with mean age of 36 years) *elderly patients (n=79, with mean age of 74 years) Investigation has showed that positive statement about ageing has been mainly demonstrated by the group of school children. That same group expressed an interesting amount of knowledge about good way of living for longevity. The nurses have the best knowledge about ageing and healthy attitude. The percentage of "wrong" answers was very high among elderly patients. There is data that children's attitudes towards old age differs from that of adults. Positive perception of ageing process is more frequent in childhood. We have expected the results of analysis of children's interviews because I was convinced that the majority of attitudes about ageing were stereotypical and full of prejudice, but children rarely have prejudice.

[23] Social Relationships and Life Satisfaction: Comparison Among Two Groups of Seniors

RESENDE, Marineia Crosara (Universidade Estadual de Campinas - Campinas,SP - Brazil). FREIRE, Sueli Aparecida (Universidade Federal de Uberlândia - Uberlândia,MG - Brazil). LEÃO JUNIOR, Roosevelt Universidade estadual de Campinas - Campinas,SP - Brazil). QUEROZ, Nelma Caires (Universidade Estadual de Campinas, SP - Brazil).

For the aging persons the activities accomplished in group can be important source of support (affective, instrumental) and satisfaction, as it has been pointed in the literature on social relationships and psychological well-being. Taking the social selectivity theory, the model of social convoy of social relationships, the studies on psychological well-being and on the support given by participants of religious (GR) or leisure (GL) groups, this study was accomplished with the following objectives: a) To investigate the hierarchical organization of the adults social relationships and participant seniors of GR and GL. b) To verify the categories of people included in the close and significant relationships. c) To verify similarities and differences in life satisfaction among participants of GR-GL. Answered the instruments (information file; Antonucci diagram; Neri's life satisfaction scale) 46 adults and seniors, participants of GR-GL. For the participants of both groups, the family relationships come as main social support, in all circles. For the GL participants the close social relationships didn't showed the members of the group, GR showed them. Regarding the general satisfaction all participants tell life satisfaction, GR (62.7%), GL (58.3%). The results agree with Antonuccis description of social convoy. The Carstenses theory is well acted in the results of GL but not in the GR. It can be cause of the number and category of people showed in each circle. It is possible that the participation in GR provides larger social-emotional support for their members. The group participation can be one of the sources of life satisfaction.

[24] From Needs to Intervention: Organising a Service to Support Family Caregivers for the Elderly

S.C.I. Pavarini, V.A.G. Varotto, E.J. Barham, A. P.R.P. Sadalla, (Universidade Federal de São Carlos, São Carlos, Brazil)

In Brazil, there is little social support or practical information available to enable family caregivers for the elderly to handle this role. Thus, the Centre for the Orientation of the Elderly and their Caregivers was created with the help of a state financing agency (FAPESP). The services offered by this Centre were developed in two stages. First, operational and organisational issues were dealt with: remodeling the physical environment, definition of goals, development of a data collection instrument, dissemination of the centre, registration of people interested in the services to be offered, selection of people currently caring for an elderly person in their home, and interviews with these caregivers. Second, a series of ten sessions (each lasting 1.5 hr) was conducted, using a group intervention format. The topics for these sessions were derived from information concerning the caregivers needs. In each session, two coordinators led the group while another two recorded the groups activities (written and photographic records), with an exchange of roles among the 10 facilitators, each week. The caregivers evaluated each session using a standardised form. The results indicate that the intervention permitted the exchange of personal experiences and the identification of coping strategies appropriate for each person through the presentation of information and discussion of topics that addressed their needs. Thus, a community service that provides a well-structured support group for caregivers of the elderly seems to be an option that is helpful to this population.

[25] Development of the support system for old people in China

P. X. Hong, Q. Y. Lu (Guangzhou Home for Old People, Guangzhou,China)

China is a developing country with 1.3 billion people. Along with the development of economics and scientific advances, the living standard and health status have improved rapidly. As a result, the mortality rate and the national birth rate have declined significantly. The aging process of population accelerates in unusual speed, much faster than developed countries. From 1985 to 2025, total population in China will increase 43%, but the aged 60 years and over will increase 24.2% in the same period. It is expected that aging population will reach 0.2 billion in 2015. The percentage of aged people will be close to 15.66% in 2020, and 23.0% in 2040. This is a serious social problem faced by our society. Therefore, development of the support system for old people is an important issue in China. The characteristics of population aging in China include the quick speed and the largest number of the aging population over 60 in the world. The education level of aged people is relatively lower. Most of them are living with family members. China will become the aging society on the relatively lower economic basis. The basic principle of the strategy for healthy aging is that "ensured by the policy and law of government, based on the community health care, relied upon family support, strengthen the consciousness of aged people for self care and disease prevention, initiate self-reliance and active participation in society, carry out the health promotion exercise in the whole population, to achieve the goal of healthy aging".

[26] Psychological Stress, Social Exchanges, and Depression in Japanese Middle-aged and Elderly People

Y. Fukukawa, C. Nakashima, S. Tsuboi, N. Niino, F. Ando, H. Shimokata (National Institute for Longevity Sciences, Aichi, Japan

PURPOSE: This study examined the relationships among psychological stress, positive and negative social exchanges, and depression in Japanese middle-aged and elderly people. METHOD: Subjects were 2,010 residents aged between 40 and 79 years old who participated in the first wave survey of the National Institute for Longevity Sciences-Longitudinal Study of Aging (NILS-LSA). The number of negative life events experienced during recent two years was adopted as the index of stressor. Positive and negative social exchanges with family members were assessed using a standardized self-report questionnaire. Depressive symptoms were measured by a Japanese version of the Center for Epidemiologic Studies Depression Scale (CES-D). Controlling for age, sex, education level, family income, and subjective health as covariables, main and interaction effects of stressor and social exchanges on depression were investigated through hierarchical multiple regression analyses. RESULTS: In addition to the significant main effect of stressor (Beta=.17), significant main effects of positive (Beta=-.20) and negative (Beta=.11) social exchanges were found (all ps<.001). The net effect of positive social exchange on depressive symptoms was then thought to be more potent than that of negative social exchange. Besides, significant (p<.05) interaction between negative social exchange and stressor was also observed; negative social exchange exerted depression-enhancing effect only at the middle or the lower level of stressor. CONCLUSION: The findings in our study suggest the unique characteristics of positive and negative social exchanges relating to psychological stress and health.

[27] Characteristics of Others in the Social Network of Japanese Senior Men

M. Nishimura, T. Ishibashi (Dia Foundation for Research on Ageing Societies, Tokyo, Japan), W. Koyano (Seigakuin University, Saitama, Japan), T. Ando (Yokohama National University, Kanagawa, Japan), T. Asakawa (Tokai University, Kanagawa, Japan)

Observed were everyday interactions, history of relationships, and characteristics of network members of Japanese senior men living in an urban area. Subjects were randomly selected men aged 60 to 79 years living in Suginami Ward, Metropolitan Tokyo. Home visit interviews were completed for 766 persons. The respondents were asked to name up to fifteen relatives, friends, or neighbors to whom they had intimate relationships, and to report their relationships with the others they named. For the characteristics of the others, the respondents were asked to evaluate each of the others with 7 items: for example, whether a person had a common interest, was tried and dependable, shared common experience, and so on. Information on the social relationships between 766 respondents and 3,590 network members was obtained through this procedure. The number of network members named by the respondents ranged from 0 to 15 with an average of 4.8. The network members were mainly senior men who had been acquainted in work place or school, had long histories of relationships, and had the same hobby, social activity, or liking. Characteristics of the others significantly differed with the beginning of relation: the others acquainted in school were likely to share the common experience, the others acquainted in work place were likely to have a common interest and have relations with family, and relatives were likely to have relations with family but less likely to share the common experience and to have a common interest.

[28] Improvement of life quality through participant activities in an aged group

Ana Moser (PUCPR, Curitiba, Brazil; USP, São Paulo, Brazil); Andréa Silveira (PUCPR, Curitiba, Brazil); Francieli Franzoni (PUCPR, Curitiba, Brazil); Gisele Delinski (PUCPR, Curitiba, Brazil); Rodrigo Tsuneta (PUCPR, Curitiba, Brazil)

Aging is a process that occurs together with development and demand of the subject being aware of losses, and earns, accepts and compensates limitations according to his own potentialities. The PURPOSE of research was improving life quality through participant activities working with self-esteem. The METHOD was experimental; participated 29 aged between 49 and 81 years old with a mensal income of utmost 4 minimum salaries, retired being that 60% do informal work (such as laundry, housemaid, farmer and trader). Were realized 23 meetings once a week during an hour and a half with about 15 participants in each one. The procedure count with pre and post test (Self Esteem Inventory of Rosenberg, 1965); in each meeting was realized warm activities and a main activity and these activities involved aspect direct or indirectly connected to self esteem and interpersonal relationship. RESULTS got were qualitative gleamed through increase of positive verbalizations like I can", "I like", "I want", "I do... because I want..." even though bigger participation in development of task and in feedback moment. It was possible to observe that after 3 years with the same participants had a raise in the participant number like wise in the acceptance behaviors of group in relation to beginners. CONCLUSION: It s possible to conclude that amplifying his self-knowledge and self-acceptance; man can decrease his defenses and establish healthier relation to the world increasing his life quality.

[29] SIMPLIFIED SCALE DEVELOPMENT TO ASSESS CAREGIVER OF DISABLED ELDERLY'S BURDEN IN GENERAL PRACTICE

KERVINIO C, REVEL V, HARITCHABALET I, SAUVANIER M, DRODE M, ALBERT D, PLACINES B, de la FOURNIERE F (Medecine Interne et Geriatrie - CHG Pau - France)

PURPOSE :The assessment of material and affective burden for disabled patient's caregivers can be carried out with the Zarit Burden Inventory. This scale enables us to intervene earlier with caregivers in order to support them and prevent a rupture in caring which is often a distressing experience . However, the inventory is composed of 22 questions with 5 answer options each. Therefore, it is relatively time-consuming and, in practice, it is used only in some specialised centres. METHOD : We propose a simplified Zarit inventory, developed firstly from a qualitative analysis of the Zarit Inventory and secondly from a statistical analysis carried out on 50 caregivers of disabled elderlies consulting in the geriatric department of the Hospital of Pau in the South-West of France RESULTS : Thus, this scale is made up of 7 questions with a choice of two answers each : repercussions on social and familial life, on work and leisure activities, on physical and mental health, financial burden, fear for ones relative future and finally wish to be helped. CONCLUSION : Provided that this study will be validated, which we intend to carry out subsequently, we think that this inventory could be used widely and particularly in general practice and could become integrated into a standard geriatric assessment.

[30] Main family carers of patients with Alzheimer's disease. The PIXEL Study

Rémy Billon centre hospitalier la rochelle Philippe Thomas centre hospitalier universitaire poitiers

Objective: To describe the human characteristics of carers in their attempt to cope with Alzheimers patients, in order to define subpopulations especially exposed to the burden of care. Methods : The PIXEL Study is countrywide survey performed in France during winter 2000-2001. A detailed questionnaire on the burden of care was given to a main family carer of patients with Alzheimers disease, during the medical assessment of the patient. 559 families answers were obtained , matched with medical information on patients cognitive status Patients were mainly outpatients. Results : Two main groups of family carers are involved : a first young group (mean age 52) cares old patients (82 years old), a second group older (mean age 71) cares patient of same ages. Burden of care and nature of complaints by carers are different according to these groups: disease acceptation of their parent, feel of guilt, difficulties to cope with incontinence are more frequent in group 1. Carers of this group reports sadness, screaming, incontinence of patients more troublesome than the carers of group 2. Conclusion : Young family carers have to cope with older demented patients, with heavier burden of care, and have more psychological problems than old family carers.

[31] Family Caregivers for the Elderly in Brazil: What they Value and the Difficulties they Face

E.J. Barham, S.C.I. Pavarini, A.P.R.P. Sadalla, V.A.G. Varotto (Universidade Federal de São Carlos, São Carlos, Brazil)

In Brazil, family members play a crucial role as caregivers of the elderly, given the lack of adequate alternatives and given that cultural norms favour intergenerational residence patterns. The objectives of this study were to identify what family caregivers do, what they value in their relationship with their elderly relative and the difficulties they face. Interviews were conducted in each respondent's home, using an interview protocol with both open and closed format items. The results show that family caregivers offer physical, social and emotional support to their elderly relatives. Positive aspects of the relationship include the opportunity to guarantee the elderly relative's well-being, valuing of the relative's special skills and presence of the elderly relative in the family context. A minority was unable to identify any benefits of this relationship, acting as caregivers out of a sense of obligation. The most frequently cited difficulties include problems dealing with the elderly relative's emotional condition, a lack of involvement on the part of other family members in dealing with the caregiving demands, a need for information about how to care for their relative, and financial limitations. These results indicate that many family caregivers need a social space in the community where they can reflect on their difficulties, obtain information and share their experiences.

[32] Gender differences in the coping strategies of caregiver in Korea

Gyounghae Han, Sung-eun Yoon, Department of Child Development and Family Studies, College of Human Ecology, Seoul National University, Seoul, KOREA.

Most of the empirical research concerning caregiving and caregivers in Korea primarily focused on caregiver's burden or stress, and relatively little attention was given to what strategies and coping behaviors caregivers used to ease the stress coming from the caregiving. Furthermore, as caregiving was usually regarded as women's work, most of the research regarding caregiving generally targeted on women caregiver. This study attempts to overcome these limitations in caregiving research in Korea. Specific research questions of the study are : 1) What are the coping strategies Korean caregivers use to ease the caregiving stress? 2) Is there a gender differences in the use of coping strategies? In order to answer these questions, data were gathered from 234 respondents(107 men and 127 women) who provided care for ill or handicapped family members or relatives. Statistical methods used for the data analysis were descriptive statistics, t-test, and regression analysis using SPSS/PC+. Results showed that main types of coping strategies were problem-solving and emotional coping and caregivers used problem-solving coping strategies more frequently than emotional coping strategies. There was no statistically significant gender difference in the pattern of coping strategies. Theoretical and policy implications of these results are discussed in the context of changing family care norms and expectations in Korean society.

[33] Primary caregiver burden of frail elderly families: A qualitative study

Sooyoun Kim, Myungcha Kim(SookMyung Women's University, Seoul, Korea)

The purpose of this study is to review the burden of primary caregiver living together with frail elderly parents and to find out alternative resources to reduce it. Data was collected by the in-depth interview to primary caregiver with open-ended questions, the participation observation and the life story analysis using the genogram and ecomap in 14 families. The major findings are: 1. Primary caregiver burden could be classified as the economic, the emotional and the service burden, the lack of space, privacy and time, worsened health. 2. Economic burden could be reduced by the assets of frail elder, economic supports from the relatives and medical care service from the community. 3. Emotional burden could be reduced by primary caregiver's affection for frail elderly parents and by appreciation from the family members and relatives, but increased by traditional norms of family and filial obligations. 4. Service burden could be reduced by supports from the family members, relatives and community. This study clarified that the formal supports such as medical insurance services for elderly diseases, home helper program and household appliance supply should be provided in addition to informal care supports from family and relatives. And it was recommended the norms of family and filial obligations should be viewed in open and realistic way.

[34] Pathways into Caregiving for Rural Custodial Grandparents

N.P. Kropf & M. M. Robinson (School of Social Work, University of Georgia, Athens, Georgia, USA).

PURPOSE: In the U.S, the increase in the number of grandparents raising grandchildren has been dramatic. To date, most research has focused on urban grandparent although estimates indicate that about 250f custodial grandparents live in rural communities. This research explored pathways into caregiving to determine how grandparents in rural communities come to assume this role, and subsequent impact on other relationships. METHOD: The study used a qualitative, semi-structured research methodology. Fourteen grandparents were included in the study, and all were involved in a multi-site statewide intervention program established for custodial grandparents. Participants were recruited from three sites that were located in rural communities across the state. The interviews were tape recorded and transcribed, and data were analyzed using QRS NUD'IST software. RESULTS: Grandparents described three pathways into caregiving. One was an Immediate Assumption of Care where no signs indicated that grandchildren would live in the household, as in a sudden death of the children's parent. A second pathway was the Co-Residential Household where all three generations resided together, until the parent moved and the children remained. A final pathway, Incremental Caregiving, occurred where the grandparent made previous, unsuccessful attempts to improve grandchildren's welfare. The assumption of care was the final resort. Subthemes within each of these pathways will be described. CONCLUSIONS: Rural grandparents assume care of grandchildren for various reasons. Depending upon the pathway into care, grandparents report different transition issues and outcomes, especially within family relationships. Rural grandparents describe few substitutions for relationships that have been severed because of caregiving demands. Loneliness, isolation, and lack of social resources are especially acute for rural caregivers.

[35] Determinants of the types and levels of sibling support on the caregiving for the elderly parents

Jeonghwa Lee, Jin-hee Kim, Gyounghae Han(Department of Child Development and Family Studies, College of Human Ecology, Seoul National University, Seoul, KOREA)

Although sibling support is assumed to be an important supportive resource for the caregiver who provides care for the elderly parents, most of the researches on caregiving in Korea focused on the primary caregiver, and overlooked the role of sibling support in parent care. Thus, we do not have enough informations about the types and the levels of sibling support and its impact on the caregiving burden. The purpose of this study is to fill some of those gaps. Main research questions of the study are: 1) What types of the supports and how much supports are given to the primary caregiver by the siblings? 2) What are the determinants of the types and levels of sibling supports? 3) Do sibling supports affect the level of caregiving burden of the primary caregiver? In order to answer these questions, data were gathered, using the structured questionnaire, from 876 daughters-in-law who lives with elderly parents and provides care for them. The statistical methods used for data analysis were descriptive statistics, cross tables, and regression analysis with SPSS/PC+ program. Results showed that siblings provide various types of supports(i.e. economic, emotional, and instrumental supports) and primary caregivers were most satisfied with the emotional supports from the siblings. Age and economic satus of the elderly parents affected the level of sibling support while the characteristics of the primary caregiver showed no significant effects. The reason of being chosen as a primary caregiver among the siblings also affect the level of sibling supports. These results are discussed in terms of changing intra-generational expectations and norms regarding parent care in Korea.

[36] Korean caregiver's perceived benefits and costs of the caregiving of elderly parents

Gyounghae Han, Jeonghwa Lee(Department of Child Development and Family Studies, College of Human Ecology, Seoul National University, Seoul, KOREA.

In spite of rapid sociocultural changes and increase of nuclear family in recent years, still quite many families in Korea have taken the extended family form where daughter-in-law provides care for the elderly parents. There have been much studies looked at the burden or costs of caregiving of these daughters-in-law while relatively little attention has been given to the positive side of caregiving. However, the nature of the intergenerational relationship in Korea is reciprocal in many regards. Thus, this study attempts to capture not only the costs but also the benefits of caregiving and related factors. For the purpose, data were gathered from 876 daughters-in-law of three generational family both in rural and urban area, using structured questionnaire. The statistical methods used for data analysis were descriptive statistics, cross tables, and regression analysis with SPSS/PC+ program. The major findings of this study were as follows: It was found that overall level of perceived benefits were higher than the costs. Marital and econimcic status of the elderly, age, job status and filial responsibility attitude of caregiver, sibling support, and coresidence duration were the significant variabes predicting the level of perceived benefits. Marital status of elderly parents, income, job status, educational level, and filial responsibility attitude of caregiver, residence region affected the level of perceived costs. The results confirm that there exist both positive and negative aspects of caregiving and the outcome of ciagaregiving are affected by the socioeconomic characteristics of caregiver and the elderly parents.

[37] Children as caregivers of older parents: a family perspective.

Marjolein Broese van Groenou, [Vrije Universiteit, SCW, dept. of Social Gerontology, Amsterdam, the Netherlands] Loes Wiggers, [Vrije Universiteit, SCW, dept of Social Gerontology, Amsterdam, the Netherlands]

PURPOSE: To explain differences in caregiving between adult children of physically impaired parents from a family perspective. METHOD: Data are collected from 136 physically impaired older parents who participated in a side-study of the Longitudinal Aging Study Amsterdam. The parents provided information on the care provision (five activities of ADL and five of IADL) and personal characteristics of each of their children (n=508; on average 3,7 children per family). Multilevel analysis is used to examine the relative impact of characteristics of the child, the parent-child relationship, the parent and the family on the intensity of care provided by the child. RESULTS: In 630f the families at least one child assisted the parent with activities of domestic and/or personal care. In 400f the families with more than one child, the tasks are shared among the children. Preliminary results indicate that the intensity of care provided by a child is significantly related to the gender of child and parent (with most care provided in mother-daughter ties), and to a lesser extent to the structural opportunities of the child (parental-, partner- and jobstatus), the family size and the marital status of the parent. CONCLUSION: The results indicate that caregiving to older impaired parents is shared among the children in many families. In addition, features of the parent-child relationship explain most of the differences in caregiving among children.

[38] The succesful care : From the analysis of caregivers of centenarians

Y.Ebihara, N.Hirose, Y.Arai, M.Takayama, K.Yamamura, S.Nakazawa, K.Yamashita, H.Shimomura, K.Nishikawa, Y.Lau (Dept of Geriatric Med, Keio University) Y.Gondoh, H.Inagaki, K. Kitagawa, Y.Masui (Tokyo Metropolitan Institute of Gerontology)

In Japan, as the elderly population is growing, the problems of caregiver's burden is becoming a wide concern. To investigate the relationship between cared and caregivers, we carried out a questionnaire survey on 110 centenarians and their caregivers, considered as representative of successful aging, who live in Tokyo metropolitan area. Level of ADL and cognitive function (COG) of centenarians, level of the quantity of care (CARE) and the exhaustion (EXH) of caregivers were investigated. ADL was ranked into 4 levels (J>A>B>C)and COG was ranked into 5 levels according to the criteria of Japan Ministry of Health and Welfare. We analyzed the effects of COG of centenarians on CARE and EXH and whether the relationship of caregivers to centenarians modified CARE and EXH. Low ADL was associated with high CARE, however, relationship between ADL and CARE was not linear; CARE of B and C level centenarians were the same. EXH of J, A and B level centenarians were similar, however, became higher in C. As COG worsening, CARE became higher, but EXH was not. The relationship of caregivers to centenarians was not associated with CARE or EXH. Any caregivers, whether they are daughter or daughter-in-law, felt the same burdens. In summary, the level of quantity of care wasn't linearly associated with exhaustion. The levels of ADL and cognitive function have different effects on quantity of care and exhaustion. It is noteworthy that the relation of caregiver to the cared wasn't associated with CARE and EXH level.

[39] The Effectiveness of a Culturally Competent Intervention for Latino Caregivers of Elderly Family Members

Blanca M. Ramos, R. W. Toseland, T. Smith (Institute of Gerontology, State University of New York at Albany, Albany, New York)

A major impact of globalization is increased international migration. Receiving countries such as the United States must help integrate new cultural groups into their new societies through culturally competent human services. This study assessed the effectiveness of HEP, a group program that includes problem solving, health education, coping strategies, and support, for caregivers of Latin American background, Latinos. To increase its cultural competency, special attention was given to cultural and linguistic factors including translating instruments into Spanish language, conducting group sessions in Spanish, hiring bilingual, bicultural staff, working collaboratively with Latino community agencies, and demonstrating sensitivity to culturally specific health beliefs, dietary practices, help seeking behaviors, and approaches to problem solving.Using a 2x3x1 randomized control group design (2 conditions, 3 times measurement, 1 group leader), 51caregivers and their frail elderly family members participated in HEP at a community-based agency. Participants were assessed on health and functional status, emotional well-being, social support, knowledge of community resources, and pressing problems one week before baseline, at eight-weeks, and at one year. Results of the baseline to eight week (data is still being collected for the 1- year measurement period) impact of HEP indicate significant positive changes in the outcome scores for HEP participants. These findings suggest Latino caregivers and care recipients benefit from culturally competent practice in health care. Multicultural competence and sensitivity are necessary to respond to the increased cultural diversity stemming from globalization particularly when providing services to ethnic minorities who like Latinos are members of disadvantaged cultural groups.

[40] Prevalence and Nature of Caregiving Among Older Persons in Nova Scotia

Kathleen M. MacPherson (Dalhousie University, Halifax, Canada)

PURPOSE: This study examines the prevalence and characteristics of caregivers aged 65+ in Nova Scotia. METHOD: The data are from the population-based 1995 Nova Scotia Health Survey (NSHS). In addition to demographic and health information, 3213 respondents indicated whether they were caregivers (definition provided). The self-identified caregivers were then asked to provide detailed information about the types and amounts of care, numbers and ages of care recipients, and degree of caregiver burden. RESULTS: There were 252 caregivers, of whom 51 (20.2%) were aged 65+. The proportion of caregivers among the age 65+ group was slightly higher for males (7%) than for females (6%). Only three (5.9%) of the older caregivers cared for more than one person at the time of the survey. The median age of care recipients was 77, and in approximately half the cases, the care recipient(s) lived with the care provider. Five (9.8%) of the older caregivers appeared to be caring for adult disabled sons or daughters, 10 (19.6%) were caring for individuals old enough to be their parents, and 36 (70.6%) were caring for age peers. Nearly all the older caregivers provided daily care (median = three to four hours per day). The majority of older caregivers reported coping well most of the time. CONCLUSION: Between 6% and 7% of older persons in Nova Scotia are caregivers, most of whom provide daily care. The risk of health problems and functional impairment makes this special group relevant to policy analysts, planners, and service providers alike.

[41] Carers of older people with dementia: assessment and the Carers Act

D. Seddon (Centre for Social Policy Research and Development, University of Wales: Bangor, United Kingdom), C.A. Robinson (Centre for Social Policy Research and Development, University of Wales: Bangor, United Kingdom)

This presentation reports the key findings of a two-year study, conducted in Wales, that evaluated the process and outcomes of assessments carried out under the auspices of the Carers (Recognition and Services) Act 1995. It describes how care managers set about assessing carers' needs and identifies some of the difficulties care managers encounter in translating into practice the policy emphasis on supporting carers. This presentation demonstrates that despite the high level of commitment to assessing carers' needs, aspects of the assessment and care management processes remain contrary to the recommendations set out in Practice Guidance. A number of organisational and procedural barriers to assessing carers' needs are identified and it is suggested that care managers lack an explicit framework to direct carers' assessments. The research that informed this presentation was completed in three phases and combined qualitative and quantitative methods of data collection and analysis. Phase One involved telephone interviews with managers in health and social services across Wales to gather information on the strategic intent of local agencies towards carer support and the implementation of the Carers Act. Phase Two involved in-depth interviews with care managers to describe how they assess carers' needs. Phase Three involved interviews with carers of older people with dementia to describe their experiences of the assessment and care planning processes. This presentation will summarise qualitative and quantitative data from the study and will outline a series of policy and practice recommendations relating to carer assessments.

[42] Determinants of Stress in Italian Professional Caregivers of Institutionalized Patients

C. Scarafiotti, M. Molaschi, P. Maina, S. Raspo, M. D. Nuzzo, F. Fabris (Medical and Surgical Department, University of Torino, Torino, ITALY)

PURPOSE: Aim of the study was to evaluate the main sources of stress in professional caregivers of institutionalized elderly. METHOD: The study included 51 subjects (15 SRN and 36 NA) working in three small institutions in Northern Italy. Data from professionals were collected using an anonymous, self-administered structured questionnaire including some personal data, the Nursing Stress Scale, and the Rosemberg Self-esteem Scale. The work load was quantified by classifying the patients with the Barthel Index and the NeuroPsychiartic Inventory. RESULTS: The overall level of perceived stress was not high (NSS mean score 37.5 +/- 13.4), and was mainly related to the domains of work load, death and dying, and lack of support. The highest level of stress was registered in the Alzheimers' Unit. Self-esteem was rather high (RSS score 57.1 +/- 8.6), but significantly lower in the subgroup working with demented patients ($p<0.001$). Professional caregivers with children showed higher levels of self-esteem, lower stress, and less conflicts with doctors and colleagues. Finally, the members of staff who chose this work were less distressed and reported a better self-esteem compared to those who entered the job by chance or because they head no other opportunities ($p<0.05$). CONCLUSION: Our data show that the work load, in particular with demented patients, is one of the main determinants of stress in professional caregivers. A proper support from the working environment, together with a steady family background and the conscious choice of this particular work can help preventing the stress.

[43] Impact of Select Contextual Variables on Inter-rater Reliability of a Caregiver Assessment Tool

Janice Keefe, and Pamela Fancey M.A.(Mount Saint Vincent University, Halifax, Canada), Nancy Guberman, (University of Quebec at Montreal, Montreal, Canada) Daphne Nahmiash, (University of Laval, Quebec City, Canada) & Lucy Barylak, (CLSC ReneCassin/University Institute of Social Gerontology of Quebec, Montreal, Canada).

Family caregivers are a central component in the care of disabled and chronically ill persons in Canada. Despite the fact that they have needs and interests which are often different from those of the care receiver, their needs are rarely assessed. Canadian research, funded by the National Health Transition Fund, has developed a comprehensive caregiver assessment tool to be used by home care professionals to systematically identify and evaluate caregivers needs. The assessment tool consists of 10 dimensions: caring work; relationship with formal agencies; housing; juggling other responsibilities; financial costs of caregiving; family dynamics; physical and emotional health; service needs; and crisis and future planning. In Spring 2000, 168 caregivers were assessed using this tool by home care assessors in eight agencies and two Provinces. The goal of this presentation is to outline the components of the assessment tool and report on the impact that select contextual variables, such as Province, rural-urban and language, have on the inter-rater reliability of the tool. Findings suggest that inter-rater reliability, as measured by Kappa, is less affected by Provincial location or language of the assessment than by being in a rural or urban setting but even here the differences are minimal. These findings are discussed in terms of the utility of tool to identify priority needs and services for family members caring for persons in different provinces, languages and settings. In addition, lessons learned from this developmental stage of the tool such as how to improve data conformity and communication are outlined.

[44] Indicator of social complexity

Vetel JM CH LE MANS FRANCE Ducoudray JM PROBTP FRANCE Leroux R CH VIERZON FRANCE

Indicator of social complexity This tool proposes an operational classification, with clear legibility, as much offered in information capture as in comprehension of results, whilst being appropriately descriptive. Notion of resources : The tool determines a hierarchised level of social timebut does not specify the persons involved Situations of future of elderly person : S1 No changes S2 Necessity of modifications : the person returns to the previous place S3 : Necessity to move out S4 : All administrative arrangements and social accompanying to be carried out before the announced decease and after. Group context : Capacity of the family group to solve problems posed above G1 Situation dealt with, completely and reliably. G2 - The group does not deal independently with the problem. G3 - The group does not effect the solutions but does not oppose them. G4 - The group is in a situation of conflict. Level of complexity : ternary quotation A : nil or negligible : information required B : average : information required, but in addition to checking and even carrying out C : high : information, checking and carrying out required, as is also negotiation and arbitration with the family group. Matrix of the 16 possible cases (crossing future and group), and the three levels of resource mobilisation. The A,B,C are distributed as follows, after validation — S1 S2 S3 S4 G1 A- A- A- A G2 A- A- A- A G3 A- B- B- B G4 B- C- C- C By effecting a section in a group of people, it is possible to determine the 0f ABC, indicating an increasing level of social work load.

[45] Acceptability of the COPE-Index in practitioners and carers of older people.

Z. B. Wojszel, B. Bien, J. Wilmanska (Department of Clinical & Social Gerontology, Medical Academy of Bialystok, Poland)

The COPE-Index is an instrument for the assessment of the negative impact, positive value of care and quality of support in carers of elderly people. It was constructed and validated in international co-operation [1], to be implemented in the routine primary practice. The aim of the study was to assess the acceptability of the instrument by carers and by practitioners. The carers evaluation questionnaire was completed immediately after COPE-Index administration in 126 family carers. Carers were identified by frail over 75 year old elderly recruited through a population study. The users evaluation questionnaire was completed by 18 practitioners, GPs and community nurses, at the end of the study. The acceptability of the COPE-Index by carers was generally good, and only every fourth carer maintained that it made the assessment process too long and complicated. Most of users would be happy to use it as part of the assessment of carers needs, but in the opinion of approximately half of them it made the assessment process too complex, too long and identified carers needs that the practitioners could not meet. On the whole, however, the COPE-Index showed to be a valuable instrument, improving the assessment process and practitioners understanding of carers needs, and at the same time making the carers feel that the practitioner is interested in their needs. [1]On behalf of the COPE group: Philp I, McKee K, Nolan M, Walker A (University of Sheffield); Lamura G, Melchiorre M G, Quattrini S, Spazzafumo L (I.N.R.C.A, ANCONA); Öberg B, Krevers B, Hässler R, (University of Linköping); Mestheneos E, Triantafillou J, Prouskas C (Sextant, Athens); Szczerbinska K (Jagiellonian University, Krakow); Chwalow J, Baudoin C (INSERM, Paris). Project funded by EC 4th Framework Biomedicine and Health Programme, Contract No: BMH-4-98-3374 and Polish State Committee for Scientific Research, Contract No: 4P05D05815

[46] Subjective burden among caregivers taking care of a YOBIYOSE-ROJIN

T.Mizuno, (School of Nursing Tokyo WOmen's Medical University) K. Takasaki (School of Allied Health Science, Tokyo Medical and Dental University)

The issue of YOBIYOSE-ROJIN or the elderly parents who were relocated to the homestead of their child due to their care-requiring condition has received widespread attention since about 1985 in Japan. In this study, to determine the favorable assistance required for these caregivers we analyzed characteristics and factors that might contribute the caregivers' burden with the elderly care. We interviewed 154 caregivers taking care of the aged over the age of 65 who moved to live with or live closely to the family caregiver within the last 5 years. The elderly who wanted to move were 28.6% and 24.00f the elderly did not know that they were going to be relocated. The elderly who had cognitive problems were 82.4% and the bed-ridden were 23.4%. As for caregiver's intention of the parents' relocation, 500f caregivers indicated their willingness. The care burden associated with mental status, aid in eating, caregiver's sleeping, caregivers' intention of the parents' relocation, physical status, caregiver-receiver relationship, length of elderly care per day and support of family members.

[47] The Family Care Network: A Partnership Model for Providing Access to Home Care and Modifications.

Elyse Salend (Partners in Care Foundation (PICF) Jim Cook (PICF) June Simmons (PICF)

Purpose: The Family Care Network assures access to community services, home care and other vital social and medical services for disabled, chronically ill, or those facing catastrophic life-threatening events. It uses short-term interventions to mobilize individuals and enable them to rise to their highest level of long term independence. It works in collaborative partnership with social service agencies and hospitals. The focus of this poster is to provide a conceptual framework and practical examples of how the Family Care Network innovative service model works and can be replicated in other communities. Method: A variety of methods used will be presented including: Partnership building, assessments, fund raising for small and large grants, client and referral satisfaction, evaluations and program development. Results: In three years of operation the FCN has served more than 2500 individuals and families. The results of the client satisfaction survey show overwhelming client satisfaction across all measures. Case mangers feel increased empowerment because they have an added resource for vital care. Conclusion: The Family Care Network fills a need for critical home care and other support services not reimbursed by other sources of funding. As such, other groups and communities may want to consider adopting its model and strategies to increase the effectiveness of the safety net for vulnerable persons that they are attempting to assist.

[48] The influence of caregiver role satisfaction and perceived control as mediating variables on caregiver stress.

M. Russell-Miller (Southern Oregon University, Oregon, USA), C. Pratt, A. Walker (Oregon State University, Oregon, USA)

A cognitive appraisal model of stress posits that mediators affect the relationship between stressors and outcome. Consistent with this model, this study investigated the influence of two mediating variables on outcomes for married adult daughters who give care to their elderly mothers. The central research question was: In married adult daughters who provide care to their dependent elderly mothers, is the relationship between caregiver stressors and the outcome of self-reported depression mediated by levels of situation-specific perceived control and caregiver role satisfaction? The stressors associated with caregiving included level of dependency, marital conflict, coresidence of mother and daughter, available income, and employment status. Sample consisted of 75 caregiving adult daughters who volunteered for a longitudinal study concerning mother-daughter relationships in adulthood. Findings indicated that caregiving role satisfaction is an important mediator between the stressors of giving care and the outcome, depression. Marital conflict had important direct effects within the model. High levels of marital conflict were predictive of lower caregiver role satisfaction and higher rates of depression. Employment status had a direct effect on perceived control with higher levels of control being associated with not being employed and lower levels associated with part and full-time employment. The hypothesized mediators of psychosocial resources of situation-specific perceived control and caregiver role satisfaction did not combine to influence outcome. However, evidence for caregiving role satisfaction as a significant mediator between stressors and outcome is an important finding and lends support to the cognitive appraisal model of stress.

[49] Analysis of Activities by Telephone line for Elder Abuse in Japan

Kinuko Takasaki, Momoe Konagaya, Taeko Chuman, Yumi chiba and Masako Tomita. (Allied Health Science, Tokyo Medical Dental University, Tokyo, Japan) (1-5-45 Yushima, Bunkyo-ku,Tokyo,113-8519,Japan)

Purpose: This study is to describe characteristics of telephone line for elder abuse by nurse in Japan. Method: The sample for the analysis was composed of 122 cases for elder abuse between August 1996 and February 2000. Qualitative studies have been made on the consultation records written by nurse. Results: Characteristic of clients: The persons who were concerned in the abuse (the abused elderly person or abuser) were 41 cases, the other persons were 81 cases. Client who called the telephone line were mostly victims daughter (42%). Characteristic of the abuser : The son and/or daughter-in-law were 49 cases. The daughter was 27 cases. The spouse was 10 cases. Characteristics of the abused elderly persons were mainly female (80%) and old (80-84 years old were 31 cases) Types of abuse were psychological emotional (68 cases), financial exploitation (46 cases), neglect (35 cases), physical abuse (32 cases). The ways of counsel on telephone line for the elder abuse by the nurse were classified into the following four: 1) To help the clients narrate satisfactorily 2) To tell how to use the social resources 3) To advise about abuse and care based on specialty knowledge 4) To maintain relationships to clients. Conclusion: If there is somebody (like a daughter) who is interested in the family, the abuse among the family should be likely to find. The function on telephone support line to elder abuse by nurse was identified.

[50] The Needs of Older Women: Services for Victims of Elder Abuse and Other Abuse.

Jacki Pritchard (Independent Researcher, Consultant Trainer) 51 Duncombe StreetWalkley, Sheffield S6 3RH, England.

Purpose: This qualitative study (funded by the Joseph Rowntree Foundation) was undertaken in three social services departments in the North of England (UK). It aimed to consider the life experiences of older women who had been victims of elder abuse, their past and present needs, and appropriate service provision. Method: Monitoring systems were set up in the three departments to collate statistics on vulnerable adults, to identify older female victims for interview and to examine practices and outcomes. In-depth interviews were conducted with 27 female elder abuse victims and focus groups were run for over 300 older people. Social workers and other social care staff were interviewed and participated in focus groups. Findings: Of all vulnerable adults identified as victims of adult abuse, older people constituted the largest service user group. Workers most frequently identified physical abuse as the main problem whereas victims gave prominence to financial and emotional abuse. The majority of female elder abuse victims had experienced abuse earlier in their lives. Victims had frequently remained in abusive situations because they did not know how and where to get the practical advice and the information they needed to leave e.g. about accommodation, money, benefits. Victims had emotional and practical needs related both to the past and the present. They emphasised the need to talk to someone, to receive practical advice and ongoing support. Conclusion: Practical help and emotional support are needed from workers in a wide range of agencies. Resources required are not always offered or are not readily made available to older victims. Effective co-ordination of specialist and non-specialist inputs of help is often seriously lacking.

[51] Elder abuse in South Africa: a not-so-hidden, but complicated shame

J.D. Joubert, D. Swart, P. Reddy, N. Mfaku (Medical Research Council, Cape Town, South Africa)

Purpose: The paper aims to provide insight into the experiences of abuse and neglect among older persons in South Africa, as found in two separate qualitative studies. Method: Study 1 was conducted among 14 persons, 55 years +, in rural Eastern Cape province during December 1997 and January 1998. Study 2 was conducted among 240 persons, 65 years +, in three different provinces of South Africa during March and April 1998. In both studies, data were collected via individual face-to-face interviews, using a semi-structured interview schedule. Results: The findings bear witness to the existence of various forms of elder abuse among the participants, i.e. material/financial abuse, physical abuse, psychological abuse, neglect, systemic abuse, lack of respect, infrastructural abuse, ideological abuse and sexual abuse/rape. It became clear that many older individuals have experienced multiple types of abuse at a given time, enacted by either the same, or different role players. Participants blamed a number of issues for the mentioned abusive behaviours and attitudes of abusers, e.g. Westernization, education, unemployment, alcohol abuse, perceived easy access to alcohol, impropriety among younger generations, the government, and lack of appreciation for parents. Conclusion: The frequency, diversity and intensity of the reported incidences of elder abuse urge serious intervention and prevention strategies in South Africa. Considering the diverse phases of South Africa's demographic transition; given the country's unique epidemiological transition; and recalling our ideological past which includes that the majority of South Africa's older persons have lived through nearly half a century of apartheid rule and discriminating policies, imply a complicated task for such strategies.

[52] Abuse of Older Adults: A Community Response Network

J. Chenier (Elizabeth Bruyere Health Centre-Geriatric Day Hospital, Ottawa, Canada) T. Cogan (The Council on Aging-Ottawa, Ottawa, Canada)

A project management committee composed of seniors, service providers, and professionals originated to investigate the need for a Community Response Network (CRN) with regard to abuse of older adults. Existing resources, agency protocols, and response models were identified and reviewed by process of a survey and interviews. Respondents estimated that older adult abuse incidents were reported to their agencies ranging from 3 to over 100 times per year. The projected increase in the number of older adults in Ottawa from 1996 to 2031 is 80,045 to 229,000 respectively; this will presumably translate to an increase in the number of older adult abuse cases. A need for a coordinated community response to abuse of older adults in Ottawa was identified and supported. Pyblic presentations, television and radio interviews, and a media briefing raised community awareness of this issue. A community workshop discussing abuse of older adults was organized; working groups initiated the process of developing a model and protocols. The CRN strives to improve the system of services in the community by creating a formal network with defined roles and responsibilities. The Ottawa CRN is defined by knowledgeable front-line workers and case managers, consistent protocols and assessments, an Interagency Consulting Service for assistance in difficult cases, and an innovative diversion program. The final component of the CRN model, the diversion program, is groundbreaking in this context. The purpose of diversion programs is to seek better resolution of offences by involving the community. In time, the expectation is increased reporting of cases of abuse, and decreased incidence of abuse of older adults based on knowledge gained through the diversion program. Partnerships with police services and the Crown Attorney are integral to the success of the diversion program.

[53] Questionnaire of living arrangement: Vitagora Concept

Carrasco Meza V.H. (Vitagora, H.U. Getafe, Madrid, Spain)
Velasco Gutiérrez J. (Vitagora, Madrid, Spain)

Purpose: Describe the population interviewed during the first 31 days of a promotional campaign related to a residential complex including standard living facilities adapted for dependent people and a social and health complex, designed for long-term care, day-care, and rehabilitation. Method: The promotional campaign was located in a commercial and leisure center (within up to 90,000 m2 constructed, with a median attendance of up to fifteen hundred people per week). People interested in Vitagora concept was interviewed, and an umbrella was given for those who responded the questionnaire. There has been no promotional campaign prior to this innitiative. Results: Data presented is related to the first 6 weeks (November-December 2000), with a total of 697 interviews (22.5 interviews/day, with 4 interviewers). 9.3% were highly interested in Vitagora concept, and 10.5% were interested, while 80.2% was not especially interested. 71.3% lived within 15 km to the commercial center (Vitagora will be located nearly next to it). Age was below 40 years in 38.6% of responders, and above 60 years in 20.8%. 13.3% were retired people, 25.4% were houseworkers and 14.3% were people working in the same complex. Conclusions: 1.- Vitagora concept has drawn a considerable attention during the first six weeks of the promotional campaign. 2.- Nearly 20% of those interviewed were interested in Vitagora concept. 3.- Though 20% of those interviewed were 60 years and over, Vitagora concept draws considerable attraction to young people (38.6% of 40 years and less).

[54] Aging affects ADL more than IADL in low stimulated nursing home residents in Southern Brazil.

M.R. Knorst, G. Messa, S. Pereira (School of Physiotherapy, Pontifical Catholic University of Rio Grande do Sul, Porto Alegre, Brazil), C. Martinelli, A. J. G. Bos (Institute of Geriatrics and Gerontology, Pontifical Catholic University of Rio Grande do Sul, Porto Alegre, Brazil)

The aim of this study is to associate the level of Activity of Daily Living (ADL) scale with the Instrumental Activity of Daily Living scale in chronic low stimulated "bed hidden" nursing-home residents. The study was conducted in 32 nursing-home residents, living for more than one year in a special ward for "bed hidden". The overall mean age was 81.3 years ± 9 (Standard Deviation - SD). The scales were conducted by trained students of Rehabilitation of the Pontifical Catholic University of Rio Grande do Sul, Brazil. 22 residents, or 69%, got the lowest grade for IADL (zero), 5 got the second lowest (one) and the remaining five got levels of 2 to 6 on the 8 level scale. The mean age of the nine residents who presented zero for both scales was 84.5 ± 8.5 while those zero IADL group with ADL higher than zero were much younger (78.3±10.7). Those who preserved some degree of IADL and ADL didn't differ much on age from the zero IADL 1 plus ADL group. We concluded that in low stimuli elderly, age is an important predicted factor ADL while IADL seems to be more rapidly affected by the amount of stimuli received by a nursing-home elderly.

[55] Aging: building and evaluating an educational unit in a PBL curriculum

Ricardo S. Komatsu, FAMEMA - Marilia Medical School, Marília-SP, BRAZIL

Background: The process to build an educational unit at FAMEMA's MD Program PBL curriculum is involving the participation of several experts from different areas: basic sciences researchers, clinical teachers, social workers, psychologists, geriatrics, nurses, working in a team to define learning objectives, to organise learning resources and practical activities, and to write educational problems. The program evaluation has been considered the opinion from students and tutors about the quality of learning objectives, educational problems, learning resources, and lectures. Objective: To describe how we built and evaluated an educational unit on ageing in a PBL curriculum at FAMEMA - Marilia Medical School, Brazil. Methods: Description of building steps, and analysis of data from evaluation forms from students (n=66), and tutors/co-tutors (n=16). Results: Learning objectives were considered satisfactory by 93.8% of tutors and 98.5% of students. The educational unit on ageing was considered satisfactory, in overall aspects, by 97% of the 66 students that answered the evaluation form. Conclusion: The introduction of an educational unit on ageing in 1999 our new PBL MD Program was plenty satisfactory.

[56] Space Efficient Universal Design Innovations

Gloria Gutman (Simon Fraser University, Vancouver, Canada) Yvette Jones (Simon Fraser University, Vancouver, Canada) Masuma Walji (Simon Fraser University, Vancouver, Canada) Mary Ann Clarke Scott (Simon Fraser University, Vancouver, Canada)

Purpose: to evaluate designs developed specifically to enhance access for elderly and people with disabilities. Research objectives included: 1. determining which of the universal design features are the most functionally appropriate based on evaluation of actual use by users with varying physical abilities; 2. dentifying and describing patterns of use of test features by users with varying abilities; 3. identifying alternative design features that may emerge from the research, and, 4. identifying the most space efficient design solutions(s) incorporating those design features. Method One hundred research participants tested and evaluated nine different household design features (seven kitchen and two bathroom configurations) by research participants with a range of mobility impairments, taking into account both relative cost, space efficiency and user friendliness, and assessing their universality. The data was quantified to identify and describe patterns related to specific activities of daily living while permitting comparisons of objective human factors task data and participants' perceived experiences. Results We found the inclusion of knee space adds to the accessibility of the design, as both ambulatory and non ambulatory participants performed well when knee space was available. Furthermore, the Lazy Susan configuration was generally a bad design for all participants, with the effects being magnified for participants in wheelchairs. Conclusion: The goal of this study was to demonstrate that specific design solutions can be evaluated and demonstrated through testing with subjects who have varying abilities in order to provide evidence for or against these design modifications. We found that performing both a quantitative and qualitative analysis on subject's behaviours led to a large amount of information that will be beneficial to existing design literature as well as lead to improved design recommendations.

[57] A Multidisciplinary Model of Evaluation in Dementia Care

M.A. Reimer, C. Donaldson, G. Currie (University of Calgary, Alberta, Canada), S. Slaughter (Bethany Care Society, Calgary, Alberta, Canada).

We report on a model for doing economic-quality of life evaluations of environments for persons with middle to late stage dementia. Most such studies have been weakened by a unidisciplinary perspective, lack of design rigour, limited power, and/or measures that failed to capture hidden costs and the experience of the persons with dementia. Key components of our model are: a multidisciplinary, multisectorial research team; combined use of utility and condition-specific quality of life measures; cost impact assessment, combining data from equivalent comparison groups as well as administrative sources; inclusion of methodological research as a component in each project; and use of local and international advisory groups. We are completing a major study in which quality of life data on 185 subjects and cost per resident per day data are being collected in experimental (pupose-built and staffed special-care facility) and comparison facilities (traditional care), controlling for levels of behavior in these facilities over a one year period. These data will be combined with data from the comparison groups on length of time in the facilities as well as with data on the uses (and costs) of other facilities visited by or used by residents. This model for doing economic-quality of life evaluations of environments for persons with middle to late stage dementia brings together the strengths of a multidisciplinary team and advisory groups for research with this challenging population.

[58] Adult Family Living: Is it a cost-effective model of care?

Donna Dosman (Department of Human Ecology, University of Alberta), Norah Keating (Department of Human Ecology, University of Alberta) Janet Fast (Department of Human Ecology, University of Alberta),

ABSTRACT Adult Family Living (AFL) is a model of care for frail seniors in which up to four people are cared for in a private home. In Canada the model is seen as attractive because of its potential to contain public costs. We have argued that reduced public costs may be accompanied by higher costs incurred by key stakeholders such as seniors and caregivers. The purpose of this presentation is to examine whether AFL is cost effective from the perspective of a key stakeholder group, AFL caregivers. Data come from a multi model evaluation of models of residential continuing care in western Canada. We draw upon several data sources: analyses of the public program costs of AFL compared to other models of residential care; administrative data including salaries and contracts; time use and focus group data from AFL caregivers. Results are that AFL models have the lowest public costs but that AFL care providers incur high levels of economic costs (capital development, home maintenance, food and household items, personal health insurance benefits, low hourly wage) and non-economic costs (social isolation, lack of privacy, little respite). We argue that the costs incurred by these self-employed formal caregivers resemble those of family caregivers and that the transfer of program costs to AFL care providers represents a privatization of public sector services. The long term viability of AFL may rest on the willingness of caregivers to sustain a family-like level of commitment to frail seniors in their care.

[59] Focusing on Environment

Sheila M. Peace & Caroline Holland (The Open University, Milton Keynes, United Kingdom); Leonie Kellaher (CESSA, University of North London, London, England).

Purpose: As part of an on-going research project, focus groups have been used within a multi-method study seeking to understand the relationship between environment and identity in later life for people living in three locations (urban/rural; village,town,city) and in different types of accommodation (age-integrated housing and age-related housing). Method: Focus groups were used in the first year to identify key issues for development within subsequent one-to-one in-depth interviews. Groups ranged from three to twelve people; in location (billiards room to church meeting room); in terms of gender and ethnicity, and these factors have influenced both the 'setting-upfi and 'developmentfi of groups. Contact has been maintained within and between groups throughout the study using a newsletter system. In a majority of cases two researchers have been present at the group meetings and they have been tape-recorded and transcribed. Results: Findings concern: the development of groups and the effects of group composition; the relationship between researchers/researched; gender issues; cultural issues and analysis of findings; identifying those factors which are more easily discussed in groups. Issues identified: privacy; security; internality/externality; community integration; visibility; adaptation; ideas relating to individual and group identity; space and place. Conclusion: The use of focus groups within a multi-methodology leads the researchers to question the emergence of different aspects of the topic under study through individual and group processes. This also leads to issues relating to analysis, and the contribution to multi-method research.

[61] Living arrangements and psychological well-being of the rural elderly in Korea

Soonduck Yoon(Rural Living Science Institute, Rural Development Administration, Suwon, Korea), Gyounghae Han(Department of Child Development and Family Studies, Seoul National University, Seoul, Korea)

In Korean society, three generational stem family has been the norm where elderly parents live with the eldest son and cared by daughter-in-law. However, there has been rapid changes in inter-generational expectations and family norms in recent years and consequent changes in the living arrangements of the elderly. Proportion of the elders who live by themselves increased dramatically in recent years. At the same time, it is often assumed that elders in contemporary Korea also prefer to live by themselves. In this study, we wants to examine the relationship between the living arrangement and psychological well-being of the elderly. Specific research questions of the study are : Does psychological well-being of the elderly differ by their living arrangement after the socio-demographic characteristics of the elderly are controlled? Are there any significant interaction effects of living arrangement and major socio-demographic characteristics, such as marital status and health? In order to explore these questions, data were gathered from 940 rural elderly who has at least one adult child in Korea using the structured questionnaire. Results from the hierarchical regression analyses shows that elders who live with their children are happier than elders live by themselves. However, living arrangement shows no such effect on the level of loneliness of the elderly parents. Significant marital status interaction effect was found on the loneliness among the rural elderly: The elderly with no living spouse reports lower levels of loneliness when they live with their adult child while no such association was found among the elders with living spouse. These results suggest the need to explore further the complex relationship between living arrangement and well-being of the Korean elderly and their preferences and expectations regarding inter-generational obligations and living arrangements.

[62] 'Hearing the voice of older people with dementia: researching empowerment in sheltered and residential care'

H.Bartlett (OCHRAD, Oxford Brookes University, Oxford, United Kingdom) and W.Martin (Oxford Dementia Centre, Oxford Brookes University, Oxford, United Kingdom)

PURPOSE In recent years there has been a significant increase in the number of people with dementia involved in social research. This not only reflects a rise in the number of people with dementia in the United Kingdom, but an underlying change in how dementia is known. Practitioners and researchers now increasingly aim to involve the older person with dementia in the decision making process and promote an understanding of their subjective experiences. The aim of this poster is to set out the research design, associated methodological issues and preliminary findings of a two-year research study about empowering older people with dementia (in partnership with Anchor Trust and funded by the National Lottery Charities Board). METHOD This qualitative study compares the decision making opportunities of older people with dementia who live in residential care and sheltered housing. The research involves focus groups with care/professional staff, interviews with older people and case studies with older people with dementia. Data was analysed using NUD:IST. RESULTS The study shows the significance of the tension between the notions of 'risk' and 'empowerment' and the multiplicity of perspectives evident when involving older people with dementia in decision making. CONCLUSIONS The findings provide insights into the identification of key decision areas for older people with dementia in different care settings. Moreover, the poster shows how the issues we were interested in - empowerment and involving older people with dementia as active participants in their own care - were mirrored in the research process.

[63] A Study on the Adaptive Behavior of the Elderly with Dementia to Environmental Relocation

Toru Kano, Seiko Suzuki Faculty of Social Welfare Iwate Prefectural University Iwate, Japan

This paper reports on the adaptive behavior of the Elderly with dementia to a new designed nursing home. We observed behavior of the elderly with dementia from morning to night both before and after the renewed nursing home. Each characteristics of nursing home are as follows; Before rebuilding: 130 residents in two floors, two-beds-rooms and 4-beds-rooms, elderly with and without dementia are mixed. After rebuilding:

130 residents in 3-care-units, one of them is a special care unit for the elderly with dementia and its bedroom is private room only. Results and Conclusion: At the start of new nursing-home, they didn't feel at home and wandered from place to place. One month from the renewal, they began to stay their room and came to the public space with their purpose or aims, for example folding and setting towels for the meal. It was not commonly observed to stay their bedroom except the case of being taken by the staffs before the renewal. They began to be able to help other residents in three month, for examples they advised how to go the toilet room. Before renewal, they could not take active behavior without staff. With a well designed environment, elderly with dementia can adapt to new environment over time, and they can develop their own way of life and own pattern of using the spaces.

[64] Effect of Environmental Change on Mental Health of Care Staffs

Seiko Suzuki (Faculty of Social Welfare, Iwate Prefectural University,Japan) T.Kano (Faculty of social Welfare, Iwate Prefectural University,Japan)

PURPOSE: In recent years, rebuilding of nursing-care facilities has been recommended in consideration of the personal care and privacy of residents in the special elderly nursing home. This study was designed to examine how the rebuilding and moving of nursing-care facility (briefly called rebuilding below) affect the mental health of care staffs. METHODS: Subjects were 29 care staffs in special elderly nursing homes, which have been rebuilt or moved recently. They filled out a questionnaire before and after rebuilding. Items questioned: 1) Stressor, 2) burnout, 3) stress-relieving factors (work morale, administrator's leadership, atmosphere of working place, and official discretion), and 4) greatness of expectation of rebuilding. RESULTS: 1. The scores of stressor and burnout were lower after rebuilding. 2. Stress-relieving factors score a higher point after rebuilding. 3. In care staffs having great expectation of rebuilding, the scores of stressor and burnout were lower after rebuilding. CONCLUSION: 1. Rebuilding tended to promote the mental health of care staffs. 2. The effect of rebuilding on the mental health of care staffs was related to the greatness of expectation of rebuilding. 3. The environmental change due rebuilding effectively worked on the mental health and work morale of the care staffs.

[65] Family Caregiving Characteristics: Predictors of Environmental Modification and Special Equipment Use

Deborah C. Messecar, (Oregon Health Sciences University, Portland,USA);Barbara Stewart, (Oregon Health Sciences University, Portland,USA);Patricia Archbold, (Oregon Health Sciences University, Portland,USA)

Purpose: The family caregiver characteristics that predict use of environmental modifications and special equipment use were studied in 106 care receiver and caregiver dyads. Method: Secondary analysis of data from the Caregiver Relief Study (Archbold, Stewart, Greenlick, & harvath, 1990). Results: Using logistic regression to control for care receiver poor health status and impairment, caregiver psychosocial variables were identified that partially explain the use of special equipment. Family caregiver characteristics did not predict use of environmental modifications. Use of special equipment in the home where a caregiver is present is mainly predicted by the caregiver's access to formal and informal supports (friends, family, and someone whose job it is) and resources (such as having enough time, energy, and money). Having resources and available help increase the odds of using special equipment in the home by 3 (95% confidence interval [CI] = 1.4, 6.2) to 4.2 (95% CI = 1.3, 13.5) times respectively. Surprisingly, having a good relationship with the care receiver decreased the likelihood of use of special equipment by 75% (odds ratio = .26, 95% CI = .08, .80), and caregiver preparedness did not predict use. Conclusion: The results indicate that some family caregiver characteristics influence the use of special equipment in the home.

[66] New Lives for Old

Bernadette Bartlam, Miriam Bernard, Simon Biggs, Paul Kingston (Keele University, Staffordshire, United Kingdom)

Housing options in later life are undergoing considerable change in Britain. One of the most recent developments is the creation of retirement communities similar to those that have been around in Canada, the United States and Europe for some time. Do these purpose-built retirement villages really herald the development of 'new lives for old people'? Or are they simply another form of institutional care? METHOD The methodology in this study builds on the findings of a completed study we undertook into one such community in Wolverhampton in 1998. Over a three year period this work is focusing on the population of older people living in Berryhill Retirement Village in Stoke-on-Trent, and is using both quantitative and qualitative methods to generate data. Using such a multi-method, triangulated approach we anticipate developing a more complete, deeper understanding of the issues involved and facilitate members of the community in determining their own, and the community's, future direction. The overall intention of the methodology is to generate a picture of the perceptions of health, identity and well-being amongst the sample population over 3 years. A number of different strategies to data gathering are being employed: · Questionnaires · Stakeholder interviews · Participant Observation · Community 'Open Space' Conferencing · Diaries · Existing documentation - minutes of meetings (staff and residents); other general data already being collected within the Village. RESULTS Preliminary findings from the initial stages of the study will be presented. CONCLUSIONS No conclusions are presently available. The study is being carried out in collaboration with The ExtraCare Charitable Trust, managers of the community, and is being funded by the National Lottery Charities Board.

[67] A Multidisciplinary Intervention to Prevent Mental Health Problems in Assisted Living Facilities

F. Whittington, C. Hollingsworth, M. M. Ball, S. V. King, V. L. Patterson (Gerontology Center, Georgia State University, Atlanta, GA, USA), S. Diwan (School of Social Work, Georgia State University, Atlanta, GA, USA), C. Rosenbloom (Department of Nutrition, Georgia State University, Atlanta, GA, USA), L. Taylor (Department of Physical Therapy, Georgia State University, Atlanta, GA, USA), & A. Neel (Restore Health Group, Atlanta, GA, USA)

PURPOSE: This paper reports preliminary results of the creation and implementation of an intervention designed by a multidisciplinary team, including a physical therapist, nutritionist, pharmacist, psychologist, social worker, and 4 sociologists, to prevent mental health and medication problems among residents of assisted living facilities. METHOD: In year 1 of the project, working in a 70-bed test facility, the team designed both the intervention and methods of evaluation. In year 2, 2 experimental and 2 control homes were selected for study. Pre-test data were collected on residents' physical function, nutrition status, medication regimens, psychological states, and social relationships. Then an intervention consisting of an exercise program, nutritional counseling, medication review, social activities, staff training, and a family support group, was implemented with residents, staff, and family members. After 6 months, the intervention will be concluded and post-test measures will be repeated in both experimental and control homes. RESULTS: Preliminary results show that residents in the intervention homes were very satisfied with the intervention overall, especially the exercise, nutrition, and medication modules. Staff and family also reported relatively high levels of satisfaction with the intervention, though staff expressed some resistance to suggested changes by team experts. Quantitative measures of change in mental health states and medication regimens will be completed after collection of post-test data. CONCLUSION: Intervention is needed to prevent, not just treat, mental health and medication problems in assisted living, and general response of residents, staff, and family members to such an intervention is favorable.

[68] Changing house conditions in the elderly: predictors and costs in a longitudinal study in Italy.

Angelo Bianchetti, Giuseppe Bellelli (Geriatric Research Group, Brescia and Ancelle della Carità; Hospital, Cremona, Italy) Federica Pignatti, Francesca Castelletti (Geriatric Research Group, Brescia, Italy) Renzo Rozzini (Geriatric Research Group and Poliambulanza Hospital, Brescia, Italy) and Marco Trabucchi (Geriatric Research Group, Brescia and University of Tor Vergata Roma; Italy)

Independence in their own homes is desirable for most people but illness and disability in later life may make this impossible unless aids are provided and adaptations made to the home and the cost of these changes may be high, expecially in the more frail elderly, such as demented people. In a longitudinal study on a sample of 1201 community dwelling elderly living in Brescia (Italy), the modifications in the living conditions, factors predicting changing and the costs were evaluated. Of the initial sample examined in 1985 (70-75 years old at baseline), 366 (78% women and 22% men) were investigated in 1997, representing the 840f the surviving. The mean age was 72.4 at the first examination and 84.6 at follow-up. At follow-up 49.30f subjects live alone, versus 72.7% at the baseline. During the period of observation 36.90f the elderly moved to a nursing home and 20 0.000000rom their own to relative's home. Cognitive impairment and disability at follow-up were the variables associated to a greater risk of changing house. Demographic variables (living with someone, level of education) and economic conditions represent protective factors. In the sample of subjects affected of AD, during the follow-up period 44.8% modified the house with a mean expenditure of 4,500 US $. Most elderly people change their living conditions and cognitive and functional status are the more important clinical risk factor. In demented people families had a considerable cost to adapt home to the their specific needs.

[69] A Gender Difference in Reporting the Need for Mobility Assistance

G. L. Jensen, J.M. Friedmann (Vanderbilt Center for Human Nutrition, Nashville, TN, USA)

This investigation was intended to characterize gender differences in the reporting of mobility limitations among community dwelling older persons. The Life Space Questionnaire (LSQ) is a self-report tool that queries the need for an assistance device or the need for help from another person to get to sequential life spaces that extend from inside the home, to outsice the home and beyond. The LSQ as well as specific queries of the need for assistance with ADLs and IADLs were mailed to 3895 participants in a Medicare managed care program. Individuals were excluded if they had expired (294), been admitted to a skilled nursing facility (35), or had switched to another health program (96). A remarkable 3014 (87%) of the remaining eligible sample returned a completed questionnaire. The analyzable sample was 54 0.000000emale and neither mean age (75 years) or body mass index (27 kg/m2) differed by gender. Women were significantly more likely than men to report needing assistance with shopping (8.6 vs 3.7%), traveling (9.6 vs 3.8%), or any IADL (10.0 vs 3.2%). The LSQ did not reveal gender differences in the need for an assistance device, but did find that women were significantly more likely to report requiring the help of another person to get outside of the neighborhood (10.3 vs 4.6%) and outside of town (12.2 vs 5.6%). Women were also more likely to report using public transportation (7.0 vs 4.2%) or travel with another person (50.8 vs 17.2%). These observations suggest that there are important gender differences in the reporting of mobility related concerns.

[69] Maximizing Independence and Consumer Choice by Offering Supportive Services in a Continuing Care Retirement Community

D.D.Rockemann (Cathedral Rock, Corp, St. Louis, Missouri, USA), M.A.Perkinson (Washington University School of Medicine, St. Louis, Missouri, USA

As residents in Continuing Care Retirement Communities (CCRCs) age in place, adult day care centers, home health care, in-home supportive services and concierge services are a practical and appealing way to maximize independence and consumer choice. The traditional model for CCRCs consists of distinct levels of care (independent living, assistant living and skilled nursing). If their health declines residents have few options other than moving to the next level of care. This study focuses on the special needs of residents living in a CCRC as they begin to age in place. Emphasis centered on creating an environment that empowered residents to make their own choices regarding any assisting care needs. Two hundred eighty self administered interviews, 60 in-depth taped interviews and three focus groups were conducted with independent living residents. Based on this needs assessment, a continuum of care model LifeChoices was created that offers resident/consumer choice in determining their own health care needs and how, when and where this care takes place. This model uses the adult day care as the central point from which all supportive services are rendered.

[70] Housing Histories and Home Pathways: negotiating the domestic environment

Caroline Holland (The Open University, Milton Keynes, United Kingdom)

Purpose: This presentation sumarises some of the findings from doctoral work on the connections between individual experiences of home, and the effects of housing choices and constraints across the life course. Method: Using an essentially grounded method, data was collected as biographical accounts, including information about present and previous housing, from a sample of 28 older women residents of Milton Keynes (mean age, 80 years). By looking in detail at the housing accounts of older migrants and long-stay residents of this English new town, the author has extended the notion of housing history, to encapsulate both functional and emotional roles in the types of homes which people create. The data was organised using Nu.dist. Results: A range of housing histories was developed from the respondentsfi narrative accounts Δ including histories of space useage, ownership, and the meaning of home. The histories show how these elements evolve over the life course, and link individual experiences with the choices and constraints afforded by national and local housing markets. An analysis of all 28 housing histories also suggested a typography of homes based on the evolving roles of home as individuals and households age. Conclusion: The presentation shows in graphic form how a biographical method has been used within a housing policy context, to advance the theoretical and methodological application of housing histories.

[71] Predictors of Relocation in the Retirement Planning of 50 - 80 Year Olds

L. Schiamberg (Michigan State University, USA), K. McKinney (University of Wisconsin, Stevens Point, USA)

This study focused on individual (e.g, age, occupation or educational level) and community (e.g, economics, safety and support services) characteristics, family factors (including the need to care for parents) and current resources (e.g, family income or current housing) as predictors to the decision to relocate at retirement. A random sample telephone survey of Michigan adults between 50 - 80 years of age (N = 573), stratified to reflect U.S. Census characteristics of age distribution, socioeconomic status and rural/urban location was used. Logistic regression of two cohort groups in the sample, 50-62 year olds and 63-80 year olds, indicated both common and different patterns of planning based on the emerging salience of retirement as a life course event. The desire to sustain or maintain friendships appears to be a particularly salient characteristic in predicting moving/aging-in-place for both the preretirement and postretirement groups, as well as for the entire sample. However, for the retirement group (63-87 years) increasing importance is given to health care needs for self and spouse as well as employment security in plans for moving or aging-in-place. Results provide a better understanding of the pattern of factors associated with retirement decision making, as well as facilitating informed community planning based on a more accurate picture of the dynamics of relocation at retirement.

[72] Living together with the elderly

M.A.Giorgi, R.C.Lopes, S.Ayama, V.B.Bruno, W.F.Lage, (Nucleo de Estudo e Pesquisa do Envelhecimento-Pontificia Universidade Catolica de Sao Paulo, Brazil)

PURPOSE: As the number of older people has been growing faster than the rate of implementation of institutional policies, care of the elderly living at home or in institutions is given by people who lack the adequate technical training or have a very low level of education. This aim of project was to teach caregivers basic notions of gerontology and care of frail elderly, while giving gerontology graduate students the opportunity to start practicing in their specific field. The starting point was a request from a home in the city of Santos, Sao Paulo. METHOD: A course comprising 18 hours of theoretical classes using visual aids, group dynamics and evaluations was developed. Enrollment was open to anyone involved in home nursing or home care services for the aged. We had a group of 35 people, residing in a popular neighborhood, many of whom had not finished elementary or secondary school. Four students of the post-graduate gerontology program at the Pontificia Universidade Católica de S.Paulo (Catholic University), from different professional backgrounds (social worker, psychologist, physical therapist and agronomist) acted as teachers, under supervision. RESULTS: Full attendance and active participation attest the students' interest in the course while the multidisciplinary team approach raised new questions about ways to care and improved work practices. CONCLUSION: Requests to repeat the course and other graduate students' interest in participating indicate that we have met the needs of caregivers, graduate students, professionals from NEPE-PUC/SP and ultimately the elderly, thus establishing the social importance of this project.

[73] Environment and desire for social contact...Do they affect the well-being of seniors

Lynn Martin, MA (Centre for Rural and Northern Health Research, Laurentian University, Sudbury, Canada) Run-Min Zhou, (Laurentian University, Sudbury, Canada)

PURPOSE:The goal of this study was to see if the well-being of the elderly was affected by their environment and their desire for social contact. METHOD: 100 seniors living in nursing homes and 100 living in apartments were interviewed in person. They answered questions concerning their sense of well-being (morale scale of the Wellness Index, Slivinske, Fitch and Morawski, 1996), their actual level of participation in social activities, and their desire for social contact. RESULTS: Desire for social contact played an important role in seniors' well being as well as in their participation in social activities. For seniors living in a nursing home, those with a strong desire for social contact participated more often in social activities than those without such a desire. For seniors with a strong desire for social contact, those living in nursing homes reported a better sense of well-being than those living in apartments. For seniors without a strong desire for social contact, there was no significant difference in well-being between those living in nursing homes and in apartments. CONCLUSION: The decision to move into a collective residence is often very difficult for both seniors and their family. While the senior's care needs and bed/apartment availability are to be considered in the decision-making process, the choice of environment should, in order to promote well-being, reflect the senior's social needs. Thus, for seniors who have a great desire to be with others, moving into a nursing home may facilitate their social activities and enhance their sense of well-being.

[74] Research on the lives of elderly Japanese people living in Germany - Particularly those who plan to stay in Germany permanently

Hiromitsu Mihara

PURPOSE: This study aims to analyse the lives of elderly Japanese who plan to reside permanently in Germany. METHOD: Questionnaires were sent to 89 Japanese people in Germany. RESULTS: The older the subjects were, the less stress they felt about, and not returning to Japan even when they entered the last stage of their lives. Most subjects did not plan on entering German nursing homes, but rather would like to stay in their own home and receive Japanese meals through a meal service program. In addition, they hoped for physical care provided by Japanese care workers or German care workers who can speak Japanese. CONCLUSION: From these results it can be seen that a Japanese meal service program and a Japanese language physical care system is desired by and must be established for elderly Japanese people in Germany.

[75] A study on Change of Residential condition in The elderly by changing of population structure -with analysis of 2% census data in 1985 and 1995-

Kim, Tae-il (Cheju National University, Cheju-Shi, Republic of Korea)

Census data is important social index to establish policies in economic field, housing field and social welfare and so on. This study is based that housing needs has been under the influence of change of Korean population. And It is aim of this study that is to understand change of residential condition in each group of population separated with 5years term as well as population structure and change of residential condition in over 65years old. 2% census data of 1985 and 1995 is used as a analysis data. Decreasing children's population, increasing population over 65years old and rapid increasing population over 50¡Δ64 years old will be influence on housing needs greatly. Person of household in 1995 has been decreasing more than person of household in 1985 and has been changing to household with three or four persons. In type of household, household with one person has been increasing and household with one or two persons over 65years old has been increasing rapidly. In case of a group over 60years old, rate of owner living in detached dwelling is high, but most of detached dwelling are very small and old. And in case of a group over 75years old, rate of rent(tenement, monthly rent with deposit in advance, monthly rent without deposit) living in detached dwelling, which residential quality is not good, is still high and also rate of living in non-house has been increasing. It is necessary to supply policy of housing for The elderly and to establish housing policy related with welfare service in order to prepare to ageing society.

[77] Homeshare: The Spread of Programs in Europe in the Context of Homeshare Development World-Wide

M. Johnson (International Institute on Health and Agein, Bristol, UK), N. Maitland (Homeshare International London, UK)

Homeshare is an exchange of housing for help. A householder offers accommodation to a homesharer in exchange for an agreed level of support. The householder ma need help with the household tasks, or income from a modest rent, or a combination of both. Homeshare also provides security and companionship. Programs appeared in Europe in the early 1990s, 20 years later than the USA. However, little information was available about their number or location. Homeshare International's research, funded by the European Union, aimed to rectify this situation. Purpose: To establish the number and features of Homeshare programs operating in Europe. Method: Telephone and desk research to identify countires and localities. Standard questionnaires to directors of all known programs. Sample personal interviews.
Results: (1) 28 Homeshare programs in 5 European countries, 86% of which are in Spain and England. (2) Homeshare more established (16 programs) and apparently sustainable in Spain than elswhere. (3) All programs established in the last decade. (4) Programs generally small, isolated, "re-inventing the wheel". (5) Most programs university-based. (6) Nature of the exchange varies widely, based on differences in culture and local needs. Conclusions: Factors determining the success and spread of Spanish Homeshare programs need further research - potentially Spain is a model for other countries of sustainable program development. The university-based model, unknown in the UK and uncommon in the USA,

may be transferrable; further research is required. There is a need for umbrella organisations. Homeshare International is confirmed to develop the network and share best practices.

[78] Health and well-being among 70-year-old migrants living in Sweden - results from the H 70 gerontological and geriatric population studies in Göteborg.

E. Silveira (Department of Geriatric Medicine, Göteborg University, Göteborg, Sweden), I. Skoog (Department of Psychiatry, Göteborg University) V. Sundh (Department of Geriatric Medicine, Göteborg University, Göteborg, Sweden), P. Allebeck (Department of Social Medicine, Göteborg University) B. Steen (Department of Geriatric Medicine, Göteborg University, Göteborg, Sweden)

Introduction: Comparative epidemiological studies in migrants in Sweden have shown increased prevalence of psychosocial morbidity in young adults, but there is paucity of information on health in older people (as those above age 65). We examined prevalence of physical and mental health problems, differentials in hospital admission and survival and associations between mental health and social factors in Swedish and non-Swedish born people aged 70 years living in Göteborg, Sweden. Purpose: To assess differences in self-reported physical health, mental health (anxiety and depression) and life satisfaction, as well as in in-patient care and mortality during the period 1992-1999 between Swedish and non-Swedish born people (migrants). Method: Semi-structured interviews were administered to 84 migrants (47 women and 37 men) with the help of bi-lingual interpreters and 409 Swedes (183 males and 226 females used as "controls"). Complementary health and social data obtained from official sources on the total sample (N=764, including non-participants in overall medical interviews and examinations) were used in comparative analyses of in-patient care and mortality. Results: Migrants - originating mainly from Estonia, Poland, Yugoslavia, Germany, Italy and Nordic countries other than Sweden - reported more dizziness, poor vision and urinary problems, and fewer gall-blader problems than natives (pı0.05). Migrants also had higher levels of anxiety and depression and bodily pain, and lower levels of general health; social and emotional functioning; satisfaction with physical health, family contacts, housing conditions and economic status than natives (pı0.05). Satisfaction with physical health was one of the strongest factors related to a lower prevalence of anxiety and depression together with family support and time spent in leisure pursuits. No significant differences in in-patient care and mortality were found between migrants and natives notwithstanding differences in self-reported health. Conclusion: The results seem to indicate poorer subjective health in migrant elders than natives in Göteborg, and also point out to a "healthy migrant" effect on survival.

[79] The effect of relocation on subjective well-being of Japanese elderly

T. Saito (Dept. of Social Gerontology, School of Health Sciences and Nursing, University of Tokyo, Tokyo, Japan) H. Sugisawa, Y. Sugihara (Tokyo Metropolitan Institute of Gerontology, Tokyo, Japan)

PURPOSE: This study examined direct and indirect effects, mediated by social contact, of residential relocation on subjective well-being of Japanese elderly. METHOD: We used longitudinal data of a national representative sample of individual aged 60 years and over (N=1,474). The initial survey was conducted in 1987, and the follow-up survey was conducted three years later. Between the surveys, 57 cases relocated to another street, municipality, or prefecture. Subjective well-being was measured with the Center for Epidemiologic Studies-Depression Scale (CES-D) and the Life Satisfaction Index A (LSIA). Social contacts were measured in terms of frequency of contacts with relatives, friends and neighbors, as well as frequency of social participation. Structural equation modeling was used to examine the effects of relocation, controlling for the initial status of well-being, social contacts, age, sex, activity of daily living (ADL), and economic hardship. RESULTS: Relocation had a positive direct effect on well-being, assessed by both CES-D and LSIA, but had a negative indirect effect mediated by decline of social contacts. CONCLUSION: Our results suggest that residential relocation indirectly has a detrimental effect on subjective well-being of the elderly through decline in social contacts, though it may directly improve subjective well-being of the elderly.

[80] Cyclical Migration among Elderly Immigrants: The Case of Taiwanese Canadians in Greater Vancouver

Jennifer Wu (The League of Welfare Improvement for Older People R.O.C, Taipei, Taiwan), G. Gutman (Gerontology Research Center, Vancouver, Canada)

This research empirically examined cyclical migration among elderly immigrants- a phenomenon not addressed previously in the gerontological literature. A convenient sample of 169 immigrant seniors in Greater Vancouver who emigrated directly from Taiwan (88 non-migrants and 81 cyclical migrants) were interviewed. It was found that elderly Taiwanese immigrants made one to two trips to Taiwan each year, with an average duration of 10.58 weeks. Timing was closely tied to the reasons for cyclical migration. For example, the high proportion of departures from Canada in the winter months from December to February reflected elderly immigrants' strong motivation of visiting family and friends during the Chinese New Year. Multiple regression analysis showed age, employment in Taiwan, homeownership in Taiwan, perceived health and having parents in Taiwan to be significant predictors of cyclical migration. Compared to non-migrants, cyclical migrants had an overall lower rate of health care utilization in Canada and showed a preference for the Taiwanese health system. This was mainly accounted for by their concerns of high costs (e.g, dental care) and barriers to accessing health care (e.g, language and long waiting lists) in Canada. Although no differences in social life were found between the two groups, cyclical migrants reported experiencing loneliness more often than non-migrants when they were staying in Canada. Based on the above findings, it is suggested that for elderly Taiwanese, cyclical migration acts as a way of fulfilling their socio-psychological, health care and economic needs after immigrating to Canada.

[81] Relationships between Social Network and Social Support among the Rural Elderly in Okinawá, Japan

Seizo Sakihara (Faculty of Medicine, University of the Ryukyus, Okinawa, Japan), Hideki Shimanuki and Hiroshi Haga (Tohoku Bunka Gakuen University, Sendai, Japan)

PURPOSE: To examine the relationship between social network and social support of the noninstitutionalized elderly. METHOD: Subjects were 767 persons aged 65 and over. Data were collected on social network and social support. Partial coefficient correlation analyses were conducted to examine whether the association between social network and social support was different by levels of instrumental ADL. RESULTS: The lower ADL group had fewer social interactions as compared with the higher ADL group. Although general notion on relationships between social network and social support was found among the higher ADL group, it was quite different for the lower level of ADL group. In later group, total score of social network ($p<.01$), relatives ($p<.01$), friends ($p<.05$), and neighbours ($p<.05$) were significantly associated to social support as a whole, but not for adult children living separately. Support getting was related to total social network ($p<.01$) and relatives ($p<.01$). Among social network members, relatives were significantly associated with support giving. Moreover, social network was strongly related to psychological well-being in the lower ADL group. CONCLUSION: Relationships between social network and social support were different by level of instrumental ADL. Social networks of the aged with lower level of ADL were partially related to social support. These findings suggest that the infirmed elderly can maintain reciprocal support system despite ADL decreased.

[82] Determinants of Voluntary Involvement & Leadership by

Community Elderly in Health Services Planning and Delivery

M. Kloseck, R.G. Crilly (Division of Geriatric Medicine, University of Western Ontario, London, Ontario, Canada)

Many older individuals volunteer their time and skills once retired, and many do not. The purpose of this study, conducted within the context of a participatory action project designed to increase elderly individuals involvement in health services planning, was to determine who volunteers and who does not, and to ascertain if there are modifiable factors that influence involvement. Elderly volunteers involved in health services planning (n=107), in a seniors apartment complex, were compared with a randomly selected group of non-volunteers (n=74). Cross-sectional survey methodology was used to measure six types of modifiable variables. Bi- and multi-variate analyses were used to determine predictors of volunteerism and leadership. Moderating effects of non-modifiable variables (age, personality, life changes, past volunteering) were examined. Volunteers were younger (M=74 years, SD=8.39 vs. M=78 years, SD=8.12, p=.005), more active (Activity Checklist: M=72.53, SD=9.36 vs. M=69.71, SD=7.51, p=.03), more satisfied with life (SHARP: M=11.11, SD=1.26 vs. M=10.70, SD=1.38, p=.05), received fewer services (chi-square=12.49, p=.002), and experienced fewer functional limitations (Likert scale: M=2.12, SD=1.21 vs. M=2.60, SD=121, p=.01). Volunteers who were extroverted, agreeable and open to change were more likely to assume leadership positions. Several interactions were found. In particular, a history of volunteering moderated the influence of health/function (r= -.43, p=.02). Functional ability most influenced involvement. Less independent individuals with a history of volunteering, however, may overcome their limitations to continue their involvement.

SESSION 21

A Falls Prevention Program

T. Grant, J. Chouinard, M. Delorme (Sisters of Charity Hospital, Ottawa, Canada)

The Bronson Pavilion Falls Clinic is a pilot project which aims to decrease the incidence of falls and fall related injuries in a high risk elderly population . The program is an interdisciplinary approach to fall risk factor assessment and reduction. Participants attend the clinic two half days per week for maximum duration of 12 weeks. Intervention includes gait and balance training, a review and management of key (fall related) medical factors and education on fall prevention. Balance performance as measured by the Berg Balance Scale has improved significantly (p<.002) in the first group of participants(N=14, mean age 73). Fall rate (# of falls/month) has decreased by 72% on average in the same group. Fracture related cost savings have been estimated at between $81,000 and $200,000 for a 6 month period. The cost of running the clinic for the same period is $ 27,000. Based on preliminary data it has been concluded that this model of care is clinically and cost effective. As follow-up data are still being collected conclusions cannot yet be made regarding sustainability of effects.

Avoiding falls: what are older people prepared to do

Janet M Simpson FCSP AFBPsS, (School of Physiotherapy, Kingston University /St George's Hospital Medical School, London SW17 0RE, UK)

PURPOSE To discover what precautions older people themselves take to avoid falling and what else they are prepared to do with help from other people. METHODS Shortly before discharge from geriatric medical wards, 6 men and 26 women (mean age (SD) 83(5.3) agreed to be interviewed. All had admitted to being at least 'slightly concerned about falling'. All lived at home: own home 26, sheltered housing 6; 59% had fallen at least once in the previous 6 months. The same experienced interviewer followed a semi-structured interview schedule to gain information in the following categories: [1] Precautions people themselves take to avoid falling. [2] Willingness to improve their own ability to withstand threats to their balance; [3] Willingness to take home safety measures,. RESULTS Within these categories responses ranged from believing no action was necessary to action taken or planned. For example: [1] 'Nothing to be done as falling is a matter of chance', 'Always hold onto something'; [2] 'I'm to old', 'Not necessary my legs are quite strong', 'Maybe if someone told me'. [3] Resentment at alterations already made, actively suggesting alterations to the authorities. CONCLUSIONS Enthusiasm to accept advice about falls prevention from other people may be guarded. Professionals cannot assume that older people will accept their advice gratefully . It is likely to be most acceptable when the proposed action is agreed with the person and it is not perceived to require much effort on the person's part or too much change in their surroundings.

Fall Prevention for Community Living Seniors

Frank MacDonald, David B.Hogan, Sheila Bricker, Barbara Delarue, Cathy Harbidge, Maggie Hunter, Barbara Metcalf [Geriatric Specialized Services, Calgary Regional Health Authority, Calgary, Canada]

Falls comprise the most common cause of unintentional injury and death for seniors. Studies have shown that at least one third of seniors fall each year. Loss of function, fear of falling, restriction of activity, and increased dependence often result from falls and persist. Fall risk factors most often identified include increasing age, a previous fall, impaired gait and balance, inappropriate medications, fear of falling, symptomatic postural hypotension, visual impairment, and unsafe environments. A randomized controlled experimental research study was conducted in the city of Calgary to test the hypothesis that a comprehensive in-home fall risk assessment followed by individually tailored recommendations will reduce the frequency of falls for community living seniors. The assessment and interventions were developed by an interdisciplinary team including a geriatrician, physiotherapists, occupational therapist, and Clinical Nurse Specialists. The protocol requires active participation of seniors in monitoring falls and following through with fall-prevention recommendations. Although fewer intervention subjects fell and fell less often, the difference did not reach statistical significance. However, in the sub-group of subjects with multiple falls (>2 falls in 3 months prior to entry), there were fewer fallers and falls in the intervention group and a statistically significant increase in the time to first fall (169 days vs. 101 days; p. 027) when compared to the control group. There were no differences in acute care utilization in the two groups.

Fall prevention program for elderly patients at discharge from a geriatric ward. Randomised interventional trial.

M.Rainfray (Centre de Gériatrie Henri Choussat - Université Bordeaux), P.Dehail (Centre de Gériatrie Henri Choussat - Université Bordeaux), I.Bourdel-Marchasson (Centre de Gériatrie Henri Choussat - Université Bordeaux), E.Dumas (Centre de Gériatrie Henri Choussat - Université Bordeaux), J.P.Emeriau (Centre de Gériatrie Henri Choussat - Université Bordeaux)

PURPOSE : Fall prevention is a major issue in geriatric medicine. Primary prevention of falls in community is non efficient and cost consuming whereas prevention in selected populations have shown some efficiency. We have tested an intervention program in elderly hospitalized fallers. METHODS : Randomised interventional trial. Eighty-one patients (86,2+/-5,2 yrs) hospitalized for fall, have been included. At discharge, after a medico-social and environmental assessment, they were randomised in two groups : Intervention or Control. In Gr I (n=37) the patients underwent an interview with a geriatrician who advised them of their medical and functionnal status, potential side effects of drugs, risk factors of falling and gave them a personalised form of guide lines. In Gr C (n=44) the usual procedure was followed. All the patients were followed during 6 months. RESULTS : Both groups were similar for age, sex-ratio, cognitive status, number of previous falls and drugs except for antihypertensive drugs which were more frequent in Gr I than in Gr C (62,1% vs 34,10<0,05). Recidive of falls occured in 21,60f the patients Gr I versus 38,6 0r C. The risk of falls was decreased in Gr I (OR=0.55; p<0.05). In a multivariate analysis, anticonvulsivant, hypnotic, antidepressant, antiparkinsonian drugs and the presence of a nurse at home were associated with a higher risk of falls whereas the ability for unipodal gait was associated with a lower one. CONCLUSION : Evaluation at discharge and elaboration of personalised guidelines prevent the recidive of falls in elderly patients.

Health Canada/Veterans Affairs Canada Falls Prevention Initiative for Veterans, Seniors and Their Caregivers

Jeannita Bernard (Health Promotion and Education Directorate, Veterans Affairs Canada, Charlottetown, Canada) and Nancy Garrard (Division of Aging and Seniors, Health Canada, Ottawa, Canada)

Health Canada and Veterans Affairs Canada recently launched a four year (2000-2004) pilot initiative in three Canadian regions aimed at developing evidence about effective falls prevention interventions directed to community-dwelling veterans, seniors and their caregivers. The serious impact of falls on Canadian seniors and veterans is evident: falls constitute 65% of all injuries, at an annual cost of $2.8 billion. Projected growth of the Canadian seniors population could accentuate the problem. Current research suggests that falls are highly preventable, and that health promotion interventions can reduce significant risk factors. Additional knowledge is needed to identify best practices, program models and community settings that are able to effectively reach the Initiative's clientele. Evaluation is a cornerstone of the Initiative, assessing outcomes for the goals of knowledge advancement, community capacity building, and delivery capacity enhancement within the two Departments. An evaluation design was developed to incorporate the experience of community projects with broad program results and stakeholder expertise. A logic model was created to maintain consistency of understanding among stakeholders, and to guide program- and community-based project development. Tools and templates are being developed to facilitate continuous reporting and congruent evaluation. The presentation will include a short description of the Initiative based on the logic model, and an exploration of the evaluation design being implemented. Particular emphasis will be placed on approaches used to integrate community project experience with a program evaluation that has national significance. A collaborative evaluation design can meet the requirements of diverse community, academic and government stakeholders.

Helping Seniors Prevent Falls at Home: A Service Learning Student Experiment

Tanya Fusco Johnson (Senior Programs University of Hawaii at Hilo)

Abstract The purpose of this research was to teach human services university students about home safety needs for older adults, train them to educate seniors about causes for falls and injuries at home, inform seniors about community services to help prevent falls, and promote better self-care in fall prevention. The method for doing this was a 12 week monitoring program in which students were matched with home-bound elderly to teach fall prevention strategies in the home. The Program Coordinator visited 71 referred or requesting seniors to conduct a room-to-toom assessment and record previous falls and helping services. Seniors were given the results of the assessment showing good conditions in the home environment as well as problematic ones. Seniors were then offered the assistance of a Home Safety Monitor for 12 weeks to educate them about the causes for falls, inform them about helping services, and encourage more pro-active self-care in fall prevention. Those accepting Monitors were the experimental group; those declining were the control group. Both groups were tracted at 6 month intervals for a year to determine whether the Monitored were safer than Non-Monitored. The results show that for the 38 Monitored, 92% had made home safety changes compared with 590f the 32 Non-monitored. While, overall, 330f the Monitored and Non-Monitored decreased falls, half the Non-Monitored increased falls compared with 330f Monitored. Therefore, we conclude that the students' monitoring intervention has helped seniors prevent falls.

SESSION 22

Global Gerontology and the IAG: History and Emerging Roles

Edit Beregi (Budapest, Hungary), Ewald W. Busse (Duke University Medical Center, Durham North Carolina) Samuel Bravo Williams (Sociedad de Geriatria y Gerontologia de Mexico, Mexico City) Gary Andrews (Center for Aging Studies, Flinders University of South Australia, Australia), Gloria Gutman (Gerontology Research Centre, Simon Fraser University, Vancouver, Canada)

The first International Congress of Gerontology met in Liege, Belgium in July 1950. In addition to the scientific program, according to the book of Nathan W. Schock, the structure of the International Association of Gerontology was formulated and the bylaws were produced. During the passing 51 years 17 International Congresses of Gerontology were organized. Interest in the field of gerontology increased, more and more topics were discussed concerning the worldwide increase of the aging population. In addition to the International World Congresses, Regional and National Congresses were also organized. The Presidents of the IAG, who are able to attend the Congress, summarize from 1983-2001 their experiences and the events during their presidency. They will analyse the past and show the future goals and trends in gerontology. The effect of globalisation on the aging research will be presented.

IAG 1983-1989

Ewald W. Busse (Duke University Medical Center, Durham, NC USA)

The six years, 1983 to 1989, were unique in a number of respects. The first was that Ewald Busse was both President of the IAG and was also responsible for the 1985 Congress in New York. This situation was the result of the resignation of Professor Hans Thomae as President of the IAG as of May 5, 1983 but actually became effective September 1, 1983. The orderly succession of vacated officers was not covered in the bylaws of the IAG. Consequently, the complexity of this situation was unusual. The situation was resolved by Professor Thomae, who recommended that Ewald W. Busse become the President. After Dr. Thomae's resignation he continued to be an active and constructive leader in the Association. An interesting arose regarding the origin of the President's chain of office which, is usually worn at all special IAG occasions. The question was resolved after careful study of the chain and the correction of misinformation that was included in a report of the 3rd Congress of the IAG. Many new developments effecting the organization and functioning of the IAG occurred during these six years. The Sandoz Lectures were established as was the Sandoz Prize. The President's Award for Young Investigators was implemented. This award was later endowed and continued as the Busse Research Award. In 1982 the United Nations held a World Assembly on Aging in Vienna. This particular event had numerous implications regarding the IAG and was strongly supported by this organization. At the conclusion of 1989 a reserve bank account was established and remains in a bank in Switzerland. Also, IAG regions were expanded and were given considerable support and the subsequent regional conferences were great successes. The relatively new impact of a great deal of research concerning aging developed during these years. It influenced program content as well as the participation of its members. Unfortunately, there were some nations that were in turmoil with the conflict between politics and science. This resulted in some representation problems particularly those participating in international congresses. A Past President Symposium was included in the program of the 1985 Congress. Each of the Presidents made presentations regarding the events during their term of office. This brief report will include some of the statements that were made by these past Presidents

The International Association of Gerontology between 1989-1993

S. Bravo (Sociedad de Geriatria Y Gerontologia de Mexico A.C.)

The XIV International Congress, held in 1989 in Acapulco, Mexico had 2577 official registrants from 74 Countries. The Regional distribution was as follows:
Region Countries Participants: Europe 26 900; North America 2 683; Latin America 21 587 ; Asia/Oceania 17 394 ; Africa 8 13
The Congress covered a wide range of areas of Gerontology. Medical and Nursing, Psychological, Social Behavioural, and Biological aspects of ageing were presented in 16 simultaneous sessions. There were a total of 73 Symposia, 85 round tables, 110 paper sessions (1200 free papers), 25 poster sessions, 5 distinguished speaker sessions, 12 Latin American and 6 Developing Countries sessions. The figures include more than 2000 presentations and represent 600 Curricular hours. While a cyclone almost cancelled a shipboard party in Acapulco Bay the XIV Congress was an unforgettable event.
As a member of the Program Planning Committee for New York'85, Acapulco'89, Hungary '93 I want to emphasize the value of IAG Congresses. No other procedure (despite such technological advances as satellites and the Internet) gives the warmth of human relationships, the ethusiasm that comes with listening to and shaking the hand of an author or of receiving in a few minutes concentrated information about gerontologic activity in different parts of the world
To assure the survival of the IAG's history, I proposed that a historical archive be established and an attempt be made to regain information from preceding Congresses and so as not to lose information from the Acapulco Congress and future events. Economic support will always be important. For economic stability, an investment in publication such as books, manuals and educational material, and active involvement in training and research are options.

The IAG Congress in Budapest. Events Thereafter: 1993-1997

Edit Beregi (Budapest, Hungary

It was a unique and exciting experience to organize the XVth International Congress of Gerontology. At the IAG Congress in Budapest, Hungary 2,973 persons from 61 countries were officially registered and 258 participants had visitor badges, exempting their registration fees. The scientific program started with the Opening Ceremony where besides the official greetings and the transfer of Presidency, the United Nations Award was presented to the IAG, followed by the presentation of the Sandoz Prize for Gerontological Research, Busse Award, and Presidential Award. The first Plenary Session took place following the Opening Ceremony, the second preceding the Closing Ceremony. At the Congress there were 46 Invited Symposia, 6 Sponsored Symposia, 42 Invited Roundtables, 36 Submitted Roundtables and 7 Sponsored Roundtables. In the Developing Countries Program, 5 Roundtables were organized. Besides, 106 Free Papers, 594 Posters, 12 Audiovisual Programs were included in the program.
Besides the scientific stimulation of the Congress due to the sponsors and registration fees, there was a profit made and from the profit the great part of the expenses of the IAG Secretariat in Budapest could be covered until 1997. Consequently, although we received from the previous Treasurer from Mexico 43,564 USD, 74,770 USD was transfered in December 1997 to Australia.
The Council Meeting during the Congress clarified IAG bylaws and their relationship to the Manual Operating Procedures, and the site of the 2001 International Congress was delcared as Vancouver, Canada. The future of the IAG will be determined by its adaptation - ability to globalize.

IAG 1997-2001

G.R. Andrews (Center for Aging Studies, Flinders University, Australia)

During the period from 1997 to 2001 the International Associating of Gerontology experienced an interesting and exciting period of evolution and transition. The IAG Regions were very active and convened a series of highly successful regional conferences including a Pan-American meeting held in San Antonio, Texas USA in 1999 that saw the effective mobilisation of the North American Committee and its collaboration with the Latin American Region in jointly hosting the quadrennial Pan-American events. The Regional activities all epitomised a renewed vigour and enthusiasm for the development of gerontological research, education, practice at all levels within nations and across the globe. International collaboration and exchange was the hallmark of this time. The advent during the period of the UN declared International Year of Older Persons was a key point around which many global initiatives were pursued and in which the IAG showed outstanding leadership and advocacy. Principle among these was the undertaking (on behalf of the United Nations program on ageing with the support of the Novartis Foundation for Gerontology) of the development of a 'Research Agenda on Ageing for the 21st Century'. This seminal effort is intended to provide a critical guide to governments, NGOs, researchers and others worldwide on priorities for investment in policy relevant research on ageing and will be included as an addendum to the Draft Revised Plan of Action on Ageing presented to the 2nd World Assembly on Ageing. 2001 heralded the 50th Anniversary of the IAG that was celebrated by an unprecedented gathering of the Executive, Regional Chairs and over 50 Presidents of constituent societies of IAG in Salsomaggiore Italy to mark the occasion and deliberate on future strategic directions for the Association. Finally work began at the beginning of 2001 on the convening of an extraordinary congress auspiced by IAG, the Valencia Forum to be held as a pre-meeting to the 2nd World Assembly in order to marshal the world gerontological research, education and practice constituency to provide the essential evidence base that will underpin the subsequent deliberations of policy makers, bureaucrats and advocates during the World Assembly itself. During the period in question the IAG has prospered, grown more active and become significantly more influential in matters of ageing on the World stage.

Expansion on the President's Inaugural Address: New Directions, New Initiatives, New Opportunities for IAG in 2001-2005

Gloria Gutman (Gerontology Research Centre, Simon Fraser University)

Using the IAG's four objectives as a starting point, this presentation describes initiatives that will be a major part of the Presidential Agenda for 2001-2005. These include serving on the Steering Committee and providing strong Executive Committee support for the Valencia Forum, an event to be auspiced by IAG, which will take place in Valencia, Spain on April 1-4 , 2002 one week before the2nd World Assembly on Ageing (WAA2). The objective of the Valencia Forum is to formulate research, educational and provider input into WAA2. Following WAA2, the President, working in concert with the IAG Regions, will endeavor to assist the UN Programme on Ageing (and individual countries or groups of countries, if invited), to implement priority research identified in the Revised International Plan of Action and/or in the Research Agenda for the 21st Century.
While the emphasis of the IAG in the prior four years has been on identifying knowledge gaps and research needed to fill these gaps in order to elaborate sound public policy on aging, major new initiatives will be proposed in the area of training. These include a collaborative effort in the area of distance education in gerontology, and the establishment of a scholarship program to facilitate faculty and graduate student exchange visits and to foster student participation in the World Congress and other IAG educational and information dissemination endeavors.
Expansion of the regional structure to establish Africa officially as an IAG Region and more generally, to strengthen and promote the IAG Regions and their activities will be a priority. Expansion of the IAG structure will also be proposed to enable the formal affiliation of international networks focused on research and/or education in gerontology.
Fostering cordial and regular communication and collaboration with other international NGOs will be another priority.
The over-arching theme for the 2001-2005 administration will be the theme of the 2001 Congress: "Global Aging: Working Together in a Changing World".

SESSION 23

Quality of Life: Trying to Know It When We See It

R. A. Kane (Division of Health Services Research, Policy and Administration, School of Public Health, University of Minnesota, Minneappolis, MN, USA). Conceptual Challenges in Measuring Quality of Life of Older People; R. L. Kane (Division of Health Services Research, Policy and Administration, School of Public Health, University of Minnesota, Minneapolis, MN, USA) Methodological Challenges in Measuring Quality of Life of Older People. I Chi and M. L. Chong (Department of Social Work and Social Administration, the University of Hong Kong) A perspective from Hong Kong. A. Ashour (Psychogeriatric Research Department, Ain Shams University, Ciaro, Egypt) A perspective from Egypt. M. Pelaez, Pan American Health Association, Washington, DC, U.S.A.) Perspectives from Latin America and the Carribean. M. MacAdam, Baycrest Center for Geriatric Care, Toronto, Canada). Perspectives from Canada.

This Symposium discusses conceptual issues, measurement approaches, and current research to define and measure the quality of life of older people, including those who live in nursing home settings and those who live in the community. Rosalie Kane will describe the issues in defining quality of life and developing a measurement strategy for a large ongoing project to measure quality of life for nursing home residents in the United States. In that project, 11 quality of life domains were identified: autonomy, individuality, dignity, privacy, enjoyment, meaningful activity, relationships, comfort, sense of security, functional competence and spiritual well-being, and efforts were made to capture a subjective report from people with substantial Alzheimer's disease. Robert Kane will briefly summarize the multifaceted measurement strategy to characterize individual quality of life and to characterize a program by the quality of life of its participants. AEach of the other panelists will react to this work in terms of the relevance of these concepts and procedures to their own regions and will summarize relevant work from their country. Dr. Chi and Dr. Chong will summarize approaches taken in both nursing home and community settings in Hong Kong.as well as indicators of quality of life that are being developed in Shanghai, an area where policy formulation and service provision for the older people has been perhaps the most well-developed among major cities in Mainland China. Dr. Ashour will present early findings on how Egyptian elders,their family carers and service providers conceptualize quality of life based on work in a nursing home and a memory clinic. Dr. Palaez will address the topic in terms of relevant developments in Latin America and the Carribean, an area that in itself is diverse enough to yield multiple conceptions of quality of life. Margaret MacAdam brings a Canadian as well as a policy perspective to the discussion. Cross-cutting themes include the tension between subjective and objective appraisals of quality of life, challenges in measuring quality of life for people with Alzheimer's disease, and ways to aggregate and use quality of life assessment to actually improve the conditions of life for older people using aging services of various kinds. The intent of this Symposium is to encourage cross-national dialogue on this issue and to identify areas of commonality and difference in conceptualizing and measuring quality of life. Prepared materials will be distributed and full audience participation encouraged..

SESSION 24

Total Care for the Aged - Models That Show the Way!

Barry Telford (Dept Veterans' Affairs - Canberra, Australia) (Home Care - A System for the 21st Century) Dave Pedlar (Departmental Gerontologist, Veteran's Affairs Canada) ("Innovations in Veteran Care in Canada") Judy Salerno (Associate Chief Medical Director for Geriatrics and Extended Care, Department of Veterans Affairs, Washington, USA) ("Extended Care - Extending a Caring Philosophy") Narelle Hohnke (Assistant Secretary, Health Care and Services, Department of Veteran's Affairs, Canberra, Australia) ("Hospital and Home - Building the Bridges") Jo Schumann (Assistant Secretary, Strategic Support, Department of Veteran's Affairs, Canberra, Australia) ("Comparing Two Cultures - Canada and Australian Perspective on Aged Care")

Issue: The main thrust of the presentation would be an international comparison of innovative and holistic approaches to care to support aged people in their homes. Australia and Canada have adopted a unique approach to caring for the veterans of all international conflicts since World War I. Structure: Senior people in the Department of Veterans' Affairs in Australia and Canada would present three short papers on their approaches to care for older people. This would preceed a Round Table discussion of the models and approaches in each country to inform policy and program development in other countries. This Round Table presents a one-off international opportunity for early discussion of dynamic approach to aged care in a changing environment faced with the challenges of increasing demands from consumers, emerging technologies in both care and communication and calls for greater coordination and efficiencies because of reducing government outlays. Content: The key features would include emphasis on: the individual's need to be in control of his/her situation; the need for independence; the mechanisms to manage the cycle of at-home and out-of-home care (eg hospital, medical, allied health services) to maximise independent living; the integration and coordination of care for older people; and the essential need for comprehensive management and Information Technology (IT) systems that underpin the delivery of a model of holistic care. The Australian Department of Veterans' Affairs unique approach to the delivery of better health outcomes for the ageing veteran community locates it among the leaders of aged care in the world. The symposium will showcase the unique approaches in recent initiatives such as community nursing, medication management and Veterans' Home Care, and demonstrate the capacity for real linkages between programs. In particular, the new Australian Veterans' Home Care program is breaking new ground in the delivery of home and community care through a purchaser/provider model and the extensive use of web-enabled technologies such as e-commerce, electronic record keeping and client assessment. The Canadian Veterans' Independence Program (VIP) addresses similar needs for home based services, in ways that best address the requirements in that country. The whole of person approach will integrate with existing services and deliver a comprehensive and coordinated approach to care for older persons. Conclusions/anticipated outcomes: There is increasing international interest in better ways of addressing the needs of aged person living in their own homes. The innovate models of care being implemented for veterans in Australia and Canada will leave a legacy for future generations of aged persons. As the 'baby boomers' age there is need to look at new and more effective models of care to meet the demands of this group. The Australian and Canadian approach have the potential to lead the way in aged care. Participants will take away from the Round Table an understanding of the approach, information on evaluation of the approaches to date, and will have the opportunity to question presenters in detail about policies and processes underpinning the approaches.

Hospital and Home - Building the Bridges

Narelle Hohnke. (Assistant Secretary, Health Services, Commonwealth Department of Veterans' Affairs, National Office, Canberra, Australia)

PURPOSE: To present an overview of innovative purchasing models used in the successful provision of appropriate health care services to meet the diverse and rapidly changing needs of the veteran community. METHOD: Since WW1, veterans have received acute and rehabilitation care through a network of Repatriation Hospitals supported by medical and dental care in the local community. During the 1990's the Department of Veterans' Affairs successfully moved from provider to purchaser of health care services for veterans, particularly through the transfer of the former Repatriation Hospitals to State Governments or sale to the private sector. RESULTS: With the veteran population at an average age of almost 80 years, the challenge has been to provide access to care which facilitates veterans ageing safely in their own home. This focus includes the contracting of both public and private sector services to provide timely and appropriate access to all health care services, including acute hospital services, rehabilitation, specialist and general practitioner services, pharmaceutical, community nursing, allied health and dental care. Emphasis is placed on discharge planning to facilitate a smooth transfer from hospital to home, supported by community nursing and Veterans' Home Care personal care, domestic assistance, home and garden maintenance, respite care. These are complemented by health promotion activities focussing on safety in the home and quality use of medicines. CONCLUSION: Most veterans can be supported within their own homes. To achieve this, the Department has needed to purchase health services both intelligently and discerningly while maintaining a focus on the individual needs and circumstances of the veteran.

Innovations in Veteran Care in Canada

David J. Pedlar PhD.

There are 357,000 veterans in Canada that represent approximately 11% of the Canadian senior population and nearly one in 4 Canadian males over age 65+. The average age of the veteran population is 79 years. Veterans Affairs Canada provides a wide range of programs and services to older veterans across Canada. The presentation will provide an overview of Veterans Affairs Canada's philosophy of senior's care that emphasizes independence and autonomy and will highlight examples of innovative programs and models of service delivery.

SESSION 26

Long-term Sequelae of Trauma in Aging Holocaust Survivors

R. Krell (University of British Columbia, Vancouver, B.C. Canada). The impact of the Holocaust on aging survivors: clinical issues. B. de Vries (San Francisco State University, San Francisco, Cal. U.S.A.) The Holocaust as a context for telling life stories. J. Lomranz (Tel Aviv University, Tel Aviv, Israel) Aintegration: Coping constructively with the long-term effects of the Holocaust. P. Suedfeld (University of British Columbia, Vancouver, B.C. Canada). Indomitable, although not invulnerable: long-term resilience and adaptation of Holocaust survivors.

ISSUE: The problems of aging are many. Are those of a Holocaust survivor any different from other elderly persons? Given the massive early life traumas, to which the survivor was subjected, it is possible that the return of early memories is particularly troubling. STRUCTURE: The session will begin with comments on clinical issues. How Holocaust survivors tell their life stories and cope with long-term effects as well as how resilience and adaptation serves their efforts to cope. CONTEXT: The traumatic life experiences of the survivor tend to recur in memory when the survivor's guard is down. Post-surgical confusion and aging are two examples where a survivor is vulnerable to confusing present day staff with uniformed personnel of another time. Earlier suffering is recalled. Numerous triggers (sounds, smells) serve as immediate pathways to the past and behaviors which are puzzling to family and caretakers not familiar with these Holocaust-driven phenomena. Comparing survivors with non-survivor Jews and non-Jews revealed differences in all three. The war marked the beginning of the life story for most survivors and war events predominated. In both Jewish groups, family births and relationship events were cited more commonly than the non-Jewish group, which identified more career, education, illness and family death events. The Holocaust determines the standard of what is told by survivors. The concept of aintegration proposes the notion that existential incompatibilities characterize life and that consistency and continuity (valued by the West) not only do not accommodate to life events but may present obstacles to life reviews and the narrative constructs of Holocaust survivors. Aintegration assumes an image of man as able to be resilient and develop and grow despite living with contradictions. And finally, a study of Holocaust survivors and control groups reveal that survivors had achieved similar success, considered life to have been meaningful and looked toward the good of future generations. However, they tended to view the world as less benevolent, were mistrustful and were more likely to have needed psychological help. While there is little difference between survivors and controls, the Holocaust had a long-term impact on some aspects of personality and attitude. COMPARING/ANTICIPATED OUTCOMES: The four studies agree that the impact of Holocaust trauma endures throughout life, sometimes with profound effects (the return of a horrifying memory) or more subtle effects such as changes of personality and attitudes. Whether or not psychological theories adequately describe the normal aging process, having gone through the Holocaust makes survivors focus on that event as primary in their life stories. The war experiences and adapting to them mark the life course of the Holocaust survivor. Nevertheless, Lomranz and Suedfeld both emphasize the survivors' resilience and ability to adapt and grow despite living with the consequences of grave trauma.

Aintegration: Coping constructively with the long-term effects of the Holocaust

Lomranz Jacob : Dept. of Psychology, Tel-Aviv University. Tel-Aviv Israel

Most adult developmental psychological theories do not describe adequately human development and coping of the elderly person and therefore do not provide us with the needed personality theories to comprehend the long term effects of trauma and the Holocaust. Existential incompatibilities characterize life. These serve as the background upon which the concept of Aintegration has been developed. Aintegration maintains that people, especially elderly, can live with contrasts, unresolved issues, inconsistencies, discontinuity and paradox and still remain in a state of well-being and mental health. Antegration, is in opposition to mainstream western values and social science which are based on harmony, Aristotelian logic, consistency and continuity. These however, do not always settle with life events. They may also present obstacles to life reviews and narrative construction of Holocaust survivors, or working through grief and Holocaust related behaviors. Aintegration bridges destructive existential states and scientific personality theory and assumes an image of man which emphasizes resilience and the ability to develop and grow despite living with contradictions. The concept of Aintegration will be presented as to its sources and research methodology. Primary research findings reveal its reliability and validity with Holocaust survivors and the relationship of Aintegration to survivors values of the world, subjective health reports, depressive symptoms, stress, PTSD and survivors' involvement's with Holocaust-related behavior and activities.

Indomitable, Although Not Invulnerable: Long-Term Resilience and Adaptation of Holocaust Survivors

Peter Suedfeld (University of British Columbia, Vancouver, Canada)

The research programme described here administered batteries of paper-and-pencil tests to individuals attending gatherings of Holocaust survivors or survivor organizations, and to control groups consisting of Jews in the same age range who lived in countries that were not under Nazi occupation or influence during World War II. In addition, quantitative content analyses of videotaped survivor oral histories were performed. Survivors had reached the same levels of occupational success as the control group and used mostly problem-oriented rather than palliative coping strategies. They considered their life to have been meaningful, and were oriented toward the good of future generations. On the other hand, they were less satisfied with their life than a control group, which consisted of Jews living in safe countries during the war;

they were relatively mistrustful of other people, considered the world to be less benevolent and controllable, and were somewhat more likely than controls to have received psychological help (but not educational, legal, or medical help). On most measures, there is little or no difference between the survivors and the controls, indicating that survivors have adapted well to their postwar environment. However, the Holocaust has had a long-lasting impact on some aspects of their personality and attitudes.

The Holocaust as a Context for Telling Life Stories

Brian de Vries (San Francisco State University San Francisco, CA 94132 USA)

The Holocaust as a Context for Telling Life Stories. Brian de Vries, Ph.D. San Francisco State University, San Francisco, CA, USA Using a narrative approach, this study explores the role of the Holocaust in the life stories of Survivors as contrasted with two comparison groups whose direct experiences did not include surviving the death camps: one Jewish and one Non-Jewish. Using the technique of the life line and measures such as number and type of life events identified as well as the events marking the beginning and ending of the life story, several differences were found between the three groups. Survivors identified an average of 10 life events, fewer than the Non-Jewish comparison group (18) and greater than the Jewish comparison group (7). Most of these events were positive, although less so for the Jewish comparison group, with very few future events identified by any of the groups. The War marked the beginning of the life story for most of the Survivors and their stories ended at an earlier age than did the stories of the comparison groups. Further, WWII events predominated in the stories of the Survivors, as did family births and relationship events (comparably seen in the stories of the Jewish comparisons). In contrast, the comparison groups, and particularly the Non-Jewish group, identified greater numbers of career, education, illness and family death events. It is proposed that the pronounced effect of the Holocaust in the life stories of Survivors (and to a lesser though still evident degree of the Jewish comparisons) serves as an anchoring and contextual influence on the nature and quality of life stories told. That is, the Holocaust sets the standard for what events merit mention and further determines the nature of the events reported and their distribution.

SESSION 28

Ageing in Egypt An Issue of Traditionalism vs. Change

Madiha El-Safty The American University in Cairoof Sociology and member of the Advisory Committee on Ageing for the National NGO Center for Population and Development (NCPD)

Purpose: The paper presents the current situation of the elderly in Egyptian Society addressing the demographic structure, relevant socio-cultural factors, available services, and the impact of social change on this segment. The paper also investigates gaps / loopholes in the system vis-à-vis the elderly population. It ends by giving a sample effort of integrating the elderly stratum in active participation. Method: This work attempts to address the transformation in the situation of the elderly in a traditional society where they enjoy a privileged status supported by strong values. However, the factors of change are now in operation. First, the demographic trend reveals an increase in the percentage of the elderly (60 +) - from 5.10 % in 1950 to 7 % in 2000. In addition, life expectancy is rising - from 52.1 in 1970 to 67 in 2000. U.N. Projections estimate this percentage to reach 11.3 in the year 2025. Second, there is the transformation in the family affecting its traditional role as provider of the care for the elderly, reflected in the increasing female employment, hence, reducing their responsibility towards the old. Labour migration of the young leaving the ageing behind; and urbanisation where residence cannot accommodate them. The paper also proceeds to survey the governmental and nongovernmental services, in the form of homes, clubs, and social security. Results: Addressing the situation of the elderly as above given has revealed inadequate coverage. Good quality homes are, for the most part, far beyond the average family's means. Pension rights are limited to employees. The poor stratum is disadvantaged. Women are the most vulnerable of the vulnerable groups. Conclusion: It is the contention of this paper that because the ageing population is not adequately covered, more efforts have to be made. One such effort is integrating the elderly in activities suited to their qualifications, especially as the legal retirement age is 60. The NCPD is working with the government and nongovernment agencies in the initial stage of a project with this objective. One area already covered is adult literacy programs. Another is the integration of homes with an orphanage, where able residents of the former can help in the latter.

Living arrangements of the old in the context of modernization.

Jacob John Kattakayam (Professor of Sociology& Director Academic Staff College University of Kerala, Kariavattom, Trivandrum)

The elderly are changing the lifestyle according to the changes that are taking place in the society. It is a common scene today that the elderly are trying to engage themselves and there is a purposeful socialization on their part so that the adjustment problem is minimum between them and the younger generation. The old within in a span of ten years has changed their outlook due to the massmedia and the overemphasis of their problem in vernacular press and the various institutions. This study looks into the various aspects that have changed the living arrangements of the old in tune with the changing circumstances of the society. The conclusion of the study show that the old can be brought as meaningful citizens who will not become the burden for the society.

Main Problems of Older Persons in Zimbabwe: Challenges and Prospects

N. Madzingira (University of Zimbabwe, Institute of Development Studies, HARARE, ZIMBABWE).

This article is based on findings of a study on support for older persons in Zimbabwe. Primary data was gathered through focus group discussions and in-depth interviews in five provinces stratified by rural urban location. A thorough literature search was also undertaken to complement the results of this study. The main problems of older persons may defined broadly as: health and health related problems, lack of economic independence, poverty, loniliness, high morbidity and mortality prevalent in communities, poor housing conditions, illiteracy and lack of information, and long distances to water points especially in rural areas. Support for older persons in this study is defined as the provision of financial assistance, meterial and emotional support, and health assistance. Complementary support to alleviate the plight of older persons is rendered by adult children, relatives, the community, the government and non governmental organisations.

Medical and Social Aspects of Gerorgian Long-Living People

N. Kipshidze (Research Institutute of Therapy. 4 Ljubliana st, Tbilisi. 380059, Georgia)

Georgia together with other republics of Transcaucasia is one of region of longevity in the world. The longevity index of the Georgian population is 28.7% on the average, ranging from 15.8% for urban population to 39.4% for rural population. Both in rural and urban populations the number of long-living women exceeds that of men. The study of geographical distribution of long-living people permitted to elaborate the map of longevity. The results of our investigations on more than two thousand long-livers show that the traditional for Georgia humane well-wishing attitude towards old people creates favorable psychological conditions for them to integrate with the society. The family status of Georgian long-livers is also conditioned by national traditions. Predominantly favorable relations in the family (87.7%) promoted maintenance of the authority of elderly people. More than two thirds of long-living people (63.5%) preserved relatively high mobility, which ensured their social activity, that is assistance to the family, society. By the Bartelly test it was determined that 84.5% of long-livers could take care of themselves. There were some nutritional peculiarities among them. CVD the leading place in the structure of pathology of Georgian long-living people (61.7%). Diseases of respiratory, digestive organs, nervous system occupy respectively 18.3%, 4.2%, 9.3%. The indices of arterial pressure were within normal range. Lipid indices were lower than in middle-aged subjects. In 93.3% of centenarians sexual potency was preserved till 60-69 years of age.

Outlook of Ageing in Asia at the Turn of the 21st Century

Mohammad Taghi Sheykhi, Department of Social Sciences, Al-Zahra University, Tehran,

The paper explores that ageing is appearing in Asia more due to the socio-demographic changes in the region. The modernizing countries of the region have undergone health and food improvements, population transition, change in their social system and life-styles—all leading to change in age structure of the population in some countries, and the rest laying the cornerstone of their ageing population in the years to come. Though currently a large portion of the Asian population is of a young age, a good number of them will get the chance to be placed at the elderly category in the future. The ageing population is emerging as probematic at the turn of the 21st century, more due to the shortage of socio-economic security for many of these seniors. As people are more under the influence social and economic development more and more people have the opportunity to be aged, thus further social security measures must be planned for, and more investments done to the elderly so as to avoid the probable challenges and controversies. Gerontologically speaking, as ageing is a new phenomenon to many of the Asian nations, further and closer network of relations must be opened up between them and the industrial world where it has earlier been experienced. Iran too, as an Asian case has been explored so far as its ageing is concerned. Some facts and figures have been given to elaborate and subtantiate this issue. Some proposals have also been forwarded in the hopes of lowering the ageing problems in Asia.

Social Networks and Disengagement: Implicatzions for Social Policy

N.K.Chadha(University of Delhi,India) , John Van Willigen (University of Kentucky,USA)

Social networks are conceptualized in terms of the size and nature of a person´s web of interaction. Social network analysis is a proven method to examine the social life of older people and can be used to show how they are situated in terms of their social interaction and does it serve their functions and satisfy their emotional needs. This paper analyses the content and meaning of social aging as it is experienced by older people in an upper middle class urban in Delhi,India looked at from the perspective of networks and to some extent from the perspective of the household. Indepth interviews were conducted on the elderly by visiting their households, Our research suggests that social involvement in old age depends upon a number of factors including marital status, income level, individual resource control and health status. Social networks provde aid and support in times of need, A person with social ties will be more known to the community. Though the network size is a good indicator of social involvement, there is also the dimension of quality.

Trends in living conditions and satisfaction among poorer older South Africans

V. Moller (Institute of Social and Economic Research, Rhodes University, Grahamstown, South Africa), R. Devey (School of Development Studies, University of Natal, Durban, South Africa)

The majority of South Africa's older population is income-poor and lives in multi-generation households. Since the first democratically elected government came into power in 1994, South Africans have been promised 'a better life for all'. A range of policies and programmes has been implemented to improve the living standards and quality of life of the poor. The paper asks how the older poor have benefited from government interventions in the period 1995-8. Drawing on data compiled from Statistics South Africa's household surveys in1995 and 1998 (n20 000 Δ 30 000 households), a set of over 35 objective and subjective indicators broken down by income is reviewed. Results show that access to services and opportunities improves systematically from poor to rich households. Major material gains for the poor during the review period include access to clean water, electricity and home ownership. In all income brackets, including the ultra-poor, households with access to services and opportunities are more likely to express overall satisfaction with living circumstances than those without. The study concludes that the most effective mechanism for poverty alleviation appears to be the non-contributory, means-tested state old-age pension, which lifts some households out of the most disadvantaged bottom income group. Policies under discussion promise further opportunities for empowering poor households with older members.

SESSION 29

Discursive Research into Ageing as a Moral Issue

Pirjo Nikander (University of TampereDept. of Sociology and Social Psychology Tampere Finland)

Pirjo NikanderUniversity of TampereDept. of Sociology and Social PsychologyFIN-33014 University of TampereTampereFinlandDiscursive Research into Ageing as a Moral IssueDiscursive and qualitative research into ageing and the life-course have, in recent years, proven the benefits of placing language use 'in situ' at the centre of analysis. The purpose of this paper is to contribute to this ongoing discussion by exploring the potential morality of everyday and institutional age discourse as an analysable issue for qualitative ageing research. Studying morality from a discursive point of view, thus, functions as a case in point that underlines the wider applicability of discursive research into ageing.Using discourse analysis, as it is conceptualised within British discursive psychology, the paper focuses on the ways in which the potential morality of any age related talk 'comes to life,' and how moral qualities of age discourse thus become analysable as a part of talk-in-interaction. Building on a detailed analysis of extracts from interviews with Finnish men and women, and on videotaped data from multi-professional meetings in charge of decisions about the elderly, the paper discusses the ways in which speakers themselves fashion their talk to address the morality of their age-related descriptions and reasoning. The paper introduces the 'provisional continuity device' as an analytical example of the recurrent means by which speakers orient to the moral implications of age discourse. It also shows, in detail, how local moral orders and moral logics are established in-and-through interaction, and how such findings jeopardise notions of post-modern fluidity of age.

Finding Meaning in Life: Older Women and Their Spirituality

Linda Foley, (Nebraska Methodist College, Omaha, Nebraska USA)

Spirituality is a broad, multifaceted,multidimensional construct that is often delineated as finding meaning in life. According to the literature, spirituality appears to increase in importance as one ages, leading to heightened meaning in life and growth toward wholeness. Spirituality of the individual is an area that is currently being reseached with increasing frequency, although knowledge about this construct is still in its infancy expecially as it relates to older women. The purpose of this research study was to explore spirituality in the lives of older women and to examine the effects of age, marital status, health, religion and education. A convenience sample of 210 older women from a variety of settings completed the JAREL Spiritual Well-Being Scale, which was developed to assess spiritual well-being in older adults. The majority of older women in this study were quite educated, healthy and living independently. Data analysis demonstrated that overall these women had a reasonably high level of spiritual well-being. Women who were healthy and educated also had higher spirituality scores. Although not statistically significant, African American women had higher spirituality scores than Caucasian women. The African American women however, made up only six percent of the total sample. As the population continues to age and life expectancies rise, considerable research in the area of spiritual well-being and its relationship to successful aging for older women becomes essential. Meeting older women's spiritual needs in the 21st century should become a collaborative challenge for all invested in their well-being.

Modern and Post-modern Narratives on Aging in Argentina: A Comparative Study

Luisa Acrich - Ricardo Iacub Universidad de Buenos Aires - Argentina

This paper examines and compares modern and post-modern narratives of aging persons as depicted in two Argentine films: Besos en la Frente and Sol de Oto. We will show how the older persons, in those contexts, position themselves in different ways. The multiple narratives currently available show these discontinuities. These are considered following philosopher Franco Crespi's statements on differences between modernism and post- modernism. Modernism strictly determined the patterns and expectations related to age, while post-modernism breaks these patterns and deconstructs them, and creates new models where discontinuities and fragmentations are constant. This is why Harry Moody states that the post-modern life course is an extension of the middle age in two senses, downwards to infancy, and upwards to the third age. We all live like young adults, an age that seems to synthesize the idea of responsibility and autonomy. This change permits the desegregation in multiple cultural identities: local and international, ethnic and cultural, age and generation. In this context, we consider narratives as stories we make of our experience which determine, model, and construct the meaning we attribute to that experience and the effects and orientations of our lives and of our relationships with significant others. Following White and Epston, every story is an arbitrary imposition of meaning to the flow of memory. Memories are social possessions, inscribed in language. With this framework we analyze both films as social representations which describe the main traits and how the above mentioned narratives appear in the particular cultural context of Argentina.

Older People's Life Experiences

Nina Chen (University of Missouri, University Outreach and Extension)

The purpose of the study is to explore older people's life experiences and how they feel about aging in Taiwan. A phenomenological research method was used to have in-depth understanding about what older people's lives look like. Twenty Taiwanese older people from 64 to 80 years of age were interviewed. The majority of them lived in an extended family and two-thirds had an elementary education. These older people were very active. They were early risers and did exercises before starting the day. They attended a variety of adult learning programs. Some of them went to evening school to complete their elementary or junior high education in their early 70's. Others helped with farming or family businesses. Filial piety was the most important component to determine their life satisfaction, however, they also needed friendship and companionship to enrich their lives. They felt being old is being sick and did not think they were old. Although age did not mean anything to them, they realized that their physical functions were decreasing and being old was not a choice. Activity, positive attitudes, and having a purpose to look forward to everyday helped them maintain a productive life. Clearly, traditional values, social interactions, and social access provided significant impacts on the quality of older people's lives in Taiwan.

Participants not Observers: Attitudes to Ageing across Cultural and Spiritual Backgrounds

Kate Barnett (Managing Director, Kate Barnett and Associates ΔHuman Services Consultants, Adelaide, South Australia)

Purpose Much has been written about the negative consequences of the ageing process, but this has not beenmatched by research identifying the positive features. There is also a considerable void in existing knowledge about attitudes to ageing, and specifically about how cultural and spiritual background can shape these attitudes and expectations of the formal aged care. Method A sample of 300 was drawn from English, Arabic, Dutch, Greek, Ukrainian, Vietnamese and Punjabi speaking people born between 1925 and 1955. These represented Buddhist, Christian, Muslim, Druze, Maronite Catholic and Sikh communities as well as people whose spiritual beliefs were not influenced by any particular religious affiliation. The sample were living in metropolitan and rural locations. Structured one-to-one interviews with open-ended questions were conducted by trained bilingual, bicultural interviewers and findings were analysed using Access data base. Results Most people hold an extremely positive view of old age which emphasises meaningful involvement on a number of levels, an active lifestyle, good health and being treated with respect. Essential to the vision of old age is being in control and having choices, while care for older people envisages a partnership between both families and service providers. (This contradicts much of the stereotyping associated with people from diverse cultural backgrounds and their attitudes to formal aged care). Conclusion Attitudes to ageing are essentially positive when good health, choice and control characterise the process. This expectation applies across cultural and spiritual boundaries, as does the vision of care for older people.

Theorising Growing and Being Older: Connecting Physical Health,Well-being and Public Health

E.Fairhurst (Manchester Metropolitan University, Manchester,England)

Meanings of health and growing older in Greater Manchester were explored in eight focus groups conducted with ten year age cohorts covering age ranges 30-79.Views on health, longevity and mortality were outlined in terms of both physical and mental health and connections were made with 'genes', diet and exercise. Talk about 'being healthy'in older age went beyond the narrow terms of the alleviation of sickness to embrace mental health in the sense of 'well being', being an active participant in life and public health concerns with the built environment such as transport, housing and neighbourhood.

SESSION 30

The Air Force Villages' Freedom House Study (FHS)

Donald R. Royall (South Texas Veterans' Health System Audie L. Murphy Division GRECC and the University of Texas Health Science Center, San Antonio, TX, USA)

This Symposium presents results from the Air Force Villages' Freedom House Study (FHS). The FHS is a longitudinal study of both the cross-sectional prevalence of Executive Cognitive Function (ECF) impairment, and the longitudinal rate of change in ECF in a cohort of well elderly residents (N=561, Age M= 78.2 ± 5.0; 59% Female) in a single (1300 bed) Comprehensive Care Retirement Community (CCRC) (the Air Force Villages). This sample is unusual in that is culturally homogeneous, highly educated (M= 15.1 ± 2.4 years), healthy (81% self-rated good-excellent; <10% diabetic or report h/o stroke) and affluent. At baseline, 92% of subjects scored/24 /30 on the MMSE. A subset (N=196) has been given an extensive psychometric evaluation that includes several putative ECF measures [e.g. the WCST, Trail Making Part B. Controlled Oral Word Association (COWA), the EXIT25, and the CLOX]. In addition, subjects receive the MMSE, and the Boston Naming Test (BOSTON), and the Mattis Dementia Rating Scale (DRS). We have obtained ApoE cDNA phenotypes on most of these cases. Three data points are available for most psychometric variables.

Apoe Phenotyping and Cognitive Test Performance in Non-Demented Elderly Persons.

D.R. Royall, A-A. Hayee, S.S. Iqbal, M.J. Polk, L. K. Chiodo, J.P. Chambers. (South Texas Veterans' Health System Audie L. Murphy Division GRECC and the 2University of Texas Health Science Center, San Antonio, TX, USA)

PURPOSE: We investigated apolipoprotein E (ApoE) expression in buccal washings of 183 well elderly retirees. METHODS: Total RNA was isolated, reverse transcribed, PCR amplified, and probed with ApoE allele specific oligonucleotides. RESULTS: Only monoallelic patterns of ApoE expression were observed. 105/183 (57.4%) expressed ApoE e3, 59 (32.2%) expressed ApoE e2 and 19 (10.4%) expressed ApoE e4. The expressed allele had significant effects on the frequency of self-reported hypertension and kidney disease (both $p < .05$). Subjects expressing e4 were more impaired on the Mattis Dementia Rating Scale Memory subscale than those expressing either other allele (both $p < .005$). These differences persist after adjusting for age and gender [ANCOVA: $F(2,117) = 4.2$, $p < .02$]. CONCLUSIONS: This pattern of expression suggests that ApoE may be genomically imprinted.

Executive Impairment: Cross-sectional Prevalence and Relationship to Level of Care.

Donald R. Royall, Laura K. Chiodo, Marsha J. Polk. (South Texas Veterans' Health System Audie L. Murphy Division GRECC and the University of Texas Health Science Center, San Antonio, TX, USA)

PURPOSE: We assessed the effects of impaired Executive Control Function (ECF) on Instrumental Activities of Daily Living (IADL's) and level of care among non-institutionalized elderly retirees with "sub-clinical" cognitive impairment. METHODS: Subjects: N= 561 residents (AGE 78.2 ± 5.0) of a single, 1500 bed, continuing care retirement community (CCRC). Methods: Subjects were examined for cognitive impairment using the Executive Interview (EXIT25), Mini-Mental State Examination (MMSE), and CLOX: An Executive Clock-drawing Test (CLOX). The CLOX is divided into executively sensitive (CLOX1) and simple constructional (CLOX2) sub-tests. RESULTS: Residents in congregate high-rises (N =301) differed significantly from those in independent living apartments (N =260) with respect to AGE, GENDER, % living ALONE, EXIT25, CLOX1, MMSE, and CLOX2 scores [all $p < .03$]. Only differences in ECF measures persist after adjusting for AGE and living ALONE [$p < .004$]. The EXIT25 [$p < .006$] and CLOX2 [$p = .02$] were associated with the use of prostheses. The differences in EXIT25 scores persist after adjusting for LEVEL and living ALONE [$p = .01$]. All instruments distinguish residents with impairment in IADL's. However, only CLOX2 ($p < .001$), EXIT25 ($p < .001$) and AGE ($p < .001$) made significant independent contributions. CONCLUSIONS: ECF has statistically significant effects on level of care and IADL impairment, even among non-institutionalized retirees. This emergent disability is not well detected by traditional global cognitive measures. Evaluation and treatment may be delayed unless ECF measures are employed.

Growth Curve Models of Longitudinal Change in ECF: Relationship to Functional Status.

Raymond Palmer, Donald R. Royall, M.D, Laura K. Chiodo, Marsha J.Polk. (University of Texas Health Science Center, San Antonio, TX and the South Texas Veterans' Health System Audie L. Murphy Division GRECC, San Antonio, TX, USA)

PURPOSE: To examine the longitudinal associations between change in ECF and functional status. METHODS: EXIT25 and MMSE scores were used to model 5 year change in functional status among n =543 FHS subjects using a latent growth curve analysis. RESULTS: At baseline, 93.4% of the subjects had a normal MMSE score. 32.2% exhibited clinically significant ECF impairment on the EXIT25. MMSE scores showed little change over time. In contrast, the rate of change in EXIT25 scores was dependent on age. There was a slow linear loss of ECF between the ages of 70 and 79 years. After age 80, ECF worsened at an accelerated rate (1.45 EXIT25 points /year). Change in the EXIT25 was a strong predictor of functional status. Unadjusted models show that the change in EXIT25 scores is strongly correlated with the change in functional impairment ($r = .69$, $p < 001$). This association remains significant (partial $r = .43$) after adjusting for age, comorbid disease, baseline physical function, and baseline level of care. The EXIT25's effect on the change in functional status is comparable to that of age, and more important than that of comorbid disease, baseline physical function, or level of care. In contrast, change in MMSE scores is not significantly associated with the change in functional impairment, either in the adjusted, or the unadjusted model. CONCLUSIONS: ECF is a strong determinant of longitudinal change in functional status among non-demented elderly persons.

Panel Discussion: Distinguishing Normal Aging from Pre-clinical AD.

D.R. Royall, Raymond Palmer, Laura K. Chiodo. (South Texas Veterans' Health System Audie L. Murphy Division GRECC and the University of Texas Health Science Center at San Antonio, TX, USA)

The FHS has detected an early and clinically significant deterioration in executive control measures among non-demented well elderly persons. This finding could easily have been missed by earlier epidemiological studies, which generally lack ECF measures. The relationship between the ECF impairments we have observed and pre-clinical Alzheimer's disease (AD) is unknown. On the one hand, it seems unlikely that the FHS has escaped AD pathology. On the other hand, early ECF impairment would seem to violate the expected patterns of cognitive decline related to Braak AD staging. Moreover, Apoe expression in the FHS is significantly related only to memory test performance, not ECF measures. The relevance of ECF to preclincal AD assessment and diagnosis will be discussed.

SESSION 31

Correlates of Senior Center Particiaption among the Korean Elderly

Seong H. Yoo (Department of Social Welfare, Sun Moon Univ. Asan City, S. Korea)

This study examines the factors related to senior center participation for the Korean elderly. A sample of 316 Koreans aged 65+ participating a senior center in Cheonan City is analysed. The results of multiple regression analysis show that gender and level of education and health are significant when the other independent variables are controlled. That is, the male Korean elderly who have higher education and better self-assessed health are more likely to participate the senior center. Gender differences are also found. In order to distinguish between the frequent users and less frequent users, a logistic regression model is estimated. There is evidence that the frequent users are persons who are more educated. These findings are not consistent with the previous geronto-logical research conducted in the U.S. in which the more frequent users are generally believed to be older and less educated with lower income. The inconsistency may be explained in part due to the short history(11 years) of senior center in Korea. Based on the findings, social policies for the elderly are discussed.

Holiday Respite for Aged Persons and their Carers: Economic and Operational Challenges

David Brous, (Impact Consulting Group, Melbourne, Victoria,

Australia), Anne Markiewicz (Anne Markiewicz and Associates, Melbourne, Victoria, Australia).

PURPOSE: As regional Australia ages, provision of residential and community care must achieve cost effectiveness despite declining community support and shrinking government allocations. Holiday respite provides positive experiences for aged persons and their carers from urban environments, reinforcing financial and operational bases of regional facilities. Hurdles include effective transfer of aged persons and continuity of care, availability of skilled staffing in respite facilities and affordability of respite by the aged and/or their carers. Maintenance of government funding to originating facilities is required to maintain operational economies. METHOD: Qualitative and quantitative social research of aged residential and community facilities in Melbourne and regional Victoria, attitudinal research of tourism operators, specification of site and physical infrastructure requirements, and financial analysis of developmental and operational costs of selected models were utilised. RESULTS: Criteria were established for appropriate siting of holiday respite services in regional locations, including impacts upon local service providers, disruption to existing regimes, enhancement of ongoing services, provision of additional, specialist staff and establishment and utilisation of accommodation infrastructure. The impact on regional tourism and the attitudes of local tourism operators was also assessed. CONCLUSION: The study shows key factors which support effective implementation of a holiday respite service in a regional environment. It provides a framework for locating aged residential care within a broader economic development context required to support ongoing viability of non-metropolitan communities with aging populations. It is relevant to First World regional communities facing a declining community base to support aging populations.

Implementation and evaluation of a culturally sensitive special needs support program for frail Chinese seniors

Daniel W.L. Lai, (Faculty of Social Work, The University of Calgary, Alberta, Canada), Liza M.Y. Chan (Calgary Chinese Elderly Citizens' Association, Alberta, Canada)

Due to language barriers and cultural differences, frail older adults from the Chinese community are often faced with various challenges in accessing day programs in the mainstream community. To address their unique cultural needs, a special needs support group program is implemented. The overall goal of the program is to help older Chinese who have deteriorating health to remain in the community as long as possible. The participants attend this program once a week. Transportation is arranged to accommodate the needs of some participants. Services offered include: social and recreational activities, culturally sensitive health maintenance and health education programs, outreach and referral services, counselling and consultation, and support services for caregivers. Outcome evaluation findings of both quantitative and qualitative nature are presented in this paper. Despite limitations in funding and program resources, satisfaction rating of the participants and family members is quite high. Achieved client benefits include: prevention of further health deterioration, enhancement of support network for the seniors, reduction of isolation, improvement in interpersonal interactions and self-confidence, establishment of support network and enhancement of knowledge and skills in caregiving among the caregivers. This program bridges the cultural gap in the mainstream service delivery system. While challenges and limitations continue to exist, understanding the context and implementation of this program will help the future development of community-based service models that fit the culturally diverse needs of older adults in Canada.

Multipurpose Centers for the Elderly - Upgrading Day Care Center Programs

David Cahn (Director, Community Services, ESHEL) Hanna Freedman (Representative, Forum of Directors of Day Care Centers for the Elderly)

This paper will describe the past 15 years of development of day care centers for the elderly in Israel, including changes in the concept and in the basket of services provided to meet the changing needs of the elderly population. The early programs were based on social clubs for the elderly, which were adapted physically in order to meet the needs of disabled elderly, and which offered meals, bathing, other personal care services, in addition to social and cultural activities. Based on these early experiences, guidebooks were published detailing the standards for construction and equipment for day care centers, and for their operation. Today, the day care centers are well-established as the center for services for disabled elderly in the community, and there is no longer any fear that the independent elderly will take over the centers, and the day care centers are expanding to serve all the elderly of the community. The larger goal is to develop a basic framework of services for all the elderly in each community, including the independent elderly, the disabled elderly, and the mentally frail elderly and their families. Each of these populations will have access to the center at specific times, or in specific facilities. These multipurpose centers will provide a variety of responses to the changing needs of the elderly population, and can provide counseling, professional and paraprofessional services, employment activities, intergenerational programs, cultural activities and other programs developed specifically for this population, and making the day care center an exclusive and attractive community center for the elderly.

Quality Service in Day Care Centres For Elderly People in Hong Kong: Users' Perspectives

Raymond Ngan, Kam Ping Kwong, Jacky Cheung (RCPM, City University of Hong Kong), Edward Leung (United Christian Hospital)

This is a community-wide programme evaluation study of Day Care Centre Services For Elderly People in Hong Kong conducted in 1999-2000 with 457 elderly service users. Although they reported high levels of quality of care in general, they also had modest perception of the quality of management in the day care center, and a low tendency for the center to consult their needs. The use of nonprofessional workers in the center tended to have significant negative effect on elderly users' perception of quality management. Data from focus group interviews showed that elderly users also preferred to have more physical rehabilitation exercises and equipment and properly trained physiotherapists in the Centre. There was, however, a mismatch among elderly users and their caregivers in regard to the duration of stay in the week and in the long run. Implications of these findings for developing excellence in quality service for day care centers will be discussed

The relationship between the old-A comparative study of the old in a neighbourhood and institutional setup

L.TharaBhai& Head Dept of Sociology Madurai Kamaraj University Madurai, INDIA

The institutional care of the old is slowly picking up in India though it is in a different perspective when compared to the other countries. The day care centers which is a new concept among the old is picking up very fast in India which not only give room for the aged to spent both within the institution and the family but also takes care of the emotional sharing between the institution and the family giving the old a mental Satisfaction. The present study compares the old people who are living in the institutions- day care centers and full time institutions. The study which analyzes 150 cases show that the most popular in the Indian context are the daycare centers because it is not giving up either the family or the culture in which they lived.

SESSION 32

Clinical, Ethical, and Legal Dilemmas in Assessing Competency: Assessor as Advocate or Adversary

M. Bay (Chair & CEO, Ontario Consent and Capacity Board, Toronto, Canada), H.M.R. Meier, MB, ChB, FRCP(C) (Head, Geriatric Psychiatry Program, Mount Sinai Hospital, Toronto, Canada), S. Marr, FRCP(C), Regional Geriatric Program, Eastern Service Area, Toronto, Canada)

Interactive discussion with panel and workshop participants followed by didactic presentation with handouts of presentation and bibliography. Presentation will focus on two areas, first a review of legal context in Ontario for assessing capacity and second it will discuss potential conflictual issues for clinicians in context of the law. Participants will gain an appreciation of the multiple factors involved in assessing competencies and acquire the skills to perform comprehensive assessments of competency.

SESSION 33

Institutional long-term care: predicting the cost consequences

Bleddyn Davies (Personal Social Services Research Unit, University of Kent, UK) Ann Netten (Personal Social Services Research Unit, University of Kent, UK), Key influences on costs and prices of institutional care. Robin Darton (Personal Social Services Research Unit, University of Kent, UK), Predicting admission to nursing home rather than residential home care Andrew Bebbington (Personal Social Services Research Unit, University of Kent, UK) Predicting the course of care for entrants to care homes.

The issue of the rising costs of institutional care of older people is a matter of international concern. While those cared for in institutions form a minority of the older people cared for, they consume the lion's share of resources. This makes this an area of particular concern for public funding bodies, insurers and those who are funding their own care. Ideally what those concerned with the funding of care need is a way into predicting the likely cost consequences of admission. The symposium brings together the results of four large-scale national studies conducted in England and Wales: · a study of 420 new users of community care tracked over five years · a survey of 2,500 publicly-funded admissions to care homes · a 42-month longitudinal follow-up of these residents; and · a cross-sectional survey of 600 homes. In order to be able to predict the cost implications we need information about the situation prior to admission, factors that affect costs on admission, factors that affect the type of home in which people are placed and factors that affect length of stay. The symposium deals with each of these in turn. Bleddyn Davies draws on the study of community care to investigate the effects of variations in services and other influences on length of time people are supported in their own homes and probabilities of admission to homes for long-term care and use of inpatient beds. Ann Netten uses the survey of admissions and cross-sectional survey of homes to identify the key factors that affect the price or unit costs of care in care homes. A key issue is clearly levels of dependency, but although dependency is associated with costs of care the main effect occurs at the point of initial placement. Under current regulatory arrangements in the UK nursing homes are much more costly and people rarely move between types of home. Robin Darton draws on the survey of admissions to identify the key factors that affect whether people are placed in residential or nursing home care. Andrew Bebbington then discusses factors that are associated with length of stay and functioning outcomes, and the hence the cost consequences of admission. Between them the studies provide a wide-ranging examination of the key factors affecting the costs of institutional care. Community service provision can reduce the need for admission to both care homes and hospital. The costs of care homes on admission are dominated by the current regulatory requirements for residential and nursing homes, a discontinuity that is set to change. Factors associated with residential care admission suggest there is further scope for diversion from this form of institutional care. The results of the prediction models emphasise the need for greater integration between residential and nursing care. Great inequality still seems to exist in access to publicly-funded care of this type.

Home and community service effects on community stays, home admission, and hospital inpatient costs

Bleddyn Davies (Personal Social Services Research Unit at London School of Economics and the University of Kent, England) Jose Fernandez (Personal Social Services Research Unit at London School of Economics, England)

PURPOSE. Reforms aimed to use home and community care services [H&Cs] to reduce inappropriate use of residential and nursing home care in a strained budgetary environment. Inpatient bed demand grew as supply fell with politically sensitive results. The paper estimates the effects of variations in H&C inputs and other influences on [a] length of community stays supported by H&CS [b] probabilities of admission to homes for long-term care and [c] utilisation of inpatient beds. METHODS. The analysis uses econometric production function and Cox hazard modelling techniques. The data are from the12-area tailor-made ECCEP study built around a cohort of 419 new community users, their caregivers and care managers followed over five years supplemented with other collections. RESULTS. Services offset 32 per cent of the negative effects of risk factors on lengths of stay in the community. Risk factors likewise influence probabilities and timing of admission to institutions. Were services for all users to be as efficiently mixed as for the best, community stays would be longer irrespective of disability and informal support, as long as prices were unaffected by variations in service volumes. Other important outcomes would be improved also. H&CS reduce hospital in-patient costs by one fifth of the costs of the community services; ie more than one half of inpatient bed costs. Risk factors greatly affect cost reductions, the reductions being greatest for the most dependent. CONCLUSIONS. Post-reform H&CS greatly extend community stays, despite big variations in efficiency. H&CS substantially reduce inpatient bed utilisation.

Key influences on costs and prices of institutional care

Ann Netten (Personal Social Services Research Unit, University of Kent) and Julien Forder (Personal Social Services Research Unit, London School of Economics, UK)

As policies seek to keep people in private households, we would expect the population of care homes to become increasingly dependent, with a consequent increase in the costs of care. The objective of the analysis was to investigate the impact of dependency on and other factors on the costs and prices of care homes in England. Regression analyses were conducted on data sets from two surveys. A survey of 2,500 publicly funded admissions conducted in the autumn 1995 and a cross-sectional survey of homes conducted in the autumn of 1996. Over 600 homes in 21 local authorities participated and information was collected about 11,900 residents. The sample of homes was designed to ensure a large enough number of homes for separate analyses for each of the major types of home: local authority, private and voluntary residential homes and nursing homes. While dependency characteristics were found to be significantly associated with the price at the point of placement and costs and prices in homes, the effect within home type was relatively flat. This was due to the fact that under the current regulatory arrangements the major cost effect of dependency is found in the higher prices charged by nursing homes. In practice the costs of care were dominated by labour market variations, with some effect from commissioning arrangements. Once other characteristics were allowed for self-funded residents were charged higher prices.

Predicting Admission to Nursing Home rather than to Residential Home Care

R. A. Darton (Personal Social Services Research Unit, University of Kent at Canterbury, Canterbury, Kent, CT2 7NF, U.K.)

Purpose: Local authorities in Great Britain vary considerably in the proportions of residents placed in nursing or residential care. This may be due to variations in demand (the type of resident approaching authorities), supply (the level and type of provision available), or policy (in terms of eligibility criteria or interpretations of need at field level). The paper will examine the pattern of admissions, the characteristics of people admitted and the relationship between these characteristics and admissions to residential or nursing home care. Method: A national longitudinal survey of 2,544 people aged 65 or over, admitted to publicly-funded residential and nursing home care, was conducted in a stratified sample of 18 local authorities between 1995 and 1999. Results: Using logistic regression analysis, characteristics of the individual explained the placement of over 80 per cent of admissions. Supply factors were statistically significant but did not improve the explanatory power. Survival among those admitted to a type of care that was not predicted by the model suggested that some unmeasured aspects of prognosis might account for some of the residual variation in placements. Conclusions: Local authorities were reasonably consistent in nursing home placement decisions, suggesting that some are more successful in maintaining people for longer at home than others. In addition to maintaining people at home to a higher level of dependency, prevention of admission to residential care is likely to be associated with interventions that address carer support, safety issues among people who are deaf, and motivation.

Predicting the course of care for entrants to care homes

Andrew Bebbington (Personal Social Services Research Unit, University of Kent, Canterbury, Kent, CT2 7NF, UK

Purpose: The primary purpose is to develop a means for predict typical length of stay, survival and functioning outcomes, and the hence the costs, for older people admitted as a publicly funded residents of care homes in the UK. Second, to use these predictors to examine variations between different locations in the service that is provided. Method. The investigation is based on a national survey of 2,500 new admissions who have been followed up 5 times over 3 years. This is based in 18 localities in the UK. Survivors are tracked to death, even if they leave the original care home. The analysis uses standard survival and healthy life expectancy methods to develop prediction models. Results. The study identifies eight key factors on admission that will determine outcomes and costs. These are: malignancy; ADL dependency; nursing needs assessment; source of admission; respiratory illness; age; gender; cognitive functioning. Survival is remarkably variable. Functioning outcomes depend on state at admission. A few people improve initially, but thereafter recovery is rare. Lifetime costs average £35,000, higher for those admitted to residential homes than nursing homes. There are remarkable variations between localities in outcomes, related more to differences in the type of person being admitted (eligibility criteria) than to the effects of care itself. Conclusion. The prediction model is a useful tool for planners. The results lay to rest myths about recent changes in survival and outcomes. They emphasise the need for greater integration between residential and nursing care. Great inequality still seems to exist in access to publicly funded care of this type.

SESSION 34

Playmaking: Theatre games to spark awareness, communication, and vitality in later life

Kathleen Weiss (Western Gold Theatre, and The University of British Columbia; Vancouver, British Columbia, Canada), and Members of "Acting Class for Seniors" (Roundhouse Community Centre, Vancouver, British Columbia, Canada)

Based on many years of experience of facilitating acting classes with seniors, this experiential workshop will demonstrate the use of theatre games to engage and stimulate the imagination and communication skills of older adults. During the workshop, participants can watch or join in a wide variety of character-based improvisations. Participants can "try on" various types of characters and explore different personas. We will work with the dramatization of dreams - both the ones which occur while sleeping and the ones through which we shape our hopes for the future. The work is fun and empowering because it uses the participants' own language and images. It has also been found to significantly increase self-esteem, self-awareness, and the ability to problem solve with others through role-playing.

SESSION 35

The role of connective tissues in the ageing process

L. Hayflick (University of California, San Francisco, CA, USA) (Ageing as distinguished from pathology.) A. Viidik (University of Aarhus, Aarhus, Denmark) (Implication of connective tissue ageing for the ageing of the organism.) A .J. Bailey (University of Bristol, Bristol, UK) (Mechanisms of age-related glycation of collagen and elastin.) M. Skalicky (University of Veterinary Medicine, Vienna, Austria) (Physical exercise and food restriction modify the collagen biomarker of ageing and mortality in rats.) H. Orimo (Tokyo Metropolitan Geriatric Centre, Tokyo, Japan) (Discussant: Clinical application of bone metabolic markers.)

Early gerontological research, when mono-cause theories of ageing were abundant, quite frequently focused on connective tissues as a cause for ageing, especially since Verzar showed that with ageing came increased stability of collagen, the main component of connective tissues and most ubiquitous protein in the body. After a period of time, when the changes in collagen were relegated to the status of epiphenomena, the importance of this protein has become increasingly obvious. The starting point of this symposium is the discussion by Hayflick, which emphasises the important distinction between normal ageing and pathological changes that increase in numbers and severity with ageing. Then Viidik introduces the spectrum of connective tissue changes with normal ageing and Bailey demonstrates the complexity of changes occurring on the molecular level in collagen and elastin. The possibility to modulate these changes by physical exercise and moderate food restriction is shown by Skalicky in an animal model. Finally, Orimo discusses the application of products of collagen metabolism as markers in clinical assessment of bone metabolism. This session does not claim that connective tissue changes are a driving force for the biological ageing processes but demonstrates the importance of these changes, and potential possibility to ameliorate them, for a number of phenomena of importance for the well-being of the ageing organism.

Aging as distinguished from pathology

L. Hayflick (University of California, San Francisco, CA, USA)

The stochastically driven systemic loss of molecular fidelity that occurs after reproductive success results in loss of physiological function, - the hallmark of aging. The long half-lives observed for maintenance of elastin and collagen molecular integrity are excellent examples of many aging phenomena that increase vulnerability to disease. The failure to distinguish age changes from disease or pathology has not only blurred our efforts to understand the fundamental biology of aging but it has profound political and economic consequences that compromise the field of biogerontology. Changes attributable to disease or pathology, can be distinguished from age changes for at least four reasons. Unlike any disease, age changes (1) occur in every animal that reaches a fixed size in adulthood given sufficient time, (2) cross all species barriers, (3) affect all members of a species only after the age of reproductive success, (4) occur in all feral animals subsequently protected by humans even when that species probably has not experienced aging for thousands or millions of years. The resolution of age associated diseases will not advance our knowledge of aging just as the resolution of the infectious diseases of childhood did not advance our knowledge of childhood development. —

Implication of connective tissue ageing for the ageing of the organism

A. Viidik (University of Aarhus, Aarhus, Denmark)

Connective tissues form the "skeletons" of all organs in the body, except the brain. Collagen is its main component and amounts to about one third of all proteins in the body. The stability of it increases with time, although there are differences between species with respect to biochemical characteristics and the speed, with which this takes place. Arteries become stiffer and less elastic, when collagen fibres stiffen and elastic fibres fragment. The fragmentation of elastic fibres in arteries and skin takes place in a parallel fashion. The connective tissue in the lungs becomes stiffer, which reduces the vital capacity and increases the residual volume. Tendons and ligaments stiffen too, although the important age-related changes in these structures are pathological lesions. Also the connective tissue in the periarticular structures stiffen with consequences for the joints. The population doubling capacity of fibroblasts decreases somewhat, but there is a reasonable reserve capacity also in the oldest old. The important phenomenon with ageing is a decreased repair capacity. While wound healing capacity in healthy individuals is not reduced to a major degree, it is drastically reduced compared to young healthy adults when the blood supply is compromised. It can be concluded that the changes in connective tissues with ageing are most often not life threatening but can add to the threat in conjunction with age-related diseases. These changes, however, also contribute to diminished well-being by reducing the functional capacity of several organs, including the lungs and the locomotive system.

Mechanisms of Age-related Glycation of Collagen and Elastin

R G Paul, D A Slatter and A J Bailey (Collagen Research Group, University of Bristol, UK)

The long biological half lives of collagen and elastin are in terms of months and years, thereby allowing the accumulation of age-related modifications. These age-related changes are deleterious and are manifest in the stiffening of the joints, the vascular system and the renal and retinal capillaries. It has long been believed that the mechanism involves intermolecular cross-linking of the proteins within the tissues but the mechanisms are only now being unravelled. It appears that cross-linking involves two different mechanisms, one a precisely controlled enzymic cross-linking during development and maturation and the other an adventitious non-enzymic mechanism following maturation of the tissue. We believe that it is this additional non-enzymic cross-linking known as glycation, involving an initial reaction with glucose, that is the major cause of dysfunction of collagenous and elastic tissues in old age. Further, the glycated collagen can stimulate breakdown of lipids releasing malondialdehyde which can then cross-link the already glycated vascular collagen. An additional indirect effect of glycation is the modification of specific amino acid side-chains, resulting in altered cell-matrix interactions. This latter aspect of glycation may be shown to be an equally important effect of ageing of collagen, particularly in basement membranes where the expression of cells may lead to an inappropriate matrix. An understanding of these glycation mechanisms is leading to the development of inhibitors of the initial glycation and compounds capable of cleaving the cross-links, thus alleviating these devastating effects of ageing.

Physical exercise and food restriction modify the collagen biomarker of ageing and mortality in rats

M. Skalicky (University of Veterinary Medicine, Vienna, Austria)

Five groups of male Sprague-Dawley rats (n =32 in each group) were kept in five groups from five to 23 months of age: (1) Free access to running wheels and food, (2) fed to pair weight with the running wheel group, (3) trained in treadmill, (4) and (5) sedentary with free access to food. The animals in groups 1-4 were housed individually while those in group 5 were housed with four animals in each cage. All animals in the running wheel group survived except two, who died in conjunction with anaesthesia. The fed to pair weight and single in case animals had the same mortality pattern, while those housed four in each cage had the highest mortality and the treadmill trained ones somewhat less. The thermal stability of collagen (which increases with age as a biomarker for ageing) was lowest in the running wheel and fed to pair weight groups. The animals that ran most had a higher value than the lazier ones. The sedentary animals housed four in each cage had the highest values. The treadmill trained animals and the individually housed sedentary animals showed an intermediate value. The differences in thermal stability of collagen were not related to levels of blood glucose and fructosamine, suggesting that the increase of thermal stability was not directly related to glycation of collagen. These results suggest that both moderate food restriction and voluntary exercise have beneficial effects. It can further be concluded that the collagen biomarker of ageing monitors these effects.

SESSION 36

219 Polymorphism of Apoe Promoter and Evolutive Course of Dementia

Fariñas F, P.Gil Gregorio, P. Lopez-Riquelme, A. Garnica (Geriatrics Service; Hospital Clínico San Carlos. Madrid. Spain.)

AIMS: To verify the association between APOE-219 polymorphisms and age-at-onset of clinical symptoms and evolutive course of Alzheimer disease (AD). METHODS: 145 patients were studied, and divided in two groups. 1) Control group (n: 73; mean age: 87.8 +/- 10.1): without clinical symptoms of cognitive impairment. 2) Study group (n. 72; mean age 83.9 +/-10.7): every patients fulfilled the criteria of dementia according to DSM-IV and NINCDS-ADRDA with an age-at-onset >or = 65 and without familiar aggregation. Cognitive Assessment MMSE and CAMCOG-CAMDEX, were used. Develop stage was assigned by Functional Assessment stages (FAST). We stabilised functional and cognitive impairment progression and CAMCOG decrease/timing of disease progression. We analyse polymorphism 219 by DGGE, previous PCR amplification. Statistical measurement includes chi-square and regression logistic analysis. RESULTS: -219 G/G variant of APOE is associated to very late onset (age >75 in 88,20f the cases, p<0.001) and show progress of AD. CONCLUSIONS: According to these results polymorphism 219 could be a genetic risk factor for very late onset and sporadic AD. The presence of this variant conditions a less aggressive clinical phenotype in the carriers.

Cognitive performance and apolipoprotein E genotypes among the very elderly living in the community

Emilio Moriguchi, Ivana Da Cruz, Flávio Xavier, Carla Schwanke, Yukio Moriguchi (Institute of Geriatrics and Gerontology of PUCRS University, Porto Alegre, RS, Brazil)

PURPOSE: Veranopolis County, Italian immigration area, located in the mountain region of southern Brazil, presents the highest longevity in Brazil (mean of 78 years old) with low incidence of cardiovascular diseases and cognitive impairment. To investigate the factors related to this longevity and the low incidence of cognitive impairment in this community, we designed a population survey to characterize the healthy people above 80 years living in this community. METHOD: 70 healthy people above 80 years old were recruited for cognitive function evaluation and apolipoprotein E genotyping (using the restriction isotyping method). Statistical analysis were done using the chi-square test. RESULTS: The mean age of the study sample was 84.4±3.3 years with 66 female and 34 male subjects. The allele frequency of apolipoprotein E in this population sample was: e2 = 0.02, e3 = 0.71, e4 = 0.26. The analysis of cognitive performance tests, in categories, in relation to apolipoprotein E alleles, showed that, even without characterizing dementia, those having e4 allele presented lower scores during cognitive tests compared to those without allele e4 ($p<0.05$). The results suggest that the presence of allele e4 may be related to decline in the cognitive performance even without the diagnosis of dementia.

Risk factors of cognitive development and genotypes in a non-demented elderly population

P. Lopez-Riquelme, P. Gil Gregorio, C. Garcia, A. Garnica, A. Sanchez-Guevara, C. Mesa and J.M Ribera Casado (Servicio de Geriatria, Hospital Cinico San Carlos,Madrid, Spain)

PURPOSE: To establish if APOE genotype is correlated with the characteristics and alterations in cognitive assessment in a non-demented elderly sample. METHODS: A prospective study door to door was done in an elderly community-dwelling population. Subjects with dementia or any organic disease which affects cognitive performance were excluded.The cognitive assessment was done by using the Folstein MMSE, CAMDEX (CAMCOG) and Ribermead test. APOE gen was analysed in a blood sample by DGGE, previous PCR amplification. Statistical analysis was done with T-student-mean comparison test for independent samples (Confidence interval 95%). RESULTS: 427 subjects (mean age 72.1±5.1 women 65.4%). Allele distribution: 2/3 (10.3%) 2/4 (1.7%) 3/4 (8.6%) 4/4 (1.7%). Presence of APOE allele: 12%. Allele Without allele p MMSE 25.8±1.5 26.8±2.1 >n.s CAMCOG 63.6±6.4 77.9±8.5 0.001 Ribermead 4.2±2.6 6.8±2 0.005 CONCLUSION: 1.- Most of non-demented elderly population have an APOE 3/3 allele distribution. 2.- Subjects with allele computed lower scores in CAMCOG and Ribermead test with significant difference than subjects without this allele, although no strong relationship was found with MMSE.

The correlation between cognitive function impairment and allele genotype of APOE among 354 apparently healthy elderly in Shanghai China.

Ma Yong-Xing, Lu Pei-Fang, Zhu Yue, Wang Chuan-Fu (Department of Aging, Antiaging and Cognitive Function, Shanghai Institute of Gerontology and Geriatrics, Huadong Hospital, Shanghai, China)

The allele genotype of APOE and cognitive function (WMS, MMSE, HDS-R) of 354 apparently healthy elderly (aged 65-85 yrs) in Shanghai were determined in order to evaluate if there were correlation between genotype of APOE and cognitive function impairment. The results (score) were as following: (1) APOE 3/3 (254 persons): MQ 94.0±16.9, MMSE 28.3±2.2, HDS-R 27.1±3.6 (2) APOE 2/3 (41 persons): MQ 91.1±19.0, MMSE 27.5±2.8, HDS-R 26.1±3.4 (3) APOE3/4 (52 persons): MQ 92.4±18.7, MMSE 27.8±3.5, HDS-R 27.1±3.9 (4) APOE2/4 (2 persons): MQ 98.5±2.1, MMSE 27.0, HDS-R 23.5±6.4 (5) APOE2/2 (2 persons): MQ 92.5±0.7; MMSE 29.0±1.4, HDS-R 26.5±0.7 (6) APOE4/4 (3 persons): MQ 92.0±16.1. No significant difference of the score of MQ, MMSE, HDS-R (F value equaling 285, 0.934 and 1.117 respectively) in various APOE genotypes were found. It is suggested that the effect of APOE as a risk factor on AD may not necessarily mediate the equal effect on cognitive function impairment in the apparently healthy elderly.

The correlation between the cardiovascular function and allele genotype of APOE among 584 elderly in Shanghai, China

Lu Pei-Fang, Ma Yong-Xing, Zhu Yue (Department of Aging, Antiaging and Cognitive Function, Shanghai Institute of Gerontology and Geriatrics, Huadong Hospital, Shanghai, China)

The allele genotype of APOE and cardiac index (CI), stroke index (SI), periphery vascular resistance (PVR) and arterial compliance (AC) of 584 elderly (65-85 years old) in Shanghai were determined in order to evaluate if there was any correlation between genotypes of APOE and cardiovascular function. The mean value of CI (L/min/M2), SI (ml/M2), PVR (dynes/S/cm-5) and AC(ml/mmHg) in various allele genotypes of APOE were as follows: (1) APOE 3/3 (416 persons): CI 1.94±0.61; PVR 2515±855 (2) APOE 2/3 (58 persons): CI 1.91±0.61, PVR 2686±1174; (3) APOE 3/4 (62 persons): CI 1.84±0.74, PVR 2740±1047; (4) APOE 2/4 (8 persons): CI 1.75±0.49, PVR 2777±1141; (5) APOE 2/2 (1 persons): CI 0.63±0, PVR; (6) APOE 4/4 (4 persons): CI 1.81±0.60, PVR 2062±160. No significant difference of the cardiac output and vascular resistance in various APOE allele phenotypes were found. It is suggested that the effect of APOE 4 as a risk factor of cardiac vascular disease may not necessarily influence the cardiovascular function of apparently healthy aged significantly, and APOE4 as a genetic factor itself is not sufficient to induce atherosclerosis.

SESSION 37

Guidelines

M. Borrie (Division of Geriatric Medicine, University of Western Ontario, South western Ontario Regional Geriatric Program, Lawson Health Research Institute, London, Ontario, Canada) L. Valiquette (Department of Urology, Centre Hospital de L'Universite de Montreal-Pavillon St. - Luc, Montreal, Quebec, Canada) D. Griffiths (Division of Geriatric Medicine, University of PIttsburgh, Pittsburgh, PA, USA) A. Saltmarche (Clinical Associate, Cross-Appointed, Graduate School, Faculty of Nursing, University of Toronto) S. Lytwynec (Geriatric Day Hospital and South western Ontario Regional Geriatric Program, London, Ontario, Canada)

Purpose To present the updated Guidelines for the Management of Urinary Incontinence in adults that are relevant to the frail elderly. Method A core committee was convened by the Canadian Continence Foundation that included clients/consumers and leading multidisciplinary healthcare professionals from Urology, Urogynecology, Geriatrics, Family practice, Nursing and Physiotherapy, a Federal government representative and an independent evaluator. The core committee decided on the 3 broad classes of clients/consumers for whom the guidelines were needed, namely men, women, and the frail elderly. The Agency for Health Care Policy and Research (AHCPR) Guidelines 1996 were accepted as a starting point for developing Canadian guidelines. These were based on a literature review up to 1995. The committee reviewed these guidelines and modified them according to a new, extensive literature search 1995-Jan 2000 that either supported them or provided new evidence for new recommendations. To develop recommendations for each assessment and treatment method, the core committee considered the quality and amount of evidence, and the consistency of findings. Canadian criteria for levels of evidence 1, 2, and 3 were very similar to the strengths of evidence A, B, C used in the AHCPR guidelines. The draft guidelines along with flow diagrams and models of care were discussed, modified, and accepted at the Canadian Consensus Conference on Urinary Incontinence, May 2000. The guidelines are now being presented to reactor panels around the country. The guidelines will be distributed at the roundtable and issues of dissemination, education, and implementation discussed.

Flow charts for management of incontinence in the frail elderly

D. Griffiths (Division of Geriatric Medicine, University of PIttsburgh, Pittsburgh, PA, USA) A. Saltmarche (Clinical Associate, Cross-Appointed, Graduate School, Faculty of Nursing, University of Toronto) M. Borrie (Division of Geriatric Medicine, University of Western Ontario, South western Ontario Regional Geriatric Program, Lawson Health Research Institute, London, Ontario, Canada) L. Valiquette (Department of Urology, Centre Hospital de L'Universite de Montreal-Pavillon St. - Luc, Montreal, Quebec, Canada) K. Moore (Faculty of Nursing, University of Alberta, Edmonton, Alberta, Canada) S. Lytwynec (Geriatric Day Hospital and South western Ontario Regional Geriatric Program, London, Ontario, Canada)

Purpose To present flow charts for management of incontinence in the frail elderly that reflect the guidelines developed at the Canadian Continence Foundation sponsored Consensus conference on urinary incontinence May 2000. Method Existing algorithms and flow charts for the management of urinary incontinence were reviewed by the core committee. The series from the 1st International Consultation on Incontinence (Monaco 1998) were based on an extensive literature review. These were modified to reflect the management of incontinence in men, women, and the frail elderly. Results The flow charts show the recommended steps in the assessment and management of urinary incontinence, and the order in which they should be considered. The flow charts appear similar but emphasize the differences between the management of men, women, and the frail elderly. An essential part of initial management is a focused history, to establish presumed etiology and to identify complex cases or serious conditions. First line management includes conservative methods using lifestyle modifications and behavioural interventions. Determining the patient's or client's expectations, is important to determine whether they want treatment, and what realistic outcomes would reflect a meaningful improvement in their quality of live. Specialized management is usually offered by a continence specialist from one of a number of disciplines. It may include more invasive urologic and urodynamic investigations. Management options include further trials of medication, devices, bulking agents such as periurethral collagen, or surgery. Conclusion The flow charts allow the health professional and client to make their own decisions in a logical way that is evidenced based.

Working Models of Continence Care in Three Settings

S. Lytwynec (Geriatric Day Hospital and South western Ontario Regional Geriatric Program, London, Ontario, Canada) K. Moore (Faculty of Nursing, University of Alberta, Edmonton, Alberta, Canada) D. Griffiths (Division of Geriatric Medicine, University of PIttsburgh, Pittsburgh, PA, USA) M. Borrie (Division of Geriatric Medicine, University of Western Ontario, South western Ontario Regional Geriatric Program, Lawson Health Research Institute, London, Ontario, Canada) A. Saltmarche (Clinical Associate, Cross-Appointed, Graduate School, Faculty of Nursing, University of Toronto)

Purpose To summarize and discuss the Canadian Consensus Working Models of continence care in 3 settings; rural/remote, small cities and urban/academic. Method The models were developed from an environmental scan of continence care and services in Canada and worldwide (Milne & Moore, 2000). A core committee convened by The Canadian Continence Foundation, included representatives from urology, urogynecology, family practice, nursing, physiotherapy, and the federal government. The core committee determined that 3 settings in the model were applicable in Canada, namely: rural/remote, small cities, and urban/academic. Important issues included definition of continence care, rationalization of health care, and the concepts of working models that could implement the updated Canadian guidelines and flow diagrams. Results The models presented at the consensus conference were reviewed by the participants, discussed in small groups, and further revised. Consensus was established by voting: over 80% representing consensus, 60-79% representing partial consensus. The proposal for working models is being sent to community reactor panels across Canada for review prior to finalization and eventual pilot testing. Conclusion Working models in three settings; rural/remote, small cities, and urban/academic provide a framework for newly developed guidelines for continence care in Canada. The working models will be illustrated using case examples and flow charts to stimulate discussion on issues of education implementation and effective ways to change practice.

SESSION 38

Caregiving and Its Psychobiology

Peter Vitaliano, (University of Washington, Seattle, WA, USA)

Caregiving and Physical Health: A Meta-Analysis of Caregivers of Persons with Dementia and Non-Caregiver Controls. David Loewenstein, (The University of Miami School of Medicine, Miami, FL, USA) Coping Style and the Prediction of Depressive Symptoms Among Cuban American and White Non-Hispanic Caregivers Mahendra Kumar, (The University of Miami School of Medicine, Miami, FL, USA) Caregiving Outcomes and Neuroendocrines. Carl Eisdorfer, M.D. (The Univeristy of Miami School of Medicine, Miami, FL, USA) General Discussant

In recent years, a significant increase in the number of elderly with dementia has been observed, thus increasing the burden on the family, particularly spouses, for caregiving. Caregiving has been found to be one of the most potent chronic stressor that can impact the mental health and endocrine systems. Moreover, chronic stress has also been related to changes cognition. These changes can bring about significant psychopathology particularly in senescence. This symposium will address mental health, neuropsychological and endocrinological functions as they are affected by chronic stress of caregiving and will propose hypotheses for future testing in order to unravel the mechanisms involved.

Caregiving and Physical Health: A Meta-Analysis of Caregivers of Persons with Dementia and Non-Caregiver Controls.

Peter P. Vitaliano, James M. Scanlan, Jianping Zhang, and Margaret V. Savage [Department of Psychiatry, University of Washington, Seattle, WA, USA]

Purpose: To provide a quantitative review of relationships of caregiving with physical health problems. Method: This presentation is based upon a meta-analysis of the papers generated from computer searches of the terms 'caregivers, dementia, health, physical health, physiology'. Results: Only 41 papers included a control group. These papers arose from 20 independent samples (N=1507 caregivers, N=1394 controls) that examined 87 (22 self-report, 65 physiological) measures grouped into 11 health (5 self-report, 6 physiological) categories. Because some research groups used the same sample to generate multiple comparisons within each category, bias was reduced by averaging effect sizes for each sample within categories. The weighted mean effect sizes (ES) (point-biserial rs) varied according to the category, namely: global self-reports (ES =.15), number of illnesses (ES = .08), number of symptoms (ES = .08), medications (ES = .09), health care utilization, (ES = .04), stress hormones (ES = .16), antibodies (ES = 16), enumerative immunity (ES = .06), functional immunity (ES = .02), cardiovascular problems (ES = -.01), and metabolic measures (ES = -.05). Conclusion: Mean effect sizes also varied according to moderators (eg, gender). We discuss these relationships in terms of the specificity of caregiver health responses to chronic stress.

Caregiving Outcomes and Neuroendocrines.

Mahendra Kumar, Adarsh M. Kumar, Drenna Waldrop, Carl Eisdorfer. [University of Miami School of Medicine, Miami, FL, USA]

Purpose: To investigate the role of the HPA axis in the development of mental health outcomes in caregivers of the elderly. Method: This presentation is based upon the design that caregiving is a model of chronic distress and would thus be related to HPA axis activity. Various published studies have been used as typical examples for this purpose and will be presented. Results: The most important mental health outcomes associated with caregiving of the elderly include depression, anxiety and psychological distress. These outcomes are related to abnormalities of the HPA axis. Conclusions: The endocrine functions in general, and HPA axis activity in particular, appear to be important mediators of mental health outcomes of caregivers.

Coping Style and the Prediction of Depressive Symptoms Among Cuban American and White Non-Hispanic Caregivers

David Loewenstein, Soledad Argüelles, Mark Rubert, Sara Czaja, Carl Eisdorfer [University of Miami School of Medicine, Miami, FL USA]

Purpose: To examine the relationship between reported depression among White non-Hispanic and Cuban American caregivers of persons with Alzheimer's Dementia and specific types of coping styles. Method: Specific types of coping styles and reported depression of 105 White Non-Hispanic and 102 Cuban American providing caregiving to spouses and parents with Alzheimer's Disease were analyzed using regression analyses. Results: For White non-Hispanic husband, wife and daughter caregivers, a coping style characterized by cognitive reframing with positive appraisal of coping resources was related to lower levels of reported depressive symptoms on the CES-D scale. Coping styles using spiritual/religious ideology and resources was also predictive of lower levels of depressive symptoms among White non-Hispanic wives. In contrast, for Cuban-American husband and daughter caregivers, lower levels of reported depression was associated with active coping strategies involving the acquisition of family-based social support and other predictors that were typically different than their White non-Hispanic counterparts. None of the patient or caregiver variables in the model were significant predictors of depression among Cuban-American wives. Conclusion: These results have important implications for determining specific types of caregivers who may be at risk for depressive symptomotology and the development of specific targeted interventions.

SESSION 39

Repartnering After Late Life Widowhood: The Gendered Perspective

K. Borell (Department of Social Work, Mid Sweden University. Ostersund. Sweden), S. Ghazanfareeon Karlsson (Department of Social Work, Mid Sweden University. Ostersund. Sweden) Living Apart Together. Balancing Intimacy and Autonomy in Old Age. J. Gierveld (Netherlands Institute for Advanced Study in the Humanities and Social Sciences (NIAS), Wassenaar; Netherlands Interdisciplinary Demographic Institute (NIDI), The Hague, Netherlands) Older women in search of egalitarian types of new partner relationships. K.Mehta (Department of Social Work and Psychology, National University of Singapore) Perceptions of Remarriage by Widowed Persons in Singapore. S. Feldman (Alma Unit for Research on Ageing, Faculty of Human Development, Victoria University, Australia) The Health and Social Transitions for Recently Widowed Older Australian Women: A Longitudinal Study. D. K. van den Hoonaard (Gerontology Programme, St. Thomas University, Fredericton, Canada) "Nobody could walk in his shoes": Older Canadian widows' attitudes toward relationships with men. Nan Stevens (Department of Psychogerontology, University of Nijmegen, Nijmegen, the Netherlands) New partners following widowhood : does gender matter?

There is a received wisdom that "women grieve, men replace" and indeed, demographic data reveal that at all ages, men are more likely than women to marry again after widowhood, and the differential increases with age. However, there is a paucity of data on late life intimate relationships of men and women following widowhood or divorce that do not lead to marriage or cohabitation. This symposium session addresses this under-investigated field in the study of ageing. Choices and constraints which influence decisions about new romantic relationships after the loss of a spouse will be explored and how these might intersect with age, gender and culture. The participants in this symposium offer a cross-cultural perspective on new partnership formation. There are six international contributions: from Northern Europe, Asia, Australia and North America. Data from primary and secondary sources will be presented and intervening factors such as health, social circumstances, life changes and transitions, same-sex friendships. The first paper examines a newly identified relationship known as Living Apart Together (LAT) and looks at choices made by older women in Sweden who do not wish to marry or live with their dating partners. The second reports on data from the Dutch NESTOR-Living arrangements and social networks of older adults survey. Longitudinal data give information about life course history and changing marital status and the paper discusses the preferences and motives to start a new intimate relationship. The third paper explores cultural differences in perceptions of remarriage for widow men and women within the Chinese, Malay and Indian populations of Singapore. The influence of family and societal values vary with religious and ethnic backgrounds and are fundamental in perceptions on the appropriateness of getting married again. Next is a paper from an Australian longitudinal study which takes older (70-75) women's health as its remit. One element is the investigation of life changes and transitions since widowhood, and this includes choices around health status, social networks and repartnering. The fifth paper reports on a qualitative study of older widows in Canada. In depth interviews reveal the ambiguity felt by many women about new partnerships and the reluctance to take on another man both out of loyalty to the deceased husband and the wish to maintain their late life independence. Finally, another paper from the Netherlands takes a gender comparative approach to new partnership formation. Interestingly, although no gender differences were identified in the quantitative analysis, the follow up qualitative study revealed that for widowers, positive well-being was associated with having a partner. In conclusion, gender, culture, family expectations, social mores and importantly, self agency, contribute to choices and constraints in establishing a new partnership whether not at all, non co-residential or living together. What is revealed from this set of papers, is a complex picture of relationship and friendship matrices which transcend the simple dichotomy of whether an older person wished or otherwise to establish another relationship after the loss of a spouse.

Living Apart Together. Balancing Intimacy and Autonomy in Old Age

K. Borell (Department of Social Work, Mid Sweden University. Ostersund. Sweden), S. Ghazanfareeon Karlsson (Department of Social Work, Mid Sweden University. Ostersund. Sweden)

The development of new intimate relationships following divorce or widowhood in later life is an under-investigated field in social gerontology. The few studies that examined dating processes in old age suggest that older individuals, especially women, do not wish to marry their dating partners. A new kind of relationship called Living Apart Together (LAT), i.e. a long-term intimate relationship in which the partners retain their own homes, represents however an increasingly popular alternative to marriage among elderly in Sweden. The purpose of this study is to explore the meaning elderly Swedish women in LAT-relationships ascribe to this kind of intimate relationships and to a home of their own. Results from structured, but not standardised, interviews with women in LAT-relationships show that a home of their own is a place in which personal control is ensured and optimised; a resource which women in LAT-relationships draw on to balance their need for privacy with their need for intimacy. On the one hand, our results indicate that for these women the home is used to facilitate space for their daily activities of choice and to limit the effects of an unequal division of domestic labour and caregiving. But on the other hand, the home represents by no means a social withdrawal. The home for the women interviewed is rather a secure base from which separate social relations are upheld: relations with friends, children and grandchildren and an intimate partner relationship depending fundamentally on the mutual satisfaction generic to that relationship itself.

New partners following widowhood : does gender matter?

N. Stevens (Department of Psychogerontology, University of Nijmegen, Nijmegen, the Netherlands)

An interesting question is whether gender influences the desire for a new partner as a strategy in the process of adaptation to loss of the partner in later life. Results of a survey and a qualitative study are described. In the survey single older persons were asked whether they would like to find a new partner; only 11% of the widowed persons replied positively. 75% were not interested in a new partner due to continued attachment to the deceased partner and satisfaction with life as a single person. There were no clear gender differences. The qualitative study revealed some interesting gender differences. Widowers were clear about whether they were interested in a new partner or not. One third had found new romantic partners or close friendships with women within 3-5 years; having a partner was associated with positive well-being. For widows, having close friendships with other women was associated with well-being. Only 8% had new partners. Desire for a partner was characteristic of widows who were lonely, who had not adapted well to their loss. Many women were ambivalent about a new partnership; they longed for companionship, love and security that a partner provides, but did not want to give up their freedom or face losing a second husband. A platonic friendship with a man was considered to be an ideal, but impossible alternative. Giving up the desire for a partner relationship appears to be adaptive for older widows, when sufficient companionship and intimacy is available in other close relationships.

Nobody could walk in his shoes: Older Canadian widows' attitudes toward relationships with men

D. K. van den Hoonaard (Gerontology Programme, St. Thomas University, Fredericton, Canada)

This presentation reports on a qualitative interview study about older Canadian widows' experiences and attitudes. Twenty-eight in-depth interviews were conducted in New Brunswick with women over 50 whose husbands had died within the previous seven years about a wide variety of issues including relationships with men. These relationships are problematic and challenging for a number of reasons. Most widows do not wish to remarry because: they feel they have already had the best possible husband, they have suffered enough with losing one husband, they do not want to schedule their lives around a new husband as they had with their previous husband, and they continue to feel a deep attachment to their deceased husbands. The continued wearing of wedding rings symbolizes both loyalty to deceased husbands and a desire not to remarry. Cautionary tales about the risks of remarriage are widespread. Norms regarding interactions between men and women are ambiguous, and widows often need to find creative new ways to interact safely with men in order to avoid misunderstandings both about their interest in remarriage or their desire or lack of desire to engage in intimate activity. In addition, the motives of men are not always clear, and changed sexual mores present challenges as do the reactions of adult children to potential relationships.

Older women in search of egalitarian types of new partner relationships

J. Gierveld (Netherlands Institute for Advanced Study in the Humanities and Social Sciences (NIAS), Wassenaar; Netherlands Interdisciplinary Demographic Institute (NIDI), The Hague, Netherlands)

A high proportion of women confronted with the loss of their partner after the age of fifty, and who are considering repartnering are deliberately planning their future life trajectory. It is especially the choice of the future type of living arrangement that becomes a 'reflexive project'. Some decide to remarry; others opt for more flexible and egalitarian types of living arrangements such as unmarried cohabitation or Living Apart and Together. We will investigate whether or not these choices are related to specific sets of motives, such as independence, religious or financial ones. Moreover the findings will be integrated and interpreted in the light of the Second Demographic Transition, and its emphasizing of an ongoing process of modernization. So, the data will be studied in a life course perspective using cohort data. Data for this study come from the Dutch NESTOR-Living arrangements and social networks of older adults (LSN)- survey. Face-to-face interviews were conducted with 4494 respondents, aged 54 to 89 years, in the Netherlands. Since the first interviews respondents have been re-interviewed after one, three, five and seven years, in cooperation with the LASA-group. Based on this dataset, life course data about e.g. partner history are available. Moreover, a group of forerunners (with new partners after late life widowhood or divorce) out the total group of respondents have been selected for in-depth qualitative interviews about the older adults' preferences and motives to start a new (type of) partner relationship. Data about the deliberately chosen flexible and egalitarian living arrangements and about the determinants and motives behind the new trend will be presented. Taking into account the ideas about the Second Demographic Transition, life course data related to cohort comparisons will elicit characteristics of the ever-changing patterns in the life course of older women born between 1903 and 1937.

Perceptions of Remarriage by Widowed Persons in Singapore

K. Mehta (Department of Social Work and Psychology, National University of Singapore)

Widowhood is a landmark transition that has socio-emotional and economic implications for the surviving spouse. The paper presents the views of widowed Singaporeans on the subject of remarriage. A quantitative-cum-qualitative methodology was employed to elicit their perceptions, which reflect three cultural groups i.e the Chinese, Malays and Indians. 237 male and female respondents took part in the survey, which was aimed at understanding the widowhood experience and their methods of coping. 25 case studies using in-depth interviews were conducted after the survey. It was found that a large majority of the respondents had negative perceptions of remarriage. Explanations given indicated that among the Chinese and Indians remarriage still carried a stigma. In the Malay culture, remarriage was more acceptable. Companionship was the main reason given by those who were in favour of remarriage. The paper discusses the cross-cultural perceptions of remarriage, highlighting the influence of family and society on the reality of remarriage as a viable option for widowed persons. Bearing in mind the fast greying profile of Singapore's population, the study has implications for services and future research.

The Health and Social Transitions for Recently Widowed Older Australian Women: A Longitudinal Study

J.E. Byles, S. Feldman, G. Mishra (Alma Unit for Research on Ageing, Faculty of Human Development, Victoria University, Australia)

The Australian Longitudinal Study on Women's Health provided an opportunity to explore and gain a broader understanding of the health and social needs of women as they age and following the death of their partner. Analysis of the baseline (cross-sectional data) from a population survey of 12,624 women aged 70-75 revealed that 4106 women were widowed. Overall, between baseline study and follow up, 700 women became widowed. This paper will present the analysis of the change in health and social outcomes for these women compared with women participants who are of the same age and remain married and those women who were already widowed at baseline. The women were asked both qualitative and quantitative questions that covered spheres of their lives, including their health, social circumstances, life changes and transitions since the death of their spouse or partner. What emerged from analysis of both quantitative and qualitative data was the identification of persistent and recurring themes of coping and transition particularly in relation to expressed needs for health support, strong social networks and physical resources. The study confirmed that the needs of widowed women who remain unpartnered go beyond a narrow definition of health, the key concerns commonly extending into more practical and social arenas. This national study has broad implications for health and for family life in both the public and private domains of the lives of older widowed women, particularly services and support that encompass a broader focus than bereavement only.

SESSION 40

Development of a simple, easy-to-use prescreening instrument for driving safety

Malcolm Man-Son-Hing (Division of Geriatric Medicine, University of Ottawa, Canada). Carole Cohen (Sunnybrook and Women's College Health Science Centre, Toronto, Canada). Frank Molnar (Division of Geriatric Medicine, University Of Ottawa, Canada). Randall Sargent (Calgary Regional Health Authority, Canada). Katharine Paddock (SCOHS, Ottawa, Canada). Neil Drummond (SWCHSC, Toronto, Canada)

The decision to disqualify a patient from driving is often the source of major difficulty for the individual concerned, the family, and for professionals. This study incorporates the exploration of the sequelae of that decision on patient/family circumstances and lay-professional relationships, with the development of an instrument which will help providers decide which patients require driving assessment.

Managing behavioural problems in a variety of care settings

Jean Kozak (Division of Geriatric Medicine, University of Ottawa, Canada). Karen Henderson (Caregiver Network, Toronto, Canada). Katharine Paddock (Research Department, Sisters of Charity of Ottawa Health Service, Ottawa, Canada). Nicole Robert (Psychogeriatric Community Services of Ottawa-Carlton, Canada). Marlene Collins (Carewest Glenmore Park, Calgary, Canada). Anne Lennox (Calgary Regional Health Authority, Canada). Frank Molnar (Division of Geriatric Medicine, University of Ottawa, Canada). Barbara Howson (Seniors Health Program, Calgary Regional Health Authority, Canada). Linda Bordage-Belanger (Ottawa-Carlton Community Care Access Centre, Ottawa, Canada). Neil Drummond (SWCHSC, Toronto, Canada)

'Problem' behaviours in community settings represent a continuing challenge for both professionals and caregivers. This study is examining why some research conducted previously into the issue has not been utilised in practice, and investigates the effectiveness of non-pharmacological methods for behavioural management, including caregiver education and support intended to combat caregiver bias against the use of drugs in behaviour management.

New medications and changing expectations

James Silvius (Divison of Geriatric Medicine, University of Calgary, Canada). Frank Molnar (Division of Geriatric Medicine, University of Ottawa, Canada) Malcolm Man-Son-Hing (Division of Geriatric Medicine, University of Ottawa, Canada). Barbara Schulman (Care of the Elderly and Rehabilitation, Sisters of Charity of Ottawa Health Service, Ottawa, Canada). Neil Drummond (SWCHSC, Toronto, Canada)

The development of new drugs for dementia (specifically cholinesterase inhibitors) may be changing both professional and lay expectations of therapy, including changes in management (such as prescribing patterns, expectations of caregivers). This study will investigate perceptions of the drugs among several groups, including families.

The effectiveness of specialized case management for dementia in the community

Neil Drummond (Sunnybrook and Women's College Health Science Centre, Toronto, Canada). Anne Lennox (Calgary Regional Health Authority, Calgary, Canada). William Dalziel (Division of Geriatric Medicine, University of Ottawa, Canada). Linda Bordage-Belanger (Ottawa-Carlton Community Care Access Centre, Ottawa, Canada). Dorothy Pringle (Faculty of Nursing, University of Toronto, Canada). Heather Brien (Toronto Community Care Access Centre, Canada). Nicole Robert (Psychogeriatric Community Services of Ottawa-Carlton, Canada). Marlene Collins (Carewest Glenmore Park, Calgary, Canada). Barbara Howson (Seniors Health Program, Calgary Regional Health Authority, Canada).

Many questions remain to be answered in relation to case management. This study is intended to broadly examine the definition of case management models across the continuum of care, seeking to explore the relative effectiveness of case management for dementia. Key questions to be examined include identifying the criteria which should determine when, and of what type, case management should be implemented for the individual client or patient, whether it is more effective to train a select cadre of professionals or to train a broader set of providers, how to involve family doctors and other health care providers in a specialised case management model, the cost effectiveness of case management, and the influence of cultural factors.

What is the experience of persons in need of a diagnosis?

Carole Cohen (Sunnybrook and Women's College Health Science Centre, Toronto, Canada) Jean Kozak (Division of Geriatric Medicine, University of Ottawa, Canada). James Silvius (Division of Geriatric Medicine, University of Calgary, Canada). Penny Ascroft, St Elizabeth Health Care, Toronto, Canada). Virginia Stewart (Bethany Care Society, Calgary, Canada). Barbara Schulman (Care of the Elderly and Rehabilitation, Sisters of Charity of Ottawa Health Service, Ottawa, Canada). Neil Drummond, (SWCHSC, Toronto. Canada)

Dementia may not be readily diagnosed in primary care settings for a variety of reasons. Little is known about the experience of the individual with dementia during the diagnostic process, in terms of identification of the problem by the individual with dementia or others, the decision to seek advice about the problem from the healthcare system or others, the diagnostic process itself including history taking, mental status exam and cognitive testing, specialised testing such as neuroimaging and neuropsychological testing,. and the process of referral and evaluation by specialists. This study will seek to identify what patients, caregivers and professionals identify as the important positive and negative experiences during the diagnostic phase.

SESSION 41

Description and outcomes of REACH, a multi-site caregiver intervention study

Richard Schulz (University of Pittsburgh, Pittsburgh, PA, USA) The Resources for Enhancing Alzheimer's Caregiver Health (REACH Project Design and Baseline Characteristics. Laura N. Gitlin (Thomas Jefferson University, Philadelphia, PA, USA) Effect of Multi-component Interventions on Caregiver Burden: The REACH Project at Six Months Follow-up. Sara J. Czaja (University of Miami School of Medicine, Miami, FL, USA) A Methodology for Integrating Psycho-Social Interventions. Steven H. Belle (University of Pittsburgh, Pittsburgh, PA, USA), Identifying Intervention Components to Reduce Caregiver Burden: Results from REACH.

Families caring for persons with dementia frequently experience burden due to behavioral dysfunction associated with the disease. Previous intervention studies to reduce caregiver burden report only minimal effects. Resources for Enhancing Alzheimer's Caregiver Health (REACH) is a NIH cooperative study involving 6 sites. Each site is testing one or more social, behavioral and technological interventions designed to strengthen family members' capacities to care for persons with dementia. The goal of this symposium is to describe the design of REACH, the population recruited, and to report six-month intervention effects on caregiver burden. This symposium is divided into five parts. The first presentation describes the design of this multi-site trial and characterizes the 1222 caregiver/care recipient dyads recruited into the study. This is followed by a report of site-specific and cross-site results on the effects of the interventions on caregiver burden. These results are based on conventional change-based site-specific and meta-analyses. In order to pool the data across sites, presentation 3 presents a methodology for characterizing the different interventions using a common metric. Presentation four shows how this metric can be used to carry out cross-site analyses. The presentation concludes with comments from a discussant, Dr. Benjamin Gottlieb. Large-scale multi-site intervention trials are still rare in the social and behavioral sciences. The REACH trial highlights both the challenges and possible solutions to conducting such trials. At a more concrete level, the findings from REACH provide guidance on the structure and content of future intervention efforts for caregivers of dementia patients.

A Methodology for Integrating Psycho-Social Interventions

Sara J. Czaja (University of Miami School of Medicine, Miami, FL, USA), Chin Chin Lee (University of Miami School of Medicine, Miami, FL, USA), Richard Schulz (University of Pittsburgh, Pittsburgh, PA, USA), Steven Belle (University of Pittsburgh, Pittsburgh, PA, USA)

Given that most real world problems are complex, health intervention studies typically implement multi-component interventions. Interventions are often not well described making it difficult to compare studies or ascribe causality to specific components of interventions. The purpose of this paper is to describe a methodology that can be used to characterize and integrate complex psychosocial interventions. The methodology is based on techniques commonly used in business and industry. The application of this methodology to the multiple interventions being evaluated in the multi-site REACH program will be described. Specifically the methodology involved the development of a comprehensive conceptual framework to link the interventions, and the use of hierarchal task analysis and the Analytical Hierarchy Process (a decision analysis tool) to describe the interventions according to this framework. The conceptual framework developed for REACH involved three dimensions - the entity and domain targeted by the intervention, and the delivery system characteristics. The results indicate that the methodology could be successfully used to map the REACH interventions to this complex conceptual framework and describe them according to a common metric. The data also indicate that high levels of consistency and reliability were achieved. These results will be discussed in terms of the cross-site analyses being conducted for the REACH project. The advantages of this methodology with respect to making comparisons across studies, and isolating causal factors that relate to desired outcomes will also be described. Finally, the application of this methodology to other types of intervention studies will be discussed.

Effect of Multi-component Interventions on Caregiver Burden: The REACH Project at Six Months Follow-up

Laura N. Gitlin (Thomas Jefferson University, Philadelphia, PA, USA); Louis Burgio (University of Alabama, Birmingham, AL, USA), Sara Czaja (University of Miami, Miami, FL, USA), Diane Mahoney (Hebrew Rehabilitation Center for Aged, Boston, MA, USA), Dolores Gallagher, Stanford University, Palo Alto, CA, USA), Robert Burns (Regional Medical Center and University of Tennessee, Memphis, TN, USA), Linda Nichols (Regional Medical Center, Memphis, TN, USA), Steve Belle (University of Pittsburgh, Pittsburgh, PA, USA), Marica Ory (National Institute on Aging, Bethesda, USA)

This paper reports the effect of 15 different REACH interventions on caregiver upset with behavioral problems following 6 months active treatment. Differential treatment effects on caregiver burden for Whites, Hispanics and Black caregivers are also examined. With-in site and cross-site meta-analyses are presented. A total of 1222 family caregivers were recruited and randomized to treatment or control group conditions across participating sites. Caregivers were interviewed using common measures at baseline, 6, 12 and 18 months. The first treatment phase occurred between baseline and 6 months. The main outcome was change (6 month-baseline score) in caregiver upset (0 = no upset to 4 = very) with 24 behavioral occurrences (8 memory, 7 depressive, and 6 disruptive behaviors) using the Revised Memory and Behavior Checklist. Average bother scores were calculated among all behaviors assigning no bother to behaviors that were not manifested. Analyses of these data reveal a promising pattern of within site and cross-site effects. Because these data have been embargoed at this time, we are unable to provide detailed results at the time of abstract submission. However, we will be able to report these data publicly at the time of the symposium.

Identifying Intervention Components to Reduce Caregiver Burden: Results from REACH

Steven H. Belle (University of Pittsburgh, Pittsburgh, PA, USA), Sara Czaja (University of Miami, Miami, FL, USA), Richard Schulz (University of Pittsburgh, Pittsburgh, PA, USA)

REACH tests different interventions at 6 sites, each of which utilizes different recruitment strategies. To enable cross-site analyses, we developed standardized measurement instruments administered under a common protocol. With interventions targeting well-defined and characterized caregiver/care-recipient dyads, a pre-planned meta-analysis was performed. However, with this approach, only broad conclusions could be reached concerning the relative success of the 9 active versus 6 control conditions. Therefore, we undertook analyses to identify intervention components associated with caregiver burden reduction. Caregiver burden was assessed by the Revised Memory and Behavior Checklist (RMBPC) which records caregiver distress related to 24 care-recipient behaviors on a 5-point scale (0-4). This measure was administered to all caregivers at baseline and to those whose care-recipients were still living at home 6 months later. Regression models used change in burden as the outcome and included baseline RMBPC score, caregiver and care-recipient characteristics, and variables derived using the conceptual framework as independent variables. While analyses have been conducted, at the time of abstract submission, data are embargoed. At the symposium we will be permitted to report data publicly. The conceptual framework provides us with the opportunity to avoid the site-intervention confound, and to be able to look more closely at aspects of the interventions associated with burden reduction.

The Resources for Enhancing Alzheimer's Caregiver Health (REACH) Project Design and Baseline Characteristics

Stephen R. Wisniewski (University of Pittsburgh, Pittsburgh, PA USA), Steven H. Belle (University of Pittsburgh, Pittsburgh, PA, USA), David W. Coon (Standford University and Palo Alto Healthcare System, Palo Alto, CA, USA), Susan M. Marcus (Thomas Jefferson University, Philadelphia, PA, USA), Marcia G. Ory (National Institute on Aging, Bethesda, USA), Louis Burgio (University of Alabama, Birmingham, AL, USA), Robert Burns (Regional Medical Center and University of Tennessee, Memphis, TN, USA), Richard Schulz (University of Pittsburgh, Pittsburgh, PA, USA) for the REACH Investigators

This paper describes the study design and sample at baseline of REACH (Resources for Enhancing Alzheimer's Caregiver Health). Established in 1995 by the NIA and the NINR, REACH was funded to test interventions for enhancing family caregiving. REACH is a cooperative study involving six different sites across the U.S. Each site is testing one or more social, behavioral and technological interventions delivered during the first six months of the study. In order to facilitate comparisons across sites, identical core measures were collected at baseline and 6, 12, and 18 months post-baseline. A total of 1222 family caregiver/car recipient dyads were recruited. The REACH caregivers are 18.4% male, with an average age of 62.5 years. Fifty-seven percent of the population is White, while 22% is Black and 20% is Hispanic. Approximately 20% of the caregivers have less than a high school education and nearly 59% are educated beyond a high school. Fifty percent of the caregivers are spouses and 43% are children of the care recipient. The care recipients are on average 78.9 years of age and 46% are men. The measures of cognitive and physical function indicate an impaired group of care recipients. The average MMSE, score was 12.6 (out of 30) and care recipients were impaired on 3.9 (out of 6) ADLs and 7.3 (out of 8) IADLs. The diversity of caregivers and care recipients in REACH poses formidable challenges in implementing successful interventions.

SESSION 42

Impact of HIV/AIDS on Older People: Experiences from Africa and Asia

S.Z. Kalula (Institute of Ageing in Africa, University of Cape Town, South Africa) Overview of Epidemiology of HIV/AIDS in Africa and Asia. R. deGraft Agyarko Ageing and Life Course, (World Health Organization, Geneva, Switzerland) Developing and alidating Methodology to Examine the Impact of HIV/AIDS on Older Caregivers in Africa. Zimbabwean Case Study. M Ferreira (Institute of Ageing in Africa, University of Cape Town, South Africa) Older Carers to Adult Children and Grandchildren Affected by AIDS : Towards Supporting the Carers. D. Wesumperuma (Asia Training Centre on Ageing, HelpAge International, Chiang Mai University, Thailand), HIV/AIDS in Northern Thailand and Older Carers: A Saga of Resilience in a Human Calamity. T. Petersen (HelpAge International, London, UK) Discussant

The impact of HIV/AIDS epidemics on older persons (50 years and over) in the Africa and Asia regions is examined in the symposium, with specific reference to the situation in three countries. First, an overview is given of the epidemiology of the epidemics in the two regions. Thereafter, findings are presented from studies conducted in (1) Zimbabwe (a quantitative/qualitative pilot study to develop and validate methodology to examine the impact of HIV/AIDS on caregivers in four African countries); (2) Sout Africa (a qualitative study of older African women as carers to adult children and grandchildren with AIDS in townships of Cape Town); and (3) Thailand (field experience and findings of studies among older carers in an urban and two rural communities of northern Thailand). Results from the studies in the African countries are similar and show that sampled older carers live in abject poverty, lack adequate food for their household, and have numerous basic physical and emotional needs which are unmet. The results of the studies in Thailand show that carers are ill-prepared to take on caregiving responsibilities towards orphaned grandchildren and experience a range of difficulties and problems, similar though to those found in the African studies. In both regions, the plight of older carers is exacerbated by poverty. Nevertheless, the presentations will demonstrate the resilience, strengths, determination and coping abilities of the carers. Discussion will be led in by a representative of HelpAge International, which NGO, through its regional offices, conducts research and implements support programmes in countries in both regions, to empower and support older carers, particularly women, in caregiving to PWAs and in their contribution to the management of the epidemics. Finally, ways will be explored in the symposium to bring the plight of older carers and the difficulties they experience to the attention of policy makers, to promote the inclusion of older persons in programmes in the regions aimed at supporting individuals affected by HIV/AIDS.

Developing and Validating Methodology to Examine the Impact of HIV/AIDS on Older Caregivers in Africa. Zimbabwean Case Study

R. deGraft Agyarko, A. Kalache, P.R. Kowal (World Health Organization, Geneva Switzerland), N. Madzingira (Institute of Development Studies, University of Zimbabwe, Harare, Zimbabwe), N. Mujuru (Ministry of Health, Harare, Zimbabwe), L. Kanyowa, R. Mupedziswa (School of Social Work, Harare, Zimbabwe), J. Matorofa (Central Statistical Office, Harare, Zimbabwe)

The main purpose of a four-country (Ghana, South Africa, Tanzania, Zimbabwe) study is to identify barriers that prevent older persons from providing adequate and fulfilling care, and to promote policies and programmes to support them as assets in the community for the care, of terminally-ill persons with AIDS (As) and children orphaned as a result of AIDS-related deaths. A mixed method of qualitative and quantitative techniques was developed and the study was piloted in Zimbabwe among a sample of 783 older persons and 23 key informants in 2000/2001. Data were collected in six provinces, in areas stratified for rural-urban, socio-economic and cultural differences, and HIV/AIDS prevalence. Preliminary findings suggest that a lack of food and basic needs not being met, such as clothing, blankets, the high cost of medical treatment for PWAs and school fees for orphans, as well as loss of economic support and diminished livelihood options are the main problems which affect the care rendered by older persons. Zimbabweans affected by AIDS were also found to have limited a ess to and low utilisation of health services, due to the high cost of health care, transport difficulties, stigmatisation of the disease and poor health-staff attitudes towards PWAs.

HIV/AIDs in northern Thailand and Older Carers: A Saga of Resilience in a Human Calamity

D. Wesumperuma (Asia Training Centre On Ageing, HelpAge International, Chiang Mai, Thailand)

The presentation is based on field experience of HelpAge International community based project with older carers and findings of two research studies in one urban and two rural communities in northern Thailand the part of the country where the AIDS infection rates are deemed highest. A combination of methods were used in the studies: in-depth interviews, review of village documents as well as district plans, PRA and focus group discussion sessions, individual semi-structured interviews and brief case studies. Impact on older people though largely indirect is hardest, particularly when they had to take up new roles as care givers to their adult children with AIDS and simultaneously taking on the responsibility in raising their grandchildren. Older people were themselves at risk of HIV infection. Most witnessed the passing of their adult children during the past five years and were unprepared to take on further responsibilities in bringing up grandchildren. They encountered a range of problems and difficulties that included physical exhaustion, over-burdened workload, financial hardships, emotional upheaval, lack of knowledge, skills and resources in dealing with adults children with AIDS, increasing conflicts with grandchildren, social stigmatism, discrimination and rejection, and exclusion from accessing appropriate knowledge and support services dealing with HIV/AIDS. Their plights were further exacerbated by their state of poverty. The burden of being a carer and the feeling of guilt and shame prevented many older people from maintaining social contacts. The project experience and studies also show their resilience, strength and determination in the face of all this. The presentation will focus on their coping ability and strengths.

Older African Carers to Adult Children and Grandchildren Affected by AIDS in Cape Town: Towards Supporting the Carers

M. Ferreira (Institute of Ageing in Africa, University of Cape Town, South Africa)

Scant, or no, attention has thus far been paid to the impact of the AIDS epidemic on older persons in South Africa, and the role and contribution of grandmothers as caregivers to persons with AIDS (PWAs) in the management of the epidemic. A longitudinal survey (over 6 months) was undertaken in four townships on the C e Flats, to gather qualitative data from 43 African women aged 50 years and older who were caring for a co-resident adult child with AIDS and grandchildren, 19 of whom had AIDS. After baseline, subjects were interviewed twice more at three-month intervals. During the study period eight PWAs died. Findings included extreme, endemic poverty in the households (half had no income, half were dependent on the subject's pension grant), and feelings of desperation and hopelessness, as well as optimism in the subject. Main difficulties experienced by subjects were a lack of money and food; the application process for social grants; transport costs to take PWAs for medical treatment; inability to pay for grandchildren's schooling; and the physical and emotional toll of caregiving and the household situation. An intervention, based on the study findings, aimed at supporting such carers, is currently under way and is described.

SESSION 43

Agitated Behaviour and Environment: Therapeutic Touch Effect on Agitation and Cortisol in individuals with Alzheimers.

D. L. Woods, M. Dimond, M. Heitkemper, M. Lentz (Department of Biobehavioural Nursing and Health Systems, University of Washington, School of Nursing, Seattle, WA), S. Elmore (Department of Psychosocial Nursing and Community Health, University of Washington, School of Nursing, Seattle, WA).

Purpose: Recent developments in neuroendocrinology suggest that the Hypothalamic-Pituitary-Adrenal (H-P-A) Axis has a role in the altered response of AD individuals to stress. Given the deleterious effects of pharmacological interventions in this vulnerable population, non-invasive treatments must be explores for their potential to mitigate hyper-responsivity to stress and attenuate detrimental cortisol levels. Method: This within-subject, interrupted time series study was conducted to test the effectiveness of Therapeutic Touch (TT) on the frequency of agitated behaviour and on salivary and urine cortisol levels in individuals with DAT. Ten subjects, aged 71-84 years and who resided in a Special Care Unit, were observed every 20 min for 10h/d, were monitored 24h/d for physical activity and had samples for salivary and urine cortisol taken daily. The study occurred in four phases: 1) Pre-treatment/ baseline (4 d); 2) Intervention/ treatment (TT for 5-7 min two x/d for 3 d); 3) Treatment effect (11 d); 4) Post "wash-out" (3 d). Results: ANOVA for repeated measures indicated a decrease in the frequency of overall agitated behaviour and in two of the six agitated behaviours (vocalization and pacing/walking) coincident with the treatment time (phase 2) and early post-treatment (phase 3). A decreasing trend over time was noted for salivary and urine cortisol. Conclusions: This study suggests that the cortisol levels in AD individuals may be mitigated by interventions such as TT, altering hyper-responsivity to stress and the quality of the social environment. In addition, TT decreases verbal agitation and pacing, two prevalent agitated behaviours.

Bio-psychosocial intervention in challenging behaviour in dementia in residential and nursing homes

E. Moniz-Cook (School of Medicine, University of Hull, UK), C. Elston, R. Pratt, J. Woodhouse, K. Richards, Tracey Warrington, Cherry Luter, Karen Jarvis, Paul Duggan (Hull and East Riding Community NHS Trust, Hull, UK)

Bio-psychosocial approaches to the management of people with dementia who challenging staff in care homes assume that the relationship between neuropathology and difficult behaviour in dementia is not necessarily causal, but that psychological and environmental factors may also contribute to the development and maintenance of this. For example, in addition to the effect of neurogenic factors, other biological aspects (e.g. infection, ill health or pain), the resident's own beliefs or experience, the social or physical environment and staff behaviour or experience may all be important in understanding and managing challenging behaviour. A bio-psychosocial algorithm for the evaluation and management of challenging resident behaviour is evaluated in 103 residents who were described 'difficult to manage' by care staff (Challenging Behaviour Score >80 = severe challenge) A bio-psychosocial analysis and the meaning behind the resident's behaviour was given to staff. Interventions included withdrawal of neuroleptics, treatment of physical health problems (infection, pain, constipation, cancer), occupation and activity support, antidepressant treatment and the following interventions were demonstrated in situ for care staff: management of aggressive resistance during self care, management of screaming and uncooperative / aggressive behaviour precipitated by frontal lobe dementia, apraxia and dysphasia. Significant reductions (pre post and follow-up) in actual resident behaviour and staff report of 'ease of management' of this, occurred in 92 residents. The success and failure of bio-psychosocial intervention and the lack of generalisation of bio-psychosocial approaches in care settings is discussed. Future case-specific bio-psychosocial intervention research within a randomised controlled design is outlined.

Decreasing Aggressive Episodes by Meeting Resident Toileting Needs

Anne Earthy (Continuing Care, Simon Fraser Health Region, New Westminster, British Columbia, Canada)

Purpose of study is to decrease aggressive episodes toward residential care staff by addressing the cause of the resident's frustration.This is a before and after study and compares results from a research group (n = 50) to a control group (n=50). In the summer of 2000 this agency received funding from the provincial Occupational Health Association to demonstrate that residents' frustration can be decreased by meeting their bodily functions in a timely manner. Funding was used to purchase electric lifts and standers, one of each per care aide assignment, so that equipment was available to assist with toileting as needed. The clinical practice guidelines on Maintaining Continence and Bowel Care were diligently implemented to individualize resident's toileting needs. Benchmarking data was collected by completing a Behaviour Checklist containing 52 behaviours, numbers and type of toileting and transfers, compliance with the 2 CPG's, skin assessments, fluid intake, bowel and skin medications, cost of briefs and linens. Number of incidents of excessive behaviours directed toward staff and muscle skeletal injuries were recorded. The anticipated outcomes include decreased episodes of excessive behaviours directed toward the careproviders. Also, an increase in the number of residents toileted at times that meet their needs, decrease in bowel and skin medications. If the resident is able to maintain their dignity and basic bodily functions it is anticipated they will be more content and less frustrated. By working together we can provide resident focused care and show that it can benefit the careproviders as well.

SESSION 45

Films and Videos on Biology and Aging

James Vanden Bosch (Terra Nova Films, Inc, Chicago, Illinois USA)

The Life and Times of Life and Times (60 minutes, released in 1998) Why do we age? Why do we live 80 years instead of 1000? This program responds to the growing public curiosity about current aging researchnot sensational pseudo-science, but serious science. A series of recent discoveries has moved aging research from the scientific margins to an exploding area of contemporary biology: Single genes which can be mutated to double the life span of experimental animals; Molecular mechanisms which limit the number of times our cells can divide; Visual identification of old cells demonstrate that, as we age, old cells accumulate in our bodies; Human genes for longevity have been found in people over 100. There is no consensus now in science as to what causes aging, and the question is being attacked on many fronts. But for the first time, the fundamental molecular mechanisms are beginning to be understood. Stylistically, The Life and Times of Life and Times blends traditional science documentary with poetic essay. Interviews with high-level charismatic researchers are intercut with nature shots, including some of the oldest creatures on earth. (Not only explanatory, these beautiful images provide a pause to reflect. After all, aging is not unique to humans.) Archival footage from old movies entertains while providing easily understandable analogies, special effects turn the television image itself into demonstrations of scientific concepts, and animation illustrates several concepts in molecular biology.

SESSION 46

Ethics Education at a Multi-level Geriatric Centre: The Baycrest Model

Michael Gordon, (Baycrest Centre for Geriatric Care, Toronto, Canada)

Abstract Purpose: To describe an innovative ethics education program at the Baycrest Centre for Geriatric Care - a multilevel academic geriatric, long-term care facility. The Centre's programs include: residential; nursing home; chronic hospital; numerous short-term programs such as rehabilitation, geriatric psychiatry, palliative care and many ambulatory, day and outreach initiatives that serve the elderly population in north Toronto. Method: The ethics program evolved under the direction of the Centre's ethics committee, which functions in an educational and consultative role. For the past three years the committee has embarked on a unit-based ethics education program. By participating in discussions on the individual clinical-care units, members of the ethics committee are able to break down barriers that often inhibit staff from referring concerns formally to the committee. Results: Following introduction of the program, a schedule of unit-based meetings was organized. In a relaxed atmosphere, members of staff present difficult cases or recurring problems. The ethics committee representatives help the staff define the problems within an ethics framework, and allow them to work through the various challenges in decision-making. Recurring themes include end- of - life decisions such as tube feeding, the withholding of treatments, DNR, as well as issues related to competency and surrogate decision-making. Principlism and other ethics frameworks are used in discussions. Case vignettes will illustrate the process. Conclusion: The unit staff prefer this module of dealing with ethics decision-making rather than the formal consultation process that is the usual way that problems are brought to ethics committees.

Ethics in Home Care

Norman Linzer, [Wurzweiler School of Social Work Yeshiva University New York, NY, USA]

Abstract PURPOSE: The purpose of this presentation is to discuss the ethical issues that arise when an elderly couple refuse home care services offered by a family agency. The social worker recommends it based on the husband's cognitive impairment, the wife's depressed state, and the apartment's unkempt condition.This case evokes the autonomy-paternalism dilemma and the decision-making capacity of elderly persons. The couple's value self-determination - appears to clash with the agency's value beneficence/paternalism. However, it is difficult to know whether the refusal is an expression of a preferred way of life or an accommodation to the travails of aging. If the former, the value appears to both coincide and clash with the agency's, which values client self-determination but also the health and social functioning of its elderly clients. If the latter, there is no ethical dilemma but a clinical challenge to maintain their viability as a family.The ethical dilemma is whether or not to respect the couple's autonomy. Is the refusal of home care the autonomous decision of "mentally competent" persons who are aware of the consequences or does it reflect a degree of mental incompetence corroborated by the physician and the social worker and the unkempt condition of their apartment? Yet, they have managed to live this way for years and are not harming anyone. Is it ethical, under beneficence, to impose services that they refuse? Perhaps even their diminished autonomy should be supported for they are able to make decisions in different areas of their lives.

Opportunities and Challenges in Becoming a Restraint Free Long Term Care Facility

Kyle Whitfield (Murray Alzheimer Research and Education Program, University of Waterloo. and School of Planning, U of W. Student)

The purpose of this qualitative study was to understand what staff of one rural long term care facility believe about the use of restraints. Several actions had been taken by the facility to significantly minimize the use of restraints ie. removal of most bed rails and taking tray tables off of geri chairs if they were not used strictly for positioning purposes. The study was designed to ask staff to evaluate the impact of these changes. The majority of staff participated in focus group interviews and in-depth individual interviews were held with managers. The results describe staff as feeling quite concerned about the safety of the residents when there is a restraint-free policy that is strict and absolute. They see a need for a policy that is flexible, individualized and involves all parties concerned about the resident, including the resident, in the decision making process. Managers were more concerned about ways to implement a no restraint policy and keep families happy about how their family member was being cared for.

Restraint use in special care units: Is it dependent on staff ratios and mix?

R. Colin Reid (Centre on Aging, University of Victoria, Victoria, BC, Canada) Neena L. Chappell (Centre on Aging, University of Victoria, Victoria, BC, Canada) Marilyn Bater (Royal Jubilee Hospital, Victoria, BC, Canada)

PURPOSE: Persons with dementia in long-term care facilities are not uncommonly restrained physically and/or pharmacologically. Pharmacologically, psychotropic drugs (anxiolytics, antidepressants, and neuroleptics) are commonly administered. Physically, bed rails, geri-chairs, lap belts, and wheel chair trays are most often used. While the vast majority of intermediate care facilities in British Columbia have a no-restraint or least restraint policy in place, most report having recently used one or more psychotropic drugs or physical restraints for the express purpose of controlling resident behaviour. Because staff shortages are a hallmark of the modern Canadian health care system, the use of restraints may depend to some extent on the availability of adequately trained personnel, in the right combination. The purpose of this study is to determine what effects staff ratios and staff mix have on restraint use in special care units. METHOD: Data are drawn from the Intermediate Care Facility Project (1995-1999). Multiple regression equations are the central methods. RESULTS: Preliminary results show that while staff-to-resident ratios are inversely related to both chemical and physical restraint use at the facility level, the relationship does not hold when examining resident-level data. Staff mix is unrelated at either level. DISCUSSION: It is concluded that because staff ratios appear to play a role in the use or non-use of both chemical and physical restraints, practitioners and policy makers may want to re-evaluate the effects of staff ratios on quality of care among long-term care residents with dementia. At minimum, a closer look at this issue is warranted.

Subtle Ethical Dilemmas in Everyday Geriatric Practice

Judah Van Dijk, Arnold Rosin

There are situations in daily geriatric practice in which subtle aspects of the ethics of autonomy are ignored, unwittingly or even with good intentions. Some examples of these dilemmas are presented here. Role reversal presents ethical pitfalls because children as caregivers are invested with a certain authority, understood but often unspoken, in dealing with their parents affairs. This sometimes extends to placement of the parent in a residential facility, ostensibly with his agreement, but often against his will. A "geriatric problem" commonly involves the family as well as the old person, leading to the question facing doctors, nurses, social workers and other professionals as to whom exactly is their responsibility and priority of management. Day Centers for disabled or demented old people contribute much to improved quality of life for patient and caregiver alike. The former is often reluctant to be taken to the facility because of its unfamiliarity or the need to leave his home for the day. The professional might have to exercise some compulsion, especially if the dependency causes significant disturbance at home, but should not co-erce. Another area open to ethical transgression is application of physical restraints or administration of tranquillisers in a nursing-home or day center for easier management of the patient. Obtaining consent from a demented patient s participation in a research trial may sometimes border on ethical inappropriateness, especially if he is partly competent. These judgemental issues demand careful situational diagnosis, often with multi-disciplinary consultation, and good communication skills with all parties concerned.

The care ethics in geriatrics

B.Placines , M.P.Labernadie(Centre de Gérontologie de Pontacq-Nay , 64800 Nay , France) , M.Wolf (Centre Hospitalier Général , 45300 Pithiviers , France), I.Haritchabalet (Centre Hospitalier Général , 64000 Pau , France)

Trough an indispensable technicality , the geriatric care tries to realise the anthropological project of the subject maintenance as the subject , that is to say to act on his own life . The french philosopher V.Jankelevitch distinguishes two faces in the ethics: an ethics of decision and an ethics of interval . If the ethics of the decision concerns particular situations , for exemple , the end of life ,the indications of the gastrostomy per cutaneous endoscopic , the choice of paraclinic investigations and treatments , the ethics of interval concerns the daily , the human relationships with the frail elderly . The ethics of interval concerns the daily , the reports with frail elderly . The role of the care team is satisfied badly with an anormality ethical , centered on the ethics of decision but concerns an ethics of interval , therefore a virtue ethics .

When Autonomy is Not Enough

Sharon Wall (Centre for Education and Research on Ageing) Sydney Australia

As in many areas of health development the aged care sector is undergoing rapid technological advances. Coupled with an increasingly ageing population this is producing situations often difficult to reconcile by law. Throughout time the law, health and medicine have had difficulty establishing a synchrony which is complimentary to all. The paradox has been created that with the rapid technological advancement in ageing and the increasing potential for continuation of life, medicine must increasingly move outside itself to solve the dilemmas and issues it presents. Through case history presentation, this paper aims to highlight some of the ethical and legal dilemmas which may arise in the care of elderly people with dementia within our community and proposes a framework for their management.

SESSION 47

Bodily Culture and Health: Narratives of Elderly Women of Ethnic Origin

Geneviève Rail (University of Ottawa, Ottawa, CANADA) Hélène Dallaire (University of Ottawa, Ottawa, CANADA) Suzanne Laberge (Université de Montréal, Montréal, CANADA) Philippe Voyer (Université Laval, Québec, CANADA)

Social scientists of health and medicine have generally focused their research on illness and have provided limited insight on issues of health per se. Analyses that did centre on health have touched on structural, social and material aspects, but have usually neglected the phenomenological ones. There lies the relevance of sociological studies within which the body and bodily practices are located individually, socially and culturally in the construction of a more or less “healthy” self. The purpose of the present study was to investigate the bodily culture as well as the perceptions of health and aging of elderly women coming from disadvantaged socio-economic milieus. A qualitative content analysis was performed using transcripts from individual interviews with 65 to 75 years-old women from the Montreal area who belong to either the Haitian or the Asian community. The use of grounded theory, as a method, favoured the emergence of results that enhance our understanding of bodily culture and health, as perceived by these elderly women. Such results enlighten the phenomenological experience of the body and the self, the place of physical activity in the lived experiences of the body, the influence of gender norms on bodily culture, and the influence of cultural norms on health and physical activity practices. * The study is funded by the Social Sciences and Humanities Research Council of Canada

Coverage of Older Women's Health Issues in Medical Journals

J. Dergal, J. Gold, P. de Nobrega, A. Misra (Baycrest Centre for Geriatric Care, Toronto, Canada), J. Clark (Baycrest Centre for Geriatric Care, University of Toronto, Canada), P. Rochon (Baycrest Centre for Geriatric Care, University of Toronto, Canada)

Purpose: To explore the coverage of issues specific to older women's health in leading medical journals. Method: We reviewed all original investigations published in the Annals of Internal Medicine, the British Medical Journal, the Journal of the American Medical Association, the Lancet, the New England Journal of Medicine, and the Canadian Medical Association Journal between January 1 and June 30, 1999. Results: Of the 553 original investigations identified, 94 articles (17%) included a women-only sample. Of these, only 18 (19%) included older women in the sample. While there was inclusion of the 'young old' (65-74 years of age) in all 18 investigations, only 4 (22%) indicated age ranges that included older women aged 75+. No studies discussed the results with respect to their impact on older women specifically. Of the 18 investigations which included older women, the topics most frequently addressed included female-specific cancers (n= 11) and hormone replacement therapy (n= 2). Of the 94 women-only sample investigations, 3 studies (3%) included older women only. All three addressed breast cancer. No investigations addressed topics related to the social, economic, or political determinants of older women's health. Conclusion: The coverage of older women's health in leading medical journals is not well represented, and tends to portray issues not specifically relevant to older women. While the younger old are somewhat represented in investigations, older women aged 75+ are rarely included in study samples. Investigations, moreover, tend to focus on strictly biomedical topics at the expense of the social, political, and economic factors that influence older women's health.

Health conditions and diseases in elderly women

Rosalina Aparecida Partezani Rodrigues (University of São Paulo at Ribeirão Preto College of Nursing, Ribeirão Preto, São Paulo, Brazil) Luciana Kusumota (University of São Paulo at Ribeirão Preto College of Nursing, Ribeirão Preto, São Paulo, Brazil) Sueli Marques (University of São Paulo at Ribeirão Preto College of Nursing, Ribeirão Preto, São Paulo, Brazil) Suzele Cristina Coelho Fabrício (University of São Paulo at Ribeirão Preto College of Nursing, Ribeirão Preto, São Paulo, Brazil)

To analyze the changes occurring to elderly women which alter senescence and senility and to identify their difficulties in daily-life activities. The subjects of this investigation were 28 elderly women whose ages ranged from 75 to 93 years and who lived in a middle-class and lower-middle-class neighborhood. The theoretical framework on aging and society proposed by RILEY was used. The methodological procedure contained a health-evaluation questionnaire with seven items and a semi-structured interview containing one inquiring question on the changes in the elderly women's lives. The data analysis was related to the framework adopted by RILEY, that is, to individual and social changes. The preserved potentialities and losses in daily-life activities and in health conditions as well as diseases prevailed in the analysis of individual changes. The morbidities that interfered the most with daily-life activities were: arterial hypertension, cerebrovascular accidents, cataract, urinary incontinence and rheumatism. This study enabled the recovery of a period of life for the elderly women, who gave accounts of the difficulties that they had faced over their lives. Thus, it favored the understanding of the aging process at the end of century in a modern society.

Older Women and Weight: The Tensions Between Health and Beauty Interpretations of the Aging Body.

Laura Hurd (Post-Doctoral Fellow, School of Social Work and Family Studies, University of British Columbia, Vancouver, B.C, Canada)

PURPOSE: To explore older women's perceptions of their aging bodies within the context of a gendered and ageist social world. METHOD: I conducted 96 hours of semi-structured interviews with 22 community-dwelling women aged 61 to 92, who varied according to class, health and marital status, and religious and ethnic affiliation. RESULTS: Today's female beauty ideal (young, thin, toned) is a potential threat to an older woman's sense that she is attractive. The majority of the women in my study express dissatisfaction with their physical appearances, particularly in terms of their weight. The women indicate that they would like to lose weight, state that they are less attractive than when they were younger and slimmer and describe having monitored or struggled to alter their weights most of their lives. Even as the women express dissatisfaction with their heavier appearances and seem to have internalized the belief that beauty is equated with youthfulness and thinness, they also tend to describe their perceived need to lose weight in terms of the health benefits rather than the appearance benefits of having a slimmer figure. The women suggest that they have reorganized their priorities such that health has become more important than beauty. CONCLUSION: There are tensions and contradictions in the meanings that older women give to weight and weight loss. While they tend to be dissatisfied with their weight, they also argue that weight loss is more important in terms of their health rather than in terms of approximating the beauty ideal.

Older Women, the Body and the Invasive Actions and (Re)actions of Others

Patricia Mitchell (Flinders University-Adelaide, South Australia

In this paper, the power/knowledge differences in what constitutes body invasion for older women are examined. The study informing the paper utilized an innovative post-modern feminist research strategy, memory-work, which allowed older women to consider the impact that relationships have on experiences of health. The choice of this methodology is significant in that it provided the opportunity for participants themselves to engage in the analysis process. The women identified Resistance as a theme to write about and this paper explores the women's responses to this theme. The memories written reflect a pattern of body invasion that cautions the need for older women to be vigilant about their bodies. The memories detailed how the significance of the body to an older woman is often unassumed or ignored. They also demonstrate how the feelings associated with the ageing body for older women are often silenced or diminished in intensity. They highlight the degree to which an older woman will go to protect herself, especially when subjected to exploitation by an 'other'. A thematic thread in the memories supports Foucault's thesis that silence is powerful and can be used powerfully. The effects of silence on others can result in the 'other' being unwittingly protected through that silence. While these older women had learned to remain silent, importantly, they had also learned to use that silence to resist the invasive action of others. The discourses analyzed in this paper reveal how the fears associated with the violation of the body linger on and are a powerful means of social control.

Subjective health in the population: Differential determinants and mechanisms between man and woman

Astrid Stuckelberger (Swiss Research Programme on Ageing, Genève, Geneva University Hospitals, Rue Micheli-du-Crest 24, CH-1211 Genève 14, Switzerland)

Longitudinal studies have demonstrated with consistency that subjective health is the most significant predictor of mortality up to 12 years of follow up, defying all objective measures of health. The mechanisms and determinants of this variable have not yet been studied. The research conducted for a thesis postulates: a) the existence of psychological mechanisms involved in the self-regulation of subjective health (coping and Health Control Beliefs), b) a sex difference in this assessment process (modelisation). A randomized and stratified sample of 744 persons (387 men and 357 women) fulfilling the selection criteria were interviewed: aged 65 and more, living at home in the Geneva canton and able to respond. The analysis, including multiple linear regression and log-linear path modeling, demonstrated the importance of psychological mechanisms and sex differentials in predicting subjective health. "Internality" (believing one can control one's health) emerged as the strongest psychological predictor of good subjective health in both sexes, with two other health indicators: functional capacity and depressive symptoms. Women use coping mechanisms (active coping and social coping) while men do not appear to use any and more so demonstrate an 'escapism' attitude. The complexity of the statistical models for women contrast remarkably with the simplicity of models for men. The study also underlines general methodological problems of population studies. The contrast demonstrated in the results using 2 different methods of analysis (weighing cases or not) calls for serious reflections in interdisciplinary research methods. On the other hand, the gender analysis method used reveals stunning differences between sexes and questions the need for adopting a statistical approach that would consider each gender as a definite and distinct population. To conclude, by proving clear gender differences in the assessment of one's health, the thesis brings new insights on sex-specific attitudes towards health and illnesses that could be a ground explanation of the constant differential in causes of mortality and life expectancy between men and women. To imagine sex-specific programs to improve those attitudes and behaviors throughout life could only bring positive effects to the longevity of men and to the quality of life of future generations.

SESSION 48

Development of a multiple intervention for older people with osteo-artritis of the hip

Patricia G.M. Staats MA (TNO Prevention and Health,Leiden, the Netherlands) Marja H. Westhoff (TNO Prevention and Health, Leiden, the Netherlands)

Purpose In 1996/1997 a multiple intervention was developed to prevent loss of mobility in people with osteoarthritis (OA) of the hip. The intervention of eight weeks consist of training on fitness-equipment, a ergonomic advice at home and a diet advice. The aim of the study is increase or stabilize daily functioning to postpone hip replacement. Method In a randomized controlled trial the intervention was evaluated in 107 community living people aged 55 years and older with OA of the hip (experimental group n=55, control group n=52. Subjects were recruited bij general practioners and by public service announcements in local media.Inclusion criteria were OA of the hip according to the clinical criteria of the American College of Rheumatology (Altman et al,1991). Exclusion criteria were if a hip replacement was indicated or performed, or people were under 55 years of age. Pre-tests, posttests and follow-up tests after three months were carried out. Questionaires were completed on, among others, hip funcion (Harris Hip Score, Harris 1969), ADL/IADL activities, and pain. Physical measurements were performed on functional ability and weight (quetelet index), An MANOVA design for repeated measures was used to test for significant differences between data of pre-, post, and follow up tests. Results A beneficial effect was found on pain that diminisched significantly (p<.04)in the experimental group compared to the controlgroup. Further effects were found on the function of the hip (p,.10), body care and movement (p<.06). No effects were found on functional ability and weight loss. Conclusion It is concluded that this multiple intervention seems to be effective in people with osteoarthritis, in particulary on a diminishing pain. The supervision of a multi disciplinary team seems to be beneficial in preventive care of osteo-arthritis. On this moment the dissemination and implementation is carry-out.

The effects of a health educational and exercise program for older adults with osteoarthritis of the hip or knee

Marijke Hopman-Rock Marja H. Westhoff, Erwin C.P.M. Tak MA. (TNO Prevention and Health, Leiden, The Netherlands)

Purpose Evaluation of a self-management program for patients with osteoarthritis (OA) of the hip or knee. The program, which consisted of 6 weekly sessions of 2 hours, included health education by a peer and physical exercises taught by a physical therapist. Methods The program was evaluated in 60 participants and 60 controls (design RCT), age between 55 and 75 years, with symptoms of osteoarthritis in the hip or knee. Questionnaires were completed about pain, behavior, knowledge, and self-efficacy. Physical measurements included quadriceps strength, range of motion of the knee or hip, and several physical function tests. A pre-test, post-test, and a follow-up test after 6 months were carried out. Results Significant MANOVA group X time effects (p< 0.05 one-side) were found for pain, quality of life, strength of the left M. quadriceps, knowledge, self-efficacy, BMI, physical active lifestyle, and visits to the physical therapist. Most effects were moderate at posttest assessment and smaller at follow-up. No effects were found for range of motion and functional tasks. Conclusion: the program seems to be effective to change behavioral as well as health variables in a desired direction. Currently, the program is disseminated and implemented in The Netherlands.

The effects of Ageing Well and Healthy, a health educational and exercise program for elderly people

Marijke Hopman-Rock Marja H. Westhoff

Purpose: to evaluate the effects of the Ageing Well and Healthy (AWH) program on the health and physical activity of Dutch elderly people. Ageing Well consists of health education by peers and a low-intensity exercise program. Method: AWH was first tested in a randomized controlled trial (n=2x25) and after that in a semi controlled longitudinal (pre-test, post-test, and follow-up) study in 400 people (control group n=156) of 65 years and older in eight different municipalities in the Netherlands. All participants were interviewed using standardized questionnaires including questions about physical activity and health (behavior). In the RCT physiological variables were measured (blood pressure, etc). Using regression-analyses, a model of behavioural determinants was tested including attitude, subjective norm, barriers, behavioural intention, and self-efficacy. Results Positive effects were found on knowledge (effect size 0.78). In women the Body Mass Index and blood glucose level was decreased (effect sizes 1.0 and 0.62). In the least active people blood pressure was lowered (effect size –0.55). AWH met the expectations of the participants. The AWH program had positive effects on the perceived health of the participants (energy/fatigue, bodily pain, and perceived change in health) but these positive effects failed to remain at follow-up 4 to 6 months later. Comparison with the results of a control group showed that the initial least active part of the experimental group (n=99) at follow-up had an average sportive activity level of 4.3 compared to 0.01 in the comparable part of the control group (ANOVA, group effect F=22.9, p 2-sided=0.02). Conclusion: The AWH program has beneficial effects on health and health behavior, is attractive, has low costs, and is easy accessible.

The impact of long-term moderate physical activity on functional performance, fracture prevalence and bone mineral density in aged women compared to controls

K.A. Ringsberg, P.O.Josefsson, P.Gärdsell, O.Johnell, I. Sernbo

The positive effects of exercise on bone mineral density, prevention of falls and fractures are well known. The aim of this study was to investigate the effects of long-term moderate physical activity on functional performance, fracture prevalence and bone mineral density in aged women comparing rural and urban age-matched women. 139 women (65 to 89 years of age) who during the last 20 years regularly and at least one hour a week participated in different groups for physical exercise were recruited from the city of Malmö, Sweden. These women were compared to two age-matched groups of controls, 139 urban women and 88 rural women. All controls were randomly selected. All patients answered a written questionnaire about their social and medical background. We analysed the fracture incidence and bone mineral density and made functional tests as muscle strength, balance, gait velocity, step length, vibration threshold. There were no difference in background factors as height, work load, milk consumption, age at menarche, number of pregnancies and smoking habits between the activity group and the urban and rural control groups. But significant differences were found in weight, alcohol consumption, help in daily activity, walking aids, health estimation and in all functional tests. Fracture incidence was significant higher in the urban group compared to the activity and rural group. No differences were found in bone mineral density between the groups. Physical active elderly women have better functional performance, lower fracture prevalence, less help in daily living and higher health estimation.

Weighted belt exercise for old women with hip fracture

N. Lindelöf, H Littbrand (Geriatric Clinic, Umeå University Hospital, Umeå, Sweden), B. Lindström, L. Nyberg (Dept. of Community Medicine and Rehabilitation, sections of Physiotherapy and Geriatric Medicine, Umeå University, Umeå, Sweden)

PURPOSE: To investigate the possibility of increasing lower limb strength, balance, and gait speed in frail older women with remaining mobility problems after hip fracture by means of a combined functional training programme with a weighted belt. METHOD: Three women aged 78-82 participated in this repeated single-subject experimental design study. They all had completed conventional rehabilitation for their hip fractures. The intervention was a functional weight-bearing exercise class performed twice a week during nine weeks. A weighted belt was used to provide additional weight loading during exercises. Isometric muscle strength was measured with a strain gauge, dynamic balance was assessed using the Step test, and gait velocity was measured over 15 meters. RESULTS: Graphical analyses showed substantial improvements of dynamic balance and gait speed, related to the intervention, in all three subjects. From end of baseline to end of intervention, gait speed improved by 16%Δ38% and Step test performance by 36%Δ67%. The subjects also increased their training intensity during the period, weight load increased by 25Δ80%. No progress was seen, however, regarding isometric knee extension muscle strength, and the control variable, hand grip strength, remained unchanged. CONCLUSION: Functional training with a weighted belt may be suitable for older women to alleviate mobility problems after hip fracture.

SESSION 50

Changing Aged Care Nursing Practice Through Research

Barbara Bowers (University of Wisconsin, Madison, Wisconsin,

USA) David Zimmerman (University of Wisconsin, Madison, Wisconsin, USA) (The Relationship Between Staffing and Quality in Long Term Care) Michael. R Nolan (University of Sheffield, Sheffield, UK) (Working with family carers: What is the basis for practice?) Susan. H Koch (La Trobe University, Melbourne, Australia) (Restraint Free Care. Is it possible?) Susie Lum (Institute of Advanced Nursing Studies, Hospital Authority Hong Kong, Kowloon. Hong Kong) Daniel Lo (Institute of Advanced Nursing Studies, Hospital Authority Hong Kong, Kowloon. Hong Kong) ("The history, development and future directions of geriatric nursing education in Hong Kong")

Issue: Increasing the research base of nursing practice in aged care. Structure: The session will involve an introduction by the Chair to set the context, followed by a presentation by each of four speakers covering relevant research in the US, UK, Australia and Asia. Audience dialogue with the panel will then be encouraged. Content: Nursing practices in aged care have been developing over recent years and examples of innovations and creative responses to long time challenges abound. Nevertheless, the extent to which practice is informed by research is not great. There are many reasons as to why practice is so often not informed by the best available evidence or indeed by any research. One reason is that insufficient research has been undertaken in the relevant areas; another is the difficulty many practitioners have in accessing, interpreting and implementing research findings. This symposium seeks to address both of these obstacles. It will highlight international research in the areas of workforce and quality, family roles in aged care, challenging practice issues and educational innovations. The integrating theme across the papers will be that of increasing the research base so each paper will preent the evidence but also illuminate how practitioners can utilise the findings in everyday practice. Conclusion/Anticipated outcomes: The anticipated outcomes for this session include increased awareness of the research being undertaken in vital areas of aged care; international opportunities for partnerships in research; understanding of how the research is applicable to everyday practice and identification of strategies that will facilitate utilisation of the research findings and improvements in quality outcomes for older people in long term care situations.

Restraint Free Care: Is it possible?

S H Koch (La Trobe University, Melbourne, Australia)

In 1996 there were thought to be about 35,000 people in Victoria, Australia with dementia, a number likely to increase to around 49,500 by the year 2011. Residential care facilities have seen an increase in the number of residents diagnosed with dementia and increased dependency levels. The changing demographics of older people in residential care facilities brings with it new care issues for nursing staff. Following two major studies undertaken by La Trobe University Gerontic Nursing Professorial Unit, the Alzheimer's Association of Australia and Alzheimer's Association of Victoria into restraint use on older people, and the abuse of older people with dementia and their carers, the outcomes of both studies indicated there was a need for nurses to change their practice. The projects provided evidence of alternative measures to the use of restraints in aged care facilities in Australia and strategies to be implemented in the prevention of abuse of older people with dementia. Nurses have a responsibility to ensure individual rights are upheld and quality care is provided. Changes to practice in restraint use and the abuse of older people with dementia is an important area of nursing practice that requires addressing. This paper will discuss how provision of best practice models can be implemented in residential care facilities to reduce the incidence of restraint use and abuse of older people with dementia.

The history, development and future directions of geriatric nursing education in Hong Kong

Susie Lum (Institute of Advanced Nursing Studies, Hospital Authority Hong Kong, Kowloon. Hong Kong) Daniel Lo (Institute of Advanced Nursing Studies, Hospital Authority Hong Kong, Kowloon. Hong Kong)

During the past fifteen years, geriatric service in Hong Kong has developed from a single geriatric unit in one regional hospital to at least one unit in all of the regional hospitals while hospital-based community geriatric assessment teams have been set up since 1994. Despite the fact that geriatric content was incorporated into the curriculum of pre-registration nursing training as one of the four specialty training for student nurses, there is an ongoing need to strengthen geriatric nursing as an area of specialization. This paper examines the development of post-registration geriatric nursing training as well as the establishment of Geriatric Nurse Specialists in Hong Kong. It argues that the nurse specialist would be able to demonstrate knowledge of rehabilitation, clinical assessment, health care assessment, knowledge of ageing processes including psycho-social perspectives, research utilization, undertaking research, pharmacology, patient-centredness and humanistic caring. With this end in view, this paper further describes strategies that might be used to achieve meaningful gains and demonstrable outcomes from the contribution of the geriatric nurse specialist practice to work towards developing user focused, outcome driven, practice based developments in geriatric nursing in Hong Kong.

The Relationship Between Staffing and Quality in Long Term Care

Barbara Bowers (University of Wisconsin, Madison, Wisconsin, USA) David Zimmerman (University of Wisconsin, Madison, Wisconsin, USA)

The purpose of this presentation is to provide an overview of research related to the staffing/quality interaction, to describe the range of ways in which the question has been approached, the findings reported from this research, and to describe the implications of such research for determining staffing in long term care settings. Efforts to monitor and enhance the quality of care in nursing homes are underway in several countries. Among the many quality issues frequently raised is the relationship between staffing and the quality of care. Although research is still insufficient to make definitive recommendations about how both the level and organization of staffing are related, recent research suggests that both the level and organization of staffing are related to the quality of care The authors will examine the quality-staffing relationship from both quantitative and qualitative perspectives . They will also present and discuss research they are currently engaging in related to the roles and relationships among staff and the implications for quality of, and the role of resident, family, and staff expectations in that relationship

Working with family carers: What is the basis for practice?

M R Nolan (University of Sheffield, Sheffield, UK)

Countries throughout the developed world are pursuing a policy of community care in order to maintain as many older people as possible within their own homes. The success of such a policy relies in large measure on the support provided to older people by family (informal) carers. Determining the best ways in which formal service systems can augment the efforts of family carers is therefore an important consideration. This paper will provide a conceptual synthesis of models of working with family carers with a particular emphasis on an empowering, partnership approach. Consideration will be given to the implications of adopting a partnership model on: the relationship between professionals, family carers and cared-for persons; assessment and intervention frameworks; indicators of outcome and success and methods of evaluation. The paper is cast within a temporal model, focusing on the most appropriate forms of support at key transition points within the caregiving career. It also raises fundamental questions about the nature of evidence, the possession of expertise, and the potential tensions between the various participants in the caregiving enterprise.

SESSION 51

Bone and Aging: An alert for Osteoporosis

Masako Ito (Dep. of Radiology, Nagasaki University School of Medicine, Nagasaki, Japan),What is aged bone? -Morphometric view of bone-, E. Schacht (Metabolic Bone Disease Unit, University Clinic Balgrist, Zurich, Switzerland), How do Alfacalcidol reduce fractures?, Tatsuhiko Tanizawa (Department of Orthopedic Surgery, Shinrakuen Hospital), Prevention of Bone Fracture by Alfacalcidol, A Retrospective Study, J.B.Lauritzen (Hip Clinic & Traumatology, Department of Orthopedic Surgery, Hvidovre Hospital, University of Copenhagen, Demmark), EFFECT OF SAFEHIP PROTECTORS IN NURSING HOME RESIDENTS AND ELDERLY ORTHOPEDIC PATIENTS.

This symposium will address current issue on Osteoporosis, which is probably the most widely known bone disorder affecting many people, the majority undiagnosed or untreated. The risk for Osteoporosis is cumulative with aging particularly in elderly woman, increasing 2-4 times in their lifetimes with a consequence of menopause. As the numbers of elderly persons increase, this brings them high risk for bone fracture with being bedridden for the rest of their lives, and also results in morbidity, mortality and associated economic costs. The focus of this session is bone and aging, particularly the risk and status of osteoporosis and hip fractures in elderly population. The first presentation will show the bone change associated with menopause or aging evaluated by micro-CT. The micro-CT is a special CT apparatus for scanning bone with high resolution. In this presentation, a stress distribution in bone will also be visualized. The next presentation will discuss the bone and aging from the physiological point of view, especially about the relationship between bone fracture and D-hormone. Alfacalcidol, a synthesized active D-hormone regulates bone remodeling, improving bone quality and prevention of falls and reducing bone fractures. This presentation will show the recent finding of alfacalcidol and its mode of action on muscle power which is unique and differentiate this form of therapy from all other antiosteoporotic drugs which all have no influence on falls. The third presentation will report the reduction of hip fracture by treatment with vitamin D metabolites and with combined therapy. The clinical study is the retrospective study in which the medeical records were inspected for the entire population over 65 yeas of age on Sado island where their life style and envioronmental factors are uniform and followed a total of 11,377 women for a 3-year period. Of these, 1,208 osteoporotic patients were treated either caocitoriol or alfacalcidol. This treatment with active vitamin D metabolites and with combined therapy showed marginally effective in preventing hip fractures and stopping the treatment clearly increased the risk of hip fractures. The last presentation will show the effective reduction of hip fracture by hip protection system, SAFEHIP in randomized three trials. These trials have revealed that SAFEHIP protectors is effective against hip fractures among nursing home residents and home dwellers, besides they seem cost-effective. The session will outline the risk and status of osteoporosis, and hip fractures increasing with aging. We are proposing an alert for osteoporosis that we should care "bone" with nutritionally balanced diet and an effective exercise, and if diagnosed as osteoporosis, we should prevent bone loss and falls with appropriate treatment. Alfacalcidol regulates bone remodeling and prevents falls, and SAFEHIP protectors reduce hip fractures with falls and these effective treatments for osteoporosis will improve the quality of life and become cost saving.

Effect of Safehip Protectors in Nursing Home Residents and Elderly Orthopedic Patients

Jes Bruun Lauritzen MD (Hip Clinic & Traumatology, Department of Orthopedic Surgery, Hvidovre Hospital, University of Copenhagen, Demmark)

SAFEHIP is the first clinical documented hip protector (see "Report on Osteoporosis in the EC-action for Prevention 1998", and Cachrane review 1999). Nursing homes SAFEHIP has been studied in three randomized in three trials. The Ekman study used copies of SAFEHIP. No of hfx / subjects Hip fix avoided Study Follow-up(mths) Intervention Control RR 95%CL No Lauritzen et al 1993 Lancet 11 8/247 31/418 0.44 0.20-0.95 10 Ekman et al 1997 Lancet 11 4/302 17/442 0.34 0.12-1. 0 7 Harada et al 2001 In press 19 1/65 8/68 0.13 - 5 Home dwellers Our controlled case cohort study among elderly orthopedic in-patients had follow-up 1 to 11/ 2 year; n 1590 (Hindso & Lauritzen, 2001). Users reported 143 falls with impact on the hip protector, and no fractures occurred. Two hip fractures occurred while the patients wore protectors, but no impact on the hip was reported. Adherence at two years was 40%. A subgroup consisted of 1,170 elderly orthopedic patients with fall or fracture. Intervention: 711 and controls: 459. The annual rate of hip fracture in controls was 5.4%. Primary acceptance was 60%. Intention to treat analysis: adjusted relative risk (RR) was 0.89 (0.52-1.5). For those still possessing protectors including seldom use to every day use (n 256) the adjusted RR was 0.71, (0.37-1.4). For those who used protectors often or every day the non-adjusted RR was 0.43, $p<0.05$ (n 131). Discussion The SAFEHIP protectors have been documented effective against hip fractures among nursing home residents and home dwellers, besides they seem cost-saving.

How Does Alfacalcidol Reduce Fractures?

E. Schacht (Metabolic Bone Disease Unit, University Clinic Balgrist, Zurich, Switzerland)

Osteoporosis is a multifactorial disease characterized by low bone mineral density (BMD), decreased bone quality and increased risk of falls. Established osteoporosis in older patients of both sexes is characterized by decoupled bone remodeling induced by sex hormone deficits and by a somatopause, but also by lack of vitamin D and, very important, by reduced synthesis of D-Hormone (Calcitriol; 1,25 (OH)2D) in kidneys and bone as well as by a lack of receptors and/or receptor affinity for D-Hormone in the target organs. As consequences of these facts there are an endocrine increase of parathormone (PTH) and a paracrine decrease of Transforming Growth Factor [TGF]-s. Parallel to the decreased bone strength there happen a loss of muscle power and an increasing risk of "intrinsic", nonsyncopal falls. It was shown a positive correlation between D-Hormone levels in serum and the proximal muscle power in the legs of elderly. These facts explain that in D-Hormone deficient patients the hip fracture risk is increased by factor 2. In Alfacalcidol therapy, D-Hormone is provided to the body in circumvention of its own regulation, by means of which much higher hormone concentrations can be achieved in the target tissues than by administration of plain vitamin D. In vitro and in vivo there is evidence that D-Hormon-Analogs normalize PTH, increase number and activity of osteoblasts, directly inhibit osteoclasts, and normalize the "high bone turnover" in the elderly osteoporotic patients ("supercoupling"). In addition it has been shown that D-Hormone-Analogs are able to increase muscle power and walking distance in elderly D-Hormone deficient patients. Besides of the known effects on vertebral fracture rate there are new clinical data confirming that D-Hormon-Analogs are reducing peripheral fractures by reducing falls. Summary: Alfacalcidol has multifactorial effects. By regulating bone remodeling, improving bone quality and prevention of falls Alfacalcidol reduces fractures. The mode of action on muscle power is unique and differentiate this form of therapy from all other antiosteoporotic drugs, which all have no influence on falls.

Preventive effects of active vitamin D metabolites and concurrent treatments in hip fractures

T. Tanizawa MD (Department of Orthopedic Surgery, Shinrakuen Hospital, Niigata, Japan)

Active vitamin D has been widely used to treat osteoporosis in Japan for the last twenty years, however its effect in preventing hip fractures is not well understood. The purpose of this study was to determine the effect of treatment with active vitamin D metabolites and other concurrent medication on the prevention of hip fractures in elderly women. We inspected the medical records of the entire female population over 65 years of age on Sado Island, and followed a total of 11,377 women for a three-year period. Of these, 1,208 osteoporotic patients were treated with either 1,25-(OH)2D3 or 1a-(OH)D3. The 765 patients who received the minimum effective dosage for more than six months made up the "treatment group". Nearly half of these patients were also treated with either elcatonin or calcium. The 443 patients who received treatment with active vitamin D metabolites, but at a dosage or for a duration that did not meet the criteria for the treatment group, were deemed the "ineffective group". The remaining 10,169 women were the "non-treatment group". Fractures in the non-treatment group occurred at a rate of 39.8 fractures/10,000 person years. The rate in the treatment group was 10.8, which was significantly lower ($p = 0.039$). Interestingly, the fracture rate after ceasing treatment was 52.1, which was significantly higher ($p = 0.002$) than the rate in patients receiving treatment. No statistical differences in the fracture rate were found between the ineffective, non-treatment and post-treatment groups. A reduction in the fracture rate was only observed in the treatment subgroup that did not also receive calcitonin ($p = 0.042$), and not in the subgroup that also received calcitonin therapy ($p = 0.333$). However, there was no statistical difference in the hip fracture rates between these two subgroups ($p = 0.157$) and the actual number of fractures was minimal (0 vs. 2). Therefore, in this study, the advantage of single treatment with active vitamin D over combined treatment with calcitonin seems to be marginal. In conclusion: 1) treatment with active vitamin D metabolites and with combined therapy may be effective in preventing hip fractures, and 2) stopping the treatment clearly increases the risk of hip fractures.

What is aged bone? Morphometric view of bone

Masako Ito (Dep. of Radiology, Nagasaki University School of Medicine, Nagasaki, Japan)

A decrease of bone mass with advancing age is a natural course in adults. However, when bone loss is accelerated beyond the physiological loss associated with menopause or aging to induce bone fragility, such a pathological loss of bone is a disorder called osteoporosis. Osteoporosis is accompanied with not only the decrease of bone mineral content but also the deterioration of bone microstructure. Established methods for analyzing microstructure indicate that cancerous bone loss in the elderly is associated with progressive reduction in the connectivity of the trabecular network, as well as change of trabeculae from plate-like to rod-like. The disconnection may explain the increased skeletal fragility. Using micro-CT, a special CT apparatus for scanning bone samples in the resolution of the level of 20 micrometer, we analyzed the age-related change of bone microstructure, and analyzed the relationship of the deterioration of microstructure with bone strength. We also evaluated the effect of medication such as alfacalcidol, bisphosphonate, PTH, and vitamin K2 both on the bone mass and microstructure for the preventing of fragility fracture. In the symposium, I will present the bone change associated with menopause or aging in vivo and in vitro, and I will give a clear and striking visual presentation of the age-related change of microstructure, such as the thinning and disappearance of the trabeculae, and a visualization of the stress distribution when the bone is loaded.

SESSION 52

Courage to Dream

Joy Coghill (Vancouver, British Columbia, Canada)

"A Midsummer Night's Dream" (Shakespeare) with actors who are sixty plus? Here is a look into the experiment that created "Western Gold" a Canadian company that attacks ageism in the market place and creates a showcase for senior professional actors. Meet trailblazer Joy Coghill and noted British director and actress Denise Coffey

SESSION 53

Clinical, Ethical, and Legal Dilemmas in Assessing Competency: Assessor as Advocate or Adversary

M. Bay (Chair & CEO, Ontario Consent and Capacity Board, Toronto, Canada), H.M.R. Meier, MB, ChB, FRCP(C), (Head, Geriatric Psychiatry Program, Mount Sinai Hospital, Toronto, Canada), Ethical and Legal Dilemmas; S. Marr, FRCP(C), (Regional Geriatric Program, Eastern Service Area, Toronto, Canada) Clinical Dilemmas.

This round table addresses the need for health care providers to increase their knowledge and skills in evaluating competencies of high-risk elderly persons. Based on case study and interdisciplinary presentations, the focus is on legal, ethical and clinical dilemmas that need to be addressed in assessing competency. This will include a discussion with presenters and participants. Handouts of presentations and bibliography will be provided. Knowledge of the areas of conflict encountered by health care professionals when assessing competency will be presented. Legal aspects, ethical framework and clinical skills will be reviewed as they relate to assessing competencies. The benefits of interdisciplinary contributions will be demonstrated. A pragmatic framework for clinical practice will be outlined. Strategies to resolve conflicting roles for the clinician and strategies to assist the clinician to continue an ongoing working relationship with the patient will be addressed. Participants will increase knowledge of the multiple factors involved in assessing competencies and acquire skills in performing comprehensive assessments of competency.

SESSION 54

[1] Tau protein of oral epithelium increases in Alzheimer's disease

Hideyuki Hattori, Masayuki Matsumoto, Hiroshi Tsuchiya, Kunimitsu Iwai, Eiji Miyauchi, Mikihiro Takasaki, Kouzin Kamino, Junichi Munehira, Yasuhiro Kimura, Kenichi Munehira, Tomoko Hoshino, Hiroshi Murai, Hajime Ogata, Hidemichi Maruyama [Department of Geriatric Medicine, Kanazawa Medical University] Hiroshi Yoshida [Diagnostic Department of R&D Center, NISSHO Corporation]

PURPOSE: Alzheimer's disease (AD) is the one of the most important diseases in an aged society like Japan, Europe and USA. A non-invasive approach is desirable for the diagnosis of AD. We detected and measured the tau protein of the oral epithelium for testing its applicability for diagnosis. METHOD: Oral epithelium was exfoliated from patients with 32 AD or 29 vascular dementia (VD), and 34 young and 33 age-matched controls. Western blot was performed for determining the molecular weight of oral tau protein. Tau protein in the cerebrospinal fluid (CSF) was measured for comparison in 29 cases among those whose oral epithelium tau protein was detected. ELIZA kit for CSF was used for determining oral tau protein. RESULTS: Western blot detected a band at 65 kDa and 110kDa each. Tau protein level in oral epithelia showed a significant positive correlation with those in the CSF($p<0.05$). The patients with AD had significantly higher levels of tau protein than the patients with VD and the controls ($p<0.01$). In patients with AD, the tau protein level were not correlated with mini mental state examination (MMSE), but patients with younger age-at-onset showed a higher level of the tau protein than patients with later age-at-onset ($p<0.05$). CONCLUSION: The tau protein in oral epithelium reflected the pathological changes as well as CSF tau. The concentration of the oral tau in AD was shown high and it seemed to be elevated from early childhood. Thus the measurement of the oral tau might be useful for screening test of AD.

[2] What is the Relationship Between Hypertension and Its Treatment in Alzheimer's Disease

W.E. DeCoteau,K. Dolgopol,F.Dudzic, A. Wilkinson (Department

of Medicine,Geriatrics, and Nuclear Medicine, University of Saskatchewan, College of Medicine, Saskatoon, Saskatchewan, Canada)

Several years ago our group commenced doing single photon emission computerized tomography (SPECT) scans on patients with chronic dementia of the Alzheimer type. We have now studied over 200 cases. In our hands, the procedure has not been very useful re: diagnosis since 20% of demented persons had a normal scan while in another 15% the changes were non-specific. Many patients did show the classic temporo-parietal pattern of Alzheimer disease, while a significant number showed the patchy pattern suggestive of vascular damage. Interestingly, this latter group basically did not differ clinically from the Alzheimer group. In particular, they did not show a so-called step-like deterioration. However, they were more likely to be hypertensive or to have a history of hypertension than were those with a classic Alzheimer scan. Therefore, this study would seem to confirm this suggestion of others that hypertension and vascular damage are important in the pathogenesis of Alzheimer disease. However, it is disturbing and provocative that control of blood pressure in one previously severely hypertensive patient normalized the SPECT scan, but was also associated with marked worsening of dementia. Thus, it appears that there is still much to be learned about the apparent association of hypertension and Alzheimer dementia. In the meantime, we urge that the treatment of markedly hypertensive elderly patients be carried out with caution.

[3] Percutaneous endoscopic gastrostomy in old patients with dementia

C. Fernandez-Viadero, N. Peña (Nursing Home for the Aged, Health & Social Welfare Service. Cantabria. Spain), M Jimenez-Sanz (Nutrition Unit, Valdecilla University Hospital, Cantabria, Spain), R. Verduga, D. Crespo (Department of Anatomy and Cell Biology, Cantabria University, Cantanbria, Spain)

To assess the advantages of use percutaneous endoscopic gastrostomy over other enteral nutrition systems. Special attention was focussed in the use of physical restrains and on the survival period after the gastrostomy procedure. METHOD: Longitudinal observational prospective study in our skilled facilited nursing home (260 beds) RESULTS: 28 patients (27 females and one male), average age of 87.3 + 5.8 years old, 14 patients have Alzheimer-type dementia. The use of physical restrain was unnecessary in all patients (0%) after gastrostomy procedure. Before, with nasoenteric-tube feeding, physical restrain was necessary in 81% (21 of 26 patients). The total observation time was 15264 days (36 to 1278 days). The overall mean survival time after gastrostomy at the end observation period was 545 days. Ten patients dead during the study, the mortality rate was 0% at 30 days after the procedure, and 11% at 90 days. CONCLUSION: The change from classic forms of enteral nutrition to percutaneous endoscopic gastrostomy in patients with dementia showed that physical restrain was not necessary, and the procedure shows for many patients a long period of survival.

[4] Environmental Conditions Associated With Agitated Behavior Among Demented Patients.

J. Aubert, C. Brochu, J. Vézina, P. Landreville, G. Primeau, S. Imbeault, C. Laplante (School of Psychology, University Laval, Quebec, Canada)

Physical and verbal agitation among institutionalized elders is a main concern for caretakers. Although the frequency of this behavior is high, the "sources" of those behaviors still remain unclear. The aim of this study is a better understanding of the environmental elements associated with the expression of this type of behavior. 15 demented patients living in a long-term care facility, showing physical agitation behavior (PAB) and verbal agitation behavior (VAB) were directly observed with an handheld computer for nearly 180 hours. The recorded observations include the frequency and duration of the agitation behavior as well as the environmental information related to the physical environment, the presence of other people, the current activities, the use of physical restraint and the time of day. Each participant was observed for 12 hours between 8 am and 8pm. PAB and VAB were respectively present 29.1% and 12% of the time. PAB was mostly displayed when patients were in their room (56.5%), not engaged in any particular activity (85.3%), were alone (54.8%) and restraint (58%). VAB was mostly displayed when patients were in their room (91.7%), not engaged in any particular activity (80.7%), were alone (79.3%) and restraint (74.4%). Agitated behavior, particularly VAB, was irregularly distributed over time. PAB was mostly observed between 3pm and 7pm (50.5%) and VAB mostly occurred between 2pm and 4pm (27.2%). More specific results were also found, indicating that certain contextual factors influence the onset of agitated behavior. (Research Funded by the Social Sciences and Humanities Research Council)

[5] Anatomofunctional approach of limb apraxia in corticobasal degeneration : an fMRI study

O. Beauchet, MD; P. Giraux, MD; F. Schneider, MD; R. Peyron, MD; F. Barral, PhD; R. Gonthier, PhD; D. Michel, PhD; B. Laurent, PhD.

PURPOSE: To determining the role of cortical and subcortical lesions in charge for limb apraxia in corticobasal degeneration (CBD, we have studied brain activity associated with sequential fingers self-paced movements while using multislice echoplanar fMRI. METHOD: Four right-handed patients aged 55-76 years (mean 64.5 years) with an upper limb apraxia compatible with a diagnosis of CBD were studied. We used an event related experimental design based on the alternation of short activation periods defined by finger self-paced movement of the right or left hand starting from an oral order (5,341 seconds) and long rest periods (21,364 seconds). Because of the marked asymmetry of clinical signs in the population studied, we used the clinical healthy side like condition controls. Functional MR images were acquired using a 1 Tesla Siemens Impact which equipped with echoplanar imaging (EPI). Data analysis was performed using the Statistical Parametric Map (SPM99)software. RESULTS: On the pathological side, activation was more significant in term of cortical surfaces, size, clusters and relating variation of signal except in cerebellum. The data also showed a reorganization of brain activity whatever the type of sequence. A weak activation was noted in controlateral premotor cortex in particular of the median part. The activation of the higher BA 5 and 7)and inferior parietal BA 39 and 40)cortex was more significant and prevail on the pathological side. A occipital activity BA 18 and 19) was also distinguished. Finally a strong participation of the prefrontal and cingulum cortex was recorded. CONCLUSION: The deficit of premotor activity seems to confirm the assumption of a preferential attack of this cerebral area in CBD. The parietal activity and the modifications which are associated pleads for a cerebral plasticity based on neuronal recruitment.

[6] Corpus callosum and Alzheimer's disease

A. Garnica, P. Gil Gregorio, N. Montero Fernández, P. López-Riquelme and J.M Ribera Casado (Servicio de Geriatria,hospital clinico San Carlos, Madrid, Spain); J.Arrazola Garcia and M. Tapia Viñé (Servicio de Radiodiagnóstico, Hospital Clinico San Carlos, Madrid, Spain).

PURPOSE:To evaluate the relationship between corpus callosum and its different regions to clinical diagnosis of Alzheimer´s disease (AD) using a magnetic resonance imaging (MRI) analysis. METHODS:A Quantitative Magnetic Resonance study was carried out in four patients with AD (meeting NINCSD-ADRDA criteria) and three age-matched non-demented subjects (ND). Total cross-sectional area and areas of five callosal subregions (AI,AII,AIII,AIV and AV) as well as cranial area were measured (mm2) from a mid-sagittal MRI slice. Neuropsychological variables collected were: CAMCOG and MMSE. Subjects were classified in stages by Functional Assessment Stages scale (FAST). Mann-Whitney test was used to analyse data. RESULTS: AD: mean age 75.5 (6.81); MMSE 18.75 (7.8); CAMCOG 55.75 (8.88); FAST 5 (0.82) and non-demented subjects: mean age 74 (3.61); MMSE 29.33 (1.15); CAMCOG 76 (10); FAST

2.67 (0.58). Mean subregional area measurements on both AD and ND showed no significant difference between the two groups. Mean callosal length and height in AD sample: 74.50 (2.08); 27.50 (3.87) and in non-demented subjects 77.33 (5.03); 28 (3.60) had no significant correlations with diagnosis. A new variable was created relating total callosal area (TCA): AD 590.50 (53.86); ND 692 (141.20) with cranial area: AD 14318 (1111.19); ND 14482 (652.61). Although it was observed a smaller proportion (TCA/CRA)*100 in AD sample (4.15%) than in non-demented group (4.77%) no significant difference was found. CONCLUSION:We conclude that in our group there was no difference between AD and ND groups in measurements of corpus callosal, perhaps due to the small number of patients of the sample.

[7] Further study on the efficacy of Reinhardt and Sea Cucumber capsule (R.S.C.) to treat age-associated memory impairment by double blind trial method in 117 cases

Wang Chuan-Fu, Ma Yong-Xing, Xie Su-Zhen (Department of Aging & Antiaging and Cognitive Function, Shanghai Institute of Gerontology and Geriatrics, Huadong Hospital, Shanghai,China)

Objective: To study the efficacy of Reinhardt and Sea Cucumber Capsule (R.S.C, Sea animal products) to treat dementia in the aged. Methods: Double blind trials were performed in 108 cases of dementia (R.S.C. 58, VD22, AD 31, VD+AD 5; placebo 50, VD 29, AD18, VD+AD 3) in the aged with MMSE. The dosage of R.S.C. and placebo were all 6 capsules (0.28g/cap) for 3 months. The effects were evaluated with MMSE, HDS and MQ(WMS). Results: MMSE increment, R.S.C. 2.880 ± 0.390, placebo 1.780 ± 0.345 ($P<0.001$). Total effective rate, R.S.C. 53.44%, placebo 28.0% ($P<0.001$) HDS increment, R.S.C. 2.450 ± 1.449, placebo 1.070 ± 1.626 ($P<0.001$) Total effective rate, R.S.C. 53.44%; placebo 30.0% ($P<0.05$). MQ increment, R.S.C. 4.190 ± 3.420; placebo 1.500 ± 3.975 ($P<0.001$); Total effective rate, R.S.C. 44.83%; placebo 20.0% ($P<0.05$). Similar effects were observed in VD and AD with slightly better results in VD. No signiicant side effects were observed. The mechanism of R.S.C. to improve cognitive function in the demented may be related to its effects to enhance neuron growth, to increase acetylcholine and to decrease glutamine level in the brain, as confirmed in cell and animal experiment, and to improve free radical metabolism and microcirculatory state confirmed clinically. Conclusions: R.S.C. is effective and safe to treat dementia (AD&VD) in the elderly.

[8] Clinical study on the efficacy of Reinhardt and Sea Cucumber capsule (R.S.C.) to treat dementia in the aged by double blind trial method in 108 cases

Wang Chuan-Fu, Ma Yong-Xing, Gu Yue-Di (Department of Aging, Antiaging and Cognitive Function, Shanghai Institute of Gerontology and Geriatrics, Huadong Hospital, Shanghai,China)

Objective: To study the efficacy of Reinhardt and Sea Cucumber Capsule (R.S.C, Sea animal products) to treat dementia in the aged. Methods: Double blind trials were performed in 108 cases of dementia (R.S.C. 58, VD22, AD 31, VD+AD 5; placebo 50, VD 29, AD18, VD+AD 3) in the aged with MMSE. The dosage of R.S.C. and placebo were all 6 capsules (0.28g/cap) for 3 months. The effects were evaluated with MMSE, HDS and MQ(WMS). Results: MMSE increment, R.S.C. 2.880 ± 0.390, placebo 1.780 ± 0.345 ($P<0.001$). Total effective rate, R.S.C. 53.44%, placebo 28.0% ($P<0.001$) HDS increment, R.S.C. 2.450 ± 1.449, placebo 1.070 ± 1.626 ($P<0.001$) Total effective rate, R.S.C. 53.44%; placebo 30.0% ($P<0.05$). MQ increment, R.S.C. 4.190 ± 3.420; placebo 1.500 ± 3.975 ($P<0.001$); Total effective rate, R.S.C. 44.83%; placebo 20.0% ($P<0.05$). Similar effects were observed in VD and AD with slightly better results in VD. No significant side effects were observed. The mechanism of R.S.C. to improve cognitive function in the demented may be related to its effects to enhance neuron growth, to increase acetylcholine and to decrease glutamine level in the brain, as confirmed in cell and animal experiment, and to improve free radical metabolism and microcirculatory state confirmed clinically. Conclusions: R.S.C. is effective and safe to treat dementia (AD&VD) in the elderly.

[9] Efficacy of Risperidone vs. Promazine in the Treatment of Behavioral Disorders in Elderly Demented Patients

P. Gareri, M. Curcio, A. Cotroneo**, U. Falconi, G. Seminara, G. De Sarro Chair of Pharmacology, Department of Experimental and Clinical Medicine "G. Salvatore", Policlinico Materdomini, University of Catanzaro; * Casa di Cura S. Vincenzo, Catanzaro; Medicine Unit, Ospedale "Maria Vittoria", Torino Italy*

The aim of this double-blind study was to evaluate the efficacy and safety of risperidone vs. promazine in the treatment of behavioral disorders in elderly patients (pts) with dementia. Pts were required to be 65 years or older, to have DSM-IV diagnoses of Alzheimer's disease, vascular dementia or a combination of both. 40 demented pts, 18 men and 22 women were selected for this study. UCLA Neuropsychiatric Inventory Scale was administered at baseline, 4 and 8 weeks; pts included had at least a score of 24 or more. The Hoehn and Yahr Scale was used for evaluating parkinsonism. After a wash-out period of 10 days, 20 pts, 9 men and 11 women, mean age 76.6 ± 6.0 years old, were randomly assigned to risperidone 1mg daily in divided doses (morning and bedtime) (group A) and 20 pts, 9 men and 11 women, mean age 77.6 ± 4.6 years old, were randomly assigned to promazine 50 mg daily (morning and bedtime) (group B). In case of lack of clinical response, after 4 weeks, dose could be increased to 2 mg/day of risperidone in group A and to 100 mg/day of promazine in group B. Repeated measures analysis of variance (ANOVA) was used for statistical analysis. A good response to the drugs was defined as the reduction of at least 50% of NPI score from baseline at 4 and 8 weeks; a partial response was defined as the reduction of NPI score inferior to 50% at 4 and 8 weeks compared to baseline. A good response to risperidone was obtained in 14 of 20 pts (70%), 6 men and 8 women; a partial response was present in 3 pts (15%) and no response was present in 2 pts. In 1 pt of female sex, the administration of the drug was interrupted at 4 weeks because of hypotension and confusion. A good response to promazine was present in 13 pts (65%), 7 men and 6 women, whilst no response was present in 7 pts (35%). Therefore, a global improvement was obtained in 85% of pts treated with risperidone vs. 65% of pts treated with promazine ($p< 0.01$). The main results were obtained on agitation, aggression and wandering. It has an efficacy either comparable or even superior to promazine, with significantly fewer side effects, since anticholinergic effects and consequent cognitive worsening are not present at the indicated dosages

[10] Influence of C-reactive protein on cognition and mobility scores

Gosch M, Talasz H, Benvenuti-Falger U, Rhomberg H.P. (Landeskrankenhaus Hochzirl Hochzirl 1 6170 Zirl Austria)

Purpose: to determine the influence of different serum levels of C-reactive protein on cognition and mobility scores Method: We included 829 patients, who were admitted to our geriatric assessment ward. Two of three patients were female. The mean age was 80.7. C-reactive-protein serum levels were measured by using a turbidimetric method of a Synchron CX5-system. We used the Mini-Mental-Score(MMSE) and the Clock Completion(CC) as cognition scores, the Mobility test of Tinetti and the Timed Up & Go test as mobility scores. Furthermore we included in our study the Geriatric Depression Scale (GDS) and the Activity of Daily Living. We proved the significance of the correlation by using the test of Spearman and Kandell. Results: C-reactive-protein serum levels have a significant influence on the cognitive and functional status in elderly people. The correlation coefficient was 0.193 for the test of Tinetti and 0.201 for the Timed Up & Go, -0.108 for the MMSE and 0.70 for the CC. The strongest correlation showed the ADL-Score with the coefficient of 0.271. We did not find a correlation between the GDS and C-reactive-portein serum levels. Conclusion: C-reactive protein serum levels have a significant influence on cognition and mobility scores, but the correlation is too weak to give clear recommendations for the interpretation of cognition and mobility scores in consideration of the serum level of C-reactive protein.

[11] Clinical course and treatment response in depressive

pseudodementia

D.Guerro-Prado, J.M.Barjau Romero, M.Vega Piñero, A. Cebollada Gracia, A. Chinchilla Moreno (Ramón y Cajal Hospital, Psychiatry Department, Madrid, Spain)

Purpose: the aim of the study is to search for treatment response and evolution in depressive pseudodementia patients, in order to distinguish if it´s a depressive symptomatology added to a previous cognitive dysfunction or if it could be consider as a clinical entity by itself. Method: We carried out a follow up of three years in a sample of seven patients with clinical diagnosis of depressive pseudodementia. We analyze sex, age, psychiatric antecedents, type of treatment received and response in clinical evolution at 3, 12 and 36 months. Inclusion criteria were: depressive affective symptomatology according to DSM-IV diagnostic criteria, acute/subacute cognitive deficit (inferior to 6 months), absence of estsblished demencial diagnosis and negative neuroimage results. Results: Mean age: 68,5 years; no patient presented psychiatric antecedents, the duration of depressive symptomatology was between 3 and 6 months (N=4) and 6 to 12 months (N=3). Total clinical remission at 1 and 3 years (N=1), partial remission (N=2), chronicity (N=4). The 3 patients who reached a total or partial response received electroconvulsive therapy (ECT) combined with antidepressants drugs; the rest of the sample, received antidepressive monotherapy. Conclusion: In spite of the limitations of the study, it could be consider that depressive pseudodementia is affective symptomatology in a clinical picture of incipient dementia. We consider that the lack of therapeutic response to antidepressants drugs during at least 12 months, like a clinical marker of poor prognosis, with later evolution to demential state in patients that present mixed affective-cognitive symptomatology. We consider ECT associated with antidepressants a possible first line treatment in this disorder.

[12] Effects of Nicergoline and Ticlopidine on Hemorheological Properties of Elder Patients with Cerebral Infarction

J. Hayashi, K. Watanabe, T. Takeichi, T. Fukushima, R. Makita, M. Yamamoto, K. Kitamoto (General Medicine, Kyorin University Hospital, Mitaka, Tokyo, Japan), J. Tokuue (TokorozawaChuoh Hospital, Saitama, Japan), N. Ishida (Tama Rehabilitation College, Ohme, Tokyo, Japan), H. Sato (TachikawaKyosai Hospital, Tachikawa, Tokyo, Japan)

To prevent re-attack of vascular occlusion in elder patients with cerebral infarction contributes to the improvement of patient's quality of life. The aim was to demonstrate beneficial effects of combination use of nicergoline and a low dose of ticlopidine on patients' properties of thrombogenesis and microcirculation. Fourteen patients over 65 years old with cerebral infarction were enrolled in this study. All of the patients complained of a headache or vertigo related to cerebral circulation impairment. They were orally administered nicergoline, an ergoline derivative, at a dose of 5 mg 3 times, and ticlopidine at a dose of 100 mg daily for 2 months. Hemorheological parameters, platelet aggregability and erythrocyte deformability, were measured prior to and after the drug administration. Adenosine diphosphate (ADP)-induced platelet % aggregation determined by the turbidimetric method revealed high in the patients as 86±8 %. Erythrocyte deformability determined by cell-flow micro-multi-channel method revealed marked impairment of erythrocyte deformability in the patients, showing corrected passing time of 9150±890 msec. At 2 months after the therapy, subjective symptoms such as headache and vertigo disappeared in all patients. ADP-induced platelet % aggregation was significantly lowered to 41±14 % ($p<0.05$). Corrected passing time was decreased to 4030±1120 msec ($p<0.05$), indicating significant improvement of erythrocyte deformability. These findings suggest that combination use of nicergoline and ticlopidine was effective to improve hemorheological disturbance, and may contribute to the prevention of thrombosis formation and microcirculation impairment in elder patients with cerebral infarction.

[13] Cerebral blood flow increases in Alzheimer's patients respond to donepezil treatment: A SPECT study

S. Mori, Y. Ushijima, M. Kondo, K. Nakajima (Kyoto Pref. Univ. of Med, Kyoto, Japan), H. Yoshikawa (Ohmihachiman Hospital, Shiga, Japan)

PURPOSE: Donepezil hydrochloride is a cholinergic agents and used for treatment for Alzheimer's disease. We evaluated the effects of the drug using a 123I-IMP SPECT. METHOD: Eight patients with Alzheimer's disease were administrated donepezil hydrochloride 5mg daily. Both cognitive function and cerebral blood flow (CBF) were evaluated before and three months after a treatment. Cognitive function was evaluated with Alzheimer's Disease Assessment Scale (ADAS-jcog). The patients were classified into two groups according to improvement of their cognition, responders and non-responders. CBF in each brain areas were measured by IMP-ARG method. RESULTS: In the responders, CBF was significantly increased in almost all brain areas, especially in the frontal lobe. In the non-responder, however, CBF was not significantly increased. CONCLUSION: These findings suggests that donepezil activates the brain diffusely, especially the frontal lobes in the patients with Alzheimer's disease and improves their cognitive function.

[14] Influence of HLA-DR4 on Alzheimer disease's course.

S. Moulias, S. Gillette-Guyonnet, F. Nourhashemi, G. Corte, S. Andrieu, B. Vellas (Department of Internal Medicine and Clinical Gerontology, Acute Unit for Alzheimer's patients, CHU Purpan, Toulouse, France).

Human Leukocyte Antigen DR4 (HLA-DR4) and rheumatoid arthritis (RA) were described to protect from Alzheimer disease (AD). The aims of this study were to investigate the prevalence of the HLA-DR4 gene in an AD population and in controls of the same area, and to follow the disease's course of those patients during two years, to see if there were differences between patients with HLA-DR4 and patients without it. Methods : we studied HLA-DR through PCR in 108 patients with AD, according to the NINCDS-ADRDA criteria, and 1000 controls. For each participant, weight, cognitive function (MMSE), autonomy level (ADL scale), ApoE genotype were also measured. Weight, MMSE and ADL were followed during two years. Results : HLA-DR4 did not show any protection for AD, only a tendency for a slower evolution, but not significant. Conclusion : HLA-DR4 does not seem to be responsible of the lowest rate of AD in rheumatoid arthritis population. But HLA results observed in a cohort must always be valid by others studies.

[15] Apolipoprotein E, body composition and Alzheimer disease.

S. Moulias, S. Gillette-Guyonnet, F. Nourhashemi, G. Corte, S. Andrieu, B. Vellas (Department of Internal Medicine and Clinical Gerontology, Acute Unit for Alzheimer's patients, CHU Purpan, Toulouse, France).

Apolipoprotein E allele (ApoE4) is associated with an increased risk of Alzheimer Disease (AD) and cardiovascular diseases. Moreover, the distribution of body fat mass to central abdominal sites is associated with diabetes, stroke, coronary heart disease and related mortality. The aim of this study is to investigate the association between ApoE, serum lipids, body composition and AD. Methods and patients : 67 women with probable AD according to the NINCDS-ADRDA criteria with a mean age of 78.7 years of age, were included. For each participant, weight, cognitive function (MMSE), autonomy level (ADL scale), ApoE genotype, blood lipids (triglycerides, cholesterol) and body composition by dual energy x-ray absorptiometry were measured. For 43 women, LDL, VLDL and HDL were also assessed. Patients were divided into two groups : 35 patients with genotype "E3/E4 or E4/E4" and 32 with"E3/E3". Results : There was no significant difference between the two groups regarding the mean age, the mean MMSE score, and the mean ADL score. Weight, fat mass and appendicular muscle mass were significantly higher in women with ApoE4. Cholesterol, triglycerides, LDL, VLDL and HDL concentrations were similar between the two groups. Conclusion : We found an association between fat mass and ApoE allele. Both of these parameters are risk factors for vascular diseases. Because vascular risk factors are related also with AD, the link between ApoE4 and body fat mass in our population could be one explanation of the high incidence of AD in ApoE4 patients.

[16] The Effects of Exelon in Alzheimer's Patients in Taiwan

Chih-Ta TAI and Ching-Kuan LIU (Department of Neurology, Kaohsiung Medical University, Kao-hsiung, Taiwan)

Purpose: The purpose of the present study is to evaluate the safety and efficacy of Exelon (SDZ ENA-713)in patients with probable Alzheimer's disease in Taiwan. Method: A total of 80 patients with mild to moderate degree of Alzheimer's disease were randomized to treatment with either Exelon or placebo for 26 weeks. Results: Among the patients enrolled for safety evaluation, the numbers of patients that suffered from serious adverse events in the Exelon and Placebo groups were 4 (10%) and 6 (15%) respectively. The mean changes from baseline in MMSE score indicated that the Exelon group improved at each time interval, whereas the placebo group worsened. The improvement of the Exelon group at Week 12 vs. baseline was statistically significant. The mean changes from baseline in Global Deterioration Scale (GDS) and Neuropsychological test (NPT) also indicated improvement in the Exelon group and deterioration in the placebo group. The differences between the two groups were marginally significant at week 26 and endpoint (P=0.062 and 0.065 for GDS; 0.050 and 0.056 for NPT). There was no significant difference between the two groups in Clinician*s Interview Based Impression of Change -plus Family Input (CIBIC-plus). Conclusion: Exelon administered at an escalating dose of 3-9 mg/day was well tolerated by Taiwanese Alzheimer's patients. It also demonstrated the efficacy of a tendency to decrease the deterioration of the disease.

[17] Association of the Apolipoprotein E e4 allele with Alzheimer's disease but not with vascular dementia

L. Traykov (INSERM U324, Paris, France), A.S. Rigaud (Hôpital Broca, Paris, France) S. Baudic (INSERM U421, Paris, France), R. Couderc (Hôpital Armand Trousseau, Paris, France), B. Lecolier (Hôpital Notre Dame de Bon Secours, Paris, France), M. Pasquet-Fevrie (Hôpital Notre Dame de Bon Secours, Paris, France), A. Smaghe (Hôpital Notre Dame de Bon Secours, Paris, France), F. Forette (Hôpital Broca, Paris, France)

While there is consensus about the association of the apolipoprotein E (ApoE) e4 allele with Alzheimer's disease (AD), the relation between this allele and vascular dementia (VaD) remains controversial. The divergent findings in the e4 allele frequency in VaD could be linked to difficulties with the clinical diagnosis of VaD and variability in the patients' selection criteria. The objective was to clarify further the relationship between ApoE alleles polymorphism and dementia. We analyzed the ApoE phenotypes of 219 patients with AD (NINCDS-ADRDA), 45 with VaD (NINDS-AIREN), 62 with mixed dementia (MD; NINDS-AIREN) and 54 age matched normal conntrols (NC). ApoE phenotyping was performed by an agarose isoelectric focussing immunoblot method. The results reveal relative overrepresentation of ApoEe 4 allele in patients with AD (33,6%) and MD (25,8%), compared with VaD (10%) and NC (8,3%). The analysis of the e4 allele frequency shows significant differences between: AD group compared with VaD ($p<0.0005$) and NC ($p<0.0001$) groups; as well as MD group versus the VaD ($p<0.05$) and NC ($p<0.005$) groups. In contrast, the frequency of the ApoE e4 allele in the VaD group did not differ significantly from that in controls. These findings corroborate the suggestion that variability of the clinical classification of cases with vascular and so-called mixed vascular-degenerative dementia may be responsible for the increased ApoE e4 frequency in previous VaD series. The results should contribute to the assessment of dementia risk profile in the elderly, indicating that ApoEe4 allele-bearing individuals have greater risk of having AD than VaD.

[18] Clinical and cerebral CT characteristics of subjects with Psychomotor Desadaptation Syndrome in comparison with patients with Alzheimer's disease

Pfitzenmeyer Pierre, Martin-Hunyadi Catherine, Mourey France, Baudouin Nathalie, d'Athis Ph, Mischis-Troussard Christelle (Service de Médecine Gériatrique. Centre Hospitalier Régional. Université de Dijon. Centre de Champmaillot. 2, rue Jules Violle. 21034 Dijon Cédex France)

Purpose: The aim of this study was to compare clinical and CT scan characteristics of patients showing Psychomotor Desadaptation Syndrome (PDS) with dementia of Alzheimer'type (DAT) patients Method : The study was conducted in Departments of Geriatric Medicine of the University Hospitals of Dijon (centre 1) and Strasbourg (centre 2), in France. Seventy-three hospitalized patients with PDS showing retropulsion as the main clinical sign (PDS group) were compared with 65 hospitalized patients with DAT (DAT group). Cardiovascular and neurological clinical characteristics, frequency of falling and assessment of postural and gait abilities, and subcortical changes on CT-scan have been recorded. Results : Orthostatic hypotension was more frequently observed in PDS group (56 % in centre 1 and 31 % in centre 2, respectively) than in DAT group (6% in each centre) ($p < 0.05$). Rigidity, akinesia, apathy and aboulia were significantly more frequently observed in PDS group than in DAT group. Falls in the past 6 months occurred more often in patients with PDS than in patients with DAT ($p < 0.05$). Patients with PDS showed significantly lower functional activities and postural abilities compared to patients with DAT ($p < 0.05$). Mean score of white-matter lesions and measurements of ventricular enlargement were significantly higher in patients with PDS than in patients with DAT ($p < 0.05$). Conclusion: PDS is characterized by loss of motor abilities and is associated with orthostatic hypotension. CT scan in patients with PDS shows usually severe white matter lesions.

[19] Neuroleptic intake reduction in patients hospitalized in specialized Long-Term-Care-Units for Alzheimer's disease

D.VASCHALDE,Y.VASCHALDE** (* Service de Gériatrie, ** Service de Neurologie, Groupe Hospitalier du Havre, BP 24, 76083 LE HAVRE cedex FRANCE)*

Four specialized Long Term Care units, twelve beds each, delivering heath services to elderly Alzheimer patients have opened, in 1996, in a geriatric ward. Their main purpose is to offer an adequate answer to those patient's needs in the sense that they permit a proper monitoring and the managment of the disease's complications. The elligible population have to comply with the following criterias : they are elderly (average 82 years old), wandering about, with an advanced or severe stage of the disease (average MMS to 5) and behaviour disorders (evaluated with Neuropsychiatric Inventory) with a mejor reduction of their autonomy (GIR average to 2). Among the 48 patients, 31 come from their private residences, 6 from a CANTOU sector in a medicalized nursing home, 11 from a long term unit. While it has been noticed an improvement of the behaviour disorders, we have also observed, restrospectively, an evident reduction of the doses of neuroleptics and even, in 16 patients, the interruption of the neuroleptic treatment. The lessening of the doses has been obtained because of a better adaptation to the environment in those structures compared to the homes or the non-specialized units that they had left. This leads us to see in Alzheimer's disease a pathology in which the frame of adaptation of someone to his environment is reduced. Neuroleptics merely offers a substitute by increasing the patient's level of tolerance or by lessening the perturbation generated when the environment cannot be modified. The institution, in an adapted environment, offers a real drugfree alternative in the procurement of care to those patients.

[20] Risk factors and clinical significance or Leukoaraiosis

M.M. Ventura (Serviço de Geriatria do Hospital do Servidor Público Estadual "Franc isco Morato de Oliveira" - São Paulo - Brasil) A.C.P.Melo (Serviço de Neurologia do Hospital do Servidor Público Estadual "Francisco Morato de Oliveira" - São

Paulo - Brasil)

Purpose: to identify the risk factors and clinical significance of leukoaraiosis (LA). Methods: were evaluated 27 outpatients of the Geriatric Unit. Mean age: 75.2 years (s.d.= 6.55). There were 11 men and 16 women. Brain images were available from all patients, submitted a Computed Tomograph (CT). The presence or not of LA was compared to age, scholarity grade (sg), application of Mini-Mental State Exam (MMSE) and the Structured Interview for the Diagnosis of Alzheimer's Type Dementia, Multi-infarct Dementia and Dementias of Other Aethiology according to DSM III-R and ICD-10 (sidam), Hachinski's scale (há), to the blood level of glucose (glu), cholesterol (col), hdl-cholesterol (hdl), ldl-cholesterol (ldl), triglycerides (try), fibrinogen (fibr), also to body mass index (bmi) and time of smoking (smk). LA was compaired to sex and the diagnosis of elevated blood pressure (ebp). Statistical Analysis: T tests for independent samples and the Fisher test. For statistical significance, p must be lower than 0.05. Results: the only item which reached statistical significance, was ebp (p=0.03). Others items analysed not reached: age (p=0.11), sg (p=0.75), MMSE (p=0.29), sidam (p=0.42), ha (p=0.2), glu (p=0.25), col (p=0.5), hdl (p=0.54), ldl (p=0.54), try (p=0.19), fibr (p=0.21), bmi (p=0.76), smk (p=0.45), sex (p=0.31) Conclusion: there was not a significant association between LA and the items analysed, except elevated blood pressure. The small sample may have influenced our results.

[21] The correlation between the cognitive function and plasma t-pa levers in 506 apparently healthy elderly in Shanghai, China

Ma Yong-Xing, Wang Chuan-Fu, Lu Pei-Fang (Department of Aging, Antiaging and Cognitive Function, Shanghai Institute of Gerontology and Geriatrics, Huadong Hospital,Shanghai,China)

The cognitive function tests (WMS, MMSE, HDS-R) and plasma level of t-PA (IU/ml) were determined in 506 apparently elderly (aged 65-85 years) in order to clarify if there was correlation between various levels of plasma t-P A and the scores of cognitive function tests. The results were as follows: (1) plasma t-PA 0.1-0.39 IU/ml group (215 persons): MQ 92.4±16.7, HDS-R 26.7±3.9, MMSE 28.1±2.9 (2) plasma t-PA 0.40-0.59 IU/ml group (231 persons): MQ 92.8±17.7, MMSE 28.2±2.8, HDS-R 27.2±0.6 (3) plasma t-PA 0.60-1.0 IU/ml group (60 persons): MQ 90.4±14.6, MMSE 27.9±2.4, HDS-R 26.9±3.1. No significant difference between various plasma t-PA levels and cognitive function states were found (F value equaling 0.475, 0.900 and 0.222 respectively). It is suggested that lower plasma t-PA levels as a risk factor in cerebral vascular disease may not necessarily influence the cognitive function in the apparently healthy elderly. It may be indicated that the drugs merely with anticoagulant effect may not be effective to improve cognitive function in the elderly.

[22] Double blind trial on the efficacy of Reinhardt and sea cucumber capsule (R.S.C.) in treatment of dementia in 136 cases of the aged and preaged

Ma Yong-Xing, Wang Chuan-Fu, Gu Yue-Di (Department of Aging, Antiaging and Cognitive Function, Shanghai Institute of Gerontology and Geriatrics, Huadong Hospital, Shanghai, China)

Objective: To study the efficacy of Reinhardt and sea cucumber capsule (R.S.C, sea animal products) to treat dementia in the aged. Methods: Double blind trials were performed in 136 cases of dementia (R.S.C. 68, VD30, AD 38; placebo 68, VD 24, AD 44) in the aged with MMSE24. The dosage of R.S.C. and placebo were all 6 capsules (0.28g/cap) tried for 3 months. The effects were evaluated with MMSE, HDS and MQ(WMS). Results: MMSE increment, R.S.C. 2.397±1.694, placebo 1.654±1.589 (P<0.01). Total effective rate: R.S.C. 54.4%, placebo 29.4% (P<0.01). HDS increment: R.S.C. 2.015±1.994, placebo 1.140±1.785 (P<0.01). Total effective rate: R.S.C. 48.60%; placebo 27.9% (P<0.05). MQ increment: R.S.C. 4.364±4.617; placebo 1.824±5.803 (P<0.01). Total effective rate, R.S.C. 48.5%; placebo 25.0% (P<0.05). Similar effects were observed in VD and AD with slight better results in VD. No significant side effects were observed. The mechanism of R.S.C. to improve the learning and retrieval function of the adult and old rats and adult mouse and cognitive function in the demented may be related to its effects to enhance neuron growth, to increase acetylcholine and decrease glutamine level in the brain, as confirmed in cell and animal experiment, and to improve free radical metabolism and microcirculatory state confirmed clinically. Conclusions: R.S.C. is rather effective and safe to treat dementia (AD, VD) in the aged and preaged.

[23] Relationship between thyroid dysfunction and cognitive impairment in geriatric outpatients.

T. Vogel, G. Kaltenbach, D. Heitz, C. Martin-Hunyadi, M. Kiesmann, F. Kuntzmann (Center of Gerontology, University Hospital of Strasbourg, France)

Clinical features of thyroid dysfunction occur frequently as unrelated symptoms in elderly. Therefore, the diagnosis is often not apparent particularly in the presence of cognitive impairment. The purpose of this retrospective study is to appreciate cognitive repercussions of thyroid dysfunction in elderly and to examine thyroid-cognition relationships. Thyroid stimulating hormone (TSH) dosage was systematically performed to 454 subjects in the geriatric day hospital .They were divided into 3 groups: hypothyroid (TSH >4.5µU/ml; n=22), euthyroid (TSH between 0.5 and 4.5 µU/ml; n=421) and hyperthyroid subjects (TSH< 0.5µU/ml; n=11). Cognitive functions are explored with the Mini Mental State Examination, and diagnosis of depression, confusion and dementia are established according to the DSM IV criteria. Age, having amiodarone, conditions of life, and weight do not statistically differ in the 3 groups even if mean weight is higher in thyroid dysfunction groups. Women have significantly more thyroid dysfunction than men (p<0.05). The prevalence of depression and confusion are similar in the 3 groups. The Mini Mental State Examination score is higher in euthyroid subjects (20.2) than in hypothyroid (17.6) and hyperthyroid subjects (13) but without significant difference. The prevalence of vascular dementia and Alzheimer disease don't differ in the 3 groups. In this study, with a limited number of subjects, we don't find any association between cognitive disturbance and thyroid dysfunction. In this old population (mean age : 81 years), other confounding factors, such as vascular factors or medications, are strongly involved to explain cognitive impairments.

[24] Double-blind trial of Huperzine-A (HUP) on cognitive impairment and dementia in 702 cases

Ma Yong-Xing, Zhu Yue, Gu Yao-Di, Xie Su-Zhen, Wang Zhan-Shun, Wang Chuan-Fu (Department of Aging, Antiaging and Cognitive Function, Shanghai Institute of Gerontology and Geriatrics, Huadong Hospital, Shanghai, China)

HUP, a new alkaloid extracted from Huperzia Serrata (Thumb) Trev, is a potent anticholinesterase with minimal toxicity and may improve the learning and retrieval function of rats. Age associated memory impairment (AAMI) treated by 0.1mg HUP PO Qid. The clinical trials were studied by double blind method on 662 patients with MQ (WMS)<100, the mean value of MQ of 355 treated and 307 control group were 84.9±13.5 and 85.8±16.1 (P<0.05), respectively. The dosage is 0.1mg PO Qid. The mean value of MQ after the treatment (the interval between pre and post tests of WMS with A and B from respectively is 2 months) of treatment and control group were 97.4±16.6 (P<0.01) and 91.8±16.9 (P<0.01), with the MQ increase of 12.5±10.2 in the treatment group, significantly higher than that of 3.9±8.2 in the control group (P<0.001). The effective rates were 62.8% and 35.5% in the two groups. No significant side effects were observed except gastric discomfort 2, dizziness 2, insomnia 3, nausea and vomiting 4 and mild exciting 1 in the treated group. Vascular dementia and Alzheimer's disease: A clinical trial of vascular dementia (25) and Alzheimer's disease (55) was conducted on 40 treated and 40 control patients with the same dosage. The MQ of treated group increased from 50.4±18.5 to 59.7±18.7 (P<0.05), that of the control group increased from 54.0±14.7 to 55.9±16.3 (P<0.05). The MQ increase of 9.4±10.4 is significantly higher than that of 1.9±10.4 (P<0.01). The effective rate of the treated group was 60%, significantly higher than that of 35% in the control group (P<0.05). No significant side effects were observed except gastric discomfort or nausea 3 and dizziness 3 in the treated group. Huperzine is an effective and safe drug to improve cognitive function in AAMI and dementia in the aged.

[25] Alzheimer's Disease Clinical Trials in 2001: A changing research environment?

V. O'Neill, H. Feldman, B. L. Beattie (Clinical Trials Program, Clinic for Alzheimer's Disease and Related Disorders, Vancouver Hospital & Health Sciences Centre - UBC Site, Vancouver, Canada)

In the era following the approval of acetylcholinesterase inhibitors as treatment for Alzheimer's disease (AD), the future of placebo controlled clinical trials has become uncertain. We want to evaluate whether the recruitment of subjects at our AD clinical trials unit has changed following the approval of donepezil in Canada, in September of 1997. A retrospective review of recruitment logs was compared for each placebo controlled clinical trial from 1992 to 1997 and then 1997-2000. Staff and recruitment strategies were constant throughout the study period. The average length of recruitment was 6-8 months. Between 1992 and 1997, there were 7 placebo controlled clinical trials conducted with a mean recruitment of 14.3 subjects per trial (SD=2.4). Following September 1997, there were 4 placebo controlled clinical trials conducted with a mean recruitment of 7.8 subjects per trial (SD=2.8). These results indicate that it has become more difficult to recruit for AD placebo controlled clinical trials and that both innovative study designs and recruitment strategies will be needed for successful progress in future clinical trials.

[26] The establishment of a dementia centre in Hong Kong

H Chiu (Department of Psychiatry, The Chinese University of Hong Kong, Hong Kong)

The establishment of a dementia centre in Hong Kong Helen Chiu Department of Psychiatry, The Chinese University of Hong Kong In South-east Asia, service development for dementia care is lagging behind developed countries. With the ageing of the population, this has become an increasingly important issue. In Hong Kong, for instance, 10.50f the general population are aged 65 or above. The paper will describe the establishment of a new dementia centre in Hong Kong. The dementia centre provides 45 day care places, 15 respite residential places, a training centre, resource library and a Dementia research unit. The objectives of the centre are: 1. to provide service for the community care of elderly with dementia, 2. to provide training on dementia care to health care professionals, 3. to train and support carers, and 4. to conduct research related to dementia care. The impact of the centre will be discussed in the light of current dementia services in Hong Kong and South-east Asia.

[27] An Applied Research Project to Improve Pain Management for Elderly Veterans in Institutional Care

M. Gibson, K. Rose, H. Neufeld-Bailey, L.Viana, D. Keast, N. Bol (St. Joseph's Health Care London and University of Western Ontario, London, ON, Canada)

PURPOSE: Epidemiological studies suggest that 70 % or more of the elderly who reside in institutions have significant pain problems. The purpose of this ongoing applied research project is to address this problem within the 370 bed Veterans Care service of a chronic care facility. METHOD: An interdisciplinary steering committee (medicine, nursing, pharmacy and psychology) is leading the project. Psychology graduate students have facilitated implementation. Multifaceted chart audits were conducted to establish a baseline for pain management practices. Audit results were compared to clinical practice guidelines to evaluate compliance. Focus groups and key informant interviews were conducted with all treatment teams and physicians to identify sources of variability that should be targeted for intervention. Educational interventions were developed collaboratively. RESULTS: Significant gaps were identified between recommended and actual pain management practices. Qualitative data clarified the contributing factors. Education was identified as a primary need. Process outcomes include the development of resources for use in patient orientation, in the patient/ family resource centre, as a visual learning aid for staff and residents, and as an adjunct to clinical intervention. CONCLUSIONS: This project demonstrates the creative use of available resources and multiple problem-solving approaches to address a complex clinical need. Clinical outcomes will be targeted in subsequent phases of this ongoing project. Through the interventions to date, care practices are becoming more closely aligned with evidence-based recommendations, while continuing to respect the unique needs of individual residents.

[28] The use of home health services by new public long-term care insurance in Japan

Nanako Tamiya, Kazue Yamaoka, Eiji Yano (Dept.Public Health, Teikyo-University School of Medicine, Tokyo, Japan)

PURPOSE: To clarify how each service under long-term care insurance (LTCI) is utilized, especially to investigate caregiver factors, which are not considered in the initial survey for eligibility and having been the important factor in the old welfare system before LTCI in Japan. METHOD: A mail questionnaire survey of the main family caregivers was conducted one month after beginning LTCI for all the applicants in Fuji-Yoshida city (n = 597). The main questions asked were: applicants sex, age, and eligible care level (0~5) decided by physical and mental status, caregivers sex, age, and relationship to the applicant, and service use: yes/no for each of the 11 home care services covered by LTCI. Multiple logistic regression was used to evaluate the effect of the independent variables on the use of each service with care level and caregiver-applicant relationship as fixed variables. RESULTS: We obtained 323 effective responses (response rate = 54%). The factor that promoted use of the most popular day service was wife caring for her husband (OR/ 95%CI=4.8/1.6-5.7) and care level was a negative factor. However, care level was a factor promoting use of all other services. For the second most popular service home help service the promoting factors were wife caring for her husband (OR/95%CI=3.8/1.0-16.8) and care level, but daughter-in-law caring for mother-in-law was a negative factor (OR/ 95%CI=0.2/0.1-0.9) CONCLUSION: Our results show that it is important to consider the caregivers situation to meet needs in LTCI adequately, especially in the transitional phase from old system into new system.

[29] Characteristics of frail elders under long-term care insurance in Japan

Yoshiharu Yokokawa(Teikyo Medical Welfare Cpllege), Ichiro Kai(University of Tokyo),Japan

PURPOSE: In order to determine the differences in social activities between frail elders and healthy elders under Long-term Care Insurance (LCI), we conducted a questionnaire survey in Japan. METHOD: Out of 1842 inhabitants aged 65 and over in a rural community of Nagano Prefecture, case group comprised all of 125 inhabitants who had been identified as needing some help for outside activities under LCI. Control group was selected from healthy elders living in the same community (N=373). A self-administered questionnaire was given in August, 2000. It included following items: instrumental ADL (IADL, 5 items), Falls Efficacy Scale (FES, 10 items) and social activities (10 items) as well as demographic factors such as age and sex. After controlling age and IADL, the effects of the group on the activities were analyzed using a logistic regression. RESULTS: 72(57.6%) inhabitants of the case group and 176(47.2Åì) of the control group completed the questionnaire individually. There were significant differences in age, IADL and FES between the two groups ($p<0.001$). After controlling age and IADL, social activities such as volunteer (odds ratio=10.09), producing fruits and vegetables to give to neighbors (3.55), communicating with friends and relatives (2.86) were more frequently observed among the control group. CONCLUSION: Our results showed living independently without help was related supportive and productive activities. Facilitating such activities as volunteer can promote healthy elders to prolong independent life. In addition, the intervention might contribute to decrease frail elders with disability.

[30] Pressure Sores in Elderly Patients Treated by a Geriatric Home Hospital Service

D. Roglia, N. Aimonino Ricauda, D. Salerno, M. Rocco, M. Molaschi, F. Fabris (Department of Medical and Surgical Disciplines. Geriatric Section. University of To)

PURPOSE: To evaluate the prevalence and the incidence of pressure sores in frail elderly patients treated at home by Geriatric Home Hospitalisation Service (GHHS). METHOD: The study was conducted in 466 patients (average age: 80.6± 9.7 DS) treated by GHHS providing diagnostic and therapeutic interventions at home, which are usually made in hospital. We evaluated demographic characteristics, nutritional, functional, cognitive status, primary diagnosis, comorbidity, presence and stage of pressure sores, mortality, length of stay. RESULTS: The primary diagnoses on admission were advanced cancer (27.7%), heart disease (16.3%), terminal dementia (10.5%), respiratory disease (6.4%). On admission 79 patients (17%) were affected by pressure sores. 330f them had Stage III- IV ulcers (NPUAP). 30.40f the 79 patients came from hospital. Only 12 patients (3.10f 386 patients treated by GHHS without sores on admission) affected by terminal illness developed sores during home treatment. 38 0eveloped Stage I ulcers and 62% Stage II ulcers. As a mean, these sores were developed 25.7±20.5 DS days after admission and 46.70f them successively healed. Patients who developed pressure sores were younger, but more functionally and mentally impaired, showing lower serum albumin levels and a greater degree of comorbidity. During treatment, the mortality rate among these patients was 66.6%, significantly higher than in patients without sores (16.3%) (p <0.001). CONCLUSION: The intervention of home hospitalization team and the collaboration with the family members may play an important role in prevention and management of pressure sores in frail elderly patients with high level of comorbidity.

[31] Neuropsychological Evaluations in the Nursing Home Population

M. Munk, P. Castro, M. Pessanha, A. Carvalho, J. Laks, E. Ribeiro Casa Gerontológica de Aeronáutica Brig. Eduardo Gomes(CGABEG) Rio de Janeiro - Brazil

Objective: An analysis of a sample population of residents in a Nursing Home (CGABEG) and the impact of age on neuropsychological evaluation scores. Materials and Methods: Our study consists of the analysis of a sample population of 106 residents, living in CGABEG. We analysed sample by age, gender, educational level and their scores in the following neuropsychological evaluations: ADL (Katz,1970), AIDL (Lawton,1982) MMSE (Folstein, 1975) and GDS (Yasavage, 1983). Results: The population studied showed the following distribution: according to gender: male 20.75%; female 79.24%. Age: 65 to 84 years old - 64.15% and >85 years old - 35.84%. Educational level: Primary (until 8 years of school) - 39.62% ; Secondary & University - 60.37%. ADL: 65 to 84 years old -severe impairment(SI) 10.44%; moderate impairment(MI)13.43% ; Full Function(FF) 76.11%. >85 years old -(SI) 25.65%; (MI) 15.38%; (FF) 58.97%. IADL: 65 to 84 years old - dependence (D) 10.44%; capability with assistance (CA) 23.88% independence(I) 67.16%. >85 years old - (D) 12.82 (CA) 48.71%; (I) 38,46%. MMSE: 65 to 84 years old (n=70) score 20.18±8.76 with 1st grade 21.05±7.09; 2nd grade and college 19.26±10.15. >85 years old(n=36) score 17.84±7.88 with Primary 17.29±8.30; Secondary & University 21.38±6.98. Comparing total score and age (t=1.34;p=0) and educational level (65-84 years old, Primary/Secondary & University t=0.84; p=0 and >85 years old Primary/Secondary & University t=0.55 ;p=0). GDS: 65 to 84 years old-normal(N) 70.14%; moderate(M) 23.88%; severe(S) 5.97%. >85 years old - (N) 66.66%; (M) 28.20; (S) 5.12% Conclusion: The variable age showed its major impact at ADL and AIDL scores. In the sample studied we could not find significant percentage depressed residents. At MMSE there's no significant variation in results, maybe due to the socio-cultural homogeneity and high educational level. This sample shows a significant high percentages in these categories: women (79.24%); age 65 to 84 years old (64.15%); educational level- secondary & University (60.37%).

[32] Depression Prevalence In A Nursing Home Population

M. Munk, P. Castro, M. Pessanha, A. Carvalho,J. Laks, E. Ribeiro, C. Moraes (Casa Gerontológica de Aeronáutica Brig. Eduardo Gomes(CGABEG) Rio de Janeiro - Brazil

Objective: An analysis of depression prevalence in a nursing home population . Materials and Methods: Our study consist of the analysis of a sample population of 106 residents, living in CGABEG. We analyzed the sample by age and using the Geriatric Depression Scale (GDS, Yesavage,1983) comparing the scores of two years. Results: The sample studied showed the following results in first year: 65 to 84 years old group(n=67), GDS : normal(N) -65.67%; moderate(M)- 28.35%; severe(S)- 5.97% . >85 years old group (n=39) : N-64.10%; M-30.76%; S- 7.69%. In second year, 65 to 84 years old group(n=67): N- 70.14%, M-23.88%; S- 5.97% and the >85 years old group (n=39) : N- 66.66%; L- 28.20%; S-5.12% . The total scores don't show the significant percentage of depression nor variation between two years. Conclusion: In this sample the prevalence of depression there's not a significant percentage. There's no variation of prevalence of depression between the two groups of age in the two years what is unusual for the elders residents in the institutions. Maybe it's due the specific characteristics and therapeutic intervention used in this institution .

[33] Reducing physical restraint in a long-term care unit

M. Michel, O. Michel, Ch. LeDu, Ch. Rouaud, V. Rigollé, V. Grevet, Ch. Roquais, M-C. Gueguen, P. Jouanny (Geriatric Medicine Departement, University Hospital, Rennes, France)

Interventions to reduce physical restraint in falling elderly are well known following OBRA'87 in the USA. This study intended to decrease our rate of physical restraints on day-time and to improve the quality of life in this frail elderly population. Method: Initially, we studied the patients with restraints at noon in two long-term units. A multidisciplinary check-up was done: capacity of posture, gait and transfers, type of restraint, falls circumstances, possibility of supervision by staff or family, fitting wheelchair, environmental management, satisfaction questionnaire about restraint. A new count was done 3 months later after multidisciplinary intervention, including physiotherapy, walking-stimulation with someone's help, safety-improvement of environment, participation of family and volunteers to the daily care-program. Results 67 patients were included, (40+27), 49 females and 18 males, age 85,4, admitted for severe dementia in 75%. Most were physically disabled: 4 could walk by their own, 17 could walk with difficulties, 21 were unable to walk (31%). Initially, 29 patients (19+10) had permanent restraint when seated on their wheelchairs (43%) Three months later, the rate of restraints lowered respectively by 58% (19 to 6) and 100 0n the two units (10 to 0), not only at noon, but all day long. For the last 6 people, with very high risk of falls, we are still trying to minimise day-times of restraint. In study time, only 3 falls occurred, without severe injury. Conclusion geriatric teams can easily change their practices concerning physical restraint with very simple multifaceted intervention. We are now working towards taking off bedrails with the same approach.

[34] Predictors of functional change in Chinese nursing home residents

Elsie Hui (Medical and Geriatric Unit, Shatin Hospital, Hong Kong), Eric MC Wong (Center of Clinical Trials and Epidemiology, The Chinese University of Hong Kong, Hong Kong), Jean Woo (Department of Medicine and Therapeutics, The Chinese Univesity of Hong Kong, Hong Kong).

PURPOSE: To identify resident- and facility-related characteristics associated with functional change in institutionalized older Chinese persons.

[35] Rasch Analysis of the Philadelphia Geriatric Center Morale Scale in Older Chinese Nursing Home Residents

Eric Wong (Center for Clinical Trials and Epidemiological Research, The Chinese University of Hong Kong, Hong Kong), Elsie Hui, (Medical and Geriatric Unit, Shatin Hospital, New Territories, Hong Kong), Jean Woo (Department of Medicine and Therapeutics, The Chinese University of Hong Kong, Hong Kong)

PURPOSE: To examine the endorsability patterns of the Philadelphia Geriatric Center Morale Scale (PGCMS), and its usefulness for older Chinese nursing home residents METHOD: The study group consisted of 230 residents (median age 79 years; 69.1 0.000000emale; median Abbreviated Mental Test (AMT) scored 9) of four nursing homes during October 1995 to March 1996. Subjects should meet the following criteria 1) aged 65 years and above , 2) Cognitive function adequate to answer the questions (i.e. AMT scored six or below), and 3) proxies were used to complete the scale. Validation of the PGCMS was based on Rasch dichotomous model, which generated item endorsability and subject agreeability measures on a common interval scale. RESULTS: Rasch residuals principle component analysis identified two constructs: unstrained affect and reconciled aging. Of the unstrained affect seven items, I take things hard was a muted item (i.e. item does not provide additional information beyond the rest of items). Of the reconciled aging eight items, Things are better than I expected was a misfit item (i.e. item does not define the same construct as the rest of the items), while As you get older you are less useful and Life isn't worth living were muted items. Rasch analysis further revealed that endorsability patterns in both constructs were quite different between male and female. CONCLUSION: The PGCMS is potentially a valid scale, which may be further revised or shortened, for Chinese nursing home residents aged 65 years and above. The use of the scale should be interpreted separately for male and female.

[36] Utility of the Nursing Home Life-Space Diameter for Assessing Resident Mobility

E.V. Cyarto & A.M. Myers (Department of Health Studies and Gerontology, University of Waterloo, Waterloo, Ontario, Canada)

PURPOSE: The Nursing Home Life-Space Diameter (NHLSD), developed by Tinetti and Ginter (1990), consists of observation ratings of residents' level of mobility ("moving around" over the past two weeks) within each of four diameters or zones (room, unit, facility, outside) categorized from 0 (never) to 5 (>3 times a day). The developers reported good inter-rater and test-retest reliability (total NHLSD scores) for two day-shift nurses across 25 residents from three nursing homes. Our study examined the influence of staff, facility layout and seasonal differences for each diameter and total scores. METHOD: Three staff (recreation, day and evening health care aides) from two facilities with different layouts were asked to rate 26 ambulatory residents at two points (7 to 14 days apart). In addition to the standard rating format, staff were asked to indicate confidence in their ratings and interviewed concerning the volitional nature of residents' behaviour (i.e, whether they went their rooms on their own), as well as seasonal variation. RESULTS: Inter-rater agreement was highest for diameter one (within resident's room), averaging 80%, and lowest for diameter three (outside unit, within facility), averaging 10%. Confidence ratings followed a similar pattern. We found differences between type of staff (the evening shift health care aides were the most consistent in their ratings, r>.90) and facility (physical layout of programs and services). Volitional behaviour and seasonal variations were also found to influence ratings. CONCLUSION: Findings indicate that the NHLSD instructions require clarification to facilitate more consistent interpretation.

[37] The acceptability of using Telemedicine for Podiatric intervention in a Residential Home for the Elderly.

H.S.Corcoran (The Prince of Wales Hospital, Hong Kong), J.Woo (The Chinese University of Hong Kong), E. Hui (Shatin Hospital, Hong Kong)

Purpose To evaluate the acceptability of using Telemedicine for Podiatric intervention from the point of view of the Elderly Client, The Podiatrist, The Residential Home Staff. To evaluate the costs and savings generated. Methods 49 Elderly clients were given a foot examination using Teleconferencing, a diagnosis was made and a treatment plan established. The findings were then compared to the results of an on-site consultation carried out within 24 hours. Active foot problems were then followed up in the same manner. In total 99 Teleconsultations and 99 on-site consultations were compared. 45 were new case consultations and 54 were follow up consultations. Results Telemedicine was found to be acceptable for use in 78.79% of cases. 71.72% of diagnoses and 74.75% of treatment plans established using Teleconference matched the on-site findings. 86.96% of clients favoured Teleconference for Podiatric intervention. HK $55,849.37 savings in transportation, escort and hospital costs were generated during the study. Conclusion Telemedicine was found to be an acceptable method of providing Podiatry service to clients of Residential Homes for the Elderly. Teleconference decreased the overall waiting time for first appointments. It was an excellent triage mechanism, and facilitated earlier identification and intervention of urgent foot problems. Wound care monitoring was particularly effective due to the slide taking facility of the equipment. Teleconference was a good medium for training the residential home staff in simple foot care and hygiene techniques. Teleconference cannot replace on-site consultation where active foot problems exist.

[38] The Influence of the Prone Position on Elderly Bedridden Patients.

Eiko Chikamori, Suzuki Manami, Kayo Kumagaya, Hisayo Taniguti, Taeko Iwasaki, Nobuko Yamaguti, Mayumi Nitou, Yosiko Inoo, Yukari Yamamoto, Chikako Oribe Kobe City College of Nursing, (JKasai Municipal Hospital, Kobe & Kasai, Japan)

The present study examined the influence of the prone position on elderly bedridden patients. Eighteen bedridden patients who were in the prone position every day were examined with regard to the change of blood pressure, heart rate, and O2 saturation. 1. After being in the prone position, the patient's blood pressure and heart rate did not change. 2. O2 saturation significantly increased after 5, 15, and 30 min in the prone position. 3. It is effective to include the prone position in the patient's program of position change for respiratory management.

[39] The Anti-depressive drugs in the elder population in a nursing home

Castro, P, Munk M, Pessanha M, Carvalho A,Laks J , Ribeiro E Casa, C. Moraes (Gerontológica de Aeronáutica Brig. Eduardo Gomes(CGABEG) Rio de Janeiro - Brazil)

Objetive: An analyzes of the use of anti-depressive drugs in elder population in a nursing home comparing with scores of depression evaluation . Materials and Methods: It was analyzed the prescriptions of anti-depressives drugs in a sample of 103 residents living in CGABEG comparing them with the scores of the Geriatric Depression Scale (GDS, Yesavage,1983). Results: In the sample of 103 residents the total scores of GDS are: normal (N)- 72,81%; Moderate(M)- 22,33% ; Severe(S)- 4,85% . Only 12 residents (11,65%) use the antidepressives drugs . According : 7 residents use triciclics (TCA) anti-depressives and GDS : N - 5 ; M-1; S- 1. Other 3 residents use selectives seratonine reuptake inhibitors (SSRI) and GDS: M- 3 to all of them. The last 2 residents use another kind of anti-depressive and the GDS : S- 2 to both of them. Conclusion: The study doesn't show any direct relation between the use of anti-depressive drugs and the low prevalence of depression in this sample, the use of anti-depressive drugs is only of 11,65% in the total sample . Maybe it due to specific characteristics and the therapeutical intervention used in this institution.

[40] A system to detect nocturnal motor activity in elderly patients in a hospital room

S. Banerjee, F. Steenkeste**, P. Couturier*, M. Debray* , A. Franco*. (*Laboratoire Interuniversitaire de Gérontologie de Grenoble (LI2G), Université Joseph Fourier, Grenoble, France;*

***INSERM : Unité 518, Toulouse, France)*

PURPOSE: To study the validity of a system of telesurveillance in elderly patients using home monitoring devices. METHOD: GARDIEN, a system of passive infra-red sensor network, is connected to a computer that is placed at a remote site from the patient. It switches on automatically every night at 9 p.m. and remains active throughout the night till 6 a.m. Data corresponding to movements are collected twice per second, and stored with indication of time when they differ. We have analysed, for a period of one month, each file that is created every night and correlated it with the reports of motor activities made by the night personels to find out whether the sequences of movements within the file correspond with the interpretation of sequences of movements by GARDIEN. We are observing the system continously to see if it is reliable enough to function independently. RESULTS: We have analysed a total of 490 possible sequences of movements made by the patient or the personels. Of these, GARDIEN is able to detect correctly 475 (96.94%) sequences that agree in time interval and 395 (80.61%) sequences that agree with the nature of movements occurred within the room. CONCLUSION: GARDIEN will be able to warn patients' caregivers in real-time by an alarm in the future. Hence, it will reduce the burden of health caregivers and consequently improve elderly patient's safety without encroaching the privacy and also without altering the lifestyle as the patient will not have to wear any device.

[41] Restraint reduction program in long-term care units : implementation and its impact on care staff

P.J. Durand, J.P. Ouellet, L. Beauchesne, A. Tourigny, R. Verreault, L. Diciare, L. Rochette (Unité de recherche en gériatrie de l'université Laval, Centre d'hébergement Saint-Augustin du Centre Hospitalier Affilié universitaire de Québec, Canada), L. Lévesque (Institut universitaire de gériatrie de Montréal, Canada), S. Lauzon (Faculté des sciences infirmières de l'université de Montréal, Canada), R. Gagnon (Centre hospitalier régional de Lanaudière, Canada)

This study aimed at (1) developing a restraint reduction program, (2) describing its implementation on long-term care units and (3) examining its effects on the perceptions and knowledge of care staff toward the use of restraints. The program was composed of three parts : consciousness-raising meeting, staff education and clinical follow-up. It was a randomized controlled clinical trial with 8 intervention care units (5 nursing homes) and 11 control units (5 other nursing homes). Care staff was surveyed at two time periods over a 7-month interval (pre-and post-test intervention ; intervention care units :N=171 [T0] and N=158 [T1] ; controls : N=181 [T0] et N=166 [T1]). The program was successfully implemented. Following the intervention, more nursing staff in the experimental care units compared with control units identified (1) seatbelts and chair with table/lap tray as restraints, (2) that restraints were likely to increase residents' level of embarrassment, and (3) that restraints were not effective to prevent injuries or falls. Results showed significant changes on the perceptions and knowledge of care staff toward the use of restraints.

[42] Some Factors Determining Length of Stay for Sub-Acute Nursing Home Admissions

M. Abbas, R.D. Kennedy (Maimonides Medical Center, New York, USA), J.Dimant (Crown Nursing Home, New York, USA), J. Kell, (Lutheran Medical Center, New York, USA)

PURPOSE: Nursing home based sub acute care is now widespread in the U.S.A.; however determinants of achieving predicted length of stay are poorly defined. METHOD: Fifty consecutive sub-acute admissions to a skilled nursing facility for rehabilitation of hip fracture, stroke and de-conditioning due to hospitalization, were identified. Using the patients' charts and Minimum Data Set (M.D.S.) predicted and actual length of stay (L.O.S.) were analyzed with respect to the following factors: age, sex, hospital pre-admission functional status, length of hospital stay, nature of disability, cognitive status, depression, pressure ulcers, urinary incontinence, number of medications, co-existing medical conditions, malnutrition, family support, and nursing home course. RESULTS: The results were calculated using Pearson's Chi square test and uni-variant and multi-variant analyses and showed that pre-hospital functional status, depression, and lack of family support were significant for prolonged LOS ($P<0.1$) and there was a trend towards significance for complicated nursing home course ($P=0.101$) and poor motivation ($P=0.104$). CONCLUSION: For sub-acute older patients referred to nursing homes for rehabilitation, significant factors for prolonging anticipated L.O.S. are pre-hospital admission functional level, depression, lack of family support, complicated nursing home course and poor motivation. When possible these indices should be factored into any estimate of L.O.S. to provide a more realistic time frame for sub-acute patients admitted to nursing homes. to provide a more realistic time frame.

[43] Community-Dwelling Adults' Attitudes Toward Nursing-Homes

Antonios Likourezos, MA, MPH Orah R. Burack, MA; Leslie S. Libow, MD (The Jewish Home and Hospital, New York, NY USA)

The purpose of the present study was to examine the relationship between nursing home attitudes, experience during visitation, and feelings about future residence in a nursing home. A secondary data analysis of a survey study examining the knowledge, attitudes, and experiences concerning nursing-homes among community-dwelling residents of the New York metropolitan area was conducted. Subjects who had never visited a nursing home and/or had lived in a nursing home were excluded from the sample. Subjects (n=748) were predominantly white non-Hispanic (85.5%), 50.0% were male, and the median age was 52.0 years (range: 18-95). Most subjects (57%) reported having a positive experience when visiting a nursing home and the majority (62%) stated that nursing home residents receive adequate care . However, over half (57%) also stated that nursing-homes hasten physical decline and death and a similar percentage (55%) had negative feeling about going to live in a nursing home. Beliefs about positive care of residents, positive experience during visitation, favorable feelings towards living in a nursing home, and disbelief that nursing homes hasten physical decline and death were all significantly positively related to each other. The results were similar after adjusting for age, gender, and race. These findings indicate possible avenues to improve societal attitudes towards nursing homes. For example, focusing on and enhancing the visitation experience.

[44] Visual Narratives: The experience of participating in a theatre group in a retirement home setting

Pamela Brett-MacLean and Krista Charbonneau (The University of British Columbia, Vancouver, British Columbia, Canada)

This poster session will explore the use of visual images within the context of a pilot study of a theatre group in a retirement home setting. Considered within the framework of a "new ethnography", the "lived experience" of long-term care residents is explored through the personal meanings they ascribe to photographs taken of the group, along with the interpretations of the researcher as participant-observer. The photographic images provide silent, evocative narratives that resist a complete or final analysis. These visual narratives invite ongoing reflection on the role of the arts in later life.

[45] The Life Space Study: Improving the Quality of Life for Nursing Home Residents Through Music

Orah R. Burack, MA, Leslie S. Libow, Patrinila Jefferson, BA (The Jewish Home and Hospital, New York, NY, USA)

Listening to music is an activity that can be easily and cost effectively provided to nursing-home residents according to their individual tastes with the use of CD-players. Most studies examining the use of music in the nursing home have focused on its effects on agitated and cognitively impaired residents. The purpose of the present study was to examine the effects of providing cognitively intact residents' with their favorite music on residents' perceived quality of life. Cognitively intact nursing home residents were individually presented with 30 minutes of taped music of their choice. Before and after the presentation subjects completed a global quality-of-life scale. Additionally, subjects responded to open and close-ended questions concerning their past music experience, music preferences, and enjoyment of the music presentation. Subjects reported listening to music significantly less often after entering the nursing home than at home, despite the importance they placed on music. Many subjects had extensive music experience and a diverse array of music preferences including jazz, popular music, opera, and rhythm and blues. No significant changes in global quality of life were found after listening to music. However, all subjects reported positive feelings in response to the music presentation and stated they would like the opportunity to repeat the intervention. The results indicate the importance of developing and providing recreational activities that cater to the individual needs and interests of nursing home residents.

[46] The Most Difficult Decision to Make: Admitting an Elder into a Continuing Care Facility

Baron, Jacqueline J.

PURPOSE: Exploration of the physical and emotional reactions of family members who recently admitted an elderly relative into a continuing care facility (CCF). METHOD: Descriptive study utilizing a questionnaire sent to 55 individuals who had admitted an elder into a CCF in the Lower Mainland of BC within the previous 6 months. RESULTS: 29 respondents to questionnaire. Most of the respondents (82.2%) were female with a mean age of 54.5 yrs. Elders admitted into the CCF were mainly the mothers of the respondents (44.8%) with a mean age of 85.24 yrs. Respondents' reactions and feelings regarding the decision-making and admission process were positive, and they reported a sense of relief following the admission. Many of their apprehensions were eased by knowing that the elder was in a safe environment and was being looked after 24 hrs. a day. Implications for nursing and recommendations for further research are proposed.

[47] Creating Success!! Serving our seniors by honoring staff

Ann Keane (Lifestyle Options/Alta. Life Care Housing Foundation, Edmonton, AB, Canada)

With the current human resource crisis challenging and threatening organizations, regions, and nations, employers are forced to embrace not only client centered but employee centered processes. By honoring those we also serve our employees, our ambassadors those who make real our missions,leaders will reap measurable, magnificent realities. Hear of drastically diminshed recuritment and retention issues of radically reduced sick time utilization and of skyrocketing employee and client satisfaction. Experience desired, measurable outcomes in seniors satisfaction by utilizing the strategies in this session to enhance not only your clients quality of life but the quality of life of your employees Come see, sense, and hear of success! Let's make this world a better place!

[48] A study on the satisfaction of care workers for their jobs in long-term care

S. Kasahara (International Buddhist University, Osaka, Japan), H. Sumii(Hiroshima Prefectual College of Health and Welfare, Hiroshima, Japan), M. Hidaka (Kobe University School of Medicine, Hyogo, Japan)

The purpose of this study is to clarify the factors of influence on the subjective satisfaction of care workers who are working at the nursing home for the aged and hospital nursing home for the elderly. Method: We send self-recording questionnaires on the satisfaction of their jobs to care workers are working at the nursing home for the aged and hospital nursing home for the elderly in Osaka Pref. in Japan. According to the analysis by the use of multiple regression analysis with SPSS, statistical software, it was shown about the relationship between the satisfied with their jobs and 1) Explanation about their facilities, 2) Approach to needs, 3) Understanding from their superior, 4) Effort on their care works, 5) Satisfaction to their income, 6) Human relationship among the fellow care workers, 7) Experience and 8) Condition of care works. Results: The significant factors from the result of multiple regression analysis consisted of 1) Understanding from the superior ($p<.001$), 2) Human relationship with among the fellow care workers ($p<.001$), 3) Explanation about their facilities ($p<.05$), 4) Approach to the needs ($p<.05$), and 5) Experience ($p<.05$). The proportion rate adjusted for the degree of freedom was 0.81, and it was significant ($p<.001$). The Summary: The care workers with high satisfaction of their care works were those who had a tendency to get the agreement about their care works from their superior , to go well with human relationship among them, to explain the content of institutional services and to have long experience in them. The consultation and the guidance system for their appropriate workplace are necessary for the care workers who is recognizing that they cannot satisfactorily explain the contents of long-term care services, go well with the interpersonal relationship within the care workers, get the understanding or the agreement from the superior, nor get more experience.

[49] Effects of Self- and Staff-referenced Congruence Among Continuing Care Retirement (CCRC) Residents

S. Green, Department of Sociology, University of South Florida, Tampa, Florida, USA, J. Parr, Foundation for Aging Research, Tampa, Florida, USA

Recent studies have examined the impact of congruence between self-assessed general health and self-reported objective health indicators (including Activities of Daily Living). Effects of congruence between self-assessed health and objective indicators reported by others have not been addressed. This study uses longitudinal survey results to examine the impact of both self-referenced and staff-referenced congruence among 122 CCRC residents. Findings of regression analyses indicate that: 1. When self-referenced categories are used, Good Health Pessimists (PHRs), Poor Health Realists (PHRs), and Poor Health Optimists (PHOs) are all more likely than Good Health Realists (GHRs) to limit activities due to health. When staff-referenced categories are used, PHRs are more likely while PHOs are less likely to limit activities. 2. Number of days spent in the CCRC's Skilled Nursing Facility (SNF) is predicted by membership in the self-referenced PHR and the staff-referenced PHO categories. Self-referenced PHRs spend more and staff-referenced PHOs spend less time than do GHRs in the SNF. 3. Self-referenced PHRs, staff-referenced PHRs and staff-referenced GHPs are less satisfied with the CCRC than GHRs. 4. Mortality is predicted only by self-referenced categories. PHRs and PHOs are more likely than GHRs to die within two years after the survey. Thus, congruence is useful in predicting outcomes among CCRC residents. The outcomes predicted, however, vary according to whether congruence is referenced by the residents' or staff members' assessments of difficulties with Activities of Daily Living.

[50] Suspicions of Discrimination in Long-term Care Settings Among Gay, Lesbian, Bi-sexual, and Trans-gender Persons

N. C. Jackson, M. J. Johnson, J. K. Arnette, & S. Koffman (Eastern Washington University, Cheney, Washington, USA)

The purpose of this study was to determine whether gay, lesbian, bi-sexual, and trans-gender persons suspect that discrimination against them is a problem in long-term care settings. 127 gay, lesbian, bi-sexual, and trans-gender persons ranging in age from 15 to 72 completed a survey that contained questions about partner status, retirement status, income, plans to reside in a care facility, and suspicions about discrimination among staff, administration, and residents of long-term care settings, among other questions. Most respondents expected that discrimination against sexual orientation was an issue among staff and residents of long-term care facilities. Virtually all respondents indicated that the development of retirement settings that cater to the needs of aging gay, lesbian, bi-sexual, and trans-gender adults was desirable. This study indicates the need to examine long-term care settings for policies against discrimination on the basis of sexual orientation and for cases of actual discrimination, and to educate older homosexuals, bi-sexuals, and trans-gender adults about social support services and community-based alternatives to long-term care.

[51] Entry to long-term care: developing a proactive response to carers of older people

D. Seddon (Centre for Social Policy Research and Development, University of Wales: Bangor, United Kingdom), M. Boyle (Princess Royal Trust for Carers, Bangor, United Kingdom)

This presentation summarises the findings from a collaborative study into the experiences and support needs of carers, living in North Wales, whose elderly relative is admitted into a long-term care facility. It depicts the complex, ambiguous nature of carers' post admission caring experiences, profiling the contribution carers make to the continued care of their elderly relative, describing the nature of carers' relationships with their elderly relative and with long-term care facility staff and identifying carers' formal and informal support networks. The study that informs the presentation was completed in three phases using qualitative and quantitative research methods. Phase One involved in-depth interviews with 78 carers whose relative had recently been admitted into nursing or residential care to identify the key factors and individuals involved in the placement decision and to describe carers' early post admission experiences. Phase Two involved semi-structured interviews with 50 professionals (health, social care and long-term care) linked to the admission of older people into long-term care to appraise current protocols and guidelines and identify examples of good practice. Phase Three involved re-interviewing a sub-sample of carers from Phase One (n=30) to describe how their post admission experiences unfold over time and to capture the temporal and dynamic nature of their support needs. A new index, PACE (Post Admission Caring Experience), devised to help the research team gather data on carers' experiences and coping strategies, will be included in the presentation. Short extracts from carers' accounts will convey the substance of the findings.

[52] A Panel Study of Older Japanese With Only Biological Daughters: Their Nursing Care Preferences

Noriko Tsukada (Nihon University Graduate School of Business, Tokyo Japan)

The purpose of this study is to explore the nursing care preferences and attitudes (and their changes over time) toward the inheritance of family homes, the child's responsibility to care for his/her parents, and the traditional way of providing nursing care, of Japanese older people who have only biological daughters. Face-to-face interviews were conducted with 10 older people who have only biological daughters in Hiroshima, Japan, in 1992, with repeat interviews in 2000. The sample was drawn with a snow ball sampling method in the 1992-interview, and the same participants except two participated in the 2000-interview. The interviews were conducted by a trained interviewer, using an interview schedule. Data were analyzed via qualitative analysis. Mean ages of the participants in 1992 and 2000 were 59.5 and 67.8, respectively. Results show that the majority of the participants exhibited a strong preference for traditional elder care styles, where older parents are provided with nursing care by their eldest daughters, though many were aware that the feasibility of their preferences was decreasing because of social forces (e.g. changing cultural values and demographic characteristics). The feelings about the social forces, however, varied from "good" to "unfair". It was also found that the participants were making efforts to shift their perceptions and attitudes to fit societal changes. The study revealed the predicament of these people as epitomized in the discrepancies between their nursing care preferences and the feasibility of the preferences and their resignation to social changes.

[53] Evaluation for Quality of Services in Nursing Homes for Elderly People in Mexico City.

Reyes-Guerrero JA,MD. Gutierrez-Robledo LM,MD. (Instituto Nacional de Ciencias Medicas y de Nutricion, Salvador Zubira, Mexico City, Mexico).

Purpose To evaluate the quality of Nursing Homes services in Mexico City Material and method: We made the evaluation of 39 Nursing homes in Mexico City, registered officially as Long term care units exclusively for elderly people. Evaluation consisted in the application of an instrument to evaluate the following areas: Geographic integration of the institution, architectural design, perception by the people into the community and around the unit; daily living activities inside the institution, institutional human and economical resources, respect to the clients, liberty and rights, and capability of the institution for future development, etc. Results: We classified the institutions in three categories according to the profile of dependence of assisted people: Institutions for autonomous people, semidependent people and total dependent. The government (public) nursing homes have the better quality of services and the most autonomous population. The private nursing homes were more numerous and they provide care for total dependent people with less Institutional and human resources. Comments: According to this study the public nursing homes are better for the elders with 850f standard requirements, however the access to this institutions is limited, in the other hand private institutions are expensive and have low quality of services with a 150f standard requirements for nursing homes. It's necessary to realize further studies to corroborate if this is a result of admission policy or is due to lack of institutional resources.

[54] Extended Care Unit - A British Experience from Warwickshire.

P. Ramesh, H.N. Desai (Department of Medicine/Geriatrics, Warwick Hospital, Warwick, United Kingdom)

Purpose Bed utilisation of acute care beds is critical in any cash limited district general hospital in Europe. Our aim was to improve this in our hospital. We describe the development, economic impact and success of an extended care unit in a community hospital attached to our acute hospital. This unit admitted those elderly patients, who were clinically stable but awaiting discharge destinations from the acute care wards. Methods 570 patients were admitted to the unit between March 1996 and March 2000, 373/570 were females, 197/570 were males. Their age was between 80 and 100 years. These patients were analysed for the purpose of this study. Prior to transfer to the eighteen bedded extended care unit, these patients were assessed in the acute wards by a nurse co-ordinator and a social worker. Results Discharge destinations from the unit were: 270/570 (47%) to their own home, 228/570(40%) to residential/nursing home, 42(7%) transferred to acute hospital, 25(4%) died, 4(0.8%) to sheltered home and 1(0.2%) to psychiatric hospital. Average length of stay was 40.5 days. A total of 22,998 bed days was saved at the acute district hospital site. Conclusions This study demonstrates that a nurse-led intermediate/extended care unit could result in resource savings in district general hospitals. The fact that 22,998 days could be saved results in shorter waiting times for surgeries and more beds available for acute admissions. This type of intermediary care has been a success and we suggest that this be adopted in community hospitals. This enables hospital resources to be utilised efficiently.

[55] Enhancement of Initiative of Nursing Home Elders by Temptation to Give Foods with Commands to Dogs

Masayoshi Niiyama, Daisuke Tokumoto, Yoko Murakami, Shigeru Morita, Harue Niiyama, Rimiko Kuroki, Shigeo Sugiyama (Rakuno Gakuen University, Ebetsu 069-8501, Japan 2 Nursing Home "Karipu Atsubetsu", Sapporo 004-0055,Japan 3 Hokkaido Asai Gakuen University, Ebetsu 069-0833, Japan)

Confirmation of improving effect on initiative of elders of tempting to command and reward dogs with foods. Three female toy dogs were exhibited for 2 hours in an acrylic pen every 2 weeks for 16 months. To increase contact with the elders, dogs were often put on a table or delivered to them who were liking for dogs. Care workers tempted the elders to put a small piece of jerky in a dish and to say commands, "sit", "wait" and "OK" to the dogs. When the commands were carried out, care workers congratulated on the elder. Actions of the dogs and the reactions of the elders were recorded on video tape. The length of their stay, frequency of voluntary actions to the dogs and their communication (conversation) were analyzed to evaluate the effects. RESULTS: Among 100 residents (average 83.4 years old), 23 elders participated. Average length of their stay increased after use of a dish from 28 to 62 minutes (end). In eighty years old man, time of stay increased from 25 to 120 minutes and number of actions of giving food also increased from 5 to 20 times. In early exhibition, the care worker led him hand in hand, but on later he voluntarily gave food to dogs with voice. From their conversation, evidences of encouragement and pressure to do for him by the neighbor were also found. CONCLUSION: To command and reward dogs with foods is very useful tool to enhance initiative of elders.

[56] High readmissions rate vs definitive institutionalitation in nursing homes.

N. Martinez-Velilla, J. Manzarbeitia-Arambarri, S. Bartolome, C. Castro, A. Areosa, F. Guillen-LLera. (Universitary Hospital of Getafe)

BACKGROUND: High readmissions rate among elderly patients and recurrent readmissions, have been reported as bad quality of care indicators. PURPOSE: To assess the relationship between acute medical care costs and those arising from definitive placement in nursing homes of high readmissions rate patients. METHOD: We took data from medical records of all the admissions during 1999. We measured the financial impact of readmissions estimating the cost of hospital care by multiplying the data on service use by the average cost for each day of care, according to every related diagnosis group. For the nursing homes we estimated the prices according to the mean costs of the hospital area. RESULTS: There were 1176 admissions of 885 patients. We focused on 291 readmissions of 175 patients. The cost of the hospital care caused by the readmissions was the 35 percent of all the service costs. The 50% of the costs originated by the readmissions were caused by the 23% of the readmitted patients. These patients had higher commorbidities, drugs, readmissions rate and geriatric syndromes. When we compared with those due to a definitive institutionalitation in nursing homes, the result was that only few patients had higher costs in the high readmissions rate group. CONCLUSIONS: -Readmission rates have limitations when used as a quality of care indicator. -Cost of hospital care of patients with higher readmissions rate should not induce to definitive institutionalitation in nursing homes in most of the patients.

[57] Quality of Life: Nursing Home and The Elderly

Nathalie FAUCHER (Hôpital Sainte-Périne, AP-HP, Paris, France), Tristan CUDENNEC (Hôpital Sainte-Périne, AP-HP, Paris, France), Michel ROGER (Hôpital Sainte-Périne, AP-HP, Paris, France), Olivier SAINT-JEAN (Hôpital Européen Georges Pompidou, AP-HP, Paris, France)

PURPOSE : Assessment of perception of quality of life in elderly population in nursing home and factors who have an influence about it. METHOD : 40 patients, with MMS >19, were asked by Farquhard questionnaire with five open questions about their quality of life. Answers were analyzed and constituted 3 groups : positive, negative or neutral quality. RESULTS : The mean age was 88.2 years (ranging from 68 to 99). Sex ratio was 0.25 (m/f). The mean MMS was 23.6 (ranging from 20 to 29). 30 0escribed the quality of life positively, 20 0escribed it negatively and 50% reported a neutral description. Positive perception was based on conservation of their way of life and their social role. Health was accessory. The social and physical environment made up for the disabilities. Negative perception was described by loss expressions, breaking of, disappointment, absences. The life experience was disagreeable and they spoke of their reduced social role. The balance between positive and negative elements made neutral quality of life. There was more resignation and death seemed to be the ultimate stage. CONCLUSION : This study demonstrates that very elderly institutionalized people are willing and able to talk about their quality of life. It will be interesting to extend the study to other nursing homes.

[58] Funding nursing home care in Canada: a comparison of regional policies and their social impacts

Robin L. Stadnyk (School of Occupational Therapy, Dalhousie University, Halifax, Nova Scotia, Canada)

PURPOSE:. This study compared the models of nursing home care funding in 10 provinces and 1 territory of Canada, focusing on the personal contributions required to fund care. The purpose of the study was to explore the relationship of the models of funding nursing home care to the everyday lives of spouses left in the community. METHOD: Using a critical ethnographic approach, the study involved a review of policy documents from 10 provinces and 1 territory, as well as key informant interviews with provincial/ territorial representative of persons implementing the policies (e.g, placement coordinators), and those affected by the policies (family caregiver support groups). Key informant interviews were analyzed for themes. RESULTS: Three models of personal contributions to funding emerged: income and asset-based, income-based, and per diem-based. Each model impacted on 1) the planning activities employed by the family 2) the placement processes and 3) the everyday life of community-dwelling spouses of those being placed. The income and asset-based model produced more themes of distress, placement problems, and worries about lifestyle of community dwelling spouses. CONCLUSIONS: Models of personal/public/nonprofit funding of nursing home placement can vary significantly within one country, even one with socialized medicine. Since demand for nursing home space is likely to increase with the aging of the population, it is important to critically examine funding policy differences, not only in terms of their characteristics, but also their impacts on the lives of people seeking placement. In this way, policy directions that support, rather than undermining, families can be identified and promoted.

[59] Facility Questions Based on Successful Aging Theory Assist in Selecting a Nursing Home

Author: Gillian Eades Telford (consultant, Bowen Island, British Columbia, Canada)

As they age in a changing world, people are seeking help in making well-informed health care choices. Selecting a nursing home is an important process in which professionals and clients working together can reach the most appropriate decision. This poster presents eight of the eighty questions that could serve as part of a helpful survey tool to use when choosing between facilities. In order for clients and families to make a selection that most effectively meets the needs of the client, certain observations need to be made and certain questions asked at each facility. The questionnaire for Directors of Care or Supervisors of facilities is designed to assist in the comparison and selection process. The observation questions were presented at the Canadian Association of Gerontology conference in Calgary in October, 2000. Presented here are selected questions to be asked about the facilities being considered. Each question is shown to be linked to theory, and many are based on accreditation standards that illustrate client-centeredness. The questions, which are straightforward, and to be answered either yes/no or by means of the Likert scale, cover physical environment, life quality within the facility, aspects of care and care delivery, and programming. The questionnaire is scored, emphasizing criteria most desired by clients, families, and care providers, as cited in the literature. The tool is being tested for validity and reliability in two provinces in Canada, and has the potential for worldwide application.

[60] Job satisfaction among private elderly home workers in Hong Kong: Effects on quality of care

YH Cheng (Department of Community Medicine & Unit for Behavioural Sciences, The University of Hong Kong, Hong Kong, China), LH Wu (Department of Nursing and Health Sciencs, The Hong Kong Polytechnic University, Hong Kong, China), LW Chu (Department of Medicine, The University of Hong Kong and

Queen Mary Hospital, Hong Kong, China), and WJ Law (Community Nursing Service, Queen Mary Hospital, Hong Kong, China)

The objectives of this study were to measure the job satisfaction of health care workers in private homes for the elderly in Hong Kong, and to explore the educational needs of these workers in the private elderly home context. Thirty-five private elderly homes located in Hong Kong Island were approached and two of them refused to participate. The survey was conducted between January and July, 1999, 162 health workers were successfully interviewed. Data collection was by means of a structured questionnaire. Results show that the level of job satisfaction among workers is not low. Similar to past studies that job satisfaction is found to be unrelated with gender, age, educational attainment, and income. However, job satisfaction is significantly related to factors such as the experience of work pressure and intention to change job. Health care workers also expressed their educational needs in terms of further training about health care for elderly in general, knowledge about common illnesses of elderly persons, knowledge about elderly persons' psycho-social needs, and communication skills. In conclusion, the findings suggest that as social change, more and more people cannot afford to take care of their frail elderly family members at home in Hong Kong, the waiting list for a place in homes funded by the government has been long. More and more of these persons to be housed in private institutes. The pre- and on-job trainings given to health care workers in these homes are crucial to the quality of care and the health of the residents.

[61] Specialised neuro-psycho-geriatric nursing home in Luxembourg: A new hope or another ghetto for elderly persons

Jean-Claude Leners (Long Term Care Centre Hospitalier Neuro-Psychiatrique Ettelbruck-Luxembourg)

Inside our neuro-psychiatric hospital of about 450 beds, a new specialised nursing home for 150 patients has been developed in order to specialise our care for neuro-psycho-geriatric patients. The challenge of this unique specialised long term care: improving the daily living conditions of the patients by establishing a network for geriatric persons. The professional help (psycho-geriatric nursing, psychiatric consultations, respite care, day centre activities, ...) will improve the well-being of the patients; on the other hand, a range of institutions will get the opportunity to consult the team. Advantages and problems will be discussed in the paper. A new kind of specialised nursing home will be described. Separation between psychiatric institutions and nursing homes will be clarified and a global luxemburgish psycho-geriatric network in which this nursing home is engaged, will show a realistic view of caring for these people.

[62] A conceptual framework for the cost-effective utilization of nursing personnel in long term care facilities

A. Perold (University of South Africa, Pretoria. Republic of South Africa)

The GOAL/PURPOSE of this recently completed doctoral study was to compile guidelines for the cost-effective utilization of nursing personnel in long-term care (LTC) facilities in the Republic of South Africa. METHOD: A combined quantitative-qualitative research approach had been applied to explore and describe the utilization of nursing personnel and caregivers in LTC. Data collection and analysis were conducted during three phases: Survey of LTC facilities (N=145), analysis of job descriptions (N=64) and focusgroup interviews (N=3). The findings of the three empirical studies were triangulated and subjected to a limited literature control. RESULTS:A conceptual framework and guidelines for the cost-effective utilization of nursing personnel in LTC were developed from the findings of this study. The conceptual framework indicates that the goal, cost-effective utilization of nursing personnel, is reached when quality care has been delivered within the constraints of the budget. The process has been described as compiling guidelines for all categories of nursing personnel regarding clinical nursing, nursing management, nursing education and non nursing tasks. The roleplayers in the process, the context of LTC and the dynamics which influence the cost-effective utilization of nursing personnel had also been presented in the conceptual framework. CONCLUSION: The guidelines which had been developed were verified by the respondents and accepted as applicable for the cost-effective utilization of nursing personnel in LTC.

[63] Teaching Family Members to be the family member of a Nursing Home Resident.

Peter S. Silin, (Diamond Geriatrics, Inc.) Vancouver, BC

Purpose: To describe an educational/ training programme for family members of nursing home residents which teaches them how to be the family member.. When a resident enters a nursing home, family members become part of a system about which they often have no understanding. They have no tools, skills, or experience to help them deal with this system. As well, they are often going through their own emotional process which they do not understand and do not know how to deal with. This affects them, their relative, and the nursing home. Nursing homes have family councils, family support groups, or family information nights, but they do not have training programs to teach people how to be the family member or about nursing homes. This poster session would be a description of a programme which does teach them that. It describes content in such areas as family and resident adjustment, how the nursing home system functions, the roles and responsibilities of the home, the resident, and the family member, and covers topics such as advocacy, visiting, abuse, grief, death and dying, and basics of dementia. Results: The intended results of this programme include: 1. faster adjustment of family to the nursing home, 2. bettter relations with staff and with the system 3. increased effectiveness as partners with the nursing home in the care of their relative.

[64] Use of Long-Term Care among Stroke Patients after Hospital Discharge

S.C. Wu, W.C.Chang, M. Chang (Graduate Institute of Health Policy and Management & Center for Health Policy Research, National Taiwan University, Taipei, Taiwan), D. Chuang (Institute of Public Health, Taipei Medical University, Taipei, Taiwan), S.H. Tang (Cardinal Tien Hospital, Taipei, Taiwan)

Access to long-term care is important to promote successful transitions of patients from hospital to home. The study monitors stroke patients' use of service and the transition among services after hospital discharge. Stroke patients hospitalized in 7 hospitals in Taipei between July 1999 and June 2000 were enrolled in the study just before discharge. Telephone interviews were conducted with the subjects at 1 month, 3 months, and 6 months after discharge. Among 598 subjects contacted in the 1st month interview, 483 subjects, suffering from ADL/IADL disabilities, are in need of long-term care while 29 have died and 86 have recovered. About 55% of them were cared for by their own family caregivers without any formal assistance. Regarding the use of formal services, 14% have been admitted to a nursing home, 7% have been cared by visiting nurses, 26% have hired an aide at home. Multiple logistic regression analysis shows that advancing age, severe ADL disabilities, cognitive impairment, and being helped by hospital staffs for discharge arrangements are significantly associated with nursing home admission. Female, severe ADL disabilities, and higher education are significantly associated with hiring an in-home aide. For those who are female, mild ADL disabilities, having more than 4 children, and not being helped by hospital staffs for discharge arrangements are more likely to be cared for by family caregivers. Further analysis for the transition of functional status and service utilization will be employed after the data of 2nd and 3rd interviews are ready.

[65] Person-centered Admission to a Long Term Care Facility: A Continuous Quality Improvement Project

Windermere Care Center (Vancouver, BC, Canada) Vancouver/ Richmond Health Board Improvement Quality Team (Vancouver,

BC, Canada)

Purpose: Historically, interdisciplinary person-centered care practice has been difficult to operationalize within the institutional context due to organizational cultures and structures. Recognizing that, the owners and management of Windermere Care Center partnered with the VRHB Quality Improvement Team to facilitate a shif toward interdisciplinary person-centered model of care through a quality improvement initiative. Method: Windermere Care Center, a 236 bet LTC facility in Vancouver, BC, identified admission to their facility as a key process for improvement and a means to initiate a change in practice. The following QI methodology was used: 1. An interdisciplinary steering committee was established to guide the process. 2. Education on team building, leadership and QI methods/tools were provided to lead participants. 3. Process Improvement Teams were developed to review key aspects of the admission process. 4. Storyboards were used to communicate progress to staff/residents and families. Partnership between Windermere staff and the VRHB QI team was crucial to the project. Evaluation was both formative and summative and consisted of pre-post surveys. RESULTS: Results from the formal evaluations are not available at this time but preliminary results indicate amove towards greater involvement and formal consultation with residents/families on quality issues, and improved teamwork amongst all disciplines. CONCLUSION: In order to effect a shift towards an interdisciplinary person-centered care model there needs to be both education and organizational strategies. This joint Windermere/QI project has been a learning experience for all and is continuing to evolve.

[66] Millenium Mental Health and the Cyberspace Senior in Nursing Homes

Norine Cooper (Seneca College, Toronto, Canada)

PURPOSE: The presentation (10 minute paper) will describe a project undertaken by Seneca College professor to introduce the frail elderly in nursing home to computers and the internet.Social Service Gerontology students and several high school students volunteered one hour per week. Now a number of residents surf the net, use email and enjoy a broadened social life and increased self esteem due to the project. METHOD: Through the use of a video, powerpoint presentation and a handout, the presenter will provide guidelines for developing a volunteer- computer program in a nursing home. RESULTS: A listing of do's and don'ts for administrators, Resident program managers and volunteer coordinators will be provided. The paper compares our results with recent research by Fiona Clarke at McGill University , Montreal Quebec. The paper concludes that the frail elderly can learn and do enjoy many of the benefits of the internet that the rest of us enjoy. The challenge is to find the resources to assist them in gaining access. Ability is not the issue - accessibility is!

[67] Cultivating Person-centred care in Nursing Homes: A Pilot Project

Carolle Sauro (Vancouver/Richmond Health Board, Vancouver), Diane Jansen (Vancouver/Richmond Health Baord, Vancouver), Joan Hibbard (Vancouver/Richmond Health Board, Vancouver, Elisabeht Drance (Vancouver/Richmond Health Board, Vancouver)

Purpose: Person-centred care is an approach that is gaining popularity within the context of nursing home care. However, for a number of reasons, care home staff have found it difficult to practice person-centred care with a resident who has dementia. Based on the literature and past evaluations, the Vancouver/Richmond Health Board's Geropsychiatirc Education Program (GPEP) embarked on a pilot project to: 1. Identify educational methods and organisational strategies that facilitate person-centred care. 2. Increase satff and family satisfaction with their involvement in care planning. Method: Three care homes were selected to participate based on pre-established criteria. The project used a longitudinal design consisting of an initial educational intervention for staff and family followed by resident care reviews using the GPEP Model. Data was collected at two points; prior to the educational sessions and at the end of the eight month project. Both quantitative and qualitative methods were used to collect the data. Results: Results indicate that 970f participants found all the educational sessions to be beneficial and that usng the GPEP Model facilitated teamwork and the development of person-centred care strategies. Overall there was an increase in staff/family satisfaction with their involvement in care planning. Conclusion: The methods used in the pilot project resulted in an increase in participants knowledge, a positive shift in attitude toward person-centred care and evidence of increased family satisfaction with their participation in care planning. Results from this project have provided direction for ongoing person-centred care iniatives in other care homes.

[68] Predictors of adverse outcomes in Chinese nursing home residents

Elsie Hui (Medical and Geriatric Unit, Shatin Hospital, Hong Kong), Eric MC Wong (Center of Clinical Trials and Epidemiology, The Chinese University of Hong Kong, Hong Kong), Jean Woo (Department of Medicine and Therapeutics, The Chinese University of Hong Kong, Hong Kong).

PURPOSE: To identify risk factors for adverse outcomes, including falls, hospitalization and death, in institutionalized older Chinese persons. METHOD: 606 subjects were recruited from institutions belonging to 4 levels of care, and assessed at baseline, 6 and 18 months. Data collected included demographics, the Abbreviated Mental Test, Geriatric Depression Scale, medical diagnoses, drugs, sensory impairment, anthropometric measurements, Barthel Index and adverse outcomes, including falls, hospitalization and death during the study period. Multiple logistic regression was used to identify subject- and institution-related characteristics associated with increased likelihood of these adverse outcomes. RESULTS: The following independent predictors were identified: Falls - age, nutritional status, history of falls, and residence in a state-financed nursing home. Hospitalization - baseline disability, functional decline at 6 months, polypharmacy and chronic obstructive pulmonary disease. Death - malnutrition, Parkinson's disease, dependency in feeding and mobility, male sex and cancer. CONCLUSION: Among the numerous risk factors for adverse outcomes identified in nursing home residents, many are potentially reversible with targeted rehabilitation programs or intervention. Efforts ahould be made to identify those at risk with standardized assessment tools, and to reverse risk factors wherever feasible.

SESSION 55

A Canadian Framework for Healthy Aging

B.C. Kennedy (Division of Aging and Seniors, Health Canada, Ottawa, Canada) A Canadian Framework for Healthy Aging. H.H. Keller (Department of Family Relations and Applied Nutrition, University of Guelph, Guelph, Canada) Nutritional risk and aging; Canadian strategies for community nutrition programs . D. Dampier (Active Living Coalition for Older Adults, Toronto, Canada) Active Living for Older Adults — A Partnership Approach to Healthy Aging. S. Powell (Division of Aging and Seniors, Health Canada, Ottawa, Canada) Preventing Injuries among Seniors: Health Canada's Contribution.

Policies to promote healthy aging can improve health outcomes and quality of life as well as contribute to management of health system pressures. Canada has developed a series of initiatives under the umbrella of Healthy Aging which target older adults in an effort to improve health and quality of life now and in the longer term. The Round Table will consist of a series of presentations on Healthy Aging by Health Canada and partner organizations. There is overwhelming evidence that much of the physical and mental decline, including several chronic diseases and injuries, that people experience as they age is due to risk factors that are both behavioural and environmental. Physical inactivity and poor nutrition are key risk factors in much age related decline and illness. As the Canadian population matures it will become increasingly important to find ways of assisting Canadians of all ages to improve healthy living practices and environmental supports to prevent, delay and reduce ill health in later life, and also to improve quality of life in the later years. This session will present the Canadian federal government's approach and over-arching framework for promoting healthy aging, followed by descriptions of specific healthy living initiatives undertaken by Health Canada and partner organizations. These describe successes, challenges and priority future actions to promote active living (Active Living Coalition for Older Adults), good nutritional practices (Dietitians of Canada), and injury prevention (Health Canada). Major gains can be achieved in later life health status, through improving behaviour risk factor elements such as physical activity and healthy eating, and by addressing physical environments. Given the volume of people approaching the critical ages of serious morbidity and mortality, serious and immediate investments in Healthy Aging is imperative. These initiatives increase awareness and discussion that are required to advance the agenda on healthy aging.

Active Living for Older Adults— A Partnership Approach to Healthy Aging

D. Dampier (Active Living Coalition for Older Adults, Toronto, Canada)

The Active Living Coalition for Older Adults (ALCOA) is a non-profit organization supported by Health Canada. ALCOA's purposes and initiatives are to promote a culture and environment that supports and motivates older Canadians to include physical activity as an essential part of daily living. ALCOA has attracted 24 national and provincial organizations involved with health, aging, physical activity and creating healthy environments. Bringing together individual strengths and a common interest in healthy aging, members have forged a collaborative partnership that is continually expanding its efforts to promote active living for all older adults. Through broad consultation, ALCOA has developed a comprehensive strategy to implement the policy and planning tool, "Moving Through the Years, A Blueprint for Action". This strategy includes working with our partners in the areas of Marketing and Communications, Influencing Policy, Communicating Research in Clear Language, Leadership and Coordination and Collaboration. This presentation will describe how ALCOA functions as a coalition and initiatives currently underway to address the goals of the Blueprint. Successes and challenges of different initiatives will be highlighted with a focus on the predicted realities and needs of the future. Active Living is an essential component to healthy aging that must be addressed by governments, seniors organizations, health providers and service deliverers. It has the potential to prevent and control numerous chronic diseases, improve mental health and physical well-being. Working together in partnership, it is possible to achieve more than individual efforts working in isolation.

Healthy Aging: A Population Health Approach to improving health status

B. C. Kennedy, (Division of Aging and Seniors, Health Canada, Ottawa, Canada)

Healthy aging is emerging as a priority focus for federal action on health. Through an intensive intra-Departmental process of research and analysis, Health Canada developed an approach and over-arching framework for promoting healthy aging, and identified determinants and risk factors with the highest impact on healthy aging, with the highest potential for effective modification through feasible interventions. The risk factors that are most amenable to change in old age and which dramatically improve functional capacity and reduce risk in a relatively short period of time are personal health practices. The strongest evidence points to physical activity, smoking cessation and healthy diet as making the most significant contribution to the prevention or delay of chronic disease and the attainment of healthy aging. Policies and programs to promote healthy aging can improve health outcomes and quality of life as well as contribute to the management of health system pressures. A multi-sectoral national strategy will produce gains beyond a narrowly defined health sector. The challenge of moving Canadians of all ages along the continuum of health requires that policy decisions at all levels and in all sectors be viewed through a healthy aging lens in order to increase the responsiveness of systems and policies to a new demographic reality.

Nutritional risk and aging; Canadian strategies for community nutrition programs.

H.H. Keller (Department of Family Relations and Applied Nutrition, University of Guelph, Canada)

This section of the Round Table session will briefly overview the known relationships between nutrition, food intake and aging in the senior population (e.g, sarcopenia). The prevalence of poor food intake and nutritional risk within North America will then be presented. Known factors that influence this nutritional risk will be discussed in the context of recent research in Canada, based on vulnerable groups of seniors. Finally, strategies employed in Canada to identify and modify this risk will be discussed. The national "Bringing Nutrition Screening to Seniors" project funded by Health Canada's Population Health Fund will be highlighted. This presentation will demonstrate that although nutritional risk is prevalent and has an impact on the health of older adults, preventative strategies including nutrition risk screening can be successfully employed.

Preventing Injuries among Seniors: Health Canada's Contribution

S. Powell (Division of Aging and Seniors, Health Canada, Ottawa, Canada)

Injuries to seniors are costly to the health system and have enormous consequences to seniors themselves. The aging of the population, with a doubling of the proportion of Canadians 65+ from the current level of 12% to 23% of the population by 2041, will significantly increase the burden of injuries in this population group if current patterns continue. Given that the causes of injuries are multifactoral, the most effective approach to preventing and minimizing the severity of injuries is one which addresses multiple factors (e.g, behavioural, biological, environmental, social) and involves a variety of sectors and disciplines (e.g, health, housing, product design). To this end, Health Canada has undertaken a variety of initiatives for the prevention of injuries among seniors. These initiatives have taken the form of public education, community based programming, research and evaluation, and policy development. While varying in nature each initiative has at its core two basic elements: addressing the multifactoral nature of injuries and building partnerships with a range of sectors. The results of these initiatives will be highlighted as will the challenges and future directions of Health Canada's approach to addressing the problem of seniors injuries. This approach is consistent with the view that overall health is determined by multiple and interrelated factors. Just as better health outcomes will result from addressing the whole range of factors that influence health so to will injuries be prevented through interventions that take into account the interrelationship of risk factors. Effective strategies to prevent injury will improve the wellness and quality of life of older Canadians and at the same time reduce demands on the health care system

SESSION 56

Ageing With A Disbility?

A. Walker (Department of Sociological Studies, University of Sheffield, UK) and C. Walker (Department of Social Policy, University of Lincoln, UK)
Age or Disability? Age-Based Disparities in Service Provision for Older

People with Intellectual Disabilities in the UK. L. Gething J. Fethney (Research Centre for Adaptation in Health and Illness, University of Sydney, Australia) Ageing with Traumatically Acquired Disability. T. Heller (Rehabilitation Research and Training centre on Ageing with Developmental Disabilities, Department of Disabilities and Human Development, University of Illinois at Chicago, USA) Research on Life-Long Caregiving Among Families of Adults with Intellectual Disabilities. R. Ngan (City University of Hong Kong, China) and M. Li (Society of Homes for the Handicapped) Community Integration of Older Adults with Intellectual Disabilities: Myths and Realities in Hong Kong.

This symposium focuses on a neglected group in research, policy and practice: those who age with a disability. The aim is to report recent research on this group and to explore some of the policy and practice issues raised by the emergence of a growing group of people who have aged with a disability. Three of the four papers focus on those with intellectual or developmental disabilities, many of whom would not have reached old age in earlier generations, and/or their family carers. The fourth paper includes those with both physical (spinal cord) and brain injuries. It is hoped, as a by-product of this symposium, to make links with other researchers in this field.

Age or Disability? Age-based disparities in service provision for older people with intellectual disabilities in the UK

Alan Walker,of Social Policy, Department of Sociological Studies, University of Sheffield, UK Carol Walker,of Social Policy, Department of Social Policy, University of Lincoln, UK

This paper focusses on the role of service providers in prescribing artificial limits to the potential of older people with intellectual disabilities. It is argued that the key factor in this social construction of dependency is the age discriminatory attitudes held by some service providers and which distinguish two different service cultures in the provision for older people on the one hand and, on the other, people with an intellectual disability. Thus the approaches adopted by care staff and the assumptions implicit within social policies can result in practices which reinforce dependency. The paper is based on two field studies conducted in the UK: a study of resettlement from three large long-stay hospitals and a follow-up study three years later. In conclusion we raise questions about the assumptions underlying the dominant model of service provision for older people and suggest that providers have something to learn from the intellectual disability field.

Ageing with Traumatically Acquired Disability

Lindsay Gething, Judith Fethney (Research Centre for Adaptation in Health and Illness University of Sydney, Sydney, Australia)

As more people survive traumatic injuries that once would have caused death, ageing with a disability is becoming an issue of worldwide importance. People with traumatically acquired spinal cord or brain injury now have a life expectancy similar to that for the general population, yet in Australia little evidence has been documented about the experiences of people aging with these traumatically acquired disabilities, in particular the factors that impinge on their health. People with spinal cord injury (n = 131, mean age 48.3, SD 13.8) and people with brain injury (n = 136, mean age 38.2, SD 11.2) were compared with a group of people drawn from the general population without disability (n = 143, mean age 42.6, SD 16.3). The three groups completed a questionnaire that included questions about general health. At all ages, people with traumatically acquired spinal cord injury or brain injury reported two or more times the number of health conditions reported by the general population. Although many of these conditions were directly related to the disability, many older people with spinal cord or brain injury also reported having to manage age-related conditions such as arthritis and sensory impairments. Many people reported this as acquiring an even higher level of disability that compromised the ability to maintain previous levels of independence. Results indicate that people with spinal cord or brain injury are entering older age with more health conditions than the general population. A rethinking of service provision is required in order to assist these people in maintaining the ability to live independently in the community.

Research on Life-long Caregiving among Families of Adults with Intellectual Disabilities

T. Heller (Rehabilitation Research and Training Center on Aging with Developmental Disabilities, Department of Disabilities and Human Development, University of Illinois at Chicago, Chicago, IL, USA)

This presentation provides an overview of research on aging family caregiving provided by the Rehabilitation Research and Training Center on Aging with Developmental Disabilities conducted over the last five years. The research has included studies of transitions in caregiving over a life-time and longitudinal studies of policy interventions. The transitions studied include developmental changes, death and illness of parents, and out of home placements. Within the context of these changes we have also examined the impact of family and individual characteristics, such as relationship of caregiver (mother, father, grandparent, or sibling), type of disability (mental retardation, autism), and available support systems (formal and informal). The intervention research has examined two types of programs; a state-wide cash subsidy consumer-directed initiative and a family future planning training and support program. In the first study the family's unmet service needs, caregiving appraisal, need for out-of home placement and the community participation of the adults with ID were examined over four years. Results indicated many benefits to participants, versus the control group, including fewer unmet needs, greater self-efficacy, less desire for an out-of-home placement, and higher increases in the community integration and monthly wage of the relative with ID. The second study has assessed the Family Futures Planning Project that uses ongoing peer and professional support to help families conduct long-term person-centered planning. The program has helped families develop letters of intent and has integrally involved the relative with ID in family future planning discussions.

Ageing With A Disbility

Raymond Ngan (City University of Hong Kong) & Mark Li (Society of Homes For the Handicapped).

How effective is the pattern of integrating older adults with intellectual disabilities in the community in Hong Kong? Whilst this has been the policy objective since 1977, the community-wide survey conducted by Messers. Ngan, Li, Yeung, Cheung & Lok in 2000 found that these older adults (N=692) showed only a modest level of social interaction, the availability of a company, and assertiveness, although the general public was receptive to their integration in the community. Despite their strong desire for community integration, these older handicapped adults showed moderate to fair levels of knowledge of their living community, and were least likely to talk with children. Adults of the moderate and severe grade Intellectual Disability showed significantly lower assertiveness, knowledge about the community and social services, and availability of a company. In particular, the older the age, the less integration and availability of a company in the community. Community acceptance, social interaction, networking and assertiveness are the areas requiring appropriate intervention. Implications of these findings in the context of community integration and isolation will be discussed in the Chinese community in Hong Kong.

SESSION 57

Biological, Behavioural and Health Care Determinants of Transitions in Health Status of Older Persons: Comparisons From International Studies

E. Dowd (World Health Organization, Geneva, Switzerland): Comparison of Healthy Life Expectancy in Adelaide, Australia, Manitoba, Canada, Italy and the USA. Betty Havens (University of Manitoba, Winnipeg, Canada): Relating elapsed time to transitions in health status in a panel of older Manitobans. C. Jagger (Department of Epidemiology and Public Health, University of Leicester, UK): Predicting activity restriction in older people: results from the Melton Mowbray Ageing Project. L. Corder (Center for demographic studies, Duke University, Durham, NC, USA): The prevalence and dimensions of disability at ages 65+ in the United States from 1982 through 1999. DJH Deeg (Department of Psychiatry and Institute for Research in Extramural Medicine, Vrije Universiteit, Amsterdam, The Netherlands): Longitudinal characterization of course types of functional limitations. Ian McDowell (University of Ottawa, Canada): Patterns of Change in Functional Ability in an Elderly Cohort over Time

ISSUE The International Network on the Methodology of Longitudinal Studies of Aging (MLSA), organized by Professor George C. Myers (Duke University) in 1997 aims at promoting dissemination of data from longitudinal studies for comparative, cross-national investigations of transitions in health, social and economic conditions of older persons. STRUCTURE In this symposium we will discuss the functional transitions of aged cohorts over time in different countries, their causal paths, and multilevel analytic modelling developed to assess how changes in one domain (e.g. changes in the economic status) affect changes occurring in other domains (e.g. changes in physical functioning). CONTENT Growing number of longitudinal studies focused on aging populations are ongoing in many countries. This reflects the importance of assessing the conditions of life of older persons and the transitions in health, social and economic well-being that accompany the aging process. The identification of biological, behavioural and environmental determinants of these transitions in older populations from different countries is the main focus of this symposium. CONCLUSIONS/ANTICIPATED OUTCOMES Comparing findings from longitudinal studies across time and cross-nationally is an efficacious step to pursue for increasing our knowledge base and devising effective policies. However, one of the major problems in achieving these goals is the lack of standardization in the conceptual design, measurement and data collection procedures of these studies. These issues will be discussed with the aim of insuring a grater coordination in future studies of this type.

Comparison of Healthy Life Expectancy in Adelaide, Australia; Manitoba, Canada; Italy and the USA

Ed Dowd, Marta Gacic Dobo (World Health Organization, Geneva, Switzerland), Gary Andrews (Flinders University,Adelaide, Australia), Betty Havens (University of Manitoba, Winnipeg, Canada): Stefania Maggi (University of Padua, Padua, Italy): Kenneth Manton (Duke University, Durham, USA)

PURPOSE: To investigate the impact of varying biological and environmental determinants in four longitudinal studies on the transitions in health status among older populations as measured by differences in Active Life Expectancy as a proportion of Total Life Expectancy METHOD: Using the Australian Longitudinal Study on Aging (ALSA), the Aging in Manitoba (AIM) longitudinal database, the Italian Longitudinal Study on Aging (ILSA) and the USA National Long Term Care Study (NLTCS) common multi-dimensional measures of functional capacity as measured by difficulties in carrying out Activities of Daily Living (ADLs) and Instrumental Activities of Daily Living (IADLs). The Grade of Membership (GOM) model computed individual difficulty scores which allowed comparison between sites and over time and which permitted the computation of Life Expectancy with four levels of functional capacity from active to frail. RESULTS: Over three follow-up periods adjusted to approximately two year intervals between 1989 and 1996, the NLTCS showed higher ratios of active to total life expectancy followed by AIMS, ILSA and ALSA. These results followed broadly differences in prevalence and development of major chronic high and low mortality disease conditions. CONCLUSION: While these findings are partially confounded by measurement differences in disease diagnosis and severity rating between studies over tihe observation period; the results confirm the differential effects of disease prevalence and their changes over time on both total and active life expectancy at later ages.

Longitudinal characterization of course types of functional limitations

DJH Deeg, Vrije Universiteit, Amsterdam, The Netherlands

Purpose Longitudinal data have provided evidence on factors that increase the risk of incidence of functional limitations (FL). However, little insight exists in course types of FL other than simple incidence. Methods This paper examines the variety of course types in survivors across the first three cycles of the Longitudinal Aging Study Amsterdam (n=1988, initial ages 55-85 years, 6 year-period covered). Using cluster analysis, five FL course types were determined: 1) 'stable low' (72.6%), 2) 'stable mild' (11.2%), 3) 'stable severe' (4.2%), 4) 'gradual increase' (4.8%), and 5) 'steep increase between T2-T3' (7.1%). Results Only 1.0% of the sample showed gradual recovery. Course type 1 was associated with younger age, male sex, higher education, and not living in an institution. At baseline, the average number of chronic diseases for each course type were: 1.0, 1.7, 2.3, 1.9, and 1.4. Among specific chronic conditions at baseline, heart diseases, diabetes, stroke, and osteo-arthritis were characterized relatively often by mild or stable severe course types. Cancer and lung diseases were not characterized by one predominant course type. Conclusions These longitudinal data show the usefulness of distinguishing between course types of FL beyond incidence.

Patterns of Change in Functional Ability in an Elderly Cohort over Time

Ian McDowell

Purpose The Canadian Study of Health and Aging has followed a cohort of Canadians aged 65 and over since 1991. The cohort was based on a representative sample of 10,263 people, including community and institutional samples, taken from 36 sampling areas across Canada. Methods The baseline study in 1991 included a health interview survey of all participants, and a clinical examination of some. Physical and cognitive disabilities were assessed. A similar approach was used at the five-year follow-up in 1996, and will be used again in 2001. Results From this study, the prevalence of physical and cognitive disabilities at the baseline will be reported, along with incidence estimates at the 1996 follow-up. Risk factors for physical and cognitive decline will be discussed. In addition, mortality has been calculated for various sub-groups defined by their initial health status at baseline. Finally, various categories of healthy or successful aging have been defined, and predictors of remaining in good health until late life will be discussed. Conclusions The CSHA represents an interesting cohort in that if offers both a representative population sample of an entire nation, and also includes both health survey data and clinical and neuropsychological examinations.

Predicting activity restriction in older people: results from the Melton Mowbray Ageing Project

C. Jagger, A.J. Arthur, N. Spiers, M. Clarke (Department of Epidemiology and Public Health, University of Leicester, UK)

PURPOSE: To investigate predictors of restriction in Activities of Daily Living in older people. METHOD: A baseline survey of a total population of people aged 75 years and older, undertaken in 1988 was linked with subsequent routine health assessments (up to a maximum of five). Activity restriction was defined as having difficulty performing on their own, requiring help or aids or not doing any one of seven Activities of Daily Living (ADLs). Socio-demographic and health factors included age, sex, marital status, living alone, home ownership, social class, difficulty managing on income, income, morale, social contact, cognitive function (assessed by the Mini-Mental State Examination and the Information/Orientation (I/O) sub-test), incontinence, self-rated health, difficulty with vision and hearing and self-report in the previous two years of: any broken bones, days ill in bed at home, visits to casualty, outpatient clinics or inpatient stays. RESULTS: Of the 1579 persons interviewed in 1988, 688 were initially independent in all ADLs. Factors associated with onset of activity restriction were increasing age, increased contact with services, lower non-family social contact, difficulty with both vision and hearing, fair/poor self-rated health and cognitive impairment (particularly orientation and visuospatial skills). CONCLUSION: Impairments in sensory and cognitive function are key factors in the onset of activity restriction. It is important that such impairments are recognised early and where possible treated, in order to help prevent a heavier burden of caring.

Relating Elapsed Time to Transitions in Health Status in a Panel of Older Manitobans

Betty Havens (University of Manitoba, Winnipeg, CANADA)

PURPOSE: To investigate whether varying elapsed time between panels, or only end states effect the transitions in health status among older Manitobans. METHOD: Using the Aging in Manitoba (AIM) longitudinal database, odds ratios of potential determinants of the transitions in self-perceived health status were calculated for the panel respondents between 1983 and 1990; 1990 and 1996; and 1983 and 1996. Similarly, odds ratios of potential consequences of self-perceived health status were calculated for the same three periods. RESULTS: The percentage of the panel experiencing any transition during the two shorter periods was less than the percentage experiencing a transition during the longer period. The odds ratios were similarly effected. CONCLUSION: These results raise the issue of temporality in longitudinal studies of health status transitions over unequal time periods even when analyses control for impact of both age and disease states.

The prevalence and dimensions of disability at ages 65+ in the United States from 1982 through 1999

L. Corder, E. Corder, K. Manton (Center for demographic studies, Duke University, Durham, NC, USA)

Purpose National Long Term Care Surveys were conducted in 1982, 1984, 1989, 1994, and most recently in 1999. Subjects are representative of Americans aged 65 years and older for each survey year. Each survey queried a core set of 27 function and performance measures (ADL, IADL) and a list of 28 health conditions. There are a total of 26735 interviews. Methods Function and performance information was used to construct model-based groups with distinct disability patterns. The modeling approach is termed grade-of-membership analysis. The prevalence of disorders was estimated for each disability group. The relative prevalence of each group was estimated for 1982, 1984, 1989, 1994, and 1999. Results Six groups best represented the pooled sample: Forty percent was not disabled (Group I). Group I tripled from 1982 to 1999. Fourteen percent had limitations for each measure (Group VI). Group VI was relatively stable over time and associated with neurologic disorders. Group II could not perform heavy work. Group III had limited range of motion and reported arthritis. Group IV could not see well enough to read the newspaper. Group V could not get in and out of bed without help. Groups II-V each decreased in frequency over time. By 1999 Groups III and IV had essentially disappeared. Conclusions Disability at ages 65 and older has become less common in the United States from 1982 through 1999. Dimensions of disability specifically involving limited range of motion and poor sight have undergone rapid decline.

SESSION 58

The Politics of Pensions Around the World

Dalmer D. Hoskins [International Social Security Administration, Geneva, Switzerland] The Politics of Pension Reform: The State of the Debate Robin Blackburn [University of Essex, Colchester, England] The Strange History of British Pension Reform 1980-2000. Eric N.A. Adjei [Social Security and National Insurance Trust, Ghana, Africa] The Politics of Pensions In Africa (In The Eye Of The Storm) Fay L. Cook [Northwestern University, Evanston, IL, USA] The Politics of Social Security in the United States

Pressures for change in public pension programs face many countries in the world. To differing degrees, the pension systems of both advanced industrial countries and developing countries confront budgetary constraints, demographic pressures, competitive priorities, and conservative critiques. The authors of the papers presented in this symposium will describe patterns of pension policy change or proposed change, the underlying causes of these patterns, and the politics of pension reform in a range of countries. The symposium will begin with a broad overview from the Secretary General of the International Social Security Administration, examining the extent to which the politics of pension reform are different in the developing countries of the world as compared to the industrialized OECD countries. Next, the focus goes to the UK and a study of the successive attempts to reform British pension arrangements. This analysis of the politics of pensions in Britain explains why pensions and pension funding is now so much closer to the center of political debate than it has ever been before. The third presentation shifts to Africa with an analysis of the difficulties Ghana experienced in setting up and maintaining the Social Security and National Insurance Trust, Ghana's national pension scheme. The final presentation examines the politics of Social Security in the United States and shows how a politics of seeming consensus has turned to a politics of dissensus with political parties, interest groups, and experts vying over sharply different definitions of the problem of Social Security and of the solutions. A cross national understanding of how countries are dealing with budgetary, demographic, and competitive pressures confronting pension policy can provide lessons to help inform debates about the future of pensions.

The New Politics of Social Security in the United States

Fay Lomax Cook [Northwestern University, Evanston, IL, USA]

This paper shows that a politics of apparent consensus about Social Security in the United States has become a politics of clear dissensus as two sets of strongly held values are pitted against each other — community versus efficiency. At center stage of the Social Security debate are policy elites who differ both on the extent of the Social Security problem and on the solution. Beginning in January, 1998, the President, first Clinton and now Bush, along with several foundations and interest groups have placed Social Security reform high on the policy agenda. First, the paper examines how policy elites use a host of factors to make their arguments for change - the demographics of an aging society, historical circumstances, and the economic climate- and construct the facts to make their arguments. Second, it examines how policy elites invoke public opinion as a way to convince the public that they are central actors in the political play on stage. Nonetheless, it appears that members of the public - as in a theater - are the spectators, removed from the stage and seated in the audience, being played to by the elites on stage. Using an agenda setting framework, the paper concludes by arguing that Social Security in the United States appears to be ripe for change.

The Politics of Pension Reform: The State of the Debate

Dalmer D. Hoskins [Secretary General, International Social Security Association, Geneva, Switzerland]

This paper analyzes why some countries succeed in enacting significant and far-reaching social security reforms while others experience successive crises marked by the fall of governments, parliamentary paralysis, and even widespread civil unrest. It describes what has been learned from the decade of the 90s when most countries with extensive social security systems undertook reform efforts to ensure both short-term financial stability and the long-term survival of the programmes in the face of demographic ageing and profound labour market changes. First, it examines the causes of the growing lack of public confidence in the future viability of these schemes, particularly among the younger population of contributors who frequently express doubts about whether they will benefit from similar levels of protection as their parents and grandparents. Second, it shows the extent to which the politics of social security reform is similar or different in the developing countries of the world from that observed in the industrialized OECD countries. The reform debate has during recent years been almost exclusively dominated by economic and fiscal considerations. Will demographic ageing eventually bring other questions to the fore, including redefining retirement and the pensionable age, the continuing vulnerability of older women as well as social security as an instrument for income redistribution and poverty alleviation among the aged?

The Politics of Pensions in Africa: In the Eye of the Storm

Eric N.A. Adjei [Social Security and National Insurance Trust, Accra, Ghana, Africa]

This paper analyzes the problems that were faced in the development of Social Security in Ghana and how these problems compare to those faced by other African countries including Uganda, Zambia, Tanzania, Zanzibar, Ethiopia, and Sierra Leone. The analysis makes clear that the International Monetary Fund (IMF) and the World Bank have played key roles in the politics of pension policy in many of these countries. Understanding the roles of the IMF and the World Bank in pension policy is central to understanding the politics of pensions in these African countries and how they differ from that of European countries and North American countries.

The Strange History of British Pension Reform, 1980-2000

Robin Blackburn [University of Essex/New University School; Colchester, England]

This paper supplies a narrative of successive attempts to reform British pension arrangements and in particular the implicit privatisation involved in cutting back on public provision while sponsoring new tax-subsidised alternatives. Margaret Thatcher's government successfully reduced state provision by indexing pensions to prices rather than earnings. The encouragement given personal pension plans set the scene for a notorious mis-selling scandal. In 1997 New Labour set out to introduce stakeholder pensions but by July 1998 the architect of its welfare reforms, Frank Field, resigned from the government. As recently as March 2000 the Labour chancellor was sticking to inflation-only rises in the state pension but the dramatic events of the next six months somehow got embroiled in pension policy and obliged him to take a different tack in November. The paper explains the arguments of the various protagonists in these developments and concludes with a consideration of why pensions and pension funding is now so much closer to the centre of political debate in Britain than it has ever been before.

SESSION 59

Improving services for people with dementia and their carers

Anne Braekus 'Evaluation of methods for assessment of dementia in primary and specialist health care' S. Cahill 'A study of design features in dementia-specific day care centres in Ireland' Tom Dening 'Improving dementia care by means of health policy: The national service framework for older people' Jane Gilliard 'The role of dementia services development centres' Øyvind Kirkevold 'Special Care Units for persons with dementia versus ordinary nursing home wards does it matter? Päivo Topo 'Improving dementia services in Finland. Has technology any role?'

ISSUE: This symposium addresses ways of improving dementia services STRUCTURE: Six ten minute presentations each to be followed by five minutes of questions CONTENT: The issue of improving dementia services is addressed from several points of view: government policy, development centres, research and innovation. The need to improve dementia services is urgent in most countries given rapidly increasing numbers of people with dementia and the impact on their families and communities. There is a parallel increase in interest in how to provide optimal care. Dissemination of research, innovation and best practice into the field is a challenge being addressed by dementia services development centres. All the presenters work in the dementia services development centres in Northern Europe. ANTICIPATED OUTCOME: An appreciation of the role and tasks of dementia services development centers especially in relation to government policy and research.

A Study of Design Features in Dementia-Specific Day Care Centres in Ireland

S. Cahill, M. Drury (Dementia Services Information and Development Centre, Dublin, Ireland), D. O'Connor, M. O'Connell (The Alzheimer Society of Ireland, Dublin, Ireland), B. Lawlor (St Patrick's Hospital, Dublin, Ireland)

PURPOSE: The careful design of day care centres for people with dementia is an area of increasing clinical, research and architectural interest. It is well established that the built environment can be used to compensate for some of the disabilities associated with dementia and can promote the individual's quality of life. The purpose of this study was to explore professional carers' attitudes to design features in the day care centres in which they were employed. METHOD: A purposive sample of care staff (N=72) from each of the 19 Alzheimer Society of Ireland Centres were included in the research and in-depth interviews were used to collect quantitative and qualitative data. RESULTS: Findings showed that while a large majority of respondents reported day care was extremely well planned and very responsive to clients' needs, much dissatisfaction was expressed about the physical size and lay out of the internal and external environment in which services were offered. In particular the need for more space (indoor and outdoor), improved lighting, a quiet room to calm clients who are agitated and a staff room where employees can take time out from caring was noted. A large majority of care staff also stated they would value additional training on design and dementia. CONCLUSION: The study is a first attempt in the Irish context to open up the debate on the topic of design and dedicated dementia care. Results from the study will contribute to the development of guidelines on accommodation and design for dementia specific day care.

Evaluation of methods for assessment of dementia in primary and specialist health care

Braekhus Anne, Engedal Knut (The Norwegian Centre for Dementia Research,Oslo, Norway)

PURPOSE: The purpose of this project was to implement and evaluate different assessments methods of dementia in primary and specialist health care service. According to Norwegian consensus, patients with suspected dementia or with mild dementia should be examined by specialiced dementia team. Due to the large amount of demented patients, patients with a mild/moderate and severe dementia should preferably be assessed in primary care. METHOD: Specialist health care services in three of Norway's 19 counties and 18 municipalities were selected for participation in this project. At the primary care level, one GP and one or two nurses formed a project group and were instructed in different ways to organize the examination and the follow-up of patients with dementia. At the specialist level, the main objective was to establish one or two dementia outpatient clinics (memory clinics) in each county. The project group from the Norwegian Centre for Dementia Research contributed with seminars twice a year, developed manuals for assessing dementia, and kept close contact with the participants. RESULT: In the three counties, five specialist teams have been established. At the primary level, three main ways of organizing has been established. 1)assessment of all the patients in the municipal by one doctor and one nurse("centralised" model), 2) the patient's primary physician and the district nurse do the assessment ("decentralised" model) and 3) the patient is assessed by their primary care physician and a specialised dementia team consisting of two nurses (combined model). CONCLUSION: Further evaluation of the project will take place in 2001.

Improving Dementia Care by Means of Health Policy: The National Service Framework for Older People

Tom Dening, Tim Brown (Department of Health, London, UK)

Older people are a Government priority in the UK. The National Health Service Plan for England emphasises four commitments delivering standards of care, ensuring fair access to services, promoting independence and improving fairness of funding for long term care. Following this, the National Service Framework (NSF) for Older People, introduced in April 2001, sets national standards across health and social care to drive up quality of care for older people. It describes service models for best practice, including for dementia. Dementia is a major health and social issue across the world. Although services for people with dementia and their carers are sometimes excellent, in practice patchy resources and variable quality are more typical. The UK Government is aware of this and is committed to bringing about change. Some policy initiatives are for older people in general, such as Better Government for Older People. Other initiatives help to support frail older people, including those with dementia, and their carers (e.g. the Care Standards Act and the Carers Act). The NSF draws much of this together to ensure that older people get better health and social care. Its underlying principles include promoting health and well being, preserving the dignity and independence of older people, recognising the crucial role played by informal carers, and fair access to services on the basis of clinical need. The NSF is improving the care and treatment received by older people from the NHS, and contributes positively for people with dementia.

Improving dementia services in Finland. Has technology any role?

Päivi Topo (National Research and Development Centre for Welfare and Health, STAKES, Helsinki, Finland)

PURPOSE: The purpose of this presentation is to describe the dementia care system in Finland and findings of a research and development project on possible uses of technology in dementia care. METHOD: The presentation is based on previous literature, national health and social care registers, and interviews of people with dementia and their family carers and formal carers. RESULTS: According to the register data the trend to emphasise community care instead of institutionalised care has continued in most of the country. According to the interviews the role of technology in dementia care is very small but there is much potential for its use in to compensation or stimulation in home care or in institutionalised care settings. Results of a qualitative study among people with dementia on their abilities to use telephone showed that ability to use telephone can be supported. A study of possibilities of using multimedia in dementia care has shown that people with moderate to severe dementia can benefit multimedia products if, in the design, their special needs are taken into account. CONCLUSIONS: Possibilities of support to informal and formal care of people with moderate or severe dementia living at home should get more attention. There are several reasons to believe that the development of dementia care in Finland should also involve developers of assistive technology or so called main stream technology. More research should be done on assessing possibilities of developing technological aids to support people with dementia and their carers.

Special Care Units (SCU) for persons with dementia versus ordinary nursing home wards - does it matter?

Kirkevold (Norwegian Centre for Dementia Research, Tønsberg, Norway), K Engedal (Norwegian Centre for Dementia Research, Oslo, Norway), A Eek (Norwegian Centre for Dementia Research, Tønsberg, Norway), Aa-M Nygård (Norwegian Centre for Dementia Research, Oslo, Norway).

PURPOSE: The aim is to analyse how organisation of wards in nursing homes influence the use of restraints and quality of care. METHOD: Data collected from two parts of a Norwegian study on use of restraints and quality of care. The study includes a survey of routines on wards for elderly (1401 wards) and data collection from 1526 patients randomly selected in various care settings. From each patient we collected CDR-score, BARS-score and PADL-score. RESULTS: In SCUs the patients more often suffered from serve dementia, the prevalence of BPSD was higher and the patients had higher level of function in ADL than in ordinary wards. SCUs were relative better staffed and they had fewer patients. There was more use of restraints in SCUs (not significant) but this effect disappears when we adjust for degree of dementia, ADL scores and behavioural scores. Conditions that reduce quality of care (8 questions about quality) were significantly more often present in ordinary wards than in SCUs even if we adjust for patient characteristics. The strongest factors that predicted conditions that reduced quality of care were patient characteristics, the type of ward, qualifications of the staff and staffing (in that order). DISCUSSION: SCUs have a positive effect on quality markers, but not on the use of restraints. Preliminary analysis of the datasets shows that different kinds of restraints are used in SCUs versus in ordinary wards.

The role of dementia services development centres

Jane Gilliard (Dementia Voice, Bristol, England & Chair, National Network of Dementia Services Development Centres)

In 1988, a centre was established at the University of Stirling in Scotland to provide support and advice to those who work with and provide services for people with dementia. Its work was unique until 1997 when further centres were established in England and the Republic of Ireland. By 2000 the National Network of Dementia Services Development Centres covered almost the entire country so that every one working in dementia care (whether at operational or strategic level) could access support and advice. This paper will present in more detail the role of dementia services development centres in the UK. The core services of these centres include: - § Dissemination of information § Training and education § Research and development § Consultancy and advice § Publications/seminars/workshops and conferences The dementia services development centres in the UK meet regularly to exchange information and ideas, to develop collaborative research proposals and to encourage new developments. Representatives from the Department of Health attend these meetings. The current policy agenda in the UK is making rapid changes to the way in which services for older people are organised and delivered. Our experience suggests that many commissioners and providers of services to people with dementia are keen to tap the expertise of the dementia services development centres.

Urinary Incontinence: Management Guidelines and Outcomes

M. Borrie (Division of Geriatric Medicine, South western Ontario Regional Geriatric Program, University of Western Ontario, Lawson Health Research Institute, London, Ontario, Canada) A. Saltmarche (Clinical Associate, Cross-Appointed, Graduate School, Faculty of Nursing, University of Toronto) S. Lytwynec (Geriatric Day Hospital and South western Ontario Regional Geriatric Program, London, Ontario, Canada) D. Griffiths (Division of Geriatric Medicine, University of PIttsburgh, Pittsburgh, PA, USA) K. Moore (Faculty of Nursing, University of Alberta, Edmonton, Alberta, Canada)

Issues that will be addressed: - Clinical practice guidelines for urinary incontinence management in elderly men and women - Decision making then diagnosis based on Canadian Consensus guidelines - Working models of incontinence management in 3 different settings Structure: The process of developing Canadian guidelines, flow charts, and models of incontinence care culminating in the Consensus conference (May 2000) was convened by the Canadian Continence Foundation. The process and conference was funded by a grant from the Population Health Fund - Health Canada, Division of Aging and Seniors. Three 15-minute presentations summarizing the results of the Canadian Consensus conference on incontinence management in adults (May 2000), relevant to the elderly. The three presentations will cover - 1. The updated AHCPR (Agency for Health Care Policy and Research) guidelines 1995-1999 2. The revised flow charts for elderly men and women 3. Three proposed working models of incontinence care Content: 1. Guidelines The AHCPR guidelines were updated from the peer reviewed literature published 1995-1999 identified through a systematic literature search using relevant keywords and the following literature databases; the Cochrane Incontinence group trial register, Medline, Cinahl, Enbase, Psychlit, ERCC, and Ageline. New or revised guideline statements were developed according to the quality and amount of evidence. The levels of evidence were assigned according to a standard published in Canadian Clinical Practice Guidelines. 2. Flow Charts These were originally developed at the 1st International consultation on Incontinence (Monaco 1998). They have been adapted to reflect the management of incontinence in men and women and the frail elderly. They provide visual representation of the recommended steps in the assessment and management of urinary incontinence and the order in which they should be considered. The flow charts appear similar but emphasize the differences between the management of the 3 different groups. 3. Working models of continence care were developed. The purpose of these models is to show how the guidelines can be put into practice in various representative settings, taking into account medical, organizational, funding and educational issues. These models suggest concrete solutions for continence care in various settings across Canada. The models were developed from an environmental scan of the models of continence care in Canada and worldwide. A care working models committee, including clients/ consumers and leading Canadian multidisciplinary healthcare professionals from urology, urogynecology, family practice, nursing and physiotherapy, and a federal government representative from the Division of Seniors and Aging of Health Canada, decided on three broad setting for which working models should be prepared: rural/remote, small city, and urban/academic. The resultant models will be briefly presented. Conclusions / Anticipated Outcomes: The presentation of the updated guidelines, flow charts, and working models will stimulate discussion on these three issues, as well as the issues of effective dissemination of education, implementation, and effective ways to influence changes in practice.

SESSION 60

Benefit of cognitive stimulation in the daily life of patients with dementia.

J de Rotrou, F Dessi, D de Susbielle, F Forette

This paper emphasises the effectiveness of a validated cognitive stimulation programme in Alzheimer outpatients. The objective of global cognitive stimulation is to reinforce residual resources of demented patients by exercises adapted to spared functions. This stimulation involves two types of factors : cognitive factors (attentional, perceptive, mnesic, verbal, intellectual) and psychological and social factors (restoration of confidence, motivation, reinforcement of social ties and feelings of belonging to a group). The exercises are organized into sessions of one hour and thirty minutes duration. The periodicity is twice weekly. Thirty patients with first stage dementia (MMS 25.4 + 3) participated in the cognitive stimulation programme for a mean period of 15 months. All the patients met the inclusion criteria for this study. Patients and their caregivers have been evaluated by means of different rating scales at the. The results demonstrate the benefit of cognitive stimulation in activities of daily living for the patients. This benefit is also demonstrated in social and psychological parametres. Regarding the caregivers, the results show that stress and burden are significantly reduced. We conclude that this non pharmacological approach appears to be parallel and complementary treatment for Alzheimer patients and their families.

Cognitive Stimulation in Elderly People

V. Diaz, C . Vasquez, M.A. Cumsille, A. Donoso, D. Nowogrodski. [HOSPITAL CLINICO UNIVERSIDAD DE CHILE, SANTIAHO, CHILE]

Objective: TO EVALUATE THE EFFICACY OF COGNITIVE STIMULATION IN A GROUP OF HEALTHY ELDER USING REUVEN FEURSTEIN METHODOLOGY. METHOD: A PROSPECTIVE, NON RANDOMIZED, INTERVENTIONAL STUDY. SETTING: COMMUNITY SENIOR CLUBS. PARTICIPANTS: 31 ELDERLY PEOPLE WITH A MINI MENTAL STATE (MMT) OVER 24. ALL OF THEM WERE EVALUATED BEFORE AND AFTER COGNITIVE STIMULATION USING YESAVAGE GERIATRIC DEPRESSION RATE (GDS), MINI MENTAL STATE (MM) OF FOLTSTEIN, BARCELONA BATTERY (BB) AND THE MMPI EXPLORATORY INSTRUMENT. INTERVENTION: 16 WORKSHOPS OF 90 MINUTES EACH ONE, TWICE A WEEK DURING TWO MONTHS. DURING THIS TIME THEY HAD MOTIVATION, SENSORY DISCRIMINATION, ORIENTATION AND ATTENTION, CONCEPT FORMATION AND REASONING ACTIVITIES, TRAINING IN EPISODIC MEMORY, MNEMONIC TRAINING. MAIN OUTCOME MEASURE: VARIATION IN THE SCORE IN GDS, MMT, MMPI USING NON PARAMETRIC METHODS AND REGRESSION ANALYSIS. RESULTS: THE MEAN AGE WAS 69 YEARS OLD (DS=6.8), MEAN OF EDUCATION WAS 5.4 YEARS OF BASIC SCHOOL (RANGE 4-7 YEARS). STATIStiCALLY SIGNIFICANT PRE TO POST TEST GAINS WERE FOUND FOR ALL THE TEST. WILCOXON SIGNED RANK PRE TO POST WORKSHOP WERE FOR MM WAS 4.84 (P=0.0001) FOR GDS 4.48 (P=0.0001); WILCOXON SIGNED RANK FOR DD WAS 3.93 (P=0.001), FOR DI=-4.16 (P=0.001), CE=-3.79 (P=0.001), TR=-4.78 (P=0.001), LW=-3.30 (P=0.001). USING REGRESSION ANALYSIS CHANGES WERE INDEPENDENT OF VARIATION IN GDS and MMT. TR WERE THE BEST PREDICTORS THE CHANGES IN THE LW, NON Dependent On AGE AND LEVEL OF EDUCATION. CONCLUSION: STIMULATION IMPROVED COGNITIVE PERFORMANCE, Controlling AGE, EDUCATION AND DEPRESSION IN ELDERLY.

Communication Breakdown, Topic Management, and Dementia of the Alzheimer's Type

B. Abbott, J.B. Orange (University of Western, Ontario, London, Canada)

Purpose: Language and communication problems, as well as memory problems, are hallmark features of dementia of the Alzheimer's type (DAT). Communication problems in individuals with DAT are specific to stage of the disease. Caregiver stress can be reduced when information is provided regarding changes in communication skills as DAT progresses. Research focusing on communication breakdowns in DAT found that the number of breakdowns increases with stage of the disease. Studies investigating conversational topic determined that individuals with DAT have greater difficulty shifting the current topic and introducing new topics. Previous studies noted the possibility of a relationship between conversation topic and breakdown, however, to date no one has empirically addressed this proposed relationship. Method: Transcripts of conversation from 18 spousal dyads (6 control, 6 early stage DAT and 6 middle stage DAT) were coded for trouble source repair (TSR) sequences and for topic initiation and maintenance parameters. Analyzes of the relationship between conversation topic and breakdown was completed using modified time series analysis. Results: Topic introductions occurred at instances of trouble source repair (TSR) sequences in the conversation of individuals with DAT. Type and manner of topic introduction were related to the TSR sequence occurrence. Frequency of occurrence of these linked variables was dependent on both stage of the disease and participant status. Conclusion: Provision of caregiver education and training programs focusing on conversational topic introduction strategies may alleviate difficulties with communication breakdown in DAT discourse.

Evolution of the writing during neurodegenerative discorders

Thomas S, Merrot s, Liagre A, Frigard B.Centre de Gériatrie - Wasquehal, France

Writing is a very precise graphic and motor action organized by brain, synthesis of a language implied by thought. It seemed coherent to study modifications of it arising during neurodegenerative disorders. 40 subjects with late-onset Alzheimer s disease (NINCDS criterias), French mother tongue, were compared with a control group (n=10, MMS 29 and 30) of equivalent age (78 years). Written and dated documents were collected for each patient, certified by the author s hand. During the visit, the patient copied out, in best possible conditions a standard sentence. In blind-study, characteristics of writing were analyzed by 3 handwritings experts, according to strict criterias (De Ajurriaguerra). A statistical analysis was performed. Alone, "movement" is the non-modified character. Premature modifications interest the characters of the line, the irregularity of the shape and the speed of the writing, as well as the broken line. Latest modifications are those of continuity, steepness, organization and signature. Irregularity of shape appears prematurely but does not increase during the disease, contrary to "unsteady" line drawing and "straining" who are deteriorated inexorably (motor apraxia deterioration?). These observations have to be compared with agraphias (left parietal lobe injury) and the spatial dysgraphias (right temporo-parieto-occipital lobe injury). In addition to classic psychometry, specifics graphological criterias can be proposed in addition to regular criterias of dementia.

Nonverbal Communication of Emotions in Patients Suffering from Moderate and Severe Dementia

J. Wilbers (Center for Psychological and Psychosomatic Research, University of Trier, Germany) A.Kruse (Institute of Gerontology, University of Heidelberg, Germany) S. Re (Institute of Gerontology, University of Heidelberg, Germany) W. Classen (Center for Psychological and Psychosomatic Research, University of Trier, Germany)

Understanding patients' actual needs and demands is a prerequisite for adequate care in institutional settings. As verbal communication about daily routines and care is no longer possible with patients suffering from moderate or severe dementia, giving meaning to nonverbal markers of emotional condition seems to be an important challenge for programs aimed to develop and improve quality standards of institutional care. Unfortunately, since contemporary research on dementia primarily focuses on the diagnosis and treatment in the beginning of the disease, expressive behavior in the case of moderate and severe dementia has not yet become a significant research topic. However, changes in demography will lead to a dramatic increase of people suffering from moderate or severe dementia. Proceeding from this background, a research cooperation was initiated to analyze nonverbal communication competencies in people suffering from moderate or severe dementia. Research results shall be used for the development of training programs for staff members and new criteria for adequate care in cases of dementia. Results from extensive psychiatric, neuropsychological and psychological examination and interviews with relatives and care givers in a sample of 40 patients from institutional services are reported. On the basis of medical and (neuro-)psychological status and relevant information about everyday-situations associated with positive versus negative affect, four persons (two suffering from moderate, two from severe dementia) were chosen as participants for a pilot study, in which participants were observed four times in positive and four times in negative situations. In this pilot study video-tapes of facial expressions of positive versus negative emotional conditions are analyzed by using a standardized coding system developed in the context of expressed emotion research.

Question Comprehension by Individuals with Dementia of the Alzheimer's type.

J.Veall, J.B. Orange (University of Western Ontario, London, Canada)

Purpose: The purpose of this study is to test the comprehension of open-ended questions and close-ended questions in indivicuals with dementia of the Alzheimer's type (DAT). Little research has looked at question comprehension in individuals with DAT. The use of close-ended (i.e, yes/no questions) instead of open-ended questions (i.e, 'wh' questions like 'when' and 'what') is frequently suggested as a strategy to reduce communication breakdowns between individuals with DAT and caregivers. Research is needed to test the effectiveness of this communication strategy. Question comprehension problems are expected in individuals with DAT due to a number of possible reasons including working memory problems, word finding difficulties, and general auditory comprehension impairments. Method: Participants (N=24) included 6 individuals with early stage DAT, 6 with middle stage DAT, and 12 normal controls. Each participant was administered a battery of standardized memory and language measures (e.g, Arizona Battery for Communication Disorders of Dementia; Bayles & Tomoeda, 1993). Further, question probes consisting of 9 question types including 5 close-ended question types and 4 open-ended question types were presented by the examiner during a mealtime context with participants in either their home or in a day program they attended. Measures of working memory, naming ability and sentence comprehension were compared to question comprehension skills for both open-ended and close-ended questions. Results: Individuals with DAT were able to answer close-ended questions significantly better than open-ended questions. Conclusion: The results suggest the effectiveness of specific question formulation to optimize auditory comprehension by individuals with DAT.

Semiotic Mediation in Alzheimer's Disease and Normal Aging

K. Lyng (NOVA ? Norwegian Social Research, Oslo, Norway), L. Bender, P. Fromholt, P. Torpdahl (Center for Gerontopsychology, Aarhus, Denmark).

The purpose of this study was to investigate the mediational properties of language in healthy old adults and old adults with Alzheimers disease. A theory of semiotic mediation states that semiotic signs (language, concepts etc.) mediate(indirectly) the relation between reality and mind. Twenty-one healthy old adults (OA), 10 persons with Alzheimers disease (AD), and 17 young healthy adults (YA) were given a selection of 12 items from Raven's Standard Progressive Matrices. Standardised verbal-conceptual hints constructed for each item were given if the subject failed to solve a given item. Two post-test without hints were given. The first was a re-test with the same items. The second consisted of a new set of items with the same principal problems. There was a considerable overlap in scores between the AD and OA when performance without hints are compared. This overlap disappeared when verbal hints were given. Young and old adults solved all items with a limited number of hints. Only a marginal gain was obtained in the AD group even when nearly all hints were given. Post-tests showed that the effects obtained for any group were not sustainable as the performance dropped back to baseline when support was withdrawn. The findings supports a position that a semiotic mediational mechanism seems to be intact in healthy old adults, but that thesame mechanisms are not working properly in Alzheimers disease. Persons with AD cannot use language as a conscious tool to control their environment and their own behaviour.

SESSION 61

Development of Services for the Aged in Israel

Hava Golander (Department of Nursing, Tel Aviv University, Israel) Yitzhak Brick (Director General, ESHEL - The Association ofr the Planning and Development of Services for the AGed in Israel, JDC. Jerusalem, Israel)

National historical overviews can illustrate the commonalities as well as the unique in the international development of services for the elderly. This study provides a historical overview of the social development of gerontological sevices in Israel which spans 150 years - beginning with early settlement in Palestine in the second half of the 19th century to the present day. Parallel with the dynamic transformations of the Jewish population in Palestine/Israel during the last 150 years, the development of services for the elderly has also been quite dramatic. Our two main data sources include historical records containing demographic information and gerontological literature. During the late Ottoman Period, the elderly comprised a relatively high proportion of the Jewish population (~13%) as many of them wished to be buried in the Holyland and immigrated to the country at an advanced age. Medical care, like all living expenses, was made possible through donations which constituted the financial basis for the establishment of various philanthropic institutions. The first old age homes developed from poor houses around the turn of the century, were gender-specific and generally catered for independent elderly. During the British Mandate, the young Zionist Jewish immigrants established mutual help organizations and community health care services. Medical services became more professional and institutionalized. Since the creation of the State of Israel, mass immigration and the natural aging of the Israeli population have served as catalysts for the development of a network of national as well as community services for the elderly. These services were planned and administered in the 60's as part of the welfare state and have undergone accelerated privatization since the 80's. The complex changes that took place within this last phase will be discussed in the light of broader processes such as modernization and globalization.

Health Behaviour Patterns of the Elderly in Osun State, Nigeria

*FAJEMILEHIN (Boluwaji Reuben, Senior Lecturer and) ODEBIYI, A. I. (College of Health Sciences and **Department of Sociology and Anthropology of Obafemi Awolowo University, Ile-Ife Osun State, Nigeria)*

This descriptive and cross-sectional study examined the health behaviour patterns of the elderly against the background of a declining economy and weakened extended family system in a society that has no formal structure of care and support for the sub group. The study was conducted using a multistage sampling procedure for the selection of the traditional core health districts and households with the elderly aged 60 years and above in ten (10) selected local government areas in Ife/Ijesa zone of Osun State. Based on the responses from the three hundred (300) respondents coupled with their primary support providers, the health behaviour profile was determined. The data generated using both quantitative and qualitative approaches were analysed utilizing multiple statistical techniques. The study revealed that coping devices among the respondents were petty trading and subsistence farming, care giving support from children, spouses and others as well as the use of individual elderly habitual orientation. It was also found that the elderly participants in this study utilized several socio-cultural and economic means to keep fit. Major among the measures are traditional health care services, self medication, maintenance of good moral conduct, leadership roles within families and communities and care-giving. Other health promoting factors are those related to cultural, religious, nutritional practices, and personal health habits. The health care orientation of the elderly respondents most importantly focused on self-medication (buying of unprescribed drugs) and use of different dimensions of traditional health care system for significant reasons such as cost and cultural beliefs coupled with values of the respondents. The study concludes that the effect of socio political and economic instability has caused serious modification and change in the cultural orientation of individuals, families and communities. The instability has no doubt weakened the already crippled state of family association and income, standard of living and quality of life.

Healthy life style and its determinants in the elderly in St. Petersburg

Pertti Pohjolainen (Kuntokallio Centre for Gerontological Training and Research, Helsinki, Finland) Ilkka Pietila (Kuntokallio Centre for Gerontological Training and Research, Helsinki, Finland)

An interview study was completed in spring 2000 in St. Petersburg as part of a project (IPSE - Improving the Planning of Medical and Social Services within Elder Care in St. Petersburg) financed by the European Commission. The study investigated the living conditions, life style, health status, functional capacity and service needs of 60-89-year-old people. This part of the study deals with healthy lifestyle and factors related to it. The research data consisted of 1216 structured interviews (412 men, 804 women). Since there were no up-to-date registers available in St. Petersburg, the sample was made by searching for appropriate people for the sample from door to door. The original sampling frame included regional lists of interviewable groups which represented the age and sex distribution of the regions. Based on the number of interviews (1216) and refusals (176), response rate (87%) could be measured after the sample was completed. Smoking was more common among men (33%) than women (4%). Among men, smoking decreased with age. Men used alcohol more often than women. Alcohol consumption decreased with age. Men who worked used alcohol more often than retired men. Married women used alcohol more often than single women, widows or divorced women. About 25% of the respondents reported they exercised at least for an hour every day. There was no gender difference in exercise activity. Background factors related to exercise activity included age, education and work/pension status among men: younger, more educated men who were still working exercised more often than others. Among women, only education was related to exercise activity.

Recycling Active Ageing Human Resources in Developing Countries

Abdul Rahim Khan USA (Panjab University, Lahore, Pakistan and Correspondent AFICS New York in Pakistan)

ISSUE: The new millennium is bequeathed with an unprecedented challenge of ageing population all over the world. More than two-thirds of the elderly people will live in the developing countries by the year 2025. Second the aged population once looked upon with reverence out of conviction, cultural norms and elderly experience are growingly looked down upon as a burden on society, a weakening appendage to the family and a victim of circumstances in the developing world. Paradoxically an aged or retired person is exemplified as a past dated newspaper. Third, global interdependencies, social change, techno-administrative developments, economic hegemony and distorted social equity are becoming formidable constraints in providing adequate quality of life especially to the ageing population. Four, there is a growing imbalance between the available and needed human resources in almost every sector in the developing countries which is exacerbated by poverty, backwardness, skill drought , crisis of ethics, confidence, honesty and patriotism and persistent skill gap particularly in the informal sector. Five, there are augmenting needs of human resources in the coming decades resulting from globalization, deregulation, market changes and competition. Six, on the other hand the added life to the older people is creating a huge pool of human resources during their active ageing, which remains untapped and contrarily is becoming a continual burden on the public exchequer. STRUCTURE: Statement outlining the organization of the session I will initiate the session through a presentation on the global perspectives of the recycling of active aging in developing countries. Three presentations on specific countries will follow to provide cross-cultural case studies. CONTENT: Summary of the presentation to be given The presentations will include demographic profiles highlighting indicants of ageing population, identify typical socioeconomic, intergenerational and societal problems from neighborhood to national level, establish parameters of human resource requirements, an assessment of active ageing population, their potentials and constraints in reengaging them and planning and programming implications. CONCLUSIONS: Statement of the conclusions, expected outcome or product of the session The deliberations will focus on the Society for All Ages goal and innovative ways to achieve it. The sectoral approach as reflected in the successive Five Year Plans will have to be replaced. In fact the concepts of development planning will have to be restructured. Carefully designed new policies and strategies will be identified. They will be aimed at promoting a new form of productive ageing, enhancing opportunities for recycling or in other words reengaging human resources during active aging, projecting the older people as assets rather than burden through the perspective of human rights, augmenting intergenerational relationships, enhancing opportunities for income generation as well as voluntary roles in the social sectors, community empowerment with their involvement in social, economic, cultural and spiritual undertakings and their engagement in a wide range of activities from micro enterprises to advisory services and nation building activities.

Social Healthy Profile and the Future of the Old Age in Chile

A. Herrera (HOSPITAL CLINICO UNIVERSIDAD DE CHILE.SANTIAGO.CHILE.)

OBJECTIVE: CHILE FINDS IN AN ADVANCE DEMOGRAPHICAL TRANSITION STAGE. IN 1998,THE OLD AGE REPRESENT 10.5% OF THE POPULATION, PROJECTING 16% FOR 2025. THE STUDY INVESTIGATION OF THE OLD AGE IN CHILE NEEDS, DEVELOP THAT 71.9% HAD A HEALTH PROBLEM, ACCORDING TO THE INDICATORS OF FUNCTIONAL AUTONOMY, 66.7% DEFINED POTENTIALLY HEALTHY, 30% FUNCTIONALLY DELICATE AND ONLY A 3.3 DEPENDENT BY SEVERE DISABILITY; THE NECESSITIES OF HEALTH AND THE ECONOMIC NEEDS WERE THE LESS SATISFIED. THE 47.5% OF THE OLD AGE WERE CARRIER OF A CHRONIC DISEASE. A MENTAL HEALTH INVESTIGATION REVEALED 5.58% TO AFFECTIVE DISORDER AND 13.3% OF COGNITIVE DISORDER. THE 10.8% ARE IN A POVERTY SITUATION, 2.3 OF THESE ARE HOMELESS AND ONLY 36.8% OF THE HOMELESS HAS ACCESS TO THE PREVISIONAL SYSTEM. THE TOTAL OF THE POPULATION OF THE OLD AGE, 79.6% HAS ACCESS TO THE PUBLIC HEALTH SYSTEM, 545% OF THESE PEOPLE, HAS THE RIGHT TO A COMPLETE FREE ATTENTION. CONCLUSION: THE CONDITIONS OF LIFE OF THE AGE DEPENDS OF THEIR ACCESS TO THE PREVISIONAL SYSTEM, FOR BEING AN ECONOMICALLY PASSIVE POPULATION. THERE IS CRISIS BETWEEN THE PUBLIC INSTITUTION AND THE PROCESS OF OLDNESS, BECAUSE OF THE ABSENCE OF CONTINUITY TO ATTEND FROM HEALTH TO DISCAPACITY, BECAUSE THE HIGHER COST ARE ASSOCIATED TO CURE AND NOT TO TAKE CARE OF. CHALLENGES: TO REORGANIZE THE CHILEAN PREVISIONAL SYSTEM. TO USE RESOURCES TROUGH THE INTERGENERATIONAL COMMON CAUSES AND TO MEDIATE ON SOCIAL ETHICS AND IMPARTIALITY. TO PRIVILEGE THE POLITICS OF THE POOR OLD AGE. TO DEVELOP INDICATORS OF QUALITY OF LIFE, MORE AMBITIOUS. A GREAT CULTURAL CHANGE MULTISECTORIAL.

The present situation and trend of care for the elderly

Jin Ling, Zhu Jiming (Shanghai Research Center on Aging, Shanghai, China)

We will discuss three kinds of older persons, the old-old whose age is 80 years old and over, the older person who is disabled, and the older person from empty nest family (there is nobody except older persons in a family). They are facing different needs of care, and we intend to point to the tendency of care services for older persons when family structure is smaller and the proportion of the old-old increases. The old-old has special physical and mental needs. The higher age makes their constitution poor and physical power weaker. Incidence of chronic disease increases with the increasing of age. The old-old need more life services provided by communities. The older disabled person has poor health and lower income; they need special care from the government and society. Small-scale family structure and increasing empty families make the role of family in life care for older persons weaken. Meanwhile the society will bring into the more and more important play. In the empty nest families, the older persons need the mental care and common life care provided by their communities. Our main point is to develop the home for destitute older persons in community and to develop the service industry for the aged. For the old old to offer services to his doorstep; for the disabled older persons to develop the aged home in their neighborhood; and for the older persons of empty nest families to provide varieties of service items to buy.

SESSION 62

Care in the Community for Dementia: a multidisciplinary, multicentred research program

Neil Drummond (Sunnybrook and Women's College Health Science Centre, Toronto, Canada) The effectiveness of specialized case management for dementia in community settings. Malcolm Man-Son-Hing (Division of Geriatric Medicine, University of Ottawa, Canada) Development of a simple, easy-to-use prescreening instrument for driving safety/ Carole Cohen (Sunnybrook and Women's College Health Science Centre, Toronto, Canada) What is the experience of persons in need of a diagnosis? James Silvius (Division of Geriatric Medicine, University of Calgary, Calgary, Canada) New medications and changing expectations. Jean Kozak, (University of Ottawa Institute on Health of the Elderly, Ottawa, Canada) Managing problem behaviours in a variety of care settings.

Issues: There are three community-based networks for the care of dementia in Canada (in Ottawa-Carlton, Calgary and Toronto), bringing together professionals from a range of disciplines with representatives of caregiver organisations. At a meeting funded by CIHR in November 2000, the three networks identified a collective research agenda, in collaboration with representatives from the research community. This consisted of five individual projects. This Round Table will discuss progress in bringing the agenda to realisation, focussing on the importance of maintaining a multidisciplinary, multicentred approach to the problems of providing care in community settings. Structure The convenor will briefly describe the development of the research program. Each of the five project leaders will then present a short description of progress in the first six months. The main body of the session will consist of an informal discussion of the program, both in terms of its overall strategic direction and its detailed content. Issues to be highlighted include methodological, ethical and practical problems associated particularly with research in community settings. We shall be particularly interested to learn of the experiences of other research groups or individuals working in similar fields or under similar conditions. Content · The effectiveness of specialized case management for dementia in community settings Many questions remain to be answered in relation to case management. This study is intended to broadly examine the definition of case management models across the continuum of care, seeking to explore the relative effectiveness of case management for dementia. Key questions to be examined include identifying the criteria which should determine when, and of what type, case management should be implemented for the individual client or patient, whether it is more effective to train a select cadre of professionals or to train a broader set of providers, how to involve family doctors and other health care providers in a specialised case management model, the cost effectiveness of case management, and the influence of cultural factors. · Development of a simple, easy-to-use prescreening instrument for driving safety The decision to disqualify a patient from driving is often the source of major difficulty for the individual concerned, the family, and for professionals. This study incorporates the exploration of the sequelae of that decision on patient/family circumstances and lay-professional relationships, with the development of an instrument which will help providers decide which patients require driving assessment. · What is the experience of persons in need of a diagnosis? Dementia may not be readily diagnosed in primary care settings for a variety of reasons. Little is known about the experience of the individual with dementia during the diagnostic process, in terms of identification of the problem by the individual with dementia or others, the decision to seek advice about the problem from the healthcare system or others, the diagnostic process itself including history taking, mental status exam and cognitive testing, specialised testing such as neuroimaging and neuropsychological testing, and the process of referral and evaluation by specialists. This study will seek to identify what patients, caregivers and professionals identify as the important positive and negative experiences during the diagnostic phase. · New medications and changing expectations The development of new drugs for dementia (specifically cholinesterase inhibitors) may be changing both professional and lay expectations of therapy, including changes in management (such as prescribing patterns, expectations of caregivers). This study will investigate perceptions of the drugs among several groups, including families. · Managing behavioural problems in a variety of care settings 'Problem' behaviours in community settings represent a continuing challenge for both professionals and caregivers. This study is examining why some research conducted previously into the issue has not been utilised in practice, and investigates the effectiveness of non-pharmacological methods for behavioural management, including caregiver education and support intended to combat caregiver bias against the use of drugs in behaviour management. Anticipated outcomes In the light of our discussion we hope to broaden participation in the program by identifying researchers and practitioners from other settings or jurisdictions who have an interest in collaborating. In addition, we anticipate using the session to help clarify a number of problematic issues. Lastly, participants at the session should derive important insights into the development of a community-based research program, which we hope will encourage similar, much needed initiatives elsewhere.

Congruence Among Elderly Mothers and Caregiving Daughters

Valerie S. Kuehne (Vice-President Academic and Provost, University of Victoria, Victoria, BC, Canada), Neena L. Chappell (Centre on Aging, University of Victoria, Victoria, BC, Canada), Deborah Hunt Matheson (Department of Psychology, University of Victoria, Victoria, BC, Canada), and M. Theresa Hunter (School of Child and Youth Care, University of Victoria, Victoria, BC, Canada).

PURPOSE: This study examined affect congruence in mother-daughter caregiving relationships. METHOD: In a series of structured and unstructured interviews, a sample of 59 elderly mothers and their caregiving daughters reported on their personal relationship, their caregiving relationship, and changes in their relationship since caregiving began. Mothers' and daughters' scores were compared to determine congruence or incongruence in affect in these three domains. RESULTS: The majority of dyads expressed positive affect congruency about their personal relationship and the caregiving relationship. Congruency was lower regarding change in the relationship since caregiving began. Of the 27 dyads that were incongruent regarding change in the relationship, more than two-thirds of the daughters reported that the relationship had improved, while a similar proportion of mothers reported that the relationship had not changed. Contextual factors appeared to be related to caregivers' affect. Specifically, daughters who had more minor children living with them tended to feel less positive about the caregiving relationship. Daughters tended to feel less positive about the personal relationship when mothers needed more care, and daughters were not the primary caregivers. CONCLUSION: The evidence indicates that the caregiving aspect of the mother-daughter relationship may have a positive effect overall on their personal relationship.

Contributions of Adult Sons/Daughters with Lifelong Disabilities to Their Aging Caregiving Parents

M. M. MacLellan, (Nova Scotia Centre on Aging, Mount Saint Vincent University, Halifax, NS, Canada), D. Norris, (Department of Family Studies and Gerontology, Mount Saint Vincent University, Halifax, NS, Canada), C. Joffres (Nova Scotia Centre on Aging, Mount Saint Vincent University, Halifax, NS, Canada)

The literature which focuses on the caregiving relationships between aging parents and adult sons/daughters with lifelong disabilities concentrates on the care provided by the parents to the adult children. This uni-directional depiction of caregiving seems plausible given the impact of disability, but it does belie the general understanding that caregiving is usually not a one-way activity in aging families. Rather, caregiving can be reciprocal. A recent qualitative study provided a means to understanding the reciprocal character of caregiving ongoing between aging parents and adult disabled offspring. This study, based on phenomenological theory, involved in-depth interviews with fifty aging families in four provinces. Through analysis, using NUD*IST software, of taped and transcribed interviews, the experiences of the parents and the meanings they ascribed to those experiences were revealed. The complexities embedded in the ongoing caregiving relationships became apparent. In particular, reciprocity emerged as a component of that complexity. For example, while it is clear that participating parents are responsible for the provision of care to their adult disabled children, it is also clear that the children offered assistance in both tangible and intangible ways. Evidence of salient intangible contributions emerged through analysis of parents' claims that their adult children positively contributed to particular intrapsychic processes such as the development and maintenance of parental self-concept, parent-child bonding, and an enhanced sense of purpose. Noteworthy is that these aspects of reciprocity varied in accordance with the etiology of the disability. Other findings which emerged included the articulation of relevant supports needed as both the parents and the offspring grow older. Marlene MacLellan Associate Director Nova Scotia Centre on Aging Mount Saint Vincent University Halifax, NS B2M 2J6 Tel: 902 457-6546 Fax: 902 457-6508 E-mail: marlene.maclellan@msvu.ca

Family Life of the Elderly in Contemporary Poland

P. Czekanowski (Department of Sociology, University of Gdansk, Gdansk, Poland), B. Bien (Department of Clinical and Social Gerontology, Medical Academy, Bialystok, Poland), W. Pedich (Department of Clinical and Social Gerontology, Medical Academy, Bialystok, Poland) , B. Synak (Department of Sociology, University of Gdansk, Gdansk, Poland).

Changes of the socio-political situation in Poland over the last ten years have had a strong impact on the economic and social situation of the elderly as well as on their family position and intergenerational relationships. The aim of this paper is to analyse the family life situation of the elderly in the contemporary Polish society. The analysis is based on the survey conducted in 2000 on the representative sample of Poles aged 65 + (1821 respondents in total), and on 600 interviews. The results of our research show that elderly people are strongly involved in family life. 73% of older people live with somebody. Almost 74% of the elderly are asked for advice concerning the important family questions. 87 % of children have an appropriate respect for their old parents. 64% of the elderly take part in family meetings at least a few times a year. More than 94 % of old parents estimate their relationships with their children as very good or rather good. If an old person was in need, he/she would turn for help mainly to some family members. The role of reciprocity is quite common in the analysed families. Apart from the tendency to decrease the percentage of old people living together with their younger family members, and some changing customs among younger generations, the family in Poland remains a stable and the most important group which satisfies psychological, social and caring needs of the elderly people. .

Investment on Children and their Care for the Elderly: An Examination of Intergenerational Reciprocity

K.nagamanickam (Bharathiar University, Coimbatore, India) S.gayathri (Bharathiar University, Coimbatore, India) U.r.kaliappan (Bharathiar University, Coimbatore, India)

The elderly in India have traditionally been assigned a place of honor and the same has been spelt out by religion, social values, norms and social and economic organizations of the society. However, the Indian family system, which has been considered as a chief source of support and sustenance for the elderly, is changing in structure and the functions because of industrialization, urbanization, modernization and occupational mobility. In this new scenario have risen many forms of institutionalized support. Apart from this, commitment to the care of elderly in different social groups varies substantially reflecting their subcultural values (Cumming and Henry, 1961). However at the micro level, even the elderly sharing religion, caste, subculture, economic status and living in the region receive differential care from family and some are entrusted with institutions. Such differences led to two research questions. What have the elderly who are taken care by the family given to their children (in early years) more than the institutionalized elderly? and what are the norms of fair exchange - balanced and generalized reciprocity - which characterize the continuing support in these families? . For this purpose data were obtained from 15 institutionalized and 15 non-institutionalized elderly from similar background by adopting control group method. The potential caregiver of each of these elderly was also interviewed in-depth. In order to minimize the element of subjectivity an assessment by key informants (relatives, neighbour etc,) was obtained. This study relied on case study for this exploratory research pursuit. The results of the present study reveal that the investment need on children has a direct bearing on the care extended to the elderly. The other factors associated with institutionalization of the elderly are discussed in detail in the paper.

Reciprocity in caregiving relations in Denmark: between elderly and family and home help

M. Lewinter (Dept. of Sociology, U. of Copenhagen, Copenhagen, Denmark)

Studies of caregiving tend to overlook the importance of reciprocity, in particular the role of elderly care recipients as givers as well as receivers. In this paper, I will analyze the role of reciprocity in caregiving relationships, and how elderly reciprocate in relation to both family and home helpers. The study is based on qualitative interviews with a random sample of home help recipients in Denmark,aged 75 years and over, plus their family caregivers and home helpers. The results indicate that reciprocating was extremely important for the elderly and occurred in ways that are often overlooked in standardized interview schedules. The paper will present several examples of this reciprocity. For instance the importance the elderly attach to remembering things like birthdays and major life events for their children, grandchildren and great grandchildren, the efforts they make to 'pay' for many of the services that family members do. As regards home help, the 'cup of coffee' that is necessary when the helper comes (which elderly call a visit) is one example of elderly reciprocating, but home helpers report that they receive much from the elderly, for instance feeling of being useful and good role models. The paper will conclude by developing a theoretical model for analyzing this reciprocity, which posits that it is a key element in preserving a sense of self-worth and integrity for the elderly.

When Caregiving Means Reciprocity: The Multiple Forms of Reciprocity in Providing Care for a Frail Relative.

J.P. Lavoie (Direction de la santé publique de Montréal-Centre and CLSC René-Cassin, Montreal, Canada), D. White, R. Zuñiga (Université de Montréal, Canada)

It is generally recognized that care provided to a frail relative constitutes a non-reciprocal relationship between caregiver and care recipient, particularly when the latter suffers from dementia. However, the preceding statement is based on little empirical evidence. Indeed, little research has been done into the question of the subjective assessment of care of a frail relative. In the context of a qualitative study involving 30 individuals from 15 families in the region of Montreal (Canada) examining the structuration of family care of a frail relative, particular emphasis was placed on the meaning attributed to care by caregivers. During semi-structured interviews, it became apparent that, contrary to the above-mentioned belief, the vast majority of caregivers consider there to be reciprocity in care. However, this reciprocity may take many forms: it may be dyadic or not, immediate, deferred or hypothetical. Four types of reciprocity were elaborated: immediate reciprocity, hypothetical reciprocity, differed reciprocity, and generalized reciprocity. While there is a connection between the type of reciprocity and the type of disability (cognitive or physical) experienced by the relative, the type of reciprocity is primarily tied to social and family norms, the quality and the nature of the relationship between the caregiver and the care recipient. The ability to see care as a reciprocal relationship seems to enable caregivers to continue involvement in the care of their relative by compensating for some of the difficulties they may experience.

SESSION 63

Adaptation of the Abbeyfield Assisted Housing Model in South Africa: An Evaluation

R. Stolze (Abbeyfield Society of South Africa, Cape Town, South Africa), M. Ferreira (Institute of Ageing in Africa, University of Cape Town, CT, South Africa)

In Africa, older persons have traditionally co-resided with kin in multigenerational households. Very few residential care facilities are available for persons who are unable to live with kin. The effects of urbanisation, industrialisation and the AIDS epidemics on family structures are resulting in a growing need for affordable, assisted housing for older individuals. The Abbeyfield Society of South Africa has thus far enabled 14 affiliated local societies to establish and own homes for elders; households that are self-supporting and overseen by local society committees. South Africa has a multi-ethnic society. Although, the UK-grown Abbeyfield model serves the country's minority Caucasian population well, a challenge has been to adapt the model to serve ethnic communities. Areas which have required special attention are fostering fundraising by local committees (to purchase housing stock) in a context of poverty; building the capacity of committees in sustainable project management; and strengthening a volunteering ethos in low-income communities. The adaptation of the Abbeyfield model to achieve sustainable, non-governmental, not-for-profit, self-supporting, assisted housing provision for African elders is examined and the South African programme evaluated, with a view to disseminating information and encouraging the replication of the model in other developing-country settings.

Aging in Place in Small African American Assisted Living Facilities

Mary M. Ball, Molly M. Perkins, Frank J. Whittington, Sharon V. King, Bess L. Combs, & Carole Hollingsworth {Georgia State University, Atlanta, Georgia

Assisted Living Facilities are non-medical, community-based living environments that provide shelter, board, and 24-hour protective oversight and personal care services to mostly elderly residents. Most residents desire to remain in these facilities as they age and increase in frailty rather than enter nursing homes or other more restrictive and higher-cost long-term care environments. Little research, however, has explored the ability of residents to age in place in these facilities. This study uses qualitative methods to examine the experiences of residents and providers in five small (6-13 residents), African American facilities for one year. Most residents were African American and low-income. Data gathering techniques included participant observation during weekly visits, informal and in-depth interviewing of residents, providers, and family members, and review of residents' records. Data were analyzed using the grounded theory method. Fifty-five residents lived in the homes over the year-long study period. Length of time spent in the homes ranged from 1 month to 20 years. Over the course of the year, five residents died and 17 were discharged. Seven of these residents went to nursing homes, four to other assisted living facilities, and six to their own homes or the homes of family members. Findings demonstrated that most decisions to discharge residents were related to increased cognitive impairment and care needs associated with dementia. Providers varied the willingness to keep residents as they aged in place. Residents able to pay higher fees as needs increased often had a better chance of remaining in the homes.

Alternative Housing For Seniors

Ron Wickman (Ron Wickman Architect, Edmonton, Alberta

Canada)

The purpose of this presentation is to identify an alternative form of housing to the larger senior's apartments, senior citizen villages and assisted living housing projects. The method used here was to build two separate single-family house projects designed to accommodate a variety of family types, including young couples with children, single parents, shared accommodations, seniors, and persons with disabilities. The built homes are designed to be flexible enough to easily adapt to a family's future needs, thus affording a family the choice to grow old in the same home and in the same community; moving to a larger seniors complex does not have to happen. The two smaller housing projects are now built with families already personalizing and adapting their dwellings. The results of these projects will continuously reveal themselves as time passes, and as the original families continue personalizing and adapting or as new families may change and adapt. The conclusion here is that good housing is designed in the beginning to allow for easier future changes, additions or adaptations. Designing a dwelling with the needs of seniors in mind is not just a technical issue that we can deal with in the future, it is a creative act that we consider now, so the future is better for everyone.

Empowerment of older people in sheltered housing and residential care: opportunities and barriers in decision-making

Helen Bartlett and Wendy Martin (Oxford Brookes University, Oxford, UK)

PURPOSE: This paper presents the first stage of a two-year collaborative study with the Anchor Trust, funded by the National Lottery Charities Board. The focus of the study is empowerment of older people with dementia. The purpose of the first stage, reported in this paper, is to map the key decision points for non-cognitively impaired older people living in residential, sheltered housing and community settings. The second stage involves in-depth interviews with older people who have dementia in these settings, to identify their perceptions of key decisions and issues of choice, and explore the opportunities and barriers in practice. METHOD: Eight focus group meetings with care/ professional staff and 32 in-depth interviews with older residents were carried out using a guide to explore potential areas of decision making. The interviews were recorded and transcribed. Data were analysed using NUD:IST. RESULTS: The key decision areas identified in stage 1 included: moving residence, money matters, personal care, domestic care, health, relationships, activities, and planning for the future. Perceived choice and control were influenced by the type of residence, health of participants, availability of family and formal help. CONCLUSIONS: The findings provide greater insight into decisions and choice and how they differ for older people living in various settings. They provide a framework for the second stage of this study to explore decision making and older people with dementia in the same settings. The outcome will be a guide for good practice on empowerment of older people with dementia.

Homeshare In Australia: Variation on a Worldwide Theme

B. Squires, W.Morris (The Benevolent Society, Sydney, Australia)

Homeshare is a program that has been established in a number of countries to help older people stay in their own homes longer. It brings together older people who need some help around the home and would benefit from having someone in the home at night, and younger people who need affordable accommodation. The younger person does about 10 hours of agreed tasks per week in return for free accommodation. The concept of Homeshare was launched in Australia at the IAG World Congress in 1997. A steering committee met in Sydney for over two years exploring a variety of options to launch the program. It was established as a service of The Benevolent Society in 2000. In other parts of the world, including Melbourne, Australia, Homeshare has been set up solely as a direct service agency. Homeshare NSW is exploring a different model: direct service, plus training and supporting others to make matches. Case managers of existing community support services will be trained and supported as they identify older people in their caseload who would benefit from having a younger person live with them. Homeshare NSW will recruit and screen suitable younger people. The program is undergoing evaluation, to see if this decentralised model will benefit a wider group of older people than a model of direct service only. The outcome will be of interest to all who are committed to increasing the choices available to older people to enable them stay in their own homes for as long as possible.

Making Real the Wellness Model in Supportive Housing

Renate K. Sainsbury, Ann Keane (Lifestyle Options/Alta. Life Care Housing Foundation Edmonton, AB, Canada, T6J 2S3)

A Wellness Model used in supportive housing brings about successful mesasurable outcomes. By utilizing wellness programs in our housing facility we have promoted wellness not illness. The programs and philosophy focus on the areas of emotional, social, spiritual, intellecutal and community wellness. We will present both quantitative and qualitative data to provide information that even though clients are frail and have numerous limitations they are still actively enagaged in life and living their life to the fullest.

Moving to a Manufactured Home: A Recipe for Reducing Older People's Fear of Crime

Sandra Woodbridge (School of Human Services, Griffith University, Brisbane Australia), Laurie Buys (School of Human Services, Queensland University of Technology, Brisbane, Australia.)

Despite statistics which indicate that older people in Australia are the least likely group within the community to become victims of crime, older people, especially women, report feeling less safe when alone in their home and fearful of becoming a victim of sexual assault or home invasion. Concerns about personal safety and security have been found to be one of the most significant factors in older people considering a move to a retirement village or manufactured home estate. This paper presents the results of a study conducted with residents of manufactured homes in South- East Queensland, The study sought to investigate the health and financial implications for older people who move to a manufactured or relocatable home park. 200 residents were surveyed and in-depth interviews were conducted. The study found a high level of satisfaction amongst residents. This high level of satisfaction was examined further and many participants nominated that a reduction in the level of fear of crime played an important part in their overall level of satisfaction. Security measures, included in the design and development of most manufactured home estates, together with reciprocity, social support and strong resident networks were vital components in reducing the levels of fear experienced by residents. In presenting the results of this study, the role of reciprocity, social support and strong resident networks within manufactured and retirement villages will be explored as will the capacity of age segregated housing such as retirement villages and manufactured homeparks to enhance older people's autonomy and independence.

SESSION 64

Vulnerability and Aging

L. Ploton & L. Israel (Laboratoire de Psychologie Clinique de la Vulnérabilité, Université Lumière-Lyon2, Bron, France) ("Retrospective study of vulnerability criteria for late adulthood depressions and Alzheimer type dementias: the ABORD Program") J. Gaucher (Laboratoire de Psychologie Clinique de la Vulnérabilité, Université Lumière-Lyon2, Bron, France) ("Vulnerabilization and vulnerability of caregivers of an older person with dementia") M. Anaut (Laboratoire de Psychologie

Clinique de la Vulnérabilité, Université Lumière-Lyon2, Bron, France) ("Factors of Vulnerability and Resilience in psychological transgenerational transmissions with the mediation of genogramme.") G. Ribes (Laboratoire de Psychologie Clinique de la Vulnérabilité, Université Lumière-Lyon2, Bron, France) ("Supportive therapy as an answer to the vulnerability") P. Cappeliez (School of Psychology, University of Ottawa, Canada) ("Functions of reminiscence and coping strategies") L. Israel & J. Gaucher (Laboratoire de Psychologie Clinique de la Vulnérabilité, Université Lumière-Lyon2, Bron, France) ("Contribution of psychology to prevention and rehabilitation of the elderly")

Clinical psychology, medical, human and social sciences, focus, as far as old age is concerned, on vulnerability. As a matter of fact, the preoccupation of elderly - as well as caregivers-highlights the importance of Vulnerability, and Vulnerabilization processes in psychogerontological clinical practices. We will present in the following symposium the researches led by an international university network connecting Lyon (France) and Ottawa (Canada). Factors, care and cure methods of Vulnerability have been studied. In this symposium the following aspects will be exposed : - Vulnerabilization process of the natural and/or professional caregiver for Alzheimer patients (J. Gaucher & al.) - Using "Family Tree Method" (Genogramme) to detect the process of Vulnerabilization and/or "Resilience" factors among relatives transmitted through generations (M. Anaut & al.) - Medical, social and psychological history of depressed and Alzheimer elderly, a French epidemiological study on the factors and indicators of Vulnerability for the elderly. (A.B.O.R.D program, L. Ploton & al.) And more precisely, concerning Vulnerability situations and for elderly: - The assessment of the place and function of supportive psychotherapy, with psychodynamical references taking into account narcissism fragility and proposing them a solution (G. Ribes & al.) - Cognitive and behavioral psychotherapy based on reminiscence which constitute a treatment method through current problem solving (P. Cappeliez & al.) - An intervention method based on memory stimulation in order to prevent cognitive impairments of the elderly. (L. Israel & al.) Those different papers result from a coherent and regular work of an international team, aiming at presenting and exploring the question of vulnerability in old age.

Contribution of psychology to prevention and rehabilitation of the elderly

L.Israel, J.Gaucher, L.Ploton, G.Ribes, J.Tyrrell, C.Biessy, H.Bruni (Laboratoire de Psychologie Clinique de la Vulnérabilité, Université Lumière-Lyon2, Bron, France)

There is a recognized need for intervention methods involving psychological approaches in the treatment of cognitive disorders of the elderly. The contribution of psychology to prevention and rehabilitation is emphasized by our local experience in this field. The rationale, goals and end-points are proposed and described. The main principle of this method is based on "transfer of training" from an artificial situation to Activities of Daily Living . This transfer represents a very positive and pragmatic achievement, allowing patients to cope with many events, and changing their negative attitudes to positive ones. Through its psychotherapeutic effects , this methodology develops aims for memory functions stimulation, arouses competence and maintains motivation to lead an active and successful life. Several techniques are used in order to combine psychotherapeutic and learning effects. An extensive choice of exercices graded by difficulty has been set up, and all levels of competence can thus be covered. This approach does not only aim to restore failing memory, but also delays its decline by putting the remaining abilities to good use. Such programs have been applied as a preventive measure in our local area, in institutions and primary care, on more than 1600 out-patients of memory clinic, as well as general practitioner's patients. It has also been applied in Geneva to hundreds of persons of the Third Age University. In other parts of France more than 2600 persons, have followed group sessions conducted by qualified psychologists specially trained during 40 hours by the author of this method.

Factors of Vulnerability and Resilience in psychological transgenerational transmissions with the mediation of genogramme

M.Anaut, J.Gaucher, L.Ploton, V.Franchi, A.Quiquandon, C.Biessy, G.Ribes, L.Israël (Laboratoire de Psychologie Clinique de la Vulnérabilité, Université Lumière-Lyon2, Bron, France)

The assessment of vulnerability in transgenerational psychological transmissions in the case of family conflicts and violence remains an important area of study and intervention method in the field of clinical psychology for the protection of elderly people. Nonetheless, this approach doesn't focus exclusively on the vulnerability model to explain the effects of psychological family transmissions. The purpose, with the mediation of a genogramme, is to examine the internal resources and protective factors that individuals and families develop in response to important difficulties or traumatisms. Seminal work on the concept of resilience has stimulated important theoretical and empirical advancements in this area. By incorporating a theoretical understanding and clinical measures to protective factors, our study can be seen as complementary to the "vulnerability approach", in regard to the care of elderly person's families. The principal hypothesis is that relational models of previous generations must influence patterns in the current generation. The study of type of adaptation and resilience which families have often experimented in precedent generations, would further enable us to develop, promote and assess new forms of care for young generations. This paper proposes to evaluate these two models of vulnerability and resilience as they apply to the care of elderly persons in France. Clinical case studies will be used to illustrate our investigations.

Functions of reminiscence and coping strategies

P. Cappeliez, V. Rivard (School of Psychology, University of Ottawa, Ottawa, Canada)

Reminiscence may serve different functions depending on life circumstances and personal characteristics. The first part of this communication will present a review of current knowledge on this topic. The second part will highlight relations between the various functions of reminiscence and specific coping strategies. We will report the findings of a study conducted with 75 older adults (M = 67 years), who indicated, on the Reminiscence Functions Scale, their frequency of reminiscence for 8 purposes (boredom reduction, death preparation, identity, conversation, bitterness revival, problem-solving, intimacy maintenance, teach/inform) as well as their stress adaptation profile according to 6 strategies assessed with the Ways of Coping (social support, wishful thinking, distanciation/emotional control, positive reappraisal, problem-solving, emotion-focus coping). The function of boredom reduction is negatively associated with problem-solving. The function of death preparation is positively associated with social support, wishful thinking, and negatively with problem-solving. The function of identity is positively correlated with social support, wishful thinking and positive reappraisal. The function of problem solving is associated with social support and wishful thinking, whereas the function of conversation is linked to problem-solving and negatively to emotion-focus coping. Results are interpreted in the context of the contribution of reminiscence to adaptation.

Retrospective study of vulnerability criteria for late adulthood depressions and Alzheimer type dementias: the ABORD Program

L. Ploton, N. Gualdo, J. Gaucher, L. Israël, J. Tyrrell, G. Ribes, C. Biessy, H. Bruni, R. Hugonot (Laboratoire de Psychologie Clinique de la Vulnérabilité, Université Lumière-Lyon2, Bron, France). L.Israel (Laboratoire de Psychologie Clinique de la Vulnérabilité, Université Lumière-Lyon2, Bron, France) Laboratoire de Psychologie Clinique de la Vulnérabilité (LPVC), Institut de Psychologie, Université Lumière-Lyon2, 5 Bd Mendès-France, F69676 Bron, France.

The ABORD Program (Alzheimer Bank of Observations, Research and

Data) represents an attempt to validate empirical observations concerning: - The development of communication techniques for use with patients suffering from Senile Dementia of Alzheimer Type (SDAT) in order to achieve a description of the disease from the patient's perspective - The affective and relational semiology of SDAT - The existence of predisposing personality factors associated with dementia. Initially this program involved the elaboration by 20 teams, of a 400 item computerized data base, designed to gather data principally on: · Medical diagnosis according to DSM-III criteria · Personal history and socio-professional antecedents · Medical, surgical, toxic and traumatic antecedents · Family history and biographical data · Personality profile and relationship data · Psychopathological background All the patients followed by 5 pluridisciplinary psychogeriatric teams who had a Mini Mental Status Examination score lower or equal to 24/30 were included in their study. The data collection lasted 5 years and allowed us to obtain 117 files of amnesic patients. We intend to present the analysis of data on SDAT patients in comparison to: - Patients suffering from other pathologies with memory impairments (essentially depressed persons) - A control sample, matched on age and gender with SDAT Significant results of this retrospective study appeared between those groups specifically when considering their childhood background.

Supportive therapy as a response to the vulnerable patient

G.Ribes, C.Joubert, C.Biessy, J.Tyrrell, H.Bruni, J.Boissin, B.Cleyet-Marel, A.Marduel, J.Gaucher, L.Ploton, L.Israël (Laboratoire de Psychologie Clinique de la Vulnérabilité, Université Lumière-Lyon2, Bron, France).

We consider as an hypothesis that the question of vulnerability is a crucial gerontological problem. The term vulnerability seems to correspond to what we call "narcissic failures". The possibilities of adapting supportive therapy appears to be a relevant response as much for the patient as for his family and medical circle. We used a questionnaire followed by an interview with practitioners working in geronto-psychology settings. We will attempt to specify the purpose, methods and results of supportive therapy concerning vulnerable patients and to understand the process of this approach. We will show how to define the purposes, methods and results of supportive therapy. We will cheek the necessity to be adapted to the patient considering the vulnerability importance: use of a mediation, involvement of the family and medical circle in the therapeutic approach. We will discuss the way of adaptating the format of therapy in relation to the level of vulnerability.

Vulnerabilization and vulnerability of caregivers of an older demented person

J. Gaucher, M. Anaut, L. Ploton, A. Quiquandon, L. Israël, A. Marduel, G. Ribes, C. Biessy, H. Bruni, J. Tyrrell. (Laboratoire de Psychologie Clinique de la Vulnérabilité, Université Lumière-Lyon2, Bron, France).

Older adults with dementia need help which is provided either by family caregivers (spouse and/or offspring) who are often lonely, or by professional caregivers who, frequently, experience important psychic suffering. The psychological profile of the caregiver, familial and/or institutional, often shows a high level of vulnerability which seems to lead him /her to the function of caregiver as well as to expose him/her to an aggravation of his/her vulnerability. This communication presents the results of two clinical investigation approaches: - By the genogram, in the case of the family caregiver, - By questionnaire, in the case of the institutional caregiver. The results of this research demonstrate the narcissic fragilization of the caregiver in contact with an older person with dementia. This narcissic fragilization could explain the increased vulnerabilization of the caregiver and his/her risk of developing depression in his/her helping role.This vulnerabilization could be linked to a longstanding and/or current problem of identification, with a parent highly demanding (devouring) and poorly gratifying (frustrating).

SESSION 65

Social Exclusion and Urban Deprivation in Later Life: The Role of Community, Gender and Ethnicity.

T. Scharf, C. Phillipson, P. Kingston and A. Smith (Centre for Social Gerontology, School of Social Relations, Keele University, UK) Conceptualising Social Exclusion and Urban Deprivation in Later Life. S. Arber and H. Cooper (Centre for Research on Ageing and Gender, Department of Sociology, University of Surrey, Guildford, UK) Gender Inequalities in Social Capital and Social Support in Relation to Older People's Health. M. Evandrou (Age Concern Institute of Gerontology, King's College London, UK) Social Inequalities in Later Life: Socio-economic Position of Older People from Ethnic Minority Groups. S. Harper (Oxford Centre on Population Ageing, University of Oxford, UK), M. Cortina Borja (Department of Paediatric Epidemiology and Biostatistics, University College London, UK), L. Kaplan (Oxford Centre on Population Ageing, University of Oxford, UK), and J. Walter (Department of Emergency Medicine, University of Chicago, USA) Social Exclusion, Urban Deprivation and Access to Health Care Services: The Case of South-side Chicago. C. Phillipson, M. Bernard and J. Phillips (Centre for Social Gerontology, School of Social Relations, Keele University, UK) Changing Patterns of Support for Older People in Urban Communities. Discussant: A. Warnes (Centre for Ageing and Rehabilitation Studies, University of Sheffield, UK).

This Symposium examines the impact of exclusion and disadvantage in the lives of older people. The issue of social exclusion and social inclusion has become an important theme in European social policy but to date has been undeveloped in relation to old age. The Symposium provides an opportunity for a major review of the operation of inequality in the lives of older people, focusing in particular on the British context. Papers will address different types of inequality, especially in regard to gender, ethnicity, and social class. An additional feature of the papers, however, will be the attempt to ground some of the main themes within the context of spatial differences, as manifest in urban and community processes. Issues for the development of social policy will also be explored. Key themes raised by the contributing papers will be explored by an invited discussant.

Changing Patterns of Support for Older People in Urban Communities.

Chris Phillipson, Miriam Bernard and Judith Phillips (Centre for Social Gerontology, School of Social Relations, Keele University, UK)

Urban environments have a major influence on the lives of older people. Urban society offers rich possibilities for social inclusion but also for social exclusion in terms of limited participation in key areas of daily life. This paper explores questions such as: how can support to older people be maintained in urban areas? To what extent is support subject to change and renewal with the arrival of new migrant groups? This study draws upon a larger research programme in three urban areas in the United Kingdom to examine these and related questions. Findings from an inner city community highlight nearly 40 per cent of older people unable to cite anyone in their street as a friend; 16 per cent having no contact with neighbours over a period of a month; 10 per cent unable to name anyone in their street by name. There is also evidence to suggest that older people experience distinctive pressures within urban contexts, with qualitative interviews indicating perceptions of neighbours as potentially hostile, and feelings of vulnerability to different aspects of economic change. To set against this, new migrant groups are offering possibilities for neighbourhoods to be renewed in distinctive ways, with the emergence of distinctive types of family and community groups. These findings are discussed within the tradition of urban sociology, and the paper underlines the importance of this area for research in gerontology. Those involved in social policy and ageing will also need a stronger urban focus to promote social inclusion for groups affected by multiple disadvantage and deprivation.

Conceptualising Social Exclusion and Urban Deprivation in Later Life

T. Scharf, C. Phillipson, P. Kingston, A. Smith (Centre for Social Gerontology, School of Social Relations, Keele University, UK)

The concept of social exclusion represents a key theme in current social policy debates. This reflects not only the deepening of social inequalities in advanced industrial nations over recent decades, but also a growing marginalisation of particular social groups and urban areas. While poverty and income inequality continue to be important elements of the social exclusion debate, a central concern refers to loss of access to important life chances, especially those that connect individuals to the mainstream of society. However, policy initiatives on social exclusion have tended, for a combination of economic and political reasons, to focus on groups such as children, young families and the unemployed. Ways in which social exclusion may affect older people have been neglected. This paper seeks to generate a better understanding of the dimensions of social exclusion that are relevant to older people. It explores social exclusion and urban deprivation in relation to three themes: participation and integration, spatial segregation and institutional disengagement. Each theme is developed with reference to empirical evidence generated through group discussions with older people living in socially deprived neighbourhoods in three English cities.

Gender Inequalities in Social Capital and Social Support in Relation to Older People's Health

S. Arber, H. Cooper (Centre for Research on Ageing and Gender, Department of Sociology, University of Surrey, Guildford, UK)

Social capital has become a key focus within research on social exclusion and urban deprivation. However, there has been a lack of research on how social capital varies between older people and younger people, or on the ways in which gender influences how differing levels of social capital are associated with the health of older men and women. This paper uses new data from the British General Household Survey, which collected an extensive set of questions on social capital and social support in 2000. Data is analysed for over 4000 people aged 60 and over. We examine how the various components of social capital vary for older people according to gender and socio-economic circumstances, as well as urban-rural context. It is expected that social capital has a greater influence on older women's than older men's health, but that this is mediated by advancing age and socio-economic circumstances. The paper argues that there is a need to develop integrated approaches which examine community level influences on older people's health together with their socio-economic and material circumstances.

Social Exclusion, Urban Deprivation and Access to Health Care Services: The Case of South-side Chicago

S. Harper (Oxford Centre on Population Ageing, University of Oxford, UK), M. Cortina Borja (Department of Paediatric Epidemiology and Biostatistics, University College London, UK), L. Kaplan (Oxford Centre on Population Ageing, University of Oxford, UK), J. Walter (Department of Emergency Medicine, University of Chicago, USA)

There has been growing international interest in emergency care for older people, which has recently started to explore not only the treatment of this older population, but also factors behind their continued use of emergency rooms as a source of care. Few studies, however, have considered in depth the social and structural factors of the communities within which these older people reside, exploring the available primary and preventative health care, social support and community based care, which may result in these emergency room presentations. This paper discusses a study of Chicago which examined these factors in the US context. Emergency Rooms of three large hospitals serving the low income ethnically mixed elderly population of south-side Chicago were studied over an 18 month period to explore the processes and events leading to presentation at the Emergency Department by older people. Attention was given to identifying preventable failure in primary and preventative health care, social support and community based care which may lead to these presentations. Demographic data was collected on some 6000 older people visiting emergency rooms, supported by 103 in-depth case studies. The study identified community based factors as being of significance in understanding older patients' use of such services. Of particular interest were the 22% who made multiple repeat visits to the Emergency Room, accounting for nearly half of all visits undertaken during the study period. Detailed analysis of this group revealed the special needs of this vulnerable population, and reasons why they chose to under-use the available community based primary care.

Social Inequalities in Later Life: Socio-Economic Position of Older People from Ethnic Minority Groups

M. Evandrou (Age Concern Institute of Gerontology, King's College London, London, UK)

There are nearly a quarter of a million individuals aged 60 years or over belonging to ethnic minority groups living in Britain. As ethnic minority groups continue to age, information regarding their circumstances in later life will be of increasing importance for the development of appropriate services and policies. This paper examines the socio-economic position of older people from ethnic minority groups in Britain, exploring different dimensions of social inequality. Using nationally representative data from the British General Household Survey, the research investigates household living arrangements, lifestyle, socio-economic status, economic resources and the experience of multiple deprivation in later life. The findings indicate that there are significant differences both between and within ethnic minority groups in access to material and social resources. Older Black Caribbeans are more likely to reside in social housing than other groups. Over a quarter of older Pakistani and Bangladeshis live in households with no central heating, and over a third live in overcrowded households. Older Pakistani and Bangladeshis are three times more likely to live in a household without a phone than white, Indian or Caribbean older people. Indian elderly persons are least likely to experience multiple deprivation, whilst just under a half of older Pakistani and Bangladeshis, two-fifths of older Black Caribbeans and a quarter of Irish elders experience medium or high levels of deprivation. Policy makers will need to explicitly recognise the multiple experience of disadvantage facing particular elderly individuals from ethnic minority groups, if poverty and social exclusion are to be tackled successfully.

SESSION 66

Application of Epithalamin in Acute Myocardial Infarction in Patients over 60

C. L. Kozlov, N. Yu. Semigolovsky (St. Petersburg Institute of Bioregulation and Gerontology, St. Petersburg, Russia)

Over the recent years, hospital lethality of myocardial infarction in elderly (over 60) and aged (over 75) patients has been 2-8-times higher than that in younger patients and equaled 16-52 % (Lerner D.J, Kannel W.B, 1986; Roig et al, 1987; Anne et al, 1988; Rybakova M.G. et al, 1998). In the Coronary Units of such a large city as St. Petersburg the percentage of deceased elderly and aged patients makes 79.3-87.7 %. It is also typical that in case of acute myocardial infarction 60 % of hospital lethality falls on the first 5 days, i.e. the term the patient stays in the Intensive Coronary Care and Resuscitation Units (Rybakova M.G. et al, 1998). Defensive action of cytomedin geroprotector Epithalamin(r) was experimentally studied on 23 patients aged 60-85 (mean age 68.7±2.5) against the background of conventional therapy (thrombolytics on prescription, nitrates, beta-adrenoblockers and/or calcium canal inhibitors, aspirin, heparin, angiotensin-converting enzyme inhibitors). 10 mg of Epithalamin were intramuscularly injected on the 1st-2nd day after acute myocardial infarction. The investigation results displayed that, compared to control group of 25 patients over 60 (mean age 67.9±2.6), the main group patients revealed a significant ($p<0.05$) decrease in hospital lethality from 12.0 to 8.6 % and reduction in retrospectively estimated term of their stay in the Intensive Coronary Care Unit from 7.5±1.0 to 5.9±1.2 days. Such promising results confirm the necessity of further studies in search of the mechanisms of the drug defensive effects, development of schemes and dosage of its application.

Association between Race and Cardiology Care for Hospitalized Older Heart Failure Patients.

A Ahmed, MPH (University of Alabama at Birmingham, Southeast Center for Excellence in Geriatric Medicine, and American Federation for Aging Research); RV Sims, MD (University of Alabama at Birmingham and Birmingham VA Medical Center); RM Allman, MD (University of Alabama at Birmingham, Birmingham VA Medical Center, Southeast Center for Excellence in Geriatric Medicine, and Alabama Quality Assurance Foundation); & JF DeLong, MD (Alabama Quality Assurance Foundation); Birmingham, Alabama, USA.

Purpose: Determine the association between race and cardiology care for older heart failure patients. Methods: We analyzed data of 1,091 Medicare beneficiaries, 65+ years, discharged from 11 Alabama hospitals in 1994 with a diagnosis of heart failure. Patients were classified as whites and non-whites (African-Americans, Hispanics and Asians) and were considered to have received cardiology care if they were admitted by a cardiologist or admitted by a generalist and received cardiology consultation. We compared demographic and other patient characteristics by race and tested statistical significance using the Chi square test. We then calculated crude odds ratio (OR) with 95Results: The study included 1,075 subjects (16 excluded due to lack of data on physician specialty), with a mean (±SD) age of 79 (±7) years, and 60% were female. Two hundred and two (19%) patients were non-white and most of these (94%) were African-Americans. Cardiologists cared for 487 (45%) patients (30% by admission and 70% via consultation). Paroxysmal nocturnal dyspnea, elevated jugular venous pressure, third heart sound, serum creatinine/2.5 mg/dL, left ventricular hypertrophy by electrocardiograph, diabetes, and hypertension were more common among non-white patients, while pulmonary edema by chest radiograph, atrial fibrillation by electrocardiograph, coronary artery disease, and chronic obstructive pulmonary disease were more common among white patients. Non-white patients were less likely to receive cardiology care (OR=0.58; 95%CI=0.42-0.80). After adjustment for various patient characteristics and hospital, being non-white was independently associated with lower odds of receiving cardiology care (OR=0.50; 95%CI=0.35-0.70). Conclusions: Older non-white Medicare beneficiaries hospitalized with heart failure were less likely to be cared for by cardiologists.

Effects of low dose anti-depression drugs on angina associated with depression in elderly

Zheng An-Lin (Department of Geriatrics,Huadong Hospital,Shanghai,China)

Objectives: To assess the effects of anti-depression drugs on angina associated with depression in the elderly. Methods: Among 96 patients with angina, confirmed by history, ECG, and radiomyocardiagraphy, 64 patients were diagnosed as angina associated with depression by CES-D (44 M, 20 F). All 64 patients maintained their original regimes together with low dose anti-depression drugs, such as doxepin, amitriptyline, chlorpromazine, prosec. The treatment course lasted 3 or 4 weeks. CES-D,ECG and the number of angina attacks were compared before and after treatment. Results: The total effective rate in terms of symptoms relief was 64.1%. The total effective rate in terms of improvement of ST-segment and T waves was 29.7%. Conclusions: The low dose anti-depression drugs have good effects on angina associated with depression. Discussion: Patients with depression always secrete excessive catecholamines which can induce coronary artery spasm and increase heart oxygen consumption. Therefore, depression can exacerbate the symptoms of patients with angina. This may be the mechanism of using low-dose anti-depression drugs in treating patients with angina.

Long term survival rate and prognostic factors of acute myocardial infarction

S.Y. Choi, M.D, C. H. Kim, M.D.(Department of Internal Medicine, Seoul National University College of Medicine. Seoul, Korea)

Purpose and Method: To identify the long term survival rate and prognostic factors of acute myocardial infarction (AMI) in Korea, total 1139 patients who presented between Jan. 1980 and Dec. 1997 were followed for an average of 115 months. 321 patients died during follow up periods 238 patients were lost and 580 patients are alive till the end of the study. Result: Overall survival rate (¡ıstandard error) were 88.2¡ı1%, 86.8¡ı1%, 85.3¡ı1.1%, 82.1¡ı1.2%, 79.6¡ı1.3%, 75.6¡ı1.5%, 73.1¡ı1.6%, 56.3¡ı2.5% at 1, 6, 12, 24, 36, 48, 60, 120 months. In univariate analysis, older, history of diabetes, higher degree of Killip class, higher peak creatine kinase level, residual ischemia on treadmill test or MIBI scan, lower ejection fraction on echocardiography or gated blood pool scan, more sever extent of coronary artery disease, lower HDL-cholesterol level at 3 months after AMI proved as poor long term prognostic factors of AMI with statistical significance ($p< 0.05$). In multivariate analysis, old age and Killip class III versus I proved as independent poor long term prognostic factors of AMI with statistical significance ($p< 0.05$). Conclusion: The mortality of AMI is composed of two components. At acute phase, within 1 month, the mortality reaches to about 12%, and at chronic phase, after 1 month from AMI, mortality increases by 3% a year for 10 years. Old patients who have poor left ventricular functions show poor prognosis.

Management of End-stage Heart Failure in Geriatric patients

J. K. Dave, A. G. Kocheril (University of Illinois College of Medicine, Urbana-Champaign, USA)

ISSUE Despite recent advances , the progression of heart failure seems inevitable. There is no consensus for the management of decompensated end-stage heart failure patients, large number of whom are symptomatic despite maximum medical therapy. STRUCTURE We present evidence-based review of etiology, pathophysiology and different treatment modalities for decompensated end stage heart failure. We discuss the global epidemic of heart failure and the role of pacemaker therapy, intermittent inotropic therapy, left ventricular assist devices, artificial heart, cardiomyoplasty and cardiac transplantation in advanced heart failure. CONTENT Congestive heart failure has been described in literature as enigma of medicine, medical hydra and Cinderella of cardiology. It is one of the leading causes of death in the developed countries. It is estimated that there are million patients in the world, (. There are 5 million Americans who have heart failure,) 700f whom are 60 years or older. It is the leading cause of hospitalization in adults more than 65 years of age. The natural history of most cardiac conditions is eventual progression to heart failure, a common problem with uncontrolled mortality and morbidity. Congestive heart failure is a major cause of the morbidity and mortality associated with cardiovascular disease. Due to increased incidence and decreased mortality of heart failure, the number of patients with advanced heart failure is escalating. In new millennium, the problem of heart failure is going to magnify due to a rapid increase in the aging population and improved management of other cardiac diseases. The prognosis of patients with symptomatic heart failure is still grim, with up to 50% mortality at 5 years. Even with increasing use of newer medications like signal modulating inhibitors and spironolactone which can potentially modify the natural course of the disease, reduce mortality and improve quality of life, the underlying pathology of disease continue to progress. The progression is due to remodeling, apoptosis, release of various neurohormones, and many unknown factors. Despite recent advances in the medical management, most patients with heart failure ultimately become resistant to pharmacological treatment although at slower rate with the appropriate treatment. With increasing incidence and decreasing mortality, the number of patients with advanced heart failure is rapidly escalating. Significantly large number of this patients are symptomatic despite maximum medical therapy. The arsenal of treatment for this group of patients with refractory advanced heart failure includes intravenous inotropes, left ventricular assist devices, dynamic cardiomyoplasty, pacemaker therapy and transplantation. Cardiac transplant remains the ultimate goal in many patients with advanced heart failure, but a limited number of donor hearts and long waiting list limits its use. The average waiting time for transplantation was 254 days in 1997. Approximately 250f patients die awaiting heart transplantation. Of patients with advanced heart failure due to cardiomyopathy who are considered to well for transplant, mortality at one year was 46%.There is a strong need of novel modes of treatment to improve quality of life as well as life expectancy in patients with advanced heart failure particularly in patients who are symptomatic on optimal medical regimen but not a candidate for transplantation We review evidence and discuss advantages, disadvantages and cost of different treatment options. We review the results of studies, which will help refining the indications, selection of patients, techniques and appropriate monitoring with different treatment options. CONCLUSION Because of the complexities of the disease process and the multifaceted nature of the management process, elderly patients with CHF require a comprehensive approach. Considering the increasing number of heart failure patients and variety of available treatment options forming a universal guideline for management of advanced heart failure patients is essential.

Rehabilitation of older patients after myocardial infarction: multicentre randomised controlled trial

Dee Jones, Robert West (University of Wales College of Medicine, Cardiff, UK)

Most previous trials of cardiac rehabilitation excluded people aged 65 or over; hence more than half of all patients admitted to hospital with acute MI. This trial included older people and evaluated a single dimension rehabilitation model. Method: We undertook a randomised controlled trial of rehabilitation among unselected MI patients in six centres. Rehabilitation programmes were developed on a psychological model. All 948 eligible patients aged >65 with confirmed MI and discharged home within twenty-eight days were admitted over two years. Baseline clinical data were collected on admission and by structured interview shortly after discharge and outcome was assessed by interview at six months and clinical examination at twelve months. Main outcome measures were anxiety, depression, morbidity, use of medication, physical activity and mortality. Results: At six months there were no significant differences between rehabilitation patients and controls in anxiety (prevalence 27% v 27%) or depression (17% v 16%) , frequency of angina, medication and physical activity. At twelve months there were no differences in clinical complications, clinical sequelae, or mortality(9.6% v 9.5%)). Conclusions: This first large multicentre trial to include older patients found little measurable benefit in those offered a psychological model of cardiac rehabilitation .Possible explanations are that the intervention was not appropriate for their Needs, that it was too little or too late. Cardiac rehabilitation for this group of patients needs to be further developed and evaluated.

Secondary prevention of acute myocardial infarction by aspirin in aged patients

Wang Yingli, Jin Wensheng, Huang Cuiyao (Department of Sanipractic, Liu Hua Qiao Hospital, Guangzhou, China)

PURPOSE: To evaluate the therapeutic efficiency effects of secondary prevention by aspirin (ASA) after acute myocardial infarction (AMI). METHODS: 221 aged patients all detained in hospital for clear diagnosis were divided into group ASA and controls in this respective study. The rates of recurrent myocardial infarction and sudden cardiac death, and the side effects were analyzed and compared between the 2 groups. RESULTS: The rate of recurrent myocardial infarction in the ASA group (6.7%) decreased significantly by 67.9% when compared to controls ($P<0.01$). Otherwise as for the rate of sudden cardiac death, even from a different event (e.g. cardiac failure, sudden death, hwart split) after AMI, it is similar between two groups ($P>0.05$). The side effect of ASA demonstrated as hemorrhage. CONCLUSIONS: If used as a long-term treatment, ASA lowered the rate of recurrent myocardial infarction but did not affect the rate of sudden cardiac death after AMI.

SESSION 67

Artworks/ Consortium for Elders and Youth in the Arts (CEYA) program (Oral, 1 hour)

Jeff Chapline, MFA (Goldman Institute on Aging, San Francisco, California, USA)

Artworks began in 1978 as one of 13 programs offered by the Goldman Institute on Aging. The Artworks program provides visual and performing art services for elder day centers and residential housing for the elderly and annually serves 500 elders at 10-15 elder centers throughout San Francisco. Recognizing the increasing physical and sociological distance between the generations and diminished benefits derived from multi-generational support systems the Consortium for Elders and Youth in the Arts (CEYA) program was initiated as part of the Artworks program in 1996. The CEYA program was designed to bridge the gap between the young and the old through engaging educational, visual and performing art collaborations, and help to keep elders connected and contributing to their communities by becoming genuine resources for youth. CEYA's objectives are to provide a solid infrastructure for planning, designing and implementing cross-generational visual and performing art projects, performances and community presentations, and to develop audiences for the work. In 1999, CEYA program was honored with the Award for Excellence in Aging Programs, presented by the United States Committee for the Celebration of the United Nations International Year of Older Persons. This presentation will provide an overview of the program philosophy and design, program personnel, planning processes, funding, as well as the extensive range of community collaborations, that have made this program a success. Examples of various cross-generational projects that have taken place across different ethnic and cultural communities will also be presented.

Celebrating Older Artists: Past and present

Robert E. Roush, EdD, MPH [Huffington Center on Aging, Baylor College of Medicine, Houston, Texas, USA]

This presentation recounts a transformational moment in the presenter's life, inspired by two art-related experiences: a visit to the Phillips Collection in Washington, DC, where he first saw Renoir's "Luncheon of the Boating Party", and his response to reading a book by Joan Hart entitled "Beyond the Tunnel: The arts and aging in America". In this book, Joan Hart shares the story about how she took reproductions of great art from the Phillips Collection to local area nursing homes where she worked with residents long thought to be demented. With Joan's art many of the residents, like Sarah, "came to life." These experiences led the Huffington Center on Aging to produce an "arts in aging" calendar featuring older artists. It is our belief that the beautiful works of aging artists are abiding reminders that older people continue to contribute to the quality of our lives. This presentation features selections from each calendar since the first one in 1996 and reveals in the words of artists exhibiting in the 2001 calendar how they feel about continuing to paint into the eighth, nineth, and even tenth decades of their life. Video clips of two artists working in their studios will be shown. The presentation will address the notion of art as "therapy" for the artists, and the use of art therapy for persons in assisted living facilities and in treatment groups for depression and dementias. It also provides a tribute to Renoir, Sarah,

Joan, and older artists everywhere, still painting, still filling our eyes with beauty and our hearts with joy.

"Rare Spirits": Our elders as subject

Jerry Grey (Artist, 15 Murray Street, Suite 101, Ottawa, Ontario, Canada K1N 9M5)

Jerry Grey's "Rare Spirits" project is a personal tribute to vintage elders. The paintings included in this project are being exhibited at the Pendulum Gallery in the atrium of the HSBC Building (855 West Georgia Street), during the World Congress. The exhibition is comprised of portraits of fifteen well-known Canadians who remained active and fully engaged in society into their eighties, such as Bill Reid and Doris Shadbolt. Each subject is portrayed in black and white and in colour, and is accompanied by an audiotape of the subject talking about his or her life and experience of aging. Jerry Grey will discuss the genesis of the exhibition which developed though her admiration of several elderly friends and her experiences in painting them. She will also comment on the responses to the work she has received when she has presented the images to seniors. She will share her insights regarding successful aging, observations about the self-image of seniors and their concerns about the physical aspects of aging, and the loss to society when we overlook the potential contributions of our elders. The exhibition opened at the Ottawa Art Gallery in November 2000 to wide acclaim. It will remain at the Pendulum Gallery in the HSBC Atrium for the month of July. A catalogue accompanies the exhibition. A book is currently in preparation.

SESSION 68

Does Declined Background Ionizing Radiation Effect Metabolic and Aging Rates?

N. Utko, A. Timchenko, Kh. Muradian(Institute of Gerontology AMSU, Kiev, Ukraine)

The negative effect and resulting accelerated aging of single-dosed, fractionated or chronic ionizing irradiation is well documented. However, little information, if any, is available concerning the background radiation (BR) with intensity lower than environmental values. The purpose of this study was to estimate the effect of various BR on aging, or to be more specific, clarify whether the declined BR will alter mortality pattern and extend life span. Material and methods: Male and female Oregon D. m. imagoes were kept on the standard medium, 12:12 dark:light cycle, and 25 °C in two succeeding series of experiments. Three environmental BR were tested: (0.10-0.12), (0.12-0.13), and (0.15-0.16) μSv/h, corresponding to the "clean" regions, Kiev city, and regions moderately contaminated by the Chernobyl accident. Flies with the declined BR were kept in a lead covered container with (0.03- 0.05) μSv/h BR, i.e. around 3-5 times lower the controls. It was found that around 70 % of the total BR was of g -, 30 % of b -, and only traces were of the a -origin. Results: No significant differences were observed when comparing the metabolic rate and survival within either the three control groups with close BR, or at the lower BR. In the first experiment, e.g, the 50 % survivals were 73 and 67 days and the last flies died on 95 and 99 days at the (0.10-0.12) μSv/h and (0.03- 0.05) μSv/h BR. In the second series, flies from both groups lived longer, revealing 50 % survivals on 80 and 84 days and the last flies dead on the 109 and 113 days. Conclusions: Despite the cherished positive effects, flies at 3-5 times lower BR revealed no detectable changes in the metabolic rate or survival. Though definitely further studies are needed, the negative effects of ionizing irradiation would hardly be "converted" into apparent positives at lower BR, at least, when D.m. life span is under consideration.

Influence of barochamber hypoxya on functioning of hypertrofed kidney of adult and old rats

Shkulyov V.V. (Karelian State Pedagogical University, Petrozavodsk, Russia)

The aim of the study was the comparison of the functioning of remained after unilateral nephrectomy hypertrofed kidneys under barochamber hypoxya depending on the rats age. The object of study was adult (over 270 days old) and old (over 690 days old) rats-females. Animals were researched under water load (2.5% from the mass of body) in normal atmospheric conditions and under the same water load in conditions of barochember hypoxia (5000 m, 3 hours). The research has found out that a single kidney of old animals did not limit the removing of liquid and almost did not distinguish from the single kidney of adult rats on this parameter. Old animals with hypertrofed kidneys under the same water load level demonstrated more intensive diurezis, than adult animals with single kidneys. However excretion of osmoticaly free water by the single kidney of old rats did not increase because of excretion growing of potassium ions. Studies in conditions of barochember hypoxia have shown the growth of all indicators (diuresis, filtration and reabsorption) in both groups of animals intensifying at this the revealed age particularities. Excretion of osmoticaly free water by the kidney of an old rat did not show the signs of increase in comparison to that one of adult rat kidney due to the growing of potassium ions excretion. Thus, the periodical influence (hypoxia) together with the permanent influence (hypertrofy) as environmental factors cause a reinforcement of manifestation of age trends of kidneys activity and old animal may lose potassium ions with water under environmental factors.

Is the optimal hypogravity an antiaging panacea in the space?

A. Timchenko, Kh. Muradian (Institute of Gerontology AMS Ukraine, Kiev, Ukraine)

Space gerontology is a newly emerging scientific discipline with remarkable past and intriguing future. At the dawn of the space era, there have been discussions whether a long-term occupation in the weightlessness would decline the aging rate due to the lower antigravity wasting, by the way, reaching up to 1/4-1/3 of the general metabolism, i.e. comparable with calorie-restrictions. Since the terrestrial evolution has progressed in the constant acceleration field of the Earth, most of the animal species never had chances for adaptation to the altered gravity. This may explain why the real energy expenditures in the weightlessness are not lower but rather exceed those on the Earth. However, the microgravity stress seems an avoidable extreme. Given the feasibility of the artificial gravity modeling in space, it is tempting to speculate that there might be a range of optimal hypogravity (OH) where the negative effects are lesser and well compensated by the positives of "antigravity savings". Though here strong confirmatory statements are far from justified, nonetheless, there are reasons to believe that OH could create a reliable background against the accelerated aging and other harmful consequences of the microgravity. Moreover, taking into account the well-known positive correlation between the rates of metabolism and aging, the expected lower metabolism in OH can decline the rate of aging and some of the age-associated diseases, tumors included. Based on results of our hypergravity study and the concept of "continuity and absence of rupture points" along the gravity axis, our approximations allow to assume that OH could correspond to 0.2-0.5 g, rendering some 10-20 % metabolic "relaxation". In a space station with 10 m in the radius, e.g, OH could be created by a 5 rpm rotation. The model allows individual adjustment of OH depending on the age and daily schedule of crew members, simply by changing the distance from the rotation axis.

Long-term effects of X-irradiation in early ontogenesis on longevity and alterations of Drosophila melanogaster DNA

V .Voitenko, A. Vaiserman, N. Koshel, T. Mozzhukhina, A. Litoshenko (Institute of Gerontology, Kiev, Ukraine)

PURPOSE: It has been shown in our previous researches that irradiation in early ontogenesis can result in increased lifespan (LS) in D. melanogaster (hormesis). The mechanism of such long-term effect is not found as yet. The study of structurally-functional changes of the D. melanogaster (line Oregon-R) DNA after X-irradiation at the egg stage was carried out for detection of "substratum of memory" about exposures. METHOD: Insects were irradiated at 1-hour egg stage with dosage 0.25, 0.50, 0.75, 1.0, 2.0 and 4.0 Gy. DNA samples were isolated from whole 5-6Δdays imago - males (200-400 flies per set, 3 sets per group). The aliquots of DNA were digested by S1-nuclease. Intact and S1-treated DNA samples were analysed by agarose electrophoresis. RESULTS: Preimaginal stage lethality was increased with increasing irradiation dose. At the same time, decrease in imaginal LS was observed only after irradiation with the greatest dose (4 Gy) only. Moreover, hormesis by LS was revealed: in males - irradiation with 0.25, 0.75 and 1 Gy significant increases in the mean LS, and with 0.25 and 0.5 Gy - the maximal LS; in females - exposures with 0.25, 0.75 and 2 Gy significant increases in the maximal LS. The densitometric assay of DNA electrophoregramms showed decrease by 39.2 % of the part of high-molecular-weight DNA in control as a result of S1-nuclease action. Samples of DNA from the irradiated flies were∫ more stable to enzyme action. The high-molecular-weight DNA content was reduced only by 16.2, 10.0 and 17.9 % in 0.25, 0.75 and 2 Gy-irradiated groups, correspondingly, (the differences from the appropriate index in the control are statistically significant, $p < 0.05$). CONCLUSION: The higher stability of DNA originated from the irradiated flies could be resulted from reparation system activation. Probably, hormesis by longevity can be also due to an increase of the reparation system power.

Radio-Induced Aging of Laboratory Drosophila Strains with Apoptosis Deregulation

Moskalev A.A, Zainullin V.G. Institute of biology of RAS, Department of Radioecology, Syktyvkar, Russia

It should be said, that the research of ionising radiation influence on life span is conducted already some decades. Nevertheless, despite the abundance of hypotheses about mechanisms of radioinduced aging, non of them has not taken any leading position. As it is known, that the irradiation is capable to induce apoptosis, in the given work investigated aging after irradiation of Drosophila strains, bearing some apoptosis defects. The strain th bears defect in the gene of inhibitor apoptosis protein Diap-1/Th. The strain 1576 is characterised by loss of a site H99 on third chromosome, bearing proapoptosis genes reaper, grim and hid. The strain P1106 is characterised by overexpression of a gene dcp-1, coding protease, participating in an induction of apoptosis effector events. Besides in the experiment two Drosophila stocks, bearing mutant alleles of a gene wingless (wg), wgl-7 / CyO and wg7L74 / CyO are used. These lines are characterised by a violation of development and increased sensitivity to an apoptosis induction. All strains were obtained from Bloomington Stock Centre and Umea Stock Centre. The research was conducted in a standard temperature and light mode. For the purpose of irradiation we used a source of gamma-irradiation, containing 226 Ra. The doze absorbed for generation was 0,6 Gy. The research was conducted in a standard temperature and light mode. For the purpose of irradiation we used a source of gamma-irradiation, containing 226 Ra. The doze absorbed for generation was 0,6 Gy. It was shown that in the strain 1576 life span after irradiation is significant increased in comparison with the control ($p < 0{,}05$). At the strain th, the reduction of life span after influence was marked ($p < 0{,}05$). The same effect was shown in the strain having an additional active copy of a proapoptosis gene dcp1 ($p < 0{,}05$). All three investigated strains are characterised by defect in so-called reaper - dependent way of Drosophila apoptosis regulation. The decrease of life span in the stock wg after effect is shown for both alleles ($p<0.001$). Thus, the received data allow assuming the important role of apoptosis deregulation in the control of radio-induced life span alteration and aging.

Simple Model to Assess the Limits of Environmental Modification of Human Aging Rate

A. Khalyavkin (Russian Academy of Sciences, Institute of Biochemical Physics, Moscow, Russia)

The solid evidences that senescence is susceptible to environmental and genetic alteration open up the good possibility that human aging could be dramatically decelerated by some genetic and environmental intervention (Finch, 1997). A lot of researchers have explored genetic intervention. Here I offer the simple model of a total environmental influence on the aging rate. It is common knowledge that reducing below a critical level the values both in the concentration of nutrients in the habitat of amoebae and the water temperature in an aquarium with hydra leads to aging of these potentially ageless creatures. This implies that by changing external conditions one can cause primitive ageless organism to age. Hence, the possibility that the same simple reason may lie at the aging base of a more complex organism with a life history that incorporates repeated reproduction should not be discounted. The more so because it is supported by the correlation between parameters of mortality statistics for different countries, the populations of which live in varying conditions. This correlation is similar to the mortality pattern for populations of potentially ageless organisms, which age in conditions preventing, to varying extents, the complete self-maintenance of the organisms. External pressure is expressed in our model by the level of the initial mortality rate Mo. Rate of aging is connected with the relative rate of the age-related M(t) growth. The above model is consistent with all available data and predicts that living conditions exist which are conducive to a significant deceleration of the human aging process. Both realization of this fact and an understanding that the human body consists of telomere-positive potentially ageless somatic stem cells make it possible to embark on a search for living conditions, physiological regimens and some means, which reduce rate of aging as far as desirable.

The effect of age on the frequency of stable chromosome aberrations in control and irradiated people.

I. Vorobtsova, A. Kanayeva, A. Semyonov, I. Zvereva.

Purpose: Stable chromosome aberrations (SCHA) are suspected to play important role in aging and carcinogenesis. Ionizing radiation is known to accelerate these processes. We compared age-response of SCHA in normal and irradiated human populations. Material and methods: Two cohorts of people at the age range of 3-80 years were studied: control (45 persons) and exposed to low doses of accidental irradiation (67 persons). FISH method was used for visualization of SCHA. Cultured metaphase lymphocytes were hybridized with biotinilated whole chromosome specific DNA probes for 1, 4 and 12 chromosomes, stained with avidin-FITC, counterstained with PI and analyzed under UV-microscope with the set of filters allowed simultaneous observation of green (FITC) and red (PI) fluorescence. Exchanges between painted (green) and unpainted (red) chromosomes were scored. Results: The frequency of SCHA in lymphocytes increased with age in both populations studied in accordance to quadratic model, being higher in exposed cohort as compared to control one. Conclusion: The frequency of SCHA is a reliable biomarker of aging and exposure in humans. Quadratic model of age-response for SCHA provides evidence that their increase is due not only to the accumulation of environmental insults but seems to reflect the genomic instability of older people. The exposure of people to low doses of ionizing radiation accelerates the age-related increase of SCHA frequency.

SESSION 69

Genetics of Aging in Model Systems

S.M. Jazwinski (Department of Biochemistry and Molecular Biology, Louisiana State University Health Sciences Center, New Orleans, USA) Multiple Metabolic Mechanisms of Yeast Aging. S. Hekimi (Department of Biology, McGill University, Montreal, Canada) The Slow Physiological Rates of clk Mutants of the Nematode Caenorhabditis elegans Are Sufficient to Increase Life Span. L. Partridge (Department of Biology, University College, London, United Kingdom) Insulin/IGF Signaling and Aging in Drosophila

The purpose of this symposium is to provide an overview of recent advances in the genetics of aging in model systems. This research encompasses studies in filamentous fungi, yeast, roundworms, and fruit flies. The genomes of the latter three have been fully sequenced. All four of these organisms combine facile genetics with short life spans, making them especially attractive as compared to vertebrate models such as the mouse. Results of studies in these model systems can inform the design of research strategies in more difficult mammalian models and in human. An important principle emerging from the genetic analysis of aging in the model systems represented in this symposium is the importance of metabolism and metabolic control for longevity. This is an especially pleasing development, because the caloric restriction paradigm has brought home the importance of metabolism in mammalian aging. H.D. Osiewacz will present his studies on the role of copper homeostasis in aging. This presentation highlights the intricate balance between energy production and oxidative damage, which is resolved in Podospora by the induction of a pathway of energy production that produces less oxidative stress. S.M. Jazwinski will detail the participation of two non-overlapping signaling pathways that adjust metabolism and result in extended longevity in yeast. These pathways, the retrograde response and caloric restriction, appear to compensate for accumulating mitochondrial dysfunction and serve to prevent the damage associated with aging, respectively. S. Hekimi will describe the isolation of additional clk mutants in the roundworm that slow physiological rates. A strict relationship exists between physiologic rate and life span in all of these mutants, raising the hypothesis that aging results from an imbalance between damage and repair mechanisms. L. Partridge will relate her analysis of the impact of the insulin/IGF signaling pathway on aging of the fruit fly. This research points to the evolutionary conservation of this pathway for regulating life span, but it indicates that certain other effects of this pathway may not be causally associated with aging. The results of all of these studies provide hypotheses and molecules that can be tested for their effects on aging in higher organisms.

Multiple Metabolic Mechanisms of Yeast Aging

S.M. Jazwinski (Department of Biochemistry and Molecular Biology, Louisiana State University Health Sciences Center, New Orleans, Louisiana, USA)

Individual cells of the yeast Saccharomyces cerevisiae are characterized by a limited capacity for generating daughter cells, termed replicative life span. Mitochondrial dysfunction triggers an intracellular signaling pathway to the nucleus, called the retrograde response, which results in alterations in the expression of metabolic genes and an extension of yeast life span. The RAS2 gene exerts part of its effect on yeast longevity through modulation of the retrograde response. Manipulation of the nutritional status of yeasts evokes a life span-extending response akin to caloric restriction in mammals. This caloric restriction can be effected through alterations of either the glucose or amino acid supply. Caloric restriction and the retrograde response operate along separate, non-overlapping pathways, which appear to interact at the level of the downstream effectors of longevity, as evidenced by the subtle combined effects on life span of caloric restriction and retrograde response mediator genes. The SIR2 gene, which is important for silencing transcription of heterochromatic regions of the yeast genome, is not required to obtain life extension through the reduction of glucose levels. This indicates that the gene dysregulation provoked by loss of SIR2 activity sustains a distinct mechanism of aging. Our studies support the existence of multiple metabolic mechanisms in yeast aging. The retrograde response appears to compensate for the mitochondrial dysfunction that accumulates with age by metabolic adaptation. Caloric restriction, on the other hand, may prevent or postpone many of the deficits of aging by adjusting metabolism.

The Slow Physiological Rates of clk Mutants of the Nematode Caenorhabditis elegans Are Sufficient to Increase Life Span

Siegfried Hekimi (Department of Biology, McGill University, Montréal, Canada)

All mutants of the nematode C. elegans that display an increased life span also display other phenotypic characteristics. For example, the long-lived clk-1, -2, -3 and gro-1 mutants have slow and deregulated physiological rates. Affected features include the cell cycle, embryonic and post-embryonic development, rhythmic behaviours, and reproduction. We have carried out genetic screens for more mutants of this type. We screened for mutants that had slow development and slow defecation cycles, but were overall healthy and anatomically wild-type. Mean life span was not used for screening. We have identified 7 new maternal-effect, and 2 zygotic mutants of this type. When life span was subsequently scored, we found that all mutants lived significantly longer than the wild type. Together with the previously identified clk genes, this represents 12 mutants for which slow physiological rates are automatically associated with a long life span. We have not yet identified a single exception to this rule. Our results support a hypothesis that suggests that aging is the result of an imbalance between processes that result in damage to the molecular constituents of cells and its repair. If the rates of both damaging and repair processes are reduced in our mutants, the total resulting damage accumulation per unit time will be reduced to the same degree. Our observations suggest that in animals that are otherwise wild-type this is sufficient to lengthen life.

SESSION 70

Negotiating Personhood and Dignity Among People with Dementia

M. Bloch (University of British Columbia, Vancouver, Canada) Establishing Advance Directives by Consensual Decision-making for the Cogntiviely Impaired Elderly. A. Carswell (University of British Columbia) Person - Environment - Occupation Model and the person with Dementia.. C. Cohen, MD (Sunnybrook and Women's College Health Sciences Centre, Toronto, Canada) Identity, Personhood, Dignity and Dementia: A Clinicians Perspective. J. Graham (University of British Columbia, Vancouver, Canada) Sufferer and Caregiver Strategies for Living with Alzheimer's Disease. C. Powell (Queen Elizabeth II Health Science Centre, Halifax, Canada) Living with Dementia: Risk? Whose? Steven Sabat (Georgetown University, Washington D.C, USA) The Role of Supporting Valued Public Personae in Maintaining Personhood and Dignity in People with Alzheimer's Disease. A. Smith (University of British Columbia, Vancouver, Canada) Medicalizing intersubjectivity: Diagnostic disclosure and its impact on the interpretation of personhood in dementia.

This is the second of a two part symposium and roundtable presentation that will extend the conceptual and methodological issues raised and developed at a recent Canadian Institute of Health Research Tri-Council workshop titled Matters on the Heart and Mind: Negotiating Personhood and Dignity Among Older people with Dementia. The specific issues to be addressed include not only how personhood and dignity are currently defined and operationalized in a variety of health care settings and in the home, but also what research agendas are necessary to truly understand these concepts and take them into everyday life and professional practice. The session will be structured around brief presentations by seven workshop participants who will highlight selected themes developed at the CIHR workshop. The content will include a discussion around critical aspects of fostering the personhood of individuals with dementia. Several papers that probe the health care system and how it shapes the dementia experience include Smith's research on diagnostic disclosure and how that legitimates selected family approaches. Moving into health care relationships, Cohen will explore generally how attending to issues of personhood impacts clinical practice. Two specific areas where personhood issues frequently surface, decision-making around living at risk and developing advanced directives, will be examined - the former by Powel and the latter by Bloch. Sabat's long standing program of research about selfhood moves the agenda forward by identifying some of the specific understandings, meanings and tools that family members and professionals need in order to sustain the person with dementia. Capitalizing on the deep knowledge that family members have about one another, Graham's paper describes the results of an ethnographic study which illuminated strategies developed by patients and caregivers for dealing with a progressive dementia. Finally, Carswell will outline and discuss a model of Person - Environment - Occupation and the powerful impact that meaningful activity can have on performance. The implications of having a perspective grounded in recognizing the personhood of the individual with dementia will be explored in terms of their impact on professional interactions as well as for family members and their interactions. Taken together, these papers suggest that the self and the identity of the person with dementia should be examined, clarified and supported. The workshop participants and the attending audience will enrich one another's understandings of the more important agendas to pursue. Participants at this session can expect to interact with experts who are moving the research agenda in new directions and hear about recent and anticipated undertakings. The outcomes of this roundtable discussion will be heightened awareness of the need for a more comprehensive, holistic and interdisciplinary approach to dementia care as well as the generation of ideas regarding furthering this research agenda.

Establishing Advanced Directives by Consensual Decsion-Making for the Cognitively Impaired Elderly

Maurice Bloch (University of British Columbia, Vancouver, Canada

Elderly persons with dementia should not have to suffer more than competent individuals who can express their own wishes about end of life decisions. Substituted decision-making is a next best method for making decisions. The substitute decision maker is required to place him/herself in the shoes of the patient and to arrive at a decision which takes into account the culture, beliefs, values and preferences of the person with dementia. Advance Directives (ADs) are documents upon which these substituted judgements can be recorded. But ADs which are established by next of kin are frequently ignored when the patient is dying. ADs established paternalistically by the physician and /or other health care providers (HCP), seldom reflect the preferences of the dying person. Decision-making must be broadened to become a partnership which includes all interested parties - namely the patient (if at all capable), next of kin and other involved family members as well as the physician and other health care providers. The protocol for decision-making must include strategies for Effective and Ongoing Communication; Participation of all interested parties; Empowerment of all parties; A Culture of Process in which the ADs are never considered final products nor ends in themselves. Consensually established ADs will result in greater satisfaction, trust and respect between the family and HCPs and will more likely be followed at the time of dying. The AD will more accurately reflect the wishes of the patient while securing the support of the family members and the HCPs

Identity, Personhood, Dignity and Dementia: A Clinician's Perspective

Carole A. Cohen M.D. Sunnybrook and Women's College Health Sciences Centre, Toronto, Canada)

In a recent workshop held at the University of British Columbia on personhood and dignity among person's with dementia three major common themes emerged out of an analysis of small discussion papers submitted by all participants in preparation for the workshop: the importance of including the perspective of the person with dementia, recognizing the impact of the interpersonal environment for fostering personhood, and understanding the dementia experience in relation to a broader socio-political context. As a clinician and teacher I can easily relate to these three major themes. In fact many participants at the symposium used clinical vignettes or personal vignettes about frail elderly family members to illustrate and ground their comments. These themes may not always be uppermost in my mind as I practice day to day. However, the opportunity to talk with others from different fields has brought a refreshing perspective to my work and teaching. This presentation will focus on a clinician's perspective and challenges in attempting to acknowledge issues related to personhood and dementia.

Living with Dementia - Risk - Whose?

Colin Powell, MD (Queen Elizabeth II Health Science Centre, Halifax, Canada)

A round-table discussion emphasizing the notion of risk in caring for older adults with dementia; with specific reference to discharge from hospital, use of physical restraints as a response to perceived risk, assessment of a patient's competency with respect to "controlling" risk; and finally recognition of the risks the professional carer undertakes.

Medicalizing intersubjectivity: Diagnostic disclosure and its impact on the Interpretation of personhood in dementia.

André Smith, (University of British Columbia, Vancouver, Canada)

Purpose: This study explores the complex familial and social dimensions in the communication and understanding of a diagnosis of dementia. While clinicians disclose diagnostic findings to inform patients and family members about the presence or potential presence of dementia, this study instead considers the ways in which this information is used to make sense of dementia in everyday life. This study also explores the role of medicalized representations in patients who do not meet criteria for dementia but subjectively experience distressing memory lapses that they attribute to a dementia disorder Method: This is a qualitative investigation of the experiences of 16 families where a relative has been evaluated at a dementia clinic. Data collection methods include in-depth interviews and observation of the clinical evaluation and disclosure of the diagnosis. Results: The results reveal that the diagnosis legitimates family members in using medicalized representations of dementia to make sense of troublesome behaviors on the part of affected relatives. More specifically, family members tend to index those behaviors to stereotypical descriptions of what people with dementia do and say that are contained in the caregiver literature or in the media. This process results in a tendency to reify the affected relative as a non-human agent being animated by pathology. Conclusion: Overall, this study draws attention to the familial and social contexts of the dementia experience. While a reliance on medicalized representations makes this experience more bearable for family members, there is the potential that they could interpret inapt efforts at signifying identity on the part of affected relatives as manifestations of pathology.

Person-Environment-Occupation Model and the Person with Dementia

Anne Carswell (University of British Columbia, Vancouver, Canada)

A model, which provides a framework for examining the interaction of a person with dementia with the environment (social, physical, cultural and institutional) and the ability to perform activities that are meaningful, is the person-environment-occupation model of occupational performance (Law, Cooper, Strong, Stewart, Rigby and Letts, 1996). This model assumes that the person, the environment and occupation interact across time and space in ways that diminish or increase performance. If we accept that part of a person's identity and self-worth is the performance of meaningful activity, which is compromised by the dementing process, then we need to understand and measure the parts of the environment the impact upon worth. As a part of the roundtable discussion this paper will present the model and discuss ways of discovering, describing and empirically testing the environmental impacts upon persons with dementia.

Sufferer and Caregiver Strategies for Living with Alzheimers disease

Janice Graham (University of British Columbia, Vancouver, Canada)

PURPOSE: This paper presents results from the Atlantic Canada Alzheimer's Disease Investigation of Expectations (ACADIE) study which focused on individualized problem areas identified by caregivers and patients with mild to moderate Alzheimer's disease (AD). Attention is given to the everyday strategies the study participants and researchers identified as successful interventions. METHOD: 108 patients and their caregivers participated in a 52 week, open-label study of an anti-dementia medication using clinical, epidemiological and anthropological methods and measures to determine treatment efficacy. Patients underwent clinical assessment and participated in extensive in-depth home interviews at 12 week intervals. Strategies identified by qualitative analysis of the subjective participant interviews were analysed alongside objective quantifiable clinical outcomes. RESULTS: Over the course of the study, specific problem areas relating to cognition, social interaction, behaviour, function, and leisure activities were identified. After initial improvements in cognition, function and leisure, patients declined by study end. Sustained improvements were observed clinically and qualitatively in behaviour and social interaction. CONCLUSIONS: Importantly, the use of ethnographic techniques afforded the opportunity to systematically collect a sample of strategies that assist the person with AD and his/her caregiver to cope with the day-to-day challenges of this progressive disease. The ACADIE study provides an evidence base for what have previously been anecdotal-based observations. An overview of the study results and examples of strategies devised by patients and caregivers to deal with the evolving problems of AD will be presented.

The Role of Supporting Valued Public Personae in Maintaining Personhood and Dignity in People with Alzheimer's Disease

Steven R. Sabat (Georgetown University, Washington, D.C, USA)

In this paper, I shall discuss the ways in which the dignity and personhood of people with Alzheimer's disease (AD) can be supported and maintained with the cooperation of healthy others in the afflicted person's social world. Specifically, I will employ aspects of Social Construction Theory as a heuristic device to illuminate (1) aspects of intact selfhood in persons afflicted with AD; (2) how certain aspects of selfhood, one's public social personae, are dependent upon the cooperation of others; (3) how the displays of such public personae are intimately related to feelings of self-worth and dignity; (4) how such displays can be limited by healthy others such that the afflicted person is consigned to a public persona of "dysfunctional, burdensome patient" resulting in a diminution of feelings of self-worth and dignity; and (5) how the behavior of healthy others can support valued public personae and thereby support the dignity and personhood of the afflicted individual. I will employ empirical data, culled from in-depth transcribed conversations with persons in the moderate to severe stages of AD, to illustrate each of these points.

SESSION 71

Elder Abuse Training Initiative: An Innovative Model in Ontario, Canada

Gloria Lattanzio, (Senior Policy Advisor, Ontario Seniors' Secretariat, Ministry of Citizenship Culture and Recreation, Toronto, ON, Canada) The Ontario Elder Abuse Strategy Diane Harris, (Performance and Training Consultant, Tillsonburg, ON, Canada) Elder Abuse Training Initiative: The Training Model Christian Awaraji, (Infomatics, London, ON, Canada) Elder Abuse Training Initiative: Innovation and Technology Paul Stolee, (aestima research, London, ON, Canada) Evaluation of a Provincial Elder Abuse Training Initiative in Community Care Carol Philbin-Jolette (Near North Community Care Access Centre, North Bay, ON, Canada) Elder Abuse Training: Practical Application and Linkage with the Coordinated Community Response Model

This symposium will describe the development, implementation and evaluation of an innovative province-wide education initiative aimed at training Community Care Access Centre (CCAC) case managers and the service providers with whom they contract to recognize and respond to elder abuse. In Ontario, CCACs provide coordinated access to a range of community services including in-home nursing, therapies, homemaking and personal support, as well as access to long-term care facility beds. The training approach placed emphasis on overall organizational and system performance and featured the development of elder abuse resource teams and the use of a website and voice chat room to exchange information. The Ontario Association of Community Care Access Centres (OACCAC) received funding from the Seniors' Secretariat of the Government of Ontario to undertake this project. The training initiative was one component of a multi-sectoral strategy undertaken by the provincial government aimed at making Ontario safer for its elderly citizens. The strategy included the establishment of the Elder Abuse Round Table, which includes 20 influential senior citizens and opinion leaders from a number of sectors. The Round Table was established to provide advice to government on the three key components of the strategy: front-line staff training, coordination of services and a public education and awareness campaign in relation to elder abuse. Susan Donaldson, the Chief Executive Officer of the OACCAC, will provide an overview of the initiative, describe the association's role in leading the project and introduce the five individual presenters. Gloria Lattanzio will discuss the Government of Ontario's Elder Abuse Strategy, and the projects funded under this strategy. Diane Harris will describe the development and implementation of the training model. Christian Awaraji will describe how technology, specifically the Internet, was used to facilitate the exchange of information throughout the initiative. Paul Stolee will discuss the evaluation of the project, including changes in practice for elder abuse identification, assessment and intervention following the training. Carol Philbin-Jolette will describe the linkage between the Elder Abuse Training Initiative and a second component of the Elder Abuse Strategy, specifically a project to develop a coordinated community response model for elder abuse. Susan Donaldson will provide a wrap-up, focusing on lessons learned and the potential applicability of this approach to other initiatives and sectors.

Elder Abuse Training Initiative: The Innovative Use of Technology

Christian Awaraji, (Infomatics, London, ON, Canada)

In any training initiative, one of the most crucial factors of success is timely exchange of information. Whether the exchange is at the level of brief communications, bulletins or even data collection, timeliness is essential for the different pieces of a project to fall into place in a well-orchestrated and professional manner. During the Community Care Access Centre (CCAC) Elder Abuse Training Initiative, the use of technology, and more specifically the Internet, has been a key component in making his happen. A web site was designed and was continuously updated to provide an accessible source of information to the participants. The web site was also used to collect data using on-line forms before, during and after the training was delivered. This process not only eliminated the unnecessary flow of paper and the cost and time lag associated with manual data entry, but also provided the evaluators with data in a format readily useable with their preferred statistical tools. Another Internet tool used was the listserver. A listserver was set up and continuously updated to be used as a means of communications with and among the participants. Also during the training, the participants were encouraged to use a voice chat room. Using Voice over IP (VoIP) technology, voice communication over the Internet can eliminate a sizeable amount of the cost associated with telephone conferencing.

Elder Abuse Training Initiative: The Training Model

Diane Harris (Performance and Training Consultant, Tillsonburg, ON, Canada)

Understanding training is not an end in itself, but a means to an end, the OACCAC elder abuse training initiative adopted a performance improvement approach, which emphasized organizational and system change and enhancing the capability of the 43 Community Care Access Centres (CCACs) and their contracted service provider agencies across the province. The training model focused on the development of elder abuse resource teams in each CCAC. Before training, CCAC teams and subject matter experts identified core competencies and gaps between current and desired practices which helped target resources to areas in which training would make a measurable improvement. These teams also described potential barriers to implementing new skills and submitted written strategies on how they would work with management to decrease these barriers in advance of training. The training design was guided by input from the CCACs and subject matter experts; this provided an appreciation of the existing work of elder abuse, and grounded the training in the day-to-day realities of the CCACs. Training sessions during May and June 2000 incorporated innovative and practical techniques to increase the likelihood that new learning would help staff address their most pressing elder abuse issues. During training, each team recorded their learning and new ideas in a team journal. They also assisted with the development of a template that would help them systematically think through the complex issues of elder abuse. After training, scheduled teleconferences, chat forums, and practical assignments supported the CCACs in applying and sharing of what had been learned.

Elder Abuse Training: Practical Application and Linkage with the Coordinated Community Response Model

Carol M. Philbin-Jolette (Near North Community Care Access Centre, (NNCCAC) North Bay, Ontario, Canada

As part of a provincial strategy aimed at reducing abuse of older persons in Ontario, Canada, the provincial government provided funding for the development and implementation of two pilot projects. One project focused on the development and implementation of a training initiative. The other project was mandated to develop and implement a locally appropriate coordinated community response model. The development and design of these two initiatives will act as a basis for a provincial framework intended to be rolled out across the province. This presentation will highlight the main components of each initiative, demonstrate how the projects interfaced with each other and what the main challenges were. As part of the OACCAC training initiative, the Elder Abuse Resource Team not only focused on training staff through educational sessions but also on developing internal structures to support an effective response to elder abuse. As well the Elder Abuse Resource Team developed external structures by linking with the project that developed the coordinated community response model. Five project components made up the main framework for the coordinated community response model. At the hub of this model is an Elder Abuse Call Centre, the Near North CCAC Elder Abuse Resource Team and fifteen primary referral agencies all working collaboratively to ensure that the community at large (including anyone who has issues or concerns about elder abuse) can easily access the system to receive information, get support or report a situation.

Evaluation of a Provincial Elder Abuse Training Initiative in Community Care

P. Stolee (aestima research, London, Ontario, Canada)

As part of a provincial strategy aimed at reducing abuse of older persons in Ontario, Canada, the provincial government provided funding to train staff of the province's 43 Community Care Access Centres (CCACs) and their contracted service agencies to recognize and respond to elder abuse. The training approach emphasized enhancement of overall organizational and system performance, and development of elder abuse resource teams. This report describes the evaluation of this initiative. Evaluation methods included measures of reaction to the training and pre-post measures of competence and confidence in elder abuse practice. The major evaluation focus was on practices for elder abuse identification, assessment and intervention. Reaction to the training was positive, and ratings of team competence and confidence were significantly higher ($p<.01$) following the training. Changes in elder abuse practice following the training included increased risk-screening and more formal assessment approaches; 63% of CCACs reported having implemented new activities aimed at elder abuse prevention. CCAC strategies to influence elder abuse practice among contracted agencies included joint teams and committees, training strategies, changes in policies and procedures, and inclusion of elder abuse criteria in requests for proposals for future contracts. Most CCACs (80%) reported increased networking among CCACs on elder abuse issues; 73% of CCACs had established new linkages with other elder abuse resources. Resource issues and workload are potential barriers to sustainability. Evaluation results indicate major improvements in elder abuse practice and are promising for the success of other training initiatives that emphasize organizational and system performance.

The Ontario Elder Abuse Strategy

Gloria Lattanzio (Senior Policy Advisor, Ontario Seniors' Secretariat, Ministry of Citizenship Culture and Recreation, Toronto, ON, Canada)

Ontario is home to 1.45 million seniors and 4% to 10% of seniors have experienced or are experiencing abuse of some kind. Elder abuse occurs in the community and in institutions, and may take different forms: physical, psychological, emotional, financial and neglect. Abusers may be family, caregivers, persons in positions of authority or strangers. By 2021, when the seniors' population will have doubled, the problem of elder abuse will become more serious if steps are not taken now to address this problem. The pain and suffering, loss of trust and loss of resources experienced by seniors will be matched by a significant cost to government and society as a whole. The Ontario government is committed to ensuring safer communities for all Ontario citizens. In keeping with this commitment, the Ontario government announced the development of a provincial elder abuse strategy. An advisory body ("The Round Table for Ontario's Elder Abuse Strategy") was established in November 1999 to provide advice to the government on the development of a provincial elder abuse strategy. The Round Table struck working groups on the three strategy priorities: raising public awareness, training front line staff and coordination of community services. These working groups developed practical, effective advice on how best to respond to the three priorities. The Government also funded two projects to address elder abuse: * A pilot project to test coordinated community response models * Training for staff of Community Care Access Centres and their contracted agencies to detect, respond and prevent elder abuse.

SESSION 72

Narrative Matters 2: Putting Stories to Work in Practice

I. R. Hallberg (Department of Nursing, Unit for Caring Sciences, Lund University, Lund, Sweden) A Narrative Approach to Nursing Care of People in Difficult Life Situations. B. de Vries and J. Blando (San Francisco State University, San Francisco, CA, USA) Guided Autobiography: A Variety of Applications. W. L. Randall (Programme in Gerontology, St. Thomas University, Fredericton, New Brunswick, Canada) Teaching Story: The Pedagogical Potential of Narrative Gerontology. P. G. Clark (Program in Gerontology and Rhode Island Geriatric Education Center, The University of Rhode Island, Kingston, RI, USA) Values and Voices in Teaching Geriatrics: Case Studies as Stories.

Narrative gerontology-incorporating various elements of biography, life review, and reminiscence-has recently captured the imagination of researchers and practitioners alike in the field of aging. Importantly, this approach offers new insights into the "inside" experience of aging that have implications for those who work with older adults and their families.

This symposium is designed to follow Narrative Matters 1: "Perspectives on Stories and Aging," which lays out the general conceptual perspectives of the narrative approach by exploring the individual, sociocultural, philosophical, and language-based dimensions of this perspective on understanding the experience of aging for the individual. This second symposium specifically explores the applied potential of narrative within clinical, community, and educational settings. The first paper, by Hallberg, analyzes the usefulness of a narrative approach in understanding "situational meaning" using interviews with leukemia patients and family caregivers. Implications of the challenges in nursing care will be explored, particularly with respect to the uniqueness of meaning and storying for patients and their care. The second paper, by de Vries and Blando, highlights guided autobiography as a specific approach, and reviews some of its many successes in academic contexts, in work with dying and bereaved individuals, and in therapeutic settings. The rewards of a sense of personal integration and empowerment, a deeper meaning in life, and the development and grounding of new relationships will be highlighted. The third paper, by Randall, explores the implications of the narrative metaphor for educators and students in educational settings. Besides offering a framework for the development of instructional applications of "life as story," this paper will make recommendations for professionals in clinical and practice-related settings. The final paper by Clark explores the instructional, clinical, and ethical issues at the root of the case study method of teaching geriatrics and gerontology. These include the relationship between "fact" and "fiction," the use of language, the perspective of the author, and the importance of how the case is to be used. Overall, the purpose of this symposium is to present specific, applied, and practical means and methods to integrate the principles and perspectives of narrative gerontology into educational, clinical, and community-based practice. These applications include interventions and programs that promise to aid those who are sick and dying, those who seek personal integration and meaning in life, those who seek to teach and learn fundamental insights into the aging experience, and those who would highlight the philosophical and value-based dimensions and dilemmas of working with older adults and their families. The intent is to give participants practical and useful tools to take back to their own practice settings that will enrich their work and the lives of those they serve as professionals in gerontology and geriatrics.

A Narrative Approach to Nursing Care of People in Difficult Life Situations

I. R. Hallberg (Department of Nursing, Unit for Caring Sciences, Lund University, Lund, Sweden)

Encountering people in difficult life situations is an everyday task for nurses. However, in professional practice there is a risk that nurses will lose sight of the uniqueness of individuals and miss their attempts to bring life events together into a meaningful story. This paper explores the usefulness of a narrative approach in understanding "situational meaning" using interviews with leukemia patients and family caregivers. Case studies will be used to illustrate significant insights gained from this narrative approach. They include a woman who was able to survive and make sense of the experience of leukemia and its treatment, in contrast to another woman who was not able to integrate the event into her life. In both cases a narrative mode was used for comforting the self, verbalizing fear, escaping from the unbearable, feeling that life was still going on in spite of the disaster, and being a part of life outside it. Findings highlight the importance of "making sense of the situation" for the development of a life-changing direction. For example, a male caregiver who had looked after his wife for fifteen years highlights the co-authoring, storying, and restorying processes, as well as how he became a guide in his wife's life. This paper will highlight the importance of the nurse-patient relationship for the patient's development of storying. Implications of the challenges to nursing care will be summarized, particularly with respect to the uniqueness of meaning and storying for patients and their care.

Guided Autobiography: A Variety of Applications

B. de Vries and J. Blando (San Francisco State University, San Francisco, CA, USA)

The Guided Autobiography is a semi-structured method facilitating the telling of life stories. It involves a written component on productive themes of life and a small group process component in which the individual life stories are shared with others. Since its introduction over two decades ago, this procedure has been used in many countries with a wide range of groups and in a wide variety of settings. This presentation is intended to highlight the Guided Autobiography and review some of these many successes. Following a description of the general process, particular attention will be directed toward the use of the Guided Autobiography in academic settings, in settings with bereaved and dying individuals, and in settings explicitly elaborating on its therapeutic potential. A novel and recent application of this procedure online (i.e, a version of the process delivered by way of the world wide web) will be reviewed. The rewards accrued from participation in the Guided Autobiography, as revealed in a growing body of literature, will be presented which include a sense of personal integration and empowerment, a deeper meaning in life, and the development and grounding of new relationships. The Guided Autobiography provides for participants, therapist, and researchers alike a prominent avenue to insights about the way life is experienced from the inside, including the experiences of growing old.

Teaching Story: The Pedagogical Potential of Narrative Gerontology

W. L. Randall (Programme in Gerontology, St. Thomas University, Fredericton, New Brunswick, Canada)

A key postmodern insight is that we think, act, and indeed "know" in terms of metaphor. Central to the conceptual framework employed in narrative gerontology is the narrative metaphor, or life as story. Thus far, however, discussions concerning this metaphor have developed primarily within the theoretical and research literature of the field. This paper will explore the unique potential—and challenge—of such a metaphor for educators in particular. Questions to be considered include: How do we teach people to bring a narrative perspective to the study of aging and related topics, such as emotionality, identity, memory, spirituality, and wisdom? What sort of "perspective transformation" are we implicitly asking them to experience? How can we help them integrate such a perspective with others that their training in gerontology invites them to adopt? Besides offering a framework for finding answers to such questions, the paper will advance a set of recommendations for professionals functioning in terms of that framework within clinical and practice-related settings. Implications for the goals of gerontological instruction in general and the role of instructors in particular will be highlighted.

Values and Voices in Teaching Geriatrics: Case Studies as Stories

P. G. Clark (Program in Gerontology and Rhode Island Geriatric Education Center, The University of Rhode Island, Kingston, RI 02881 USA)

The use of case presentations in clinical settings and instructional case studies in educational contexts is commonplace in gerontology and geriatrics. Reliance on them to highlight the multifaceted and complex health-related needs of older adults is widespread, and their appeal in illustrating the clinical complexity and moral conflicts in working with older persons is obvious. This is especially the case in teaching the value of interdisciplinary teamwork. So popular is the use of case studies, however, that their uncritical adoption may become the problem. This paper explores the instructional, clinical, and ethical issues at the root of the case study method in geriatrics and gerontology. Following a survey of the literature describing their uses and applications in such methods as problem-based learning (PBL), this paper will develop an analytic framework—based on life narrative theory in understanding aging—within which to explore several issues in case study approaches. These include: the relationship between "fact" and "fiction," the use of language, the perspective of the author, and the importance of how the case is to be used. Illustrations will be drawn from actual case studies, and recommendations will be developed as guidelines for those who write, present, and use case studies in clinical and instructional contexts.

SESSION 73

Complex Causal Processes in Research on Population Health: Interactions Among Psychosocial, Behavioral and Health Factors

V. Didelez (Department of Statistical Science, University College London, England) A Comparison of Graphical Chain Models and Logistic Regression for Application to Health Studies. E. Stoller (Department of Sociology, Case Western Reserve University, Cleveland, OH, USA) Qualitative Approaches to Research: Exploring Lay Perspectives on Health and Illness in Late Life. D Brauer (School of Nursing, University of Minnesota, Minneapolis, MN, USA) Evaluating Scales Used in Research with the Elderly: Classical Theory and Item Response Theory Methods. S. Henly (School of Nursing, University of Minnesota, Minneapolis, MN, USA) Evaluating Scale Performance Using Item-Response Theory: A Comparison of Two IRT Models.

Recent years have witnessed an accumulation of inconsistent and contradictory bodies of research findings about the causal influence of many factors correlated with disease and longevity. It is recognized that methodological problems affecting both the measurement of variables and the analysis of data contribute to confusing information about many factors that are believed to exert influence on health. This symposium will present findings from international and interdisciplinary collaboration on methodological issues affecting research on complex causal relationships. It is well documented in health research conducted by a range of disciplines that diseases seldom develop from single causes. The relative capacity of disease agents to overcome host defenses is determined by complex causal processes that operate at different levels of causal influence. Yet, most health research is focused on specific factors, often, but not always, "controlling" for other types of influences. Research specially focused on interactions among social, psychosocial, behavioral and health variables is rare. One reason for this is that quantitative health research is seriously constrained by the limited availability of analytic techniques that elaborate interactions among different levels and types of variables. Another reason is the strong schism between qualitative and quantitative health research. The first paper will discuss methods for elaborating complex statistical relationships among types of causal influences. In the second paper, qualitative methods and their role in understanding complex causal processes will be discussed. Measurement is the basic building block in all fields. It determines the validity and soundness of research findings. Data collected with complex measurement instruments are often used in health research to represent psychosocial and behavioral concepts. It is known that psychosocial, behavioral and health variables can be confounded in measurement scales. Variables that do not validly measure concepts or that measure more than one concept are another source of contradictory information about health. The third and fourth papers will present findings illustrating methodological aspects of measurement and alternative strategies and statistical models used for validating measurement scales.

A comparison of graphical chain models and logistic regression for application to health studies

V. Didelez (Department of Statistical Science, University College London, England), I. Pigeot, (Institute of Statistics, University of Munich, Germany), A.Wister, K. Dean (Gerontology Research Centre, Simon Fraser University, Vancouver, Canada)

Quantitative research has been seriously constrained by the limited availability of analytic techniques that elaborate interactions among social, psychosocial, behavioral and health variables. A newly developed statistical technique, graphical interaction modeling, has considerable potential for providing new knowledge about relationships among different types of variables. With graphical models, conditional independence properties are derived from the analysis and presented in interaction graphs. Merits of graphical models for analyzing multivariate data will be explored using an empirical study on coping with chronic illnesses as a function of interrelationships among three types of influences affecting coping: social situational variables, illness context variables and four self-care practices. In order to reveal direct and indirect dependencies, a graphical chain model is selected from the data based on an appropriate selection strategy. We contrast the results with those obtained from a standard main-effects logistic regression model where interactions are generally not identified and indirect effects are not taken into account. As anticipated, some findings are consistent across the two analyses, but there are important differences. For example, perceived seriousness affects how self-care practices influence coping. There is evidence of other interactions as well. It was found that the type of illness assumes an important role as a mediating variable and that gender has an indirect effect on coping which could not be revealed by the logistic regression. In conclusion, this comparative case study demonstrates that, while graphical modeling is no panacea, it provides an important new option for elaborating the inherent multidimensional nature of influences shaping health and aging, and thus responds to the need for methodological developments that can better capture associations in complex systems.

Qualitative Approaches to Research: Exploring Lay Perspectives on Health and Illness in Late Life

E. Stoller (Department of Sociology, Case Western Reserve University, Cleveland, OH, USA)

Qualitative strategies enable researchers to explore cultural meanings and lay explanatory models of disease, to elucidate the decision processes accompanying treatment and management of disease, and to examine the process through which individuals integrate the disruption of illness into their autobiographies. Qualitative researchers encourage research participants to share their understandings and experience with disease in their own words. This approach provides insights into the lived experience of illness, an insider's (or "emic") perspective that can be masked by research designs that impose the perspective of the researcher or clinician on the patient's story. Qualitative strategies thus promote the identification and deeper understanding of complex behavioral and psychosocial influences that affect disease and aging processes. This presentation will focus on the application of techniques for generating and analyzing qualitative data (e.g, in-depth interviews, illness narratives, focus groups) for studying the experience of illness from the perspective of older adults. Special attention will be focused on how this methodological approach can generate an insider's perspective on lay explanatory models and lay management strategies among older adults with chronic conditions. The importance of incorporating an emic (or insider's approach) in health research and clinical interventions in gerontology will also be discussed.

Evaluating Scales Used in Research with the Elderly: Classical Theory and Item Response Theory Methods

D. Brauer, K. Dean, S. Edwardson (School of Nursing, University of Minnesota, USA)

Since measurement is the basic building block in all fields, it must be assured that variables constructed to represent theoretical concepts are valid measurements. In health and gerontological research, data collected to represent complex psychosocial and behavioral concepts are frequently used to construct measurement scales. When multiple dimensions are represented, psychological or social variables other than the intended theoretical concept may be represented in the scale. This can result in serious confounding in results of multivariate statistical analysis as well as measurement bias with regard to subgroups of the population. This paper presents comparative findings from validating a measure of social network support with methods derived form Classical Test Theory (CTT) and Item Response Theory (IRT), the two major theoretical perspectives used to evaluate measurement scales in social science research on health. Since differences in model assumptions and methods have generated debate regarding the strengths and weaknesses of the alternative approaches, it is important that researchers in the field are informed about the issues and the information obtained using the two options. The results of the comparative analysis in this study indicate that the measure of social support cannot be considered a valid measure of that concept. Both CTT and IRT methods detected problems in the scale. However, there are important differences in the information provided by using methods derived from the two measurement perspectives. It is concluded that the IRT methods provided more useful information about measurement problems in the scale.

Evaluating Scale Performance Using Item-Response Theory: A Comparison of Two Models

S. Henly, K. Dean, D. Brauer (School of Nursing, University of Minnesota, USA)

Research in aging populations often depends on data collected with complex measurement instruments. Potential confounding of psychosocial, behavioral and health variables in measurement scales can misrepresent individuals on study variables and distort the results of multivariate analyses. Understanding the performance of measurement scales is therefore essential for obtaining valid findings and for interpretation of results. Many researchers refer to published data on the reliability and content validity of instruments without investigating their performance. Since instruments often function differently in different populations, examining the performance of a published scale is critical. Scale evaluation methods based on Item Response Theory are appearing more frequently in the literature. Yet information about alternative IRT methods is extremely limited. This paper compares the results of validating an instrument with the two most commonly used IRT models. The Positive Emotionality (PEM) and Negative Emotionality (NEM) scales are part of the Multidimensional Personality Questionnaire, a 300-item, 14-subscale instrument developed in a college-age population using classical-test theory methods. There is evidence suggesting that PEM and NEM influence health outcomes in healthy young adults. The purpose of this study was to examine the performance of this instrument in a sample of 325 chronically ill, predominantly older adults with chronic rheumatic illnesses. The 14 MPQ subscales were evaluated using 1-parameter and 2-parameter IRT models. Findings are compared to show similarities and differences produced by the two models. Implications for evaluation of research instruments is emphasized. This type of methodological study demonstrates the importance of measurement issues in research with aging populations and illustrates potential barriers to the rigor needed to advance scientific knowledge.

SESSION 74

Supportive Housing Around the World: Programs, Policies and Prospects

S. Golant (Department of Geography, University of Florida, Gainesville, FL, USA) The Potential of Assisted Living Facilities as a Solution to Canada's Long-Term Care Crisis. J. Pynoos (Andrus Gerontology Center, University of Southern California, CA, USA) Home Modification Problems, Policies and Programs in the United States and Japan. P. Liebig (Andrus Gerontology Center, University of Southern California, CA, USA). Housing Options and Issues in India. V. Regnier (School of Architecture, University of Southern California, CA, USA), A New Look at Northern European Assisted Living for Older People). Discussant: G.Gutman (Gerontology Research Centre, Simon Fraser University, Vancouver, Canada)

With the globalization of aging, a key concern of all societies is how to help older persons age in place in their own homes and communities by creating and maintaining housing environments that support elders psychologically, functionally and socially. In general we know far more about senior housing solutions in North American and Europe, and far less about Asian approaches. Additionally, our knowledge is largely based on case studies of programs and policies in individual nations, rather than on cross-cultural/cross-national comparisons and contrasts. This symposium draws on the research conducted by four Fulbright Scholars in Canada, India, Japan, the Netherlands and Scandinavia. The purpose is to describe assisted living, home modification programs, and board and care home practices in these several nations and to make comparisons with the United States and other countries. The policy context and eldercare relevance of programs and practices will be analyzed and lessons to be learned by these various approaches will be emphasized by all presenters and the discussant.

A New Look at Northern European Assisted Living Housing for Older People

V. Regnier (School of Architecture and Andrus Gerontology Center, University of Southern California, CA, USA)

In the next 3 to 5 years the US and the world will see unprecedented growth in the number and percentage of people over the age of 85. Northern European countries like Sweden have already experienced rates of growth (17.2% over 65+) that are 1.5 times greater than the US. This presentation will focus on the lessons learned from a 1999 site visit research analysis of 100 housing projects for the older mentally and physically frail in 5 northern European countries (Sweden, Denmark, Norway, Finland and the Netherlands). In these projects, the design of the environment plays a very significant role in encouraging physical exercise, supporting social exchange and friendship formation and encouraging independence and autonomy. Some of the best assisted living and housing with services projects in Europe and North America will be used in this session to illustrate design features that make the environment more accessible, encourage independence, develop interesting landscape views, encourage informal social exchange, invite family interactions, support therapeutic programs, embrace the needs of residents living in the surrounding community, build physical competency and balance the community and privacy concerns of residents. Concepts will be grouped into 8 categories that deal with topics such as unit clusters, indoor/outdoor relationships, designing for dementia, daylighting treatments, exercise and physical therapy, informal social settings, interior design and accessories, mixed-use programming strategies, and settings that support affect and sensory stimulation.

Home Modification Problems, Policies and Programs in the United States and Japan

J. Pynoos, K. Makigami(Andrus Gerontology Center, University of Southern California, Los Angeles, CA, USA)

The aging of older persons in industrialized countries has led to the development of new types of supportive housing options such as assisted living and service housing that provide physically supportive environments coupled with a range of services. However, there is a growing recognition that the supply of this purpose-built housing will be limited by its expense and that attention needs to also be placed on assisting older persons to stay in their own dwelling units, their strongest preference in relation to housing options. Most of the conventional housing in which older persons live, however, was not built to facilitate aging in place. In fact, it contains features that make it difficult to carry out activities, impede caregving, limit accessibility and create hazards. Especially troublesome are entrances, stairways and bathrooms. Comparing the United States and Japan, this presentation will identify the types of housing problems that older frail persons face in their own homes and analyze the home modification policies and practices that have evolved to assist them in aging in place. Particular attention will be placed on how well modifications meet cultural needs of residents and the role of home modifications in broader strategies of community-based care.

Housing Options and Issues in India

P. Liebig (Andrus Gerontology Center, University of Southern California, USA)

Housing options for the aged in India differ from those in more developed nations. Familial co-residence remains the primary living arrangement for elders, especially in rural areas. However, old-age homes have existed for more than 250 years, primarily for destitutes The number of homes are increasing, in part due to urbanization, to grants from the national and state governments to non-governmental organizations and to a growing demand from the middle-class for paid homes and assisted living. Still, less than 1% of India's 57 million elders live in old-age homes (OAHs), some of which house other groups. This paper reports on a 1997-98 study of 48 OAHs by comparing types of homes (for-pay, free). Topics addressed are geographic location, age- segregation, size, privacy features and common areas, health care and help with activities of daily living, expenditure patterns, reliance on inkind donations, staffing and administration, and philosophies of care (therapeutic environments, resident mutual care). The paper ends with a discussion of India's recent (1999) National Policy on Older Persons that concentrates on general housing issues of elders, rather than on age-specific housing, in keeping with eldercare traditions. These policy measures are contrasted with those of the United States and other Asian nations.

The Potential of Assisted Living Facilities as a Solution to Canada's Long-Term Care Crisis

S. M. Golant (University of Florida, Gainesville, Florida, USA)

Canada's steadily growing older population is becoming top heavy with persons in their late 70s and 80s who are at increased risk of chronic health problems and physical and cognitive impairments that threaten their ability to maintain independent households. All Provinces and Territories offer publicly-subsidized home-based services, but demand for this assistance now outstrips supply, especially by elders with chronic disabilities that require continuous personal care and nursing services. The backbone of Canada's organized response to elder frailty, its publicly-subsidized nursing homes, are also in short supply and a significant percentage of existing facilities are of poor quality. Provinces and Territories, worried about the increasing costs of nursing home care, are also beginning to restrict admittance to only the most frail elders. Yet government leaders have offered no new strategies for dealing with the care burden of frail seniors who will no longer be eligible for publicly-subsidized nursing homes. A relatively new shelter and care option in Canada, the assisted living facility, offers promise as one solution. Already widely available in the United States, it is primarily developed by for-profit developers and targeted to upper middle- and high-income seniors. Canada's for-profit sector is beginning to provide these newer shelter and care facilities, but various social, economic, and political barriers now impede their efforts. This paper examines the factors influencing the status and growth of for-profit assisted living facilities in Canada and the urgency for proactive initiatives by both the private and public sectors.

SESSION 75

The role of geriatrics and gerontological societies in the century of the elderly

Gerald Bennet (St. Bartholomew's and the Royal London School of Medicine and Dentistry, London, England) (Discussant) R Maia Guimarães (Hospital da Universidade de Brasília, Past President; Brazilian Geriatrics Society, Brasília, Brazil) (Ageing in Latin America: Getting Old Before Getting Rich) K Brummel-Smith (Providence Health System, President, American Geriatrics Society, Portland, OR, USA) (The Present and Future of Geriatrics in the United States) Young-Soo Lee (Asa Medical Center, President, Korean Geriatrics Society, Seoul, Korea) (New Role of Korean Geriatric Society in the 21st Century)

This symposium intends to discuss the role of the geriatrics and gerontological societies in the 21st century: "The Century of the Elderly". It will present the views from three different societies, namely USA, Korea and a Latin American overview. The focus of this session is on future trends of the scientific societies related to ageing. Apart from the cultural and economical differences it is predictable that a great demand for social and health assistance will face a scenario of shrinking financial support. The geriatrics and gerontological societies will be involved on the planning and discussion of innovative care delivery and also on technical and ethical issues involving the elderly, mainly the more vulnerable. It is expected that a minimum agenda of action could be achieved to provide IAG with a panorama for its future global planning.

Ageing in Latin America: Getting old before getting rich

R. Maia Guimarães (Hospital da Universidade de Brasília, Brasília. Brazil)

A fast demographic transition is on course in Latin America. The economical scenario in the region is far from ideal for attending the increasing social and health demands of an aged population. However Cuba and Costa Rica, notwithstanding opposite political regimens, are developing countries that achieved a good standard of care of the elderly despite limited financial resources. Brazil and Mexico, the largest countries and greatest economies in Latin America have not so far implemented an adequate policy for the elderly. In all countries, but mainly in those in where gerontology and geriatrics are less developed and human resources scarce, the role of the societies is essential. In some, advocacy for the elderly will be more relevant and in all the discussion of basic and conceptual aspects are mandatory. It seems opportune to support basic actions like primary care and the development of informal and family care. The Gerontological and Geriatrics Societies should be deeply involved in education of lay people and also on training family and community doctors. In the other side the societies will permanently discuss alternatives of care and support and also therapeutic and any other interventions in the ageing process. Despite the extraordinary progress science will achieve in coming years, the commitment of Gerontology and Geriatrics Societies should be to the more vulnerable and fragile elderly. Any intervention in the ageing process should be offered not only to those who can afford it but also to as many as possible who will benefit from it.

New Role of Korean Geriatric Society in the 21st century

Young-Soo Lee, (Asian Medical Center, Seoul, Korea; President, Korean Geriatrics Society)

Dramatic increase of the elderly population and change of the old culture and improvement of the medical technology, the government has difficulty to provide enough financial support to the elderly care not only outpatient care but also term care and developing new medical policy for the geriatric medicine to educate and train the geriatrician for the new century for the elderly. However, a national health delivery system has been established, and Korean Geriatric Society also has been established 33 years and its members have been very active to study and develop the geriatric medicine for the Korean elderly. In Korea, geriatric medicine is relatively new but the demand is increasing rapidly, so the governmental health department and geriatric society and it's members are under the tremendous pressure to renovate the health delivery system and educate the physician to care the increasing number and needs of the elderly in the 21 century in the Republic of Korea.

The Present and Future of Geriatrics in the United States

Kenneth Brummel-Smith, (Providence Health System, Portland, OR, USA; President, American Geriatrics Society)

Abstract: Purpose: To describe the current state of geriatric health care in the United States and to discuss the challenges and opportunities that are likely to be faced in the next 30 years Method: This presentation will review the literature regarding health care provider supply in the United States, innovative approaches to care used, and opportunities for new development in the field of health services for the elderly client. Results: Despite a rapidly growing need, the number of geriatric fellows, geriatric nurse practitioners, and other geriatric-trained health care providers has remained stagnant over the last 4 years. Many physicians in the community are finding it difficult to manage a practice that is focused on older patients. Medicare reimbursement has remained low creating additional disincentive to practice geriatrics. In addition, new drugs and technologies are rapidly driving up the cost of care. These new developments are often marketed directly to the older population, creating large demand for their use. However, a number of innovative care delivery systems have been developed to meet the need. The Program for All-inclusive care of the Elderly, the Social HMO, EverCare, new activities within the Veterans Affairs department, and model senior clinics are being developed. Conclusion: We can expect there to be competing demands for a rising population and a relative shrinking US dollar directed to health care. Support for increased geriatric training is needed. Consumer demands are likely to play a larger role in expanding geriatric health services in the future.

SESSION 76

Emerging Patterns of Community Care in Newly Industrialized Societies

A. Chong (Department of Applied Social Studies, City University of Hong Kong, Hong Kong) Community Care in Hong Kong. K. H. Phua (Department of Community, Occupational & Family Medicine, National University of Singapore) Emerging Patterns of Community Care Financing in Newly Industrializing Societies. X. Zhang (Department of Social Work and Social Administration, the University of Hong Kong) An Exploratory Study of Community-based Care for the Frail Elderly in Urban China. S. Yan (Department of Sociology, Peking University) The Influence of Urban Growth on Community Care in Newly Urbanized Areas in Mainland China. Y. Koh (Graduate School of Social Welfare, Kangnam University) Home Care Policy and Programs for the Aged in South Korea.

ISSUE: Most of the newly industrialized societies in Asia are experiencing rapidly aging of population and reducing family support functions in care for their senior citizens. In order to maintain the frail elders to continue staying in the community, most of these societies are developing community care programs for their senior citizens. Although the Western experiences are useful to the Asian countries in developing community care services, different background in history, political and economic development, and culture leads to very different concerns and patterns of community care derived from these societies. In particular, financing community care for the ageing population has surfaced as a critical issue in many newly industrializing societies. STRUCTURE: The symposium draws upon policy analyses in different newly industrialized societies to understand the emerging patterns of community care. CONTENT: Hong Kong has adopted community care policy since 1970s and this policy is still upheld by the Government. Chong reviews the experiences in implementing the community care policy in Hong Kong. China has seen a rapid urban growth since 1980s, especially in the periphery of the big cities. However, the urban expansion is achieved in different ways across big cities. How different ways of urban growth are associated with different potential community care patterns for the elders in China would have policy implications. Yan examines the differences, between before and after the local areas being transformed from rural into urban through different ways. Zhang examines the existing pattern of the community-based care for the frail elderly in urban China, and to explore the major features of China's practice compared with that in the West. Phua discusses the current trends of the changing age structure and its tremendous implications for the employment, financial security and care of the aged. As the ageing population is expected to intensify the demand and expenditure for health care, it is necessary to plan for appropriate and cost-effective services for the increasing number and proportion of elderly persons. Hence the urgency for bold and innovative approaches to the organization and financing of community care against the pressures of increasing health care costs. Koh will examine the rationale, objectives, activities, and outcomes of the volunteer-based home help service in Korea, which later had a positive influence on the home care policies and programs of the government and become a model program for the care of low income frail elders in South Korea. CONCLUSIONS: The symposium will provide a unique overview of the emerging patterns of community care in newly industrialized societies in Asia.

An Exploratory Study of Community-based Care for the Frail Elderly in Urban China

Xuetai Zhang (Department of Social Work and Social Administration, University of Hong Kong)

This research aims to examine the existing pattern of the community-based care for the frail elderly in urban China, and to explore the major features of China's practice compared with that in the West. It is a qualitative study, which adopted two main research methods: a document analysis and a case study, which has different levels of focus and serve as complementary evidence. The document analysis part focuses on the elderly care policies at central and city levels. The focus of the case study is on the four individual street offices with a quite high percentage of old people in Guangzhou and Shanghai. It is found in this study that except for the "Three Nos" elderly the community-based care for the frail elderly with family members is almost completely provided by their families because of the lack of formal care. It is also found that China's community-based elderly care has its own characteristics different from that in the West while they share the same. The findings imply that a more explicit family support policy should be taken into consideration on concerned departments' agenda while retaining as far as possible the traditional roles of the family and community in supporting their elderly.

Community Care in Hong Kong

Alice Ming-lin Chong (City University of Hong Kong, Hong Kong)

Hong Kong has become an ageing society since 1980's. In 1999, 10.7% of its total population or 734,100 aged 65 and above. The ageing population is expected to increase greatly, especially among the 80+, which was 12.6% in 1996, and which will increase to 16.8% in 2016. Community care has always be the cardinal principle in the provision of welfare services for older people in Hong Kong. But there has been a change in the rationale behind. Under the British rule (i.e. before 1997), community care has often been taken as an actualization of filial piety. In reality, it has been used as an excuse to shift the responsibility of taking care of the older generation upon the family, or literally upon the woman. With the great increase in the number of old-old and the recognition of the incapability of the family to take care of the increasingly frail or demented older people, the government is now more ready to face the ageing issue squarely. The Elderly Commission, which is a high-level advisory body, has been set up since 1997 to advice the government on policy formulation and programme monitoring. Several new initiatives are launched to facilitate ageing in place, e.g. services to carers, project for demented elderly. While this change of rationale is in the right direction, the planning effort is still rather piece-meal and reactive. Some initiatives are launched without careful consideration. Comprehensive and forward planning is, therefore, recommended if Hong Kong aims at effective community care.

Emerging Patterns of Community Care Financing in Newly Industrializing Societies

Kai Hong Phua (National University of Singapore, Singapore)

Financing community care for the ageing population has surfaced as a critical issue in many newly industrializing societies that have undergone rapid demographic and epidemiological transition. Current trends of the changing age structure will have tremendous implications for the employment, financial security and care of the aged. As the ageing population is expected to intensify the demand and expenditure for health care, it is necessary to plan for appropriate and cost-effective services for the increasing number and proportion of elderly persons. Hence the urgency for bold and innovative approaches to the organization and financing of community care against the pressures of increasing health care costs. Women generally outlive and therefore outnumber men in the older age structure of populations. The community care problems of the ageing population are consequently more reflected in the conditions and needs of a growing proportion of elderly women. As the common pattern in Asia continues for an older male to be cared by a younger spouse or female member of the family, this would not pose more problems for the care of the elderly male than for the elderly female person. Widowhood, one-parent (maternal) and one-person (female) households are usually associated with reduced income, increased poverty and enhanced risks of morbidity for the survivors. In addition, population shifts due to housing and employment patterns can exacerbate the situation when an increasing proportion of elderly women already require assistance for their well-being. Typically, women have much shorter periods of paid employment in the labour market and lower levels of earnings than men. Further development of social security and health care systems will need to take these factors into account. To avert both the gender and intergenerational problems posed by rapid population ageing, a mix of three pillars to support the basic functions of old age security redistribution, insurance and savings, have been proposed. As community care needs are projected to be greater in the rapidly ageing societies of newly industrializing Asia, a similar mix of financing methods are recommended to offer more protection while promoting economic growth. These considerations have formed the basis for the emerging systems of integrating old age security and health care financing in some newly industrializing societies of Asia, including recent plans for the financing of long term care in Japan and Singapore. Some elements of a diversified health care financing system based on a combination of savings, social insurance and taxation, will continue to be strengthened further to include greater integration with community care for the growing number and proportion of the elderly population in Asia.

Home Care Policy and Programs for the Aged in South Korea

Yang-Kon Koh (Graduate School of Social Welfare, Kangnam University, South Korea)

Korea is aging rapidly. Recent economic growth and improved living conditions have extended life expectancy and increased elderly population, while modernization process of industrialization, urbanization, and nuclearization of the family has weakened the care functions of the family. And yet, government programs are not fully developed to provide the needed care for the elderly who are suffering from poverty, poor health, role loss, and social-psychological isolation. Recognizing the serious problems of older Koreans, in 1987 HelpAge Korea has initiated a pilot program of "volunteer-based home help service", which later had a positive influence on the home care policies and programs of the government and become a model program for the care of low income frail elders in South Korea . This paper will examine the rationale, objectives, activities, and outcomes of the volunteer-based home help service in Korea. Impact of HelpAge Korea's model for other developing countries will be also discussed.

The Influence of Urban Growth on Community Care in Newly Urbanized Areas in Mainland China

Shengming Yan (Dept. of Sociology, Peking University, Beijing, & Dept. of Social Work and Social Administration, University of Hong Kong, Hong Kong, People's Republic of China)

China has seen a rapid urban growth since 1980s, especially in the periphery of the big cities. However, the urban expansion is achieved in different ways across big cities. How different ways of urban growth are associated with different potential community care patterns for the elders in China would have policy implications. Using survey data in the newly urbanized areas of four big cities in mainland China (Beijing, Shanghai, Suzhou, and Guangzhou), this paper examines the differences, between before and after the local areas being transformed from rural into urban through different ways, in the contact of the old persons (aged 60 or above) with their informal support networks (children and grandchildren, other relatives, friends or neighbours), the relationships between them, and when dependent on others in their daily activities the care for the elders from families, friends or neighbours, as well as community services. Results indicated that different patterns of urban expansion have significant impact on the changes in these aspects, even after the effects of the characteristics of the older respondents are controlled. Implications for the potential patterns of community care in these areas, which resulted from different ways of urban expansion, are discussed.

SESSION 78

Films and Videos on Alzheimer's Disease

James Vanden Bosch (Terra Nova Films, Inc, Chicago, Illinois USA)

A Thousand Tomorrow's: Intimacy, Sexuality and Alzheimer's (30 minutes, released in 1996) One of the major changes that Alzheimer's Disease brings to a spousal relationship is how it affects intimacy and sexuality. Through candid interviews with spouse caregivers, and where possible, the spouse who has Alzheimer's, this video explores this often unspoken issue, looking at: The blurring of roles between caregiver and intimate partner as the need for caregiving increases; Changes in behavior that affect intimacy between the partners; Mismatch of sexual desire and attraction. Accompanied by an extensive viewer's guide, A Thousand Tomorrow's helps remove some of the difficulty that many people have in comfortably discussing the effects of this disease on a couple's intimate life. // He's Doing This to Spite Me: Emotional Conflict in Dementia Care (22 minutes, released in 2000) Those who are close to someone who has dementia often find it hard to deal with the erratic and difficult behaviors that result from the disease. They may interpret these behaviors as intentional. This, combined with the stress of caregiving and a lack of understanding of the effects of the disease, may cause the caregiver to respond with frustration, impatience, even anger. Three caregivers openly share their experiences and frustrations as they interact with their loved one who has dementia. These scenes are integrated with comments and guidance from professionals in the field of dementia care. The result is a video that teaches caregivers how to reframe the caregiving dynamic into one that is more comfortable and productive for both the caregiver and care-receiver.

Films and Videos on Mental Health and Aging

James Vanden Bosch (Terra Nova Films, Inc, Chicago, Illinois USA)

Depression in Older Adults: The Right to Feel Better (30 minutes, released in 1998) This video confronts misunderstandings about depression, and gives a clear message that it can be accurately diagnosed and effectively treated, leading to an improvement in quality of life. The video explores case examples of three older adults who either have dealt with or are currently dealing with depression. These cases are augmented by comments from professionals in the field, such as Dr. Dan Blazer, author of Depression in Late Life. Covers several topics related to depression in older adults, including: Prevalence, Causes, Treatments, Suicide Risk, Issues for Nursing Homes, Public Policy. // Choice and

Challenge: Caring for Aggressive Older Adults Across Levels of Care (22 minutes, released in 1998) Staff working in long-term care facilities must often deal with aggressive behaviors from residents who are suffering with cognitive disorders. Aggressive behavior is perhaps the most troublingand often, least understoodof all behavioral problems. Developed during a year-long project sponsored by the American Psychiatric Nurses Association, this training package consists of a 22-minute video and reproducible print materials and handouts. Taped in three actual long-term care settings, the video shows real life episodes of aggression, and discusses strategies for preventing or defusing such episodes. The video focuses on the importance of empathic understanding, therapeutic communication, and assessment in the personalization of care. A workbook accompanies the video.

SESSION 79

Assessment and Intervention for High-Risk Seniors in the Emergency Department: Cross-National Perspectives

J.McCusker(St.Mary's Hospital Center,Montreal, Canada)ISAR: A Short Self-Report Emergency Department Screening Tool to identify Seniors at Increased Risk of Adverse Outcomes. J.Verdon (Cité de la Santé de Laval,Montreal,Canada) ISAR II: Development of a Brief Standardized Nursing Intervention for High-Risk Seniors in the Emergency Department. P.Jacobs ISAR II: Cost-Effectiveness of a 2-Stage Intervention for High-Risk Seniors in the Emergency Department. G.A.Caplan(Prince of Wales Hospital, Sydney, Australia) Risk of Admission within Four Weeks of Discharge of Elderly from teh Emergency Department-The DEED Study. G.A.Caplan (Prince of Wales Hospital,Sydney,Australia)Discharge of Elderly From the Emergency Department-The DEED II Study. S.W.Meldon (Department of Emergency Medicine, MetroHealth Medical Center, Cleveland, Ohio) Case Finding of At-Risk Elders in the Emergency Department

ISSUE:An emergency department(ED)visit appears to be a sentinel health event for seniors, associated with high rates of functional decline and other adverse outcomes following the visit. However, high risk patients are rarely identified in the ED, and many do not receive appropriate care or follow-up in the community after the visit.STRUCTURE:This symposium will present work conducted by 3 groups, in Canada, Australia, and the U.S. aimed at improving the care of older patients, during and after an ED visit. CONTENT: The Canadian group has developed and evaluated a 2-stage intervention: screening and assesement. The screening tool, ISAR, was first developed and validated as a brief-self report questionnaire that can be administered during the ED visit and identifies patients at increased risk of functional decline, repeated ED visits, and high rates of hospital utilization. A brief, nursing assessment and referral tool for high-risk patients was then developed and has been evaluated in a randomized trial (ISAR II). The Australian group has also identified risk factors for admission among older patients 4 weeks after discharge from the ED (DEED). The DEED II study was a randomised trial of a comprehensive geriatric assessment intervention delivered at home with 24 hours of discharge from the ED. Finally,the SIGNET project from the U.S. is a 2-stage (screening and assessment) intervention that has undergone substantial feasibility testing in a large multi-site study. CONCLUSION/ANTICIPATED OUTCOMES: The symposium will highlight similiarities and differences in the approaches taken, and make recommendations for implementing similar programs in other settings.

Case Finding of At-Risk Elders in the Emergency Department

S.W. Meldon (MetroHealth Medical Center, Cleveland, U.S.A), L.Mion,(Cleveland Clinic Foundation,Cleveland,U.S.A) R.PalmerCleveland Clinic Foundation,Cleveland,U.S.A), C. Emerman(MetroHealth Medical Center, Cleveland, U.S.A), D.Bass (Benjamin Rose Institute, Cleveland,U.S.A

OBJECTIVE: Study of community-dwelling elderly ED patients to examine feasibility of 1) RN case finding for common risk factors for unplanned ED visits, hospitalizations or nursing home placement; 2) subsequent referral to community agencies. METHODS: Prospective cross-sectional design. Setting:4 EDs: tertiary referral center; public hospital; community hospital; HMO setting. Subjects: All elderly ED patients over 18 month period. Variables: Demographics, presence of 6 risk factors (yes/no) assessed by RN screen: confusion, no caregiver, recent ED use/hospitalization, polypharmacy, falls/difficulty walking, RN concern. Patients with positive screen (confusion or >1 risk factor) were assessed by geriatric nurse specialists (GNS). Identified health or social needs were referred to appropriate health service. Prevalence of variables, positive screens, and referrals (analyzed by Chi square) are reported. RESULTS: 28,437 (72%) patients screened; average age 77 yrs (range 61-102); 67% women; 69% white. Prevalence of individual risk factors: 370olypharmacy, 34 0ifficulty walking, 27% RN concern, 26% recent ED/hospitalization, 21o caregiver, 12CONCLUSION: The ED is a feasible site for geriatric case finding. One-half of at-risk elders, detected by simple RN screen, were felt to need referral after GNS assessment. ED case-finding resulted in significant increases in community services referrals.

Discharge of Elderly From the Emergency Department -The DEED II Study

G.A.Caplan, P.Timmiss, K.Abrahams, A. Brown (Post Acute Care Services, Prince of Wales Hospital Sydney,Australia)

PURPOSE: To describe DEED II trial results. METHODS: We conducted a randomised controlled trial of a comprehensive geriatric assessment (CGA) and multidisciplinary intervention within 24 hours of discharge from the ED for patients aged 75 years and over. Patients randomised to the intervention group were seen at home within 24 hours and assessed by a nurse. The patients were discussed at a multidisciplinary case conference and referrals were made as appropriate for medical, nursing and allied health interventions. RESULTS: 739 patients were enrolled over a 17 month period from a single ED. There were no differences in baseline characteristics between the two groups. There was no difference to mortality. On average 1.65 new problems were found and addressed in each patient. Patients randomised to the intervention group maintained a greater degree of physical and mental function (Barthel Index [/20] change from baseline at 6 months: -0.25 v. -0.75; p<0.001; Mental Status Questionnaire [/10] change from baseline at 12 months: -0.21 v. –0.64; p<0.001) and had a longer time to first emergency admission (382 v. 348 days; p=0.01). There was also a lower rate of total admissions to hospital during the first month (16.5 versus 22.2%; p=0.048). For the intervention group, compared to the controls, there was a non-significant tendency for patients to remain living alone at home. CONCLUSIONS: CGA and multidisciplinary intervention can improve health outcomes of older people at risk of deteriorating health and admission to hospital. Patients over 75 discharged from the ED should be referred for CGA.

ISAR: A Short Self-Report Emergency Department Screening Tool to Identify Seniors at Increased Risk of Adverse Outcomes

J. McCusker (St. Mary's Hospital and McGill University, Montreal, QC, Canada), F. Bellavance(École des Hautes Etudes Commerciales,Montreal, Canada), S. Cardin (Centre de Recherche du CHUM,Montreal,Canada)J. Verdon (Cité de la Santé de Laval, Montreal, Canada)

PURPOSE: This presentation will review the development and validation of a 6-item self-report screening tool, ISAR, that predicts functional decline and other adverse outcomes during the 6 months after an emergency department (ED) visit in patients aged 65+. METHODS: In phase 1 of the project, 27 potential screening questions were developed based on a literature review of risk factors for mortality, institutionalization, increased functional dependence, and high rates of use of hospital and ED services. In phase 2, the screening tool itself was tested in the ED in a multi-site cohort with 6-month follow-up after the index ED visit. Outcomes were collected by interview and from administrative databases. Scale development and selection methods included logistic regression, receiver operating characteristic curves, and expert judgment. RESULTS: Among 1673 patients who completed the follow-up measures, 488 (29.2%) had an adverse health outcome (mortality, institutionalization, or increased functional dependence). The proposed screening tool (ISAR) comprises six self-report questions on functional dependence (premorbid status and acute change), recent hospitalization, impaired memory and vision, and polymedication. The tool performed well in the total cohort aged 65 and over, and in sub-groups defined by disposition (admitted or released from ED), language of questionnaire administration (French or English), information source (patient or other), and other characteristics. ISAR also predicts repeat ED visits, and high inpatient hospital utilization. CONCLUSIONS: The ISAR is a short self-report questionnaire that can quickly identify elders in the ED at increased risk of several adverse health outcomes and detect those with current disability.

ISAR II: Cost-Effectiveness of a 2-Stage Intervention for High-Risk Seniors in the Emergency Department

J.McCusker (St.Mary's Hospital Center and McGill University, Montreal, Canada), P.Jacobs (University of Alberta, Edmonton) N.Dendukuri (St.Mary's Hospital Center, Montreal, Canada)P.Tousignant(Régie Régionale de la Santé et des Services Sociaux de Montreal-Centre), E. Latimer (Douglas Hospital, Montreal,Canada)

PURPOSE: To evaluate the cost-effectiveness of a 2-stage (screening and assessment) intervention for seniors in the emergency department (ED) METHOD: Community-dwelling patients aged 65+, at risk of functional decline, and ready to be released from the EDs of 4 Montreal hospitals, were randomized to the intervention (n=178) or usual care (n=210). Data collected during the 4-month follow-up period included: health outcomes for patients and caregivers (physical and mental health measures), and use and cost of health services (based primarily on administrative databases). The perspective of the cost-effectiveness analysis is societal, including patients, caregivers as well as the formal health care (government)funded system. Costs include post emergency room care, including hospitalization, physician services, community care, outpatient drugs, as well as patient and caregiver costs. Cost items were measured with a self-reported questionnaire. Unit costs for these items were either province-wide rates or else were estimated direct using provider data. Cost effectiveness is assessed in qualitative terms, such that outcomes and costs are separately compared. RESULTS: The intervention reduced the risk of patient functional decline at 4 months (adjusted odds ratio 0.53,95% CI 0.31, 0.91), but did not affect the other health outcomes. Based on chart review, a larger proportion of intervention than control group patients were referred to local community health centres (13.0% vs 5.3%, p<.01)or their family physician (24.9% vs 14.4%, p<.01). Based on administrative data, intervention group patients were more likely to receive home care services after their visit, controlling for previous use (OR 1.65, 95% CI 0.89, 3.08). More intervention than control patients (26.8% vs 17.7%, p=.05) reported that they contacted their family physician as a result of their ED visit. CONCLUSIONS: The beneficial effect of the intervention appears to be explained by a modest increase in referral to and contact with primary and home care services. The cost-effectiveness of the intervention will be discussed

ISAR II: Development of A Brief Standardized Nursing Intervention for High-Risk Seniors in the Emergency Department

J.Verdon (Cité de la Santé de Laval, Montreal,Canada) J. McCusker (St.Mary's Hospital and McGill University,Montreal, Canada), L Poulin de Courval,(CLSC Côte-des-Neiges, Montreal,Canada) P Tousignant (Régie Régionale de la Santé et des Services Sociaux de Montréal-Centre, Montreal,Canada)

Objective : To describe the standardised nursing assessment tool used in the ISAR-II trial, the geriatric problems identified, and the interventions that were implemented. Methods: A standardised nursing assessment tool was developed for use with patients aged 65+, with an ISAR score of 2+, who are ready to be released from the emergency department (ED). The assessment checklist focuses on new problems and on uncompensated old problems and handicaps, requiring either a medical intervention, a new or increased level of home care or other service, or comprehensive geriatric assessment. After completing the assessment, the intervention nurses consulted with hospital ED and geriatric staff and made referrals, as needed, to the primary physician, the local community health center, the geriatric outpatient clinic, or other community services. Results: Among the 147 intervention group patients, the average duration of the assessment was 28.0 (SD 12.57) minutes. Overall, 61.2% had one or more new or uncompensated problems. The problem categories most frequently checked were: physical (37.4%), ADL (22.5%), medical (22.5%), behavioral or affective (20.4%), and social (16.3%). This assessment resulted in a consultation or medical intervention in the ED among 46.50f cases, 2 admissions to hospital, referral to the primary physician for specific follow-up (28.6%), and to the community health center for services (31.3%). Conclusion: Brief standardised nursing assessment in the ED allowed identification and intervention on new or uncompensated problems in 61.20f seniors identified at risk by the ISAR tool.

Risk of Admission within Four Weeks of Discharge of Elderly from the Emergency Department -The DEED Study

G.A.Caplan, A.Brown, W.D.Croker, J.Doolan (Prince of Wales Hospital, Sydney Australia)

PURPOSE: To identify risk factors for admission for patients aged 75 years and older after discharge from the Emergency Department (ED). METHODS: Prospective evaluation of Discharged Elderly from the ED (DEED) who were followed up after four weeks. Setting: ED of a teaching hospital for one year. Subjects: Patients aged 75 and over discharged from the ED to their home or hostel. Main outcome measures: Demographic data, indices of function and cognitive status and admission to hospital within four weeks. RESULTS: 468 patients aged 75 and over (mean age 81.7 years; range 75-98) who were sent home from the ED were enrolled; 80 patients (17.1%) were admitted to hospital during the subsequent four weeks. Risk factors for admission included dependence in the following activities of daily living (relative risk). CONCLUSION: Older patients are at increased risk of readmission within four weeks of being sent home from the Emergency Department. It is possible to identify high risk patients by a questionnaire. This allows targeting of these patients for more intensive follow-up in an attempt to ameliorate further deteriorations in their health.

SESSION 80

Developing and Implementing Community-Based Fall Risk Reduction Programs: Sharing the Hurdles and Highlights.

Courtney Hall (Center for Successful Aging, California State University, Fullerton, CA. USA) The ABCs of Developing and Implementing a Community-Based Fall Risk Reduction Program. N. Lemon (Center for Successful Aging, California State University, Fullerton. CA. USA) Fallproof: A Community-Based Fall Risk Reduction Program. Debra J. Rose (Center for Successful Aging, California State University, Fullerton, California, USA) Analyzing the Effectiveness of Fallproof: A Community-Based Fall Risk Reduction Program. C. Jessie Jones (Center for Successful Aging, California State University, Fullerton, CA. USA) Community-Based Applied Research: Lessons Learned.

This symposium will address the hurdles and highlights associated with the development and implementation of a model fall risk reduction program in multiple community-based facilities throughout Southern

California. The externally funded research project to be described was implemented in 18 community-based facilities over a three-year period. Older adults at moderate to high risk for falls were first identified and then entered into the eight-week training program that operated two days per week (one hour per session). Each group-based program was taught by one trained instructor with the assistance of 3-5 peer mentors (i.e, healthy older adults) recruited from the community and then trained with and by the instructor. In the first presentation, Hall will outline the multiple steps and hurdles associated with initiating and implementing an applied research project of this magnitude. Some of the important steps to be described will include such things as surveying the needs of the community, establishing community partnerships, selecting appropriate community sites, establishing procedures, responsibilities, and timelines with facility directors, developing program content, training instructors and peer mentors, and scheduling regular assessments designed to evaluate the overall effectiveness of the program. The second presentation by Lemon will describe each of the core components of the implemented program and the accompanying theoretical rationale. The four core components of the program will be described. They include center of gravity control training, postural strategy training, multisensory training, and gait pattern enhancement and variation training. The third presentation in this symposium will be devoted to a discussion of the short- and long-term outcomes of the three-year research project. Rose will discuss the program s overall effectiveness as it relates to observed changes in the underlying impairments of balance and mobility, functional performance, level of disability, balance-related self-confidence, and actual fall risk reduction. The major variables that best predict successful program outcomes in this community-based older adult sample will also be identified. In the final presentation in this session, Jones will share the lessons learned from this ambitious project. What to do, what not to do, and, what to do when the unexpected happens will be the focus of this presentation. The highlights associated with implementing community-based fall risk reduction programs will also be shared with the audience, in addition to a number of important recommendations intended to better prepare individuals interested in developing and implementing fall risk reduction programs within the community in the future. Finally, Rose will describe additional resources currently being developed to provide potential instructors and peer mentors with the specialized knowledge needed to successfully implement fall risk reduction programs of this type within their immediate community. These include a comprehensive instructor-training manual, accompanying instructional software, and an instructor and peer mentor certification-training program scheduled to begin operating in September, 2001.

Analyzing the Effectiveness of Fallproof: A Model Community-Based Fall Risk Reduction Program

Debra J. Rose, (Center for Successful Aging, California State University, Fullerton. CA. USA)

The purpose of this presentation will be to discuss the preliminary program outcomes associated with Fallproof, a community-based fall risk reduction program that has been implemented at multiple sites over a three-year period. The effectiveness of the program was determined using multiple tests designed to measure changes at multiple levels of physical function (i.e, impairment, functional performance, disability). In addition, multiple psychological measures were also used to determine whether positive short- and long-term changes in balance-related self-confidence, depression, and perceived quality of life occurred as a function of program participation. The degree to which program compliance influenced fall risk and actual fall incidence rates was also determined. Repeated measures multivariate analyses of variance conducted revealed significant differences between groups (i.e, control, experimental) in multiple measures of impairment (i.e, maximum excursion, maximum velocity, sensory organization), functional performance (i.e, Berg balance scale score, Up and Go time, gait speed, 30 second chair stand), and disability (i.e, composite physical function score). Significant improvements in balance-related self-confidence, perceived quality of life, and level of depression were also demonstrated for the intervention group only. Moreover, participants in the high compliance group demonstrated a significantly higher reduction in fall risk when compared to a low compliance group, and the control group. Fall risk was reduced by approximately 35-40% in the high compliance group. Preliminary analysis of fall incidence rates in a sub sample of participants six and twelve months post-program also yielded a decline in the number of injurious falls sustained.

Community- Based Applied Research: Lessons Learned

C. Jessie Jones, (Center for Successful Aging, California State University, Fullerton. CA. USA)

Identifying ways to promote active life expectancy and reduce the onset of physical frailty has become a major goal for gerontology researchers and health fitness practitioners throughout the world. The rapid growth in the aging population, and the rising cost of medical care, makes it necessary to provide more cost-effective community-based exercise programs, especially programs that specifically address the increasing risk for falls among older adults. However, conducting applied research in a community setting, especially with the more frail older adult can be quite challenging. The purpose of this presentation is to share the "lessons learned" from the development and implementation of multi site community-based fall risk reduction programs. Although the programs have resulted in significant improvements in multiple dimensions of balance and mobility and an overall reduction in fall risk, many lessons have been learned and will be shared during this presentation. "What to do", "what not to do", and "what to do when the unexpected happens" will be discussed. Additional topics to be addressed include applied research design and analysis issues, fundraising, public relations, community partnerships, instructor and peer mentor recruitment and training, and program implementation and expansion. Future recommendations and directions in program and resource development will also be presented.

Fallproof: A Model Community- Based Fall Risk Reduction Program

N. Lemon, (Center for Successful Aging, California State University, Fullerton. CA. USA)

The purpose of this presentation will be to describe the core components of Fallproof, a model fall risk reduction program currently operating in 18 community-based centers in Southern California. This innovative program specifically targets impairments within the postural control system identified through a comprehensive balance and mobility assessment conducted prior to entry into the program. The program is theory driven and focuses on the systematic manipulation of the individual s intrinsic capabilities, the goals of the task being performed, and the constraints of the practice environment. Each of the screening tests administered will be described and the dimension of balance and mobility addressed discussed. The four core components of the program will then be described and the theoretical rationale for their inclusion provided. The core components to be discussed include center of gravity control training, postural strategy training, multisensory training, and gait pattern variation and enhancement training. Video footage of specific exercises associated with each program component will also be presented during this presentation. How the various exercise progressions and/or the practice environment is structured to address the individual capabilities of each participant within a group setting will also be discussed.

The ABCs of a Community-Based Fall Risk Reduction Program

Courtney Hall, PT (Center for Successful Aging, California State University, Fullerton. CA. USA)

Due to the realities and limitations of the current medical system in the United States, and the difficulties associated with diagnosing balance disorders, older adults who are repeatedly falling often experience difficulty accessing appropriate medical treatment for their condition. Moreover, capitation currently limits the length of time an older adult, even with a diagnosis and medical insurance, can receive treatment for a diagnosed balance disorder. Community-based fall-risk reduction programs could provide two important ancillary services: (a) extended treatment time for patients who have been discharged, but still require additional balance and mobility training, and (b) early identification of individuals at risk for falls and targeted programming designed to prevent injurious falls. In an effort to address this need, researchers at the Center for Successful Aging at California State University, Fullerton developed and implemented a model fall-risk reduction program in 18 community-based centers. The purpose of this presentation is to identify and describe 12 basic steps involved in developing a successful program. The basic steps to be discussed include 1) surveying community needs, 2) raising external funds, 3) establishing community partnerships, 4) selecting appropriate community sites, 5) establishing procedures, responsibilities, and timelines with facility directors, 6) developing program materials, 7) training and supervising instructors and peer-mentors, 8) ordering and providing equipment, 9) developing and scheduling regular balance and mobility assessments, 10) providing individual and group feedback, 11) conducting an external evaluation of the program, and 12) marketing and disseminating program outcomes.

SESSION 81

Advancing Gerontological Education in Nursing (AGEIN): The Challenge for the Future

M. Nolan (University of Sheffield, Sheffield, UK) An Introduction to the AGEIN Project. J. Brown (University of Sheffield, Sheffield, UK) Creating a Conducive Clinical Learning Environment for Nursing Students. S. Davies (University of Sheffield, Sheffield, UK) Qualified Nurses' Experiences of their Educational Preparation to Work with Older People. J. Keady (University of Wales, Bangor, Wales) Mental Health and Older People: Values, Beliefs and Future Opportunities. J. Nolan (University of Sheffield, Sheffield, UK) Students' and Qualified Nurses' Views of Older People

Issue Nurses provide significant amounts of care for older people yet studies from several countries suggest that such work is often the least preferred career option. With prevailing demographic trends, and the increasing complexity of health care, the education of nurses at all levels must equip practitioners with the knowledge, skills and attitudes necessary to provide high quality care to older people. Crucially work with older people must be accorded value and status so that nurses are attracted to, and remain in, the specialty. Structure The AGEIN Project is a 3 year multi-method longitudinal study of nurse education relating to older people and is the largest ever undertaken in the UK. This symposium comprises 5 papers which highlight key issues arising from the study and consider their implications for the education of nurses within the UK and beyond. An international perspective is provided by discussants from Australia (Professor Rhonda Nay), the US (Professor Barbara Bowers) and Sweden (Dr Ulla Lundh). Content The first paper provides an overview of the project, its methodology and phases. Particular attention is given to a conceptual synthesis of over 3000 references addressing the practice of nursing with older people in 6 areas: acute and rehabilitative care; community care; continuing care; learning disability; mental health and palliative care. Paper two focuses on the characteristics of a positive learning and clinical environment as identified by pre-qualifying student nurses. Data were gathered using longitudinal focus groups and individual interviews with cohorts of students at 4 sites. Students were tracked through their nurse training, and the influence of the clinical environment on their attitudes and feelings towards work with older people explored in-depth. Paper three provides a complementary perspective considering the educational experiences and preparation of qualified practitioners. Using the same 4 sites as in paper 2 data were gathered from practitioners completing programmes relating to work with older people and those undertaking training for community nursing. Paper four turns attention to mental health in older age and describes the results of both a literature synthesis and an empirical case study of the ways in which qualified practitioners develop the skills required to work with older people with mental health problems. The final paper focuses on the perceptions pre-qualifying and qualified nurses hold of older people. Data were gathered from large samples of both groups (n = 1000+) using a knowledge-based quiz and an attitude towards work with older people questionnaire. This paper highlights important similarities and differences between the samples and considers the implications of the results for the education of practitioners. Anticipated Outcomes The symposium considers a disparate number of conceptual, methodological and practical issues relating to the education of nurses for work with older people. Although data emanated from the UK the results have far wider relevance, with the implications being considered by the international discussants. The symposium provides a conspectus on key issues and the basis for a consensus on the way forward for nurse education in the New Millennium.

Advancing Gerontological Education in Nursing (AGEIN): An Overview

N. Nolan (University of Sheffield, Sheffield, UK)

Purpose This is the first paper in a symposium considering a 3 year multi-method longitudinal study of the perceptions of nurses towards work with older people in the UK. The ultimate aim is to develop an epistemology of practice and education for such work in a range of health care settings. Method A multi-method triangulated design was adopted including literature and empirical components and comprising intensive (in-depth case studies) and extensive (national postal surveys) elements. Results This paper provides an overview of the AGEIN Project describing the theoretical and methodological rationale. The main emphasis, however, is given to the literature synthesis which involved the analysis of over 3000 references in order to identify key elements of nursing care with older people. This paper focuses on a framework for considering person-centred care which has been termed the 'senses framework'. This is used to highlight and distil the essential components of person-centred care as described in the literature, these include creating a sense of: security; belonging; continuity; purpose; achievement and significance. Conclusion Based on an extensive review of the relevant nursing and gerontological literature this paper proposes a new framework within which to conceptualise and begin to isolate the essences of person-centred care. The framework has a number of far reaching implications for work with older people and for nurse education and practice.

Creating a Conducive Clinical Learning Environment for Nursing Students

J. Brown (University of Sheffield, Sheffield, UK)

Purpose To explore how clinical learning environments influence student nurses' attitudes towards, and predisposition to work with, older people and to identify the characteristics of environments which stimulate positive perceptions of older people. Method Cohorts of students (130 informants) were followed longitudinally throughout their 3 year training in 4 case study sites. Data were collected using focus group interviews every 6 months and students were also asked to identify those clinical placements in which they had a positive experience. Such placements were visited and data gathered from in-depth interviews with key staff members, usually the ward leader. Data were subject to content analysis in order to identify key themes. Results The results indicate that positive clinical learning environments are the product of a complex set of factors which influence the degree to which students feel: safe to explore practice; they belong to the ward; there is continuity between theory and practice; they are able to have a sense of purpose and achievement; they can make a meaningful contribution to patient care. These factors are examined and discussed. Conclusion This component of the AGEIN Project provides important new insights suggesting the type of relevant experiences to which the students should be exposed if they are to develop positive attitudes towards work with older people.

Mental Health Nursing and Older People: Values, Beliefs and Future Opportunities

J. Keady (University of Wales, Bangor, Bangor, UK)

Purpose The mental health needs of older people are poorly addressed by service providers and policy makers in the UK with a recent national report drawing attention to inconsistencies and the lack of integrated care pathways. Within nursing education the absence of a suitable epistemology of practice is mirrored in the devalued status of older people within pre-qualification education and the limited opportunities available for post-qualification training. Method A comprehensive review of the literature in the area was conducted, resulting in the identification of over 900 separate items addressing important aspects of mental health nursing with older people. Complementing this empirical work involved a series of telephone interviews with qualified mental health nurses completing programmes of education for work with older people over a period of one year, together with visits to their areas of practice. Results >From the literature review three themes emerged: 1. Developing an integrated policy and service framework 2. Creating a new vision for professional assessment and intervention 3. Reconfiguring professional training and role identity These will be discussed and illustrated by relevant examples from both the literature and the empirical data. Conclusion This component of the AGEIN Project takes an important first step in articulating an epistemology of practice for mental health nursing and older people. The presentation will be grounded in policy and educational contexts for nursing which, while emanating from the UK, are of far wider relevance.

Qualified Nurses' Experiences of their Educational Preparation to Work with Older People

S. Davies (University of Sheffield, Sheffield, UK)

Purpose Older people are the major users of health care in the UK and a plethora of standards for such care is now appearing. These initiatives, together with a policy of community care, are having a major impact on the educational needs of practitioners. Student nurses are also undertaking placements in new areas including nursing and residential homes and require support and mentorship, placing further demands on qualified practitioners in these settings. Method This phase of the AGEIN Project explored the perceptions and experiences of nurses enrolled on specialist post-qualifying programmes designed to prepare practitioners to meet the needs of older people. Four educational sites were selected for intensive case study, providing access to students commencing programmes in the care of older people and community programmes. Semi-structured telephone interviews were undertaken with students at intervals during and following completion of such programmes, complemented by a small number of focus group interviews and the observation of selected teaching sessions at each site. Results/ Conclusion The data provide telling insights into the challenges of nursing older people within a changing health service. The difficulties of combining study with full-time employment and family commitments were also vividly described. However, there are indications that the recent restructuring of post-registration nursing education within the UK is beginning to bear fruit in terms of enabling practitioners to develop the specialist knowledge and expertise they need in order to provide high quality care for older people. Key themes are identified and their implications for nurse education considered.

Students' and Qualified Nurses' Views of Older People

J. Nolan (University of Sheffield, Sheffield, UK)

Purpose Although there have been several surveys of nurses knowledge of or attitudes to older people these have usually been small scale, non-random, or both. Moreover, the instruments used have either been generic or of questionable relevance. This paper describes the results of surveys of student and qualified nurses in the UK using specially designed instruments. Method New instruments were designed assessing nurses' knowledge of older people and their attitudes towards working with older people. These were administered to samples of students and qualified nurses (n = 1000+ in both samples). Extensive volumes of qualitative data were also collected. Analysis was undertaken using SPSS and content analysis. Results Currently data are being loaded for statistical analysis and content analysis has started. Preliminary content analysis suggests that nurses are generally favourably predisposed to work with older people but that enthusiasm wanes following early negative experiences of such work. This hypothesis is examined further in the statistical analysis which also provides insights into the levels of awareness that practitioners have of the situation of older people in the UK, indicating whether they can accurately gauge their likely future care needs. Conclusions The surveys represent the largest body of data ever collected in the UK and provide a comprehensive view of the current situation. Although the quiz is based on the UK its format is easily adapted for use elsewhere and the attitudes instrument has potentially widespread applications which will be addressed in this paper.

SESSION 82

[1] Nurses understanding of the assessment process with older people

Pauline Ford, (Royal College of Nursing, London, England.)

This paper will present emerging findings from an ongoing study that aims to explore through interpretation how nurses understand the process of assessment and how this is influenced by use of the 'RCN Nursing Older People Assessment Tool'. Within an overarching philosophy of multiagency working, there is an ongoing need for nurses to demonstrate their contribution to the continuing health care of older people (Ford, 1995, 1997; UKCC, 1997). Furthermore, with the emphasis on assessment on current national policy work, studies exploring the contribution of particular professional groups to a person centred assessment are needed. Working within a framework of person centred practice, the emerging issues that reflect the challenges of achieving a person centred approach to assessment will be addressed. Issues relating to nurses' understanding of assessment, the context of practice and societal influences will all be considered.

[2] Adherence to Recommendations of Community-Based Comprehensive Geriatric Assessment Programs: A Comprehensive Review of Literature

F. Aminzadeh, (Regional Geriatric Assessment Program of Ottawa Carleton, Canada)

PURPOSE: Non-adherence with the recommendations of short-term community-based consultative comprehensive geriatric assessment (CGA) programs is a significant threat to the effectiveness of these programs. This paper synthesizes the literature on patient and physician adherence to recommendations of community-based CGA programs. METHOD: Papers cited were identified by an English language literature search of MEDLINE, Health Star and CINAHL databases from January 1980 to November 1999. This search was supplemented with literature identified from the reference sections of relevant publications. RESULTS: Patient adherence rates in these settings ranged from 46% to 76% which approximates the rates for the consulting physician adherence (49%-79%). Many characteristics of patient, treatment, care provider and clinical setting were identified to influence adherence. The beginning understanding of these factors has led to the development of some adherence enhancing strategies (i.e, developing treatment plans based on an understanding of patient beliefs and resources, using a combination of methods to communicate the plan, simplifying the plan, and creating a continuum of formal and informal support to carry out the plan). However, without systematic evaluations it is difficult to evaluate the relative effectiveness of these interventions. CONCLUSION: Further research targeting more representative samples, using validated assessment tools and multiple data collection methods are needed to expand our knowledge of patterns and predictors of adherence and to evaluate the relative effectiveness of adherence enhancing intervention strategies.

[3] Content Validation of a Frailty Checklist Derived From Comprehensive Geriatric Assessment

Rolfson D (University of Alberta, Edmonton, Canada) Majumdar S (University of Alberta, Edmonton, Canada) Tahir A (University of Alberta, Edmonton, Canada) Tsuyuki R (University of Alberta, Edmonton, Canada)

PURPOSE: Comprehensive geriatric assessment (CGA) is well suited to identify markers of frailty in seniors and thus anticipate further decline. We were interested in the development and content validation of a checklist to determine frailty after CGA. METHOD: Established concepts of frailty were summarized based on a structured search of existing literature. A checklist, which allows the identification of geriatric syndromes, and the rating of each concept of frailty was constructed. An expert panel comprised of geriatric medicine specialists determined the degree to which the checklist and its items encompass each concept of frailty. Redundancy and acceptability of the checklist were also evaluated. Finally, the items were ranked according to their relative importance in the overall concept of frailty. RESULTS: Four key concepts of frailty emerged from the literature: sarcopenia, homeostenosis, functional frailty, and dynamic frailty. Nine chronic and five acute geriatric syndromes were included in the checklist. The expert panel found that the checklist and its items adequately encompassed each concept of frailty. The checklist was only slightly redundant and was easy to understand. Problems with cognition, burden of illness, balance and mobility, continence and social support were deemed to be more important chronic syndromes than problems with mood, nutrition and medication issues. Delirium, falls and immobility, and functional decline were valued over weight loss and urinary incontinence as acute markers of frailty. CONCLUSION: The frailty checklist appears to have excellent content validity in translating the results of CGA to an estimation of frailty by specialists in geriatric medicine.

[4] Depressive symptoms in patients of a geriatric medicine outpatients clinic and the Geriatric Depression Scale

R. Rigo, E. Ferriolli, J. C. Moriguti, C. E. Paiva, J. S. Marchini (Division of General Internal and Geriatric Medicine, School of Medicine of Ribeirao Preto, University of Sao Paulo, Ribeirao Preto, SP, Brazil), A. Dalacorte (Neurosciences Department, Pontificial Catholic University of Rio Grande do Sul, Porto Alegre, RS, Brazil)

This study was intended to determine the prevalence of depressive symptoms in patients aged 60 years or over of a university geriatric medicine tertiary care outpatients clinic and to correlate this finding with the score of a worldwide employed scale for the detection of depression, the Geriatric Depression Scale (GDS - Yesavage). The structured clinical observation records of 45 consecutive patients (30 female and 45 male, mean age 74.3 years and 73.2 years, respectively) admitted to a tertiary care university geriatric medicine outpatients clinic were reviewed. Twenty (44.4%) of the patients had depressive symptoms, with no significant difference between genders. The mean GDS score of patients with and without depressive symptoms were 13.4 and 7.6, respectively ($p = 0.001$). Agreement between the presence or absence of depressive symptoms and the GDS score (cut-off score = 11) was 72.2%. There was no correlation between the educational level and the presence of depressive symptoms. Sleep complaints, but not memory complaints, were more frequent among patients with depressive symptoms. Cigarette smoking and alcohol intake were not significantly associated with the presence of depressive symptoms. Depressive symptoms were highly prevalent in this sample of clinical patients and the Geriatric Depression Scale showed good sensibility for their detection.

[5] Inter-Rater Reliability of the Assessment of Living Skills and Resources (ALSAR) in Community-Dwelling Seniors.

Suzette Wilson (Mount Saint Joseph Hospital, Vancouver, Canada) Suniti Seth (Mount Saint Joseph Hospital, Vancouver, Canada) Edith Yu (Mount Saint Joseph Hospital, Vancouver, Canada) Christine Schiller (Saint Vincent Hospital, Vancouver, Canada) Debra Morgan (Mount Saint JOseph Hospital, Vancouver, Canada)

Accurate evaluation of elderly clients' skills and resources for managing instrumental activities of daily living forms the basis of the ALSAR (Assessment of Living Skills and Resources)level of risk score. The degree of inter-rater reliability, that was established in the original study, was low for Resources, and was gleaned from therapists trained at a basic level. The purpose of this study was to determine whether the accuracy of ALSAR Skill and Resources scores improved with enhanced therapist training. Five occupational therapists trained at a basic level administered three non-intrusive ALSAR items to a convenience sample of twenty geriatric day hospital clients. A further twenty clients were evaluated following enhanced therapist training. Intra class correlation coefficient (ICC) and percentage agreement was used to measure agreement between raters. Enhanced training did improve reliability at post-intervention for both skills and resources for two ALSAR tasks. Overall reliability for resources however was low (ICC = .305 - .475). Eight contributing factors were identified. Current ALSAR administration guidelines are not sufficient to support acceptable inter-rater agreement for Resource scores for the three selected tasks in this study. Further research is required.

[6] Reliability and validity of functional movement scale: A new clinical measure of functional limitations

S. Usuda (Gunma University School of Health Sciences, Maebashi, Japan)

PURPOSE: The Functional Movement Scale (FMS) is a new clinical measure for evaluating the functional limitations of elderly. The purpose of this study was to assess the reliability and the validity of the FMS. METHOD: The FMS consists of eleven items: sitting balance, reaching down to floor in sitting, lie-sitting, sitting-standing, standing balance, transfers, reaching down to floor in standing, turning, walking, sitting on floor-standing, stair climbing. Each task is scored on a five-point scale (0-4). Fifty stroke patients (mean age, 65.8 +/- 8.8 yr) were assessed for impairments, functional independence and FMS. Motor and sensory impairments were scored on a three-point scale. Cognitive impairment was measured by the revised version of Hasegawa dementia scale (HDS-R). Reliability of the measure was assessed through the ratings of three physical therapists. RESULTS: The intraclass correlation coefficients measuring the inter- and intra-rater reliability for the test as a whole were .93 and .91 respectively. There was a high degree of internal consistency, a Cronbach's alpha of .95. The Scale correlated moderately with impairments and functional independence. Path analysis revealed that the Scale mediates between impairments and functional independence. CONCLUSION: The FMS has demonstrated high reliability and clinical validity. This tool is easy to administer and score and has measurement properties that are useful in clinical practice and research.

[7] A non-discriminating geriatric assessment on the surgical wards in a Spanish District General Hospital. A pilot study.

C Trescoli, JA Avellana, A Belenguer, I Salvador, V Palop and C Tejero (Geriatric Assessment Unit, Hospital de la Ribera, Alzira, Spain)

Hospital de la Ribera is a 250-bed hospital with most of the Surgical Specialities. It has performed more than 15000 inpatient surgical operations during this year. Elective surgery is often cancelled because prolonged hospital stays secondary to post-operative complications and worsening of known medical pathologies. The Spanish Health System (Insalud) publishes national data of the number of patients, type of surgical procedure and hospital-stay: total and by each procedure. A Surgical Geriatric Assessment Team (mixture of the American Hospitalist model and the classical Geriatric assessment team) was created to prevent unnecessary hospital stay. All surgical inpatients older than 65 were assessed by our team during the first 24 hours and only were actively followed-up if necessary. 629 consecutive inpatients (mean age: 74.5 years) were admitted for the most common 27 surgical operations during one month period. Our surgical inpatients older than 65 had total mean stay of 5.0 days. The mean hospital stay for Insalud surgical-inpatients was 8.3 days for all ages (42% reduction) for the same period. All surgical procedures had a shorter hospital stay. An early non-discriminating geriatric assessment to all surgical inpatients older than 65 can have a reduction in surgical inpatient stay by: 1) Creating an early discharge plan by identifying social, functional and cognitive problems that could be barriers to rehabilitation and discharge. 2) Close collaboration with the surgical, nursing and rehabilitation team. 3) Identifying, preventing and treating medical problems during the pre and post-operative period.

[8] Reliability of wound assessment in the elderly using high quality digital images

M. Debray, P. Couturier, F. Greuillet, S. Banerjee, C. Hohn, A. Franco (Centre Hospitalier Universitaire, Grenoble, France)

Purpose : The transmission of digital wound images through internet could be a useful tool to permit remote assessment among elderly patients living far away from a referral centre. However, the validity of remote assessment using digital wound images has not been studied before. With this aim, we studied the reliability between bedside and remote wound assessment. Method : 12 elderly in-patients with pressure sores (NPUAP III or IV) or leg ulcers were recruited after they gave informed consent. Each patient had two examinations, i.e, bedside and remote, using standardized wound digital images coupled with clinical data. Wound assessment included : size, bed colour, edges and undermining assessment, infection status. The reliability between the two assessments was measured using Cohens Kappa for qualitative variables and correlation (Spearman test) for continuous variables. The hypothesis that there was no difference between the two assessments was tested using McNemar test for dichotomous variables. Results : Kappa were fair to moderate for bed color (0.49) and edges assessment (0.3). There was a highly significant correlation for estimated wound size and correlation coefficients were respectively for length and width: 0.93 and 0.97. There were no significant differences between remote and bedside examination for the assessment of undermining and wound infection. Conclusion : The reliability between remote and bedside assessment was similar to the reliability reported in the literature between two physicians assessing wound during a bedside examination. Therefore, the use of digital images to assess wound did not worsen the reliability between two physicians.

[9] Bedside Swallowing Assessment in Elderly Patients with Chronic Cerebral Infarction and Their Outcome

T. Iwamoto, J. Koshibu, M. Kikawada, Y. Yoneda, M. Uno, M. Takasaki (Department of Geriatric Medicine, Tokyo Medical University, Japan)

To estimate the usefulness of the bedside swallowing assessment proposed by Smithard et al, we studied the outcome of 102 elderly patients with chronic cerebral infarction after assessment of swallowing by this test and brain computerized tomography (CT). All patients were admitted on a long-term medicare basis with motor disturbance. They were divided into two groups according to the findings: the positive group (n=33), who showed any of the listed types of difficulty in swallowing water, and the negative group (n=69). Followed up to 2.2 years, their outcome were studied. CT findings were studied on type of infarction, number and laterality of infarction, grade of periventricular lucency (PVL), presence of ventricular dilatation (VD), and severity of cortical atrophy (CA). The mean age was 76.4 years at registration and 61 were men. Eighteen patients died during the observation period and 15 of those were in the positive group, indicating higher annual death rate. All of the 15 patients in the positive group died of pneumonia. CT findings showed high incidence of multiple infarction, bilateral hemispheric lesion, severe PVL, VD, and severe CA in the positive group. These findings indicated that this evaluation method was useful in screening swallow function for elderly patients with cerebral infarction in the chronic phase. Furthermore, CT findings suggested that severe white-matter lesion, VD, and severe CA as well as multiple infarction seen in bilateral hemisphere was related to dysphasia, probably due to multiple factors involving pyramidal- and extrapyramidal-tracts with higher brain function.

[10] Energy Expenditure of "Get up and Go test" in elderly with Psychomotor Desadaptation Syndrome: Preliminary study

C. Mischis, F. Mourey, P. Mankoundia, P. Pfitzenmeyer (Centre de Gérontologie de Champmaillot Dijon, France).

Purpose : Psychomotor Desadaptation Syndrome (PDS) is characterized by postural abnormalities. From our experience in rehabilitation of frail elderly with PDS, we have thought that these abnormalities could be linked with an high energy expenditure. The aim of this study was to compare the energy expenditure in patients showing PDS with control group during Get up and Go test. Method: The Get up and Go test has been performed in 21 volunteer females, 10 with P D S (group 1) and 11 control (group 2) who have been matched on age (mean age:85 +/- 7.32 vs 83.36 +/- 6.48 years respectively). Subjects with cardiorespiratory decompensation and subjects showing MMSE < 18 were excluded. For all, energy expenditure was measured by indirect respiratory calorimetery during a resting period, a Get up and Go test and a recuperation period. The energy expenditure was calculated by the integration of the area under the curve representing oxygen consumption as a function of time. Results: Duration of the Get up and Go test was found significantly different between the 2 groups, (55.50 +/- 19.19 sec in group 1 vs 40.55 +/- 13.85 sec in group 2). The results showed that Vo2 (ml/min) was higher in group 1 compared with group 2 (368.73 +/- 342.8 vs 188.25 +/- 227.9, respectively) during the 3 periods, but the difference was not statistically significant. Conclusion: This first results showed the feasibility and the interest of this study. In order to determine the modifications of the energy expenditure in elderly with PDS, the sample size would be increased.

[11] Unique Demographic Characteristics of a Vancouver Geriatric Program and the Implications for Care Provision

Hill AJ MD (University of British Columbia, Vancouver, Canada), Smith G (University of British Columbia, Vancouver, Canada) , Jang G MSN (University of British Columbia, Vancouver, Canada).

Purpose: The Mt St Joseph's Geriatric Programis a community based program providing comprehensive geriatric assessment and short term management to frail community dwelling ethnically diverse elderly. We wanted to better characterise these patients in terms of age, presenting problems, years of education and language. This data would inform our practice and provide the basis for subsequent research on aging and ethnicity. Methods: At admission all patients have a standard database entered for clinical purposes. We retrospectively reviewed this database. Results: 634 patients were registered in a 5 month period. Of these patients 345 had English as a second language. 312 needed interpreters to gather clinical information. The languages spoken were English (311), Chinese (233), Punjabi (52), Italian (26) Vietnamese (14) and a further 7 languages. 201 patients had 0 years of formal education and a further 127 had < 6 years of formal education. The patients attending this program tended to be younger and less educated than an equivalent patient population in a less ethnically diverse neighbourhood. Conclusion: The impact of ethnicity on aging remains a complex and poorly studied area. This program is in a unique position to analyse how care is provided to this group with particular attention to language and literacy. The characteristics identified have an impact on care provision and should be identified in programs providing care to ethnically diverse elderly.

[12] The impact of the celing effect in evaluating comprehensive geriatric assessment.

Hill AJ MD (university of British Columbia, Vancoouver, Canada), Smith GN (University of British Columbia, Vancouver, Canada), Malone M MD (University of British Columbia, Vancouver, Canada.)

Purpose: Outcome studies in geriatrics have difficulty identifying outcome measures that capture the heterogeneity of the population and the range of problems identified in geriatric assessment. Studies use global scores which lack sensitivity or a range of instruments in domains that are not abnormal in all patients. To assess the significanceof the ceiling effect we reevaluate previous data excluding patients within the normal range Methods: Mobility (TUG, Berg Balance Test), cognition (MMSE, Clock Drawing Test), ADL's (Barthel), iADLs (ALSAR) and quality of life (Life Satisfaction Index, GDS) were assessed at admission and discharge in patients who attended day hospital for >5 visits. Initial analysis included all patients who were eligible for the study. Subsequent analysis includes only patients who performed outside the normal range for an instrument. The difference between these two sets of results is analysed. Results: 105 patients completed admission and discharge assessment. Statisitically significant Improvements in ADL, IADL function, mobility and mood were identified on initial analysis however improvements had questionable clinical value. When analysing only impaired patients the changes were more marked. Conclusion: Outcome evaluation of comprehensive geriatric assessment cannot be adequately analysed by including all patients in the analysis regardless of admitting scores or diagnosis. Contrary to current practice we suggest that only patients who are impaired in a particular domain should be included in the analysis of that domain. Programs can include sensitive instruments in multiple domains to capture the heterogeneity of the population without diluting their results by a ceiling effect.

[13] Functional disability among low income elderly: evidence from Chile.

PP Marin, R Kornfeld (Geriatric and Gerontological Center PUC, Chile, Pontificia Universidad Catolica de Chile, Santiago,Chile), SP Wallace (School of Public Health, University of California-Los Angeles, USA),

PURPOSE: To determine the prevalence of functional disability in two poor districts of Santiago, Chile and to identify whether conditions associated with functional impairment in developed nations also apply in this context. METHODS: Cross sectional, observational study. The three primary care clinics in low-income districts of Santiago, Chile. Between 1997 and 1999, 1337 clinic users age 65 and over were screened using a closed choice questionnaire; the last 386 were asked an extended version. A binary outcome measure was constructed using seven questions concerning functional status that relate to lower-body disability. Logistic regression was used estimate the odds of independent variables predicting disability. RESULTS: Lower body related disability was reported by 10.5% of respondents. The rates of poor tested vision, self reported depression, and self reported poor memory are remarkably high (78%, 70%, 61% respectively). Depression, poor hearing, having no children, declaring one's health worse than age-peers, taking more than three medications daily, being age 75 or older, incontinence and overweight each significantly increased the odds of having disability. Gender, poor vision, poor memory, falls and hospitalization were not associated with disability. CONCLUSIONS: Most of the predictors of functional decline identified in developed nations are associated with lower body disability in this population. Many conditions are amenable to relatively low-cost interventions that could potentially reduce disability levels are well improve the quality of life of older persons.

[14] The Walking Velocity: Is it a Predictor Factor of Losing Functionality in the Elderly?

Herrera, P. (National Institute of Geriatric. President Eduardo Frei Montalva Santiago. Chile) Mascayano M. (National Institute of Geriatric. President Eduardo Frei Montalva;. Santiago. Chile) Melián, H. (National Institute of Geriatric. President Eduardo Frei Montalva Santiago. Chile) Meroni, M. (National Institute of Geriatric. President Eduardo Frei Montalva Santiago. Chile) Silva, J. (National Institute of Geriatric. President Eduardo Frei Montalva Santiago. Chile.)

OBJECTIVES: To validate a simple test to get an early detection of the risk of losing autonomy in the elderly. METHOD: 1. The walking velocity of 282 healthy elderly 60 years and over, was measured applying the Normal walking velocity test which was chronometered, performed twice on a three meters distance (the average was considered). We defined as a functionality risk factor those average velocities equal or lower than 0.4 m/seg. 2. A Geriatric Evaluation was performed on people with low rank of walking velocity: Functionality Measurements: Katz, Lawton & Brody and get up and go tests. Cognitive evaluation. This geriatric evaluation classified this population as: 1. Functionally Altered 2. Functionally Normal: with /without risk of losing autonomy. RESULTS: We observed in these 282 elderly, that only 37 had a walking velocity equal or lower than 0.4 m/sec. (13.1%) which were considered on risk of losing their autonomy, and then we performed the Geriatric Evaluation on this same 37 volunteers: GERIATRIC EVALUATION: (n=37) 18 functionally altered (48.64%). 18 functionally normal but at risk (48.64%). 1 functionally normal, without risk (2.7%). CONCLUSION We conclude that the walking velocity test is a highly reliable instrument to detect risk of losing functionality in the healthy elderly population, which is an easy, fast and low-cost way to be applied in the community, as a proper screening test.

[15] Impact of a Specialized Geriatric Medicine Unit on Subsequent Emergency Room Visits

D. Maher and R. Ikuta (Acute Geriatric Program, Lethbridge Regional Hospital, Lethbridge, Canada)

Specialized inpatient acute geriatric units targeting the frail elderly patient with complex medical problems should decrease the number of subsequent emergency room (ER) visits. A preliminary retrospective, descriptive study was undertaken to examine the above assumption. We chose two months in different quarters of the year, October 1999 and March 2000, and examined the number of ER visits in the six months prior to admission to our Geriatric Assessment and Rehabilitation Unit (GARU) and six months after discharge. In October 1999, there were 16 discharges from GARU and of those 16, there were 20 ER visits overall prior (average 1.25 ER visits, range 0-3 of which 3 patients had no ER visits). After discharge from GARU, there were 14 ER visits overall and the average dropped to 0.88 (range 0-7 of which 10 patients had no subsequent ER visits). The average number of days to the first post-discharge ER visit was 67 days (range 5-161). In March 2000, there were 19 discharges from GARU and of those 19, there were 35 ER visits prior (average 1.84, range 0-6 of which 4 patients had no ER visits). After discharge from GARU, there were 14 ER visits overall with a decrease in the average to 0.74 (range 0-4 of which 9 patients had no subsequent ER visits). The average number of days to the first post-discharge ER visit was 85 days (range 8-145). After admission to GARU, there were 6 fewer ER encounters in October 1999 and 11 fewer in March 2000. In conclusion, in the appropriately targeted frail elderly patient with complex medical problems, admission to a specialized geriatric medicine unit reduces subsequent ER visits.

[16] Tympanic and rectal body temperature in elderly men and women

Märtha Sund-Levander, and Lis Karin Wahren, (Department of Medicine and Care, Faculty of Health Sciences, University of Linköping, Sweden)

BACKGROUND: A subset of seniors might demonstrate a lower body temperature compared with younger subjects. However, data on normal body temperature in seniors are sparse and few studies focus on their tympanic and rectal measurement. OBJECTIVE: To study tympanic and rectal body temperature with a view to predicting factors of low body temperature in non-febrile seniors. METHODS: Elderly women (n=159) and 78 men, aged >65 years, living in community residents homes were included in the study. Data on chronic diseases and medication were collected from medical records. Tympanic and rectal temperature was measured twice daily; once at 9 am and then at 6-8 pm. In addition, body mass index (BMI), activities of daily living (ADL-status), as well as details regarding dementia and malnutrition were recorded. RESULTS: The variation in tympanic and rectal temperatures ranged between 33.8 °C to 38.4 °C and 35.6 °C to 38.0 °C respectively. ADL- status, dementia, BMI and analgesic significantly influenced tympanic temperature in women, and dementia the rectal temperature. In men, dementia, related to rectal temperature, was the only predictive variable. CONCLUSIONS: ADL-status, BMI and dementia shall not be overlooked when assessing temperature in seniors. It is vital to record the time as well as the method used. More research is needed to clarify predictive factors of low normal body temperature in seniors.

[17] Foot Pain and Disability in Older Persons

Guarniere A.P, Santos F.C, Bellinazzi V.R, Ramos L.R (Discipline of Geriatric Medicine, Federal University of São Paulo / Brasil)

Purpose: This study examines the foot pain and disability in older persons Method: Interviews with thirty elderly with foot pain were carried out. The questions would be sensitive to identify individuals with a range of disabilities associated with their foot pain. of people of people Results: The median age of this people was 75 years old (17% male and 83 0.000000emale). The percentage of people reporting foot pain to walk was 86.6%, foot of people pain during the rest was 33.3%, using shoes was 7.3% and to the orthostatic position was 20.0%. The percentage of people with foot pain reporting disability to walk distances was 96.6%, to walk inside home was 16.6%, staying to the orthostatic position was 70.0% and reporting falls was 40.0%. The percentages of disability to activities of daily liying and to the leisure time were 30.0% and 56.6% respectively. To the self-hygiene was not observed disabilities. Some adaptations because the foot pain were reported: 96.6 Conclusions: Greater use of the foot pain and disability interviews should lead to a much better understanding of the debilitating impact of painful foot conditions.

[18] Frail assessment of elderly people in emergency department by using a simple clinical scale: a pilot study.

R. Gonthier, MD; S.Farce, MD; MA. Banchon, MD ; C. Girtanner, MD; R. Gonthier, PhD.

PURPOSE: The number of elderly people which are hospitalised in emergency department is increase. It represent a heterogeneous group in term of pathology, autonomy and social environment. The objective of this study is to individualize the frail elderly adults using a simple clinical assessment to adapt their orientation and assumption. METHOD: We prospectively followed over 3 months the hospital course of 176 older patients aged other 75 years (mean age 83,5 +/- 6 SD) and admitted in an emergency department. For distinguishing two groups according of frailty, we chose 9 clinical parameters which were easy to collect in short time (instrumental activity of daily-living, more than 3 drug including one psychotropic, other 78 years old for man and 83 for women, more than 2 interventions in residence per week by a professional of health, depression or dementia, proven denutrition, postural instability, social or environmental isolation, hospitalization in the previous year). RESULTS: The patients aged other 75 years accounted for 110f all hospitalised subjects during the follow-up. The increase number of frail parameters was correlated with a increase in duration of stay (21,6 +/- 4,3 days for 2 parameters, 22,7 +/- 4,6 days for 3 parameters, 23,5 +/- 4,9 days for 4 parameters, 25,5 +/- 5,7 days for 5 parameters). The number of patients who involved to a chronic loss of autonomy which leading to institutionalization was more important if they had 4 parameters and more than 3 and less (31,4 % versus 9,5%; p<0,01). CONCLUSIONS: The assessment of frailty may be possible with a simple clinical scale in emergency department. The threshold of 4 parameters seems to predict orientation and assumption of frail patients.

[19] Risk Assessment in the Community Setting

R. Cumming, J. Andruschak, C. Au, S. Coady, D. Duncan, J. Lochbaum, B. Lye, C. Rauscher, T. Zacco, (Vancouver Richmond Health Board, Vancouver, B.C, Canada)

Abstract: Purpose: A risk assessment tool was developed to provide a consistent, collaborative approach to the assessment of risk for individuals perceived by care professionals, families or significant others to be living at risk in the community. Method: A multidisciplinary committee with representation from all Community Health Centres in the Vancouver region of the Vancouver Richmond Health Board reviewed tools for assessment of risk in the community setting. Results: The Risk Assessment and Care Planning Tool directs clients, caregivers, and health professionals to assess a client's strengths, areas of risk and the resources that are available (currently or potentially) to provide safe care in the home environment. If consensus about risk factors is not reached this is easily identified. Risk is assessed in the areas of personal factors (including functional, mental and health status, and risk taking behaviors), external factors (social and environmental conditions and medications prescribed by physicians) and additional factors that may exist. In each area clients are identified as being at no risk, tolerable risk or intolerable risk. Intolerable risk indicates that intervention is required. Conclusions: The VRHB Risk Assessment Tool provides community health professionals, their clients and caregivers with the foundation for a comprehensive assessment of risk, realistic goal setting, and care planning in the community setting.

[20] Thermal treatment for elderly in a Spanish and French balneary

A.Cerrada, J.M. Casado, S. Palomo, J.M. Ribera (Geriatric Department, Hospital Clínico San Carlos, Madrid, Spain), P. Diestro (Department of Hidrology, Balneary of Baños de Montemayor, Cáceres, Spain), C. Herisson (Functional Reeducation Central Service, Hôpital Lapeyronie, Montpellier, France), R. Carbonnel (Service of Thermal Medicine, Balaruc les Bains, France).

PURPOSE: To assess the profile of the patients, main diseases, drug intake and objective and subjective evolution in elderly patients attending balnearies in two countries: Cáceres (Spain) and Balaruc (France). METHOD: Randomized selection of the elderly attended at the balneary, 52 patients in Spain and 76 in France. Information was obtained through an interview first and last day of the cure evaluating: gender, age, social statment, main disease, medication before and after the cure and subjective and objective evolution. Descriptive statistical analysis comparing results between both groups. RESULTS: In Spain: women: 67%, married:67%, widowed:27%. Mean age: 71 years (58%>70). Reumathological problems (98%), respiratory diseases were present in 33%. Drug intake: 3.2/day,with a reduction of 6% and supression of 2% after the cure. Mobility increased in 85% of patients and 80% improved respiratory symptomatology. Nearly 100% referred positive subjective evaluation and satisfaction and would repeat the program. In France: women: 63%, married: 79%, widowed: 9% divorced: 9%. Mean age: 61.4 years (71%<65). 100% had reumathological problems. Drug intake: 2.1/ day with an increase of 4% after the cure. Objective evolution in terms of mobility increased in 61% of the cases. Positive subjective evolution was perceived in 64% (290 reat majority). CONCLUSION: Spanish patients are older, with greater drug compsumption and higher percentage of widowed. Respiratory problems are frecuent and also treated. Positive subjective and objective evolution is higher in this group with no increase of drug intake. Social statment differs slightly in French with more married and divorced. No significative difference in terms of sex and main disease; female with chronic reumathological problems. French balnearies are more selective on one pathology.

[21] Resoluteness in clinical geriatrics: the geriatrician as the

manager of elderly patients health care

Matheus Roriz Silva Cruz, Elisabete Michelon (Instituto de Geriatria e Gerontologia - PUCRS, Porto Alegre, Brazil)

PURPOSE: Resoluteness is the capacity of doctor to resolve problems without recurring to consulting services. We described the resoluteness of an inpatient geriatric service. METHOD: All medical charts of patients admitted to a geriatric ward during 1999 were reviewed. Data collected included: the number of admission in the period, the number of diagnoses in each admission and the clinical and surgical services consulted. Resoluteness was calculated considering both the total and clinical consultations per admission and per number of diagnoses. RESULTS: There were 323 admissions in the period. The mean age was 76 years and 56% were women. The total number of consultations required was 301, 40% of these to clinical and 43% to surgical specialties. The most frequently consulted clinical specialties were neurology (n= 25), cardiology (n= 23), gastroenterolgy (n= 20) and oncology (n= 15). The surgical specialties most frequently consulted were general surgery (n= 41), urology (n= 26), orthopedics (n= 18) and vascular surgery (n= 15). The resoluteness per admission was 36.2% for all consultations and 90% when considered only the clinical ones. The mean number of diagnoses was 3.4 per admission. The resoluteness per diagnoses was 89.4 %. CONCLUSIONS: Clinical resoluteness of a Geriatric Inpatients service was 90% per admission and 89.4% per diagnosis. The results of this study endorsees the importance of a Geriatric team in the integral management of the elderly.

[22] A Comprehensive Geriatric Assessment in Community-Dwelling Elderly of Easter Island

A. Brizzolara, C. Letelier, V. Duk, L. Delgado, C. Ovalle (Chilean Air Force Hospital,Santiago,Chile), JL Ballester (Hanga Roa Hospital, Easter Island,Chile)

A Chilean Air Force health operative performed a frailty elderly diagnosis. We enrolled subjects aged 65 yrs or more, who presented changes in the last year in their functional status in accordance with the criteria of local health workers. Fifty two elderly (15 M/37 F) were evaluated with the following: Pfeiffer SPMMSQ , Yesavage GDS short, Barthel ADL, Reuben Test (RT) for complex functions (24/24 points), Sensory evaluation (Rosenbaum chart; 1-2 KHz audiometer), Body Composition, FAT, FFM and TBW (Biodynamics (r), Impedance Analysis), Calcaneus Bone Ultrasonometry (Achilles Express(r)), QOL with COOP-WONCA charts, Social Risk (SR) and Comorbidity Index (CI). Statistics: Non parametric for the mean differences between groups. Results: Groups of M/F: Age(yrs) 75.9±0.7; 74.8±0.7 (ns), BMI(Kg/m◊) 25.7± 1.3; 26.9 ±0.9 (ns); ADL(%) 75.8±7.6; 97.9±0.6**, SPMMSQ 3.6±0.7; 1.9±0.4*, GDS 3.2±0.8; 3.1±0.6 (ns), RT 16.6±1.7; 20.9±0.7*, FAT(Kg) 20.7±1.8; 25.7±1.5 (ns), FFM(Kg) 49.1±2.5; 42.5±1.0**, TBW(%) 78.8±0.9; 75.8±0.4**, Bone Stiffness 91.7±6.9; 75.5±2.8* (*p<0.05; **p<0.01). No differences between genders were obtained either for CI, SR, Sensory and COOP-WONCA. Conclusion: Reduction in lean body mass and subsequently in mass cell and bone have been proposed as the clue of the aging frailty model and/or disability. Gender differences in functionality and cognition found in this sample of comparable age community-dwelling elders cannot be fully explained with the classical model. Indeed, the female group has shown a better performance in the aging process, independently of the body composition changes and irrespective of GDS, QOL perception, sensory, SR and CI. (Thanks to Merck Sharp Dohme for their cooperation).

[23] Maximizing Specialized Geriatric Care to Impact Population Health of the Older Adult

M. Carr (Simon Fraser Health Region, Burnaby Hospital, Burnaby, B.C, Canada), B. Bailey (Simon Fraser Health Region, Queens Park Care Centre, New Westminster, B.C, Canada), P. Roy (Saint Mary's Hospital, New Westminster, B.C, Canada)

Specialized Geriatric Services Program has traditionally serviced the complex, frail elderly population in a specified unit or location. In a health region which covers 2450.22 sq. km and 505,300 people, the Simon Fraser Health Region and St. Mary's Hospital Specialized Geriatric Services Program Team (SGPT) are challenged to assure maximum care outcomes with minimal expert resources for older adults. SGPT collaboratively developed an innovative service delivery model. The model encompasses the full spectrum of health/illness services: preventive, promotive, supportive, curative, rehabilitative and palliative domains. SGPT is composed of core clinical interdisciplinary experts. The SGPT is the assessor of needs, developer and implementer of service programs utilizing principles of best practice. SGPT members provide direct care and centrally evaluate macro and micro effectiveness of services. The opportunity to evaluate the effectiveness of this model is an ongoing collaborative endeavour in partnership with academic institutions.The uniqueness of the model is the interactive accessibility and dialogue between SGPT, the front-line health care and community service providers and the older adult population. Based upon the literature and regional health indicators, SGPT selected falls, depression and incontinence as three target foci. Each foci was developed and implemented throughout the domains of health. Documents and preliminary research results such as "The First Step: Fall Prevention Starts with You", "Coming Out of the Water Closet: Continence" and clinical practice guidelines for depression and incontinence. SGPT continues to dynamically evolve a truly seamless spectrum of approach to assure the overall well-being of the older adult.

[24] Adult's health chronic condition - a concept analysis by Maria Célia de Freitas

Maria Célia de Freitas (Graduate student in the doctoral´s program in nursing at University of São Paulo at Ribeirão Preto College Nursing, Ribeirão Preto, São Paulo, Brasil) Maria Manuela Rino Mendes (University of São Paulo at Ribeirão Preto College Nursing, Ribeirão Preto, São Paulo, Brasil)

The purpose of this study was to define the concept of adult's health chronic condition presented in nursing, medical, psychological, anthropological and sociological literature. Considering the volume of publications, authors analyzed periodicals published from 1994 to 1998. Authors applied an evolutionary perspective of concept analysis according to RODGERS (1989, 1993), emphasizing the essential attributes, the antecedents, consequences, related concepts and a case model, outlining the meaning units of the concept studied. The adult's health chronic condition was expressed by characteristics that configured the essential attributes, such as permanence, irreversibility, residual incapacity, incurability, degeneration and long time. The most frequent antecedents were: the genetic heritage, old age, congenital causes, tobaccoism and use of food with saturated fat. Regarding the consequences, authors found: physical, social and psychological changes, disabilities, changes in life style, adaptation and coping needs in social and health contexts. With respect to the related concepts, authors emphasized: non transmissible diseases, functional disability, limitations and disease lasting longer than three months. Finally, the authors concluded that the health chronic condition is a complex construction of concepts defined as a force capable of modifying life process. Therefore, it is really relevant for the development of new research confronting concepts such as oldness/aging.

[25] A model multidimensional assessment to evaluate a health of elderly living in the Brazilian community

Gislaine Flores, Alexandre Manica da Cruz, Carlos Frentzel, Monica Nascimento, Emilio Moriguchi, Ivana Da Cruz

PURPOSE: To develop a multidimensional model of geriatrics assessment to evaluate a health profile of elderly living in the community. METHOD: Cross-sectional, descriptive study in the Gravatai , RS Brazil, from 345 volunteers with >60 years, both genders, and free living. An instrument of assessment that broaches the principal aspects related with global health of the elderly that could be applicable in Public Health Policies was developed, consisting of 86 questions, distributed in 6 sections: identification, socioeconomic profile, nutritional behavior, evaluation of general health, biochemical profile and body measures. RESULTS: The time of application was 21.15 ± 9.10 min. The concordance index of the data was 97.9 % among interviews. In the sample, 79.1% were women, was 67.24 ± 6.14 years old. The median monthly family income was 2.32 ± 0.78 Brazilian minimum wages, 76.6% lives in their own house and 74.1% were retired. 67% had a lower education level. The familiar profile was: 51.3% widowed, 4.26 ± 3.03 children/elderly, and 97.7% with regular family relationship. 35.1% showed lower nutritional risk, 24.6 % were smokers. 44.9% of the elderly told to be healthy and 64.6 % told to be a good quality of life. 72.9% were independents for their activities of daily living. The were cardiovascular diseases were the morbidity more frequent. The results gave rise to a feasible and acceptable model, named Elderly Simplified Multidimensional Profile (ESMP) which can be used to evaluate the global health of elderly that live in developing country.

[27] Suffering, Satisfaction and Entropy

B.Z. Aminoff (Geriatric Deptartment and Memory Clinic, Sheba Medical Center, Israel)

Life, from the moment of ovulation to the development of the fetus, birth and adulthood is a gigantic step in the organization of material in the most orderly advanced manner, ultimately expressed in terms of beauty, power, intelligence and a desire to conquer the world. In sum it is a process of the depression of entropy. With the first smile of a baby and with every subsequent achievement and progress, whether physical or intellectual, establishing a family or a career, all contribute to the diminishing of chaos and entropy, thus creating foundations for satisfaction, happiness, joy, pride and other positive emotions. The secret of life lies in the constant motivation of a living creature to advance, improve, acquire and conquer the world without any limitations so as to reduce the level of entropy and consequently experience pleasure. The incentive to acquire positive emotions is the engine of all progress and creativity in science, art, economics, sport or all else. Alternately: a loss of power, beauty, knowledge or property in the present, past or in the future, causes a shallowing of entropy depression, and is the source of negative emotions and suffering. Thus with aging the entropy depression becomes shallower and disease and death become more likely. Entropy is a measure of disorder. As disorder increases, so does entropy. At the end of a patient's life any medical, functional, cognitive and social deterioration is the result of an increased level of disorders and entropy that causes an increased level of suffering.

[28] Multidimensional Assessment of Health and Risk Factors of the Elderly

Lj.Kozareviæ-Vuèièeviæ, N.Vojvodiæ (Institute for Gerontology Home Treatment and Care Belgrade, Yugoslavia) Dj.Kozareviæ (Center for Multidisciplinary Study, University of Belgrade, Yugoslavia), L.Israel (Institute of Psychology, University Lyon 2, France)

Multidimensional Assessment of Health and Risk Factors of the Elderly. Multidimensional assessment of health status of the eldery population including risk factors is elaborated with the aim of determining the most adequate approaches in research and comprehensive health care of the elderly. Three main topics are presented: (1) concept of health, (2) investigation of health status and risk factors, and (3) problems of assessment in clinical and epidemiological practice. Among the six dimenstions of health i.e. physical, mental, social, subjective, functional and spirrtual health, the focus is on subjective health and functional ability, as the most important ones for the elderly especially their quality of life. Findings from the study on health and functionalk ability of the elderly in Belgrade, theYugoslavia Cardiovascular Disease Study and current practice in home care of the elderly in Belgrade, are used to ilustrate importance of multidimensional assessment, especially of functional ability in relation to other health dimenstions. In the conslusion, as a model, are indicated approaches of importance for further rationalisation of assessment instruments and determination of more effective preventive and medical services needed for the comprehensive care of the elderly.

[29] Online Networking and Support: An Effective Resource For Nurses?

Selena Santi (Simon Fraser University & The Vancouver/Richmond Health Board) Vancouver, British Columbia Canada

Purpose: Internet usage has increased in popularity, but little is known about the impact of this technology on health care practices within residential care. In response to this gap in knowledge, a Website Needs Assessment Survey was developed and implemented by the Geropsychiatric Education Program (GPEP) of the Vancouver/Richmond Health Board (V/RHB). The purpose of the Needs Assessment was to determine health care providers' access, usage and needs related to the Internet.

[30] Need for gerontology education in China

Sun YingXin (Dalian Vocational and Technical College. Dalian. China) Chang Li (Dalian University of Technology Secretary to the President. Dalian, China)

There are many factors leading to the backwardness of the study of gerontology in China. However, in the aging society, the study of gerontology is needed urgently. Thus, China needs to pay attention to the study of gerontology as much as possible. There is a need for gerontology education in China. In this article, the research was centered on the population ageing situation and the work for the aged in China by way of statistics, comparison, analysis, and induction. Through the comparison with those in China, a point was made that it was necessary for China to devote much more money in major and research systems in universities and colleges . At the same time, the program of Service and Management on the Aged should be set up in the Advanced Technological college in order to cultivate the special talented people and train the service people already working in this field. Only by doing this can the gap between the developed and the developing countries be narrowed and diminish at last. This is to meet contemporary needs.

[31] The Rights of the Elderly in Brazil

S.C.I. Pavarini, V.A.G. Varotto , A. P.R.P. Sadalla, E.J. Barham (Universidade Federal de São Carlos, São Carlos, Brazil)

The Brazilian Constitution of 1988 guarantees all citizens the right to health, shelter, education, transport, work, and leisure. In addition, the Brazilian elderly have rights specific to their age group. The aim of the National Policy on Ageing (Bill 8842/94) is to secure the rights of the elderly, creating conditions to promote their autonomy, social participation and integration. The objective of this project was to raise the awareness of the local population concerning the rights of the elderly. To this purpose, the Federal University in São Carlos, Brazil, in partnership with the Ministry of Justice, offered an extended education course, Rights of the Elderly. One of the course activities involved interviewing members of the community belonging to one of three groups: service providers in institutions and community groups for the elderly (n = 21), the elderly who use these services (n = 36), and elderly who do not use these services (n = 19), to identify what they know about the rights of the elderly. The results indicate that, although most respondents say they are satisfied with the legislation, they were unfamiliar with many of the rights for the elderly. The legislation of rights is only effective if the wider society respects these rights in daily practice, creating social conditions that are just and developing caring relations with the elderly. Thus, two informational brochures were prepared to disseminate information about the rights of the elderly and about organisations for the elderly that operate in the city.

[32] Project Masibambisani (Helping each other to carry): participation of South African elderly in educational development.

Jacobus Retief Hoffman (Witbank Society for the Aged, Witbank, Republic of South Africa)

Purpose: Project Masibambisani is an intergenerational program integrating older persons in relevant developmental issues in their communities - sharing skills and expertise as well as positively addressing the ageist notion that they are mere passive beneficiaries of care. The more than 100 000 poverty-stricken children under the age of fifteen in the district of Witbank (South Africa), highlight education as one of the most urgent developmental needs. Method: Older persons in partnership with the Dutch Reformed Church, the Mpumalanga Department of Education and local teachers identified six of the least developed primary schools in both urban and deep rural areas. A major shortcoming identified after visits to these schools, is the lack of educational aids to enhance a stimulating learning environment. Older persons consequently implemented the project by collecting used and remnant materials (plastic bottles, fabric off-cuts, old tennis balls, etc.), recycled and creatively adapted it to be used as educational aids within three learning areas of Curriculum 2005 (Communication, Literacy and Language Learning; Life Orientation; Numeracy and Mathematics). At a workshop to illustrate the utilization of the different items, each school received an educational aids kit. Results: Fifty-five elderly participated and contributed to the process of reconstruction and development, while schools are enquiring about possible participation in the next program - all in all enhancing the status of elderly as active contributors in the community. Conclusion: Development practitioners should take note: Older persons have the potential to be critical developmental agents - social problems and challenges will only be successfully addressed through an integrated and intergenerational approach.

[33] The Socialization of Nursing Students in Academia to Prevent Ageism: An Action Theory Approach

Beth de la Rue [University of Southern Queensland, Toowoomba, Queensland, Australia]

PURPOSE: The aims of this study, funded by the Queensland Nursing Council, are in Bachelor of Nursing [BN] final year students: explore their attitudes towards ageism; explore issues arising out of practicing ageism in clinical practice; and empower them to come to terms with these issues to prevent a replication of ageism in their future practice as a Registered Nurse. METHOD: Participatory action research provided the theoretical directions for this study. 10 final year BN students at the University of Southern Queensland volunteered to participate. Data collection was over 6 months and was collected by survey, focus group meetings, and clinical diaries containing reflections about nursing the older person while on clinical experience in a range of health care agencies. RESULTS: Findings indicate that these students had an acute self-awareness of what ageism was and its implications on professional practice. It was also revealed that there was a fear of the ageing process itself and what might happen when one is older and requires health care. They were profoundly influenced by both positive and negative role models in all health professionals. It was revealed that younger patients have more time spent in rehabilitation and are given more information about community resources on discharge. CONCLUSIONS: Recommendations as resolutions focused upon including ageism throughout the BN curricula; more exposure to explore attitudes towards ageism through such strategies as reflective practice and self-directed cd-roms; clinical decision-making scenarios in aged care simulations; focus groups with Registered Nurses who are professional role models in aged care; and more clinical practice during their BN program in aged care settings.

[34] Teaching Interdisciplinary Dementia Care: Challenges and Opportunities in Program Development

B. Purves (School of Audiology and Speech Sciences, University of British Columbia, Vancouver, Canada), D. O'Connor (School of Social Work and Family Studies, University of British Columbia, Vancouver, Canada), and J. Perry (School of Nursing, University of British Columbia, Vancouver, Canada).

Poster with small table near outlet for lap-top computer The purpose of this project was to develop and evaluate an interdisciplinary CD-ROM learning module for student health professionals about interacting with people with dementia. The module, drawing on literature from nursing, social work, and speech-language pathology, is designed to supplement coursework in all three programs. It focuses on the impact of cognitive and communicative deficits on human interaction and on strategies to limit the consequences of such deficits in caring for people with dementia. A fundamental premise of the program is that meaningful interaction is critical to supporting personhood of individuals with dementia, and is accordingly an essential component of care across most health professions. The module gives students opportunities for guided independent study. The interactive multi-media format, structured around the development of a single case example, creates an intermediate step between classroom and clinical practice. Interdisciplinary issues concerning differences in language, focus, and goals have been addressed within a view of interdisciplinarity acknowledging that while disciplines share areas of overlap and common concern, each has unique knowledge and expertise. Results from students' assignments and evaluations of the program reveal several points of convergence and divergence in responses of undergraduate and graduate students in different health disciplines. These findings offer suggestions for ways in which the module can be integrated into and supported by coursework in each discipline to enhance student learning both about interaction with persons with dementia and about other disciplines. They also offer preliminary guidelines for applicability of the module in continuing staff education.

[35] The National Summer Institute in Geriatrics: Ten Years of Experience

C. van Ineveld (University of Manitoba, Winnipeg, Manitoba, Canada), K. Fruetel (University of Western Ontario, London, Ontario, Canada), L. Beattie (University of British Columbia, Vancouver, British Columbia, Canada)

Undergraduate medical students in Canada make career choices early in the course of training, usually in their third year. For faculty members, fostering and maintaining an interest in working with the elderly in medical students is a challenge. The National Summer Institute in Geriatrics brings together 30 to 35 first and second year students from across the country for a one week interactive curriculum. The program is held in alternate years and moves between universities. Five institutes have been held in 3 sites. On average 13 of Canada's 16 medical schools participate. Topic areas include successful aging, ageism, clinical giants, ethics, preventive health and research. All institutes have been highly rated by participants. At the end of the 1999 Institute, all participants felt they had a positive attitude towards aging and working with the older persons and all would strongly recommend the program to their peers. Interaction with seniors and clinical teams were the most highly rated aspects of the program. Challenges in organizing the Institute are securing stable funding and establishing a system for longitudinal follow up of participants.

[36] Interprofessional advanced education in dementia studies: educating champions of change

M. S. Parsons (Oxford Dementia Centre, Oxford, England)

Major developments have taken place in the integration of health and social services for older people with dementia underpinned by social models of disability and person centred values espoused by professionals championing such changes. Further service development, however, depends to a large extent on the specialist skills and knowledge of managers and practitioners and on their capacity to work together across different agencies. In response to the need for continuing professional development, Oxford Brookes University is offering the first interdisciplinary Master's Degree in Dementia Studies in England and Wales which has attracted over 50 students from statutory and voluntary agencies across health, social work and housing services. The course has been designed by a group including representatives from health and social services organisations, university research centres in memory and ageing, and academics from the university Schools (faculties) of architecture, biology and molecular science, nursing, social work, and psychology. Professionals can exit at three different levels but Master's Degree is of most interest. Following completion of foundation modules in dementia, students choose established modules offered by various Schools or new interdisciplinary modules in housing, design and dementia, or food, nutrition and dementia. Part time university attendance for one day a week over two years is manageable for busy professionals, but an on line version of the course is being developed. In future, those championing change in health, social services and housing for older people with dementia

[37] Visualizing the Future of Geriatric Education

J. Tomkowiak, A. Gunderson (Southern Illinois University School of Medicine, Springfield, Illinois USA)

Southern Illinois University School of Medicine has developed a curriculum that focuses on the process of healthy aging, preventitive medicine and the developmental tasks of aging including ethical, biomedical and psychosocial aspects of aging. The purpose of this poster is to describe the content of this dynamic new curriculum and illustrate the process used to integrate the geriatric curricular components into the overall medical school curriculum. The overall goal of this educational program was to encourage medical students to develop knowledge, attitude and skills that proactively support the senior population and successful aging, while effectively and efficiently addressing health concerns. The new curriculum was seamlessly integrated into a small group, case based curriculum, and includes problem based learning cases, standardized patient experiences, self assessment, clinical encounters, continuing education and a three year Geriatric Mentor program. Students were administered two surveys prior to participation in the curriculum, and again after the completion of the first year. Pre and post curricula comparisons reveal an increase in geriatric knowledge as well as an improvement in attitude toward caring for the geriatric population. This curriculum provides direction for the future of geriatric medical education at SIU and other educational institutions.

[38] A SURVEY OF HIGHER MEDICAL TRAINING IN GERIATRIC MEDICINE IN THE UNITED KINGDOM

U. K. SINHA, (Department of Integrated Medicine, Princess of Wales Hospital, Coity Road, Bridgend, U.K.) M. HASAN (Senior Lecturer Geriatric Medicine, Llandough Hospital, Penlan Road Penarth, Cardiff, U.K.)

Purpose This study attempts to obtain the trainees' views on a 'Specialist Registrar Training Programme' in the United Kingdom. Method Postal questionnaire survey of 100 Specialist Registrars in Geriatric Medicine. The questions were related to career choice, training supervision, study days, research and overall perception of training Result Seventy-four (74%) Specialist Registrars responded. Reasons given for the choice of career are genuine interest [58(78%)], better future prospect [26(35%)] and less competition at the point of entry [21(29%)]. Sixty-four (86%) have study days organised by the deanery. Thirty-four (46%) have three monthly appraisal by their educational supervisor. Fifty-eight (78%) get either one or two sessions for audit and research every week. Twenty-five (34%) have no proper access to research facilities like computer and the Internet. Thirty-five (47%) do not get adequate supervision for research. Sixty-one (82%) find it very difficult to get funding for research. Thirty-seven (50%) feel the training is inadequately supervised and 17 (23%) feel it is service orientated. Fifty-four (73%) are satisfied with their training. Conclusion Genuine interest, better future prospect and less competition are main reasons for making a career in Geriatric Medicine. Most deaneries regularly organise and generally trainees do not have problems attending them. Lack of regular appraisal by the educational supervisor, inadequate research supervision and lack of research facilities are important areas of deficiencies. It is also more focussed towards service.

[39] Gerontological and geriatric nursing: From the state of the art in Brazil to a proposal for undergraduate teaching

Maria Manuela Rino Mendes (University of São Paulo at Ribeirão Preto College Nursing, Ribeirão Preto, São Paulo, Brasil) Lisete Diniz Ribas Casagrande (University of São Paulo at Ribeirão Preto Faculty of Philosophy and Sciences, Ribeirão Preto, São Paulo, Brasil)

Starting with the questioning from nursing students during practical and theoretical activities with adults in a hospital, we tried to characterize the state of the art in gerontological and geriatric nursing in Brazil. Literature on the subject was reviewed (from 1951 to 1988) as well as some undergraduate and graduate programs in nursing schools (1985). The nursing practice with older persons was also observed in a hospital unit. The results obtained from this study were the basis for elaboration of a proposal of gerontological and geriatric nursing education. Goals, contents and experiences were included in the context of the courses that constitute the minimum curriculum in nursing undergraduate programs. The suggested strategy is in accordance with legal determination; however, it will require interdisciplinary mechanisms, since assistance to the elderly is an interface for multiple specialties. In 1996, this study was partly updated as to the characterization of research in geriatric and gerontological nursing in Brazil for the period from 1989 to 1995.

[40] Transforming Gerontology Education to Meet the Needs of 21st Century Health Professionals

Mahony, M.J, Russell, C, Shaw, T, Sefton, A, Ryan, G. & Barnet, S.

Ageing (and its implications) is one of the hottest topics in continuing professional education across the spectrum of health professionals. Demand for knowledge and skills in this area is coupled with the demand to be able to learn at one's own choice of time, place and pace. Use of on-line learning has become necessary but in itself is not sufficient to meet these demands. Sound educational design must lead the use of technology. A whole system approach to design and support of the learning environment is also required to ensure a suitable, robust and sustainable learning system. This poster reports on a collaborative research and development project to marry these elements in a new approach to gerontology education. All faculties in the University of Sydney's College of Health Sciences are contributing to this innovative project aimed at delivering continuing professional education opportunities seamlessly articulated into a graduate program leading to the Master of Health Science (Gerontology) degree to a multi-professional audience. Web-supported learning is the core delivery mechanism for a curriculum based on constructivist principles, judicious use of a case-based approach and commitment to placing the learner at its centre. The poster will present the resulting system design, details of the underpinning theory, and an assessment of strengths and weaknesses in the approach to date.

[41] Nursing Standards for nursing geronto-psychiatric patients

I. Göschel; A. Besendorfer, BScN (FADO-Fortbildung für Altenpflege aus Dortmund, Dortmund, Germany)

The most important for quality-securing in nursing for geronto-psychiatric patienten are nursing standards.

[42] A Strategic Plan for Educating California Healthcare Providers about Elder and Dependent Adult Abuse

D.C. Francis, C.H. Hirsch, D. Koin [UC Davis, Sacramento, CA, USA], D. Schneider [UC San Diego, San Diego, CA, USA], L. Mosqueda [UC Irvine, Irvine, CA]

Through enabling legislation, the California Office of Criminal Justice and Planning in 1997 funded the creation of 2 Medical Training Centers (MTC), whose mission is to develop standardized training programs for healthcare providers in California that will teach them to recognize, assess, report, and collaboratively manage the various forms of family violence, including elder and dependent adult abuse (EDAA). A parallel objective of the Elder Abuse Domain has been to catalyze discussions among policy makers of models for integrating the activities of Adult Protective Services (APS), law enforcement, and clinicians in the management of EDAA. The MTC have used education experts to design systematic approaches to course development that span each domain. In EDAA, academic geriatricians, plus an expert in the Child Protection Center model, collaborated to identify a core content that has formed the basis for the development of basic, advanced, and specialized courses on EDAA that target nurses, primary-care physicians, psychiatrists, and geriatricians. To date, the courses have been piloted as traditional lectures and workshops, attracting relatively small numbers of attendees. To reach larger numbers, the MTC are working with stakeholder organizations, and will translate the basic courses to video and distance learning formats. The widespread education of healthcare providers about EDAA is a formidable challenge, yet critical to the management of this immense social problem. The State of California is innovatively meeting this challenge by using legislation and State agencies to spur academic institutions to develop and disseminate the courses that will train the State's healthcare providers.

[43] Incorporating Geriatrics into Medical School Curricula

G. Paul Eleazer,MD; Victor A. Hirth,MD; Ellen Roberts,PhD; Darryl Wieland,PhD; Rebecca Boland, MA. [University of South Carolina School of Medicine, Nine Richland Medical Park Drive, Suite 630, Columbia, SC 29208, USA]

Purpose: The Aging of the population of the United States has led to a call for increasing the amount of geriatric related content in medical school curricula. Herein, we describe a successful program at a community-based medical school, which has utilized multiple methods to increase curriculum content in geriatrics. Methods: Through the use of a vertical curriculum in geriatrics, aging related content is inserted into and tracked in multiple different medical school courses vertical curriculum format. Through the use of learning objectives, geriatric content in specific courses is directed following national recommendations. A recent longitudinal patient care experience exposes medical students throughout all four years of medical school. Each of these approaches will be described in detail. Surveys of curriculum content have been conducted every 2 years since 1990. Results: Ongoing analyses has indicated a significant increase in curriculum content in geriatrics as documented by time allocated to geriatric topics as well as test questions and learning objectives related to geriatrics. Time allocated to geriatric material has more than doubled since 1990. Course learning objectives related to geriatrics have increased significantly. Conclusion: A multifaceted approach to increasing curriculum content in geriatrics has been successful in this community-based medical school.

[44] Development of Gerontology in Russia: the Role of International Collaboration

O. N. Mikhailova (St. Petersburg Institute of Bioregulation and Gerontology, St. Petersburg, Russia)

Foundation of the Gerontological Society of the Russian Academy of Sciences started a new epoch of the Russian gerontology in 1994 following the USSR disintegration. The Society immediately established good contacts with international and national gerontological organisations and was admitted to the IAG at the 16th World Congress of Gerontology in 1997 (Adelaide, Australia). Russian gerontologists actively participate in international meetings on gerontology and geriatrics. Joint programmes on ageing biology, medical and social care for the elderly are launched. St. Petersburg Institute of Bioregulation and Gerontology collaborates with Italian National Institute of Ageing, NIA Gerontological Research Centre (Baltimore, USA) and Paris University. St. Petersburg Geriatric Centre participates in joint educational and training programmes with Finnish, Swedish, American and British geriatricians. A Russian representative co-develops the UN Research Agenda on Ageing for the 21st Century. International conferences have been organised in Moscow, St. Petersburg and Samara. Decision to conduct the 2nd European Congress on Biogerontology the first major gerontological event conducted in Russia - in St. Petersburg in 2000 was partly explained by comprehended necessity to integrate the Russian science with the world scientific community despite financial impediments. While isolation of the Soviet science chiefly resulted from political controversy, it is more an economic matter today. The Congress summoned about 350 Russian and foreign researchers to provide efficient communication and knowledge exchange on every aspect of gerontology. Intensified collaboration of the Russian and international gerontologists will definitely contribute to the development of gerontology, medical and social care for the elderly worldwide.

[45] A Multidisciplinary Research Programme On Aging In Finland

M. Jylhä (The School of Public Health, University of Tampere, Finland), M. Saarenheimo (The School of Public Health, University of Tampere, Finland

A central challenge of scientific communities in the aging societies is to open up new innovative perspectives and to create opportunities for collaboration between different diciplines, on one hand, and between research and practice, on the other hand. In Finland, a multidisciplinary research programme was opened in the beginning of year 2000. The programme consists of 21 projects. The general objective of the Research Programme on Aging is to produce information that can help contain the problems and challenges thrown up by the ageing of the population. The programme addresses two main types of questions: The first cluster of questions concerns the basic processes of ageing as a biological, psychological, social, cultural and societal phenomenon. The second cluster of questions addresses the challenges presented to individuals, communities and society at large by the processes of ageing. The programme will be promoting cooperation between different lines of inquiry both in the context of multidisciplinary research projects and through more open dialogue between different themes and disciplines. Ageing is here understood in broad terms, without setting out any specific definition. The research projects aceepted to the programme represent a large variety of disciplines and methodologies and also different universities and research institutes. The projects range from basic neurobiological research to applied social science and from large epidemiological projects to small qualitative studies. The programme is jointly financed by the Academy of Finland, the Social Insurance Institution, the Finnish Work Environment Fund, the Ministry of Social Affairs and Health, the Ministry of Education, the Ministry of the Environment, the Association of Finnish Local Authorities and the Statistics Finland. The forms of cooperation in the programme include seminars and workshops on differet themes and a a web site with administrative and topical information and opportunities for discussions and publications. We also encougrage informal research networks and organise researcer training in cooperation with existing doctoral programmes.

[46] A new teaching model of geriatrics and gerontology at Prague medical faculty

Z. Kalvach [1-st medical faculty, Charles University, Prague, Czech Republic], B. Maskova, J. Stepan [@-nd medical faculty, Charles University, Prague, Czech Republic]

Drawing on 6 years of teaching experience in the field of geriatrics and gerontology we present our two-module model of geriatric gerontological teaching at medical faculties. Basic principles: 1. Geriatric topics in traditional courses [e.g.. physiology, surgery] 2. Introductory course (e.g. general gerontology in first two years) common for students of medicine, nursing, occupational therapy, physiotherapy and so on to support team spirit and interdisciplinary experience. The course outlines demographical, biological, psychological and social aspects (e.g. ageing and old age, successful aging, long term care), but it is mainly focused on communicative skills and reflection of the elderly as human beings with special risks, limitations and needs. 3 The advanced synthetic part of the medical training provides space for a specialised course of multidisciplinary geriatrics focusing on clinical differences, atypical manifestations and special problems [falls, delirium, immobilisation]. According to our experience in advanced stage of medical training, students prefer to discus the proper medical topics [differential diagnosis, treatment], while they enjoy the communicative and social approach in the early stage.

[47] Outcome Assessment: Enhancing Educational Development in Geropsychology.

Gail F. Hicks, [Eastern Washington University, Cheney, WA USA] poster, see #1 above for title Jan M. Kaschmitter, M.S. [Grant County Mental Health, Coulee City, WA USA] poster, same as above Theresa J. Martin, [Eastern Washington University, Cheney, WA USA] poster, same as above

Abstract Purpose of the study was to assess student learning and develop assessment method for feedback to instructor of Psychology and Adult Life and Aging Method. Instructor feedback included student (1) knowledge of aging, (2) attitudes toward aging, specifically attitudes consistent with the concept of successful aging, and (3) intellectual development and learning preferences that would facilitate decision making about instructional methods, course content, and expectations of students. Assessment included three pre- posttest measures and a student evaluation. Results: Student performance data suggest content mastery was significant at .05 for the overall test and two texts. Pre-Post administration of Tollett/Adamson Aging Attitude Scale demonstrated movement toward positive attitudes (.01 level). Employing the Learning Environment preference Scale of intellectual development, students assessed at Perry's position three. Conclusion: Data indicate that this approach to outcome assessment has merit in providing instructor feedback for student performance and course modification. Recommendations for course modification and outcome assessment are provided.

[48] Experiences in developing a Learning Network for delivery of Geriatric Curriculum Materials

John Puxty, (Queen's University, Kingston, Canada)

Economic and manpower restraints and accessibility to learners challenge our ability to prepare health professionals for their future roles in relation to an aging population. In 1995 we embarked on the creation of a learning network structure and resources to augment delivery of both undergraduate and graduate geriatric education at Queen's university. Methodology: The strategies evolved over the last five years and included creation of computer-based core resource materials, standardization of tutorial presentations, posting of materials and power point presentations on an intranet and development of multimedia case scenario illustrating common health care challenges of the elderly used. Results: Our evaluations indicate a high level of acceptability and ease of use by learners based on utilization data (71-93% users), patterns of use, and their subjective reports on the utility of materials (content, relevance, ease of use, and areas for improvement). Educational benefits were seen in terms of inter-activity at tutorials and lectures and, impact on learner's knowledge acquisition, comprehension, application to practice and self-perceived confidence in caring for the elderly. Conclusion: Our experience suggest the creation of a learning network of geriatric curriculum resources had benefits in terms of inter-activity, flexibility of learning, enthusiasm of learners, and is at least as effective as other forms of learning technology delivery. Economically it offers real advantages to the user but has a high development cost to the provider that may be prohibitive.

[49] Revision and problems of an educational course for certified care workers under the care insurance

Mika KUNISADA (Fukuyama municipal Women's Junior College) Kimiko YAMAOKA (Niimi public junior college) Michiko HIGUCHI, Kumi HIKIGI (Kinki welfare university) Masami HIDAKA (Kobe University, School of Medicine) Hiroshi SUMII (Hiroshima prefectural health welfare university)

Certified Social Worker and Certified Care Worker Law was enacted in May 1987 and education of certified care worker (CCW) was begun at 1988. Meanwhile, the social environment for CCW has changed greatly. Majority of these changes, the basic concept of welfare was changed from care service in facilities to care service at home. The curriculum for CCW was revised in 2000. Care insurance started at this time and included to curriculum for CCW. In this change required educational aspect on home care. The point of curriculum revised. (at two years course) 1) Total educational time was increased from 1500 hours to 1650 hours. 2) Enactment of the main teacher qualification - One person or more is had CCW licensed in proper teacher. 3) Require of visit care practice Relationship between Care insurance and visit care practice - In the care insurance, the visit care service is classified into the body care, housework help, and the combined type. However, we want to educate the aspect of evaluate all life of individual persons who needed care in the pre-practice orientation for student. Problem in the future - We explain the care insurance system and the revision of the curriculum for CCW. However, many problems both will have been still left in the future. Especially, the difficulty of the work is actually felt in the visit care practice. It will be necessary to make the manual which considers the attitude, view point and meaning of the visit care.

[50] A Comparison of Enrollment Patterns of Older Students in College Classes : an Ongoing Longitudinal Study

W.C. Hays [Gerontology Program, School of Community Affairs, Box 135, Wichita State University, Wichita, KS 67260-0135]

PURPOSE: This research analyzes 18 cohorts of older students who were enrolled at a Midwestern University during the period of 1982 - 1999. This research is part of an ongoing investigation of students 60 and over who enroll for credit and as auditors in regularly scheduled college courses. METHODS: Cross cohort comparisons are used to analyze enrollment changes through time both between and within cohorts. The research uses curve fitting and time series analysis to show the enrollment pattern of each cohort. Emphasis is placed upon graphical presentation of the data. RESULTS: Findings include a trend toward enrollment increases in successive cohorts and a consistent pattern within cohorts similar to classic survival curves. CONCLUSIONS Over the almost twenty years of gathering data older students have show consistent interest in taking a variety of college courses. Patterns of enrollments of cohorts over time are fairly consistent, although specific courses in which students enroll has changed over time.

[51] Medical Students Facilitate Pursuit of Healthy Lifestyle for Geriatric Community

A. Gunderson, J. Tomkowiak (Southern Illinois University School of Medicine, Springfield, Il. USA)

Healthy lifestyle habits have a documented role in successful aging. The purpose of this poster presentation is to introduce the concept of a medical student facilitated community education event and discuss the opportunities and challenges of this type of approach to geriatric education. Second year medical students involved in a new geriatric curriculum at SIU School of Medicine formed a collaborative partnership with faculty and geriatric mentors to design and host a community-wide Geriatric Health Fair. The working group completed a needs assessment to determine the education, information and interest needs of the older adult community and created a day long event to meet the identified health promotion objectives. The event included mini health seminars provided by the students, safety education, risk screenings, community services and information displays by area health providers. The results of this event are broadly represented in the acquistion of knowledge by both students and geriatric participants, and an improved attitude of the students to health promotion activities for the older adult population. The findings also support research conclusions that health promotion and disease prevention activities are beneficial at any age.

[52] Older People's Knowledge of the Emergency Telephone Number and CPR Training in Australia

M.Clark, E. Enraght-Moony, K. Balanda, M. Lynch, T. Tighe, G. FitzGerald (Australian Centre for Prehospital Research, Queensland Ambulance Service and University of Queensland, Australia)

Purpose: Cardiovascular disease is a major public health issue in Australia. Cardiac arrest is most likely to occur in those aged over 60 years, occur in the home and is usually witnessed. Community members assist survival from out-of-hospital cardiac arrest by contacting emergency medical services and performing cardiopulmonary resuscitation (CPR) prior to the arrival of the ambulance. In Australia there is a paucity of population based information about the extent to which community members, including older people, know the emergency telephone number and are trained in CPR. This study examines these two issues with a view to targeting training. Method: A telephone survey of randomly selected Queensland adults (n=4,490) was conducted to ascertain current knowledge and recency of CPR training. Results: Although most respondents (88.3%) could correctly state the Australian emergency telephone number, significant age differences were apparent ($p<0.001$). Just over half the respondents (53.9%) had completed any form of CPR training and only 12.1% had current training. Older people were more likely to have never participated in CPR training than younger adults and males were more likely to have engaged in CPR training than females. Additional demographic and socioeconomic differences were found between those never trained in CPR and those who were trained. Conclusion: The results emphasize the need to increase CPR training in those aged 60 years and over and particularly in older females. A need to increase awareness of the emergency telephone number among older people was identified. A community based education strategy is described.

[53] Smile 10, Health 100 - An Odontogeriatric Educational and Preventive Program

M.A. Brondani (IGG-Geriatric and Gerontology Institute, PUC University, Porto Alegre, Brazil)

Purpose: The Smile 10, Health 100 program objects, by a simple and useful method, to highlight the value of active learning and reinforcement of behavior change in older learners, and show and support the need to integrate, by education, oral health knowledge with health promotion and with social function. The program attempts to give bases and behavioral approaches to educating community-dwelling elderly about general and buccal health, thereby enhancing their self-social position as active persons. Finally, it proposes continuous dental and denture care (buccal hygiene) not just for oral health, but even more importantly, related and associated with the body health that culminates in an integrated feeling well status. Method: One day educational/informative class-like seminars focused on oral health issues and its integration with general health is proposed. Separated 20 older people groups are suggested to attempt the seminar. Slides were developed to be used on a 35mm projector, poster-format papers to help the explanation and a 24 pg folder to be handed to the people. During the seminars 3 areas will be discussed and taught: 1) Knowledge of buccal diseases, buccal, dental, and denture care (brush, flossing, etc.) and their implications for whole body will be transmitted. 2) Dentures and prosthesis rehabilitation will have special attention, as well as their functional need, maintenance, and aesthetic factor. 3) Buccal cancer, alcohol and tobacco use have to be very well explained due to their high incidence of consumption and related problems during the aging process. At the end of each seminar, a little folder will be distributed to each person. This folder shows, in a minimized size model, all the aspects seen during the presentation. It includes: photos, illustrated pictures and a simple and objective written part.

[54] Quality of care process for the elderly : criteria for team auto evaluation of good clinical practice (GCP)

R. Moulias, Y. Wolmark, M. Guesnier (AP-HP, PARIS FRANCE)

Elderly patients are often victims of malpractices due to routine, poor information or absence of coordinated care. Method. Working group composed of physicians, hospital directors, nurses, other medical auxiliaries, psychogists have prepared selection of criteria for GCP. Two types of files were tested for auto evaluation by voluntary geriatric teams. 1- Criteria concerning one clinical issue as gait disorders, cardiovascular disorders, iatropathology, hygiene, staff formation, pressure sores, nutrition, 80 y.o. patients medical examination, swallowing disorders, nursing home entrance and so on. Each of these groups of criteria could be studied in team by the staff to auto evaluate and to improve its practice in one field or more. 2 - A selection of key criteria from each "field" was made to permit a rapid auto evaluation of the care process, to select stronger and weaker points, and to choose first priorities for improvement of the care given by the team. These critera were validated by testing them in different geriatric wards in numerous places disseminated over all the country. Results. This evaluative tool was accepted as a tool for detecting poor care and for improving, step by step, the quality of care. Collective auto evaluation permits an appropriation of the quality process by all the staff and restores a sense for the care. Conclusion. Auto evaluation of GCP is a useful tool for quality process in geriatrics

[55] The French Society of Geriatric and Gerontology Handbook for Good Quality Care of Elderly Patients

Y. Wolmark,R. Moulias , M. Guesnier (AP-HP, PARIS FRANCE)

The objective was to elaborate quality criteria for the care or elderly patients.These criteria must be applied in geriatric hospital wards. The Geriatric Quality Handbook includes criteria for hospital geriatric structures, care organization and clinical practices. Method. Working group including physicians, hospital directors, nurses, other medical auxiliaries, psychogists have prepared selection of quality criteria. All quality crieria were tested for auto evaluation by 40 voluntary geriatric teams.The quality standards deal with the following subjects : 1- Adequate structure and organization of the geriatric network including hospital facilities and ambulatory care. 2- Process of hospital welcome, patients information 3- Conditions of housing and feeding 4- Security of care includig prevention of intra-hospital infections 5- Dementia and behaviour desorders 6- Criteria concerning one clinical issue as gait disorders, cardiovascular disorders, iatropathology, hygiene, staff formation, pressure sores, nutrition, 80 y.o. patients medical examination, swallowing disorders, nursing home entrance and so on Results. After validation of each file by geriatric teams this tool has been accepted as national standard and will faclitate accreditation procedure for geriatric wards. Auto evaluation is useful for geriatric teams and works toward a global improvement of quality of care. The French Geriatric Quality Handbook will be available on the French Society of Geriatric and Gerontology web site. Conclusion. The French Geriatric Quality Handbook is a validate, simple, evolutive, didactic tool for evaluation and improvement of quality care.

[56] Description of a Geriatric Crisis Outreach Service in Vancouver, British Columbia.

B. Shatzko, L. Bauming, D. Byres (Vancouver / Richmond Health Board - Vancouver Community Mental Health Services, Vancouver, British Columbia, Canada

Purpose: Elderly individuals who suffer both mental illness and physical illness require immediate response to any psychiatric or behavioural crisis they experience as well as assistance linking to appropriate resources in hospital or in the community. Method: A project was developed to fill this gap in service by creating a nursing position that could respond in a timely manner to the client and their caregivers during a crisis. The nurse provides an on-site assessment and / or expert consultation and education over the phone as well as short term management and linkage for these elderly individuals and their caregivers. Results: The Geriatric Crisis Outreach Service has been successful in diverting elderly clients from use of the hospital emergency rooms and in maintaining these individuals in their home. Physicians have given positive feedback about the program as have staff in geriatric programs operating out of local mental health teams. Since the program's inception in May 1998 the Geriatric Crisis Outreach Service has responded to 2, 020 requests for urgent assistance of which 620 involved emergent on-site assessments. The majority of referrals to the service come from mental health teams, police, health units, hospitals and family or friends. To date less than four percent of clients responded to were transported to hospital.

[57] Medical manpower needs for geriatricians in Quebec

Guy Lacombe Maurice St-Laurent and Jacques Morin (Association des mÈdecins gÈriatres du QuÈbec,Sherbrooke, P.Q,Canada)

The ´Association des MÈdecins GÈriatres du QuÈbec[a] groups together geriatricians, a recognized medical speciality in Quebec since 1987 and an independent body since 1996. In 1998 the organization responded to a provincial consultation concerned with determining physician manpower requirements. The report, entitled ´A medical manpower plan for geriatricians in Quebec, new perspectives in response to new problems[a], addressed the current state of this medical speciality in Quebec and in Canada, the evolution of manpower, and its distribution in Europe. The evolution of medical knowledge demonstrates the need for a specialist who is attentive to the specific requirements of this population, as well as the need for educating geriatric specialists. Furthermore, the importance of first line medicine in regard to older persons is also underlined. Three modalities are proposed through which geriatric specialist needs can be evaluated from a population needs perspective: 1. Canadian, American (U.S.) and British objectives, 2. projections guided by the current Quebec care structure and the role of the geriatric specialist, 3. ratio of geriatrician / older population published in those countries in which geriatric specialists currently practice. These analyses indicate that Quebec should have between 118 and 160 geriatric specialists within a collaborative and complementary orientation with key groups of general practitioners involved in the various services for the elderly.

[58] Motivation for study and feelings of elderly students at the UTA in Slovakia

Nadezda Hrapkova (University of the Third Age at Comenius University Bratislava, SLOVAKIA)

Purpose of our presentation is to show possibilities of study for elderly in Slovakia, to present results of research about motivation for study and feelings of elderly students at UTAs. The results were recovered from study of opinions of elderly students, from questionnaires, interviews and by comparative method of results from geriatric depressive scale of four groups three groups of elderly students (from Slovakia, Austria, Poland) and one control group non-students at UTA (Slovakia). The results have confirmed better health, good feelings and less depressions of students in comparison to non-students. Elderly are motivated different but most of them are motivated by desire to get knowledge, to improve their quality of life and for filling of necessity of social contact. The aims of education in old age are characterized in many levels. Most important is creating substitutive life programme for elderly and positively influencing the ageing process and quality of life by education.

[59] Evaluation of a Regional Geriatric Outreach Program

J. STANBURY, K.BELL (NORTH SHORE HEALTH REGION, NORTH VANCOUVER, B.C,CANADA)

The purpose of this poster presentation is to provide information regarding the implementation of a regional interdisciplinary geriatric outreach program. The north shore geriatric outreach program (nsgop), established in 1995, is designed to address the complex health needs of older adults residing in the community through the short-term intensive involvement of an interdisciplinary team of health care professionals. A primary goal of the nsgop is to assess and treat recent, unexplained health concerns that threaten the ability of an older adult to remain in the community. The primary focus of this poster session is on the clinical outcome measures obtained through analysis of data following nsgop intervention. These measures include; the pre-post test results of the physical, social, psychiatric and functional status of participating clients as well as the impact on professional and informal caregivers. Data regarding the impact on health service utilization such as acute care bed utilization, family physician office visits and admission to long term care facilities will also be presented. Evaluation of the effectiveness of the north shore geriatric outreach program to-date reveals statistically significant results for its participants and for the north shore health region.

[60] Role of the Internet and Telephone in Care Management of Older Veterans

JG Ruiz, AG Golden, S Dang, L Veras, O Rodriguez, B Roos (VA Medical Center & University of Miami School of Medicine, Miami, FL, USA)

PURPOSE: To determine whether telecare (care coordination incorporating telephone and Internet-based data collection) can improve quality of life and/or reduce resource utilization in older veterans with a high rate of hospital, emergency room, and clinic visits. METHOD: In a quasiexperimental design, we are comparing quality of life and resource utilization of a subgroup of elderly veterans (60 years and older) whose total cost to the medical center was greater than $20,000 over the prior year with a similar subgroup of high utilizers without telecare. For inclusion, veterans will have specific DRGs (chronic obstructive lung disease, coronary artery disease, congestive heart failure, and diabetes mellitus) and/or 2 emergency room visits or 2 hospitalizations within the 6 months before enrollment in telecare. RESULTS: Since initiating telecare in May 2000, a total of 3,011 charts have been screened and 83 patients (82 men/1woman, average age 72) have been enrolled with principal diagnoses of HTN(38), DM(28), COPD(13), and CHF(4). Patient satisfaction with telecare is high, and telecare technology is well accepted. Thus far, it appears that patients are more reassured and comfortable with receiving home care; ER visits have already diminished. It appears that telecare surveillance instills confidence in patients that a health care worker is watching them all the time. CONCLUSION: In frail older veterans, telecare appears to improve access, continuity, and/or coordination, probably with reduced costs to the institution.

[61] Post-Operative Mortality Rate in an Orthopedic Hospital

L.E.G Garcez-Leme,; C.R Carelli;; M.M Amatuzzi,; I Suzuki; G.T Sguizzatto,; C.A Souza,; F Kitadai,; M. E Furlanetto; E Takeda,; I Ferreira; I Momiy,; M.J Silva; M.P Liranço,; L Cassimiro; L Guerreiro - (Geriatric Unit /Orthopedic Institute/ University of São Paulo School of Medicine/São Paulo/Brazil)

To study the impact of a structured geriatric team in the mortality rate of elderly people admitted to surgical treatment in the Orthopedic Hospital from the University of São Paulo School of Medicine (Brazil), we analyzed mortality rates of people older than 60 years, in comparison with the rates of mortality for the same age group and surgical procedures in the level of the whole country, state and city of São Paulo, in the years of 1998 and 1999. The team includes orthopedists; geriatricians, anesthetists, nurses, nutritionists, social workers, psychologists, physiotherapist and occupational therapy professional. In comparison with the post-operative mortality rate for surgical procedures in elderly in Brasil (3.69%) and in the state of São Paulo (4.45%) in the same period, the post-operative mortality rate in our service was 1.57%. The results show us the benefits of a structured geriatric team in provide security in orthopedic procedures in elderly people.

[62] Findings and Characteristics of Nonagenarians at Hospital Admission

B. Boga, I. Csák, K. Pecze (Károlyi Sándor Hospital, Budapest, Hungary)

In a general medical department of a district hospital in Budapest in 2ooo we treated 1631 patients, among them 43 (2,6%) were 9o years old or over (female: 31, average age: 92,o yr). We analyse their symptoms and status at admission and we try to find some characteristics of this age group. The causes of admission were in 19 cases: general weakness, in 8: confusion, in 6: falls, in 4: dyspnoe, in 4: cough, in 4: vertigo, in 3: angina, in 3: abdominal symptoms.The objective findings were in 9 cases pneumonia or bronchitis, mostly without fever, in 11: diabetes (only 1 required insulin), in 7: malignancy, in 6: marked ischemic ECG signs (in 3 subendocardiac infarction), in 12: atrial fibrillation (in 6 tachyarhythmia),in 2: severe cardiac pump failure, in 4: cholelithiasis. Noticeable laboratory findings were as follows: mild anemia: 7 (Hb: 9,5-11 g/dl , 1 extreme), mild azotemia: 11 (se- kreatinin: 1oo-17o umol/l , 1 extreme), kation diversion: 8, increased Cl-level: 7 (1o7-117 mmol/l). Blood pressure was in 33 normal or acceptable (12o/8o-16o/95 Hgmm), in 5: lower (min. 9o/6o), in 5: higher (max.19o/9o). Mean length of stay: 8,9 days(1-27 days), for all patients: 9,8 days, mortality rate: 7/43 (16%), 9 required long-term care. As conclusion we can say that this age group of patients presented on the one hand a relative stability: few and mild deviations in the blood pressure and laboratory data, few cardiac failure, no stroke, no significant diabetic disturbance and on the other hand general frailty and cognitive impairment appeared more frequently as the consequence of several coexistent disorders.

[63] Hospitalization rate in the elderly in the Czech Republic 1981-1998

Z. Kalvach [1-st medical faculty, Charles University, Prague, Czech Republic]

To assess efficiency of health care system, above all hospital services from gerontological point of view. Data have been analyzed about hospital stays and nursing home stays in the Czech Republic in 1981, 1986, 1992, and 1998. Changes in medical technologies and strategies as well as transformation of the health care system after 1989 have changed consumption of hospital services and hospitalization rate dramatically in the group of young people but not in the group of the elderly above all the women. Consumption of hospital days per capita increased in women over 75 from 6.110 [1986] to 6.741 = 110.3% [1998], while it decreased in the whole population from 2.677 to 1.862 [69.5%]. There was substantial increase of hospitalization rate in the elderly because of early rehospitalizations and incorrect removals of unpleasant interdisciplinary geriatric patients floating between the traditional departments. Hospitalization rate in the whole female population increased on 110.9% [233.71] but in the group of women over 75 on 171.7% [529.71]. Development of appropriate geriatric care and services, including hospital acute geriatric units, a more efficient long term care and home care systems, seems to be necessary in the Czech Republic.

[64] Influence of Local Heating on Skin Microcirculation in Healthy and Damaged Aging Skin

V. Schubert (Department of Clinical Neuroscience, Occupational Therapy and Elderly Care Research, Huddinge University Hospital, Stockholm, Sweden)

The aims of this prospective, controlled study were to evaluate the local skin blood flow (SBF) and tissue oxygenation of a pressure ulcer and compare the results with undamaged skin, and to estimate basic values which can be used when evaluating the efficacy of different therapies. Two complementary techniques, laser Doppler fluxmetry and transcutaneous oxymetry (tcPO2), were used together in a combined probe to simultaneously evaluate the influence of heat stress at 44°C on skin microcirculation, at the same time and in the same area of the ulcer edge. Twenty-eight patients (mean age 85 years) with stage 2 and 3 pressure ulcer were enrolled. Compared with undamaged skin, the total SBF of the ulcer was increased at rest before the heating. It increased even more in a biphasic manner during the heat-induced hyperemia, showing a first short peak superimposed on a gradually increasing response. The tcPO2, on the other hand, was significantly reduced, mirroring a capillary ischemia. The hypothesis is that the main parts of the SBF in a pressure ulcer pass through thermoregulatory vessels in subpapillary tissue layers. Interactions between the increased blood flow and metabolic activity at the ulcer edge may be oxygen-consuming, leading to reduced oxygen diffusibility from the capillaries to the skin surface, contributing to tissue ischemia. Disturbances of the local SBF and tissue oxygenation at the ulcer edge, where the epithelialization part of the healing starts, will influence the ulcer healing rate and may affect the ulcer healing progress in aging skin.

[65] Predictors of 6-Month Mortality in Hospitalized Elderly People

M. Zanocchi, M. Ponzetto, C. Scarafiotti, F. Francisetti, B. Maero, P. Maina, F. Fabris (Medical and Surgical Department, University of Torino, Torino, ITALY)

PURPOSE: Aim of the study was to evaluate risk factors for mortality 6 months after hospitalization in elderly patients. METHOD: We evaluated the outcome by telephonic interview in 395 patients (mean age 77.9 ± 8.2 yr, 202 men and 175 women) admitted to University Geriatric Ward in Torino (Italy). We considered as predictive variables age, gender, marital status, schooling, functional status (ADL, IADL), cognitive status (SPMSQ), affective status (GDS), medical dependence evaluated by Dependence Medical Index (DMI), prevalence of chronic diseases, patient's clinical severity according to APACHE II scale, presence of electrocardiographyc alterations, Body Mass Index, systolic and diastolic blood pressure and some hematological parameters (albumin, hemoglobin, Tcholesterol, creatinine, sodium, potassium). RESULTS: The total rate of mortality was 20.2%, 25.5 0n men and 13.7 0n women. Died patients were older (88.4± 8.2 yr.) than survivors (77.2 ± 8.5) ($p<0.05$). Independent predictors of 6-month mortality were: male gender (RR 2.31; IC 95% 1.31-4.07), DMI score (RR 2.28; IC 95% 1.31-3.99), low serum albumin (<2.8 g/dl) (RR 2.39; IC 95% 1.16-4.89), impaired IADL score (RR 1.89; IC 95% 1.01-3.56), cancer illness (RR 3.40; IC 95% 2.01) and APACHE II score <13.7 (RR 1.45; IC 95% 1.27-1.65). CONCLUSION: In our study the predictive factors for mortality cover distinct domains: demographic, functional and clinical. The identification of risk factors for post-hospital mortality is essential for planning medical and caring interventions in frail elderly.

[66] Change in Barthel index during hospitalization predict survival in older adults

R.Rozzini, P.Barbisoni, T.Sabatini, S.Boffelli, M.Ferri, N.Travaglini, M. Trabucchi. Medical Unit for the Acute Care of the Elderly, (Poliambulanza Hospital) and Geriatric Research Group, via Romanino 1, 25122 Brescia, Italy

Functional status impairment in elderly patient is widely considered a strong predictor of poor outcome. Moreover the issue of functional stability or instability (homeostasis) in the context of an ill older adult goes back to the concept of frailty. Frailty still escapes an operational definition, but some authors have suggested that the loss of homeostasis might be a good indicator of frailty. In this perspective, the inability to remain functionally stable after an acute illness (i.e. the loss of function) might be the consequence of frailty. We would like to contribute with some personal data to the discussion of the role of function on the outcomes of elderly patients. The study has been done in an ACE Medical Unit (ACE-MU), Poliambulanza H, Brescia (Italy) on 801 patients (67 0.000000emales) consecutively admitted from thee first time (completely dependent patients; patients admitted for a stroke and those died in hospital were excluded). Admission to the ACE-MU is mainly (70%) through ER and 30% after outpatient clinic visit. The most prevalent diagnoses on discharge were: heart diseases (19%), COPD (18.5%), and GE disease (21.1%). The mean LOS was 6.7+1.8 days. Changes in functional status was defined as the difference between Barthel score at discharge and on admission; failure to improve was considered as a marker of frailty. Six months mortality was the outcome measure of our analysis. After controlling by age, sex, serum albumin, COPD, liver cirrhosis, renal failure, GE disease, and premorbid functional status (all of which are associated to mortality in univariate analisis) failure to improve in function is independently associated with greater mortality (RR: 2.2,

95%C.I. 1.2-3.9). We hypothesize that failure to improve during hospitalization might mirror a broader condition of inability to react to treatment or to act synergistically with the "vis medicatrix naturae".

[67] A clinical analysis of 741 cases of acute abdomen of surgery on elderly

Liu Yuesong (Nanjing Red Cross Hospital,Nanjing,China)

PURPOSE: To study the clinical feature and pathogenic state of acute abdomen surgery on elderly. METHOD: The multiple clinical factors were analyzed in this report of 741 cases of acute abdomen surgery on elderly. RESULT: The categories of disease that produce the acute abdomen on elderly include: (1) three hundred and twenty-seven cases of acute cholecystitis and cholelithiasis (44%); (2) three hundred and nineteen cases of acute appendicitis (43%); (3) sixty-nine cases of mechanical intestinal obstruction(9.3%); (4) seventeen cases of acute pancreatitis (2.2%); (5) nine cases of gastric perforation and intestinal perforation (1.2%). Five hundred and thirty-nine cases were cured, one hundred and seventy-nine cases improved, and twenty-three cases died. The mortality rate was 3.2%. CONCLUSION: Aged patients with acute abdominal surgery present the follow clinical features: (1) abdominal pain with rather long duration; (2) abdominal pain of unknown etiology; (3) many non-typical cases and high misdiagnosis rate; (4) severe morbidity and mortality. It is very difficult to diagnose and treat acute abdominal surgery on elderly because it is a complicated disease. Treating the complicating disease and preventing complications after operation could control mortality of the aged patient with acute abdomen of surgery. It is highly important to make, as soon as possible, a definite diagnosis and accurately treat the aged patient with acute abdomen of surgery.

[68] Effect of the hospitalization on ADL in Acute Care Unit in Mexico.

Reyes-Guerrero JA, Gutiérrez-Robledo LM, (Instituto Nacional de Ciencias Médicas y Nutrición Salvador Zubirán México city México).

Objective: To measure prospectively the impact of the hospitalization over the activities of daily living (ADL) in elderly people Material and method: In a period of six months we evaluated all patients of 70 years old or more who were admitted into the hospital for care in acute unit. Mental status (MMSE) and ADL during the hospitalization period of all the patients were done. The evaluation consist in measurement of capability for ADL at admission, during and discharge and one month before of the hospitalization. The evaluations consist in HARP (Hospital Admission Risk Profile), Katz and Lawton scales for ADL. The information was recollected by direct interrogatory. Results: Functional decline occurring as a result of acute illness is not rare. We made the identification and evaluation of all elders who have been hospitalized in acute care unit during 3 months (n= 203). The mean age was 76(± 10); years old. 60 0.000000emale. Using the Wilcoxon test we obtain the following results. PERIOD RATED Z P One month previous/ admission -6.78 <0.00001 One month previous/ discharge -6.95 <0.00001 One month previous/ one month after -3.09 <0.0019 admission/discharge 0.82 0.41 Admission /one month after discharge -1.81 0.06 Discharge / one month after discharge -3.66 0.002 Conclusions: It is possible to identify the subjects in risk of functional decline and lack of capacity for ADL early at admission. Functional decline is a result of the acute illness. It is more significant comparing the admission respect to one month before hospitalization discharge.

[69] Risk Factors and Incidence of Delirium in Geriatric Inpatients of an Urban Mexican Teaching Hospital

Villalpando-Berumen JM, Pineda-Colorado AM, Palacios P, Reyes-Guerrero J, Gutiérrez-Robledo LM (Geriatric Clinic, Instituto Nacional de Ciencias Médicas y Nutrición Salvador Zubirán; Mexico City, México)

We determined the incidence, risk factors, outcome and probable causes of delirium in elderly inpatients of an urban teaching hospital in Mexico City. >From June to December 1995 we evaluated patients hospitalized for more than 24 hours, excluding individuals with delirium upon admission, those sedated, intubated or unable to speak. Twelve percent developed delirium, diagnosed by daily Confusion Assessment Method; 50% was attributed to two or more causes, 10% to inadequate pain control, metabolic problems in 7.5% and infection in 7.5%. Each case was randomly compared with three non-paired patients without delirium from the same cohort. We found a significant increase of delirium in individuals over 75 (p<0.001), with low scholarship (p= 0.04), greater number of comorbid conditions (p<0.001), more days hospitalized (p=0.02), hematocrit <30% (RR 2.1 [1.2-4.1]) and glucose >140 mg/dl (RR 2.1 [1.2-3.6]). Surgery and indirect malnutrition indexes were not significant risk factors. We found no difference in hospital-related deaths due to a low mortality rate (4 with delirium, 5 without), although 5-year follow-up showed a significant (p= 0.03) increase in mortality for those who developed delirium during hospitalization. In our Latin American elderly population, the incidence of delirium is similar to that reported worldwide, and it is associated with longer periods of hospitalization and increased mortality. Greater number of comorbid conditions, age, low scholarship, high glucose levels and low hematocrit were associated with a higher incidence. The frequency of delirium attributed to pain show the importance of ensuring adequate pain control in the hospitalized elderly.

[70] Urinal incontinence of elderly women

L. Vértes (Chief physician, President of Gerontological Section of Hungarian Association of Rehabilitation, Budapest, Hungary)

Ours is a geriatrics department where we mostly heal and rehabilitate the aged patients of the VI. district of Budapest. This time we gathered data on "aged" women as defined by the World Health Organization (aged 65-74). We questioned urinal incontinence patients hospitalized for various reasons on the second week after their check in. We only considered one aspect, a clear state of mind. We asked patients how much time after the occurrence of the first symptoms they had consulted a physician and who they had consulted first. We asked the reasons of a delay to be explained. Among others it is characteristic of aged patients that they suffer from several (according to international literature, on the average 8) diseases simultaneously. Our aged patients were referred to our department for various reasons from there area (home) or another health-care or social institution. The data of table one are most shocking. Of 100 of our patients suffering from urinal incontinence, this fact was indicated on the documents of only 9 say nine! at the time of check-in! (However, the "trendy" and "general", but very unlikely and unjustified „art. scler. univ." was stated in almost every case!) Assigning person/ institution All cases Indication of urinal incontinence (n) Family physician 36 2 Urology department 4 2 Gynaecology department 2 1 Other department 58 4 Total 100 9 Table 1 The indication of urinal incontinence on the family physician's referral, clinic closing report (among the diagnoses or in the epicrisis) Let us review the data of the "other side". The truth is, it does not reflect a more favorable situation. The ladies are very patient they even waited 3,4,5 years!!! Physician first consulted Years after the first symptoms 1 1.5 2 2.5 3 3.5 4 4.5 5 Family physician 1 2 4 3 2 2 1 1 1 1 Nephrologist - - - - - 3 3 - - - Gynaecologist 3 8 5 1 14 17 19 6 1 2 Table 2 The consulting of doctors by aged female urinal incontinence patients Why did you put off seeing a doctor? Some answers: I am old, there is no help anyway, my mother and my grandmother had the same trouble, too, I have been operated several times already, I have nobody I could talk to about this, I was not sent for a check-up, I was not accepted for an operation. All these of course may only be excuses but there is no denying that it is also a sign of the lack of health education, the not so optimistic state of doctor-patient relationships. As a physician involved in this issue I was, however, pleased that several of our patients stated that they used TENA pads, with which they were very satisfied and rated it as the best product. Almost all of our aged patients suffering from urinal incontinence asked for or proposed the publication of information booklets relating to this issue on early symptoms, complaints, and 34 of them asked why there was no screening examination, why was the screening not compulsory, why were family physicians not involved in the issue. Several of them believed that there is shame relating to the position of the disease, this is why it is a "taboo" both in families and in the mass media.

[71] Mortality predictors in nonagenarians admitted to an acute geriatric medical ward.

N. Martínez-Velilla, L. Rodríguez-Mañas*, N. Morón-Carande**. * Hospital Universitario de Getafe, Madrid, Spain ** Hospital Central de la Cruz Roja, Madrid, Spain*

PURPOSE: This study examined several variables in order to assess the relationship between them and death in nonagenarians. METHODS: Data were retrospectively collected in all patients admitted to the acute geriatric ward during 1999. Nonagenarian patients who died during the study period were assessed for demographic characteristics, cardiovascular risk factors (diabetes, blood pressure, pulse pressure), ischaemic heart disease, cardiac failure, stroke, dementia, cancer, chronic obstructive pulmonary disease and functional status. Control group was randomly selected between nonagenarian patients who remained alive at discharge. Logistic regression analyses (crude and adjusted) was the statistical method used. RESULTS: There were 1176 admissions of 885 patients to the acute geriatric ward during 1999. 37 nonagenarian patients died during the admission. Distribution by age (93.1 +/- 2.62 vs 93 +/- 2.4) and gender (2:1; women:men) were similar for case and control groups respectively. Multiple logistic regression analyses identified relationship only in patients with diabetes (OR 9.07 (1.56-52.4)) and functional status OR(12.7(2.45-66.3)). The remaining variables did not show any significative relationship. CONCLUSIONS: - Functional status was the best predictor of mortality in nonagenarians admitted to the acute geriatric medical ward during the admission. - Diabetes was the only medical diagnosis with prognostic reliability.

[72] Appropriatemess of Admissions to a Typical Acute Gerontology Department In a U.K. District Hospital

Makinde, K, Thomas, P. (Prince Philip Hospital, Llanelli, United Kingdom)

PURPOSE: Given scarce resources and rising demand in the State Funded Health Service: to establish if elderly medical acute admissions were appropriate as assessed against the A.E..P. standard (Europe) and explore the reasons for inappropriate admissions . METHOD: Retrospective study over a two month period (one winter, one summer); review of the clinical notes as described by Gertman1 et al 1981 of all admissions to an age related Acute Gerontology Unit. 1Gertman P and Restuccia J, The AEP. Med Care 1981;19:855-871 RESULTS: Total sample size 192 patients Male:Female 1:1 Median age: 80 years 17% were inappropriate admissions The main reason was social causes - 52% Dementia - 12% Muscular skeletal pain - 9% The reference of inappropriate admissions were:- Family Physician - 52% A&E - 30% Of those inappropriately admitted:- 18% had length of stay of over 17 days 36% had lengths of stay of 6-16 days 46% had lengths of stay of less than 5 days CONCLUSION: Substantial numbers of patients admitted for inappropriate reasons, mainly social. A large number of bed days are blocked in a system which is under pressure. It would appear that a more intense holistic assessment of patients before admission and improved access to Social reviews could reduce the problem.

[73] Readmission in hospital of elderly patients and the perception of nursing teams about hospital discharge organization

Marcia Regina Martins Alvarenga (University of Marília at College Nursing) Maria Manuela Rino Mendes (University of São Paulo at Ribeirão Preto College Nursing)

An epidemiological and descriptive study on the readmission of elderly patients in a medium-sized general hospital located in the city of Marília, São Paulo, Brazil in 1996 and 1997. Purposes: 1) to characterize the re-hospitalizations of patients residing in the municipality, considering variables such as sex, age, marital status, origin, profession, main and secondary diagnoses, time of hospitalization, type of discharge, financing source, type of procedure and interval among hospitalizations; 2) to analyze the nursing registrations in the patients' records concerning their conditions during admission and discharge; 3) to describe the perception of the nursing team regarding the reasons for re-hospitalizations and the organization of discharge. A database about the hospitalizations was created using Epi-Info 6 so as to analyze these events. A semi-structured interview guide was applied to the nursing team, the answers to which were submitted to data analysis. Seven hundred sixty-four records were investigated, which represented the hospitalization of 262 elderly patients and 502 re-hospitalizations. Thirty-two percent of such patients had been re-hospitalized and 55% had returned to the institution in less than 60 days. The average period of hospitalization was of 5.71 days. Among the causes for re-hospitalizations, the family's social, economic and cultural conditions, the patients' physical and emotional conditions can be pointed out. In such patients, circulatory and respiratory chronic diseases predominated. The analysis of records and accounts shows the usual organization of discharge, the nursing activities related to the decision of discharge and steps taken for the elderly's release. Follow-up after discharge lacks.

[74] Risk Factors of Re-Hospitalisation in the Elderly (over 75) in a General Hospital: A Longitudinal One Year Follow-Up

E. Alix , B. Pichot-Duclos , O. Thomas , F. Foubert, P. Bourrier , Y Lannéhoa , JM. Vetel . Centre hospitalier du Mans - FRANCE

Purpose: to determine and validate relevance of eight risk factors, assessed in a cross sectional study [1] of elders aged 75 and over, previously admitted in a general hospital via emergency unit, to predict risk of multiple hospitalisations in a follow up of one year. Method: longitudinal study of one year. Sample exposed (E) when 2 or more risk factors (R.F.) (previous hospitalisation, social stress, fall >2, pathologic behaviour, active diseases, loss of autonomy, eating difficulties, and drug-induced iatrogenia) are identified. Collection of data at end point, one year after inclusion (i.e. living-place, isolation, number, date, place and duration of eventual hospitalisation, and death) is made with G.P.'s help. Results: 554 elders were alive after first hospitalisation (deceased, n = 58), 2 were lost sight of. The sample (E) is composed of 344 persons vs 205 (NE), (deceased n = 118 , p < 10-3). (E) are affected 2 time more by changing living-place and death and multiple hospitalisations. Number of hospitalisation is one (60,3%), two (28,4%), three (7,5%). Distribution of re-hospitalisation is 12,6% the first month, 25% the third and 53,2% at the end of the study. Statistical analysis use discriminant canonic functions to test a model with eight items (previous hospitalisation, iatrogenic disease, falls, loss of autonomy, age at admission, number of active diseases, mental disorder). Results of this model reach 60,10f well classified. A seven items model using A.G.G.I.R. (a european autonomic scale) and excluding mental disorder reach 62,5%. Conclusion: We selected a frail population, with increased risk of multiple hospitalisation and death. A preventive action of geriatric assesment should be conducted at first amission in emergency unit when 2 or more risk items are present [1] Risk factors of multiple hospitalisations in the elderly over 75 in a general hospital: Results of a cross sectional study (same authors)

[75] Risk Factors of Multiple Hospitalisations in the Elderly >75 in a General Hospital: Results of a Cross-Sectional Study

E. Alix1 , B. Pichot-Duclos1, O. Thomas2, F. Foubert2, P. Bourrier3, Y Lannéhoa3, JM. Vetel1. Address: 1 Geriatric department, C.H. Le Mans 2 Medical information department. C.H. le Mans 3 Emergency unit CH Le Mans

Purpose: to determine prevalence of several items selected as risk factors in the literature, in a sample of patients aged 75 and over, admitted in an emergency acute unit. Method: Cross sectional study to establish prevalence of eight risk factors: previous hospitalisation, social stress, fall >2, pathologic behaviour, active diseases, loss of autonomy, eating difficulties, and drug-induced iatrogenia. Selection of the sample was realised at admission with hazard allocation table Risk exposure was determined by the presence of 2 and more risk factors (R.F.). Results: Of

1852 elders, 620 (29,75%) were selected. 5 were excluded. Only 447 had complete assessment in medical unit because of a short-term stay in hospital. Mean age was 83 ± 5,7. Sex ratio was 0,39. Exposed elderly were 65 % (403) of the sample (same sex-ratio [ns]). Incidence of death during hospitalisation was 9 % (58). Mean number of R.F. in exposed patients was 2,97 ± 1,02. Distribution of R.F. is 2 (25%), 3 (21%), 4 (11%), 5 (5%) and 6 (0.9%). Most observed RF was: multiple pathology, previous hospitalisation, and loss of autonomy. In the exposed sample, mean age is higher (p < 10-3), cognitive disease (p< 0,05), depressive illness (p < 0,02), loss of autonomy (p < 10-3), and social intervention (p < 10-3) are more frequent, increasing risks of rehospitalisation. Conclusion: The exposed population appeared to be frail and vulnerable with a potential risk of multiple hospitalisation. Mean duration stay in hospital is 2,73 days greater than the unexposed population (p < 0,01). Longitudinal follow-up within one year has been designed to confirm relevance of R.F. to be strong descriptive items of rehospitalisation.

[76] The Medical Complications of Ischemic Stroke in the Elderly and their Effects on Outcome

L.Denti, A. Cecchetti, S. Perelli Ercolini, L. Marchini, M.F. Merli, A. Giordano, M. Sacco' and G. Valenti (Chair of Gerontology and Geriatrics, University of Parma, Parma, Italy)

Medical complications of acute stroke are likely to affect the outcome, causing death and delaying rehabilitation. In this study, we intended to assess the predictive value of medical complications on mortality and functional outcome in a representative sample (inception cohort) of hospital-referred aged patients. 121 patients, aged 82.3+/-7.1, consecutively admitted to a Geriatric Ward with acute stroke, were enrolled into the study. Complications, both neurological and medical, were monitored prospectively during in-hospital stay, and recorded according to pre-specified clinical definitions. They were related to poor outcome, defined as severe disability (Barthel index < 60/100) or death, at 1 month (or at discharge) and at 3 months. Medical complications were significantly related with poor outcome, independently of other clinical covariates, such as admission neurological impairment (assessed by NIHSS), neurological complications, therapy and pre-morbid functional status (OR of poor outcome at discharge and 3 months, for the occurrence of at least 2 medical complications, 12.7, 95%IC 2.72-31.5 and 12.3, 95% IC 2.5-59.2). Among the single medical complications, a significant and independent association with outcome was found for fever, dysphagia and urinary incontinence. In conclusion, our study confirmed that medical complications of acute stroke influence the outcome, independently of neurological impairment. These results suggest that, to set up stroke services for elderly patients, a multidisciplinary stroke team, possibly including a geriatrician, can deliver a far better care that a single group of specialists (usually neurologists).

[77] Hospital Geriatric Diseases

Enrique de Mestral (National Faculty of Medicine, Asunción Δ Paraguay, Past-president of the Paraguayan society of geriatrics)

Purpose: study the most frequent hospital geriatric diseases. Method: We present a prospective, observational, transversal study of different diseases in 159 patients older than 60 yrs. seen at the Hospital de Clínicas. Data were taken from physical examination and current laboratory studies, EKG and chest X-Ray. Results: Cardiovascular system diseases are predominant, followed by infections, metabolic, central nervous system, urogenital, respiratory, hematologic, digestive, toxic, ophthalmologic, surgical, osteoarticular, dermatologic and neoplastic diseases. The most used medications are antibiotics, enalapril, aspirin, furosemide, ranitidine, parenteral hydration, enoxaparine, bronchodilators, vitamins, anti TBC drugs, atenolol and prednisone. Conclusion: We have placed particular interest in the study of arterial hypertension and we conclude that the treatment of even isolated systolic pressure is of greatest importance, because of its significant morbidity.

SESSION 83

Empowering Future Generations for Peace: The Elder's Role

Lt. Gen. Romeo Dallaire (RET) (Quebec City, Canada, former commander of the United Nations Observer Mission in Uganda and Rwanda "Transmitting Fundamental Values to Younger Generations Through the Healing of Painful Memories")Jacob Lomranz, (Tel Aviv University, Tel Aviv, Israel "Constructive Aging: Elderly as Promoters of Peace")Astrid Stuckelberger, (Swiss Research Program on Aging, University of Geneva, Geneva, Switzerland"Generations of peace or war: Role and Responsibility of Elders")Discussant: Gloria Gutman, (Gerontology Research Centre and Programs, Simon Fraser Univ, Vancouver, Canada and President, IAG)Chair: Carl Taillon, MD FRCP(C), (Quebec City, Canada)

The forces underlying a culture of war and a culture of peace are opposed. Nevertheless, the wounds provoked by conflicts and wars create and engender the necessities of a culture of outer and inner peace. Today the strife observed in the world implies and concerns the whole society. In this context, the elders are key to the promotion of the culture of peace and of war by the simple fact that, throughout their lives, they are witnesses of History at the personal as well as at the family and society level. Through living the history of their own nation, the elders have experienced the profound impact of war on the society and their family. The way the collective memory of war and peace process is transmitted to the next generations is a powerful factor of social transformation: (i) Either by encouraging a spirit of forgiveness and of reconciliation within society (political) or/and within the family (socio-genealogical) and within the self (psychological), (ii) or on the contrary, by increasing the hatred and the will of revenge of one generation on to another one, through daily attitudes, behaviors and words e.g. through informal education of war. The participants in this symposium will present and reflect on (i) how the psychological and spiritual dimension of the individual can be pre-conditions to a dignified, significant and harmonious aging and exitus, (ii) and more so - on how elders can empower future generations to transform conflict into peace. One way to overcome discord, egoism and hatred is through the commitment of ageing individuals to be role models representing key values of forgiveness, reconciliation and peace. Those issues and the implications of these models at the individual and socio-political level will be discussed. The symposium aims at giving an impulse to the creation of a Forum on the humanitarian role of the elders in the ever more Global Village and to enclose this issue in the UN Plan of action of the 2nd UN Assembly on Aging in Madrid in April 2002.

Participants: Lt. Gen. Romeo Dallaire's presentation will offer a perspective on the impact of war as it relates to aging. In order to look at the experiences of today's seniors, he will draw in part on his own experiences and suffering during his military career. Dallaire will reflect on how war has affected his values and views on peace - how it has changed him - and how it has helped him discover the true value of peace. Together with his personal views, he will weave in and discuss the impact war has had on today's seniors survivors of other wars including WWII - and the way they view their relevance and ability to be meaningful contributors to the community and what we can learn from them.

Prof. Jacob Lomranz, President, Israel Gerontological Society, Founder and ProDirector, The Herczeg Institute on Aging in Aviv University. The Professor Lomranz will discuss aspects of his clinical work with post-war trauma patients as well as the result of researches with Auswitchz's victims. He will elaborate on the atrocities experienced by those victims of the holocaust and their repercussions all through the life course, the consequences in old age. An important component of the results is to discuss and highlight which mechanisms of adaptation lead or not an individual to elaborate his peace of mind. Prof. Lomranz will share with the participants the characteristics of the ageing of persons affected by genocide or by war and underline the factors playing a role in their hope to enjoy their life and maintain serene values as well as the awareness of passing those to their descendants.

Dr. Astrid Stuckelberger, Ph. D. President of the Swiss Society of Gerontology, Co—founder Geneva International Network on Ageing, Geneva coordinator for the Peace Summit of Religious and Spiritual Leaders. Dr. Stuckelberger will address the role and responsibilities of elders in building and promoting a culture of peace or war within the family and the 'global village' they live in. From their own inner/outer peace-making process - through memories and actions, through reporting the 'history' linked to war/peace - the elders set models of how to engage or not in the peace process: either through building reconciliation or through perpetuating conflicts. The responsibility of elders in leaving behind them a legacy of peace or war can empower their children, grand-children and society as a whole. Thus, subtle and powerful models of behavior (life and death) are influencing future generations - an area that has very rarely been addressed or investigated. As an illustration, Dr Stuckelberger will also present the emerging role of senior religious and spiritual leaders in world affairs and their recent common commitment to peace at the UN.
Given the worldwide increase in longevity, policy on ageing should enable the elders to bring their human expertise in improving the state of the world not only for tomorrow but also for the generations to come.

Constructive Aging: Elderly as Promoters of Peace

Jacob Lomranz (Department of Psychology. Tel Aviv University, President: Israel Gerontological Society)

This talk brings together three theoretical and existential areas: (1) Long-term effects of trauma, (2) adult development and aging and (3) positive gerontology. The long-term effects of trauma will be considered in light of the studies on Holocaust survivors. Together with the comprehension the detrimental and psychopathological effects of Nazi atrocities, attention should be paid to the, not studied enough, coping abilities, strength, resilience and astonishing human powers of adjustment of the Holocaust survivors during the atrocities as well as when they aged. Research and a model of comprehending such long-term effects will be presented, as will research on the related concept of Aintegration. Adult developmental theory is needed to understand the aging survivor as well as the total aging population. Major adult developmental theories will be noted as will the deplorable position of many elderly, survivors and the general aged population, living without meaning or personal and social roles. However, admits the social-cultural situation, specific late developmental tendencies and abilities, such as; wisdom, values, spirituality, the search for meaning, increased humanitarian concern, interiority, postformal thinking, cognitive abilities, more mature defences, and creativity, develop in the process of aging. Such process and factors should play a major role as we consider critical gerontology leading to paradigmatic shifts in our thinking, which I term "positive gerontology, and to the utilization of the wasted potential of many aged in that conceptual framework. It is in that framework, which concentrates on building on strength, that the characteristic abilities of many elders should come to fore and thus enable systematic propositions for the "elderly as promoters of peace."

Generations of peace or war:: Role and Responsibility of Elders

Astrid Stuckelberger, (President of the Swiss Society of Gerontology, Co—founder of the Geneva International Network on Ageing, Geneva coordinator of the Peace Summit of Religious and Spiritual Leaders)

Facts and figures today in the majority of countries show that while fertility rates drop below replacement level, the number and proportion of elders up to centenarians has increased. The population structure has expanded from '2-3 generations' to the possibility of finding '4-5 generations', especially in the developing world where the age of the mother at child birth is lower. In this context, the importance of the dynamics between generations emerges as a key component in sustaining social and human development. Thus the role of elders within the global agenda will need to be addressed.
Today, the elderly are getting organized as a political force and although some local groups are already involved in humanitarian actions, the elder's identity is still marked by ageism with a lack of recognition for their influence and possible 'mission' in Society. In fact, the elderly are, consciously or not, engaged in the role of being the models or anti-models for the next generations and in particular inter-generational models of peace-making and peace-building.
The contribution of transmitting values and beliefs sustaining peace or war from grand-parents to parents to children to grand-children is not thoroughly considered and too often underestimated. Cultivating a culture of peace in whatever situation the elder lives can empower future generations with the image and lessons of the past as opposed to a culture of war which perpetuates resentment and hatred.
The presentation will address two aspects involved in the empowerment of future generations: i) At the individual level: the concept of aging goes far beyond the mere fact of "fulfilling one's life and living a retiree life", it also includes the notion to reconcile with oneself, with one's life, to find peace of mind and to get prepared to die well leaving an image of serenity. ii) At the societal level: aging is inseparable from the notion of social participation and responsibility of the elders towards the next generations. The cultural and spiritual inheritance that the older generations leave behind them is in a way the state of the world they have collectively co-created. The younger generations are living by the example of life and through being educated in a spirit and a culture of war or of peace.
Traditional cultures and faiths have long recognized the role and responsibilities of elders towards future generations. The recent role played by elder religious and spiritual leaders by jointly signing a 'committement to Global Peace' at the UN could certainly strengthen the common purpose of supporting the peace efforts locally, regionally and globally. Knowing the call of time at the United Nations is to bring civil society in all aspects of the World affairs and preserve the "Human Touch" in the face of globalisation, one could imagine that a 'Senior civil society for World Peace' would be a driving force in promoting respect of all forms of life, dignity, right, kindness, love and peace.
In April 2002, the 2nd UN World Assembly on Ageing will take place in Madrid (Spain). The opportunity to bring the older generations into the global picture of today's priorities is unique.

SESSION 84

Bio-demography of Longevity

(1) S. J. Olshansky (School of Public Health, University of Illinois at Chicago, Chicago, Illinois, USA), B. A. Carnes (NORC / Center on Aging, University of Chicago, Chicago, Illinois, USA) and R. N. Butler (International Longevity Center, New York, NY, USA) If humans were built to last. (2) J.M. Robine (INSERM, Montpellier, France) A new biodemographic model to explain the trajectory of mortality (3) C. Cebula (Full Spectrum Medicine Inc, Littleton, MA, USA) and R. Klatz (American Academy of Anti-Aging Medicine, Chicago, IL, USA) Date mining: A model for acquisition and management of multidisciplinary proactive preventive health parameters. (4) E. Crimmins (Andrus Gerontology Center, University of Southern California, Los Angeles, CA, USA), M. Wong (Andrus Gerontology Center, University of Southern California, Los Angeles, CA, USA) and T. Seeman (Division of Geriatrics, UCLA School of Medicine, Los Angeles, CA,USA) Allostatic load and cognitive functioning: A biopsychosocial approach to understanding SES differences in cognitive change. (5) M. Poulain (Universite Catholique de Louvain, Belgium) Are demographic variables linked to longevity: some recent results from Belgian centenarians

In recent years demographers have increasingly incorporated biology into their theoretical models and empirical analyses of mortality and intermediate health outcomes associated with aging. This incorporation of biology into the traditional demographic approach has been termed biodemography. Current biodemographic analyses address questions such as what is the potential for longevity or life expectancy and healthy life expectancy in the human population and how and why might these change. Five papers linking biology and health outcomes will be presented in this session. The first two (Olshansky et al. and Robine) will present theoretical approaches to the biodemography of longevity. Olshansky et al. recognize that the anatomical features of the human body are the basis of common health problems of old age. Robine proposes a biodemographic model that explains human mortality trajectory with measures of current conditions and the aging process. These will be followed by a paper documenting the characteristics of a particularly long-lived group on the island of Sardinia (Poulain et al.). The final two papers (Cebula and Klatz and Crimmins et al.) reflect current biodemographic work which links indicators of biological well-being to the health problems of old age for aging individuals. This work extends current demographic approaches in that biological indicators are joined with more traditional indicators of socioeconomic status, health behaviors, and psychological characteristics collected in population surveys to predict the likelihood of avoiding health problems in old age or the likelihood of living to a very old age. Cebula and Klatz describe an approach to producing data to further work in the biodemography of health outcomes while Crimmins et al. apply a biodemographic approach to the loss of cognitive ability, one of the major health problems of old age and one that differs across social groups. This session will provide an overview of some of the most important current biodemographic research.

f Humans Were Built To Last

S. Jay Olshansky (University of Illinois at Chicago; Bruce A. Carnes - NORC/Center on Aging, University of Chicago; Robert Butler,(International Longevity Center, USA)

Bulging discs, fragile bones, fractured hips, torn ligaments, varicose veins, cataracts, hearing loss, hernias and hemorrhoids: the list of bodily malfunctions that plague us as we age is long and all too familiar. Why do we fall apart as we reach the prime of life? We deteriorate because we were not designed for extended operation and because we operate the living machines we call our bodies beyond their warranty period. As we push further into our post-reproductive years, anatomical features of the human body that worked well at younger ages, become transformed into design flaws, revealing themselves as the common health problems of an aging body. In evolutionary terms, we harbor such flaws because natural selection, the force that molds our genetically controlled traits, aims neither for perfection nor for a long, healthy life. Had our bodies been crafted from scratch, we would have fewer design flaws capable of making us miserable in our later days. Evolution does not work that way, however. Instead, it cobbles together new features by tinkering with existing ones. In this manuscript we describe how various anatomical features of the human body were poorly designed for extended operation, why such structures lead to many of the disorders associated with aging, and what the human body might have looked like had selection optimized for a healthy old age rather than for reproduction early in the lifespan.

A new biodemographic model to explain the trajectory of mortality

J. M. Robine (Sante and Longevite, INSERM, Montpellier, France)

Since Buffon's time (1749), biologists and demographers have repeatedly stated that a man in good health will live to be 90, 100, or 110 years but not longer. This paper seeks to link the approaches of biologists and demographers in understanding potential human longevity. For demographers, mortality measures essentially the current conditions: the quality of the ecological and social environment. For biologists, mortality measures mainly the ageing process. The biodemographic approach links these two approaches taking into account that human beings spend the greater part of their time improving the quality of their physical and social environment, making it more and more favorable to the realisation of their potential longevity. This paper proposes two measures of the quality of this environment: first, an age when individuals are the most robust and resistant to environmental hazards, indicated by the lowest mortality rate recorded; second, the age when individuals become frail because of the passage of time, with no or extremely little resistance to environmental hazards, indicated by a constant mortality rate among the oldest old. Between these two measures of the quality of the environment, mortality measures the ageing process leading young vigorous individuals into frail senile elders.

Data Mining: A Model for Acquisition and Management of Multidisciplinary Proactive Preventive Health Parameters

Catherine Cebula [Executive Vice-President, Full Spectrum Medicine, Inc, Littleton MA USA / Project Administrator, LEXCORE, Chicago IL USA] Ronald Klatz [President, American Academy of Anti-Aging Medicine, Chicago IL USA]

PURPOSE: We present an orientation on the burgeoning clinical specialty of anti-aging medicine (an overview of demographics, trends, and predictions), setting the stage to review the design of a unified program for measuring a set of multidisciplinary health parameters that has been constructed specifically to standardize the data collection efforts for LEXCORE (Life Extension Core of Information), an unprecedented longitudinal study of how and why we age, sponsored by the American Academy of Anti-Aging Medicine (A4M) (Chicago, IL). METHOD: Based on the Health Risk Appraisal (HRA) model, a novel computer application solution designed for LEXCORE modernizes the acquisition of subjective and objective parameters of health, reflecting the multi-disciplinary approach that forms the basis of wellness-based proactive preventive healthcare. The resultant compilation permits longitudinal management of patient data for both clinical and research purposes. RESULTS: This presentation reviews the multitude of health parameters involved in the contemporary assessment of individual health. Segments of data resident at LEXCORE's on-line data repository will be shared to demonstrate how the centralization of information creates a valuable collective research database. CONCLUSION: A wellness-based, patient-centered model for clinical healthcare delivery is poised to become the preeminent mode of healthcare in the 21st century. We present a method that modernizes to collect a breadth and depth of patient data to promote delivery of effective healthcare, while compiling data to perform outcomes analysis in a longitudinal research setting. The construct of LEXCORE and its standardizing data collection platform, and the lessons learned in solutions to research design considerations, can provide valuable insights to those teams interested research in implementing similar technology.

Allostatic load and cognitive functioning: A biopsychosocial approach to understanding SES differences in cognitive change

E. Crimmins (Andrus Gerontology Center, University of Southern California, Los Angeles, California, USA), M. Wong (Andrus Gerontology Center, University of Southern California, Los Angeles, California, USA) and T. Seeman (Division of Geriatrics, UCLA School of Medicine, Los Angeles, California, USA)

Changes in cognitive functioning are a major health problem at the oldest ages and cogntive loss is more common among those of lower SES. Major declines can result in a loss of independence and need for personal care. Cognitive change is related to change in a number of physiological systems. This paper investigates the predictive power of "allostatic load" or systemic biological load as a predictor of the differential cognitive change experienced by SES. Data used for this analysis come from the MacArthur study of successful aging: a three-wave longitudinal study of high-functioning persons 70-79 at baseline living in the communities of New Haven, East Boston, and North Carolina. Multivariate analytic approaches are used to relate allostatic load at the initial interview to later cognitive state and cognitive decline. We find that cognitive decline is greater among those with higher biological load but that this relationship is limited to selected aspects of cognitive decline. Allostatic load differences are mediators of the cognitive change experienced by SES groups. A set of biological predictors is important in understanding differential cognitive aging among socioeconomic groups.

Are demographic variables linked to longevity: some recent results from Belgian centenarians

Michel Poulain, Michel Foulon, Dany Chambre GeDap

First we intend to come back on the problem of data reliability and completeness when analysing longevity and more particularly centenarians. Age misreporting, double-counts and other problems that affect the reliability of data are more numerous when dealing with centenarians. Therefore we will shortly present the data sources we have in Belgium and the way we organize the data collection in order to achieve exhaustivity in our centenarian data base. The Belgian Centenarian Data Base covers all centenarians living in Belgium and born between 1870 and 1899, that means more than 6000 cases. More information about demographic variables are only available for sub-groups of centenarians, e.g. the centenarians of the region of Tournai as far as information on parents and great parents are needed and the centenarians who are 104 and more when the marital status and living arrangement are concerned. The main objective of this contribution is to enhance the links between longevity and some demographic variables. Here is a list of these variables and for each of these we will check if there is a correlation or not with longevity. Please note that for most variables longevity and longevous persons are considered through centenarians while non or less longevous persons are ordinary persons who are supposed to die around 70 or 80 at usual modal age at death. 1. Year of birth: is longevity increasing with time? 2. Month of birth: is longevity varying with season of birth even 100 years later? 3. Sex: is longevity related to sex and is this relationship constant in time? 4. Marital status: Have single a larger probability to become centenarian compared to married or widowed persons? 5. Living arrangement: Are centenarians living alone, in couple, with their children or in a nursing home? 6. Age at death for parents and great parents: such a link should indicate clearly that longevity has a genetic component. 7. Age of parents when the centenarian was born: this is a possibility to check the Gavrilov's hypothesis 8. Age at death for brothers and sisters: here also the genetic component is important but the common environment has also to be considered. 9. Number of children and age at last offspring for female centenarians. This list is probably not exhaustive but there is definitively too much variables to be examined in a single presentation.

SESSION 86

Prevention and Therapy of Coronary Heart Disease: Effectiveness of Lipid Lowering Therapy

S. Maggi (Center on Aging, National Research Council, Padova, Italy): Epidemiology of modifiable risk factors in the elderly. The ILSA Study. P. Jonsson (Landspitali University Hospital, Landakot, 105 Reykjavik, Iceland): The Major Vascular Risk Factors in midlife are associated with Impaired Cognitive Function in the Elderly. G. Masotti (Geriatric Clinic, University of Florence, Florence, Italy): Management of older patients with CHD: from intensive care to rehabilitation E.Manzato, (Department of Internal Medicine, University of Padova, Italy): Diabetes, dyslipidemia and CHD

Atherosclerosis is a multifactorial condition, with important clinical consequences, coronary heart disease (CHD), stroke and other cardiovascular diseases (CVD). Some of the most important risk factors for atherosclerosis are well identified and their modification results in a decrease in the morbidity and mortality associated with CVD. However, there are several questions that need further evaluation, in particular the management of the different risk factors in the elderly and the cost-benefit associated with interventions. STRUCTURE In this symposium we will discuss the epidemiology of major modifiable risk factors for CVD in the elderly (Maggi and Jonsson) and the therapeutic approaches used for the prevention and treatment of CHD in the elderly (Manzato and Masotti) CONTENT Age is one of the most important predictors of vascular risk, therefore many drugs would be prescribed in older subjects, especially in those with several concomitant risk factors. In patients with clustered risk factors a global risk approach seems to be very important, in order to establish a therapeutic goal to prevent CVD. It is clear that in this group of patients multidisciplinary therapeutic management is also indicated in order to modify their life style. Stop smoking, improving their dietary habits and reinforcing the practice of physical activity are the cornerstone for the management of these individuals, especially in the older groups of the population, as well as drug treatment for hypertension and high cholesterol. CONCLUSIONS/ANTICIPATED OUTCOMES In the old age, high blood pressure and high cholesterol in some conditions are important modifiable vascular risk factors, therefore drug treatment is indicated. For example, several studies in secondary prevention in middle aged and old subjects at high risk demonstrate that statin therapy decreases CVD morbidity by about 30%.

Diabetes, Dyslipidemia and CHD

E. Manzato (University of Padua, Italy)

Purpose: The prevalence of diabetes mellitus is increasing worldwide due to the increasing proportion of elderly subjects and to the increasing prevalence of overweight. Macroangiopathy is the most frequent complication in type 2 diabetes. Diabetic dyslipidemia is one of the causes of the increased atherogenesis in diabetic patients. In the well treated and non hyperlipoproteinemic type 2 diabetic patients attending our clinic body weight is related to the lipoprotein levels while glycemic control or the type of hypoglycemic treatment are not. Hypertension, microalbuminuria, obesity, and impaired extrahepatic insulin sensitivity are associated with lipoprotein abnormalities and altered lipoprotein physical properties in type 2 diabetic patients. Method: We have evaluated the role of some lipoprotein alterations as risk factors for macroangiopathy in a 9-year follow-up prospective study in patients with type 2 diabetes. Results: In type 2 diabetic patients the risk of atherosclerotic vascular complications is not present in the whole population but it is limited to those patients who have at the same time high blood pressure, increased extrahepatic insulin sensitivity, and lipoprotein abnormalities. The patients who died from macroangiopathy complications more frequently than all the other patients were smokers, they had baseline symptoms of macroangiopathy, and they had higher age, higher fasting plasma glucose, lower fasting C-peptide, lower apo AII, apo CII, apo CIII, and apo E. Conclusion: In some recent large intervention trials the hypolipidemic therapy in diabetic patients seems more important than the degree of the metabolic control to prevent coronary events. Diabetic dyslipidemia is therefore one modifiable vascular risk factor.

Epidemiology of Modifiable Risk Factors in the Elderly. The ILSA Study

S. Maggi, N. Minicuci, C. Destro, G. Crepaldi (Center on Aging, National Research Council of Italy, Padova, Italy), G. Farchi (National Institutes of Health, Rome, Italy)

Purpose: The aim of this study is to evaluate the relationship between modifiable risk factors and CHD in the elderly. Method: Information on vascular risk factors including systolic and diastolic blood pressures, total and LDL cholesterol, triglycerides, fasting glycemia, and on life style risk factors, such as current smoking and obesity were analyzed in the Italian Longitudinal Study on Aging in about 5,000 individuals and their association with CHD was evaluated Results: We have estimated about 76.000 new cases of Myocardial Infarction (MI) in the population 65+years of age in Italy, in 1998. In the general older population, about 46% of men and 39% of females are overweight and about 15% and 37% are obese, more than 60% are hypertensive and about 13% have diabetes. A significant association was found with all these factors and the incidence of MI. Conclusion: The prevalence of risk factors is still very high and selected interventions for health promotion and disease prevention could have a major impact on the health of older Italians. There has been a substantial decline in most of the western countries in the CVD mortality rates in the last 30 years and it is estimated that 80% of the decline in CHD mortality could be due primarily to improvements in hypertension and dyslipidemia control, as well as to other medical and surgical interventions and to the changes in life style (decreased smoking habit, better diet, increased physical activity, etc.), adopted by most western countries' populations in the second half of this century.

Major Vascular Risk Factors in midlife are associated with Impaired Cognitive Function in the Elderly.

Bjorn Einarsson, M.D.(Icelandic Heart Association - Heart Preventive Clinic, and Dept. of Geriatrics, Landspitali, University Hospital, Reykjavik, Iceland, Palmi V. Jonsson, M.D. (Dept. of Geriatrics, Landspitali, University Hospital, Reykjavik, and University of Iceland, School of Medicine, Reykjavik), Nikulas Sigfusson M.D, Ph.D (Icelandic Heart Association - Heart Preventive Clinic), Helgi Sigvaldason, (Icelandic Heart Association - Heart Preventive Clinic), Anders Wallin, M.D, (Institute of Clinical Neuroscience, Göteborg University, Sweden), Vilmundur Gudnason, M.D, Ph.D (Icelandic Heart Association - Heart Preventive Clinic, and University of Iceland, School of Medicine, Reykjavik)

The aim of this study is to evaluate the longitudinal and cross-sectional relationship between vascular risk factors and cognitive function in the elderly. Method: Vascular risk factors including systolic and diastolic blood pressures (S/DBP), total cholesterol (T-Chol), triglycerids (TG), fasting (f-BG) and 90 minutes (90-BG) blood glucose tolerance test, and current smoking (c-Sm) were registered at six stages in the Reykjavik Study over 26 years for 584 men and 846 women and compared with cognitive impairment (CI) on the MMSE and DSST tests in stage VI, when the participants were between 70 and 86 years of age. Results: Longitudinally, SBP was a significant risk factor for CI in men (Odds ratio (OR) 1.12 & 1.13; $p<0.01$ for MMSE & DSST respectively; per 10 mm Hg) and women (OR 1.09 & 1.15; $p<0.001$). DBP was also a risk factor in men for DSST (OR 1.22; $p<0.01$). According to MMSE, T-Chol. was a risk factor in women (OR 1.03; $p<0.01$; per 10 mg/dl), TG for men (OR 1.03; $p<0.01$; per 10 mg/dl) and women (OR 1.04; $p<0.001$; per 10 mg/dl)), F-BG in men (OR 1.10; $p<0.001$; per 10 mg/dl), 90-BG in women (OR1.05; $p<0.001$; per 10 mg/dl), and C-Sm.for women (OR 1.42; $p<0.01$). Cross-sectional analysis showed reversal of many of these relationships. Conclusion: The classic vascular risk factors in mid life are associated with cognitive impairment in old age, but once cognitive decline sets in these relationships are apparently reversed.

Management of Older Patients with Coronary Heart Disease: from Intensive Care to Rehabilitation

G. Masotti, N. Marchionni, F. Fattirolli, S. Fumagalli, M. Di Bari, M. Chiarlone (Unit of Gerontology and Geriatrics, Department of Critical Care Medicine and Surgery, University of Florence and A.O. Careggi, Florence, Italy)

Purpose. Coronary patients (CHD pts) with life-threatening conditions, and survivors of acute myocardial infarction (MI) who deserve rehabilitation, are remarkably numerous at older ages. Nevertheless, elderly pts are usually excluded from life support technology and cardiac rehabilitation (CR). We analyzed the results of: 1) in-hospital cardiopulmonary resuscitation (CPR) of CHD pts experiencing a cardiocirculatory arrest (CA); 2) CR after MI. Methods. 1) Analysis of the 245 pts receiving CPR over 10 years. 2) Randomized controlled trial testing the efficacy of 8 weeks of outpatient, hospital-based (OCR) or home-based (HBCR) CR vs. usual care (UC) in middle-aged (45-65 years), elderly (66-75 years), and old-old (76-85 years) pts with MI. Results. 1) Older pts had a lower immediate survival (<70: 52.6% vs. 70+ years: 39.4%; $p<0.05$). Ventricular tachycardia/fibrillation bore the lowest mortality as compared with asystole or electromechanical dissociation ($p<0.001$). At multivariate analysis, mechanism of CA, acute MI, heart failure (HF), and need for mechanical ventilation, but not age, predict mortality. Long-term survival was also independent of age and associated with HF. 2) Of 773 eligible pts, we enrolled 270 without HF, cognitive impairment or disability. Old-old pts were more likely excluded. Exercise tolerance (ExTol) increased in each age-group only with CR. The improvement with OCR and HBCR was similar. HRQL improved in all the middle-aged and elderly pts, while in the old-old only with CR. Conclusions: 1) Prognosis after CPR is independent of age. 2) Improvement in both ExTol and HRQL with CR suggests that HBCR is more cost-effective than OCR.

SESSION 88

Improving Primary Care Physician Response to People with Dementia and Their Families

Suzanne Cahill (Dementia Services Information and Development Centre, Dublin, Ireland) Sharing the Diagnosis of Dementia: What Do General Practitioners Say and Whom Do They Inform? Murna G. Downs (Bradford Dementia Group, University of Bradford, England) An Intervention to Improve Primary Care Practitioners' Response to People with Dementia and Their Families. Richard H. Fortinsky (University of Connecticut Center on Aging, Farmington, CT, USA) Dementia Care Partnerships between Primary Care Physicians and Local Alzheimer's Association Chapters. Steve Iliffe (Primary Care, Royal Free and University College London Medical School, London, England) Educational Issues in the Recognition and Management of Dementia in Primary Care. John Keady (School of Nursing and Midwifery, University of Wales, Bangor, Wales)

ISSUE: The prevalence of Alzheimer's disease and other types of dementia is projected to increase dramatically over the next several decades. Primary care physicians throughout the world will be faced with the increasingly common prospect of detecting, diagnosing, and managing dementia in their older patients. At the same time, these patients and families will present in the physician's office with growing demands for knowledge and action, thanks to remarkable advances in computer access to health information and in pharmaceutical science. This symposium will highlight current barriers reported by primary care physicians that prevent them from responding optimally to the challenge of providing high-quality dementia care. Presentations will also feature completed and ongoing interventions undertaken to improve the response of primary care physicians to people with dementia and their families. STRUCTURE: This symposium will feature four presentations based on original research, followed by a discussant who will comment on all presentations. CONTENT: The opening presentation will focus on current dementia care practices of physicians based on a recent survey of general practitioners in Australia. Results from this survey reflect the current state of knowledge and practice among primary care physicians in other countries where surveys have been conducted. The next two presentations will describe an ongoing intervention in Great Britain designed to educate general practitioners about detecting and managing dementia in the primary care setting. This study is designed as a randomized trial; one presentation will focus on characteristics and pre-intervention experiences of physicians and family caregivers enrolled in the study, and the second presentation will describe the three educational interventions. The final presentation will describe two trials of a different type of intervention, designed to create a dementia care partnership between primary care physicians and local Alzheimer's Association chapters in the USA. The first trial demonstrated promising benefits of this type of intervention, and final results will be presented. The second trial, using a randomized design in a different geographic region of the USA, is currently underway and interim results will be presented. Finally, the discussant will comment on implications of the presented studies, with special focus on necessary enhancements to educational curricula and community-based services to improve the response of primary care physicians to persons with dementia and their families. CONCLUSIONS/ANTICIPATED OUTCOMES: This session will provide detailed information about challenges facing primary care physicians as they care for patients with dementia and their families, as well as promising interventions grounded in extensive pilot work designed to improve primary care for this growing population throughout the world. Informatio exchanged in this session will be very useful to practitioners, educators, and researchers concerned with improving dementia diagnosis and management practices through direct educational strategies as well as organizational partnerships at the local community level.

An Intervention to Improve Primary Care Practitioners' Response to People with Dementia and their Families

Murna Downs (Bradford Dementia Group, University of Bradford, UK), Steve Iliffe (University College London, UK), S Turner and M Bryans (Centre for Social Research on Dementia, University of Stirling, Scotland) and J Wilcock (University College London, UK)

PURPOSE: The aim of this paper is to present an overview of an ongoing educational intervention study designed to improve diagnostic and management knowledge and behavior by primary care practitioners for people with dementia and their families. METHOD: The study employs a randomised controlled design to test the differential efficacy of 3 educational interventions with 40 primary care practices in London, England and Stirling, Scotland. Outcomes include practitioners' knowledge of, and adherence to, evidence-based guidelines in the primary care management of dementia (Eccles et al, 1997) and family carers' satisfaction with primary care and knowledge about dementia and available services. RESULTS: To date, 83 GPs, 19 nurses, and 110 family carers representing 20 practices have been recruited into the study. The mean age of GPs is 37 with 61% male. Nurses are all female with an average age of 44 years. Most family carers are female and on average 66 years of age. The paper will present a wide range of baseline data findings for GPs, nurses, and family carers, including family carers' experience and satisfaction with primary care, and GPs' and nurses' knowledge of dementia, recommended guidelines, and available services for people with dementia and their families. CONCLUSION: The educational intervention is expected to improve practitioners' dementia care knowledge and behavior, and family carers' satisfaction with care and dementia knowledge. Baseline results will be discussed with reference to previous work in this area, and in the context of implications for evidencing change in outcome measures due to the intervention.

Dementia Care Partnerships between Primary Care Physicians and Local Alzheimer's Association Chapters.

Richard H. Fortinsky (University of Connecticut Center on Aging, Farmington, CT, USA).

PURPOSE: This presentation summarizes two interventions to improve the capacity of primary care physicians and family caregivers to manage persons with dementia. Both interventions feature partnerships between primary care physicians and local chapters of the Alzheimer's Association in Ohio and Connecticut, USA. >METHOD: In the Ohio study, 29 physicians referred 59 family caregivers to a care coordinator at the local Alzheimer's Association chapter. The care coordinator designed individualized care plans for families, and shared care plans and follow-up information with referring physicians. Outcomes included family caregivers' self-efficacy for managing dementia, and physicians' satisfaction with and knowledge of community-based services. The ongoing Connecticut study, a randomized >trial with similar intervention and outcomes, includes 68 primary care physicians in 43 sites. Physicians randomized to the intervention group will refer 100 family caregivers to a care coordinator at the local Alzheimer's Association chapter; 100 family caregivers will receive usual care from physicians randomized to the control group. RESULTS: In the Ohio study, family caregivers reported a statistically significant increase in self-efficacy for managing dementia from pre-intervention to post-intervention measurement points. Participating physicians reported increased satisfaction with, and knowledge of, community services. Complete results will be presented from the Ohio study; baseline results from the Connecticut study. CONCLUSION: The Ohio study yielded promising results, suggesting that partnerships between primary care physicians and local Alzheimer's Association chapters could benefit physicians and family caregivers. The Connecticut study is employing a more rigorous evaluation design to further test this intervention.

Educational Issues in the Recognition and Management of Dementia in Primary Care

Iliffe S, Wilcock J, Walters K, Rait G (Primary Care, RFUCLMS, London, England), Downs M (Bradford Dementia Group, University of Bradford, England), Turner S, Bryan M (University of Stirling, Scotland)

PURPOSE: The early diagnosis and continuing management of dementia challenge primary care practitioners. The best approach to enhancing professional skills is not yet known, but is being tested in a trial ofeducational interventions in Great Britain. METHOD: A core curriculum for dementia training was developed from evidence-based guidelines by a multi-disciplinary group. A review of the literature on professional learning identified three approaches to promoting professional knowledge and skill with potential, and these were developed as training packages, validated and field tested for acceptability. RESULTS: The three packages are: a workbook and training schedule for small group learning; a decision support system inserted into the electronicmedical record, for use during consultations; and an electronic tutorial on a CDRom, for individual study. Excerpts from these packages will be demonstrated. CONCLUSION: A core curriculum for training primary care professionals in the early diagnosis and continuing management of dementia can be developed and expressed as different educational packages, guided by adult-learning principles. The three packages are currently the subject of a randomised trial to test their impact on professional practice.

Sharing the Diagnosis of Dementia: What do General Practitioners say and Whom do they Inform?

S. Cahill, (Dementia Services Information and Development Centre, Dublin, Ireland)

PURPOSE: This study was designed to explore approaches used by general practitioners (GPs) in diagnosing and managing dementia. Method: A self-administered questionnaire was mailed to a sample of GPs (N=198) who belonged to the Aged Care Assessment Team's database, at an Australian (Brisbane) city hospital. A total of 101 GPs agreed to participate in the study, yielding a response rate of 51%. RESULTS: Findings demonstrate that while most respondents considered dementia diagnosis a GP responsibility, more than half failed to use standardised assessment tools such as the MMSE or Clock Drawing Test. Most GPs competently identified the diagnostic features of dementia, however, findings showed a wide variation in practice regarding the type and amount of information disclosed at diagnosis, and to whom this information was conveyed. Some GPs reported focussing on broad non-specific discussions about prognosis and future care planning, while others reported talking more frankly about Alzheimer's Disease, related dementias and their aetiology. A large minority stated they avoided using words like "dementia" or "Alzheimer's Disease", talking instead about memory and problem behaviours, brain atrophy and ageing. GPs readily identified problems encountered when attempting to diagnose dementia; nearly half reported they would welcome post-graduate training in this area. CONCLUSION: This research expands on earlier Australian work (Brodaty et al, 1994) by reporting on the medical and non-medical services recommended by GPs at diagnosis, and how dementia information is communicated by medical practitioners to patients and their principal caregivers. Plans for designing interventions to address study findings will be discussed.

SESSION 89

Age-Related Bone Loss in Normal Population of Ukraine: Data of Ultrasound Bone Densitometry

V. V. Povoroznjuk

Bone tissue state in the residents of Ukraine, subjects of both sexes, was studied. The total of 1866 persons (1364 women and 502 men; 2089 years old) were included. The heel bone examinations were performed by means of an ultrasound bone densitometer "Achilles+" (Lunar Corp, Madison, WI). The speed of sound (SOS, m/s), broadband ultrasound attenuation (BUA, dB/MHz) and a calculated "Stiffness" index (SI, %) were measured. It was found out that the ultrasound parameters characterizing state of spongy bone tissue, and its density decrease after 45 years old in women and after 70 years old in men SI lower than the fracture threshold was found in: 2,4% men; 13,4% women in age group of 5059 years; 9,6% men; 24,6% women in age group of 6069; 22,6% men; 50,0% women in age group of 7079 years, 20,1% men; 53,3% women in age group of 8089 years. Thus, while aging the ultrasound parameters characterizing bone tissue state decrease significantly and number of the examined with indices lower than the fracture threshold increases

Calcaneum ultrasound bone measurement in a geriatric long stay department

N. Schwald, Y. Boudali, A. Chahwakilian, S. Debray-Meignan

This study includes 117 patients (mean age : 86,7 years) living in a long stay department. The evaluation of bone mineral density was based on calcaneum ultrasound measurement. The studied parameters were : age, weight, physical activity, hemiplegia or not, diagnosis known to affect bone metabolism (i.e. hyperthyroidism ...), medications and osteoporosis traitements. The biology of the calcium metabolism, the nutritionnal balance, and the thyroid activity were noted. Hip, vertebral or limb fractures were searched. Then 12 monthes later, we noted patients with new fractures. The 18 valid patients (group V)(13%) with no fracture nor hemiplegia history had a higher bone density than the other ones (group A): right T score of group V : -1,89 versus A : -2,87, p<0,0008 ; left T score group V : -2,19 versus A - 2,85, p<0,002. The 27 patients (23%) with one or two hip fracture had a lower bone density (T score : -3,34, p<0,0001) than valid patients. It was similar for the 40 patients (33%) who had at least one limb fracture (T score : -3,56, p<0,0001). The 16 patients with left hemiplegia (13,6%) had a lower bone density on the stroke side (T score : -3,56, p<0,0001) ; the results was different with right hemiplegia. Four patients (3,4%) had suffering a new fracture during the next year ; they had a lower bone density than the others patients (right T score : -3,55, p<0,005 ; left T score: -3,67, p<0,008). The results showed a low bone density in case of fracture or hemiplegia with a difference between the side of stroke. Ultrasound measurement could make a simple evaluation of bone density in elderly people.

Determinants of bone loss at the femoral neck in elderly Japanese women. JPOS Cohort Study

M. Iki , A. Morita, Y. Ikeda, H. Aihara, A. Yura (Knki U Schl Med, Osaka-Sayama, Japan), S. Kagamimori (Toyama Med Pharmac U), Y. Kagawa (Kagawa Nutr U), T. Matsuzaki (Inst Comprehens Com Hlth Care), H. Yoneshima (Kasukabe-Shuuwa Hosp) and F. Marumo (Tokyo Med Dent U) (for JPOS Study Group)

PURPOSE: To clarify determinants of bone loss at the femoral neck in elderly Japanese women. METHODS: In Japanese Population-based Osteoporosis (JPOS) cohort study, we selected 1,850 women aged 15 to 79 years randomly from 3 municipalities located north, middle and south parts of Japan. The baseline study and the follow-up study which was conducted 3 years after the baseline comprised bone density measurement by dual-energy X-ray absorptiometry at the spine, hip (QDR4500A, Hologic Inc, USA) and distal forearm (pDXA, Norland/Stratec, USA/Germany), and interviews on medical history and on various lifestyle factors including smoking, drinking, exercise and diet habits. RESULTS: Among 1,628 women who underwent the baseline study, 1,285 (78.9%) completed the follow-up study. In 10-year age grouping, the greatest bone losses at the spine and forearm were observed in the subjects with age 50-59 at baseline. At the femoral neck, however, the greatest loss occurred in those with age 70-79. We examined which biological or lifestyle factors affected the bone loss at the femoral neck in this age-group of subjects. We found that the subjects with heavier weight, higher physical activities, and greater intakes of milk and fermented soy beans (natto in Japanese), and without smoking habit showed smaller bone loss at the femoral neck. CONCLUSION: To prevent hip fracture through reducing bone loss at the femoral neck, we recommend the elderly women not to lose weight, not to smoke, to be active in life and to take more milk and natto.

Hormonal status and its relationships with bone mineral density and bone turnover markers in women.

Blain H 1, Vuillemin A 2,3, Guillemin F 2, De Talance N 4, Doucet B 5, Durant R1, Jeandel C1 (1 Antonin Balmès Gerontology Center, Montpellier, France; 2 Faculty of Sport, Nancy, France ; 3 School of Public Health, UPRES EA 1124, Faculty of Medecine, Nancy, France; 4 Laboratoire de biologie cellulaire, Explorations fonctionnelles métaboliques, CHU-Brabois, Vandoeuvre-les-Nancy, France ; 5 Laboratoire central de chimie, Hôpital central, Nancy, France).

PURPOSE: The study's aim is to determine across different aged women the interrelationships between hormonal and growth factors serum level, bone turnover markers and femoral neck, lumbar spine and total body bone Mineral density (BMD). METHOD: The relationships between bone turnover markers and hormonal factors, measured by radioimmunoassay, and femoral neck, lumbar spine and total body BMD, measured by dual energy x-ray absorptiometry, were studied in univariate and multivariate regression models in 196 women aged 18 to 90 (56.0 ± 18.4 years). RESULTS: Leptin was significantly correlated with bone alkaline phosphatases, osteocalcine and urinary cross-laps and independently of age and menopause associated with total body, femoral and spine BMD. Estradiol was significantly positively correlated with total body and lumbar spine BMD and with bone alkaline phosphatases, osteocalcine. Estradiol and lumbar spine BMD relation disapeared when leptine was introduced in the logistic model. DHEA and IGF-I were positively correlated with BMD at the 3 sites (p<0.001) disapearing with age-adjustment. After age-adjustment, osteocalcin and urinary Cross-Laps were significantly negatively associated with total body BMD, femoral neck BMD and lumbar spine BMD. CONCLUSION : leptin is positively and independently associated with BMD. Estradiol level appears positively correlated with total body and lumbar spine BMD and negatively with markers of bone remodeling, the relation between estradiol and lumbar spine BMD being due partly to leptine. Correlation between DHEA, IGF-I and BMD is explained by their age-related decline. Osteocalcin and cross-laps appear as potential markers of osteoporosis.

Iranian menopausal women's life style and osteoprosis

Shayesteh Jahanfar(Iran University of Medical Science; National Research Centre for Reproductive Health, Deputy Research Ministry of Health), Fahimeh Ramezani Tehrnai(Gazvin University), Mehdi Sadat-Hashemi(Tarbiat Modaress University)

Purpose: To obtain early and late meopusal complications of menopausal women. Method: Using cluster sampling, 435 subjects were interviewed at their home. A standard questionnaire was filed out and they were sent to Bone Mas Densitometry. Results: The results suggests that the level of calcium intake is a 1/3rd of westeners. Exercise is not a major part of an Iranian women's life style. Mild to moderate osteoprosis was found to be relatively high in copmparison with other studies. Femoral and vertebral osteoprosis were found to be associated with duration of reproductive age, number of children, calcium intake, and the pattern of exercie.

The relationship between diabetic osteoporosis and the biochemical markers of bone metabolism in the elderly

You Chuanyi, Chen Fan, Wu Shufen

Objective: In order to investigate the mechanism of diabetic osteoporosis the bone mineral density and bone metabolic biochemical markers in diabetes in the elderly were measured. Methods: The bone mineral density using dual-energy X-ray absorptiometry was observed in the 55 cases of type II diabetes. Serum bone special alkaline phosphatase (B-ALP), Osteocalcin (BGP), Tartrate resistant acid phosphatase (TRAP), pyridinoline (Pyr) and deoxypyridinoline (D-Pyr) level were measured by ELISA methods. Results: In comparison with control group, the level of serum B-ALP and BGP were normal ($p<0.001$). Conclusions: The manifestations of abnormal bone metabolism in diabetes were low bone formation and increase of bone resorption. These changes are earlier than the onset of osteoporosis. So the biochemical markers of bone metabolism are more sensitive in predicting osteoporosis.

SESSION 90

A Study of Health Care Patterns in Elderly with HIV in Nakhon Pathom Province, Thailand

R. Sasitorn & C. Kannikar (Faculty of Nursing, Christian College, Nakhon Pathom, Thailand)

The purpose of this ethnographic study was to explore, describe and interpret individual understanding of HIV infection and the perception of health and patterns of health care in HIV patients in Nakhon Pathom province, Thailand. Data collection involved formal and informal interviews, and field notes. Since not many elderly have HIV infection only four people gave their consent to join in this study as 'informants'. Data was analyzed by using content analysis. The elderly indicated that having HIV carried a stigma in society. They identified their health as good or bad according to their signs and symptoms. They used both modern medicine and alternative treatments to make them get better. It was found that being optimistic helped them cope with the illness. The patterns of care in those patients were similar in all the subjects. They changed their health behavior especially concerning food, avoiding seafood, bamboo shoot, and mushrooms. Besides, they gave special care to their skin because the skin changes would make other people know of their illness. In addition, they had more rest, enough exercise, tried to put their mind at peace, and monitored their changes of illness in order to see a doctor before their condition deteriorated. In conclusion, they admitted that they would follow those patterns of care to keep their health good and to be able to enjoy the rest of their lives.

An Information Sheet on HIV/AIDS and Aging

Michael MacLean (Faculty of Social Work, University of Regina, Regina, Saskatchewan, Canada) and Chris Clapp (Canadian Association on Gerontology, Ottawa, Ontario, Canada)

The purpose of this presentation is to highlight the issue of HIV/AIDS with people aged 50 and over who have the disease and for people aged 60 and over who are caring for people with the disease by showing how an Information Sheet on the topic was developed. The goal of the Information Sheet is to outline challenges faced by older adults infected with HIV/AIDS and to help older adults who are caregivers of those infected with HIV/AIDS. This Information Sheet was developed from considering the literature on the topic of HIV/AIDS and aging, having a questionnaire completed by several Canadian AIDS Service Organizations (ASOs) and organizing a workshop on the topic at a national conference on HIV/AIDS to develop recommendations for older adults, family members, friends , health care and social service providers and volunteers on how to meet the challenges related to HIV/AIDS and aging. The results of this consultation on this topic is an Information Sheet that considers general issues, health issues, myths and realities about aging, unique challenges faced by older adults with HIV/AIDS such as social support, housing, income, education and prevention, and the challenges that older caregivers for people with HIV/AIDS have to face. The Information Sheet concludes with several recommendations about how to meet the challenges of HIV/AIDS and aging.

Assets and Needs of Older Hiv-Affected Caregivers

Cynthia Cannon Poindexter [Boston University School of Social Work, Boston, MA, USA]

purpose: This qualitative study explored the assets and needs of 7 older HIV-affected caregivers in Boston to determine their lived experiences. methods: Two open-ended interviews were conducted with 7 older HIV-affected caregivers in the Boston area between February and September of 1998. Although specific questions about their needs and assets were not asked during the interviews, analysis of the data through grounded theory principles generated this framework. results: It appears that the stresses and blessings are often two sides of the same coins. For example, family is both a strength and a need; the reciprocity with the adult or child with HIV is both a joy and a burden; when they have services it's a help; when they don't, it's a problem; they had some extraordinary emotional resources, but also faced some incredible emotional pressures; and their coping was helped if they and their family members went public and fought for justice; yet stigma, ignorance, and discrimination took a toll. conclusion: When allowed to tell their stories in an unstructured ways, elderly HIV-affected caregivers describe the burdens and joys of caregiving in similar terms. Researchers, advocates, and practitioners should recognize that the experiences of caregivers are contextual and complex. Formal supports should be developed and offered to help them maximize their existing resources and minimize their challenges.

HIV in Older Adults: Its Transmission, Prevention and Impact on Those Living with the Disease

Jane P. Fowler [National Association on HIV Over Fifty, Kansas City, MO, USA]

Abstract: PURPOSE: To call attention to the fact that the Human Immunodeficiency Virus (HIV) does exist in the aging community; to explain how HIV impacts older adults in ways that differ from their younger counterparts; to discuss the need for dissemination of accurate information to elders on transmission and prevention of HIV. METHOD: In this presentation, the speaker a 65-year-old retired journalist will share her personal story, summarizing the turn of events that transformed her from press interviewer into media interviewee, from private person to public activist for the issue of HIV/AIDS in older adults. As co-chairperson of the National Association on HIV Over Fifty (NAHOF), she will describe her work as a public spokesperson and educator, imparting information on the subject of the virus as it relates to elders.<?xml:namespace prefix = o ns = "urn:schemas-microsoft-com:office:office" />RESULTS: Session participants will learn that, in the United States, 11 to 15 percent of the AIDS cases are in people over age 50 and those figures are expected to rise as infected persons of all ages survive longer due to treatment advances; that older adults are not generally perceived as being at risk for HIV because of the myth that they are no longer sexually active; that adults aging with HIV are often invisible, isolated and ignored. CONCLUSION: It is imperative that the aging community and its health care and social service providers be educated about the impact of HIV/AIDS in elders in order to reduce the incidence of the virus and improve care and treatment for those already infected.

HIV/AIDS and the Older Adult: Access to Medical and Social Services

Teresa Fritsch (Simon Fraser University, Vancouver, British Columbia, Canada)

Purpose: A qualitative comparison of experiences with accessing HIV/AIDS related medical and social services and perceptions of service requirements was conducted with men and women aged 30 to 65. It was expected that older adults experience difficulty accessing services compared to younger adults and that service availability for their age group was limited. Methodology: Individuals participating in the one-on-

one interviews were recruited via flyers and posters located within supporting HIV/AIDS service organizations. Results: Older adults (50+) indicated sufficient access to, and positive experiences with accessing medical and social services noting that HIV and aging stereotypes had little influence on access. More than half proposed the need for targeted medical services indicating that none were in place. Although realizing benefits in mixed age support groups, most older adults indicated the need for age specific, yet non-traditional social programming currently lacking. Individuals 30-49 also reported positive experiences with accessing medical and social services. More than half of those 40-49 but less than half of those 30-39 felt medical services should target individuals 50+ specifically. All participants between 30-49 indicated the need to target social programs to older adults however, only half of the 30-39 group felt that social programming should be different from other age group social programming. Conclusion: Older and younger adults did not differ in their ability to access HIV/AIDS related medical and social services. As age increased from 30 to 65, a greater need to provide both medical and social services specific to the older adult was indicated.

Stigma as experienced by grandmothers raising HIV-positive grandchildren

Cynthia Cannon Poindexter [Boston University School of Social Work, Boston, Massachusetts, USA]

Purpose: The purpose of the qualitative study was to ascertain how stigma is experienced by grandmothers who are raising HIV-positive grandchildren Methods: Eight grandmothers in Chicago and Boston who are raising HIV-infected grandchildren participated in open ended interviews which generated qualitative data. Using the framework of associative stigma, internalized stigma, and stigma management, the presenter highlights the voices of the research respondents and draws implications for gerontologists, child care workers, HIV professionals and health care providers. Results: Findings were that disclosure, confidentiality, and trust of formal services are profound concerns for grandparents who are raising HIV-positive and HIV-affected children. Stigma has implications for the caregivers which are personal, and interpersonal, and socio-political. Unlike their peers who are caring for relatives with less stigmatized conditions, HIV-related elder surrogate parents are highly vulnerable to secrecy, shame, isolation, complicated grief, and stigma, which contributes to emotional stress and isolation Conclusion: Grandmothers not only manage stigma, they rise above it. There is a mixture of ageism and AIDS phobia which creates an atmosphere of isolation, invisibility, and discrimination for the population of HIV-affected grandparents. They are being neglected both by the Aging Service network and the AIDS Service network. In order to right this gap, practitioners, policy-makers, and researchers need to highlight the realities of HIV-affected grandmothers and help to lessen the stigma which keeps them hidden.

SESSION 91

Access to care: the impact of disability, health infrastructure, and social characteristics of the neighborhood

Joan F. Van Nostrand, DPA (Office of Rural Health Policy; U. S. Dept. of Health and Human Services, Rockville, USA)

While much is known about the impact of personal characteristics and health infrastructure on the access of older persons (65+) to health care, little is known about the impact of the neighborhood. This research examines the impact of disability and other personal characteristics, the U. S. health care infrastructure, and the social structure of the neighborhood on access to health care. The data source was the 1994 National Health Interview Survey. Problems with access were defined as needing but not receiving medical, dental or mental health care; prescription drugs; or eyeglasses. The survey was geocoded by adding information on block groups (neighborhoods) to match to the 1990 census to obtain data about the social characteristics of the neighborhood. Logistic regression, using SUDAAN and controlling for age, gender, and race, was conducted. Older persons with increased risk of access problems were those with severe disability, in poverty, without private insurance to supplement government-funded insurance (Medicare), and in non-metropolitan areas. Low physician to population ratios did not increase the risk. Older persons at lower risk of access problems lived in neighborhoods with a greater concentration of elderly and a common ancestry, ethnicity, or heritage. These results suggest that strategies to improve access to care should look beyond the physician-patient-family relationship and toward the community. Building inter-disciplinary collaboration between physicians and key community stakeholders of social and advocacy organizations is a strategy that can improve access and, thereby, the health of older persons.

Encouraging Elders to Stay in Their Own Home and Community: The Israeli Experience

Tamar Paltiel, RN, BA, MPH, [Assistant of the National Head Nurse of Public Health Services, Ministry of Health, Jerusalem, Israel]

Keeping elders in their own home and neighborhood, as long as they can carry on their normal life, is known to be the most appropriate elderly care policy. To meet this goal the Israeli legislator has adopted the long-term care insurance law. The implementation of this 1988 law is carried out by nationwide government employed community health nurses. They conduct a personal assessment at the elderly person's home. Standard, well-defined, structured assessment procedures guarantee that the services are provided on equitable basis. Community Health nurses have been chosen to conduct the assessment because: 1. They are familiar with the needs of the older population, and are used to recognizing their needs. 2. They are well aware of the possible alternatives within the family and the community such as day clubs, or supportive organizations. Thus, nurses are able to suggest most adequate solutions for the person and his family. 3. The Community Nurses are not associated with agencies that provide the home care service. Hence no conflict of interests may exist. Eligibility entitles the elder assistance by nurse aid in his/her ADL paid for by the National Insurance Institute. The law, the tests and evaluation carried out by the public health nurses and the actual nurse aid support resulted in: 1. Fewer families request for hospitalization of their elderly family member in nursing homes. 2. Improvement in the quality of life of the eligible elder able to stay in his/her own home and community.

Housing for an Aging Population: Planning Implications (HAPPI)

V. Burholt (Centre for Social Policy Research and Development, University of Wales, Bangor, UK), J. Clifford-Jones (Age Concern, Caernarfon, Gwynedd, UK), K. Doughty (Technology in HealthCare, Menai Bridge, Gwynedd, UK), P. Elliston (Institute of Medical and Social Care Research, University of Wales, Bangor, UK), E. Evans (Department of Housing and Public Protection, Caernarfon, Gwynedd Council, UK), A. Lloyd-Jones (Social Services for the Elderly, Caernarfon, Gwynedd Council, UK), E. Owen (Care and Repair, Penygroes, Gwynedd, UK), R. Tudor-Edwards (Institute of Medical and Social Care Research, University of Wales, Bangor, UK), G. Windle, (Centre for Social Policy Research and Development, University of Wales, Bangor, UK).

This paper reports on a study entitled Housing for an Aging Population: Planning Implications (HAPPI) which examines the housing needs and preferences of the aging population in Gwynedd, UK. The study aims to predict levels and types of housing required at the beginning of this century and the impact that this would have on community social and health care. It compares the perspectives of people age 70+ (N=500) with the preferences of people aged 50-60 (N=50). The sample was drawn from a diverse range of areas: a dispersed farming community, a retirement destination, an ex-quarrying community, an urban area, a concentration of difficult to let sheltered housing and a market town. Quantitative data were collected for respondents aged 70 and over, through the administration of a structured interview schedule. The quantitative data includes the opinions, attitudes and choices of a broad range of Gwynedd residents regarding housing and services. Qualitative data were collected for respondents aged 50-60 through the administration of vignettes. These were structured in order to fit the personal situation, or perceived future situation of the respondents. Given that we knew that most people would respond that they desire to age in place, the key question in the in-depth interviews was What changes in personal circumstances would force you to consider leaving your home? The data for the two age groups are compared to show the differences between housing preferences of people aged 70 and over and people aged 50-60.

Living Environment, Self-image, and Self-esteem Among Older Persons in Different Housing Types in Hong Kong

Oi-ling SIU, Gemma Wong (Lingnan University, Hong Kong)

PURPOSE: The purpose of the study is to investigate the relationship between living environment, self-image and self-esteem among older persons living in different types of housing in Hong Kong. METHOD: A face-to-face interview methodology using a structured questionnaire was adopted for the study. The questionnaire consists of sections measuring living environment (14 items on satisfaction of size, design of environment, living arrangement, complexity and other people), self-image (6 items from Chow & Kwan [1985]), and self-esteem (10- item Rosenberg's Self-Esteem Scale). A total of 60 older persons (12 females, 48 males; 58 aged above 60 years old) with 34 living in private housing and 26 in bed spaces (called "caged housing") in an old urban district in Hong Kong were interviewed. The interviews were conducted by the same interviewer, with the presence of one of his friends, during all the interview processes. RESULTS: The results showed that satisfaction of living environment was statistically significantly related to self-image ($r=.50$, $p < .01$) and self-esteem ($r=.52$, $p < .01$) among the respondents. Furthermore, the respondents living in private housing scored statistically significantly higher in self-image ($t=8.33$, $p < .001$) and self-esteem ($t=6.07$, $p < .001$) than those living in bed spaces. CONCLUSION: Living environment and housing type are predictive of older persons' self-image and self-esteem in a Chinese sample in Hong Kong. These findings corroborate previous findings in Western societies.

Presenting An Alternative Person-Environment (P-E) Framework To The Lawton and Nahemow (1973) Ecological Model of Aging

Y. Cvitkovich, A. Wister (Simon Fraser University, British Columbia, Canada)

This paper presents a modified Person-Environment (P-E) framework to Lawton and Nahemow's (1973) Ecological Model of Aging. The principal contribution of our revised approach is measurement of older individuals' differential prioritization of key environmental domains. It is based on the assumption that well-being and adaptive behaviour is influenced to a greater degree by the person-environment balance or mismatch in those areas deemed more important by the individual. Using data (N= 174) drawn from a local study carried out in Vancouver, P-E fit is summed across several domains (structural environment, social support, and formal services) with domain scores weighted according to the participant's appraisal of priority of needs for maintaining well-being. Results from this research indicate that the prediction of well-being is significantly improved over that predicted by the Lawton and Nahemow model. The alternative framework plots the weighted subjective appraisal of P-E fit over time for research participants. The framework incorporates most of the features of the ecological model but nonetheless can be used with longitudinal research to determine changes in P-E fit and changes in priority of needs over time. This framework can be particularly useful as a planning and service allocation tool targeting seniors.

Some policy implications of very old people remaining in homes of their own

A. Tinker and J. Askham (King's College London, Age Concern Institute of Gerontology, London, England)

Abstract Purpose: This paper presents some policy implications of a study of very old (85+) people in the UK. The objective was to examine how some very old people remain in homes of their own, what enables them to do so and the circumstances in which they do so umproblematically or not. Method: The research consisted of secondary analyses of a number of large scale national data sets, including the Census, and qualitative interviews with 42 people aged 85 and over and their carers. Results: Currently 75% of people aged 85 and over live in homes of their own. Nearly all resist a move to an institution. Reasons include a strong desire for independence, control and continuity. Marital status plays a role and married people were found to be unlikely to be in an institution even if very old or ill. Important factors in enabling very old people to remain at home include their self perceptions of independence, the role of housing and the involvement of family members. Conclusion: Although generalisations are dangerous there a number of factors which need to be taken into account for future policies. These include changing family patterns, changes in housing tenure and the role of assistive technology. Policy implications include a rethinking of the role and costs of community care, consideration of their housing (including particularly the role of sheltered housing and adaptations), and primary health care, a need to support and acknowledge the role of professionals and families and an greater emphasis on preventive services

SESSION 92

Association of memory complaints, depression and life-events with cognitive change. The Longitudinal Aging Study Amsterdam

M.G.Dik (Vrije Universiteit, Institute for Research in Ex-tramural Medicine, Amsterdam, The Netherlands), H.Comijs (Vrije Universiteit, Department of Psychiatry, Amsterdam, The Netherlands), M.J.Aartsen (Vrije Universiteit, Faculty of Social Gerontology, Amsterdam, The Netherlands) and D.J.H.Deeg (Vrije Universiteit, Department of Psychiatry, Institute for Research in Ex-tramural Medicine, Amsterdam, The Netherlands),

ISSUE: Researchers in the field of cognitive aging agree that, on average, cognitive functioning declines with aging. However, major individual differences in rate and onset of decline are observed. The individual variability in cognitive change suggest that cognitive decline is not only determined by age, but also by other factors. The studies presented in this symposium focus on the influence of memory complaints, depression and stressful life-events on change in cognitive functioning, in a longitudinal sample of older adults in The Netherlands. STRUCTURE: This symposium will start with a short introduction by the convener, in which the general design of the Longitudinal Aging Study Amsterdam (LASA) will be presented. After this, four researchers of LASA will present their findings. After the presentations, the discussant Mike Martin (The German Center for Research on Aging, Heidelberg, Germany) will discuss the presented papers. CONTENT: Miranda Dik, focuses on the association of memory complaints with cognitive decline and the extent whether this association is affected by a biological risk factor (ApoE). She concludes that both memory complaints and ApoE independently predict cognitive decline. Hannie Comijs focuses on the association between the exposure to depression and cognitive decline in non-demented oder persons. She examines if duration of exposure and severity of depression are related to cognitive decline over a period of six years. The results suggests that depression is associated with decline in speed of information processing, but not with decline in memory function. Marja Aartsen presents a LISREL-model, used to estimate relationships among four different stressful life-events on cognitive functioning at follow-up. Severe illness of a relative was found to enhance maintenance of cognitive functioning, independent of the effect of depression. The positive effect was found only among respondents who had a confidant and/or a high level of mastery. More serious life events, such as death of partner or relatives, or illness of the partner did not affect cognitive functioning. Dorly Deeg presents some findings of the consequences of an airplane crash on the Bijlmer suburb on cognitive functioning and anxiety. Her conclusion is that although in older persons living in the area closest to the crash, changes in physical and emotional health over time are more unfavorable than in older persons living farther away, their cognitive functioning appeared to improve. CONCLUSION: On general, large individual differences in cognitive change were observed. Rate and onset of cognitive decline appeared to be the result of a complexity of influencing factors, such as memory complaints, depression and stressful life-events.

Contrasting changes in emotional and cognitive functioning after the air plane crash on the Bijlmer suburb

D.J.H. Deeg (Vrije Universiteit, Department of Psychiatry, Institute for Research in Extramural Medicine, Amsterdam, The Netherlands), A Huizink (Institute for Research in Extramural Medicine, Amsterdam, The Netherlands), C Jonker (Vrije Universiteit, Department of Psychiatry, Institute for Research in Extramural Medicine, Amsterdam, The Netherlands), A.T.F. Beekman (Vrije Universiteit, Department of Psychiatry, Amsterdam, The Netherlands)

PURPOSE In October 1992, an air plane crashed into a high rise apartment building in the Bijlmer suburb of Amsterdam. This study focuses on intra-individual changes in physical and mental health in relation to residen-tial distance from the crash. METHOD Data from the Longitudinal Aging Study Amsterdam (initial ages 55-85 years) include one pre-crash (t0) and two post-crash observation cycles (t1, t2). Three groups are distinguished: those living within a radius of 1 km from the crash (initial n=34), those living 1 to 2 km from the crash (initial n=64), and those living in the rest of the city of Amsterdam (initial n=968). Data on physical health, including self-reports of functional ability, are availa-ble for all three cycles. Measures on anxiety symp-toms, and test-based cognitive perform-ance are avail-able for the two post-crash cycles. RESULTS Participation in the follow-up cycles was lower in the 1 km group (t1: 71%, t2: 47%) than in the other groups (t1: 81%, t2: 66%), which was partly explained by a raised mortality in the 1 km group. Moreover, functional ability showed a greater decline from t1-t2 in the 1 km group. Those without functional limitations in the 1 km group showed a relatively great increase in anxiety. By contrast, fluid intelligence which was stable in the other groups showed an increase in the 1 km group. Also, in those without functional limitations, information proces-sing speed which declined in the other groups did not decline in the 1 km group. CONCLUSION Although in older persons living in the area closest to the crash, changes in physical and emotional health over time are more unfavorable than in older persons living farther away, their cognitive functioning appeared to improve.

Memory complaints and ApoE add to the rate of cognitive decline in cognitively normal elderly

M.G. Dik, C. Jonker, H.C. Comijs, L.M. Bouter, J.W.R. Twisk (Vrije Universiteit, Amsterdam, The Netherlands), G.J. van Kamp (Vrije Universiteit Medical Centre, Amsterdam, The Netherlands), D.J.H. Deeg (Vrije Universiteit, Amsterdam, The Netherlands).

PURPOSE: This study in cognitively intact elderly, selected from a population-based study, investigates to what extent subjective memory complaints and Apolipoprotein E (ApoE) predict future cognitive decline, evaluating their separate as well as their combined effects. METHOD: We selected 1,562 subjects, aged 62-85 years, with no obvious cognitive impairment at baseline (Mini-Mental State Examination>24) from the Longitudinal Aging Study Amsterdam (LASA). Memory complaints and ApoE phenotypes were assessed at baseline. We studied cognitive decline using the Mini-Mental State Examination (MMSE), the Auditory Verbal Learning Test (memory: immediate and delayed recall) and the Coding Task (information processing speed). Follow-up data were collected after 3 and 6 years. Data were analyzed with Generalized Estimating Equations (GEE), adjusted for age, sex, education and depression. RESULTS: Baseline memory complaints were reported by 26.3% of the cognitively intact elderly. Overall, 26.2% were carrier of at least one ApoE E4 allele. Memory complaints were significantly associated with a greater rate of decline on all cognitive measures, except on immediate recall. Also, ApoE E4 carriers showed a greater rate of decline on MMSE and information processing speed after 6 years. The effects of both memory complaints and ApoE were additive, with an almost two times higher decline compared to subjects without both factors. CONCLUSION: Both memory complaints and ApoE E4 predict cognitive decline at an early stage. This implies that subjective memory complaints are well-founded and that they should be taken seriously, especially in elderly with ApoE E4 since they carry an additional risk.

The association between the exposure to depression and cognitive decline in non-demented elder persons.

Hannie C. Comijs, Sandra W. Geerlings, Aartjan T.F. Beekman (Institute for Research in Extramural Medicine, Vrije Universiteit, Amsterdam, The Netherlands)

PURPOSE: Studies on the relationship between depression and cognitive decline have shown varying results. We examined if duration of exposure and severity of depression are related to cognitive decline in a six year follow-up period. METHOD: The study is based on a sample of 327 depressed and 325 non-depressed older persons from the Longitudinal Aging Study Amsterdam. Depression was assessed by means of the Center for Epidemiological Studies Depression scale (CES-D) in eight successive waves. Cognitive functioning was assessed with the Mini-Mental State Examination (MMSE), the Coding Task and Rey's Auditory Verbal Learning Test (AVLT). RESULTS: In our sample of non-demented persons 45% was not depressed at baseline and did not become depressed in the subsequent tree years, 20% had a changeable course of depression and in 18% the depression was chronic. No associations were found between the course of depression and subsequent cognitive decline. An association was found between severity of depression (high mean-score on CES-D) and decline in information processing speed. No such associations were found with the MMSE and AVLT. The Coding Task measures information processing speed, but includes components of memory. Therefore it is a sensitive measurement for cognitive decline. However, as we found no association with decline in memory performance our findings does not suggest global cognitive decline but an isolated decline in information processing speed. CONCLUSIONS: The interpretation of our results may be that depression and decline in information processing speed share a common underlying central nervous-system disorder, such as subcortical white matter pathology.

The role of resistance resources in the relation between stressful life-events and cognitive change

Marja J. Aartsen (Vrije Universiteit, Faculty of Social Gerontology / LASA, Amsterdam, The Netherlands), Carolien H.M. Smits (Trimbos Institute, Utrecht, The Netherlands) and Theo van Tilburg (Vrije Universiteit, Faculty of Social Gerontology /LASA).

PURPOSE: Stressful life-events have been found to increase feelings of depression. Depression may negatively affect cognitive functioning. Thus, a negative effect of stressful life-events on cognitive functioning is to be expected. However, some studies observed that stressful life-events resulted in higher levels of cognitive functioning. It may be that resistance resources (i.e. having a confidant, high level of mastery) play a role in this relationship. METHOD: The study is based on 759 married adults, aged 62-85 years at baseline, participating in LASA. Four stressful life-events were selected; severe illness of relatives, severe illness of the partner, death of one or more relatives and death of the partner. Cognitive functioning was assessed with the 15 Words Task and Raven's Colored Progressive Matrices. Depression was assessed on the symptom level with the Center for Epidemiologic Studies Depression Scale. A Structural

Equation Model was developed to test the effect of life-events on cognitive functioning three years later, taking into account the effect of baseline cognitive functioning, depression, and resistance resources. RESULTS: Severe illness of a relative was found to enhance maintenance of cognitive functioning, independent of the effect of depression. The positive effect was found only among respondents who had a confidant and/or a high level of mastery. More serious life events, such as death of partner or relatives, or illness of the partner did not affect cognitive functioning. CONCLUSION: Seriousness of life-events and resistance resources partly determine whether life-events affect cognitive functioning.

SESSION 93

Changes in the Prevalence of Dementia in the U.S. Age 65 and Older Population from 1982 to 1999

E. H. Corder, K. G. Manton (Center for Demographic Research, Duke University, Durham, NC, U.S.A.)

Background. We examined changes from 1982 to 1999 in the prevalence of severe dementia in the U.S. population aged 65+. The data used were from the five National Long Term Care Surveys conducted in 1982, 1984, 1989, 1994, and 1999. Each survey was a nationally representative population sample. Surviving subjects were included in subsequent surveys along with newly selected subjects. The same survey instruments, sample design and field methods were employed each year. Methods. Dementia prevalence rates for 1982, 1994, and 1999 were calculated by summing the sample weights for the demented subjects and dividing by the size of the age 65+ population for that year. Tests for trend were conducted using t-tests of changes in proportions over time. Results. In absolute terms the number of severely demented persons declined from 1.3 to 0.9 million persons - a highly significant decline, from 4.7 to 2.5 percent of the U.S. elderly population (t-test = -11.6). A larger numerical decline, from 1.4 to 0.9 million persons, was found adjusting the 1982 age structure to that in 1999. The age standardized 1982 rate of 5.25% would predict a total of 1.9 million cases for the larger 1999 population instead of the 0.9 million found. Conclusion. The dramatically lower prevalence of severe dementia in 1999 compared to expectations based on the 1982 rates has profound implications for the levels and types of long-term care services which will be used in the U.S, especially of intensive nursing home care, in the future.

Cognitive profile in an elderly community-dwelling population

C. Osuna, P. Gil Gregorio, C.Garcia, P. López-Riquelme, C. Osuna, P. Alonso-Fernández and J.M. Ribera Casado.(Servicio de Geriatria,Hospital Clinico San Carlos,Madrid,Spain).

PURPOSE: To know the cognitive performance of a non-demented elderly community-dwelling population. METHODS: A prospective study door to door was carried out in a rural population. Subjects with dementia or any organic illness that could affect cognitive performance were excluded.The following data are collected: age, gender, years of education, illness and drugs used. Cognitive assessment was done using the cognitive section of CAMDEX (CAMCOG), Ribermead test and Forward and Backward Digit span. In all of these test appropriate cutoff were defined for cognitive impairment. Statistical analysis was performed with T-student-mean comparison test (Confidence interval 95%). Spss statistical software was used. RESULTS: 427 subjects (mean age 72.1±5.1,women 65.4%). MMSE: 26.8±1.7, MMSE<23: 14.1. CAMCOG: 77.8±5.9, CAMCOG >70: 20%. Ribermead: 7.5±2.5, Ribermead < 5: 25%. Forward digits: 4.9±1.1, Backward digits: 2.7±0.9. CONCLUSION: Twenty five percent of community-dwelling elderly have memory disorders.

Cumulative incidence of dementia and other mental symptoms related to formal support - a 25 years follow-up in a total cohort

G. Samuelsson, (Gerontology Research Centre, Lund, Sweden), G. Sundström, (Institute of Gerontology, Jönköping, Sweden), O. Dehlin, (Department of Community Medicine, Malmö, Sweden), B. Hagberg, (Gerontology Research Centre, Lund, Sweden).

PURPOSE: The overall purpose of the study was to analyze the aging process in terms of its medical, psychological and social components and to identify predictors of health, survival, well-being, and life satisfaction. METHOD: The study population was based on one entire cohort (N=192) persons of newly retired persons comprising all men and women born in 1902 and 1903 and living in a Primary Health Care district. All subjects went through an interview, psychological testing and a standardized medical examination. The sample has been followed since 1969 (from age 67) with eight examinations. Further all contacts and diagnoses from Primary Health Care as well as formal social support were registered. RESULTS: The cumulative incidence of dementia and other mental symptoms between 67 and 92 years of age for alive at age 92 and for persons dead before 92 showed that there was totally 61% without any mental diagnosis. Corresponding figures for persons with dementia diagnoses was 10.5% and persons with other type of mental symptoms was 23% and persons with a combination of dementia diagnoses and other mental diagnoses was 5%. There was no significant differences between survivors and dead persons regarding the different diagnose groups. Among the survivors at age 92 65% was mentally well, 18% had an dementia diagnose and 18% had other forms of mental disorders and none had an combination of dementia and other mental diagnoses. Formal support between 67 and 92 related mental disorders showed that persons with mental diagnoses including dementia were over-represented among those who got formal support comparing to mentally healthy persons. The frequencies of persons receiving home help and being relocated to institutions increased with age and the increase is specially strong for persons with mental diagnoses. However, as many as 37% among the demented did not receive any formal support during the 25 year period and more than 50% among the mentally healthy persons. Persons who only got home help were rare among demented. CONCLUSIONS: The incidence rate of other mental disorders then dementia were higher comparing to dementia during the 25-year period. Formal support was as expected much higher among persons with mental diagnoses. However, as many as 37% among the demented did not receive any formal support but was supported by the family.

Prevalence of Dementia and Mild Cognitive Impairment in Subjects 65 Years or Older in Mexico City. An Epidemiological Survey.

Gutiérrez-Robledo LM, Ostrosky F, Sánchez L, Juárez S, Villa A. (Instituto Nacional de Ciencias Médicas y Nutrición Salvador Zubirán *Facultad de Psicología Universidad Nacional Autónoma de México*

Main objective: Estimation of dementia and mild cognitive impairment (MCI) prevalence in the urban area of Mexico City in free living individuals 65 years or older. Methodology: A sample of 4,047 subjects was obtained through a two-stage cluster sampling design . The sample was obtained from the bureau of the census' 1995 population count. The sample was: tested for cognitive impairment with the Mini-Neuropsi instrument (Mexican version of the CASI), and the primary caregiver was asked to fill the Pfeffer test, they received the Brief Geriatric Depression Scale and were asked for socio-demographical information. Those who screened positive received a neuropsychological battery with the Neuropsy inventory (Ostrosky et al.), and a standardized clinical examination according to the CERAD clinical evaluation protocol including lab testing and CAT scan. A sub-sample of those screening negative also received the neuropsychological and clinical exam. Dementia was defined using two independent sets of diagnostic criteria. Final diagnosis was determined by a panel (neurologist, geriatrician and neuropsychologist). Results:The non-response rate was 12% and 3% were discarded according to elegibility criteria. Mean age was 72.4 years (72.3 males and 72.4 females) 32.6% were males. Mean number of years at school was 4.37 years. 48% were illiterate. Prevalence of cognitive impairment is

10.1% (dementia 3.9%, MCI 5.5%, depressive pseudodementia 0.7%). Prevalence of dementia and MCI increases with age and is higher in women. Alzheimer's disease represents 66 0f dementia cases, vascular dementia was recognized in 23% Parkinson's dementia in 2.5%, post-traumatic in 2.5% y alcoholic in 5.2%.

Reliability of the etiologic diagnosis of dementia in the elderly: agreement with neuropathology

Dina Zekry, MD; Charles Duyckaerts, PhD; Robert Moulias, MD; Joël Belmin, PhD; Jean-Jacques Hauw, MD Laboratoire de Neuropathologie Raymond Escourolle (Drs D. Zekry, C. Duyckaerts and J.-J. Hauw), Hôpital de la Salpêtrière, INSERM U 106 and 360, Association Claude Bernard, Pierre et Marie Curie University, Paris, France; Hôpital Charles Foix (R. Moulias), Ivry-sur-Seine, France and Hôpital René Muret (J. Belmin), Sevran, France.

Purpose: To examine the faculty of clinicians and the accuracy of clinical criteria to distinguish between Alzheimer's disease (AD), and vascular (VaD) or mixed dementia (MD). Methods: Prospective clinico-neuropathological study in hospitalized elderly patients. We studied 33 patients over 75, who had a clinical evaluation, in whom the criteria and scores of DSM III, NINCDS-ADRDA, Loeb and Gandolfo (Loeb), ADDTC, NINDS-AIREN, and the HIS were applied, and who were autopsied. We assessed the agreement between the pre-mortem diagnosis and the neuropathological diagnosis, considered as the gold standard. Results: The highest agreement was found between the Loeb and the HIS (K=0.92). and the lowest one between the clinical evaluation and the NINDS-AIREN (0.47). When comparing clinical criteria and neuropathology, the agreement was moderate for the HIS (0.50) and the Loeb score (0.43), substantial for the ADDTC (0.63) and the NINDS-AIREN (0.67). When excluding MD, the agreement between all clinical criteria and scores and the pathological diagnosis rose to 0.88 (almost perfect). The HIS was the most sensitive (0.89) and the NINDS-AIREN the most specific (0.86) for the diagnosis of VaD. All sets of clinical criteria significantly distinguished pure AD from VaD. In contrast, MD cases diagnosed pathologically had been classified as VaD in 50% by the HIS and the Loeb, 36% by the ADDTC and 22% by the NINDS-AIREN. Conclusion: Pure cases were diagnosed with high accuracy by all clinical criteria, and MD was underestimated. This may be of interest when clinical criteria are used for assessing the etiology of dementia.

The incidence of dementia in England and Wales

MRC Cognitive function and ageing study (www.mrc-bsu.cam.ac.uk/cfas) (Writing committee Fiona E Matthews, MRC Biostatistics Unit, Cambridge UK and Carol Brayne, Institute of Public Health, Cambridge UK)

PURPOSE: To estimate the incidence of dementia in a population based sample in England and Wales. METHODS: The Medical Research Council cognitive function and ageing study (MRC CFAS) is a multi-centre two-phase two-stage cohort study. One of its primary aims was the estimation of the incidence of dementia within a community setting. 13,004 individuals from five centres across the UK (Cambridge, Gwynedd – Wales, Newcastle-upon-tyne, Nottingham and Oxford) participated in interviews two years apart. At each wave more detailed interviews were undertaken of cognitively frail individuals and a random sample of all others, stratified by age 65-74 and 75 and over. The aim was to sample 2,500 individuals from each centre, and get more detailed cognitive information (including AGECAT organicity diagnosis) from 500 of these. RESULTS: Incidence of dementia by age shows the expected increase with male rates slightly lower than female rates. The rates increase almost exponentially from less than 10 per 1000 person-years per year in the youngest ages to more than 100 in the oldest old. The 10 fold increase seen is similar in both the men and the women. Not much variation is seen in rates in each of the five centres. CONCLUSION: Incidence of dementia is a substantial community problem within the oldest of our society despite their high mortality. The long term effects of the exponential increase seen will have increasing importance as old age becomes an increasingly achievable goal within society.

The prevalence of dementia among older people in long-term care institutions in Jerusalem, Israel

T. Dwolatzky, L. Feldman (Shaare Zedek Medical Center, Jerusalem, Israel), A.M. Clarfield (Herzog Hospital, Jerusalem, Israel and the Division of Geriatric Medicine, Sir Mortimer B. Davis- Jewish General Hospital, McGill University, Montreal, Canada) J. Brodsky, Y. King (JDC-Brookdale Institute of Gerontology, Jerusalem, Israel)

PURPOSE: Institutional care for the elderly in Israel is categorized according to the cognitive, functional, medical and nursing needs of the patient. There are homes for the independent and frail elderly, wards for nursing and skilled nursing care, and units for the cognitively impaired. The prevalence of dementia among the residents of these facilities is unknown. We studied the prevalence of dementia in long-term care institutions in Jerusalem to determine whether the services provided meet the needs of this group of patients. METHODS: A representative sample of residents in each type of facility was randomly chosen. A single physician (LF) examined all of the study patients, including history and physical examination, laboratory investigations, functional state and mental status examination (using 3MS questionnaire). RESULTS: A total of 311 patients were interviewed, representing 11.40f the 2716 residents in 34 institutions in the Jerusalem area. Among the study patients, the mean age was 83.9 years, and 75% were women. The diagnosis of dementia appeared in the medical records of 500f patients. However, 77cored less than 77 on the 3MS test (consistent with cognitive impairment). In the independent and frail departments, 58 0.000000ailed the 3MS, compared to 97 0n nursing wards, and 100 0n skilled nursing and mentally frail units. CONCLUSION: There is a high prevalence of dementia in long-term care institutions in Jerusalem. The majority of the residents of these institutions are cognitively impaired. This finding necessitates the restructuring of services for the institutionalized elderly in Jerusalem.

SESSION 94

Aging as Creative Reconstruction

Kenneth J. Gergen, (Swarthmore College, Swarthmore, Pennsylvania, USA); Mary M. Gergen, (Penn State University - Delaware County, Media, Pennsylvania, USA)

The metaphor of "aging as decline" is an unfortunate byproduct of a modernist worldview equating personal worth or value with production. More promising for the present century is a conception of aging as creative reconstruction. This first entails the positive reconstruction of the image of aging, as an alternative to the negative stereotypes long pervasive in western culture. Also entailed is the innovative reconstruction of the forms of life open to the aging population, as an alternative to the constricting modes of life and the disenchantment of the world currently invited by "maturity." And finally, required is the improvisational reconstruction of ongoing relationships, as an alternative to the fixed and routinized byproducts of convention. The major means to creative reconstruction are located within the realm of the arts. The arts are particularly rich in offering opportunities for experimenting with realities, with identities, with expressive potentials, and with relational possibilities. At the same time, however, "the arts" should not be circumscribed in terms of place and time, but rather, offer a mode of being that can be fully integrated into the normal activities of daily life. In effect, when aging is creative reconstruction, art and life converge.

SESSION 95

Role of Antioxidants in the Progress of Aging

Jim Joseph (Laboratory of Neuroscience, USDA-HNRC at Tufts University, Boston, USA) ("Fruit Polyphenolics, Brain Aging, and Neurodegenerative Disease) Koji Uchida (Laboratory of Food and Biodynamics, Graduate School of Bioagricultural Sciences, Nagoya University, Nagoya, Japan) ("Modulation of Intracellular Oxidative Stress By Anticarcinogenig Antioxidants) Takahito Kondo (Department of Biochemistry and Molecular Biology in Disease, Atomic Bomb Disease Institute, Nagasaki University School of Medicine, Nagasaki, Japan) ("Impairment of Glutathione Synthesis In the Progress of Aging") Keiichiro Suzuki (Department of Biochemistry, Hyogo College of Medicine, Osaka University Medical School, Osaka, Japan) ("Oxidative Stress and No Induce HB-EGF, A Potent Mitogen in Aortic Smooth Muscle Cells)

OVERVIEW: We always face to stresses such as oxidants from both outside and inside the body. Reactive oxygen species (ROS) is a kind of major oxidants produced during respiration of oxygen and, further more, from food, sun beam, ionizing radiation, chemical substances, smoking and so on. We possess scavengers to reduce toxicity of ROS. It has been believed that vulnerability to ROS may increase in aging, providing a fertile environment for the development of aging, neuronal and vascular degenerative diseases, and cancer. Glutathione (GSH) and its related enzymes, such as glutathione peroxidase (GPX), function as scavengers for ROS. Then, progress of numerous disorders reflecting increased oxidation was believed as a result of an abnormal GSH metabolism. However, mechanisms of impairment of these antioxidant activities often found in physiological and pathological aging are not fully elucidated. It is appreciative if we can uptake antioxidants from dietary supplementation, which serve as antioxidants themselves otherwise stimulate the activity of antioxidants. In this session, we first address to introduce the preventive effect of antioxidants from dietary supplement on the progress of aging or degenerative diseases. J. Joseph shows effect of polyphenolics from fruits and vegetables on brain aging, and neurodegenerative diseases. The speaker also shows evidences the polyphenolics have a positive effect on tumorgenesis and cardiovascular diseases. K. Uchida shows that 4-hydroxy-2-nonenal, a potent electrophile, is a marker of products of endogenously produced oxidation. He also shows evidence that natural antioxidants, such as quercetin and the polyphenols possess chemoprotective effect on the intracellular oxidative stress. Reduction of mitochondrial damage by ROS is also found in rat liver treated with quercetin and the polyphenols. Secondly, it is introduce how antioxidants are impaired in pathological aging. gamma-Glutamylcysteine synthetase (g -GCS) is a rate-limiting enzyme for the synthesis of GSH. The activity of g-GCS is important to maintain the level of GSH, and the cellular redox potential (reduction/ oxidation state). T. Kondo shows that the concentration of GSH and the expression of g-GCS are impaired in cells treated with hyper-glucose or oxidized low-density lipoprotein. Under such conditions the cells loss scavenger activity and redox regulation of intracellular signal pathways. K. Suzuki reports that GPX, a potent antioxidant enzyme, is inactivated by NO and glycated intermediates. Such inactivation of GPX further induces the expression of heparin-binding epidermal growth factor-like growth factor, which may closely relate to atherosclerosis. As conclusion, aging is accelerated by impairment of cellular function by ROS: the loss of scavenger activities and redox potential. On the other hand antioxidants from dietary supplement can cause protection of aging, neuronal disorders, vascular diseases and carcinogenesis.

Fruit Polyphenolics, Brain Aging, and Neurodegenerative Disease

J.A. Joseph, B. Shukitt-Hale, D. Fisher, A. Martin, K. Youdim

Research indicates that vulnerability to oxidative stress (VOS) may increase in aging, providing a fertile environment for the development of neurodegenerative diseases [(e.g, Alzheimer's disease (AD) or vascular dementia (VAD)]. Previously, we showed that there are increases in aged Fischer 344 rats both in vitro (increased hydrogen peroxide-induced decrements in striatal synaptosomal calcium buffering) or in vivo (motor and cognitive deficits after dopamine infusion into the zona compacta) experiments. Since there has been good success with respect to the positive benefits of dietary fruits and vegetables on cancer and cardiovascular disease, we believed the age-related increases in VOS could be antagonized by dietary supplementation (SPPL.) with fruit (strawberry, blueberry, BB) or vegetable (spinach) extracts high in antioxidants. Results showed that the SPPL were effective in forestalling or reversing several parameters of aging (e.g, cognitive behavior and neuronal signaling). One of the most striking changes involved reversals of motor behavioral deficits in BB SPPL senescent rats, that were coupled with decreased evidence of oxidative stress and inflammatory markers (leukocyte invasion) in the gastrocnemius and quadriceps, as well as decreases in lysosomal protease activity and increases in neurogenesis. It may be that these reversals are systemic and involve both peripheral and central sites by a multiplicity of polyphenolic activities. These beneficial effects may be especially beneficial in forestalling or reversing neurodegeneration in AD and in VAD with the polyphenolics found in fruit and vegetables having the same positive effects with respect to CNS aging as has been seen with tumorgenesis and cardiovascular disease.

Impairment of Glutathione Synthesis in the Progress of Aging

Takahito Kondo, Department of Biochemistry and Molecular Biology in Disease, Atomic Bomb Disease Institute, Nagasaki University School of Medicine, Nagasaki, Japan

Glutathione (gamma-glutamylcysteinyl glycine, GSH) is synthesized via two ATP-requiring steps catalyzed by gamma-glutamylcysteine synthetase (GCS), a rate-limiting enzyme for the synthesis of GSH, and GSH synthetase. The activity of GCS is important to maintain the level of GSH. GCS is composed of a heavy subunit, which is catalytic, and a light subunit, which is regulatory. GSH and its related enzymes, such as glutathione peroxidase, glutathione reductase, and glutathione S-transferase function as scavengers for reactive oxygen species, and progress of numerous disorders reflecting increased oxidation was believed as a result of an abnormal GSH metabolism. Another important function of GSH is to maintain the redox potential within cells. In the present study, we show evidence that the concentration of GSH and the expression of GCS are impaired in macrophages treated with hyper-glucose or oxidized LDL, concomitant reduction of the activities of GSH-related enzyme. GCS is upregulated by TNF-alpha and IL-1beta or oxidative stress mediated by MAPKs to stimulate NF-kappaB or AP-1. Under high concentration of glucose, the cells lost responsibility to these cytokines or oxidatives stress, suggesting that the redox regulation of the intracellular signal pathways by GSH is impaired. Thus, it seems likely impairment of GSH metabolism participates in progress of diabetic or atherosclerotic complications leading progress of aging.

Modulation of intracellular oxidative stress by anticarcinogenic antioxidants

Koji Uchida, Laboratory of Food and Biodynamics, Graduate School of Bioagricultural Sciences, Nagoya University, Nagoya 464-8601, Japan

Oxidative stress has been implicated in the pathogenesis of numerous diseases, including cancer. In the present study, the chemoprotective effect of natural antioxidants, such as quercetin and tea polyphenols, on intracellular oxidative stress was studied. In rat liver epithelial RL34 cells, 4-hydroxy-2-nonenal (HNE), a potent electrophile endogenously produced during oxidative stress, dramatically induced the production of reactive oxygen species (ROS) and a highly mutagenic aldehyde acrolein, which correlated well with the reduction in cell viability. We found that quercetin and tea polyphenols, such as epigallocatechin gallate and theaflavins and their gallate esters, significantly inhibited the HNE-induced ROS production and cytotoxicity. In addition, HNE induced a transient decrease in the mitochondrial membrane potential, which was also retarded by the antioxidants. These data suggest that the antioxidants, such as quercetin and tea polyphenols, are potential inhibitors against mitochondrial ROS production induced by HNE.

Oxidative stress and NO induce HB-EGF, a potent mitogen in aortic smooth muscle cells

Keiichiro Suzuki, Young Ho Koh, and Naoyuki Taniguchi**

Glutathione peroxidase (GPx), a major peroxide scavenging enzyme is inactivated by various oxidative stress such as an NO, methylglyoxal, or 3-deoxyglucosone. The SNAP or peroxynitrite induces the expression of the heparin-binding EGF-like growth factor (HB-EGF) through the inactivation of GPx and the accumulation of peroxide. HB-EGF, a potent chemoattractant and mitogen for smooth muscle cells, is initially synthesized as a membrane-anchored precursor (pro-HB-EGF), which then undergoes proteolytic cleavage to give the mature soluble form (s-HB-EGF). This induction is accompanied by JNK and c-Jun/AP-1 activation. The blocking of the HB-EGF induction by curcumin, c-jun antisense oligonucleotide and a dominant-negative mutant of JNK1 provides support for these results. A longer pretreatment of rat aortic smooth muscle cells (RASMC) by SNAP induces HB-EGF and reduces the TNF_+actinomycin D-induced apoptosis. This protection is blocked by antisense HB-EGF s-oligonucleotide. These findings indicate that the induction of HB-EGF by NO would be an adaptive response as an autocrine protective factor against apoptosis by NO in RASMC. HB-EGF is regulated by both oxidative stress and shear stress, and closely related to atherosclerosis.

SESSION 96

Hypothalamus and Aging

V. Bezrukov (Institute of Gerontology, Kiev, Ukraine) (Chronic electrical stimulation of lateral hypothalamic area increases viability of old rats) T. Dubiley (Institute of Gerontology, Kiev, Ukraine) (Hypothalamus, aging and age-related pathology) T. Kvitnitskaya-Ryzhova (Institute of Gerontology, Kiev, Ukraine) (Effects of aging and stress on the morpho-functional characteristics of different hypothalamic nuclei) A.V. Everitt (Department of Physiology, University of Sydney and the Centre for Education and Research on Aging) ("Hypothalamus, pituitary, food intake and aging")

The symposium addresses the morphological, electron microscopical and functional changes in the hypothalamus, hypothalamic mechanisms of age-related pathology, age changes in emotional behaviour, and life extension due to stimulation of lateral hypothalamic area. Neuronal loss and ultrastral changes in various hypothalamic nuclei were irregular. In SON, PVN and VMN the neuronal and glial number was stable in aging, whereas in LHA it declined 1.4-fold. When comparing the ultrastructural and ultracytochemical changes in VMN and LHA, it was found that they developed earlier in LHA than in VMN. In SON and PVN we did not observe any expressed neuronal loss in aging. The ultrastructural analysis and karyometry of neurosecretory cells testified to an adequately preserved high level of secretory activity in old age. Using two stress models, emotional-painful stress (EPS) and dehydration, the EPS caused mainly destructive changes in the negative emotiogenic area (VMN), being more pronounced in old animals. The amounts of gliocytes decreased 1.3-fold in adult and 1.4-fold in old rats, whereas their amounts in LHA were reduced by 1.3 times only in old animals. Under dehydration the volumes of neurosecretory cell nuclei in SON and PVN were much more increased in adult vs. old animals. Thus, the anterior and middle hypothalamic nuclei displayed essential differences in the rate, degree, character and pronouncement of the structural signs of aging as well as the limited reserves and, as a consequence, an age-associated decline of their response to stress. Age-related metabolic (transmitters content and turnover) and functional changes (integral electrograms, electroexcitability, sensitivity to humoral factors, control of autonomic functions, etc.) varied in different HN. LHA self-stimulation was accelerated in the majority of old rats, while its deceleration was found in the majority of adult animals. BP increase due to chronic stimulation of VMH (rabbits) was higher and BP increase after ouabaine microinjection into VMH (rats) was higher and developed more often in old animals as compared with adults. VMH electrolytic lesions induced less developed insulin hypersecretion and body mass gain (obesity) in old rats compared with adults. Due to chronic stimulation of LHAp, the survival and life-span of old rats increased, the rewarding function of LHAp improved, memory and immunological processes enhanced, the pain sensitivity reduced, the metabolism decreased, with no change seen in metabolism activation at stress. Thus, chronic electrical stimulation of LHAp increases the viability of old rats. Thus, changes in hypothalamic nuclei are an important mechanism for development of age changes in the metabolism, functions, age-related pathology and aging proper. Activation of positive emotiogenic zone of hypothalamus may lead to increase in viability and adaptability of an aging organism and to life extension.

Chronic electrical stimulation of lateral hypothalamic area increases viability of old rats

V.Bezrukov, T. Dubiley, I. Pishel and Yu. Rushkevich (Institute of Gerontology, Vyshgorodskaya st. 67, 04114 Kiev, Ukraine)

Two series of experiments were performed in the Wistar rats (age=29 mo),involving an implantation of monopolar electrodes in the posterior part of lateral hypothalamic area (LHAp). The stimulation was performed by cycles: 4 days of stimulation (one 15 min session per day) followed by 3 days of break. The age-matched intact rats were used as control. Chronic 1-3 mo stimulation of LHAp improved the survival of old rats. An increment in the remaining maximal life-span of stimulated animals was 33% compared to control. Chronic 1 mo stimulation of LHAp resulted in increases of: self-stimulation frequency, retention index of avoidance response, latency of tail-flick response, and PHA-stimulated proliferative activity of splenocytes, compared to control animals. A decrease in oxygen consumption at rest was registered in stimulated versus control animals, while the stimulation had no effect on the increase of this index during cold stress. Due to chronic stimulation of LHAp, the survival and life-span of old rats increased, the rewarding function of LHAp improved, memory and immunological processes enhanced, the pain sensitivity reduced, the metabolism decreased, with no change seen in metabolism activation at stress. Thus, chronic electrical stimulation of LHAp increases the viability of old rats.

Effects of aging and stress on the morpho-functional characteristics of different hypothalamic nuclei

T.Kvitnitskaya-Ryzhova and S.Mikhalsky (Institute of Gerontology, Vyshgorodskaya st. 67, 04114 Kiev, Ukraine)

This work aimed to study age-related changes in the hypothalamus areas involved in various regulatory processes in aging and under stress conditions. Using light and electron microscopy, morphometry and ultracytochemistry, we examined the ventromedial nucleus (VMN), lateral hypothalamic area (LHA), supraoptic (SON) and paraventricular nuclei (PVN) of adult (8 mo) and old (24-26 mo) Wistar rats. Two stress models were used: emotional-painful (EPS) - for examining different emotiogenic area (VMN - negative emotions; LHA - positive) and water deprivation - for the areas involved in osmotic regulation (SON and PVN). In VMN the neuronal and glial number was stable in aging, whereas in LHA it declined 1.4-fold. The ultrastructural and ultracytochemical analysis has also shown that age changes developed earlier in LHA than in VMN. In SON and PVN we did not observe any expressed neuronal loss in aging. The ultrastructural analysis and karyometry of neurosecretory cells testified to an adequately preserved high level of secretory activity in old age. The EPS caused mainly destructive changes in the negative emotiogenic area (VMN), being more pronounced in old animals. The amounts of gliocytes decreased 1.3-fold in adult and 1.4-fold in old rats, whereas their amounts in LHA were reduced by 1.3 times only in old animals. Under dehydration the volumes of neurosecretory cell nuclei in SON and PVN were much more increased in adult vs. old animals. Thus, the anterior and middle hypothalamic nuclei displayed essential differences in the rate, degree, character and pronouncement of the structural signs of aging as well as the limited reserves and, as a consequence, an age-associated decline of their response to stress.

Hypothalamus, aging and age-related pathology

T. Dubiley, Yu. Rushkevich, V. Bezrukov (Institute of Gerontology, Vyshgorodskaya st. 67, 04114 Kiev, Ukraine

Emotiogenic zones of the hypothalamus change irregularly with aging. Study of the metabolic and functional changes in the hypothalamic nuclei (HN) was performed in experiments with adult and old rats and rabbits. Methods: light and electron microscopy, electrogram recording, electric stimulation of hypothalamic nuclei via implanted electrodes, intracerebral microinjections of catecholamines, acetylcholine and ouabaine, changes in autonomic functions due to electrical and chemical stimulation of HN, hypothalamic models of arterial hypertension and obesity, self-stimulation of lateral hypothalamic area, avoidance reaction due to VMH stimulation, reproducing morphine dependence. Age-related metabolic (transmitters content and turnover) and functional changes (integral electrograms, electroexcitability, sensitivity to humoral factors, control of autonomic functions, etc.) varied in different HN. LHA self-stimulation was accelerated in the majority of old rats, while its deceleration was found in the majority of adult animals. BP increase due to chronic stimulation of VMH (rabbits) was higher and BP increase after ouabaine microinjection into VMH (rats) was higher and developed more often in old animals as compared with adults. VMH electrolytic lesions induced less developed insulin hypersecretion and body mass gain (obesity) in old rats compared with adults. Thus, uneven, irregular changes in hypothalamic nuclei are an important mechanism for development of age changes in the metabolism and function and age-related pathology.

Hypothalamus, Pituitary, Food Intake and Aging

A.V. Everitt (Department of Physiology, University of Sydney and the Centre for Education and Research on Aging, Concord Hospital, NSW, Australia)

The hypothalamus controls the intake of food and the secretion of pituitary (hypophyseal) hormones, both of which affect aging processes in the rat. The purpose of the study was to compare the anti-ageing effects of food restriction and the removal of pituitary hormones by hypophysectomy in the rat. Male Wistar rats were hypophysectomised at age 50 days, food restriction was begun at age 50 days, and a third group of ad-libitum fed controls were used. Measurements were made at various ages of food intake, body weight, urinary protein excretion, kidney histology, hind leg muscle histology and collagen fibre breaking times. The life duration of all rats was recorded. Both hypophysectomy and food restriction abolished body growth, halved food intake and retarded aging in kidney, collagen in tail tendon and hind leg muscles of the rat. Hypophysectomy had a greater anti-aging effect on almost all parameters than food restriction. Since food restriction inhibits the secretion of almost all pituitary hormones (except ACTH) it is proposed that the anti-ageing effect of food restriction is due to the reduced secretion of pituitary hormones. Hypophysectomy shortened life duration, but glucocorticoid therapy restored life expectancy to normal. Food restriction prolonged life about 30%. Thus the hypothalamus, acting through the pituitary hormones and the intake of food, influences the rate of aging in the rat and determines its duration of life.

SESSION 97

The Aging Mind: Cognitive and Biological Perspectives

Professor Patrick Rabbitt [University of Manchester, Manchester, United Kingdom]: What do we see when we Remove Practice and Drop-Out Effects from Longitudinal Data? Helen Christensen, [Australian National University, Canberra, Australia]: The Nature of the "Common Factor" and its Association with Education, Gender, APOE and Age Stuart W. S. MacDonald [University of Victoria, Victoria, British Columbia, Canada]: Relations Between Physiological and Cognitive Function in Older Adults Shu-Chen Li, [Max Planck Institute for Human Development, Berlin, Germany]: Co-Evolving Fields: A Theoretical Path from Deficient Neuromodulation to Dedifferentiated Cortical Representations to Cognitive Aging Deficits Alan A. Hartely, [Scripps College, Claremont, California, USA]: Age and Attention to Higher-Level Processing: Who is Most Affected, the Executive or the Worker?

The aging mind is often associated with loss - of speed, capacity, and flexibility. Certainly, considerable research has revealed that the average trajectory in many domains of cognitive functioning is characterized by decline or even accelerating decline. Recent research has also drawn attention to individual differences in cognitive change and the ways in which declines in some areas may be offset by assets in others. Although such descriptive conclusions represent an important first step, considerable work remains to be done to provide a coherent explanation for the cognitive changes that are associated with aging. One research theme that has re-emerged in recent years is the extent to which cognitive change in aging can be understood by integrating behavioral and biological levels of analysis. Although this focus is not new, renewed attention has been prompted by theoretical efforts in cognitive aging such as the common cause hypothesis and advances in other fields such as genetics and behavioral neurology. Research on linking these domains has also been advanced by the greater availability of longitudinal data on cognitive functioning in later life and methodological advances in statistical analysis, network modeling, and neuroimaging. The broad goal of this symposium is to provide an update of research focused on the general issue the biological basis of cognitive functioning in aging. Particular stress was placed on studies based on longitudinal data. Five papers are presented. In the first paper, Patrick Rabbitt presents an analysis of practice and drop-out effects from a 17-year longitudinal study of cognitive functioning in middle-aged and older adults. The analysis suggests age-related decline tends to be underestimated and draws attention to the need to focus on individual differences in change and sample variability rather than sample means. The second paper by Helen Christensen uses longitudinal data from the Australian National study to examine the existence of a "common factor" of cognitive aging and its relationship to age, gender, education and genetic structure. The third paper presented by Stuart MacDonald reports results from the Victoria Longitudinal Study examining relations among multiple indicators of physiological functioning and cognitive change in late adulthood. In the fourth paper, Shu-Chen Li presents an integrative theory linking cognitive aging deficits with deficient neurotransmission causing noisier information and less distinctive cortical representation. Neural network models are presented to illustrate the theory. The final paper by Alan Hartley focuses on attention to higher level processing associated with executive functioning. Alternate models for age-related models in executive function are presented drawing on experimental and neuroimaging research.

Age and Attention to Higher-Level Processing: Who is Most Affected, the Executive or the Worker?

Alan A. Hartley [Scripps College, Claremont, California, USA]

Attention commonly refers to the selection of a location in space for preferential processing. However, we can also speak of attention to processing. Maintaining a focused stream of cognitive processing, e.g, to hold something in working memory, can also be described as an expression of attention. In current parlance, this higher-level attention is often said to involve executive functions. Preliminary evidence from neuroimaging shows that the dorsolateral prefrontal cortex (DLPFC) is actively involved in these executive functions such as subvocal rehearsal, inhibiting competing information, scheduling subtasks, and maintaining task goals. The functions may be carried out there but more likely DLPFC coordinates processes that are delegated to other areas such as polar PFC, inferior lateral PFC, anterior cingulate cortex, basal ganglia, and the cerebellum. There is strong evidence for age-related impairment in tasks requiring executive functions. The impairment in higher-level attention may be due to age changes in the coordinating executive process, in the subordinate processes, or both. I will present elaborated models for each of these possibilities, review the available evidence, and suggest new directions for research.

Co-Evolving Fields: A Theoretical Path from Deficient Neuromodulation to Dedifferentiated Cortical Representations to Cognitive Aging Deficits

Shu-Chen Li [Max Planck Institute for Human Development, Berlin, Germany]

Gradual declines in many fundamental aspects of cognition pervade the aging process. Related fields of cognitive aging research have been advancing rapidly, but mostly independently, at different levels. Behaviorally, people's abilities to briefly keep information active in mind (working memory), attend to relevant information and process information promptly are compromised with age. Biologically, brain aging involves structural losses in neurons and synaptic connections along with declines in various neurotransmitter systems. Explanations for cognitive aging deficits have also been postulated at various levels. Some assume age-related reduction in information processing resources, such as working memory capacity, attention regulation and processing speed. Others hypothesize age-related increase in neuronal noise or dysfunction of the prefrontal cortex. To facilitate integration, in this presentation along with reviewing biological and behavioral aspects of cognitive aging, a recent integrative theory linking cognitive aging deficits with deficient neurotransmission causing noisier information processing and less distinctive cortical representation is described. Modeling age-related attenuation of catecholaminergic modulation by lowering a neural network parameter to reduce the signal-to-noise ratio of information processing account for benchmark phenomena, ranging from age differences in learning rate, asymptotic performance and interference susceptibility to i nter- and intraindividual variability and ability dedifferentiation. Although details of the theoretical path from neuromodulation to the distinctiveness of cortical representation to cognitive aging deficits await further empirical validation, cross-level theorizing of the kind illustrated here provides frameworks for related fields to co-evolve through cross-level data synthesizing and hypothesis testing.

Relations Between Physiological and Cognitive Function in Older Adults

S. W. S. MacDonald, R. A. Dixon (Department of Psychology, University of Victoria, Victoria, British Columbia, Canada)

A growing body of research has explored a variety of biological markers of cognitive aging. Relations among indicators of physiological status and cognitive performance were examined in a cross-sectional (455 adults aged 61 to 95) and several longitudinal samples (125 adults aged 67 to 95 spanning 12 years and 455 adults aged 61 to 95 spanning 6 years) from the Victoria Longitudinal Study (VLS). Multiple physiological indicators were considered including systolic and diastolic blood pressure, peak expiratory flow, visual and auditory acuity, body mass index, and grip strength. Cognitive measures included reasoning, processing speed (perceptual, semantic), and memory (working, episodic, semantic). We examined cross-domain relations both concurrently (VLS sample 2 wave 3 and sample 1 wave 5) and across the preceding 6-year (3-wave) and 12-year (5-wave) periods. Regression methods (hierarchical regression and hierarchical linear modeling) were used to examine physiological-age and physiological-cognition relations. Cross-sectional findings indicated that physiological status significantly predicted level of cognitive performance independent of age. Moreover, significant relations between physiological status and cognitive performance among adults aged 83 to 95 were greater in both number and magnitude compared to those aged 67 to 82. In contrast, longitudinal findings demonstrated few independent or unique contributions of physiological indicators as predictors of cognitive performance. Impaired physiological status was generally associated with poorer cognitive performance. Results point to the role of physiological status as a correlate of concurrent level and, to a lesser extent, longitudinal change in cognitive functioning of older adults.

The Nature of the 'Common Factor' and its Association with Education, Gender, APOE and Age.

H. Christensen, A. J. Mackinnon, and A. F. Jorm [Australian National University, Canberra, Australia]

A prominent hypothesis in cognitive aging is the existence of a common factor that is responsible for age-related deterioration in cognitive and non-cognitive processes. Using data primarily from longitudinal studies, we examine the nature of this common factor, its relationships to age, gender, education and the APOE genotype. The findings suggest that a number of specific processes operate concurrently with any 'common cause' factor.

What do we see when we Remove Practice and Drop-Out Effects from Longitudinal Data?

Professor Patrick Rabbitt [University of Manchester, Manchester, United Kingdom]

We report data from a 17 year longitudinal study of changes in cognitive performance in two samples of 2600 people who were aged from 49 to 92 years when first seen between 1982 and 1985. The results illustrate powerful practice effects during longitudinal studies which have been neglected in all previous reports. They also illustrate the power and the nature, of "drop-out" effects. When practice and drop-out effects have been taken into consideration it is evident that age related decline is accelerated, occurs at different rates on different tasks, and varied so markedly between individuals, that increases in sample variability rather than decline in sample means are the most interesting characteristics of longitudinal data. The data allow some adjustments to our understanding of differences between "primary" and "secondary" ageing".

SESSION 98

Postural stability and fall prevention

M. Schroll (Copenhagen University Hospital, H:S Bispebjerg, Denmark) ("Diagnostic Work-Up") Lillemor Lundin-Olsson (Department of Geriatric Medicine, University of Umea, Sweden) Pertti Era (Metitur Oy, Jyvaskyla, Findland) ("Assessment of Postural Control and Risk of Falling") Chris Todd (University of Manchester) Clemens Becker (Geriatrisches Zentrum) ("Psychological, Social and Educational Aspects of Postural Stability and Fall Prevention") Sirpa Hartikainen (University of Kupio) Sirkka-Liisa Kivela (University of Turku, Clinical Sciences) ("Postural Stability, Fall Prevention by Exercise and Training Balance and Strategies in Intervention Studies")

The EU Commission Research Directorate General by the External Advisory Group for the Key Action Ageing has held an exploratory workshop to define the scope of four subsequent workshops and a finale in 2001. The purpose is to stimulate the design of an integrated initiative for research on postural stability and fall prevention in the elderly population. The chairmen of the four EU workshops will present the content of their respective workshops to open the discussion. Much research has been done regarding single factors: intrinsic as well as extrinsic. Future research should be focused on the interplay between the opportunity (environment-related), the functional abilities of the person in question and the individual's own perception of his/her capacity.

Assessment of postural control and risk of falling

Lillemor Lundin-Olsson (Depertment of Geriatric Medicine, University of Umeå, Sweden) Pertti Era (Metitur Oy, Jyväskylä, Finland)

The general objective of a European series of workshops is to stimulate Pan European co-operation in order to design an integrated initiative for improving postural stability and preventing falls in the elderly population. The overall aim of the third workshop was to explore measurements of postural stability, their usefulness, validity and possible role in indicating a risk of falling. The first half of the workshop focused on the technology based methods to measure balance and mobility. The new technologies are based mostly on accelerometers and gyroscopes connected to portable data loggers and they enable the registrations of various aspects of gait, postural transitions (including falls), balance and mobility. The clinical assessment of posture control was discussed in terms of functional approach, systems approach and instrumental evaluation. The second half of the workshop concentrated on the evaluation of performance-based clinical measurements and field tests of balance and moving ability. In addition, the dual or multitasking concept in balance assessment as well as relations between perceived and actual balance were discussed. During the final discussion it was concluded that at present no single measure or scale is capable to fulfil the demands of a sensitive, valid and reliable tool to measure postural balance and indicate future fall risk. A major challenge is to find and develop measures and tasks that are ecologically relevant and posses a clear relationship with the performance of tasks in the actual environmnet.

Diagnostic work-up

M. Schroll (Copenhagen University Hospital, H:S Bispebjerg, Denmark)

Prevention of falls is dependent on targeting of high risk individuals, but differently in the community and in institutions. The purpose of the third EU workshop has been to outline simple guidelines for geriatricians who meet the faller as patient. A systematic diagnostic work-up is based on knowledge about biological mechanisms involved in postural control: Senses, judgement, musculoskeletal control. A structured multidisciplinary comprehensive assessment can be outlined. Multimorbidity and polypharmacy leads to interacting impairment related functional limitations in the elderly, whereof postural instability is a major one. That emphasizes an interdisciplinary geriatric approach. The doctor's role is leader of the team, coordinator of actions and responsible for identification of the medical diagnoses and medical intervention and follow-up. Clinical trials have shown that streamlining of referral of fallers by easily detectable predictors of further falls, and implementation of comprehensive medical assessment programs in geriatric clinics, focusing on fallers, are able to prevent falls and also cost-effective.

Postural stability, fall prevention by exercise and training balance and strategies in intervention studies

Sirpa HartikainenSirkka-Liisa Kivelä

Prevention of falls is dependent on targeting of high-risk individuals, but differently in the community and in institutions. The fourth EU workshop has two purposes. First is to outline guidelines for muscle and balance exercises for geriatricians and general practitioners to prevent falls in communities and in institutions. The other purpose is to outline good intervention strategies for studies in falls prevention. Falls prevention can base only on the knowledge about risk factors (multimorbidity, weak muscle strength, polypharmacy, weak sight. etc.) and mechanisms involved in postural control: senses, judgement, musculo-skeletal control. A structured multidisciplinary comprehensive assessment of the elderly can be outlined. To exercise muscle strength and balance can be one possibility to prevent falls among the elderly. Intervention strategies in falls prevention are different depending on the population involved and the place of intervention (a home or an institution). The intervention can have whole elderly population as a target or can be targeting a smaller group of elderly with high risk. The community-based intervention has whole elderly population as a target but these interventions are often low in intense and seldom effective. The interventions concerning the elderly in high risk for falling can be more intensive and seem to be more effective than community based interventions.

Psychological, social and educational aspects of postural stability and fall prevention.

Chris Todd (University of Manchester, Manchester, UK) Clemens Becker (Geriatrisches Zentrum, Ulm Germany)

PURPOSE: The presentation reviews the deliberations of an European Commission Expert Workshop convened to consider psychological, social and educational aspects of posturalcontrol and fall prevention amongst older people. METHOD: The workshop overviewed areas of research on falls amongst elderly people. RESULTS: Topics reviews are presented for: psychological research into fear of falling (Yardley), social learning theory underpinnings for behaviour change interventions (Diederiks), effects of visual impairment (Wahl), psychotropic drug use (Weyerer), use of internet resources in education to promote activity amongst older people (Carls). It is clear that previous research into fall and fracture prevention has not been informed by psychological theory of behaviour change. Social cognition models predict, explain and give basis for programmes to change health related behaviours (Sutton). The Theory of Planned Behaviour (TPB) provides such a theoretical perspective and is applicable to fall prevention. TPB predicates a series of steps in development of an intervention strategy and these are described. CONCLUSIONS: Future research needs to embrace lessons from psychological theory, to strengthen interventions, ensure adherence and make interventions consonant with expectations, attitudes, fears, and goals of the target population. Multi-factorial interventions used in future RCTs will need to take account of these issues as well as assessing nature and level of impairments and medication use that have been the grist of endeavours to date. In preparation for a definitive RCT a series of feasibility and pilot studies are to be proposed under the EC Fifth Framework Programme 2002 as a Thematic Network.

SESSION 99

A Typology of Resident Abuse

S. Hirst (Faculty of Nursing, University of Calgary, Calgary, Alberta, Canada).

Research has identified the presence of resident abuse within long-term care facilities. However, resident abuse has not come under the same scrutiny, as have other aspects of abuse against older adults. This is due, in part, to the difficulty in defining this phenomenon. The purpose of this study was to articulate a definition of resident abuse as perceived by registered nurses working in long-term care institutions. Those who work within long-term care institutions are viewed as members of this culture. Since cultural members use language to convey particular meanings and experiences, it is important to identify how it or variants of it are used when studying resident abuse. One qualitative approach to studying language is ethnoscience, which is the systematic study of the way of life of a designated cultural group in order to obtain an accurate account of how they perceive and know their universe. This uncovering process is done through analysis of answers provided by participants to the researcher's questions. Data is constructed into a taxonomy, which describes a system of different contrastive sets about a given phenomenon such as resident abuse. The five major identified categories of characteristics (perception of hurt felt by older residents, acts of omission or commission, context of care, intentional or unintentional, and behavioural clusters) reflect the richness of the descriptions given by participants. Findings suggest that the definition of resident abuse used by cultural members differs from that used by individuals who are not members of this culture.

Elderly Abuse

Rabindra Nath Sabat(Friends'Association for Rural Reconstruction,LL/3, Civil Township, Rourkela-769004, Orissa, India)

The elderly feel abused or that they are neglected by way of not providing them with sufficient food and other facilities, comforts, necessary elementary services of health care and hygiene etc. A random sampling of 1262 families affected by the super cyclone was taken in a district through structured questionnaires and interviews focusing on the basic economic needs like food, shelter, cloths and other health needs. Elderly abuses in the family in the domestic situation are rising very fast as percieved by the elderly people. Deprivation of love, care, concern, understaing and neglecting the health needs as well as other economical and emotional needs are increasing on the elderly by their own family members. The elderly as a vulnerable group in the cyclone affected areas feel that their own family members do not need them. The family members are forgetting whatever they have done for their family. The decline of the human values has further deteriorated the socio economic condition of the elderly people.

Emerging Issues in Elder Abuse: Implications for Prevention and Intervention

J.I. Kosberg, B.L. Torgusen (School of Social Work, The University of Alabama, Alabama, USA)

Given population aging in both developing and developed nations, it is projected that the problem of elder abuse worldwide will increase. Two general explanations for elder abuse have been cited, inappropriate caregivers and caregiving burden. There are additional current and emerging issues leading to elder abuse that have been recently identified around the world. This presentation, based upon empirical studies and practice experience, will include discussion on elder abuse resulting from (1) decreasing levels of marital satisfaction by a spousal caregiver, (2) high rates of divorce and remarriages resulting in confusing caregiving responsibilities, (3) resentment in the care of a parent-in-law, (4) increased gender equity resulting in caregivers who are either angry wives or inexperienced husbands, (5) women in the workforce interrupting their careers due to caregiving responsibilities, (6) family disharmony caused by the misconception that quantity of family members increases quality of care, (7) mobility of adult children who reluctantly must take their elderly parents with them, (8) economic challenges of an adult child dependent upon an elderly parent, (9) increased life longevity of dependent, mentally and physically impaired children living with elderly parents, (10) the increased likelihood of grandparents caring for abusive grandchildren, and (11) threats against an elderly person's pet. The conclusion to be reached is that there is a need (1) to be aware of such contemporary problems adversely affecting the elderly in a country and (2) to initiate programs and policies to help both elderly care recipients and also their family caregivers.

Ethical issues identified by Practitioners in Elder Abuse

Marie Beaulieu (UQAR, Rimouski, Québec, Canada) Lyse Montminy (U. Laval, Québec City, Québec, Canada) Jocelyne St-Arnaud (U. of Montréal, Montréal, Québec, Canada)

Ethical issues in practice related to elder abuse is a growing area of concern. To be able to influence and accompany practitioners in changing their practices, we need to better understand all the difficulties that their are facing in their practice. There difficulties are often much more subtle than basic knowledge, they are related to ways that practitioners are able to identify confrontation and dilemmas between their personal values, their professional values , the values of the service in which they practice and the values of the client (being here the older adult, the abuser or both). This study, financed by SHSRC is based on 20 in-depth interviews conducted with practitioners working in two areas in Québec (Québec city an urban area) and Bas-Saint-Laurent (a semi-rural and rural area). Ten practitioners work in public services (government agencies) while the others are in community services. Results show that many ethical dilemmas are experience by practitioners. In their professional judgement and actions they are encouraged or discouraged by the support their receive from their institution as well as their possibility to share a certain number of values with their client. This paper will insist on the value of autonomy which is a central value in practice with older adults. Beside a general reflection on this key issue we will nuance our results by area, organisation, sex and professional background.

Korean Elder Abuse; how can we say who is victim and who is perpetrator

Han, Dong Hee Research Institute of Science for Better ALiving for the Elderly #1102 Samwhan Officetel 830-295, Bumil-dong, Dong-gu, Busan 601-060 Korea

The purpose of this paper is to explore some of the major situation with elder abuse and to understand both elderly victims and adult perpetrators in Korea. One of the confounding aspects of abuse of elders by adult children is that it is not always possible to separate the victims from the perpetrators. The meshing of personalities combined with a long history of intimate interaction often obliterates clear-cut distinctions between the abused and the abuser-victim or perpetrator. To achieve the aim of this study, data was collected from 15 abused elders and 15 adult caregivers who have been felt exhausted and stressed and who didn't have any choice and coping strategy by using the in-depth interview. Hence this study point both of situational elderly and adult children. To us wildly understand the reason of elder abuse in Korea. Also research in elderly abuse has pointed out the reason that abused elders become as a third vulnerable population among family violence. Under this circumstance, this study approached the problem of elderly abuse through examining its causal relationships and situation ; personal factors, family situational factors, socio-cultual factors, socio-politic factors. KEY WORDS : elder abuse, individual factors, family situational factors, socio-cultural factors, socio-political factors, victim, perpetrator

Making the Connection - Elder Abuse and Animal Cruelty

E. Podnieks (Ryerson Polytechnic University, Toronto, Canada)

The Ontario Network for the Prevention of Elder Abuse (ONPEA) and the Ontario Society for the Prevention of Cruelty to Animals (OSPCA) are currently conducting a pilot project to examine the relationship between animal cruelty and elder abuse. Much anecdotal evidence supports the link between animal cruelty and elder abuse, however, currently there is little Canadian research or data available. OSPCA conducted research on the relationship between domestic violence and animal cruelty and found similar conclusions to U.S. research; abusers often harm and threaten their victim's beloved companion animals in order to maintain control in abusive relationships. We suspect the same dynamics may play out in elder abuse. This project consists of three phases: research, development of education and cross-training materials, and a province-wide education campaign for the public and those who work with elders and animals. The goal of this pilot project is to develop training models that will include cross-training and cross reporting components. Animal investigators will be taught to recognize elder abuse and those working with elders will be taught to recognize animal cruelty. All workers will learn how and where to report suspected abuse and neglect. Once models have been developed a provincial education campaign aimed at the public and those working with elder and animals will be implemented. Joint efforts between ONPEA and OSPCA to recognize, record, and report incidents of abuse and neglect will provide opportunities for earlier intervention, and eventually, violence prevention in the area of elder abuse and animal cruelty.

Perceived Importance of Elder Abuse as Compared to Other Problems of Community Living in Israel

S.M.Neikrug (Tel-Hai Academic College, Upper Galilee, ISRAEL)

PURPOSE: This paper evaluates the perceived importance of elder abuse as compared to other Problems of Community Living in Israel. We also evaluate the congruence between the importance of elder abuse to older Israelis and perception of its importance to professionals in agencies serving the aged. METHOD: An instrument indicating 19 major problems of community living, including abuse by strangers and abuse in the family, was developed by a panel of older persons. This instrument was administered to a sample of older Israelis (60+) living in the community (n= 1164) and human service professionals (n= 443) serving the aged. RESULTS: The results indicate differences between older persons and professionals regarding the nature and the severity of the problem. The findings indicate that professionals serving older adults often feel that neither they nor their agency have resources to deal with elder abuse. CONCLUSION: Many professionals are personally committed to a client centered approach, but those in agencies sampled, were limited in terms of their knowledge of the importance of elder abuse. Preventing elder abuse and neglect is essentially tied to combating isolation so elders know that they live in supportive communities. For professionals, a commitment to quality of service and concern for client's quality of life requires that they be equipped with solutions for clients' problems. Older clients must know that help is available for their problems.

Risk factors for Chinese elderly abuse in Hong Kong

E.C.W, Yan & C.S.K, Tang (The Chinese University of Hong Kong, Hong Kong, China)

The present study attempted to explore the risk factors for physical, verbal and social abuses among Chinese elderly. A total of 276 elderly Chinese (90 males and 186 females, age ranged from 60 to 91) were sampled from local community centers and recreational areas. All participants completed a questionnaire without monetary reward. Of the 276 participants, 27.8% (N=75) suffered at least one incident of abuse in the past year. Verbal abuse was most prevalent among the three types of abuses, accounted for 26.8% (N=74) in the present sample. Physical and social abuses were relatively rare, accounted for 2.5% (N=7) and 1.8% (N=5) respectively. Participants' age, visual ability, presence of chronic illness, memory, and their dependence on caregivers were correlated with abuse generally (r ranged from .149 to .256, p<.05), indicating elder individuals having poor visual ability, chronic illness, poor memory, and dependence on their caregiver were more likely to be abused. This trend was mainly observed in verbal abuse and physical abuse. Analysis of logistic regression suggested participants' dependence on their caregivers and their caregivers' dependence on them as the two most salient predictors for abuse. Specifically, verbal abuse was best predicted by participants' visual ability, memory, dependence on their caregiver and caregivers' dependence on them, while only the latter two were useful in predicting physical abuse, and social abuse was better predicted by participants' age.

SESSION 100

Networking About Older Women's Networks

N. Manap (Vice President for Programme Development and International Affairs, Tsao Foundation, Singapore)

The objectives of this session are to inform and present an update on the Asian Older Women's Health Network and to network with other older women's network initiatives internationally. The network was formed at the end of the first international conference on the health of the older women in asia held in 1999, entitled - Women's Health - The Nation's Gain: An International Conference with a Special Focus on Older Women In Asia. The network was formed with the mission of enabling older women in Asia to achieve better physical, mental and social well-being through collaborative health promotion activities. Among its key objectives include : -the sharing of information on research, policies, events and innovative programmes related to older women's health; -to advocate and raise awareness about health and health promotion issues of older women in Asia; -to advocate for the empowerment of older women's involvement in health promotion.

SESSION 101

Assessing Outcomes In A Case Management Program For Community-Dwelling Frail Older Adults

Glenna A. Dowling (Goldman Institute On Aging, Goldman Research Center, San Francisco, USA Eva M. Schmitt .(Goldman Institute On Aging, Goldman Research Center, San Francisco, USA

PURPOSE: This paper describes the impact of a case management program, Multipurpose Senior Services Program (MSSP) on community dwelling frail older adults. METHOD: The Goldman Institute on Aging in San Francisco is conducting an ongoing outcomes project to evaluate the impact of a MSSP on depression and health care service utilization. Depression is assessed using the Geriatric Depression Scale (GDS) and health care service utilization is tracked by case managers. Assessments occurr at enrollment, 6 months and 1 year. RESULTS: General Linear Model analysis revealed a significant increase in physician and clinic visits (p< .001, n=52) and a significant decrease in the number of hospital and nursing home admissions (p< .001, n= 52) during the year after enrollment. On average, participants did not show signs of depression at enrollment and were stable over time (n= 43). However, participants whose GDS scores at enrollment indicated a possible clinical depression improved significantly (p< .05, n= 17). CONCLUSION: These results support the contention that MSSP improve outpatient health care for participants and decrease nursing home and hospital admissions during the year after enrollment. These outcomes show that MSSP enables participants to remain in the community and thereby avoid or delay institutionalization.

Case-Management: Setting Up a Medico-Social Network from a Proximity Hospital

M. Habrias (Centre Hospitalier de Bourganeuf, France)

A proximity hospital organised a gerontological network in order to provide a comprehensive management of the problems of the elderly population living in the area. The purpose was to set up the public hospital as a main support to aging in place, by making available for the elderly, their families and all the parties involved in community maintaining, a hospital competence and logistics.The means :A coordination team was put in place in the hospital, based in the geriatric care department, using part- time of geriatrician, Head nurse, social worker and secretary, aiming at monitoring all the parties involved outside hospital : family, social, medical, care providers.The hospital logistics was made available : offices, referent interlocutors, computers, meeting rooms, meal home delivery, home care, housing and/or hospitalisation. Now six years old, this coordination groups together all the actors involved in a global management, and also acts preventively, including a watch structure well organised : for this purpose, the home aides, housing technicians, postmen, policemen, legal guardians and volunteers were given a specialised training and attend the monthly, up to date, comprehensive adjusting meeting.This way of working could be used not only as a gerontological management. It can be integrated in other networks (pain, cancer&) and participate to public health issues.

Case/Care Management in Berlin - A Comprehensive System of Coordinating Centers from Community-based Rehabilitation

S. Hensse (The Geriatric Research Group, Virchow Clinic, Medical Faculty of the Humboldt University of Berlin, Germany) M. Ruhnau-Wuellenweber (The Coordinating Center "All Around Aging", The Protestant Geriatric Center in Berlin, Germany) E.M. Schmitt (Goldman Institute on Aging, Goldman Research Center, San Francisco, USA) H. Gerecke (Department of Work, Welfare and Women, Berlin, Germany) P. Wissmann (Albatros e.V, Berlin, Germany) E. Steinhagen-Thiessen (Medical Director, the Protestant Geriatric Center in Berlin, Medical Faculty of the Humboldt University of Berlin, Germany)

As of 1999, the city of Berlin has 12 government funded community-based coordinating centers for rehabilitation providing care management services to the city's older adults as well as (family) care-takers of demented, frail or disabled elderly. The evaluation of model projects in 1988 to 1991 led to regular government funding of these centers. The goal of the coordinating centers is to enable older adults to remain in, or return to, their own homes and reduce the number of involuntary nursing home placements and unnecessary hospital admissions. The coordinating centers are a response to the lack of coordination and cooperation between the intersection of different systems of care (hospital, community-based), which often results in inappropriate care, especially for the disabled elderly, as they move from one system to the other. In addition, the confusing diversity and obscurity of available services results in these services not being known or used. The primary methods used are support-management, rehabilitation planning, and counseling of older adults, their relatives, as well as professionals and institutions. Each center is responsible for a defined geographic area, is familiar with the services available therein and for providing and updating this information for a central databank available to all coordinating centers. This approach has shown to be effective in preventing unnecessary nursing home placements, prolonged hospitalizations, care-giver burn-out syndrome, and crisis situations in home-care settings.

Cost-effectiveness analysis of a case management project for community-frail elderly in Hong Kong

Leung AC, Liu CP, Yau DCN, Wu YM (Aged Care Research & Development Unit, Haven of Hope Christian Service, Haven of Hope Hospital, 8 Haven of Hope Road, Tseung Kwan O, Hong Kong)

This is to measure cost-effectiveness of our case management intervention on community-dwelling frail elderly in Hong Kon. 130 hospital discharged patients were randomly assigned to experimental and control group respectively in July 2000. A case manager with consultation from a multidisciplinary team provided interventions to clients in the experimental group only. Clients¡≈ mean age was 74.9 (SD=7.2, range=60-96) and 54.6% of them were male. After intervention, the average unplanned hospital readmission rate in 5 months was reduced by 43.4% and 27.3% in experimental (P=0.004) and control group (p=n.s.) respectively. The average number of bed-days in hospitals in 5 months after intervention was decreased by 48.2% and 31.3% in experimental (P=0.009) and control group (p=n.s.) respectively. The average number of bed-days in acute hospitals was reduced by 56.2% in experimental (P=0.007), and 15.5% in control group (P=n.s.). The average number bed-days in rehabilitation hospitals was reduced by 39.1% in experimental (p=n.s.), and 50.9% in control group (P=0.02). The average cost of bed-days in hospitals reduced US$2430 in experimental group (P=0.005), while the average cost reduced US$940 in control group (P=n.s.) in comparison of 5 months before and after the study. In conclusion, well-planned case management intervention could significantly reduce frail elderlies¡≈ unplanned hospital readmissions and length of stay in hospitals. Adequate and well-coordinated community and home-care services are important for its success. The burden of informal carers should also be addressed. This model of care is a step forward to enable frail elderly to age in place in their familiar environment.

Efforts to Use Managed Care to Improve Care Coordination

R.L. Kane (University of Minnesota School of Public Health, Minneapolis, USA)

This paper will examine data from several demonstration projects designed to use managed care to improve care coordination for older persons covered by Medicare and Medicaid, i.e, people who need both long-term and active medical care. The basic underlying principle is that pooling resources will allow more flexibility and innovation and encourage coordination of medical and social care. The programs examined include Minnesota Seniors Health Option (MSHO), Wisconsin Partnership Program (WPP), and Program for All-Inclusive Care of the Elderly (PACE) The approaches applied vary in the extent of their reorganization of the medical system. Some involve active efforts at case management. They vary in their ability to capture physicians' active attention. Most rely on physicians who have only a small proportion of their practices enrolled in these efforts. The results have been generally disappointing. There is not clear progression in benefit based on the extent of change in the underlying care system. The approach of layering on another level of case management does not produce coordinated care. The case mix of enrollees varied somewhat, but after adjustments, there was little difference in unmet needs or satisfaction with care. Utilization data is still being analyzed, but will be ready by the time of presentation.

Is the decision the problem or making the decision? The Science of Decision-making applied to Case Management.

Karen Parent (Queen's University) and Malcolm Anderson (Queen's University Kingston, Ontario Canada)

Purpose: To discuss the science and complexity of case management decision making in home care in the wake of health system reform and deficit reduction. Method: Using a grounded-theory approach, qualitative data was collected from case managers working in home care from several jurisdictions across Canada. More specifically, data was collected on resource allocation and decision-making under constraint. Results: A model of key dimensions was developed to depict the complexity of the dynamic interactions among controllable, uncontrollable, environmental/ structural constraints, and possible outcome variables. It was found that decisions made by case managers were often influenced by their own values as well as by the cultural, political, legal and philosophical underpinnings of the organization. It was also found that the nature of the decisions was affected by the case manager's assessed or perceived risk of the client and family caregiver. A further level of analysis reveals that case managers are faced with two distinct challenges: the decision itself as well as the decision-making process. To understand these challenges, principles from applied management science have been incorporated to develop appropriate and valid strategies in response to the challenge of making good strategic decisions in the home care environment. Conclusion: Making decisions in today's home care environment can be challenging at best when resources, both fiscal and human, are limited. To ensure that case managers make the best decision for clients, their families and the organization they work for, decision support tools need to be developed and tested.

Making decisions about long-term care for older people: the role of a multi-disciplinary panel

Pat Le Riche and Mark Hughes (Goldsmiths College, London, United Kingdom)

This paper examines the development of a multi-disciplinary panel used for making decisions to place older people into residential and nursing home care in the London Borough of Greenwich. The paper draws on a quantitative analysis of 1375 panel documents and on semi-structured interviews with panel members and social workers. In 610f cases older people moved directly from hospital into long-term care, with an average waiting period (from panel to placement date) of 21 days. In 180f cases older people moved directly from a respite bed into long-term care (often remaining in the same facility). Consequently many older people are involved in decisions to enter long-term care while in temporary living arrangements and often during a time of crisis and physical ill health. Interviewees noted that strategies to involve older people in assessment and decision-making processes are often inconsistently applied and it is notable that service users, relatives or advocates are not allowed to attend the panel meeting itself. The paper concludes with an evaluation of the role of the multi-disciplinary panel in decision-making processes. This evaluation will include strategies for involving older people and their carers in assessment and decision-making processes and the position of panels in long term placement and rehabilitation strategies.

The Development of Expert Systems for Japanese Care

Management
Eiji Kitajima, (Tokai University, Isehara, Japan). Keiko Fujibayashi (Toyo University, Tokyo, Japan) Akio Nishimura, (National Institute of Health Services Management, Ministry of Health and Welfare). Shinichi Okada, (Osaka Cty University, Osaka). Mari Okada, Ed.D. (Hanazono University, Kyoto, Japan).

PURPOSE: The objective of this study is to develop the Expert System for the Japanese Care Management. METHOD: The Care Management practitioners were asked to make the assessments and plannings for the care services. The logics of the assessment and planning practices were studied. RESULT: The practitioners did not make the assessment and the planning in distinctive ways. They seemed to make the assessments and the plannings interactively. CONCLUSION: It was found that the application of the neural computing and fuzzy logics were useful for the development of an computer-assisted Expert System of the Japanese Care Management.

SESSION 103

The financing of the care of the older person with DRG and similar systems.

Baeyens J.P, (AZ Damiaan, Oostende, Belgium) (Introduction to the problem of financing geriatric care with DRG.) Ceulemans S, Petermans J, Baeyens J.P, Wauthy I, Swartenbroeckx N, Closon M.C, (Hôpital de la Citadelle, Liège ; AZ Damiaan, Oostende ; UCL, Bruxelles, Belgium) (Can we improve DRG Case-Mix for geriatric patients?) Topinkova E, Neuwirth J, Haas T, (Departments of Geriatrics, 1ste Medical faculty, Charles University and Insitute for Postgraduate medicale Education, Prague; 3rd Department of Internal Medicine, 1st Medical Faculty, Charles University, Prague, Czech Republic.) (Resource Utilization groups (RUG) A suitable case-mix system for geriatric long-term care.) Baeyens J.P, Ceulemans S, Petermans J, Mets T, (AZ Damiaan, Oostende, Hôpital de la Citadelle, Liège, UZ VUB, Brussel, Belgium) (Methodology to find out what are real essential data to have a good case-mix.)

ISSUE: In many countries the financing of the care of geriatric patients is very difficult, because the classic DRG system that is very useful for younger patients is in reality not fitting the situation of geriatric patients. We have to find something to replace the DRG system in the geriatric departments. STRUCTURE: After an introduction by the convener, two studies (a Belgian and a Czech) will be presented and a starting study in Belgium will be presented. CONTENT: DRG alone are not sufficient as explanation of the length of stay (LOS) and may not be used as a basis for prospective payment. Specific geriatric characteristics should be considered: dependency, social characteristics as geriatric intervention. Another way to improve the DRG case mix is improving coding diagnosis procedure. Case-mix system RUG-III explains resource variance for defined patient groups in chronic post-acute care. This system has been validated in countries with different institutional setting and health care systems. Its implementation permits fair distribution of resources on the health system level. On the facility level it can improve staffing and budgeting decisions. RUG-III provides data for analytical and comparative research on national and international level. The starting study in Belgium will be presented on a very practical way, with all the details en practical problems. ANTICIPATED CONCLUSIONS: We hope and are sure that an interesting discussion will follow and that the discussions started up at the European Congress of Berlin in 1999 will be continued. OUTCOMES: an international collaborative project.

Can we improve DRG Case-Mix for Geriatric Patients?

** CHR de la Citadelle bd XII e de Ligne - 4000 Liège - Belgium ** AZ Sint Joseph - Nieuwpoortsesteenweg - Oostende - Belgium *** CIES - Ecole de Santé Publique - UCL - Clos Chapelle aux Champs - 1200 Bruxelles - Belgium*

Purpose: Diagnosis Related Groups (DRG's) are used for prospective payment in different countries, but DRG are poor predictors of cost or length of stay (LOS) in acute geriatric units. Method : We evaluated the role explanatory factors of LOS : DRG's, demographic characteristics (age, sex), Katz score on admission and before discharge, social characteristics, geriatric procedures (physical therapy, occupational therapist, speech therapy, social and nutritional assessment). Statistics: Non-parametric tests (Wilcoxon and Kruskall) for univariate analysis and a stepwise regression for multivariate analysis. Results: 4332 acute geriatric stays in 17 Belgian hospitals were analysed. Mean age is 81 years, sex ratio is 2.5 Female/Male. Mean LOS was 21 days (Q25: 12 days, Q75: 75 days). Before admission, 70% of the patients were living home, 28.5 % were admitted from long-term care facilities. Mortality was 12.7%. 46% of the patient were home discharged. Univariate analysis comparing LOS showed a correlation ($P< 0.0001$) between: patient impaired autonomy on admission (Katz score H, K), physical therapy, procedure like naso-gastric tube, transfusion, urinary catheter, physical therapy. Discharge to an nursing home was related to an additional LOS ($P< 0.001$). Multivariate analysis showed a positive role of Score H or G on the Katz scale on admission, surgical DRG, DRG related to orthopaedic surgery, DRG with major complication, nursing home discharge, naso-gastric tube placement. This variables explained 26% of the variance of LOS of our geriatric population. Social and nutritional assessment by dietitian and physical therapy decreased LOS Conclusion: DRG alone are not sufficient as explanation of LOS and may not be used as a basis for prospective payment. Specific geriatric characteristic should be considered: dependency, social characteristics as geriatric intervention. Another way to improve the DRG case mix is improving coding diagnosis procedure.

Methodology to find out what are real essential data to have a good case-mix.

Baeyens J.P. (AZ Damiaan Oostende Belgium), Ceulemans S and Petermans J. (Hôpital de la Citadelle, Liège, Belgium), Mets T. (UZ VUB, Brussels, Belgium)

PURPOSE: A lot of data can be recorded about geriatric patients. Some of them are essential to have a good case-mix. What are this corner data? METHOD: The full list of recorded data in the Belgian starting study will be presented and explanation will be given. RESULTS: We hope to organise a good discussion on what data are really very important to collect and how. CONCLUSION: could be an international collaborative project, with the Belgian study as model, to have an international validated system.

Resource Utilization Groups (RUG) a suitable case-mix system for geriatric long-term care

E. Topinková, J. Neuwirth (Department of Geriatrics, 1st Medical Faculty, Charles University and Institute for Postgraduate Medical Education, Prague, Czech Republic), T. Haas (3rd Department of Internal Medicine, 1st Medical Faculty, Charles University, Prague, Czech Republic)

Institutional long-term care (LTC) represents a costly segment of health care services in developed countries. Until recently, quantitative policy research addressing cross-country differences in institutionalization rates, structure of LTC facilities and relative costs was unavailable. The newly developed RUG, version III case-mix system enables to define facility performance in economic and quality terms, particularly to classify nursing home residents according to their clinical characteristics and determine their relative use of resources. Brief history and characteristics of RUG-III will be given. Differences between RUG-III and Diagnosis Related Groups (DRG) case-mix systems will be discussed. Results of international validation of RUG-III will be presented. A total of 14,152 residents of LTC facilities in 8 countries (Czech Republic, Finland, Japan, Spain, United Kingdom, and USA) were evaluated using RUG-III items of Minimum Data Set and measurements of staff time for 24 hours were performed. Coefficients of variance for resource use ranged from 33.4% (UK) to 64.0% (Spain). Cross-national correlations between case-mix indexes for total samples and selected RUG-III groups were statistically significant. In all countries, RUG-III groups hierarchy has been followed. Conclusions: Case-mix system RUG-III explains resource variance for defined patient groups in chronic post-acute care. This system has been validated in countries with different institutional setting and health care systems. Its implementation permits fair distribution of resources on the health system level. On the facility level it can improve staffing and budgeting decisions. RUG-III provides data for analytical and comparative research on national and international level.

SESSION 104

Building Communities that Promote Successful Aging: The Experience Corps Model

Marc R. Freedman (Civic Ventures, Inc, San Francisco, USA) Transforming the role of older adults in society Linda P. Fried (Johns Hopkins Medical Institutions, Baltimore, USA) The Experience Corps: A social model for health promotion, generativity and decreasing structural lag for older adults Thomas A. Glass (Johns Hopkins Medical Institutions, Baltimore, USA) Experience Corps: Design of an Intergenerational Health Promotion Program Kevin D. Frick (Johns Hopkins Medical Institutions, Baltimore, USA) The Costs and Benefits of the Experience Corps Program

Issue: Community-level approaches could support successful aging through social institutions that improve health and well being of our aging society. If these approaches were also designed to provide opportunities for productivity and to direct the substantial source of social capital to address unmet social needs, such approaches would simultaneously meet a range of needs for both older adults and of society. Structure: This symposium presents four talks and a concluding panel discussion with the audience. Content: This symposium addresses the broad issues and opportunities associated with taking an international approach to societal organization to support successful aging, and then describes a new model of senior service, which was designed to meet goals of both generativity and health promotion: the Experience Corps. There is a need for social institutions that offer meaningful and productive roles on a large social scale, to permit older adults to remain engaged in society and to contribute post-retirement. Scientific data indicates that such engagement is beneficial to health and function and protects against mortality. Additionally, remaining physically active and, perhaps, cognitively engaged, are also important roles, could be designed to help address unmet social needs. If such a program could include a critical mass of older adults at both local and national levels, this could bring underused human capital to help resolve such needs. We have designed such a model, called the Experience Corps, which brings older adults to public elementary schools in a program designed both for high impact and health promotion. This symposium describes the Experience Corps program, the results of a national demonstration project and the pilot for a randomized trial, and its potential import and cost-effectiveness. It concludes with a discussion with the audience as to the levels of evidence needed to warrant the fiscal expenditures and sustainability at local and national levels.

Experience Corps: Design of an Intergenerational Health Promotion Program

Thomas A. Glass (Johns Hopkins Medical Institutions, Baltimore, USA) George Rebok (Johns Hopkins Medical Institutions, Baltimore, USA) Joel Hill (Johns Hopkins Medical Institutions, Baltimore, USA) Michelle Carlson (Johns Hopkins Medical Institutions, Baltimore, USA) James Tielsch (Johns Hopkins Medical Institutions, Baltimore, USA) Scott Zeger (Johns Hopkins Medical Institutions, Baltimore, USA) Kevin Frick (Johns Hopkins Medical Institutions, Baltimore, USA) Linda K. Fried (Johns Hopkins Medical Institutions, Baltimore, USA)

PURPOSE: The Experience Corps project is a community-based health promotion intervention designed to create purposeful social roles for seniors in school-based settings. Our team is currently conducting an extended pilot test involving 131 older adults deployed in 6 Baltimore elementary schools. The program is intended to prevent physical and cognitive disability in older adults and to promote improved academic performance in children. The purpose of this presentation is to describe the Experience Corps intervention design with particular attention to theoretical and practical considerations learned during several years of pilot study. METHOD: A community-based health promotion program will be described. RESULTS: Few opportunities exist for older adults to find meaningful productive engagement. Such roles will be especially needed in the coming decades. The Experience Corps represents a multidisciplinary intervention approach that combines several key elements including a) intergenerational relationships, b) generativity and productive activity, c) organizational development, d) volunteerism, and e) health promoting components. A theoretical model of Experience Corps will be presented which draws on elements of activity theory, as well as an Eriksonian perspective on the importance of generativity in late life. The structure and design of the main components of the Experience Corps program will be described. CONCLUSION: The Experience Corps model is a potentially cost-effective, high impact model of health promotion that may have wide applicability in many organizational settings. Its effectiveness should be evaluated through a randomized trial.

The Costs and Benefits of the Experience Corps Program

Kevin D. Frick (Johns Hopkins Medical Institutions, Baltimore, U.S.A.) Linda P. Fried (Johns Hopkins Medical Institutions, Baltimore, USA)

PURPOSE: To estimate the costs of the Experience Corps program, monetary values of some of the program's benefits, and discuss effects for which monetary values are difficult to estimate. Potentially negative effects on other organizations for which the older individuals volunteer are of interest. METHOD: Project records and anticipated program changes are used to project future costs. In a small randomized pilot study, the changes experienced by the intervention and control groups during a short intervention period were compared. Volunteer activities at baseline and recent activities in the follow-up were assessed. RESULTS: With 30 volunteers per school, the program is projected to cost over $100,000 per school. Changes in the intervention group were more frequently in the right direction, although not always statistically significantly greater than changes for the control group. The number of other activities in which the older individuals participated did not go down, although the time spent in each activity could not be assessed. CONCLUSION: A program like the Experience Corps requires infrastructure development and a change in the social contract and is likely to be expensive. This program tends to attract older individuals already doing some volunteer work, although it does not appear to interfere with the continuation of other volunteer activities. Evidence suggests that the program leads to functional benefits that may result in long run cost savings. The policy issues that could be addressed through formal cost-benefit analyses of new social programs such as the Experience Corps will be discussed.

The Experience Corps: A Social Model for Health Promotion, Generativity and Decreasing Structural Lag for Older Adults

Linda P. Fried (Johns Hopkins Medical Institutions, Baltimore, U.S.A.) Marc R. Freedman (Civic Ventures, Inc, San Francisco, U.S.A.) Tom Endres (AARP, Washington DC, U.S.A.) George W. Rebok (Johns Hopkins Medical Institutions, Baltimore, U.S.A.) Michelle Carlson (Johns Hopkins Medical Institutions, Baltimore, U.S.A.) Teresa Seeman (University of California, Los Angeles, U.S.A.) Jim Tielsch (Johns Hopkins Medical Institutions,

Baltimore, U.S.A.) Thomas A. Glass (Johns Hopkins Medical Institutions, Baltimore, U.S.A.) Barbara Wasik (Johns Hopkins Medical Institutions, Baltimore, U.S.A.) Kevin D. Frick (Johns Hopkins Medical Institutions, Baltimore, U.S.A.) Scott Zeger (Johns Hopkins Medical Institutions, Baltimore, U.S.A.)

Scientific evidence has accumulated to indicate the potential for important social approaches to health promotion for older adults including the creation of new institutions that provide productive and meaningful roles post-retirement. Such roles are desired by older adults, and their lack has been termed a serious structural lag. Evidence also indicates that remaining physically, cognitively and socially active is beneficial to health. Finally, there is substantial experience in the optimal models for senior service from which to draw. We have designed a new model for productive engagement and simultaneously, health promotion of older adults, which creates high impact volunteer roles for older adults on a large scale in public elementary schools, based on current evidence as to best practices. This presentation describes the design and rationale for that model. The Experience Corps program places a critical mass of older adults in public elementary schools, performing roles identified by Principals as the most significant unmet needs for the schools. These often include literacy support, library programs, conflict resolution, and other academic and enrichment programs. Program design requires a commitment of 15 hours per week: participants work in teams, in a critical mass in the school, and receive reimbursement for expenses. The program design and rationale, and changes in health and function observed in a national demonstration project and a randomized pilot study will be presented.

Transforming the Role of Older Adults in Society

Marc R. Freedman (Civic Ventures, Inc, San Francisco, USA)

America, like much of the developed world, is in the midst of a demographic revolution. This vast increase in the number of older adults, and the vitality and longevity of this population, comes at the precise time when many social scientists are convinced that the country is facing a social capital crisis—a decline in civic involvement so essential for the functioning of many non-profit and community organizations. A potential solution to this crisis exists in the time, talent, and experience of the aging boomer population, provided they can be engaged to perform a wide range of volunteer and paid tasks that promise to enrich their lives, enhance their health and well-being, and contribute needed social capital to the community. A key factor in realizing this untapped potential will be to rectify structural lag that currently exists—in short to correct the mismatch between the interests and capacities of the new generation of older adults, and the opportunities for meaningful participation offered by the majority of civic organizations. Fortunately, this gap is being closed by a group of social entrepreneurs who are inventing new institutional arrangements with the potential to transform the role of older adults in society. This talk will describe the aforementioned movement, analyze its scope and prospects, and offer recommendations for future research and policy directions.

SESSION 106

Innovations in Gerontological Education

C. Tompkins, D. Stepp (Association for Gerontology in Higher Education, Washington D.C. USA), S. Kunkel (Miami Univ. of Ohio, USA), J. Hendricks (Oregon State Univ. USA), and D. Peterson (Univ. of Southern California, USA) Gerontology Comes of Age in the U.S. P. A. Holtsberg and L.W. Poon (University of Georgia, Athens, Georgia USA) Best Practices In Gerontological Distance Education in the U.S. A. Kruse (Institute of Gerontology, University of Heidelberg, Germany) Courses Of Study In Gerontology At German Universities. M. Luszcz, G. Andrews, J. Lawrence, and S. Cody (Flinders University, Adelaide, Australia) Graduate Certificate In Applied Gerontology in Australia. H. Shibata (Obirin University, Japan) Gerontological And Geriatric Education In Japan. B. Hagberg (Gerontology Research Centre and University of Lund, Sweden), B. Johansson(Institute of Gerontology and University College of Health Sciences, Jönköping, Sweden) Recent Development In Gerontology Education In Sweden.

This symposium brings together gerontological educators from different countries to examine and discuss recent innovations in the teaching of gerontological courses in higher education. Topics include national gerontological education effort, distance education, as well as curriculum, certificate, and disciplinary development.

Best Practices in Gerontological Distance Education in the U.S.

P. A. Holtsberg and L. W. Poon (Gerontology Center, The University of Georgia, GA, USA),

Gerontology educators in the USA have been experimenting with distance education technologies to present their academic courses for more than one decade. Current trends suggest a continuing and possibly accelerating proliferation in gerontological distance education. Unfortunately, relatively little attention has been devoted to sharing past experiences and lessons learned with these technologies so that current and future programs can implement "best practices" to maximize the educational experiences of future distance learners. This paper summarizes lessons learned and best practices from the most well-established and innovative USA programs, including the Distance Learning Partnership in Gerontology sponsored by The University of Georgia Gerontology Center. Since its inception in 1995, more than 1000 advanced undergraduates and graduate students from 10 universities located throughout Georgia (USA) have matriculated in one or more of 4 core courses (Survey-, Biology-, Psychology- and Sociology-of-Aging) taught by more than 35 faculty.

Courses Of Study In Gerontology At German Universities

A. Kruse (Institute of Gerontology, University of Heidelberg, Germany)

Since processes of development over the life span and the life situation in old age are of interest for many scientific disciplines, theories and findings from contemporary Gerontology are also significant topics in the education of students in other scientific disciplines. Consequently, at German universities, many institutes do offer seminars on gerontological research questions for students, who have finished their basic courses. For some disciplines, focusing on gerontological research is offered as one possibility for specialization and consolidation of scientific knowledge for graduate student. For studying regular courses in Gerontology at German universities, it is a prerequisite that the student has already made an exam in at least one discipline of social or medical sciences, especially in Sociology, Psychology, Medicine, Education, Social Work or Economics. Curricula of contemporary courses in Gerontology are conceptualized on the basis of a mean duration of 4-5 semesters, including diploma examination and degree dissertation. In accordance with gerontological theory, research and praxis, it is the aim of gerontological education at German universities to integrate perspectives and findings from numerous disciplines, i.e. to focus on the interdisciplinary character of Gerontology. Consequently, from the early beginning, participating in empirical gerontological studies is an integral part of education in Gerontology at German universities. The participation of students in gerontological research has proven to be useful for both, the students and the research staff, since the scientific competencies the students acquired in their basic disciplines do enrich research questions and designs. Since interdisciplinarity and research practice contribute to an attractive qualification, university graduates are in great demand at the German labor market.

Gerontological and Geriatric Education In Japan

H. Shibata (Obirin University, Japan)

Geriatric education is available in 19 medical schools in Japan. However, there is no interdisciplinary training in gerontology. Gerontological education is markedly behind those available in the U.S. However, comprehensive graduate education in gerontology consisting of health and social sciences are being launched in Japan.

Gerontology Comes of Age in the U.S.

C. Tompkins and D. Stepp (Association for Gerontology in Higher Education USA), S. Kunkel, (Miami University of Ohio, Scripps Gerontology Center USA), J. Hendricks (Oregon State University USA), D. Peterson (University of Southern California USA)

This paper will include an historical presentation of gerontological education in the United States, a discussion of how the field has evolved, and an exploration of what the future holds. Important steps such as the creation of national standards and guidelines for gerontological education and the Program of Merit review process have led to gerontological education "coming of age" in the United States. An overview of gerontological programs including specializations, certificates, undergraduate degrees, masters and doctoral degrees will be presented. Participants will have the opportunity to examine various educational resources such as AGHE's Standards and Guidelines, Careers in Aging: Consider the Possibilities and the Directory of Educational Programs in Gerontology and Geriatrics. Innovations in, and challenges for, the field such as critical pedagogy and credentialing and accreditation debates will also be discussed.

Graduate Certificate In Applied Gerontology in Australia.

M. Luszcz, G. Andrews, J. Lawrence, and S. Cody (Flinders University, Adelaide, Australia)

This presentation will focus mainly on the development of a Graduate Certificate in Applied Gerontology at Flinders University. This web-based program is done in conjunction with the Faculty of Social Sciences, the Centre for Ageing Studies and Novartis Foundation for Gerontology. The course aims to meet the professional development needs of graduates involved in the delivery of policy, planning or delivery of services to older people. The first intake will be for Semester 1, 2001. The program will be associated with educational opportunities and innovations available through other Universities in Australia.

Inovation on Gerontological Education - Recent developments in Sweden

B. Hagberg (Gerontology Research Centre and University of Lund, Sweden), B. Johansson(Institute of Gerontology and University College of Health Sciences, Jönköping, Sweden)

As a multidisciplinary subject, gerontology has had difficulties finding its place in ordinary curricula's within the university programs. The solution most often has been to be focused in one discipline such as sociology, psychology, geriatrics or nursing and reach out and incorporate competencies from other relevant areas. This might very well work in basic training sacrificing depth for breadth while difficulties with breadth becomes troublesome on the PhD level and for specialist training. Education has mainly developed outside the main university system by foundations of certain institutes/centres, the Institute of Gerontology in Jönköping (1970), the Gerontology Research Centre in Lund (1974), and the Stockholm Gerontology Centre (1986). Although these centres have a main focus on research, there have been significant educational spin-off effects, for example by BA, MA, and PhD thesis completed at these sites. A full undergraduate program in gerontology is, however, only offered at the Institute of Gerontology, University College of Health Sciences in Jönköping and a PhD program for gero-psychologists is given at the department of Psychology, Lund University. The Gerontology Centre in Lund plays a major role offering an advanced internordic gerontology course for university/college faculty. This strategic course provide research updates from various field of gerontology and has the potential of attracting more students to the field. A formal specialisation is nowadays possible in geriatric medicine, for RNs, social workers and psychologists. In order to meet the demands from professionals, conventional classroom teaching is more frequently combined with outreach education systems, using TV broadcasting and the Internet.

SESSION 107

Care and Support for Older People: from the Centre to the Periphery

Herman J Sixma (Netherlands Institute for Health Services Research, Utrecht, The Netherlands) Older people's perceptions of quality of care. Rachel Seymour (University of Portsmouth, Portsmouth, UK) Systematic analysis of carer-elder interactions: A multi method approach. Kevin J McKee (University of Sheffield, Sheffield, UK) Carer and Care-receiver perceptions of dependency for activities of daily living in informal care of older people: negative impact of disagreement on outcomes of care. G. Lamura (INRCA, Ancona, Italy) Elderly care and respite services: main results of a survey on 400 dependent elderly and their carers living in Central Italy. Lena Dahlberg (Dalarna Research Institute, Falun, Sweden) Public and voluntary organisations Δ support for caregivers. Monika Reichert (University of Dortmund, Dortmund, Germany) Discussion.

ISSUE: The topic of how society might best support its older citizens is becoming increasingly pertinent due to widespread population ageing. Much research has been carried out, but there has been little attempt to harmonise and synthesise this work. Such a task is complex, because support for older people is provided by a number of different actors and organisations, and the research in this area is performed by groups with different disciplinary backgrounds and interests. There is a need to integrate research, so that an overview can be generated of how the net of care and support for older people might best operate. This symposium brings together a group of individuals from different disciplinary backgrounds and from different European countries. Each will focus on a different aspect of research on caring for older people. In this way, a broad perspective on this topic will be developed with potential for integration. STRUCTURE: The symposium contains five individual papers and a sixth paper provided by a discussant. CONTENT: The papers are arranged so that a continuum of perspective on care for older people is generated. The first paper in the symposium, by Herman Sixma, describes the development of a new instrument measuring quality of care from the perspective of elderly people. The next two papers concentrate on the nature of the caregiving relationship. The first of these papers, by Rachel Seymour, describes an observational study of care and other interpersonal behaviours in the homes of older people being cared for by a relative. The second of these papers, by Kevin McKee, describes a study on how carers' and care-receivers' disagreement over care-receivers' level of dependency for activities of daily living impacts on a range of carer and caregiving outcomes. The fourth paper in the symposium, by Giovanni Lamura, then extends the focus on the caregiving relationship to include formal service provision, in a report of a study that examines the impact of caregiving on relatives of frail elderly, and formulates suggestions regarding care and respite services. The final paper in the symposium, by Lena Dahlberg, then brings this examination of the net of care to its broadest level, by considering the relationship between the public sector and voluntary organisations in the delivery of support to relatives who care for older people. The discussant, Monika Reichert, will then present an overview of how disparate aspects of research on care for older people can inform each other, and suggest prospects for future caregiving research. CONCLUSIONS/ANTICIPATED OUTCOMES: This symposium provides a forum for integrating different aspects of research on care for older people, allowing cross-disciplinary insights and the opportunity for consolidation of existing work. An overview should emerge of how the net of care and support for older people might best operate. The cross-European perspective will allow for an awareness of the cultural influences on care for older people, sensitising researchers to the need to take account of location and history. An agenda for future research is another potential outcome of the symposium.

Carer and Care-receiver perceptions of dependency for activities of daily living in informal care of older people: Negative impact of disagreement on outcomes of care.

Kevin J McKee (University of Sheffield, Sheffield, UK), Ian Philp (University of Sheffield, Sheffield, UK), Brian Ballinger (Royal Dundee Liff Hospital, Dundee, UK), Mary M L Gilhooly (University of Paisley, Paisley, UK), David S Gordon (Lanarkshire Health Board, Hamilton, UK), William J Mutch (Ashludie Hospital, Dundee, UK), Janice E Whittick (Chamberlain Consultants, Edinburgh, UK)

PURPOSE: This study sought to determine how carers' and care-receivers' disagreement over care-receivers' level of dependency for activities of daily living impacts on a range of carer and caregiving outcomes. METHOD: Older people (65+ years) resident in the community were identified through general practice records and recruited to the study (N=115). Through interview, family caregivers were also identified. Structured questionnaire-based interviews were carried out separately with the older person and his/her carer, focusing on reported dependency for activities of daily living and incorporating a range of measures of psychological well-being and relationship functioning. After two years, the surviving members of the sample were contacted and re-interviewed, and changes in health status and place of residence of the older person noted. RESULTS: Bivariate analyses within the cross-sectional data demonstrated significant relationships between levels of carer/care-receiver disagreement and outcomes. Total disagreement between carer and care-receiver was correlated with carer self-reported stress ($r=.39$, $p<.001$), carer willingness to continue caring ($r=.190$, $p=.042$), carer acceptance of institutional care ($r=.21$, $p=.025$), and carer-receiver's social death ($r=.18$, $p=.049$). Longitudinal analyses demonstrated similar relationships over time, while different patterns emerged relative to whether the carer or care-receiver perceived higher dependency in the care-receiver's activities of daily living. CONCLUSIONS: Much caregiving research has concentrated on the carer, whereas less research has focused on the relations between carer and care-receiver as a determinant of outcomes of caregiving. This study demonstrates the importance of assessing the nature of the carer/care-receiver relationship, and provides important information for potential supportive interventions.

Elderly care and respite services: Main results of a survey on 400 dependent elderly and their carers living in Central Italy

M. G. Melchiorre, C. Sirolla, S. Quattrini, G. Lamura (INRCA, Ancona, Italy)

PURPOSE: Main results of a study carried out in Central Italy are presented, aimed at identifying the impact of caregiving on relatives of frail elderly, and formulating suggestions regarding care and respite services. METHOD: A random sample of 400 elderly users of the Home Care Services delivered in 6 local Health Districts has been recruited, together with the relatives providing most care. Both were administered a structured questionnaire including questions on the use of existing health and social care services. RESULTS: Elderly care relies in Central Italy still heavily on family based support. Health care is mostly provided by means of GPs and of hospitals, while social care is delivered mainly in terms of monetary transfers. Community care is rarer, and mainly providing home services for basic medical tests (such as blood or urine tests), nursing care, physioterapic care, transportation and household care. Existing care services are however not always taken advantage of, due to aversion or lack of information among potential users. Nursing homes, in particular, have a negative image, which could improve remarkably if they were able to accept "temporary" patients. Volunteer organizations are known and used only by a minority of users, while care provided by foreign immigrants is more widespread, often for cohabitation purposes. CONCLUSION: A more holistic approach to the needs of the frail elderly and their caregivers could improve the supply and use of existing formal care services, by providing more flexible and personalised "respite" solutions for caregiving relatives, who today have to rely for this mainly on informal resources.

Older people's perceptions of quality of care

Herman J. Sixma (Netherlands institute for health services research, Utrecht, The Netherlands)

PURPOSE: User views on quality of care are generally assessed by patient satisfaction questionnaires. However, doubts have been cast on the validity and reliability of such instruments. Aims of this paper are: (1) to describe the development of a new instrument measuring quality of care from the perspective of elderly people, (2) to examine the potential of the new instrument in quality assurance (QA) and quality improvement (QI) studies. METHODS: A combination of qualitative and quantitative research methods was used to develop the QUOTE-Elderly instrument. Focus group discussions about older people's perceptions of quality of care preceded a postal survey, which was completed by 338 elderly people. Explorative and confirmative factor analyses and reliability analysis were applied to evaluate the taxonomy and feasibility of the instrument and the internal consistency of (sub)scales. RESULTS: Using scale optimisation, a new self- administered questionnaire was produced, including generic quality aspects and category-specific aspects particularly relevant for elderly people. Feasibility tests of the QUOTE-Elderly, in which importance and performance ratings were combined into quality impact indices, showed considerable differences in the functioning of general practitioners, hospital consultants, home helps and home care agencies as perceived by elderly people. CONCLUSIONS: The QUOTE-Elderly is an assessment instrument for quality of care from the perspective of cognitively intact, non-institutionalised elderly people. The instrument can be regarded as a method, more than a fixed set of items. The conceptual framework underlying the new instrument can also be applied in other, more specific groups of elderly people.

Public and Voluntary Organisations - Support for Caregivers

Lena Dahlberg (Dalarna Research Institute, Falun, Sweden)

PURPOSE: Extensive public sector activity is often said to have a suppressive effect on voluntary activity. However comparative studies have shown that this is not always the case. For example, in Sweden voluntary activity is quite substantial, even though public welfare is well developed. The activity of voluntary organisations can, though, often differ from that of public organisations, being less nursing oriented. During the 1990s cut-backs have been made in Swedish public care for older people, especially in the area of social support. In the same period, municipalities have made efforts to cooperate with voluntary organisations and are sometimes even encouraged to do so by the state. The purpose of this study was therefore to investigate the relationship between the public sector and voluntary organisations. METHOD: The study was carried out within the area of support to relatives caring for older people. It was based on a survey of 80 municipalities and 358 voluntary organisations. The response rates were 89% and 72% respectively. RESULTS: The study shows that all of the municipalities and one third of the voluntary organisations are offering various kinds of support to relatives. Moreover the study shows that the public activities did not have any suppressive effects on the voluntary activities. CONCLUSION: This study indicates that it is possible to develop both public and voluntary activities in the same area at the same time. Moreover, the municipalities have great potential to stimulate and encourage the activities of voluntary organisations.

Systematic analysis of carer-elder interactions: A multi method approach.

Rachel Seymour (University of Portsmouth, Portsmouth, UK),Anthony Gale (University of Portsmouth, Portsmouth, UK), Paul Morris (University of Portsmouth, Portsmouth, UK)

PURPOSE: The aim of this novel research was to document care and other interpersonal behaviours in the home of older people being cared for by a relative. METHODS: The senior author lived with 8 families for a minimum of 3 days as a participant observer. Circa 150 page transcripts were produced for each family. Expressed emotion interviews were also conducted with the caregiver and older person. RESULTS: Data include categorical analyses of: i) care behaviours; ii) emotional ethos of the household (initiated and received positive, neutral and negative affect); iii) behaviour of individuals (profiles of emitted and received interaction process scores, (Borgatta, 1962)); and iv) dyadic, triadic etc interactions (sociometric diagrams of the rate and direction of behaviours among family members and professional carers). Minuchin (1974) structural maps and methods based on distance regulation theory (Kantor and Lehr, 1975) described family dynamics. The geographical layout of the home was shown to have causal relationships with caring arrangements. The 8 families were then ranked on several dimensions on the basis of the primary data and multidimensional analysis. The observer also conducted repertory grids to elicit her own constructs of the family within a principal components analysis. CONCLUSIONS: This in- depth research on a handful of families enables us to create a framework within which to conceptualise caring behaviours in the home. It enabled convergence between four methodologies: observation, transcript analysis, interview and repertory grid. Comparisons are drawn between these data and those derived from more conventional techniques, highlighting the validity of the present methodology.

SESSION 108

Balance impairment - Test for tendency of falling using virtual reality - A pilot study

Gustaf Bucht (Dept of Geriatric Medicine, Umeå, Sweden) Lillemor Lundin-Olsson (Dept of Geriatric Medicine, Umeå, Sweden) Lars Nyberg (Dept of Geriatric Medicine, Umeå, Sweden) Anders Backman (VR-lab, Umeå, Sweden)

Purpose: To assess how attention-demanding and unexpected events influence older people's capacity to control balance and movement in a virtual reality environment. Background: Falls and the resulting injuries constitute a large health problem in the elderly population. Most falls occur during walking and turning and the fall risk increases when the person divides his attention to external stimuli. Method: The person is walking on a normal floor and is fed a known environment in VR and is exposed to some unexpected events. The hardware in the system consists of HMD, 9 trackers, and two SiliconGraphics computers. The software consists of the presentation of computer graphics and registration and handling of movement data. Results: Eight persons took part in the experiment. They were walking with and without the HMD and with and without unexpected external stimuli. Evident disturbances of walking pattern such as changes in speed, stride-length and balance reactions like slipping where observed when the persons were exposed to the unexpected event. Two persons experienced symptoms of cyber sickness. Conclusion: There is a potential use for balance impairment assessment in a safe virtual reality environment and it may be used to create individualized training programs.

Big steps for fall prevention: Effect of age and step size on ability to recover balance by stepping.

E. Hsiao (Biomechanics Laboratory, Department of Orthopaedic Surgery, University of California, San Fransisco, California, U.S.A.), P. Stotz (Injury Prevention and Mobility Laboratory, Simon Fraser University, Burnaby, British Columbia, Canada), S. N. Robinovitch (Biomechanics Laboratory, Department of Orthopaedic Surgery, University of California, San Fransisco, California, U.S.A. and Injury Prevention and Mobility Laboratory, Simon Fraser University, Burnaby, British Columbia, Canada)

PURPOSE: Previous studies indicate that elderly individuals are less able than young at recovering balance by stepping. The present study examined (a) whether step length affects young and elderly females' ability to recover balance through a single forward step, and (b) whether, for a given step length, recovery ability differs between young and elderly. METHODS: Ten elderly and ten young women (of mean age 75±3 (SD) and 28±4 yrs) participated in experiments where they were suddenly released (by means of a tether and electromagnet) from a forwardly inclined standing position. Subjects were instructed to recover balance by taking as large and quick a step as possible, or by stepping to floor-level targets located a horizontal distance of 15, 25, or 35% body height in front of the toes. For each condition, we determined the maximum release angle where this could be achieved in two consecutive trials. RESULTS: For both young and elderly, the maximum recoverable angle increased with increasing step length ($p<0.001$). However, mean values of the maximum recoverable angle were smaller for elderly than young at step lengths of 25%BH (13.5±1.8 vs. 17.5±3.8 deg; $p=0.01$) and 35%BH (14.3±2.7 vs. 21.6±4.0 deg; $p<0.001$), and in the unrestricted step length condition (16.8±2.5 vs. 27.5±2.5 deg; $p<0.001$). CONCLUSIONS: While step length affects ability to recover balance with a single forward step, additional variables contribute to age-related declines in recovery ability. These seem related to control of downward rotation before step contact, and the magnitude of foot contact forces generated during step contact.

Effect of footwear on static and dynamic balance in young and elderly subjects

U. Lindemann, S. Scheible (Bethesda Geriatric Hospital Ulm, Germany), B. Najafi, K. Aminian (Federal Institute of Technology Lausanne, Switzerland) , T. Nikolaus, C. Becker (Bethesda Geriatric Hospital Ulm, Germany)

PURPOSE: It has been proposed that footwear is important for stability and fall prevention strategies. Especially lateral stability is hypothesized to be improved by ankle stabilizing footwear. Most studies so far have been conducted with males. METHODE : Laterally reinforced boots (LRB) were tested against standardized sport shoes and socks. 14 frail elderly women (mean age = 86 years) with severe gait impairment and 15 young subjects (mean age = 31) were examined. Mean velocity of center of pressure in lateral direction on a force platform was measured as a parameter of static balance. Habitual and maximum gait speed were tested in addition. RESULTS : In young subjects LRB provided more lateral stability than socks ($p = .0229$). No effect of footwear on static balance and gait speed was seen in the elderly. The tested footwear had no elevated heels as the elderly women were used to wear. All women complained about fear of falling backwards. The test persons were unwilling to wear boots for daily activities. CONCLUSION: Footwear with lateral reinforcement was able to improve lateral stability in younger subjects. Flat soles and ankle supporting footwear were not accepted in elderly women. Furthermore heel height should be considered as a major confounder in balance and mobility assessment of elderly women. Further research is needed to evaluate the effect of proper footwear on balance with slightly elevated heels versus flat soles.

Effects of Age and Gender on Maximum Hip Flexion Power

C. Smeesters, J. A. Ashton-Miller (Biomechanics Research Laboratory, University of Michigan, Ann Arbor, MI, USA), N. M. Cole (Biologic Engineering Inc, Dexter, MI, USA)

The ability to move a leg rapidly enough to complete a compensatory step in time to arrest a fall requires the hip muscles to develop a large value of mechanical power (defined as the product of hip joint torque times leg velocity). Currently, measurements of muscle power output are made at relatively low velocities (usually < 250 deg/sec). Although it is well known that significant losses occur with age in hip flexor strength, the effects of age and gender on maximum hip flexor power at higher velocities remain to be quantified. We therefore tested the null hypothesis that neither age nor gender will significantly affect maximum hip flexor power in healthy adults. Maximum hip flexion power output was measured in 40 healthy subjects: 20 young (18-27 years old) and 20 old (65-84 years old) with equal numbers of males and females in each group. Measurements were made in the gravity-free plane at 5 resistance levels, spanning the range of attainable velocities, using a custom dynamometer. The maximum attainable hip flexion power decreased with increasing age (ANOVA, $p < 0.0005$) and female gender ($p < 0.0005$). Maximum attainable hip flexion velocity at zero resistance level also decreased with increasing age ($p < 0.0005$) and female gender ($p < 0.0005$). This age-related reduction in older adult hip flexor muscle power may underlie the diminished ability, especially in older women, to take a sufficiently rapid step to arrest a forward fall (e.g, Thelen et al. 1997, 2000).

Strength and flexibility influences on age-related changes in Functional Reach.

Q. Liu (Orthopaedic Biomechanics Laboratory, Department of Orthopaedics & Rehabilitation, Oregon Health Science University, Portland, Oregon, U.S.A.), J. Graham (Biomechanics Laboratory, Department of Orthopaedic Surgery, University of California, San Fransisco, California, U.S.A.), R. S. Hall (Injury Prevention and Mobility Laboratory, Simon Fraser University, Burnaby, British Columbia, Canada), S. N. Robinovitch (Injury Prevention and Mobility Laboratory, Simon Fraser University, Burnaby, British Columbia, Canada)

PURPOSE: Functional reach, which is the maximum forward distance one can reach without stepping or losing balance, is a commonly used index of postural stability. Our aim in the present study was to determine the biomechanical cause of age differences in functional reach. METHOD: We measured body segment positions and used inverse dynamics to estimate corresponding torques at the hip and ankle as subjects (20 elderly, aged 65-87 yrs and 10 young, aged 23-38 yrs) executed maximum forward reaches. RESULTS: When compared to young subjects, elderly subjects had smaller average values of maximum forward reach (13 ± 4 (SD) vs. 20 ± 2 percent body height; $p=0.015$ by independent samples t-test). They also reached with smaller average values of ankle plantarflexion rotation (-1.1 ± 1.9 vs. 2.5 ± 3.1 deg; $p=0.001$), hip flexion rotation (22.9 ± 7.9 vs. 38.1 ± 9.5 deg; $p<0.001$), ankle plantarflexor torque (0.63 ± 0.26 vs. 0.82 ± 0.23 Nm/kg; $p<0.001$), and hip extensor torque (0.73 ± 0.22 vs. 1.11 ± 0.24 Nm/kg; $p<0.001$). However, in both groups, peak joint rotations at the ankle and hip were well within available ranges of motion. Furthermore, reach distances correlated more strongly with hip extensor torques than ankle plantarflexor torques ($r=0.75$ vs. $r=0.59$; $p<0.001$ for both correlations). CONCLUSION: These results suggest than declines with age in functional reach are due to reductions in hip extensor strength (and to a lesser extent, ankle plantarflexor strength) and not reductions in joint flexibility.

SESSION 109

Australian Longitudinal Study of Ageing: International Comparative Perspectives

G. Andrews (Centre for Ageing Studies, Flinders University, Adelaide, Australia) (An Overview of the Australian Longitudinal Study of Ageing.) Du Peng (Peoples Univesity of Beijing, Peoples Republic of China), G. Andrews (Centre for Ageing Studies, Flinders University, Adelaide, Australia) and M. Clark (Rehabilitation and Ageing Studies Unit and Centre for Ageing Studies, Flinders University, Adelaide, Australia) (Successful Ageing: a Chinese and Australian Comparison.) S. Davis and G. Andrews (Centre for Ageing Studies, Flinders University, Adelaide, Australia) and K. Anstey (Prince of Wales Medical Research Institute, University of New South Wales, Randwick, Australia Impact of Social Activity on Mortality an American and Australian Comparison.) J. Dowd and M.Gacic Dobo (Evidence for Health Policy Programme, World Health Organization, Geneva, Switzerland) (Patterns of Disability in a Panel Study of an Old Old Population.) P. S. Kent, M. A. Luszcz (School of Psychology, Flinders University, Adelaide, Australia) (Preclinical Signs of Naming and Constructional Ability in a Community Sample.) A. L. Byers, C. van Doorn, S. V. Kasl, and B. R. Levy (Department of Epidemiology and Public Health, Yale University, New Haven, Connecticut, USA) (Paternal Attachment as a Risk Factor for Depression in Older Women.)

The Australian Longitudinal Study is a cross-disciplinary prospective study of adults aged 70 years and over that began in Adelaide, Australia in 1992. It is a population based bio-psycho-social and behavioral study of 2087 older adults residing in the community and in residential care. The study is being conducted by the Centre for Ageing Studies of Flinders University of South Australia. The Center for Demographic Studies, Duke University, Durham, North Carolina, USA, has collaborated in the study and partial funding was obtained for the first four rounds from the National Institute of Aging. The general purpose of this research is to gain further understanding of how social, biomedical, and environmental factors are associated with age-related changes in the health and well-being of persons aged 70 years and older. Emphasis is given to the effects of social and economic factors on morbidity, disability, acute and long-term care service use, mortality and successful aging. The aim is to analyze the complex relationships between individual and social factors and changes in health status, health care needs and service utilization dimensions. The sample for the Australian study was randomly generated from within the Adelaide Statistical Division using the State Electoral Database as the sampling frame. The sample was stratified by gender and the age groups 70-74, 75-79, 80-84, and 85 and over. Both community and institutional dwelling individuals were included in the list of specified persons. An additional component was that spouses aged 65 and over of specified persons also were invited to participate, as were other household members aged 70 years and over. Data from ALSA has been progressively archived with Inter-university consortium for Political and Social Research (ICPSR). Subsequent follow-up has been conducted using both telephone and face to face assessments over an eight month period. Extensive analyses utilizing the baseline and longitudinal data will continue, and have been carried out in both Australia and the United States. Active groups of collaborators are analyzing data relating to ADL/IADL performance, cognitive function, co-morbidity, cardiovascular disease and risk factors, dental health, diet and nutrition, diabetes, exercise and physical activity, family relationships and support, formal service use, hearing function, injuries and falls, mortality, sensory function, social activities, social interactions between couples, successful aging and other parameters. This Symposium examines a series of locally conducted and international comparative efforts using the ALSA data sets. Analyses range over several arenas and their correlates including successful ageing, morbidity, disability, social activities, cognition and depression. Both cross-sectional and longitudinal analyses are illustrated. This symposium demonstrates the value of international collaborative work done in relation to major studies undertaken in a particular location.

An Overview of the Australian Longitudinal Study of Ageing

G. Andrews (Centre for Ageing Studies, Flinders University, Adelaide, Australia)

The baseline data collection for the Australian Longitudinal Study of Ageing began in September 1992. Components included a comprehensive personal interview, conducted via Computer Assisted Personal Interview, a home-based assessment of physiological functions, self-completed questionnaires, and additional clinical studies. Personal interviews were carried out at this first wave for 2,087 participants. Clinical assessments were obtained for 1,620 of the participants. After an interval of one year respondents were re-contacted by telephone. These interviews included questions regarding changes in domicile, current health and functional status, new morbid conditions, changes in medication, major life events, general life satisfaction, and changes in economic circumstances. In Wave 2, 1,779 participants were re-interviewed. The third wave of the study began in September 1994. This phase was a complete reassessment, with face-to-face interviews, clinical assessments, self-completed questionnaires, and other clinical and laboratory studies. Data collection for the fourth wave began in November 1995. Wave 4 is a short telephone interview similar to Wave 2. 1,504 interviews were completed. A fifth wave of telephone interviews was conducted during February 1998 resulting in 1,171 completed interviews. In addition to the primary data collection from respondents, ancillary data collection has been ongoing since the initiation of the study. Data has been collected from a range of secondary providers. Lists of ALSA participants are compared biannually with the agencies' lists to determine the prevalence and incidence of receipt of services from these organizations. A sixth wave of data collection involving comprehensive face-to-face re-interviews, and clinical assessments has recently been completed.

Impact of Social Activity on Mortality: An American and Australian Comparison

S. Davis and G. Andrews (Centre for Ageing Studies, Flinders University, Adelaide, Australia) and K. Anstey (Prince of Wales Medical Research Institute, University of New South Wales, Randwick, Australia)

Previous research has clearly demonstrated the benefits of physical activity for the health and well-being of older people. Physical activity is often seen in the context of exercise and other fitness activities. Yet, there is a range of activities outside of this realm which also generate benefits for older people and may lower the risk of mortality. Analysis of data from a US population based study identified social and productive activities that involved little or no enhancement of fitness but still lowered the risk of all cause mortality as much as fitness activities did. The Australian Longitudinal Study of Ageing has followed over 8 years a cohort (2070) of persons aged 70 years and over at baseline (including spouses aged 65 years and over) . This paper reports on an analysis of that data which examined the association between physical, social and productive activity and seven year survival in older South Australians and compares findings with the American study.

Paternal Attachment as a Risk Factor for Depression in Older Women

A. L. Byers, C. van Doorn, S. V. Kasl, and B. R. Levy (Department of Epidemiology and Public Health, Yale University, New Haven, Connecticut, USA)

Research is needed to understand why women are at greater risk of depression than men. According to Jung’s Electra complex (counterpart theory to Freud’s Oedipus complex), females develop a stronger attachment to their fathers than their mothers. This study examined whether paternal attachment influenced the likelihood of depression among women (N=487) aged 70 and older in the Australian Longitudinal Study of Ageing (ALSA). The association of interest was analyzed using weighted multiple logistic regression and baseline data surveyed beginning in 1992. As hypothesized, we found that women whose fathers died at a younger age than their mothers were over twice as likely to report depression as women whose fathers died at an equivalent or older age than their mothers. The final model resulted in an odds ratio of 2.29 (p=0.009; 95% CI=1.23, 4.26), adjusting for age, education, self-rated health, number of medications, and Activities of Daily Living. Also, as predicted, the opposite-sex effect was stronger in women than in men (p= 0.01). These findings suggest that attachment theory is a possible explanation for increased risk of depression in adult women who lose their father before their mother.

Patterns of Disability in a Panel Study of an Old Old Population

Patterns of Disability in a Panel Study of an Old Old Population J. Dowd and M.Gacic Dobo (Evidence for Health Policy Programme, World Health Organization, Geneva, Switzerland), G. Andrews (Centre for Ageing Studies, Flinders University, Adelaide, Australia)

Using Grade of Membership (GOM) analysis participants in the Australian Longitudinal Study of ageing were studied over five successive waves of investigation. A combination of 15 ADL and Nagi disability items were used to define a series of four GOM profiles through a range from healthy (profile I) to frail (profile IV). The effect of transitions between disability profiles over time and mortality incidence was explored. This form of analysis allowed the complex dynamics of ageing, function, morbidity and mortality to be studied and the effects of a variety of independent variables including age, gender, education, social support, co-morbidity and change in domicile to be identified. a): While there is a tendency toward transition to increasing severe disability profiles between rounds due to age, there is evidence of return to less severe patterns in some population groups with advantageous changes in environmental or health status indicators; b): Stable or increasing prevalence and incidence rates of both fatal and nonfatal chronic diseases lead to transition to more severe disability profiles between rounds; c): The transitional effects of morbidity and co-morbidities show differences by age, gender, education, housing, self-rated health and presence of a confidant. These results demonstrate the influence of morbid and co-morbid changes on the development of functional disability over time in a population 70 years of age and above. Also shown are the positive and negative effects of socio-economic, environmental and social support variables on functional status change.

Preclinical Signs of Naming and Constructional Ability in a Community Sample

P. S. Kent, M. A. Luszcz (School of Psychology, Flinders University, South Australia).

Early symptoms of dementing illnesses include naming or constructional difficulties. We classified participants from a population-based sample of community dwelling older adults (aged 65 to 89) on these abilities to identify individuals with preclinical signs of possible impairment. Naming was assessed using 15-item versions of the Boston Naming Test (BNT15); construction using the pentagon copy task of the Mini-Mental State Examination (MMSE). Three groups, equivalent in age, gender and education level, were compared. The impaired naming group (n=25) and impaired construction group (n=23) comprised people with scores >2 SD below the mean for their age group on the respective task, but intact scores on the alternative task. The control group (n=38) scored in the normal range on both tasks. Verbal fluency, abstract reasoning, speed of processing and memory were also investigated; impaired groups performed equivalently on them, and did not differ from controls on memory or speed. Impaired naming, but not construction, also differed from controls on reasoning and fluency. Results suggest that (a) differential deficits in naming or construction can be identified in a community sample; (b) naming impairment is accompanied by parallel decrements on other language tasks (c) deficits occur in the absence of impaired memory. Data currently being collected will enable us to (a) determine if these cross-sectional deficits differentially predict cognitive, especially memory, decline (b) whether individuals with constructional impairments show differential deficits for other constructional tasks and (c) if individuals showing either impairment are at risk for mortality or dementia.

Successful ageing: A United States, Chinese and Australian comparison

Du Peng (Institute of Population Research, Peoples University of Beijing, Peoples Republic of China) G. Andrews (Centre for Ageing Studies, Flinders University, Adelaide, Australia) M. Clark (Rehabilitation and Ageing Studies Unit, Flinders University, Adelaide, Australia)

The MacArthur studies of successful ageing in the United States examined data from participants aged 70-79 years drawn from three community-based populations. High, medium and low functioning groups were identified using physical and cognitive criteria. Cross-sectional analyses demonstrated that these groups differed in their sociodemographic characteristics, health status, cognitive performance, physical functioning, mental health, lifestyle, health conditions and health care utilisation. These findings have been replicated and extended using cross-sectional data from the Australian Longitudinal Study of Ageing. Criteria comparable to those employed in the MacArthur studies were again used to define high, medium and low functioning groups. The current paper seeks to extend these analyses by introducing a longitudinal dimension, and by examining the value of the MacArthur model cross-nationally. Data are drawn from the Australian Longitudinal Study of Ageing and the Beijing Longitudinal Study of Ageing. Hierarchical logistic regression is used to model the association of baseline healthy ageing status with subsequent status on a range of health, social and economic factors. Baseline healthy ageing status is defined using the MacArthur criteria, while outcomes at selected intervals after baseline are successively modeled. These analyses are conducted using parallel data from the Australian and Beijing studies. The results indicate the extent to which the MacArthur classification retains its predictive value with the passage of time, and permit a preliminary evaluation of the cross-national value of the MacArthur model by contrasting the findings obtained with the Australian and Chinese ageing populations.

SESSION 111

Films and Videos on Art and Elderhood: Amargosa, Academy Award Finalist

James Vanden Bosch (Terra Nova Films, Inc, Chicago, Illinois USA)

Amargosa, distinguished as an Academy Award finalist in its film category, tells the story of dancer-choreographer-painter Marta Becket who found that her life in New York didn't allow her the freedom to pursue her dreams as a dancer and artist, and that instead a vacant auditorium in Death Valley provided her with a blank canvas to create her own brand of dance theater. At age 74 her performances and artwork still draw audiences from hundreds of miles away. Her story is told with cinematic beauty, poetic narrative and a stunning musical score. Amargosa is a testament to dreams and creative endeavors everywhere

SESSION 115

Progress in Managing Cardiovascular Disease in the Elderly

Ferenc Follath (Universität Spital, Zürich, Switzerland) (Treatment of heart failure in the elderly) Charles Cline (Malmö University Hospital, Malmö, Sweden) (Nurse led clinics for the older patient) (Interventional cardiology in the elderly) (Antithrombotic therapy and thrombotic bleeding risk in the elderly; Atrial fibrillation)

The management of cardiovascular disease in general is well documented but little account has been made how modifications in terms of treatment and delivery need to be implemented for the older patient. Older patients have been largely excluded from clinical trials of treatment. This session is organised to address major cardiovascular diseases affecting older people and how our treatment approach requires adaptation to take account of the multi-disabled older patient. Presentations cover management of heart failure, the value or otherwise of interventional cardiology in the elderly, a discussion of the pros and cons of antithrombotic therapy and, finally, how other professionals can facilitate the delivery of better health care to the older patient. Attendees will be able to modify their own clinical practice to benefit their older patients.

Nurse led clinics for the older heart failure patient

Charles Cline

Chronic heart failure is a major disease in developed countries affecting at least 2% of the population with an increasing incidence, in contrast to other cardiovascular diseases. It seriously affects mortality, morbidity and quality of life. Also it is the cause of considerable health care expenditure and accounts for 1-2% of the total health care budget in some European countries. Importantly heart failure is a disease of the elderly and most patients are over 70 years. In order to improve outcomes, as well as curtail health care costs, increasing attention has been paid the management to the management of heart failure. In this context observational and randomised trials have been performed in which nurse led clinics have been shown to be a valuable instrument. Ideally the aim of such a clinic is to educate patients and their families in heart failure, to teach patients the elements of flexible diuretic self-management, to up titrate angiotensin converting enzyme (ACE) inhibitors, angiotensin receptor blockers (ARB's) and betablockers, to provide easy access for evaluation in case of increasing signs and symptoms of heart failure hereby preventing emergency room visits and hospitalisations and to encourage long term compliance to prescribed medication. Ideally all data on patient weight, prescribed medication, signs and symptoms of heart failure should be recorded in a patient diary which can regularly be review by a heart failure nurse. This approach has been shown to be effective resulting in over 80% reduction in admissions in non-randomised studies and 36-44% reduction in randomised studies. These benefits have been found to be combined with improvements in quality of life. However, studies on nurse led clinics have been relatively small, often short term and performed at single centres. There is a need for larger studies with longer follow up. The possibility that nurse led clinics in combination with easy access could lead to increased health care utilisation cannot be overlooked however no published studies have shown any negative effects. In a study of the clinical implementation of a nurse led clinic for heart failure no evidence of detrimental effects was found.

The treatment of heart failure in the elderly

F. Follath (Department of Medicine, University Hospital Zurich, Switzerland)

Heart failure (HF) is one of the major health problems in the elderly population with a prevalence reaching more than 10% in the age group >75 years. The cause of HF is coronary artery disease in the majority of male patients, while non-ischaemic HF, such as hypertensive heart disease, is more frequent in females. Associated with a higher age is an increasing incidence of co-morbid conditions, which has an important impact on prognosis and efficacy and tolerance of drug treatment of HF. The Charlson co-morbidity index is directly related to mortality after myocardial infarction and HF. Reduced renal function, in particular, is a frequent and clinically relevant negative prognostic factor. Since many essential HF-drugs (e.g. enalapril, lisinopril, captopril, digoxin) and antiarrhythmic agents (e.g. sotalol) are eliminated in a pharmacologically active form by the kidney, dosage adaptation to measured/estimated creatinine clearance values is essential. An additional problem in the elderly HF patients is the simultaneous use of other non-cardiac drugs resulting in a higher risk of interactions and side effects. For these reasons therapeutic guidelines for HF - often derived from studies in highly selected patient groups - have to be adapted for the elderly. Symptomatic improvement may become a more important therapeutic aim than prolongation of long-term survival

SESSION 116

Inequalities in Old Age: Theoretical and Empirical Developments in Race, Class, and Gender

Stephen Crystal, (Institute for Health, Health Care Policy, and Aging Research; Rutgers University; New Jersey, USA) Cumulative Advantage, Public Policies, and the Distribution of Resources in Later Life. Julie Ann McMullin, (Department of Sociology; University of Western Ontario; London, Ontario, Canada) Theorizing Inequality: Diversity, Structure, and Agency. Sol Encel, (Social Policy Research Centre; University of New South Wales, Sydney, Australia) Age Discrimination in Australia. Toni Calasanti, (Department of Sociology; Virginia Tech, Virginia, USA) Making Citizenship Real: Citizenship, the Life Cycle, Equality and Inequality.

Inequalities in old age is an important theoretical and empirical arena for the pursuit of studies in race, class, and gender. This session is devoted to the exploration of: 1) Cumulative advantages, public policies, and the distribution of resources in later life 2) Theorizing inequality: diversity, structure, and agency 3) Age discrimination 4) Citizenship, the life cycle, equality and inequality 5) Gender, race, ethnicity, class, sexuality, etc.: Age relations In the United States, economic inequality is higher among persons over 65 than among younger adults. This reflects a process of cumulative advantage and disadvantage over the lifespan as individual lifecourse events (such as the delayed impact of early human capital investments, savings behavior, and the onset of disability) interact with social policies (such as the design of retirement income systems). This presentation will review the "cumulative advantage" concept and explore the way in which societal choices concerning retirement income systems affect later-life distributional outcomes in the U.S. and in other economically developed countries, particularly with respect to differences in outcomes by race, gender, and educational attainment. It will also touch on the ways in which health care financing choices affect distributional outcomes.

Age Discrimination in Australia

S. Encel, Social Policy Research Centre, University of new South Wales, Sydney, Australia

Legislation to ban age discrimination, especially in employment, was enacted in all States and Territories of Australia in the 1990s. In each case, the implementation of the law is entrusted to a statutory board or commission. The effectiveness of such legislation has been examined by a number of commentators, and is also the subject of an extensive review by the Law Reform Commission of the State of new South Wales. The most common criticism is that the system is excessively legalistic and should be reformed to give the various boards the power to be more proactive. The system is also being examined in a British study which compares the Australian experience with anti-discrimination legislation and practice in Canada and the United States, as a prelude to the possible enactment of legislation in the United Kingdom. The present writer is a contributor to this study, which is sponsored by the Joseph Rowntree Foundation.

Cumulative Advantage, Public Policies, and the Distribution of Resources in Later Life

Stephen Crystal, (Institute for Health, Health Care Policy, and Aging Research; Rutgers University, New Jersey, USA)

In the United States, economic inequality is higher among persons over 65 than among younger adults. This reflects a process of cumulative advantage and disadvantage over the lifespan as individual lifecourse events (such as the delayed impact of early human capital investments, savings behavior, and the onset of disability) interact with social policies (such as the design of retirement income systems). This presentation will review the cumulative advantage concept and explore the way in which societal choices concerning retirement income systems affect later-life distributional outcomes in the U.S. and in other economically developed countries, particularly with respect to differences in outcomes by race, gender, and educational attainment. It will also touch on the ways in which health care financing choices affect distributional outcomes.

Gender, Race, Ethnicity, Class, Sexuality, Etc.: Age Relations

Toni Calasanti, (Department of Sociology, Virginia Tech, Blacksburg, VA, USA)

Despite recent attention to how race/ethnicity, class, gender, and (less so) sexuality influence old age, theorists of aging generally have not adressed age relations as a unique form of inequality—they have not explicity theorized age relations. The goal of my presentation, then, is two-fold. First I will extend recent arguments concerning the importance of theorizing age relations. I suggest that, by focusing on successful aging we reinforce ageism, even when we acknowledge that ability to age successfully varies by social location. Such a focus not only emphasizes individual, and not structural factors, but also keeps us busy trying to treat or ameliorate old age, or demonstrate that the old are, in fact, more like the young, rather than theorizing old age as a political location. As a result, we end up treating the old, and old bodies, as deviant. Second, I want to suggest some ways in which we can use a feminist approach to understanding race, ethnicity, gender, class, and sexual preference to begin to theorize age realtions and old age as these intersect with other social inequalities.

Theorizing Inequality: Diversity, Structure, and Agency

Julie Ann McMullin, (Department of Sociology, University of Western Ontario; Ontario, Canada)

In the literature on aging and the life course, most theories of inequality tend not to focus on human agency. Instead, such theories place emphasis on macro processes and structures. This paper explores the intersections between structure and agency and discusses how research on inequality might benefit from considering these intersections. I discuss how agency and key structural bases of power and diversity (e.g. class, age, gender, and ethnicity/race relations) are intertwined and develop several concepts and mechanisms that may usefully link structure and agency in theories of inequality.

SESSION 118

Are Future Medical Doctors Being Prepared to Care for Older Persons?

Alexandre Kalache, (World Health Organization, Geneva Switzerland, Facilitator) Ingrid Keller,(World Health Organization, Geneva Switzerland) Gerry Bennett (Academic Department of Health Care of Older People St Bartholomew's and the Royal London School of Medicine and Dentistry, London) Carlos Alberto Cano Gutierrez (Associated Proffesor, Faculty of Medicine, Director Institute of Ageing, Pontificia Universidad Javeriana, Bogotá, Colombia) Emilie Marinoni (President, International Committee of the Swiss Medical Students' Association, Université de Genève, Switzerland) Ahmad Halwani (National Officer for Medical Education 2000/01, Lebanese Medical Student Association, American University Beirut, Beirut, Lebanon)

Issue: Due to rapid population ageing, coming generations of medical doctors will see more and more older patients. However, are they being trained to adequately deal with their problems? Such training is overwhelmingly important not only for the future generations: increasingly practice of medicine requires sound knowledge of medical care in old age. The WHO, in collaboration with the IFMSA, conducted a worldwide survey among medical students, to collect data about if and how geriatric medicine is included into the national as well as local medical curricula. The outcomes of this survey and future implications for curriculum development will be addressed. Structure: Chair: Alexandre Kalache, MD, Ph.D. Each participants will give a short presentation on his/her experience from the "teaching" and from the "being taught" point of view. Active participation of the audience will be sought. Content: Ingrid Keller, M.Sc, MPH World Health Organization Geneva Brief overview of the "Teaching Geriatrics in Medical Education" Study, including the results about if and how geriatric medicine is taught in medical schools from some 80 countries on all continents. Some cases of multi-disciplinary geriatric teaching programmes with a life course perspective will be highlighted. Professor Gerry Bennett Academic Department of Health Care of Older People St Bartholomew's and the Royal London School of Medicine and Dentistry, London, UK Education for medical undergraduate students in geriatric medicine in the UK Professor of Geriatric Medicine from developing country: Teaching geriatric medicine from the point of view of a developing country Medical student from a developed country: The students' point of view of being taught geriatrics in a developed country Medical student from a developing country: The students' point of view of learning about older persons' care Anticipated outcome: In collaboration with professors of geriatric medicine and interested students, WHO aims to develop a minimum core curriculum for geriatric medicine, applicable globally and flexible enough in such a way as to respond to local needs. This symposium will provide an overview of the work done so far as well as seek comments from the audience on the way forward Δ particularly in the relation to curriculum development. The symposium should also give an opportunity for identification of partners for future activities in the field of medical education, lead by WHO. Ingrid Keller Overview of the "Teaching Geriatrics in Medical Education" Study This study was carried out as a collaborative project between the WHO and IFMSA (International Federation of Medical Students' Associations) from December 1999 to February 2001. Data obtained through an e-mail survey about the inclusion of geriatric medicine into national curricula were analysed. In addition we obtained complementary information on curricula of medical schools. Some 280 schools from 70 countries were surveyed. Selected results about if and how geriatric medicine is included into local medical curricula and how it is taught, will be presented. Some cases of multi-disciplinary geriatric teaching programmes with a life course perspective will be highlighted. In many countries, even those with an already high percentage of older persons among the population, geriatric medicine does not form part of the undergraduate curriculum of medical education. Strategies to be adopted for the inclusion of geriatric medicine into the medical curricula will be discussed. Professor Gerry Bennett Education for medical undergraduate students in geriatric medicine in the UK International demographic changes are making almost all doctors into reluctant geriatricians. The UK was once seen as not only the birthplace of modern geriatric medicine, but also the repository of the knowledge base via its geriatricians with international reputations. An innovative project involved the development of study guides (tutorials in print) in the core subjects of geriatric medicine, gerontology, stroke, elder abuse, ethics, confusion, Parkinson's disease, etc. These were positively evaluated and peer reviewed. The development of new problem based learning curriculum and a survey indicating a strong bias towards computer based information focused on transforming the paper based guides into an interactive CD-ROM format. The first three CDs are in their final phase of development. They will provide a flexible teaching programme providing the key knowledge base and the minimum data set for examination purposes. It brings geriatric medicine back to the forefront of medical education at a crucial time for the subject. Professor Carlos Alberto Cano Gutierrez Teaching geriatric medicine from the point of view of a developing country Older people are the age group increasing the fastest in many developing countries. Good training in care of older persons is urgently needed for future medical doctors. Some model curricula are available for example from Colombia, but often geriatric medicine is not recognised in the national medical curricula. The focus must be on inter-disciplinary and community based training. Emilie Martinoni Geriatric training from the point of view of a medical student from a developed country Medical students in many developed countries receive training in geriatric medicine. However, training per se may not be enough. It is the attitude of medical students today which will influence the medical treatment of older persons tomorrow. Bearing in mind that the majority of the students from developed countries are brought up in nuclear families, and they may see only extremely frail older patients during their training, it is crucial for them to have contact with healthy older persons during their training. Multi-disciplinary and community-based training can make an essential contribution to equip future medical doctors with appropriate knowledge and shape their attitudes positively towards older persons. Ahmad Halwani Geriatric training from the point of view of a medical student from a developing country In many developing countries, the topic of ageing has not yet come to reach a place high on the national agenda, or even public awareness. As one consequence, medical students are not trained in old age care, even though it would be timely. Despite the fact that the need for geriatric specialists will remain limited, the need for well trained general practitioners who can attend older persons on the primary health care level is much more urgent.

SESSION 119

Geriatric Patients and Their Drugs: Assessment of Correct Intake

I. Findl, E. Lehner, K. Welsch, G. Pleiner, K. Klaushofer, K. Koller (Hanusch-Hospital, Vienna, Austria)

The purpose of this study is to identify risk patients with difficulties in drug management, using the 'Drug Assessment Test (DAT)' in order to organize support for them at home. The study involved 200 geriatric patients, 159 women and 41 men with a mean age of 78.9 years. The assessment included social, demographic and clinical data and a series of standardized tests: Mini Mental State Test, Syndrom Kurz Test, Activity of Daily Living, Geriatric Depression Scale and the Drug Assessment Test which we have recently developed and validated. Statistical analysis included factor analysis, item analysis, multiple regression analysis and logistic regression analysis. The DAT includes three factors: 3 cognitive, 3 motor and 3 complex functional motor tasks. Only 45 patients (23%) performed all tasks correctly. The significant predictors for the DAT performance were cognitive competence and functional mobility. When relating support at home to performance, the data showed that 38% of the patients received too little support, especially those living alone and those with reduced functional mobility. The treating doctors assessed the patients' performance in drug management better than the patients themselves. About half of the patients and a quarter of the doctors overestimated the patients' competence. Without having performed the DAT at least a quarter of the patients would have been discharged without the necessary support at home. The Dat is a new instrument that closes a gap in the geriatric assessment program. By this tool we can improve the patients' care after stay in hospital.

Predictors of antidepressant medication among elderly patients in long-term institutional care

Finne-Soveri Harriet (Stakes/Kustaankartano, Helsinki, Finland), Noro Anja (Stakes, Helsinki, Finland), Björkgren Magnus (Chydenius-Institute, Kokkola, Finland)

To analyse the predictors of antidepressant medication among elderly patients in long-term institutional care (LTIC). METHOD: The subjects were driven from database including 2400 RAI (Resident Assessment Instrument) assessments of elderly residents in LTIC. The data was collected during April to September in 2000. Logistic regression was used as the analysis method. The dependent variable was classified as 0 if there were no antidepressant and 1 if any antidepressant use. As predictors were used symptoms of depression, as dummy variable, the reference being no symptoms, the first included one or two symptoms, and the second included 3 or more symptoms, and gender, age, length of stay (LOS), previous history of mental diseases, diagnoses of depression and type of institution. RESULTS: Of the residents 38.1% had an antidepressant, 73% were women, average age 82 years, average length of stay 2.4 years, 13% had diagnosis of depression, less than 1%

had bipolar depression, 15% had previous history of mental diseases. No symptoms of depression were discovered in 28%, one to two symptoms in 32%, and more than 3 symptoms in 40%. In logistic model those who were younger and those with longer LOS used seldom antidepressants, and those who had three or more symptoms had more often antidepressants (OR=1.6). Both depression diagnosis (OR=6.3) and bipolar depression (OR=3.2) predicted antidepressant use. No difference between the types of institution was found. CONCLUSION: Symptoms of depression occur vary frequently in all levels LTIC. However, proper diagnosis, the targeting of the medication and appropriate length of it needs attention.

Quality Use of Medicines in Residential Aged Care: Issues Affecting Implementation of Best Practice Guidelines

A. Gilbert (Quality Use of Medicines and Pharmacy Research Centre, University of South Australia, South Australia, AUS), J. Cheek (Centre for Research into Nursing and Health Care, University of South Australia, SA, AUS), L. Sansom (School of Pharmacy and Medical Sciences, University of South Australia, SA, AUS), A. Ballantyne (Centre for Research into Nursing and Health Care, University of South Australia, SA, AUS), R. Penhall (Department of Geriatric and Rehabilitation Medicine, Royal Adelaide Hospital, SA, AUS) J. Jones (Centre for Research into Nursing and Health Care, University of South Australia, SA, AUS)

Despite the existence of best practice guidelines for achieving quality use of medicines (QUM) in residential aged-care facilities (RACFs), there is ample evidence of poor compliance with the guidelines. This study identified factors influencing the implementation of best practice, and developed methods to implement guidelines for achieving quality use of medicines in RACFs. The multi-method descriptive and exploratory study, conducted in 12 RACFs in South Australia, comprised three stages. Stage One used three data collection methods; Critical Incident Technique interviews, Focus Groups and Nominal Groups, involving views of people such as general practitioners, pharmacists, nurses, allied health professionals, residents, facility managers and owners to ensure a comprehensive analysis of issues. Stage Two, using Participatory Action Research, built on data collected in Stage One to develop a range of strategies which could also be used to address issues identified in the previous stage. Stage Three drew on data obtained from Stage One and Two to develop recommendations for changes at policy, structural, organisational and individual levels, to support QUM. Evidence from Stages 1 and 2 indicated the need to assist RACFs to interpret the best practice guidelines and develop standard operating procedures for a range of situations surrounding medication use. The establishment and facilitation of a Medication Advisory Committee (MAC) in each facility appeared to be an essential component of implementing QUM in RACFs. Of the 12 facilities, 11 have established a functional MAC, each with acceptable Terms of Reference and a strategic plan.

the use of psychotropic medications as chemical restraints in nursing homes - a nurse's perspective

Lisa Clinnick (Hepburn Health Service, Daylesford, Victoria, Australia)

A research study using a grounded theory approach explored nurses' perceptions on the use of psychotropic drugs as chemical restraints within nursing homes. Four nurses currently working in aged care were interviewed using an in-depth collective approach for data collection. Data analysis was completed and identified three main categories that represent for this group the use of psychotropic drugs as chemical restraints within nursing homes. These included knowledge, the role of the registered nurse, and the ability to influence outcomes. From the analysis it would appear that the nurses interviewed perceived that through increased knowledge nurses are able to expand their role and their ability to influence outcomes regarding the prescription and administration of psychotropic drugs as chemical restraints.

Working Collaboratively to Minimise Medication Misadventures in Aged Care Facilities

Kay Price RN, (Centre for Research into Nursing and Health Care, University of South Australia, Adelaide, Australia) Lyn Hepburn-Brown (Managing Director, Nursing Agency of Australia, FULLARTON, SOUTH AUSTRALIA, AUSTRALIA)

PURPOSE: In Australia there have been nationally disseminated documents that state for example that residential aged care facilities can minimise the risk of medication misadventure by ensuring systems are in place that contribute to the quality use of medicines (Australian Pharmaceutical Advisory Council, 1997). At the same time, changes in both funding to residential aged care facilities and staff arrangements of these facilities necessitates the need to engage the services of an agency to provide relief health care personnel. Indeed, up to 20% of staff working in the aged care sector are agency staff. As such, it seems reasonable to suggest that agencies that supply relief staff in turn have an obligation to ensure that agency staff provided have the required skills to perform that work required in accordance with legislation and professional standards and codes. The research study has been funded by the Commonwealth Department of Health and Aged Care through the Pharmaceutical Health and Rational Use of Medicines (PHARM) - Quality Use of Medicines (QUM) Evaluation Program. METHOD: Where people want to understand and improve their situation, an appropriate research approach of choice is Participatory Action Research [PAR]. PAR is change oriented, interventionist, and is informed by a critical concern to identify issues and collaborate so as to reflect upon practice to systematically reconstruct it. RESULTS: The Nursing Agency of Australia takes seriously its responsibilities related to medications management, yet requests for agency staff, particularly in what are termed low level aged care facilities, engenders debates about legislative and professional standards. Commercial and budgetary realities of aged care facilities significantly influence developments related to the quality use of medicines. CONCLUSION: Minimising medication misadventures requires residential aged care facilities and agencies working in collaboration to ensure that legislative and professional standards be put in place. It is imperative that health service research continues to address difficult areas of practice to ensure that QUM is not a rhetorical practice.

SESSION 120

A Case-control Study of Spousal/Consortial Homicide-Suicide in Older Persons

D. Cohen, J.E. Malphurs (University of South Florida, Tampa, Florida, USA)

Purpose: To identify factors that differentiate older married perpetrators of homicide-suicide and suicide only. Method: A total of spousal/ consortial homicide-suicide were ascertained in florida in 1998-1999. Two suice controls were matched to each homicide-suicide case by age, race, method of death, and district. Over 250 variables were coded from medical examiner records and law enforcement reports. Groups were compared using chi-square and Fisher's exact test. Case-control comparisons were made using McNemar's procedure. Results: Homicide-suicide perpetrators had significantly more domestic violence than suicide controls or were caregivers in contrast to suicide perpetrators who were care recipients. There were no differences in autopsy findings or sociodemographic factors but both groups had significant depression. Conclusion: Depression plays a role in both homicide-suicide and suicide, but the associated factors may be different: cargiving in homicide-suicide and receiving care for health problems in suicide. Marital strife is a significant factor in another type of homicide-suicide.

Older Persons, Gambling Problems and in-home responses

E. McKee (COPA, Toronto, Canada)

There is a preponderance of information that indisputably demonstrates the aging of our society. At the same time, there is growth in the gaming industry, and the specific targeting of older persons. This targeted marketing of a potentially vulnerable and growing population has raised concerns among those in the fields of addiction treatment for older persons. There is little research attention paid to older adults relative to younger persons with gambling problems. However, as mentioned, there is recognized significant growth in both the numbers, and in the accessibility of gambling venues. Since 1983, COPA's primary objective with its funding from the Ministry of Health remains to provide outreach assessment and treatment in the home setting. COPA offers home assessments, treatment planning and case management to residents of the former West Toronto Health District who are age 55 or older, making COPA's expertise accessible to all, even the cognitively and mobility impaired. The objective is to assist them, when appropriate, to remain in their community through treatment, advocacy and support. Consistent with the findings of the former Donwood, COPA found that about 10% of its clients who were receiving treatment for substance use problems also had gambling problems. Using its home-visiting harm reduction approach, COPA has obtained some note-worthy successes in reducing the harmful effects of gambling. This presentation will focus on two of those successes, with detailed case presentations that review the treatment and outcomes. Discussion will then focus on the application of this approach to problem gambling treatment to other areas.

Problem Gambling Prevention for Seniors

Richard Govoni (University of Windsor, Windsor, Canada) Deana Johnson (Council on Aging, Windsor-Essex County, Windsor, Canada)

With the increase in gambling availability over the last three decades, there has come a growing awareness that gambling is a potentially addictive behaviour similar to drugs and alcohol. Prevention programs designed to meet the needs of seniors and which receive input from the target group have an increased chance of success. The purpose of this study was to test the applicability of the Participatory Action Research (PAR) methodology to the development of a gambling prevention program. PAR treats participants as co-researchers and involves them in the development of solutions. The techniques of random telephone surveys, key informant interviews and focus groups were used to develop an understanding of the nature of the problem and to develop possible solutions. Late onset addictions have a different etiology than do addictions in the general population and seniors are particularly vulnerable to the financial consequences of problem gambling. Based on the research, a non-heirarchical group process, Syntegration, was conducted involving broad-based community members. This process produced a framework for the development of a community gambling prevention program for seniors that can be applied to other jurisdictions.

States Treating Elder Inmates

J. M. Mattern (John Carroll University, Cleveland, Ohio, U.S.A.)

This is part of a pilot study undertaken to provide preliminary background information for a large federal grant. The U.S. can be considered the worlds foremost jailer with an inmate population of nearly 1.7 million (Maker, 2000). U.S. prison inmates are growing in numbers and aging in place. Numbers of inmates aged 50+ are likewise increasing due to the trend of increased incarceration, anti-crime legislation, and longer sentences. By the year 2030, the U.S. Census Bureau estimates that 1/3 of U.S. prison population will be 55+ years of age (James, 1992). Like community-dwelling elders, incarcerated elders will become high-volume users of health care (Rylander, 1996). They may exhibit age-related conditions sooner and are less healthy than their community-dwelling counterparts. Elder inmates also exhibit different medical and social needs than their younger counterparts (e.g, legal assistance, privacy). Elder inmates have a legal right to appropriate and adequate health care. This study surveyed various state correctional departments and determined how elder inmates are housed and treated. The data shows that some states have been effective in reducing costs of prison health care spending and staff appear to be somewhat educated about the aging process. Many states do not employ SCUs or age-appropriate services and programs (e.g, special diets, 24-hour nursing care) for their elder inmate populations. Older inmates pose unique and costly problems for prisons already struggling to manage outdated, overcrowded, and under-funded prisons (Maker, 2000).

SESSION 121

Gender, Identity and the Home in Later Life

Cherry Russell (The University of Sydney, Sydney, Australia)

The home has always been a central concern in discussions of older people, and it has been identified as having particular significance in the life worlds of older women. This paper draws on in-depth interviews with older Australians in which they were asked to talk about the meaning and significance of home in their lives. I describe the study of 66 older Sydney home dwellers and outline the sociological framework used to analyse the interview data. The findings suggest that, in important ways, the experience of home in later life is a gendered phenomenon. Emotional attachment to one's home appears to mean different things to older women and men. At the same time, feelings of strong attachment to home were by no means universal, even among women. Overall there was considerable diversity in the centrality of 'home' to the construction of personal meaning and identity in later life. This diversity raises issues of conceptual and practical significance in social gerontology. These include implications for housing research, where an overly romanticised view of the home as the core of an older person's identity may lend credence to minimalist approaches to public resource allocation.

Home as a Site for Long-Term Care

P.C. Kontos (University of Toronto, Ont, Canada) P.D. McKeever (Home Care Evaluation and Research Centre, University of Toronto, ON, Canada), J. Angus (University of Toronto, Ont, Canada)

PURPOSE: Publicly funded Home Care programmes have proliferated throughout Canada as health care institutions have either closed or reduced their range of functions. Consequently, the "home" has become the primary setting for formal health care and social support service provision. The largest proportion of home care services are provided to the aged afflicted with chronic illnesses, disabilities or other related frailties. The "Hitting Home" Project provides the first comprehensive description of the living and working conditions of Canadian households which function simultaneously as personal dwellings and as sites for the labour intensive work of health care professionals and paraprofessionals. METHOD: In-depth qualitative case studies of 20 households were conducted in urban, remote and rural regions of Ontario. RESULTS: Data consisting of housing circumstances, use of space, distribution of responsibilities, working conditions and social relations, challenges the presumption that contemporary homes are suitable sites for caregiving/ receiving. In many instances, household spaces are not designed with long-term care in mind, and their use as sites of care necessitates physical and social adjustments that result in sub-optimal environments for care and/or personal life. CONCLUSION: The devolution of health care into Canadian homes is changing the meanings, physical conditions and spatio-temporal ordering of both domestic life and health care work. The social and spatial relations, and the material conditions that characterize long-term home care, point to the need to improve both home care and housing policy, whereby services are provided and received under circumstances that do not compromise important aspects of Canadian cultural life.

Living differently: home, space and bereavement

Author: B. Penhale (University of Hull, UK)

Living Differently: home, space and bereavement Purpose: This paper will provide an overview of recent research concerning the use of space by older people following bereavement. Method: The growing numbers of widowed people over 75 years represent not only an increasingly visible proportion of the population who access leisure facilities, but also a population at risk of social isolation within domestic space. Their response to the death of a long-term spouse or partner may be either an increased use of public space or a withdrawal into the privacy of their home. There is little current research on changing adaptations to the spaces of home and locality following crucial life events of this kind. In the light of the gendering of public and private space, bereavement of an opposite sex partner is likely to confront men and women with different sets of challenges. An overview of the issues concerning older people, use and experience of space and bereavement will be provided. Presentation of the findings from a small qualitative study consisting of interviews of both women & men in relation to their experiences following bereavement will be included. Results: The findings of the research in relation to specific themes of spatialised memory, health and continuing relationships with the dead partner will be presented. Possible future developments will be examined. Conclusion: The need for further research such as potential effects on health status and continuing bonds will be emphasised.

The Meaning of Home among Elderly Immigrants: Directions for Future Research and Theoretical Development

F. Ahmadi Lewin (Department of Sociology, Uppsala University, Uppsala, Sweden)

The paper discusses the notion that, in research on elderly immigrant housing, it is not enough to delineate the residential geography of different elderly immigrant groups or to study the economic and social reasons for their segregated habitations and exclusiveness. It is also necessary to understand, in the spatial context, the degree of integration and the differences between groups. In explaining these differences, we should take into consideration each elderly immigrant group's own value system, norms and preferences. It is argued that one necessary task in this endeavour is to gain knowledge about different elderly immigrant groups' understandings of what a home symbolises - what home means to them in the context of their particular ways of thinking and culture. From this point of view, the paper concludes that, when investigating the meaning of home among elderly immigrants, an integrative theoretical approach based on an experiential perspective and a phenomenological and developmental perspective are deemed appropriate to be adopted.

SESSION 122

Flexible Retirement: Policies and Practices

M. A. Hardy & L.E. Hazelrigg (Pepper Institute on Ageing, Florida State University, FL, USA) ("Readjusting Retirement Policy in the US: Risking Flexibility") Tony Mallier & David Morris (Coventry Business School, Coventry University, Coventry, United Kingdom) ("Flexible Retirement in Britain: Problems and Prospects") Gerhard Naegele (Institute of Gerontology, Dortmund University, Germany) ("Flexible Retirement in Germany: Policies and Practice") Eskil Wadensjo (Swedish Institute for Social Research, Stockholm University, Stockholm, Sweden) ("Flexible work: the demise of the Swedish partial pension system")

Issue: Flexible retirement as a policy option is a concept which is now receiving attention from governments and the social partners at the level of the enterprise. The objective of the symposium is to examine, and evaluate, the differing approaches towards flexible retirement which are evolving in a number of nations. Structure: While a 1998 OECD study, "Maintaining Prosperity in an Ageing Society" reported demographic ageing "has so far posed no major economic or social problems for our societies" (p.10), older citizens in OECD countries have in the final quarter of the last century often sought to leave their employment before their previously anticipated retirement age. The papers being presented to the symposium will focus on alternative policies which have been developed to encourage, and facilitate, the continuing employment of older workers and seek to evaluate the level of success these policies have achieved. Content: The interest in flexible retirement as a policy option arises in part from the recognition that in the recent past many older workers have often withdrawn involuntarily from the labour force at an earlier age than was the case of earlier generations. Simultaneously, it has been increasingly recognised by governments and employers that many older workers are able, and willing, to continue to make positive contributions to the economic well being of society in the years subsequent to their normal retirement age. Further, amongst, and in addition to, this latter group there are older people who desire to perform a caring role or wish to undertake unpaid voluntary work in the community.Against a background of demographic ageing it is questionable whether society can continue to afford to forego the potential offered by older mature workers although it is acknowledged some ageing employees, because of mental or physical characteristics and/or personal preferences, may desire to retire prior to the normal retirement age. Conclusion: The introduction of flexible retirement policies, for example 'a decade of retirement', would enable employees to retire either fully or partially at any point within a defined age range and receive a pension which is proportionately lower the earlier, and proportionately higher the later, they retire. Such strategies would enable older workers to gain a greater control over their lives by permitting them to continue to contribute their employment skills while simultaneously allowing them to determine when, within a defined age range, they retire from the labour force.

Flexible Retirement in Britain: Problems and Prospects

Tony Mallier & David Morris (Coventry Business School, Coventry University, Coventry, United Kingdom)

Published statistical data indicates that as a consequence of structural changes in the British economy in the latter part of the twentieth century a significant proportion of older people withdrew from the labour force on the grounds of early retirement and ill-health. There are no indications that either employers, trade unions and/or older people sought alternative strategies to total withdrawal as the size of industrial workforces declined even though this strategy often resulted in subsequent social exclusion and represented a waste of human capital. However, demographic factors are now more favourable to older people and the need for their continuing contribution to employment is increasingly recognised. If this is to take place in a form other than conventional full-time employment, for example through flexible retirement, there will be a need for changes in: * the pension framework to allow for greater retirement flexibility, * government and employer policies to counter age discrimination, * the provision of training programmes to enable older people to contribute to the economy. The establishment of an employment environment by government which recognises the potential value of older people is an essential pre-requisite for action by employers who will need to re-assess their practices with respect to older people especially where there is a desire to introduce flexible retirement strategies. However, for the above changes to be effective the attitudes of older people, for whom early retirement has become socially acceptable, to employment will also require to change.

Flexible Retirement in Germany: Policies and Practice

Gerhard Naegele (Institute of Gerontology at the Dortmund University, Dortmund, Germany)

In Germany, public gradual retirement schemes (Altersteilzeitgesetz) were introduced in 1996 in order to replace the hitherto prevailing practice of early retirement. Although the number of persons who are entitled to gradual retirement schemes has risen significantly in the past the actual utilization rate is quite low. When gradual retirement schemes are used at all they are used as a "block model", i.e. workers in practice misuse the concept in order to continue with early retirement. The aim of this paper is first to describe how the original concept of gradual retirement has been transformed into a new form of early retirement and second, to analyse the respective reasons. Based on this, thirdly, some evaluative considerations are made and recommendations are given on how the concept of gradual retirement can be made more successful in the future.

Flexible work: the demise of the Swedish partial pension system

Eskil Wadensjo (Swedish Institute for Social Research, Stockholm University, Stockholm, Sweden)

Sweden has had a special partial pension scheme since 1976. It has been one of three part-time pension schemes. These three schemes have been: 1) a partial disability pension; 2) a partial early old-age pension (leading to a lower pension after 65); 3) a special partial pension scheme (which does not lead to a lower pension after 65). The possibility of combining a pension and work is a part of the general expansion of the Swedish welfare state and also a part of the strong commitment to the work principle. The special partial pension scheme became very popular with a high take-up rate and was criticized for being too expensive. As a part of the decision on the old age pension scheme in 1994, the partial pension scheme was made less generous. It was also decided that the scheme will be totally abolished from the year 2001. The other two options for combining work and receiving a pension will continue. The far less generous rules from 1995 led to a reduction in the take-up rates of partial pensions. The pressure on existing full-time early exit pathways increased. The number of people who take a partial early old age pension has not increased to a large extent, and the take-up rate of the part-time disability pensions has been stable among those aged 60 to 64. The main effect for older workers has been that fewer of them work part-time and more work full-time or are outside the labour market.

Readjusting Retirement Policy in the US: Risking Flexibility

Melissa A. Hardy & Lawrence E. Hazelrigg (Pepper Institute on Ageing, Florida State University, FL, USA)

For the majority of older workers, the timing of retirement has been heavily influenced by the eligibility requirements for receiving benefits from the federal and employer-sponsored pensions. Although flexibility was initially located primarily with employers, federal regulations gradually increased workers' flexibility in determining when and how they retired. An historical analysis of U.S. policy demonstrates how worker flexibility in retirement has increased in the latter part of the twentieth century. In large part, this trend toward increased worker flexibility has been manifested through policies that strengthen workers' pension rights, allow greater variation in work histories in determining Social Security benefits, remove barriers to the hiring and retention of older workers, and encourage increased heterogeneity in the timing and financing of retirement. The trend toward defined contribution pension plans in lieu of traditional defined benefit plans, proposals to privatize (partially or entirely) Social Security, the age discrimination in employment act, and the removal of the earnings test for Social Security beneficiaries exemplify this trend. However, the increase in flexibility has been accompanied by a shift toward individualization, increased uncertainty with regard to retirement planning, and increasing income inequality in old age. In this paper, we examine the two faces of increased flexibility and the projected consequences for the institution of retirement in the U.S.

SESSION 123

The Interaction of Sensorimotor and Cognitive Functioning in Aging

P. Baltes Δ Opening remarks (Center for Lifespan Psychology, Max Planck Institute for Human Development, Berlin, Germany) N. Teasdale (Université Laval, Division de kinésiologie, Département de médecine sociale et préventive, Québec, Canada) Why do elderly persons need to allocate specific attentional resources to the control of their posture? K. Li (Centre for Research in Human Development, Concordia University, Montréal, Canada) Walking while memorizing: The use of attention to maintain walking performance. S. Kemper (University of Kansas, Lawrence, KS, USA) The Costs of Doing Two Things at Once for Younger and Older Adults. S. Lord (Prince of Wales Medical Research Institute, Sydney, Australia) Sensorimotor and balance factors associated with aging and falls in older people. R. Krampe - discussant (Center for Lifespan Psychology, Max Planck Institute for Human Development, Berlin, Germany)

The purpose of this invited symposium is to convene a multi-disciplinary group of researchers who study the relationship of sensorimotor and cognitive aging. Current theories of balance, walking, and aging, indicate a greater reliance on attentional capacity as sensorimotor ability declines. This in combination with age-related cognitive decline creates a "scarce resources" scenario in which one resource domain (sensorimotor, cognitive) might trade off in importance with the other. This dynamic relationship between domains is the focus of the symposium. The group will present findings that address this "attentional hypothesis" using a variety of methods. Several issues will be raised: If a cognitive load is imposed during balancing or walking, does balance invariably suffer? To what extent do older adults adopt a conservative strategy to successfully prevent falls while walking? Is cognitive status a significant determinant of falls in the elderly? The symposium is structured as a series of four research papers, introduced by co-convenor P. Baltes. The findings from the research papers will be integrated by R. Krampe, discussant. Teasdale's paper describes the impact of attentional load on specific features of balance control: the variability and slowing of postural recovery. Notable is his use of everyday balance scenarios in an experimental setting. Teasdale's influential use of dual-task methodology to study the role of attention in balance is adopted in several of the papers (Teasdale, Li, Kemper). The paper given by Li describes a dual-task study in which walking on a narrow track is performed while memorizing word lists. Across several task difficulty manipulations, older adults were found to favour walking at a cost to memorizing performance. A similar pattern was found when external walking and memory aid use was measured. Kemper reports a study in which younger and older adults performed a walking task while speaking. Speaking was also measured when concurrently performed with less complex motor and cognitive tasks. By measuring walking and speech quality, it was determined that older adults maintain the same quality of speech output regardless of the difficulty of the concurrent task. This paper also suggests that older adults adopt a conservative strategy to manage concurrent walking and cognitive tasks. The final research paper given by Lord utilizes a different methodological and theoretical approach. The focus of Lord's paper is the prospective determination of falls frequency, and incorporates cognitive / attentional status as one of many possible predictors. Lord's clinical background and multivariate approach help to situate the attentional hypothesis in a larger functional and theoretical context. His findings indicate that among several physiological measures (e.g, sensory status, muscle strength, body sway), reaction time serves as a significant and independent predictor of falls frequency. Lord's paper also discusses potential applications of such multiple-measure assessments in designing interventions for the prevention of falls. It is expected that together, the research papers can be integrated to derive a broader understanding of the dynamic relationship between sensorimotor and cognitive aging.

Sensorimotor and Balance Factors Associated with Aging and Falls in Older People

S. Lord (Prince of Wales Medical Research Institute, Sydney, Australia)

The purpose of the study was to determine normative values for simple assessments of vision, vestibular function, peripheral sensation, lower limb muscle strength, reaction time and balance in community-dwelling older people, and to determine whether impaired performances in these tests individually and cumulatively predict falls in this group. Large populations of older people participating in the Randwick Falls and Fractures Study (RFFS) and the Dubbo Osteoporosis Epidemiology Study (DOES) underwent the assessments. Twelve-month falls incidence in both groups was also determined. In both studies, each physiological measure showed a significant age-related decline. Falling was associated with low contrast visual acuity and contrast sensitivity, poor vibration sense and proprioception, reduced lower limb strength, slow reaction time and impaired balance, as indicated by sway tests and two clinical stability measures. In the RFFS study, discriminant function analysis identified visual contrast sensitivity, proprioception in the lower limbs, quadriceps strength, reaction time, and sway on a foam rubber mat as significant and independent risk factors for falls. This procedure correctly classified 75% of the participants into multiple faller or non-multiple faller groups. We are now using the normative data to derive profiles for individual subjects which outline impairments in the physiological systems that contribute to stability, and use this information to target interventions for improving vision, strength and balance and reducing falls risk. A physiological profile approach is useful for identifying overall falls risk in older people and for identifying impairments in specific sensorimotor and balance domains. This information can provide the basis for targeting falls prevention interventions effectively.

The Costs of Doing Two Things at Once for Younger and Older Adults

S. Kemper, R. Herman, C. Lian (University of Kansas, Lawrence, KS, USA)

Young and older adults were asked to provide language samples in response to elicitation questions while concurrently carrying out a variety of different tasks (walking, simple finger tapping, complex finger tapping, listening to concurrent noise, listening to concurrent speech). The language samples were scored on a variety of dimensions including measures of fluency, syntactic complexity, and semantic content. The participants' performance on the concurrent tasks is also coded. The goal was to assess whether concurrent task demands have differential effects on young and older adults' speech; the hypothesis that working memory limitations restrict older adults to a simplified speech register was tested by comparing their speech during a baseline condition with that produced while concurrently performing memory-demanding tasks. The results indicate that dual task combinations affected the fluency and grammatical complexity of young adults' speech but had little effect on the semantic content of young adults' speech. In contrast, older adults have developed an optimized speech register that is buffered from effects of dual tasks. Older adults' fluency and grammatical complexity were unaffected by dual task combinations as was their semantic content.

Walking while memorizing: The use of attention to maintain walking performance

K. Z. H. Li, (Centre for Research in Human Development, Concordia University, Montreal, Canada), U. Lindenberger, (Developmental Psychology Unit, Saarland University, Saarbrücken, Germany), A. M. Freund, & P. B. Baltes (Center for Lifespan Psychology, Max Planck Institute for Human Development, Berlin, Germany)

This study was designed to address current theories of attentional demand in the maintenance of balance and walking in old age. The increased allocation of attention to sensorimotor performance is seen as developmentally adaptive, reflecting two processes (loss-based selection and compensation) that are featured in the selection, optimization and compensation theory of successful development (Baltes & Baltes, 1990). Concurrent walking and memorizing were evaluated to determine if task priority varied across younger and older adult groups. Cognitive (memorizing) and sensorimotor (walking a narrow track) performance were measured singly, concurrently, and when task difficulty was manipulated. Compensatory aid use was measured to provide another index of task priority. Before dual-task testing, extensive training was carried out on each component task and external aid. Age differences in dual-task costs were greater in memory performance than in walking, suggesting that older adults prioritized walking over memory (loss-based selection). When given a choice of external aids to use, older adults optimized walking whereas younger adults optimized memory performance. The results have broad implications for theories of cognitive and sensorimotor aging, and the costs and benefits of assistive devices and environmental support for older populations.

Why do elderly persons need to allocate specific attentional resources to the control of their posture?

N. Teasdale, P. Corbeil, M. Simoneau (Université Laval, Division de kinésiologie, Département de médecine sociale et préventive, Québec, Canada; Northwestern University, Department of Physical Therapy and Human Movement Sciences, Chicago, USA)

Using the simple task of maintaining an upright standing posture, we have described in a series of experiments how aging imposes greater reliance upon cognitive levels of control. This imposes a challenge to the postural control system of the elderly because, with aging, cognitive levels are characterized by an increased slowness and variability. The purpose of the present experiment is to examine how these two characteristics impinge on the postural stability of elderly persons. A model was developed to examine how slowness and variability of the postural responses (delays in the onset of the ankle muscular torque, decreased ankle rate of torque development and amplitude of ankle torque) impose constraints on the postural stability. The model integrates known characteristics of the postural behavior of elderly males and females. Small and daily life postural contexts are simulated. The effects of aging on the feasible temporal and torque boundaries of postural stability are determined. The temporal and torque boundaries found highlight that delays in ankle torque onset and slow rate of torque development observed with aging diminish the repertoire of responses allowing balance recovery. Elderly females are particularly affected. With aging, postural responses are more dependent upon cognitive processes and are affected by attentional demands. Slowness in postural response observed with aging, constrains significantly the repertoire of postural response that can be used to regain balance. This highlights the importance of considering how aging affects the dialogue between sensory-motor and cognitive systems.

SESSION 124

An Innovative Approach to Working with Long Term Care Facilities to Improve the Quality of Life of Residents

Kyle Whitfield 9Murray Alzheimer Research and Education Program, University of Waterloo) and School of Planning - University of Waterloo(PhD. Candidate)

The Murray Alzheimer Research and Education Program (MAREP) works with six Long Term Care facilities in Ontario using a participatory action research model to enhance the quality of life of residents with Alzheimer disease and related dementia. This presentation will describe MAREP research initiatives at the Innovation Centres, the approach used to implement findings and the benefits and challenges of this model. The benefits of this kind of an approach is the level of collaboration created between the researchers and the facility staff. A challenge is ensuring research is action focussed in a time when fiscal restraints limit staff availability for participation in research activities. A further challenge is implementing research findings to ensure they are relevant and applicable for front line staff.

Canada's First Comprehensive Provincial Alzheimer Strategy

Elizabeth Esteves (Ontario Seniors' Secretariat, Toronto, Canada)

There are more than 100,000 people living with Alzheimer Disease and related dementias in Ontario. This number is expected to grow to more than 150,000 by the year 2011 when the first of the baby boomers reach 65 years of age. The Ontario government recognized the necessity of responding in a coordinated manner to the needs and concerns of people whose lives are affected by Alzheimer Disease and committed $68.4 million over five years to the implementation of a 10-point plan of action. With the announcement on September 10, 1999 of Ontario’s Strategy for Alzheimer Disease and Related Dementias: Preparing for Our Future, Ontario became the first province to initiate a comprehensive response to Alzheimer Disease and Related Dementias. Ontario’s Alzheimer Strategy was designed to improve the quality of life of people with Alzheimer Disease and to provide support to their caregivers and families. The ten components of the strategy are as follows: 1. Staff education and Training 2. Physician Training 3. Increase in Public Awareness, Information and Education 4. Planning for Appropriate, Safe and Secure Environments 5. Respite Services for Caregivers 6. Research on Caregiver Needs 7. Advance Directives on Care Choices 8. PyschoGeriatric Consulting Resources 9. Co-ordinated, Specialized Diagnosis and Support 10. Intergenerational Volunteer Initiative In this presentation, the speaker will provide an overview of the development of Ontario’s Alzheimer Strategy, the implementation process and the status of the ten initiatives.

Cultural and Socio-economic Aspects of Demented Elderly Caretaking in the World

Valerie Wenner (Hopital) Georges Clemenceau (Assistance Publique-Hopitaux de Paris(AP-HP)Service du Docteur BIZIEN91750-CHAMPCUEILFRANCE) Alec Bizien (Chef de service Hopital) Georges Clemenceau (AP-HP91750-CHAMPCUEILFRANCE) R. Moulias (Centre de gerontologie "l'Orbe"Hopital Charles FOIX AP-HP94205-IVRY SUR SEINEFRANCE)

The twenty first century is going to be marked by an unprecedented world ageing.This ageing characterized especially by an increase of elderly aged above 80 years,involves the development of new chronicles pathologies physical and/or psychic. To the forefront of psychic dependence;the dementia who is all the more frequent as the person is old. This work based on the demented elderly care taking in the World,intervenes therefore in a context of topicality.This work is the outcome of: -a bibliographical research -an exchange with some geriatrics correspondents of the whole World joined by postal mail and/ or electronic. It results from this study that: -the developed countries confronted with this demographic transition since approximately a century,except Japan(a quarter of century)have already,mostly,developed a policy for the elderly(northern developed countries especially) -the developing countries,mostly,had to or will have to face up this transition rapidly,India and China especially,but still remain unprovided with means place in position by the governments. Africa sub-saharian seems for the moment not to be concerned. This study allows to envisage: -human solutions:reminiscence therapy in Japan,group homes in Sweden,etc... -economic solutions:the new gold plan in Japan,the plan of social action in China,the insurance dependence in Germany,etc... Certainties appear: -there is no universal care taking of demented elderly so cultural,historical and economic differences are numerous; -a real difficulty for governments to set up a policy for demented elderly,for lack of human and economic means; -a need to make increasingly international exchanges so as to find solutions always more adapted to demented elderly.

Dementia Advice and Support Service

Jayne Lingard, UK Service Development Manager, Mental Health Foundation. Alisoun Milne, Lecturer in Social Gerontology (Tizard Centre, University of Kent, Canterbury & Programme Consultant, Mental Health in Later Life, Mental Health Foundation, London, UK)

Late in 2000, the Mental Health Foundation launched its 'Dementia Advice and Support Service'. The core component of the programme is the development of six early intervention schemes for people with dementia and their carers. This initiative reflects the Foundation's concern with the inconsistency of support available for people in the early stages of dementia as well as a recognition that, although dementia cannot be reversed, access to advice and support services at an early point can benefit both users and carers (Milne et al, 2000). Whilst the specific nature of each scheme differs, all six offer home-based support, information, advice and befriending to older people and their carers. The key service aims are to: delay or prevent the use of mainstream services, improve user and carer quality of life, support carers, provide access to advice and information and help users and carers plan for the future. The schemes are funded for two years; they reflect a range of locations and populations and are led by a number of different care agencies. The Foundation is keen to reflect a range of service types whilst also ensuring that the programme retains coherence and evaluability. This paper will describe the aims, nature and success of this unique programme of early intervention services. It will also include the initial findings of the independent programme evaluation, which runs in parallel with the development of the schemes.

Evaluating Dementia Care Networks in Ontario

Chambers LW (McMaster University, Hamilton, Canada), Lemieux-Charles L (University of Toronto, Toronto, Canada), Kevin Brazil, McMaster University, Hamilton, Canada), Rhonda Cockerill (University of Toronto, Toronto, Canada, Susan Jaglal (University of Toronto, Toronto, Canada

PURPOSE: To report results from four communities with dementia care networks. METHOD: Our multiple case study design used key informant, focus groups, survey questionnaires to providers, caregivers and individuals with dementia (70 per network), and reviews of agency documents (15 per network). RESULTS: Network effectiveness is being considered at the network level (meeting network's goals, collaboration among members), from the providers' perspective (meeting agency's goals and collaboration with other members) as well as caregivers' and individuals' with dementia views on satisfaction with care. Network analysis described the relationships between agencies in each network. Review of administrative links across agencies within networks enabled comparisons within and among the four communities on whether agencies shared staff/volunteers, facilities, training programs/workshops, and administrative information. Data on service delivery within networks focused on referrals sent, referrals received, case coordination, joint clinical programs, service contracts, and shared client-related information. Assessment of network structure revealed the extent of centralization of control of services and the concentration of services in one or more agency within networks. Operational processes reviewed focused on administrative coordination and task integration across agencies within networks. CONCLUSION: This project with the provincial Ministry and dementia care networks is designed to increase their capacity in locating, appraising, summarizing and applying research to policy making and management of evidence-based decision-making about the organization of dementia care.

SESSION 125

Characteristics of Stroke Rehabilitation Patients Associated With Discharge to a Residential Home

Rasvan E. Lalu (Gerontological-Economic Research Organization - GERO, Kreuzlingen, Switzerland)

PURPOSE. This study explores characteristics on admission and respectively on both admisssion and discharge related to discharge to a residential home in elderly stroke patients. METHODS. Data from 3275 consecutive inpatients of a geriatric rehabilitation unit have been used to test multiple logistic regression models of being discharged to a home for aged persons on following variables at admission, respectively at admisssion and discharge: having a limitation in bathing, respectively dressing, using the toilet, walking, eating, bladder and bowel control, having 3 to 7 ADL limitations, using ambulation devices, suffering of one or more out of 12 comorbiditiy categories, having 2 to 5 comorbidities, being 75 years old or more, being married. RESULTS. On admission, needing help in using the toilet and being urinary incontinent are associated with increased risk of institutionalization (OR = 7.27; CI = 3.37 - 15.68 resp, OR = 2.57; CI = 1.40 - 4.73), while being married and using an orthopedic device are negatively related to institutionalization (OR = 0.10; CI = 0.04 - 0.26, resp. OR = 0.44; CI = 0.22 - 0.88). When discharge data are taken into account, some additional factors appear to be associated with discharge to a residential home: pulmonary diseases (OR = 2.71; CI = 1.33 - 5.50), arrhytmia (OR = 1.94; CI = 1.19 - 3.18) and LOS greater than 45 days (OR = 1.40; CI = 1.10 - 1.78). DISCUSSION. The findings confirm the association between using the toilet, bladder incontinence and being married with institutionalization and suggest that the use of orthopedic devices, pulmonary diseases and arrhythmias are also related to institutionalization.

Comparison of two functional independence scales as outcome measures in geriatric post-stroke rehabilitation

J. Desrosiers, A. Rochette (Centre de recherche en gérontologie et gériatrie, Institut universitaire de gériatrie de Sherbrooke, Québec, Canada), L Noreau (Rehabilitation Department, Laval University, Quebec, Canada), G. Bravo, R. Hébert and C Boutin (Centre de recherche en gérontologie et gériatrie, Institut universitaire de gériatrie de Sherbrooke, Québec, Canada).

PURPOSE: Functional independence is an important outcome measure in post-stroke rehabilitation. The objective of the study was to compare two scales measuring this concept, the Functional Autonomy Measurement System (SMAF) and the Functional Independence Measurement (FIM), with stroke patients involved in an intensive rehabilitation program. METHOD: Participants were evaluated with the SMAF and the FIM during the rehabilitation period (T1: admission; T2: discharge; n = 132) and twice after discharge (T3 = two weeks; n = 118; T4 = six months later; n = 102). At T3 and T4, a handicap measure, the Life Habit Assessment (LIFE-H), was added to the data collection. RESULTS: Results showed that: 1) the total scores of the SMAF and the FIM are strongly correlated at each measurement time (r = 0.93 to 0.95); 2) the SMAF total score is statistically more responsive than the FIM total score (SRM: 1.20 vs 0.97; $p < 0.01$) and most of this difference is due to the instrumental activities of daily living category of the SMAF; and 3) in general, the strength of association with the LIFE-H is of a similar magnitude for both instruments, but in some life habit categories, the SMAF is more strongly correlated with this handicap measure. CONCLUSION: This study suggests the usefulness of the SMAF in post-stroke rehabilitation.

Prevalence of poststroke depression undetected in primary care

F. Eto (Department of Rehabilitation Medicine, University of Tokyo Hospital, Tokyo, Japan) T. Sakata (Social Survey Research Information, Tokyo, Japan)

PURPOSE: To explore how properly primary medical doctors detect depressive states of their patients in chronic cerebrovascular disturbances. METHODS: A mail survey was conducted to elucidate the influential factors on health-related quality of life after cerebrovascular disease. Questionnaires for clinicians and their patients were mailed to 2587 hospitals with more than 100 beds, which had at least one of the following departments: neurosurgery, neurology, psychiatry or rehabilitation. Each mailing contained a request to the clinicians and questionnaire for 5 cases. Among voluntary respondents from the clinicians and the patients, 378 valid paired replies were collected. The questions for the physicians included items on diagnosis, duration of illness, psychiatric symptoms such as depression and so forth. The questionnaire for the patients was composed of items from the EuroQol clinical version, Geriatric Depression Scale short form (GDS) and so on. RESULTS: Among valid respondents 333 poststroke patients completed GDS. Using a cut-off value of >6 to indicate clinically significant depressive symptoms in GDS score, 150 patients (45.0%) were defined as in depressive states. Their doctors in charge answered on psychiatric symptoms of 266 patients, and then, identified only 24 of 119 depressive state patients defined by the self-administered GDS. As for proper identification rates among four medical specialties psychiatrists showed the best, 0.67 and others did less than 0.2. COCLUSION: These results suggest that considerable numbers of medical doctors underestimate the depressive state in poststroke patients. Further educational program may be essential for primary care.

Quality of Life after Stroke: Dimensions and Measurement

Adelheid Susanne Esslinger (Friedrich-Alexander-University Erlangen-Nuremberg, Department of Business Administration, Nuremberg, Germany)

This paper introduces and applies a three-step research design measuring the specific quality of life aspects of post-stroke patients. The research motivation results from the fact that the aging society and its multi-morbidity is generating an increasing population of post-stroke patients. In a first step, semi-structured interviews with 20 patients out of the 1,200 patients containing database of the University of Erlangen's Stroke Unit were held and audio-recorded. In a second step, the interview results were examined regarding such aspects, which are specifically relevant for post-stroke patients but not covered by already existing quality of life assessments. Several yet underrated post-stroke quality of life dimensions were summarized by a questionnaire containing 25 questions with mostly Likert-scaled answer choices. In step three, 33 post-stroke patients were confronted twice with this newly developed standardized questionnaire. The second response took place one month after the first. The empirical analysis of 28 questionnaires returned suggests that the following six dimensions of quality of life of post-stroke patients deserve prime consideration: activities of daily living and mobility, social role-taking, communication, cognition, coping, and future-vision. Further exploration of the quality of life impacts of post-stroke patients promises to improve care management and rehabilitation.

SESSION 126

Supporting Emotional Health - A Counselling and Psychoeducational Model for Elders in the Community

Joy Barkwill (Century House, New Westminster, Canada) The Organizational Challenges of Expanding Community Health Promotion Initiatives from a Seniors' Centre Perspective; Dot Josey, Beryl Petty (Century House, New Westminster, Canada) Senior Peer Counselling: The Role of a Paraprofessional Volunteer in the Continuum of Emotional Health Services; Beryl Petty, Heather Whiteford (Family Services of Greater Vancouver, New Westminster, Canada) Vital Connections: A Professional Counselling Service for Older Adults in the Community; Bill Munn (Geriatric Services - New Westminster Mental Health, New Westminster, Canada) Sharing Insights on Emotional Wellness

Issues: There are many challenges in later life that can adversely affect the older person's emotional health. Although there are services in place for those requiring psychiatric support, there are few services for those who are mildly or moderately depressed. The older population can be described as "needy but resistant." Often it is difficult for the older person to reach out and accept help, especially with personal concerns. There are some older people who have no one with whom they feel comfortable talking to about everyday worries or even more inner core issues. A supportive network is health promoting in that it provides a buffering effect to life's negative events. The challenge for mental health service providers is to explore ways of engaging senior clients in therapeutic involvement. This requires the adaptation of existing counselling approaches and the exploration of new methods for a more senior friendly approach toward providing emotional support. Specific organizational strategies can help to establish a supportive community to promote the service. Structure: Overview - a seniors' centre perspective An Emotional Health Service design Phase I Peer Counselling Phase II Professional Counselling Phase III The psychoeducational program Each presentation will be 20 minutes with questions and comments following didactic information. Video excerpts highlight aspects of the presentation. One experiential exercise will be used. Content: This session will focus on challenges in providing accessible and acceptable emotional support to older adults living in the community. Based on fifteen years of service experience in a seniors' recreation centre, this session will discuss the originally defined needs and the successful evolution of a volunteer paraprofessional service that was augmented by professional counselling, and subsequently adding a psychoeducational component in the form of prevention focused community forums. The success of this continuum of care will be explained as a result of cooperative plans and community structure. Conclusions/Anticipated Outcomes: - Participants should have enhanced information on emotional health issues of seniors, a better understanding of the concept of preventative interventions in mental health and increased awareness of counselling strategies for the older population. - Participants will have the descriptions of three working models of emotional support programs that can be operationalized in other settings. - Participants will be sensitized to the varied challenges of evaluating psychologically focussed programs for older adults.

Senior Peer Counselling, The Role of a Paraprofessional Volunteer in the Continuum of Emotional Health Services

Dot Josey (Century House, New Westminster, British Columbia, Canada), Beryl Petty, (Century House, New Westminster, British Columbia, Canada)

As the new millennium challenges the health care system to provide more with less, there is a greater interest in exploring the potential of the volunteer sector as a resource. With an expanding aging population, the need for efficient and cost effective ways of providing service to the older population has never been more important. Senior Peer Counselling is one such program that utilizes the volunteer skills and abilities of older people, a relatively untapped resource, to reach out to their peers who do not have family or other support services to help them with everyday concerns. With similar life experience, and a common language, older persons, even those most skeptical about accepting any type of supportive service, are often more likely to accept help from a peer. Senior peer counsellors are selected and recruited under specific guidelines prior to having an extensive 52 hours of training in communication skills and gerontology. An informal evaluation of the impact of Century House senior Peer Counselling of New Westminster, B.C, a program that has assisted over 800 clients since its inception in 1985, reported benefits to both the giver and receiver of the service. Client outcomes were based on self-reports of stronger coping skills. The community professional who referred clients to the program also reported positive outcomes. Senior peer counselors enjoyed increased self confidence, greater abilities to deal with difficult people in their personal lives, and became more active as community leaders.

Sharing Insights on Emotional Wellness

Bill Munn (Geriatric Services - New Westminster Mental Health, New Westminster, British Columbia, Canada)

An educational component is a vital part of any preventative endeavour There is perspective and information with regard to emotional health that older people can share, towards mutual enhancement of their coping skills. An educational milieu may attract individuals who are not comfortable with, or in need of, counselling. Their queries, fears may be addressed or validated in a group setting, and the open discussion reduces the stigma usually attached to emotional health issues. This presentation reports on one such educational program. Elders in a community seniors' centre were asked to define emotional health, and discuss issues and strategies in a facilitated focus group format. A core group then went on to plan a series of public educational forums throughout the year, covering emotional health topics directed at seniors. Mental health professionals facilitated these sessions, with the goal of producing an interactive combination of presented ideas and concepts, and participant response and contribution. A four year program, Sharing Insights On Emotional Well Being, will be presented, including topics chosen by participants, attendance and reported benefits.

The Organizational Challenges of Expanding Community Health Promotion Initiatives from a Seniors' Centre Perspective

Joy Barkwill (Century House, New Westminster, British Columbia, Canada)

Recreation centers for senior citizens play an integral role in supporting the well being and independence of older adults. The importance of physical health care services for older adults has long been recognized but there was a gap in the care of their emotional health. The seniors centre was often the first one to notice an emotional health decline in daily participation patterns. Being aware that older adults don't reach out easily for help with their personal concerns more accessible senior-friendly options were explored. Century House, is a city owned and operated seniors recreation centre in New Westminster - a Vancouver suburb, with a membership of 2000 representing approx. 20% of the 50+ age group in the community. It is in this setting that we initiated the following programs. Initially there was a senior peer counselling program followed up with a one to one professional counseling, and shortly after a prevention/education program that has resulted in an all encompassing battery of services based out of this centre. The success of this service model is based on three organizational components: - the service is provided in a non-medical accessible and acceptable setting - the consumer age group assisted in the design and delivery of service, and continues to assist with securing funding to sustain it while advocating for improvements as needed - community support has been firmly established as a result of advisory committees, the co-operative partnering of service delivery and most importantly the quality of the service that the client receives.

Vital Connections - A ProfessionalCounselling Service for Older Adults in the Community

Beryl Petty (Family Services of Greater Vancouver, New Westminster, British Columbia, Canada), Heather Whiteford (Family Services of Greater Vancouver, New Westminster, British Columbia, Canada)

Despite increased attention to preventative interventions in addressing the mental health of older adults, there are few clinical counselling opportunities for those who experience persistent distress associated with age-related loss. These individuals, who are often mildly to moderately depressed, may require greater guidance than a paraprofessional, but they do not meet the criteria for psychiatric service. Their unique psychological needs are often not recognized or addressed adequately in traditional health care settings. Older adults may not seek help from traditional counselling agencies in the community, nor do such agencies provide special outreach to the older population. This presentation describes a counselling service which has, as its primary focus, prevention, early detection and intervention in the emotional challenges of the older population. Adaptations to traditional counselling practice that made it more acceptable to seniors included: improved accessibility physically and emotionally; structuring counselling sessions to provide more choice, flexibility, openness and informality; and the use of a multi-generational treatment modality, which was appropriate to the developmental life stage tasks of finding meaning, and dealing with unfinished business. Client profiles, referral sources, and reasons for service utilization, are described in 82 clients. Implications for practice include the need for a more comprehensive period of engagement for an older client, extension of services to provide greater flexibility and individually centered service; and attention to the availability and non-intrusiveness of the therapist.

SESSION 127

Respect for The Elderly: Cross-Cultural Perspectives

N. Chow (Department of Social Work & Social Administration, The University of Hong Kong, Hong Kong) The Practice of Filial Piety among the Chinese in Present-Day Hong Kong. B. Knight (Andrus Gerontology Center, The University of Southern California, Los Angeles, California, USA) Familism and Caregiving Burden and Distress in U.S. Ethnic Population. T. Ogawa (Human-Environment Studies, Kyushu University, Fukuoka, Japan) Older Persons Living with their Children in Japan. G. Garrusso (Andrus Gerontology Center, The University of Southern California, Los Angeles, California, USA), D. Feng (Department of Human Development, Texas Tech University, Lubbock, Texas, USA), and M. Silverstein (Andrus Gerontology Center, The University of Southern California, Los Angeles, California, USA) Parent-Adult Child Affection and Consensus: Cross-Generational and Cross-Ethnic Comparison. K. Sung (School of Social Work & Andrus Gerontology Center, The University of Southern California, Los Angeles, California, USA) Elder Respect: Exploration of Ideals and Forms in East Asia.

This symposium addresses researches on respect for the elderly in different cultures. The focus of the symposium is on how younger generations treat the aged in changing times in terms of care and support for the elderly. It is expected to provide information on similarities and differences between cultures in terms of change and continuity of tradition of elder respect, changing expressions of elder respect, future projections regarding elder respect, and issues of concern to be explored by gerontologists and policy makers.

Elder Respect: Explorations of Ideals and Forms

K. Sung (School of Social Work & Andrus Gerontology Center, The University of Southern California, Los Angeles, California, USA)

This presentation introduces the result of a study of the forms of elder respect practiced in East Asia. The study distinguishes a comprehensive set of 14 forms of elder respect ranging from care respect to ancestor respect. Traditional Confucian teachings associated with respect for parents and elders were reviewed, forms of elder respect practiced by Asians are explored based on findings from recent studies conducted in Asia, and the meanings of the forms are summarized. These forms are compared with forms of elder respect found among young adults in the U.S. Changing expressions of elder respect and its continuing influence, and cultural differences and similarities are discussed.

Familism and Caregiving Burden and Distress in U.S. Ethnic Populations.

B. Knight (Andrus Gerontology Center, The University of Southern California, Los Angeles, California, USA)

Familism values are generally thought to be high in non-White U.S. populations and theoretically should be related to lower appraisals of caregiving as stressful than are found in White caregiving groups with higher individualism values. Drawing from several studies by Knight and colleagues, the results appear more complex. African American caregivers, Hispanic caregivers, and Korean-American caregivers have all be found to have high ratings of familism values. As compared to White caregivers in the U.S.: African-Americans have lower burden, but equal emotional distress outcomes; Hispanic caregivers have about equal levels of burden and distress; and Korean-Americans have higher levels of burden and distress. The relationship of familism values, burden appraisals, and emotional outcomes of caregiving appear to be much more complex than expected. Path models suggest that the influence of cultural values may be counterbalanced by other variables affected by ethnic group status, or be attenuated by intervening variables

Older Persons Living with their Children in Japan

Takeo Ogawa (Faculty of Human-Environment Studies, Kyushu University, Fukuoka, Japan)

Purpose: In the traditional Japanese family system, older persons enjoyed their later life with supports from their children. Many older persons maintain a sense of filial piety for thinking about their later life. But social changes are affecting their actual life. Japanese sub-regions, 47 prefectures, on 22 social indices, are evaluated with traditional life style in that older persons live with their child. Method: Factor analysis and correlation analysis are applied to the analyses of 47 cases and 22 indices. Results: 5 factors are extracted after varimax rotation. Factor 1 is composed of demographic properties. Factor 2 is composed of household traits. Factor 3 is composed of working situation. Factor 4 is composed of social attitudes. And factor 5 is composed of primary industry for older persons. Conclusion: Although gerontocracy is strongly correlated with ancestor worship and respect for old parents, it will decrease with emigration, and increase a positive sense of social welfare. Filial piety is no more a fundamental factor for sustaining traditional family. The more people emigrate from local communities, the less ancestor worship will be, and the more dependent on nursing homes. Japanese sub-national areas are diverged from the traditional family system.

Parent-Adult Child Affection and Consensus: Cross-Generational and Cross- Ethnic Comparison

R. Giarrusso (Andrus Gerontology Center, The University of Southern California, Los Angeles, California, USA), D. Feng (Department of Human Development, Texas Tech University, Lubbock, Texas, USA), and M. Silverstein (Andrus Gerontology Center, The University of Southern California, Los Angeles, California, USA)

Euro-American parents' affection for their adult children has been found to be significantly greater than their adult children's affection for thema phenomenon known as the "intergenerational stake phenomenon." However, it is unclear whether this cross-generational difference In affection exists for all gender dyad configurations (mother-daughter, mother-son, father-daughter, father-son) or for ethnic groups with a more collectivistic orientation. The purpose of this study is to compare levels of affection and consensus for Euro-American and Mexican-American parents and their adult children. The data for this study come from two samples (1) 131 Euro-American parent-child dyads from the USC Longitudinal Study of Generations, and (2) 375 Mexican-American parent-child dyads from the Study of Three-Generation Mexican American Families. The results revealed that Euro-American mothers and fathers have significantly greater affection for their daughters than their daughters have for them; however, this gap was not found for sons. Among Mexican-Americans, sons have significantly greater affection for their fathers than their fathers have for them, a pattern opposite to that predicted by the "intergenerational stake hypothesis." Whereas Euro-American mothers perceived significantly greater consensus than their children perceived, there were no significant differences in consensus among Mexican-American parents and children of any gender dyad type. Analyses of Covariance revealed that when children of either ethnic group perceived themselves to be similar in attitudes and values to their parents, the gap between parents' and children's level of affection was significantly smaller. In addition, Mexican-American children's level of acculturation was a significant predictor of the magnitude of the gap in affection, even after controlling for perceived consensus. The results are discussed in terms of the limited generalizability of the "intergenerational stake hypothesis."

The Practice of Filial Piety among the Chinese in Present-Day Hong Kong

N. Chow (Department of Social Work & Social Administration, The University of Hong Kong, Hong Kong)

With more than 98 percent of the population in Hong Kong being Chinese and having returned to become part of China in 1997, the issue of the practice of filial piety has once again been raised in the formulation of a policy to support the elderly by the new Hong Kong Government. The presentation reports on a study conducted in 1998 to look at the actual practice of filial piety by the Chinese in Hong Kong. According to Confucius classics, the practice of filial piety can be differentiated into three levels: to provide for the needs of elderly parents, to adhere to their advices, and to bring to them honor and pride. By operationalizing the three levels into some common activities, more than a thousand respondents were interviewed for their extent of practicing them. Though Confucius might be disappointed, results showed that the majority of the Chinese in Hong Kong still adhered to his teachings, at least in spirit

SESSION 128

Bridging the Gap Across the Atlantic: Researching an Inner-City Intergenerational Mentoring Programme

Sally Newman (University Center for Social and Urban Research. University of Pittsburgh, PA 15260-5907) Stephen W Ellis (Manchester Metropolitan University Institute of Education. Crewe. Cheshire. UK CW1 5DU)

Rapid social change over the last two decades has brought into sharp focus new relationships that exist between different generations. Because of social factors driving our cultures i.e. geographic separation among a family's generations and segregated living patterns, children and young people may well lose contact with older generations, both within their family networks and within the wider community. Against this background this paper will seek to explore the impact that older people have in an educational setting and, examine the mutual effect this has in developing and promoting intergenerational understanding. This cross cultural action-research study was conducted over a period of 3 years in inner-city schools both in the USA and in the UK. The study sought to elicit the views and experiences of children, older mentors and teachers involved in an intergenerational mentoring scheme and to examine any cultural differences that might impact our findings. The research reveals that there have been significant personal and educational gains for children, older mentors and teachers involved in the scheme. Evidence suggests the mentors have become a wise advisor, friend and a teacher to identified individuals and groups of children in the class setting. This unique USA/UK study concludes that this evaluation should act as a baseline towards some extended research into the sustainability of older mentors working in schools, and the humanizing effect this has within school level in terms of improving intergenerational perception, understanding and cooperation.

Elderhostel: Who attends and why

Jill Hayes , RN,C (North Georgia College & State UNiversity, Dahlonega, GA USA)

Purpose The United States (U.S.) is currently experiencing a dramatic change in demographics, reflected most significantly in the rising numbers of older adults (Hooyman & Kiyak, 1996). It is estimated that by the year 2035, the cohort age 65 years or older, with equal 200f the American population. Current cohorts of adults age 65 years and older are characterized as having higher educational levels, and more financial resources than previous cohorts of similar age (Atchley, 1997). This trend is predicted to continue and will include additional characteristics of a pursuit of productive retirement lifestyles, improved health status, and a desire for more personal growth (Kaplan, 1981). According to Murk (1992), older Americans are on the move and the pursuit of personal growth within the context of educational settings, both formal and informal, is becoming increasingly popular. Method Participants of an elderhostel experience in the heast Georgia mountains were surveyed to identify common demographic characteristics, along with motivational factors for attendance. Participants were also surveyed to ascertain their satisfaction with the program and whether the program met their expectations. Results Findings revealed similarities and differences between this population and those populations represented in the literature. These findings are discussed as to their implications for program planning for future cohorts of older adults, and for the development of programming to meet the needs of more diverse populations of older adults. Conclusions There is a dearth of current literature on educational experiences such as elderhostel programming. Yet this country and the world are experiencing a dramatic increase in the numbers of well, productive, well educated, and financially stable older adults. In addition, society increasingly recognizes the value of higher education and frequently promotes lifelong learning. Universities are more and more developing outreach activities to lure nontraditional students into the academic environment, both as educators and consumers. Further research is needed to confirm the demographic characteristics of the new old population and their needs and desires for post-retirement activities. Programming aimed at promoting education and life enhancement in older populations must be carefully planned relative to content and delivery to attract participants and meet their needs.

Planning and Developing of the University of The Third Age in Jakarta/ Indonesia

Titus Kurniadi (Chairman of Wulan's Foundation & Board of the Indonesian Society of Gerontology in Jakarta); and Tony Setiabudhi PhD. (Trisakti Medical School/ Indonesian Society of Gerontology Jakarta/ Indonesia)

During the First National Congress of Older Persons; which was officially declared by the Indonesian Vice President (Megawati Sukarnoputri) it was also announced that a National Institute Centre on Ageing Studies was also founded (31 January 2001). This institute is actually a manifestation of a close cooperation between Indonesian Society of Gerontology and Trisakti Foundation. While Trisakti Foundation is a welknown foundation in Indonesia because it's establishing the biggest private university which become a famous community based institution and nowadays it is very popular and knowned as "Campus of Reformation". While on the other hand; Trisakti Medical School with the cooperation of Jakarta Municipal Health Divison, since a few years ago is concerned on improving the skills of older persons and started with some courses for this group (e.g. hydrophonics and entrepreneurship). Since we noticed that this kind of courses is now being felt to have a positive impact for the retirees as well as for the other groups of older persons we want to start with a better program including to conduct the "PRE-RETIREMENT" plan for pre-elderly groups in all of the provinces through-out Indonesia.

Senior Adult Education In India - Exploring the Options

I.J. Prakash (Bangalore University, India)

The concept of Senior Learning Centers is still new in India. An exploratory study was carried out to examine attitudes of people toward establishing Senior Adult Learning Centers (SALC), people's opinion about Who, Where, How SALC should be organized and What should be the content of teaching, was carried out in Bangalore. 350 people from different walks of life- educators, opinion leaders, students, professionals and senior citizens themselves were interviewed. There is general agreement as to the need for SALC. People differ, however, in who should organize SALC and How. Several factors are outlined as facilitating and preventing participation of elderly in SALC.

Showcasing a senior driven fifteen year experiment in third age learning.

Catherine Marcellus M.A. (Lifetime Learning Centre Society,

Mission, BC, Canada), Diana Muntigl, (Lifetime Learning Centre Society, Mission, BC, Canada)

The traditional paradigm for empowerment of third age learners is the sharing of power between formal institutions of education and the seniors served by third age programs. Lifetime Learning Centre Society is a new paradigm based on a 15 year experiment in third age education which is controlled and directed by seniors without any formal institutional or on-going municipal support. The study is a comprehensive evaluation of this delivery model for third age learning. The study examines the model against accepted criteria and goals for third age learning to establish if the model has had a significant impact on changing the meaning of "learning" in the post retirement years and if the model makes a significant contribution to the field of third age learning. Utilizing a method of participatory research, the study examines the impact the model has on quality of life issues, on health and aging, on the responsiveness of programs to personal and community issues, and on program planning. The study shows that the model has a qualitative impact on quality of life and health and that there is high support for continuing education and wellness programs for people in their retirement years. The study indicates that senior driven participation in third age adult education increases relevance of programs which adds to socialization, personal well-being, and community activity. Comments from people involved in these programs include "You have opened so many doors for us"; "The very best learning of my whole life". The book group over the years has been a great thing in my life"; "Thank you for all the pleasure you have brought me". The study indicates that the programs have generated mental and physical fitness, social and cultural interconnectedness, community activism and heightened awareness of community history. Through involvement with and management of programs such as Lifetime Learning, participants are more stimulated, socially active and connected to the community as a whole; and through health programs such as third age fitness and Osteofit, individual lives are made more interesting and participants have a feeling of well-being and social cohesiveness through lifelong learning.

SESSION 129

A Psychometric Assessment of Caregiver Burden: A Cross Cultural Study

Kuei-Ru Chou (Director of Research Development Committee, School of Nursing, National Defense Medical Center, Taipei, Taiwan, R.O.C.)

PURPOSE: The purpose of the study was to examine the psychomtric properties of a Chinese translation of the Screen for Caregiver Burden (SCB) in 150 primary caregivers of relatives with dementia. METHOD: A descriptive cross-sectional design with 150 primary caregivers of relatives with dementia in Taiwan was used. The psychomtric properties of this instrument have been established through three investigations. The first investigation evaluated the consistency between the Chinese and English version of the SCB through asymmetrical translation and back-translation. The second investigation established the internal consistent reliablity and test-retest reliability. The last investigation used hypotheses testing and contrast group technique to establish the SCB's construct validity. RESULTS: Across three investigations, the Chinese version of the SCB demonstrated appropriate internal consistency and good stability. SCB scores were significantly related to caregiving involvement, caregiver's health status, and the quality dyadic relationship between the caregiver and care-receiver. Sujbective burden scores were also significantly higher for caregivers than for controls. CONCLUSION: The preliminary evidence suggests that the Chinese version of the SCB is an appropriate instrument for measuring caregiver burden of relatives with dementia in Chinese populations.

Development of a Carer Screening Tool

D. Rembicki (Eastern Domiciliary Care Service, Adelaide, Australia), R. Penhall (Eastern Domiciliary Care Service, Adelaide, Australia), R. O'Connor (School of Health Services Management, University of New South Wales, Sydney, Australia)

PURPOSE: The primary purpose of this present study was to develop and validate a brief Carer Screening Tool. The aim of the screen is to identify carers who are at risk of suffering a reduction in their well being as a result of their caring role. The screen would enable assessors and service providers to target comprehensive and expensive assessment processes only to those carers who are in need of assistance from the formal support sector. METHOD: Items for the screen were developed by utilising a focus group methodology with carers and community assessors/service providers, and from a review of the literature in relation to carer burden. RESULTS: Results revealed a number of variables in relation to the care recipient [difficult or challenging behaviours, crisis in their health status], the carer and the caring role [sleep disturbances and associated fatigue, age, disability status and health of the carer, new carers, knowledge and information deficits, constancy of the caring role and the inability to leave the care recipient alone, and the carer's sense of loss] and external factors [other roles and commitments of the carer, including employment]. CONCLUSION: Draft items for inclusion in the screen have been identified and will be further refined via the use of an Expert Panel and continued field trials by community care agencies in Adelaide.

Family caregiver complaints about about outpatients with dementia (Pixel Study)

Ph Thomas (University Hospital of Poitiers;France) ; C Hazif Thomas (University Hospital of Poitiers;France) ; Montagne(President of Association des Neurologues libéraux de langue Française;JP Clement (University Hospital of Limoges;France; JP Belmin (University Hospital of Bobigny;France)

Objective. The aim of this study is to look at the relationship between the family complaints facing demented outpatients behavioural disorders and the stages of the disease. Methods. The multicentre study was performed on 408 outpatients with different types of dementia, mainly Alzheimer's, as well as on their main caregiver. After agreement of the patients and of the family, a specialist medical doctor, neurologist, psychiatrist or geriatrician assessed the patients. At the same time, a self administred questionnaire was given to the patients' family caregivers, concerning a list of complaints scored from 1 to 3 relating to various patients disorders. Results. 408 patients were included (76.5 year old +/- 0.36): 172 men, 236 women. Senile dementia of Alzheimer's type concerned 344 of them. The mean score at Folstein's MMS was 14.7 +/- 0.39. The first family complaint at any stages of the disease relates to loss of motivation, from 60% at the eartly ones to 77 0.000000or the severe stages. A weak cognitive status is accompagnied by a high score of family complaints. Conclusion. Family complaints about demented patients concern mainly the negative symptoms of the disease.

Positive Appraisal Resources in the Alzheimer's Caregiver Situation

Nancy Blume (Nursing Department, Fort Hays State University, Hays, Kansas, USA)

There is a paucity of information about potential positive aspects of caring for a person with Alzheimer's disease. A theoretical model of positive appraisal resources and their effect on caregiver's well-being was examined in a descriptive relationship-seeking study of rural elderly caregivers (N=45). The variables of hope, finding meaning through caregiving, and coping were the positive resources examined in relationship to sense of coherence as the outcome variable. Subjects who had been in the caregiving role for three years or more and were age 60 and older were recruited from Alzheimer's support groups in the rural areas of a midwestern state in the USA. Data were collected through individual in-home visits using questionnaires and analyzed using correlation coefficients, regression analysis and path analysis procedures. Results of the study showed that even though caregivers were coping at a low level, nearly 69% found positive aspects of caregiving. Levels of hope, coping and finding meaning significantly contributed to a sense of coherence for caregivers F 4.36 ($R2 = .2491$, $p=.0094$). A test of the theoretical model in which insignificant paths were removed showed a path linkage from hope to meaning to coherence. Hope, a sense of doing good, was a precursor to meaning. Caregivers found meaning through positive attitude and choice as well as ultimate meaning in their spiritual valuing and beliefs while provisional meaning came from the day-to-day tasks and giving of self. Coherence came from being able to comprehend the situation so that it was manageable in some way.

SESSION 130

Gerontology Education Needs in Developing Countries

Miguel Angel Acanfora (Argentinean Society of Gerontology and Geriatrics, Buenos Aires, Argentina), (Training Human Resources for Healthy and Active Aging in Latin America.) (2) Mark Gorman (HelpAge International, London, United Kingdom), (Gerontology in Africa Priorities for Education, Training and Research: An NGO Perspective) (3) Vinod Kumar (St.Stephen's Hospital, Delhi, India), (Gerontology Educational Needs in the Indian Subcontinent) (4) Joseph Troisi (International Institute on Aging, United Nations Malta, Valletta, Malta), (Meeting the Challenges of Population Aging through the Training of Personnel) (5) D. Wesumperuma (Asia Training Centre on Aging, HelpAge International, Chiang Mai, Thailand), (Disadvantaged Older Men and Women in Asia and Gerontology Education)

The aging of population is a world wide phenomenon affecting regions with different levels of intensity and with far-reaching consequences. The increase will be much more dramatic in the less developed regions, where the older population will be multiplied more than nine times from 171 million in 1998 to 1,594 million in 2050. As the rate of aging in these regions is more rapid, developing countries will have less time to adapt to the consequences of population aging. The need to respond to the prospects of an aging world was comprehensively canvassed during the World Assembly on Aging held in 1982. The Vienna Plan of Action on Aging established broad recommendations on how to meet the challenges of population aging. During the past 18 years, a number of governments started becoming increasingly concerned to formulate policies to respond to the fundamental changes resulting from the aging of their populations. Similarly, a number of care programmes and delivery services aimed at meeting the needs of older persons started emerging. The success of all these efforts did not often meet the expected results. One of the reasons behind this failure is the fact that, very often the very people who are directly involved in the delivery of these services lacked the basic skills and orientation to carry out their roles competently. The presentations covering Africa, India and South America corroborate this. Each presentation, in its own way, emphasises the necessity that every government not only recognises the underlying importance for health manpower development but provide appropriate continuing education and training. The standard of care provided depends on the personal qualities of the carers as well as on their professional preparation. However important the role of the State and that of Non-Governmental Organisations, it is equally important to identify, promote and support the role of older persons themselves and that of Associations of Older Persons. They are the best advocates of their own cause. HelpAge International is succeeding in tapping the resources of older people as trainers in self-care and as focal points for community based training. The International Institute on Aging, United Nations-Malta (INIA) provides multi-disciplinary education and training in Gerontology and Geriatrics at various levels to personnel mainly from developing countries. In order to maximise the efficiency and effectiveness of practical training, INIA has designed and implemented innovative training strategies and techniques oriented towards persons who are working or who intend to work in the field of aging. These, in turn, promote the multiplier effect in their respective countries through the dissemination of the information, knowledge and skills acquired. The challenges ahead of us, especially in the next thirty years are huge. In order to meet the special needs of the rapidly expanding older population, training of personnel at all levels has become a major issue which needs to be tackled with emergency. The time has come for societies in developing countries, the State, the NGOs, the family, the community, and the older persons themselves to have the necessary training lest events overtake history.

Disadvantaged Older Men and Women in Asia and Gerontology Education

D.Wesumperuma (Asia Training Centre on Ageing, HelpAge International, Chiang Mai, Thailand)

The needs of disadvantaged older persons in Asia are complex and diverse. Results of a series of Participatory Needs Assessments and workshops involving professionals, policy makers, researchers and practitioners as well as older men and women conducted by HelpAge International-Asia in Bangladesh, Cambodia, Lao, Philippines, Thailand and Vietnam highlight the alienation of older persons from mainstream social life particularly the adverse impact of socio-economic political exclusion, negative attitudes, stereotyping as well as health and livelihood issues. Gerontology educators need to address these wide-ranging issues of the disadvantaged. Some innovative training interventions initiated by several community-based NGOs in the HelpAge network in Asia have come up with encouraging results by directly engaging older people to tap their capabilities in meeting many of these challenges. In the Philippines an NGO project trains older persons as community gerontologists. In Vietnam, older persons are trained as trainers in self-care in the community. In Cambodia, Thailand and in Bangladesh, older persons are trained to run income generation projects to help meet livelihood needs. In Vietnam and in Thailand, the Older Peoples' Associations are focal points for community based training for peer help, social involvement, access to information and self care. In Bangladesh, an NGO is exploring how Traditional Birth Attendants could be oriented to include in their work basic health care of older persons. In Thailand and Vietnam, initiatives have been taken to train older persons as volunteers in home help/care. This presentation shows how community based participatory training programme interventions aimed at empowering disadvantaged older persons deserve careful study by educators in gerontology.

Gerontology Educational Needs in the Indian Subcontinent

Vinod Kumar (St.Stephen's Hospital, Delhi, India)

The Indian subcontinent contains a significant part of the world's population. Despite many variations in the region, there are many prevalent positive determinants. These include: the joint family system, the traditional home caring of older persons, and social and spiritual enrichment. Parallel to these are a number of negative determinants including illiteracy, double disease burden, lack of awareness of the aging process. Millions of India's elderly suffer from hearing problems, poor vision, hypertension, coronary artery disease and diabetes. Health services are inadequate available and utilised. Recent socio-demographic changes have necessitated a re-thinking on gerontology educational needs. Educational objectives, guided by principles of primary care including community participation, inter-sectoral action, domiciliary approach and cost effectiveness, must ensure adequate social, psychological and health care training so as to provide good quality of life in later years. Equally important is the need to ensure motivation of trainees and avenues for their utilisation. Educational programmes based on knowledge, assessment and care should be so designed as to incorporate field practices in addition to physical, socio-economic, psychological and spiritual aspects. Care of the severely ill elderly, exposure to available schemes and programmes, health promotion, physical therapy, nutrition and an understanding of determinants of health need to emphasised. The re-orientation of national public policies in the field of aging also determine the success of these educational programmes. This presentation outlines the aims, principles and contents of gerontology training and quality and scope of utilisation of trainees in keeping with the factors influencing old age care in the subcontinent.

Gerontology in Africa Priorities for Education, Training and Research: An NGO Perspective

Mark Gorman (HelpAge International, London, U.K.)

The field of gerontology in Africa, is relatively new . However, it is fast gaining significance as the issues of the mainstream development agenda are increasingly seen from an ageing perspective. Poverty, material security, gender, the impact of HIV/AIDS, as well as the impact of social forces such as globalisation and its outcomes, are all becoming the subjects of age-related research, training, education and action. This paper examines these developments in African gerontology and analysis some of the key future priorities for educating and training the rising generation of gerontologists on the continent. From an NGO perspective, it aims to highlight the key future research/education, practice links

Meeting the Challenges of Population Aging through the training of Personnel INIA's mandate.

Joseph Troisi (International Institute on Aging, United Nations Malta, Valletta, Malta)

Although almost 20 years have passed since the World Assembly on Aging, the results achieved in the implementation of The Vienna International Plan of Action on Aging have been less than expected. One of the reasons behind this failure is reflected in the pronounced scarcity of trained caregivers. The Plan of Action had emphasised that several of the recommendations made could not be implemented unless each country had trained personnel in the field of aging. To this effect, Recommendation 57 urged that "Practical training centres should be promoted and encouraged ... to train such personnel especially from developing countries, who would in turn train others" As a result of resolution 1987/41 of the UN Economic and Social Council, the United Nations signed an official agreement with the Government of Malta to establish a United Nations Institute on Aging aimed at helping developing countries to prepare for the inevitable consequences of population aging. This Institute was inaugurated on 15 April 1988 by the then UN Secretary General, Mr.Javier Perez de Cuellar. INIA's mandate is tripartite in nature, namely: 1) to train personnel from developing countries who are working or who intend to work in the field of aging or with the elderly; 2) to act as a practical bridge between developed and developing Countries in the area of information exchange in the field of aging; and 3) to provide advocacy to developing countries in matters concerning aging and older persons.

Training Human Resources for Healthy and Active Aging in Latin America

Miguel Angel Acanfora (Argentinean Society for Gerontology and geriatrics, Buenos Aires, Argentina)

The majority of the world's elderly population is living in developing countries. A lot needs to be done to ensure the implementation of the concept of Healthy and Active Aging while at the same time improving the Quality of life of older persons in these countries. By and large, the health systems and programs of care in these countries are mainly, if not exclusively, based on "assistance". Medical care is only provided in acute situations. There is a lack of a health promotion and prevention "conscience". Housing for older persons and long term care are only a "theoretical reality". The majority of these countries do not have trained personnel in the field of aging. There are a lot of volunteers, but they do not have the required knowledge or basic training. It is essential that those working with older persons should have the needed "basic knowledge". At the same time, scientific Gerontology associations and universities must assume a real social participation and partnership and not remain enclosed in pure research. There is an urgent need to work inside society in a partnership with the beneficiaries. This presentation discusses various efforts being made in this regard by different countries in Latin America.

SESSION 131

Films and Videos on Independence & Aging

James Vanden Bosch (Terra Nova Films, Inc, Chicago, Illinois USA)

94 Years and One Nursing Home Later (33 minutes, released in 2000) Family had always been important to Belle Greenberg. How, then, did she come to be alone and isolated from family at the end of her life? In this video, Laurel Greenburg, Belle's granddaughter, sets out to uncover this question. Laurel's search delves into the relationships and changing roles within the family as parents age. It reveals how difficult it can be, and yet how important it is, for families to communicate with each other around issues of aging and aging care. By example, the story shows that even in a loving and close family, miscommunication can and does occur. The video touches emotions we all feel, and leaves the viewer with a deeper understanding of family ties and the role they play in late life well-being. // Fear of Falling: A Matter of Balance (17 minutes, released in 1995) Older people often restrict their activities because they think it will reduce risk of falls. However, this restricted activity can lead to physical de-conditioning that can actually increase fall risk. This video and facilitator's manual combination provides step-by-step strategies for helping elders to 1) overcome the fear of falling and 2) take active steps to reduce the risk of falling. This program has been formally evaluated in a randomized field trial, and participants who completed the program reported: reduced fear of falling; increased confidence in managing falls; increased level of intended activity; increased mobility control.

SESSION 132

Family-Centered Practices in Long Term Care

M. Seymour (Medicine Hat College, Medicine Hat, Canada) Family Partnership: The Foundation to Quality Caregiving. B. Gorchynski (BG Healthcare Consulting) Family Experiences of Admitting an Elder to a Care CentreM. Osis (Osis Consulting Services, Calgary, Canada) Partnering with Families.

This Round Table discussion will present two studies exploring the experiences of families when an aging member moves into a Care Centre and a project designed to enhance family-staff relationships in long-term care. The discussion will begin with a presentation on the conceptual frameworks, methods, including instruments used, and findings of these two Canadian studies followed by a presentation of the evaluation of the clinical project. Participants will be invited to discuss the findings and explore the possibilities of implementing interventions that family members found to be of benefit. Family caregiving and support both prior to and following transition into continuing care, is recognized as a valuable contributor to the health and well being of the elder. Increasingly, families are expressing desire for involvement in the daily life and activities of the resident. Given the increased demands in the face of reduced resources for long-term care, supporting these families is more than a 'nice thing to do': it is imperative to meeting the needs of the elder, the family and the system. The first study presents the perceptions regarding staff responses to family input into care. Participatory action research was used to allow the researcher and the participants to work together to analyze a social system (Cormack, 1991). The results show that families were initially treated with respect and felt a true partnership with staff. This changed when the resident began to demonstrate difficult behaviors. In the second study, the Placement Response Scale (Dellasega and Nolan, 1999) was used to identify stressors and corresponding family responses throughout the placement process. The results support the assumption that the process of placing an elder in a Care Centre is a stressful and often overwhelming event. The findings of these studies and project provide some strategies to facilitate the process at all stages, which have implications for health care professionals working with family caregivers before, during and after admission to a Continuing Care Centre. This discussion will provide an opportunity for participants to debate the role of families in care within an institutional environment and the impact of care centre placement on the caregiving relationship. Exploration of approaches that family caregivers perceive to be of benefit will be facilitated. The discussion will provide a forum to share protocols for legitimized and meaningful family participation.

Family Experiences of Admitting an Elder to a Care Centre

B. Gorchynski (BG Healthcare Consulting, Calgary, Canada)

The purpose of this study was to examine caregiver experiences before, during and after admitting an elder to a care centre. The Placement Response Scale (Dellasega and Nolan, 1999) was used to identify the stressors and corresponding family responses throughout the placement process. Identification of these issues is an important first step in determining strategies that could be used at specific points in time to reduce both immediate and long-term negative outcomes for caregivers. Specifically, this study applies the Placement Response Scale in an interview setting to identify common events/feelings at each stage in the placement process as well as the families' degree of stress as related to those events/feelings. Demographic and contextual data was examined in relation to these caregiver responses. Results of the study also provide reliability data to the developer of the Placement Response Scale to further refine the instrument as well as providing important pilot data for future studies. The results of this study support the assumption that the process of placing an elder in a Care Centre is a stressful and often overwhelming event. As well, the continued involvement of the family caregiver throughout the process and after admission is confirmed. Qualitative feedback provides simple strategies to facilitate the process at all stages, which has implications for health care professionals working with family caregivers before, during and after admission to a Continuing Care Centre. This project has identified areas for further study particularly related to the interventions family caregivers perceived to be of benefit.

Family Partnership: The Foundation to Quality Caregiving

M. Seymour (Medicine Hat College, Medicine Hat, Canada)

This study was designed to explore the perceptions that family members have related to the respect demonstrated to them regarding their input to care by the formal caregivers after institutionalization. The methodology used was participatory action research as this method is a way of doing research and working on solving a problem at the same time (Cormack, 1991,p. 155). The method allows researcher and participants to work together to analyze social systems with the view of changing them. Action research is a process containing both investigation and the use of its findings(Smith, 1986 cited by Cormack, 1991, p. 155). The initial interview demonstrated the premise that hardiness is a major component of family caregivers personalities. These families further reported that on admission to a continuing care facility each felt a partnership with the health care team. However when their loved one began demonstrating behaviors such as resistance to care each reported a sense of loss of this partnership. All participants who experienced changed behaviors with their loved one reported less eye contact with the formal caregivers and an authoritarian tone used. What may be learned from this small sample study is that there continues to be a need on the part of the family caregivers to be actively involved in the care of their loved one based on their hardy personality trait. The formal care providers need to recognize these caregivers strengths. Through negotiation, family members may find meaningful roles.

Partnering with Families

M Osis (Osis Consulting Services, Calgary, Canada)

Partnering with Families is a project designed to enhance family-centered processes and relationships between staff in long-term care centres and their residents families. For family members, caregiving does not end with placement into a centre. Traditionally, families have not been viewed as members of the team but relegated to the roles of visitor, informer, or supporter and too often seen as interfering with institutional care/ practices. The social system of the care centre fosters a pragmatic and problem-oriented approach toward eldercare. Breaking away from this paternalistic approach is a major challenge. Three care centres participated in this six-month demonstration project to address this challenge. Through education, role modeling and consultation staff were encouraged to develop sensitivity to the issues and concerns of family caregivers and to enact family-centered practices to enhance a partnership model. Fifteen families were invited to receive brief therapy (up to 5 sessions) for distress related to the aging member's health status or for family conflicts. Through this project, we learned that assisting families to draw on their strengths, to learn new approaches to problem solving, and adapt to loss and disappointment are achievable goals. This presentation will provide an opportunity for participants to discuss the project design, the problems and surprises that occurred and explore the possibilities of achieving similar outcomes in their settings.

SESSION 133

[1] The effect of reminiscence program on the elderly with dementia-a randomized clinical trial

Etsuko Tadaka, The University of Tokyo,Tokyo,Japan Katsuko Kanagawa, Ishikawa Prefectural Nursing University,Ishikawa,Japan

Purpose: To examine the effect of an intervention of group care program consisting of reminiscence and reality orientation to prevent the decline of cognitive function and daily living activities in the community elderly with dementia(AD or VD a according to DSM-IV) in a randomized clinical trial. Method: Subjects were randomly assigned to either intervention group or control one. For the intervention group, a group care program was provided, on the other hand, for the control one, the usual day care program was provided once a week for 10 consecutive weeks. Result: 1) There was a significant difference in cognitive function between the intervention group and the control one of VD subjects, the total MMSE scores and orientation score in the intervention group increased, while that of the control one decreased. 2) There were significant differences in withdrawal and vitality between the two groups of AD and VD subjects, the intervention group showed improved these function, while the control one showed a loss of function. 3) The group process review suggested that the improvement of interpersonal relationship were seen in the intervention group. Conclusion: the group care program can be effective for improving cognitive function and daily living activities on community elderly with dementia. It is suggested, however, that sustained intervention may be necessary to maintain the effect over time.

[2] Medical ethical issues of Alzheimer's disease of the aged

Ma Yong-Xing (Department of Aging, Antiaging and Cognitive Function, Shanghai Institute of Gerontology and Geriatrics, Huadong Hospital, Shanghai, China)

Combined and brief case report of four patients of Alzheimer's disease (AD). Their names were Gu (Male), Wang (Female), Xu (M), Chen (M). Age: 60~80 years old. Sex: three male, one female. Occupation: two doctors, two vice directors of administrative unit. They were still working in the early period of AD. Their family members all have eagerly hoped that the hospital does not give the AD diagnosis to their directors for various reasons in certain period and do not tell the patients they have suffered from dementia. So we only told the patient, and even the family the patients suffered age-associated memory impairment (AAMI), but required treatment and care. The report of CT do not use the term "atrophy", but only the °senile change of brain". After some months, or even longer, the slow deterioration of the disease progressively occurred. We gradually obtained the understanding between the doctor, family and their organization, and even the patients themselves.

[3] Second National Survey on Measures for People with dementia in Norwegian municipalities.

Arnfinn Eek & Aase-Marit Nygård (The Norwegian Centre for Dementia Research, Tønsberg/Oslo, Norway

This is the second national survey of the services provides for people with dementia in Norwegian municipalities. The first survey was carried through in 1996/97. One of the goals is being able to register changes in these services throughout the time period 1996-2000 in relation to the increased effort put into health and social care for the elderly during this period. METHOD Data has been collected through a distribution of questionnaires to all of the Norwegian municipalities and subsequent follow-ups via telephone to those that either did not return the questionnaire, or returned it incomplete. In the survey from 1996/97, all of the municipalities (435) were represented, something we wish to accomplish again with this new survey. RESULTS In 1996/97, the results of the survey showed that only 14 % of nursing-home beds were in special care units for people with dementia, while in fact over 70 % of the patients suffered from dementia. Neither did any other service institutions for older people have an adequate service program for people with dementia. Only 2 % of these patients outside an institution received the offer of specialized day care-centres. The stat s increased focus on care for elderly has brought on a significant development on the services provided for old people in general, and this survey will show whether this development is also shown through better services for patients with dementia. Data from the last survey will be ready in March/April 2001, and will be presented and discussed at the congress.

[4] Management of dementia in primary care knowledge and attitudes of Czech general practitioners

E. Topinková, J. Neuwirth (Department of Geriatrics, 1st Medical Faculty, Charles University and Institute for Postgraduate Medical Education, Prague, Czech Republic), T. Haas (3rd Department of Internal Medicine, 1st Medical Faculty, Charles University, Prague, Czech Republic)

Demographic ageing, improved diagnosis and treatments will increase number of demented patients. By the year 2030, 30% increase is expected in the Czech Republic. Primary care physicians will play a key role in diagnosis and management of dementia. The aim of the study was to examine general practitioners' (GP) attitudes to and knowledge of dementia. A sample of 450 Czech GPs from 4 regions were sent questionnairs. Overall return rate was 71.6%. GPs consider dementia an important part of their clinical practice (85.4%) and are willing to take part in diagnosis and management. However, more than a half is aware of late/incorrect diagnosis and only 25-40% of dementia patients are diagnosed by Czech GPs. Alarmingly, it seems that 48.6% of GPs do not evaluate cognitive functions in elderly patients at all/only exceptionally. Another 18% would do that but do not know how or do not have time (12.1%). Standardised tests are used only by 8%. None of GPs rated their knowledge as very good, only 21.1% as sufficient. Reasons for misdiagnosis were: dementia diagnosed as ageing cognition, lack of time, missing patient's complaints, lack of practical screening instruments, lack of knowledge, reimbursement reasons. Conclusions: Czech GPs are willing to take the role of case finders and managers of dementia patients in the community. There is considerable lack of knowledge and poor care practices in diagnosing dementia in primary care. Training, availability of practical instruments and economic stimuli are seen as the most important factors to improve dementia management.

[5] SOCIAL MEALS PROGRAM

Rosemary Dunne, RT (Adanac Park Lodge, Vancouver, BC) Jessica Bryant, RT (Youville Residence, Providence Health Care, Vancouver, BC)

PURPOSE: To decrease the risk of dehydration and malnutrition for individuals living with dementia. To reduce the stress around the dining experience in the areas of meal consumption, environment and social interaction. To maintain or re-familiarize individuals life long learned dining / social interaction skills. To increase confidence and self esteem. To increase food and fluid consumption to help create a buffer weight for end stages of dementia. To demonstrate the importance of a genuinely normalized, calm dining environment. To demonstrate the imperative nature of having one who is not impaired coach, cue, support, interact and dine with the participants as they eat independently. To demonstrate that we, as caregivers, due to our task focus and time awareness disable residents prematurely by taking over due to slowed functional abilities. METHOD: Participant weights, MMSE scores, significant life events (death of a loved one, falls, ulcers), frequency of UTI's, were documented. Additionally, quantity and quality of food and interaction outside of the program was monitored in a checklist format. Participants (3-5) and their facilitator dined in an area outside of the hectic resident dining room of the special care unit. Video footage of facilitator methods of cueing and management of the dining environment as well as social interaction was documented. A list of specific behaviours around which there were serious concerns was developed for each participant. This is reflected upon and compared against the noted changes resulting from the program. These are evaluated to demonstrate change and positive outcomes. With the intention of promoting the implementation of Social Meals Programs (SMP) in dementia care environments, we propose to demonstrate the outcomes of a successful two-year informal study of three participants in the SMP. RESULTS: All three participants have both improved and maintained their weights within their Desired Weight Ranges (DWR). Participants in the program consume complete meals, using utensils independently, when in the program. Frequently outside of the program, they refuse nourishment or are overwhelmed so much by the environment (perhaps) that caregivers take over the task of self-nourishment by 'feeding' the person hurriedly. All three participants have experienced positive outcomes, in spite of the continuation of the dementing process, when a comparison is made with the lists of referred reasons (specific behaviours and concerns noted for evaluation) for participation. CONCLUSION: The concept of the Social Meals Program is a valid and valuable one. The program not only protects individuals against premature physical, social and cognitive decline but it also serves to create a sense of community amongst the participants. Participants have not only gained and maintained weight, increased fluid intake significantly and self-nourishment skills but also friends. It is not uncommon to see the participants interacting, protecting and supporting one another outside of the program when on the unit. There is a significant level of trust and rapport build between participants and facilitator such that the facilitator is recognized and sought out for support. There is also a more significant level of willingness to comply with requests of care providers than previously seen. For example, participant L. who repeatedly refused to have her weight taken is now fully cooperative. There is no doubt that by the implementation of this program, the quality of care and the quality of the special care environment is dramatically improved. As a result, participants in the SMP are able to live to the best of their ability both happily and in a state of optimal health.

[6] Measuring Quality of Life of Persons with Dementia in Three Types of Care Settings

Daniel Kuhn (Mather Institute on Aging, Evanston, IL, USA) Perry Edelman (Northwestern University and Mather Institute on Aging, Evanston, IL, USA) Roseann Kasayka (Heather Hill Institute, Chardon, OH, USA)

Purpose: A number of tools and methods for assessing dementia-specific quality of life (QOL) have recently become available but data documenting the reliability and validity of these instruments is limited. Without measures to assess QOL, determinants of desirable outcomes for people with dementia cannot be identified and efforts of administrators, program directors, and frontline staff to improve QOL in care settings will be hampered. Method: This study tested three methods and several tools to assess QOL of people with dementia in three types of care settings: two adult day centers, two assisted living facilities, and two nursing homes. Demographic information and data regarding severity of dementia, depression rating, functional status, and comorbid conditions was collected to determine the comparability of sites and to control for these characteristics in certain analyses. Results: Methods including observation, direct interviews with people with dementia, and staff proxy questionnaires present their own statistical and methodological strengths and weaknesses. Conclusions: A combination of these three methods may be most useful in assessing QOL. Practical considerations may rule out more time consuming methods and thus choosing the most appropriate method and tools must be consistent with organizational aims.

[7] The effect of group work program for elderly people of mild cognitive impairment

Yukari Morita, Kiyohito Okumiya, Masanori Nishinaga, Daisuke Kuzume, Yoshinori Doi, Toshio Ozawa (Kochi Medical School, Kochi, Japan), Kozo Matsubayashi(Kyoto University, Kyoto, Japan)

PURPOSE: We evaluated the effect of group work program for elderly people of mild cognitive impairment. METHODS: The subjects of mild cognitive impairment were assigned to an intervention group and a control group. The intervention group consisted of ten people, 79.0 years old and the control group consisted of twelve people, 79.3 years old. We programmed the group work for four months. The each group work was held weekly for three hours. The program consisted of music therapy, art therapy (poem, handicrafts), reminiscence, cooking, interchanges between elderly and children and so on. We evaluated the effect of group work by cognitive and neurobehavioral function and QOL (life satisfaction index). RESULTS: The control group significantly deteriorated in Kohs block test but the intervention group did not change. There was no difference between two groups in other cognitive or neurobehavioral functions. The QOL of intervention group ameliorated significantly. CONCLUSION: we showed the effects of group work program for elderly people of mild cognitive impairment in improvement of QOL and prevention from deterioration of cognitive function.

[8] Cognitive and Functional Evaluation of Centenarians By Convectional Methods

Casarotti D, Muzzoni B, Albertelli N, Cravello L, Magri F, Rossi G, Ferrari E. (Department of Internal Medicine and Medical Therapy, Chair of Geriatrics, University of Pavia, Italy)

The aim of this study was to evaluate the predictive role of the convectional geriatric assessment in peculiar condition such as in the extreme segment of live. We studied two groups of subjects: 89 free living healthy old subjects (aged 72-92 yrs, mean 79.98 +/- 0.52 SEM) and 48 free living or living in a nursing home centenarians (aged 100-107 yrs, mean 101.2 +/- 0.22 SEM). In every subject we evaluated: the cognitive performances (MMSE), the functional state (ADL and IADL), the behaviour (GDS) and the comorbility (CIRS). In the whole group the subject s age was significantly correlated negatively with both the MMSE score and the ADL and IADL evaluation and positively with the CIRS severity and comorbility score; furthermore the MMSE score and each of the six domains were strongly related to the ADL and IADL dependence. These relationships were also present, even if at a lower degree of significance in the group of old subjects. On the contrary, in the group of centenarians, the MMSE score did not show any correlation with ADL and IADL, whereas it was negatively related to the CIRS score. Only some MMSE domains, i.e. language and praxia, maintained a good relationship with the ADL and IADL score. In spite of the deeper impairment of the functional and cognitive performances, the centenarians were basically satisfied with their life. Furthermore, the poor performance of ADL and IADL tasks were not related to a depressed mood, unlikely from "younger" old subjects. The conventional instruments seem to lost sensitivity and specificity in this selected population; therefore new approaches seem to be necessary.

[9] Memory Assessment Clinics Self-rating Scale (MAC-s). Spanish validation in a clinic elderly sample

M. Izal, I. Montorio, M. Márquez, A. Losada (Autonoma University of Madrid, Madrid, Spain)

Memory self-perception is useful for memory assessment (Larrabee & Crook, 1994), because of its relation with objective measures, the possibility of being compared with the the latter ones, and because self-efficacy and perceived competence influence performance. Finally, identifying specific memory problems in daily life allows a situacional and functional analysis that can contribute to determine ways of intervention (Tobiansky et al, 1995). The Memory Assessment Clinics Self-Rating Scale (MAC-S; Winterling et al, 1986) was elaborated to overcome existing limitations in this kind of instruments. The 49 items that compose the MAC-S are divided in two subscales, efficacy and frequency, and four global questions more. The results of the Spanish adaptation of this scale, administered to 240 patients of the Cantoblanco Memory Unit in Madrid, are presented. Results show that the internal consistency is adequate for both subscales (0.88 for efficacy and 0.86 for frequency). Also, statistically significant differences were found in scores obtained by four groups of subjects (normal, age-associated memory impairment, dementia and affective disorder). Finally, the score profiles based on MAC-S shows special utility for the diferential clinical diagnostic of dementia, since using it together with memory performance tests, self-rated depression (GDS), and family interview, successfully contribute to discriminate between initial dementia stage, age-associated memory impairment and cognitive decline related with mood disorder.

[10] CERAD Word List Normative Data for Nondemented Controls

Ross Andel (Andrus Gerontology Center, University of Southern California, USA), Margaret Gatz, Amy Fiske (Psychology Department, University of Southern California, USA)

Purpose: Word List tasks are in wide use for dementia assessment, with Delayed Recall found especially sensitive to mild dementia. Impairment is inferred by contrasting performance to norms developed from nondemented samples. In this study, we compare previously reported means for the CERAD Word List tasks with means obtained from two new nondemented samples. Method: The first sample included 79 Swedish Twins (mean age = 75.4 years) from the population-based Study of Dementia in Aging Twins, some of whom were co-twin partners to dementia cases. The second sample included 52 volunteers (mean age = 76.9 years) recruited from senior organizations in Los Angeles. On average, participants in the twin study attained less than high school education, while the Los Angeles volunteers finished college. Results: On average, the twins scored 17.2 (SD=4.4) on Learning, 4.9 (SD=2.4) on Delayed Recall, and 68.1 (SD=29.2) on Savings (a percentage of verbal information from Trial 3 retained in Delayed Recall). The Los Angeles volunteers scored a mean of 19.5 (SD=3.5) on Learning, 5.1 (SD=2.2) on Delayed Recall, and 73.8 (23.6) on Savings. Conclusion: Delayed Recall and Savings scores were markedly below mean scores for a university-based dementia registry normative sample reported by Welsh et al. (1994). Learning scores were somewhat lower, even after taking education into account. These results indicate that the scores for normal older adults on the CERAD Word List tasks may set too stringent a standard.

0Supported in part by a grant from the National Institute on Aging (AG08724).

[11] Behavior Problems in Dementia: Measurement and Comparison of Daily and Weekly Reports

E. E. Femia (Gerontology Center, Pennsylvania State University, PA, USA), S. A. Leitsch (School of Social Work, University of Michigan, MI, USA), S. H. Zarit (Gerontology Center, Pennsylvania State University, PA, USA), and M. A. P. Stephens (Kent State

University, OH, USA).

PURPOSE: The Daily Record of Behavior (DRB) is a measure that assesses the daily frequency, duration, and perception of 12 behavioral domains commonly exhibited by persons with dementia. The Weekly Record of Behavior (WRB) is a similar measure of the same domains over a week long period of time. In this study, we examined the rates of behaviors and their fluctuation throughout the day and over a 2-day period. We then compared the DRB with the WRB to uncover potential differences between the daily and weekly reports. METHOD: Participants included 72 family caregivers (51pouses; 46% adult children) residing with the person with dementia. During an in-home interview, caregivers completed the WRB, and during 2 telephone interviews in the same week, they completed the DRB. Caregivers were called 24 hours after a target day, in which he/she observed the behavior, memory, and mood of the care recipient throughout 4 phases of the day (morning, afternoon, evening, overnight). RESULTS: Memory problems, naps, and mood/anxiety problems occurred most frequently. Naps, reality problems, sleep, and eating problems were the longest lasting, while bathing, sleep, disruptive, and reality problems were the most upsetting. Problems occurred most frequently in the morning compared to the afternoon and evening periods. However, as the day wore on, behavior problems were perceived as more upsetting. Generally, these daily results were consistent over a 2-day period and with the weekly reports; however, behaviors reported in the WRB had a longer duration and some were reported to be more upsetting.

[12] Does Dementia Explain A Subsequent Physical Disability

C. Sauvaget, M. Yamada, S. Fujiwara (Radiation Effects Research Foundation, Hiroshima, Japan) H. Sasaki (Hiroshima Atomic Bomb Casualty Council Health Management & Promotion Center, Hiroshima, Japan) Y. Mimori (Hiroshima University School of Medicine, Hiroshima, Japan)

Cognitive impairment and disability are strongly and consistently related in cross-sectional studies. However, results based on longitudinal studies are more accurate since they allow the establishment of a temporal relationship between exposure (dementia) and outcome (physical disability). A group of 1358 atomic-bomb survivors aged 61 years old and over who lived in Hiroshima City, Japan, were followed for four years. Most of them lived in the community, and 3% lived in institutions. At baseline, the diagnosis of dementia was comprehensively assessed by a series of cognitive tests, neurological examination, as well as magnetic resonance imaging and computer tomography scan for some subjects. Diagnosis of dementia was made according to DSM-III-R criteria. At baseline and at the follow-up survey, the functional status of the subjects was examined through basic activities of daily living (BADL), and instrumental activities of daily living (IADL). The results showed that incidence of physical disability in BADL and IADL increased with age. At the multiple logistic regression analysis, dementia was a strong predictor of physical disability for the incidence of BADL (odds ratio (OR) = 14.0 (5.4-36.3)), and of IADL (OR = 3.9 (1.8-8.3)), after adjustment for age, sex, and medical history of stroke. Dementia was an important determinant of functional status after four years. The risks were higher for self-care tasks (BADL) than for more intermediate and complex tasks (IADL) suggesting that other factors than cognition, such as motivation, or perceptual, sensory and motor abilities are involved in IADL performances.

[13] Music therapy and sensory integration therapy in severe dementia: a randomised controlled study

Tiziana Metitieri, Angelo Bianchetti, Alessandra Marrè (Geriatric Research Group, Brescia and Ancelle della Carità, Hospital, Cremona, Italy) Gialuigi Perati (Vismara-DePetri Geriatric Instutute, San Bassano, CR, Italy) and Marco Trabucchi (Geriatric Research Group, Brescia and University of Tor Vergata Roma; Italy)

The efficacy of music and psychomotor therapy to decrease behavioural problems of individuals with moderate to severe Alzheimer disease living in a Special Care Unit (SCU) was assessed. A randomised controlled study was conducted in a SCU for patients with moderate to severe dementia with relevant behavioural disturbances. Eighteen subjects were randomly assigned to a 3-week rehabilitative programme (a music individualised therapy or a psychomotor individualised therapy programme). They were randomly scheduled for observation of a wide range of behavioural symptoms during the day (morning, lunch time and night) for three months (the month before, during and after the intervention). Cognitive function was assessed with the Mini-Mental State Examination (MMSE) and behavioural symptoms with the Neuropsychiatric Inventory (NPI). The patients, 3 men and 15 women, (mean age=76.2±9.9 years; mean MMSE score=7.4±2.9; mean NPI total score=59.3±22.6), were randomly assigned to the two conditions (9 patients in each group). In the post-treatment assessment the following change was observed from baseline: the music therapy condition reduced significantly the frequency and the severity of anxiety and apathy ($p<0.05$) on the individual symptoms NPI score; the psychomotor condition showed a significant decrease of the frequency of anxiety ($p<0.05$), and the severity of apathy ($p<0.05$). Music therapy was more effective than psychomotor therapy in reducing the daily frequencies of the observed behavioural disturbances and in enhancing communication skills. Music therapy and psychomotor therapy may be effective in reducing anxiety and apathy in moderate to severe demented patients living in an instituzionalized setting.

[14] Effects of a short course on memory on memory self-efficacy of actively learning older adults

Richard D. Tucker (University of Central Florida, Orlando, FL)

Purpose: With increased awareness of Alzheimer's Disease in the general population, older adults have developed an Alzheimer's phobia. This is characterized by negative self-statements regarding everyday memory, excessive concerns with current memory lapses as indicators of impending dementia, and low memory self-efficacy. Research on memory self-efficacy has confirmed these characteristics among populations of community-based older adults. The purpose of this study was to assess the effects on memory self-efficacy of a short course on the myths and realities of memory changes in aging actively learning older adults. Method: Participants were 44 older adults (mean age 73.1 yrs.)who were attending a five-day Elderhostel program. The group consisted of 27 women (mean age 71.4 yrs.) and 17 men (mean age 75.7 years). The 15 item Memory Self-Efficacy Scale has four factors: Descriptive Memory (DM), Judgment of Memory (JM), Memory Concern (MC), and Self-efficacy (SE). The six-hour course consisted of a presentation of research on normal vs. abnormal memory changes; discussion by participants of their memory concerns; an AARP video Memory: The Long and Short of It; and suggestions for keeping mentally active. Results: Pre and Post test comparisons revealed no differences in DM, but significant differences ($p<.05$)showing less MC and more favorable JM. SE showed a modest but insignificant difference. There were no significant differences across factors by gender. Conclusion: Results are discussed in terms of the assessment of memory self-efficacy among active older adult learners, and the impact of an information program on memory.

[15] Generalized Slowing in Cognitively-Impaired-Not-Demented Patients and Healthy Adults

K.R. Peters, P. Graf (Department of Psychology, University of British Columbia, Vancouver, B.C, CANADA), S. Hayden (Clinic For Alzheimer's Disease and Related Disorders, UBC Hospital, Vancouver, B.C, CANADA)

This research examined whether a widely accepted theory of normal cognitive aging —the Generalized Slowing Hypothesis— can explain cognitive deficits in individuals with cognitive impairments. The Generalized Slowing Hypothesis stipulates that age-associated declines in high-level cognition are mediated by reductions in processing speed. We examined this hypothesis is 55 Cognitively-Impaired-Not-Demented or CIND adults (M age = 66.47; SD = 9.44) and in 42 age- and sex-matched healthy adults (M age = 59.41; SD = 9.86). Processing speed was measured by three tests: Finger Tapping, Simple Reactions, and Card Sorting. The California Verbal Learning Test (CVLT) and Rey-Osterrieth Complex Figure test (ROCF) were used as measures of high-level cognition. Hierarchical regression analyses were performed in order to determine the ability of age to predict performance on the CVLT (total words correctly recalled during trials 1 to 5) and on the ROCF test (immediate recall) before and after statistically controlling for the influence due to the three measures of processing speed. The generalized slowing hypothesis was supported in the CIND group. The degree of attenuation in the predictive ability of age after statistically controlling for processing speed did not differ significantly between the two groups for either the CVLT (control = 44%; CIND = 58%, p >.05) or the ROCF test (control = 67%; CIND = 48%, p >.05). These findings suggest that the cognitive deficits of CIND patients can be partially explained by processes that are involved in normal cognitive aging.

[16] Memory changes across the adult lifespan: The formation of gains and losses

Monica Mori (Concordia College, Moorhead, MN, USA)

This study employed a cross-sectional design to examine memory changes across the adult lifespan. In a verbal report task, 162 adults whose ages ranged from 16 to 83 years were asked to describe a series of color photographs, and following a delay, were asked to re-describe the pictures from memory. Participants' verbal reports were transcribed and coded for the number of references to things depicted in a picture, called given information, and to things that are not depicted in the picture per se but related to things in the picture, called beyond information. The most important findings were that: 1) memory for given information showed the expected age-related decline and memory for beyond information showed no age-related change, and 2) memory performance on the verbal report task was related to study performance. Results are discussed in terms of maturational changes in schema structure, the developmental notions of selective optimization with compensation and loss in the service of growth (Baltes, 1987; Labouvie-Vief & Schell, 1982) and the use of the verbal report task as an age-free measure of memory.

[17] The cognitive function of the Japanese centenarians: Estimating Memory and Executive function using the MMSE.

H. Inagaki, Y. Gondo, Y. Masui (Tokyo Metropolitan Institute of Gerontology, Tokyo, Japan), K. Kitagawa (Komazawa University, Tokyo, Japan), N. Hirose, Y. Arai, M. Takayama, Y. Ebihara, K. Yamamura, S. Nakazawa (Keio University, Tokyo, Japan), K. Yamashita, H. Shimomura, K. Nishikawa, Y. Lau (Keio Junior college of Nursing, Tokyo, Japan).

PURPOSE: We report the result that estimated the Japanese centenarians Memory and Executive function using the MMSE. Rabbitt & Lowe (2000) reported, using the subject below 80 years, that memory declined with ageing but executive function was maintained. We investigated the cognitive functions that decline and maintain until the extremely old period, comparing young-old and old-old. METHOD: The 207 subjects (65-105 years) who live in Tokyo Metropolitan were performed MMSE. Range of total MMSE was 18-30 of 65-91 aged and 0-27 of centenarians, furthermore 50% of the 65-91 aged scored 27 or above. So we selected the subjects scored 18-25 (that was mean (26.7) minus 0.5 SD of 65-91 aged group) from both 65-91 aged and centenarians. Then we grouped three by age, and analyzed the data of 25 young-old (65-74), 18 old-old (75-89) and 16 centenarians (100-103). RESULTS: Using one-way ANOVA, we compared the score of Memory (Registration, and Recall) and Executive function (Repeat, Listen & Obey, Read & Obey, and Write Sentence) among 3 age groups. In result, centenarians Recall score was lower significantly than young-old ($F(2,56)=4.34$, $p<.05$). There was no significant difference on other items. CONCLUSION: The centenarians maintained their executive function and declined the Recall comparing young-old and old-old. This result corresponded the report of Rabbitt & Lowe (2000). Its shown the ageing affect to cognitive function appears locally, and there is the function that maintains until extremely old period.

[18] Prevalence of Cognitive Impairment in Santiago, Chile. The SABE Project

Albala C (Nutrition and Food Technology Institute; University of Chile, Santiago, Chile), Garcia C (Nutrition and Food Technology Institute; University of Chile, Santiago, Chile), Marín PP. (Fac of Medicine, Catholic University of Chile, Santiago, Chile), Vio F (Nutrition and Food Technology Institute; University of Chile, Santiago, Chile), Arroyo P (Fac of Medicine, University of Chile, Santiago, Chile), Peláez M (Pan American Health Organization, Washington DC, USA).

Purpose: To estimate the prevalence of cognitive impairment in Santiago, using a diagnostic test previously validated, consisting in a short version of MMSE and the Pffefer Activities Questionnaire (PFAQ). Methods: Cross sectional survey in a random, representative sample of 1306 subjects aged 60 and over, living in the city of Santiago. Cognitive impairment was defined by a score below 13 on the short MMSE (maximum score 19) and above 5 (maximun score 33) in the PFAQ. In all the subjects, a short version of MMSE was applied and when scoring >13, PFAQ was applied to a surrogate. Results: MMSE was positive in 12.5% of the total sample (8.5% men and 13.9% women) from whom 45% were illiterate. PFAQ was negative in 27% of those who scored <13 in MMSE giving a positive screening in 9.0% of the total sample (7.3% men and 11.7% women). There was a significant increase with ageing ($r2= 0.82$), that reached 30% of positives in people aged 85 or over. All the items of MMSE were affected by age, but not by gender. The interaction between gender and age resulted in a higher prevalence in women. Cognitive impairment was significantly higher in less educated subjects. Conclusion: Total prevalence of cognitive impairment was 9.0% in Santiago, the more frequent the older and the less educated.

[19] A short test to evaluate cognitive impairment based on Folsteins MMSE

Albala C, Icaza G, Vio F, Garcia C. (Nutrition and Food Technology Institute; University of Chile, Santiago, Chile), Marín PP. (Fac of Medicine, Catholic University of Chile, Santiago, Chile), Quiroga P, (Fac of Medicine, University of Concepción, Concepción, Chile), Palloni A (University of Wisconsin, Madison, USA), Peláez M (Pan American Health Organization, Washington DC, USA), Branch L and Fillenbaum G (Duke University, USA).

Purpose: To develop a short cognitive test based on the MMSE previously validated in Chile, feasible for extensive health surveys, harmonized to the Latin American culture. Method: The analysis was based on preexisting data of the WHO project. Age associated dementias done in 2318 people aged 60 and more living in Concepcion. From the original data file, 50% of subjects were randomly selected for a reduced model to explain the MMSE score (maximum score 30, cut point 22). The other 50% of subjects was used to validate the predictive model. The statistical analysis, run on SAS, included multiple regression and ROC analysis. Results: The first selected variable to explain the total score of MMSE was orientation followed by attention/concentration, delayed recall, comprehension, registration and visual/spatial capability. The adjusted model with these six variables was validated in the test file. The final model explaining 93.5% of the total MMSE variability, follows: Orientation (date, month, year, country) Registration (tree, table, plane) Attention/Concentration (1-3-5-7-9), Delayed Recall (tree, table, plane) Comprehension (to fold a paper...) Visual-Spatial Ability (to draw circles). Maximum Total score is 19. The best sensibility and specificity (93.8 and 93.9) plotted in a ROC curve, selected 13 as the score corresponding to cut-off point of 22. The concordance of both tests had a Kappa index of 0.83 (95% CI: 0.80 0.87). Conclusion: The study provided a good, easy and short time consuming test for cognitive impairment to be applied in health surveys.

[20] Bright Light and Behaviour in Dementia: An Observation Study

M. Dimond, M. Lentz, R. Burr (University of Washington, Seattle,

WA, USA)

PURPOSE: To describe the effect of evening bright light on agitated behaviors in cognitively impaired, institutionalized older adults. METHOD: Design: a randomized crossover experimental design with pre- and posttests of the effects of evening light with repeated measures. Sample: N=63. Settings: 8 special care units (SCUs). The Agitated Behavior Rating Scale (ABRS) was used to observe behaviors. Pre-test/ Post-test: 4 days of every 20 minute observations between 8am-12noon and 3-7pm each day. The intervention was evening bright light for 14 days. The sham treatment consisted of having the residents' room configured with lights and a control box, but the lights were not turned on. A 2-week washout was followed by crossover to either light or sham. Hypothesis: Bright light will diminish the frequency of selected agitated behaviors. RESULTS: Two subscales of the ABRS were included in the analysis: manual manipulation (MM) and vocalization (V). Results of two-tailed t-test pre-post light for both am & pm observation periods were mixed. In both the light and the sham arms reductions and increases in MM and V occurred. Increased MM and V behaviors occurred more often after the light treatment, while decreases in MM and V behaviors occurred more often in the sham arm. Therefore, the hypothesis was not supported. These findings are contrary to previous reports of the effect of light on agitated behavior. CONCLUSION: The mixed findings may be due to the timing of the administration of the light, variation in cognitive impairment, and environmental variability among the SCUs.

[21] Influence of Personal and Environmental Characteristics on Circadian Activity in Persons with Dementia.

R. Burr, M. Lentz, M. Dimond (University of Washington, Seattle, WA, USA)

PURPOSE: Changes in level and timing of activity are often seen in persons with dementia although it is unclear what factors contribute to the activity patterns. The purpose of this study was to examine the contributions of individual characteristics of age and cognition (MMSE) and environmental characteristics of ambient light (lux) and structure (nursing home special care unit, SCU) to the circadian rhythm of activity. METHOD: Data were obtained over four days on a sample of 8 men and 49 women, ranging in age from 63 to 102 (mean+/-SD=85.4+/-9.0) years old with a diagnosis of dementia residing in SCUs in eight nursing homes. Subjects continuously wore an activity sensor in a specially designed vest underneath their usual clothing. Light measurements and behavioral observations were made every 15 minutes during four hour blocks each morning and afternoon. RESULTS: The circadian activity pattern was related to patient age (24 hour cosinor mesor: r = -.60; p=.000; cosinor magnitude: r=-.534, p=.000), MMSE score (mesor: r=.35, p=.007; magn.: r=.340, p=.01), percent daytime awake (mesor: r=.15, NS; magn.: r=.35, p=.007), and average daytime illumination (mesor: r=.265, p=.046, magn.: r=.410, p=.006). The activity pattern was also influenced by SCU (Pillai's Trace=.556, F=1.853, df=(18,147), p=.024). Controlling for age did not alter the relationships of activity with MMSE total score and SCU. CONCLUSION: In this study, younger subjects with higher MMSE scores, taking less daytime naps, and exposed to more daytime light, had more consolidated circadian activity patterns. Care setting contributed significantly even after controlling for these factors.

[22] To what extent is dementia reported on medical care records?

G. Fillenbaum, M. Tyrey, G. Cook (Center for the Study of Aging and Human Development), B. Trapp-Moen (School of Nursing), C.F. Pieper (Division of Biometry, Department of Community and Family Medicine), A. Heyman (Division of Neurology, Department of Medicine) (all Duke University Medical Center, Durham, NC)

PURPOSE: Dementia tends to be under-diagnosed in primary care practice and in hospitalized in-patients. The present study examines the extent to which there is underdiagnosis of clinically assessed older epidemiologic study participants. METHOD: We examined 178 primary care practice, hospital and nursing home records for the previous five years for 153 participants in a study of the prevalence and incidence of dementia, and compared reports of dementia on these records with study-based clinical determination of a dementing disorder. RESULTS: Of the 153 participants, 57 (37.2%) were white, 96 (62.7%) were African American, with mean age 74.2 (sd=3.6) years and mean education 7.0 (sd=3.6) years. On clinical evaluation 84 (54.9%) received a study diagnosis of dementia and 69 (45.1%) did not. The 178 medical records included 86 (48.3%) primary care, 69 (38.8%) hospital and 23 (12.9%) nursing home records. Dementia was noted for only 52.5% of those with a study diagnosis of dementia, and for 5.9% of those in whom dementia had not been identified. For those with study identification of dementia, this condition was reported on 82.5% of the nursing home records, but on less than 50% of the primary care and hospital records. Logistic regression analyses indicated that accurate reporting of dementia was not associated, separately or in combination, with age, sex, race or education. CONCLUSION: Based on record review, identification of dementia appears to be related to location of service (which may be a marker for severity of disease) rather than to demographic characteristics of the individual.

[23] Driving and Dementia Toolkit: Development and Evaluation

Anna Byszewski, University of Ottawa, Sean Marshall, The Rehabilitation Centre, Lynn Hunt, The Rehabilitation Centre, Clarissa Bush, SCO- Elizabeth Btuyere, D. Guzman, SCO-Elizabeth Btuyere, Kathy McKinley, The Alzheimer Society, Malcolm Hing, University of Ottawa, Ian Graham, University of Ottawa, Stephanie Amos, University of Ottawa, William Dalziel, University of Ottawa,Ian Richardson, OTTAWA, ONTARIO

Purpose: With the increasing population of elderly who have cognitive loss and drive, resources are needed to assist in the evaluation and management of this aspect of dementia care. Method/Results: Under the auspices of the Dementia Network of Ottawa, a toolkit was developed to address the gap in this area. The primary target group are family physicians who care for the older patient. This descriptive poster will present how the toolkit was produced with focus group input and the contents which include: an algorithm of resources, facts on driving and dementia, the legal responsabilities of physicians, how to assess the condition, what and how to inform the patient/caregiver and required forms/documentation. (The printed form of the toolkit will be available for viewing) In the evaluation stage, a pre and post questionnaire was used to assess knowledge and confidence gained. Conclusion: A toolkit can be used to address the need for information in dealing with this highly sensitive and important domain of dementia care.

[24] Using Goal Attainment Scaling to Evaluate a Health-Related Community Development Project with Seniors

R.G. Crilly, M. Kloseck (Division of Geriatric Medicine, University of Western Ontario, London, Ontario, Canada)

Goal Attainment Scaling (GAS) is a versatile, under-utilized evaluation tool that actively involves community members and stakeholders in the evaluation process. We have used GAS in a participatory action project with seniors to evaluate seniors involvement in the planning of their own health services. GAS provided a methodology for setting goals, a way of creating a scale (-2, -1, 0, +1, +2) to objectively measure the degree of achievement, over- or under-achievement of goals established for various components of the project, and a way of combining goal achievement scores for an overall project score. For example, using the formula: GAS = 50 + 103(wixi) %(.73wi2) + .3(3wi)2 the overall GAS score for community capacity building goals (one component of the project) increased from 22.62 at baseline to 50.00 at year 1. This poster will demonstrate the use of GAS in (1) creating and tracking goals to demonstrate involvement in health planning by seniors and improvement in a community s capacity to bring about change, (2) measuring progress toward goals by setting and achieving interim goals at various stages throughout the evaluation process, (3) establishing a hierarchy of goals, where the amalgamation of the achievement of lesser goals becomes a measure of the achievement of greater goals, and (4) maintaining a project "score card", with GAS being used as an ongoing measure of the performance of the project. GAS was found to be very "user-friendly" and readily understandable by elderly individuals and health professionals not familiar with program evaluation.

[25] Reevaluating the driving skills of elderly drivers: assessment practices

T. Audet (Centre de recherche en gérontologie et gériatrie, Institut universitaire de gériatrie de Sherbrooke, Université de Sherbrooke, Sherbrooke, Canada) and M. D'Amours (Centre de recherche en gérontologie et gériatrie, Institut universitaire de gériatrie de Sherbrooke, Université de Sherbrooke, Sherbrooke, Canada)

Along with the aging of industrial societies, an increased number of elderly drivers will be on the road. As a group, elderly drivers have one of the highest crash rates per vehicle mile of travel. A decline in sensory, cognitive, and physical capacities during the aging process is often associated with some reduction of the ability to drive safely. The general goal of this study was to describe and evaluate assessment practices of different countries in regard to enhanced safety for maturing drivers. The study was based on 90 legislations (canadian, american, european, oceanian, and asian). Firstly, the different practices whose aim is to assess driving skills in elderly drivers were surveyed. Secondly, the efficiency of those practices was examined based on their scientific value, popularity, and capacity to correctly detect elderly drivers at risk. Analyses indicated that the decision to reevaluate driving skills of elderly drivers is usually linked to specific procedures in license renewal or is made following reports by medical staff, police officers, family members or employees of licensing agencies. No more than 35% of legislations surveyed have procedures based solely on the age of drivers. Although many practices have sound scientific bases and are popular among legislations from different countries, it is more difficult to prove that they really are enhancing safety by pointing out the impaired elderly drivers. More research is needed to insure that the mobility and security of elderly drivers are well served by current assessment practices.

[26] Right Foot Behavior of Elderly Persons while Driving in a Simulator

V. Cantin, N. Teasdale, F. Sergerie (Université Laval, Division de kinésiologie, Département de médecine sociale et préventive, Québec, Canada), J. Blouin (Université de la Méditerranée, Marseille, France)

PURPOSE : The aim of this experiment was to examine the driving behavior of elderly persons at intersections, and more particularly the right foot movements. METHOD : Twenty five elderly persons (mean age = 66, range of 61-79) and 15 young adults participated. All elderly were active drivers (on average, 150 km/week with more than 35 years of driving experience). They all scored 25 or higher on the Mini Mental Test. They drove an 8-km practice run to familiarize themselves with the simulator and a 16-km experimental run through a simulated neighbourhood (STISIM Inc. instrumented with a mid-sized sedan with automatic transmission). For the experimental run, 27 events consisting of crossings with a stop sign or crossing lights were presented. All subjects were instructed to drive as normally as possible and to avoid any accident. RESULTS : On average, the elderly were slower than young adults to complete their experimental run (on average, 26 min vs 23 min). An interesting between-group comparison concerns the stereotypical breaking behavior of the young adults compared to the varied pattern observed for the elderly. The deceleration of the vehicle was characterized by irregular and jerky pedals' behavior (for both the breaking and accelerator pedals). This yielded less consistent stopping distance for the elderly than for the young adults. CONCLUSION : A main issue that remains is to determine whether the observed behavior for the elderly results only from a perceptual or also from a motor problem. Supported by the MAIF and NSERC Canada.

[27] Prevalence and correlates of subjective memory complaint in Mexican elders >65.

Fachinelli M.P. Gutiérrez-Robledo LM, Sánchez L. Juarez S. Villa A. (Instituto Nacional de Ciencias Médicas Salvador Zubirán Ostrosky F, (Facultad de Psicologia Universidad Nacional Autónoma de México).México D.F. México

Objective : prevalence estimation of subjective memory complaint (SMC) and its correlates in subjects older than 65 in Mexico city. Methods : A representative sample of 4000 subjects living in the community in Mexico city was obtained through the bureau of the census. All were examined with Folstein MMS, brief GDS, Minineuropsi (an standardized minimal neuropsychological assessment developed for Mexican population) and socio-demographic and health status data. Results: prevalence of SMC is 55 % . Recent forgetfulness in 90 % and remote in 20 % . Mean age of cases was 73 vs 71 in controls (p 0.000). Risk of SMC increases with age: 75 -79 OR=1.33 (p=0.001), 80 -84 OR= 1.28 (p=0.029) , 85 -89 OR = 1.86 (p=0.000) , 90- 94 O.R. = 1. 94 (p= 0.014) , over 95 O.R. = 3.66 (p=0.012). It is more frequent in women OR = 1.2 (p= 0.000) , and in less educated people: 1 to 6 years O.R. = 1.24 (p= 0.000) widowhood increases the risk: O.R. = 1.33 (p= 0.000), as does impaired sight O.R = 1.52 (p= 0.000), impaired hearing OR =3.1 (p=0.022), low self perception of health: OR=3.21 (p= 0.000) and depression, OR = 3.6 (p= 0.000). Conclusions : Aged, female gender, widowed and poorly educated people are at a higher risk of SMC. Depression , visual and hearing impairment, were associated as well with SMC.

[28] The factors associated with cognitive decline in the community-dwelling elderly Japanese.

M. Fujisawa, F. Ando, N. Niino, S. Tsuboi, Y. Fukukawa, C. Nakashima, and H. Shimokata (Department of Epidemiology, National Institute for Longevity Sciences, Obu, Japan)

PURPOSE: Cognitive decline is a serious problem among the elderly. The purpose of this study is to determine the factors associated with cognitive decline in the community-dwelling elderly Japanese. METHOD: The subjects were 307 Japanese men and women aged 60 to 79 years who participated in the NILS-LSA (National Institute for Longevity Sciences-Longitudinal Study of Aging). They were random samples from a community-dwelling population who were followed up 2 years. Blood pressure, blood chemistry (glucose, HbA1c, triglyceride, total cholesterol), body mass index (BMI), smoking history, and periventricular hyperintensity (PVH) on brain MRI were examined. Cognitive function was assessed by Mini-mental State Examination (MMSE). The subjects were divided into two groups according to change in cognition: cognition-declined group (MMSE score decreased 3 points or over during 2 years) and cognition-unchanged group. Each of the baseline data was classified into two categories and associations with change in cognitive function were analyzed. RESULTS: During two years, cognitive function declined in 26 subjects (mean age 68 years). There was no difference in mean age and gender distribution between cognition-declined group and cognition-unchanged group. The incidence of cognition decline in the group of baseline systolic blood pressure (SBP) >= 160mmHg was 23.5%, which was significantly higher than that in baseline SBP<160mmHg group (7.6%) (p<0.05). The incidence of the cognition decline was higher in moderate to severe PVH group (13.9%) than no to mild PVH group (p<0.1). CONCLUSION: High SBP may predict cognitive decline and PVH on MRI may also relate to cognitive decline.

[29] Clinical features and risk factors of institutionalization Alzheimer's Disease in a regional memory clinic in Hong Kong

KC Chiu (Division of Geriatric Medicine, University Department of Medicine, Queen Mary Hospital, the University of Hong Kong, Hong Kong SAR), LW Chu (Division of Geriatric Medicine, University Department of Medicine, Queen Mary Hospital, the University of Hong Kong, Hong Kong SAR), CP Chung (Division of Geriatric Medicine, University Department of Medicine, Queen Mary Hospital, the University of Hong Kong, Hong Kong SAR),

Wayne Hu (Division of Geriatric Medicine, University Department of Medicine, Queen Mary Hospital, the University of Hong Kong, Hong Kong SAR)

Introduction: Symptomatology of Alzheimer's Disease (AD) and risk factors of institutionalization have been widely reported in the Caucasian populations. Local data are lacking in Hong Kong. Objectives: To review the clinical features of Alzheimer's disease and examine factors associated with institutionalization. Design: A retrospective case series analysis Setting: A regional Memory Clinic in Queen Mary Hospital Methods: Case records of all consecutive patients attending the Queen Mary Hospital's Memory clinic from 1/1/1997 to 30/6/2000 were reviewed. All patients who had probable AD (i.e. AD) by NINCDS-ADRDA criteria were recruited. Demographic data, presenting symptom, cognitive and non-cognitive symptoms, vascular risk factors, cognitive assessment scores, functional status and place of residence were documented and analysed. Results: 96 AD patients were recruited. 72.9% were female. The mean age at first visit was 77.3 years (s.d.= 6.55 years). The interval between symptom onset and first visit was 3.1 years (s.d.=2.0 years). 90.60resented to the clinic because of poor short-term memory. History of getting lost was associated with disorientation in place, moderate to severe severity of dementia, history of wandering, and formal education. 83.3% had non-cognitive symptoms at clinical presentation. These included behavioural changes (59.4%), perceptual/ psychotic changes (51.0%), sleep (27.1%) and mood (24.0%) changes. Institutionalized AD was characterized by an older age at first visit, being widow, had atrial fibrillation, lower MMSE scores, more advanced stages of dementia, lower BADL and IADL scores, more unusual behaviours, poorer comprehension of language and more comorbidities. . Multivariate logistic regression analyses reviewed that marital status, the number of comorbidities and IADL scores were independent risk factors associated with institutionalization. The mean time from symptom onset to institutionalization was 36.8 months (s.d.=29.3 months). Conclusions: The clinical features of AD among Chinese elderly in a regional Memory Clinic in Hong Kong share many common features to those reported by Caucasian studies. Several risk factors were found to be associated with institutionalization in our AD patients.

[30] Cognitive impairment and survival in elderly people.

J.C. García, J.L. Torres, L.M. Gutiérrez-Robledo, A. Villa. (Geriatrics Clinic, National Institute of Medical Sciences and Nutrition, Mexico City)

PURPOSE. Determine the influence of cognitive impairment in the survival of elderly people. METHOD. We analyzed the data from elderly patients during the initial comprehensive geriatric assessment made from 1994 to 1999 in the outpatient and the inpatient setting of a tertiary care center. We measured the score in the mini-mental state examination and formed three groups: 1. Without cognitive impairment (MMSE 24-30); 2. mild cognitive impairment (MMSE 18-23); and 3. severe cognitive impairment (MMSE 0-17). We document survival from the charts in July 2000. The odds ratios, survival analysis and regression analysis were performed controlling variables such as demographic and associated diseases. RESULTS. 2351 patients were evaluated, 874(37.2%) male and 1477(62.8%) female patients. There were 1057(45%) deceased patients. In the group 1 were evaluated 1654(70.4%) patients with a median survival of 59.96 months; in the group 2: 415 (17.7%) patients with a median survival of 25.32 months, OR 1.96 CI 95% 1.58-2.44; and the group 3 with 282(12%) patients, median survival 14.76 months, OR 3.06 CI 95% 2.34-3.99. The functional status assessed through the Katz, Lawton; associated illnesses: ischaemic heart disease, cancer, pneumonia, liver disease and undernutrition were also related with mortality in the proportional hazard models, also being in the inpatient setting increase the risk Exp B 1.82 (CI 95% 1.55-2.13). The MMSE sustained its risk for mortality Exp B 1.29 (CI 95% 1.19-1.40) after adjusting for the variables in consideration. CONCLUSION. The findings support that even mild cognitive impairment is related with mortality in elderly people.

[31] Sensorial Disorders in Elderly Patients with Dementia and their Offspring

M.Covic, G.Prada, C.Ciucurel(Ana Aslan National Institute of Gerontology and Geriatrics, Bucharest, Romania), T.Covic (Carol Davila University of Medicine and Pharmacy, Bucharest, Romania)

The purpose of our study was to identify the characteristic sensorial disorders in elderly patients with vascular dementia and Alzheimer dementia, as well as in their offspring. We selected only elderly patients with offspring and presenting early forms of Alzheimer dementia and vascular dementia as diagnosed by DSM IV criteria and psychological tests. On all patients we also performed auditory, visual and olfactory tests. We divided the elderly subjects into two groups of 30 patients each: Alzheimer dementia group and vascular dementia group. We noticed the predominance of olfactory disorders in Alzheimer dementia group, and of visual and mainly auditory (100%) disorders in vascular dementia group. Analyzing the offspring of the two groups of elderly patients we noticed the presence of olfactory disorders in children of patients with Alzheimer disease as follows: 62 0.000000or unpleasant odors, 37 0.000000or pleasant scents, and 8 0.000000or odorless substances. The changes in olfactory perception were encountered only in offspring of Alzheimer dementia patients. This could be considered a predictive factor for the development of this type of dementia and could trigger early measures for the possible future patients.

[32] Management of Behavioural and Psychological Symptoms of Dementia: Utilisation of Spiritual and Religious Methods

Nilamadhab Kar, DPM, DNB; (Department of Psychiatry, Kasturba Medical College, Manipal, 576119, India ; and Geriatric Care and Research Organisation, 130, Ratnakar Bag, Bhubaneswar, 751002, India)

Abstract: Purpose: Behavioural and psychological symptoms constitute and essential component of dementia syndrome. The stress of the caregiver is increased by the behavioural disturbances and these are often the cause for which demented patients come in contact of psychiatric services for the first time. We intend to assess the behavioural and psychological symptoms of dementia (BPSD) and to find out the affect of religious and spiritual intervention in these symptoms especially agitation. Method: We assessed the behavioural and psychological symptoms of dementia in 50 patients using a semistructured questionnaire filled with the help of primary caregiver and the observation of the clinician. The appropriate medicinal, psychological and behavioural treatment methods were available for the BPSD to the patients. In addition the patients were encouraged to spend more time in religious activities at home and at religious places; and attending spiritual discourses relevant to their faith/ religion. Spending time and continuing the rituals were stressed more. Their BPSD were ascertained in the follow up and were compared with that of ones who did not use the spiritual and religious methods. Results: A significant proportion of dementia patients (n=32) , mostly ladies (n=21), reported utilizing the methods suggested for more time and with greater regularity. The activities included religious activities at home, attending temples/mosques/ churches, spending more time there, listening to religious discussions and spiritual discourses. It was found out that with clinical interventions both groups of patients improved. However the patients who practiced the religious rituals remained more calm and accepting; and less agitated, abusive and disruptive than before. Care givers' reported that they were more manageable, communicative and with good emotional responses. Caregivers of these patients were more in control, had less frustration, dejection and anger. Conclusion: Religious and spiritual activity may continue to have meaning in a person's life even in presence of gross cognitive deficits. The religious symbols and life long ideals may have lasting impressions on the behavior of the persons. These may be integrated to the management methods of BPSD in patients in late life.

[33] Elderly patients with depression and dementia - An outpatient geriatric unit in São Paulo, Brazil

E. L. Klein, Y. M. Garcia, R. M. R. Funari, T. D Gonçalves, C. Z.

Pereira, V. C. Aranha, L. L. Mansur, S. G. Rasquel, C. Amaral, E. M. S. Gonçalves (Disciplina de Geriatria Δ Medical School of São Paulo University, São Paulo, Brazil)

PURPOSE: Depressive and cognitive disorders are common diagnoses in geriatric practice that benefit from an interdisciplinary approach. This presentation describes a group that develops this concept in a controlled practice. METHODS: Patients attending to a short-term ambulatory from the discipline who had a diagnosis of depression or dementia are referred to this group, where an multidisciplinary team sees them. They are submitted to conventional assessment plus specific tests regarding those diagnoses, belong to both sexes and are elderly older than 60. Their evolution was reviewed after 6 months. RESULTS: 68 patients have been included up to now. After 6 months of follow-up, 56 patients had been seen, ages varying from 62 to 92 years, mean age=75.4. 27.3% were married, 54.5% widowers, 10.9% single and 5.4% divorced. Initial diagnosis was depression in 33 patients, dementia in 14, depression plus dementia in 7. In 12 patients first diagnosis was not correct, and in 4 depressed ones symptoms disappeared. There were 2 deaths, and 2 patients abandoned treatment. The inclusion of new patients on the following 2 months did not cause remarkable changes on results. CONCLUSIONS: Depression was the most frequent diagnosis; initial diagnosis was frequently modified after a more careful evaluation; a small number of depressed patients became asymptomatic in this short period of time, but the improvement of the demented ones was not so noticeable.

[34] Training staff to reduce agitation in the nursing home: A preliminary study

Philippe Landreville (Université Laval, Québec, Canada) Louise Dicaire (Hôpital Jeffery Hale, Québec, Canada) René Verreault (Université Laval, Québec, Canada) Louise Lévesque (Institut universitaire de gériatrie de Montréal, Montréal, Canada) Vital Bouchard (Hôpital de l'Enfant-Jésus, Québec, Canada)

Agitation is verbal, vocal, or motor activity that is inappropriate or disruptive. It includes non aggressive behaviors, such as wandering and repetitive questioning, as well as aggressive behaviors, such as swearing and hitting. Behavioral techniques aimed at modifying environmental antecedents and consequences have been shown to be effective in reducing agitated behaviors. We conducted a preliminary study of the impact of training nursing home staff to use a behavioral approach for managing agitation. All nursing staff (n=25) of all working shifts of a unit located in a large nursing home and the 21 residents of this unit participated in the study. Eleven residents (50%) had a diagnosis of dementia. Residents and staff were assessed before and after the two-month training program. The program emphasized the development of behavioral skills for the assessment, prevention, and reduction of both aggressive and non aggressive agitated behavior. It included eight hours of inservice training followed by eight hours of weekly supervision by the trainers. Complete data on both assessments were obtained for 960f staff and 900f residents. Results indicate a reduction in the number and frequency of agitated behaviors in residents following staff training. Moreover, staff members were more knowledgeable about behavioral approaches, used behavioral techniques to a greater extent and felt more effective in managing agitation after training. More than 900f staff members were satisfied with the training program. These findings suggest that staff training may be useful for reducing agitated behaviors in nursing home residents and justify further research in this area.

[35] Educational Level and Age influences in MMSE scores in the Elderly

P. Castro, Laks J , Munk M, Belusci LN, Hermolin MK, Pessanha M, Engelhardt E CDA/IPUB UFRJ e Casa Gcrontologica de Aeronáutica Brigadeiro Eduardo (CCABEG), RJ - Brasil

Objective: An evaluation of cognitive state of residents living in a nursing home and comparing the results by age and educational level . Materials and Methods: A sample of elders residents in CGABEG (n= 106) was evaluated using the Mini-Mental State Examination (MMSE, Folstein et al, 1975) by age groups: 65-84 years old and >85 years old and by educational level (illiterate , primary until 8 years of school, secondary/university: >8 years). A cut off for cognitive impairment defined according educational level (13 points to illiterate, 18 points to primary and 26 points to secondary/university). Results: The group 65-84 years old (n=70) has a score of 20.18± 8.76. The scores by educational level: Primary are 21.05±7.09 and Secondary/University are 19.26±10.15. The group >85 years old (n=36) has a score of 17.84± 7.88 and by educational level: Primary are 17.29± 8.30 and Secondary/university are 21.38± 6.98. There's no significant difference in total score results of this sample when we comparing them by age (t=1.34; p=0) as well comparing by educational level 65-84 years old, secondary/university and primary (t=0.84;p=0) and >85 years old, secondary/university and primary (t=0.55; p=0). Conclusion: In this sample of residents living in the CGABEG, the cognitive performances measured by MMSE doesn't show a progressive down related about educational level and age as others studies about that. Maybe these results are due to the special characteristics of this population like socio-cultural and educational level homogeneity .

[36] Implementation of a Regional Dementia Care Program

NORTH SHORE GEROPSYCHIATRIC INITIATIVES GROUP, NORTH VANCOUVER, B.C. CANADA

Purpose: The focus of this poster presentation is to provide information about the implementation and outcomes of a regional educational program designed for interdisciplinary caregivers using an abilities enhancing framework. The abilities enhancing framework provides direction for individualized care in congruence with the retained abilities of persons with dementia. The abilities assessment tool facilitates the identification of retained abilities in the ares of self-care, social, interpretive and interactional abilities. The north shore health region gero-psychiatric initiatives group (representatives of consumer and professional groups within the north shore health region) sponsored the program. Sponsorship included speaker and consultation fees, wage replacement costs of interdisciplinary staff, and a formal evaluation of the program. The education program initially targeted indisciplinary staff from the regional special care units and adults day programs. The professional staff attended a 2 day workshops, and non-professional staff attended a 1 day workshops. Each facility and adult day care center were utilized three-4 hour consultation sessions with the workshop presenter. This is an ongoing education program that continues to target indisciplinary staff throughout this region which includes community and residential services and acute care. For the purpose of this poster presentation, the focus will target the educational methods and outcomes of special care units and adult day programs.

[37] Rates of Cognitive Decline in Alzheimer's Disease and Lewy Body Variant

Edward Helmes (Edith Cowan University, Perth, Australia), John Bowler (Royal Free Hospital, London, England), Harold Merskey (University of Western Ontario, London, Canada), David Munoz, Vladimir Hachinski (University of Western Ontario, London, Canada)

More research has been directed recently to the Lewy body variant of dementia. We compare the rates of cognitive decline over time in three groups with dementia from the University of Western Ontario Dementia Study: Alzheimer's disease, Lewy body variant, and a group with both Alzheimer's disease and Lewy bodies. All diagnoses were verified by autopsy. Cognitive impairment was measured with the Extended Scale for Dementia (ESD). Members of each group with dementia were age- and sex-matched with individuals without dementia. The 15 cases of Alzheimer's disease, seven cases with Lewy bodies and eight cases with both conditions were all free of significant vascular disease. Linear regression was used to determine rate of change in ESD scores over time in months. The number of observations ranged from 4 to 18 over a period of 2 to 9 years. All three control groups showed regression lines that approximated horizontal lines, reflecting no change in cognitive status over time. As expected, all groups with dementia showed progressive cognitive impairment. Analysis of the slope parameter showed that all groups deteriorated at the same rate of approximately 2 ESD points per month. Results suggest that the final rate of cognitive decline in dementia may not necessarily reflect the underlying cause

[38] Agreement between patients' and proxies' reports of quality of life in Alzheimer's disease

JL.NOVELLA and C.JOCHUM and F.BLANCHARD(Department of Internal Medicine and Gerontology, hôpital Sébastopol Rheims, France) JOLLY D (Department of Medical Information, hôpital Maison Blanche, Rheims, France) MORRONE I (Department of reeducation, hôpital Sébastopol, Rheims, France) ANKRI J (hôpital Sainte Perine, Department of Gerontology, Paris, France)

Purpose: The study was an interrater reliability study in which the Health Related Quality of Life (HRQL) scores of elderly persons with Alzheimer's disease were compared with HRQL scores as provided by two different proxies. Method: Agreement between self reports and proxy reports of HRQL was examined in a sample of 76 patients with mild to moderate Alzheimer's disease and their proxies. Recruitment took place in hospitals and institutions in four French-speaking European countries (France, Belgium, Luxembourg and Switzerland). Patients and proxies completed an '17-item Duke health profile'. The items were rephrased for the proxy. Results: The proportion of exact agreement between patients and proxies on the 17 items ranged from 26.3% to 52.6%. Results reveal poor to moderate agreement (the intraclass correlation coefficient ICCs from 0.00 to 0.61 for 10 subscales) between patients' and proxies' reports. Agreement was higher for measures of function that are directly observable (physical health, disability) and relatively poor for more subjective measures. Proxy reliability varied according to the relationship of the proxy to the index subject. Spouses and nurses agreed more closely with index subjects than did children or nurses' aides. Agreement decreased with increasing severity of dementia. Statistically significant differences in mean scores were noted for several dimensions, with proxies tending to rate the patients as having a lower HRQL than the patients themselves. Conclusion: This study indicates the importance of considering the information source of patient's HRQL. However, for individual level assessments proxies should be used with caution.

[39] Measuring General Health Status in Dementia: practical and methodological issues in using the SF-36

JL. NOVELLA and C. JOCHUM and F. BLANCHARD (Department of Internal Medicine and Gerontology, hôpital Sébastopol Rheims, France) D.JOLLY(Department of Medical Information, hôpital Maison Blanche, Rheims, France) I. MORRONE(Department of reeducation hôpital Sébastopol, Rheims, France) J. ANKRI(Department of Gerontology, hôpital Sainte Perine, Paris, France)

Purpose: This study examines the measurement properties of the Medical Outcomes Study short form 36-item (SF-36) health status measure in a representative sample of dementia patients. Methods: A total of 138 subjects with dementia were evaluated with the SF-36. They were recruited from 16 European's centers, including 7 university hospital centers. Dementia severity, demographic variables, comorbidity and functional limitations were also measured. The measurements obtained were compared by source of information (patient, family proxy, and care-provider proxy). Results: Thirteen patients refused to complete the questionnaire. Help from the interviewer was necessary in 72,80f the cases. The average completion time was 18,8 min. Missing data exist on the average in only 5.60f the cases on average, except among patients with severe dementia (Mini Mental State Examination < 10). For reliability, internal consistency was acceptable (Cronbach's coefficient = 0.5 Δ 0.7) when the role emotional (0.45) and social functioning (0.49) measures were eliminated. Reproducibility as measured by test-retest scores was moderate to good (intraclass correlation coefficient: r = 0.51 Δ 0.81) except for role emotional (0.17), bodily pain (0.47) and mental health (0.45). The SF-36 has a good construct validity in our study. Intraclass correlation coefficient suggests that proxies are a poor substitute for capturing a patient's perspective of his/her health status. Conclusion: The SF-36 is unsuitable for severe dementia, because severity of disease mainly affected the feasibility, acceptability, and reproducibility of the instrument. But this study confirms that it is possible to question subjects with mild to moderate dementia on their health status.

[40] Identifying Cognitive Impairment in the Frail Elderly - the MMSE and the Clock Test

Smith GN (University of British Columbia, Vancouver, Canada), Hill AJ MD (University of British Columbia, Vancouver, Canada),

Purpose: A range of cognitive screening instruments are used for assessment of the elderly. The MMSE is the most widely reported however its sensitivity is questioned. Authors have adjusted cut-offs according to patient age and education to improve diagnostic accuracy. This study compares raw and adjusted scores of the MMSE with the Clock Test (Schulman et al, 1993) and with neuropsychological evaluation. Method: 83 participants (age =81+/- 7; range =65-93) attending a Geriatric Day Hospital referred for neuropsychological assessment. 5 live in facility, 41 with family or spouse and 37 alone. Diagnosis based on medical history and neuropsychological testing were Alzheimer's disease (AD) -35, vascular and mixed dementia (Va D) -24, Impaired but not dementia (InotD) -17, not cognitively impaired -7. Results: MMSE scored < 24 in 510f AD, 330f VaD, 60f InotD and 00f unimpaired individuals. 11 patients who scored >24 on the MMSE had severe memory loss (Clinical Dementia Rating=2). Age and education adjustments (Bravo et al.) did not improve the diagnostic accuracy - MMSE impaired in 400f AD, 330f VaD, 120f InotD. The Clock Test correlated with diagnosis of dementia better - impaired in 740f AD, 630f VaD,650f Inot D and 1 of the unimpaired patients. Conclusion: The MMSE failed to identify cognitive impairment in >500f our sample. Age and education adjustment did not increase the sensitivity of the MMSE. The Clock Test proved superior to MMSE but failed to identify >330f patients with dementia

[41] Correlates of caregivers' awareness of cognitive deficits in mild demented patients.

Alessandra Pezzini, Angelo Bianchetti, Tiziana Metitieri, Giovanna Cipriani, Giuseppe Bellelli (Geriatric Research Group, Brescia and Ancelle della Carità Hospital, Cremona, Italy) Marco Trabucchi (Geriatric Research Group, Brescia and University of Tor Vergata Roma; Italy)

Factors related to caregivers perception of the change in mental status of demented patients have not been extensively studied and might be influenced by several elements. In this study variables influencing awareness of cognitive symptoms among caregivers of mild dementia patients were examined in a group of 71 mild demented patients (&& 0.000000emales, mean age 74.2±8.7; mean MMSE 21.7±4.1) who were referred to our outpatients clinics in Italy. In a correlation analysis only MMSE, controlled association for category (FPC) and Digit Span Backwards were significantly correlated with caregivers' awareness of patients' cognitive deficits (p<0.01). Moreover, variables evaluating non cognitive symptoms, and functional status proved significantly correlated with caregivers' awareness of patients impairment in cognitive functions. In a multiple linear regression model, only behavioral symptoms, FPC and functional status result independently correlated with caregivers cognitive anosognosia. Anxiety and caregiver burden are independently related to caregivers cognitive anosognosia, also when patients; characteristics are included in the multivariate analysis (p<0.001). Our data indicate that cognitive symptoms are recognized by relatives only when they interfere with daily functions or modify the usual behavior of the patient. Moreover, psychological status of caregivers, and in particular anxiety and burden are independently related to caregivers cognitive anosognosia. Among caregivers; characteristics only psychological variables were correlated with recognition of patients cognitive deficits and not educational variables.

[42] Use of objective scales for assessing pain when the elderly patient is unable to communicate

Use of objective scales for assessing pain when the elderly patient is unable to communicate B. Verlhac, B. Dieudonne, B. Forette (Hopital Sainte Perine, Association Claude Bernard, 75016 Paris, France).

Assessing pain in the elderly patient becomes difficult or impossible when verbal communication is impaired. To overcome this, several objective scales have been developed. We looked for the specificities of three of them which seemed particularly adapted. The study was conducted for 6 months on 120 demented elderly patients hospitalized in a long-term care unit. Every patient showing any unusual manifestation which could be possibly related to some kind of pain was assessed with pain scales. We used 3 different objective pain scales that we describe: DOLOPLUS 2, ECPA and ECSP. Assessment was performed on 32 patients and, in 13 of them, revealed a pain that disappeared with analgesic treatment. In the 19 others cases, the unusual manifestations were sensitive to psychotropic treatment. In a control group of 40 matched patients who did not exhibit any unusual manifestations the scores were in the normal range for the three scales. Each scale had its own specificity: DOLOPLUS 2 was global and well-adapted to institutionalized patients, ECPA was well-suited to bed-ridden patients, ECSP was very easy to use for a rapid systematic screening. In conclusion: Each objective pain scale has its own specificity for pain assessment in each elderly patients who are unable to communicate.

[43] Cognitive Status in Elderly Hospitalized Subjects

M. Ponzetto, M. Molaschi, E. D'Agostino, D. Gangemi, F. Russo, P. Maina , F. Fabris (Medical and Surgical Department, University of Torino, Torino, ITALY)

PURPOSE: Aim of the study was to evaluate cognitive status and in-hospital mortality in elderly patient. METHOD: In 1745 elderly patients (971 men and 774 women), consecutively admitted to University Geriatric Ward in Torino (Italy), we considered age, gender, schooling, cognitive (SPMSQ) and functional (ADL) status, number of pathologies, length of hospital stay, in-hospital mortality. The study group was divided by gender and by level of cognitive impairment (moderate-severe: more than 4 errors on SPMSQ, mild: 1-4, no impairment: 0 errors). RESULTS: Subjects affected by moderate-severe cognitive impairment were older (80.7 ± 8.0 yr.) than patients with mild deterioration (79.5 ± 7.8 yr.) and patients without cognitive problems (75.3 ± 8.3 yr.) ($p<0.001$). In the entire study group and in men the prevalence of subjects who completed only primary school was higher among patients with moderate-severe cognitive impairment ($p<0.001$). In the total sample and in men, more subjects affected by moderate-severe cognitive deterioration were living with assistance before hospitalization ($p<0.001$). The prevalence of functional impairment was higher (70.9%) among patients with moderate-severe cognitive impairment ($p<0.001$), without gender differences. In-hospital mortality was higher (21.2%) among patients with moderate-severe cognitive deterioration ($p<0.001$), without sex differences. CONCLUSION: The evaluation of cognitive status in elderly patients allows to individuate frail subjects needing specific care plans.

[44] Does Mini Mental State Exam help differentiate normal versus demented patients with low grade scholarity?

M.M. Ventura (Serviço de Geriatria do Hospital do Servidor Público Estadual "Francisco Morato de Oliveira" - São Paulo - Brasil) A.C.P.Melo (Serviço de Neurologia do Hospital do Servidor Público Estadual "Francisco Morato de Oliveira" - São Paulo - Brasil)

Purpose: evaluate if is possible for the Mini Mental State Exam (MMSE) to diferentiate between normal and demented patientes with low grade scholarity. Methods: 64 patients with low grade scholarity in our Geriatric Unit were examined. They looked for our service because of memory problems. There were 49 women, 15 men. Mean age: 76.4 years (sd: 6.96). From these patients, 38 were diagnosed as having Alzheimer's disease (AD), 26 were non demented (nd) - normals, or were classified as mild cognitive impairment. To everyone, the MMSE was applied. Statistical Analysis: T tests for independent samples. Statistical significance is reached when p is less than 0.05. Results: Every item analysed showed statistical significance when comparing these two populations: MMSE total points ($p=0.01$); MMSE temporal orientation ($p=0.001$), MMSE spatial orientation ($p=0.01$), MMSE registration ($p=0.01$), MMSE attention ($p=0.01$), MMSE recall ($p=0.01$), MMSE language ($p=0.04$). Conclusion: MMSE could help us in differentiating between normal and demented patients with low grade scholarity.

[45] A Randomized Controlled Trial of Home Hospitalization Services for Elderly Patients with Dementia

D Salerno, N Aimonino Ricauda, V Tibaldi, D Amati, M Molaschi, F Fabris (Department of Medical and Surgical Disciplines. Geriatric Section. University of Turin)

PURPOSE: To assess the feasibility of home hospitalization for elderly patients with advanced dementia and a relevant degree of comorbidity - to identify benefits of this care setting compared with general medical care in reduction of the caregiver's stress and the requirement for long-term institutional care. METHOD: The study was conducted on 100 randomized patients with advanced dementia: 50 managed in a General Medical Ward (GMW) and 50 at home by Geriatric Home Hospitalization Service (GHHS) that provides at home diagnostic and therapeutic interventions which are usually made in hospital. GHHS team includes geriatricians, nurses, physiotherapists and social workers. Both groups were examined using the same protocol and were evaluated on admission and discharge. RESULTS: Demographic characteristics, comorbidity, duration of dementia, behavioural disturbances, nutritional, functional and cognitive status on admission were not different in the two groups. No significant differences between the two groups were observed on admission for the characteristics and the level of caregivers' stress. Mortality was not significantly different in the two settings of care. On discharge the use of antipsychotic drugs was significantly reduced in the GHHS patients. Only one patient of GHHS group was transferred in nursing home versus twenty of GMW group ($p < 0.001$). Caregivers' stress on discharge was significantly reduced only in the caregivers of GHHS patients ($p < 0.001$). CONCLUSION: GHHS is a feasible alternative to hospitalization in patients with advanced dementia and it reduces the requirement for long-term institutional care.

[46] Magnetoencephalographic characterization of the memory impairment in Alzheimer's disease.

F. Maestu, A. Frenandez-Lucas, C. Amo, T. Oriz-Alonso (Centro MEG Complutense, Madrid Spain) P.Gil Gregorio, A. Garnica, P. Lopez-Riquelme (Servicio de Geriatria, Hospital Clinicao San Carlos, Madrid, Spain)

PURPOSE: to characterize the magnetic brain activity of AD patients during a memory task. METHOD: We have done an study with MEG in three different groups. Patients with Alzheimer's disease (9), mild cognitive impairment (7) and control subjects (7). All have done a short-term memory task during and MEG recording. Two kind of stimuli were presented: a target and non target letters. RESULTS: Our preliminary results are as follow: the AD is the group with less number of dipoles on both hemispheres, showing the same amount of dipoles to the target than to the non-target stimuli. The next group in order of the number of dipoles were the mild cognitive impairment group. As the opposite than the AD, this group had less dipoles to the non-target than to the target stimuli. The control were the group which have got the higher quantity of dipoles and the maximum diferencies between target and non-target stimuli. CONCLUSIONS: This preliminary results could indicate a different pattern of magnetic activity in function of the cognitive impairment.

[47] Alzheimer's disease: Functional and cognitive decline associated with APOE polymorphism

Fariñas F, Gil P, Bullidos M.J, Sánchez-Guevara A, Valdivieso F, Ribera J.M. (Geriatrics Service; Hospital Clínico San Carlos. Madrid. Spain).

AIMS: To know the contribution of differents polymorphims of APOE gen (codificant region and promoter) described and risk factors to clinical features. METHODS: 145 patients were studied and divided in two groups: 1) Control group (n: 73; mean age: 87.8 +/- 10.1): without clinical symptoms of cognitive impairment. 2) Study group (n: 72; mean age: 83.9 +/- 10.7): every patient fulfilled the criteria of dementia according to DSM-IV and NINCDS-ADRDA with an age-at-onset < or = and without familiar aggregation. Cognitive assessment MMSE-Folstein and CAMCOG-CAMDEX were used. Develop stage was assigned by Functional Assessment Stage (FAST). We stabilised functional and cognitive impairment progression indexes from FAST/period of disease progression and CAMCOG decrease/period of disease progression. Polymorphisms -491, -427 and +113 and those from codificant region were analyzed by RFLP and DGCDE, previous PCR amplification. Statistical measurements include chi-square and regression logistic analysis. RESULTS: No relationship was found between APOE genotype and progression indexes of AD, but it was found with the age at onset of clinical symptoms. Genotype ApoE 4/4 is associated with an earlier onset (<75 years, 66.7%) and 3/3 with later onset (>75 years, 65.1%). No evidence of association between polymorphisms and type of onset and progression of AD was found. Polymorphism +113 was associated with later onset (>75 years, 72.7%). CONCLUSION: No strong relationship between the studied polymorphisms and clinical course and odds-ratios develop AD was found.

[48] Introduction to the Poster Symposium Highlighting the Canadian Study of Health and Aging

Ian McDowell (University of Ottawa, Ottawa, Canada), Joan Lindsay (Centre for Chronic Disease Prevention and Control, Health Canada, Ottawa, Canada) Background and Objectives of the Canadian Study of Health and Aging (CSHA). Ian McDowell (University of Ottawa, Ottawa, Canada) Study methods and data collected in the CSHA. Ian McDowell (University of Ottawa, Ottawa, Canada), Joan Lindsay (Centre for Chronic Disease Prevention and Control, Health Canada, Ottawa, Canada) Prevalence and incidence of dementia in the CSHA. Réjean Hébert (Université de Sherbrooke, Sherbrooke, Canada) Incidence of vascular dementia. J. Lindsay (Centre for Chronic Disease Prevention and Control, Health Canada, Ottawa, Canada), D. Laurin, R. Verreault (Université de Québec, Québec, Canada), R. Hébert (Université de Sherbrooke, Sherbrooke, Canada), B. Helliwell, G. Hill, I. McDowell(University of Ottawa, Ottawa, Canada) Risk factors for dementia of the Alzheimer type. Danielle Laurin, René Verreault (Université de Québec, Québec, Canada), J. Lindsay (Centre for Chronic Disease Prevention and Control, Health Canada, Ottawa, Canada), Éric Dewailly, Bruce J. Holub (Université de Québec, Québec, Canada) Omega-3 polyunsaturated fatty acids and dementia in elderly persons. Danielle Laurin, René Verreault (Université de Québec, Québec, Canada), Joan Lindsay (Centre for Chronic Disease Prevention and Control, Health Canada, Ottawa, Canada), Kathleen MacPherson, Kenneth Rockwood (Dalhousie University, Halifax, Canada) Physical activity and risk of dementia in elderly persons. Gerry Hill (Kingston, Ontario), Joan Lindsay (Centre for Chronic Disease Prevention and Control, Health Canada, Ottawa, Canada) The impact of dementia on the expectation of life of elderly Canadians. PD St. John, PR Montgomery, B Havens, (University of Manitoba, Winnipeg, Canada), E Kristjansson (University of Ottawa, Ottawa, Canada) Marital status and gender effects on mortality and institutionalisation. H. Payette, M.-J. Kergoat, B. Shatenstein, V. Boutier, S. Nadon (Institut universitaire de gériatrie de Montréal) Validity of self-reported height and weight estimates in cognitively-intact and impaired elderly individuals. Janet L. Ingles, John D. Fisk, Heather R. Merry, Kenneth Rockwood (Dalhousie University, Halifax) Dementia defined by neuropsychological test performance: predicting the outcomes. Holly Tuokko, Robert Frerichs (Centre on Aging, University of Victoria, Canada) Best methods for assessing neuropsychological change in cognitively intact older adults. N. Silverberg, H. Tuokko, R. Frerichs (Centre on Aging, University of Victoria, Canada) The clinical detection of cognitive impairment across normative data sets. R.E.Steenhuis & S. Schwartzberg (University of British Columbia, Vancouver, Canada) Neuropsychological performance in Canadian seniors with depression and cognitive dysfunction. Edward Helmes (Edith Cowan University, Perth, Australia), Truls Østbye (Duke University, Durham, NC, U.S.A.) Personality Change in Older Adults with Dementia from CSHA: Effects of Severity of Cognitive Impairment. A. Colantonio, P. Clarke (University of Toronto, Toronto, Canada) Characteristics of Elderly Community Dwelling Wheelchair Users: Results from the Canadian Study of Health and Aging. Elizabeth Sykes (University of Ottawa, Ottawa, Canada), Truls Østbye (Duke University, North Carolina, USA), Steinar Hunskaar (Norway) Predictors and incidence of urinary incontinence in elderly Canadians: a 5-year follow-up. Marie-Jeanne Kergoat, Bryna Shatenstein, Sylvie Nadon (Institut universitaire de gériatrie de Montréal) Nutritional aspects of the Canadian Study of Health and Aging: longitudinal study of dementia. Carole A Cohen, Angela Colantonio, Lee Vernich (University of Toronto, Toronto, Canada) Positive Aspects of Caregiving: Results from CSHA-2. A. Colantonio, A. Kositsky, C.Cohen (University of Toronto, Toronto, Canada) What support do caregivers of elderly want? Results from the Canadian Study of Health and Aging.

ISSUE: Detailed information on the epidemiology of dementia is required for evidence-based policy-making. The Canadian Study of Health and Aging (CSHA) is one of the largest epidemiologic studies of dementia; it began in 1991 and ran follow-up studies in 1996 and 2001. STRUCTURE: This suitee of posters describes the CSHA, its origins, the data collected, and provides an overview of the range of results obtained. CONTENT: The posters are clustered into 6 groups: (i) study origins, objectives and methods; (ii) core findings on prevalence, incidence and risk factors for dementia in Canada; (iii) the impact of dementia on people and on health services delivery; (iv) methodological issues in studying dementia; (v) findings on other health conditions, and (vi) caregiving. CONCLUSIONS/ ANTICIPATED OUTCOMES: More than 130 jopurnal articles have so far been published from this study, which has contributed not only to our understanding of dementia, but also more broadly to understanding the population health of elderly people. This poster presentation will offer a showcase of this important study in an international forum.

[49] Background and Objectives of the Canadian Study of Health and Aging (CSHA)

Ian McDowell (University of Ottawa, Ottawa, Canada), Joan Lindsay (Centre for Chronic Disease Prevention and Control, Health Canada, Ottawa, Canada)

PURPOSE: The Canadian Study of Health and Aging is a multicenter, population-based cohort study of dementia and other health topics. This poster will describe the origins and objectives of the study, and will give an overview of its design, organization and data collection methods, to provide an introductory background for the other posters in the series. METHODS: The CSHA has followed a representative population sample of 10,263 participants aged 65 or over. Field work began in 1991, and follow-up studies were undertaken in 1996 and 2001. CONCLUSION: The study has achieved broad objectives, and currently over 130 papers have been published to describe the results of the study.

[50] Study methods and data collected in the CSHA

Ian McDowell (University of Ottawa, Ottawa, Canada)

PURPOSE: This poster will provide a more detailed explanation of the study methods used in the three phases of CSHA. The study design will be described, indicating how the design reflected the study objectives. METHODS: The study drew representative samples of people aged 65 or over from the community and institutions across Canada. Thirty-six sampling areas were used in a stratified cluster design; sampling weights were developed to provide population estimates. The sample included 9,008 people aged 65 or over from the community, and 1,255 from institutions. Data collection included interviews and questionnaires, clinical and neuropsychological examinations, physical measurements and blood collection, and access to public records such as death certificates. RESULTS: The study results are being presented in the other posters in this series. CONCLUSION: The CSHA forms one of the leading epidemiological studies of dementia in the world.

[51] Prevalence and incidence of dementia in the CSHA

Ian McDowell (University of Ottawa, Ottawa, Canada), Joan Lindsay (Centre for Chronic Disease Prevention and Control, Health Canada, Ottawa, Canada)

PURPOSE: To summarize the prevalence and incidence of dementia, including Alzheimer's disease, in contemporary Canada. METHOD: Clinical and neuropsychological examinations were used in 1991 to identify prevalent cases of dementia, and again in 1996 to identify incident cases. Dementia was defined using the DSM-III-R criteria; Alzheimer's disease was defined clinically using the NINCDS-ADRDA criteria. RESULTS: Our prevalence estimates suggest that 8.0% of all Canadians aged 65 or over met criteria for dementia: a total of 252,600 people (95% CI = 244,500 - 260,700). These are roughly equally divided between the community and institutions; the female:male ratio is 2:1. The prevalence rises from 2.4% among those aged 65-74 years to 34.5% among those aged 85 or over. These estimates will be compared to those from other international studies. Incidence rates were estimated, based on the 1991 population, and included data on those who died between the first and second phases of the study. 960 incident cases were identified; the overall age-standardized incidence rates were 21.8 (women) and 19.1 (men) per thousand undemented persons per year. This translates into 60,150 new cases of dementia per year in Canada. The logarithm of the rates rises linearly with age, but suggests a slight slowing of growth in incidence in the highest age-groups. CONCLUSION: These rates lie toward the upper end of the range of incidence estimates found in other studies. Nonetheless, we calculate that several factors may have biased our estimates downward, suggesting that the incidence of dementia may be higher than many studies have reported.

[52] Risk Factors for Vascular Dementia

R. Hébert (Université de Sherbrooke, Sherbrooke, Canada), MF Dubois (Gerontology and Geriatrics Research Centre, Sherbrooke), J. Lindsay (Laboratory Centre for Disease Control, Health Canada, Ottawa), R. Verreault (Laval University, Québec), K. Rockwood (Dalhousie University, Halifax), G.Hill (Sisters of Charity of Ottawa Health Service Inc, Ottawa).

PURPOSE: Very few population-based studies have examined risk factors for Vascular Dementia (VaD) using incident cases. METHOD: The Canadian Study of Health and Aging identified 105 incident cases of VaD over the five-year period of follow-up. Cases were defined using the NINCDS-AIREN criteria. A total of 802 control subjects were also randomly selected from the same cohort. Exposure was determined using a risk factor questionnaire administered to the subject or a proxy at the beginning of the study. RESULTS: Significant risk factors were: age (OR=1.05), residing in rural area (1.86), living in an institution (2.22), diabetes (2.01), depression (2.44), stroke (6.15), hypertension for female only (2.19), heart problems for men only (2.34), taking aspirin (2.42), occupational exposure to pesticides or fertilisers (2.22). Protective factors were: eating shellfish (0.45), smoking cigars (0.20), and regular exercise for women only (0.45). There was no relationship with gender, education, and alcohol. CONCLUSION: The role of depression, pesticides, fertilisers and shellfish need to be further investigated. VaD as an adverse effect of aspirin raises concerns about this widely used medication in atherosclerotic patients.

[53] Risk Factors for Institutionalisation of Demented Subjects

Réjean Hébert, Marie-France Dubois (Institut universitaire de gériatrie de Sherbrooke), Christina Wolfson (McGill U, Montreal), Larry Chambers (McMaster University, Hamilton), Carol Cohen (University of Toronto)

PURPOSE: In Canada, half of people with dementia are living in institutions. Factors leading people to use this expensive resource should be identified in order to implement strategies for decreasing the need for admitting demented patients in an institution. METHOD: Informal caregivers of 326 demented elderly living in the community were interviewed at CSHA-1. The date of institutionalisation was obtained at CSHA-2, that is five years after the baseline interview. Survival analysis using clinical data from the demented subjects and data from the interview with their informal caregivers were carried out using Cox proportional hazard modelling to estimate the Hazard Ratio (HR). RESULTS: Over the five year period, 166 subjects (50.9%) were institutionalised. From the multivariate analysis, the factors significantly associated with institutionalisation were: type of dementia (Alzheimer's disease, HR: 1.87), level of disability (total impairment, HR=4.63), caregiver's age (HR=1.02), caregiver is someone other than spouse or child (HR=1.55), extreme caregiver's burden (HR=1.68). The caregiver's burden was associated with the demented subject's behavioural disturbance (r=0.63) and the caregiver's depressive mood (r=0.61). CONCLUSION: Screening caregivers for burden and depression and designing interventions to decrease the consequences of behavioural disturbance on the caregiver would be relevant avenues to explore to decrease institutionalisation of demented patients

[54] Incidence of vascular dementia

Réjean Hébert (Université de Sherbrooke, Sherbrooke, Canada)

PURPOSE: To describe the incidence of vascular dementia in Canada. METHODS: Vascular dementia was diagnosed, using Hachinski criteria (and other criteria, for purposes of comparison). Incidence rates were estimated, based on the 1991 population. Rates have been computed by age-group and sex and these will be compared to rates found in other countries. RESULTS: Particular attention will be paid to the interface between vascular dementia and Alzheimer's disease, as our understanding grows of the involvement of vascular factors in AD.

[55] Risk Factors for Dementia of the Alzheimer Type

J. Lindsay (Centre for Chronic Disease Prevention and Control, Health Canada, Ottawa, Canada), D. Laurin, R. Verreault (Université de Québec, Québec, Canada), R. Hébert (Université de Sherbrooke, Sherbrooke, Canada), B. Helliwell, G. Hill, I. McDowell(University of Ottawa, Ottawa, Canada).

PURPOSE: This poster covers the prospective analysis of risk factors for Alzheimer's disease (AD) based on the CSHA data. METHOD: Of 6,434 cognitively normal participants aged 65 or over in 1991 (CSHA-1), 4,615 were alive in 1996 and participated in CSHA-2. Their cognitive status was re-assessed in 1996 (CSHA-2) in a screening interview, followed by a clinical examination where appropriate. A case-control analysis was conducted, including 194 AD cases and 3,894 cognitively normal controls. RESULTS: Increasing age, fewer years of education and apolipoprotein E å4 were significantly associated with increased risk of AD. Use of non-steroidal anti-inflammatory drugs, wine, coffee and regular physical activity were associated with a reduced risk of AD. No statistically significant association was seen with family history of dementia, sex, history of depression, estrogen replacement therapy, head trauma, antiperspirant or antacid use, smoking, high blood pressure, heart disease or stroke. CONCLUSION: The protective associations we observed warrant further study. In particular, regular physical activity has the advantage of protecting against many other diseases, and is a modifiable behavior.

[56] Who Ages Successfully? Insights from the Canadian Study of Health and Aging

B. Kristjansson, I. McDowell, and R. Aylesworth (University of Ottawa, Ottawa, Canada), G. Gutman (Simon Fraser University, Vancouver, British Columbia)

PURPOSE: It is commonly assumed that as Canadians live longer there will be an increased social burden, since the elderly account for a large proportion of health care use. However, by no means all of those who survive to old age become sick; in fact many older people are active and healthy. Older people are a valuable resource for society; many work, help family, participate in sports, do crafts, and volunteer. A fuller understanding of those who grow old successfully may suggest ways to promote healthy aging. The Canadian Study of Health and Aging (CSHA) offers an excellent opportunity to study healthy, or successful, aging in a cohort of 10,250 elderly people.

[57] Omega-3 polyunsaturated fatty acids and dementia in elderly persons

Danielle Laurin, René Verreault (Laval University, Québec, Canada), J. Lindsay (Centre for Chronic Disease Prevention and Control, Health Canada, Ottawa, Canada), Éric Dewailly, Bruce J. Holub (University of Guelph, Canada)

PURPOSE: It has been suggested that ù-3 polyunsaturated fatty acids (PUFAs) could be involved in the preservation of the cognitive function. The main objective of this analysis is to determine the relationships between plasma concentrations of ù-3 PUFAs in the phospholipid fraction, and the risk of dementia in elderly persons using data from the Canadian Study of Health and Aging (CSHA). METHOD: Blood samples taken at baseline, from subjects that were clinically examined during both phases of CSHA were available for 174. Of these, 79 were initially with no cognitive impairment, 43 were diagnosed as having cognitive impairment-no dementia (CIND), and 42 with dementia. Among the 79 non-demented subjects, 27 were diagnosed at follow-up as having cognitive impairment or dementia. Two separate analyses were performed. RESULTS: No difference in relative concentrations of N-3 PUFAs was observed between controls, and both prevalent CIND and dementia cases. Unexpectedly, higher eicosapentaenoic acid concentrations were observed among incident cognitively impaired and dementia cases as compared to controls. Higher docosahexaenoic acid concentrations were found in subjects with dementia. CONCLUSION: The protective effect of ù-3 PUFAs on cognitive impairment or dementia is not confirmed by these results

[58] Physical Activity and Risk of Dementia in Elderly Persons

Danielle Laurin, René Verreault (Laval University, Québec, Canada), Joan Lindsay (Centre for Chronic Disease Prevention and Control, Health Canada, Ottawa, Canada), Kathleen MacPherson, Kenneth Rockwood (Dalhousie University, Halifax, Canada)

PURPOSE: Little attention has been paid to the identification of modifiable lifestyle habits for its prevention. The main objective of this analysis is to determine the association between physical activity and the risk of cognitive impairment and dementia in elderly persons, using data from the Canadian Study of Health and Aging (CSHA). METHOD: Physical activity was assessed at baseline by combining two questions from a risk factor questionnaire, regarding frequency and intensity of exercise for subjects who reported regular physical activity. RESULTS: Of the 6434 subjects presumed with no cognitive impairment, 4615 completed the 5-year follow-up. Among them, 3894 remained without cognitive impairment, 436 were diagnosed as having cognitive impairment-no dementia (CIND), and 285 with dementia. Significant trends for increased protection with greater physical activity were observed. Compared with no exercise, physical activity was associated with lower risks of cognitive impairment, Alzheimer's disease, and dementia. High levels of physical activity were associated with significant reduced risks of cognitive impairment (OR=0.58; 95% CI 0.41-0.83), Alzheimer's disease (OR=0.50; 95% CI 0.28-0.90), and dementia (OR=0.63; 95% CI 0.40-0.98). CONCLUSION: Regular physical activity could represent an important and potent protective factor for cognitive decline and dementia.

[59] The impact of dementia on the expectation of life of elderly Canadians

Gerry Hill (Kingston, Ontario), Joan Lindsay (Centre for Chronic Disease Prevention and Control, Health Canada, Ottawa, Canada)

PURPOSE: To determine the life expectancy, with and without dementia, for Canadians aged 65, and to estimate the effects of reducing or postponing the incidence of dementia, and of reducing the excess mortality of those with dementia. METHOD: A two-state model was used, with sex-age-specific incidence and mortality rates obtained from the CSHA. Life expectancies at age 65 were calculated for women and men separately, and for a combined cohort using the sex ratio at age 65. RESULTS: With current incidence and mortality rates a cohort of 1,000 Canadians aged 65 would experience 18,205 subsequent person-years of life: 16,837 without dementia and 1,368 with dementia. eliminating dementia completely would increase the total years lived to 20,338. Eliminating the mortality differential would produce the same increase in total years lived, but the years lived with dementia would increase to 3,501. Postponing the incidence of dementia by 5 years would increase the total years lived to 19,004, adding 1,317 to the years lived without dementia, and subtracting 518 from the years lived with dementia. CONCLUSION: The simple two-state model provides a convenient method of estimating the potential benefits of prevention and treatment of dementia.

[60] Marital Status and Gender Effects on Mortality and Institutionalisation

PD St. John, PR Montgomery, B Havens, (University of Manitoba, Winnipeg, Canada), E Kristjansson (University of Ottawa, Ottawa, Canada)

PURPOSE: Married persons have a lower mortality than persons who have never been married, divorced or separated. It is less clear if there are differences between men and women in this protective effect. OBJECTIVE: 1. To determine if marital status predicts mortality or institutionalisation in men and women. 2. To determine if these effects are independent of potential confounders. METHOD: Secondary analysis of the Canadian Study of Health and Aging, a longitudinal, population-based study conducted between 1991/2 to 1996/7. We used data from 8474 community-dwelling seniors in all Canadian provinces. Predictor variables were: marital status (never married, married/common-law, and divorced/widowed), gender, education, self-rated health (good, not good), score on the modified Mini-Mental state examination. Outcomes were nursing home placement, and death, Bivariable analyses were conducted and logistic regression models were constructed. Interactions between marital status and gender were sought. RESULTS: Never married and previously married persons were more likely to die or be institutionalised than married persons. This was true for both men and women. In multivariable models, marital status did not predict mortality in men or women. Married men were less likely to be institutionalised. Married women were not less likely to be institutionalised than never married or previously married women. CONCLUSION: Associations between marital status and mortality may be accounted for by other factors, such as education (or social class), and health status. Marital status appears to predict institutionalisation in men but not in women, even after accounting for the effect of age, education, and health status.

[61] Validity of self-reported height and weight estimates in cognitively-intact and impaired elderly individuals

H. Payette, M.-J. Kergoat, B. Shatenstein, V. Boutier, S. Nadon (Institut universitaire de gériatrie de Montréal)

PURPOSE: A high prevalence of undernutrition has been observed in the elderly, particularly in cognitively impaired or demented individuals. Self-reported height and weight were tested as simple and non-invasive methods to efficiently screen individuals at risk. METHOD: A subset of subjects (n=465) participating in CSHA-2, including cognitively intact and impaired individuals as well as demented subjects. Self-reported values of height and weight were compared to direct standard measurements using Pearson's correlation coefficients and linear regressions by cognitive status. Estimation bias was determined using paired Student t-tests. Sensitivity and specificity of body mass index (BMI) derived from self-reported data were calculated. RESULTS: Self-reported and measured weights were highly correlated (r>.90) in all three categories of cognitive status. A tendency to underestimate their weight was observed in cognitively impaired (r=.86) and demented (r=.85) subjects. A systematic overestimation of recalled height was observed, particularly among individuals of short stature. Self-reported BMI showed excellent sensitivity (>93%) in detecting underweight individuals in all three categories. CONCLUSION: Self-reported height and weight data can be obtained in normal and cognitively-impaired elderly persons as well as in mild or moderate cases of dementia and can be used as a valid tool to screen for risk of undernutrition.

[62] Dementia Defined by Neuropsychological Test Performance: Predicting the Outcomes

Janet L. Ingles, John D. Fisk, Heather R. Merry, Kenneth Rockwood (Dalhousie University, Halifax)

PURPOSE: To assess the predictive validity of different case definitions for cognitive impairment and dementia by comparing rates of adverse outcomes for five diagnostic groups: individuals who had neuropsychological test results indicating dementia without otherwise meeting dementia criteria (NPDementia), those who had a traditional dementia diagnosis (of mild and moderate-severe severity), those who had cognitive impairment but no dementia (CIND), and those who had no cognitive impairment (NCI). METHOD: The Canadian Study of Health and Aging is a prospective, cohort study of 10,263 randomly selected community- and institutional-dwelling persons aged 65 years or older. Our sample comprised 1659 of these participants who had completed a neuropsychological assessment. Participants were reassessed 5 years after the original study. RESULTS: Rates of institutionalization and death for those with NPDementia and CIND were significantly higher than those with NCI and less than those with mild (for death rates only) and moderate-severe dementia. Rates of progression to dementia were also increased in NPDementia and CIND groups, relative to the NCI group, and those in the NPDementia group were less likely than those in the CIND group to revert to a diagnosis of NCI at the 5-year follow-up. CONCLUSION: Individuals with NPDementia and CIND have substantially worse outcomes over five years than those with NCI, and the case definition of NPDementia identified individuals with a more stable form of cognitive impairment that is unlikely to resolve.

[63] Best methods for assessing neuropsychological change in cognitively intact older adults

Robert Frerichs, Holly Tuokko (Department of Psychology and Centre on Aging, University of Victoria, Canada)

PURPOSE: Serial neuropsychological assessments are becoming increasingly important for clinicians who are interested in detecting early cognitive changes. The purpose of this study was to examine the utility of several models for measuring normal cognitive change over a five year interval in a sample of 208 adults over age 65. METHOD: The models included a standard deviation (SD) method, the reliable change index (RCI), with and without correction for practice effects, and models based upon simple and multiple regression. Participants had completed a neuropsychological test battery and had been identified with No Cognitive Impairment (NCI) during consecutive waves of the Canadian Study of Health and Aging (CSHA). The neuropsychological test battery included measures of memory, language, abstraction, judgement, constructional abilities, and psychomotor processing speed. Participants' test-retest performances on each neuropsychological measure was categorized as deteriorated, not changed, or improved for each model. The models were also compared in terms of the width of the prediction interval. RESULTS: Although the SD method is typically used in clinical practice and yielded the narrowest prediction intervals, it was the least accurate for measuring cognitive change over time. The RCI method with correction for practice effects was as accurate as more sophisticated regression-based models. CONCLUSION: These findings highlight the importance of accounting for measurement unreliability as well as practice effects in the determination of cognitive change in older adults.

[64] The clinical detection of cognitive impairment across normative data sets

N. Silverberg, H. Tuokko, R. Frerichs (Department of Psychology and Centre on Aging, University of Victoria, Canada)

PURPOSE: An essential aspect of the decision-making process in any assessment of cognitive functioning is the selection of appropriate normative data sets for interpreting test results. The availability of normative data for older adults has increased over the last 15 years, but most data sets do not account for the effects of age, education, and gender. The purpose of this study was to examine the extent to which discrepancies arise when different sets of normative data are used to identify cognitive impairment in older adults. METHOD: The test scores values indicative of performances falling 1 and 2 standard deviations (SDs) below the mean for sets of published norms for a variety of neuropsychological measures were examined in comparison to a normative data set that adjusts for the effects of age, education and gender. RESULTS: In all cases, there was correspondence between the data sets with respect to the identification of very poor performances (i.e, -2 SD). However, a lack of correspondence between the adjusted and unadjusted normative data sets was frequently observed for scores falling 1 SD below the mean. Education level was the most important variable with respect to observed discrepancies. CONCLUSION: Although these findings are reassuring with respect to the identification of severe impairment, they raise concern about the utility of some normative data sets for the identification of mild cognitive impairment, especially for older adults with high levels of education.

[65] Neuropsychological performance in Canadian seniors with depression and cognitive dysfunction.

R.E.Steenhuis & S. Schwartzberg (University of British Columbia, Vancouver, Canada)

PURPOSE: Depression is thought to influence cognition, especially mental efficiency. METHOD: Seniors from the second phase of the Canadian Study of Health and Aging were examined. Participants (n=38) who received a consensus diagnosis of cognitive impairment not dementia (CIND) where depression was the presumed cause of the cognitive dysfunction were matched on demographic variables to seniors found to have 1) no cognitive impairment, 2) CIND considered related to conditions other than depression, and 3) dementia. RESULTS: Neuropsychological test performance for persons with CIND and depression fell significantly below (p<.05) that of persons without cognitive impairment for sustained attention, memory, oral fluency, conceptual thinking and visuoconstruction. Neuropsychological test performance did not differ on any measure for persons with CIND and depression and those with other causes of CIND. Participants with CIND and depression had higher scores than those with dementia for orientation, memory, naming, oral fluency and language comprehension. CONCLUSION: The findings showed the pattern of cognitive dysfunction differed when comparing seniors with CIND and depression to those with dementia and to those without cognitive impairment. However, there was no unique pattern of cognitive dysfunction differentiating CIND where depression was the presumed cause from CIND associated other etiologies.

[66] Personality Change in Older Adults with Dementia from CSHA: Effects of Severity of Cognitive Impairment

Edward Helmes (Edith Cowan University, Perth, Australia), Truls Østbye (Duke University, Durham, NC, U.S.A.)

PURPOSE: Personality change is frequently described in dementia, and is one of the criteria for dementia in some diagnostic systems. Changes in personality do, however, also occur as part of the normal aging process. METHOD: We address whether the occurrence of personality change is a linear function or an inverted U-shaped function of the severity of cognitive impairment in a sample of 1132 older people with dementia from the Canadian Study of Health and Aging. A group of 921 older people from the same study, without cognitive impairment, provided a comparison of the frequency of personality change without dementia. In the consensus diagnosis of personality change, CAMDEX summary rating, seven CAMDEX variables from a knowledgeable informant and 6 Behavior Rating Scales were used to evaluate personality change. Rates of personality change were compared across measures, and all indices showed more extensive change in the group with dementia than in the cognitively unimpaired group. RESULTS: The least difference was shown on the Rating Scale measure of Impulsivity; the greatest difference was shown for Reaction to Encouragement. CONCLUSION: There was greater evidence of a linear increase in the frequency of personality change with increasing cognitive impairment than for an inverted-U function.

[67] Positive Aspects of Caregiving: Results from CSHA-2

Carole A Cohen, Angela Colantonio, Lee Vernich (University of Toronto, Toronto, Canada)

PURPOSE: Researchers have begun to explore the positive aspects ofcaring and how they relate to the negative consequences of caring such asburden and depression. The purpose of this study was to examine the positiveaspects in a national sample of caregivers derived from the Canadian Studyof Aging-2. METHOD: This study used a sample of caregivers derived from the Canadian Study of Health and Aging (part 2) to identify positive aspects of caregiving and examine how they determine caregiver outcome. Two hundred and eighty-nine caregivers caring for seniors living in the community were questioned about their caregiving experience. They were asked if they could identify any positive aspects related to their role and the number of positive aspects. A stage stepwise multiple regression approach was used factoring background/ contextual variables, stressor variables (3 MS score, ADL limitations) mediator variables (positive aspects of caregiving, number of services used) and outcome variables (depression as measured by CES-D score, burden and self-assessed health measures). RESULTS: Two hundred and eleven caregivers (73%) could identify at least one specific aspect of caregiving. An additional 20 (6.9%) could identify more than one positive aspect. Positive aspects of caregiving determined a significant proportion of the outcome variables: CES-D score ($p<0.01$), burden score ($p<0.001$) and self assessed health ($p<0.001$). CONCLUSION: The authors suggest that clinicians should inquire about the positive aspects of caregiving if they are to fully understand the caregiver experience and identify risk factors for negative caregiver outcomes in those caregivers who cannot identify any positive aspects of caring.

[68] Predictors and Incidence of Urinary Incontinence in Elderly Canadians: A 5 Year Follow-up

Elizabeth Sykes (University of Ottawa, Ottawa, Canada), Truls Østbye (Duke University, North Carolina, USA), Steinar Hunskaar (Norway)

PURPOSE: Urinary incontinence is more than a physical problem. It has widespread psychological and social effects, such as isolation, feelings of loneliness and disturbed relationships with friends and relatives. It also increases the demand for nursing and home services. METHOD: Cross sectional analyses of data from CSHA-1 reported baseline prevalence of incontinence as well as cross sectional correlates of incontinence at baseline. We analyzed CSHA-2 data to document the risk, among those elderly who were continent at baseline, of developing incontinence within a five year period, and to determine the importance of sociodemographic and medical factors and cognitive and functional status as predictors of the development of urinary incontinence. RESULTS: The incidence of urinary incontinence increases by age in both men and women. Incontinence increases dramatically with severity of dementia, less so with physical immobility. Diabetes mellitus was related to development of incontinence in men but not in women; prior stroke was related to development of incontinence in both sexes.

[69] Nutritional aspects of the Canadian Study of Health and Aging: longitudinal study of dementia.

Marie-Jeanne Kergoat, Bryna Shatenstein, Sylvie Nadon (Institut universitaire de gériatrie de Montréal)

PURPOSE: Description of anthropometric parameters in an elderly population, examining their evolution during aging and in light of cognitive deficits, and identification of predictors of nutritional risk. METHOD: We conducted secondary analyses on anthropometric data in community and institution subsamples of CSHA1 and 2 participants. Height and weight were measured in 1464 community participants and among 963 in institutions. Variables with nutritional interest included weight loss, appetite, eating autonomy, difficulty in meal preparation, perception of health status, daily activities of living, depression, and sociodemographic variables. Nutritional risk was defined by 3 categories of weight loss. Separate analyses were conducted for community and institutional participants, producing univariate, bivariate (unpaired t-tests, chi2 tests, ANOVA, MANOVA) and multivariate analyses (multiple linear and logistic regression). RESULTS: Both weight and height were lower in institutional compared to community-dwelling participants, and in women and among the oldest subjects. These parameters decreased further as severity of cognitive disorders increased. Average weight loss over 5 years was 2 kg in both groups; height decreased by 2 cm in institutional participants and 1.4 cm in the community-dwelling. In institutions, predictors of weight loss were increasing frailty, measured on a 7-point scale ($\beta=-1.23$, $p=0.04$) and difficulty eating alone ($\beta=4.24$, $p<0.001$). In the community, weight loss was predicted by a stated loss of interest in life ($\beta=4.24$, $p<0.001$). CONCLUSION: Body weight and stature declined with aging in elderly Canadians participating in the CSHA, particularly among the very elderly and those suffering from Alzheimer's dementia. Several predictors of nutritional status as determined by anthropometric indicators could benefit from (therapeutic) interventions.

[70] Characteristics of Elderly Community Dwelling Wheelchair Users: Results from the Canadian Study of Health and Aging.

A. Colantonio, P. Clarke (University of Toronto, Toronto, Canada)

PURPOSE: Few studies have profiled elderly wheelchair users based on data from representative national samples of elderly. METHOD: This paper describes sociodemographic, health and function characteristics of wheelchair users using data from the second wave of the Canadian Study of Health and Aging (n=5389) where approximately 5% of the community living participants reported using a wheelchair. We performed ANOVAs and chi square analyses to describe the characteristics of wheelchair users in relation to those who did not use wheelchairs in the community. RESULTS: Our findings showed that wheelchair users were more likely to be older, female, and unmarried ($p<0.001$). They were more dependent in all activities of daily living and had a significantly higher number of chronic health conditions ($p<0.001$). A large proportion (70%) reported having arthritis and 20% reported having a stroke or the effects of stroke in the last year. We also report on the prevalence of other chronic conditions and functional limitations in this population. CONCLUSION: The implications of these findings in relation to the provision and design of assistive technology for the elderly in the future are discussed.

[71] What Support Do Caregivers of Elderly Want? Results from the Canadian Study of Health and Aging

A. Colantonio, A. Kositsky, C.Cohen (University of Toronto, Toronto, Canada)

PURPOSE: This study concerns support strategies among caregivers of elderly persons. METHOD: We used data from the Canadian Study of Health and Aging caregiver questionnaire which included 43 informal caregivers of elderly persons living with dementia and 145 informal caregivers of elderly persons not living with dementia. Outcome variables included interest in attending support groups, receiving telephone support from either a professional or a fellow caregiver, receiving a newsletter, volunteer support, and support via computer. RESULTS: There were no significant differences between the two groups with regard to interest in any of the support services. There was substantial interest in receiving telephone support by a professional and fellow caregiver (44.9% and 41.0% respectively) and 44.2% of the dementia caregivers expressed interest in receiving a newsletter. Relatively less interest was displayed for support groups (10.4%), volunteer help in caring for the care-recipient (24.2%), and computer support (16.7%). CONCLUSION: Implications for program delivery are discussed.

[72] Psychiatric steroid related complications in elderly patients with temporal arteritis

AL Fauchais V Boivin E Hachulla ph U Pasturel M Lambert V Queyrel PY Hatron B Devulder PhMD Internal medicine Department, University Hospital of Lille, France

Purpose : to analyse psychiatric related complications in aged (>65 years old) with temporal arteritis Method : retrospective cohort study Results : in a cohort of 126 elderly patients with a diagnosis of TA and followed with a mean period of 64 month, clinical and biological manifestations, outcome and corticoïd adverse effects were recorded throughout the follow=up period. Twenty patients (16%) (mean age 73 +/- 7.9 years, male n = 6) exhibited corticoid related psychiatric complications. Symptoms appear to be dose dependant and generally begin during the first month of treatment. psychiatric disorders were as follow : mood disturbances (n = 8), depression (n = 6), mania (n = 3), anxiety neurosis (n = 2) and dementia (n = 1). Three patients were hostitalized in psychiatric units and 2 in nursing home. Psychiatric adverse affects appears to be more frequent with prednisone than prednisolone (p<0.05). In conclusion, steroid psychiatric related complications in elderly are frequent and exposed this group of patients to disability and dependancy.

[73] Aging and predictive reasoning: The influence of personal variables in the performance of older adults.

Castaneda, Sanchez, Quintana, and Gonzalez. (Facultad de Psicologia, Universidad de la Laguna, La Laguna, Tenerife, Spain)

The influence of personal variables on the performance of older adults in predictive reasoning with stereotyped contents was analysed. Our specific aims were to know: a) if there were gender differences in sensitivity to masculine and feminine stereotyped contents; b) the relative strength of gender-stereotyped contents in relation to the task data; and c) the type of verbal explanations given for categorical choices. Personal context variables such as motivation, self-capacity and familiarity with the task were taken into account. The sample included 43 participants over 65 years old. The task varied in the content of the base rate information (masculine and feminine stereotypes) and in the congruence or incongruence of the individuating data. Base rate choices, confidence scores and explanations of the choices were registered. Results indicated that older adults were able to build one-dimensional models with both types of content, which varied under congruence/incongruence between sources of information, as well as in rationales for the different choices, in the same way as children and adults in previous research but with a greater influence of personal variables in the participants' performance levels. The stereotyped content was not important in predicting an outcome. The main conclusion is that older adults have a similar pattern of cognitive performance with predictive reasoning tasks when compared with other age-groups. They update and integrate all the information into a plausible model of the problem but more in relation to personal contextual variables than from a pattern determined by biological aging of cognitive functioning.

[74] Psychosocial Correlates of Reminiscence Functions in African and Caucasian American Adults

Michele L. Norman (The University of Memphis, Memphis, USA)
Joyce L. Harris (The University of Memphis, Memphis, USA)
Jeffrey Dean Webster (Langara College, Vancouver, Canada)

PURPOSE: Very little is known about the interrelationships among aging, culture, and cognition (e.g, Park, Nisbett, & Hedden, 1999) particularly when the cognitive dimension under consideration is reminiscence (e.g, Webster, 2001). Merriam's (1993) study is the only published report we are aware of, and she found that African Americans scored higher than Caucasians on reminiscence dimensions related to understanding themselves and passing on life lessons to others. METHOD: In this study, we extend and elaborate on Merriam's work by investigating differences in reminiscence functions, family memory dynamics, and generativity in African American and Caucasian adults (N = 33). Participants ranged in age from 18 to 75 (M age = 43.5) and completed the (1) Reminiscence Functions Scale (RFS), (2) the Family Memories Index (FMI), and (3) the Loyola Generativity Scale (LGS). RESULTS: Results indicated that (a) African Americans scored higher on the total RFS ($t = 2.64$, $p < .05$) and on the specific factors of Identity, Intimacy Maintenance, and Teach/Inform; (b) African Americans scored higher on the LGS ($t = 2.03$, $p < .05$); and (c) the RFS factor of Bitterness Revival negatively correlated with both the FMI ($r = -.435$) and the LGS ($r = -.395$) and the RFS factor of Teach/Inform was positively correlated with the LGS ($r = .436$). CONCLUSION: Results indicate that cultural variables, such as a strong oral tradition, may influence the expression of individual memories consistent with certain ethnic/racial values and goals which has implications for both theories of reminiscence and clinical applications.

[75] Age Differences in Level and Intraindividual Variability of Perceived Competence and Control

Judith Levy-Bencheton, David F. Hultsch, Michael A. Hunter, and Esther Strauss [University of Victoria, Victoria, British Columbia, Canada]

Theorists have suggested that beliefs about competence and control are important mediators of performance and well-being in a variety of domains. These beliefs can be examined both globally and with reference to a particular domain (e.g, memory). It has also been suggested that short-term variability in beliefs may be as important as absolute level of perceived competence and control. We examined level and intraindividual variability of both global perceptions of competence and control and specific beliefs with regard to memory functioning. Participants consisted younger (n = 20; 20-33 years) and older (n = 33; 70-84 years) adults tested weekly over 10 occasions. At each occasion, participants were administered a beliefs questionnaire before and after a series of cognitive tasks. In the case of global beliefs, the younger participants showed greater internal locus of control than the older adults. Within the memory domain, the older adults had a more positive view of their present ability and expected less inevitable decrement than the younger individuals. Intraindividual variability results indicated that the younger participants were more variable on both global locus of control and potential improvement across the 10 weeks. Memory- specific beliefs were influenced by exposure to the cognitive testing across a given session. Older participants declined more than the younger participants in both competence and ability. The younger participants showed a greater decline in inevitable decrement than the older individuals. The results suggest that older adults may have more stable and differentiated beliefs about competence and control, particularly with respect to memory functioning, than younger adults.

[76] Determinants of self perception in the elderly

José Luis Vega Vega (Department of Developmental and Educational Psychology, University of Salamanca, Spain), Belén Bueno Martínez (Department of Developmental and Educational Psychology, University of Salamanca, Spain) and Placidia Franco Suarez-Barcena (Department of Developmental and Educational Psychology, University of Salamanca, Spain)

In March of 1999 it was carried out a study of the people over 60 years of age in the city of Salamanca. It was selected a sample of 501 elderly people (294 women and 207 men). The sample was stratified by sex and age on the base of the census of the city of Salamanca. One the objectives of the study was to know the factors upon which depends the positive and negative shelf perceptions. A broad interview was carried out collecting sociodemographic data and data about health, ADLs, caring and other basic needs, social network and support, evaluation of social services, educational and social activities carried out by elderly and, as well, information about attitudes, image and values. Of the whole population of the city of Salamanca (160.000 inhabitants) 23.5% have more than 60 years, 7.93% have more than 75 years and 4.4% have more than 80 years. The results reflect that the positive self perceptions are observed more frequently than the negative ones. The people over 60 years are more frequent to perceive themselves as amusing (65%) and less frequent to perceive themselves as inactive (26%), sick (27%), sad (25%) and annoying (10%). The women and the people of advanced age (over 75 years) and those with the lowest educational level have more negative self perceptions. Significant statistical differences in self perceptions were also found, on one hand, in function the ADL level, the perceived state of health and the illnesses they suffer and, on the other hand, in function of the social network and the social support that they receive.

[77] Structured Reminiscence and Gestalt Life Review: Group Treatment of Older Adults for Late Life Adjustment

Steven D. Koffman, Assistant Pofessor of Clinical Psychology Department of Psychology Eastern Washington University Cheney, WA 99004 USA

Professionals in gerontology often promote reminiscence because they believe that it is a "good thing" for old people to tell their stories and to be listened to. Anecdotal dynamics have come to be associated with this process such as developing acceptance, a sense of serenity, ego integrity. It is appropriate to wonder about the significance of the life review process on quantifiable aspects of psychological well-being. The integration with the structured reminiscence model of Gestalt and other process-experiential techniques has strong theoretical support but lacks clinical trial and empirical support. Outcome evidence measuring the effectiveness of two psychological group interventions, the Structured Reminiscence (SR) and Gestalt Life Review (GLR), is essential to determine the actual value of treatment by these models. A randomized trial of the two interventions, with pre and post measures, was undertaken. Participants (N=36, mean age = 72.6 years) were assigned to one of three treatment levels: SR and GLR groups which met concurrently for an eight week period and a Wait List Control (WLC) condition. Although neither of the two treatments had a statistically significant effect on "trait-related" variables, evidence of a trend emerged suggesting that participants in the GLR group showed significant improvement ($p < .05$) on five "state-related" variables of symptom report: depression, somatization, hostility, interpersonal sensitivity, positive symptom report. This contrasted with those in both the SR and WLC conditions for whom no changes were shown.

[78] The Importance & Role of Elderly People' Stress Confronting Resources / Capabilities

Adelina Bojan (Ana Aslan National Institute for Gerontology and Geriatrics, Bucharest, Romania)

The purpose of this study, carried out on a group of 143 elderly Romanian people (with an average age of 68), is to analyze the role of the resources / capabilities variables (Coping Resources Inventory, Hammer, A.L. & M.S. Marting) within the adaptive equation individual-situation according to the transactional pattern of stress: the results of the study prove that it is the cognitive resources that contribute to maintaining a positive self-image , having beneficial effects on the efficiency of the social integration through a correct evaluation of the intensity and consequences of the stressing events. The cognitive resources are highly appreciated by the elderly studied (even a little exaggerated in self-evaluation). They are perceived as the main capabilities on which the elderly rely in confronting psychotraumatizing events. The elderly studied associate the cognitive resources mainly with the social and physical resources, less with the emotional ones, and not at all with the spiritual Δ philosophical ones. The physical resources are also highly appreciated, though being realistically evaluated as less representative.

[79] Reminniscence Training and Activity Programmes for Informal Carers: A Cross-Country Study of Effectivess

PAM SCHWEITZER (AGE EXCHANGE, LONDON, UK)

The purpose of the study was to pilot reminniscence training and activity programmes with small groups of informal carers in 10 different European countries, to share results and to test the effectiveness of this particular intervention in improving understanding, ability to cope and quality fo communication of people with demnentia and those who care for them. Three underlying objectives were: 1) to maximise remaining intact memory (often long term) of people with dementia and provide opportunities for them to succeed. 2) to create opportunities for pleasurable reminiscence work in groups made up of people with dementia and their family carers. 3) to promote positive attitudes to dementia care based on valuing, listening to and involving the individual as fully as possible. Weekly meetings of carers and people with dementia (sometimes together and sometimes in separate spaces) developed friendships and understanding through arts-based reminiscence activities. We used before and after testing through several questionnaires against a randomised control group. The results showed an improvement in self perception on the part of people with dementia and a reduction ion relative stress. The conclusion was that families benefitted greatly from the meetings and developed new ways of coping with dementia at home. The international pppilot project was very thoroughly documented and then disseminated in the form of an illustrated user-friendly manual for carers, now available from Age Exchange in the UK.

[80] Meaning of illness and coping strategies among cancer patients

T. Huard, F. Lavallée, J. Baillargeon (Université du Québec à Trois-Rivières, Trois-Rivières, Québec, Canada)

It has been demonstrated that when exposed to a stressful event such as a disease, certain individuals adopt a more efficient coping profile than others to diminish anxiety and depressive symptoms. It was also demonstrated that the way the individual evaluates the stressful situation has an important influence on his/her coping profile. The objective of the present research was to verify if the personal meaning attributed by cancer patients to their illness could be associated with some specific soping strategies. The sample includes 52 women and 18 men (mean age = 64 years) with a diagnostic of cancer. They were met individually to complete a French adaptation of the Ways of Coping-Cancer and to identify and classify according to their importance for them a list of 8 categories of illness meaning. The results indicated that 3 of the 8 categories of meaning were associated with the use of different coping strategies. People who see their illness as a strategy were using significantly more often the social support strategy. Those who see their illness as value were using social support and focusing on the positive strategies. Finally, participants who consider their illness as a loss were using the cognitive escape avoidance strategy. These findings should help the health care personnel a better understanding of the cognitive and behavioral processes that diminish the distress among patients dealing with cancer.

[81] Intraindividual Change in Extraversion and Neuroticism in Old Age

Ilka Lißmann (Free University Berlin), Jacqui Smith (Max Planck Institute of Human Development, Berlin) & Paul B. Baltes (Max Planck Institute of Human Development, Berlin)

Purpose. The proposed study addresses changes in personality in old age. Intraindividual change in two personality dimensions is examined: "neuroticism", and "extraversion". Previous cross-sectional research suggests that these two dimensions show mean level negative age differences from 20 to 60 years. Whether these trends continue in very old age or not is an open question. Hypotheses. In addition to an expected increase in neuroticism and decrease in extraversion over time, it is hypothesized that age will be a significant covariate of the trajectories of neuroticism and extraversion. Method. Three waves of longitudinal data on neuroticism and extraversion from the Berlin Aging Study (BASE) are analysed. The BASE sample initially consisted of N=516 persons (aged 70-103 years, stratified by age and gender). N=206 individuals participated in a second assessment four years later, and N=132 in a third measurement point six years later. Sample attrition was primarily due to mortality. Neuroticism and extraversion were assessed on all occasions with selected items from the NEO (Costa & McCrae, 1985a). Individual growth curve modeling are used to examine hypotheses about trajectories of change over a six-year period of old age. Results. Initial results indicate that neuroticism increases over six years and extraversion decreases over six years. Age is a significant covariate. Conclusion. There are intraindividual changes in personality over time in old age.

[82] The use of engagement and disengagement coping strategies among older adults.

Dalton, C.L, Chaikelson, J, Conway, M, Basevitz, P, & Pushkar, D (Center for Research in Human Development, Concordia University, Montreal, Canada)

Research generally suggests that the use of disengagement coping strategies is associated with negative consequences. Some researchers, however, have suggested that disengagement may lead to positive consequences under some circumstances. This may occur when disengagement strategies are used in combination with other coping strategies. This hypothesis, however, has not been tested. The purpose of the present study was to determine if the use of disengagement strategies is associated with positive motivational, belief and affective consequences when used in combination with engagement strategies. The sample consisted of 150 community-dwelling seniors aged 65+ who completed questionnaires assessing dispositional coping style, desire for control, beliefs of control and affect. Using median splits, older adults were classified into four coping groups based on the tendency to engage or disengage from coping situations: 1) high engagement and low disengagement 2) high engagement and high disengagement, 3) low engagement and low disengagement, and 4) low engagement and high disengagement. Results from Manova showed that higher levels of engagement strategies were related to more positive consequences, including high desire for control, high levels of perceived control, and low levels of negative affect, regardless of the use of disengagement strategies. Higher levels of disengagement strategies, in contrast, were associated with more negative consequences if accompanied by low levels of engagement. On the other hand, higher levels of disengagement strategies were associated with more positive consequences if accompanied by high levels of engagement. These results underline the importance of considering the use of different coping strategies in combination.

[83] Need related Personality Characteristics of Indian Elderly Women

Reeta Kumar (Dept. of Psychology, Banaras Hindu University, Varanasi, INDIA) Aradhana Srivastava (Agrasen Kanya P.G. College, Varanasi, India) Manju Devi(Govt. College, Gyanpur, India)

Need related personality characteristics of elderly women , who have either been or are still in teaching profession and homemakers of same age, have been explored. It is a cross-sectional study designed to assess the effects of Age (2 levels) and professional status (2 levels) and their interaction effects, if any. The sample consisted of 60 women in teaching profession (TP) and 60 home makers (HM). Each of these sub group included 30 Ss in Age range of 50-60 yrs. (Yo) and 30 aging 60 years (Oo). Significant of Age Oo scoring higher than Yo women was found for n-O order, n- Abasement and n-Affiliation and with Oo scoring lower than Yo on n-Heterosexuality. Significant of professional status was obtained for n-Abasement with HM scoring lower than TP women at both Age levels. Interaction effects could be observed for n-Achievement, n-Exhibition and n-Deference with TP scoring higher and younger age level but lower at older age than HM. None of the effects were significant for n-Intraception, n-Succorance, n-Dominance, n-Nurturance, n- Change, n-Endourance, n-Aggression. Implications of the results have been discussed in context to Indian sociocultural setting.

[84] The personality traits of Japanese centenarians: Evaluation by the family

Y. Gondo, H. Inagaki, Y. Masui (Tokyo Metropolitan Institute of Gerontology, Tokyo, Japan), K. Kitagawa (Komazawa University, Tokyo, Japan), N. Hirose, Y. Arai, M. Takayama, Y. Ebihara, K. Yamamura, S. Nakazawa (Keio University, Tokyo, Japan), K. Yamashita, H. Shimomura, K. Nishikawa, Y. Lau (Keio Junior college of Nursing, Tokyo, Japan).

PURPOSE: Recently, along with the expanding life span, the number of centenarians are increasing in the world. Researchers believe that some personality traits may contribute to their longevity. Investigating long lived survivor's personality helps us to know the good strategy or behavior to manage stress. In this study we explore the personality trait of centenarians by the five-factor personality inventory (NEO-FFI). METHOD: Sixty items of NEO-FFI was included as a part of the questionnaire for the mailing survey to investigate the quality of life of the centenarians living in the Tokyo Metropolitan. We asked the family member to evaluate personality of centenarians. One hundred five (83 women and 22 men) valid answers were analyzed. Mean score of five domains, Nuroticism (N), Extraversion (E), Openness (O), Agreeableness (A) and Conscientiousness (C) were compared with the self reported answer of 232 elderly (AGE 67-87) and 247 students (AGE 19-23). RESULTS: N and O are lower in centenarians compare to the elderly and students. However, C is higher in centenarians. E and A were the same as students but different with elderly. E was higher and A was lower than elderly. CONCLUSION: Decline of Nuroticism, Openness and increase Conscientiousness in centenarian seems to be a natural changes according to the aging process. In contrast, the same level of Extraversion and Agreeableness seem that sociable, active, cheerful, optimistic behavior of Extravart and egocentric and skeptical behavior of disagreeable person may contribute to the survival of centenarians by reducing stress.

[85] The influence of the personality and culture in the perception of the aging

Geraldine Alves dos Santos (Pontifícia Universidade Católica do Rio Grande do Sul - PUCRS - Porto Alegre, Brasil) Nair Mônica Ribascik do Nascimento (Instituto de Geriatria e Gerontologia da PUCRS) Cícero Emídio Vaz (PUCRS) Gilson Luis Da Cunha (PUCRS) Maria Cristina da Silva Sant'Anna (PUCRS) Ivana Beatrice Mânica da Cruz (PUCRS) Yukio Moriguchi (PUCRS)

Purpose: To analyze the correlation between self-thinking about aging with cultural and personality aspects of the elderly with successful aging. Method: 119 subjects of Southern Brazil, older than 70 years, without compromising antecedents of personality, were evaluated. Instruments used included the Rorschach and a Questionnaire about sociocultural aspects and perceptions of aging. The Pearson Correlation Test was used. Results: Successful aged people demonstrated correlation between the perception of the aging as the best phase of life and considered family the most important (0,205), paranoid defenses (-0,231), to modify the habits (-0,215), presence of primary relationships with decrease of the adaptation capacity (-0,216); the family life is more intense although impoverishment of the relationships occurs, due to the absence of affective lacks and the safety provided by the family. The idea of considering aging as a good phase, like any other, but that demands changes is correlated with: the importance given to the family by the parents (-0,221), the relevance given to the respect for the other people by the parents (0,194), affective-emotional conditions (-0,229) and depression (-0,193). Aging as a difficult phase: parents demanded obedience without discussion (-0,189), decrease of the capacity to establish primary relationships, showing more flexibility (0,188) and a more critic view of reality. Conclusion: The way the aging is lived doesn't affect the existence of successful aging, although it stimulates alterations in the perception of this experience.

[86] Clinical Profiles of Patients in a Specialized Memory Clinic in Hong Kong

W. Mok, K.C. Chiu, L.W. Chu, C.P. Chung, W. Hu, S.L. Hui.(Division of Geriatric Medicine, University Department of Medicine, Queen Mary Hospital, Hong Kong SAR)

Purpose: Analysis of the disease subtype statistics in our population with the aim of identifying the baseline characteristics of the population. Method: Case records of 288 consecutive patients, who have attended the Memory Clinic of Queen Mary Hospital in H.K. from 1/1/1997 to 30/6/2000, were reviewed. Results: Among the 288 subjects in this cohort, 242 (83.7%) were diagnosed to have dementia according to the DSM-IV criteria. 43 subjects had other diagnoses:- 26 (9.0%) mild cognitive impairment (MCI); 12 (4.2%) depression; 3 (1.0%) epilepsy; 1 (0.3%) delirium. One subject had normal cognition. Of the 242 patients with dementia, 118 (48.8%) were diagnosed as probable AD according to the criteria of the National Institute of Neurological and Communication Disorders and Stroke ¡V Alzheimer¡¦s Disease and Related Disorders Association (NINCDS- ADRDA); 76 (31.4%) Vascular Dementia (VaD) according to the criteria of the National Institute of Neurological Disorders and Stroke ¡V Association Internationale pour la Recherche et l¡¦ Enseignement en Neurosciences (NINDS-AIREN). 25 (10.3%) Mixed AD & VaD type. Other subtypes included cerebral tumors or trauma (2.1%), normal pressure hydrocephalus (1.7%), Parkinson¡¦s disease with dementia (0.4%), frontal-temporal dementia (0.4%), dementia with lewy body (0.4%) and other dementias (1.7%). Diagnosis was uncertain in 3(1% out of 288 patients that have been assessed.) because of incomplete assessment or investigation results. Among the 118 probable AD patients, 13 of them were found to have coexisting vitamin B12 deficiency . Conclusion: This is the first and largest case series analyses of dementia presenting to a specialist multi-disciplinary Memory Clinic in Hong Kong.

[87] A University-Government-Advocacy Group Initiative to Promote More Effective Utilization of Mental Health Services

C. Norris-Baker [Galichia Center on Aging, Kansas State University, Manhattan, Kansas, USA], D. Altus [Washburn University, Topeka, KS], M. Carman [Prairie View Inc, Newton, KS], N. Trout [Johnson County Mental Health Center, Olathe, KS], E. Schwartz [Kansas Department on Aging, Topeka, KS]

In states such as Kansas, where rural areas have high proportions of elders and limited access to services, the need for information on mental health and aging is acute. A cooperative initiative among a mental health advocacy group, university researchers, and the State of Kansas addressed this problem through a project to develop, disseminate and evaluate a mental health guidebook and related materials. Objectives included providing comprehensive, easy to access information about mental health services and resources and enhancing coordination of care for older Kansans experiencing mental disorders. Year I focused on developing the 96-page guidebook, written for a paraprofessional and consumer audience. Approximately 7,500 copies were distributed state-wide to community mental health centers, area agencies on aging, long-term care facilities, healthcare providers, county extension offices, academic institutions, public libraries, and advocacy groups. A total of 1576 service providers received surveys asking them to evaluate the impact of this guidebook, with a return rate of19%. Approximately 98% of respondents believed the guidebook would improve knowledge about mental health services, while 67% believed it would improve coordination of care. Respondents overwhelmingly believed (97%) the guidebook would benefit older Kansans and their families. Based on the success of the initial project, 20,000 additional guidebooks were printed, and the partners expanded their dissemination strategy in Year II. A poster, bookmarks, brief fact sheet, slide show and speaker's bureau have been developed to compliment the guidebook, and evaluation of their efficacy will be presented as well.

[88] Melatonin secretion and aging

F. Magri, S.B. Solerte, M. Fioravanti, S. Chytiris, I. Engaddi, B. Muzzoni, M. Corino, L. Busconi, E. Ferrari (Department of Internal Medicine and Medical Therapy, Chair of Geriatrics, University of Pavia, Italy)

Since melatonin circadian rhythm may be considered as a coordinating signal for several biological functions we studied the pineal secretion in 52 healthy old subjects (66-92 y), in 42 old demented patients (69-91 y), in 20 healthy centenarians (100-107 y) and in 22 healthy young controls (19-43 y). Plasma melatonin was measured in blood samples collected every 4 h during the day and every 2 h during the night in old and young healthy subjects and in patientswith senile dementia; the 6-hydroxymelatonin sulfate (aMT6s) excretion was evaluated in two different urine samples collected from 08:00 to 20:00 and from 20:00 to 08:00 in healthy centenarians. Elderly subjects, demented or not, exhibited a clearly flattened circadian profile of plasma melatonin, due to the selective impairment of the nocturnal peak. An age-related decline of the circadian amplitude of melatonin rhythm occurred in old subjects, and especially in demented ones, when compared to young controls. Furthermore, the melatonin nocturnal peak was significantly correlated with the severity of the cognitive impairment (MMSE score). The aMT6s urinary excretion also declines with age. However, likewise to young controls, in centenarians the aMT6s excretion was significantly higher at night- than at day-time. In conclusion, the pineal secretion can be affected by age and by the degree of cognitive impairment. In a selected population like centenarians the maintenance of the circadian organization of melatonin secretion may suggest that the amplitude of the nocturnal peak and/or the persistence of a prevalent nocturnal secretion may be an important marker of biological age and of health status.

[89] The relationship between sleep disturbance and the pulmonary function and symptoms in the elderly.

Sang-hyun Lee, M.D, Moon Jong Kim, M.D. (Department of Family Medicine, Inha University, Inchon, Korea. Department of Family Medicine, Jungmun Medical University*, Korea.*

Purpose: Sleep complaints are common among the elderly. Among the illness associated with disturbed sleep, respiratory symptoms and functions may be improved by the proper treatment. The improvement of respiratory symptoms and functions may affect better effect on sleep. The purpose of this study was to assess the relationship between sleep disturbance and the pulmonary function and symptoms in the elderly. Method: We investigated 590 people aged 60 years or older who visited Health Care Center of Inha University Hospital in 1998. Sleep disturbance and the pulmonary function and symptoms were evaluated. Result: The prevalence of disturbance maintaining sleep (DMS) was 21.3 0n men and 40.1 0n women whereas the prevalence of disturbance initiating sleep (DIS) was 2.8 0n men and 7.2 0n women. The frequency of DMS was significantly higher in the elderly men with dyspnea than those without dyspnea. We could not find the relationship between DMS and the other respiratory symptoms such as cough. There was no difference of pulmonary function according to DMS. Through multiple logistic regression analysis, DMS seemed to be associated with factors such as gender, dyspnea. There was no association between DMS and factors such as age, body mass index, cough, smoking, exercise, FEV1 and FVC. Conclusion: DMS was more common in the elderly women than the elderly men. DMS seemed to be associated with dyspnea in the elderly men. But there was no relationship between the pulmonary function and DMS

[90] Use Of An Individualized Music Protocol to Promote Sleep Onset in Older Women

J.E. Johnson (University of Nevada, Reno Orvis School of Nursing, Reno, USA)

The purpose of this study was to describe the impact of an individualized music protocol on the time to sleep onset in older women with chronic insomnia. Inclusion and exclusion criteria were established using the International Classification of Sleep Disorders. Names of potential participants were obtained from physicians and nurse practitioners. Using a pre/post test design, a convenience sample of 52 women with a mean age of 80.5 years participated. They lived in their own homes. Each selected the music they wished to use in the study. Data were collected using an investigator constructed questionnaire designed to determine the subjective assessment of time to sleep onset and level of satisfaction with sleep before and after the use of music, and level of satisfaction with the use of music to promote sleep onset. Interviews were conducted to further explore the subjective experience of using music to promote sleep onset. Questionniare data were collected for 10 nights each in the pre and post test phases. Participants received explicit instructions on the use of music. Data were analyzed with t-tests and conceptual coding. Results showed that music signficantly reduced the time to sleep onset and increased sleep satisfaction. Participants were very satisfied with the use of music. Themes included "Fond Memories," "A Miracle," and "Relaxation and Contentment." The use of an individualized music protocol is a useful intervention for older women experiencing difficulty falling asleep.

[91] Impaired Nocturnal Melatonin Output in Nondipper as Opposed to Dipper Hypertensive Patients

Jonas M, Grossman E (Department of Internal Medicine D, The Chaim Sheba Medical Center, Tel-Hashomer), Laudon M (Neurim Pharmaceuticals Ltd, Tel Aviv), Garfinkel D (Aging Research and Department of Internal Medicine E, The E. Wolfson Medical Center, Holonand Maccabi Healthcare Services, Israel)

Objective: To evaluate whether melatonin plays a role in the circadian rhythm of blood pressure. Methods: Twenty-four hour ambulatory blood pressure was measured in 16 elderly patients with essential hypertension. According to nocturnal fall in the mean arterial pressure, patients were defined as dippers (n = 8) or nondippers (n = 8). Urinary excretion of 6-sulfatoxymelatonin (6SMT), the main metabolite of melatonin, was determined by ELISA assay in two separate collections, during daytime (12h) and during the night (12h). Results: Both groups were similar in regard to age, sex and mean daily blood pressure. During the night, the mean arterial pressure decreased by 10.2% in the dippers and increased by 8% in the nondipper patients. 6SMT excretion was comparable during the day in dippers (3.28 0.87 g/12h) and nondippers (2.31 0.68 g/12h). However, while the dippers presented the physiological nocturnal increase in urinary 6SMT excretion (mean 8.19 1.68 g/12h), this nocturnal surge in melatonin excretion was missing in nondippers (mean 2.56 0.79 g/12h). Conclusions: Unlike dipper hypertensives, nondipper patients do not exhibit the normal nocturnal increase in melatonin secretion. Melatonin may play a role in the circadian rhythm of blood pressure.

[92] Quality of sleep reported by elderly outpatients of the Group of Attention of Elderly Health (GRASI).

M.F. Ceolim, M.J.D'E. Diogo, F.A. Cintra (Departamento de Enfermagem, Faculdade de Ciências Médicas, Universidade Estadual de Campinas, Campinas, SP, Brasil)

The purpose of this study was to describe sleep quality and characteristics of elderly outpatients of the GRASI, a group from Hospital das Clínicas (HC) of Universidade Estadual de Campinas (Unicamp, SP, Brasil). This group is conducted by nursing teachers of Unicamp School of Nursing and its main focus is health promotion and education of the elderly who attend the group. In this research, a specific instrument to assess sleep quality, the Pittsburgh Sleep Quality Index (PSQI), created by Buysse and col. was used. Eight men and 12 women, volunteers, who took part in the activities developed at GRASI in 1998, were the subjects of the study. Fifteen subjects (75%) reported bad sleep quality according to PSQI. Most frequent disorders were: nocturia, night sleep interruptions, early wakening and low sleep efficiency. Napping was reported by 60% of the subjects, and 90% of them napped unintentionally. The results suggest that gerontological nurses should include detailed assessment of sleep patterns in their routine, in order to help the elderly properly choose non-pharmacological treatment alternatives, or seek medical care if necessary.

[93] Prevalence and factors associated with insomnia in Brazilian elderly: The Bambuí Health and Ageing Study

F. L. Rocha1(4), E. Uchôa(2,3,4), H. L. Guerra(2,4), J. O. A. Firmo(2,4), P. G. Vidigal(2,3,4), M. F. F. Lima e Costa(2,3,4) (1Medical Residency of Psychiatry, Institute of Social Security of the Civil Servants of Minas Gerais, 2 Oswaldo Cruz Foundation Rene Rachou Research Institute, 3 Federal University of Minas Gerais Medical School, and 4 Research Group on the Epidemiology and Anthropology of Ageing (REGEA), Belo Horizonte, MG, Brazil).

Purpose - Population-based studies of insomnia among older people residing in communities in developing countries are rare. The objectives of this population-based study were to determine the prevalence and factors associated with insomnia among older adults (60 years and over) living in a Brazilian town with 15,000 inhabitants (Bambui, MG). Method: All 1,742 residents in this age group were selected for a structured interview and blood tests. From these, 1,516 (87.0%) participated in the study. Results: The prevalence of insomnia was 38.9%, being higher among women (45.3%) than among men (28.8%). The use of sleeping pills was reported by 380/1513 (25.1%) of the participants; 186 (49.0%) of these complained of insomnia, suggesting that their treatment should be reassessed. Factors independently associated with insomnia were: female sex (OR=1.78; 95%CI=1.41-2.24), dissatisfaction with free time arrangements (OR=1.88; 95%CI=1.28-2.77), self rated health as reasonable or bad/very bad (OR=2.02; 95%CI=1.50-2.72 and OR=3.12; 95%CI=2.21-4.39, respectively), history of previous medical diagnosis of some chronic conditions (OR=1.38; 95%CI=1.10-1.73), inability to perform routine activities due to a health problem in the previous 2 weeks (OR=1.54; 95%CI=1.10-2.15), and staying in bed in the previous 2 weeks (OR=1.61; 95%CI=1.04-2.48). Conclusion: The prevalence of insomnia was high, indicating that this was a public health problem for older adults living in the study community. Our results emphasize the necessity for further investigations about insomnia among older people living in small communities in Brazil and other developing countries.

[94] Does cholesterol intake relate to depression in Japanese elderly?

F.Ando, T.Imai, Y.Fukukawa, S.Tsuboi, C.Nakashima, N.Niino, H.Shimokata (National Institute for Longevity Sciences, Obu, Japan)

PURPOSE: Some studies have suggested that low serum cholesterol concentration by diet induces depression. In the present study we investigated the relation of cholesterol intake and serum cholesterol level with depressive state in Japanese elderly. METHOD: Subjects comprised 391 males and 378 females aged 65 to 79 years who participated in the National Institute for Longevity Sciences Longitudinal Study of Aging (NILS-LSA). Depressive state was estimated using Japanese Version of the Center for Epidemiologic Studies Depression Scale (CES-D). Cholesterol intake was assessed by 3-day dietary record (3DR) and serum total cholesterol level was measured after overnight fast. Subjects were divided into three groups according to their intakes of cholesterol and serum cholesterol levels. CES-D scores were compared among three groups (low, middle and high cholesterol intakes or serum cholesterol levels). RESULTS: The mean scores of CES-D, the means of cholesterol intake and serum cholesterol were 7.4 ±6.9, 370.0 ± 143.9 mg/day, 210.5 ±32.8 mg/dl in males and 8.6 ±7.2, 310.9 ± 128.0mg/day, 232.6 ± 35.2mg/dl in females. CES-D scores showed a trend to increase as the decrease of cholesterol intake even after adjusting for total energy intake. However serum cholesterol level did not relate significantly with CES-D score even though there was a positive significant relationship between cholesterol intake and serum cholesterol level. CONCLUSION: Cholesterol intake but not serum cholesterol level relates with depressive state of elderly in this study.

[95] Existential meaning and depression: One study with attendants Pucpr's

Cloves Amorim (PUCPR Curitiba - Brazil) Ana Maria Moser (PUCPR/UNIVALI / USP Curitba - Brazil) Auristela Moser (PUCPR Curitiba - Brazil) Margareth Favile (UTPR Curitiba - Brazil)

In Brazil, it is estimated that the population with age superior to 60 years old is 15 million. Some researches show the incidence of depressive symptoms in 15% of this population. The objective of this research was to evaluate the incidence of depression on women attending the Universidade para Terceira Idade da Pontifícia Universidade Católica do Paraná (Pontifícia Catholic University of Paraná's University for Third Age). 35 women took part with ages between 54 and 79 years old. 74% think that it is good to be alive, that life is not empty and that they feel themselves useful too; 95% feel themselves full of energy, searching for social contacts, and only 8% do not feel themselves well waking up in the morning. It is emphasized that in all the questions it was not verified scores indicating a depressive state. These data are referred to a portion of the population, economic distinguished, since they attend a private institution and have good physical health. The conclusion is that the Universidade da Terceira Idade's programs facilitate the healthy aging process while providing the companionship, the self-esteem development and room for new social roles, re-meaning their existential perspective.

[96] Differential Predictors of Depression and Anxiety in Nursing Home Residents

L. Dalzell, C. Konnert (University of Calgary, Calgary, Canada)

There is a high prevalence of depression and anxiety in the nursing home population, and difficulties arise when attempting to differentiate these mental health problems. The present study was designed to determine the differential predictors of depression and anxiety, with the goal of obtaining two different predictive models, one that specifically predicted depression and another that specifically predicted anxiety. The following predictors were examined: (1) indices of physical health and sensory functioning, (2) cognitive status, (3) primary and secondary appraisal and anticipatory coping, (4) dysfunctional thoughts, (5) perceived control, and (6) indices of social support. The predictors were selected because of their relevance to theories of depression and anxiety developed on younger adults. The predictors were measured with scales that had previously been used with an elderly population, and many that were designed specifically for nursing home residents, or physically frail elderly. The sample consisted of 70 nursing home residents (mean age = 81.4, ranging from 61-98). Results indicated that the first predictive model accounted for a significant amount of variance in depression (39%), but not in anxiety (4.5%). The second predictive model accounted for a significant amount of variance in anxiety (21.6%) and depression (20.3%). Thus, these models enabled the differentiation of depression from anxiety, but not the differentiation of anxiety from depression.

[97] Depression in Geriatric Patients

Marcos Garcia Pastoressa, Felipe Ricardo Lopez Garcia, Jorge Luis Diosdado Salazar, Enrique Sanchez de la Barquera, Rosa Emma Maldonado Rodriguez, Manuel F. Barrientos Suarez, Eydid Alvarado Davila. (Hospital General de Zona No. 13, Norberto Trevino Zapata, IMSS. Hospital General Alfredo Pumarejo. SST. H. Matamoros, Tamaulipas, Mexico)

Introduction. Depression among geriatrics patients is one of the most common psychiatric diseases, is a disabling mood disorder that impairs one's well-being and may ever threaten a sufferer's life, however depression is a treatable illness. Many symptons of geriatric patients are attributed to the aging process or to medical disorders. Objective. To estimate the prevalence of depression and associated sociodemographic factors in Mexican geriatric patients. Research design. A descriptive, prospective and transversal study. Setting. Internal Medicine Departments of two Hospitals in H. Matamoros,Tamaulipas, Mexico. Method.Hamilton Depression Rating Scale (HDS) was used to measure depression and a 37 items questionary about sociodemographic variables. Results. They were 187 patients, 118 (63.1 %) females and 69 (36.9 %) males.Mean age was 65 years. 89 (47.6 %) were married, 152 (81.3 %) had incomplete elementary school, 97 (51.9 %)with USD 300.00-600.00 income per year, 74 (42.0 %) living in son's house. The symptoms of depression were founded in 95 patients (50.8 %). Associated variables to depression were: diabetes mellitus, annual low income and to be male. Conclusion. Prevalence of depression was high (50.8 %), this mental disorder is an important health problem among our geriatric patients. Depression was greatest among those with low income, less support from family and less institutional support. Finally, this mood disorder often is under-diagnosed and under-treated, therefore we need to improve its diagnosis using clinical screening instruments during initial contacts in primary care sector.

[98] Influence of Psychological Independence on the Relationships between IQ and Depressive Symptoms

C. Nakashima, Y. Fukukawa, S. Tsuboi, N. Niino, F. Ando, H. Shimokata (National Institute for Longevity Sciences, Aichi, Japan)

PURPOSE: To clarify the effects of psychological independence and change in IQ on depressive symptoms in middle-aged and elderly Japanese. METHOD: Subjects were 605 men and women from a community living population aged 40 to 79 years followed up two years. The effects of psychological independence at the initial survey and 2-year longitudinal change in IQ on the subsequent depressive symptoms were examined. Psychological independence was measured by the Locus of Control Scale (Wakabayashi et al, 1995). Depressive symptoms were measured by Japanese version of the Center for Epidemiologic Studies Depression Scale (CES-D). IQ was estimated by the Wechsler Adult Intelligence Scale-Revised Short Forms. Subjects were classified into three groups by the 2-year longitudinal change in IQ (Decline, Invariable, Increase) and also into three groups by psychological independence score at the initial examination (Low, Middle, High). RESULTS: Analysis of covariance controlled for age, gender, and CES-D at the initial survey revealed no significant main effects of psychological independence and change in IQ on CES-D at the second survey, but there was significant interaction effect between psychological independence and change in IQ ($p<.05$). This interaction indicated that there was no significant effect of psychological independence on CES-D in IQ Invariable or Increase group, while, in IQ Decline group, CES-D in Low independence group (CES-D: 10.6) was significantly ($p<.05$) higher than those of Middle(7.3) and High(6.6) independence groups. CONCLUSION: The findings in our study suggest that psychological independence may have some effects on the relationship between change in IQ and depressive symptoms.

[99] Depressive symptoms and mortality in elderly people.

M.Trabucchi, T.Sabatini, P.Barbisoni, M.Ferri, N.Travaglini, S.Boffelli, R.Rozzini. Medical Unit for the Acute Care of the Elderly, (Poliambulanza H) and Geriatric Research Group, via Romanino 1, 25122 Brescia, Italy

Aim of the study is to evaluate if depression in elderly is an independent risk factor for mortality in community residing older adults. The data were obtained in a multidimensional study carried out in a community-dwelling population aged 70 and over living in the rural city of Ospitaletto, Brescia, Italy. Of a total number of 613 over 70, valid questionnaires available were 549 (89.60f the eligible population). In addition to demographics (gender, age, years of education), mood was assessed with the short version of the GDS and cognitive performance with the MMSE. Patients with a MMSE between 14 and 24 were considered as cognitively impaired; 25 subjects with a MMSE lower than 14 were excluded from the study. The study has been performed on 524 persons. Depression was stratified into three GDS levels: no depression (0-2), mild (3-5), and moderate to severe depression (higher than 5). Physical health was assessed as the number of chronic conditions, and disability by Katz's BADL scale. Disabled were defined those with 1 or more BADL functions lost. The mean age of the 524 elderly subjects (173 males and 351 females) was 76.6+5.1 years. They had 4.6+1.9 years of education, were affected by 3.5+2.2 chronic conditions; 134 (24.4%) lived alone and 149 (27,1%) had 1 or more BADL functions lost. MMSE and GDS mean scores were 25.8+3.6 and 3.7+3.0 respectively. Vital status was assessed for each subject 60 months from the baseline analysis. One hundred and twenty nine persons (24.6%) died during the follow-up period. Obtained data show that in the crude and adjusted Cox regression analysis depressive symptoms are associated with 60-month mortality, indicating a dose dependent association between depressive symptoms and mortality even when mental impairment and disability were taken into account (RR: 1.6 95% CI 1.1-2.5 and RR: 1.5 95% CI 1.2-2.8 respectively).

[100] Is depression being detected in elderly patients?

V. Spinola Dias Neto, C. K. Hübner, F. J. Turrini, L. C. Gabas, M.B. Lopes, P. K. M. S. Machado (Centro de Ciências Médicas e Biológicas da Pontifícia Universidade Católica, Sorocaba, Brasil)

Purpose: In population over sixties the incidence of major depression is around 15%, this present geriatric research is engaged in diagnostic and treatment of this disease in no psychiatric services. Method: During the period from October to December, 2000, 33 patients over 60 years or more ward of the Leonor de Barros Hospital, Sorocaba and 36 from the pre-surgery wing of the Regional Hospital (States Hospitals), Sorocaba were availed in their bed about depressive symptoms and their cognitive capacity, using respectively the Hamilton scale for depression (21 item) and the Mini Exam of mental state (Mini-Mental). The score of 14 points was adopted as the limit number for Hamilton test and for Mini-Mental the score was 17, both in agreement with the literature. Patients without verbal communication, with psychiatric disorders established or with dementia were excluded from the present study. Drugs of any kind in use at the moment of the examination were investigated. The software EPI-INFO 5.0 has been used to compute the results. Results: In the ward were found 39.3% of patients with symptoms of major depression, in the surgery service this rate was 36.1%, this difference represents no meaning according to statistics. Among these illness patients only 2.89% had the diagnosis of depression and current treatment for this disease. Conclusion: This study concluded that it' s worried the rates of incidence of major depression in hospitals is high, and there no diagnostic, and which is not receiving effective treatment.

[101] Support Groups for Depressed Elderly Patients with Parkinsons Disease

V. D. Berentsen (Geriatric Outpatient Unit, Department of Medicine), I. HogenEsch (Department of Neurology), G. S. Havag, L. Johansson (Therapists Department, Haugesund County Hospital, Haugesund, Norway)

Purpose. To work out a method for undertaking and evaluating support groups for depressed elderly patients with Parkinson s disease. To investigate the effect on symptoms of depression and Parkinsonism. Patients. Eight patients were included. All had depression, Parkinsonism, and additional diseases. Method. Depressed patients were recruited from the local Parkinson patients organisation. Patients were examined by nurse, neurologist and physiotherapist before start and after 6 and 12 months. The following rating scales were used: Unified Parkinson s Disease Rating Scale (including Hoehn and Yahr state and ADL-score), Mini Mental State, Geriatric Depression Scale, Montgomery and Asberg Depression Rating Scale, Barthel-index, Nottingham Health Profile. Social network, living conditions, and drug consumption were noted. The physiotherapist prepared individual training programs. The meetings took place every second week for one year and were chaired by a nurse, a physiotherapist, and the hospital s priest. Each meeting lasted for 1 hr 20 min, using the first 20 min for Parkinson-trim . The conversation concentrated on living with Parkinsonism, making everyday life more comfortable, and reminiscences of grief and pleasure. Results. All patients attended most meetings. Patients enjoyed participating, and contacted each other spontaneously outside the group setting. Some scores from rating scales improved, but the numbers were too small to produce statistically significant differences. Discussion. It is easy to organise and perform support groups for depressed elderly patients with Parkinsonism. Patients may benefit from participating and feel more happy and comfortable. The economical costs are low. The method is feasible and should be investigated in further studies.

[102] Effectiveness of physical therapy in the treatment of Parkinson Disease.

Giuseppe Bellelli, Cathrine Bellwald, Marco Ponte, Angelo Bianchetti, (Geriatric Research Group, Brescia and Ancelle della Carità, Hospital, Cremona, Italy) Marco Trabucchi (Geriatric Research Group, Brescia and University of Tor Vergata Roma; Italy)

Physical therapy (PT) is considered an important therapeutic option in Parkinson disease (PD). With the aim to evaluate the usefulness of a standardized program of PT a study was conducted on 30 PD at different levels of severity (mean age 75.0±10.2, 50 0.000000emales, Hohen & Yahr scale from 2 to 5 (mean 3.2±1.1), mean MMSE score 20.2±8.5). PD patients were admitted to our rehabilitative Unit from October 1999 to October 2000. All the patients underwent a standardized program of PT, on the basis of the severity of the disease and the symptoms, for 1.5 hour/day consecutively for 4 weeks. After the treatment period a statistically significant improvement in gait and balance (Tinetti scale for gait from 3.8±3.7 to 8.0±3.7 and Tinetti scale for balance from 4.2±5.4 to 10. ±4.6, p<0.001) and in functional status measured with Barthel Index (from 39.8±29.9 to 70.9±28.8, p <0.0001) was observed. Also the symptoms of the disease measured with the UPDRS scale showed a statistically significant improvement, even cognitive and affective symptoms (from 7.5±4.3 to 4.8±3.9, p<0.001) and complications (from 4.7±5.8 to 2.7±3.4, p<05). The more significant improvement was observed in the sample of more severe patients (H&Y 3 to 5). No significant changing of pharmacological therapy was carried out during the period of rehabilitation program. Our data shows that PT represent an important opportunity for PD patients, also in the advanced stages of the disease, with effects not only on the motor symptoms, but also on affective status and global functional status.

[103] Sensitivity and specificity of clinicaldiagnosis of idiopathic Parkinson disease in the elderly

VERNY M (Centre de Gériatrie et INSERM U360, Hôpital Salpêtrière PARIS, France), BONNET A-M (Fédération de Neurologie, Hôpital Salpêtrière PARIS, France), BEINIS J-Y (USN, Hôpital Charles Foix, IVRY, France), PIETTE F (La Triade, Hôpital Charles Foix, IVRY, France), GALLINARI C (Gérontologie 2, Hôpital Charles Foix, IVRY, France), LAURENT M (L'Arche, Hôpital Charles Foix, IVRY, France), MEAUME S (L'Orbe, Hôpital Charles Foix, IVRY, France), HAUW J-J (Laboratoire de Neuropathologie et INSERM U360, Hôpital Salpêtrière PARIS, France) DUYCKAERTS C (Laboratoire de Neuropathologie et INSERM U106, Hôpital Salpêtrière PARIS, France)

PURPOSE: Diagnosis of Parkinson's disease in the elderly remains difficult

The validation of clinical diagnostic criteria by neuropathological examination has rarely been obtained. The aim of this study was to determine specificity and sensitivity of clinical diagnostic criteria in cases of Parkinson's disease (Hughes et al, Neurology, 1992) and to identify the items most useful to the diagnosis. METHOD: The inclusion criterion was parkinsonism, apparently due to a neurodegenerative disease. From 1993 to 1999, 103 patients living in long term care units at Charles Foix Hospital (Ivry, France) fulfilled that condition. They were clinically examined once a year. Seventy-two patients died and autopsy could be performed in 40 cases. RESULTS: These preliminary results concern 21 clinicopathological cases: 7 were men, 14 women; mean age: 83 years (+/ - 2,5) at death. Ten cases had neuropathological lesions of Parkinson's disease and 5 had a sufficient number of cortical Levy bodies to endorse the diagnosis of dementia with Levy body. Four of these cases also had vascular lesions and in 3 other cases, Alzheimer's lesions were present. Four cases had neuropathological lesions of progressive supranuclear palsy. The sensitivity of the clinical diagnosis of Parkinson's disease at the inclusion was 90%, the specificity was 64%. Rest tremor and asymmetric Parkinson syndrome at the onset of the disease had a high specificity (82% for each). Sensitivity was respectively 50% and 70%. The absence of gait disturbances at the onset had a high sensitivity (90%) but specificity was 45%. CONCLUSION: Parkinson's disease is overdiagnosed in the elderly. Progressive supranuclear palsy and Alzheimer's disease with parkinsonism were, on the contrary, underdiagnosed. Associate lesions are frequent in this population.

[104] In-Shoe Pressure Monitoring - A Pilot Study In Parkinson's Disease

E.Waldie (Department of Geriatric Medicine, Princess Alexandra Hospital, Brisbane, Australia), B.Dinh (Department of Podiatry, Princess Alexandra Hospital, Brisbane, Australia), D.Purdie (Department of Social and Preventive Medicine, University of Queensland, Brisbane, Australia), D.Le Couteur (Department of Geriatric Medicine, The Canberra Hospital, Canberra, Australia)

PURPOSE: In-shoe pressure monitoring has been useful in a number of disease processes that affect gait. This pilot study investigated the use of this technology in Parkinson's disease, a significant cause of gait disturbance in the elderly. METHODS: 10 people with clinically mild Parkinson's disease and 10 age, sex, height and weight matched controls were studied using the EMED PEDAR(Novel gmbh) system of in-shoe pressure monitoring. In-shoe pressure monitoring was performed over an 8 metre walking distance at three speeds - fast, medium and slow. For each recorded step, the foot was divided into thirds for separate analysis - heel, midfoot and forefoot. Data from left and right feet was pooled at each speed for each study group and average values obtained for comparison between groups. RESULTS: Values for contact time, peak pressure, maximum force, contact area, pressure time integrals and force time integrals were compared between groups. The Parkinson's group compared to controls showed a significant increase in forefoot and midfoot contact time and significantly decreased forefoot maximum force and heel peak pressures. These differences occurred at all walking speeds, becoming more marked as gait speed increased and would be consistent with the well-described shuffling, flat-footed gait pattern of Parkinson's disease. CONCLUSION: In-shoe pressure monitoring can be used to discriminate gait abnormalities in Parkinson's disease. Further research to better delineate these differences and to determine whether they are measurable at a very early stage in the disease is indicated.

[105] Muscle changes in Alzheimer's type dementia

P. Prokopova [Institute of pathology, 1-st medical faculty, Charles University, Prague, Czech Republic], Z. Kalvach [1-st medical faculty, Charles University, Prague, Czech Republic], M. Zeman [1-st Department of surgery, 1-st medical faculty, Charles University, Prague, Czech Republic]

To assess muscular changes in patients with Alzheimer's type dementia, including histochemical changes reported to afflict not only brain but also peripheral nerves and muscles, in connection with clinical experience of muscle weakness in this kind of patients. Clinical investigation including nutritional condition, stand up and go test, histochemical investigation of biopsy from muscular gluteus medius in patients with Alzheimer's disease and hip fracture treated by surgery. The study is in progress and it is to be finished before the congress takes place. Preliminarily we have found significantly more serious muscle weakness in patients with Alzheimer' s type dementia than in patients with vascular dementia in age over 65 years. There was also histochemical positivity of antitau and beta amyloid precursor protein antibodies and lower activity of anti acetylcholine antibodies in several muscle samples of demented patients with hip fractures, diversing from muscle samples of non-demented patients. Muscles could be interesting tissue for diagnostic process in demented patients. From clinical points of view muscle weakness can be an underestimated impairment of serious importance in demented patients.

SESSION 134

Cross-national comparisons of perceptions of inter- and intra-generational communication

K.A. Noels (University of Alberta, Edmonton, Canada), H. Giles (University of California, Santa Barbara, U.S.A.), A. Williams (University of Wales, Cardiff, Wales), H. Ota (Aichi Shukutoku University, Japan), E. Ryan (McMaster University, Hamilton, Canada), S.H. Ng (Victoria University of Wellington, New Zealand), L. Somera (De La Salle University, Manila, Philippines), T.-S. Lim (Kwangwoon University, Seoul, South Korea)

Positive intergenerational communication has been suggested to predict older adults' subjective well-being. Unfortunately , much research conducted in Western nations suggests that intergenerational communication is often problematic. The cultural value of filial piety in East Asian nations, might lead to the expectation that intergenerational relations would be more positive in East Asian than in Western nations. Accordingly, this study examined young adults' perceptions of intergenerational communication in six Pacific Rim nations. Participants from three Western (Canada, U.S.A. and New Zealand) and from three East Asian (the Philippines, Korea and Japan) nations completed a questionnaire regarding their perceptions of interactions with family elders, non-family elders and same-age peers. Analyses of variance compared the six nations' perceptions of the three target groups' communication behaviours, and self-perceptions of obligation to be respectful towards the other person and positive emotions in the interaction. Nonfamily elders were generally perceived as less accommodative than family elders. Participants in both cultural groups indicated an obligation to be most deferential towards nonfamily elders, followed by family elders, followed by same-age peers. Whereas both groups perceived interactions with the same-age peers more positively than the two older groups, the Western group perceived the older age groups more positively than the East Asian group did. Thus, contrary to expectation, intergenerational communication appears to be more problematic than intragenerational communication and this pattern is more evident in East Asian than in Western nations on some variables. Implications for a pancultural model of positive intergenerational communication — with family and nonfamily elders — are discussed.

Enhancing Communication With Older Adults to Promote Health

K.A. Noels (University of Alberta, Edmonton, Canada), H. Giles (University of California, Santa Barbara, U.S.A.), A. Williams (University of Wales, Cardiff, Wales), H. Ota (Aichi Shukutoku University, Japan), E. Ryan (McMaster University, Hamilton, Canada), S. H. Ng (Victoria University of Wellington, New Zealand), L. Somera (De La Salle University, Manila, Philippines), T.-S. Lim (Kwangwoon University, Seoul, South Korea), Cross-National

Comparisons of Perceptions of Inter- and Intra-Generational Communication Sik Hung Ng (City University of Hong Kong, Hong Kong, China), How Might Inter-generational Communication in the Family Be Enhanced to Promote Seniors' Well-being? M. L. Hummert (University of Kansas, Lawrence, U.S.A.) & E. B. Ryan (McMaster University, Hamilton, Canada), Impact of Family Communication During Decision-Making about Age-Related Predicaments Helen Edwards (Queensland University of Technology, Brisbane, Australia), Family Caregiving: Promoting Health Through Everyday Conversations M. K. Pichora-Fuller, A. J. Carson, L. M. Dillon Edgett (University of British Columbia, Vancouver, Canada), Living with Hearing Loss: How One Person's Experiences Influence Another's

According to the Communication Predicament of Aging Model, older adults are at risk for experiencing stereotype-based conversational interactions that undermine their self-esteem and well-being. This symposium will address the communication predicaments of older adults from a cross-cultural perspective. Secondly, within the framework of the Communication Enhancement Model, positive strategies are highlighted for more effective intergenerational communication, especially between older adults and their family members. The Chair will introduce the two communication models initially and will lead the discussion among participants and the audience following the five individual presentations. Noels et al. highlight barriers to intergenerational communication satisfaction across both Western and Eastern cultures of the Pacific Rim both within and outside the family. Young adults from six countries perceived interactions with same-age peers as less problematic than with both family and non-family elders. Contrary to expectation, this pattern was even more evident in the East Asian countries. Ng discusses findings from self-reports and analyses of family converstaions in terms of how intergenerational communication may be enhanced. Self reports indicated three types of factors: internal motivation, behaviors in accord with Communication Accommodation Theory, and behaviors in accord with Politeness Theory. Conversational analyses revealed instances of communication brokering where the middle generation mediated a meaningful dialogue between their children and their aging parents. Hummert & Ryan turn the spotlight specifically on family interactions during decision-making occasions when the older adult's need for autonomy conflicts with the adult child's sense of responsibility. They review how the decision process unfolds and feature those strategies most likely to achieve mutually beneficial outcomes. Providing evidence supporting the family communication predicament, Edwards demonstrates how, in everyday conversations, paternalistic communication patterns develop between care providers and older care receivers. These negative communication patterns impact on the mental health of the care receiver. Two types of communication enhancement strategies are proposed: preventative strategies aimed at challenging the stereotypes of caregiving where the care receiver is seen as a passive recipient of care; and intervention strategies aimed at managing the content and process of communication between family caring dyads. Pichora-Fuller et al. shift to social influences on how older adults deal with a hearing impairment. Three interview three studies indicate that it is more challenging for older adults to live with a hearing loss when others living in the same situation also experience communication challenges. The other person also plays an important role in whether or not the individual seeks and benefits from audiologic rehabilitation. These findings suggest that family-focused rehabilitation might be more beneficial than the traditional individual-focused interventions. The focus on communication within the family extends the domain of the two communication models beyond interactions with service providers. We anticipate that future research within these conceptual frameworks can further elaborate the potential of various communication enhancement strategies to promote greater intergenerational communication satisfaction and thereby to support older adults as they strive for positive aging.

Family Caregiving: Promoting Health Through Everyday Conversations

Edwards, Helen. (Queensland University of Technology) Brisbane, Queensland, Australia

Most older people who require care because of health problems are cared for by their family. Commonly, family care is provided by spouses or by adult children who find the caregiving stressful and report poor mental health. Although most research has focused on carers, older care receivers also report poor mental health. As a caring process, family caregiving requires the carer and care receiver to discuss and negotiate many issues. From a communication perspective, paternalism can develop and the carer responds to the physical and role limitations of the older care receiver, highlighting the 'sick role' of the older person and the care provider's status of the carer. Evidence supporting the family communication predicament will demonstrate how, in everyday conversations, paternalistic communication patterns can develop and affect the mental health of the older care receiver. Because of the intimate, long term relationships inherent in family caregiving, it is important to maintain positive communication patterns. Using the communication enhancement model, two types of health promoting communication strategies between older people and their family carers will be proposed: preventative strategies aimed at challenging the caregiving stereotype of the care receiver as a passive recipient of care, and intervention strategies aimed at managing the content and process of communication between family caring dyads. These strategies will facilitate health promoting communication which, in turn, will improve the physical and mental health of family carers and older people for whom they care. A framework for health professionals working with family caring dyads will be presented.

How Might Inter-generational Communication in the Family be Enhanced to Promote Seniors' Well-being

Sik Hung Ng (City University of Hong Kong, Kowloon, Hong Kong)

Earlier research has shown that older adults' subjective well-being (life satisfaction, satisfaction with health, etc.) is correlated with the quality rather than the frequency of contact with their children. In the present paper, I summarize a number of studies from self reports and family conversations, to show how the quality of inter-generational communication may be enhanced. Self reports indicate three major enhancing factors: internal motivations (I talk to elders because I want to) and conversational behaviors that accord with Communication Accommodation Theory and Politeness Theory. Analysis of family conversations was carried out by tracking the turn-by turn social interaction among grandparents, parents and grandchildren. The results unravel some beautiful sequences of ‘communication brokering' in which parents attempt to broker a meaningful dialogue between grandparents and grandchildren. These results point to areas in inter-generational communication, particularly those within the family, that can be harnessed to promote the well-being of seniors (and other family members).

Impact of Family Communication During Decision-Making about Age-Related Predicaments

Hummert, Mary Lee (University of Kansas, Lawrence, Kansas, U.S.A.) & Ryan, Ellen Bouchard, (McMaster University, Hamilton, Canada)

Throughout the life span, the parent-child relationship experiences many changes as its members shift between states of dependence, independence, and interdependence. As parents age, they often find themselves increasingly dependent on their children. In some cases, parents' declining health requires that they make important decisions about health care, place of residence, driving, and other aspects of daily life. Adult children may find themselves participating in this decision process. Both parents and children face these decisions with trepidation, recognizing that the outcomes of such decisions have profound implications for parents' self-esteem and quality of life as well as for intergenerational relationships. This trepidation arises in large part from a tension between parents' need for autonomy and children's corresponding need for paternalism (i.e, a desire to protect parents). In this presentation, we consider how parents and children can best approach this decision-making process. Using the Communication Enhancement Model as a frame, we review how this decision process unfolds in families and highlight those strategies that hold the most promise of achieving mutually beneficial outcomes for parents and children.

Living with hearing loss: How one person's experiences influence another's

M.K. Pichora-Fuller, A.J. Carson, L.M. Dillon Edgett (University of British Columbia, Vancouver, Canada)

The prevalence of hearing loss increases with age, with the majority having clinically significant impairment by age 75. Despite the high likelihood that one older person with hearing loss will live with another older person with hearing loss, audiologic rehabilitation has traditionally focused on the individual rather than on the person in the context of the family or community. The results of three studies concerning the effect of the experience of others on one's own experience of hearing loss will be presented. The first study investigated how 30 residents in a home-for-the-aged experienced hearing loss in everyday situations before and after a full-time on-site audiologic rehabilitation program was provided. The second study investigated how seven older women and their family members living in the community experienced hearing loss before and after their first audiologic assessment. The third study investigated how hearing loss was experienced by older adults taking group audiologic rehabilitation classes in the community. The interviews from all three studies indicate that it is more challenging for older adults to live with a hearing loss when others living in the same situation also experience communication challenges. The other person also plays an important role in whether or not the individual seeks and benefits from audiologic rehabilitation. The advantages of offering family or group interventions is highlighted.

SESSION 135

A Summary of the Current Research Activities on Elder Abuse in Japan: A Preliminary Report

T. Tatara (Shukutoku University in Chiba, Japan)

The purpose of the study is to find out the nature and extent of elder abuse research activities in Japan. A review of the research reports and published materials on elder abuse is being conducted, and in addition, personal interviews are also being conducted with several researchers who have done elder abuse research. The preliminary findings show that there has been a great deal of progress in understanding the nature and dynamics of the problem in Japan, thanks mainly to researchers. Yet, there has still been little information about the prevalence and incidence of elder abuse in Japan. Thus, we have little idea about how serious the problem is in our country. Additionally, there are no systems, to speak of, which can prevent and treat elder abuse in Japan, and most social workers are not trained in elder abuse intervention.

Elder abuse and neglect in residential settings in Germany

Thomas Goergen, (Institute of Criminology at Giessen University, Giessen, Germany)

The study aims at collecting data on types and frequency of elder abuse and neglect in German nursing homes, analysing conditions leading to abusive/neglectful behaviour, and examining prevention and intervention by police, courts and other authorities. METHOD: The study chooses a multimethod approach, combining qualitative interviews in nursing homes, questionnaire surveys among nursing home staff, and analyses of cases known to courts, police, nursing home control agencies, and other relevant institutions. RESULTS: In a pilot study among nursing home staff, 79% of subjects report having abused or neglected at least one resident during the last 12 months. Different types of neglect and verbal/psychological abuse are most common. Subtypes of elder abuse and neglect show differential correlation patterns with measures of work stress. Subjects attribute abuse and neglect not only to staff shortage and work overload but also to a number of factors in the offender's personality and at the political and social level. Data collected in co-operation with nursing home control agencies supply information about the ways in which these authorities control and examine residential facilities; deficiencies are mainly detected in the fields of insufficient care and psychosocial neglect. An analysis of public prosecutor's files points at prototypical cases and raises questions as to the limits of controlling elder abuse and neglect by criminal prosecution. CONCLUSION: Multimethod approaches seem appropriate both to measure up to the complexity and heterogeneity of elder abuse and neglect and to enhance researchers' chances of gaining sufficient access to the field.

Elder Abuse: New Directions in Research and Practice

Rosalie Wolf (UMass Memorial Health Care, Worcester MA, USA) The National Elder Abuse Report Survey 2000. Toshio Tatara (Shukutoku Universuty in Chiba, Japan) A summary of the Current Research Activities on Elder Abuse in japan. Thomas Goergen (Institute of Criminology at Giessen University, Giessen, Germany) Elder abuse and neglect in residential settings in Germany. Margot Schofield (University of New England, Armidale, Australia) Vulnerability to elder abuse: predicting health outcomes among older Australian women.

Globalisation allied to fast communications systems allows academic and practitioner knowledge to become dispensed rapidly around the world. Over the last 5 to 10 years countries world wide have been exposed to an emerging literature around the phenomena of elder abuse and neglect. However, it is also clear that different countries socially construct social problems in different ways. Therefore, empirical knowledge alone is insufficient to legitimate a social problem: the political climate needs to be receptive for that social problem to be addressed in social policy terms. This invited symposium brings together researchers from the UK, USA, Germany, Spain, Australia and Japan. Within each of these countries elder abuse has been acknowledged; however, the empirical knowledge base varies. The aim of this symposium is to expose recent research to a wider global audience, allowing comparisons and contrasts to be made cross-culturally. There will be 5 presentations of 15 minutes duration followed by a 15 minute discussion. Dr Rosalie Wolf will consider the findings of a 1999 nation-wide survey of Adult Protective Services to estimate the number of complaints and substantiated cases . The data also detail types of abuse, sources of referrals, demographics of victims, penalties for failure to report, time frame for investigation, changes in legislation. Dr Thomas Geoergen will report the findings of a multi-method study aimed at collecting data on the types and frequency of elder abuse and neglect in German nursing homes using qualitative interviews and surveys. In a pilot study among nursing home staff, 79% of subjects report having abused or neglected at least one resident during the last 12 months. Dr Schofield reports on the first large scale Australian community study to examine longitudinally the relationship between vulnerability to abuse and health outcomes among older women. A nationally representative sample of over 12,000 older women were screened in 1996 for vulnerability to elder abuse, using a brief self-report screening measure. The purpose of the study reported by Dr Toshio Tatara is to find out the nature and extent of elder abuse research activities in Japan through a review of research reports, published materials, and interviews with elder abuse researchers. The preliminary findings show that there has been progress in understanding the nature and dynamics of the problem but little information about the prevalence and incidence. Additionally, there are no systems. to speak of, which can prevent and treat elder abuse in Japan. Dr Bazo reports the first results of a research in progress about elder neglect and mistreatment in Spain. A sample of 98 abused elderly suffering from some sort of health problems and dependency are examined. 111 mistreatment cases have been detected by the home workers among 2,351 persons assisted by the Community Services (4.7%). Three main conclusions emerge: a) the nature of mistreatment differs by types; b) neglect and mistreatment may be associated with dependence; and c) gender, i.e, being a woman, may be a more influential risk factor than being dependent.

The experience of conflict and ambivalence in intergenerational exchange.

P. Kingston, J. Phillips and M. Ray (all Keele University, UK)

In this paper we discuss the role of conflict and ambivalence between parents and their adult offspring. Numerous scholars have argued that intergenerational family conflict has been an enduring facet of Western history. A discourse of ambivalence can be traced through for example, policy debate in relation to older people and the future of the welfare state and welfare 'rationing'. However, research which attempts to conceptualise and operationalise conflict and ambivalence in the context of intergenerational relations is in its genesis. This study attempts to take the current knowledge base further. We explore as preliminary hypotheses that intergenerational relationships in cultures increasingly influenced by 'job culture' will inevitably be coloured by ambivalent feelings. Further, we speculate that ambivalence will be experienced by older people receiving support and care from younger family members focused on a discourse of burden and loss of independence. Younger and older family members providing regular care and support to other family members are more likely to experience ambivalent feelings about notions of duty set against increasingly complex and diverse roles and responsibilities. At this stage, our results and discussions are inevitably preliminary. We make use of initial analysis of questionnaires administered to participants (N=1200) in each of five participating countries (Israel, Spain, Norway, Germany, UK). We focus attention on the components of the questionnaire which specifically address conflict and ambivalence. In addition, we present analysis from qualitative data which, using both biographical approaches and vignettes asking participants to reflect on their experiences and attitudes about family values in relation to intergenerational exchange and support.

The National Elder Abuse Report Survey 2000

Rosalie S. Wolf (UMass Memorial Health Care, Worcester, MA, USAA) Eva Kutas (National Association of Adult Protective Services Administrators, Salem, OR, USA) Paula Mixson (Texas Dept. of Protective & Regulatory Services, Austin, TX, USA)

PURPOSE: This survey is a follow-up of earlier efforts to estimate the number of elder abuse reports nationwide investigated and substantiated by Adult Protective Services programs (APS). METHOD: A mailed (emailed) survey questionnaire was completed by the 50 state APS program directors, plus the District of Columbia and Guam. RESULTS: Over 350,000 complaints were investigated in 1999 and 131, 206 validated (based on 33 states). Friends were most often the source of reports followed by law enforcement and health care professionals. 48% of reports were for self-neglect and 17.8% for caregiver neglect,11.5% for physical abuse and financial exploitation, 9.7%, emotional abuse, and 1.4%, sexual abuse.. Other information dealt with the demographics of victims, penalties for failure to report, time frame for investigation, changes in legislation, settings where APS has authority for investigation, . CONCLUSION: The findings underscore the difficulties in trying to obtain a national picture from 50 different state programs. They also point out the need for better APS data management information systems and national standards.

Vulnerability to Elder Abuse: Predicting Health Outcomes Among Older Australian Women

Margot J. Schofield (University of New England, Armidale Australia), Gita D. Mishra (Cambridge University, Cambridge, UK).

Purpose: The Women's Health Australia study is the first large scale community study to examine longitudinally the relationship between vulnerability to abuse and health outcomes among older women. This presentation examines relationships between baseline vulnerability scores and health outcomes three years later. Methods: A nationally representative sample of over 12,000 older women in the Australian Longitudinal Study on Women's Health were screened in 1996 for vulnerability to elder abuse, using a brief self-report screening measure. This was part of a mailed survey comprising over 200 items covering demographic, psychosocial and health variables. There was a three year follow-up mailed survey with a telephone follow-up to maximise cohort retention. Results: Validation of the baseline abuse screening measure identified four factors, each of three items, representing the following domains: 'vulnerability', 'dependence', 'dejection' and 'coercion'. This presentation examines the relationships between baseline vulnerability factor scores and follow-up measures of physical and mental health, including the SF-36 quality of life survey, and measures of health conditions and health service use. The predictive validity of the 12-item screening instrument and a shorter 6-item version controlling for potential demographic, psychosocial and health confounders will be reported. Conclusion: The valuable policy and service delivery implications of this large community cohort study will be discussed.

SESSION 136

Validation of an exceptional male longevity area in Sardinia

Michel Poulain

A recent genetic study on Sardinian centenarians has shown figures where the prevalence of centenarians in Sardinia was very high and the sex ratio very low. As an example, in the Nuoro Province, Deiana and al. (1999) present data with 2.4 centenarians per ten thousand inhabitants and a sex ratio of 1.1 female centenarian per male centenarian. That was the starting point of a large validation process and demographic analysis developed during the year 2000 and the results will be presented for the first time during this symposium. The first presentation by Michel Poulain will report on the full validation process of all data related to the Sardinian centenarians. Thereafter he will demonstrate that the prevalence is totally inappropriate to estimate the longevity within a given population where migration flows are important as it is the case in Sardinia. Therefore he introduces as longevity index the proportion of new born that reach the age 100 in the cohorts born between 1880 and 1899 in a given place. This index shows an exceptional male longevity compared to similar data in Belgium and Denmark. We calculate an longevity index as high as 135 centenarians per million new born compared to 124 in Denmark and 60 in Belgium. When calculating the same calculation at communal level it appears that the longevity index may be as high as 700 in a group of 9 communes located in a mountain area in the Province of Nuoro. In this particular area we have identify 33 male centenarians for only 23 female centenarians all of them were born in these villages between 1880 and 1899. These numbers are to be compared with the expected numbers of centenarians based on Danish longevity index: 6 males and 20 females. By extending this approach to all Sardinian communes, we will identify an area in the central mountainous part of Sardinia with a population experiencing an exceptional longevity. All previous reports of exceptionally longlived populations have been invalidated by careful demographic research, including Abkhazia in Caucasia, the village of Vilcabamba in Ecuador, the Hunza population in Kashmir, and the Japanese island of Okinawa (e.g, Mazess and Foreman 1979; Palmore 1984). Age exaggeration was often observed in past populations and still is commonly observed in populations without careful civil registration. Age misreporting generally increases with age and is usually more often observed among males than females. And finally we will point out for the longevity area similar survival probabilities after 50 years for male and female with in consequence similar numbers of male and female centenarians and a sex ratio close to one. As a conclusion this exceptional male longevity definitively launches the explanatory research suggesting that complex gene-gene and gene-environment interactions are responsible for the longevity phenotype, together with socio-economical and other contextual characteristics.

Some bioclinical and genetic characteristics of the Sardinian centenarians

Gianni PES

In the third contribution, Gianni PES will present some bioclinical characteristics of the Sardinian centenarians based on the results of the AKEA study. Thereafter the results of various biochemical investigations in blood samples as well as in cells, will be presented based on routine haematological test, markers of inflammation (cytokines, coagulation factors), other specific tests, including a full endocrinology assessment, bone markers, cardiovascular risk markers (lipids & lipoproteins, Lp(a), plasma homocysteine, markers of endothelial damage), plasma redox status, antioxidants and vitamins. Considerable research has been done to identify candidate genes. As reviewed by DeBenedictis, Jeune, Christensen, Vaupel, Yashin et al. (in press), 13 genes with polymorphisms associated with longevity had been reported in at least one study by the middle of the year 2000. The best known of these genes and the one with the largest impact is ApoE. Even this gene, however, has a modest impact on mortality. Studies in several countries are consistent with the conclusion that the ApoE2 polymorphism may lower annual death rates at older ages by about 10% and the ApoE4 polymorphism may raise rates by about 10%. A genetic characterisation of the centenarians will be presented in order to identify the genes responsible for the high longevity rate and the unique F/M ratio of Sardinian centenarians.

The AKEA research project and two male supercentenarians alive in Sardinia

Ciriaco CARRU

In the second contribution, Ciriaco CARRU will present the AKEA research project based on 141 sardinian centenarians with the survey questionnaire and the different analysis that have been developed. Thereafter he will summarize the data collected on the two male supercentenarians alive in Sardinia : Antonio TODDE born in January 1889 living in Tiana and declared by the Guinness last year as the oldest validated man living in the world and Giovanni FRAU born in December 1990 and living in Orolli. First of all it is remarkable that there are no female supercentenarians (aged 110+) in Sardinia while among a hundred of supercentenarians alive around the world, at least four out of five are females. Moreover these two male supercentenarians are living in the longevity area within a total population of approximately one hundred thousands inhabitants. These elements confirm the exceptionality of the male longevity in this area. A comparative presentation of the two supercentenarians will be presented mainly on a bioclinical and genetical points of view but also on socio-economic characteristics, nutrition habits and living arrangements.

Towards a more integrated analysis of the male exceptional longevity in Sardinia

Claudio FRANCESCHI

The fourth contribution will be delivered by Claudio FRANCESCHI will be based on the identification of a longevity area in the mountainous part of Sardinia with the hope that this identification will contribute to the first preliminary explanations of this high male longevity. Genetic factors, epidemiologic variables, socio-economic indicators and all life course demographic information will be taken into consideration in order to understand this exceptional and unique situation around the World as up to now no other longevous population has been fully validated. A key question is whether the explanation for this longevity is at the individual level, with heterogeneous populations in all areas of Sardinia, but with some areas having a greater proportion of individuals with the influential attributes. Or are there more or less homogeneous areas, with everyone in some areas having a relatively good chance of surviving from 80 to 100. That is, are there some people with a 25% chance of surviving from 80 to 100 whereas most people only have a 1% chance? Or, alternatively, are there areas where almost everyone has a 10% chance and other regions where almost everyone has a 2% chance.. The male advantage after age 80 in the central region of Sardinia, if confirmed, would be unique. All other regions of allegedly high male longevity have been shown to be artifacts of bad data or inappropriate analysis. Even if the males on Sardinia or some region of Sardinia do not have an advantage over females after age 80 but suffer death rates close to female levels, this would be of great interest. Low male mortality at oldest-old ages could be due to some factor that helps males survive but does not (much) improve female survival chances. Alternatively, there could be some factors that help both males and females, coupled with some deleterious factors that only females suffer. At what age does the male survival advantage in the central region of Sardinia start? Is this advantage a recent development? Can the male advantage be linked to earlier cohort selection or debilitation or is it a period phenomenon? Which causes of death contribute to the differential between male and female survival? Which environmental, economic, and social characteristics of communes are linked with survival? Can a particular pattern of age-specific, sex-specific, cause-specific, area-specific and perhaps period or cohort-specific mortality in the central region of Sardinia or for Sardinia as a whole be identified? Early-life events have a major impact on late-life survival. Very little information is available, however, that connects early-life events with exceptional longevity. And the precise nature of the early-life events that affect adult survival is still controversial and not fully understood (e.g, Kannisto et al. 1997; Christensen et al. 1995; Vaupel et al. 1998). Furthermore, data are available on the environmental, economic, and social characteristics of all the communes of Sardinia, so studies can be done on which ecological factors may affect longevity. In the ongoing AKEA research project we will gather demographic information about survival rates, archival data about early-life events, questionnaire data about individual characteristics, medical data, genetic information, and ecological data about the environmental, social, and economic characteristics of the places the subjects live. We want to analyse these data in an integrative, coherent way to explore possible determinants of longevity and particularly this exceptional male longevity.

SESSION 137

Injury Prevention Programs for Older Drivers: Preventing Injuries, Promoting Mobility

Allen R. Dobbs, (DriveABLE Assessment Centres and University of Alberta, Edmonton, Canada) Bonnie M. Dobbs, (University of Alberta, Edmonton, Canada)

The private automobile is the most common means of transportation for seniors. In fact, seniors rely more on the private automobile for transportation than do people in younger age groups. Unfortunately, aging is associated with an increased probability of illness and even the best of drivers can become unsafe when medical conditions impair abilities requisite for driving safely. It has been especially difficult to judge when a driver is no longer safe to drive when the medical conditions affect mental abilities. The decision is especially difficult if the persons mobility, independence, and access to services would be negatively affected, especially if the criteria for continued fitness-to-drive are determined only by consensus judgements. This suggests that progress toward fair and effective injury prevention programs needs to address two issues: Mobility for those who are no longer safe to drive, and assessment criteria that go beyond expert opinion. A program addressing both of these issues will be described. Research-based driver assessment procedures form the core of the program. These assessment procedures are consistent with recent judicial decisions and have become the standard for medically at-risk drivers in one Canadian province and are accepted in several others.

Older drivers, health and mobility

D O'Neill (Trinity College Dublin, Ireland)

This presentation will give an overview of ageing, health and personal transportation. It will provide essential background to the development of scientific inquiry in the area. This will include data compiled for a 2001

OECD report as well as a 2001 report from the United States Transportation Research Board. This will include the delineation of the most important question, the impingement of personal transport options by age-related disease. A secondary area is the appreciation of the undue importance given to risk in the literature on the older driver. This is the basis of screening programmes (widespread in the European Union) which may negatively impact on the personal liberty, mobility and health of older people.

Older drivers, health and mobility

K Tallman, BL Beattie (University of British Columbia, Canada)

Will present data about the evaluation of fitness to drive using our data emphasizing performannce based evaluation from our data and the negotiation of transportation alternatives

Older drivers, health and mobility needs

D O'Neill (Trinity College Dublin, Ireland)

This presentation will give an overview of ageing, health and personal transportation from differing perspectives, including government, older drivers, geriatricians and neuropsychologists. Older drivers are the safest group of drivers and show themselves to be very responsible in their approach to driving. however, they suffer disproportionately from their frailty if involved in crashes. The challenge to society is to enable older people to be maximally mobile in a manner determined by themselves. This symposium will draw on new research examining how personal mobility needs can be best met in the 21st century.

Understanding problems of older drivers

Patrick Rabbitt, Paul Sutcliffe, Dianne Parker and Loraine Macdonald

We describe a 5-year longitudinal questionnaire study on 340 drivers aged from 60 to 82, and a larger study in which 1900 drivers in this age range completed a questionnaire listing difficulties they encounter while driving and the Cornell Medical Inventory, 500 of these completed 41 different laboratory tests that have been widely used as predictors of driving competence, and 200 of these were twice tested for driving competence on the road. The results suggest that older motorists are sensitive to changes in their own competence, and that most such changes are associated with changes in general health status, and performance on tests of physiological integrity, rather than with calendar age, per se.

SESSION 138

MENTAL FITNESS FOR LIFE: The Key to Vital Aging.

W.J.A. Thompson (Simon Fraser Health Region, New Westminster, Canada) Moderator; J. Blaine (Century House, New Westminster, Canada) Giving your Brain a Mental Fitness Warmup; S. Cusack (Simon Fraser University, Vancouver, Canada); MENTAL FITNESS FOR LIFE: Assessing the Impact of an 8-week Mental Fitness Course; J. Ebert (Century House, New Westminster, Canada) CREATIVE THINKING: Getting out of the Box; B. Guttmann-Gee (Century House, New Westminster, Canada) GOALSETTING: Aging with Purpose and Passion; F. Hogg (Century House, New Westminster, Canada) Enhancing Learning and Memory; G. Hurst (Century House, New Westminster, Canada) CRITICAL THINKING: Erasing and Replacing Limiting Beliefs; D. Josey (Century House, New Westminster, Canada) Developing a Positive Mental Attitude (PMA); E. Keilbart (Century House, New Westminster, Canada) GOALSETTING: Getting Where You Want to Go; P. Mowat (Century House, New Westminster, Canada) MENTALLY FIT FOR LIFE: New Research with a Positive View of the Aging Brain; K. Warner Schaie (Pennsylvia State University, University Park, USA) Respondent.

ISSUE: The challenge of population aging is to embrace the extended lifespan as an unprecedented triumph and to develop the human potential for continuing purposeful, productive engagement to the end of life, whether that comes at 80, 90, or 120. Recent research on the brain and cognition suggests that mental decline is not inevitable — indeed, mental abilities can continue to develop to the end of life, when stimulated and challenged. Inspired by the work of American researchers such as Marion Diamond, Mark Pippenger, David Nussbaum, Arnold Scheibel, K. Warner Schaie, and David Snowdon, the research and development of Mental Fitness programs for seniors spans a period of seven years. The purpose of this symposium is (1) to describe the research and development of programs; (2) to outline the seven critical components of Mental Fitness and (3) to summarize the benefits of the program from the perspective of (a) participants, and (b) the analysis of pre and posttest scores on measures of healthy aging. Results from standard measures of health suggest the Mental Fitness program has a significant effect on memory, self-esteem, and confidence.

STRUCTURE OF THE SESSION: Mental Fitness participants, (ages 65 to 87) will introduce the critical components of the" Mental Fitness for Life" program, drawing on personal experience to explain practical application and benefits. J. Blaine leads a mental fitness warmup exercise; S. Cusack summarizes research that suggests a Mental Fitness program has a powerful impact on healthy, productive aging; J. Ebert introduces the topic of creativity and describes a personal "out of the box" experience; B. Guttmann-Gee takes a lifespan perspective on goalsetting and its relationship to purpose and health; F. Hogg describes her personal experience with learning and memory; G. Hurst defines critical thinking as a method for creating change; D. Josey explains how she got PMA; E. Keilbart outlines a process of goalsetting and achieving; P. Mowat highlights research that is optimistic and empowering; K. Warner Schaie responds to the panel presentations, suggesting implications for future research and practice.

CONCLUSION: Our primary objective is to showcase a uniquely Canadian model of lifelong learning, the Mental Fitness for Life program, which is research-based, empowers seniors, and emphasizes an optimistic view of healthy aging. In taking a grass roots approach and including the personal experience of senior advocates, we expect to reach a broad audience of professionals and seniors from around the world. We intend to make vital connections that lead to future collaborations and partnerships and serve to move third age education higher on the international agenda.

Giving Your Brain a Mental Fitness Warmup

J. Blaine (Century House, New Westminster, Canada)

Like physical fitness, the way to become mentally fit for the rest of your life depends on vigorous exercise. Every mental fitness class provides a variety of games and puzzles that are designed to give the brain a workout. The mental fitness word game is designed as an interactive opener for a mental fitness class. It is a warm-up exercise for the brain comparable to warm-up stretches that are recommended before physical activity. The Mensa Group, an organization founded in the UK for and by people with intelligence quotients in the upper 5th percentile, is a source of puzzles and games that work well for a mental fitness class of participants with diverse educational backgrounds. In the beginning of an 8-week Mental Fitness for Life program, the questions are easier to ensure that every participant will experience success. The emphasis is on participation rather than knowledge. As the weeks go by, the exercises become increasingly more difficult. The purpose of this presentation is to give World Congress participants a brief mental fitness warmup.

MENTAL FITNESS FOR LIFE: Assessing the Impact of an 8-week Mental Fitness Course

S. A. Cusack (Simon Fraser University, Vancouver Canada), K.J.Oakley (University of Ottawa Institute on Health of the Elderly, Ottawa, Ontario, Canada) and W.J.A. Thompson (Simon Fraser Health Region, New Westminster, Canada).

The research and development of Mental Fitness programs spans seven years beginning with a grass roots research project in the context of Century House, a 2100-member seniors recreation centre in Western Canada. This paper briefly describes the evolution of programs in six phases, outlines the seven critical components of Mental Fitness, and summarizes the benefits of the program based on (a) anecdotal evidence derived from participant observation records, focus groups, written evaluations, and (b) pre and post test scores on four standard measures of health. The focus is on 18 participants (aged 62 85, average age 72) who completed the most recent 8-week introductory program, (Cusack & Thompson, 2000). The program includes the following topics, goal setting, critical thinking, creative thinking, positive mental attitude, speaking your mind, learning and memory. As in previous programs, anecdotal evidence attests to improved memory and self-confidence, enhanced self-esteem, and more positive attitudes. In addition, pre and post program measures on Rosenberg's Self-esteem Scale, Oakley's Self-confidence Scale, Bradley's Depression Subscale, and Cusack-Thompson's Mental Fitness Self-assessment Scale support anecdotal evidence, that the Mental Fitness for Life program has a statistically significant positive effect on self-esteem, self-confidence in their mental abilities, and improved memory. Depression scores did not reach significance, due to the substantial increase in one of the depression scores and small sample size. In conclusion, developing mental fitness exercises body, mind, and spirit and we believe it is the key to vital aging in the 21st century. Future directions include adapting and piloting the program in other contexts (e.g, persons with early stage Alzheimers) and other countries; and further testing of the effect of a mental fitness program on various measures of healthy aging.

CREATIVE THINKING: Getting out of the Box

J. Ebert (Century House, New Westminster, Canada)

Creative thinking is the third critical component of mental fitness, and it follows logically from critical thinking. Participants are encouraged to eliminate old ways of thinking about aging and replace them with new knowledge that serves them well. Creativity is the result of new and unique ways of expressing oneself in the world. A tradition of scientific research suggests that creativity peaks at the height of mental powers, in your 30's, 40's, or 50's, depending upon what you are creating. However, new research links creative self-expression with healthy aging. Thinking and acting "out of the box" is now a positive activity that has many benefits to individuals and groups at all stages of the lifecycle. Puzzles and games that are part of a mental fitness class give participants the courage to climb out of the box and think and act in unique and delightful ways. This brief presentation describes a unique "out of the box" experience that had positive emotional benefits, bringing joy, vitality, and an enhanced willingness to take new risks.

CRITICAL THINKING: A Process for Erasing Limiting Beliefs.

G. Hurst (Century House, New Westminster, Canada)

Critical thinking is the second component of mental fitness, and it is a method or process for building a sound knowledge basefor vital aging. Many older adults have grown up and grown old with beliefs about declining mental abilities with age. Critical thinking is a process for calling into question the underlying customary ways of thinking and acting. Critical thinking is a process, not an outcome. Being a critical thinker entails a continual questioning of assumptions as we begin to reinterpret our past actions and ideas from a new vantage point. Manifestations of critical thinking vary according to the context in which it occurs. Some attitudes that are necessary preconditions for being critical include curiosity, flexibility, skepticism and honesty. It is the ability to distinguish bias from reason and fact from opinion. The emotions emotional responses, sensing, intuition are all part of critical thinking in adult life. Critical thinking is triggered by positive as well as negative events. It is a lived activity, not an abstract academic pastime. As our beliefs are generally self-fulfilling prophecies, the ability to think critically is a logical process that helps us establish strong, positive ways of thinking and being in the world.

Developing a Positive Mental Attitude (PMA)

D. Josey (Century House, New Westminster, Canada)

Generally, the purpose of educational programs is to build new knowledge, skills, and/or attitudes. Developing knowledge requires that we exercise our learning skills: building new skills requires practice and commitment. Often, we believe that changing attitudes will follow new knowledge and skill development. We used to believe that some people are born with a positive attitude and others have a negative attitude. That's just the way we are. Now we know that optimism, like pessimism, can be learned. Seligman's work on "learned optimism" is used to change negative attitudes that have been developed over a lifetime to positive attitudes about our own aging and possibilities for continued personal development. This brief presentation describes the evolving positive mental attitude of one member of the program. It also attests to the benefits of PMA to mind, body, and spirit. PMA may also assist the individual in making a speedy recovery from an illness. With PMA, the individual is always anticipating better things ahead.

GOALSETTING: Aging with Purpose and Passion

B. Guttmann-Gee (Century House, New Westminster, Canada)

Goalsetting is arguably the most important component of the Mental Fitness program and new research suggests that setting goals is related to healthy aging. The roots of research on goalsetting are found in McClelland's early work on achievement motivation; and more recently Lapierre et al. (1997) focused on the relationship between longterm projects and a sense of meaning in life. Strong correlations are reported between purpose in life and psychological well-being. Goalsetting is a thread that runs through every workshop in the Mental Fitness for Life program. Goals can be simple and short term, and they can be grand and related to one's personal purpose or mission in life. Goals that class participants have undertaken include short term goals such as quitting smoking, losing weight, keeping a journal, exploring creativity through the arts, developing a more positive attitude, memorizing poetry, becoming a standup comedienne, researching one's family tree. What is missing in the literature is a lifelong perspective on setting goals in the context of an individual life — the purpose of this presentation is to describe one woman's experience with goalsetting, large and small, across the life span.

GOALSETTING: Getting Where You Want to Go.

E. Keilbart (Century House, New Westminster, Canada)

Goalsetting is an exercise and a process for getting where you want to go. Many older adults have had goals throughout their lifetime, and others never set goals. Many older people today have survived by living from challenge to challenge, from day to day, responding to what was expected of them. Goalsetting is not something they may have practiced throughout their earlier years, and they may need to experience what a dynamic tool it is for getting things done. It's a 10-step process for getting where you want to go. Goals are like maps, they keep you on course and help you to clarify what is important in your life. Goals are like magnets, they attract things and people that help to get them accomplished. Accomplishing a goal that you have set for yourself feels good, and gives you the confidence to achieve more than you ever thought you could.

MENTAL FITNESS FOR LIFE: Enhancing Learning and Memory

F. Hogg (Century House, New Westminster, Canada)

The sixth and seventh critical components of Mental Fitness are learning and memory. You may wonder why they are introduced as topics at the end of a Mental Fitness program. You may also wonder why they are introduced in the same workshop session. All of the elements of mental fitness are intimately and intricately interconnected, but learning and memory are inseparable. If you don't remember something, you probably have not learned it. Good learning skills and habits ensure that we remember what we have a mind to. The purpose of this presentation is to show how concentration helps us learn, which subsequently strengthens memory. The speaker draws on personal experience to illustrate the concentration required to learn successfully, so that memory remains vital. Scenarios are drawn from personal experiences in civic and organizational contexts, extensive travels, and success in embracing the new technological age. By using all of the components of mental fitness, goalsetting, critical thinking, positive thinking, and creativity, and taking personal risks, she was more secure in her ability to learn and remember. Ultimately, life is enhanced and empowered by a greater confidence and ability to meet the future.

MENTAL FITNESS FOR LIFE: New Research with a Positive View of the Aging Brain

P. Mowat (Century House, New Westminster, Canada)

We can all agree that all kinds of exercise is necessary if we want to go on living to a healthy old age. That's certainly true for physical fitness. But its an effort to be disciplined enough to plan and maintain an exercise program. The thought of it is so boring. Who wants to do anything just because it's "good for you". Throughout our lifetime, we have been taught to expect a steady decline in our mental abilities as we age. Once we get to our 80's, we can expect to "lose it". Now we know that was wrong. Totally wrong. The best news has come to us through recent scientific research into the function of the brain. It is common knowledge that we only use a very small portion of our brain cells. If cells are injured or die, we are limited, sometimes to the degree of helplessness. Recent news tells us that the brain is capable of alerting new channels, growing new dendrites, to parts of the brain that have not as yet been activated. I picture this organ (the brain) like a vast musical instrument awaiting its own motivation to play upon it, to exercise it, to learn to draw forth beautiful music even to compose new tunes. In a mental fitness program, we are researching ourselves, exploring new frontiers, taking new risks, and achieving new goals. And we stand before you as living testaments that the program works.

SESSION 139

Cardiovascular Disease in the Elderly: Update in the Management

Choel-Ho KIM(Seoul National University,Seoul,Korea - "Current status of cardiovascular diseases in Korean Elderly") Masaru Yanai and Hidetada Sasaki(Tohoku University ,Sendai,Japan - "Prevention and treatment of pneumonia in the elderly")Seungbum KIM and Yasuyoshi Ouchi (Tokyo University,Tokyo,Japan - "Cardiovascularaging as a cause of cardivascular disease in old age") Yoshinosuke Fukuch (Juntendo University,Tokyo,Japan - "Greater burden of COPD in Japan")

This symposium will address the issues of the practical approaches in cardiovascular/pulmonary disease in the elderly. The speakers will first discuss cardinal features of age changes associated with physiological aging,followed by most updated diagnostic/therapeutic modalities in both the heart and the lung illness.

The structure of the symposium will follow concise and clear-cut descriptions regarding those main issues as mentioned above. Each speaker is asked to present their lectures in 15 minutes with additional discussion in 5 minutes. Dr.CH KIM will review the current status of cardiovascular disease in the elderly in Korea. Epidemiology and treatment strategy commonly adopted in his country will be discussed with some provisional proposals regarding future improvement. Dr.Yanai and Sasaki will present both basic and clinical evidence of pharmacotherapy for aspiration pneumonia. He will try to convince the audience that brain disorder is responsible in the majority of micro aspiration causing life threatening pneumonia in old age. Drs.Sb KIM and Ouchi will demonstrate significant influences of aging on cardiovascular functions at macro/micro levels. They will provide some of the evidences that may increase the incidence as well as the magnitude of cardiovascular diseases commonly found in the elderly. Dr.Fukuchi will tackle the issue of prevalence of COPD in Japan that has been reported to be very low as compared to other industrialized countries with comparable smoking rate. Multicenter population based prevalence study for COPD was completed recently in Japan.The result disclosed that COPD is found in more than 5 million of Japanese over 40 years of age,in nearly 9 % of the population of this age blanket. This will urge the medical community of Japan to be more concerned about great health burden of the illness .

At the end of the symposium,the audience should be better informed and equipped with most updated modalities in diagnosis as well as management of cardio/pulmonary diseases in the elderly.

SESSION 140

Oral Taking of Medicines by the Elderly

Babberih Y, Merrot S, Pivion M-C, Frigard B, Centre de Gériatrie - Wasquehal, France

Oral taking of medicines is concerning too by elderly subjects dependance and leads frequently staff to use subterfuges to make sure of the effective grip of the therapeutic. This study has for objective to estimate frequency, modalities, documentary evidences of this practice and pharmacocinétics repercussions. A "given-day " inquiry gathered 11 hospitable structures (768 subjects, 82y.) A phone inquiry was at the same time led with the pharmaceutical industry. 14,6 % take themselves their therapeutics. For others it is inevitable to déconditionner, what is legally forbidden. For 21,7 % galénic modification is usual by the opening of capsules or by crushing pills. Pharmacocinétic is affected by this practice and more still when "mixture" is incorporated into food or warm liquids (coffee, soup,...) tepid or cold (yoghourts, gel water, compotes...). This practice is not correlated to medicines number (sometimes very high). To justify this custom, staff evokes the certainty of taking, gulp disorders, confusionnel state, opposition, rapidity of administration. Errors are so committed for the forms to prolonged liberation, real "errors of taste" are provoked, as for the pharmacocinétique... Even the consulted laboratories can not define the half-life of a capsule "effect-delay" opened and mixed in a (sometimes) boiling coffee... It only remains to convince pharmaceutical industry to find an oral presentation better adapted to this population and to persuade authorities to appreciate importance of time past male nurse daily for these essentials tasks.

Medication-Related Problems in the Elderly, Defining the Issues, Identifying Solutions

William Simonson (President, American Society of Consultant Pharmacists) (Alexandria, Virginia, USA)

Purpose: Only recently has the impact of medication-related problems (MRP)in the elderly been fully appreciated. Negative outcomes include decreased quality of life, and increased morbidity and mortality. The economic impact of MRP in elderly nursing home residents has been estimated at more than $4 billion per year and a total of more than $80 billion per year in the outpatient population. Method: Using a power point presentation, the speaker will review the types of MRP that may occur in the elderly and will assess their potential impact on health, quality of life and economics. The management and prevention of these problems through an interdisciplinary effort will be reviewed. Results: It has been found that through interdisciplinary cooperation between pharmacists, other health professionals, and family members, medication-related problems can be assessed, understood, modified, and corrected. This presentation will review medication-related problems and their impact in the elderly and will explore how caregivers and family members can work in an interdisciplinary approach to improve drug therapy, minimize adverse outcomes, and enhance the quality of life in the elderly. Conclusion: The speaker will discuss resources that are available to solve potentially complex medication-related problems and will provide practical guidelines on how caregivers and family members can work together to improve drug therapy of the elderly

Overdosage of oral anticoagulant treatment in the elderly: a retrospective study of 83 cases

C. Perret-Guillaume (Médecine B, CHU Nancy, France), B. Hanesse (Médecine B), M. Frédéric (Médecine H, CHU Nancy, France), O. Cézard (Médecine B), M.C. Schmal-Laurain (Médecine B), C. Schmidt (Médecine H), D. Wahl (Médecine H), F. Paille (Médecine B), J.D. de Korwin (Médecine H), F. Pénin (Médecine B), G. Thibaut (Médecine H).

Our purpose was to study characteristics of patients older than 65 years old presenting an oral anticoagulant overdosage (excluding first week of treatment) in two different internal medicine units. We wanted to determine factors influencing the severity of bleeding. We retrospectively analysed 83 cases during 14 years. A major bleeding was defined as: neurologic or digestive bleeding, hematoma, shock, death or necessity of blood transfusion. The mean age of patients was 80.4 years (7.9 SD), with a sex ratio of 1.8 female / 1 male. The mean INR was 9.1. No bleeding was observed in 21.7% of cases, a minor bleeding in 24.1% and a major bleeding in 54.2%. We noted an ecchymosis in 16 cases, hematuria in 12, digestive hemorrhage in 20, hematoma in 16, death in 8. The oral anticoagulant was definitively stopped in 48.2% of cases. Patients received vitamine K1 in 47% and a blood transfusion in 37.3% of cases. In univariate analysis comparing minor and major accidents (Pearson Chisquare and analysis of variance) a statistic link was found between the occurence of a major hemorrhage and an history of gastrointestinal bleeding ($p=0.05$), a longer APTT ($p=0.02$) or a lower protidemia ($p=0.04$). In multivariate analysis a longer APTT and a lower protidemia remained statistically linked to the severity of bleeding. Oral anticoagulant treatment overdosage is severe in the elderly (death in 9.6% of cases in our study). The severity of bleeding seems much linked to APTT than PTT prolongation. We noted the importance of an history of gastrointestinal bleeding or denutrition.

Particular Aspects of Digoxin Intoxication in Patients of Different Ages

C.R.Revnic (U.M.F."Carol Davila", Bucharest, Romania) G.Onose, F.Revnic, ("Ana Aslan"N.I.G.G,Bucharest,Romania) C.Zeana (Emergency Hospital,Bucharest,Romania)

Introduction: Many innotropic agents have been experimented in patients with cardiac disases.Nevertheless cardiac glycosides represent one of the most common and safe drugs.Digitalis overdosage is frequently found in medical practice.this isresponsable sometimes for patient death. elderly patients have an increase sensitivity towards digitalis especially because of the cardiac amiloidosys and the tendency towards arithmias.The aim of our study was concerned with investigation of clinical and paraclinical manifestations of voluntary digoxin intoxication as well as in elderly patients with overdosage of digoxin. design and methods:Two groups of patients have been taken in our study:groupA(17 cases:15 female and 2 male)related with the observation of clinical and paraclinical manifestations of voluntary intoxication with digoxin on healthy heart and on group B(7 cases) has the aim of investigating clinical and paraclinical manifestations of digoxin overdosage comparatively in patients withlong term treatment with digoxin with different associated pathologies over a three years period.Digoxinemia has been estimated with a fluoroimmunoassay method involving monoclonal antibodies with a DELFIA Research Spectrofluorimeter 1234 and the results have been processed with a FIA program. Results and discussion:Both,the acute intoxication with Digoxin in healthy subjects as well as the digoxin overdosage is characterised by a complex symptomatology represented by gastrointestinal visual as well as neuropsihic perturbations,besides the cardiac ones.Between the manifestation of intoxications with digoxin (suicide tentative with (unique and high doses)and the clinical picture of therapeutical intoxication are great differences.From cardiotoxic point of view ,in the first category are included severe conduction perturbations.In voluntary intoxications EKG modifications appear late,long time after dessapearance of clinical signs(sometimes at two weeks).The main cause of overdosage has been related with renal insufficiency with fixed nitrogen retention unknown by the patient and becouse of nonadjustement of digoxin dose according with kidney state.An increase in plasma K^+ and Mg^{++} has been noticed in voluntary intoxication ,due to their massive liberation from tissues.In the case of therapeutical overdosage ,hipoK^+ as well as hypo-Mg^{++} lowers serum level of digoxin at which appear toxic phenomenos.Overdosage manifestations being nonspecific,digoxinemia can clarify the origin of some perturbations contributing to diagnosis establishment. Neurological and dyspeptic symptoms are frequently seen in digitalis intoxication and represent main indexes of drug toxicity not related to EKG data.The patients with main dyspeptic symptoms seem to be older than the neurological ones Although,gastroenterical disturbances are often difficult to be discriminated in elderly,these symptoms deserve particular atention in monitoring digitalis therapy.

Quality Pharmaceutical Care: A Key Contributor to the Resident's Quality of Life and Comfort

Netha Dyck and Penny Murray (Winnipeg Regional Health Authority, Winnipeg, Manitoba, Canada)

The quality of pharmacy services provided to the residents by 38 personal care homes (PCH) in Winnipeg and the 5 contracted pharmacy services was assessed to facilitate optimum pharmaceutical care and promote resident comfort and quality of life. The standards review process included self-assessment by each PCH, using a tool based on current pharmacy standards, an analysis of drug utilization and cost, a site visit, and a detailed report for each of 38 PCHs. Several quality indicators were established and are being monitored. This review process provided data for analysis, and benchmarking for the pharmaceutical effectiveness of the pharmacy providers. The site visit provided opportunity for direct interaction with staff and included an audit of medication practices. The comprehensive report summarized the findings of the self assessment and site visit, and detailed the PCH position in relation to other PCHs within Winnipeg. Results revealed a high level of compliance with the established Manitoba Standards for Pharmacy Service in PCHs in Winnipeg. Drug utilization statistics have revealed variable usage in expected areas of behaviour management and specific disease areas. Average cost factors have also been tracked. Quality indicators are being monitored across the PCH Program and quality improvement opportunities have been identified. In conclusion, the standards review process has revealed best practices, and facilitated identification of quality improvement opportunities for all PCHs within the Winnipeg region.

The Incidence and Severity of Side Effects of Drugs in the Elderly

C. M. Gavrilescu, D. Munteanu, S. Iliescu, J. Hurjui (University of Medicine and Pharmacy Iassy, Vth Internal Medicine Clinic, Iassy, Romania)

PURPOSE: To verify if there appears alonger number of side effects to drugs in the elderly. METHOD: Clinical descriptive study which surveyed all the side effects appearing to drugs used in an Internal Medicine Clinic,

The C. F. University Hospital on a period of six years (1994 1999). RESULTS: The total incidence of side effects was almost equal in young or old patients. In the elderly there appeared more often neurological, cardiovascular and metabolic side effects. The high frequency of some side effects didn t reflect their importance, for example: · The respiratory side effects were more frequent in young people, but severe obstructive syndroms appeared more often in the elderly. · The psychiatric side effects, more frequent in young people, manifested in their case as sleep disturbance and depressive symptoms, while in the elderly they manifested as confusional and pshychotic states. The medicaments which determined more often side effects in the elderly were: nonsteroidal antiinflammatory drugs, converting enzyme inhibitors, digitalics, psychotrops and oral antidiabetics. Serious side effects were present in 3,8 % of the patients (out of which 56,91% were aged). In young people the greatest risk of side effects was present in men (74,3%), while in the elderly the risk was approximately equal for men and women. CONCLUSION: The incidence of the side effects of drugs in the elderly wasn t significantly higher. Yet, their appeared a different profile of the clinical manifestations and of the severity of the side effects in the young and in the old patients.

The Role of the Interdisciplinary Team in Managing Geriatric Drug Therapy

William Simonson (President, American Society of Consultant Pharmacists) (Alexandria, Virginia, USA)

Issue: Geriatric drug therapy is complex. Medications have a variety of beneficial pharmacologic effects including prevention of age-related conditions, control of symptoms, or cure of disease, but negative outcomes may also occur. The use of prescription and non-prescription medications may also result in a variety of medication-related problems, ranging from adverse drug reactions and interactions, to excessive prescribing. Drug therapy also has financial and social implications that impact on caregivers, family members and friends. Structure: In senior care environments optimal drug therapy must be a team effort. The responsibilities of some team members, such as pharmacists and physicians are well defined by practice standards, legislation and regulation. Other members of the team may play a less recognized but non-the-less important role. Still other members of the team may have indirect, but still important, responsibilities pertaining to the senior patients drug therapy. Content: This round table will explore the role of each member of the interdisciplinary health care team relating to their responsibility with a senior patients drug therapy. Discussion will include what is expected of each discipline and how they can most effectively provide appropriate input to optimize the patients drug therapy. Conclusion/Anticipated Outcome This roundtable will help to identify the role of the role of the various members of the interdisciplinary team in drug therapy of seniors. The discussion will help define the role of the interdisciplinary team members in optimizing drug therapy in the senior population

SESSION 141

Dissolving the Divide: The Amalgamation of the Two Tier System of Long Term Care in Australia

Diane Gibson (The Australian Institute of Health and Welfare, Canberra, Australia)

Purpose: To examine the consequences of amalgamating the two tier institutional long term care system in Australia into a single system. Method: Time series analysis of the national institutional long term care database derived from administrative systems in Australia. Results: Until 1997, long term care in Australia was provided in hostels (low care) and nursing homes (high care), two separate systems with separate funding provisions. This dual system of residential care is found in a number of other countries. The 1997 reforms led to the amalgamation of the two systems, a development which was intended to increase the flexibility and equity of the long term care system, and facilitate 'ageing in place' for people living in facilities which were previously categorised as hostels. Time series analysis shows that ageing in place has indeed occurred, along with an increase in dependency levels of long term care residents, and consequent increases in expenditure on long term care. Conclusion: It is argued that the move to a single system has indeed increased flexibility and equity, and facilitated ageing in place for residents. A tradeoff has been apparent in increases in resident dependency and in the costs associated with the system of care. The implications of these findings are considered in the context of current policy directions in other OECD countries.

Identified Funding Issues Issues in Long Term Care Facilities

Dan Levitt,, CHE Administrator Jackman Manor Aldergrove, B.C. Canada Derek Morton, M.Div, C.G.A. Administrator Blenheim Lodge Vancouver, B.C. Canada

Purpose: Funding issues are at the forefront of residential care facilities' concerns. Financial pressures continue to impact the level and quality of services provided to seniors. The goal of this paper is to enhance the quality of life of residents living within residential care facilities by advocating on their behalf for adequate funding. Method: This report is based on the impact of funding constraints experienced at residential care facilities. The document was prepared and circulated to all continuing care facilities and all health authorities in British Columbia. Results: 1) Transfer Payments - to residential care facilities are not sufficient to provide quality care; 2) Resident Issues - challenge staff as there are increasing demands from a frailer population; 3) Staffing Issues - the actual cost of salaries is higher than funding allocations; 4) Administrative Isssues - cost pressures decrease the time available for direct care. Conclusion: With the increasing number of long stay patients in acute care beds and the increasing length of community wait lists, it is critical that priority be given to stable funding to ensure quality services to residents.

Long term care, who are we? (French thoughts over worldwide concerns)

P. Rumeau [service de gérontologie L'Orbe, Hôpital Charles Foix, Ivry sur Seine, France], S. Moulias [service de médecine gériatrique, Hôpital Charles Foix, Ivry sur Seine, France], P. Senet [service de gérontologie L'Orbe, Hôpital Charles Foix, Ivry sur Seine, France], M. Rumeau [centre de gérontologie, CHU La Grave, Toulouse, France], S. Meaume [service de gérontologie L'Orbe, Hôpital Charles Foix, Ivry sur Seine, France], R. Moulias [service de gérontologie L'Orbe, Hôpital Charles Foix, Ivry sur Seine, France].

Abstract Purpose In those cost conscious times comes back the question of the need to care for sick, disabled, elderly people. We, gerontologists, working in long term care units, cannot spare a reflection on our goals and usefulness in the society. Method Those ideas are coming from ours experimenting with trying to explain our job to acute care doctors, families, social workers, speaking with economists, and lobbying politicians. Results, We care for people with polypathology and polydisability. 80% of our patients are demented. Nearly 50% are lonesome, and 90% need social aid to pay for the hostelry part of their hospitalisation bill (the rest is paid by medical insurance). We need 1.3 caregiver for each patient for a fair quality of life and of care, average pension of our patients is below half the payroll of those who care for them. Our patients expect from us a daily pertinent medical and nursing care, life comfort in spite of disabilities, respect of their human dignity. Conclusion Long term cares are for people who, because of their disabilities and diseases, needs the help of an important number of professionals caring for them to optimise their comfort. Our economic responsibility is to be as efficient as possible with as little costs as possible, but also to say "stop!" when funding gets too low to achieve our goals. It's then the choice of the nation to know if it wants to care for its elders as for "normal" citizens.

The Case of Ontario's Long Term Community Care Market: Who's Choice is it Anyway

Tamara Sussman (M.S.W, C.S.W, Candidate, University of Toronto, Faculty of Social Work, Toronto, Ontario Canada

A review of Ontario's long term community care policy reveals that seniors with chronic health care needs do not have the 'choice' this commodified system promises to consumers. Further, other major stakeholders: government agencies, service providers and family members lack 'choice' in this market system. It is recommended that 'choice' be removed from current discussion as it's presence has served to detract from more important debates in community long term care policy such as, government responsibility, service equity and family obligation.

SESSION 142

Transition in Environmental Supports: Evaluating Options

Doris L. Milke (The Capital Care Group, Edmonton, Canada) A prospective analysis of residents discharged to a nursing home from an Alzheimer Care Centre. Connie Wark and Doris L. Milke (The Capital Care Group, Edmonton, Canada) Aging-in-place: Ways to make it happen. Barbara M. Gfellner (Brandon University, Brandon, Canada) Community movers: functional change over eight years. Kate Oakley (University of Ottawa Institute on Health of the Elderly, Ottawa, Canada) Explicit and implicit reasons for joining a seniors centre reveal QOL.

This symposium examines a spectrum of living environments and supportive services designed to accommodate the diversity of needs Δ from community living to long term care - found in our contemporary aging population. The four presentations involve evaluative research and include several longitudinal studies. Each presentation identifies specific areas for preventive planning, program development and intervention with regard to a particular target population. In the first paper, Milke (A prospective analysis of residents discharged to a nursing home from an Alzheimer's care centre) examines factors leading to discharge of clients from an Alzheimer's care centre to a personal care home. In comparison to reduced mobility at the time of discharge, progressive declines in socializing and health at 3-month intervals over the next nine months were associated with this relocation. The second presentation (Wark and Milke: Aging-in-place: ways to make it happen in long term care) underscores the substantial rate of moves among clients in nursing homes and goes on to examine alternatives to personal care home placement where long term care clients can age-in-place. The third paper (Gfellner: Community movers: functional changes over eight years) is an eight-year follow-up of older adults who changed residence (mostly to seniors housing complexes) within the community. Relocators reported declines in health, some functional abilities, transportation and social activities in comparison with non-movers, with more serious mobility limitations among those who moved a second time. Nevertheless, personal control and well-being remained consistent for both movers and non-relocators. In the final paper Oakley (Explicit and implicit reasons for joining a seniors' centre reveal QOL) reports that some older adults' reasons for involvement in a Seniors' Centre are related to personal well-being as well as specific health conditions. The findings presented in this symposium offer insight into some of the particular concerns and ramifications of environmental contingencies on the functional well-being of older adults in a variety of settings. Discussion will focus on how these results can be adapted and applied to other situations.

A prospective analysis of residents discharged to a nursing home from an Alzheimer care centre

Doris L. Milke (The Capital Care Group, Edmonton, Canada)

Dementia-specific residential long-term care settings do not routinely care for persons throughout the final stages of dementia. This study examined how residents fare while in the residence and at 3, 6, and 9-months after discharge to a nursing home. METHOD: Status was examined via the Mini-Mental Status Examination (MMSE), Brief Cognitive Rating Scale, Multidimensional Observation Scale for Elderly Subject (MOSES), Functional Independence Measure (FIM), Cohen-Mansfield Agitation Index, and a clinical interview with the caregiver. Of the 43 participants, only 18 were discharged during the study. The discharged residents' mobility had declined by the time of discharge and continued to decline at 3, 6 and 9-months after discharge. This was evident in FIM and MOSES scores. A substantial proportion had a heart problem at discharge and this proportion increased at 3 and 6-months following discharge. However, in the clinical judgement of caregivers, the most important factor in the decline of those discharged was Alzheimer's disease, not falls, or other diagnoses. MMSE scores of those discharged and not discharged were not different at discharge, but differed significantly by 3 months post-discharge. For those discharged, large changes in social interaction were seen post-discharge. Relocation main effects indicated that those discharged were more likely than those not discharged to have declined in physical health. Their decline continued post-discharge, whereas no similar decline was evident in those not discharged.

Aging-in-place: Ways to make it happen in long term care

Connie F. Wark & Doris L. Milke (The Capital Care Group, Edmonton, Canada)

Popular lore suggests that the last move for elderly persons seeking to meet their service needs is a move into a long-term care (LTC) centre. A recent study, however, indicates some persons keep moving within the LTC system. METHOD: Evaluative research. Discussion with 51 family members indicated that the majority (51%) of their relatives in LTC had been moved once, 16% had moved twice, 7% moved three times, and 7% had moved four times. Approximately half (24) could expect one more move, either because increasing needs for care were expected to demand more staff time than could be provided, or because a key reason for admission would diminish (e.g, wandering). A healthcare campus with a continuum of services still requires residents to move. Thus, 18 residents had been moved within one organization's centres, with 30% moving once, 7% had moved twice, and 5% moving three times. This suggests the LTC system needs to examine aging-in-place. The CAPITAL CARE Group has been developing centres where LTC clients can age-in-place. For example, Laurier House is a life-lease LTC centre where residents receive nursing home level care in their studio, single-bedroom, or two-bedroom suite, instead of in a semi-private bed, like most nursing homes. A spouse or friend who does not require care may live within the suite, just as they would in an apartment. An evaluation confirmed the overwhelming success of this model. Now the organization is piloting an aging-in-place centre for dementia clients. Both centres will be described in terms of aging-in-place.

Community movers: Changes in functional abilities and well-being over eight years

Barbara M. Gfellner (Brandon University, Brandon, Canada)

Self-reported change in health, functional abilities, mobility, social activities, caregiving as well as quality of life indices were examined among older adults who relocated and changed residential settings within the community. There were 165 participants (400f the original sample interviewed six years previously) including 56 recent relocators (M = 80.1 years; 45 women) and 109 non-relocators (M = 76.8 years; 81 women). The groups were consistent for marital status (49% widowed, 38% married); 200f the movers and 30f the non-movers subsequently relocated again. Movers tended to relocate to seniors' housing (63%) or apartments (25%) while more non-movers resided in their own houses (45%) and seniors' housing (41%). Movers had lived on an average, 6 years in their current domicile; 15.1 years for non-movers. During home interviews participants rated the extent of change they experienced since they were previously interviewed for 16 areas of functioning and completed measures of ADLs, health, service needs, life satisfaction, involvement with family and friends, stress, life control, physical and psychological well-being. Relocators showed significant declines for health, ability to do heavy chores, transportation, getting to places out of walking distance, visiting family in comparison with non-movers. Alternatively, subsequent movers indicated more substantial declines in mobility at home and decreased caregiving responsibilities and assistance needs. Although ADLs were greater among movers than stayers, measures of well-being were similar for both groups. However, movers reported significantly higher ratings in the past for health, life satisfaction, and socializing in comparison with non-movers.

Explicit and implicit reasons for joining a seniors centre reveal QOL

Kate Oakley (University of Ottawa Institute on Health of the Elderly, Ottawa, Canada)

This study investigated whether seniors who join a Seniors Centre for explicit services (e.g, type and variety of programs) have higher levels of well-being (QOL) than individuals who join primarily for the implicit services (e.g, opportunity for social interaction). A questionnaire was administered to 295 seniors to obtain data on demographics, specific reasons for joining a centre, social, educational and physical activity levels, as well as QOL variables. Three sub-groups of individuals emerged: seniors who joined primarily for the type and variety of specific programs offered (active=57.4%), seniors who joined because they were lonely and needed someplace to go (lonely=19.8%), and seniors who cited both reasons (lonely proactive=22.7%). Data support the hypothesis that individuals who joined the centre for implicit reasons (e.g, to reduce loneliness) yielded lower QOL scores than those who joined for explicit reasons (i.e, type and variety of activities). Individuals in the lonely but proactive group obtained QOL scores in the mid-range but data were similar to individuals in the lonely group in terms of factors that negatively influence well-being (e.g, anxiety, depression, health problems). Both lonely and lonely proactive groups differed from the active group on three physical health problems only: high blood pressure, stroke, and circulation problems). Interestingly, the lonely proactive group more closely resembled the active group on positive factors associated with well-being (e.g, positive affect, having a confidant). Evidently, reasons for joining a centre reveal important information about well-being and can guide the development of specific programs geared to implicit needs.

SESSION 143

Narratives of Control and Coping by Middle-aged and Older Cancer Survivors

T. O. Blank, B. N. Singlevich, C. D. Stelle, K. E. Belizzi, and S. Shaperow [University of Connecticut, CT, USA]

PURPOSE: The role of control processes in coping with both acute trauma and chronic health conditions is well established. Yet, because most studies are quantitative and scale-based, little is known about varieties and domains of control experiences. Thus, the purpose of this research is to explore spontaneous expressions of control-related thoughts in narratives about surviving cancer. METHODS: Twenty autobiographical books by cancer survivors or spouses were surveyed. Instances of control-related ideas were marked and coded. Age at diagnosis ranged from 36-70 (M=54; SD=9.27); 14 males and six females. Open coding led to a taxonomy of control-related thoughts. RESULTS: Expressions of control, loss of control, and desire for control were related to several major domains: physical aspects of one's body and pain, psychological aspects of emotions or thoughts, activities and lifestyle, and control related specifically to treatment decisions. Most commonly mentioned areas concerned psychological aspects, pain, and sense of mortality. There were almost two times as many expressions of loss of control as feelings of being in control. Control references were especially apparent in the early post-diagnosis period and dissipated after one had reached a new normal following treatment. There were wide ranges in number and type of references to control across authors. CONCLUSION: In free narratives, cancer survivors regularly express thoughts and feelings related to control, especially loss of control, especially soon after diagnosis. Thus, exploring ways to maintain and enhance sense of control is important to the well-being and coping of cancer survivors.

Reactivated Trauma: The Holocaust Survivor Copes With Cancer

S.Hantman (Bob Shapell School of Social Work, Tel-Aviv University, Israel)

The purpose of this paper is to shed light on the effect that exposure to prior trauma has on the ability to adapt to present trauma. Specifically, Holocaust survivors adaptation when confronted with a life-threatening illness, namely Cancer. The sample consisted of 200 elderly Cancer patients, 150 of whom were Holocaust survivors and a control group consisting of 50 Cancer patients who had not been in the Holocaust and were of similar demographic background. The subjects were administered a battery of questionnaires that included the PAIS, SCL-90R, Posttrauma Inventory, SOC and Survivors' Coping Patterns with the Holocaust (constructed by the author). In comparing the two groups results point to a slightly higher level of PTSD in the Holocaust group. However, when comparing the Holocaust survivors amongst themselves, three styles of adaptation were found: Those who failed to adapt, those who adapted successfully by expressing Holocaust memories, and those who adapted successfully by repressing Holocaust memories. Patterns of adaptation were found to be positively associated with psychosocial adjustment to cancer.These results suggest the long-range effect that coping outcomes have on recurrent exposure to stress. In addition, the study showed that a strong Sense of Coherence was associated with less psychopathology, which resulted in a better adjustment to cancer.These findings suggest that a strong Sense of Coherence may play an important role in protecting against long-term negative effects by promoting mental health. These results point to a resemblence between the psychosocial adaptation of Holocaust survivors to cancer and their adaptation in the aftermath of the Holocaust. This supports the Crisis-Resolution perspective that claims that the quality of prior coping patterns with traumatic stress will shape future coping patterns with stress.

Social Comparison Processes In Autobiographies Of Midlife And Older Cancer Survivors

K.M. Bellizzi, C.E. Oakes, C.D. Stelle, & T.O. Blank [University of Connecticut, Storrs, USA]

PURPOSE: Social comparison theory has been used to explain how individuals cope with having cancer. Previous research shows that persons with cancer tend to affiliate with people who have already experienced the disease, for informational or comparison purposes. However, findings have been mixed in respect to whether upward or downward comparison is the most common and/or effective strategy for good psychological adjustment. Also, the literature is unclear about whether or when cancer survivors engage in parallel (shared fate) comparisons. METHOD: The goal of this study was to explore the usage of three social comparison styles (downward, upward, and parallel) of midlife and older cancer survivors using an in-depth content analysis of 20 autobiographical books. The sample in the study consisted of 14 males and 6 females ranging in age from 36-70 (M=54, SD=9.27). Of the 20 subjects in the study, 55% had prostate cancer, 20% had breast cancer, and 25% had other forms of cancer. RESULTS: Subjects used significantly more parallel comparisons than upward and downward comparisons ($t = 4.215$, $p = .000$). Further, subjects used significantly more upward comparisons than downward comparisons ($t = 3.133$, $p = .005$). CONCLUSIONS: Thus, although cancer survivors used all three forms of social comparison, these data suggest that cancer survivors, and perhaps an aging population dealing with major health issues, prefer to interact with others who were similar to themselves or faring better. Findings will be discussed with respect to situational and individual factors that influence the three different social comparison styles.

The Lived Experience of the Older Adult with Cancer: An Ongoing Critical Incident

Marty Pentz (Indiana University East, Richmond, IN, U.S.A.)

Purpose: The purpose of the study was to investigate the lived experience of the older adult with cancer to enable social workers to better serve this population. Method: Qualitative grounded theory methodology with in-depth interviews was used. Seventeen older adults with cancer were interviewd along with a focus group of five oncology social workers. Results: What emerged from the data was the grounded theory of cancer being an ongoing critical incident. The themes that brought this conclusion were: 1) importance of internal and external activity, 2) coping (how they coped), 3) coping (what brought on the need to cope, 4) importance of attitude in resilience and quality of life, 5) emotions, and 6) working through all that a cancer diagnosis brings on. Conclusion: The author concludes that more research needs to be done on the ongoing nature of cancer, the need to increase social works role with this population, the importance of listening to how they cope, listening to how they define meaningful activity, and the importance of attitude in the quality of life of the older adult with cancer.

SESSION 144

Trends in Physical Activity -Linking Research, Program Development, Policy and Practice

Y. Netz (Gerontological Studies, Zinman College at the Wingate Institute, Israel) Physical Activity for Older Adults-An Area of Academic Specialty in a College of Physical Education and Sports Sciences and International Collaboration. T. Tzuck (The Association for the Planning and Development of Services for The Elderly in Israel, Tel Hashomer, Israel) Education and In-service for Teachers and Instructors to Develop Professional Manpower. Y. Ben Moshe (The Association for the Planning and Development of Services for The Elderly in Israel, Jerusalem, Israel) Physical Activity Programs on Local and National Level. Y. Dantziger (Ministry of Health, Tel-Aviv, Israel) Improving Physical Activity in Day Care Centers

This symposia will describe a holistic approach of a common effort of researchers , clinicians and policy makers in Israel to get older adults to exercise and maintain their exercise behavior. The benefits of exercise in old age influence a wide variety of diseases and conditions affecting both physical and mental health. A fruitful collaboration between researchers and service providers developed an infrastructure that provide programs which are geared to ensure for availability and accessibility of opportunities to exercise in old age. The symposia will highlight the development of professional manpower and facilities, the services tailored for different target groups, the mass programs aimed to arouse awareness and knowledge on opportunities to exercise. Specifically the symposium will describe the following programs: An academic program "physical activity for older adults-an area of specialty in a college of physical education and sports sciences" and international collaboration to promote new area of specialization. Education and in-service courses for teachers and instructors including special training for working in fitness rooms with elderly. Physical activity programs on the local level "service package" including a variety of courses to meet the needs of different groups, at a low cost and special services like fitness rooms designed specifically to meet elderly needs; activating elderly volunteers as health promoters and as walking leaders' groups; day care centers improving physical activity service for frail elderly both physically and mentally; national mass events "exercise activity days of the elderly" aimed to increase awareness and knowledge on programs. The anticipated outcome of the common effort -an increase in the percentage of elderly people exercising on a regular basis in Israel to 40%.

Continuing education and in-service training of physical education in services for the elderly in Israel.

Tali Tzuk, Director, Human Resources Development and Training, ESHEL, Israel.

Within the framework of a national collaboration towards the enhancement of an infrastructure of services to promote physical activities among seniors, ESHEL Human Resources department undertook its role as a vehicle for levering the standards thru the development of a series of educational opportunities which will upgrade the level of existing knowledge and raise the interest of teachers to work in old age home, day care centers and community clubs. Between 1996-1999, we initiated a series of short term courses for certified teachers in the community. This initiative was carried out in collaboration with the Ministry of Education, the Ministry of Health and Wingate College of Education. Two major programs dealt with such contents: 1. Working in general fitness courses for elderly persons. 2. working in fitness rooms. The contents of these programs will be described along with some dilemmas encountered.

Improving Physical Activity in Day Care Centers

J. DANZIGER, CHIEF PHYSIOTHERAPIST (MINISTRY OF HEALTH, TEL-AVIV, ISRAEL)

In most of the day care centers physiotherapists are equal members of the team. The main role of the physiotherapists is in prevention, health promotion and instructing the staff in daily life activities. It was decided by the Ministry of Health and ESHEL to develop a program to improve physical activity of the healthy elderly and handicapped elderly visiting the day care centers. The program was developed by a physiotherapist together with a physical education teacher. The program included active exercises to improve muscle strength and endurance balance exercises in sitting standing and walking. In order to examine the effectiveness of the program a study was carried out in two day care centers. A tool to assess the base line capacities of the healthy and handicapped elderly was developed. Both the physiotherapist and the physical education teacher examined visitors and established their abilities. The program was taught to the members of the staff, who carried it out and worked with the visitors. Results: the examination tool and the program served to improved physical activities of the visitors participating in the activities.

Physical Activity for the Aged - an Area of Specialty in a College of PhysicalEducation and Sports Sciences

Yael Netz Ph.D(Zinman College of Physical Education and Sports Sciences at the Wingate Institute, Israel)

Specialty of physical activity for older adults in a physical education department and on the courses to be included in the program. At the Zinman College we have developed an area of specialization " Physical Activity" for Older adults".The program includes theoretical and practical courses as well as student teaching practicum. "The Aging Cardio-respiratory System and Typical Diseases" is an example of a theoretical course and "Fitness Room Activity for Older Adults" is an example of a practical course. Students enrolled in the program are trained, in addition to their major training as physical education teachers in schools, to work with the elderly in community centers, retirement centers and nursing homes. In addition we conduct research related to exercise behavior and exercise prescription in old age. As the head of gerontology studies at the Zinman College I will discuss typical issues related to this area of specialization.

Physical Activity Programs on the Local and National Level

Yosefa Ben Moshe MPh (ESHEL, The Association for the Planning and Development of Services for the Elderly in ISRAEL, Jerusalem)

Physical activity programs can make a significant difference in the quality of life of the elderly by encouraging the introduction of a variety of physical activity programs into the local community for the elderly. Seniors often do not participate in physical activities because they do not have access to organized programs and do not know how to begin an exercise program themselves. Physical activity programs need to be 1) located close to home 2) inexpensive 3) varied enough so that everyone can find something to of appeal. Physical activity programs are operated both by professionals and by volunteers. Certain physical activity programs must be operated by trained instructors (fitness rooms), while other programs may be operated by volunteers (walking groups). ESHEL's physical activity project encourages local municipalities to coordinate physical activity programs for seniors, with professional instructors. Recently, much attention and efforts were invested in setting up a program of building fitness rooms specially designed and adapted for the elderly all over Israel, mainly in conjunction with day care centers for disabled and frail elderly. Special emphasis was also placed on walking as an activity accessible to everyone, providing training programs for elderly volunteers as walking group leaders (offered to all ethnic groups and socioeconomic strata). Over 5,000 elderly took part in the Jerusalem March in September 1999, one of the annual National Physical Activity Day for the Elderly. The annual activity days for seniors generate publicity for the different programs and showcase the benefits of physical activity in old age. The target to achieve: 40% of the elderly people exercise on regular basis

SESSION 145

Technology: Findings from the Center for Research and Education on Aging and Technology Enhancement (CREATE)

Sara J. Czaja (University of Miami, Miami Fl, U.S.A.) An Overview of the Center for Research and Education on Aging and Technology Enhancement. Wendy A. Rogers (Georgia Institute of Technology, Atlanta, GA, USA) Enabling Older Adults to Successfully Use the World Wide Web. Arthur D. Fisk (Georgia Institute of Technology, Atlanta, GA, USA) Enhancing Performance with Environmental Support: Age-Related Differences. Neil Charness (Florida State University, Tallahassee, Fl, USA), Sara J. Czaja (University of Miami, Miami, FL, USA) Enhancing the Usability of Telephone Menu Systems for Older Adults. Sunkyo Kwon (Discussant) (Technical University of Berlin, Berlin, Germany) Summary and Implications of the CREATE Findings

The rapid infusion of technology into most setting implies that most people need to use technology on a regular basis to perform routine tasks. In order to function independently, people of all ages must learn how to assimilate technology into their lives. This represents a challenge for many older people as the literature indicates that older people typically have difficulty learning to use and operate technical systems. The Center for Research and Education on Aging and Technology Enhancement (CREATE) is multidisciplinary, collaborative Center, funded by the National Institute on Aging, dedicated to solving the problems of aging and technology. The focus of this symposium will be on describing the goals and activities of CREATE and presenting some findings from the initial research projects. The projects that will be discussed relate to a variety of technologies. Initially an overview of the structure and purpose of CREATE will be provided (S. Czaja). This overview will include a discussion of the conceptual approach and methodologies being adopted by CREATE to examine the issue of aging and technology. This will be followed by findings from a study concerned with enhancing the usability of the World Wide Web W. Rogers). The focus will be on sensory, motor, and cognitive changes that occur with age that may influence the ability of older people to interact with the Web. Data from two studies that focus on search strategies and navigational aids will be presented. The next presentation (A. Fisk) will focus on how the provision of environmental support may facilitate the ability of older people to use technical systems. The concept of environmental support will be discussed relative to task strategies. This presentation will present findings from two studies that demonstrate how the provision of environmental support may improve performance and the implications for system design. The next project (N. Charness) will discuss input device design may constrain the ability of older people to use technology. Data from a study examining pointing and clicking devices for pointing tasks will be presented. The findings suggest the type of input device that may be most suitable for older adults to minimize age differences with graphical user interfaces. The final study (S. Czaja) will discuss the usability of telephone menu systems (IVR systems). Data from a study examining age differences in the use of these systems as a function of speech rate and menu complexity will be presented. Preference data from older and younger adults will also be presented. The implications of these findings for the design of IVR systems will be reviewed. The final presentation (S. Kwon) will summarize the findings from the research and discuss the implications with respect to the broader issue of aging and technology. The goal of the symposium is to provide an overview of some of the issues relate to aging and technology and highlight some findings from current research in this area. An additional goal is to demonstrate how findings from applied research projects can be translated into guidelines for design interventions.

An Overview of the Center for Research and Education on Aging and Technology Enhancement (CREATE).

Sara J. Czaja (University of Miami, Miami, FL. USA)

Information technology is integral to work, education, and daily life. Simple tasks such as fueling an automobile, banking, shopping, or locating a book in the library typically involve the interaction with some form of technology. In order to function independently people of all ages must lean how to assimilate technology into their lives. Currently, the needs of older people have largely been ignored in the design of technical systems and older people often have difficulty learning to use and operate technology. This presentation will provide an overview of the newly established Center for Research and Education on Aging and Technology Enhancement (CREATE). CREATE is a multidisciplinary, collaborative Center, funded by the National Institute on Aging, dedicated to solving problems of aging and technology. The conceptual framework and methodological approaches being adopted by CREATE will be presented. The specific objectives of CREATE are to develop a comprehensive database on aging and technology that will consist of information regarding: user preferences and needs, problems with existing systems, and efficiency of design solutions. These issues are being examined across a broad range of technologies and tasks using protocols directed towards practically relevant research. The conceptual framework for CREATE is based on Human Factors Engineering and Cognitive Psychology. The research projects focus on distinct but complimentary aspects of the human/technology interface. This presentation will describe the CREATE research program and how the findings from CREATE will contribute to the literature on aging and everyday competence and the development of design guidelines for technical systems.

Constrains on Interacting with Computer Systems as a Function of Adult Age: Input Devices

Neil Charness, Patricia Holley, and Jeff Feddon [Florida State University, Tallahassee, FL, USA]

In 2000, over 50% of USA households owned computer systems. Given normative age-related changes in perceptual, cognitive, and psychomotor ability, in what ways do current computer systems tax the ability of older adults, particularly in terms of input devices? We examine ability to interact with computer systems using point and click interfaces with pure pointing tasks, as well as with mixed pointing and typing tasks. To assess the loss of use of a preferred hand to disease or injury, we also required participants to perform the menu-selection task with their non-preferred hand. In the first experiment, 24 young, middle-aged, and older adults who were experienced mouse users performed a menu selection task with mouse and lightpen input devices. Results showed that older adults were generally slower than middle-aged and younger adults though the type of device used interacted with age. The lightpen, a direct positioning device, was significantly superior to a mouse, an indirect positioning device, particularly for older users. Use of the lightpen also significantly minimized hand differences in performance. Preference for device did not correlate significantly with performance with the device, suggesting that letting users configure their own interfaces may not lead to optimal performance. For pure pointing tasks, a direct positioning device should be preferred to an indirect one in order to minimize age differences in performance with graphic user interfaces.

Enabling Older Adults to Successfully Use the World Wide Web

Wendy A. Rogers, Aideen Stronge, and Richard Pak [Georgia Institute of Technology, Atlanta, GA, USA]

There are more individuals today over the age of 65 than there have ever been and the number is expected to continue to grow. Consequently, this is a user population whom web designers must accommodate. We will review studies of age-related differences in web usage patterns and usage difficulties. Older adults are interested in using the web, and many of them do; however, evidence suggests that older users have more difficulty finding information, they are slower, they make more errors, and are likely to get lost while navigating. As a method of understanding the potential source of these difficulties, we will elucidate the characteristics of older adults that must be considered in the context of web design. The focus will be on sensory, motor, and cognitive changes that may influence interactions with computers in general, and the web in particular. We will also present data from two studies. One study focused on assessing age-related differences in web searching strategies by experienced users. The other study assessed the interaction between spatial ability and use of a navigational aid for young and older adults. Together these the data from studies provide design suggestions as well as recommendations for training older adults to use the web.

Enhancing Performance with Environmental Support: Age-Related Differences

Arthur D. Fisk and Timothy A. Nichols [Georgia Institute of Technology, Atlanta, GA, USA]

Supportive information in task environments can be presented in many different ways, such as the coloring and underlining hyperlinks on the Web or the arrangement of items on one's desktop. However, age-related differences are often found in individuals' ability to utilize the supportive information in a task. Discerning why these differences exist can be complicated. We investigated two explanations for this age-related failure to utilize and benefit from environmental support. One formulation of the environmental support hypothesis is based on the concept of limited resources and additional age-related deficits in resources. Thus, the amount of available processing resources may be pivotal in determining whether an individual will utilize the pattern information. An alternative explanation for the age-related differences in utilization is related to strategies. Older adults may adopt inefficient strategies or may be unable to utilize an optimal strategy for this task. We report results from two experiments. Using a resource manipulation with younger adults, we found that increasing the memory set size increased the benefit of providing environmental support. Using the same task, we assessed the role of strategies in older adults' use of environmental support, via an instructional manipulation. The pattern of results has implications for the theory of environmental support as well as for the use of environmental support from a system design perspective. Finally, the results have implications for specifying enduring versus labile effects of cognitive aging. These latter three points will be discussed.

Enhancing the Usability of Telephone Menu Systems for Older Adults

Sara J. Czaja and Joseph Sharit [University of Miami, Miami, FL, USA]

Telephone voice menu systems (IVR systems) are increasingly be used by business and service organizations. Many of these applications, such as on-line banking, are complex and users are required to navigate through a myriad of submenus in order to obtain information or perform a task. Furthermore, it is assumed that users will be able to use these systems without any training. Finally, there are no existing standards to guide the development of these systems so there is a lack of consistency across applications. Given that older adults are generally less familiar with technology than are younger people and there are cognitive and perceptual changes which occur with age. The use of IVR systems may be especially problematic for older people. This paper will present findings from a recent study examining age and the usability of IVR system. The overall of the presentation is to demonstrate how design factors such as speech rate and menu complexity impact on user performance and acceptance of these systems. The finding indicate that older adults find these systems difficult to use especially with high rates of speech compression. They also take longer, on average, than younger people to complete activities. These findings will be discussed in terms of strategies which can be sued to enhance the design of these systems.

SESSION 146

Connecting Older People Across the World

R. Adler (People & Technology, Cupertino, California, USA). Connecting Older People Across the World: The SeniorNet Experience. R. Foskey (Institute for Rural Futures, University of New England, NSW, Australia). Crossing Boundaries - Technology and Older People, An Australian Experience. D. King (Seniors' Education Centre, Centre for Continuing Education, University of Regina, Regina, SK, Canada). Creating Connections - In Canada and Across the World. K. Williamson (Information and Telecommunications Needs Research (ITNR), Monash University, Victoria and Charles Sturt University, Wagga Wagga, NSW, Australia). Enabling Older People with Disabilities to Connect With Others Across the World: An Australian Perspective.

Abstract Aging and technology are two phenomena that are converging in the 21st century. As the world's population continues to age and as learning technologies continue to develop rapidly, older adults are becoming one of the largest groups of users of computers and the Internet. Not only are older persons taking to technology, they are using it more for communication, information, and entertainment.The purpose of this symposium is to present the interesting and unique ways older people from various cultures, backgrounds and life situations across the world are using technology to be connected in their daily lives. The first presenter will discuss the continued growth of SeniorNet in the United States and internationally, including its "Learning Centers," online activities, and volunteer involvement. The second presenter will give an overview of a newly established national e-mail listserver called the EAT Network (education, ageing and technology), the use of technology to create and improve links between older people that bridge geographic and cultural barriers, and other developments in Australia. The third presenter will describe the various facets of a multi-year technology and urban/rural older adult project in Canada involving work with First Nations,Metis, and other rural people, the use of everyday technologies (bank machines, automated telephone services) and the creation of a bilingual, Canadian network for third age learning, CATALIST. The fourth presenter will address the special challenges faced by older people with disabilities who wish to access online services by discussing the findings of two projects which indicate the initiatives that can be taken. The symposium will also highlight the connections being fostered between older people in different countries. It is expected that this session will bring a greater understanding of national and international efforts by and for older people across the world to be and to remain connected via technology in a fast changing world.

Connecting Older People Across the World: The SeniorNet Experience

Richard P. Adler (People & Technology, Cupertino, California, USA)

SeniorNet is a San Francisco-based non-profit organization whose mission is to create a community of computer-using seniors in the U.S. and internationally. When it was founded in 1986, SeniorNet's initial goal was to build an online community for older adults. But it quickly became apparent that the great majority of seniors lacked both the equipment and the skills necessary to get online. So SeniorNet began establishing a network of local "Learning Centers" to provide older adults with a friendly introduction to computers and online communications tailored specifically to their needs and interests. Today, there are more than 200 SeniorNet Learning Centers operating in senior centers, community centers, public libraries, shopping centers, and on college and university campuses in 36 states. To date, more than 100,000 adults over age 50 have been trained by SeniorNet. SeniorNet also operates what is now one of the longest-running, most active communities online. SeniorNet's website (www.seniornet.org) site hosts literally hundreds of discussions on topics ranging from travel and gardening to health and politics and adapting to retirement. While most participants are U.S. residents, others participate from as far away as Australia, Israel, and Japan. Some come for social interaction or to get emotional support, others are drawn by the opportunities for learning and intellectual stimulation. Organized online activities include book discussion groups, bereavement support groups, and intergenerational forums. Almost all of the online activities are moderated by volunteers. Volunteers have also organized a series of events that have allowed participants who originally met online to meet in the "real world." Events scheduled for 2001 include a meeting in Washington, DC and a group trip to Europe. SeniorNet is continuing to grow. It is opening approximately 25 new Learning Centers each year and adding new features to its online network. In 1999, it merged with ElderWeb, which provides resources online for professionals in aging. SeniorNet is also expanding internationally, with a major initiative in Japan in 2001.

Creating Connections - In Canada and Across the World

Donald A. King (Seniors' Education Centre, Centre for Continuing Education, University of Regina, Regina, SK, Canada)

Abstract This paper will examine the various ways the Seniors' Education Centre, Centre for Continuing Education, University of Regina, Saskatchewan, Canada is involved in creating connections via technology with and for urban and rural older adults, including First Nations and Metis persons. The multi-year technology and older adults initative carried out by the Centre in cooperation with various national and international partners will be discussed. The design, delivery and evaluation of effective ways of using learning technologies for the benefit of third age learners will be examined. Electronic networking, Web page development, online courses and online discusssions are some of the strategies that will be outlined. Some emerging themes from focus groups, workshops and town hall meetings on the impact of everyday technologies - banking machines, automated telephone services - on the day-today lives of older people will be shared. The creation of CATALIST, a unique bilingual (French, English) Canadian network for third age learning will be described. Issues dealing with starting a national online organization and its value as a possible model for other countries will be explored. International cooperation will also be touched upon. The presentation will provide an opportunity to look at: (1) how the multi-year initiative has been timely and innovative, contributing to third age learning in Canada and elsewhere; and (2) how the initiative offers older adults the possibility of increased access to lifelong learning and a better quality of life.

Crossing Boundaries - Technology and Older People, An Australian Experience

Roslyn Foskey (Institute for Rural Futures, University of New England, Armidale, NSW, Australia 2351)

During 1999 the University of New England in Armidale, Australia hosted an International Year of Older Persons event titled 'Making the Connections: Non-metropolitan Older People and Technology', which consisted of a seven week online conference/video-conference based workshop in six rural communities and a more "traditional" two day conference at the University. Making the Connections brought together people interested in issues surrounding the use of technology by older people from across both Australia and the world (notably the Seniors' Education Centre, University of Regina, Saskatchewan, Canada). One lasting outcome from Making the Connections has been a national e-mail list server called the eat network (education, ageing and technology) managed through the Institute for Rural Futures at the University of New England. This list brings together over 80 participants from across Australia and elsewhere in the world in an environment in which ideas and issues can be discussed and information exchanged. The list has been able to draw together people from a range of backgrounds who share a common interest in ensuring that technology has a positive influence on the quality of life for older people regardless of where they live. In addition to managing the eat network, the Institute for Rural Futures has continued to explore the potential for innovative use of technology to create and improve links between older people that bridge geographic and cultural barriers. In May 2000 Aboriginal elders from the Armidale area were linked via vido-conference for a discussion with members of the Intercultural Grandmothers Uniting Program at the University of Regina, Saskatchewan, Canada.

Enabling Older People With Disabilities to Connect With Others Across the World: An Australian Perspective

Kirsty Williamson (School of Information Management and Systems, Monash University, Victoria and School of Information Studies, Charles Sturt University, Wagga, Wagga, NSW, Australia)

Research indicates that few older people were using the Internet in the mid-1990s in Australia. While there has been a considerable change in this situation, there are still major barriers to be broken down, especially for older people with disabilities. The paper will discuss two recent studies which examined issues concerned with assisting people with disabilities to use online services, particularly the Internet. While neither study was limited to specific age groups, the majority of participants in one project and over one-third of those in the other project were over the age of 55. The former project focussed on the potentialities of the Internet to assist blind and sight-impaired people. The latter project included three key objectives: the selection of a core set of adaptive equipment, suited to people with a range of different disabilities for use in public settings, particularly in public libraries; the development of related training for users and librarians alike; and the identification of standards and policies for achieving appropriate levels of online public access by disability groups. The findings of both projects indicate that there is a great deal that can be done to assist older people with disabilities to share more easily in the brave new world of instant information and communication offered by the Internet. The paper will discuss these findings and conclusions which were made about the initiatives that can be taken. These include the adaptive equipment which was found to provide the easiest access and was most favoured by older people - especially in public settings - as well as policies and strategies which can be put in place by organizations such as public libraries and governments to maximise access and participation. Issues of Web design, universal design and training will also be highlighted.

SESSION 147

Music for Health, Learning and Community in Later Life

Terence Hays (School of Curriculum Studies, University of New England, Armidale, NSW 2351, Australia) The Meaning and Importance of Music in the Lives of Older People. Brunhilde Arnold (Giessen, Germany) A Retired Social Gerontologist as an

Older University Student in Music: Experiences and explanations. Wendy Watts (George Derby Centre, Burnaby, British Columbia, Canada) The Making of a Professional Recording: Music therapy at work.

This symposium will address the importance of seniors having music in their lives to provide meaning, social contact with others, personal artistic expression and ongoing learning and personal growth. The symposia opens with an Australian study that researches the impact and meaning of music in older people's lives. The presenter gives an overview of the benefits and relevance that music has had with over thirty seniors who live in the community. His study demonstrates how participation in music is crucial in supporting well-being and in enhancing identity, self-esteem and social contact with others. This study is followed by a personal experience of a retired gerontologist studying music as an older learner. Her personal narrative considers the attitudes of her intergenerational peers and professors, and describes the personal benefits she has gained. The third presenter is the director of a musical "combo" in a veteran's facility. She will describe the therapeutic benefits that the combo members have received through performing and recording a CD, as well as how the combo has inspired and motivated others to experience a "creative community" within the long-term care facility. Through the presentation of qualitative studies, personal stories and shared experiences of seniors with music, it will be shown how participation in music can help to connect seniors with their past, as well as foster a meaningful connection with both the present and the future, and provide opportunities for meaningful learning and creative self-expression.

A Retired Social Gerontologist as an Older University Student in Music: Experiences and explanations

Brunhilde Arnold (Giessen, Germany)

The aims of learning as an older, no longer employed person are various and reach from passing time, private enhancement to the change in a new field of activity. My strategy was to qualify for a field which would open to me possibilities to be active in music as well for older persons as for myself. My paper is based on my own experience, so it is a qualitative study from a member of the European Older Students Research Group. It will - besides general remarks on learning in our "third life" - answer questions: What does it mean to study music among younger students, who are coming already very well educated in the field of music to university? What are the attitudes of professors in seminars as well in individual classes towards the student over sixty? Preparation and endurance of tests. What personal resources of happiness and benefit do develop?

Music Therapy at Work: The George Derby Residents' Combo and the making of a professional recording

Wendy Watts (George Derby Centre, Burnaby, British Columbia, Canada)

This session will describe the evolution of the George Derby Residents Combo, from it's creation in 1995 as a music therapy program at George Derby Centre (a Veterans Affairs funded continuing care residence) to the professional recording and release of a "Greatest Hits" compilation on CD. The presentation will focus on the therapeutic results that occurred as a result of practicing music therapy in this way. The presenter will examine how the production of professional recording helped to influence a reshaping of attitudes regarding notions of creativity and ability in later life. Other positive outcomes will also be described, including the therapeutic benefits experienced by the participants, and how the project inspired other resident members of the facility, and helped to engender a more positive culture within the facility. Comparisons will be made to other types of music therapy programming with the elderly in long-term care, and criteria for resident membership will be discussed. The objective of this session is to share an understanding of how this type of music therapy program can educate, motivate and inspire residents to achieve their potential. The George Derby Resident Combo CD is a symbol of the potential that elderly people have for growth and learning and artistic expression.

The Meaning and Importance of Music in the Lives of Older People

Terrence Hays (School of Curriculum Studies, University of New England, Armidale, NSW 2351, Australia)

This presentation describes the impact and meaning that music has in the lives of older people and discusses ways in which it can be used to gain a better understanding of the lives, identity and experiences of older people. Using a grounded theory design, this study utilized in-depth interviews and focus group interviews to analyze the relevance and significance of music in the lives of 30 older people living in the community. The findings suggested that music for many older people is crucial in supporting a sense of well-being. The data shows that the role of music is varied and can be used recreationally, educationally, socially, emotionally, therapeutically and spiritually. The importance and relevance of music depends on the life experience of the older person and has a major impact with regard to making meaning, self-esteem, and social contact with others. The data also reveals how people have incorporated music in their lives and how this process is important to their current identity. This study demonstrates that participation in music connects the past with the present and future and provides a forum for continuity in life. The study supports the proposition that music can enhance older people's quality of life by facilitating the maintenance of self-esteem and identify, assisting in the development of friendships, aiding in the sharing of memories, and maintaining social interests. Recommendations for how health professionals can use music more effectively are provided.

SESSION 148

Cultural Perspectives on Longevity: Five Country View Points

Robert N. Butler (International Longevity Center-USA, New York, USA, "Cultural Perspectives on Longevity: The United States View Point"); Sally Greengross (International Longevity Center-UK, London, England, "Cultural Perspectives on Longevity: The English View Point"); Françoise Forette (International Longevity Center-France, Paris, France, "Cultural Perspectives on Longevity: The French View Point"); Rosy Pereyra (International Longevity Center-Dominican Republic, Santo Domingo, Dominican Republic, "Cultural Perspectives on Longevity: The Caribbean View Point"); Yukiko Kudo (International Longevity Center-Japan, Tokyo, Japan, "Cultural Perspectives on Longevity: The Japanese and Asian View Point")

This symposium will explore how the Japanese, French, English, Caribbean and the North American cultures define longevity. The ISSUE to be addressed is how the different cultures relate to and adjust to similar issues that arise from an aging population. Each country addresses a social, economic, cultural issue from a different point of view. These papers highlight those points of view. The symposium STRUCTURE will have a moderator, R. Butler, who will introduce each of the speakers and field the questions. Each representative, including the moderator, will give an overview of his or her paper. The time for each speaker will be equal, leaving ample time for questions and answers from the audience and each other. The CONTENT of each paper to be presented will include: the culture's conception and definition of longevity; the distinctive changes in each cultures' attitudes toward longevity and the rising expectations of still greater longevity; the emergence of "anti-aging" medicine and its contrast with the development of geriatric medicine; the degree that prejudice with respect to aging or ageism is operative each country; the differences in the treatment and portrayal of older people in each society; and the employment of age prejudice in medicine, language and imagery. The CONCLUSIONS/ANTICIPATED OUTCOMES of this symposium is to highlight the differences and similarities in cultural attitudes towards longevity. It is anticipated that each country's representative and those of the audience will create an open dialogue and explore deeper values and conflicts that could exist with increased longevity. Through an open dialogue we can realize our assumptions of other country's cultural attitudes towards longevity and learn new ways of viewing longevity within our own country. Discussant: Julia T. Alvarez, Ambassador to the Dominican Repbulic

"Cultural Perspectives on Longevity: The Caribbean View Point"

Rosy Pereyra (ILC-DR, Santa Domingo, Dominican Republic)

The PURPOSE of this paper is to highlight the cultural attitudes towards longevity in the Caribbean. The METHOD will be to give a brief overview of a paper that explores: the Caribbean's cultural conception and definition of longevity; the distinctive changes in each cultures' attitudes toward longevity and the rising expectations of still greater longevity; the emergence of "anti-aging" medicine and its contrast with the development of geriatric medicine; the degree that prejudice with respect to aging or ageism is operative each country; the differences in the treatment and portrayal of older people in each society; and the employment of age prejudice in medicine, language and imagery. The RESULTS of the paper is an assessment of the impact of longevity on the cultural and social issues in the Caribbean that will provide an understanding of the progress the Caribbean has made or needs to make in order to integrate our aging population. The CONCLUSION creates an open dialogue and explores deeper values and conflicts that exist with increased longevity and creates a recommend agenda to meet the needs.

"Cultural Perspectives on Longevity: The English View Point"

Sally Greengross (ILC-UK, London, England)

The PURPOSE of this paper is to highlight the cultural attitudes towards longevity in the United Kingdom. The METHOD will be to give a brief overview of a paper that explores: England's cultural conception and definition of longevity; the distinctive changes in each cultures' attitudes toward longevity and the rising expectations of still greater longevity; the emergence of "anti-aging" medicine and its contrast with the development of geriatric medicine; the degree that prejudice with respect to aging or ageism is operative each country; the differences in the treatment and portrayal of older people in each society; and the employment of age prejudice in medicine, language and imagery. The RESULTS of the paper is an assessment of the impact of longevity on the cultural and social issues in England that will provide an understanding of the progress England has made or needs to make in order to integrate our aging population. The CONCLUSION creates an open dialogue and explores deeper values and conflicts that exist with increased longevity and creates a recommend agenda to meet the needs.

Cultural Perspectives on Longevity: The French View Point

Françoise Forette (ILC-France, Paris, France)

The PURPOSE of this paper is to highlight the cultural attitudes towards longevity in France. The METHOD will be to give a brief overview of a paper that explores: France's cultural conception and definition of longevity; the distinctive changes in each cultures' attitudes toward longevity and the rising expectations of still greater longevity; the emergence of "anti-aging" medicine and its contrast with the development of geriatric medicine; the degree that prejudice with respect to aging or ageism is operative each country; the differences in the treatment and portrayal of older people in each society; and the employment of age prejudice in medicine, language and imagery. The RESULTS of the paper is an assessment of the impact of longevity on the cultural and social issues in France that will provide an understanding of the progress France has made or needs to make in order to integrate our aging population. The CONCLUSION creates an open dialogue and explores deeper values and conflicts that exist with increased longevity and creates a recommend agenda to meet the needs.

Cultural Perspectives on Longevity: The Japanese and Asian View Point

Yukiko Kudo (ILC-Japan, Tokyo, Japan)

The purpose of this paper is to highlight the cultural attitudes towards longevity in Japan and Asia. The method will be to give a brief overview of a paper that explores: Japan's cultural conception and definition of longevity; the distinctive changes in each cultures' attitudes toward longevity and the rising expectations of still greater longevity; the emergence of "anti-aging" medicine and its contrast with the development of geriatric medicine; the degree that prejudice with respect to aging or ageism is operative each country; the differences in the treatment and portrayal of older people in each society; and the employment of age prejudice in medicine, language and imagery. The results of the paper is an assessment of the impact of longevity on the cultural and social issues in Japan that will provide an understanding of the progress Japan has made or needs to make in order to integrate our aging population. The conclusion creates an open dialogue and explores deeper values and conflicts that exist with increased longevity and creates a recommend agenda to meet the needs.

"Cultural Perspectives on Longevity: The North American View Point"

Robert N. Butler (ILC-USA, New York, USA)

The PURPOSE of this paper is to highlight the cultural attitudes towards longevity in the United States. The METHOD will be to give a brief overview of a paper that explores: the North American's cultural conception and definition of longevity; the distinctive changes in each cultures' attitudes toward longevity and the rising expectations of still greater longevity; the emergence of "anti-aging" medicine and its contrast with the development of geriatric medicine; the degree that prejudice with respect to aging or ageism is operative each country; the differences in the treatment and portrayal of older people in each society; and the employment of age prejudice in medicine, language and imagery. The RESULTS of the paper is an assessment of the impact of longevity on the cultural and social issues in the United States that will provide an understanding of the progress the United States has made or needs to make in order to integrate our aging population. The CONCLUSION creates an open dialogue and explores deeper values and conflicts that exist with increased longevity and creates a recommend agenda to meet the needs.

SESSION 149

A randomised controlled trial of psychological intervention with dementia spouse caregivers - five year follow-up

E. Moniz-Cook, M. Wang, (School of Medicine, University of Hull, UK), C. Elston (Hull and East Riding Community NHS Trust, Hull, UK), S. Agar (Department of Clinical Psychology, University of Sheffield, UK)

Chronic stressors associated with caregiving and depressed mood appear to be risk factors of poor health and mortality in older spouses of people with dementia. A randomised controlled trial of psychosocial intervention for 54 informal caregivers was compared with 59 'usual care' recipients. People with moderate to advanced dementia and their informal caregivers were referred to community EMI teams, by their family physician and randomised to experimental or control Community Psychiatric Nurses (CPNs). Experimental CPNs were trained and supervised in the following 'caregiver experimental intervention': support to attend to physical health complaints, problem solving, anxiety and depression management, training in family communication and arranging practical / respite services. At 18 and 24 month follow-up, experimental caregivers reported: significant reductions in their relative's problem behaviour; significantly lower perceived burden and depression. Here we report mortality follow-up (average 4.5, range 4 - 5 years) of the original sample. 54% (610f the experimental group / 47 0f the control group) were spouse caregivers. Mortality status was taken from health records with 100 0.000000ollow-up ascertainment. Although there was no difference in health status between groups at baseline, mortality in spouse (but not other) caregivers was significantly higher in the control group. This study, although underpowered, suggests that individualised psychosocial intervention targeting anxiety and depression, may have an impact on health status in spouse caregivers. Conceptualisations from emerging psycho-immunological intervention research in cancer care are used to outline potential intervention research with spouse caregivers of older people with dementia.

Hope and Alzheimer's Disease: An Education Program in Support of the Family Caregiving Journey

L. Barrett (Centre for Health Promotion Studies, University of Alberta, Edmonton, Canada), D. Barrett (Alzheimer Society of Edmonton, Alberta, Canada) and W. Edey (Hope Foundation of Alberta, Edmonton, Canada)

PURPOSE: The Caregiver Educat on Program is designed to augment coping skills and quality of life for caregivers of relatives with Alzheimer's disease and their families early in the caregiving journey. As such, its aims are to enhance caregiver capacity to avoid crises and to remain active participants in the community, to maximize the well-being of persons with dementia living at home, and to assist all involved to envision a future with hope and meaning. To that end, the purpose of the present study was to evaluate the pilot test of this program and to make recommendations for implementation. METHOD: Delivered in small group format, program information and materials on the development of effective skills and techniques in caring for a senior as well as on access to community resources, are intertwined with exercises that build personal support mechanisms. Specific attention is paid to integrating messages of hope and to caregiver sharing of personal experiences. Thus, evaluation strategies focused on caregiver knowledge, skill and attitude changes related to assisting with meaningful daily living and personal care activities, problem solving abilities, management of personal stress, and identification and use of community resources. RESULTS: This paper reports caregiver changes related to the caregiving role on completion of the program. Specific attention is directed to identifying changes in caregiver confidence, competence and hope. CONCLUSION: Drawing from the quantitative and qualitative findings, the paper concludes with recommendations for program implementation.

Pre-Post Mood, Burden, and Coping Assessment: Effectiveness of Support Groups for Dementia Patients and/ or Caregivers

M. Gorman (Queen Elizabeth II Health Sciences Centre - QEIIHSC, Halifax, NS, Canada, and P. Myers (QEIIHSC & Acadia University, Wolfville, NS, Canada)

This presentation examines the use of the Profile of Mood States, the Zarit Burden Inventory, and the Coping Inventory for Stressful Situations in measuring the effectiveness of the 8-week QEIIHSC support group for dementia patients and/or their caregivers. Dementia is an adaptational challenge that may elicit negative emotions and attempts to cope for both the patient and their caregiver. Although problem solving or task-oriented coping is generally considered to be healthiest, dementia presents a number of uncontrollable situations that may require alternate coping strategies. Furthermore, caregivers of dementia patients are also faced with the burden of coping with a chronic and deteriorating situation that may threaten their own physical and mental health. The QEIIHSC support group uses a structured approach to providing information about the nature of dementia, training in developing balanced coping skills, and the availability of social support and resources. A realistic appraisal of what can and cannot be controlled in dementia is expected to yield positive changes in the outcome measures: the alleviation of negative moods and some aspects of burden, and more appropriate use of coping skills and resources. This study reports changes in moods, aspects of burden, and coping skills as indicators of program effectiveness in five groups with an average of 11 participants per group.

The Circle Model: Support for relatives of people with dementia (A model carried out in Sweden)

Britt Almberg (The National Board of Health and Welfare and The Karolinska Institute, Sweden.)

t is necessary that family caregivers receive considerable support and assistance on an individualized basis to prevent them from being overburdened, and to prolong the time the person with dementia can remain at home. Indeed, effective interventions that will fit the preferences of the family caregivers are increasingly needed to reduce the stress of caregiving. For these reasons, a model - The Circle model - was developed, tested and evaluated in six places in Sweden. Participants were relatives of people with dementia, volunteers and parish deacons. The model is unique in that family caregivers and volunteers were educated together in study circles and their training the volunteers replaced the caregivers in their homes regularly. It provides the caregivers with necessary training and regular time-off from the day-to-day care relative care of a relative with dementia. An advantage with the model is training proceeding the care replacement period. These phases provide the necessary knowledge for dealing with the complexity and severe nature of dementia. It also provides an insight for those providing the respite care into what family caregivers are experiencing. Another advantage of this model is that persons suffering from dementia can remain in their homes, in an environment, which is familiar to them. The Circle Model is going to be developed into a national study in Sweden.

The evaluation of a personalized phone call intervention conducted with family caregivers of individuals suffering from Alzheimer's disease

C. Dubé, J. Vézina (School of Psychology, University Laval, Quebec, Canada)

This study's objective is to evaluate the efficacy of a personalized phone call intervention aimed at lowering depressive symptoms, anxiety, burden and family caregivers' desire to institutionalize the family member suffering from Alzheimer's disease presenting with non-aggressive behavioral disturbances. The sample included 50 family caregivers and an equivalent number of individuals suffering from Alzheimer's disease. The family caregivers were divided in two groups: the treatment group (n=25) and the control group (n=25). The results suggest that caregivers who participated in the intervention significantly reduced their depressive symptoms in comparison to the control group. Similar results were also found with anxiety levels since a significant decrease was noted amidst the treatment group. Finally, caregivers who participated in the intervention reported a significant decline in their intentions to institutionalize their kin. Overall, the results indicate the pertinence to create personalized call intervention programs that are based upon behavioral therapies and that primarily take into account the behavioral disturbances of individuals suffering from Alzheimer's disease.

The systemic support to the caregivers in Alzheimer's disease: interest of the Calgary model

M.P.Labernadie , B.Placines (Centre de Gérontologie de Pontacq-Nay , 64800 Nay , France) , F.Canton (Centre de Gérontologie de Pontacq-Nay , 64530 Pontacq , France) , M.Tastet (Centre de Gérontologie de Pontacq-Nay , 64800 Nay , France), M.N.Lannette (Centre de Gérontologie de Pontacq-Nay , 64800Nay , France), M.A.Jareno (Centre de Gérontologie de Pontacq-Nay , 64530 Pontacq , France)

The support to the caregivers is now integrated in the therapeutic program proposed in the case of Alzheimer 's disease . The constitution of the support group , the systemic familial therapies in wich finds the patient with Alzheimer's disease . The proces presents: the first one , the pre-therapeutic phase concerns the familial evolution with the genogram , the ecomap , wich allow to know the social network of the subject and the pattern of circular communications allowing to know the sentimental modalities and the ideic of the interindividual exchanges; the second one , the therapeutic phase is realised by a nurse through semi-directive interviews: after the evaluation of the pretherapeutic phase , different hypothesis are elaborated and some questions rise up; these last one allow the evolution of familial system . The objective is to help , on the hand the principal caregiver in difficulty to exploit the ressources of familial system in order to become a source of support and a collaborator in the therapeutic project; on the other hand to develop the Familial system in order to improve the patient's and caregiver's quality of life.

SESSION 150

Creative Housing Solutions for Older Adults

Malgosia T. Zlobicki, [School of Architecture, Interior and Industrial Design, Queensland Univ. of Technology, Brisbane, Australia] (Graduate Education in Design for Aging Through Flexible Delivery) Satoshi Kose [Building Research Institute, Tsukuba, Japan] (Housing for an aging society: adapting housing design toward universality) Satya Brink (Gerontology Research Centre, Simon Fraser University, Vancouver, Canada) (Housing for Successful Aging - A trade-off between location, services and technology for acceptable housing cost) Ad van Berlo [Smart Homes Foundation, The Netherlands] (Smart Homes: Security and comfort for older people) James T. Sykes [Department of Preventive Medicine, Univ. of Wisconsin, Madison, Wisconsin, USA] (Proposed Public Initiatives to Provide Assisted Living Services to Frail Elders in Subsidized Housing) Juan F. Hitzig [Adolfo Hirsch Home and Hospital, Buenos Aires, Argentina] (Impact of the Environment on Health, Aging and Dementia: "From Cell to Habitat")

The abstract ISSUE: Design and policy for optimal solutions to housing and services for the elderly STRUCTURE: statement outlining the organization of the session. After a brief initial presentation by the convenor introducing subjects and participants, each of them will address the audience in turn. At the end the convenor will draw the conclusions. CONTENT: summary of the presentations to be given. We were able to gather, as required, six leading experts in the field of education, research, policy, design, technology, security, economy and health. They will talk about their experiences in education and design for housing and services for the elderly. CONCLUSIONS/ANTICIPATED OUTCOMES: statement of the conclusions, expected outcome or 'product' of the session. The main goal is to raise the issue of the necessity of integrating different kinds of expertise in order to solve adequately the growing problem of providing appropriate housing and services for older adults. Due to demographic reasons, it is necessary to educate the population, especially professionals and policy makers, on the multiple social, economic, and technical knowledge required to solve the problems addressed.

Graduate Education in Design for Aging Through Flexible Delivery

MT Zlobicki (School of Architecture, Interior and Industrial Design, Queensland University of Technology, Brisbane, Australia)

From late 1997, the School of Architecture, Interior and Industrial Design, Queensland University of Technology, commenced to develop Australia's first postgraduate course in design for aging. This process was preceded by a continuing professional education complement on design for aging over two semesters. The new course, to be known as Graduate Certificate in Built Environment (Design for Aging), is to comprise four core units: Design for Aging Criteria, Design for Aging Performance, Design for Aging Evaluation, and Design for Aging Realisation. The principal aim of the course is to provide designers and aged care professionals with the opportunity to rapidly advance their knowledge of innovative design for aging practices and trends applicable to their work-related activities. Participation is expected from local, national and international targets. An expression of interest in the course from designers and aged care professionals is being monitored through a preliminary enrollment form. By 2000, over 50 pre-enrollments were received. The course is to be offered through a two-week 'compact' of intensive lectures and group-work, as well as via e-mail/Internet tuition. It is to encompass such disciplines as architecture, interior/industrial/urban design, and landscape architecture. Australian and overseas experts from diverse backgrounds have been consulted on the most favourable course content. It is likely that in the future, the course will be expanded by a further four core units to become a Graduate Diploma in Built Environment (Design for Aging).

Housing for an aging society: Adapting housing design toward universality

Satoshi Kose (Building Research Institute, Tsukuba, Japan)

Purpose: The whole globe is aging, and it is of vital importance to solve problems related to the trend. The Japanese Construction Ministry started a five-year research project on design for the aging society in 1987. Design for All Ages was set as the key concept. It is a clear departure from age segregation that has been the idea of sheltered housing scheme. It assumes that residents will age in place, and that the dwellings should be able to respond to the changing needs of residents. Method: It has been tried to integrate existing knowledge with new ideas derived from experiments, etc. Basic concepts for dwellings that have been finally adopted are: Safety; accessibility; usability; and affordability. The above can be interpreted as follows in terms of design guidelines: 1) Basically flat floor, no door sills, no step differences, unless vitally necessary. 2) Handrail installation at critical places, such as stairs, bathroom, toilet, and entrances. 3) Wider corridors and doors. Results: The final Guidelines are based on the discussions of effectiveness, design and economic feasibility, climatic conditions, and cultural tradition. To put them into practice, the Japan Housing Loan Corporation took a decisive step to ask barrier-free or energy conscious design to be eligible for lowest interest rates, starting fiscal 1996. Conclusion: Along with the issuance of Guidelines, consumer education was also done through various measures. These new moves will work to promote construction of barrier-free dwellings, and the majority of newer dwellings will be basically barrier-free in the long run.

Housing for Successful Aging - A trade-off between location, services and technology for acceptable housing cost

Satya Brink [Gerontology Research Centre, Simon Fraser University, Vancouver, Canada.]

Housing decisions taken by seniors are more complex than previous ones and they have major implications for quality of life. While earlier housing decisions are based on size and location for acceptable housing cost, seniors have to make trade-offs between design, location, services and technology. If homes are not designed for aging, additional costs may be required for renovation. Because home care is not universally available in Canada and equally well distributed across the country, the majority of seniors depend on informal care by members of their families. In weighing their options, seniors must determine, whether it is better to move to a more central location where there are more services and amenities which can be accessed without driving, or whether they should move closer to their children, who most likely being of child rearing age, live in the suburbs. Data shows that most seniors live in homes with more space per person than younger families. Most seniors do not move, since they own their homes free of mortgage and they can continue to rely on their existing network. Houses in which seniors have aged in place are older and therefore, rarely hard-wired for technology. The introduction of wireless technology may be positive.

Impact of the Environment on Health, Aging and Dementia: From Cell to Habitat

Juan F. Hitzig [Adolfo Hirsch Home and Hospital, Buenos Aires, Argentina]

The purpose of this paper is to state the influence of the environment over the person, based on experiences held with 150 residents at the Adolfo Hirsch Home and Hospital in Argentina. By creating prosthetic and therapeutic environments we stimulate our patients' autonomy and noticeably reduced accidents and disabilities. The built environment was complemented with stimulation based on physical, psychical and spiritual activation programs; this contributed to reduce institutionalization stress and to improve the quality of life, thus delaying some effects of aging. Recreating "spaces" and "moments" increased the performance of cognitively deteriorated patients. Health, illness and the rhythm of aging are the result of an eco-psycho-neuro-immune endocrinologic interaction. We are partly a product of environment, which is itself an extension of ourselves. The latest knowledge about neurotransmitters, stem cells and Neuronal Growing Factor lead us to believe that the central nervous system is not as hostile to neuronal regeneration as it was once considered. We may conclude that health is the result of person-environment interaction, particularly in patients with cognitive pathology. Designing environments does not only mean to create safe and functional surroundings for daily life. It also means to create a physical area and an atmosphere which generates emotions and perceptions whose neurochemical translation will improve health and slow down aging. Assisted homes, residences and nursing homes may become the ideal providers of these concepts. Examples will be shown.

Proposed Public Initiatives to Provided Assisted Living Services to Frail Elders in Subsidized Housing

James T Sykes [Department of Preventive Medicine, Univ. of Wisconsin, Madison, Wisconsin, USA]

The abstract Where one lives is the single most compelling fact of one's life, and that is increasingly true as people age. With longevity the probability of disability increases; fortunately, when one has assistance, lives in an accomodating affordable apartment, and practices self-help, despite disabilities, one may remain in one's home for many years. Recently, the Elderly Housing Coalition, a coalition of US voluntary organizations with an advocacy mission, issued a white paper, written by James T. Sykes, urging the Departments of Health and Human Services and Housing and Urban Development to provide the benefits of assisted living in subsidized housing programs by funding service coordinators, physical adaptation of apartments and facilities and enabling community service providers to utilize space within housing projects to deliver supportive services to frail residents - in effect bringing services to frail residents rather than transporting people to the services. Based on state and national research findings that document the effectiveness of service coordinators, co-located services providers, and limited physical facility adaptation, the report is being used by housing advocates to urge priority attention to the need for expanding programs to enable frail elders living in subsidized housing to remain in their homes, with the services they need, and at a reasonable cost to individuals and to the nation. This presentation will highlight efforts to focus public attention on social problems vulnerable to public policy interventions and to apply comprehensive evaluation research to inform and urge public policy initiatives.

Smart Homes: Security and comfort for older people

Ad van Berlo, M.A. [Smart Homes Foundation, The Netherlands]

The abstract: Smart home technology in the integration of technology and services through home networking for a better quality of living. As demonstration projects, in the Province of North-Brabant in the Netherlands, five apartment blocks with in total 120 apartments were built for older people. From the beginning they were involved to express their wishes and needs. During the year 2000 all five projects have been finished and older citizens are living now in the houses. Applications with smart technology include: Central access to the building and to the individual apartment is allowed with an electronic card. There are emergency, intruder and smoke alarms, but also automatic alarming at too long periods of inactivity. All lights, temperature and blinds can be controlled via normal buttons on the wall or by remote control. The electric stove is automatically de-activated when leaving the apartment (using the switch at the front door) or going to sleep. Above the bed, there is also a panic button and there is the switch for switching off the inactivity measurement when going to sleep. The five demonstration projects with home automation for older people have learnt what older people themselves find very important to live comfortably and secure. First reactions of most residents are very positive. Of course there have been problems with using all equipment and sometimes difficult to use interfaces. Now, most residents don't want to miss all technology and are very proud on it.

SESSION 151

Caregiving Needs of Chinese Stroked Elderly Families in Hong Kong

Regina Lee (The Hong Kong Polytechnic University, Department of Nursing & Health Sciences, Hong Kong Special Administrive Region, China

This study aimed to fill the gap services by identifying the perceived difficulty in handling tasks among Chinese family caregivers of stroked elderly using Caregiver Tasks Inventory (CTI), developed by Clark and Rakowski in 1983, which was derived from clustering points of consensus from an intensive literature review. CTI consisted of 45 items with three subscales: direct care, intrapersonal tasks, and intrapersonal ties. A descriptive, cross-sectional survey method was employed. 85 family caregivers of stroked elderly were recruited to investigate the caregivers' needs in this study. The ratio of female to male was 13:4. The majority (51%) aged between 60 and 86, 20% aged between 50 and 60, and 10% aged between 24 and 50. Most of the elderly (58%) were Comprehensive Social Security Assistance Scheme recipients. Results indicated that the perceived level of difficulty in handling the three main aspects of tasks were different: direct care (Mean = 1.67), intrapersonal tasks (Mean = 1.51), and interpersonal ties (Mean = 1.42) and caregivers who had a shorter duration of caregiving perceived greater difficulty especially in direct care and intrapersonal tasks ($p < 0.05$). These findings indicated the need for nurses, and other health care providers, to establish appropriate interventions, programs, and services for these caregivers.

Caring For The Carer: an Australian Survey of Carer Needs

Jane E Gallagher (Carers Association ACT, Canberra, Australia)

In Australia (population 18.3 million), 500,000 people have the prime caring responsibility for a family member, usually a partner or parent. Carer respite is funded by the Federal Government, but provided by State-based non-profit organisations. A national network of Carer Respite Centres has been established to coordinate the provision of emergency, short term, and residential respite care. This paper presents the findings of a recent survey of primary carers' needs conducted by the Canberra Respite Care Centre in the Australian Capital Territory. Method: 100 consecutive clients of the Canberra Respite Care Centre completed an interviewer-administered needs-assessment questionnaire. Results: Carers who were still in paid work (20% of respondents) wanted the Canberra Respite Care Centre to organise electronic networks (e.g. e-mail, chatrooms) and teleconferencing opportunities so that they could communicate with other carers and with the respite care providers. Older carers (age 65/+) (66% of respondents) indicated that their need for respite care generally began when their own health began to deteriorate or when the medical condition of the person they were caring for began to deteriorate. Carers from non-English-speaking countries (12% of respondents) indicated a lack of professional support within their own communities and therefore wanted the Canberra Respite Care Centre to work with their own ethnic associations to establish carer support groups and provide carer education sessions. Conclusion: Providing respite care is not a simple matter. Different groups have different needs and respite care coordinators should regularly survey their clients and potential clients to ascertain their respite needs.

Services for Family Caregivers in the Context of Reduced Hospital Stays: Two Paradigms

F. Ducharme (Researh Centre, Institut universitaire de gériatrie de Montréal, Montreal, Canada), G. Pérodeau (Université du Québec, Hull, Canada), M. Paquet (Régie Régionale de la Santé et des Services Sociaux de Lanaudière , Joliette, Canada), J. Dufour (Association des Hôpitaux du Québec' Montreal, Canada), D. Trudeau, A. Legault (Research Centre, Institut universitaire de gériatrie de Montréal, Montreal, Canada)

The purpose of this study was to explore the perceptions and expectations of family caregivers and health care administrators towards services offered to caregivers of the elderly in the context of the shift towards ambulatory care. A qualitative ethnographic method was used to document the standpoints of these two groups considered as informants of the lay and technocratic sub-cultures. Focus-group were conducted in rural and urban areas with caregivers and administrators separately using semi-structured interview guides. A comparative content analysis of transcribed verbatim of group interviews showed divergent perceptions: 1) caregivers perceive a lack of services and a poor fit between their values, needs and available services; they expect the development of new adequate and accessible services in the context of their increased responsibilities in home care; 2) in contrast, hospital and community centres administrators perceive caregivers as resources for the health care system rather than actual clients of services; they believe that a proper structure of services and a variety of adequate multidimensional services are implemented in hospitals and in community settings. These results suggest different paradigmatic views which may explain, in part, the low use of services by caregivers and the slow development of innovative services for caregivers as co-clients of the health care system. Stakeholders' paradigms are important socio-cultural determinants of services; this study emphasizes the importance in sharing perceptions between two key-players. It also unveils the need for a stronger interconnection between formal and informal networks frames of reference with regard to health care services. These conditions are prerequisites for implementing adequate services as the health care reform imposes larger responsibilities to families for the care of the elderly population in many developed countries.

The COPE Index: an innovative instrument for a first stage assessment of needs in informal carers

K. McKee, I. Philp, M. Nolan (University of Sheffield, United Kingdom), G. Lamura, L. Spazzafumo (INRCA, Ancona, Italy), C. Prouskas (SEXTANT, Athens, Greece), B. Öberg, B. Krevers (University of Linköping, Sweden), B. Bien (Medical Academy of Bialystok, Poland) and the COPE group (1) (1): J. Chwalow (INSERM, Paris, France); E. Mestheneos, J. Triantafillou (SEXTANT, Athens, Greece); M.G. Melchiorre, S. Quattrini, C. Sirolla (I.N.R.C.A, Ancona, Italy); K. Szczerbinska (Jagiellonian University, Krakow, Poland); Z. B. Wojszel, J. Wilmanska (Medical Academy of Bialystok, Poland); B. Politynska (University of Bialystok, Poland); R. Hassler (University of Linköping, Sweden); C. Abrams, K. Meadows (University of Hull, United Kingdom); K. Lothian (University of Sheffield, United Kingdom).

In this presentation the main features of the Carers of Older People in Europe (COPE) Index are described. This is an innovative instrument for the assessment of carers' needs which is based Δ unlikely most of the currently used, mainly burden-related tools Δ on an evaluation of both positive and negative aspects of caregiving. Five countries collected data from informal carers of older people (N=577) via a common protocol, which had undergone previous cross-cultural linguistic validation. Data included a) the COPE index, a 17-item instrument collecting carers' perceptions; b) a questionnaire on demographic and caregiving circumstances, and c) three instruments for the criterion validation of the COPE Index: the General Health Questionnaire, the Hospital Anxiety and Depression Scale, and the World Health Organisation Quality of Life-BREF. Principal Component Analysis showed that two emergent components, negative impact and positive value, were common across countries, while a third component, quality of support, was not. Negative impact and positive value scales were internally consistent and significantly associated with the criterion validity measures. Four items from the quality of support component were also associated with the criterion measures. These items and the two scales were retained in the final version of COPE Index. The evaluation of the factorial structure, internal consistency, and criterion validity of the COPE Index allows to say that, while further testing is required, this instrument can currently be considered a useful alternative to existing instruments which are usually administered for a first stage assessment of informal carers' needs.

The need for family care for seniors in Shanghai City in the 21st century

Gui shixun (East China Normal University , Shanghai, China)

Rapid social change is characteristic of Shanghai as it is within other places in China and other countries around the world. Family care is a particular interest, given traditional cultural notions of filial piety within China. Based on the 1998 survey of Shanghai elderly population, the author analyzes health needs of seniors in Shanghai, taking into account their functional disability and their family situation. Projections are made about the family care that will be needed in the first 50 years of the 21st century and policies suggested for improving family care. Suggestions include: promoting education on respect, support and assistance of seniors; gradual implementation of the policy permitting a couple to have two children; developing community services that support family care; promoting prevention; encouraging young healthy retired seniors to participate in family care; strengthening the training of those people who provide family care; improving coordination of public welfare services and public health services; requiring family care; and providing appropriate policies and sufficient funds to support family care.

SESSION 152

Multi/Inter-disciplinary research in Gerontology ideals and realities

Vidik (University of Aarhus, Aarhus, Denmark). Multidisciplinary research a biologist s view. L.W. Poon (University of Georgia, Athens, Georgia USA), I. C. Siegler (Duke University Medical Center, Durham, North Carolina USA). Interdisciplinary gerontology: Looking back and forward. N.L. Chappell. (Center on Aging, University of Victoria, Victoria, British Columbia, Canada). Multidisciplinary Research: Achieving the Promise. G. Samuelsson (Gerontology Research Center, Lund, Sweden. Multi-disciplinary research in gerontology -reflections from 30 years of experiences. Discussant: L. Tornstam (University of Uppsala, Uppsala, Sweden)

In most handbooks in gerontology it is stressed that gerontology, in its nature, is inter-disciplinary. In the practice that seems not to be fulfilled. This symposium, with participants from North America and Europe will cover following topics: 1. What is the main features of the policy for multi-/inter-disciplinary research from a political, research foundations, and a professional perspective during the past years? What are the main obstacles to multi-/inter-disciplinary research when analyzed from a structural perspective (i.e. research foundations, proposal reviewers, university structure) as well as from the individual researchers point of view (furthers one's career, training and incentives)? 3. What can be done to strengthen the multi-/inter-disciplinary research, according to both a structural and individual perspective?

Interdisciplinary gerontology: Looking back and forward

L.W. Poon (University of Georgia, Athens, Georgia USA), I. C. Siegler (Duke University Medical Center, Durham, North Carolina USA)

This paper will examine the development of gerontology beginning with the early uni-disciplinary emphases, obstacles in academic institutions toward multi- and inter-disciplinary gerontology, examples of inter-disciplinary programs, as well as what must be done in order for gerontology to be recognized as a discipline.

Multi-disciplinary research in gerontology -reflections from 30 years of experiences.

G. Samuelsson (Gerontology Reserach Center, Lund, Sweden)

"..we has a mountain of information but little integration across disciplines and phenomena" and ...Gerontology is islands of knowledge" according to Birren (1999). Looking for a definition of Multi-disciplinary Research in different encyclopedias in Gerontology nothing was found. Is that a reflection of the interest and strength of Multi-disciplinary research in Gerontology? Scrutinizing multi-disciplinary research from a University perspective it was and is still in Sweden and many other countries impossible to get through a dissertation with a multi-disciplinary perspective - the University structure is still not ready for a break through of that. The training in Gerontology have features of multi-disciplinary research knowledge but when it come to writing a dissertation the University reality is not ready to accept it. How to strengthen successful multi-disciplinary research? On the structural level there is a need to reorganize the Research Foundations and my suggestion to set up special sections for multidisciplinary research with experienced multi-disciplinary researchers as reviewers. Regarding the University structure there is a need to set up special departments with multi-disciplinary research as the main goal with possibilities for one or more colleagues to produce dissertations with multi-disciplinary perspectives. My experiences is also that there exists a big gap between the political expectations on research to be more integrated and holistic in its performing. However, political pressure on the scientific society is a very controversial suggestion but perhaps a must to strengthen the integration of different disciplines. A last suggestion is also to start up projects about multi-disciplinary research to collect experiences from the field.

Multidisciplinary research: A biologist's view

A. Viidik (University of Aarhus, Aarhus, Denmark)

Some biologists tend to have solutions to most problems. The best example is the completion of the mapping of the human genome - it has been claimed that the results are just for harvesting. Further, the solution to the enigma of the ageing process might be just around the corner, especially since biologists already can double the life span of roundworms. Hype claiming this has been voiced in the popular press. But, the genome of the roundworm contains about 19,000 genes and the human one about 100,000. This suggests a much higher degree of complexity in the human genome. And the gene-manipulated roundworm is no longer fit for life outside laboratory glassware. Further, having a map of the human genome does not mean that the functions of the genes and the gene products are known. Many years of work, which cannot be done by automated sequencing machines, thus remains. This leads to the question how research on the enigma of the biological ageing process should proceed, keeping the deliberations within a reasonable degree of reality. One must realise that the biological processes of ageing do not act alone. There is a multitude of interactions, both positive and negative, from a variety of sources that confound the "clean" models studied in the controlled and protected environment of the laboratory, such as lifestyle factors as well as influences derived from psychological and social mechanisms. One example is the death of an old husband or wife the surviving old partner has an increased risk of death, partly due to immunosuppression initiated by psychological mechanisms and mediated by the hypothalami-adrenal axis. Multidisciplinary research, combining the knowledge and methods available in biology, epidemiology, medicine, psychology and sociology, could be the solution. Such research can be conducted in several modes (some at times called interdisciplinary research). One mode is a protocol, in which every discipline conducts its part and the synthesis of the results is made by statistical analyses. The outcome is a bunch of correlations, which not necessarily show causative relations, especially if the participating scientists are not aware of limitations and ambiguities of the from different disciplines derived set of research tools. Another mode seems more appealing. The members of the team of scientists from different disciplines speak, so to say, each other's languages and together analyse the strong and weak points inherent in all research tools used. The analyses of the set of results will then probably point with more confidence towards causative relation. The work to achieve this common "working language" is much harder than just chasing the statistical significances that more guarantees publishability than enhances our knowledge of the mechanisms of human ageing.

Multidisciplinary Research: Achieving the Promise

N.L. Chappell. (Center on Aging, University of Victoria, Victoria, British Columbia, Canada).

Although some researchers have been engaged in multidisciplinary research for many years, funding agencies have just recently recognized this approach and now often require it. Frequently, unfortunately, multidisciplinarity appears only on paper and is not translated into the interaction among those involved. Often, many names are put on a proposal and each is provided with their own monies and each proceeds to conduct their own research from their own disciplinary perspective as they always have. This talk discusses what happens in reality and why it happens, and then goes on to discuss the ideal or the promise and how to achieve that promise. Achieving the ideal of multidisciplinary research implies that there is sufficient understanding of one another´s approach in order to ensure a dialogue between different perspectives; it requires commitment from those involved, and it requires time. Furthermore, multidisciplinary research among differing academic researchers is different from multidisciplinary research which incorporates applied perspectives from non-academics, such as different levels of government or seniors´ organizations. Finally, amidst the current popularity of multidisciplinarity, it must be remembered that we require and will always require strong disciplinary research upon which the foundation of multidisciplinarity is built.

SESSION 153

Changing Attitudes to Filial Piety in Asian Cultures

S. J. Choi (Seoul National University, Seoul, Korea), J. C. B. Leung (The University of Hong Kong, Hong Kong, China), J. Lubben (School of Public Policy and Social Research, UCLA, USA), Y. Yokoyama (Hokusei Gakuen University, Sapporo, Japan)

This symposium deals with the attitudes of original Asian countries' people and Asian immigrants to America toward filial piety in modernizing contemporary societies, their practice of the value in their societies, and ways to promote the value as a more universal one across the culture. Three presenters from Hong Kong, Japan, and South Korea speak on their observations on their original countries' people, and one presenter from America speaks on his observations on Korean Americans living in Los Angeles. Prof. Leung from Hong Kong, China reviews recent studies on filial piety and family support for the elderly in China, and shows to what extent the cherished value and practice of filial piety have been eroded by demographic shift and modernization. The results of his reviews shows that filial obligations are still intact and the majority of the elderly still live with and are cared by their children. With longer life expectancy more healthy elderly prefer to live independently from their children, whereas more frail elderly people have to move into institutional care. He argues that there is an urgent need to have an objective appraisal of the changing family values toward the care of the elderly, and formal home-based and community-based social services should be developed to facilitate family support. Prof. Yokoyama from Japan says that most of Japanese people still believe the value of filial piety as a virtue in Japanese culture and as a respectable social moral even in modern Japanese society. He argues that the changing sense of filial piety forces Japanese elders to become less dependent on their children regarding the matter of care-giving, on the other hand, it makes them suffer from the feeling of being abandoned by their children. Prof. Choi from South Korea addresses the dimensions of, and attitudes to, practice of filial piety in modern Korean society and suggests some underlying beliefs that can promote modern practice of filial piety as a more universal social value across the culture. Three dimensions were identified in practicing filial piety: behavioral, emotional and familial dimensions. He argues that some new relational beliefs between parents and children that can promote modern practice of filial piety may be equality, reciprocity and virtue. Prof. Lubben from America examines confirmation of filial piety norms among Korean Americans contrasting those data with that collected from a comparison group of non-Hispanic white Americans. His findings are that there are more intergenerational social supports exchanges among Korean American elders and their offspring than among the comparison group, and they are much more likely to live with adult child or grandchild than their comparison group. He argues that filial piety norms might explain some of the family social support differences observed. These presentations are expected to come up with finding positive functions of practicing filial piety in modern society and suggesting some new practice guidelines to promote the value of filial piety as a more universal social value across the culture.

Changing Attitudes and New Dimension of Filial Piety in Modern Japanese Society

Y. Yokoyama (School of Social Welfare, Hokusei Gakuen University, Sapporo, Japan)

The value of filial piety is still appreciated and its practice is considered to be important in modern Japanese society. Filial piety comes from Confucianism and the Japanese people learn the value at home or school. However, practicing filial piety in modern Japanese society has become difficult because of social change in Japan. The first purpose of this study is to describe current attitudes toward the value of filial piety among Japanese people in modern Japanese society. The second purpose is to describe a new dimension of filial piety conducted by Japanese people in the present Japanese society. The third purpose is to describe how the changing attitudes to filial piety in modern Japanese society affect social support for Japanese elders. This study was done by literature review and library research. The results are as follows: (1) Most of Japanese people believe that the value of filial piety is a virtue in Japanese culture. The filial piety is also considered to be a respectable social moral even in modern Japanese society. (2) Some young Japanese people do not much appreciate the sense of filial piety and they believe that elderly people are a sort of social burden. Thus they feel that aged people should be taken care of by the society, not by the family. (3) Changing sense of filial piety forces Japanese elders to become more independent from and less dependent on their children regarding the matter of caregiving. One the other hand, they are suffering from the feeling of being abandoned by their children.

Changing Attitudes to, and Promotion of Filial Piety in Modern Korean Society

S, J. Choi (Seoul National University, Seoul, South Korea)

How to uphold the value of filial piety in modern society has been one of the recurring issues in modernizing Korean society. Koreans generally show relatively wide consensus in maintaining the spirit of filial piety (respect for, love of, care for, and obedience to parents); however, they tend to show relatively negative attitudes toward its practice guideline that has been traditionally prescribed. This presentation is concerned with investigating practical dimensions of and attitudes to filial piety, and tries to find some relational beliefs between parents and children that can promote modern practice of filial piety as a social value in modern Korean society. This study was done through library research and the results are as follows. A review of literature reveals that there are three dimensions in the conduction of filial piety: behavioral, emotional and familial dimensions. These practice dimensions seem to have been formulated based on the underlying beliefs of patriarchal, authoritative, and unilateral relationship between parents and children. Because of these beliefs modern Koreans seem to show negative attitudes toward the prescribed practice guidelines of filial piety in traditional sense. This presentation suggests some new relational beliefs of equality, reciprocity and virtue that modern practice of filial piety can be based on in both familial and societal level. This study argues that filial piety might be promoted as a more universal value across the culture if we could create some new relational beliefs between parents and children, and between the elderly and the society by revising practical guidelines fitting modernizing society.

Family support and filial obligations in China: Change and continuity

J. C. B. Leung (The University of Hong Kong, Hong Kong, China)

For centuries, it has been a cherished Chinese tradition for the elderly people to be supported and cared by their offspring, and formal social services for the aged were often regarded as not necessary. This presentation reviews recent studies on family values and family support for the elderly in China, and shows to what extent the cherished values and practice of filial obligation have been eroded by demographic shift and modernization. This review is based on two sources of data. First, the presentation reviews major studies in China on family support for the elderly in recent years. Second, data are derived from a random sampled opinion survey on welfare attitudes, carried out by the author in a Chinese city in 1998. Evidence shows that filial obligations are still intact, and the majority of the elderly still lived with and are cared by their children. With longer life expectancy, more healthy elderly people are preferring to live independently, whereas more frail elderly people have to move into institutional care. The implications of these findings are that family care based on traditional values cannot be taken for granted as natural and without limits. There is an urgent need to have an objective appraisal of the changing family values toward the care of the elderly, and formal home-based and community-based social services should be developed in China to facilitate family support.

Indicators of Filial Piety among Korean Americans living in Los Angeles

J. Lubben (School of Public Policy and Social Research, UCLA, USA)

This study examines confirmation of filial piety norms among Korean American populations residing in Los Angeles, California and contrasts those data with that collected from a comparison group. Randomly selected Korean American (n=223) and non-Hispanic white American (n=201) adults age 65 years and above were interviewed regarding social support networks, intergenerational exchanges and attitudes towards aging. All Korean elders in this study were immigrants who had lived in the United States for an average of only 11 years whereas the comparison group was mostly born in the U. S. (86%). There were more intergeneraltional social support exchanges among Korean elders and their adult offspring than among the comparison group. The Korean American were three times more likely to live with a child and five times more likely to live with a grandchild as the non-Hispanic white American comparison group. There is some evidence to support Asian American scholars who suggest that filial piety norms might explain some of the family social support differences observed. The paper discusses some of the reasons for these differences and possible consequences on levels of social integration with friends and neighbours.

SESSION 154

Using Indicators to Measure Well-Being: An International Perspective

Kristen Robinson [National Center for Health Statistics, Hyattsville, USA] Older Americans 2000: Key Indicators of Well-Being; Martha Pelaez [Pan American Health Organization/World Health Organization, Washington, USA] Latin American and Caribbean Indicators of Aging and Well-Being; Alan Lopez [World Health Organization, Geneva, Switzerland] A Cross-National Comparability of Data on the Health Status of Older Persons; Kathryn Wilkins [Statistics Canada, Ottawa, Canada] The Impact of Excluding Institutionalized Elderly from Survey Data.

ISSUE: General indicators of social and economic well-being are typically employed to provide benchmark information for measuring future progress within a particular population group. For the older population, such key indicators are generally measured in the areas of population size and growth, socioeconomic status, health status, health care utilization, and urban/rural residency. By examining a broad range of indicators, researchers, policymakers, and service providers can better track those areas of well-being that are improving for older people, as well as highlight those priority areas which require more attention and effort. STRUCTURE: The symposium will consist of papers from four individuals who will discuss the indicators of aging and well-being their organizations use to evaluate the status of older populations in select countries. The presentations will include brief discussions on the indicators selected to assess aging and well-being, the data used to construct the indicators, key findings derived from the data, and the data needs that still exist. A discussant will summarize the findings of these papers and briefly comment on the data needs of an aging world. CONTENT: In an effort to describe the overall status of the U.S. population age 65 and older, the Federal Interagency Forum on Aging-Related Statistics (Forum) recently released a new report Older Americans 2000: Key Indicators of Well-Being (Older Americans 2000). The report is divided into five subject areas (population, economics, health status, health risks and behaviors, and health care) and includes 31 key indicators carefully selected by the Forum to portray aspects of the lives of older Americans and their families. To stimulate discussion on these important measures of well-being, the Forum organized this symposium to present a cross-national comparison of the indicators used to measure the status and well-being of older populations around the world. The panel members consist of study directors and project officers from international organizations who are currently involved in collecting and analyzing data on older populations. CONCLUSIONS/ANTICIPATED OUTCOMES: The outcome of this symposium will be a cross-national comparison of key indicators of aging and well-being. It will include an overview of elder well-being across the participating countries, a discussion of the disparities revealed by these indicators, and a review of the data needs identified by each of the panel members. The Forum will produce a compendium of these papers that will be used to revise, update, and improve the indicators in the next edition of Older Americans 2000. In addition, the Forum hopes this symposium will promote cross-national research and encourage greater international collaboration

A Cross-Population Comparability of Data on the Health Status of Older Persons

Alan D. Lopez and Chris Murray [World Health Organization, Geneva, Switzerland]

PURPOSE: Cross-national comparisons contribute important findings to the study of health and well-being in older populations. Until recently, however, little has been done to improve the "cross-population comparability" of the survey instruments used to collect and monitor indicators of health and well-being. Identification of various methods and parameters to achieve cross-population comparability will improve both the quality and utility of cross-national data. METHOD: The World Health Organization analyzed over 60 representative national health surveys for the estimation of disability-adjusted life expectancy for World Health Report 2000. During this project, researchers found a large number of survey instruments were being used to evaluate health status across countries. There was no single survey instrument being commonly used by all (or most) of the countries to collect, evaluate, and monitor health status. RESULTS: Evaluation of the cross-population comparability of data on the health status of older persons has shown that comparability problems relate not only to differences in survey design and methods, but much more fundamentally to unmeasured differences in expectations and norms for health. CONCLUSION: The results of this research are relevant not only for international programs concerned with measuring and monitoring the health of older populations across countries, but also for national programs that have diverse older populations living within their borders.

Latin American and Caribbean Indicators of Aging and Well-Being

Martha Pelaez [Pan American Health Organization/World Health Organization, Washington, USA], Alberto Palloni [University of Wisconsin-Madison, Madison, USA] and Guido Pinto [Pan American Health Organization/World Health Organization, Washington, USA].

PURPOSE: In an effort to document the status of aging research in Latin America and the Caribbean (LAC), the Pan American Health Organization has developed sub-regional databases for planning, monitoring, and evaluating the well-being of elders. METHOD: The databases include information from the Health and Well-being Study on Aging in seven urban centers in LAC; statistical data available from national surveys and administrative data sources; and qualitative data obtained from work done with key informants and focus groups of older persons. The presentation will: a) explain the different approaches taken for the development of the databases; b) present the indicators selected by each sub-regional committee grouped around five main topics — population, economics, health status, health risks and behaviors, and health care; and c) discuss the implication of this work for policy making. RESULTS: Accessibility to adequate data proved to be one of the major problems encountered during this project. Specifically, it was difficult to construct measures of inequality relating to well-being and gender, age cohort, socioeconomic status, and urban/rural residency. In addition, the unprecedented demographic changes occurring in the Region have made it clear that researchers must measure not only the current well-being of elders, but also develop a system for measuring the health inequities and disabilities of the diverse cohorts of elders during the next 20+ years. CONCLUSION: There is a great need for the development of core data on aging and health across developing countries. Specific recommendations will be discussed.

Older Americans 2000: Key Indicators of Well-Being

Kristen Robinson [National Center for Health Statistics, Hyattsville, USA]

PURPOSE: The global population is aging at a rate unprecedented in history. In the United States, the population age 65 and older is expected to double by 2030. To better understand this diverse population, the Federal Interagency Forum on Aging-Related Statistics produced Older Americans 2000: Key Indicators of Well-Being. This comprehensive report provides a valuable tool for tracking the condition of the older population and for making policy decisions that will affect them. METHOD: While many U.S. Federal agencies provide data on various aspects of the challenges confronting older Americans, it is sometimes difficult to understand how this group is faring overall. For the first time, the U.S.

Federal statistical system has come together to pool their data and provide a unified picture of the overall health and well-being of older Americans. RESULTS: Older Americans are healthier, wealthier and better educated than ever before. However, despite decades of progress, older minorities still lag behind in many of the indicators highlighted in this report including education, self-rated health status, and net worth. CONCLUSION: While this report provides substantial information on the population age 65 and older, it is important to note that there remain several important areas where more data are needed to support research and policy efforts. Some of these areas include gathering information on older minorities, improving measures of disability, and including the institutionalized population in national surveys.

The Impact of Excluding Institutionalized Elderly from Survey Data

K. Wilkins, M.P. Beaudet, G. Catlin [Statistics Canada, Ottawa, Canada]

PURPOSE: Health-related indicators such as health status, dependency, and health risks and behaviors are important measures of well-being for the older population. However, the data sources used to construct these indicators often exclude the institutionalized population (i.e, people in nursing homes, psychiatric hospitals, and long-term care facilities) from the base populations used for sampling. METHOD: Using data from Canada's National Population Health Survey (NPHS), this study expands on previous work related to the effects of excluding the institutionalized population on various health-related estimates for the elderly population. The specific variables studied are self-reported level of health, restriction in activities of daily living (ADLs), health status, prevalence of arthritis, dementia, heart disease, incontinence and smoking. Age groups examined include the young-old (65-79) and the old-old (80+). Estimates of the differences in prevalence of selected indicators are derived from two NPHS samples: one composed of the household sample only and the other composed of the household plus the institutionalized population. The technique used to determine the statistical significance of the difference between the prevalence estimates takes into account the design effect of the surveys and the overlap between the samples. RESULTS: The findings in this study build on previous work that found in people aged 65 or older, 7% of the household population are dependent on others for carrying out ADLs, but in the total population of this age group, 11% are dependent. CONCLUSION: These findings indicate the importance of including institutionalized persons when deriving prevalence estimates for the elderly.

SESSION 155

Case Management in Evolving Health Care Systems

Carol Austin (Calgary, Alberta Canada Canadian Perspectives on Case Management in the Evolving Health Care System) Donna Smith (Edmonton, Alberta Canada Canadian Perspectives on Case Management in the Evolving Health Care System) Jenny Brodsky (Jerusalem Israel Improving the System of Care for the Elderly in a Changing Health Care Environment) Walter Leutz (Waltham, MA U.S.A. U. S Health Care Developments) Elizabeth Ozanne (Melbourne, Victoria Australia The Role of Case Management in Health Reform: An Australia and New Zealand Comparison)

Issue: One challenge in the provision of health and social services to older Adults is the fragmentation of delivery systems, producing care that lacks continuity, reduces efficiencies and affects the quality of services, Case management has emerged in a number of countries as a common response to this challenge. National variations in the provision of case management reflect the specific policy and programmatic contexts. Structure. Presentations will focus on the provision of case management in five countries (Israel, Australia, New Zealand, the United States and Canada). Speakers will discuss the evolution of case management in the various health care systems, emerging issues and approaches that have been implemented and their development or modification. Summary: Israel has addressed fragmented service delivery through demonstration projects and national committees that have developed recommendations. Findings from these initiatives suggest the need to critically analyze these experiences, to identify common themes in the data and to revisit the original policy goals. Since the early 1990's U.S. initiatives focused on managed care state programs designed to link acute and long term care. Findings from the S/HMO, PACE, state dual eligibility programs and a Kaiser Permanente HMO demonstration will be reported. The recent emphasis on continuity of care, services integration and case management in Canada will be presented. A research project designed to retrieve and analyze experiences (at system and consumer levels) in six integrative strategies (LINCS) will be presented. Findings from the Coordinated Care Trials will be presented in the larger context of Australia's aged care policy. New Zealand's recent experiences with restructuring its approach to aged care and health services will be reported. Conclusions I Anticipated Outcomes: This symposium will provide cross national comparisons of how the case management function has evolved in various health care systems. Outcomes will include identification of context specific impacts and common trends across national boundaries.

Canadian Perspectives on Case Management in the Evolving Health Care System

D. Smith (University of Alberta, Canada) C. Austin (University of Calgary, Canada)

This paper reports on a project funded by the Canadian Health Services Research Foundation which is designed to examine the status of service integration in health care. Six integration strategies are the focus of the research (a community based geriatric outreach program, a mental health triage program for seniors, the minimum data set for community and continuing care, integrated assessment and case management for community and continuing care, pre-hospital and emergency care and an adult health clinical teaching unit). These strategies are embedded in three regional health authorities in Alberta and Saskatchewan. A multi-method approach (contextual information, documents, client and cost data- bases, interviews with key informants, clients and caregivers) is used to collect data from these sites. The SASI tool (Self Assessment for Systems Integration) has been adapted to assess the extent to which systems integration is present. While several systems integration components are in place (governance, identification of high risk populations, case management and client involvement) other elements are less well developed (management strategies, information technology systems, financing systems, a full array of services and seamless service delivery across settings and over time). Case management alone cannot enhance continuity of care for seniors.

Improving the System of Care for the Elderly in a Changing Health Care Environment

J. Brodsky (JDC- Brookdale, Jerusalem, Israel)

In Israel, as in many other countries, one of the major shortcomings of the system of care for the elderly is its fragmentation. As a result of recent reforms in the health care system and the sharp increase in the need for long-term care, different models have been proposed in Israel to improve the integration of services for the elderly. The purpose of this paper is to summarize lessons from the experiences in the Israeli system, based on demonstration programs and analysis of recommendations of national committees. The discussion will make an effort to identify areas where there seems to be more consensus and convergence- i.e. efforts to improve coordination and develop the appropriate case management mechanisms to ensure continuity of care and areas in which there is less consensus-such as organizational and financial integration among different components of the system. It will analyze prerequisites, advantages, disadvantages, implications and consequences expected from different directions. Based on our analysis, we conclude that the different models should be critically examined in an attempt to determine if there is a consensus regarding the goals of changing the system, beyond the desire to simplify it and reduce bureaucratic complication. Is reducing the financial burden on families a goal? Is increasing level of expenditure a goal? Whatever the model selected, there should be a holistic approach to its organizational and financial components. Most importantly, it will be necessary to examine the implications for the appropriateness of care of the elderly, for the equity of the system and for costs.

Role of Case Management in Health Reform: An Australian/ New Zealand Comparison

Elizabeth Ozanne (The University of Melbourne, Australia)

Australia and New Zealand are both countries that have undertaken major health system reforms in the last decade, opening their substantially public systems to market pressures while maintaining universal access. New Zealand implemented their reforms with an NHS-style integrated model of finance and service delivery. Australia has a mixed system, with national health insurance for primary-care services, and an integrated system for acute and tertiary services. New Zealand undertook its first wave of reforms in the 1980's, introducing area health boards which integrated many health services under a common geographic structure. In the 1990's it created a purchaser/provider split which evolved into a funder/provider arrangement after the 1996 election with the partial corporatisation of publicly owned health enterprises. In the mid-1980's, Australia began experimenting with performance-based hospital financing and competition between public and private hospitals. Case Management has played a varying role in these reforms and this paper seeks to explore the nature of that role both in the Case mix and Coordinated Care Programs implemented in Australia and across the two phases of health reform in New Zealand.

U.S. Health Care Developments

W. Leutz (Brandeis University, Waltham, MA; U.S.A.)

When Bill and Hillary Clinton proposed a managed competition model for health reform in the early 1990's, there were explicit provisions for fair treatment of citizens with chronic illnesses and disabilities. There was even a new benefit for personal care. Since the Clinton plan failed in 1993, the US health care system has charged ahead with privatized, unmanaged competition. Government has responded with payment and regulatory changes, but not with efforts to make mainstream managed care work better for the frail. Rather, several demonstration programs - Social HMOs, PACE, and state dual eligible initiatives - have tried to carve out special managed care options for citizens with disabilities. These programs include richer benefits, chronic illness care, and case management for coordinating acute and long-term care. This presentation reviews the progress of these initiatives, including barriers to their success in the current environment. Also considered will be findings from a recent demonstration in the Kaiser Permanente HMO, which tested a less ambitious but perhaps more feasible approach to linking acute and chronic care.

SESSION 156

Social Policy for the Elderly in Developing Countries

Vijaya Kumar,S (Council for Social Development, Hyderabad, India Social Policy for the Elderly in Asia-sub Region. Iurdaya Rajan, S (Centre for Development Studies, Trivandrum, India Financial & Social Security for Older Women : A Case Study from India Nalini, B (Dept. of Sociology, Madurai Kamaraj University, Madurai, India Health Programmes & Policies for the Elderly in India Prakash Rao, A (Population Research Centre, ISEC, Bangalore, India Social Security Policies for Elderly in India : Gaps between Policies Implications and Needs. Narayana Reddy, V (Dept. of Anthropology, S.V.University, India Social Policies in Sri Lanka, Bangladesh and Nepal : A Cross Cultural Analysis. Changmei He (China National Committee on Ageing) Aging Issue and Its Social Policy in Rural China)

Aging issue and its policy choice in rural China

Changmei He (Survey and investigation department, China National Committee on Ageing, Beijing, P.R.China) Xiaochun Qiao (Institute of Population Research, The People's University of China, Beijing, China)

Purpose: Proposing social policies in context of the aging problem triggered by the rapid shrinking of family size and the reform of socioeconomic institution. Method: Using the method of population projection to estimate the change of age structure and the change of family size in the first half of the 21st century. Combining the related social economic data with projected demographic data to estimate the extent of the problem of aging. Results: 1. The elderly population (60 and over) is 1283 million in current China. It is expected to reach 4000 million in the middle of the 21st century. Its corresponding proportion will increase from 10% to 28%. 2. The average number of children per elderly family will decrease from current 6.1 to 1.8 in the middle of the 21st century. 3. The family care for the elderly will be clearly inadequate due to lack of the number of children (especially male) and the number of children living together with their old parents because over 100 million adults from rural areas will migrate to urban areas. 4. Following the increase of life expectancy, the health expectancy of the elderly have no intensive increase. 5. There are no social security for most people in rural areas. Now less than one percent of adults have participated in social insurance plans in rural areas under the condition that the social relief institution in the conventional planning economic system has been eliminated. 6. The benefit to the people who have participate in the social insurance are so tiny that it is unable to guarantee the living for the elderly. Conclusion: 1. The conventional virtue of the family care in China will no longer exist due to lack of support of children. 2. The appearance of the serious problems of aging will happen from the year of 2010 3. Government will take a responsibility for the aging after the people have taken responsibilities on curbing family size. 4. It will be late to settle the problem of aging if the government and people don't take any action on that now.

Financial and Social Security for Older Women : A Case Study from India

S. Irudaya Rajan

In recent years, the concern for financial and social security is deeply influencing the social and economic policy of the developed as well as developing countries. Social security, stated in terms of assistance and insurance is not a new one for India. For instance, in August 1995, a scheme to protect the poor elderly was announced titled: National Old age Pension Scheme. The numerical ceiling is 5.4 million elderly above 65 years and the qualified amount is Rs. 48020 lakhs. Kerala is the first State in Indian to complete the demographic transitions and also in initiating the social security policies for the elderly women. Apart from central assistance, in Kerala State there are couple of State based social security schemes which is catering the felt needs of the elderly women and most of the schemes are becoming the model for other states in India. The present paper discuss the State based social security programmes for elderly women in Kerala in detail.

Health Programmes and Policies for the Elderly in India

Balasubramaniam Nalini

A scrutiny of health policy and programmes of the government reveal that very little focus is being made on the health care of the elderly population. The elders have never fixed as the target group of any health scheme but, are found to be only a section that can avail the benefits of some schemes. This negligence is due to two reasons firstly increase in life expectancy is a new phenomenon in India and second aging issues are mostly considered to be the concern of the family and not the state. The present research aims to bring out schemes of the State government, that cover the elderly population, analyse the socio-economic variables that operate in the utilisation of these schemes, and to suggest strategies to improve the effectiveness of policies for an age-integrated society. These objectives were carefully examined in the paper and the finally suggested certain policy oriented recommendations.

Social Policies in Sri Lanka, Bangladesh and Nepal : A Cross Cultural Analysis

V. Narayana Reddy and S. Vijaya Kumar

Most of the subregional countries in Asia subregion - India, Sri Lanka, Bangladesh and Nepal are developing countries with underdeveloped economy. Under the trends of globalisation these countries are to some extent experiencing economic crises. However, as a constitutional obligation all these countries are having Social Security and Welfare Policies to cater the needs of the people. Some of these policies are doing much better than others, however, since the societies are in transitional stage certain reforms are essential to the age-old policies which were framed on traditional way. By examining the existing Social Security Policies in India, Sri Lanka, Bangladesh and Nepal, policy oriented comprehensive suggestions were highlighted in this paper.

Social Policy for the Elderly in the Asia-Sub Region

S. Vijaya Kumar

Social security is currently going through a crisis globally and many countries have undertaken to reform their social security policies and systems in order to cope with the crisis. Developed countries are one step ahead than Developing countries in this matter. Considering this silent crisis China started reforming its social security policies and India too proceeding in this direction. The other Asia sub regional countries such as China, Bangladesh, Sri Lanka and Nepal are yet to think about this and for that matter their social security policies are in the infancy stage. The present paper highlights the existing social security policies in Asia sub regional countries and critically examines the gaps and suggests the viable methods for reforming the policies in a felt need basis and sustainable way.

Social Security Policies for Elderly in India : Gaps between Policies, Implementation and Needs of the Elderly

A. Prakash Rao

Social Security Policies are in vogue in India since many years, despite these policies the coverage of the aged population is limited across the states, and regions. Gender disparities are also affecting the implementation procedure. To examine the gaps between the social security policy, implementation and the needs of the elderly, a study was undertaken in Karnataka State which has been a pioneering State in India in implementing the social security policies for the elderly in particular. A need assessment out comes, policy implications, gaps and methods to fill the gaps were extensively discussed in the paper and the final section suggests how to build a model of viable social security policy for the elderly in India.

SESSION 157

Transformative Learning and Leadership Development in Health Promotion

M. Shaw (The Institute for Transformative Learning, Vancouver, CANADA) Conceptional Framework of Transformative Learning: Life Review and Guided Autobiography in Leadership Development M. Westwood (Department of Educational and Counselling Psychology, University of British Columbia, Vancouver, CANADA) Life Review Program for Canadian World War II Veterans and Peacekeeper Veterans. D. Kuhl (Palliative Care, Providence Health Care, Vancouver, CANADA) Lessons Learned About Living from the Dying: Transforming Leadership in Palliative Care G. Turner (St. Andrews-Wesley Church, Vancouver, CANADA) Faith and Meaning Making in Post Modern Culture: Servant Leadership and Transforming Our Stories B. de Vries (Department of Gerontology, San Francisco State University, California, USA) Discussant

This symposium explores a model of transformative learning using life review and the guided autobiography method (de Vries, Birren & Deutchman, 1995) for health promotion. Guided autobiography provides a narrative lens to focus on life review, life stories, leadership development and organizational transformation. The focus of this exploration is on the conceptual framework, along with emphasizing interdisciplinary applications of this model in research and practice. The implications for leadership and organizational transformation will be emphasized. For leaders faced with challenges and changes learning through reflection and dialogue as hermeneutic inquiry, in the autobiographical format, can contribute to new knowledge, meanings and wisdom to inform decisions and actions. This model adds a positive new dimension in leadership development, health promotion and the aging paradigm. The first presenter (Shaw, M.) focuses on the conceptual framework of transformative learning (Mezirow, 1991, 2000) and suggests that the guided autobiography method provides a focus for reflection, dialogue and communicative learning, for leaders in health promotion. The second presenter (Westwood, M.) describes the Life Review Program for Canadian World War II Veterans and Canadian Peacekeeper Veterans emphasizing leadership development in this application of guided autobiography in the counselling context. The third presenter (Kuhl, D.) explores the application of guided autobiography in palliative care. A qualitative case study highlights the potential for resolving end of life issues, through personal integration and transformation. The importance of leadership development and interdisciplinary collaboration is highlighted. The fourth presenter (Tuner, G.) focuses on faith development and meaning making in life stories in postmodern culture. Meaning making is one of the salient themes in autobiographical life review. Focusing on servant leadership and the Jazz Vespers service(s), clarifies the connection of faith, meaning and stories, in the transformation of church culture. The discussant (de Vries, B.) summarizes the presentations identifying strengths and limitations of using this model of transformative learning in leadership development and health promotion. Suggestions for future research and practice conclude this symposium. We anticipate that this symposium will spark interest in adding this new dimension this model of transformative learning to existing models of health promotion. The guided autobiography method is only one approach to facilitating reflection, dialogue, and action learning. We hope that symposium participants will suggest other interventions and ways to refine this model. The application of guided autobiography developed in an education setting has been used in the military culture and palliative care. In both examples, guided autobiography was effective in leadership development and organizational transformation. However, we anticipate that this model will meet with scrutiny. Guided autobiography and life review is not for everyone. For leaders of organizations inner work is a challenge because (a) the inner self may be considered private and not for public disclosure, and (b) the outer self can be highly successful in power relationships in the organization. We welcome discussion, suggestions, and questions as these questions and challenges actually serve as a catalyst for transformative learning the very model we promote.

Conceptional Framework of Transformative Learning: Life Review and Guided Autobiography in Leadership Development

M. Shaw (The Institute for Transformative Learning, Vancouver,

CANADA) Conceptional Framework of Transformative Learning: Life Review and Guided Autobiography in Leadership Development M. Westwood (Department of Educational and Counselling Psychology, University of British Columbia, Vancouver, CANADA) Life Review Program for Canadian World War II Veterans and Peacekeeper Veterans. D. Kuhl (Palliative Care, Providence Health Care, Vancouver, CANADA) Lessons Learned About Living from the Dying: Transforming Leadership in Palliative Care G. Turner (St. Andrew’s-Wesley Church, Vancouver, CANADA) Faith and Meaning Making in Post Modern Culture: Servant Leadership and Transforming Our Stories B. de Vries (Department of Gerontology, San Francisco State University, California, USA) Discussant

The purpose of this presentation is to explore the conceptual framework of transformative learning and the guided autobiography method of life review as it relates to leadership development and health promotion. Transformative learning is defined as the process of effecting change in a frame of reference and is an interdisciplinary, meaning centered, contextual model of learning (Mezirow, 1991, 2000). The guided autobiography provides a method to bridge stories and individual and/or social change. Focusing on the interpretation and meanings the hermeneutics in life stories brings the voices and visions of leaders into the aging paradigm. Learning from contradictions and questions in our stories, through reflection and dialogue and the transformation often inherent in this process can contribute to personal integration, leadership development and organizational transformation. The Method: I used an ethnographic approach with a focus on reflexivity, in a case study with six leaders to explore transformative learning and life review in the group counselling context. The Results: Four process themes and two content themes emerged that imply transformative learning. These themes include: reflexive reconstruction of the self; co-construction of the meaning of experience; moral betrayal and breaking a covenant; the importance of leadership in creating a democratic spaceaction planning and life planning; and dreams as a template for action. The Conclusion: This model of transformative learning is one way to address contradictions and engage in reflection and dialogue, to promote leadership development in health promotion. However, guided autobiography is not for everyone. Inner work for leaders is a challenge. Protection of privacy is a major consideration. More research is necessary to evaluate and refine this model of transformative learning.

Faith and Meaning Making in Post Modern Culture: Servant Leadership

M. Shaw (The Institute for Transformative Learning, Vancouver, CANADA) Conceptional Framework of Transformative Learning: Life Review and Guided Autobiography in Leadership Development M. Westwood (Department of Educational and Counselling Psychology, University of British Columbia, Vancouver, CANADA) Life Review Program for Canadian World War II Veterans and Peacekeeper Veterans. D. Kuhl (Palliative Care, Providence Health Care, Vancouver, CANADA) Lessons Learned About Living from the Dying: Transforming Leadership in Palliative Care G. Turner (St. Andrews-Wesley Church, Vancouver, CANADA) Faith and Meaning Making in Post Modern Culture: Servant Leadership and Transforming Our Stories B. de Vries (Department of Gerontology, San Francisco State University, California, USA) Discussant

This presentation focuses on meaning making and transformation in life stories in post-modern culture. Meaning in life is one of the salient themes in the guided autobiography method of life review. In the transformation of stories, the faith dialogue is viewed through triangulation of Jesus story, our story, the others story, with particular emphasis on the cultural context. Transformation in church culture, through exploration and questions emerging from the biblical stories the narratives of Jesus are put into practice in faith development in planning retreats for the church council. Servant leadership is highlighted in the model of meaning making and transformation. The Method: Transforming meaning in stories through dialogue with the Christian story and the focus on servant leadership is applied in an innovative Jazz Vespers service held every Sunday afternoon at St. Andrews-Wesley Church. The Results: As a leadership model in story telling and story listening this service attracts some of the best Jazz musicians in Vancouver and has an ever increasing number of faithful followers Jazz Vespers has transformed this faith culture. The Conclusion: The Jazz Vespers Service has transformed the church culture. It attracts an audience and musicians from many faith and spiritual traditions. Many who profess to having no faith come for the music and the word. Jazz Vespers is an inclusive community for transformative learning and leadership. It clarifies the connection of faith, meaning and stories in the transformation of church culture.

Lessons Learned About Living from the Dying: Transforming Leadership in Palliative Care

M. Shaw (The Institute for Transformative Learning, Vancouver, CANADA) Conceptional Framework of Transformative Learning: Life Review and Guided Autobiography in Leadership Development M. Westwood (Department of Educational and Counselling Psychology, University of British Columbia, Vancouver, CANADA) Life Review Program for Canadian World War II Veterans and Peacekeeper Veterans. D. Kuhl (Palliative Care, Providence Health Care, Vancouver, CANADA) Lessons Learned About Living from the Dying: Transforming Leadership in Palliative Care G. Turner (St. Andrew’s-Wesley Church, Vancouver, CANADA) Faith and Meaning Making in Post Modern Culture: Servant Leadership and Transforming Our Stories B. de Vries (Department of Gerontology, San Francisco State University, California, USA) Discussant

Purpose: To explore spiritual and psychological issues at the end of life, along with highlighting the implications for leadership development and transformation in palliative care. Method: A qualitative method, namely, existential phenomenology was implemented to interview 21 people who knew they had a terminal illness, either cancer or AIDS. Questions were based on life review themes from the guided autobiography method. Results: Ten themes emerged as significant to the experience of living with a terminal illness: communication, iatrogenic suffering, pain, touch, time, life review, truth, longing to belong, who I am, and transcendence. Conclusion: Service to those who are that end of life would be enhanced in addressing specific psychological and spiritual needs, training of care providers would best incorporate methods to support those who are experiencing psychological and spiritual distress at the end of life, and research is necessary to evaluate specific interventions.

Life Review Program for Canadian World War II Veterans and Peacekeeper Veterans.

M. Shaw (The Institute for Transformative Learning, Vancouver, CANADA) Conceptional Framework of Transformative Learning: Life Review and Guided Autobiography in Leadership Development M. Westwood (Department of Educational and Counselling Psychology, University of British Columbia, Vancouver, CANADA) Life Review Program for Canadian World War II Veterans and Peacekeeper Veterans. D. Kuhl (Palliative Care, Providence Health Care, Vancouver, CANADA) Lessons Learned About Living from the Dying: Transforming Leadership in Palliative Care G. Turner (St. Andrews-Wesley Church, Vancouver, CANADA) Faith and Meaning Making in Post Modern Culture: Servant Leadership and Transforming Our Stories B. de Vries (Department of Gerontology, San Francisco State University, California, USA) Discussant

The Life Review Program for Canadian War Veterans focuses on transformative learning, applying guided autobiography and group enactments for health promotion in the counselling context. The Life

Review Program developed at the University of British Columbia is a joint venture with Veterans Affairs Canada and the Royal Canadian Legion. Life review promotes health by contributing to personal integration and life span development for participants, along with promoting leadership development and organizational transformation. The Method: Six groups of veterans in Vancouver and Victorian participated I the Life Review Program. One group was comprised of Canadian Peacekeeping Veterans. Each group met once a week for six weeks. The guided autobiography method was used for groups of World War II Veterans. Group enactments were added to promote trauma repair for Peacekeeper Veterans. Professionally trained leaders facilitated all groups. The Results: suggest the following benefits of life review for Canadian Veterans: Validation of life experiences; integration of war events; facilitation of repair; reconcilliations of past events; identification of achievements; effective coping strategies and contributions to their country; consolidation and development of future focus and life goals. The Conclusion: The life review program contributed to personal integration for participants. For Veterans new knowledge, meanings and wisdom emerged from sharing their stories. This implies that this model of life review contributed to transformative learning. Action planning was a salient theme with implications for individual, leadership and organizational transformation. World War II veterans indicated a strong desire to serve as mentors to Peacekeepers. Leaders had a greater understanding and appreciation for Canadian Veterans. And Veterans Affairs Canada and the Royal Canadian Legion adopted and expanded this program.

SESSION 160

Successful Aging: Current Perspectives and Future Outlook

P. Perrig-Chiello, W. Perrig, and A. Uebelbacher (University of Berne, Switzerland) Physical and Psychological Resources of Functional Autonomy in Old Age. V. Menec (University of Manitoba, Winnipeg, Canada) Activity and Successful Aging. D. Jopp (Research Group on Psychological Gerontology, Free University of Berlin, Germany) and J. Smith (Max Planck Institute for Human Development, Berlin, Germany) Successful Aging in Old and Very Old Age: On the Dynamic Interplay Between Resources and Life-Management Strategies. K. A. Wallace (University of Montana, Missoula, MT, USA) and C. S. Bergeman (University of Notre Dame, Notre Dame, USA) Personal and Support Resources as Protective Factors in Later Life: Implications for Successful Aging Outcomes. Ronald P. Abeles (Special Assistant to the Director Office of Behavioral and Social Sciences Research Office of the Director, National Institutes of Health) and Carolyn M. Aldwin (Dept. of Human & Community Development University of California, Davis) Discussants.

During the last decade, successful aging has become a topic of growing interest. Many different concepts have been developed to describe the process of aging well. Several determinants have been identified as promoting successful aging. These include personal characteristics, behavioral strategies, and attitudes or beliefs. This symposium emphasizes on these different perspectives on successful aging. A central goal of the session is to review and to update recent theoretical and empirical developments in the field and to discuss future outlooks. Individual presentations focus on specific resources, strategies, and other protective factors that enhance successful aging of old and very old adults. P. Perrig-Chiello and colleagues investigated the role of personal resources in the successful aging context. More specifically, they examined the predictive power of physical and psychological resources on functional autonomy as a central condition of successful aging. Data from the Basel Interdisciplinary longitudinal Study on Ageing provided a cross-sectional and a longitudinal perspective. Results revealed differential predictive patterns: activities of daily living (ADLs) were better predicted by physical than by the psychological resources, whereas memory variables and health control beliefs had a higher predictive value for instrumental activities of daily living (IADLs). In her presentation, V. Menec focuses on activity as determinant of successful aging. Results of the longitudinal Aging in Manitoba study suggest that the number of activities individuals' engaged in is a significant predictor of successful aging outcomes. More detailed analyses indicated that participation in social activities particularly visiting friends was related to aging well. In contrast, more solitary activities such as watching TV or reading showed no comparable interrelationship to optimal aging. These findings support the assumption that remaining active in later life is beneficial to successful aging. D. Jopp and J. Smith studied the dynamic interplay between personal resources and life-management strategies. Their results suggest an age-differential pattern in the prediction of interindividual differences in satisfaction with aging. In the Young-Old, resources and SOC-life management strategies had both unique effects in predicting aging satisfaction, whereas in the Oldest-Old the importance of resource possession increased and the influence of SOC-strategies decreased. Here, the interaction between resources and life-management strategies explained a substantial amount of variance, indicating that old-old persons with few resources profited most from using SOC-life management strategies. K. Wallace and C. Bergeman explored the pathways through which psychosocial attributes such as personal and familial/community support resources promote successful aging. Their study extends the perspective on successful aging by taking into account specific life circumstances such as dealing with critical events by including life events and perceived stress in their models as well as successful aging outcomes. Path analyses indicated that perceived stress mediated the relationship between events and personal resources and partially mediated the relationship between life events and successful aging. Results demonstrate that the investigation of successful aging can profit from including other well-established psychological concepts such as the stress theoretic perspective. Individual presentations will be discussed by R. Abeles (National Institutes of Health) and C. Aldwin (University of California, Davis).

Activity and Successful Aging

V. Menec (Department of Community Health Sciences, University of Manitoba, Winnipeg, Canada)

PURPOSE: This longitudinal study was designed to examine the role of activity in successful aging. METHOD: 1537 participants of the 1990 and 1996 waves of the Aging in Manitoba study were included in the analyses. Individuals were classified as having aged successfully in 1996 based on four criteria: good functional, physical and mental status and positive health perceptions. The role of activity in 1990 (participation in 16 activities, such as visiting family or friends or reading) in successful aging was examined using logistic regressions, with age, gender, education, ADLs/IADLs, self-rated health, health status and disability status, assessed in 1990 being controlled in all analyses. RESULTS: A summary score of the number of activities individuals' engaged in was significantly related to successful aging (adjusted odds ratio [AOR] = 1.08, $p < .01$). Subsequent analyses indicated that participation in social activities, particularly visiting friends (AOR = 1.69, $p < .01$), albeit not phoning friends/relatives, was related to successful aging. None of the more solitary activities (such as watching TV or reading) was related to successful aging. CONCLUSION: These findings support the view that remaining active in later life is important to successful aging. That visiting, but not phoning friends emerged as a predictor of successful aging suggests that it is not merely talking with others that is beneficial, but that face-to-face interaction outside of one's home affords additional stimulation. Providing seniors who are isolated, such as individuals living in remote rural areas, with the means to interact with others therefore seems important.

Personal and Support Resources as Protective Factors in Later Life: Implications for Successful Aging Outcomes

K. A. Wallace (University of Montana, Missoula, USA), C. S. Bergeman (University of Notre Dame, Notre Dame, USA)

The present study considered the pathways through which various psychosocial attributes promote successful aging outcomes. Relationships were examined between Personal Resources (self-esteem, hardiness, optimism), Familial/Community Support Factors (community support, family environment, friend support), Life Events, Perceived Stress, and Successful Aging Outcomes (life satisfaction, depression, physical health). Mail-out questionnaires were completed by 286 individuals (ages 60 - 97). Path analyses revealed that Perceived Stress mediated the relationship between Life Events and Personal Resources and partially mediated the relationship between Life Events and Successful Aging. Both Personal Resources and Familial/Community Support partially mediated the relationship between Perceived Stress and Successful Aging. Exploratory analyses were conducted to examine the proposed model by groups. Participants were divided by stress and successful aging outcome, resulting in four groups (nonoptimal, successful, vulnerable, resilient). Compared to the model in which parameter estimates across groups were constrained to be equal, a more relaxed model in which directional paths were free to vary provided a significantly better fit. These exploratory results indicated that for individuals in the vulnerable group, both Personal and Support Resources mediated the negative effect of Perceived Stress on Successful Aging, whereas for resilient individuals, only Personal Resources significantly predicted Successful Aging. Results emphasize the importance of appraisal in the stress process and suggest that protective attributes may be of particular importance for individuals who are vulnerable. Although longitudinal research using larger samples is needed, the present study provides a more global view of resiliency in later life.

Physical and Psychological Resources of Functional Autonomy in Old Age

P. Perrig-Chiello, Walter Perrig & Andreas Uebelbacher (University of Berne, Switzerland)

Functional autonomy is a core condition of successful aging. To maximize autonomous functioning is not only a claim of social policy but primarily an individual need. Part of the challenge in preventing unnecessary dependence in old age is to recognize the large diversity among the elderly and the different availability, utilization and interaction of their physical, psychological and social resources. This presentation focuses on functional autonomy (ADL, IADL and both together as basic competence in accordance with the two-component model of Baltes et al, 1996). The aim of our research was to examine the predictive power of physical resources (objective and subjective health, physical mobility) along with psychological resources (objective and subjective memory, personality, health control beliefs) on functional autonomy in a sample of 441 healthy elderly persons from the Basel Interdisciplinary longitudinal Study on Ageing (IDA-Study), aged 65 to 95 years in a cross-sectional and longitudinal perspective. Structural equation models were calculated. Results suggest that ADL were better predicted by physical resources than by the psychological ones, but for IADL the inverse was the case, here memory variables and health control beliefs played a dominant role. Contrary to other results (Baltes et al, 1996) basic competence was better predicted by memory parameters than by physical mobility and health measures. More research is needed to test the reliability of these data. In addition, experimental intervention studies are requested to prove the validity of such models on the interdependence of physical, psychological and social resources and different levels of autonomy.

Successful Aging in Old and Very Old Age: On the Dynamic Interplay Between Resources and Life-Management Strategies

D. Jopp (Research Group on Psychological Gerontology, Free University of Berlin, Germany), J Smith (Max Planck Institute for Human Development, Berlin, Germany)

Successful aging in old and very old age is investigated by focussing on the dynamic interplay between resources and life-management strategies. As the possession of resources has been shown to be no guarantee for positive aging, we explore whether optimal resource utilization as captured by SOC life-management strategies promotes successful aging. 156 elderly between 70 and 90 years of the Berlin ALLEE study (M. Baltes & Lang, DFG-Ba-902/11-2) were investigated to answer this question. As expected, young-old persons had more resources available than the oldest-old. SOC life-management strategies did not differ between age groups. The criterion aging satisfaction showed no age differences as well. Multiple hierachical regression analysis indicated that interindividual differences in aging satisfaction were predicted by resources and SOC strategies. Separating young-old and old-old, the explained variance in aging satisfaction was comparable in size in both groups. At the same time, analyses also revealed that the predictive pattern was age-differential: In the younger group, variance in aging satisfaction was accounted for by unique effects of resources and SOC strategies. In the older group, the proportion of explained variance by resources increased, and the resources-by-SOC interaction accounted for the rest of the variance. SOC strategies lost their unique contribution at that age group indicating that strategy use becomes increasingly dependent on resource status. Especially in very old age, elderly are profiting from the buffering effect of SOC when resources are low. Data also proposed that very old persons with high resources and low SOC are most vulnerable over time.

SESSION 161

Build-a-Case and Dementia: A Brand New CME Technique that is Peculiarly Familiar

**Jocelyn Charles, M.D. Director of Cognitive Support Services, Sunnybrook and Women's College Health Sciences Centre, University of Toronto. *Bernard Marlow, M.D. - Director of CME, Department of Family & Community Medicine, University of Toronto *Barbara Liu, M.D. Geriatrician & Clinical Pharmacologist, Sunnybrook & Women's College Health Science Centre, University of Toronto. * David Ryan, - Interdepartmental Division of Geriatrics, University of Toronto. Director, Education in Aging & Health, Regional Geriatric Program of Toronto.*

Build-a-case is a promising new format for CE that will be familiar to practitioners of case and problem-based learning. Build-a-case predicates itself on a simple fact: with the right process of inquiry, building teaching cases provides a rich context for learning. Treating the case building process as a learning event offers several advantages. First, the cases that are built represent high levels of contextual nuance which match the practice contexts of physicians, contexts which may often be quite diverse and different from those of CE professionals. Second, during the build-a -case process, physicians describe their different approaches to practice and the recognition of these differences provides an opening for consideration of guidelines. Third, the process generates cases that can be used in future case based learning and as we know "case-based learning eats cases". Finally, inasmuch as the the process challenges educators to facilitate physician learning armed primarily with a process of reflective inquiry than with a body of knowledge, build-a-case is entirely in keeping with several principles of adult learning. The round-table will begin with a brief overview of problem based learning. Next, using the stages of dementia care as a focus the build-a-case process will be facilitated. A review of our research with the method and the conceptual framework we have built around the process will be examined before a final discussion of applications and research issues.

SESSION 162

Policy into Practice: Organisational Difficulties and User Perspectives

M. Fellows (BCOP - Broadening Choices for Older People, Birmingham, UK) Implementation Process: Striding the Hurdles.

A. Ritch and M. Ehtisham (City Hospital, Birmingham, UK) Intermediate Care: Trendy Name or New Animal. A. Abrahams (University of Central England, Birmingham, UK) Consumer Led Health Care: Involving Older People in Nurse Education. A. Withnall (University of Warwick, Coventry, UK) Learning for Healthy Ageing.

The symposium will outline current policy developments in the UK relevant to the organisation of care for older people. Local examples of how these policies are being put into practice will be discussed in the areas of education, institutional and community care. Presentations will focus on major issues within these developments. Organisational difficulties which may have interfered with the achievement of predicted outcome objectives will be discussed in each of these areas. The views and perspectives of users of services in each of these areas will be explored and the effect to which they might have been able to influence effective outcomes. Presentations will cover the following issues. The barriers to effective policy implementation in an organisational setting will be outlined as well as examples of ways of overcoming them. They include lack of clarity and consultation, poor communication, difficulty in gaining willing participation, unrealistic expectations and excessive bureaucracy. The recent development of the concept of intermediate care will be explained. Though the precise definition of intermediate care is still unclear it involves services which facilitate the transition from hospital to home and from acute illness back to functional independence. The emphasis is on providing in other than acute hospitals those services which are beyond the scope of the traditional primary care team. Some will involve resources from both sides of the health and social care boundary and raise such issues as individuals being required to contribute financially to what has previously been free health care. Attitudes of health care providers will need to change if a more consumer- orientated service is to be achieved. The involvement of older people in nurse education aims to promote positive attitudes which may help the implementation of user involvement in health care. The promotion of lifelong learning gives the opportunity to improve health education for older people. Initiatives at national and local level demonstrate both the value of educational activities in which older people can take part and how they can develop the skills required to influence the promotion of healthy ageing. It is expected that the outcome of the session will be a greater understanding of the degree to which the views of users are able to influence the development of new projects and their involvement in educational programmes is able to affect change across the age range. An appreciation of the influence of a consumer led approach on service objectives will be gained.

Consumer Led Health Care: Involving Older People in Nurse Education

A. Abrahams (University of Central England, Birmingham, UK)

The need for user participation in various aspects of health care has attracted considerable interest since the beginning of the National Health Service. This is now being further reflected at all levels in the government's NHS Plan launched in July 2000 which promises a 'consumer-orientated' NHS. Health care providers are the obvious force by which such attitudinal change may be effected, and the case of nurse education is used to explore how such policy approaches are reflected in practice. A case study involving older people in both the presentation and teaching of older adult care to student and post-registration nurses is examined, in the context of traditional teaching approaches and their level of user involvement. The aim of this innovative approach is to increase user participation and promote positive attitudes among student nurses towards older people.

Implementation Process: Striding the Hurdles

M. Fellows (BCOP - Broadening Choices for Older People, Birmingham, UK)

Managers often question why some policy implementation appears to work effectively with little effort, while others labour until they die. The care of older people within an organisational setting requires little or no difference in its analysis when considering such a question. In understanding the reasons why policy implementation works or fails, we must be clear about the barriers that exist. In summary these can be recognised as lack of clarity; poor communication; consultation; gaining support and willingness to participate; unworkability - unrealistic; organisational culture; bureaucracy; external pressures. Within the symposium the speaker will consider each of these barriers in turn, offering solutions and examples where they have been overcome.

Intermediate Care: Trendy Name or New Animal

A. Ritch (Secretary, Institute of Ageing and Health - West Midlands, Birmingham, UK), M Ehtisham (City Hospital, Birmingham, UK)

As part of the development of services for older people the concept of intermediate care arose in the mid 1990s. While it is difficult to give a precise definition, the original idea revolved around facilitating patients' recovery from illness, enabling them to achieve functional independence after acute illness. It covers the period when traditional medical care is no longer required and so began to be thought of as a means of shortening length of stay in acute hospital beds or even reducing the numbers of older people admitted to acute hospitals as medical emergencies. Intermediate care should involve the provision of rehabilitation and so may be no different from existing services in secondary care, but it may or may not include specialist medical care. A rehabilitation unit was developed in Birmingham within a Social Services residential home mainly to allow easier discharge from the nearby acute hospital although admissions from home are possible. Nursing and therapy staff are funded by the health authority, but are not available at weekends, so excluding those with higher levels of dependency. On moving from a hospital bed to the unit, patients become liable for the financial charge levied on all short stay residents in Social Service homes. Low bed occupancy has been a persistent problem. Once in the unit, clients actively participate in the process of assessment of need and the setting of rehabilitation goals. Arrangements are in place for a formal assessment of service effectiveness and patient acceptability.

Learning for Healthy Ageing

A. Withnall (University of Warwick, Coventry, UK)

The promotion of lifelong learning and better health in the ageing population are both pressing policy issues in the UK. This suggests the creation of a major opportunity to improve the delivery of health information and health education for older people. However, current institutional arrangements often coupled with stereotypical views of older people's ability to learn may militate against the provision of appropriate and easily accessible health promotion work. At a national level, work by the DfEE funded "Older and Bolder" development project is attempting to change traditional perceptions about older people and learning by showing the sheer range of educational activities in which older people in a range of situations take part and the positive outcomes learning can have for their lives. At a local level, the example of the Beth Johnson Foundation's health and health promotion work with seniors in the area of North Staffordshire over a number of years has demonstrated how different groups of older people can develop the necessary skills to make their voices heard in the area of health and health promotion. It is concluded that more work could be done to ensure that educationalists can work alongside health promotion professionals and older people themselves at the local level to ensure the promotion of healthy ageing right across the life course.

SESSION 163

Community Advisory Committee Shaping a Study: Mexican-American Elders' Under-Using Skilled Home Health Nursing

Janice Crist, [University of Arizona, Tucson, USA]

This paper discusses how a community advisory committee shapes community studies. Impaired functional ability requires skilled home health nursing in the home. Nationally, Hispanic elders use skilled home health nursing (SHHN) services only half as often as Anglo elders. The research aims were to identify predictors of use of SHHN services by Mexican American elders in the Tucson area and to establish whether under-use is problematic and differs from national literature. Ten people, more than half Mexican American, were asked to participate on a Community Advisory Committee, to meet quarterly. Fifty-nine providers of SHHN and other community services, 9 Mexican American elders and 9 Mexican American family carers were interviewed. Six themes: expectations of discrimination, lack of knowledge about services, expectations embedded in familism, traditional health practices, lack of health insurance and neglect/abuse, were validated by a community advisory committee. Results enhance extant national knowledge about under-use and in partnership with community advisors will determine interventions. The process of finding, recruiting and retaining key informants, primary informants, and community leaders and other representatives to form a community advisory committee require personalismo, respeto, frequent reminders, and reciprocity, are complex, delicate and essential.

Generational differences in attitudes towards public home help for the elderly: The case of Sweden

G. Hammarstrom (Department of Sociology, Uppsala university)

In comparison to most Western countries, Scandinavian countries have developed a more active state involvement in help and care programs for the elderly. In Sweden, over the past decade, alternatives to the hitherto dominating public programs have been suggested in order to reduce, or at least limit, public expenses. This study aims to find out the degree of Swedes' commitment to public involvement in the help and care of the elderly. The underlying assumption has been that younger people have more positive attitudes towards alternatives to public programs than middle aged and elderly people. For this purpose a survey has been carried out with a representative sample of the population born between 1910 and 1975. Using three hypothetical care-needs situations, differing in type and duration of care, the respondents have been asked who they wish would provide their own home help care and how it should be financed. In addition they have been asked who should organize the elderly care. The results show that in general, the majority prefer public solutions. There are however some generational differences, mainly between those born in the 70's and those born in other decades. The oldest respondents prefer public home help provision, which is financed and organized by the state. The so-called Swedish baby-boom generation - that is, those born in the 40's - would consider private alternatives to a certain extent. In contrast, those born in the 70's prefer a public-private mix of alternatives.

Home Based Care in Indonesia

Tony Setiabudhi PhD. (Trisakti Medical School/ Indonesian Society of Gerontology Jakarta/ Indonesia)

In 1998; UN-ESCAP (United Nations' Economic and Social Commission for Asia and the Pacific) ask the author to write an Indonesian report in line with : "The Development of Community Based Organizations Serving Older Persons in Indonesia". During his presentation at Bangkok (December 1998) the author got some suggestions and he tried to improve and he asked to himself : "what can be carried out in a better way in Indonesia ?"Later on; at some point of the HelpAge Regional Conference which was held in New Delhi last September 2000 ASEAN NGO's Coalition meet HelpAge KOREA and discussed about the possibility that South Korean Government is eager and willingly to assist and support these kind of project and amplifying it into a bigger program. Most of the ASEAN NGO's Coalition is trying their best to improve the : HOME BASED CARE PROJECT; because it is expected that it will grow into the right direction. We hope that it can be adopted as one of the best plan for our region. This paper will present the PUSAKA's Activities (Home-Care Program from Indoneia) in one hand and compare it with the latest recommendation from Seoul's meeting (April 2001)

Japanese workers' collective associations specializing in services for the elderly

M.Oka (Economic Research Institute, Yokohama City University, Yokohama, Japan)

A unique cooperative association specializing in services for the elderly was inaugurated in 1989 as the first experiment of Japanese cooperative movement. The association named the Welfare Club has successfully organized ordinary people as the bearer of the service in so-called workers' collectives in which all members take part in investment, management and work aiming at fulfilling the needs of their own community. This report presents the results of a questionnaire survey conducted in the spring of 2000 on the workers' collectives. According to the 36 valid replies followed up by in-depth interview survey, the workers' collectives were consisted of about 50 members in average, mostly middle-aged housewives with a few experts and qualified persons. They provided mainly the home help service, the meal cooking/delivery service, and the transportation service by driving of a car together with various additional service needed to support the daily life of the elderly. The service was provided for a cheap charge. Other costs were covered by subsidies, donations, etc. In 1997 the annual average income of the workers' collectives was about US $91,000. It was not large, however, they provided 6,300 hours of service for 2,300 cases in average, a considerable contribution for the elderly. Most of them were working in cooperation with a local government and other non-profit organizations. The Welfare Club and the workers' collectives suggest a possibility of civil initiative toward a welfare community based on active participation of ordinary people.

Not only time, talk, and patienceâ¤≈ The very old patients evaluate their doctors.

V. Garms-Homolova (Institut fuer Gesundheitsanalysen und soziale Konzepte e.V, Berlin, Germany)

Purpose: In the seventies the so called "consumerism in medicine" was identified. It was recognized that patients were no longer humble when interacting with doctors, but demanding the best service and high expertise. The elderly occurred as the only exception: as patients who remained self sufficient, and who easily were satisfied by doctors who listen and who have time. The purpose of the presentation is to examine how far this picture is still correct. Method: 25 "old old" patients of GPs were repeatedly interviewed in the course of 10 months. The qualitative semi-structured interviews were transcribed and analysed. The results of this qualitative content analysis were compared with findings of a study with 19 patients realized in 1989. Results: The very old patients determined decisively the course, content and form of their communication with GPs. Particularly the degree of personal involvement in the interaction was controlled by the patients. Time, listening, and attention were still seen as important quality dimensions of the GP-patient-interaction, but the interviewee also articulate demanding expectations towards the "professional expertise" of their GPs. They differentiated strictly between the "good doctor" (highly professional physician, who give and use all available information) and the "nice doctor" (a pleasant person, who had less skills). Characteristics of doctor's office (location, staff) influenced whether the GP's service was evaluated positively or not. Conclusion: The comparison of this study with the results from 1989 showed that today old patients more often required specialized therapy, exact information and professional communication skills.

The current state of home care in a city in Southern Finland

Seija Muurinen, RN, (health care), (Herttoniemi Hospital, Helsinki, Finland) Ritva Raatikainen, RN, DSocSc, (Dept. of Nursing Science, University of Tampere, Finland)

The purpose of the study was to clarify the current state of home care for the purposes of quality improvement. The goals were to analyse the clients independent initiative, need for help and helping action from the viewpoint of clients and care workers. Of the clients (N=231), 135 were randomly selected to participate in the study, and all the care workers (N=49) were included in the study sample. Of the clients, 97 (74%) were interviewed, and 38 (78%) care workers completed a questionnaire. The data were analysed mainly by statistical methods. Nearly all the clients (89%) felt it was important that they were able to take care of their daily activities independently. However, 37% of the care workers responded that none of the clients had the possibility of increasing their activity status through rehabilitation. Half the clients coped poorly with home activities, e.g. running errands and moving about outside. About a quarter of the clients (27%) experienced fear or anxiety and nearly half (43%) felt lonely. The clients had often received help in many physical activities, but the help was weaker in mental and social activities. Some differences were found in the clients and care workers responses. In prevention, acute illness and rehabilitation and in all mental and social activities the care workers mentioned that they had helped a larger proportion of clients than what was the proportion of those who had received help.

The spectrum of home-based care

Iudomyr Mykyta (Western DomCare, Adelaide, Australia)

Purpose: To provide practical suggestions for the implementation of home care services. Method: The author draws on the experience of a large Regional Aged and Extended Care Service, which has been operating since 1971, and has assisted over 50,000 clients in that time. Conclusions: The paper examines the reasons for the current trend towards home-based care in health and aged care. The advantages and disadvantages of home care solutions across the care continuum, from acute care, through rehabilitation to long term care and primary care are discussed. Practical suggestions for implementation of home care schemes are offered.

SESSION 164

Bridging Gaps between Research and Practice: Successful Dissemination of Roybal Center Research Interventions

T. Prohaska, J. Warren and S. Hughes (University of Illinois at Chicago, IL, USA) Sustaining Exercise Research Interventions in Older Populations: Issues in Program Dissemination and Diffusion. S. Hughes, T. Prohaska, and M. Angiolillo (University of Illinois at Chicago, IL, USA) Dissemination Efforts at the Midwest Roybal Center for Health Maintenance. S. Tennstedt (New England Research Institutes, Watertown, MA, USA), V. Quinn and A. Jette (Boston University, Boston, MA, USA) From Research to Practice: Dissemination of a Group Program to Reduce Fear of Falling. K. Ball and V. Wadley (University of Alabama at Birmingham, AL, USA) and D. Roenker (Western Kentucky University, Bowling Green, KY, USA) Disseminating Research Results on Older Drivers to Applied Settings. R. Mockenhaupt (Robert Wood Johnson Foundation, Princeton, NJ, USA)

The Edward R. Roybal Centers for Research in Applied Gerontology have been funded by the National Institute on Aging (USA) to translate basic behavioral and social research theories and findings into practical outcomes for older adults. This symposium will report on the work of three Roybal Centers to disseminate health promotion strategies tested previously at the respective institution. The symposium begins with a discussion of theoretical, conceptual, and programatic issues associated with the perpetuation, dissemination, and diffusion of research interventions in community settings. The exercise interventions designed and tested at the Midwest Roybal Center for Health Maintenance are used to illustrate these issues. Investigators from this Center continue with a presentation of their dissemination strategies, describing the formation of the Senior Health Alliance Promoting Exercise (SHAPE) and associated activities. Investigators from the Roybal Center for Late-Life Enhancement in Boston then describe the dissemination of a group program shown efficacious in reducing fear of falling and associated activity restrictions. This intervention program has been successfully adapted to community-based health promotion programs in a wide range of settings across the U.S. Finally, the UAB Center for Research on Applied Gerontology discusses how its research on driving skills and behaviors of older adults is being used in a model screening program to identify older drivers at risk of crash involvement for subsequent intervention. Robin Mockenhaupt of the Robert Wood Johnson Foundation is the discussant.

Disseminating Research Results on Older Drivers to Applied Settings

K. Ball (the University of Alabama at Birmingham, Birmingham, Alabama, USA), V. Wadley (the University of Alabama at Birmingham, Birmingham, AL, USA), D. Roenker (Western Kentucky University, Bowling Green, KY, USA)

Visual and cognitive impairments contribute to increased disability in older adults. A measure of the Useful Field of View (UFOV(r)) has been shown in many prior research studies to be an effective predictor of crash risk in this population. The Maryland Department of Motor Vehicle Administration, the National Highway Traffic Safety Administration and the National Institute on Aging are collectively supporting a large sample (N=5000) field trial in driver licensing facilities of a brief screening battery, including an abbreviated form of UFOV(r), designed to identify older drivers who are at risk for crash involvement. A model driver screening program has been proposed for the assessment of risk factors with the goal of referring at-risk drivers for appropriate intervention within a variety of health care settings. One of the key remaining activities in this program is the evaluation of dissemination approaches designed to inform both the public, as well as health care providers, of prior research findings, changes in public policies regarding older drivers, and the benefits of new programs of evaluation and re-training. Issues involved in the dissemination of this information will be presented.

Dissemination Efforts at the Midwest Roybal Center for Health Maintenance

S. Hughes, T. Prohaska, M. Angiollilo (University of Illinois at Chicago, Chicago, Illinois, USA)

In order to facilitate the dissemination of findings from the four randomized trials currently under way at the Midwest Roybal Center in Chicago with funding from the National Institute on Aging, we have partnered with a number of organizations that provide services to seniors in Cook County IL. Specifically, we have developed the Senior Health Alliance Promoting Exercise (SHAPE) alliance which is attempting to promote awareness among seniors of the importance of enhanced participation in physical activity. Dissemination activities conducted to date include the development of an inventory and guide regarding existing exercise opportunities for seniors in Cook County, the development and implementation of an interactive ShapeChicago.com website, and the inauguration of an annual Senior Health and Fitness Walk that is held in May along Chicago's beautiful lakefront (1,000 seniors participated last year and 3,000 are targeted this year). Critical partnerships and barriers and facilitators to this type of innovative dissemination activity will be described.

From Research to Practice: Dissemination of a Group Intervention to Reduce Fear of Falling

S. Tennstedt (New England Research Institutes, Watertown, MA USA), V. Quinn and A. Jette (Boston University, MA, USA)

This paper discusses the methods of dissemination of a group intervention to reduce fear of falling and associated activity restriction in community-residing older adults. The intervention was designed and its efficacy established in a randomized controlled trial conducted by the Roybal Center for Late-Life Enhancement at Boston University. Successful dissemination of this group program was launched with a conference for area practitioners and providers and continued with strategic alliances with providers. Initially, these providers included hospitals, state and local health departments, home health agencies, and senior service organizations. Further dissemination via the world wide web has expanded both the range of providers and geographic area. The group program has been implemented in a wide range of settings with different target populations. Replication trials of the intervention have been planned in the U.S. and the Netherlands.

Sustaining Exercise Research Interventions in Older Populations: Issues in Program Dissemination and Diffusion

T. Prohaska, J. Warren, S. Hughes (University of Illinois at Chicago, Chicago, Illinois, USA)

While there is considerable documentation on the benefits of exercise in older adults, relatively little research has explored how to translate innovative health promotion interventions into self-sustainable community based exercise programs to diverse older populations across community settings. As part of the organizational structure of the Roybal Centers, we developed a Core Dissemination component designed to help translate effective and innovative exercise research programs for older adults into sustainable community owned and directed programs. This paper identifies the theoretical, conceptual, and pragmatic issues associated with the perpetuation, dissemination and diffusion of exercise research interventions in community settings. Gaps in the transition from research to practice are offered from the perspective of the researcher and community practitioner. These gaps include delays in the research process, limitations in the communication of research findings, differences between the researcher and practitioner in the use of theory and outcomes of success, the unidirectional nature of the transition, and constraints inherent in program application. Solutions are offered that require the researcher, the community and practitioners to recognize the need for collaboration and mutual responsiveness to needs.

SESSION 169

[1] Evaluation of the Alternative Level of Care Management Initiative (The Carelinks Program)

Marcus Hollander, Hollander Analytical, Victoria, B.C, Canada Valerie Embree. KPMG Consulting, Vancouver, B.C, Canada Pat Light, Simon Fraser Health Region, New Westminster, B.C, Canada

Goal was to determine the impacts on the patient, family and health system of the redesigned process for assessing and coordinating appropriate community services for individuals identified in acute Hospitals (Emergency Department, in-patient units) but not requiring acute care. Evaluation used a prospective study of clients from both study and control sites at 3 and 6 weeks post-discharge; information from informal care providers, physicians and other service providers; reviewed acute versus non-acute days in hospital using a standardized tool; and evaluated administrative databases for cost information. Clients receiving services via the new process reported improving health over time while the control group reported worsening health status over time. Re-admission rates to hospital were similar for both groups. Physicians, service providers, and informal caregivers reported satisfaction with the new process. There was a net savings of approximately $985,000 as a result of the Carelinks implementation and the concurrent closure of 30 hospital beds.

[2] Using the Biographical Approach to Enhance the Care of Older People

E. Hanson (Sheffield University School of Nursing and Midwifery, United Kingdom and Gothenburg University Department of Nursing, Sweden), A. Clarke (Sheffield University School of Nursing and Midwifery, United Kingdom), and H. Ross (Sheffield University School of Nursing and Midwifery, United Kingdom)

PURPOSE A qualitative study to investigate whether the biographical approach may be used to enhance person-centred care for older people in hospital. METHOD Focus groups were undertaken to ascertain staff's perceptions of biography before and after they had used the approach. Wherever possible, interviews were also carried out with patients and relatives concerning their thoughts about telling their stories both before and after they had worked with biography. Support workers were given a dedicated day to initiate the biography with patients; they then continued working on it alongside their everyday work activities. Patients were encouraged to talk about their past and present lives and their stories were recorded in a book, which remained their property, together with any photographs, and other personal items that they wished to include. RESULTS Findings revealed that the approach: assisted staff to view the patient as a person and to understand their needs more fully; enabled them to develop closer relationships with the patient's relatives; increased job satisfaction. Staff also recognised several considerations regarding the use of the approach: it was not suitable for everyone, in particular, those individuals who were more reserved or who had painful past experiences; the importance of privacy and confidentiality in sharing personal information; the importance of getting to know the patient. Staff wished to continue working with biography once the project was finished. CONCLUSION The biographical approach made a considerable contribution to the overall job satisfaction of staff and in so doing led to a more person-centred approach to nursing care.

[3] Home, home with help or hospital admission, decision making through presenting client characteristics.

Robert McKim and Teresa Genge (both are from Northeast Community Health Centre, Edmonton, Alberta ,Canada)

This study compares the clinical characteristics of clients who are assessed by a multidisciplinary team in an outpatient senior's clinic for discharge to home, home with enhanced services and inpatient placement. Method: A retrospective study looking at data collected over a three-year period is reported. A total of 1967 clients referred for an acute change in medical, social, and or functional status were reviewed and their discharge disposition were monitored. Clients were assessed and grouped into three possible categories. Those who could go home with additional services (n=1236), those who could go home with enhanced services (n=546), and those requiring hospitalization (n=191). An ANOVA and Chi-Square tests were used to determine statistically significant differences in characteristics between groups. Results: Significant differences in demographic features were noted between those clients who went home without enhanced services versus those who were referred for admission. Assessment tools including the BARTHEL, ALSAR, MMSE, BCRS, Clock score, CAM, GDS, difficulties in medication management all showed significant differences between groups. Social support and living conditions showed minimal differences. Differences in medical morbidity were also noted. Conclusions: The presence of delirium and functional decline, especially abilities to manage IADL and ADL, and low cognitive status are strong predictors of discharge disposition. Social support and medical morbidity showed less predictability. The relevance of these findings to service provided from a Community Health Center will be discussed.

[4] The Geriatric - Oncologic Boom Catastrophe: An Incentive for Developing Better Palliative Care Services

Doron Garfinkel, (Society for the Inhibition of Age-related Processes, Aging research & Department of Medicine E, Wolfson Medical Center, Holon, ISRAEL)

Throughout history, the average life span has been increasing slowly in an estimated pace of one year per century. However, the average life span leaped by 30 years in the 20th century reaching 77- 80 years in developed societies. Unfortunately, this trend and improved curative medicine create an exponential increase in the incidence and complexity of all chronic, age - related diseases and an increased portion of non-healthy non curative patients in the general population. The economic burden on the rest of the healthy productive population may become unbearable and represent a ominous fate for the independent existence of the society as a whole. The global number of new cancer patients has almost doubled since 1975. US Medicare expenditures for the elderly have increased 40-50 fold since 1967 and are expected to double in ten years. Ethical and legal restraints forbid physicians from denying care for patients suffering from specific illnesses. The social implications are ominous and our children may have to decide whether to treat their parent or to invest in their children's future. We must increase awareness of this problem in both government and in the general public in an attempt to divert more resources to preventive medicine and for research on inhibiting the age-related processes. The more means we find to slow processes of aging, the more we will be able to keep adults healthier for a longer period of time while reducing the time and cost of palliative care. The ratio between disabled people and the rest of the population will also be reduced. At the same time, we must improve cost effectiveness of our palliative care.

[5] Grandparents Parenting Grandchildren: An Exploratory Study to Assess Mental Health, Parental Stress and Social Supports

F.Butler, N.Zakari (George Mason University, Fairfax, VA USA)

The purpose of this research is to describe the emotional health of grandparents raising grandchildren and to determine the level and source of stress produced by the caregiving role. A sample of grandparents who are primary caregivers for their grandchildren and reside within a three-state metropolitan area in the US were interviewed over a fifteen month period. The design employed both qualitative and quantitative data collection methods and analyses to assess health status, level of stress, economic difficulties, family support and social interaction. Scores on key mental health indicators and self-perceived changes in mental health indicated high anxiety, moderate depression and inadequate social relationships in half of the participants. Parental Stress Index scores revealed that 47 percent of participants had high total stress scores (greater than 260) in the child domain subscales. High attachment subscale scores occurred in 15 percent of caregivers, indicating a lack of emotional bonding. Within the parent domain, role restriction was the most prevalent high score, occuring in 30 percent of the caregivers. This study showed an urgent need for professional counseling for at risk grandparents. Policy implications to support the grandparent caregiving role which emerged from the study, include income support, health insurance for the children, transportation to special programs, teacher education and access to support groups. Recommendations regarding areas of practice and education include accurate caregiver and family assessments, formal and informal suports, appropriate referrals and close monitoring for at risk grandparents.

[6] Hospitality in Continuing Care - Implementing a Social Model

Debra F. Elm (The Good Samaritan Society, Edmonton, Canada)

The Good Samaritan Society (GSS), a multiple site continuing care organization where multiple levels of services are provided, implemented a social model of providing services called the Hospitality Model. The model was developed using Henri Nouwen's writing on hospitality as an approach to relationships and The University of Toronto's work on "Quality of Life". The main goal of the model is to provide a safe place where both residents/clients and staff alike have the freedom to "be", "belong" and "become". Organizational structures were put in place to accommodate the model. The structures include definition of the purpose of the resident/client assessment of need process and format, definition of service, and definition of the roles of both staff members and the residents/clients. Outcomes and indicators were identified. A roll out plan was determined which included education of the staff, focus groups, role modeling by the leaders of the organization and the introduction of the assessments and service processes. Although GSS is at the beginning stages of implementation, roll out barriers have been identified and recommendations have been made.

[7] Examining health system reorganisation and cancer diagnoses and treatment procedures in British Columbia (1990-1999)

Brackley ME, Allan DA, Penning MJ (University of Victoria, Victoria, Canada)

PURPOSE: Over the past decade, provincial and territorial governments across Canada shifted health care funding allocation and organisational foci toward a community-based population health model. Regionalisation, defined as the transfer of decision-making power from provincial to community levels, was adopted to achieve this aim. This presentation is a part of a larger project designed to assess effects of regionalisation on allocation of health care resources, utilisation of health care services, and health outcomes. Here, we assess patterns of cancer diagnosis and treatment in three regions of British Columbia, representing rural and urban communities, before and after major health system reorganisation in 1997. METHODS: Data (1990-1999) are drawn from the British Columbia Linked Health Data resource (http://www.chspr.ubc.ca/); access to the resource is allowed through the British Columbia Ministry of Health. Files are hospital separation and medical service plan records. Data include a 10ample of the entire province, and 100amples from Capital, Okanagan-Similkameen and Upper Island/Central Coast health regions. Age-standardised rates for cancer diagnoses and treatment procedures are assessed and compared between rural and urban regions both prior to and after 1997. RESULTS AND CONCLUSIONS: Preliminary results suggest few differences in diagnoses for particular cancer groupings between rural and urban regions, or between dichotomous time periods. Further analysis of treatment procedures, as well as time series results, will be presented.

[8] Social Work and Family Medicine: Geriatric Research Partners

A. W. Roy, [School of Social Work, Springfield College, Springfield, MA, U.S.A.] J. Lesser [School of Social Work, Springfield College, Springfield, MA, U.S. A]

The purpose of this study was: (1) to pilot test a Social Support/ Health Behavior survey with a low-income, multicultural sample of elders and (2) to facilitate interdisciplinary collaboration between social work geriatric research and Family Medicine practice. Using a convenience sample (N=34, mean age 72)face-face interviews were conducted utilizing a multi-dimensional questionnaire. Using a reliability program in SPSS for PC, we found that two out of three health behavior scales were reliable: Cancer Detection Practices (alpha=.67) Risk Avoidance Behaviors (alpha=.41) and Promotive Health Behavior (alpha=.12). As well, the Social Network Questionnaire (SNQ) (alpha=.30), the Multidimensional Scale of Perceived Social Support (MSSP)(alpha=.86) and Inventory of Socially Supportive Behaviors(ISSB) (alpha=.86) were internally consistent. Feedback from our interviewers in terms of survey length and item clarity revealed that elders received the survey favorably, lending evidence for face validity, that is, the survey appears to have measured what it was intended to measure. The second objective, to promote integration of social work research within Family Medicine practice, will be examined in terms of ethical issues, confidentiality and recruitment of elders. This was a successful pilot of a social support/health behavior instrument, as well as a positive collaboration between Family Medicine and Social Work research. It is hoped that the integration of these two disciplines may yield greater understanding of elders' health needs and improve our ability to deliver preventive medial care to under-served elders.

[9] Improving the Planning of Medical and Social Services within Elder Care in St. Petersburg

L.Lenskaya, I.Zalmanov (St.Petersburg City Geriatric Centre, Russia), V.Dorofeev (St.Petersburg Committee for Statistics, Russia), E.Lomakina (Public Health Committee of St.Petersburg, Russia).

The purpose of the project was to improve the elder care planning by producing a study of elderly people's service needs based on survey material of structured face-to-face interviews and by composing a development plan for the elder care services on the basis of the study and situational analysis. The IPSE survey study was based on World Health Organisation's ELSA - European Longitudinal Study on Ageing research programme. The survey study was addressed to gain reliable information on living conditions, health status, functional ability and service needs on the elderly population. The data collection of the IPSE survey study was carried out in St. Petersburg in April, 2000 covering 1.216 60-89-year-old respondents from 13 districts of St. Petersburg city. One of the key problems in planning elder care services in St. Petersburg is the lack of exact information of, firstly, service needs of the elderly and, secondly, the functioning of the elder care system. According to the results of the IPSE survey study, 1 % of the aged population are in need of daily help in their everyday tasks. On the population level this means that there are approximately 97.000 elderly people in St. Petersburg who need assistance in daily living. This need for help in daily living does not concern to a large extent medical professionals, but the assistance can be provided by professional social workers and to some extent by volunteers, family members and friends.

[10] Financial Analysis of Outpatient Geriatric Care Management Program

Victor A. Hirth, MD [University of South Carolina School of Medicine, Nine Medical Park Drive, Suite 630, Columbia, SC 29203, USA]

PURPOSE: The purpose of this study is to determine the potential financial performance of a Geriatric Care Manager (GCM) program. GCM is geared to assist the older patient in navigating through the complexities of the US health care system. Functions of the social worker acting as GCM include, developing a comprehensive care plan which includes evaluating the elder's level of function and special needs as well as long term care issues, monitor service delivery, maintain contact with out of town family members and counseling and support. This service is not covered by Medicare. METHOD: A financial model, based on a 5 physician geriatric outpatient practice, was developed using known fixed overhead expenses and variable social workers' salaries expense with estimates of hourly GCM activity at a rate of $75/hour. Hourly activity needed to break even, and estimates of year one and three income were calculated. RESULTS: The GCM program is projected to lose $925 in the first year of operation, based on 50 cases requiring 15 hours per case per year, but by year three to generate income of $71,541 annually (150 cases @ 15hrs/case). The break even point, at which the program would be budget neutral, would be 3.0 hours per day of GCM activities. CONCLUSION: On the basis of these projections the GCM program would break even shortly after the first year and by year three contribute $71,541 to net income of the practice. This favorable financial performance supports the implementation of the GCM program.

[11] Care Needs influencing Discharged Patients and Their Families

Yumi Chiba and Kinuko Takasaki (Schoolof Allied Health Science, Tokyo Medical Dental University, Tokyo, Japan)

Purpose: This study was to clarify the structural factors of care needs to discharge for the patients and their families with cerebral vascular disease. Methods 1) Pre-test: ten families of discharged patients were interviewed in order to make the categories of necessary care needs to discharge. 2) One hundred forty four discharged patients who were hospitalized during April 1997 to September 1998 at S Hospital, Saitama prefecture in Japan, were chosen. The self-administrative questionnaire with the structural 41 items and other related questions for discharge. Returned samples were 87(60.4%). The factors of care needs were analyzed between two groups, 40-64 years (n1=41) and over 65 years (n2=46) through t-test, chi- square test and Kruskal-Wallis test. Result s: 1) The result of pre-test for care needs to discharge was summarized into 41 items; consisted of 35 items of common care needs (4 factors) and 6 items of rehabilitation care needs(1 factors). Cronbachs alphas in both were 0.95. 2) With the comparison of two groups, significant answers were 20 items. The contents of the items were kind of cerebral vascular disease, history of hospitalization and heart disease, rehabilitation (PT, ST) in hospitalization, handicaps of ability to listen, anxiety in the future, family type, working, income, public services including care needs. Conclusion: The study indicated care needs for assessment of individual discharge planning in addition a screen tools of care needs in order to carry smoothly to discharge for the elderly patients.

[12] Counseling and Coordinating Services at the Protestant Geriatric Center in Berlin - A Case of Care Management

S. Hensse (The Geriatric Research Group, Virchow Clinic, Medical Faculty of the Humboldt University of Berlin, Germany) M. Ruhnau-Wuellenweber (The Coordinating Center "All Around Aging", The Protestant Geriatric Center in Berlin, Germany) E. Steinhagen-Thiessen (Medical Director of the Protestant Geriatric Center in Berlin, Medical Faculty of the Humboldt University of Berlin, Germany)

The counseling and coordinating services of the protestant geriatric center in Berlin, Evangelisches Geriatriezentrum Berlin gGmbH (EGZB), have been available to the residents of Berlin since February 1994 and are geared towards the elderly, interested friends and relatives, care-takers of impaired or frail elderly, and geriatric professionals. One of the major goals of this coordinating center is prevention: preventing inadequate and inappropriate placement of (impaired) elderly in nursing homes, preventing unnecessary hospitalzations and frequent rehospitalizations, preventing burned-out syndromes and the development of crisis situations that can lead to unintentional violence and elder abuse in home-nursing, etc. Evaluations of questionares from over twelve hundred counseling cases show that there are significant differences in the counseling and support requirements of (family) care-givers as opposed to persons not primarily or directly involved in home nursing. Also, the assistance needed by persons already involved in home nursing varies considerably form persons pending such a step. The results regarding initiating situations that led to taking up contact with the center, types of information and support requested, and outcomes confirm that care-givers need sufficient qualified information and support to dealing with existing or anticipated problems. Since elderly persons and their relatives often seek help from family physicians and other health care professionals, a greater focus must be placed on providing these professionals with necessary information.

[13] Social work with older people: continuity, change, and challenge in the twenty first century.

M. S. Parsons (Oxford Dementia Centre, Oxford, England)

Welfare pluralism and care management have changed the nature of social work which faces further challenges from the integration of health and social services for older people in England and Wales.These developments prompted a large English local authority to commission an evaluation of the quality of care management for older people, identifying good practice, barriers to its consistent achievement, and possible improvement. The research design was highly participatory. providing opportunities for reflection on social work practice. Care managers completed 'simulated' assessments and care plans for older people using case studies. Teams pooled individual responses and reflective practice accounts. Formative results from this data were fed back to teams and senior managers who met in focus groups to discuss implications for social work with older people. Findings showed social work with older people being redefined in different ways.

Bureaucratisation of social work practice and introduction of contract culture have affected the capacity of social workers to maintain values in practice. However, demands for skilled decision making in increasingly complex perennial dilemmas of care/ control and rights/ risks involving older people and their carers are being met by social workers, who are also re forging traditional networking skills in response to the need for effective inter professional and inter agency collaboration. Responding to social diversity, policy shifts, time and resource constraints, social workers demonstrate a capacity for continuity and adaptation to change in striving to achieve the best possible outcomes for older people and carers.

[14] Practitioners' Self-Evaluation in Care Management Practice of Japan

C. Hata, S Okada and M. Shirasawa (Graduate School of Human Life Science, Osaka City University, Osaka, Japan)

Purpose: In this study, the authors attempt to evaluate care management practice for the elderly of Japan by using a practitioners' self-evaluation method. Method: The sample was recruited from the participants in care management professional workshops. Survey was mailed to all of the participants (N=287). Of these, 79.1% completed the survey. The survey included two self-evaluation measures as well as several demographics. The measures are self-rated performance and self-confidence concerning care management process. The care management conceptual process includes: (1) intake, (2) assessment, (3) care planning, (4) linking and implementation, and (5) monitoring. Results: The data indicated that the measures were reliable as evidence by the high internal consistency (alpha >0.90). Factor analyses suggested that the five conceptual factors mentioned above were retained in the self-confidence measure and that in the self-rated performance measure, several items loaded onto different factors from the factors posed in the conceptual process. However, there was a strong correlation between the two measures. Analyses of variance revealed that the significant factors affecting the two self-evaluation measures were: (1) the number of cases, (2) the existence of assurance mechanism for site visiting, (3) the existence of a supportive supervisor, (4) the involvement of interdisciplinary conferences, and (5) the experience of professional training. Conclusions: The survey results revealed that each process factor of actual care management practice might be implemented in a manner of nonlinear dynamics and that work environment was crucial in improving care management practice.

[15] Older people from South Asia: Cross-national sample selection in India, Bangladesh and the United Kingdom

V. Burholt (Centre for Social Policy Research and Development, University of Wales, Bangor, UK), G. C. Wenger (Centre for Social Policy Research and Development, University of Wales, Bangor, UK), A. Biswas (Shahjalal University, Sylhet, Bangladesh), P. Dave (Maharaja Sayajirao University of Baroda, Fatehgunj, Vadodara, Gujarat, India), M. Ehtisham (City Hospital NHS Trust, Birmingham, UK), S. Guthrie (Centre for Social Policy Research and Development, University of Wales, Bangor, UK), S. Sodhi (Patiala, Punjab, India), S. Soneja (HelpAge India, Delhi, India).

This paper reports on a cross-national study which focuses on the impact of migration of family members on sources of help and support to older members of Gujarati, Punjabi and Sylheti families living in the United Kingdom, India and Bangladesh. The paper focuses on the initial stages of the project, that is sample selection in each of the countries. Comparable samples of people aged 55 and over were drawn in the UK (N=300) and Asia (N=300): 100 each of Sylhetis, Gujaratis and Indian Punjabis. Previously studies in South Asia and of immigrants from some of these countries have had difficulties in achieving adequate representation of women. This paper will discuss the methods that were employed in order to overcome this problem, such as gender-matched interviewing and stratification of the sample by gender. The UK sample was drawn from Gujarati, Punjabi and Sylheti elders in Birmingham via contacts established through local ethnic associations and the use of 'snowball' technique. This technique will be discussed with regard to the benefits over other sampling techniques in this instance. In Asia the sample was drawn from villages identified as primary sources of migration to the UK. The paper would discuss the principal investigators' entry points to the communities through village leaders. This paper will draw on evidence collated for popular reports for villagers in South Asia and migrant groups in the UK. The paper will present profiles of each community using photographs of older people, living conditions, and village views, as illustration.

[16] Japanese research trends in social gerontology

Yoshiko Someya,(Shukutoku Univ Chiba-city,Japan) Tatsuya Fujino,M.A,(Shukutoku Univ, Chiba-city,Japan)

This research analyzes research trends in the field of social gerontology. The Foundation of Social Development for Senior Citizens conducted the research project from January to May in 2000. 4835 reports were collected throughout Japan dating from 1987 to 1998 and divided into 9 fields. Social welfare research occupied 30.8 %, followed by social and opinion survey (26.9%), psychology (9.3%), housing and environment (8.9%), public health (8.6%), family and family life (6.6%), economy and employment (5.7%), foreign issues (2.2%), and demography (1.0%). Because the Japanese government welfare policy for the aged, so called the Gold Plan, was enacted in 1989, the volume of publication peaked in 1990. 60.9% of the total publications were published in the Kanto district where the Tokyo metropolitan government is located. In conclusion, more research reports on gender related issues and publications outside the metropolitan areas are expected to be published in the future.

[17] Aging in Peru : An open agenda

Dante I. Gazzolo (School of Psychology,Universidad Ricardo Palma , Lima ,Perú)

This paper address the advancement of gerontological work in Peru in the last 18 years. Despite the elderly population has increasing its number from 4.6% to 7.2%, there is simply a slight advance in this area. In the government area, the task was to create different older adult clubs in many cities of the country with a recreational focus. The Ministry of Health does not have an up to the moment office related to aging issues. Only the Ministry of Women Affairs and Human Development, created in 1996, has a small dependency with two professionals. However, since last July we have National Policies for older adult population. The Ngo's have focused their work to organize this people in different areas. They have established a Network that do a great job with poor older adults in some places of the country. The Third Age concept is now more known in the civil society. The Peruvian University has made good efforts. Geriatrics is now being taught in at least four schools of Medicine. Gerontology is only being taught in one school of Psychology in all the country. Research has been done mainly in Medicine, Psychology, Nursing and Social Work. We point out the great need to push governmental efforts to make visible the aging agenda and in this point, our University Ricardo Palma is doing its best effort through research and gerontological programs in the community.

[18] The Behavioural Urgent Service (BUS) Pilot Program: A Collaborative Initiative to Enhance Care

C.A. McAiney (Division of Geriatric Psychiatry, McMaster University, Hamilton, Canada), J. MacLeod (Rehabilitation and Senior's Health Program, Hamilton Health Sciences Corporation, Hamilton, Canada), J.K. Le Clair (Geriatric Division, Department of Psychiatry, Queen's University, Kingston, Canada), A.S. Luthra Rehabilitation and Senior's Health Program, Hamilton Health Sciences Corporation, Hamilton, Canada), K. Saperson (Division of Geriatric Psychiatry, McMaster University, Hamilton, Canada)

The Behavioural Urgent Service (BUS) pilot program was designed to provide a more integrated delivery system of care to elderly individuals with complex needs and urgent behavioural problems. The primary goals of the BUS Program are to: (1) enhance the response to urgent behavioural problems in long-term care facilities and the community, (2) reduce inappropriate admissions to emergency departments, and (3) enhance the capacity of health care providers within the system. The BUS Program was evaluated to determine the impact on clients as well as the larger system. The evaluation goals included: characterizing the client population, determining client dispositions after referral, and examining the impact of the program on clients, referring agencies and other partners. Over 110 clients were referred to the BUS Program in the first year. 500f these individuals were from long-term care facilities and over 75uffered from dementia. Approximately 400f clients were able to be maintained in their place of residence, and almost 50% were linked with the appropriate specialty service without the need for transfer to hospital. The program was highly valued by referral sources, specialty services, and emergency department staff. The program was also found to help reinforce and enhance training in geriatric mental health that had recently been conducted. The BUS pilot program has been successful in providing a quicker and more appropriate response to individuals with complex needs and urgent behavioural problems. It has reduced inappropriate transfers to emergency departments and has helped to enhance the capacity of service providers.

[19] Evaluation of nurse-led case management of older patients in general practice

J. Hodgkinson, M. McKinnon, J. Townsend, R. McGurk (Centre for Research in Primary and Community Care, University of Hertfordshire, Hatfield, UK)

PURPOSE: To evaluate the effectiveness of nurse-led case management of older adults in primary care, using developed practice guidelines and agreed care pathways, in improving patient quality of life, health status and satisfaction with practice care and cost effectiveness in health service usage. METHOD: Ten practices in urban and rural areas of England were randomly assigned either to intervention of nurse-led case management or to continued usual care using a randomised controlled trial design. Following training in case management, the GP, Practice Nurse, District Nurse and Social Service workers in intervention practices met regularly to agree care pathways and undertake regular review of care for 18 months, using specially selected and adapted evidence-based guidelines in the case management meetings. The effectiveness of case management is assessed in terms of mortality and morbidity rates, consultation rates, and number and length of hospital stays, collected from practice records and health authorities. Information about patient perceived quality of life and patient satisfaction with care is obtained from 40 in-depth qualitative interviews and through three questionnaires, which incorporate EuroQol and the Geriatric Depression Scale, at different points in the trial. RESULTS: The mid-point questionnaire (N=866) found intervention practice patients were significantly more likely to report higher health status, higher functional independence (self-care and preparing meals), and higher satisfaction with practice care than control practice patients ($p<0.05$), but there was no baseline difference. CONCLUSIONS: Nurse-led case management appears to have a positive impact on patient self-perceived health, quality of life and satisfaction with practice care.

[20] Advance Care Planning Among Residents in a National Sample of U.S. Nursing Home Residents

W. J. McAuley, S. S. Travis (College of Nursing and Health Professions, UNC Charlotte, North Carolina, USA)

The U.S. Patient Self Determination Act requires that individuals admitted to U.S. nursing facilities receiving Medicare and Medicaid reimbursement must be informed of their right to accept or refuse medical care and receive written information regarding advance directives (AD). The purposes of this presentation are to: (a) describe the prevalence of advance planning of various types in nursing homes, and (b) describe variables that predict having any form of AD, and that differentiate between two levels of AD: "basic" (living will, do not resuscitate (DNR)), and "progressive" (do not hospitalize, and no feeding/medication/other treatment). Data were derived from Public Use File 1 of the Medical Expenditure Panel Study Nursing Home Component, which was designed (with the application of appropriate weights) to produce valid national estimates of U.S. nursing home residents in 1996. Tabular and logistic regression analyses were employed to examine the prevalence and predictors of advance care planning. Less than half of residents had any AD, with DNR being most common. Most individuals with a progressive directive also had at least one basic AD. Significant predictors of having any AD include being White, female, and older, and having a diagnosis of Alzheimer's disease or cancer. Among individuals with any AD, variables predictive of having a progressive versus a basic directive include longer residence in the facility, and diagnosis of peripheral vascular disease or emphysema/COPD. We discuss the implications of the results for an emergent conceptual framework of factors influencing decisions to employ advance care planning in long-term care.

[21] An Evaluation of Consumer Protection Provisions in Long Term Care Insurance

A. Scharlach, B. Robinson (Center for the Advanced Study of Aging Services, University of California, Berkeley, CA, USA)

This study examined the adequacy of consumer protection policies and practices in long-term care insurance (LTCI). The qualitative analysis included longitudinal case studies and detailed case record reviews of 35 consumers participating in the California Partnership for Long Term Care, an innovative public-private partnership between long-term care insurance carriers and Medi-Cal (Californias health care program for the poor). Data collection included multiple interviews with policyholders, family members, care managers, and insurance company representatives, over a six-month period. Participants generally were found to be satisfied with the services they received from care managers and from direct service providers. Consumers; basic service needs appeared to be met in most cases, although two-third had at least some unmet needs. One-third of consumers did not utilize all of the services identified in their care plans, while one-half utilized services other than those listed in their care plans, suggesting the need for additional assistance with care plan implementation. While most participants understood the general types and amount of coverage their LTCI policies provided, few knew what criteria needed to be met for eligibility, how to file an appeal, or that their long-term care insurance policies included a unique asset protection feature. These findings suggest the need for more comprehensive care monitoring and service coordination activities, as well as enhanced consumer education. The findings also suggest a number of other specific improvements in quality assurance and consumer protection procedures that could be implemented by government agencies, insurers, and care management organizations, in order to better protect the rights and meet the needs of elderly consumers under long-term care insurance.

[22] Cluster Care Model for Cost-Effective and Quality Home Support Services

Gwen Fillippelli Case Manager White Rock Continuing Care South Fraser Health Region White Rock, BC, Canada Patricia Neale Case Manager Langley Continuing Care South Fraser Health Region Langley, BC, Canada Linda Bell Executive Director Delta Home Support Service South Fraser Health Region Delta, BC, Canada

Cluster Care is a model of integrated service delivery that provides a multidisciplinary team to enhance the health, well being, and quality of life of clients in the community. Cluster Care has the potential to improve the quality of services by increasing availability / access to the right care between clients and care providers and provide a cost-effective service. A seven month Cluster Care Pilot project was carried out in the South Fraser Health Region to determine the extent to which a different approach to allocating home support services could benefit clients while making better use of available resources. The project was designed to provide information on among other thingswhether shorter, but more frequent visits (e.g. to monitor medications or nutritional intake) rather than one longer visit, would translate to better care and more efficient service. KEY FINDINGS · 71% of clients were more than 80 years old · 88.4% women · clients used 75% of the maximum authorized hours · cluster care is suitable for majority of clients requiring home support · increased visibility improved access, helped identify new clients · prompt response to client needs · effective care coordination · close monitoring allowed clients to remain at home LESSONS AND CHALLENGES · ensure sufficient lead time 6 month · choose appropriate site Ø high density geographic area Ø clients receiving large number of hours · promote a shared vision among care providers team work is essential, involve all team members in team meetings · insure policies and procedures are supportive not obstructive · assign one Home Support Agency to the cluster · ensure that care levels and care plans are current · promote the Program vigorously Ø clients and family, other tenants, apartment manager Ø service providers including HSWs

[23] Supporting family care systems for the elderly with cerebrovascular accident from a holistic health perspective

Oséias Guimarães de Andrade (University of Maringá at Maringá College Nursing, Maringá, Paraná, Brazil) Rosalina Aparecida Partezani Rodrigues (University of São Paulo at Ribeirão Preto College Nursing, Ribeirão Preto, São Paulo, Brazil)

This work aimed at understanding the reality of the family care system for the elderly with cerebrovascular accident (CVA) and at implementing support to such system by means of conceptions based on a holistic health framework. Five families who cared for their elderly relatives with CVA in their own homes participated in the research. Based on the participant research-action methodology, we shared the care system with the families for an approximate period of six months. During such time, we developed the technique of Drawing-Story Procedures with a Theme and Participant Observation as instruments for data generation. At first, these data were thematically analyzed, which made it possible for us to identify three themes: 1) the major caretaker as a focus of the family care system for the elderly with CVA; 2) the environment of the family care for the elderly with CVA, which revealed a context of complexities and singularities and 3) the nature of holistic thinking in the reality of the family care system for the elderly with CVA. These data were then submitted to a process of synthesis which favored the understanding of the reality involving the care system for the elderly with CVA. This allowed an interaction with such families, which became a support for a holistic health perspective. Its implementation contributed to the elderly's lives with their families in addition to showing the need to re-think our culture as to the valorization of women, their caretaker role, the elderly, humane care and, therefore, life itself.

[24] Model for Participation of Seniors in the Public Health System

Bonnie Lillies, Bernadet Ratsoy, Gerald Hickey (Vancouver/ Richmond Health Board, Seniors Population Health Advisory Committee, Vancouver, Canada)

PURPOSE: To present a model for seniors participation in the development and delivery of health care services for seniors. DESCRIPTION: The Ministry of Health in British Columbia, Canada moved to a regional model for health care delivery in the 1990 s. The Vancouver/Richmond Health Board (V/RHB) is one of 11 regional boards administering health care under the new system. That board established eight Population Health Advisory Committees (PHAC s) to provide input from historically under-represented or under-served populations. Seniors formed one of these populations. The MANDATE of Seniors PHAC is: ·to liaise between the seniors population and the V/RHB ·to advise the V/ RHB regarding the concerns, needs and priorities of seniors ·to develop recommendations regarding research, policy, planning, resource allocation, services and programs, and educational activities for seniors ·to review the development, implementation and evaluation of health policies and programs to ensure health needs of seniors are addressed RESULTS: Since its inception, the Seniors PHAC has influenced health care delivery for seniors in the Vancouver/Richmond Health Region. Priorities the Seniors PHAC identified, promoted, and monitored include: ·increasing community based services ·increasing access to health services ·coordinating elder abuse programs ·enhancing mental health services ·enhancing education, training, and support for informal caregivers ·increasing respite care ·providing affordable appropriate seniors housing. CONCLUSION: Seniors in the Vancouver/Richmond health region have a new and effective structure that has formalized and enhanced their participation in the development of health services for seniors in this region.

[25] An introduction of the honorary organization of the aged

Wang Chuguang (The Central Research Institute of Culture and History Beijing China)

The paper would like to introduce the organization of the elderly intellectuals in China by the name of Research Institute of Culture and History. It is scattered all over the country from the Capital city of Beijing to municipalities. The elderly intellectuals enjoy a happy and meaningful life by participating in various activities of the institute.

[26] Randomized Controlled Trial of Home Hospitalization Services for Elderly Stroke Patients: A 6-Month Follow-Up

D. SALERNO, N. AIMONINO RICAUDA, M. BO, D. AMATI, V. TIBALDI, M. MOLASCHI, F. FABRIS (Department of Medical and Surgical Disciplines, Geriatric Section, University of Turin, Italy)

PURPOSE: to assess the feasibility of hospital at home for elderly patients after ischemic stroke, to evaluate the hospital readmission rate and the requirement for long-term institutional care six months after stroke. METHOD: the study was conducted on 120 randomized patients aged over 70 years (average age: 81.6±7.4 years), with ischemic stroke, admitted to the Emergency Department of our hospital: 60 patients were treated in the general medical ward (GMW), 60 were managed at home by the Geriatric Home Hospitalization Service (GHHS). GHHS provides diagnostic and therapeutic interventions at home which are usually made in hospital. GHHS team includes geriatricians, nurses, physiotherapists, occupational therapist, speech therapist and social worker. Patients were assessed on discharge, at 3 and 6 months after stroke. RESULTS: the functional and cognitive recovery in survivors continued to occur within six months, in both groups. Mortality was not significantly different in the two groups. Six months after stroke GHHS patients presented a more significant improvement in depression score evaluated by Geriatric Depression Scale-GDS (mean± SD, GHHS patients 8.4±6.3, GMW patients 13.0±9.6; $p<0.001$). At follow-up, 950f GHHS patients were still living at home versus 66.70f GMW patients ($p<0.001$). Six months after discharge there was a significant difference between the number of hospital readmissions among GHHS patients and GMW patients (chi-quadro 24.3, df 2, $p<0.0001$). CONCLUSION: GHHS is a possible alternative to routine hospital care and reduces the hospital readmission and the requirement for long-term institutional care for elderly patients with ischemic stroke.

[27] Pragmatic Randomised Trial of Home Visits by Nurses to Elderly People with Hypertension in Mexico

Carmen Garcia-Peña (Medical Research Unit on Ageing, Research Coordination. Mexican Institute of Social Security, Mexico City, México), Margaret Thorogood (Health Promotion Research Unit. London School of Hygiene and Tropical Medicine, London UK), Ben Armstrong (Environmental Epidemiology Unit. London School of Hygiene and Tropical Medicine, London UK), Sandra Reyes (Medical Research Unit on Ageing, Research Coordination. Mexican Institute of Social Security, Mexico City, Mexico) and Onofre Muñoz (Research Coordination. Mexican Institute of Social Security, Mexico City, Mexico)

Purpose: To assess the effectiveness of nurses home visits in reducing blood pressure in elderly people. Methods: Randomised Controlled Trial. The intervention group where offered nurse visits over six months with blood pressure checks and negotiated lifestyle changes. The control group continued to receive usual care. Setting: Family Medicine Clinics of the Mexican Institute of Social Security. Participants: 718 hypertensive participants aged 60 years and over, residents of Mexico City. Main outcome measures: Change in blood pressure, weight, salt intake, self reported physical activity from baseline. Results: After six months, 36.5% of the intervention versus 6.8% of the control group had a blood pressure of less than 160/90 mm/Hg. The difference in the mean change in systolic blood pressure was 3.31 mm/Hg (p=0.03, 95% CI 6.32, 0.29). For change in diastolic blood pressure the difference was 3.67 mm/Hg (p=0.00, 95% CI 5.22, 2.12). Weight and sodium excretion reduced more in the intervention group, but not significantly. Conclusions: Nurse home visits are effective in reducing blood pressure in hypertensive patients aged 60 years and over.

[28] Prevalence of Neuropsychiatric Diseases in Dependent Elderly in a Home Care Setting

R.D.Miranda, A.M.Z.Gagliardi, V.R.Bellinazzi, L.R. Ramos (Geriatric Division, Federal University of Sao Paulo - UNIFESP)

PURPOSE: We have now in Brazil a great increase in elderly population, and we expect to have in 2 or 3 decades the sixth elder population of the world. With the increase in the life expectancy there is also the increase in the chronic degenerative diseases, among them the neuropsychiatric ones can be highlighted. Home care becomes fundamental to the assistance of such patients who have difficulties moving around. It also becomes very important to use scales that are easily administered and have good reliability to assess both cognitive and mental health functions. Our objective is evaluate the prevalence of neuropsychiatric diseases in elderly patients in a home care setting. METHOD: This is a cross sectional study of the group (n=38) of elderly in home care. The neuropsychiatric diagnosis was based on the history, clinical examination and screenings for mental health problems and cognitive impairment. RESULTS: The prevalence of cognitive deficit was 50%, of mental health problems was also 50%, stroke 23.7%, Parkinson's disease 15.7% and cancer in the central nervous system 5.2%. CONCLUSION: There was a large prevalence in neuropsychiatric diseases among dependent elderly in a home care setting. That is the reason why it is always very important to carry out active search of these diagnoses in this group of patients.

[29] "Care of the seriously ill in the community". An overview of a program of research

Kevin Brazil (Department of Clinical Epidemiology and Biostatistics, McMaster University, Hamilton)Tom Abernathy (Central West Planning Information Network, Hamilton) Paul Krueger (Department of Clinical Epidemiology and Biostatistics, McMaster University, Hamilton) Lynne Lohfeld (Department of Clinical Epidemiology and Biostatistics, McMaster University, Hamilton) Patrick Critchley (Hospice of Windsor, Windsor) Michel Bedard (Lakehead Psychiatric Hospital, Thunder Bay) Kathleen Willison (Victorian Order of Nurses, Hamilton-Wentworth, Hamilton) Gayle Edward (St. Joseph s Health Care System Research Network, Hamilton)

This report will provide an overview and status report on a three-year longitudinal study of both informal and formal palliative care services that are accessed by the terminally ill and their family caregivers. Study objectives include: 1. Describe the pattern of informal and formal care used by the terminally ill and their caregivers. 2. Describe family caregivers reactions to providing care, bereavement and bereavement care. 3. Determine the factors which influence family caregiver s satisfaction with community services. Family caregivers (n=500) are being recruited to be interviewed at two points in time when the terminally ill person is designated as palliative in a community nursing agency, and six months subsequent to the first interview. Ontario Ministry of Health data bases are being used to describe service utilization patterns of the terminally ill in the study locations. A sample of caregiver and terminally ill dyads (n=12) will be recruited from the participants of the family caregiver survey to participate in-depth interviews. Study locations will include the catchment areas of five Community Care Access Centres (CCAC); Hamilton-Wentworth CCAC (urban base);Brant CCAC (urban/rural mix), Haldimand-Norfolk CCAC (rural base); CCAC of Waterloo region (urban/ rural); CCAC of Wellington-Dufferin. Funding for this project is provided by the Ontario Ministry of Health and the Canadian Health Services Research Foundation.

[30] Evaluation Method of Action Plan and Implementation Based on Clients Outcome in Home Care

Kumiko Fujiya, Setsu Shimanouchi (Tokyo Medical and Dental University, Tokyo, JAPAN) Yoko Shimizu (The Japanese Red Cross College of Nursing, Tokyo, JAPAN)

The purposes of our study were to determine a frame of reference for outcome improvement and to describe the evaluation method of action plan and implementation. We studied 552 subjects living in the community who were 40 years old or older at 7 Visiting Nursing Stations located in Japan. A client assessment form was made up of demographic items and outcome measures. Outcome measures were composed of 35 items. Clients' outcome data was collected 2 times on September and November in 2000. The rate of outcome improvement was calculated and each Visiting Nursing Station decided some target outcomes, then action plans were determined and implemented. Based on these results, ability of staffs and power of organization were evaluated. A frame of reference for ability of staffs had 5 categories (assessment, plan, implementation of the plan, monitoring, care effect). And a frame of reference for power of organization had 3 categories (information sharing, cooperation, role). In both indexes, each category was composed of 5 subcategories. These were monitored 2 times, before and after implementation of some action plans. This study suggested that using a frame of reference facilitated to evaluate of care effect and it was useful to improve the ability of staffs and power of organization.

[31] Health care restructuring: Impact on home care service utilization among older adults in British Columbia

Penning MJ, Allan DE, Brackley, ME (Centre on Aging, University of Victoria, BC, Canada)

Purpose: Over the past decade, provincial governments across Canada have restructured health services by transferring decision-making authority from provincial to regional levels, in recognition of the importance of community-based population health models. The intent is to alter focus from institutional care towards community-based services such as home care. This presentation assesses the extent to which such a shift is occurring, whether it entails expansion or redirection of home care services, and implications for older adults in one Canadian province, British Columbia. Method: Analyses are conducted using data (1990-1999) drawn from hospital separation and long-term care files available within the British Columbia Linked Health Data resource, and from the BC Ministry of Health. Samples include 10% of those living and using services in the province as a whole, as well as 100% of those living in and using services within three specific regions of the province during each year. Changes over time in service utilization rates, standardized by age and sex, are examined. Results and Conclusion: Preliminary results reveal declines over time in hospital and home support service utilization (number of clients served and hours of service provided) together with increases in the intensity of service provided and in client levels of care. Changes in the age distribution of those receiving services are also evident. These findings are discussed in terms of the increasing medicalization of community-based care.

[32] An Analysis of Home and Community Based Care Programs in Central and Eastern Europe

C.A. Emlet (University of Washington, Tacoma, Tacoma, Washington, USA), M.C. Hokenstad (Case Western Reserve

University, Cleveland, Ohio, USA), C. J. Nicols (Ridgemont Terrace Nursing Home,Port Orchard, Washington, USA)

PURPOSE: Few studies have examined the development of home and community based care programs in Central and Eastern Europe. This project analyzed 97 community based care projects from 20 countries throughout Central and Eastern Europe. METHODS: Projects were examined to determine levels of service delivery. Projects were categorized into service delivery models by adopting the conceptual framework developed by Chernesky (1999). RESULTS: Projects fell into four distinct categories: client centered, intergenerational, educational and organizational. Client centered projects consisted of direct services such as day care programs, home care and meal programs. Intergenerational programming included services such as intergenerational camps, homes for orphans and elders and programs that utilized mid-life individuals to assist older adults. Educational programs focused primarily on health care providers including physicians, nurses and social workers, while including volunteer and empowerment for older adults themselves. Organizational projects included developing cooperatives of NGO’s, creating governmental structures for hospice care and providing NGO’s with technical assistance. Thirty-nine projects were client centered with the next most common categories being educational (38) organizational(12) and intergenerational (8). Estonia, Russia and Romania implemented the largest number of client centered projects with seven, six and five respectively. Lithuania has focused significant resources into educational programs implementing eight, while Estonia implemented seven and Romania and the Czech Republic five each. CONSLUSION: As home and community based care programs become more established and common in Central and Eastern Europe, it will become necessary to further develop an organizational focus of care for the elderly.

[33] Chinese styled household old age care

Chen Yong (Policy Research Department China National Committee on Aging Beijing China)

This paper will discuss the current situation of the old age care in China, focusing on the household care of the elderly, its status, possible future development and implications on the support system in China. Further, the author would discuss the policies and measures to support the old traditional household care of the elderly in China.

[34] Current Conditions of Home Helpers in Urban Japan

T. Ishibashi, Y. Yamada, M. Nishimura (Dia Foundation for Research on Ageing Societies, Tokyo, Japan), W. Koyano (Seigakuin University, Saitama, Japan)

Home-help services are assigned to the core of home care services in the Japanese new long-term care system started in 2000. However, the conditions under which home helpers are working have not yet been fully explored. The purpose of the present study was to scrutinize the current conditions of home helpers. A questionnaire survey was carried out in a suburban city of Tokyo, and 886 home helpers working there responded (response rate was 87%). About 90% of home helpers were women, mainly aged 40 to 60 years, who had completed child bearing; the remaining 10% were men, mainly aged 60 years or older, who started to work in home-help services after their retirement from career job. 95% of the respondents were part-time employees working 2.8 days a week in average. For nearly 70% of the respondents, the average monthly income was less than 50,000 yen (about US $450); only 10% obtained 100,000 yen or more. Nevertheless, 70% of the respondents did not want to obtain more income from their current job. 45% of home helpers had less than 2 years of experience in home-help services; 30% had not received professional training at all and did not have any qualification. It is frequently told that home helpers are to be well-trained professional workers. However, the current conditions of Japanese home helpers are far from the ideal: not only employment status and wage, but also helpers, self-identity and attitudes seem quite different from those of professional workers.

[35] Factors Related to Refusal to Use Home-Based Care Services in Japan

M. Okada (College of Social Sciences, Ritsumeikan University, Kyoto, Japan), K. Fujibayashi (Faculty of Sociology, Toyo University, Tokyo, Japan), S. Okada (Graduate School of Human Life Science, Osaka City University, Osaka, Japan), H. Koyama (National Institute of Health Services Management, Tokyo, Japan)

PURPOSE: This study aimed to clarify factors leading to refusal to use home-based care services that were essential to meet the normative needs of the elderly and their family. METHOD: We mailed the self-administered questionnaire to 500 home-based care centers which were randomly selected from 4307 centers across Japan. The response rate was 61%, and 305 care managers completed the questionnaire. The questionnaire included the items regarding demographics, the number of refusal cases, the kind of refused services, and the supposed causes not to use services in one case retrospectively chosen by the respondents. RESULTS: Of the respondents, 83.6% had refusal cases in the past one year. By a factor analysis, we extracted 11 factors related to refusal cases. The results of t-test revealed that the family caregivers had higher scores in negative self-evaluation due to service use, inappropriate accessibility of services, and feelings of burden due to service use than the elderly. On the other hand, in feelings of loss of freedom due to service use, incomplete understandings about services and their circumstances, and difficulties in communicating with others, the elderly had higher scores than the family caregivers. CONCLUSION: This study implied the strategies to reduce the number of refusal cases in home-based care. For family caregivers, the target is to reduce self-blame and to increase the tendency of positive thinking. For the elderly, the one is to enhance appropriate understandings about service and to enable the elderly to develop a sense of control even using services.

[36] The Differences in Managerial Perspectives among Home Care Providers

M.Shirasawa,T.Enomoto,H.Lim,N.Shimamura,M.Tokoro,S.Okada,A.Ozawa,Osaka City University,Graduate School of Life Science,Osaka,558-6868,Japan

Purpose: In Japan, the public long-term care insurance was introduced from April 2000. Under the insurance program, home care service providers must be certified in order to obtain the insurance payment, and non-profit and profit agencies are eligible for the certification. The purpose of this study is to clarify the differences in managerial perspectives among managers of three types of home care agencies under the new insurance system as follows: (1) Non-profit Social Service Agencies(NSS), (2) Non-profit Health Service Agencies(NHS), and Profit Human Service Agencies(PHS). Methods: The sample was all managers of home care agencies in Osaka Prefecture (N=1,099). Survey was mailed to all of the managers. The response rate was 28.5%. The survey includes several measures concerning managerial perspectives and several demographic measures. Results: Factor analyses revealed that seven factors were extracted in managerial perspective measures. Analyses of variance indicated that managers in PHS were more sensitive to user's needs, service evaluation, consumer-driven policy, and workplace environment in their managerial perspectives than the other managers. On the other hand, managers in NSS had a stronger sense of community development than the others. Conclusions: Under the public long-term insurance system, managers of home care providers should be aware of and sensitive to internal and external conditions. The results indicated that managers in NSS and NHS should be more sensitive to user's needs, service evaluation, consumer-driven policy, and workplace environment than the counterpart and that those in PHS and NHS should be aware of communicating with community members around the agencies.

[37] Recommendations for Pest Management in Health Care Facilities

Donnie E. McIntosh (Good Samaritan Society) Edmonton, AB, Canada

PURPOSE: A review of pest management practices in one care setting led to the discovery that routine application of pesticides on a monthly basis occurred whether pests were evident or not. This paper will summarize the development of a collaborative effort to achieve effective pest management in Health Care Settings which best reflects Best Practice standards, and the approach used in one community to share the information with other care settings. METHOD: A review of existing practice and subsequent consultation with the best practice nurse, the pesticide industry, and the regulatory agency resulted in the development of a policy and procedure for Health care settings. This information was presented to provincial health representatives, public health inspectors, occupational health and safety officers and physical plant directors via a community health sponsored information workshop. RESULTS: Information was shared from the perspective of the stakeholders. Representatives from acute care, continuing care, community health and environmental services participated in a half day education forum, resulting in the sharing of a mutually agreed upon approach which best serves the needs of the residents in health care settings. This project, which originated in a Continuing Care site with contributions from Alberta Environment, and the Structural Pest Operators Industry, demonstrates how a united approach from stakeholders can result in an effective model for pest management. CONCLUSION: The Best Practice approach to controlling pest populations in health care environments is that of Integrated Pest Management. Regular monitoring, preventive measures, evaluation of sanitation practices and responsible use of chemicals and other alternatives can be achieved with effective communication between health care facilities, Regulatory agencies, and the Structural Pest Operators Industry. Administrators in health care facilities are encouraged to review pest control programs with provincially certified pest operators to assure the program implemented incorporates Integrated Pest Management. A sample Policy and Procedure format is provided.

[38] Ten Ways in Which Dying Changed in the U.S. During in the 20th Century

Mercedes Bern-Klug (Center on Aging, Univ of Kansas Med Center, Kansas City, KS USA)

ISSUE: The 20th century witnessed unprecedented improvements in life expectancy. With these improvements have come changes in the way in which most people will die: in old age; with multiple chronic conditions; in an institution; without their dying recognized as such. Accompanied by back ground demographic data and figures, this poster presents 10 comparisons for changes in the end of life that occurred in the U.S. during the 20th century. The poster also lists ideas for consideration by health professionals as they interact with older adults at the end of life, to enhance the experience of aging and of dying. These ideas include: aggressively securing information about prognosis and likely future health decisions; working to combine the medical, social and spiritual contexts of the patient and his/her loved ones to build a firm understanding of the context of treatment decisions; advocating for broader choices for community-based long-term care/end-of-life care; helping patients and families understand that with some diagnoses, it is not always clear when the end of life is close.

[39] Blurring the boundaries: Facilitation and promotion of hospice care and pain treatment

J. Kenneth Arnette (Department of Psychology, Eastern Washington University, Cheney, WA, USA)

The hospice movement has exploded in recent years, providing advanced pain treatment for terminally ill patients. Yet, there continues to be resistance on the part of physicians, patients, and their families to hospice care. There are at least two reasons for this: first, a potential hospice patient must renounce all curative treatments; second, a pysician must certify that the patient has six months or less to live. These factors essentially require that all parties involved admit "defeat," that is, the inevitability of death. The result is that, for example, in the state of Colorado, as many as 80% of terminally ill patients do receive hospice care, but the average length of that care is a mere two weeks. This situation denies effective pain treatment to the patient for the vast majority of time during the disease process. The present work proposes a model for pain management that effectively blurs the distinction between palliative care and pain treatment during the curative phase of the disease process. The goal is to provide a team of pain treatment professionals, following an interdisciplinary, biopsychosociospiritual model, that works with the patient prior to the terminal phase and continues treatment following the decision to admit the patient into hospice. The consistency, personal relationships, and trust built among the treatment team, referring physician, patient, and family are crucial in allowing the discussion of end-of-life options and facilitate the choice of hospice care early enough to be helpful to the patient seeking a "good death."

[40] Site of death and caregivers satisfaction of the elderly patients in domiciliary terminal care

Katsunori Kondo (Nihon Fukushi University, Aichi, Japan), Kyoko Higuchi (Gifu University, Gifu, Japan), Hiroaki Sugimoto (Nihon Fukushi University), Junko Kuze (Nihon Fukushi University), Kazuaki Miyata (Nihon Fukushi University)

PURPOSE: To analyse the associations between the site of death and family caregivers satisfaction of elderly patients in domiciliary terminal care. METHOD: We analysed data from home-visit nursing care stations in Japan concerning 1305 patients (>65 years old, mean 82.8 years) who had died in the last three months. The nurses in charge estimated the family caregivers satisfaction using a global 5-point score. RESULTS: (1) The rate of death at home was 50.4% while 18.5% were admitted to hospital within the last week mainly for medical reasons.(2) The estimated caregivers satisfaction score, from 5 (satisfactory) to 1 (unsatisfactory), was distributed as follows; 21.8%, 34.2%, 27.9%, 12.5% and 3.6%, respectively.(3) The caregivers whose preferred site of death was identified (n=799) were divided according to the preferred/observed site of death; home/home, home/hospital, hospital/hospital, hospital/home. The mean estimated caregivers satisfaction for each group showed significant differences ($p<.01$), 4.2, 3.7, 3.4 and 2.8, respectively.(4) In a multiple regression analysis, the following 6 factors were significantly correlated with greater caregivers satisfaction ($p<.001$, R2=0.33): the extent of meeting patient's desire, the appearance of critical symptoms, the patient's age, physician's positive attitude towards domiciliary terminal care, caregivers firm intention to care at home, being informed about the predicted terminal courses. However, the site of death was not included. CONCLUSION: These results suggest that the management process, such as the assessment of caregivers preferences, rather than the observed site of death should be focused on for developing better quality of domiciliary terminal care.

[41] The need for Palliative Care in Aged Home

PT Lam, TC Sim, MF Leung (Dept. of Medicine & Geriatrics, United Christian Hospital, Hong Kong)

Purpose: To study the prevalence of advanced incurable cancer in aged home residents and to assess their palliative care needs. Method: A cross-sectional survey was conducted between 1 - 30 September 2000 in 23 aged homes in Kwun Tong District. These comprised all government licensed aged homes in the district. All residents with diagnosis of advanced incurable cancer were identified and interviewed by a nurse or a specialist using a standard questionnaire. The analysis used descriptive statistics to summarize the quantitative data. Results: A total of 49 seniors, including 20 males (41%) and 29 females (59%), with mean age 79.1 (SD8.2) years were identified from 2042 residents of the 23 aged homes; with cancer prevalence 2.4%. Among these 49 seniors, 15 (30.6%) were cared by hospice professionals. 23(46.9%) were suffering from either physical or psychological symptoms and 7(14.3%) were suffering from both. 4(8.2%) were clinically depressed. Pain (12, 24.5%) was the most common complaint, followed by fatigue (8, 16.3%) and anorexia (5,10.2%). Overall, 11(22.4%) had poor to fair symptom control, and 28(57.1%) expressed need for extra psychosocial support. Conclusion: A significant number of aged home residents suffering from advanced incurable cancer had unmet needs, with inadequate control of physical symptoms and inadequate psychosocial support. However, less than one third received care from hospice service. There is a strong need to develop palliative care service in aged homes locally. Ongoing needs for training of aged home staff and liaison between aged homes and specialized palliative care service should be identified.

[42] Supporting Terminally Ill Patients who Wish to Live out Their Lives at Home

Israel S. Berger and Doron Garfinkel and Israel S. Berger (Maccabi Healthcare Services, Home Care Unit - Dan District, Givataim, Israel)

Background and Purpose: Due to improved medical technology in the last decades, the average length of survival since a terminally ill patient is first classified as "non-curative" until death, is increasing all the time. For some patients who prefer to live at home even in the presence of severe debilitating disease, hospitalization may represent a severe impairment of their quality of life. Paradoxically, in an attempt to relieve the heavy medical and legal responsibility, physicians and health professionals sometimes pressure these patients to spend their last period of life outside home even if there is no apparent advantage of hospital over home care. However, comprehensive palliative approach insists on helping patients at every stage of their disease according to their individual wishes, by relieving physical suffering but also attempting to alleviate mental, familial, social and financial problems. Patients and Methods: Over the past year, several dozens of our Home Care Service terminally ill patients died, most of them in an institutional setting. Fifteen families requested that the patient live at home until death. In each case, there was a consensus between family and patient that the later should stay at home even if the situation worsens, symptoms aggravate or death occurs. We enabled them to accomplish this by providing a 24 hour medical availability. Results: The patients suffered from advanced cancer, ALS, end stage pulmonary fibrosis, end stage liver failure and dementia. The age upon death ranged from 63 to 93; there were 11 men, four women, most of them were living with a spouse who also served as the primary care giver in about half of them. In all patients, only palliative care was given and most of them had very few distressing symptoms during the last days of their life. The Home Care physician was available 24 hour a day and was present at the time of death and signed the death certificate. Conclusion: a proper medical support group can enable patients and families who wish to die at home, to do so with dignity while experiencing a reasonable quality of life before death.

[43] End-of-life care: Formal and informal care in the last three months of the lives of elderly people

G. Visser, M.I. Broese van Groenou (Department Sociology and Social Gerontology/ Longitudinal Aging Study Amsterdam (LASA), Free University Amsterdam, The Netherlands), M. Klinkenberg (Department Social Medicine/ Longitudinal Aging Study Amsterdam (LASA), Free University Amsterdam, The Netherlands) D. Willems (Department Social Medicine, Free University Amsterdam, The Netherlands)

PURPOSE: 1: To acquire more insight into the use of informal and formal care in the last three months of the lives of indepently living elderly in the Netherlands. 2: To provide more insight into the informal caregivers, and the size, length and nature of their caregiving tasks. METHOD: This study involved a sub-sample of the Longitudinal Aging Study Amsterdam. Relatives of deceased LASA-respondents were interviewed (n=270). For the elderly who lived at home three months before they died (n=167) descriptive methods were used to make a distinction between four caring arrangements: no care, formal care, informal care, and both informal and formal care. The relatives who provided informal personal care received a written self-administered questionnaire (n=46). Descriptive methods were used to focus on size, length and nature of their caregiving tasks RESULTS: A majority of independently living elderly (77%) received some form of care in the last three months of their lives: 61 elderly received informal and formal care, 54 received informal care, 13 received only formal care and 39 elderly received no care at all. The results showed that differences between groups are found regarding the need for care and availability of a spouse. The results for elderly who received informal personal care (n=46) showed that their informal caregivers were mostly spouse (n=23) or child (n=17). They provided informal personal care, like washing or help with taking medication. In many cases they also provided household and management care, like organizing - or financial care. CONCLUSION: There is a considerable need for care in the end-of-life and informal care plays an important part during this period.

[44] End of Life Decisions: A Jewish Perspective

Rabbi M Avrum Ehrlich (Mandelbaum House, University of Sydney, NSW Australia) &Frederick Ehrlich (UNSW & St. George Hospital, Sydney, NSW Australia)

Debates about the extent to which intervention should be applied or withheld in prolonging or shortening life are often influenced by the dictates of religion. In the industralised Western "First World", Christianity has been a dominant influence, albeit with significant inter-denominational differences. Judaism, however, has also developed a position, after debates extending over more than 2000 years, and its conclusions are relevant. Jewish religious and legal texts were searched for relevant material including the Bible, Talmud, and The Shulchan Aruch as well as modern responsa and rabbinic writings. The results, rather surprisingly for some, show the Jewish position to be very close to the emerging consensus on this subject in Western countries. Whilst recognising that at each border of this emerging consensus there are some who advocate preservation of life with every possible effort to the very last moment whilst others offer assisted death almost on request, the broad middle-of-the-road practice in most institutions happens to correspond fairly closely with the Jewish position. This insists on defining the condition of the dying individual with some precision, but forbids interfering with the dying process. Orthodox Judaism allows the withdrawal of treatment and even basic sustenance but prohibits active measures to accelerate death.

[45] Integrating ethical decision-making into practice for community health care professionals.

The Vancouver/Richmond Health Board Ethics Support Group (Vancouver/Richmond Health Board, Vancouver, B.C, Canada)

ABSTRACT Purpose: The Vancouver/Richmond Health Board Ethics Support Group recognized that professionals in community practice were articulating a need for support with ethical decision-making. Scant literature or research was available describing or supporting an ethical decision-making process for community practice involving professionals who are participating in care with population-based and age-based groups, agencies, programs, or disciplines. Method: The Ethics Support Group, a cross-agency, cross-discipline group, has developed a unique ethical decision-making framework as well as a process for implementation with community professionals. The process, when integrated into practice for all professionals through discussions of specific complex care situations, has incorporated appropriate literature, and promotes a collaborative approach for making ethical decisions. This process includes the client and their support system, and recognizes the contributions of partnering health care providers across the continuum. Results: This approach is in its early implementation phase and has not yet been fully evaluated. Evaluation will continue through 2001. Preliminary results may be available in June 2001. Conclusion: The Vancouver/Richmond Health Board Ethics Support Group recommends a consistent and transparent process to ethical-decision making; an integrated approach supporting client-directed care delivery in community settings.

[46] The study of regimen of the Taoist school and the social security in the aged population

Jin Bing, Feng Yue Peng , Li Jia Jie (China Taoism Health

Reservation, Beijing , China)

The Taoist school is an ancient Chinese skill developed to preserve good health and longevity. This skill of preserving good health and longevity is a major part composing the Tacist culture and has been considered to be a gem in the thesaurus of Chinese traditional culture. Mr. Jin Bing, who is a successor to the skill of preserving good health and longevity of the Taoist school, has for many years committed himself to the cause of carrying on, researching and disseminating this skill. His job is intended to achieve good health and long life-span of the human race, especially the health of the elderly. Mr. Jin Bing chose the research and development of the skill of preserving good health and longevity of the Taoist school as his lifelong pursuit and ends. The skill of preserving good health and longevity of the Taoist school is made possible by self-cultivation which is supposed to be helpful in preventing diseases, extending the coming of senescence and promoting people's physical conditions. The skill is of great advantage to protect "the Five Major System", e.g. heart, liver, spleen, stomach and kidney of the human body and to keep people in good health.

[47] Develop elder service industry to provide assistant for the elder living at home

Zhu jiming, Shou lili (Shanghai Research Center on Aging, Shanghai, China)

Today China is experiencing the great changing process from planned economy to market economy. Meanwhile, the population is aging, more and more elderly should be provided. In recent years, many researchers and government officers put forward the concept of °aging project industrialization", as the main method to solve the aging problem. It is to say, at the aspects of elder's economy guarantee, health care, and social service, etc, when the government's function weakening, various industry behavior should be introduced to maintain elder's living standard. In this paper, we will analyze Shanghai's social economy development and the elder industry's actuality and problems, and bring forward the contention that elder service industrialization's condition has been ripe, and it should be the forerunner at all of the elder industries. Shanghai's family size is being smaller and smaller, and more and more family has simply old people, elder service industry may provide many kinds of help for elder living at home, ensure their living quality not to decline.

[48] Are Age and Chronic Medical Conditions Good Predictors of Work Loss Days?

Margaret Wan (Department of Gerontology, University of South Florida, Tampa, Florida, U.S.A.), Sandra L. Reynolds (Department of Gerontology, University of South Florida, Tampa, Florida, U.S.A.)

A major barrier to the employment of older workers is the employer’s perception that they are often sick and absent. This study explored demographic, health, and social factors that might be predictors of work loss days of workers aged 18 to 70. It examined data from the United States National Health Interview Survey, 1998. Face-to-face interviews were administered among a probability sample of the civilian noninstitutionalized population to compile information about the health and other characteristics of respondents. Among other questions, respondents were asked about chronic illnesses, occupations, and their work loss days during the past 12 months. The subset of data here consisted of respondents that had a job during the week prior to the interview and for whom data required for this study were available (N=15,771). Ordinary least squares regression estimated the effects of potential predictors. The results show that age has no significant effect on work loss days. Among 11 chronic medical conditions frequently associated with age, only angina pectoris and stroke are significant predictors of work loss days. Occupation and certain health factors are important, such as self-rated health and visits to physicians in the past 12 months. The findings suggest that age and chronic medical conditions are not good predictors of work loss days. Recognizing the predictors reveals opportunities for the prevention of work disability and the improvement of productivity of workers of all ages. Work ability assessment instruments and test protocols should be utilized to evaluate functional capacity related to actual workplace settings.

[49] Tax Reform and Its Impacts on Midlife and Older Americans

John R. Gist [AARP Public Policy Institute, Washington, DC]

PURPOSE: Income tax reform became a subject of intense debate in the US in the 1990s, with proposals for a flat tax or a national sales tax or other consumption taxes to replace the income tax. This paper will estimate the impacts of four recent tax reform proposals (flat tax, a consumed income tax, a retail sales tax, and a 10% income tax) in terms of age, income, and marital status. METHOD: The method used to analyze tax impacts is microsimulation, using a tax model that merges data from the US Census Bureau's Current Population Survey and the Internal Revenue Service Statistics of Income data file. RESULTS: The analysis shows that the flat tax would reduce effective tax rates by more than four percentage points, the consumed income and 10% income tax would reduce it by about one percentage point, and the retail sales tax would increase it by over two percentage points. The flat tax is the most generous to those over age 65, the consumed income and retail sales taxes tax those over 65 more heavily than younger ages, and the 10% tax is the most neutral with respect to all ages. The consumed income tax and retail sales taxes treat couples less favorably than singles. The flat, consumed income, and retail sales taxes all are regressive, while the 10% income tax is more neutral regarding income. CONCLUSION: The flat tax appears most generous to the oldest age group, but consumption tax reform would generally be harmful to lower income groups regardless of age.

[50] Modelling costs alongside studies of effectiveness: a case study of alternative living arrangements for people with middle to late stage dementia

Gillian Currie, Cam Donaldson, Munsoor Mirza, Marlene Reimer, Susan Slaughter, (University of Calgary, Calgary, Canada)

PURPOSE: To determine the efficiency of different treatment options in health care, we must measure costs as well as effectiveness. Here, we describe a study of the costs of alternative living arrangements for people with dementia being undertaken as part of a controlled trial in Calgary, Alberta. METHOD: In the study of effectiveness, residents in the experimental facility have been matched with residents in two control groups; those residing in (A) any other facility in the region and (B) another facility within the same organisation as the experimental facility. The cost study combines data from the trial with those from administrative databases. To compare costs of residents in the experimental facility with those of control group B, a cost/resident/day (including operating costs and capital costs) will be calculated for each facility. As not all residents are participants in the trial, data on case mix of those in and out will be collected to ensure comparability. Data on cost/resident/day will be combined with data from the trial on length of stay in each facility from admission to the study until death or the end of data collection. Use of other services (ie. doctor visits or hospital admissions) has been collected via chart review and will be added to facility costs for each resident. The procedure for group A is similar, except data on charges will be used instead (due to confidentiality of financial data). CONCLUSION: As well as outlining the cost study model, preliminary data from this study will be presented.

[51] Illness of the Elderly in Thailand and Its Implied Economic Loss

Wathinee Boonchalaksi and Yupin Vorasiriamorn (Institute for Population and Social Research, Mahidol University, Nakhon-Pathom, THAILAND)

The aim of the study was to investigate the duration of illness of the elderly and the cost of care.The Survey of the Elderly in Thailand was used; it covered 7,713 of the elderly samples.Descriptive statistics were ultilized such as percentage and mean. The outcome of the study shows that on the average, the elderly aged 60 and over became sick twice a year and each sick period was 12 days. As for the impaired elderly, the average period of sickness was 59 days. The average cost per person for those hospitalized was 10,897 Baht per year. It can be estimated from the study that in the future if the number of elderly reaches 11 million, the government will bear extremely high expenses because 80% of the sick elderly need care from government hospitals.

[52] Distribution of vasopressinergic and oxytocinergic neurons in the hypothalamus of the senescence accelerated mouse.

R. Verduga, D. Crespo, M. Herreros, M. Megias (Department of Anatomy and Cell Biology, Cantabria University, Cantanbria, Spain), C. Fernandez-Viadero, (Nursing Home for the Aged, Health & Social Welfare Service. and Department of Anatomy and Cell Biology, Cantabria University, Cantabria, Spain)

PURPOSE: The senescence-accelerated mouse (SAM) is considered a murine model of accelerated aging. Two different strains of SAM with respect to the process of aging were used in this study, SAM-P8 (prone), and SAM-R1 (retarded). To determine the features of the neurons in the SAM hypothalamus that synthesize the neurohormones oxytocin (OXT) and arginine vasopressin (AVP), we used antisera for both hormones. The results in the SAM were compared with those for other mouse strains. METHOD: animals perfused and fixed by standard methods. The following staining procedures and hystological methods were performed: thionin, AVP, or OXT immunocytochemistry, NADPH-diaphorase, electron microscopy and Dil tracer. RESULTS:The observations suggest that there are no differences in the hypothalamus of these mice with respect to the topography of the supraoptic (SON) and paraventricular (PVN) nuclei. The outstanding observation in the SAM hypothalamus was the consistent presence of a well-developed arrangement of neurosecretory neurons that formed the mouse accessory cells (MAC). The MAC appeared bilaterally in close proximity to the third ventricle wall. It was present in males and females, and its morphology and cellular features were similar in young and aged SAM. Most of the MAC neurons synthesize AVP, a few produce OXT, and some are positive for the enzyme NADPH-diaphorase. The tracer Dil revealed that these neurons project into the neurohypophysis. CONCLUSION: The presence of this nucleus suggests that the SAM could present greater neurohormone synthesis than other mice. This, in turn, may play a deleterious role in the overall process of adaptation to the effects of aging.

[53] Age-related peculiarities of cholinergic regulation of adrenal glands reaction on the influence of single irradiation

Gorban E.N, Topolnikova N.V, Bobrovnitsky J.A, Osipov N.V. (Institute of Gerontology Acad. Med. Sci. Ukraine, Kiev, Ukraine)

PURPOSE: To study influence of single roentgen irradiation (X-irradiation) on cholinergic regulation of adrenal glands (AG) glucocorticoid function in adult and old animals in early terms after irradiation. METHODS: Experiments have been conducted on Wistar male rats 8 and 26 mo of age. To study peculiarities of nervous regulation of AG glucocorticoid function M-cholinolytic atropine. Atropine was injected intraperitoneally twice a day for 3 days in a dose 10 mg/kg body weigh. Since 24 hours after last atropine administration animals were subjected to single X-irradiation in a dose 3,52 Gy. Animals were tested in an hour after irradiation. Glucocorticoid function of AG was determined by intensity of 11-oxycorticosteroid (11-OCS) secretion by isolated AG. Level of 11-OCS in blood and incubation media was measured by fluorometric method. RESULTS: Chronic administration of atropine led to sound activation of 11-OCS secretion by isolated AG in adult animals, didn't influence greatly this index in old rats. It is demonstrated that an aging is accompanied by decrease in M-cholinergic regulation of AG glucocorticoid function. Since an hour after X-irradiation in adult rats in contrast to old ones it was noticed an increase of 11-OCS secretion by isolated AG. It means that during aging primary reaction of AG cortex on since an hour after single irradiation is decreased. CONCLUSION: It can be suggested that in old rats the cause of changes in early reaction of AG cortex on single irradiation is age-associated decrease in nervous control over glucocorticoid function of AG cortex.

[54] Body composition changes after oral hydration in Brazilian elderly determined by Bioeletrical Impedance Analysis (BIA)

Machado, J.M.T.; Machado, D.T.M.; Berkenbrock, I. (Serviço de Clínica Médica - Pontifícia Universidade Católica do Paraná - Curitiba - Brazil) Saad, V. (Departamento de Biotecnologia Eletroanálitica - Intensimed Serviços Médicos - Curitiba - Brazil) Varga, J.; Gajardo, R.C.; Monte, O.; Dias, A.A (Departamento de Ciências Fisiológicas - Fac. de Ciências Médicas da Santa Casa de São Paulo - Brazil)

Purpose: Evaluate changes in bioeletrical parameters and components of body composition after oral hydration in Brazilian elderly. Methods: We recruited 35 healthy subjects (70 -90 years old) and we also advertised of following protocol: all subjects are submitted a medical interview and physical examination, we measured weight (kg) arterial pressure and heart rate before and after ingestion of 400 ml of water. Subject characteristics are listed in Table 01. Single frequency BIA was performed at 50 kHz and 800 mA (BIA101-Q, R.J.L. Systems Inc.) with standard tetrapolar lead placement. Both Resistance (R) and Reactance (Xc) were determined in Ohms (W), before and after oral hydration. Phase angle (PA) was calculated conform this formula: PA (q) = a tan (Xc/R) in degrees. Body composition parameters were determined with programs Fluids and Nutritional Analysis and Weight Manager (R.J.L. Systems Inc.). Were determined: Total Body Water (TBW), Extracellular Water (ECW), Intracellular Water (ICW), Lean Body Mass(FFM) and Body Fat (BF) in percentage of body weight. Table 01: subjects n Age (y) Weight (kg) Height (cm) Total 35 76.3 +/- 5.8 69.7 +/- 16.9 158 +/- 10.0 Male 10 74.3 +/ - 5.44 78.8 +/- 25.5 168.7 +/- 5.9 Female 25 77.1 +/- 5.9 65.8 +/- 9.2 152 +/ - 7.6 Results: Arterial Pressure (both systolic (SAP) and diastolic(DAP) and heart rate are listed in Table 02. Table 02: systolic arterial pressure (SAP), diastolic arterial pressure (DAP) and heart rate (HR). Total Male Female SAP: Mm Hg Before 133.7 +/- 15.0 134.4 +/- 15.4 132.0 +/- 14.0 After 136.8 +/- 16.8 138.5 +/- 17.4 131.9 +/- 13.7 DAP Mm Hg Before 80.4 +/- 9.5 81.0 +/- 10.5 80.0 +/- 6.3 After 82.3 +/- 9.3 81.9 +/- 9.6 83.1+/- 8.3 HR Before 81.3 +/- 10.9 82.4 +/- 10.9 77.4 +/- 9.9 After 81.7 +/- 8.7 86.0 +/- 8.6 77.6 +/- 7.8 The bioeletrical parameters (R, Xc and PA (q)) are listed in table 03. Table 03: resistance, reactance and phase angle Total Male Female R Before 482.0 +/- 65.3 502.4 +/- 62.1 431.0 +/- 40.6 After 500.1 +/ - 61.1 519.0 +/- 54.5 452.9 +/- 52.2 Xc Before 48.0 +/- 6.7 49.7 +/- 6.5 43.7 +/- 4.7 After 47.7 +/- 6.3 48.5 +/- 5.9 45.6 +/- 6.9 AF Before 5.71 +/- 0.57 5.67 +/- 0.57 5.81 +/- 0.60 After 5.47 +/- 0.11 5.37 +/- 0.63 5.74 +/- 0.47 The components of body composition are listed in Tables 04 and 05 Table 04: total body water, extracellular water and intracellular water Total Male Female: TBW Before 51.2 +/- 7.3 49.0 +/- 5.6 59.4 +/- 5.5 After 51.2 +/- 6.2 48.3 +/- 3.7 58.4 +/- 5.4 ECW Before 46.5 +/- 3.4 48.3 +/- 2.0 42.1 +/- 1.9 After 47.2 +/- 3.7 48.8 +/- 2.1 43.1 +/- 3.5 ICW Before 53.6 +/- 3.6 51.9 +/- 2.5 57.9 +/- 1.9 After 52.7 +/- 3.4 51.2 +/- 2.1 56.6 +/- 3.0 Table 05: body fat (BF), lean body mass (LBM), body cell mass (BCM) and extracellular tissues (ECT). Total Male Female: BF Before 26.9 +/- 10.5 30.1 +/- 8.7 18.9 +/- 10.4 After 28.5 +/- 8.45 31.8 +/- 4.8 20.1 +/- 9.7 LBM Before 72.3 +/- 9.6 68.8 +/- 6.6 81.1 +/- 10.5 After 71.15 +/- 8.5 68.2 +/- 4.8 79.9 +/- 9.7 BCM Before 30.7 +/- 6.2 27.9 +/- 4.4 37.8 +/- 4.2 After 29.6 +/- 5.3 27.2 +/- 2.9 35.7 +/- 4.8 ECT Before 37.9 +/- 6.4 34.9 +/- 4.2 45.3 +/- 4.5 After 38.0 +/- 6.3 35.5 +/- 4.9 44.2 +/- 4.7 Conclusions: 1) There were no differences in clinical parameters evaluated. 2) There was a difference in resistance measured before and after oral hydration but there were no differences in reactance or phase angle 3) There were differences in the extracellular water and intracellular water but there was no difference in the total body water.

[55] Variation of composition in aging determined by bioeletrical impedance

Dias, A.A Saad, V. ; Varga, J. ; Gajardo, R.C. ; Monte, O. (

Departamento de Ciências Fisiológicas - Faculdade de Ciências Médicas da Santa Casa de São Paulo - Brazil) Machado, J.M.T.; Machado, D.T.M.; Berkenbrock, I.(Serviço de Clínica Médica - Pontifícia Universidade Católica do Paraná - Curitiba - Brazil)

PURPOSE: To compare parameters of body composition determined with Bioeletrical Impedance Analysis (BIA), between young (athletes and sedentaries) and elderly people. METHOD: Subject characteristics are listed in Table 01. Single frequency BIA was performed at 50 kHz and 800 mA (BIA101-Q, R.J.L. Systems Inc.) with standard tetrapolar lead placement. Both Resistance (R) and Reactance (Xc) were determined in Ohms (W). Phase angle (PA) was calculated conform this formula: PA (q) = a tan (Xc/R) in degrees. Body composition parameters were determined with programs Fluids and Nutritional Analysis and Weight Manager (R.J.L. Systems Inc.). The following were determined: Total Body Water (TBW), Extracellular Water (ECW), Intracellular Water (ICW), Lean Body Mass (FFM) and Body Fat (BF) in percentage of body weight. Table 01: subjects n Age (y) Weight (kg) Height (cm) Elderly Total 37 76.3 +/- 5.8 69.7 +/- 16.9 158 +/- 10.0 Male 12 74.6 +/- 5.2 78.0 +/- 24.6 168 +/- 5.9 Female 25 77.1 +/- 5.9 65.8 +/- 9.2 152 +/- 7.6 Young Total 176 20.4 +/- 1.6 67.18 +/- 12.2 173 +/- 9.2 Male 112 20.5 +/- 1.7 72.5 +/- 10.3 177 +/- 7.3 Female 64 20.3 +/- 1.4 57.8 +/- 9.2 165 +/- 6.7 Athletes Male 31 19.9 +/- 1.6 66.8 +/- 8.4 175 +/- 6.5 RESULTS: The measured parameters (R and Xc) and calculated PA are listed in tables below: Table 02: resistance, reactance and phase angle R Xc PA Elderly Total 482.38 +/- 64.48 47.89 +/-6.45 5.70 +/- 0.58 Male 426.58 +/- 41.26 43.75 +/- 4.60 5.88 +/- 0.56 Female 509.16 +/- 55.91 49.88 +/- 6.28 5.61 +/- 0.58 Young Total 533.93 +/- 57.58 62.73 +/- 7.58 6.79 +/- 0.86 Male 491.40 +/- 62.29 61.31 +/- 7.17 7.16 +/- 0.73 Female 608.36 +/- 70.19 65.20 +/- 7.65 6.15 +/- 0.69 Athletes Male 438.83 +/- 70.19 58.70 +/- 12.27 7.58 +/- 0.69 Table 03: total body water, extracellular water and intracellular water TBW EEW EIW Elderly Male 51.72 +/- 7.03 46.72 +/- 3.35 53.42 +/- 3.52 Female 59.81 +/- 5.83 42.55 +/ - 1.72 57.90 +/- 1.67 Total 48.16 +/- 3.85 48.56 +/- 1.96 51.44 +/- 1.96 Young Male 56.16 +/- 5.83 41.01 +/- 1.09 58.99 +/- 1.09 Female 58.54 +/- 5.06 40.34 +/- 0.69 59.66 +/- 0.64 Male 51.99 +/- 3.81 42.18 +/- 0.54 57.82 +/- 0.54 Athletes Male 65.48 +/- 4.64 40.87 +/- 0.73 59.13 +/- 0.73 Table 04: lean body mass and body fat BF LBM Elderly 27.22 +/-10.17 72.05 +/- 9.23 M 18.36 +/- 10.42 81.64 +/- 10.42 F 31.12 +/- 7.17 67.84 +/- 4.10 Young 19.91 +/- 7.07 81.09 +/- 7.07 M 16.70 +/- 6.65 83.30 +/- 10.42 F 22.79 +/- 6.05 77.20 +/- 6.05 Athletes M 9.40 +/- 4.01 90.59 +/- 4.01 CONCLUSIONS: 1) There were differences in R, Xc and PA between young and elderly (p<0,001) and between sex in elderly (p<0,001). 2) With aging are progressive decline in Phase Angle (p<0,000001). 3) The experimental data also confirms differences between groups in the TBW, EEW, and ICW.

[56] Changes in bioeletrical parameters after oral hydration of elderly as determined by Bioeletrical Impedance Analysis (BIA)

Dias, A. A, Varga, J, Gajardo, R.C, Monte, O. (Departamento de Ciências Fisiológicas - Faculdade de Ciências Médicas da Santa Casa de São Paulo - Brazil) Machado, J.M.T, Machado, D.T.M, Berkenbrock, I (Serviço de Clínica Médica - Pontifícia Universidade Católica do Paraná - Curitiba - Brazil) Saad, V. (Depto Biotecnologia Eletroanálitica - Intensimed Serviços Médicos - Curitiba - Brazil)

PURPOSE: Evaluate changes in bioeletrical parameters in whole body and segmental Bioeletrical Impedance Analysis after oral hydration in Brazilian elderly. METHOD: We recruited 35 healthy subjects (70 -90 years old) and we also advertised of following protocol: all subjects are submitted a medical interview and physical examination, we measured weight (kg) before and after ingestion of 400 ml of water. Subject characteristics are listed in Table 01. Single frequency BIA was performed at 50 kHz and 800 mA (BIA101-Q, R.J.L. Systems Inc.) with standard tetrapolar lead placement (wrist and ankle in right side), segmental impedance were performed in arms (A), legs (L) and infraclavicular (IC) regions both right and left sides. Both Resistance (R) and Reactance (Xc) were determined in Ohms (W). Phase angle (PA) was calculated conform this formula: PA (q) = a tan (Xc/R) in degrees. Table 01: subjects n Age (y) Weight (kg) Height (cm) Idosos Total 35 76.3 +/- 5.8 69.7 +/- 16.9 158 +/- 10.0 Male 10 74.3 +/- 5.44 78.8 +/- 25.5 168.7 +/- 5.9 Female 25 77.1 +/- 5.9 65.8 +/- 9.2 152 +/- 7.6 RESULTS: The measured parameters are listed in Table 02 Table 02: measured bioeletrical parameters R Xc PA Whole Body Before 482.37 +/- 64.48 47.72 +/- 6.46 5.69 +/- 0.59 After 499.08 +/- 61.66 47.50 +/- 6.29 5.42 +/- 0.56 Right Arm Before 297.58 +/- 37.24 31.48 +/- 4.39 6.10 +/- 0.79 After 286.87 +/- 49.13 30.54 +/- 5.58 6.08 +/- 0.62 Left Arm Before 313.42 +/- 39.79 32.08 +/- 4.89 5.89 +/- 0.76 After 305.48 +/- 46.11 32.55 +/- 5.52 6.05 +/- 0.68 Left Leg Before 130,90 +/- 32.70 14.72 +/- 4.45 6.39 +/- 0.97 After 133.18 +/- 24.82 17.70 +/- 3.83 6.61 +/- 1.34 Right Leg Before 131.59 +/- 22.72 16.44 - 4.66 7.22 +/- 2.01 After 134.06 +/- 26.21 15.20 - 4.77 6.27 +/- 0.97 Right IC Before 95.72 +/- 27.19 11.53 +/- 3.40 6.97 +/- 1.54 After 92.26 +/- 19.90 13.32 +/- 3.53 7.64 +/- 1.81 Left IC Before 87.13 +/- 17.25 9.96 +/- 1.40 6.69 +/- 1.28 After 95.00 +/- 16.08 12.14 +/- 3.05 7.35 +/- 1.62 CONCLUSIONS: 1) There are no differences between measures of Resistance (R) and Reactance (Xc) after oral hydration . 2) There are differences in the Phase Angle in right leg, and both infraclavicular segments (p<0,05) (probably showing alteration in bioeletrical parameters of thorax or lungs).

[57] Body Weight and Life Duration of Conventional Wistar Rats from 1952-1990

A.V. Everitt (Department of Physiology, University of Sydney and the Centre for Education and Research on Ageing, Concord Hospital, NSW, Australia) D.Willis, N.Seedsman (Department of Physiology, University of Sydney), E.Polikevics (Concord Hospital)

During the 20th century human populations have progressively increased their body size and life duration due to improvements in nutrition, public health and medical care. This study investigated equivalent changes between 1952 and 1990 in body weight and life duration of the conventional male Wistar rat. Data were obtained from records of rats born in 1952, 1967, 1977 and 1987. Food intakes were estimated in young adults aged 200 days and urinary protein outputs in middle age at 500 days. Age at natural death was recorded. Body weight at age 50 days increased from 118g (N=33) in 1952 to 183g(N=20) in 1987, and the maximum at about 500 days also increased from 406g (N=68) in 1952 born rats to 512g (N=20) in 1987 born. Mean life duration was also extended from 726 days (N=68) in the 1952 cohort to 826 days (N=72) in the 1987 cohort. The maximum life duration was 1084 days in the 1952 rats and 1130 days in the 1987 group. Food intake at 200 days was 21.3g/day (N=100) in 1952 rats decreasing to 19.8g/day (N=25) in 1987. Protein excretion in middle age decreased significantly from 32.7mg/day (N=52) in the 1952 cohort to 13.9mg/day (N=17) in the 1987 cohort. Thus, conventional male Wistar rats significantly increased their body size and mean life duration between 1952 and 1987. The severity of renal disease was also reduced.

[58] UVB-induced premature senescence of human diploid fibroblasts

F. Chainiaux, J.-P. Magalhaes, F. Eliaers, J. Remacle and O. Toussaint (Unit of Cellular Biology and Biochemistry, University of Namur, Namur, Belgium)

In this work, we show that repeated stresses with UVB (290-320 nm) induce SIPS (Stress-Induced Premature Senescence) of human diploid skin fibroblasts (HDFs). HDFs at early cumulative population doublings were exposed 3 or 5 times to increasing subcytotoxic doses of UVB with 1 stress/day. After two days of recovery, several biomarkers of replicative senescence were established. First, there was an increase in the proportion of cells positive for the senescence-associated ß-galactosidase (SA ß-gal) activity. Second, there was a loss of replicative potential assessed by a very low level of [3H]-thymidine incorporation. Third, the steady-state level of the mRNA of two senescence-associated genes, e.i. fibronectin and apolipoprotein J, was also increased in fibroblasts at 72 hrs after 3 exposures to UVB. In conclusion, these results suggest that it is possible to induce SIPS in HDFs after repeated exposures to subcytotoxic doses of UVB. Acknowledgments : F. Chainiaux is a research assistant and O. Toussaint is a research associate of the FNRS, Belgium

[59] Longitudinal Studies of Biomarker of Aging in Humans

E. Nakamura (Dept. of Life Science, Faculty of Integrated Human Studies, Kyoto University, Kyoto, Japan), L.M. Ueno, Y. Yamashita (Laboratory of aging Studies, Graduate School of Human and Environmental Studies, Kyoto University, Kyoto, Japan)

The present study was conducted to identify biomarkers of aging based on a 7-year longitudinal study of the Japanese women, and also to investigate to what degree the biomarkers identified based on cross-sectional data agree with those based on longitudinal data. The subjects of this study consist of two groups of cross-sectional (N=981) and longitudinal samples (N=112). Based on a stepwise logical method, 6 variables of FEV1.0, SBP, glucose, MCH, calcium, and albumin/globulin ratio were finally selected as biomarkers of aging. These biomarkers assured the following criteria: 1) evidence of change of with the passage of time, and 2) directness and regularity of age-related changes. This variable set showed substantial covariance along one principal component related to chronological age. Thus the first principal component was used as a global aging index (BAS). The mean slopes of the regression lines of BAS by three age groups (age<45, 45<age<65, 65<age) were 0.091, 0.076, 0.164, respectively. An analysis of these mean slopes for three age groups by one-way analysis of variance detected a significant difference [$F(2, 107)=7.589$, $p<0.01$] . Pair-wise multiple comparisons by Scheffe method showed significant difference between groups of age<45 and 65<age ($p<0.01$); groups 45<age<65 and 65<age ($p<0.01$). These results suggest that the rate of aging in elderly women becomes about twice compared to those in young adult and middle-aged women.

[60] Assessment of Bone Changes of Salmon Calcitonin Microspheres in ovariectomized rats

Mi Jung Kim, Si Bok Park, Sang Gun Lee, Il Gyu Park(Dept. of Rehabilitation Medicine and Clinical Pathology, Hanyang Univeristy Hospital, Seoul, Korea), Yong Gu Park(Dept. of Pathology, Kyung Hee Hospital, Seoul, Korea), Kang Choon Lee3(Drug Targeting Laboratory, SungKyunKwan University, Suwon, Korea)

Purpose: To assess bone changes of salmon calcitonin microspheres against osteoporosis in ovariectomized rats. Methods: Salmon calcitonin (sCT) microspheres were prepared by a solvent extraction/evaporation method from a hydrophilic 50:50 poly (lactide-co-glycolide) polymer (PLGA); MW 10,000. The bone changes of sCT microspheres were studied in ovariectomized (OVX) rats. OVX rats were injected s.c. with blank microspheres and sCT microspheres (14 and 7 mg/kg as sCT) weekly, and free sCT (4 mg/kg) on alternate days. Sham-operated control rats and the remaining OVX rats were injected s.c. on alternate days with saline vehicle. The treatment was initiated on the first day after surgery and continued for a period of eight weeks. Bone measurements were performed in the distal femoral metaphysis and L5 vertebrae with DEXA. Plasma osteocalcin, calcium, alkaline phosphatase, phosphate, and deoxypyridinoline in urine were measured as biochemical indices. Results: Both vehicle and blank microsphere treated OVX rats lost substantial amounts of bone relative to sham-operated control rats. Bone density in OVX rats treated with high dose of sCT microspheres was significantly higher than that of free sCT-treated OVX rats, but less than that of sham-operated control rats. The protective effect of sCT microspheres in the distal femur was apparent compared with other skeletal sites. Amounts of plasma osteocalcin in OVX rats treated with free sCT and sCT microspheres were greater than that in vehicle-treated OVX rats. Conclusions: Salmon calcitonin microspheres were assessed for protection against bone loss in ovariectomized rats. This research was supported by the grant from the Ministry of Health and Welfare (HMP-98-D-2-0020), Korea.

[61] Elemental Analysis of Bones by Recoiling Atoms in Heavy Ion Beams

L.Brazdes (National Institute of Gerontology and Geriatrics, Bucharest,Romania), M.Petrascu (National Institute for Physics and Nuclear Engineering, Bucharest, Romania)

An increasing demand for accurate elemental analysis of biological materials has become more important since knowledge of their mechanisms and of their impact on human diseases has significantly progressed. A quantitative method for elemental analysis of bones ,based on detection and identification of recoiling atoms in a 100 MeV Iodine beam accelerated at the Bucharest TANDEM has been worked out.In the developed method it was possible to resolve each element between Z=3 (Lithium) and Z=38 (Strontium) A (delta E,E) ionisation chamber was used to asses differences in light elements depth gradients, concentrations and ratios.For energy calibration of the delta E ionisation chamber and of the Silicon detector, special runs with Oxygen and Si beam have been undertaken.With this method it is possible to get absolute values for the concentrations of different elements,provided the matrix is well defined. In our case,since the matrix itself (Calcium)is subject to variations from sample to sample ,only the ratios: Ca/P, Ca/ Sr, Ca/Mg, Ca/Li, Mg/Li , Sr/Li of different human femoral bone compartment: cortical bone and trabecular bone,in normal bone or in osteoporosis could be relevant. From our data two main conclusions can be drawn:1. In osteoporosis,in trabecular and cortical samples the ratio Ca/Mg is two times less than in the case of the normal samples;2.The concentration of Lithium in the trabecular samples, in osteoporosis, is by far higher than in trabecular normal samples. It seems to be worth to undertake a systematic study over a large number of samples.

[62] Age-related changes in human fetal skin fibroblast migration and signal transduction

H. Kondo and Y. Yonezawa (Dept. Cell Recognition, Tokyo Metropolitan Institute of Gerontology, Tokyo, Japan)

We demonstrated previously that the migration of human skin fibroblasts into a denuded area declined during in vitro and in vivo cellular aging. In addition, we found that the migration of fetal skin fibroblasts was stimulated by an autocrine factor, bFGF whereas the migration of adult- and old-donor skin fibroblasts was stimulated by a paracrine factor, PDGF. To find out the cause of age-related decline in human fetal skin fibroblast migration, we studied the signal transduction pathway. We attempted to clarify it by comparing with a previously reported bovine endothelial cell migration stimulated by bFGF, in which the bFGF signal was mediated by phospholipase A2 (PLA2)-coupled G-protein and PLA2 via arachidonic acid. Cell migration into a denuded area was determined by Stenn's method (1980). We first studied whether cell migration was suppressed by a neutralizing anti-bFGF antibody, PLA2-coupled G-protein blocker or PLA2 inhibitor. Further, we studied whether arachidonic acid release was inhibited by them. The results indicated that human fetal skin fibroblast migration was mediated by PLA2 via arachidonic acid without the involvement of pertussis toxin-sensitive G-protein, different from endothelial cell migration. In addition, the cell migration suppressed by a neutralizing anti-bFGF antibody or PLA2 inhibitor was restored by arachidonic acid addition. Then, we studied whether arachidonic acid addition restored cell migration decreased by in vitro cellular aging. The results indicated that age-related decline in cell migration was not restored by arachidonic acid addition, suggesting that it was caused by the events involved in downstream of arachidonic acid.

[63] Single-stranded G-rich telomeric DNA ends activate p53 and trigger a senescence-like arrest

Gabriele Saretzki, Thomas von Zglinicki (Dept of Gerontology, University of Newcastle, UK)

PURPOSE: The distal end of telomeres is a G-rich single-stranded (ss) overhang which is normally protected by loop formation and intercalation in the double-stranded telomere. Telomere shortening in human somatic cells leads eventually to replicative senescence via activation of p53- and pRb-dependent pathways. How this activation occurs is not known. Recent data suggest that a certain treshold telomere length cannot induce senescence by itself. We hypothesised that exposure of free overhangs might be the trigger to activate p53. METHODS: ss oligonucleotides of varying sequence and G/C content were transfected into human fibroblasts and U87 glioblastoma cells being either wild-type for p53 or overexpressing a dominant-negative mutant p53. Cell growth was monitored by clonogenic assay and DNA staining/FACS, p53 and p21 expression was measured by Western blotting and ELISA, and telomerase activity was estimated by TRAP assay. RESULTS: G-rich ss oligonucleotides, and most efficiently those of telomeric sequence, activate p53/p21 and block the cell cycle in a p53-dependent manner. C-rich ss oligonucleotides have no effect. Cells which overcome the block activate telomerase and elongate their telomeres. CONCLUSION: The existence of free G-rich ss telomeric overhangs in the nucleoplasm, i.e. the disruption of telomeric loops, is an efficient trigger for a senescence-like cell-cycle arrest.

[64] Poly(ADP-Ribose) Polymerase Activity as a Correlative Parameter in Gerontological Studies

G. A. Shilovsky, A. N. Khokhlov (Evolutionary Cytogerontology Sector, School of Biology, Moscow State University, Moscow, Russia), S. I. Shram (Institute of Molecular Genetics, Russian Academy of Sciences, Moscow, Russia)

In 70-80s many data published showed a strong positive correlation between DNA repair level and poly(ADP-ribose) polymerase (PARP; EC 2.4.2.30) activity. Moreover, the specific PARP inhibitor, 3-amino benzamide, suppressed the DNA repair. It has been proposed that PARP is a DNA repair pathway enzyme However, Lehmann in 1995 showed that although poly(ADP-ribosyl)ation took place during DNA repair, it was a kind of by-process. It also has been shown that PARP-lacking mice do not demonstrate any problems either with DNA repair capacity or longevity. So, the role of PARP in the cell is still rather unclear. A. Buerkle investigated the PARP activity in leukocytes from 13 mammalian species. The data obtained showed that the level of gamma-radiation-induced PARP activity had a strong correlation with species life-span. He proposed that the higher poly(ADP-ribosyl)ation capacity of long-living animals (as compared with short-living species) allowed them to decrease the rate of unrepaired DNA damage accumulation with age. The data about the age-related changes of PARP activity had also been obtained, but they were rather contradictory. Our own investigations on the «stationary phase aging» cultured cells also demonstrated the lack of a strong relationship between PARP activity and cell aging. We assume that histone protein's poly(ADP-ribose) modification around the DNA strand break works as a damage marker or «alarm signal». In conclusion, we want to say that PARP activity is just a correlative parameter, not an aging trigger or mediator. It means that it is necessary to be much more careful in interpretation of detected enzymatic activity changes and their role in the deteriorative aging processes. The work is supported by Russian Foundation for Basic Research (grant 00-04-48049).

[65] Okadaic acid-induced neurodegeneration

DongHo Kim, Woo-Kyoung Koh, HeaNam Hong (Department of Anatomy and Cell Biology, College of Medicine, University of Ulsan, 388-1 PoongNap-Dong, SongPa-Gu, Seoul, Korea)

Alzheimer's disease (AD) is characterized by regional deposition of senile plaques, neurofibrillary tangles, and extensive neuronal cell death. Although the extent of neuronal death and synaptic loss is most directly linked to the severity of clinical disease, the mode and mechanism of neuronal cell death remain unclear. Okadaic acid is currently used in models of AD research to increase the phosphorylation of tau and neuronal death. To investigate neuronal cell death mechanism, we used okadaic acid on tau phosphorylation and neurodegeneration in vivo and in vitro cortical neuron culture. In cultured neurons, okadaic acid induced tau phosphorylation as early as 6 h after treatment, evoked dendritic damage and distal axon like dystrophic neurite formation. Using immunocytochemistry and fluorescent study, we found that markers of oxidative activity such as nitrotyrosine, c-jun, 2-dichlorofluorescein diacetate (DCF), and heme oxygenase-1 (HO-1) were altered in okadaic acid-treated neuronal culture. Immunoreactivity of nitrotyrosine and c-jun, and DCF-oxidation were increased in degenerating neurons, while HO-1 expression was increased in astrocyte in response to okadaic acid. The data suggest that tau phosphorylation and oxidative damage be implicated in okadaic acid-induced neurodegeneration.

[66] On the Simplicity of Mammalian Ageing

de Magalhaes, Joao Pedro (University of Namur (FUNDP), Namur, Belgium)

Ageing's incidence and magnitude is considerably greater in mammals than in their amphibian and reptilian ancestry; for example, all studied mammals age after the sexual peak while amphibians and reptilians are classes composed of several apparently non-ageing species. The defended hypothesis is that mammalian ageing evolved together with the first mammals and persisted in all mammalian species until present; it's proposed that primordial mammals were species with high mortality rates leading to the loss of oocyte regeneration capacity and eventually senescence; alternatively, antagonistic pleiotropy might be at work, meaning that mammals have certain functional advantages over their ancestry that as a by-product cause ageing. In addition, mechanisms behind mammalian senescence might be much simpler than we think; the ageing changes of most mammalian species appear to be the same phenomenon only timed at different rates; other observations such as evolutionary theory, progeroid syndromes, mathematics, and life-extension procedures are used to support the hypothesis. Finally, experiments capable of testing this hypothesis and its potential implications are discussed.

[67] Analysis of Correlations between the Life Span of Animals and Some Cell Proliferation Parameters

L. Prokhorov (School of Biology, Moscow State University, Moscow, Russia)

Estimate of correlations between the maximum life span of animals (birds, fishes, reptiles, amphibian) and cell roliferation parameters: cell doubling number and mean rate of doubling of these cells during embryogenesis or for the time from zygote formation to growth termination. Mathematical analysis of reference data and results of own investigations. We showed earlier that the maximum life span of mammals is proportional to the cell doubling number and inversely proportional to the average rate of doubling of these cells, during mbryogenesis or for the time from zygote formation to growth termination (Prokhorov, 1999a,b). We found now that there are the same correlations for animals of other types: birds, fishes, reptiles, amphibian. We founded the maximum life span of birds, fishes and reptiles to be proportional to the number of cell doublings, and inversely proportional to the rate of duplication of these cells during embriogenesis (except fishes) or for the time from zygote formation to growth termination. For amphibian these correlations are not so good. The discovered correlations can explain the mechanism which determine the life span of animals. It will help to predict if the preparation or any effect can to decrease the cell proliferation rate and not decrease saturation density in culture it can increases the life span of animals.

[68] Correlations between the Life Span of Animals and Cell Proliferation Rate and Metabolism Level

L. Prokhorov (School of Biology, Moscow State University, Moscow, Russia)

To answer a question: why do the many different and heterogeneous factors increase the life span of animals? We used the transformed Chinese hamster cells growing without subcultivation and medium change. We have made the analysis of reference data for various substances influence on the life span of animals. The decrease of the medium temperature from 37 to 27 degrees Celsius or the introduction of

BHT (30, 50 mkg/ml) and ethanol (1 or 2%) in growth medium induce the decrease of the proliferation rate of cells and increase the life span of the cultures more than twofold. The antioxidants (BHT, epigid) in the concentrations which increase the life span of animals, decrease the cell division rate in cultures. In some studies it was shown that the decrease of temperature induces the decrease of metabolism rate (Frolkis, Muradian, 1988) and increases the ontogeny periods (Loeb, Northrop, 1917). The reducing growth rate of animals during restricted feeding is explained by the slowing down cell proliferation rate (Nikitin, 1984). The hydrocortisone increases the life span of Human fibroblast cultures and time of cell division of these cells (Cristofalo, Sharf, 1975; Macieira-Coelho, 1975). We suppose that practically all factors which increase the life span of animals decrease the average cell division rate and metabolism rate at the growth period of organism and slowing down metabolism rate after growth termination.

[69] The comparative analysis of the health and disease in 1005 old people with different occupations.

Huanzhi Ma, Qiuling Zhang (Department of Geriatrics, Xiehe Hospital, Tongji Medical College, Huazhong University of Science and Technology, Wuhan, China) Erkang Zeng (Departmant of Gerontology, Tongji Medical College, Huazhong University of Science and Technology, Wuhan, China)

Purpose: The study is to survey if people's occupation could affect their aging process and cause senile diseases Method: 1005 elderly were selected as subjects. Among them 563 were male and 442 were female; 945 subjects were aged 60 to 89, the others were beyond 90. Subjects were divided into 5 groups according to categories of occupations, namely: workers, numbered 471; farmers, 127; intellectuals, 206; cadres, 81; and housewives, 120. They have worked for more than 20 years in their occupations. The data collected were using standardized format and method. The items for each subject include: (1) face to face interview; (2) medical history; (3) physical examination, and (4) laboratory test. Results: (1) generally, body height and weight decreased with their age (2) the prevalence rate of hypertension had no significant difference (SD) ($P>0.05$) among 5 groups. (3) plasma lipid had remarkable SD among 5 groups, it trends that mental labors were higher than manual labors. (4) The immunity function had SD for lymphocyte transformation rate ($P<0.05$), E-R($P<0.05$) and IgM ($P<0.01$). (5) Senile disease had no SD. Conclusion: Occupation had some effects on health of elderly.

[70] Mathematical model of the whole diagram of age mortality

V. Dontsov (National Gerontology Center, Moscow, Russia)

Purpose: By the purpose of assay was the simulation of regulatory influences on the process of cells regeneration as the probable central mechanism of ageing for self-renovated tissues of mammals. Material and methods: The theoretical computer simulation method was used. Results: Let level of renovation in multicellular organism be depended on concentration of some stimulated renovation factor "F" - the product of special positive regulator cells "D". For time-depended growth during some years it is necessary the positive F-factor gradient. The well-known biological mechanism for this situation realization is time-dependent natural death of negative regulator cells "I": the balance D - I = F is resulting in stimulation of growth or its restriction. If the "D" cells is non-renovated, there is period of ageing as result of decreasing of "D" cellsnumber due to formula: $dD/dt = - Kd*D$, $dI/dt = -Ki*I$, ($Kd < Ki$). The age mortality is presented here as log (1/F) due to general theory of ageing as decreasing of "general vitality" (as function of cell renovation intensity). Anyone may see the well coincidence of theoretical curve and any experimental and demographic real age mortality curves (For optimal: Do=Io=100, Kd=0.01, Ki=0.05, c=10, $M=Ln(1/(F+c)*100) * 100$). Conclusion: The results is coincident with regulator group theory of aging and the main mechanism of aging as the decreasing of renovation intensity ofdifferent regenerated units in organism.

[71] Model of aging taking into account packing of cells

V. Chernilevsky (Moscow State University of Medicine and Dentistry)

Purpose: The numerical experiment was carried out on a model of organism for valuation mechanisms of aging. The cells (C) were substituted for deformable spheres in limited volume. Proliferetion simulated by the doubling of C with the given coordinates. The moments and quantity of divisions, coordinates of C and form of limiting surfaces varied since a stage og zygota; connections of calculated points described by graph of conditions (GC) with tops - coordinates of the centres of C after the next division; the position of C calcucated in accordance with the locally maximum dence packing as condition with a minimum potentinal energy; distrophy, braking of C, apoptosis and telomeric effects (TE) simulated by absence of division in zone with critical density of C or with above critical number of divisions; the destruction of C exempted volume for the subsequent divisions in stages of morphogenesis; variants of GC without a possibility of divisions meant how death, the immortality simulated at presence stem C at the expence of packing effects, the GC life span optimizated at an expenditure of stem C as resource. It is established: death of C changes the packing, that prolongs GC at the expence of next divisions; initially lethal effects (LE) for C prolong the GC life, apoptosis compensates LE of proliferation, TE compensates LE of limiting surfaces, the variants of packing determine length of GC and explain the difference in species life span, unlethal variants of packing were not revealed. These data allow to explain the effects of aging by regulator hypothesis.

[72] Lowering metabolism - a possible method of human life span

V. Chernilevsky (Moscow State University of Medicine and Dentistry)

Purpose: The method is based on the data that at many mammalia in state of hypobiosis basal metabolism is lowered (BML) very much and aging is delyed independently from the mechanisms, and after hypobiosis the process of self-renovation of tissues has been activated. In addition the life span of some species (Microtus, Soricidae etc.) is able to increase in several times. In the experiments on life prolongation of mice, don't flowing into hypobiosis, us have been success BML by hypoxi-hypercapnic gaseous medium. In that work possibilities of BML in man have been investigated with aim of longevity. It is known that in man during sleep decrease the respiration and puls rate, body temperature, oxygen consumption (VO2) and carbon dioxide discharge (VCO2). On the background fool muscular relaxing and starvation (BFMRS) it causes BML for 20%. The further BML during sleep is possible for training of respiration on the BFMRS. Such trainings are known in active state. The first economy of respiration has been reached by limitation depth of breath and expiration. Then the decrease of respiration rate has been working by training in breath holding and stepped respiration on the BFMRS. For the time the slow respiration has been automating. It is established that in such respiration VO2 and VCO2 are lowering twice, oxygen utilisation coefficient is increasing, stability to hypoxia and resistance of organism to different diseases are working, viability is raising. The BFMRS relives respiratory training, makes them more effective and allows BML twise. Application of automatic rhythm 2 respiration a min on the BFMRS for 7-8 hr sleep essentially should BML and delay aging. After sleep processes of self-renovation should be intensified by training widening of reserve possibilities of organism.

[73] Antioxidant Action of Crenotherapy by Sulphured Mineral Water and Peloids on Human Beings: Changes in Urinary Levels of Tbars

Hernández-Torres A.; Ramón-Giménez J.R.; Cuenca-Giralde E.; Márquez-Montes J. (Agency of Health Technology Assessment of National Health Institute "Carlos III". Universitary Hospital "Clínica Puerta de Hierro". ASEPEYO. Madrid. SPAIN)

PURPOSE: The measurement of urinary elimination of Thiobarbituric Acid

Reactant Substances (TBARS) from an homogeneous population (within a control environment) provides us with a huge amount of information about the process of human lipoperoxidation or aging. The sulphur absortion from the mineral water increases the -SH radicals included in the gluthation tripeptid. These -SH radicals work like free radicals scavengers. METHODS: Prospective clinical study in humans, in a Spanish spa of sulphured mineral waters and peloids, evaluated the change obtained in human oxidative balance before and after crenotherapy administration with sulphured mineral water and peloids. 110 volunteers, 55 men and 55 women, (age: 68.5±0.5), were included in our study in a Spanish spa. Controlled variables were: habits, medical conditions, solar radiactions received during treatment, age, diet, smoking, etc. The urinary samples from volunteers were analyzed following the usual method for detection of TBARS, analyzing the influence of Crenotherapy over the variables mentioned above, in elderly population samples, weighting each variable in the final results (Stepwise backwards). The treatments were baths: 37.5-39°C, 15 minutes, jets, peloid application, and inhalatory therapies, followed by 30-45 minutes rest, to improve the organic reaction. Mineralization water: 10.4 mg H2S/l In the statistical analysis performed, the means were compared using Student's "t" Test and ANOVA and, performing at the end of the statistical analysis a multiple linear correlation to weight (Stepwise backwards) each variable mentioned above, in elderly population samples, in the final results. RESULTS: There was a decrease in the lipid peroxidation process and in the urinary elimination of TBARS, obtaining ssd in the Crenotherapeutic Effect, (CE) which was clearly antioxidant and independent of sex. The daily urinary elimination of TBARS was ssd ($p<0.01$); The difference, CE, was lower in women than men, although both showed a good correlation between Basal and Post-treatment results. In other words, the post-treatment results and CE were conditioned by basal elimination of TBARS. The Crenotherapy using sulphured mineral waters decreases the urinary elimination of TBARS. It occurs either in men or women, or in both (when they are studied together). Therefore, the TE is not related to sex. This suggests a shift of the patient's oxidative balance towards the antioxidant side. The topical treatment administration was very important to achieve a satisfactory results in front of the inhalatory approach. The treatment produced an important vassel dilatation and a transcoutaneous absortion around 10 ml.cm-2.h-1. It was a direct relatioship between TBARS elimination and solar radiations, being more important in women. The urinary elimination of TBARS decreases on the three groups of age: (61-65, 66-70, 71-75); We found a trend to decrease the productions of TBARS in patients, (men and women) between 61-75 years old, higher in men after crenotherapy ($p<0.01$). CONCLUSIONS: 1.- The Crenotherapy using sulphured mineral waters decreases the urinary production of TBARS . It occurs either in men or women, or in both studied together). CE is not related to sex. This suggests a shift of the patients oxidative balance towards the antioxidant side. 2.- The technique used to analyze TBARS is not invasive and it is also easy to use. It allows us to know the patients oxidative situation by simple urinary measurements (before and after the treatment). 3.- There is a positive linear correlation between TBARS urinary levels from patients (that just arrived to the spa) and CE achieved. The basal production of TBARS affects the CE. 4.-The smokers rate in our study population is under the average in the Spanish smokers rate. It shows that the spa users have a high health understanding and special worrys about their health status. There was not difference in the production of TBARS among smokers and no smokers. The topical treatment is only effective and must be longer than seven days and certainly after 14 days. There is a direct relatioship between TBARS urinary elimination and solar radiactions (which vary among sex). There was not dependence among the TBARS elimination, CE and age. There is a tendency to decrease the urinary TBARS elimination related to age (61-75 years), more significant among men, This suggests a shift of the patients oxidative balance towards the antioxidant side. The CE in women, does not depend of the age and it does in men.

[74] Estimating stature from knee height in elderly Egyptians.

Nayera E. Hassan, Ashraf H. Shaalan and Aly A. El-Nofely (National Research Center, Cairo, Egypt)

Stature is difficult or impossible to be measured in the non-ambulatory elderly persons, and its value may be spurious if measured in those elderly persons with certain skeletal deformities e.g. excessive spinal curvature. Hence, the objective of this study is to re-emphasize the correlation between knee height and stature, to develop prediction equations for stature depending on knee height and age based on anthropometric measurements of the Egyptian elderly, and to validate the applicability of prediction equations of stature as presented by Chumlea et al. (1985) on Egyptian elderly. A cross-sectional study was performed on 307 Egyptian subjects (129 males and 178 females), older than 60 years of age, including both institutionalized and non-institutionalized, ambulatory, free from physical deformities and all are residents in Cairo and Giza cities. Stature and knee height were measured following the formal descriptions, using standard instruments by qualified anthropologists. The results revealed that knee height is significantly and positively correlated to stature in both sexes (r: 0.64, $p<0.001$ for males and r:0.59, $p<0.001$ for females). Age-dependent statistical models for prediction of stature from knee height were developed specifically for each sex. These are: Stature of males = 103.37 + (1.36 x knee height measurement in cm) Δ (0.102 x age in years) and Stature of females = 98.09 + (1.35 x knee height measurement in cm) Δ (0.14 x age in years). When tested, these models proved to be more precise in predicting heights of Egyptian elderly than those developed on other populations.

[75] Aurintricarboxylic acid as a putative anti-aging agent

Vadim Fraifeld, Alexandra Lichtenstein, Ilana Nathan (Ben-Gurion University of the Negev, Beer-Sheva, Israel), Natalie Utko, Albert Timchenko, and Khachik Muradian (Institute of Gerontology, Kiev, Ukraine)

Purpose: Cell-protective properties of aurintricarboxylic acid (ATA) demonstrated in a variety of in vitro systems, could be integrated in a multicellular organism, offering the potential for anti-aging activity. We tested this possibility, using Oregon-R Drosophila melanogaster as a model system. Materials and methods: The study included 1) follow-up the survival of flies maintained on a standard cultural medium with or without ATA, starting from the second day of eclosion; 2) estimation of the effect of ATA on metabolic rate (CO2 production); 2) assessment of the capacity of ATA-treated flies to withstand the stress. The flies were exposed to a high ambient temperature (38 °C for 90 min) or to a low level of oxygen (less than 1 0.000000or one hour). Antihypoxic activity of ATA was also examined in cultured cells. Results: It was found that (a) long-term treatment with ATA (0.5 mM) improves D. melanogaster imagoes' survival, especially at a late period of life. This effect was not apparently related to a reduction in metabolic rate, since the level of CO2 production in ATA-treated flies was similar to that in controls; (b) one-week maintenance of fruit flies on the medium, containing 1 mM ATA, increases their resistance to diverse stress insults, including heat shock and hypoxia; (c) ATA at concentrations of 25-100 ?M significantly abrogates cell death in an in vitro model of chemical hypoxia caused by ATP-depletion. Conclusions: Life-span extension effect and the ability to enhance resistance to stress, supports the suggested anti-aging activity of ATA.

[76] Muscular Histochemistry, Performance, Physical Function & Exercise Training in Older Adults

ME Cress (University of Georgia, Athens, GA, USA), SW Stevenson (Calif. State Polytech Institute, Pomona, CA, USA), PC Esselman University of Washington, Seattle, WA, USA), SA Jubrias (University of Washington, Seattle, WA, USA) KE Conley (University of Washington, Seattle, WA, USA)

Muscular Histochemistry, Performance, Physical Function & Exercise Training in Older Adults ME Cress (University of Georgia, Athens, GA, USA), SW Stevenson (Calif. State Polytech Institute, Pomona, CA, USA), PC Esselman University of Washington, Seattle, WA, USA), SA Jubrias (University of Washington, Seattle, WA, USA) KE Conley (University of Washington, Seattle, WA, USA) Purpose: Fitness is an underlying determinant of function. Methods: 39 volunteers (69 ± 4 yr; M ± SD) participated in 6 mo. of moderate (3 x/wk) endurance (ET) or resistance training (RT) or no formal exercise (CON). Electron microscopy of biopsies of the m. quadriceps femoris, and whole muscle volume from MRI were used to calculate mitochondrial (MITOVOL) and myofibrillar (MYOVOL). Physiological capacity outcomes: isokinetic knee extension (KE) strength (60 deg * s-1) and aerobic power (VO2peak); Functional outcomes: the Continuous-Scale Physical Functional Performance (CS-PFP) that yields an overall score (PFP-TOT), a lower body strength score (LBS), stair-climbing power (SP), and a 6 min walk distance (WD). Results: PFP-TOT= 58 (scale 0-100) and VO2peak was 29 ml*kg-1*min-1 indicate relatively high initial fitness and function. MITOVOL and MYOVOL, but not QF correlated with aerobic power (101 ± 35 W) and KE torque (82 ± 29 Nm) ($r = 0.62 - 0.89$). MYOVOL correlated with SP; $r = 0.52$ ($p < 0.05$). KE strength relative to body mass (N * kg-1) correlated with function ($r = 0.33 - 0.40$). Change in aerobic power did not correlate gains in functional measures ($p > 0.05$). The RT increased QF volume (8.7%) and training-specific strength (leg press; 66%), but not KE torque. ET improved aerobic power (16%; $p < 0.05$), but not MITOVOL or function. Conclusions. : Moderate exercise training that elicits mode-specific adaptations may enhance physical reserve but not measurably affect functional performance older adults whose initial fitness is over the physiological thresholds.

[77] The immunomarker of aging and the modulatory effect of Chinese medicinal herbs on the dysfunction of lymphocytes in the elderly

J.L. Zhang, J.D. Liu (Beijing Hospital, Institute of Geriatrics, Beijing, China)

This study examined an immunomarker of aging and evaluated the modulatory effect of Chinese medicinal herbs (CMH) on the immune function of lymphocytes in the elderly. Forty-seven elderly and fifteen young persons were selected as study subjects. Peripheral blood lymphocytes (PBL) were isolated by Ficoll-Hypaque gradient centrifugation. The responsive proliferation was investigated by means of the 3H-TdR incorporation procedure. The phenotype and receptor of lymphocytes were measured using indirect immunofluorescence. Both Rg1 and Gy-P significantly increased the responsive proliferation of lymphocytes in the elderly, $p<0.001$ and $p<0.05$, respectively. Rg1 also had a stimulatory effect on the receptor, CD25, and phenotype, CD45RA, CD45RO, in lymphocytes in aged persons. The immunomarker of aging was established by multiparametric indications on the basis of study at the cellular and molecular levels. The possibility exists that a lowered immune function can be reversed with modulation. In the near future, a highly purified, nontoxic, and more effective immunomodulator could be produced from CMH as an antiaging drug.

[78] Terminal treatment of elderly chronic dialysis patients

S. Saima, Y. Akiyama, N. Miyauti, H. Yamada, Y. Nakamura (International Medical Center of Japan , Tokyo, Japan)

Japan has the highest number of patients on dialysis in the world, however, there has scarcely been any discussion on how long dialysis must be continued as life-sustaining therapy in elderly patients on chronic dialysis who are terminally ill with renal failure and various complications, or senility. In the present study, we performed a retrospective analysis on how elderly dialysis patients actually face death in relation to such problems. The study included the cases of 31 elderly patients who had been on chronic dialysis for at least a year before death and who were at least 75 years of age at death (median : 82.1 years). Among these, 90% faced a slow death; the final period of hospitalization was under 30 days in 60% of the subjects. During the year before death, the subjects showed a marked decrease in the degree of independence in the activities of daily living and increase in the severity of dementia. One month before death, 75% of the subjects were bedridden and at least 50% had moderate to severe dementia. Dialysis had been discontinued in 9 patients. In other patients, the interval between the final day of dialysis and the day of death was less than 2 days in 65%. In many of the subjects who had received adequate care at home until almost the end, the decision was made to stop the dialysis during the short period of hospitalization before death, since due to aging, it has become difficult to administer to treatment to these patients.

SESSION 170

A Study on the Factors Influencing the Efforts and Duration of the Elderly Welfare Agency Sponsorship

Hyekyung, Suh(Graduate School of Social Welfare, Hallym University, Seoul, Korea

The purpose of this study was to offer the data for effective management of sponsors by analyzing the factors that influence the duration and effort of the charitable giving in the welfare agency for the older adults. Data were obtained from the response to the questionnaire which were administered on 335 sponsors of three elderly welfare agencies. The major findings were as followings: (1) those who have the more educated and more stable occupation tend to maintain the charitable giving more; (2) older people have a tendency to maintain the sponsorship longer;(3) the sponsors who contribute to the another social welfare agencies tend to maintain the sponpsorship more and longer; (4) the more direct relationship with recipients have, the longer duration of the charitable giving expect; (5) among the independent variables, such as demographic, socio-economic, sponsorship behavior, and agency-related characteristics, 'agency-related' factors were found to be the best predictors of the effort and duration of the charitable giving giving in the elderly welfare agency. These results would be of substaintial value to charitable organization seeking to understand and eventually influence the behavior of potential sponsors. From variables related to different donating bahavior, fundraiser in non-profit sector can develop strategies and models of whether an individual is likely to give a particular form of charity appeal.

Arguments about Care: Current Theories on Aged Care and Their Implications for Policy and Research

Michael Fine (Department of Sociology, Macquarie University, Sydney, Australia)

Controversy surrounds aged care. While population aging is advanced as a justification for expanding aged care provisions by many advocates, it is seen by others as a demographic and economic threat which makes it imperative to cut expenditures. Neither is there agreement on the form that care should take and the balance that needs to be struck between acute care, long-term institutional facilities and home and community provisions; the role of case management; the efficiency of public and private systems of delivery; the balance between familial based care and formalised professional provisions; the availability and role of informal caregivers, or the extent to which social divisions based on gender, income and culture need to be taken into account in the formulation of aged care policy. Although the assumptions and theoretical models are rarely made explicit, these controversies are reflected in the different theories and perspectives adopted by experts and policy makers. Using the methods of comparative theoretical analysis, this paper reviews the major theories of care from social science, economics, medicine and gerontology and draws out their implications for policy and research. The results suggest that the absence of normative consensus in theory reflects real struggles for control and use of resources in the public domain. It is concluded that current theories are fragmented and particular, and that to better engage with policy a more complex and interdisciplinary approach to the theory of care is needed.

Community Care - Harnessing Human Resource in Elder Care

I.J. Prakash (Bangalore University, India)

In India, families were the traditional care givers. In recent years, there is a desperate search for alternatives to family care which is not always available to every older person. In Bangalore, several innovative efforts are being made to provide quality care to older people in a community setting. Though most of them are still in experimental stage, the results are encouraging. Day care, Young old as carers for old - old, day centers, old age clubs are being used to encourage volunteerism among the people and involve neighbourhoods in elder care. This paper describes some such approaches seen in Bangalore.

Enabling elders to age in place: the provision of enhanced home & community care services by HKSAR GOVT

Eliza Leung Wong Kwok-shing, JP Assistant Director of Social Welfare (Elderly) (Social Welfare Department The Hong Kong Special Administrative Region Government, The People's Republic of China

The core principles of the Hong Kong Special Administrative Region Government in the provision of care and support services for our senior citizens are 'ageing in place', 'care in the community' and 'continuum of care'. A range of community support services including home help service, day care centres, social centres, multi-service centres, support teams for the elderly and respite services for the elderly is provided to assist older persons to continue to live in the community. In 1999, we have re-engineered the traditional form of home hlep service and set up home care and meal service teams to strengthen personal and nursing care services to elders and enable service providers to deploy their resources flexibly. To enable frail elders of moderate impairment level to continue to live at home, we have designed and developed an integrated form of enhanced home and community care services which will be launched in March 2001. The services will be a package of intensive home and community-based care and support services for the elders and their carers, and nursing and para-medical support to be provided according to individual's needs. In performance monitoring, the emphasis is on output and outcome measures. This new initiative will be closely monitored and will provide the basis for benchmarking and development of an improved inter-sectoral/organizational cooperation to meet needs of clients. Development of this initiative from home help service will be highlighted and discussed in this presentation.

Healthy Aging Project

Michael Stones, Lee Stones, Christine Knight (Lakehead University, Thunder Bay, Canada

The Healthy Aging Program aims to promote healthier aging based on individualized assessment and programming. The assessment is delivered on the internet to facilitate access in rural regions, and contains a validated screening tool followed by further assessment of triggered problems. Paraticipation in Healthy Aging Program Modules is recommended based on assessment outcomes. These are standardized and tested interventions not readily accessible in most communities, and delivered by trained facilitators. Early findings on the development of the project are described.

Social Support for the Elderly in Malta: Is it Sustainable?

R. Bonello (Maltese Association of Gerontology and Geriatrics, University of Malta, Malta)

Purpose: The presenting scenario in the Maltese Islands, whereby the majority of the services are heavily subsidised by the Government, is one which has disturbing implications for continuing sustainability for future services. Method: The focus of this paper is a critical analysis based on findings from a national survey, demographic data and existing social policy. Results: The Ageing of the population in Malta has not only changed the very structure and composition of the total population but has also altered the structure and composition of the elderly population in itself. Moreover, family patterns have changed. The number of informal carers have been drastically reduced resulting in a higher burden on the state. Moreover, there is no monitoring of the efficiency and accountability of services. Consequently, one questions whether they are really fulfilling a need. Whether those in need are really being catered for. One also questions whether these services are creating a dependent older generation thus contradicting the notion that older persons should remain active for as long as possible. Conclusions: Government needs to make services more sustainable based on the fundamental principles of solidarity and equity. This can be brought about by: a) Better co-ordination of service provision. b) Encouraging an increasing proportion of the public to choose private services. c) Strengthen existing strategies and devise sustainable new approaches that can compensate for the decline in support division brought about by the dynamics within the family.

SESSION 171

Basic and Intervention Research on Stress Moderators among Older Adults

Karl Pillemer (Dept. of Human Development, Cornell University, Ithaca, USA), Jill J. Suitor (Dept. of Sociology, Louisiana State U, Baton Rouge, USA); Susan Folkman [University of California, San Francisco, USA]; Alex J. Zautra, Mary Davis, and John Reich (Arizona State University, Tempe, USA); S. H. Zarit, E. E. Femia, (Gerontology Center, Pennsylvania State University, University Park, USA), A. Townsend (Case Western Reserve University, Cleveland, USA), and M. A. P. Stephens (Kent State University, Kent, USA).

ISSUE: This symposium reports on new developments in theory and intervention concerning the stress and coping process. Specifically, it addresses issues related to the role of coping not only in mitigating negative moods states, but also in maintaining positive emotions. It also addresses issues related to the planning of interventions for family caregivers that moderate their stress and improve their health and life quality. STRUCTURE: Following introduction of the panel members and an overview of the symposium by the convenor, the panelists will each make 15 minute presentations, and the symposium will conclude with a 15 minute commentary by the discussant and a 15 minute question and answer period with the audience. CONTENT: Two of the presentations focus on basic research and its implications for theory and intervention, and two focus on intervention research. The former two papers place their emphasis on evidence gathered from older adults and from AIDS caregivers that coping serves the dual functions of maintaining positive emotions, not only mitigating distress. The latter two papers examine the power of two different interventions to moderate particular stressful demands faced by family caregivers. One intervention involves the provision of respite services to the family caregivers of persons with dementia, whereas the other involves a highly structured program aimed to reduce tensions between family caregivers and the staff of nursing homes in which the caregivers' relatives have recently been placed. CONCLUSIONS: The symposium will convey information about the measurement of coping and its outcomes among older adults, with an emphasis on the dynamic nature of coping and attendant emotions. The symposium will also highlight key issues in the planning and evaluation of strategies of intervention on behalf of family caregivers, including the intensity and duration of the intervention and the dimensions of stress that are ameliorated by different intervention protocols.

Do Respite Services Moderate the Stress of Family Caregiving?

S. H. Zarit, E. E. Femia, (Gerontology Center, Pennsylvania State University, PA, USA), A. Townsend (Case Western Reserve University, Cleveland, OH, USA), and M. A. P. Stephens (Kent State University, Kent, OH, USA).

There is growing evidence that the stresses associated with care of a person with dementia can be ameliorated through a variety of psychoeducational and respite services. Successful treatment outcomes depend on several factors, including provision of adequate amounts of treatment, and consideration of the mechanisms of treatment, including the specific domains on which treatment will have an impact and whether there are mediating or moderating effects. In this paper, we explore the benefits associated with adult-day care use by family caregivers of people with dementia. The treatment group consisted of 121 family caregivers enrolling their relative in participating adult day care programs for a period of 3 months or longer in a US state with a large network of day care programs. The control group were 203 caregivers from another state with a very limited network of day care programs serving people with dementia. Caregivers were primarily spouses (44%) or adult children (42%) of the person with dementia. Measures were divided into those assessing the direct impact of day care on the caregiver's daily routine (primary subjective stressors) and more generalized indicators of well-being. Use of adult day care had a direct effect on both sets of measures of caregiver distress. After 3 months of day care use, caregivers reported lower scores on two measures of primary subjective stress, overload and strain, and on two measures of well-being, depression and anger. There was no evidence of mediating or moderating effects of treatment.

Effects of Cooperative Communication Intervention on Stress of Family Members of Nursing Home Residents

K. Pillemer (Dept. of Human Development, Cornell University, NY, USA), J. J. Suitor (Dept. of Sociology, Louisiana State U, Baton Rouge, LA, USA)

Research has demonstrated that caregivers typically maintain close ties to institutionalized family members. However, many family members experience distress regarding the relative's transition to the nursing home, largely due to difficulties relating to facility staff. Little is known, however, about the most effective ways to reduce the stress of family members. The Partners in Caregiving project conducted a randomized, controlled intervention study of a program designed to increase cooperation and effective communication, and to reduce conflict, between family members and staff. Participants included 932 relatives recruited from 20 New York nursing homes, who were assigned to treatment and one of two control conditions. Parallel training sessions on communication and conflict resolution techniques were conducted with families and staff on the intervention units. A pretest interview and two posttest interviews were conducted to measure outcomes. Main effects were found for the intervention, including: 1) Family members in the intervention group increased in their perception of positive behaviors by staff; 2) Family members in the intervention group demonstrated decreased scores on the CES-D depression scale relative to controls. Important effects on other outcome variables were revealed in one subgroup: caregivers to residents with dementia. Among dementia caregivers, caregiver burden was found to significantly decrease in the treatment group relative to controls; and dementia caregivers improved on a scale measuring the degree to which staff members are seen as understanding and empathetic increased relative to controls. Implications for future intervention work on this issue are discussed.

Moving Along: Modifying Coping Theory and Implications for Intervention

Susan Folkman [University of California, San Francisco, US]

PURPOSE: This presentation will show how findings from basic longitudinal research on coping and emotion led to modifications in coping theory, and how the modified theory in turn suggests new directions for intervention, especially for caregivers of seriously ill individuals. METHOD: 253 caregivers of men with AIDS were followed for up to five years between 1990 and 1997. Participants were interviewed bi-monthly for two years and semiannually for three additional years on stress and coping processes and psychological well-being. RESULTS Findings (reported elsewhere) show that positive mood was sustained throughout caregiving and bereavement, despite high levels of depressed mood. Data from other studies showing a similar pattern indicate this finding is not an aberration. Analyses of both quantitative and qualitative data indicate that the psychological and social processes that support positive mood differ to a certain extent from those that regulate distress, and depend in large part on beliefs, goals, and values that infuse the immediate context with meaning. These findings led to a revision in coping theory that takes into account the role of positive emotion in the coping process. CONCLUSION: Although both caregiving and bereavement are associated with increases in morbidity and mortality, most people survive, resume their role responsibilities, and regain a sense of well-being. A key to resilience may rest in the observation that people have the capacity to experience positive emotions during intensely stressful times. Interventions can help reinforce psychological and social processes that support positive mood.

Stress, Chronic Illness, and Emotional Health: The Many Colored Days of Older Adults

Alex J. Zautra, Mary Davis, and John Reich (Arizona State University, Tempe, AZ, USA)

PURPOSE: This presentation suggests that a focus on the dynamics of emotional health may benefit gerontological research. New approaches championed as positive psychology urge practitioners and researchers alike to attend more to sources of human strength and resilience and less to human frailties and deficiencies. We urge that attention to both positive and negative affective realms of human engagement will contribute greatly to our knowledge of how elders resolve the challenges that they face as they age. Further, affective experiences are dynamic rather than static conditions of the mind, influenced strongly by degree of stress in the person's life. We will present data indicating that greater attention needs to be paid to both the breadth and depth of emotional life. METHOD: We will rely on findings from two extensive studies of older adults: a longitudinal investigation of 265 elder men and women, and a study of 300 women over 50 years of age, interviewed weekly for 4 to 5 months. RESULTS : We found clear evidence of separate dimensions of affective health through factor analytic studies of emotion terms rated by the study participants. These affective dimensions were associated with different adaptation challenges. Further, we found evidence that the degree of independence between these dimensions varies as a function of life stress. CONCLUSION: We discuss how research and interventions for elders may benefit from adopting a dynamic two-dimensional approach to emotional health.

SESSION 172

Osteoporosis and Quality of Life in the Elderly

Edison Rossi- Brasil- Pathophysiology and diagnosis of Osteoporosis. Giovanni Passeri- Dept.of Internal Medicine and Biomedical Sciences, University of Parma, ItalyBone and fractures in Centenarians. Pawel Szulc- INSERIM 403, Research Unit, Nosptial Herriot, Lyon, France- The prediction of fractures in elderly women. Takao Suzuki- Tokyo Metropolitan Institute of Gerontology, Tokyo, Japan.- Consequences of fall and fractures in the Elderly. Ernesto Palummeri-Dpert.of Geriatricas, Gelliera Hospital, Genova, Italy- Rehabilitation and social intervention in hip fractired Elderly. Neil Binkley- Geriatric Section, University of Madison, Wisconsin, U.S.A.- Pharmacological Prevention and therapy of fractures in the elderly.

The Symposium underlines the worsening of the quality of life in the elderly in the consequence of osteoporotic fractures and deals firstly with the pathophysiology and diagnosis of osteoporosis (particularly in the eldest ones- centenarians).the causes of fractures and lastly the possibility of prevention, therapy and rehabilitation. A good quality of life in the elderly depends on a variety of physical, functional, psychologic and social factors. Among them, physical/mental self-sufficiency is of great importance, together with the possibility of self-care and deambulation; for the latter, the integrity of the skeleton is of pivotal importance. When permanent skeletal lesions take place, self sufficiency and consequently a good quality of life may be permanently and heavily compromised. These pathophysiology and the diagnosis of involutional osteoporosis (a situation debilitating bone structure and exposing the skeleton to fracture risk following a minor trauma (usally a fall)) are firstly exposed. Among the fracture producing permanent disabling outcomes, vertebral and more hip fractures have to be considered. Hip fracture have heavier consequences, because they may permanently impair self-sufficiency and cause serious nursing and social burden. About one quarter of 75 ys. plus hip fractured subjects remain disable and a number of them ask for institutionalization. Deambulation impairment undermine social relationships and thereafter psychical stimulation, favouring the decline of cognitive ability. Life expectancy increment and widespreading of civilization will induce a noteworthy increment of this lesions in the decades to come, with a consequent heavier impact on the elderly's quality of life. Prevention and care of fractures and at least rehabilitation and social intervention are necessary.

Bone Loss, Fractures and Disability in Centenarians.

G. Passeri, (Dep. Internal Medicine & Biomedical Sciences, University of Parma, Italy), G. Pini, (INRCA- Italian National Research Center for Aging, Ancona, Italy, Dep. Experimental Pathology, University of Bologna, Italy) , L. Troiano (Dep. Biomedical Sciences University of Modena), R. Vescovini, (Dep. Internal Medicine & Biomedical Sciences, University of Parma, Italy), P. Sansoni, (Dep. Internal Medicine & Biomedical Sciences, University of Parma, Italy), M. Passeri, (Dep. Internal Medicine & Biomedical Sciences, University of Parma, Italy), R. Delsignore, (Dep. Internal Medicine & Biomedical Sciences, University of Parma, Italy), N. Giuliani, (Dep. Internal Medicine & Biomedical Sciences, University of Parma, Italy), M. Pedrazzoni, (Dep. Internal Medicine & Biomedical Sciences, University of Parma, Italy), C. Franceschi (Dep. Experimental Pathology, University of Bologna, Italy, INRCA- Italian National Research Center for Aging, Ancona, Italy).

Centenarians are examples of "successful aging", however, little is known regarding their skeleton, despite the importance of the prevention of fractures and disability in this frail population. 104 centenarians were visited at home or in retirement facilities. After a complete clinical assessment (history, physical, cognitive and performance tests), blood was drawn to evaluate bone metabolism and phalangeal (DBMSonic, IGEA, Italy) or calcaneal (Sahara, HOLOGIC, USA) ultrasonography was performed. 30 subjects were self-sufficient, 38 were disable for both cognitive and/or physical impairments. 50 subjects were able to walk either unassisted (19) or with supports (31). In the year prior to our visit, 38 centenarians suffered, at least, one fall. 38 subjects sustained a total of 55 fractures; among them, 22 sustained 28 hip fractures, 14 of these had occurred within the last 5 years. Only 2 of the 22 hip-fractured were walking self-sufficient after the event. 25OH vitamin D was detectable in only 5 centenarians, and below the sensitivity of the method in the other 99. Mean serum calcium was 8.60.7 mg/dl, and below 9 mg/dl in 75% of them. Mean PTH was increased (123±108 pg/ml), and above normality in 64%; serum cross-laps (CTX), marker of bone resorption, was elevated in 90% of the subjects. Serum IL-6 was elevated in 81% of the centenarians, being positively correlated with PTH ($p=0.019$) and CTX ($p<0.001$) and negatively with calcium ($p<0.001$). Phalangeal (62 subjects) and calcaneal (28 subjects) ultrasonography showed that most centenarians had markedly low values, indicating a severe state of osteopenia, a severe risk factor for fragility fractures. Ultrasonographic parameters were significantly correlated with resorption markers: phalangeal UBPI was negatively correlated with PTH ($p=0.032$) and with CTX ($p=0.036$), calcaneal SoS with CTX ($p=0.05$). These findings indicate that extreme longevity is characterized by vitamin D deficiency, secondary hyperparathyroidism, increased bone resorption, and severe osteopenia. It is evident that an appropriate prevention of bone loss, by simple supplementation of calcium and vitamin D, has to be considered in the oldest olds, in order to prevent further bone fractures and the following disability

Pharmacological prevention and therapy of fractures in the elderly

Binkley Neil (University of Wisconsin-Madison, WI, U.S.A.)

Recently, the pharmacologic treatment of osteoporosis has substantially improved. Specifically, excellent prospective randomized trials in postmenopausal women demonstrate fracture reduction efficacy with alendronate, risedronate and raloxifene. Additionally, smaller studies observe fracture reduction in osteoporotic postmenopausal women receiving nasal salmon calcitonin and in men receiving alendronate. However, the role of gonadal steroids in osteoporosis treatment remains controversial in both genders. Currently, most available pharmacologic agents act via osteoclast inhibition; i.e, are anti-resorbers, and are thereby limited in the amount of bone mass increase they achieve. However, "anabolic" agents which stimulate bone formation, may soon receive regulatory approval. It is reasonable to expect that these agents will have a profound impact on fracture reduction. An additional recent advance in osteoporotic fracture treatment is the injection of bone cement into compressed vertebral bodies. This technique, percutaneous vertebroplasty, may dramatically and rapidly reduce pain and improve function. Unfortunately, pharmaceutical trials have largely excluded frail elderly individuals, including residents of long-term care facilities. In these individuals who are at high fracture risk, the role of anti-resorptive agents, singly or in combination, remains uncertain. Studies of current, or soon to be available, agents which increase bone mass are urgently needed. Additionally, the possibility that agents exist which not only increase bone mass, but improve muscle strength in frail elderly people, must be explored.

Rehabilitation and social intervention in hip fractured elderly

E.Palummeri, (S.C. Geriatria, E.O.Ospedali Galliera, Genova, Italy), G.Pioli, (S.C. Geriatria, E.O.Ospedali Galliera, Genova, Italy), S.Trasciatti,(S.C. Geriatria, E.O.Ospedali Galliera, Genova, Italy), A.Barone, (S.C. Geriatria, E.O.Ospedali Galliera, Genova, Italy F.Vallone (Servizio di Recupero e Rieducazione funzionale, E.O.Ospedali Galliera, Genova, Italy), G.B.Andreoli (Direzione Sanitaria, E.O.Ospedali Galliera, Genova, Italy), G.Barban, S.C. Geriatria, E.O.Ospedali Galliera, Genova, Italy), A.Cella,(S.C. Geriatria, E.O.Ospedali Galliera, Genova, Italy), V.Curiale,(S.C. Geriatria, E.O.Ospedali Galliera, Genova, Italy), P.Scarpaci,(S.C. Geriatria, E.O.Ospedali Galliera, Genova, Italy), G.Zunin, (S.C. Geriatria, E.O.Ospedali Galliera, Genova, Italy), A.Giusti,(S.C. Geriatria, E.O.Ospedali Galliera, Genova, Italy)

Hip fractures are a major cause of mortality and disability in the elderly. The overall mortality rate ranges between 4.5 and 6.5% during hospital stay and reaches to 20% at 6 months from fracture. Almost 20% of survivors become heavily dependent in performing the activities of daily living and need a nursing home care. Complete recovery from dependency at one year from fracture varies from 40 to 70% of patients. In hospital complications are variable according to pre-operatory length of stay, total lenght of stay, and co-morbidity. Almost 10% of patients develop failure to recover. In order to improve this dramatic picture several intervention models were developed adopting a multidisciplinary team approach including early evaluation and intervention by a multidisciplinary team. According to several model proposed, the interventions were developed during hospital stay and/or at home after discharge form orthopedic or geriatric or rehabiltation ward. Intra-hospital models (ortho-geriatric units, geriatric-orthopedic rehabilitation units) generally show a reduction in total length of stay, in number of complications, in drug use, and in institutionalization rate compared with control groups. Home care interventions result in better functional outcomes than nursing home care at moderate or no additional cost. Few examples in literature are of integrated models (in hospital and home-care). Recently (september 2000) we developed a model in which orthogeriatric experience is joined with a home-care intervention (hospital-at-home). To provide continuity of care the home-based rehabilitation protocol is performed by the staff of the geriatric ward in cooperation with primary care physician and includes a daily visit of physiotherapist and, if necessary, skilledd geriatric nurse, assistant nurse and consulting services. Preliminary data show a reduction in length of stay, in mortality rate and in recovery of functional status.

Risk Factors of Osteoporosis

P. Szulc (INSERM Research Unit 403, Lyon, France)

Osteoporosis is characterised by enhanced bone fragility and a consequent increase in fracture risk. In clinical practice, postmenopausal osteoporosis is most frequent. Loss of ovarian function and a rapid decrease of estradiol secretion result in an activation of bone resorption which is not matched by bone formation. This leads to a rapid bone loss especially in the trabecular compartment. In men, decreased testosterone secretion also results in a decreased bone mineral density (BMD). However, decrease of testosterone secretion develops later in age, is progressive and less compared with the menopause in women. Therefore, bone loss is less and has different profile in the trabecular and cortical compartments in elderly men compared with elderly women. In the elderly, vitamin D deficiency and secondary hyperparathyroidism are major mechanisms of bone loss mainly in the cortical compartment. Vitamin D deficiency is observed particularly in institutionalised or home-bound persons. There are a lot of risk factors of secondary osteoporosis. Among them, prolonged corticotherapy with doses higher than 7.5 mg prednisone daily is probably the most frequent clinical problem. Other hormonal risk factors include congenital and acquired hypogonadism, hyperthyroidism, Cushing's disease, hypopituitarism. Gastrectomy and other gastrointestinal diseases may result in malabsorption which contributes to bone loss. BMD can also decrease during treatment with certain medicines as heparin, loop diuretics, immunosuppressors, antiandrogens, thyroid hormones. Several lifestyle factors like smoking, ethanol abuse, low sunlight exposure, or sedentarity can also give rise to bone loss. Genetic factors play a very important role in the pathogenesis of osteoporosis mainly as determinants of peak BMD.

SESSION 173

From Seniors' Concerns to Government Action: Bridging the Gap

I. Cumming (British Columbia Seniors' Advisory Council, Victoria, Canada) Successes and Challenges Experienced by Seniors Attempting to Influence Public Policy. M. Kloseck (Division of Geriatric Medicine, University of Western Ontario, London, Canada) Current State of Seniors' Involvement in Program and Policy Development: What the Evidence Tells Us. Geri Hinton (Office for Seniors, B.C. Ministry of Health & Ministry Responsible for Seniors, Victoria, Canada) Linking Seniors with Government: The British Columbia Experience.

This session will (1) address the current state of seniors' involvement in health planning and policy development, and the successes and challenges experienced, (2) identify gaps in current procedures which prevent seniors' concerns from being translated into government action, and (3) collaboratively develop potential action strategies to address these gaps so that seniors can more successfully influence the formation of public policy. These issues will be addressed from an international perspective, using research methods and findings and the personal experiences of seniors. Prior to the 2001 World Congress a letter, accompanied by a formal questionnaire, will be mailed to ____ seniors' organizations representing _____ countries. The letter will explain the purpose of the session, encourage international seniors to attend, and ask seniors to share their experiences by completing the enclosed survey. Cross-sectional survey methodology will be used to gather information regarding seniors' linkages with government, their degree of involvement in policy development, and any successes and challenges experienced. Survey data will be analyzed in advance of the 2001 World Congress and findings will be used to generate questions for the focus groups which will be held as part of the session. The session will begin with two brief presentations designed to set the context for the focus groups. The first will highlight survey results and research-based findings on factors influencing seniors' involvement in planning and policy development. The second will be a combined presentation by the B.C. Seniors' Advisory Council and the Office for Seniors and will describe the experiences and outcomes of initiatives to influence public policy in British Columbia. The introductory presentations will be followed by formal focus groups involving all session participants. The focus groups will be facilitated by trained seniors using focused discussion and applied research techniques (Krueger, 1994; Krueger & King, 1998). Qualitative analysis will be used to examine focus group data and to identify trends, gaps in current processes designed to link seniors to government, document ideas from participants about what works here and elsewhere, and guide future action. Following the 2001 World Congress the presentation material from the two speakers, along with the results of both the survey and the focus group session, will be compiled into a formal document that will be made available to all participants and other interested individuals. This scientific approach is an attempt to move beyond the typical informal round table discussions generally conducted by seniors organizations, and identify clear steps to bridge the gap between seniors' concerns and government action. Action strategies can then prioritized and implemented using other suitable scientific techniques that take into account theories of aging, and involvement and community empowerment theories. (Word Count = 435, Characters = 2437)

SESSION 174

International Comparison of Education in Geriatric Medicine

Yusuke Suzuki [Department of Geriatrics, Nagoya University, Nagoya, Japan] (Title : Pre and Postgraduate Education in Geriatric Medicine in Japan) Miguel Ramos [Department of Geriatric Medicine, St. Luke's Medical Center, Manila, Philippines] (Title: Status of Geriatric Medicine in Asia) Patricia P. Barry [Merck Institute of Aging & Health, Washington DC, USA] (Title : Geriatric Medical Education in the United States) Philippe Huber [Department of Geriatrics, Geneva University, Geneva, Switzerland] (Title : New Experience of Teaching Geriatrics in Switzerland) L.M. Guttierez (Instituto Nacional de Ciencias Medicas y Nutricion "Salvador Zubiran") ("Geriatric undergraduate education in South America")

ISSUE: As most nations are currently experiencing aging of society, there is a growing demand of training healthcare professionals engaged in care of older patients. However current educational system of geriatric medicine for medical students, residents and practicing physicians is not yet well established. The symposium aims to provide geriatricians with the opportunity for discussing the issue of how integrated geriatric education can be incorporated into conventional medical educational system. STRUCTURE: The symposium consists of presentation by four speakers and discussions by all attendants. Each speaker features current status and raises agenda of geriatric education in each country including overall review and introduction of new experiences. CONTENT: Dr. Yusuke Suzuki from Nagoya University will present current status of pre and post graduate geriatric education in Japan. Necessity of establishing integrated and continuous educational curriculum of geriatric medicine has been urged as a forerunner of aging population. The obstacles for implementation of integrated geriatric education will be introduced and also the agenda for fundamental reform will be proposed. Dr. Miguel Ramos from St. Luke's Medical Center will introduce status of geriatric medicine in Asia based on investigation carried out by Geriatric Medicine in Asia Working Group (GMAWG). It is suggested that the difference in demographic status bears diversity in development of geriatric medicine and the barriers to the development of academic geriatrics are raised from socioeconomic, perceptive and educational perspectives. Dr. Philippe Huber from Geneva University will introduce new experiences of undergraduate geriatric training, which was implemented from 1995 as a new integrated problem-based curriculum. It is aimed to foster a positive and multidisciplinary approach of the care of the elderly. By implementation of the new curriculum, positive evaluation of student's knowledge, skills and attitudes were confirmed, which necessitated a substantial increase in the teaching time of geriatricians. Professor Patricia Barry from Merck Institute of Aging & Health will present US activities in geriatric education reviewing medical education literature and ongoing project for practicing physician education. The increase in amount of educational materials in geriatric medicine and the possibility of changes in medical practice in the care of older patients by innovative techniques for education were suggested. CONCLUSIONS: With increasing demand of geriatricians as a specialist in order to meet growing numbers of elderly patients. It has become an urgent issue to establish desirable curriculum of geriatric education, which is characterized by multidisciplinary and problem-based approaches. However there still exists obstacles for implementation of integrated geriatric education feasible within framework of existing medical education. Further communication among educators of geriatric medicine will enhance quality of education for improvement of healthcare of the elderly.

Geriatric Medical Education in the United States

Patricia P. Barry, MPH [Merck Institute of Aging & Health, Washington, DC, USA]

PURPOSE: to present US activities in geriatric education for medical students, residents, and practicing physicians METHOD: descriptive reviews of 1) US medical education literature and of 2) an ongoing US project for practicing physician education in geriatric medicine RESULTS: 1) There has been an increase in the amount of educational material in geriatric medicine presented to US medical students, trainees and practicing physicians. 2) The use of innovative techniques for education of US practicing physicians is feasible and more likely to result in changes in medical practice in the care of their older patients. CONCLUSION: Although significant amounts of material in geriatrics are presented in US medical education programs, more is required. Many US physicians still have inadequate preparation for the increasing numbers of older adults that will be seen in the practice of medicine in the next 20-30 years.

Geriatric Medicine Education and Training: Asian Perspective

Miguel Ramos Director, Geriatric Centre, St. Luke's Medical Centre Quezon City , Philippines Masafumi Kuzuya Department of Geriatrics, Nagoya University Graduate School

Purpose: Identify issues in the development and growth of geriatric medicine as a specialty in Asia. To compare various existing geriatrics education and training programs and identify barriers in the growth of academic geriatrics in the different parts of Asia . To formulate collaborative strategies for future directions. Methods: Collaborators in the field of geriatric medicine in the various parts of Asia were searched and identified. Each provided loca data through a self administered questionaire. Results: Collaborators from China, Hong Kong, India, Indonesia, Japan, South Korea, Singapore, Taiwan (Formosa), Thailand and the Philippines participated in this study. Brief historical perspectives showed variable levels of growth and development of geriatric medicine in each participating places in Asia Demographics and health care programs relevant to older people were variable, there is however reported shortage of geriatricians even in aged population like Japan, Singapore and Hong Kong. Conclusion: Geriatric Medicine is at various stages of development in the different parts of Asia. A collaborative effort among the geriatricians in the region could be an effective strategy to meet the

Geriatric undergraduate education in South America

Luis Miguel Gutierrez Robledo

INTRODUCTION: Teaching of geriatrics in every South American medical school is an urgent need. Three main obstacles for introducing teaching of geriatric medicine at the undergraduate level were identified: - lack of an agreement about what has to be taught - crowded curriculum - virtual absence of dedicated professorship in the field OBJECTIVES: To establish a consensus of the basic geriatric knowledge needed by primary care physicians. METHODS: - Review of the existing teaching programs, postal interview of medical school deans, questionnaire addressed to existing teachers and students. - Consensus meeting. RESULTS: The results of the various analysis were presented to a group of representatives of 33 out of 57 existing medical schools. Group discussions with these representatives and conducted by board certified geriatricians proposed a consensual undergraduate curriculum. Then, a teaching guide was produced and a written consensus statement was distributed to all medical schools. A program directed to faculty development on geriatrics is ongoing throughout specific faculty development actions receiving support from PAHO, AMFEM and the geriatrics societies. Conclusions: Teaching of geriatrics in every medical schools is a necessity and shall be mandatory included in their curricula. It must be independent and specifically evaluated. A program is proposed to promote teaching of geriatrics in Mexican medical schools, but an urgent need of geriatric medicine teachers exists.

New experience of teaching geriatrics in Switzerland

Huber Ph, VU Ch, Michel JP

Description and evaluation of a new integrated problem-based curriculum at the University of Geneva school of medicine in 1995, which offered the opportunity to design an innovative longitudinal curriculum in geriatrics as a part of the core undergraduate curriculum. METHOD: Evaluation of the new geriatric program, implemented from the second to the fifth year of medical training, which attempts to foster a positive and multidisciplinary approach of the care for the elderly. During the pre-clinical training, geriatric objectives (theories of aging, cellular mechanism of aging) are integrated in basic sciences problems. At the same time Clinical Skills and Community-Oriented Skills programs prepare the students to cope with behaviour/communication difficulties and public health challenges. The clinical training includes a 12-weeks"integration" unit followed by 11 mandatory clinical clerkships. Seminars focused on frequent clinical problems in older persons (stroke, dizziness, fall and dementia) allow the acquisition of geriatric assessment techniques including mental examination and nutrition status. -All students are exposed for a one week period to the home care of frail elderly and one third spend 8-weeks internal medicine clerkship in the University geriatric hospital. RESULTS: The positive evaluation of the student's geriatric knowledge, skills and attitudes confirm the importance of the implementation of this innovative geriatric program, which necessitated a substantial increase in the teaching time of geriatricians. CONCLUSION: The most important positive effect of this geriatric innovative program would be a long term positive attitude toward the oldest living in the community and better care for the most frail patients.

Pre and Postgraduate Education in Geriatric Medicine in Japan

Yusuke Suzuki, Department of Geriatrics Nagoya University Graduate School of Medicine, Nagoya, Japan

PURPOSE: 1) to review current status of pre and postgraduate education in geriatric medicine in Japan. 2) to raise agenda for further improvement in teaching by introducing ongoing reform. METHOD: descriptive reviews based on the results of investigations carried out in all medical schools who have department of geriatrics. They consist of interpretation and analyses of the results of questionnaire to teaching staffs of geriatric departments and medical students. RESULTS: The results of the questionnaire to teaching staffs of geriatric medicine showed that time spared for teaching of geriatric medicine is not sufficient to cover the broad range of knowledge and experience required. Majority of the staffs felt that bedside teaching is more important than lecture-oriented education to pregraduate medical students. The necessity of integrated curriculum incorporating basic science of aging was suggested. It also became evident that the number of teaching staffs engaged in teaching geriatrics has not yet reached its sufficiency. CONCLUSION: Because of difference of aspects from organ-oriented subjects of internal medicine, there is an urgent need for fundamental reform of education in geriatrics. Curriculum focusing on common symptoms of the elderly and problem-based approach have to be emphasized in teaching.

SESSION 175

Is Hardening of the Arteries Back? A Symposium on Vascular Risks for Neurodegenerative Dementias

Kenneth Rockwood (Dalhousie University, Halifax, Nova Scotia, Canada) (Is hardening of the arteries back? A symposium on vascular risks for neurodegenerative dementias) Susan Kirkland (Dalhousie University, Halifax, Nova Scotia) ("Estrogens, statins and the risk of Alzheimer's disease") Howard Feldman (University of British Columbia, Vancouver, B.C.) (Vascular risk factors to common vascular and neurodegenerative dementias) Chris MacKnight (Dalhousie University, Halifax, Nova Scotia) ("The Missed Diagnosis of Cerebrovascular Disease: Dementia with Clinical and Neuroimaged Stroke Yet Normal Neuropathology")

ISSUE: This symposium will include addresses on four topics that explore various aspects of the relationship between vascular risk factors and neurodegenerative dementias, and will highlight data from the Canadian population-based and clinic-based cohort studies. The objectives are to review the relationship between vascular risk factors and dementia, to examine the classification of mixed dementia, and to explore the impact of indication bias on the claims of causal relationships between vascular risk factors and dementia. STRUCTURE: Four presentations, synthesizing old data and presenting new information. Panel discussion and question-and-answer to follow. CONTENT:Overview: the changing face of vascular risk factors and dementia. K. Rockwood, Dalhousie University, Halifax NS Canada. For many years it was held that as people became old they became "senile" and that this was due to "hardening of the arteries". With an appreciation of the importance of neurodegenerative diseases, especially Alzheimer's disease, as entities distinct from the effects of aging, there arose an operationally sharp distinction between neurodegenerative and vascular dementias, notwithstanding the classification of so-called "mixed" dementia. Recent data from a number of fronts (clinical, epidemiological and neuropathological) have served to undermine this distinction. CONCLUSION:This session will outline important contributions to that debate, and present empirical data in support of a new clinical and radiographic classification of the types of vascular cognitive impairment and mixed dementias.

Estrogens, statins and the risk of Alzheimer's disease

Susan Kirkland (Dalhousie University, Halifax, Nova Scotia, Canada) Estrogens, statins and the risk of Alzheimer's disease

Purpose:Following initial enthusiasm for the apparently protective effect of estrogen on incident Alzheimer's disease have come the more disappointing results of intervention studies, which showed no impact on progression of dementia in randomized trials. Method:These findings are discussed in the light of recent experience with estrogen and cardiovascular disease. Result:Despite many observational studies showing an apparently protective effect of post-menopausal estrogen supplementation, intervention studies have failed to replicate this benefit. A likely explanation appears to be indication bias in the observational studies, i.e. women who self-select to take estrogen tend to be healthier than those who do not. Hence their better outcomes might reflect their better baseline health status. Lately, statins also have been shown in observational studies to be associated with a lower risk of dementia, with a relative risk reduction similar to that seen in cerebrovascular disease. Conclusions: Using data from the Canadian Study of Health and Aging, the possibility of indication bias will be examined in this context.

The Missed Diagnosis of Cerebrovascular Disease: Dementia with Clinical and Neuroimaged Stroke Yet Normal Neuropathology

Chris MacKnight and Kenneth Rockwood (Dalhousie University, Halifax, Nova Scotia, Canada) The Missed Diagnosis of Cerebrovascular Disease: Dementia with Clinical and Neuroimaged Stroke Yet Normal Neuropathology

Purpose: Despite the common assertion that vascular dementia is the second most common form of dementia, neuropathological series typically find few cases of pure vascular dementia. Most clinically-diagnosed cases are found at autopsy to have either no infarct and/or significant co-existing Alzheimer's changes. Method: Case review. Results: Two cases will be presented where the patient had a clinical diagnosis of stroke, supported by physical examination and neuroimaging. Both patients met NINDS-AIREN criteria for probable vascular dementia, and had large cortical infarcts. Neuropathology in both patients was normal, showing no changes of vascular disease or Alzheimer's disease. Conclusions: The 'gold standard' of neuropathology appears not to be as appropriate in vascular dementia as in Alzheimer's disease. Current clinical criteria also are lacking. A new, phenomenological approach is required.

Vascular risk factors in relation to common vascular and neurodegenerative dementias.

Howard Feldman (University of British Columbia, Vancouver, BC, Canada) Vascular risk factors in relation to common vascular and neurodegenerative dementias.

Vascular risk factors are seen commonly in people with dementia. This presentation will report data from two clinic-based cohort studies (The Consortium to Investigate Vascular Impairment of Cognition and A Canadian Collaborative Cohort Related Dementia) to contrast the role of vascular risk factors in vascular dementia, Alzheimer's disease, dementia with Lewy bodies and frontotemporal dementia. The CIVIC and ACCORD data underlie the argument that the concept of mixed dementia should be expanded to include all neurodegenerative dementias seen in the presence of expressions of cerebrovascular disease, but that mixed dementia cannot be diagnosed simply on the basis of neurodegenerative dementia in patients with vascular risk factors.

SESSION 176

Adhesion molecule MAC-1 and Blood pressure measurement in Elderly subjects in BELFAST study.

I.M.Rea(Department of Geriatric Medicine, Queens University, Belfast, UK), M, Armstrong, H.D.Alexander (Haematology Laboratory, Belfast City Hospital, UK) S.McMillan (ImmunoBiology Laboratory, Royal Victoria Hospital, UK).

PURPOSE: Loss of endothelial function is associated with sustained hypertension and although mechanisms are poorly understood, putative mechanisms include pro-inflammatory responses induced by mechanical stretching with cytokine release and up-regulated expression of endothelial adhesion molecules. There is some evidence that the integrin adhesion molecule MAC-1, important in tethering monocytes and neutrophils to endothelium, is up-regulated when endothelial damage is initiated. Because blood pressure increases with age, we measured MAC-1 on neutrophils, monocytes and lymphocytes to assess if there was any association with atherosclerotic risk factors including blood pressure. METHODS: In a pilot study of 33 elderly subjects (70-90+ years), selected for good health by Senieur protocol and randomly selected from the BELFAST study, baseline MAC-1 expression on monocytes and neutrophils was associated with systolic blood pressure (p=0.04) and with diastolic blood pressure for lymphocytes (p=0.05). Serum cholesterol and LDL cholesterol were associated with baseline and TNF-a stimulated MAC-1 expression on lymphocytes while measures of renal function were negatively associated with MAC-1 expression. Serum TNF-a was associated with down regulation of MAC-1 expression on lymphocytes only. CONCLUSIONS: These preliminary findings suggest that adhesion molecule expression may be differently regulated on monocytes, neutrophils and lymphocytes, that individual interpersonal factors may influence their expression but do lend support to the putative suggestion linking pro-inflammatory mechanisms to atherosclerotic risk factors.

Arterial Hypertension in an Elderly Population. Prevalence among a Third Age Open University Students

R. A. Lourenço, R. P. Veras {Rio de Janeiro State University, Rio de Janeiro, Brazil}, N. A. S. Silva {Rio de Janeiro Federal University, Rio de Janeiro, Brazil}

Purpose: The major objective was to find the prevalence of arterial hypertension among elderly students. The secondary objectives were to study the prevalence of others cardiovascular risk factors, and verify the relationships of constitutional, social, economical, and biochemical variables with blood pressure levels. Method: From a random sample of sixty years old and older students, stratified by sex, three hundred subjects (216 females) responded. The diagnosis of hypertension was based on current use of antihypertensive drugs and/or the average of 3 blood pressure measures >= 140x90mmHg. The statistics was done by Chi-square and Student's tests, and logistic regression analysis. Results: The prevalence of hypertension in the total sample was 53.3%, 48.8% males and 55.1% for females. The obesity prevalence (BMI=27kg/m2) was 44.3%, and hypercholesterolemia (TSCh=200mg/dl) was 74.9%. The prevalence of diabetes mellitus was 7.0%. The final logistic model suggested that systolic pressure was influenced by height, sex and marital state; and diastolic pressure by age, sex and marital state. Conclusion: When compared with other brasilian results our population has similar prevalence of hypertension, and lower prevalence of diabetes mellitus and tabagism; the disease awareness, treatment adhesion, and blood pressure control were similar to those found in developed countries. The logistic model explained just a little part of the total variability of blood pressure levels. However, we have to be attentive to the association between cardiovascular risk and the high prevalence of hypertension, obesity and hypercholesterolemia. This conclusion appoint to the need to create risk factors detection programs among our students.

Arterial stiffness is associated with orthostatic hypotension in elderly subjects

Jacques BODDAERT 1, Joel BELMIN 2 1 Department of Medecine Interne Geriatrique, Hopital Pitie-Salpetriere, Paris, France. 2 Department of Medecine Interne Geriatrique, Hopital Rene-Muret-Bigottini and University Paris-Nord,Sevran, France.

PURPOSE We made the hypothesis that the age-related arterial stiffeness could interfere independantly of other factors in the haemodynamic response to orthostatism. METHOD Between January and July 1998, 57 elderly patients (mean age 86, 68-98 years-old), 8 men and 49 women adressed for falls were assessed with classical method for orthostatic hypotension (OH) defined as a fall of 20 mmHg or more in systolic blood pressure (SBP) 1, 2 or 3 min after standing. The carotido-femoral and carotid-brachial pulse wave velocities (PWV) were measured using Complior device (Colson). Twenty-six young pathology-free subjects (mean age 33, 28-38 years-old) were selected to obtain reference data. RESULTS Baseline characteristics showed a higher prevalence of hypertension (63%, 48% and 0% respectively) in the elderly subjects with OH (n=33) compared to elderly subjects without OH (n=24) or young subjects (n=26). Carotid-femoral and carotid-brachial PWV were significantly higher in elderly patients with OH (respectively 16.25 +/- 2.66 and 10.98 +/- 1.05 m.sec), as compared to elderly patients without OH (14.29 +/- 2.79 and 8.55 +/- 1.95) (p<0,01) and young subjects (8 ;38 +/- 1.39 and 8.71 +/- 1.29) (p<0,01). In variance analysis, an effect of axis and group was found (p<0.0001). The difference between supine and 1 min standing SBP was significantly correlated with carotid-brachial PWV(p<0.05). CONCLUSION Our study shows that upper limb arterial stiffness was increased in elderly patients with OH as compared with young and elderly patients without OH. Arterial stiffening might intervene in the baroreflex alteration in advancing age and OH.

Body mass index, skinfold thickness and subcutaneous fat patterning in hypertensive vs. normotensive elderly Egyptians.

Ashraf H. Shaalan and Aly El-Nofely (National Research Center, Dokki, Cairo, Egypt)

Body mass index (BMI), skinfold thickness and subcutaneous fat patterning were investigated in hypertensive versus normotensive elderly Egyptians. A cross-sectional sample was chosen from institutionalized and non-institutionalized subjects in Cairo and Giza cities, whose blood pressure during physical examination is either lower than or equal to 140/90 m.m.hg. (normotensives), or higher than or equal to 160/95 m.m.hg. (hypertensives), their blood pressure history either constantly low without antihypertensive drugs intake (normotensives) or usually high with or without antihypertensive drugs intake (hypertensives), and clinically free from other diseases that might affect blood pressure. They comprised 309 subjects, of whom 132 males (79 normotensives and 53 hypertensives) and 177 females (81 normotensives and 96 hypertensives). Body weight, stature and skinfold thickness at triceps; subscapular and suprailiac areas were measured following the formal descriptions and usuing standard instruments. Three derived variables were calculated; mean of skinfold thickness as and index of total body fat, mean of subscapular and suprailiac skinfold thickness as an index of trunck fat and BMI as an index of overall adiposity. Although age was not significantly different in both normotensive versus hypertensive males and females, BMI and mean skinfold thickness were significantly lower in normotensive than hypertensive groups in both males and females. There was significantly higher deposition of peripheral fat in hypertensive males, and of central fat in hypertensive females than in normotensive males and females respectively. This conclude an association between body mass, body fat and fat patterning with blood pressure of eldrely Egyptians.

Hypertension and cardiovascular risk factors clustering in a Brazilian community. The Bambui Health and Ageing Study.

S. M. Barreto, V. M. A. Passos, J. O. A. Firmo, H. L. Guerra, P. G. Vidigal, M. F. F. Lima e Costa (Federal University of Minas Gerais Medical School, Oswaldo Cruz Foundation René Rachou Research Centre, Belo Horizonte, Brazil)

PURPOSE: The baseline data of a population-based prospective study of the aged were analysed in order to: a) determine the prevalence of hypertension in a small town; b) investigate the clustering of other cardiovascular risk factors among hypertensive individuals and c) verify whether the elderly differed from younger adults in the overall pattern of clustering. METHOD: The data comprised the whole population aged 60+ years and a representative sample of people aged 18-59 years residing in Bambui, Brazil. The independent association between hypertension (blood pressure>140/90mmHg) and other cardiovascular risk factors was investigated using multiple logistic regression. RESULTS: Hypertension is highly prevalent in this community (24.8%), especially in the elderly (61%), being positively and significantly associated with physical inactivity, overweight (BMI>25kg/m2), hypercholesterolemia, hyperglycemia and hypertriglyceridemia. Only 7% of hypertensive individuals were not exposed to other metabolic or lifestyle risk factors. The combined prevalence of selected metabolically linked risk factors increased as the population aged, both in hypertensive and normotensive individuals, but prevalence was greater among those with hypertension at all age groups. The coexistence of hypertension with four or more cardiovascular risk factors occurred six times higher than expected by chance, after adjustment for age and sex (OR=6.3;95%CI:3.4-11.9). CONCLUSION: Hypertension is variably hazardous depending on the number and severity of associated risk factors. The important clustering of cardiovascular risk factors found among hypertensive individuals has therapeutic implications, especially for the elderly because of the high prevalence of manifest atherosclerotic diseases in this group. Results reinforce the need to improve individual's global risk profile.

Intraindividual reproducibility of postprandial hypotension

F. Puisieux, D. Court, E. Baheu, H. Bulckaen, A.L. Fauchais, P. Dewailly. (Service de Médecine Interne et Gériatrie, CHRU Lille, 59037 Lille Cedex, France)

Background: Postprandial hypotension (PPH) is increasingly recognized as a common cause of falls and syncope in the elderly. No studies have addressed the variability of PPH. Objective: To assess the intraindividual reproducibility of PPH. Methods: 50 patients (42 women and 8 men; mean age: 83*8) were included in the study. To evaluate PPH, we measured blood pressure (BP) before and every 15 minutes for 90 minutes after the start of a standardized mixed meal (Jansen and Lipsitz Ann Intern Med 1995;122:286-95). PPH was defined as a decrease in systolic BP of 20 mmHg or more. Three sets of BP were obtained for each subject on two successive days: (1) in the morning of the first day between 8:00 and 10:00 a.m.; (2) in the afternoon of the first day between 4:00 and 6:00 p.m.; (3) in the morning of the second day between 8:00 and 10:00 a.m. Results: 32 participants (64%) experienced PPH on at least one test. Among them, 19 (38%) had PPH in the morning of the first day, 16 (32%) had PPH in the afternoon of the first day, and 21 (42%) had PPH in the morning of the second day. Kappa statistics indicated that intraindividual reproducibility of PPH was correct when the two morning tests were compared together (day-to-day variability; kappa value=0.6), but was low when the morning test was compared with the afternoon test (within day variability; kappa value=0.08). There was also a strong positive correlation between preprandial BP and meal-induced BP decline. Conclusions: Because of the relatively correct reproducibility of meal-induced BP changes, we conclude that the diagnosis of PPH may be based on a single standardized test, on the condition that the test was performed under circumstances (time of the meal) similar to those in which the symptoms occurred.

Isolated Systolic Hypertension in a Multiracial, Elderly Population

YC Chia (Department of Primary Care Medicine, Faculty of Medicine, University of Malaya, Kuala Lumpur, Malaysia), P srinivas (Gleneagles Hospitle, penang, Malaysia) P Poi (Department of Medicine, University of Malaya, Kuala Lumpur, Malaysia), S Ebrahim (Department of Public Health, University of Bristol, Bristol, England)

Background and Aim Isolated Systolic Hypertension (ISH) is associated with a high mortality and morbidity. The aim of this study was to examine the prevalence of ISH and its relationship to other cardiovascular risk factors in a multiracial elderly population. Methods A survey was conducted amongst 1414 elderly persons aged 55 years and over.The prevalence of known hypertension and smoking were derived from history. Measurements of blood pressure, weight, height, waist and hip circumference and blood chemistry were performed on all subjects. Age, sex and race were also examined in those found to have ISH i.e. systolic blood pressure of equal and >140 and diastolic of <90 mm Hg. Results 26.8% and 25.6% subjects were found to have ISH and conventional hypertension (BP>140/90 mm Hg) respectively on measurement. Only 19% of those with ISH knew they had hypertension. The mean age of those with ISH was 66.8 while normotensives was 64.6 ($p<0.001$). The male to female ratio was 50.4:49.6 ($p=0.88$). 45.6% were under 65 years while 54.4% were over 65 ($p=0.001$). There was no difference in the prevalence of ISH amongst the 3 racial groups (Malays, Chinese and Indians; $p>0.05$) Those found to have ISH had significantly higher cardiovascular risk factors than normotensives (mean cholesterol 5.7 v 5.6, serum glucose 7.3 v 6.3 ,BMI 22.9 v 22.1, waist-hip ratios 0.93 v 0.91,) and this was also true for smoking. (all $p<0.05$). Conclusion: The prevalence of ISH amongst the elderly was very high. The majority were not aware they had hypertension. They also carried higher cardiovascular risk factors than normotensives. In the light that ISH should be treated, greater efforts should be made at detecting ISH.

The Morning Changes of Blood Pressure as Risk Factors of Cardiovascular Events

Bonacasa R, Carbone P, Falvo F, Cantatore A, Cravello L, Ferrari A, Ferrari E. (Department of Internal Medicine and Medical Therapy, Chair of Geriatrics, University of Pavia, Italy IRCCS, "S. Matteo" Polyclinic, Preside of Belgioioso, Pavia Italy)*

The aim of this study was to evaluate the influence of age on the rate of rise (slope) of blood pression during the early morning hours in normotensive and hypertensive subjects. Ambulatory blood pression and heart rate measurements were performed by the Spacelabs 90207 monitor in 20 normotensive old subjects (mean 85 ± 2 ys), 11 untreated hypertensive old subjects (mean 89 ± 3 ys) and 18 healthy young controls (mean 44 ± 3 ys). Systolic and diastolic slope of blood pression from 06:00 to 09:00 was significantly higher in young controls where compared with normotensive old subjects (9 ± 1 mmHg/h vs 3 ± 1 mmHg/h, $p< 0.01$; 7 ± 1mmHg/h vs 4 ± 1mmHg/h, $p< 0.05$). The rate of rise of systolic blood pression from 06:00 to 09:00 was significantly greater in untreated hypertensive old subjects, by comparison to normotensive old subjects (7±1 mmHg/h vs 3±1 mmHg/h, $p< 0.05$). A significant age-related decline of systolic blood pression slope occurred in normotensive subjects ($p< 0.05$). Since it is well known that the early morning hours are characterized by a peculiar incidence of acute cardiovascular events, the evaluation of the slope of blood pressure and heart rate in this time may be particularly useful for the assessment of the risk factor for catastrophic cardiovascular events.

Predictors of the Atrial Fibrillation in Old and Senile Age

N.N.Kiphidze; T.G.Zubiashvili; G.A.Donadze. (Research Institute of Experimental and clinical Therapy, Tbilisi, Georgia)

The aim of the paper was to study the cause of arising the atrial fibrillation (AF) in patients of old and senile age. The results of the examination of 112 patients with the diagnosis of paroxysmal form of AF and 30 patients with constant form of AF (disease began after physical lading), old (60-74y) and senile (75-89y) entered the given work. Both men and women underwent examination. Period of disease from 1 to 6 years. Patients underwent clinico-instrumental complex examination, including anamnesis, objective investigation, ECG, 24h ECG monitoring, test with physical load on the veloergometre and echocardiographic investigations. As a result of the carried out investigations the atrium extrasystolia (AE) was fixed in 83.90f patients on ECG in a repose. In some cases extrasystolia had the allorhytmic character. After 24h of ECG monitoring AF paroxisms were observed in 82.90f patients with initial AE, while before the beginning of AF paroxisms, increase of AF frequency was observed. Test with phisical load provoked arising of AF paroxisms, which always arised after activation of AE. In patients with AF, significant increasing of left atrium sized and left atrium/aort index was noted (especially in patients with constant form of AF) in comparison with patients without AE. Hence, presence of AE can be marker of AF arising.

SESSION 177

Control and rights: Quality of life and quality of care in institutional care

Susan Tester (University of Stirling, Stirling, Scotland, United Kingdom) Gill Hubbard (University of Stirling, Stirling, Scotland, United Kingdom)Murna Downs (University of Bradford, England, United Kingdom)

The paper presents early findings of a current three year study Exploring perceptions of quality of life for frail older people during and after their transition to institutional care, funded within the UK ESRC Growing Older Research Programme. The main aim of this study is to contribute to understanding of the meaning of quality of life for frail older people. One specific objective, addressed by this paper, is to examine links between quality of life in institutional care and quality of care. The study takes an ethnographic approach, giving priority to the views of frail older people. This paper draws on two early stages which developed themes for later fieldwork with individual residents. First, six focus groups with older people and carers in the community explored the group members' perceptions of life in nursing homes, based on their experiences of visiting homes. Second, researchers undertook general observation in six nursing homes, over 24 hours, using qualitative methods with a framework based on focus group findings. Key themes from initial findings concerned frailty, strength and control, identity and rights. Focus group members perceived that older people lost control over daily activities as nursing home residents, but that, however frail, many were able to maintain some physical or mental strength and the ability to assert control. They observed that although nursing home residents lost aspects of their identity, some identities could be maintained through exercise of rights and choices. The paper concludes that professional carers have an important role in enabling residents to exercise control and rights; it stresses the importance of verbal and non-verbal communication and emotion in promoting quality of life; and identifies the findings' implications for care policy and planning.

Effects of Empowerment Strategies on Veterans' Satisfaction with Food Quality and Service in Long Term Care

C. Lovett-Smith & M. Gorman (Queen Elizabeth II Health Sciences Centre, Halifax, NS, Canada)

The purpose of this study is to explore the issue of quality of life and satisfaction re food quality and food services in a Veterans' Long Term Care facility. Food is considered to be pivotal quality of life issue with such residents and thus can represent contentment with their current "home" environment as well as being a vehicle of control within the same environment. This study extends its quality assurance evaluation by including staff perceptions of veterans' satisfaction levels. Results from repeated questionnaires in 1997, 1999, 2000 (and 2001) show that satisfaction with both food quality and delivery improves with an increase in the use of empowering strategies: (a) direct involvement (e.g, regular weekly meetings between staff and veterans), (b) enhancement of delivery style (e.g, bulk food with hostess present) and (c) in general, management attempts to respond to veterans's concerns and ratings of satisfaction. The Satisfaction Survey as well as unobtrusive measures of weight change, "clean plates", and food wastage are used to triangulate data to show that Veterans are increasingly more satisfied than in 1997 and that these empowering methods all contribute to the veterans' greater quality of life. Discussion includes the pragmatics of budgetary responsibility and the need to balance this with the degree of satisfaction possible (or dissatisfaction tolerated) given that "food " can be considered a control device for the veterans.

Health outcomes for people living in long term care facilities.

L. Robichaud, P. J. Durand (Geriatric Research Unit of Laval University, Quebec city, Canada), R. Bédard (CLSC-CHSLD Haute-ville Des Rivières, Quebec city, Canada) , J. P. Ouellet (CLSC-CHSLD Les Sources, Quebec city, Canada)

This project aimed to explore the quality of life outcomes as perceived by residents and familly caregivers. The qualitative study was undertaken with 27 participants from five nursing homes in Quebec city, between 1998 and 1999. Semi-structured individual interviews were used for this grounded theory study. Theoritical sampling was used to select participants including equal numbers of residents and familly caregivers from each nursing home. Eligibility for the study was restricted to residents over the age of 65, able to communicate. Interviews were tape-recorded, transcribed and checked for accuracy. Trustworthiness techniques relevant to the study were selected from four criteria, (Guba 1981) : credibility, transferability, dependability and confirmability. The findings relate the characteristics of an optimal living environment. The main quality of life outcomes are : possibility of taking care of peers, feeling of being part of a group, self-respect (for both residents and caregivers), feeling of reciprocity within the relationships, emotional support within the physical assistance, competence, open-minded and flexible organization, well adapted services and activities to the needs of physical and mental health and well adapted environment to the needs of care and self-realization. These outcomes will be discussed first as essentiel for caregivers to reinforce their human attitudes and second as usefull for researchers to develop or adapt measures of quality of life. In conclusion, the Maslow pyramid of needs is still essentiel to guide the human development from the physiological to the self-realization needs.

How do residents appreciate their quality of life in old people's home.

Merrot S, Randoux L, Thomas L, Frigard B. Centre de Gériatrie - Wasquehal, France

What glance do the residents fit to their old people's home and daily? How do they smell integrated in this home? Do they feel affected by the functioning of their institution? We conducted an inquiry concerning old people's homes in the North of France. All residents were subjected to MMS and to a depression scale. A prolonged interview was offered to every person in the aim to transcribe it on a detailed and systematized questionnaire. There is an evident indifference with regard to general and official texts, since they do not concern the daily. The weak investment of the resident is usual : most of them are satisfied by state of their old people's home, very few (20%) suggest solutions or improvements. Family win back to a place which was lost, the decline related to multifaceted ageing is more dreaded than death. The felt fatalism don t have to incite to resignation : efforts should be pursued so that the residents got involved about their own life in institution and not conceived as simple spectators. What to suggest? The placing being dreaded more by fatalism than by spontaneity, an important effort should be spread by an efficient psychological approach during the months preceding the admission : this waiting period (always insufficient) is indispensable. Progressive contact of institutions allows to future resident to observe its pace of life with impartiality, specially to be integrated in a dynamic way and provided projects.

Interests and Needs of Long-term Care Residents-Study and Practical Application

P. Andrews (Vancouver Hospital and Health Sciences Centre Δ VGH Site, Vancouver, BC, Canada), J. Clark (Vancouver Hospital and Health Sciences Centre - UBC Site, Vancouver, BC, Canada), R. Wang (Three Bridges Community Health Centre, Vancouver Richmond Health Board, Vancouver, BC, Canada)

This study was initiated to explore needs and interests of a specific geriatric population in an institutionalized setting. A random group of 20% of the facility's residents were surveyed. Participation was determined on a probability basis through systematic sampling. Data from these residents was collected in seven categories Δ rise/retire schedules, dressing/bathing, meals, mobility, interests, social and general topics (including spirituality). The survey process was adapted to meet the needs of individual residents. In addition, an anonymous staff questionnaire solicited staff perceptions of these same topics (response rate: approx. 20%). After data correlation, fundamental similarities and differences emerged. Examples of parallels: (1) the value of support from caring staff; (2) the problem of repetition and lack of variety in diet; (3) the negative impact of lack of privacy. Noteworthy inconsistencies included: (1) the greater importance placed by residents (vs. staff) on opportunities for excursions outside the facility; (2) the belief by a significantly greater percentage of staff than residents that there is a need to enhance the weekend/evening activity schedule. As it is the underlying philosophy of long-term care that each facility is the residents' home, it is essential that the needs and preferences of this population be respected. The study provided a baseline and valuable data, as well as insight and benefits to the long-term care setting. The results of the surveys have been used to make changes to the residents' environment, arrange appropriate staffing schedules, enhance program planning and have been effective in improving resident/family relationships.

Quality of Long-Term Institutional Care Frm the viewpoint of Informal Caregivers and Nursing Personnel

ML.Perälä, O.Räikkönen (National Research and Development Centre for Welfare and Health, Helsinki, Finland)

PURPOSE: Despite of the emphases of the Finnish health and social policy the quantity of institutional care was not been able to reduce due to insufficient home care services and the increased number of the elderly people. Concurrently qualified services in long-term institutions were demanded. In this study the quality of long-term institutional care was described and explained from the viewpoint of patients informal care givers (relatives) and nursing personnel. The focus was the sufficiency of help received, patients self-determination and patients collaboration with personnel. METHOD: The queries were answered by 2441 relatives who visited patients in institutions during two weeks at the end of 1998 and by the nursing personnel of study institution (n=2969). The data was cross-tabulated (chi-square) and analysed using the analysis of variance. RESULTS: The results of informal care givers and nursing personnel were parallel. The quality of care was best in the private service houses and private nursing homes, and worse in heath centres and public nursing homes. The more in need of care that the patient was, the less the relatives were satisfied with the sufficiency of care given and with the collaboration with health care personnel. Spouses and daughters of the patients were most dissatisfied and older relatives and the relatives of older patients were the most satisfied with the care. Patients were rather well-informed about their care issues. Especially elder relatives and patients who were less in need of care were satisfied. Willingness to participate seems also closely related to patients ability to decide and participate. However, the possibilities to participate were related to patients' willingness.

What's Important to Residents in Aged Care Facilities?

D.P. Boldy and S. Chou (Department of Health Policy and Management, Curtin University of Technology, Perth, Western Australia)

The residential aged care standards and accreditation process in Australia identifies consumer (resident) satisfaction as a key component of quality improvement and an expected outcome of care. However, only a limited amount of relevant research has actually been undertaken from the resident's perspective. This paper will describe such a study, which uses valid and reliable questionnaires. The overall purpose was to develop a method of measuring resident satisfaction in aged care facilities and to explore the relationship of 'satisfaction' to: (1) organisational factors (such as size, age and location of a facility); (2) staff factors (such as job satisfaction, experience, staffing level, and mix); and (3) resident factors (such as age, sex and dependency level). The ultimate aim was to provide information for eventual improvement in residential aged care services. The study involved a total of 70 aged care facilities, 983 staff and 1146 residents. Key findings from the study include the fact that satisfaction with staff care has a significantly positive impact on all aspects of resident satisfaction and that staff satisfaction itself is also significant. This latter aspect appears to be more important than actual care hours provided. The staff recruitment and training implications of these and other findings will be discussed within the wider framework of aged care funding and regulation processes in Australia.

SESSION 178

Canadian and Korean Stereotypes about Communication Skills in Old Age

Ellen Bouchard Ryan (McMaster University, Hamilton, Canada), Young-sun Jin (Kyung Pook National University, Taegu, South Korea) and Ann P. Anas (McMaster University, Hamilton, Canada)

This cross-cultural study examined whether stereotypes of the communication skills of older adults would be more positive among Korean adults than among Canadians, especially among older respondents. Recent research suggests that traditional norms of filial piety and honoring elders may not currently be as strong in the East as once thought, but little of this work has incorporated the views of the old. The sample (N = 448) consisted of young and older adults from both Canada (Mean ages = 19.7 and 71.8 years) and South Korea (Mean ages = 20.5 and 64.9). Respondents rated either a typical 25-year-old target or a typical 75-year-old target on a variety of communication skills designed to elicit both negative and positive stereotypes of aging. Young targets were viewed more favorably with regard to the hearing-memory factor by all four country/age groups while old targets were rated higher in terms of the storytelling factor among all but the older respondents from Korea. No overall target age effect was observed for social skills, but a predicted ingroup effect revealed for both countries that the young and older participants each gave higher ratings to their own age group. No target age effects were observed for the other factors, benevolence and complaining. These data highlight the universality of pro-young stereotypes about hearing and memory and the variation of positive pro-old stereotypes among country and participant age groups. The findings are interpreted in light of direct assessments of filial piety norms.

DO CANADIAN SENIORS INVEST OR DIVEST IN FINANCIAL, SOCIAL AND HUMAN CAPITAL

Satya Brink, (Gerontology Research Centre, Simon Fraser University, Vancouver, Canada)

This research tests the validity of the popular view that seniors cease to accumulate financial, social and human capital after their working lives and that they are consumers rather than contributors. Indicators of financial , social and human capital were examined based on national survey data from Statistics Canada. Analyses showed that, despite variation, Canadian seniors continue to invest, rather than only divest, in all forms of capital. Financial capital may be held in non-liquid assets, such as housing, but seniors also have liquid assets and continue to save as well as pay taxes. About a fifth of assets is held on average as investments. Eighty percent of seniors made financial donations and they were larger on average than for other sub-populations. Despite the loss of the work context, human capital development measured in learning and new skills continues. In 1996, 20,000 were enrolled in a formal education program. They are the fastest growing group in the use of computers, doubling the percent of users in the year 1997. Social capital activities also persist with a quarter of all seniors engaging in volunteer activities, and contributing more hours than other age groups. Over a third provide assistance to family and friends while over eighty percent received assistance. These indicators show an increasing trend for seniors cohorts over time but tend to fall with age.

One Day I'll Be Old Too!

T. A. Seedsman, S. Feldman, H. Mahoney (Alma Unit for Research on Ageing, Victoria University of Technology, Melbourne, Australia)

This two-stage research project aimed to measure children's perceptions of ageing and to combine that information with the views of their teachers and older people working with them to develop sustainable curriculum initiatives to strengthen intergenerational relations. The study involved eight primary schools, two of which were control schools. Pre- and post-tests were given to children in Grade 4 (N=288) using the survey instrument Children's Views on Aging by authors Sally Newman and Ronald Marks. The pre-test was followed by an intervention and the children were then post-tested to determine if their attitudes toward older people or ageing had changed. Qualitative evaluations from the adults (55+) involved in the interventions (N=18) and the teachers (N=19). The curriculum initiatives were developed within a partnership program between Victoria University's teacher training and one of the experimental schools. Data analyses generated two main themes: first, children value their relationship with older people; and second, while they value this relationship, they have a negative view of the physical, social and emotional effects of ageing. The children's attitudes toward older people and their own ageing selves was not altered by the intervention. The older adults and teachers felt the interventions had been beneficial to themselves and the children. The children valued older people, however they did not view the ageing process favourably. Teachers and older adults believed in the value of older people being involved in children's learning activities. Sustainability of this intergenerational initiative was found to be dependent upon a centralised infrastructure.

Taking the time to age with excellence

J.A. Frederick, (Statistics Canada, Ottawa, Canada) J.E. Fast (University of Alberta, Edmonton, Alberta)

PURPOSE: Society's views of aging are clouded by a layer of myths that would have us believe that the aged are sick, demendted, frail, weal, disabled powerless, sexless, passive, alone, unhappy and failing. Like most myths, the ones about aging are a bewildering blend of trth and fancy. METHOD: This paper uses Statistics Canada's 1998 General social survey on time use ot examine the lifestyles and perceptions of quality of life of about 1000 respondents age 70 and over. RESULTS: Findings suggest that only a small group of seniors, those who are unattached and living with others, fit the myth. They had the most leisure time of all, so much so thay they also reported having time on their hands that they didnt know what to do with. They slept more than other seniors and spent the least time on unpaid work—domestic work, family care and volunteer work. They also were the most stressed and least satisfied with their health, finances and life overall. CONCLUSION: The vast majority—married seniors living with a spouse and widowed seniors living alone—were generally health, active, independent, socially integrated and happy.

Tom, Mick or Esther? How the British media patronises older people and ageing issues

S.B.Burke (Daycare Trust, London, UK)

Purpose: This paper examines British media coverage of older people and ageing issues to identify the impact on older people, policymaking and public understanding Method: The author was communications consultant for the British Society of Gerontology and the Better Government for Older People programme in 1999-2000. The paper focuses on three stories which attracted media coverage then: a) older people as 'mystery passengers' testing the quality of London buses b) recommendations to Government to tackle ageism and improve the image of older people c) research on religious attitudes as people age The media coverage has been analysed for its messages, portrayal of older people and implications for Government. The author interviewed older people about the coverage and policymakers about its effect. Results: All three stories received substantial coverage. But older people were portrayed as 'undercover spies' with sinister, snide overtones; Tom Jones, Mick Jagger and Esther Rantzen were identified as role models for the new generation of older people; and older people were presented as inflexible despite evidence of changing opinions. For older people, this coverage reinforced negative feelings towards the media. For policymakers, it deterred and delayed Government from responding to recommendations challenging these perceptions of older people. Conclusion: British media often trivialise ageing issues, patronising older people as 'old, helpless and grey' with a knock-on effect on policymaking and public attitudes. The paper highlights the need for a campaign by older people, Government and media to change the image of older people and the way the media reports ageing issues.

Who Cares? Growing Old in an Ageing World

Haim Hazan (The Herczeg Institute on Aging Tel Aviv University Tel Aviv, Israel)

Who Cares? Growing Old in an Ageing Country Haim Hazan Viewed within a socio historical context, growing old in Israel is unfolded as a cultural narrative exteding from invisibility to visibility. The disourse of visibility alters in correspondence with societal transformations such as demographic changes. globalization. ethno-religious orientations and post-Zionist trends. Three case studies are analyzed to demonstrate the effects of these processes on alternative conceptions of the status of the old. It is suggested that the seemingly diverse patterns of care for the old in Israeli soceity are embedded in a collective mode of exchange. Care for the old in Israel is thus interpreted in terms of generalized reciprocity applying to both the Zionist nation-state and to its post-modern era. Notwithstanding the differences in social identity, memory and selfhood, old age is perceived by elderly and non-elderly alike as ambivalence consisting of the invisibility of the excluded other and the visibility of collective conscience. This contradiction is sustained by sponsored settings for the old promoting both exclusion and inclusion.

SESSION 179

Being at risk of dementia: fears and anxieties of older adults

Lynne Corner (Centre for Health Services Research, University of Newcastle, Newcastle upon Tyne, UK)John Bond (Centre for Health Services Research, University of Newcastle, Newcastle upon Tyne, UK)

PURPOSE: The purpose of the study is to identify the knowledge level of older adults about dementia and to determine the fears and concerns of older people about getting dementia. METHOD: The prevalence of dementia rises markedly with age. 18 million people worldwide have dementia and in 25 years, 34 million people will have dementia (Alzheimer's Disease International, 2000). As part of a study exploring what quality of life means for people with dementia and their carers, the views of older adults without dementia are also being sought using qualitative methods. RESULTS: Preliminary findings reflect a negative discourse about dementia. Participants expressed confusion over diagnosis of dementia and how this differed from 'normal' ageing. Their narratives reinforce negative sterotypes and assumptions about the experience of dementia. Uncertainty about possible genetic links and environmental causes was a source of considerable anxiety. The perceived stigma surrounding dementia, uncertainty over and anxieties about admission to long term care are also key themes. CONCLUSION: Understanding the concerns of older adults will inform what information older people need to receive from statutory and voluntary organisations.

Continuing constructions of the self: biographical approaches in dementia care

Jonathan Parker and B. Penhale (University of Hull, UK)

Purpose: This paper will explicate some of the ways in which older people with dementia continue to develop identity and ascribe meaning to aspects of their lives through the processes of reminiscence and biography. Methods: The paper is based on the authors' research into reminiscence and biographical work with older people with dementia. This research was conducted using a range of qualitative techniques designed to give voice to the experiences of older people and maximise opportunities for participation. The study included a European dimension as it was conducted over three sites (UK, Sweden, France), and was continued in further work in the UK. Results: Qualitative methods were employed and, therefore, results remain at a (rich) descriptive level. Increased verbalisation, participation and social activity were recognised across all study sites. Benefits for those involved were found in terms of increased quality of life (across subjective dimensions), and in relation to matters of identity (re)formation. Conclusion: The methods and results indicate that biographical and reminiscence methods can be used effectively with people with dementia. The implications for education and training in the fields of social and health care practice are evident. The paper will conclude with a call for greater attention to the processes involved in creating an active partnership with people with dementia in an attempt to maximise social inclusion in care practices.

Correlates of Personal Concerns about Developing Alzheimer's Disease among Middle-Aged Persons

S. J. Cutler (Dept. of Sociology, University of Vermont, Burlington, VT, USA), L. G. Hodgson (Dept. of Sociology, Quinnipiac University, Hamden, Ct, USA)

This study examines correlates of personal concerns about developing Alzheimer's disease (AD) among middle-aged persons. The data are from telephone interviews with two subsamples of respondents, 40-60 years of age: (1) adult children who have a living parent with a diagnosis of probable AD (N=108); and (2) a matched comparison group of persons with no parental history of AD (N=150). The dependent variable is a single item asking respondents to indicate along a 4-point scale how concerned they are about personally developing AD. Using stepwise regression, predictors measuring subjective perceptions of memory functioning, overall family history of AD, knowledge of AD, and demographic and socioeconomic characteristics were entered into models for the total sample and each of the subsamples. For all respondents, being an adult child of a parent with AD, being worried about one's ability to remember, being female, having greater knowledge of AD, and being married emerged as significant predictors (adj. R-squared=.360). Among the adult children, only two predictors were significant: being worried about one's ability to remember and having higher levels of education (adj. R-squared=.160). For the comparison group, being worried about one's ability to remember and having greater knowledge of AD, poorer assessments of everyday memory functioning, and lower levels of education were significant (adj. R-squared=.193). These results indicate that worries about memory functioning play a consistent role in personal concerns about developing AD across both groups, but that additional pathways to personal concerns differ among individuals having and not having a parent with AD.

Dementia: A Complex Journey of Transitions

Susan Slaughter (Bethany Care Society, Calgary, Canada) and Jane Bankes (Calgary Regional Health Authority, Calgary, Canada)

In this session we will outline a model which describes the progressive, dynamic nature of dementia and the ongoing impact of the disorder on the functional abilities of persons who experience dimentia. The model suggests a range of abilities possible for persons at any given point within the illness trajectory. This range of abilities may be influenced by excess disability. Information and support is necessary for staff, families and the older person as they learn and adjust to various transition points. The goal in using this model is to optimise functional ability of the person experiencing dementia, and to support the work of families and care providers.

Insight and quality of life in dementia

John Bond (Centre for Health Services Research, University of Newcastle, Newcastle upon Tyne, UK Lynne Corner (Centre for Health Services Research, University of Newcastle, Newcastle upon Tyne, UK)

PURPOSE: The medicalisation of insight labels the person with dementia as lacking functional, psychological and social competencies. The process of labelling influences the behaviour and practice of the person with dementia and their informal caregivers, particularly their perceptions of risk. The purpose of this analysis is to investigate the impact on the quality of life of people with dementia of being labelled as having loss of insight. METHOD: Qualitative data from participant observation and focused interviews with people with dementia and their informal caregivers. RESULTS: Qualitative data illustrate the extent to which individuals' lives are controlled by different perceptions of risk. We report case studies of older people with dementia and their informal caregivers which highlight the way that the activities pursued by people with dementia are controlled by caregivers protecting their 'loved ones' from perceived risks resulting from lack of insight. CONCLUSION: Understanding how caregivers perceive and value risks will inform the development of suitable educational methods and materials. Catherine Brennand Centre for Health Services Research 21 Claremont Place University of Newcastle upon Tyne NE2 4AA UK Tel: +44 (0)191 222 7046 Fax: +44 (0)191 222 6043 Email: C.M.Brennand@ncl.ac.uk

Perspectives on Embodiment and their Implications for Understanding Alzheimer's Disease

P.C. Kontos (University of Toronto, Ontario, Canada)

PURPOSE: There has been a proliferation of texts in the social sciences and humanities under the paradigm of embodiment that share the assertion that culture, power and discourse are embodied phenomena rendering the body intimately related to, and, to differing degrees, constituted by the social nature of human life. Drawing on Pierre Bourdieu's concept of "habitus" and Margaret Lock's concept of "local biology", I explore an alternative way of conceptualizing Alzheimer's disease, one that transcends the mind/body dualism, by granting the body creative and intentional capacity for perceiving and experiencing. METHOD: The literary texts Scar Tissue, by Michael Ignatieff, and Elegy for Iris, by John Bayley, are treated as sources of data to analyze the relationship between biology, intentionality and the physical/cultural surroundings in Alzheimer's disease. RESULTS: The narratives of these texts illuminate a notion of agency that is an attribute of the body and not inferred necessarily from consciousness. They offer evidence of the notion of a bodily consciousness, separate from mental consciousness. This notion challenges the biomedical discourse on Alzheimer's disease which assumes that only the mind relates us to the world and, consequently, that cognitive impairment implies a body that has no intention or identity. CONCLUSION: Approaching Alzheimer's disease within a paradigm of embodiment recognizes that bodily consciousness is an integral part of who we are as sentient beings. This alternative theory of the body illuminates aspects of human existence that are hidden if the study of Alzheimer's disease is approached only with the tools of biomedicine.

Social World of Dementia: Inner Experience and Cognitive Loss

R.Goodman (Baycrest Centre for Geriatric Care, Toronto, Canada)

A pilot ethnographic study was conducted with a group of elders with moderate cognitive loss, residing in a long-term care facility, to ascertain how they construct their social world. When ways of knowing and remembering begin to falter for older people with cognitive loss, dynamic processes emerge. These processes of negotiations between self and social environment is the focus of a qualitative study that examines the construction of meaning of self, of life, by older people as they sustain increasing cognitive loss. Through interviews and participation-observation of a therapeutic women's group, insight into their social world emerges. Feelings and emotions bound up with salient themes in their narrative are explored. A sense of purpose in life, the meaning of experiences, are given voice in daily interactions. A person's relational abilities, awareness and interest in others, tendency to trust others, all contribute to how an "impaired" person experiences institutional living. Elements of personhood need validation through opportunities to exercise competencies. Enhancing subjective meaning related to quality of life issues, highlights the critical importances of understanding the social world of the older person with cognitive loss.

The Exploration of Self-determined Behavior and Activity

Vignettes in Residents Experiencing Senile Dementia

D. Marcy-Edwards, N.K. Grant (Faculty of Nursing,The University of Calgary), S. Slater (Father Lacombe Nursing Home)

Abstract Purpose: To describe the behaviors of 54 residents living in a nursing home suffering from SDAT (senile dementia of the Alzheimer type) or related dementias during interactions with vignettes. A vignette (Hiatt, 1994) is a designated area within the residential care setting which contains clusters of objects designed to both attract attention and encourage interaction / exploration. Method: Vignettes were created to reflect areas of interest residents may have experienced in the past. Four separate vignettes were designed and included a gardening centre, a dressing table, an office / desk centre and a craft table. They were located in a position in the environment which was easily viewed and accessed by residents. Each vignette remained in place for 7 days and was immediately followed by a new vignette. The vignettes went through a second rotation, with data being collected for a total period of 56 days. Three camera, 24 hour video surveillance was used to monitor the vignette site and provide the data for the study. Basic demographic data collected included gender, age, previous occupation, and hobbies. Cognitive ability was assessed using the MMSE, and the single question geriatric depression assessment evaluated depressive behavior. Results: Residents who brought themselves to the vignette spent less time than residents who were brought by a staff member, family member or volunteer (mediators). Time spent at vignettes sites was dependent upon the type of mediation that occurred at the vignette. The mediator who interacted with the resident and objects, and who encouraged resident interaction with the objects, significantly increased time spent at the vignette site. Residentfis whose mediators only interacted with the objects in the vignette and did not encourage resident interaction with objects spent less time, and residentfis whose mediators merely brought the resident to the site and interacted with neither the resident nor the objects spent similar amounts of time as those who were self mediated. Objects selected for interaction were commonly bright in colour, unusual in shape and size, offered texture or were previously unknown to the user i.e. glove stretcher, feather boa. Conclusion: Vignettes attracted residents with moderate to severe congitive impairment, time spent at vignettes was influenced by mediation, and objects selected for manipulation were bright, textured, required manipulation and often unusual.

SESSION 180

Ageing in 2020: What Prospects for Future Elderly Cohorts in Great Britain?

Maria Evandrou (Age Concern Institute of Gerontology, Kings College London, UK), Jane Falkingham (Department of Social Policy, London School of Economics, UK).

The number of persons aged 65 and over living in Britain will increase by 50% between 2000 and 2020. Little attention, however, has been paid to the likely socio-economic characteristics of the post-war 'baby boom' generations in Britain in the twenty-first century, and how they may differ from previous cohorts of elderly people. This paper examines the demographic, social and economic experiences of four different birth cohorts over the period 1974-1998 using data from the British General Household Survey. The experiences of two cohorts currently in old and late-middle age (born in the period 1616-20 and 1931-35) are compared with those of two younger cohorts, taken to represent those entering retirement in 2020-30 (born in the 1940s and 1960s). The analysis focuses on three key areas - living arrangements, health, and resources. Changes in demographic behaviour have implications for the continued reliance on the family as a source of social care for tomorrow's elders, with a decline in the potential supply of care from spouses and children of the 1960s Baby Boomers. The evidence on the health of future elders is mixed; it may be premature to assume that tomorrow's elders will be healthier. Successive cohorts of men both enter the labour market later and leave earlier, and have lower overall participation rates at any given age. In contrast, women from the 1960s cohort experience higher rates of participation at any given age than earlier cohorts and longer working lives, thus increasing their potential pension entitlements.

Aging processes in China and Canada: Similarities and differences

Jacques Légaré and Mo Long Centre interuniversitaire d'études démographiques Département de démographie, Université de Montréal Montréal, Canada

Purpose : To show, by a case study, that even if all countries of the world will age intensively during the XXI century, processes will vary from one to the other. Method: Using information on ages structures for a descriptive comparative analysis. Results: According to official UN projections, both Canada and China will have near 300f their total population aged 60 and over in 2050. Such tresholds will have been reached through very different processes in terms of timing and speed. Conclusion: Even if both countries will try to limit their population aging, policies used will differ. Canada will mainly recourse to migration policies while China will have mainly to revise its fertility control measures.

Comparative Analysis of Rates of Aging of the Populations in the Crimea, Kyiv and Western Ukraine Based on Biological Age

L.Ena, N.Akhaladze, A.Tokar, I.Belaya (Institute of Gerontology Academy of Medical Sciences, Kiev, Ukraine)

The rates of aging of the following three populations were studied: the aborigenal population of Western Ukraine (367 persons, sample I), Southern Ukraine - migrants from Russia (364 persons, sample II), Central Ukraine - Kyiv (424 persons, sample III) based on definition of biological age (÷A). METHOD: The following parameters were assessed and correlations with calendar age made: systolic pressure (SP), diastolic pressure (DP), pulse pressure (PP), vital lung capacity (VLC), breath holding after exhalation (BhE), body weight (BW), hearing threshold (HTh), static balance (SB), subjective scoring of health (SSH), Veksler test (VT), ECG indeces (R-R, Q-T). Interpopulational comparisons were carried on using the formula of ÷A, which had been developed by a method of multiple linear regression. Development of such formula was one of the research objectives. RESULTS: the formulas for definition of ÷A have been developed: ÷A (men) =57.964 + 0.056* PP - 0.0069* VLC - 0.126*SB + 0.614*SSH + 0.131*BW; R2=0.56 BA (women) =28.800 + 0.099*BW + 0.1216*SP + 0.1087*PP - 0.1014*SB + 0.767*SSH - 0.0074*VLC; R2=0.55 The coefficients of simple regress between ÷A and calendar age reflect the speed of age changes. I: Man ÷A = 0.974* age (R2 = 0.965) Woman ÷A = 0.975* age (R2 = 0.959) II: Man ÷A = 0.943* age (R2 = 0.921) Woman ÷A = 0.936* age (R2= 0.946) III: Man ÷A = 0.972* age (R2 = 0.959) Woman ÷A = 0.958* age (R2 = 0.947) The allocation of groups of persons with varying rate of aging has shown that interpopulational distinction consisted of prevalence two extremes, i.e. slowed down (11-21 % of population) and accelerated (8-14 % of population) rates aging. Factor analysis has shown varying contribution of separate parameters in ÷A formation in populations. CONCLUSION: The population of Southern Ukraine is characterized by an accelerated rate of aging, and that of Western Ukraine by a decelerated rate. This findings correlates with the average life expectancy. Each population was found to be heterogenous, including people with decelerated normal and decelerated aging.

Demographic aspects of ageing population in Albania

Fiqiri Sherri, Fatmir Mema (Albanian Association of Demographers, Tirana, Albania)

Purpose: The need for a real strategy for protection, socioeconomic development, and health care of an ageing population in Albania during the difficult transition period. Being sensible not only of central and local governments but also increasing the level of participation of civil society in helping the ageing population. Method: Collection of information from different sources, field survey through questionnaires, and socioeconomic analyses of the real situation and problems of the ageing population. Results: Until now, the ratio of economic dependence of the ageing population has been very low, but it is not a less difficult feature because of a high level of unemployment within the country. The health care is at a low level mainly based on the very low pension. The high level of emigration during the last decade has had an impact not only on the age structure of the entire population, but also on the composition of Albanian family, especially on the ageing population. The problems are more troublesome in the rural areas compared with urban areas. Conclusion: The situation is going to become worse because the ratio of economic dependence will increase around 50% within the year 2020 and will be 2.5 times higher within the year 2050. The change of the demographic structure of the ageing population will be a factor for changing the profile of morbidity. An additional factor will be the epidemiological transition based on the socio-economic changes and standard of living.

Demographic Situation and Process of Ageing in St.-Petersburg

V.Dorofeyev (St.-Petersburg Bureau of Medical Statistics, Russia), I.Piettila (Kuntokallio Foundation, Finland)

This analysis has been prepared within the frameworks of the IPSE Improving the Planning of Medical and Social Services within Elder Care in St. Petersburg project of the European Commission s Tacis. The demographic situation was in a base for starting the IPSE project. Demographic ageing in St.-Petersburg is proceeds under influence of combined factors. Birth rate occupies a last place amongst all subjects of Russia. Population pyramid to 1999 has gained strongly pronounced retrogressive type. The most negative situation is noted in death-rate of persons of able-bodied age. From 1981 to 1999 absolute number of persons 60 years old and over in St.-Petersburg was enlarged on 31,2%, including at an age 85 years and over - more then in two times. At that number of total population of city was enlarged on 1,0% only. On the forecast to 2011 number of population over able-bodied age will increase on 8% else and total number of population of city will decreased on 6%. Thus, in perspective the dependency ratio for persons of elderly age will increase that will deepen economic and social problems. During 1981-1999 was noted yearly increasing of old age coefficient, average age of population, coefficient of ageing and longevity coefficient. For this period a number of persons 60 years and over was enlarged on 38% quicker, than number of rest part of population. For the last 5 years average future lifetime for the elderly had increased on 11,2%-15,6% in different age groups, life expectancy for newborns was enlarged on 7,9%. Thus, in St.-Petersburg is noted sharply denominated process of population ageing which has certain consequences in demographic, economic and social aspects.

Growing from a copy to an original. Increasing nominal scale dispersion in ageing populations.

Bo G. Eriksson (Department of Sociology, University of Göteborg, Sweden)

Purpose: It is a common assumption in many gerontological textbooks and research publications that individuals compared to each other in an ageing population become more and more unique. The validity of this assumption is rarely documented. Such documentation is even more rare when it comes to properties measured on nominal scales. The purpose of this paper is to present a set of dispersion measurements and an application of one such measurement first, in a the total Swedish population and secondly in a longitudinal population study of 70-years-olds in Göteborg, Sweden Method: First, a set of measurements is presented and a measure that is suited for statistical inference from a sample to a population is chosen for the study. The property studied in the total population is marital status. The property studied in the sample constituting the longitudinal population study of 70-years-olds is type of housing. Results: There is an increased dispersion in marital status in the total ageing population with two maxima followed by a decrease in the oldest part of the population. There is an increasing dispersion in type of housing in the sample studied. Conclusion: There is a good measurement of nominal scale dispersion. These two examples show that for different properties there is no support for a general assumption of increasing dispersion in ageing populations.

The Demographic change Δ how can societies face the challenge? Main Results and Recommendations of the Federal Parliamentary Study Commission on Demographic Change in Germany

Gerhard Naegele (University of Dortmund/Institute of Gerontology at the University of Dortmund, Germany)

Because Germany will - like many other countries - undergo a dramatic demographic change, the Federal Parliament established a special „Study Commission on Demographic Change„ in 1992. The purpose of this commission is to analyse the consequences of this change for the individual as well as for the society, draw conclusions, and develop political recommendations for the forthcoming decades. The work of the commission, whose members are scientists and Members of the Parliament of all fractions, covers the following topics: ? family relations and other social networks, ? intergenerational relationships, ? labour market and migration policy, ? the long-term financial stability of the social security systems (statutory health insurance, statutory old age income security systems, long-term care insurance) , ? statutory health and care policies, ? social and care services on the community level, ? living conditions and environment, ? the utilisation of skills and potentials of an ageing society. In the meantime, two interim reports have been published (1994, 1998). The final report which will include political recommendations will pass parliament in spring 2002. This paper provides a prelimenary insight into main results and recommendations regarding the above mentioned topics which might be also useful for the policies of other countries. In addition, the paper discusses the chances these recommendations have to be put into action.

SESSION 182

Cardiovascular risk factors and prevention of dementia by calcium-channel inhibitor based antihypertensive treatment. New evidence from the Syst-Eur trial

F Forette,ML Seux,O Hanon (Department of Geriatrics, Hôpital Broca, University of Paris V, France) JA Staessen, L Thijs(Department of Molecular and Cardiovascular Research, University of Leuven, Belgium) on behalf of the Syst-Eur Investigators.

Besides age, genetic factors and level of education, vascular factors have been identified as risk factors for dementia. The Syst-Eur vascular dementia project investigated whether antihypertensive drug treatment could reduce the incidence of dementia in older patients with isolated systolic hypertension. Eligible patients were non demented, at least 60 years old, and had a sitting blood pressure (BP)ranging from 160 to 219 mm Hg systolic and below 95 mm Hg diastolic. Active treatment consisted of nitrendipine (10-40 mg/day) with the possible addition of enalapril (5-20 mg/day), hydrochlorothiazide (12.5-25 mg/day) or both drugs titrated or combined to reduce the sitting blood pressure by at least 20 mmHg to below 150mmHg. Cognitive function and diagnosis of dementia were based on the Mini Mental State Examination(MMSE) the DSM-III-R criteria and the Modified Ischemic Score with brain imaging. The median MMSE score at randomisation was 29 in both treatment groups and the median systolic/diastolic blood pressure was 173/86 mm Hg. The incidence of dementia was reduced by 50%, from 7.7 cases per 1000 patient-years in the placebo group (n=1180) to 3.8 cases in the active treatment group (n=1238) (21 vs 11 patients, p= 0.05). After termination of the double-blind phase, all patients were offered active trial medication. The mean follow-up increased from 2 to 3.9 years and the number of dementia cases from 31 to 64. BP in the former placebo group remained 3.3/3.9 mm Hg higher than in the former active group. Long term active treatment reduced the incidence of dementia by 55% (43 versus 21 patients, p= 0.0008). Alzheimer type dementia was reduced as well as vascular or mixed dementia. Halving the incidence of dementia may have important public-health implications and underlines the high interest of treating hypertension in the elderly.

Dehydrepiandrosterone (DHEA) does not improve cognitive function in healthy elderly.

F Forette, J de Rotrou, AS Rigaud, (Department of Geriatrics, Hôpital Broca, University of Paris V, France) V Faucounau (Fondation Nationale de Gérontologie) S Legrain (CHU Bichat) EE Baulieu (INSERM U448 and College de France) on behalf of the DHEAge trial Investigators.

The decrease with age of secretion and blood levels of DHEA and its sulphate (DHEAS) raises the issue of a possible compensation of declining function by replacement of the steroid. In spite of doubts as to its efficacy and safety, DHEA is largely used because of its commercial availability outside the regular pharmaceutical network. The DHEAge study aimed at investigating the safety and efficacy of a one year administration of 50 mg DHEA in elderly. This paper presents the results on cognitive function. The double-blind study was run on 280 healthy subjects aged 60 to 79 years. Subjects were randomly allocated 50 mg/day of DHEA or matching placebo for one year. Cognitive function was assessed using a battery of validated tests measuring immediate and delayed recall, logical memory, code learning, verbal fluency and executive control. There was no correlation at entry between cognitive scores and DHEAS levels. After 12 months, there was no difference between the placebo-group and the active group in the cognitive scores in spite of the increase to young adult values of DHEAS levels in the latter. In patients whose baseline DHEAS were below the first quartile of the DHEAS distribution, no difference was seen between the two groups. A one year administration of 50 mg/day of DHEA does not improve cognitive function in healthy elderly people. The promising properties of DHEA as a neurosteroid must lead to further controlled studies using larger populations and a longer follow-up period. Meanwhile, uncontrolled use of DHEA should be discouraged.<?xml:namespace prefix = o ns = "urn:schemas-microsoft-com:office:office" />

Double blind trial on the efficacy of Reinhardt and Sea Cucumber capsule (R.S.C.) in treatment of age-associated memory impairment (AAMI) in 168 cases

Ma Yong-Xing, Wang Chuan-Fu, Xie Su-Zhen (Department of Aging, Antiaging and Cognitive Function, Shanghai Institute of Gerontology and Geriatrics, Huadong Hospital, Shanghai, China)

Objective: To observe the efficacy of Reinhardt and Sea Cucumber Capsule (R.S.C. Sea animal products) in treatment of age-associated memory impairment (AAMI). Methods: Double blind trials were performed in 168 cases of AAMI in the aged and preaged with MQ<90(WMS). The dosage of R.S.C. and placebo were all 4 capsules (0.28g/cap) tried for 3 months. The effects were evaluated with MQ(WMS). Results: The mean value of MQ(WMS) before and after treatment were 81.35±7.51 and 90 64±8.98 (P<0.001) in 83 cases treated with R.S.C. and 84.34±6.80 and 88.60±7.40 (P<0.001) in 85 cases in placebo group respectively. Significant difference of mean value of MQ increment between R.S.C. 9.30±6.46 and placebo 4.31±5.29 (t=5.49, P<0.001) were observed. The total effective rate of the R.S.C. and placebo were 62.65% and 23.53% respectively (P<0.001). No significant side effects were observed. The mechanism of R.S.C. to improve the learning and retrieval function of the adult and old rats and adult mouse, and memory function in the aged and preaged persons with AAMI may be related to its effects to enhance neuron growth, to increase acetylcholine and decrease glutamine level in the brain as confirmed in cell and animal experiments, and to improve free radical metabolism and microcirculatory state confirmed clinically. Conclusions: R.S.C. is rather effective and safe to improve memory and cognitive function in the elderly.

Estrogen therapy and mild cognitive impairment in old postmenopausal women

A Dutruc (Hopital Broca Paris, France), L. Traykov (Unite INSERM 324, Paris, France), F. Latour (Hopital Broca, Paris, France), F. Moulin (Hopital Broca Paris, France), O. Hanon (Hopital Broca Paris, France), M.L. Seux (Hopital Broca Paris, France), H Barei (Hopital Broca Paris, France), F. Forette (Hopital Broca Paris, France), A.S.Rigaud (Hopital Broca, Paris, France)

Some authors have suggested that estrogen replacement therapy in women has a beneficial effect on cognitive performance, reduces the risk of subsequent dementia and increases response to anticholinesterasic therapy in Alzheimer's disease (AD) (Yaffe K et al. JAMA 1998). However the benefit of estrogens in the prevention of mild cognitive impairment (MCI), a pathological condition at risk for the development of AD, is still unknown. The objective of this retropective study was to determine whether estrogens have a beneficial role in the prevention of MCI in old postmenopausal women. We studied 252 women (mean age 69±7 years) including 149 with normal cognitive functions and 103 with MCI, consecutively recruited between January 1997 and December 1999 in a day care hospital. Cognitive status was evaluated with the Mini Mental State Examination (MMSE) and a screening neuropsychological battery. Women were evaluated by detailed recording of medical history, including age of menopause, type and duration of previous estrogen therapy, physical examination, brain computed tomography and laboratory tests. Our results showed that women with normal cognitive functions treated with estrogens have significantly higher neuropsychological performances than non treated women (p=0.005). Similarly, in estrogen treated women with MCI, cognitive scores were significantly higher than in non treated women (p=0.02). These results suggest the benefit of estrogen therapy in the prevention of MCI in old postmenopausal women. However further investigations are required to elucidate the specific cognitive domains that may respond to estrogen.

Indication of olanzapine in the behavioral and psychological signs and symptoms (BPSD) in Alzheimer' disease

B. Placines (Maison de retraite Saint-Joseph , 64800 Nay , France), C.Geny (Centre Hospitalier Général ,6400 Pau , France), J.P. Duviau (Maison de retraite Saint-Joseph , 64800 Nay , France) F.De La Fournière (Centre Jean Vignalou , 64000 Pau , France),

The olanzapine (ZYPREXA) is a new anti-psychotic drug with a particular pharmacological profile: a selectivity for the serotoninergics receptor 5 HT2A and 5 HT2C is higher than the dopaminergics receptors D2 .This non-controlled trial presents 15 patients with AD who are treated by Olanzapine for the BPSD . The evolution of the BPSD describes in accordance to the Sydney consensus in 1995 of the American Psychogeriatric Association .The result at 32 weeks are encouraging , with a behavioral regulation and cognition Improvements . The necessaries doses oscillate between 5 and 7.5 mg per day. This encouraging results have to can allow to envisage double-bind placebo and Haloperidol controlled study , of the patients with moderate to severe AD with BPSD , on the semiologic lecture with the American Consensus dated of 1995 .

Naftidrofuryl and Vascular or Mixed Dementia : Results of a Multicenter, Double-Blind Trial

Jean-Paul Emeriau (Department of Internal Medicine-Geriatrics, Xavier Arnozan Hospital, C.H.U. Bordeaux, France),Philippe Lehert (Department of Statitical Analysis, University of Mons, Mons, Belgium),Michel Mosnier (Medical Department, Cardiovascular Unit, Lipha Santé, Lyon, France)

Background : Dementia is a cerebral disorder resulting in a progressive deterioration of intellectual function that compromises the patients’ability. The diagnostic criteria for dementia are primarily clinical and are based on the Diagnostic and Statistical Manual of Mental Disorders, Fourth Edition. The Hachinski score and computed tomography of the brain help distinguish between degenerative and vascular dementias. Purpose : to examine the efficacy of naftidrofuryl in patients with vascular or mixed dementia Methods : A multicenter, randomized, double-blind study compared naftidrofury 600mg/d with placebo for 1 year in patients with vascular or mixed dementia. A preliminary 2-month washout period allowed selection of patients who were compliant with treatment. The end point was change in the scores on the Alzheimer Disease Assessment Scale cognitive subscale and the Mini-Mental State Examination. Results : 84 patients were assessable on an intent-to-treat basis, and 74 were assessable for the per-protocol analysis (on treatment). Statistically significant improvements in cognitive and global function were observed in patients receiving naftidrofuryl. Naftidrofuryl was well tolerated and produced no clinically significant abnormalities in laboratory test results. Conclusion : The results suggest that Naftidrofuryl is effective and well tolerated in treating the symptoms of vascular and mixed dementia

Synergistic action of pharmacological and nonpharmacological approaches in senile dementia

M.Giordano, A.Uttuso, F.Muratore, L.J.Dominguez, M. Barbagallo (Institute of Internal Medicine and Geriatrics, University of Palermo, Italy, Alzheimer Center, AUSL-6, Ospedale Ingrassia, Palermo, Italy)

PURPOSE: Use of acethylcholinesterase inhibitors is a promising therapeutic strategy against cognitive impairment and functional disability. Reality orientation therapy (ROT) is a type of cognitive rehabilitation particularly indicated for mentally deteriorated patients with temporal-spatial disorders. The efficacy of the association of the two therapies has not been adequately studied. METHODS: 100 elderly subjects (mean age 78.4+4.32 yrs) with Alzheimer disease were studied. All subjects were treated with an acethilcholinesterase inhibitor (donezepil, 5 mg/day) and subsequently divided in two groups, group A (62 subjects) that underwent a 3 weeks, daily nonpharmacological training program with ROT and physical reactivation sessions, and group B (38 subjects) that did not receive any additional nonpharmacological therapy. All subjects were tested at baseline with MMSE, ADL, IADL and were re-evaluted after 3 weeks (T=21d, end of the training program) and 2 months after the end of the training (T=2m). Control group subjects were also evaluated at the same time points. RESULTS: Group A had a MMSE of 17.1+3.1 at baseline, 19.6+2.4 at T=21d and 20.8+1.7($p<0.01$) at T=2m; ADL increased from 4.0+0.8 to 5.3 +0.8($p<0.01$); IADL increased from 8.2 +2.0 to 9.1+2.5($p<0.01$). In the same time period, no significant differences were found in group B. CONCLUSIONS: Our results suggest a synergistic efficacy of a combined approach with pharmacological and nonpharmacological therapies. However, longer studies are needed to verify whether the better results scored by the patients that underwent a nonpharmacological program is a net gain or an acceleration of the benefits of the acethilcholenesterase inhibitors.

The safe dosage range of Huperzine: An intraventricular administration in rats and Rhesus Monkeys

Cheng Pu, Xu Zhao-Zhong, Ma Yong-Xing (Department of Aging, Antiaging and Cognitive Function, Shanghai Institute of Gerontology and Geriatrics, Huadong Hospital, Shanghai,China)

Huperzine A is one of the newest cholinesterase inhibitors which is effective for the treatment of Alzheimer's diseases in oral and IM administration. So we consider that higher concentration of Huperzine A in CSF after intraventricular injection may have better effects with less toxicity because of the decreasing dosage. The safe dosage is titrated in twenty-four rats and four Rhesus Monkeys (R.M.) in order to find the minimal dosage without significant side effects compared with Control. The animals were randomly divided into two groups (test and blank group). After intraventricular intubation, the investigator gave drugs through the tube then carefully observed the vital signs (TPR), pupil reaction to painful stimulation, and peripheral cholinergic effects (drooling and fasciculation) for 10 minutes. Based on the results of the observation, it is concluded that the safe dosage range is 1-2g for rats and 2g/Kg - 8g/Kg for R.M.

SESSION 183

Creative Storytelling with People with Dementia: The Time Slips Project

Anne Basting (Fellow, Brookdale Center on Aging; Project Director, The Time Slips Project, Center for Creative Aging; Brooklyn, New York, USA)

Creative storytelling relieves the pressure to "remember" and opens new channels of communication with people with Alzheimer's disease and related dementia. Above all, creative storytelling is a joyful, meaning-making activity that can bring staff, clients, and families closer together. This presentation will provide an overview of some approaches to creative storytelling, with clients or with loved ones based on experience with the Time Slips Project

Enriching Presence and Possibility in Later Life: Living History Theatre and Conflict Resolution Theatre

Susan Perlstein (Director, National Center for Creative Aging/ Elders Share the Arts (ESTA), Brooklyn, New York, USA)

A broad range of approaches to older adult theater groups across a variety of settings schools, colleges, community centers, neighborhoods, residential communities and health care institutions can be used to support and enhance relational connections between seniors, and their families, friends, neighbors, and others in their communities. In this session, participants will be introduced to "Living History Theater" as a model which invites older adults to celebrate and share their life stories. Participants will learn about oral history and life review interviewing techniques, and then learn how to transform the life stories into storytelling and living history theater. The structure for designing, planning, implementing and evaluating both projects and programs will be discussed. The focus of the theater work will be on improvisational techniques emphasizing life cycle themes and issues that concern seniors. A variety of presentation formats will be described, along with different approaches that can be used with both well and frail seniors, and intergenerational groups. Illustrations will also be given that point to the power of theatre in relation to conflict resolution and engendering understanding and connection across different groups.

Partners Through the Years: Prevention of elder abuse through drama

Satwinder K. Bains (Abbotsford Association for Healthy Aging, Abbotsford, British Columbia, Canada); Barbara Tollefsen

Partners Through the Years involved an innovative, community development approach that used theatre to increase awareness of elder abuse, and sensitivity toward ageist and sexist stereotypes among children and teenagers. The goal was to teach youth about how abuse happens to prevent them from falling into disrespectful patterns and becoming abusers themselves. Three planning/working groups were set up in an elementary, junior and senior high school with each group composed of students, a teacher advisory, program coordinators and two senior women-turned-actors volunteers. Through a process of information exchange and education each group created plays appropriate for their age group, and developed the plays into presentations with accompanying age-appropriate discussion materials. The productions challenged the students to identify stereotypes and then develop a script and other dramatic approaches to engage the audience in questioning their acceptance of ageist and sexist stereotypes. Each school, although given identical information and training on the topic of elder abuse, used different dramatic vehicles to engage consideration and concern about the issue of elder abuse. Drama proved to be a powerful tool to help young people reflect on their relationships with seniors.The project demonstrated that an intergenerational approach based on drama and performance can be used to effectively to address serious social issues facing the seniors. As members of each group worked together to develop the r plays and skits, they learned more about each other and through tł at process challenged the stereotypes they held of one another.

SESSION 184

Carcinogenesis and Aging

V.N. Anisimov (N.N. Petrov Research Institute of Oncology, St.Petersburg, Russia) Carcinogenesis and Aging: The Role of genetic and environmental factors. L. Balducci (H. Lee Moffitt Cancer Center, Tampa, FL, USA) Cancer in the Elderly. Y. Suh (Seoul National University; Seoul, Korea) Cell Signalling Pathways of Cytotoxic Stress in Cancer and Aging. S.V. Ukraintseva (Max Planck Institute for Demographic Research, Rostock, Germany. J. Vijg (University of Texas Health Science Center and Institute for Drug Development, Cancer Therapy and Research Center, San Antonio, TX, USA) Genome Deterioration in Relation to Aging

Cancer in the elderly is an increasingly common problem accounted for by carcinogenesis at molecular, cellullar and organism levels. This symposium will review a problem from the point of views of studies in clinical oncogerontology, epidemiology, molecular biology and experimental carcinogenesis stucies. Being a clinician, Prof. L. Balducci will discuss a problem as a relation between "seed" and "soil" effects in the tumor-bearing organism. The "seed" is the cancer cell and the "soil" is the older tumor host. Dr. S. Ukraintseva will present an overview on the typical patterns of cancer age-specific incidence rate in human populations, including a plateau, a wave, and an accelerated increase with age. She subdivide individual age-associated changes into three components, having different influence on cancer meorbidity: basal, ontogenetic and time-dependent. Prof. J. Vijg will discuss a genomic instability as a major cause of both cancer and aging. Using a transgenic mouse model with a chromosomally integrated lacZ mutation target gene, he has shown an accumulation of mutations with age in an organ-specific manner. Dr. Y. Suh will present an evidence that the capacity of a tissue to activate the stress activated protein kinases may involve in the protective response against carcinogenesis, presumably by inducing apoptosis to eliminate alkylation-damaged cells after exposure of animals to an alkylating agent. Prof. V. Anisimov will present an overview on the role of genetic and environmental factors in age-related susceptibility to carcinogenesis.

Cancer in the Elderly

Lodovico Balducci (H. Lee Moffitt Cancer Center & Research Institute, Tampa, FL, USA)

Cancer in the elderly is an increasingly common problem accounted for by carcinogenesis, and cellular and molecular changes. Carcinogenesis is a time consuming process and older people live long enough to develop cancer. Cellular and molecular changes of age make older persons more susceptible to environmental carcinogens and to the growth of cancer. The biology of certain tumors may change with the age of the patient. Breast cancer appears more indolent, while acute myelogenous leukemia (AML), large-cell non-Hodgkins lymphoma (NHL) and ovarian cancer appear more aggressive. In this change of biology, we should recognize a "seed" and a "soil" effect. The "seed" is the cancer cell, the "soil" is the older tumor host. In AML, we have mainly a "seed" effect: the leukemic blasts becomes more drug-resistant with age. In NHL, we witness a "soil" effect as age is associated with an increased concentration of circulating I1-6 that is a lympatic growth factor. In breast cancer, we see both a "seed" and "soil" effect . Tumor cells are better differentiated and richer in hormone-receptors in older women, and at the same time, decreased production of estrogen and decreased mononuclear cell reaction render the "soil" less favorable to the growth of breast cancer. Management of cancer in the older patient should include primary prevention of cancer, including chemotherapy. Age is not a contraindication to surgery, although surgical mortality increases with age, this is accounted for by emergency surgery mostly.

Cancer in the Elderly

Lodovico Balducci (H. Lee Moffitt Cancer Center & Research Institute, Tampa, FL, USA)

Cancer in the elderly is an increasingly common problem accounted for by carcinogenesis, and cellular and molecular changes. Carcinogenesis is a time consuming process and older people live long enough to develop cancer. Cellular and molecular changes of age make older persons more susceptible to environmental carcinogens and to the growth of cancer. The biology of certain tumors may change with the age of the patient. Breast cancer appears more indolent, while acute myelogenous leukemia (AML), large-cell non-Hodgkins lymphoma (NHL) and ovarian cancer appear more aggressive. In this change of biology, we should recognize a "seed" and a "soil" effect. The "seed" is the cancer cell, the "soil" is the older tumor host. In AML, we have mainly a "seed" effect: the leukemic blasts becomes more drug-resistant with age. In NHL, we witness a "soil" effect as age is associated with an increased concentration of circulating I1-6 that is a lympatic growth factor. In breast cancer, we see both a "seed" and "soil" effect . Tumor cells are better differentiated and richer in hormone-receptors in older women, and at the same time, decreased production of estrogen and decreased mononuclear cell reaction render the "soil" less favorable to the growth of breast cancer. Management of cancer in the older patient should include primary prevention of cancer, including chemotherapy. Age is not a contraindication to surgery, although surgical mortality increases with age, this is accounted for by emergency surgery mostly.

Carcinogenesis and aging: the role of genetic and environmental factors

V.N. Anisimov (N.N. Petrov Research Institute of Oncology, St.Petersburg, Russia)

It is reasonable to suggest that the risk of spontaneous tumors development should increased in long-live species and strains in comparison with short-live ones. However, no significant positive correlation between life span and tumor incidence was found in animals of different species and inbred mice of different strains. It seems that genetic factors were much more responsible for the variation in spontaneous tumor incidence, localization, and histological type, than the length of life span of animals in various populations. Much more important the correlation between the life span and spontaneous tumor incidence in different groups (populations) of animals of one strain or stock. Our data have shown that more "rectangular" pattern of survival curves directly associated with increased rate in development of fatal tumors in rats of the same strain. The exposure to some mutagens, chemical carcinogens and ionizing radiation was followed by acceleration of aging in vivo. Exposure to carcinogenic agents and tumor promoters at different age has demonstrated age-related accumulation in different tissues of cells which have been randomly exposed to carcinogens and, as a result, are pass at least one stage before complete malignant transformation. Significant differences in age-related changes in the sensitivity of various tissues to the action of different carcinogens have been identified. The analysis of the available data on transgenic and mutant mice has shown that only few models represent examples of life span extension. As usual, the incidence of spontaneous tumors in these mice was similar to those in controls, whereas the latent period of tumor development was increased. Practically all transgenic models of accelerated aging show the increased tumor incidence and shortening of tumor latency. This phenomenon has been observed both in mice which display phenotype more resemble to the natural aging and in mice showed only partial features of normal aging process. Available data have shown that tree types of genes are involved in control of aging: genes which control cell proliferation and death directly ("gatekeepers"), DNA repair genes that maintain the integrity of the genome ("caretakers") and "homeostatic" genes. Gatekeepers directly regulate the growth of tumors by inhibiting growth or promoting cells. In contrast, inactivation of a caretaker gene leads to genetic instability which result in increased mutation of all genes, including gatekeepers. The important role in tumor promotion and progression plays genes involved in tissue metabolic and growth pathways and immune signaling genes, acting as "homeostatic" genes. It is clear, that both aging and carcinogenesis are complex multifactorial processes that can have many causes. In that sense new transgenic and knockout mouse models with prolonged or reduced longevity will be an important instrument for evaluation the role of involved in aging genes in mechanisms of carcinogenesis.

Cell Signaling Pathways of Genotoxic Stress in Cancer and Aging.

Yousin Suh, Kang-Ae Lee, and Sang-Chul Park. Department of Biochemistry and Molecular Biology, Seoul National University, College of Medicine,

Unrepaired or misrepaired DNA damage has been implicated in both cancer and aging. Alkylating agents represent one of the most abundant chemical sources of DNA damage in our environment and are known to cause cancer in an organ-specific manner. Using rat as a model system, we demonstrated very distinct organ-specific patterns in the activation of the stress activated protein kinases and induction of apoptosis in rats treated with a direct acting alkylating agent, Methyl methanesulfonate (MMS). Our data strongly suggest that the capacity of a tissue to activate the stress activated protein kinases may involve in the protective response against carcinogenesis, presumably by inducing apoptosis to eliminate alkylation-damaged cells after exposure of an intact animal to MMS. It has been suggested that changes in apoptosis may be an important factor in aging. However, whether apoptosis plays a role in the protective response to genotoxic agent in aging has yet been demonstrated in vivo. We demonstrate that the efficiency of apoptosis in response to MMS is significantly decreased in aged rat tissues compared to young counterparts. To understand the mechanisms underlying the impaired apoptotic responsiveness in aging, we are currently studying changes in major apoptotic signaling pathways during aging after MMS treatment.

Genome Instability, Aging and Cancer

Jan Vijg,

Genomic instability has been implicated as a major cause of both cancer and aging. Using a transgenic mouse model with a chromosomally integrated lacZ mutational target gene, mutations were found to accumulate with age in an organ-specific manner. Depending on the organ, many of the accumulated mutations were genome rearrangements rather than point mutations, some of them involving millions of basepairs. It is hypothesized that these large rearrangements find their origin in misannealing of DNA double-strand breaks during error-prone repair. They may lead to aging by affecting normal regulation, i.e, through gene dosage or position effects. In humans, allelic variation at loci controlling genome stability, i.e, genes involved in double-strand break repair, could contribute to the observed individual variation in life span and cancer risk. To explore this possibility a novel gene-scanning system, two-dimensional gene scanning (TDGS), was used to search for haplotypes of polymorphic variants in genes involved in maintenance and repair of the nuclear genome in human centenarians, i.e, people with extremely high survival and an apparently low cancer risk. In these association studies significant differences were observed in haplotypes of the breast cancer susceptibility gene BRCA, which is involved in recombinational repair, between centenarians and control groups. These results will be discussed in terms of the possibility to extend health-span, i.e, cancer- and disease-free survival, by the manipulation of genome stability pathways.

On the Role of Individual Aging in Cancer Morbidity Patterns

S.V. Ukraintseva (Max Planck Institute for Demographic Research, Rostock, Germany)

There are observed three typical patterns of cancer age-incidence rate in human populations. Those are a plateau, a wave, and an accelerated increase of the incidence rate with age. Typical traits of total cancers morbidity include higher morbidity in early childhood, lower morbidity during a reproductive period, an accelerated increase of morbidity near to the end of a reproductive period, and the deceleration in this increase (or even the decrease) at oldest old ages. This late deceleration in the increase of cancer incidence rate looks paradoxical. The role of differential selection in this phenomenon has been well studied. However, a possible contribution of individual aging to the shape of a cancer morbidity curve has not been studied so far. Here we specify most common patterns of age-associated changes in an individual organism and discuss their possible influence on cancer morbidity patterns in population. We subdivide the individual age-associated changes into three components ((i) basal, (ii) ontogenetic and (iii) time-dependent), which have different influence on cancer morbidity. Basal changes are related to the universal decrease in the rate of living during an individual life. As a result, some phenotypic effects of aging may accumulate in an organism at a slower rate with age. The basal changes are likely to contribute to a late plateau of a cancer morbidity. Ontogenetic component is connected with a change of the stages of ontogenesis (e.g. the growth, the reproductive period and the climacteric) during an individual life. The ontogenesis-related changes may be partially responsible for often observed wave-like patterns of a cancer morbidity. Time-dependent changes in an organism are related to a long time of exposure of the organism to different harmful factors rather than to the age per se. These changes are most likely to contribute to the acceleration of a cancer morbidity with age. We discuss how the different components of individual aging may interact in a human organism and influence cancer morbidity in population.

SESSION 185

Primate Models of Age-Related Disease: Opportunities to Test Anti-Aging Interventions

Patrick McGeer [University of British Columbia Vancouver, BC Canada] Primate Models of Neurodegenerative Disease Mary Lou Voytko [Wake Forest University School of Medicine, Winston-salem, North Carolina, USA] Estrogen Enhances Cognitive and Neurobiological Profiles of Monkey Models of Menopause Angela Black [Laboratory of Neurosciences, National Institute on Aging, Baltimore, MD USA] Long-term Calorie Restriction in Rhesus Macaques: Measures of Skeletal Health and Reproduction Function Julie Mattison [Laboratory of Neurosciences, National Institute on Aging, Baltimore, MD USA] Calorie Restriction and Aging in Primates: The NIA Study in Review

This symposium will focus on nonhuman primate models of age associated disease and strategies for intervening in these disease processes and the biological changes that occur with aging. Due to similarities to human physiology, behavior and endocrinology, the use of nonhuman primates as animal models of age-related disease in humans has witnessed a steady increase in recent years. Nonhuman primate models of neurodegeneration, cardiovascular disease and diabetes are particularly well described. Nonhuman primate models have also been utilized for studies of various interventions targeting aging processes including hormone therapy and studies of caloric restriction a nutritional paradigm that extends lifespan and retards aging in short-lived species. This symposium will focus on primate models of neurodegenerative disease including Alzheimer's disease. Effects of estrogen replacement therapy on neurobiology and behavior in older female monkeys will also be explored. This session will also include an overview of recent findings from an ongoing trial of caloric restriction in rhesus monkeys. Findings from over 14 years of study show that this nutritional intervention reduces several risk factors associated with cardiovascular disease and diabetes and may reduce overall morbidity, particularly the incidence of neoplastic disease in rhesus monkeys. Effects of this nutritional intervention on bone and skeletal health and reproductive function will also be presented.

Calorie Restriction and Aging in Nonhuman Primates: The NIA Study in Review

J.A. Mattison, G.S. Roth, D.K. Ingram, M.A. Lane (National Institute on Aging, NIH, Baltimore, USA)

Caloric restriction (CR) is the best known intervention for delaying aging, maintaining function, and extending lifespan. From flies to rodents, the benefits of CR have been demonstrated in over 70 years of research, but have yet to be established in long-lived species. For 14 years, the NIA has been investigating the CR paradigm in nonhuman primates to determine the applicability of this practice to humans. Approximately 200 monkeys, primarily rhesus (Macaca mulatta), with a small number of squirrel monkeys (Saimiri sciureus), aged across their respective lifespans, were randomly assigned to a diet group. The CR group receives approximately 30 0.000000e+00ss than control-fed, adjusted for age and body weight. All monkeys receive two meals per day of a diet supplemented with extra micronutrients such that the only substantive variable is the number of calories consumed. Although there is evidence of reduced mortality in the CR group, no statistical conclusions can be drawn at this time of the study. However, beneficial effects consistent with a slower rate of aging are apparent. Monkeys restricted while very young had delayed skeletal and sexual maturation, which did not affect adult bone mineral density or reproductive hormone function. Moreover, the age-associated decrease in DHEAS levels was attenuated in the CR group. Restricted animals exhibit several indices of improved health. Preliminary findings indicate a reduced incidence of proliferative diseases such as cancer and endometriosis; better cardiovascular health indicated by lower blood pressure and lipids, and elevated HDL; and improved glucoregulatory function such as lower insulin levels and increased insulin sensitivity which could protect against diabetes. These results suggest that CR may be a relevant anti-aging intervention in humans.

Long-term calorie restriction in rhesus macaques: Measures of skeletal health and reproduction function.

A. Black, D.K.Ingram, G.S, Roth, and M.A. Lane [National Institute on Aging, National Institutes of Health, Baltimore, USA]

Purpose: Calorie restriction (CR) extends lifespan and slows aging and age-related disease in short-lived mammalian species. Although a wide variety of physiological systems have been studied using this model, little is known regarding the effects of long-term CR on the skeleton and reproductive axis. Methods: Data were collected from 43 females (8-28y, 23 CON, 20CR) and 48 males (14-36, 26CON, 22CR) starting when they had been restricted at 300f ad lib tum for 6 and 11 years, respectively. Results: CR male monkeys had lower bone mineral density (BMD) and bone mineral content (BMC) values but this was accounted for by adjusting for differences in age and body weight. CR did not alter BMD or BMC in female monkeys at any skeletal site. Markers of bone turnover, vitamin D and PTH concentrations were not altered by CR. No effects of CR were observed on reproductive hormone concentrations in male or female monkeys. Similarly, CR did not alter menstrual cycling in females. The total number of menstrual cycles over 3 years, and the percent of normal menstrual cycles (24-34 days) was lower in older than younger monkeys. Endometriosis was diagnosed in 5CR and 1CON female. Hormonal determination of ovulation is currently being studied in these females. Conclusion: Long-term CR does not negatively impact bone mass in female monkeys but appears to reduce bone mass in males via a physiologic normalization to a smaller body size. Chronic CR has, thus far, not affected indices of reproductive function in this population, although it may reduce the incidence of endometriosis in females.

SESSION 186

Alternative Models of Care and Shelter

A.Tinker (Age Concern Institute of Gerontology, King's College London, England) Long Term Care: The Recent Experience of the United Kingdom. A. Howe, (Consultant Gerontologist, Brunswick, Australia) 'Ageing in Place' Or in Many Places? Lessons from Australia L. Wagner (The University Hospital Centre for Nursing and Care Research, Copenhagen, Denmark) Frail Elderly People in Denmark - Preventive Work in Home Care Shows Results.

Abstract ISSUE Policies to enable older people to remain in their own homes are worldwide in response to the wishes of older people but also as a response to the problems of institutions. These include the cost, problems of obtaining staff and effects of institutionalisation. The main issues are what alternatives can be provided. These concern policies across a range of services foremost being those to do with care and shelter. Many countries have had long-standing policies and services while some have experimented with new ones. The focus of this Symposium is on the experiences of the United Kingdom, Australia and Denmark. STRUCTURE Three short papers. Participants in the Symposium are invited to share the experiences of their countries. CONTENT In the UK the 1999 Royal Commission on Long Term Care provided a focus for debate about alternatives to institutions. The author and colleagues undertook the major empirical piece of research examining alternative models of care and housing together with policies for health which need to underpin ageing in place. The importance of rehabilitation, prevention and good basic services were stressed. A particular focus was on sheltered housing with care, intensive domiciliary support, co-resident care and assistive technology. Innovative services were examined and evidence presented about the success of these schemes including costings. This research will be presented together with the current policy background and a discussion of what has happened since the Royal Commission reported in terms of policy, practice and research. In Australia 'Ageing in place' has been applied narrowly in formal policies in attempts to integrate hostels and nursing homes. Likely changes include: • policies to loosen care linked to specific accommodation • provider responses to funding uncertainties and to expand community care • initiatives outside formal government programmes • demand and preferences of a segmented older population, with a generally high level of home-ownership but differing capacities to participate in housing markets. While policies have created conditions favourable to activity outside formal government programmes, these consequences are not well recognised for formal services. A better understanding of these dynamics requires a fuller account of the models of care including combinations of different forms and intensities, the characteristics of residents and their patterns of movement between different kinds of care. In Denmark an evaluated scheme in Skaevinge Municipality together with the national policy context is discussed. This was one of integrated health care based on principles of self-care. The original goals were: • a common set of municipal health services for all regardless of their type of residence • priority to be given to preventive measures • nursing homes to be changed into health centres (with rented appartments for elderly people and a 24 hour integrated care service available for the whole municipality) • staff to be educated to understand the value and effect of self-care. The evaluation showed an improvement in self evaluated health, staff felt a sense of ownership and responsibility, operating costs remained the same, and the number of days for people aged 75+ in hospital fell. CONCLUSIONS The identification of common solutions. worconab

'Ageing in Place' Or in Many Places? Lessons from Australia

A. Howe (Consultant Gerontologist, Brunswick, Australia)

PURPOSE: Ageing in place has been applied in a narrow sense in formal and aged care policy in Australia, in attempts to integrate the two levels of residential care (hostels and nursing homes). But 'ageing in place' covers a much wider range of options for care and accommodation. The increasing diversity of options in recent years prompts questions about the factors underlying these trends, and this paper canvasses four sources of change: METHOD: Analysis of policies and research on options RESULTS: These changes have taken place: policy changes have loosened previous bundles of care that were only provided in specific accommodation settings; providers have responded to funding uncertainties both as regard government funding and user payments in standard residential care programs and to incentives to expand community care; there have been initiatives outside formal government programs notably in a growing and diverse private retirement housing sector; the demand and preferences of a segmented older population have led to differing expectations for care needs and how they should be met. CONCLUSION: These developments have many implications for formal services, reducing demand for some kinds of support, but generating increasing demand for others. A better understanding of these dynamics requires a fuller account of models of care that includes all the combinations of different forms of accommodation and different intensities of care that are provided within and between them, and of the characteristics of residents in each and their patterns of movement between kinds of care.

Frail Elderly People in Denmark - Preventive Work in Home Care Shows Results

L. Wagner (University Hospitals Centre for Nursing and Care Research, the National Hospital of Denmark, Copenhagen, Denmark)

PURPOSE: This paper presents an account of an evaluated scheme in one area together with the national policy context. It was one of integrated health care based on principles of self-care. The original goals were: a) a common set of municipal health services to be available to everyone regardless of their type of residence b) priority to preventive measures to support and strengthen an individual's own health and quality of life c) nursing homes to be changed into health centers (with rented apartments for elderly people and a 24 hour integrated care service available for the whole municipality) d) staff to be educated to understand the value of self-care. METHOD This project took place from 1984-87 in Scavenge Municipality and was evaluated 10 years later by the Danish Institute of Health Care. The objective of the evaluation was to compare the older people with those in the rest of the County and nationally. RESULTS: A questionnaire to older people in 1997 showed that their self-evaluated health was better compared with an equivalent age group in 1987. Staff felt a sense of ownership and responsibility. Despite an increase of 30% in the age group 75+ operating costs remained the same between 1986 and 1996. The number of days for people aged 75+ in hospital fell to 2 to 3 days compared with the county and nationally. A long and thorough period of preparation was felt to contribute to the success of the project. CONCLUSION: A successful scheme.

Long term care - the recent experience of the UK

A. Tinker (King's College London, England)

Abstract PURPOSE The purpose of this presentation is to outline the research which was undertaken by the author and colleagues for the 1999 Royal Commission on Long Term Care on alternatives to institutions followed by an account of what has happened since the Royal Commission reported. This will include the policy options being put forward by the various political parties and current provision by housing, health and social service agencies. METHOD The research examined alternative models of care and housing together with policies for health which need to underpin ageing in place (Tinker et al, 1999). A particular focus was on very sheltered housing (sheltered housing with care), intensive home (domiciliary) support, co-resident care and assistive technology. RESULTS The importance of rehabilitation, prevention and good basic services was stressed. The four services outlined above were assessed in terms of feasibility, acceptability, outcomes and costs. It was concluded that the needs of older people on the margins of institutional care are complex and depend on many different factors. There is no general rule about whether care and housing at home cost more or less than alternatives. It all depends on the amount of care provided CONCLUSION Caring for older people in their own homes is a realistic option but the costs (economic and social) need to be taken into account and more research is needed. Tinker, A, Wright, F, McCreadie, C, Askham, J, Hancock, R, and Holmans, A (1999) Alternative Models of Care for Older People, Royal Commission on Long Term Care, Research Volume 2, The Stationery Office, London vansymat

SESSION 187

Lessons from the Field: Subject Recruitment in Social Support Intervention Research with Seniors

L. Barrett, M. Stewart. A. McKinnon, A. Neufeld, L. Liu, S. Warren, P. MacCracken, J. Triscott, N. Letourneau, G. Rueck, A. Barnfather (Centre for Health Promotion Studies, University of Alberta, Edmonton, Canada)

PURPOSE: Implementation of intervention research in the field of social support for seniors requires specific practical knowledge and skill for achievement of study goals. Underlying processes such as subject recruitment, enrollment protocols, and follow-up procedures across multi-sited projects are essential to the effective completion of such research. METHOD: This paper uses our recently completed multiple site RCT, on dyadic family caregiver telephone support to those caring for seniors with chronic conditions, as a case in point to report practical experiences related to the establishment and maintenance of these underlying processes. RESULTS: Specific attention is directed to identification of key facilitators and challenges as well as key strategies to enhance or overcome these factors in subject recruitment and other related processes. CONCLUSION: Discussion of these and related issues could be of help to others pursuing social support intervention research goals with seniors. Implications for practice, policy and research are summarized.

Recent developments in caregivers support in Sweden

Lennarth Johansson(National Bord of Health and Welfare, Stockholm, Sweden)

The 1990s implied a breakthrough in policy and practice in recognizing family carers and their need of support in Sweden. New legislation has been enacted, which urge local authorities to develop caregivers support. This has been followed by State grants to the local authorities, in order to stimulate and enable them to develop supportive services. During 1999 to 2001 a State grant of 300 million SEK has been dissiminated to the local authorities on a per capita basis as to be used to develop and extend new services for carers. A condition to receive the grant was that a local action plan, addressing caregivers support was established, based on collaboration with voluntary organisations. The National Board of Health and Welfare was commissioned to follow up and evaluate the effects of the State grants and report back to the national government annualy. The first two years of experiences show a country wide increased alertness in caregivers support issues, improved and extended service possibilities and a newborned interest in and understanding of voluntary work as a measure to support caregivers. New and extended services, especially respite services and support groups for carers, is now availbe in almost the entire country. In conclusion: Recent developments in caregivers support show an interesting progress. However, there is still far to go before caregivers support has been integrated in the supportive services for the elderly and their families in general. Issues regarding access, quality and timing of supportive services prevails and need to be addressed and elaborated on further.

The Changing Relationship: A Structured Approach to Providing Support to Caregivers of the Frail Elderly

R. Climans (Baycrest Centre for Geriatric Care,Toronto,Canada),A. Consky (Baycrest Centre for Geriatric Care, Toronto, Canada),L. Patterson (Baycrest Centre for Geriatric Care, Toronto, Canada).

Purpose: Social work practice in all developed countries is facing new challenges in meeting the needs of growing numbers of caregivers of the frail elderly. Results from an evaluation of a structured graduated approach to caregiver self- and peer support are presented. Method: The evolution of a unique group model demonstrating a parsimonious use of social work services yielding good outcome is discussed. It was created to meet the distinct needs of spouses/partners living in the community experiencing the complex issues related to aging and disease processes. Initial focused content for six weekly sessions includes companionship and intimacy, challenging behaviours, community resources and future-care planning. Following the intensive six- week group, members have chosen to join a monthly alumni group facilitated by a social worker. In the third stage of the model, members move towards a mutually self-supportive group with minimal involvement of the social worker. Measures of perceived helpfulness of content, leadership and group process were taken. Results: The results indicated that group members improved in their ability to manage in their personal situations as they have become less isolated and more informed and supported in their role as caregivers. Conclusions: This structured approach to increasing self-sufficiency and mutual support of family caregivers appears to be an effective way to teach and empower caregivers of the frail elderly. It has implications for social work practitioners and managers in all settings who are faced with increasing numbers of frail elders and limited professional social work resources.

The Quality of Life of the Families, Partners in Care

Edouard Behets Wydemans (Belgian Association Cantous, Rixensart Belgium) Robert Devilers (Belgian Association Cantous, Rixensart Belgium)

The Belgian Special Care Unit for disorientated elderly stands for the creation of a common living environment in a nursing home where people with a decreasing autonomy can find a community where communication, mutual help and relationships are promoted through the participation in the activities of daily life. Together with professional caregivers, the family is expected to become actively involved in each project in order to stimulate the residents to make full use of their present resources. One of originalities of The Belgian Special Care Unit for disorientated elderly lies in fact on the active involvement of the family in the care-taking of the needs of the group. We'll present the results of some research realized in collaboration with the "catholic university of Louvain" that evaluate the quality of life of the family members involved in the care-taking of their parents. We show that by being encouraged to do such simple tasks as helping a loved one at mealtime or accompanying a resident to an activity, family members feel more needed and experience less guilt. This research confirms that a real involvement by giving relatives a more active role in their loved one's care helps to curb frustration and helplessness . This research shows the need to develop educational Programs for families on a variety of financial, legal and health issues. It shows also the satisfaction of the relatives about the Special Care Unit (Activities, design, relation with the caregivers, well-being of their loved ones, ...). We show that the involvement contribute to decrease anxiety, nervousness, fatigue and pessimism of the families.

The Well-Being of Family Caregivers at Home: An Introduction to a 15-session Group Program.

L. Lévesque (Centre de recherche de l'Institut universitaire de gériatrie de Montréal), J. Vézina (École de psychologie de l'Université Laval), C. Gendron (Centre de recherche de l'Hôpital Douglas de Montréal), F. Ducharme (Centre de recherche de l'Institut universitaire de gériatrie de Montréal), R. Hébert (Centre de recherche de l'Institut universitaire de gériatrie de Sherbrooke), J.-P. Lavoie (Direction de la Santé publique Montréal-Centre), Michel Préville (Centre de recherche de l'Institut universitaire de gériatrie de Sherbrooke), Louis Voyer (Centre de recherche de l'Institut universitaire de gériatrie de Sherbrooke)

Family caregivers who take care of a demented person at home are likely to be exposed to disruptive behaviors. Studies have shown that those disruptive behaviors have deleterious effects on the psychological well-being of family caregivers. Although many programs exist to alleviate stress, a critical review of outcomes studies have indicated modest positive effects. Apart from some methodological limits of the outcomes studies (e.g, small sample size), there is a lack of theoretical underpinnings to guide the development of support groups, and their short duration precludes discussion on the various topics during sessions. Taking into account these observations, a group program to promote the caregivers' well-being has been developed by a team of researchers. Also a multisite randomized control trial on a sample of 160 caregivers is ongoing to test the efficacy of the program. The aim of this paper is to present the key theoretical elements of the program. The program is based on Lazarus and Folkman stress and coping theory (1984). The intent of the program is to focus on teaching caregivers the process of breaking down a global situation into specific stressors and to practice three coping strategies according to the nature of the stressor: problem solving for changeable stressors (problem focus), reframing for unmodifiable stressors (emotion focus), and how to seek formal and informal help (problem and emotion focus). Assignments that caregivers do alone at home are means through which coping strategies are learned and practiced. (Research Funded by : le Fonds de la recherche en santé du Québec, le Conseil québécois de la recherche sociale et la Société Alzheimer du Canada)

SESSION 188

Aging and Individuals with a Developmental Disability (Mental Retardation)

S. Keshen and S. Stemp (Reena, Thornhill, Ontario, Canada)

PURPOSE: For the first time in history individuals with developmental disabilities (mental retardation) are aging. This positive change in their life span, however, has exposed a gap in support services between health care and social services. Reena (a community agency working with developmentally disabled adults in the Greater Toronto area) has identified this as a major issue and has begun a community development initiative in the province of Ontario. The scope of this new aging trend, the current issues, the provincial project and its' outcomes will be discussed and explored in this presentation. METHOD: A partnership was developed with Health Canada to sponsor a series of symposia throughout the province. Implementation occurred through a community development process that ensured relevance, built on the strengths of the community and provided a framework to sustain their outcomes. The outcomes for each process were community-based and founded on the principle of relationship building for future partnerships and community linkages. RESULTS: The second phase of this project was completed by April 2001, with a total of 5 geographic communities engaged in working towards systemic change. This has occurred through inclusion into existing senior services as well as the creation of new and creative support models. CONCLUSION: The issue of seniors with a developmental disability is an exciting new challenge. When partnerships and collaboration are developed and supported, they will have the ability to provide a quality of life for individuals with a developmental disability growing older for the first time in history.

Aging & Homelessness: An educational intervention

Sylvia Davidson (University Health Network, Toronto, Canada), David Ryan (Regional Geriatric Program of Toronto and the University of Toronto, Toronto, Canada), Linda Meneelly (Women's Residence, Toronto, Canada)

Homeless seniors are a silent epidemic and it is not uncommon to find 80 and 90 year-old homeless men and women in the shelters of Toronto. Across Canada, there may be as many as 6,000 homeless seniors.

Supported by the Regional Geriatric Program of Toronto, a learning needs survey of the staff of two of the largest shelters in Toronto was completed. As expected, the profile of learning needs was very similar to that obtained in facilities and services whose role is solely the care of seniors. A program of learning interventions was planned and delivered and the results of the year long program of educational intervention were evaluated. The profile of learning needs, the program it generated and its evaluations are the focus of the present paper. Enduring outcomes of the program include the integration of a workshop on aging in the Toronto Hostel's Certificate Program in Service Provision to the Homeless, an Aging and Homelessness Project Website, and increased levels of service to homeless seniors.

Aging in a Healthy Community: Master Planning for the 21st Century

Max B. Rothman (SE Florida Center on Aging, Florida International University, North Miami, Florida, USA

The abstract must not exceed 1,600 characters (250) words.... This developing project is intended to address a broad range of interconnected issues affecting the relationship between any community and a growing older adult population. Individuals plan for personal aging but communities typically do not. Developed in collaboration with United Way of Miami-Dade County and major community organizations and institutions, this pilot project provides a framework within which communities throughout the world can identify and analyze the specific needs and issues of their own unique older adult populations. Major areas of concern include healthy aging and new roles and opportunities, the economic implications of an aging society, and services and long term care. An overarching issue is the articulation of values and goals of an aging community. The methodology is based on various types of needs assessments and analysis of best practices, community-wide strategic planning involving public and private sectors, cost benefit analysis of resources allocation options, and the development of targeted strategies around priority areas. The project will produce four specific outcomes: community specific data that addresses all major issues; creation of new leadership partnerships among major community organizations; workable strategies for building healthy communities; and documentation through a final report that can serve as a model for wide-spread replication. The project is in the early stages of development. The presentation will focus on the concept and major developments and issues identified as of the date of the conference.

Canadian Community Action for Seniors and Alcohol Abuse

C. Spencer (Gerontology Research Centre, Simon Fraser University, Vancouver, Canada; D. Bradshaw (Seniors Well Aware Program,Vancouver, Canada)

Between 138,000 and 220,000 older Canadians experience alcohol or other drug problems. Yet in a given year, less than 3% receive assistance through mainstream or senior specific treatment programs. The Seniors Well Aware Program has begun a three year national project funded by the National Population Health Fund to increase the local and regional capacities across Canada to address alcohol issues among seniors. This paper describes the national project and the processes by which it is (1)raising issue awareness among various service providers and volunteers at the community level; (2)bringing together key informants from across Canada to identify best practices on how to reach seniors and aid them; (3)developing action strategies to address this health problem effectively from a community development perspective; (4) building consensus, developing and disseminating information on best practices across Canada; and (5) building and enhancing networks for sustained information sharing. The project brings together the knowledge and insights of seniors, health care and other service providers, and specialists in aging and addictions from across Canada to share strategies and best practices. The project involves ongoing sharing of information and peoples experience through focus groups, joint action meetings, and network development at the national level to raise knowledge levels, improve skills’ bases, foster positive attitudes and enhance resource/networking capacities of people who are in contact with seniors within their local communities.

How Do They Fare: The Foodways of Marginalised Ageing Men

Cherry Russell, Denise Touchard (The University of Sydney, Sydney, Australia)

This paper describes the practices, venues and cultural meanings associated with the acquisition and consumption of food by low income, non-married men living alone in the inner city of Sydney, Australia. It draws on findings from the Ageing Men's Health Project, a three-year ethnographic study that has generated 1200 hours of field observations and in-depth interviews with 67 men aged 50+ years. A key aim of the project is to examine how ageing men outside middle-class suburbs and nuclear families manage their daily lives, particularly in the face of declining health, what supports are available to them, and what their attitudes and experiences are in relation to the receipt of assistance. Findings suggest that virtually all of these men experience some degree of food insecurity and that housing and health status play a significant mediating role. Men in all non-institutional housing types patronised emergency food aid centres but largely rejected mainstream community services such as meals on wheels and shopping assistance. It is argued that eating is not merely an instrumental survival strategy but an interpretive practice through which ageing men maintain social relational continuities and negotiate an independent identity.

Older People Taking Action - successful models of engaging with older service users

Hilary Bath (Age Concern England, Northampton, United Kingdom)

PURPOSE To outline the UK's Better Government for Older People (BGOP) programme, in particular from a voluntary and community sector perspective and to share the success factors which lead to the engagement of older people in decisions that affect their lives and their communities To share the best practice developed by Age Concern within its "Involving Older People" programme, including older people in consultation programmes and training of older people, by older people in participation skills To share Age Concern's work on older people as community activists and animateurs. METHOD 2 year action research partnership programme, lead by UK government, national and local, in partnership with older people and the voluntary, community and statutory sectors 2 year community development programme between Age Concern bodies and older people and their organisations RESULTS 28 recommendations targeted at government, central and local, health authorities, voluntary and community groups and older people from BGOP in 5 thematic areas: * Combating Age Discrimination * Engaging with Older People * Better Decision Making * Better Meeting Older People's Needs * Promoting a Strategic and Joined-Up Approach Partnership approach between older people and decision makers and takers leads to the most effective decision making, but older people and their organisations need time, energy and resources to enable this to happen. CONCLUSION Every stakeholder benefits when the voices of older people are heard and acted upon and when older people are motivated to get involved in their communities and in the decisions that affect their lives.

Older Peoples Participation in a bid for a Healthy Living Centre: focus group findings

K. Emslie (Southport and Formby Primary Care Group, Southport Merseyside, U.K.) B.Wademan, J. Ledwitch (Older Volunteers (S and F. PCGp Southport UK) J.James older volunteer (S and F PCGp Sothport UK)and research student (University of Lancaster UK)

Older people were consulted to inform a bid to The New Opportunities Lottery Fund in Britain for a 'Healthy Living Centre' (H.L.C.) in a retirement area with a large ageing population. Twelve Focus Groups were held involving 89 people. These were facilitated by a group of trained older volunteers. The groups discussions were taped with consent and transcribed verbatim. Care was taken to include people with a wide age range, socio-economic background, and health status. After initial modification the Topic Guide was systematically followed. Our findings were that health, very broadly defined, was considered most important for quality of life and well being. Next in importance was prompt access to good quality health care when the individual themselves considered it necessary.Barriers were identified: lack of information, fragmentation of and lack of clarity about provision, patronizing professional attitudes and age discrimination. Difficulty with transport was also an issue. A significant proportion of our sample expressed strong fears about personal safety. An interesting division of opinion was identified about the quantity and quality of existing service and leisure provision (Excellent/Absent). The division appears to be between long standing residents and those people who have retired to the area. In general, it was thought that a H.L.C. would be a 'good thing', although there was some scepticism. It would need to be well publicised, central, with multiple methods of access, open at week ends and bank holidays. Staff should be informed and friendly, neither patronizing nor prescriptive and preferably mature.

Screening by the Elderly for the Elderly

Y. Ben-Moshe (EHEL- The Association for the Planning and Development of Services for the Aged in Israel, Jerusalem, Israel)

Screening can identify many problems in old age which can cause functional decline. Risk factors for decline can be detected by screening and referred for treatment. Programs run by trained elderly volunteers, which are aimed at providing screening services the local level, will be discussed. These programs are activated at the grassroots level in five different areas, which include: vision, hearing, environmental risk factors for falls, balance, nutritional risk factors.The presentation will deal with the rationale of services based on elderly volunteers; training process; screening tools; organizational setting; dissemination of the programs; programs results and the development of anational policy which grows out of local initiatives national policy which grows out of local initiatives.

Seniors Quality of Life Project

Mary Hill, Patrick McGowan (UBC Institute of Health Promotion Research, Vancouver, BC, Canada); Lillian Baaske, Mary Brown, Patricia Fulton, Mary Hill, Mohinder Grewal, Tom Kinloch, Anne Kloppenborg, Simon Oosterhuis, Mish Vsadasz (Vancouver and Richmond BC).

The goal of this Participatory Research project was to obtain seniors' perspectives on factors that influence their quality of life and to initiate action to address these factors. Eight Canadian cities partiicpated in the project. In Vancouver, project activities were overseen by a seniors coordinating committee and guided by a larger community advisory committee. In phase one of the project (i.e, the information gathering phase) eleven focus group meetings were conducted primarily with seniors, but also with service providers and health care professionals. Meeting notes were transcribed and analyzed using QSR Nud.ist. The themes were not pre-determined but arose out of the focus group data. Altogether, 18 separate themes were identified and those identifiied as problems in six groups or more related to: health care problems, products and services, financial constraints, diversity, housing, safety, recognition-representation, transportation, care facilities, home care, social network, macro-economic and social forces. In addition to posing problems, focus group participants also suggested potential solutions. In Phase two of the project (i.e, the action phase) committee members planned and implemented a variety of strategies that included: making presentations to the regional health board and City of Vancouver Seniors Advisory Committee; submitting briefs and action statements to candidates in the Federal election and to elected members and staff in municipal and provincial government. Members of the project coordinating committee will discuss the strengths and weaknesses of the various methods used in the project to get government to address seniors' issues.

SESSION 189

THIRD AGE EDUCATION AND LEADERSHIP: Program Models, Benefits, and Future Challenges.

L. Jest (Capilano College, North Vancouver, Canada) Moderator; Alan Aberbach (Simon Fraser University, Vancouver Canada) The Seniors Program at Simon Fraser University: Addressing Lifelong Learning Needs of the Opsimath; R. Kornfeld (Catholic University of Santiago, Santiago, Chile) Interactive Gerontology Course for Professionals: A New Use for Distance Television; L. Veelken (University of Dortmund), Dortmund, Germany) Aspects, Results, and Efficiency of an Integrated Model of Senior Studies; R. Veras (University of Rio de Janeiro, Rio de Janeiro, Brazil) Open University Studies on the Elderly: An innovative program in Brazil; Alexandra Withnall (University of Warwick, Coventry, UK) Developing Third Age Program Models in the UK; Respondent (TBA).

ISSUE: The concept of the "Third Age" has both an individual and a societal definition. Individually, it refers to the third phase of a life following compulsory work and/or raising a family. Beginning as early as 50 years, the third age is characterized by relative freedom to pursue personal interests and to engage in fulfilling activities. Thus, a society in the "Third Age" is characterized generally as having an aging population as well as a certain level of affluence. The challenge is to extend the period of vitality and productivity to the end of life, thus eliminating the fourth phase of dependence for the majority of people. The term, "Third Age Education", is preferred to that of retirement, senior, or older adult education, because it has a positive, adventurous connotation suggesting the freedom, vitality, and creativity that describes older persons in the 21st century. Third Age Education, however, is a serious enterprise deserving public support because it is a means for developing the human resource potential of an aging population through individual and collective empowerment. Those in the third age who engage in learning/ education for personal development and self-interest tend to contribute more productively through paid and/or unpaid work. Education is a pathway to leadership and service. A Third Age Education Program will, therefore, reflect a range of opportunities for learning and for contributing through service (i.e, as volunteers) to the academy and wider community.

STRUCTURE: This symposium brings together a panel of international leaders in the field of Third Age Education who represent a variety of program models in the context of Higher Education. A moderator will introduce the panel. Participants will present brief introductions to their programs with respect to (a) sociocultural context; (b) history; (c) client group; (d) courses and programs offered; (e) role of the Academy in curriculum and instruction; and (f) leadership of senior volunteers. Discussion will focus on common evolutionary trends, benefits to students, university, and society; present and future challenges. A respondent will summarize the presentations, highlighting strengths and future challenges.

CONTENT: A. Aberbach reviews the 25-year evolution of the Seniors Program at Simon Fraser University; R.Kornfeld will outline an innovative interactive Distance Education Program in Chile; L. Veelken describes an integrative intergenerational model of Seniors Studies at the University of Dortmund, Germany; R. Veras introduces the Open University Studies on the Elderly at the University of Rio de Janeiro in Brazil; Alexandra Withnall (University of Warwick, Coventry, UK) will describe two different models of third age learning in the UK (1) the Seniors Studies Institute at the University of Strathclyde, Glasgow, Scotland, and (2) the University of the

Third Age in Pembrokeshire, Wales. Respondent (TBA).

CONCLUSIONS: Through dialogue and publications, we plan to foster a greater appreciation of the value of Third Age Education to the health and wellbeing of all members of society. We anticipate new insights into Third Age Education based on discussions of different models, strengths and challenges. We intend to produce a collection of papers to be published in English and Spanish that summarizes challenges and future directions to be continued at the next World Congress in Brazil in 2005.

Aspects, Results and Efficiency of an Integrated Model of Senior Studies

L. Veelken (University of Dortmund, Dortmund, Germany)

For 20 years exists a model of further education for seniors in the university of Dortmund. The elements are: integration in the university; learning of young students and senior students together as an Intergenerational Program; learning in groups, in connection with Gerontology and Geragogy/Gerontagogy; five semesters study program; preparation for senior volunteers; certification; international network. The method is interviews, attending observation and analysis of documents. Results are the sociopolitical effort, the training for activities in Non-Profit Organisations and the intergenerational learning. The effort is: the socio-political significance of the academic studies program, discovering and practicing in new areas of interest in socially relevant fields and gaining applying knowledge and individual empowerment. After their certificate seniors are working in the field of social work; in leisure, sports, and education; in social and political participation; in multimedia; and in international cooperation and networking. The development of both generations offers participants the opportunity to learn from each other and gain a new perception about other generations. The seniors get in touch with another way of life and the young students see their own view of age changing. In this field takes place cooperation with the UNESCO international research program (Intergenerational Programmes (IP), the International Consortium for Intergenerational Programs (ICIP) and an international master study project between universities in Canada and Europe. Necessary for third age education are longer, integrated, intergenerational study programmes as a training for senior volunteers in an international network.

Developing Third Age Education Program Models in the UK

A.Withnall (University of Warwick, Coventry, UK)

The purpose of this paper is to discuss the programs of the Senior Studies Institute at the University of Strathclyde, Glasgow, Scotland and the University of the Third Age in Pembrokeshire, Wales, both of which have developed a range of opportunities for Third Agers to take part in educational programs. They represent two contrasting locations - urban and rural. A series of semi-structured focus groups discussions were held with groups of 8-10 learners at each location as part of a wider research project investigating older people's choices and experiences of lifelong learning activity. The SSI students take part in a taught program with a range of study options and are encouraged to become involved in, and to take the lead in a variety of innovative community projects. The U3A is technically a voluntary organisation but students regard themselves as attending a University in the sense of "a community of scholars" and are very much involved in designing their own learning activity rather than simply responding to what is offered by an educational institution. Members of both groups felt that participation in learning helped them increase and maintain self worth and confidence, engaged their minds and helped them to be creative. Education in the Third Age also offered opportunities for "indulgent" learning. Higher education institutions could therefore have a bigger role to play in enabling older people to take the lead in both contributing to the wider community and in developing and managing their own learning opportunities in the Third Age.

Interactive Gerontology Course for Professionals: Distance Television

Rosa Kornfeld, Pedro Paulo Marín, Carlos Isaac (Pontifical Catholic University, Santiago, Chile)

An interactive course for working professionals was developed in 1999 using a multidisciplinary perspective on gerontology designed to assist them with their professional duties. It was specifically designed to reach professionals in isolated areas of the country where continuing education opportunities are rare. The general public (especially older adults) also benefited since they were able to watch the course and learn more about aging. METHOD: 12 television programs of 25 minutes each were produced by the academic staff of the Program for the Elderly of Pontifical Catholic University (PAM-PUC) in collaboration with Educational Television of Catholic University (TELECUC). PAM-PUC maintained an academic tutorial center where enrolled participants could ask questions about the materials via e-mail, fax, and toll-free telephone. Participants were provided with a custom designed textbook, manual, workbook, prepared lecture notes, test booklets, and final project guide. The program was financed by the Chilean government with additional private sector support. RESULTS: 1,800 professionals enrolled throughout the country who received the materials and participated in the course. A substantial number of the general public also watched the course without enrolling (the Peoplemeter rating was 6, approximately double the viewership of previous general television continuing education courses). Most participants reported that they would apply the material from the course in their professional work. CONCLUSION: This method of distance education can provide continuing education to large numbers of professionals in hard to reach locations. The basic materials can also be easily modified so that they are appropriate for educating older adults about the aging process.

Open University Studies on the elderly: an innovative program in Brazil

Renato Veras (Third Age University Open University - Rio de Janeiro State University, Brazil)

The Open University for Studies on the Elderly (UnATI) aims to contribute to the improvement of physical, mental and social health levels of the elderly using the existing capabilities in the university, so as to become a center of public health, sociotherapy, delivery of community services, ergotherapy, research, and gerontological action within the institution. This broad mandate has been implemented in the State University of Rio de Janeiro (UERJ) due to the present availability in the university of personnel whose interests focus on the theme and activities of both servicing and research. This is further stressed by the fact that the state of Rio de Janeiro and the city of Rio de Janeiro in particular harbor the largest share of elderly people in Brazil. The purpose of such a center in a university is to offer health care and other services related to the university's academic and scientific perspective. Its main purpose is, therefore, to develop cultural and intellectual activities within a holistic approach, integrating physical and health care, social contact and participation in the learning process. All activities at UnATI are carried out within this same approach. Consequently, the range of activities must be wide enough to include the full diversity of the social and cultural context. The structure of UnATI is based on three areas - Teaching, Extension, and Research - which encompass all activities of the project. Teaching: Over one hundred and ten courses are being offered each semester, in many different areas both for seniors and professionals along specific programs, designed to provide personnel qualification for those who work with the third age. Extension: There is a multidisciplinary sector of health care for the elderly at the University Hospital, including juridical assistance. Research: UnATI supports and stimulates professionals who work there to develop research projects with the aim of investigating a number of aspects of the third age in Brazilian society. After seven years as a regular unit, more than three thousand people have already enrolled at UnATI's courses, and more than two thousand were assisted by the outpatient service. These numbers attest the success of the project with the target population.

The Seniors Program at Simon Fraser University: Addressing Lifelong Learning Needs of the Opsimath

Alan Aberbach (Simon Fraser University, Vancouver, Canada

Simon Fraser University opened its doors in 1965, and within ten years the university created the Continuing Studies division, designed to link the university with the Greater Vancouver community. In the year of its inception, a Seniors Program became a necessity to insure its mandate. The purpose of Continuing Studies at Simon Fraser University is, "to help adults achieve their intellectual, professional and cultural goals through programs for lifelong learning that build on the strengths of the University and the resources of the community." In particular, "Continuing Studies will ensure the widest possible access to programs and expand outreach in order to respond to community needs." SFU's Seniors Program helps fulfill that mandate. The program is unique in British Columbia: It is the only university that offers a year round Seniors Program consisting of both credit and non-credit courses. Those enrolling in the university may work for an undergraduate degree or may qualify for a Seniors Certificate upon the completion of thirty credit hours. To encourage lifelong learning, all credit courses are tuition free. Thirty intellectually stimulating, non-recreational, credit-free courses are offered each year. In addition, the popular Seniors Forum brings together seniors in a monthly lecture/discussion format on timely subjects. Over 1000 seniors have participated in the Seniors Program, and in 2000 the program celebrated its Silver Anniversary Year by expanding and enhancing its already ambitious program.

SESSION 191

Evidence Based Practice: International Elder Abuse Initiatives

S. Aziz (WISE Senior Services, Santa Monica, California, USA) Combating Elder Financial Abuse in the United States: Two Model Programs. C. McCreadie, A. Tinker (Age Concern Institute of Gerontology, King's College London, UK) and G.C.J. Bennett (St. Bartholomew's and the Royal London School of Medicine and Dentistry, London, UK) Elder Abuse: Do General Practitioners Know or Care? G.C.J. Bennett and M. Vogel (St. Bartholomew's and the Royal London School of Medicine and Dentistry, London, UK) Elder Abuse - A CD-ROM Education Tool. E. Podnieks (Ryerson Polytechnic University, Toronto, Canada) Elder Abuse: A Challenge for the Compassionate Church. J. Pritchard (Independent Researcher, Consultant, Trainer, Sheffield, England) Male Victims of Elder Abuse: A Taboo Subject.

A defining goal of the International Network for the Prevention of Elder Abuse has been to share innovative and creative practice, policy, program and professional approaches with other countries. The Symposium is an example of this commitment. Lia Daichman (convenor) has brought together a group of international experts whose eclectic views and visions are on the cutting edge of elder abuse intervention. Financial abuse is widely acknowledged as a major threat to the safety and security of older adults. A paper by Aziz focuses on the success of a model program in California. She explores peer counseling as a viable intervention strategy. Bennett and McCreadie address the perceptions of family physicians in the management of elder abuse. Their two papers examine the critical role played by physicians in the community who are ideally positioned to provide service to older adults and their caregivers. The first presentation will describe a CD-ROM teaching tool for physicians and the second will provide insight into the actual knowledge and awareness of elder abuse of these practitioners. One largely untapped community resource for raising awareness about elder abuse is religious institutions. Research has shown that older women go to their faith community for guidance and support when they have been abused. What help is available to them? Do faith leaders respond to the disclosure of abuse? Podnieks presents a new paradigm for discussion. We have a good understanding of elder abuse as a women's issue, but how much do we know about male victims? Some surprising findings are revealed by Pritchard. The discussant, Ariela Lowenstein, will highlight points of convergence and divergence across the papers and reflect on the implications of these questions for the area of elder abuse, both present and future. Clearly, the papers in this symposium bring new information and interpretation to many different aspects of elder abuse and neglect. In doing so, they contribute to the body of knowledge that will guide us in developing successful prevention and treatment programs.

Combating Elder Financial Abuse in the United States: Two Model Programs

S. Aziz (WISE Senior Services, Santa Monica, California, USA)

The incidence of elder financial abuse is growing in the United States. Loss of an elder's financial assets can result in increased morbidity and mortality. In Los Angeles County, California, two volunteer-based programs, aimed at combating the rising tide of elder financial abuse and operated through collaborative public/private partnerships, are serving as national models. The Los Angeles County Area Agency on Aging Fiduciary Abuse Specialist Team (FAST), created in 1993, is a multidisciplinary consultation and training team that provides consultation on difficult-to-resolve cases of elder financial abuse to protective services and other caseworkers and provides education and training to service providers, members of the financial community and the public. Accomplishments include recovering or preventing the loss of millions of dollars in client assets and improving the ability of member agencies to intervene in financial abuse cases. The model has been successfully replicated. The Telemarketing Victim Call Center (TVCC), created in 1998, conducts peer counseling by trained volunteer "fraud fighters" to known victims of telemarketing fraud. The TVCC has contacted over 50,000 targeted victims nationwide, has reached and provided peer counseling to almost 8,000 of those individuals, and has generated 70 resulting law enforcement investigations annually. Preliminary findings show that peer counseling has resulted in a significant reduction in the willingness of victims to respond to fraudulent sales pitches over the telephone. The presentation will describe these two model intervention programs and their impact in stopping elder financial abuse, preventing further victimization, and enhancing collaboration and coordination of services.

Elder Abuse - A CD-ROM Education Tool.

G.C.J. Bennett, M. Vogel (Academic Department of Health Care of Older People, St. Bartholomew's and the Royal London School of Medicine and Dentistry, UK)

Elder abuse, the physical, psychological, financial or sexual mistreatment of older people is an increasingly important subject that needs to be taught to medical and other multi-disciplinary students. One education tool, a Study Guide (tutorial in print) was positively evaluated at two United Kingdom medical institutions; St. Bartholomew's and the Royal London School of Medicine and Dentistry and the Queen's University, Belfast. The study guide on elder abuse forms the core material in a new education tool - the teaching CD-ROM. This tool has been educationally evaluated at each stage of development and the product Elder Abuse: An introduction for students includes; definitions, prevalence, indicators, clinical issues in history taking and examination, interventions, institutional features and an advice section. It was developed in co-operation with Action on Elder Abuse, the United Kingdom's leading organization on the topic and uses international data with hyperlinked websites, e.g. INPEA (International Network for the Prevention of Elder Abuse), to give the student as wide a perspective as possible. The tool includes referencing, summaries, questions and answers, basic and intermediate level databases enabling students of differing capabilities to navigate a complex subject. The concept map at the beginning of the CD-ROM, allied with clear graphics and images as well as evidence-based, peer reviewed content make this, the authors believe, a unique educational tool in teaching and dissemination of the current knowledge base concerning elder abuse.

Elder Abuse - A CD-ROM Education Tool.

G.C.J. Bennett, M. Vogel (Academic Department of Health Care of Older People, St. Bartholomew's and the Royal London School of Medicine and Dentistry, UK)

Elder abuse, the physical, psychological, financial or sexual mistreatment of older people is an increasingly important subject that needs to be taught to medical and other multi-disciplinary students. One education tool, a Study Guide (tutorial in print) was positively evaluated at two United Kingdom medical institutions; St. Bartholomew's and the Royal London School of Medicine and Dentistry and the Queen's University, Belfast. The study guide on elder abuse forms the core material in a new education tool - the teaching CD-ROM. This tool has been educationally evaluated at each stage of development and the product Elder Abuse: An introduction for students includes; definitions, prevalence, indicators, clinical issues in history taking and examination, interventions, institutional features and an advice section. It was developed in co-operation with Action on Elder Abuse, the United Kingdom's leading organization on the topic and uses international data with hyperlinked websites, e.g. INPEA (International Network for the Prevention of Elder Abuse), to give the student as wide a perspective as possible. The tool includes referencing, summaries, questions and answers, basic and intermediate level databases enabling students of differing capabilities to navigate a complex subject. The concept map at the beginning of the CD-ROM, allied with clear graphics and images as well as evidence-based, peer reviewed content make this, the authors believe, a unique educational tool in teaching and dissemination of the current knowledge base concerning elder abuse.

Elder Abuse: A Challenge for the Compassionate Church

E. Podnieks (Ryerson Polytechnic University, Toronto, Canada)

Churches play a critical role in the prevention of elder abuse and neglect through fostering public awareness and providing services for families at risk for being abusive. Unfortunately, although research indicates that clergy are one of the most likely groups of caregivers to encounter cases of elder mistreatment, they are also least likely to refer abuse or neglect cases to helping agencies and have not been effective at treatment intervention. Training clergy to recognize and respond to elder abuse is imperative. A project is underway in Ontario to educate and raise awareness of elder abuse in faith communities. The project seeks to provide basic information, referral sources and alternatives that victims, religious leaders and service providers need to know in order to work effectively and sensitively with elder abuse. The project seeks to address both safety and relationship needs in harmony with religious belief systems. It aims to generate and enhance the formation of new partnerships among faith leaders and community services. The faith community needs to be open to and explore community resources. At the same time, the secular community needs to develop a new respect for religious values that may influence intervention. A spirit of collaboration must be fostered in order for these groups to work together. Outcomes include the reduction of harm to older congregants, a more informed clergy, empowerment of senior members of faith communities and mobilization of faith communities' ability to respond effectively to elder abuse.

Elder Abuse: Do General Practitioners Know or Care?

C. McCreadie and A. Tinker (Age Concern Institute of Gerontology, King's College London, UK), G.C.J. Bennett (St. Bartholomew's and the Royal London School of Medicine and Dentistry, London, UK)

Two surveys of General Practitioners' knowledge and awareness of the abuse of older people are reported. The first took place in Tower Hamlets, a deprived borough in London in 1997; and was replicated in the much larger and more diverse city of Birmingham in 1999. The findings in both areas were remarkably similar. Just under half the respondents (73 GPs in Tower Hamlets, and 291 GPs in Birmingham) had diagnosed a case of elder abuse in the previous year; around 85% identified having a patient in at least one risk situation (out of a possible twenty) and around 40% identified having patients in five or more risk situations. Regression analysis of the combined data sets (n=363) indicated that the strongest factor predicting GP diagnosis of abuse was knowledge of five or more risk situations. Other independent variables were not significant, including the amount of home visiting, the number of older people on a GP's list, or characteristics of the GP such as age and gender. Questions about training indicated that although very small proportions of GPs had had any training about elder abuse, 70% in both areas would find it helpful. The findings suggest that research-based education and training would help GPs become better at identifying and managing abuse

Male Victims of Elder Abuse: A Taboo Subject

J. Pritchard (Independent Researcher, Consultant, Trainer, Sheffield, England)

Whilst undertaking a qualitative research study on the needs of older women who were victims of elder abuse, older men started to disclose to the researcher about the abuse they were currently experiencing or had experienced in childhood or earlier in adulthood. Consequently, the focus of the inquiry broadened to include male victims. The research project was undertaken in three social services departments in the North of England (UK). Monitoring systems were set up to identify the number of vulnerable adults who were being abused. In-depth interviews were conducted with 11 older men who were victims of elder abuse and focus groups were run for over 300 older people. Social workers and other social care staff were interviewed and participated in focus groups. Over one fifth of victims of elder abuse identified in the three departments were male. In these cases 51% of the abusers were female. Financial abuse was the most common form of abuse identified. The main needs of male victims identified were: place of safety; continued/regular contact with professionals; permanent accommodation; personal safety; permission to talk; assessment; loyalty and duty; protection of the abuser; practical advice; company; dealing with losses and bereavement; cultural; police involvement. The abuse of males should be defined in a wider context and not solely in terms of the previous definitions of abuse commonly used in child abuse and domestic violence work. The present study found that carer's stress was not a causal factor in the abuse of the men.

SESSION 192

Comparative perspectives on living arrangements and health of older adults in the developing world

Zachary Zimmer (Population Council, New York, USA) and John Bongaarts (Population Council, New York, USA), Living arrangements of older adults in the developing world: An analysis of DHS household surveys. Kathryn M. Yount (Emory University, Atlanta, USA) and Emily Agree (Johns Hopkins School of Hygiene and Public Health, Baltimore, USA), Gender, health, and informal support: Challenges of population aging in the Middle East. Angelique Chan (National University of Singapore, Singapore), Elizabeth Frankenberg (RAND, Los Angeles, USA) and Mary Beth Ofstedal (University of Michigan, Ann Arbor, USA), Stability and change in living arrangements of older adults in Southeast and East Asia. Manisha Sengupta (Johns Hopkins School of Public Health, Baltimore, USA), Gender differences in self-reported disabilities among the elderly in India. Rebeca Wong (Georgetown University, Washington, USA), Health, utilization of health care, and aging in Mexico.

Population aging is occurring across the developing world, yet in comparison to the West, the consequences of tehse age structure changes have been understudied. In an attempt to broaden our understanding of aging in the developing world, the current symposium concentrates on investigations of living arrangements and health of older adults using large representative surveys that allow for comparative analyses. Comparative approaches are essential to gerontological and demographic research, though it is more common to compare effects across socio-demographic groups than across countries, regions, or other subgroups in non-Western environments. Yet, such analyses have great power in determining effects that are universal versus those that subject to cultural, regional or subpopulation variation. The symposium is organized around five papers that begin with the broadest possible comparative view of living arrangements and health across global dimensions. This is followed by examinations first on a regional and then on a countrywide basis. In this fashion, comparative research will be offered at various levels of analysis. Zimmer and Bongaarts first examine differences in patterns of living arrangements across 43 countries using data from Demographic and Health Surveys. Although these data were collected to study maternal health and fertility, household composition can be determined based on the relationship of household members to the household head. This data is used to examine how household structures differ regionally and across macro level characteristics that describe countries, such as life expectancy. Yount and Agree will explore how gender and living arrangement patterns are related to health outcomes across four countries in the Middle East. They use data from the WHO Collaborative Study on Social and Health Aspects of Aging. Chan, Frankenberg and Ofstedal will move the discussion to Asia in order to examine correlates of living arrangements across three countries that are, or will soon be, experiencing rapid population aging: Taiwan, Singapore and Indonesia. Sengupta’s paper will keep the discussion geographically in Asia, but examines regional variation in India using data from northern and southern states of the country. The aim of this paper is to determine how gender disparities in health differ across broad regional divisions of India, and how these are further influenced by living arrangements of older adults. Wong will compare health and health care utilization in Mexico across subgroups of age and socioeconomic status employing a sample of over 60,000 individuals responding to a Mexican Ministry of Health survey conducted in 1994. By focusing on comparative approaches, each presentation offered in this symposium examines how living arrangements and/or health of older adults in the developing world is a function of a broader environment, be it regional, national or cultural. As such, this group of papers, taken together, will assist in establishing an understanding of the ways in which health and living situations of older adults are differentially determined across diverse settings of the developing world.

Gender differences in self-reported disabilities among the elderly in India

Manisha Sengupta (Johns Hopkins School of Public Health Baltimore, USA)

The purpose of this paper is to evaluate gender disparities in physical disabilities in the population age 65 and over in India, and examine how these disparities differ across regions of India and across living arrangements. Gender differences in disabilities among older adults have been well studied in developed countries, but there is very little information in developing countries, especially those in South Asia. On balance, past research, including some studies conducted in Bangladesh and Egypt, shows that females report greater functional limitations than do males, but the significance of gender is reduced as other sociodemographic variables are added into equations. The male - female disparity has been attributed to differential reporting and greater prevalence of disabling diseases among women. In the current paper, these hypotheses are tested using data from the National Family Health Survey conducted in India in 1992-93. Northern and southern states of India are distinguished in order to determine whether there are regional differences in the way in which gender discriminates in physical health. Logistic regression techniques analyze the gender differentials and its relation to living arrangements, while at the same time controlling for age, education and asset ownership. The results show that gender disparities exist in disability status, even after controlling for socioeconomic status. These gender differences are more pronounced in the north, where they reflect the historical gender bias in society.

Gender, health and informal support: Challenges of population aging in the Middle East

Kathryn M. Yount (Emory University, Atlanta, USA) and Emily Agree (Johns Hopkins School of Hygiene and Public Health, Baltimore, USA)

Declines in fertility and mortality have caused unprecedented population aging in the Middle East. While evidence from more developed countries suggests that elderly men and women experience differential protective effects from marriage and social networks, the effects for the Middle East remain unknown. This dearth of information persists despite a known female disadvantage in health status and access to care at other ages. Distinguishing features of marital and parental life in the Middle East suggest that the effects of social support in later life that have been observed elsewhere may not be the same in this setting. To explore these questions, this study uses data on the health status and living conditions of non-institutionalized men and women 60 years of age or older from four countries: Bahrain (n = 799), Egypt (n = 1,179), Jordan (n = 1,193), and Tunisia (1,236). The data are a part of the 1989 World Health Organization Collaborative Study on Social and Health Aspects of Aging. First, basic gender differences in self-assessed health, functional disability, and access to care are explored. Next, the differential effects of marriage and social support on health and access to care are formally tested to assess the mechanisms by which gender inequality in these outcomes emerges in later life. Based on findings, policy and programmatic responses to meet the needs of growing numbers of older women and men in the region are discussed.

Health, utilization of health care, and aging in Mexico

Rebeca Wong (Georgetown University, Washington, USA)

The paper examines the patterns of morbidity and health care utilization in Mexico, comparing between the elderly and those of younger ages. The overall hypothesis is that the elderly exhibit distinct illness and utilization patterns such that future aging of the population may represent increasing demands for health care. The empirical analysis uses data from a national household survey completed by the Mexican Ministry of Health in 1994. The sample consisted of 61,500 individuals, asking demographic and socioeconomic data, illness reports, and health services used for each household member. Multivariate models are estimated for: the presence of illness report, use of health care services, and choice of provider. Preliminary results are consistent with the notion that the elderly and women report more illness than the young. The elderly do not use health services differently than other adult age groups. Although the poor use less health care than the rich, having health insurance coverage closes the gap in utilization that is found between the rich and poor. And adult age groups, including the elderly, tend to use better quality of services than children. In conclusion, the preliminary analyses indicate that the observed differentials in the propensity to use health care services by older age or higher income groups in Mexico seem largely a result of differences in health care coverage. Differences in health care utilization, largely, do not seem to result from differences in the disease patterns observed across the age groups.

Living arrangements of older adults in the developing world: An analysis of DHS household surveys.

Zachary Zimmer (Population Council, New York, USA); John Bongaarts (Population Council, New York, USA)

Studies of living arrangements of older adults in developing countries tend to employ country-specific data and are therefore limited in comparative scope. In an attempt to add a global dimension to research on living arrangements, the current study employs data from Demographic and Health Surveys (DHS) conducted in 43 countries in Latin America, Asia and Africa. Although these surveys are normally employed to examine fertility and maternal health issues, information that is gathered allows for the determinations of the structure of a random sample of households in each country. The paper begins by examining differences in household structure patterns across diverse geographic environments employing countries as the unit of analysis. This includes looking at differences in size, headship and composition among households containing older adults. Following is an examination of macro level determinants where variables such as life expectancy, percent with education and percent urban are used to distinguish living arrangement patterns across countries and regions. Emphasis here is placed on the percent of older adults who coreside with adult children and on the gender ratio of coresident children. Results indicate that coresidence, household size, and living alone all correlate with indicators of socioeconomic development. There are also strong regional variations in living arrangement patterns. We conclude that although there is no standard household structure for older adults in the developing world, strong consistencies exist across regions and across countries with similar levels of economic and social development.

Stability and change in living arrangements of older adults in Southeast and East Asia

Angelique Chan (National University of Singapore, Singapore), Elizabeth Frankenberg (RAND, Los Angeles, USA) and Mary Beth Ofstedal (University of Michigan, Ann Arbor, USA),

This paper explores the correlates of living arrangements of older adults (age 55 and older) both at one point in time and over time, drawing on newly available panel data from three countries: Singapore, Indonesia and Taiwan. The theoretical framework that guides the analysis hypothesizes that intergenerational coresidence is influenced by needs, preferences, and opportunities of both older parents and their children. As indicators of these three dimensions, the analysis focuses on the effects of availability and attributes of children, as well as demographic, socioeconomic and health characteristics of older parents, on concurrent living arrangements and change in living arrangements over a 3-4 year period. We use binary logistic regression models to estimate effects of these factors on parent-child coresidence in the baseline survey, and multinomial logistic regression models to estimate effects on transitions in coresidence over time. Results show that the percent of older adults living with one or more children is high in all countries, ranging from 86% in Singapore (1995) to 73% in Taiwan (1996) and 62% in Indonesia (1993). Living arrangements appear to be fairly stable over a 3-4 year period; over four-fifths of respondents in each country had the same living arrangement in both survey years. Preliminary results of the multivariate analysis suggest that both need and opportunity factors influence intergenerational living arrangements cross-sectionally and over time. The results also reveal a number of similarities and several interesting differences in results across countries that are highlighted in the discussion

SESSION 193

Looking Inward, Looking Outward: Review of Three Dementia Networks in Canada

B. Howson (Seniors Health Program, Care in the Community, Calgary Regional Health Authority, Alberta, Canada) The Calgary Dementia Care Network Experience. W. Dalziel (Regional Geriatric Assessment Program, and Care of the Elderly, SCO Health Service, Ottawa, ON, Canada) and B. Schulman (Care of the Elderly and Rehabilitation Program, SCO Health Service, Ottawa, ON, Canada) The Dementia Network of Ottawa-Carleton Experience. C. Cohen (Sunnybrook and Women's College Health Science Centre, Toronto, ON, Canada) The Dementia LINCΔToronto Experience and Review of a Framework for Network Development and Evaluation.

The objectives for the session are: to describe the experience of developing three Canadian dementia networks, to review their range of activities and accomplishments, and to discuss with participants the comparisons and contrasts of international approaches and possible models for networks. In recognition of the unique challenges faced by health and social service providers to individuals with dementia and their families, a number of networks have developed across Canada focusing on dementia care. While each network has focused on different aspects of dementia care, all of the networks were spearheaded because of concerns and gaps in the organization and delivery of dementia care services such as fragmentation of services, poor coordination of services, long waiting times, inappropriate referrals and inconsistent standards of care/service or guidelines for practice. The networks also recognized the need for improvement and developing opportunities for coordinated education and research. The session will highlight the evolution and experience of three community-based dementia networks (Calgary, Ottawa and Toronto) formed between 1997 and 1999 in two different Canadian provinces. The presenters will discuss the concept of networks (also known as alliances, consortia, partnerships), the origins of the networks, the stakeholders, their mandate and objectives, demographics of the regions being served, their successes, challenges and lessons learned. The presentation will describe the accomplishments of the networks, e.g. an inventory of Dementia Care Services and the production of a Dementia Services Directory (Calgary), the development of a competency profile for the Dementia Support Worker (Calgary), identified the continuum of services required by individuals living with dementia and their caregivers (Toronto), the development of a dementia caregiver database (Toronto), development of a common referral form for assessment and treatment services (Ottawa), and the development of a local resources guide on driving (Ottawa). The presenters will also outline the scope of their respective and conjoint research and evaluation endeavours. A framework for network development and evaluation will be provided to facilitate information exchange and discussion among the attendees about their experiences. Elements of the framework will include setting up a dementia network, components of a network, mandate, goals and objectives, membership, leadership, resources, sustainability, service delivery, education, research, evidence-based outcomes, and evaluation. It is hoped that participants will learn from the international experience of others at the session and how they compare and contrast with the Canadian experience.

The Calgary Dementia Care Network Experience

B. Howson (Seniors Health Program, Care in the Community, Calgary Regional Health Authority, Alberta, Canada)

This presentation will provide an overview of the origin of the Calgary Dementia Care Network, its stakeholders, mandate and objectives, its activities and accomplishments, lessons learned and challenges that lie ahead.

The Dementia LINC Toronto Experience and Review of a Framework for Network Development and Evaluation

C. Cohen (Sunnybrook and Women's College Health Science Centre, Toronto, ON, Canada)

This presentation will provide an overview of the origin of the Dementia LINCΔToronto, its stakeholders, mandate and objectives, its activities and accomplishments, lessons learned and challenges that lie ahead. This presentation will also describe a framework for network development and evaluation to facilitate information exchange and discussion among the attendees about their experiences internationally.

The Dementia Network of Ottawa-Carleton Experience

W. Dalziel (Regional Geriatric Assessment Program, and Care of the Elderly, SCO Health Service, Ottawa, ON, Canada) and B. Schulman (Care of the Elderly and Rehabilitation Program, SCO Health Service, Ottawa, ON, Canada)

This presentation will provide an overview of the origin of the Dementia

Network of Ottawa-Carleton, its stakeholders, mandate and objectives, its activities and accomplishments, lessons learned and challenges that lie ahead.

SESSION 194

Films and Videos on Intimacy and Aging

James Vanden Bosch (Terra Nova Films, Inc, Chicago, Illinois USA)

The Personals (37 minute, released in 1999) The longing for love, sex, and relationships does not end as we grow older. The Personals is a touching film that follows a group of older adults as they rehearse and perform an original play about their quest for dates through the personal ads. The material for the play is drawn from the comedy and drama of their own lives, and the film follows them into their homes to further explore their thoughts and feelings about intimacy in their elder years. Winner of a 1999 Academy Award for Best Short Documentary, and also awards from over 20 International Festivals. // For Better or For Worse (55 minutes, released in 1993) In this video, five culturally diverse couples, each together fifty years or longer, draw on rich storehouses of wisdom and experience, and recount colorful stories of their shared journeys. The couples discuss topics such as conflict resolution, love and sex, aging, and the inevitability that one will die before the other. Their stories are remarkably frank and open-minded. In a time when marriage has become much more difficult to sustain, For Better or For Worse offers wise, refreshingly down-to-earth insights into what may still be one of the most rewarding undertakings in life.

SESSION 195

Everyday Life and Social Integration of Older Adults in Rural Areas

N. Keating (Department of Human Ecology, University of Alberta, Canada), J. Keefe (Department of Family Studies and Gerontology, Mount Saint Vincent University, Canada) and B. Dobbs (Department of Psychology, University of Alberta, Canada) Addressing the Everyday Life of Rural Elders: Rural Communities and Support to Seniors. C. Norris-Baker (Galichia Center on Aging, Kansas State University, USA) Applying the Behavior Setting Approach to Rural Aging in the United States: Lessons Learned. T. Scharf (Centre for Social Gerontology, School of Social Relations, Keele University, UK), G.C. Wenger, V. Burholt (Centre for Social Policy Research and Development, University of Wales, Bangor, UK) and F. Thissen (Amsterdam Study Centre for the Metropolitan Environment, University of Amsterdam, Netherlands), Social Integration of Older People in Rural Europe: Findings from the OPERA study. H. Mollenkopf , S. Baas and F. Oswald (The German Centre for Research on Ageing, University of Heidelberg, Germany) Exploring Outdoor Mobility and Activities of Older Adults in Rural Areas of East and West Germany: A Diary-based Approach. I. Ruoppila, T. Suutama and K. Salminen (Department of Psychology, University of Jyväskylä, Finland) Social Relations and Interest-Based Activities of Older People in Rural Finland. H.-W. Wahl (The German Centre for Research on Ageing, University of Heidelberg, Germany) Discussant.

This symposium brings together researchers and data-sets capable of illustrating the potential for considering the "real" day-to-day lives of older people living in rural areas of a range of nations. Contributors to the symposium will address elders' opportunities for social integration, taking into account prevailing national conditions. The symposium opens with a conceptual paper that emphasises the continuing need for data on social integration relating to the everyday life of older people, and identifies why the need for such data is especially relevant in rural contexts (N. Keating et al.). Second, a classic approach to daily life contexts, i.e. the behavior setting approach first used by Barker and Barker with elders in 1961, is stressed by C. Norris-Baker. Third, the dominant concerns and opportunities for social integration of elders in the UK/Wales, The Netherlands, Germany (East and West), Poland and Hungary are explored with reference to a comparative data-set generated at the beginning of the 1990s (T. Scharf et al.). Fourth, H. Mollenkopf et al. present findings deriving from the analysis of detailed diary-based records of older people's outdoor behavior in two rural regions of Germany. Fifth, data from Finland, representing the European country with the most pronounced differences between urban and rural areas, are presented by I. Ruoppila and associates. Finally, H.-W. Wahl discusses findings generated by the range of studies incorporated into the symposium. The discussion identifies advantages and limitations associated with attempts to gather data as near as possible to the 'lived experiences' of older people living in rural areas, and notes lessons to be learned from these data in terms of social integration.

Addressing the Everyday Life of Rural Elders: Rural Communities and Support to Seniors.

N. Keating (Department of Human Ecology, University of Alberta, Canada), J. Keefe (Department of Family Studies and Gerontology, Mount Saint Vincent University, Canada), B. Dobbs (Department of Psychology, University of Alberta, Canada)

A stereotype of rural life is that residents are embedded in close-knit, supportive networks of kin and friends. In this paper we argue that this 'rural idyll' masks the potential diversity in support networks of rural seniors. Canada is used as a case example from which 3 types of rural communities are discussed that may differ substantially in availability of social networks. Farming communities have a high proportion of seniors who have aged in place with longstanding friend networks but small kin networks because of out-migration of young people. Retirement communities also have high proportions of seniors but most will have no longstanding kin or friend networks since seniors move into these communities after they leave the labour force. Remote communities have small proportions of seniors who have small social networks because of reduced life expectancy and out-migration of young people. The potential for social integration/social isolation of seniors in each of these communities and of the relationships between these types of support networks and informal caregiving networks are considered. In many countries, rural areas have disproportionate numbers of seniors. Yet rural diversity would suggest that some communities have informal systems that will buffer seniors from negative health outcomes and risk of isolation, whereas in other rural communities, a lack of informal support networks may place seniors at risk for negative health outcomes and isolation. Data on social integration relating to the everyday lives of older people could help considerably in deconstructing the 'rural idyll'.

Applying the Behavior Setting Approach to Rural Aging in the United States: Lessons Learned.

C. Norris-Baker (Galichia Center on Aging, Kansas State University, Manhattan, Kansas, USA)

This paper uses a transactional environment-behavior framework to consider the impacts of rapid changes in the cultural, social, and physical dimensions of the rural environment on the daily life experience and social integration of older residents living in small towns. Case study data are drawn from experiential field research conducted in four rural Kansas communities over a ten year interval. Methods included in-depth interviews with older residents, participant observation, behavior setting identification, photo-documentation, and archival research. Based on the behavior setting concepts of behavioral focal points, underpopulation and understaffing, and historical and temporal contexts, the presentation traces the history of several key setting transformations and their short and longer-term consequences at the individual and community level. The importance of lacking physical-social structures, declining population, and threats of setting loss are highlighted. Different strategies for sustaining everyday activities and maintaining place, self, and community identities in the face of environmental change and deculturation are reported. Conclusions address the importance of recognizing the complex roles behavior setting dynamics play in maintaining social integration among older residents of small rural communities, as well as creating, sustaining, and preserving settings that serve these older residents and support aging in place in rural communities in the U.S.

Applying the Behavior Setting Approach to Rural Aging in the United States: Lessons Learned.

C. Norris-Baker (Galichia Center on Aging, Kansas State University, Manhattan, Kansas, USA)

This paper uses a transactional environment-behavior framework to consider the impacts of rapid changes in the cultural, social, and physical dimensions of the rural environment on the daily life experience and social integration of older residents living in small towns. Case study data are drawn from experiential field research conducted in four rural Kansas communities over a ten year interval. Methods included in-depth interviews with older residents, participant observation, behavior setting identification, photo-documentation, and archival research. Based on the behavior setting concepts of behavioral focal points, underpopulation and understaffing, and historical and temporal contexts, the presentation traces the history of several key setting transformations and their short and longer-term consequences at the individual and community level. The importance of lacking physical-social structures, declining population, and threats of setting loss are highlighted. Different strategies for sustaining everyday activities and maintaining place, self, and community identities in the face of environmental change and deculturation are reported. Conclusions address the importance of recognizing the complex roles behavior setting dynamics play in maintaining social integration among older residents of small rural communities, as well as creating, sustaining, and preserving settings that serve these older residents and support aging in place in rural communities in the U.S.

Exploring Outdoor Mobility and Activities of Older Adults in Rural Areas of East and West Germany: A Diary-based Approach

H. Mollenkopf, S. Baas, F. Oswald (The German Centre for Research on Ageing at the University of Heidelberg, Heidelberg, Germany)

The purpose of this paper is: (1) to describe and compare the conditions for outdoor mobility in rural settings in eastern and western Germany; (2) to explore the everyday walks and journeys of older adults in these areas, as well as the motives underlying them; (3) focus is placed on certain well-defined activities in order to compare the social integration of men and women in eastern and western areas. The empirical basis is a survey conducted in 1999 in rural areas of eastern and western Germany with a sample of 412 persons aged 55 years or older, collected in a random route procedure, and disproportionately stratified by gender and age. Respondents completed a standardised questionnaire assessing individual and environmental aspects of mobility and activity. In addition, they kept a specially designed diary which comprehensively described the trips they went on over a three-day period. Both individual and environmental aspects of mobility differed significantly between the eastern and western regions, including the availability of shops and services, the proportion of respondents who actively drive a car, number of leisure activities, and satisfaction with the outdoor environment (all items W >E). In both areas, walks and journeys mainly took place in the immediate neighbourhood. The western German elders proved to be more mobile and showed a larger diversity of activities than eastern Germans of the same age. The correlation of activity patterns and socio-demographic aspects or individual aspects enabled us to identify well-integrated groups of older people as well as those who are at risk of social exclusion.

Social Integration of Older People in Rural Europe: Findings from the OPERA Study

T. Scharf (Centre for Social Gerontology, School of Social Relations, Keele University, UK), G.C. Wenger, V. Burholt (Centre for Social Policy Research and Development, University of Wales, Bangor, UK), F. Thissen (Amsterdam Study Centre for the Metropolitan Environment, University of Amsterdam, Netherlands)

This paper considers the social integration of older people in rural areas of six European nations. Particular emphasis is placed upon integration in intergenerational relationships and in local communities. The paper uses data collected within the context of the Older People in Europe's Rural Areas (OPERA) study, designed to compare the situation of older people in some of Europe's most rural areas. Quantitative data, collected in between 1988 and 1991, using comparable questionnaires, are presented. In relation to integration within intergenerational relationships, the paper presents data on household and family structure, neighbours and friends, levels of contact, expectations of informal help and respondents' attitudes to personal relationships. Community integration is analysed with reference to older people's institutional ties, social activities, and affective attachment. All variables of interest show significant differences between the countries. In terms of integration in intergenerational relationships, an important difference is the proportion of older people in rural areas who live in multi-generation households. This factor appears to influence many of the other findings on family life and contacts with non-kin. The importance of informal non-kin relationships differs, reflecting settlement types and distances between households. The paper reveals great variability in the nature of community integration between European nations, suggesting that such integration is closely associated with a range of individual and household characteristics.

Social Relations and Interest-Based Activities of Older People in Rural Finland

I. Ruoppila, T. Suutama, K. Salminen (Department of Psychology, University of Jyväskylä, Jyväskylä, Finland)

The purpose is to describe social relations and interest-based activities of older people living in rural areas of Finland and compare them with those living in urban areas. Method: The data is based on two representative stratified (age 75-79, 80-85/89; gender) samples of persons living in central Finland. The first sample included one urban and 7 rural municipalities (participation rate 69%; n=200). The second sample was drawn from three remote rural municipalities (participation rate 81%; n=150). Both data sets were generated in the 1980's by home-interviews. Results: The economical resources were lower in rural than urban areas. Rural older persons lived more often with another person in their household. The rural subjects had more children and grand-children and more frequent interaction with them, and they evaluated their inter-generational relationships to be more positive than did the urban subjects. They also had more siblings and more frequent interaction with them. The urban subjects felt more often to be forgotten, although there were no differences in feelings of loneliness. Urban older people devoted more time to physical activities and reading and less to different handicrafts than rural persons. Participation in interest-based activities was higher among the urban subjects. There was a trend of less social interaction and participation in activities among the older age-groups. Men had better health and more interest-based activities than women; women had more social relationships and engaged in more social interaction than men. Conclusion: The 75-89-year-old Finns living at home have a rather high or at least moderate level of social functioning showing, however, some differences between rural and urban persons.

SESSION 196

The Myths and Realities of Aging: Analysis Across Time and Across Cultures

N. Cutler (National Council on the Aging, Washington, DC, USA) and S. Cutler (University of Vermont, Burlington, VT, USA), Cohort Changes in Health as a Personal Problem: 1974-2000. N. Whitelaw and N. Cutler (National Council on the Aging, Washington, DC, USA) Predictors of Vital Aging: Factors that Compensate For Less Health and Wealth. F. Forette (ILC-France, Paris, France), Y. Kudo (ILC-Japan, Tokyo, Japan), N. O'Brien (ILC-USA, New York, NY, USA) International Myths and Realities on Aging: A Five-Country Comparison. Discussants: M. Mettler (Healthwise, Inc, Boise, ID, USA, and R. Pereyra (ILC-Dominican Republic, Santo Domingo, Dominican Republic).

ISSUE: In the context of increasing older age longevity around the world, the systematic and continuing assessment of public response to the aging of self and to the aging of society is fundamental to the development of sound social policies and practices. STRUCTURE: The Myth and Reality of Aging in America conducted by the National Council on the Aging in 1974 was a landmark national study that provided baseline measurements of the attitudes of younger and older people toward the issues, the problems, and the very definitions of aging. A quarter-century later American Perceptions of Aging in the 21st Century repeated many of the questions from the original research to measure the impact of twenty-five years of societal aging on these fundamental attitudes and perceptions. At the same time a core set of the questions was asked in surveys in four additional countries. These year 2000 projects extend the research in two key ways: a focus on the measurement and meaning of vital aging as citizens around the world anticipate living to age 75 and older; and a core set of responses to the questions measured concurrently in five countries. CONTENT: This Symposiums three papers include: (1) A twenty-five year cohort analysis, 1974 to 2000, examining the degree to which change and continuity in perception of health as a personal problem is a function of aging, of generational cohort, or of secular trend. (2) A cross-sectional analysis of patterns of vital aging and personal optimism about living to age 75 or age 90, with a focus on family, friends, community involvement, and health and financial literacy and efficacy as possible compensatory factors in producing positive feelings about vital aging in the face of declining health and income. (3) A comparative cross-cultural analysis of the core Myths and Realities response patterns from a concurrent set of surveys fielded in the Dominican Republic, France, Japan, the United Kingdom, and the United States. CONCLUSION: It is apparent that as individuals recognize that older-age longevity is increasing, their concern with health as a key element of their personal aging is also increasing. Even if health and income decline, however, vitality in older age is enhanced by continued productivity and involvements with family, friends, and community, and robust levels of health and financial literacy and efficacy. The Symposium is organized by the National Council on the Aging in collaboration with the International Longevity Centers in five countries.

Cohort Changes in Health as a Personal Problem: 1974-2000

N. Cutler (National Council on the Aging, Washington, DC), S. Cutler and M. Johnson (University of Vermont, Burlington, VT, USA)

PURPOSE: Recent research has noted an improvement over the past two decades in the health status of the older population. This study examines whether cohort changes over the period 1974-2000 in personal perceptions of health as a problem show evidence of such an improvement. METHOD: Data are drawn from three nationally representative surveys of the U.S. population 18 years of age and older: the 1974 and 2000 Myths and Realities of Aging Surveys conducted for the National Council on the Aging and the 1994 Images of Aging Survey conducted for the American Association of Retired Persons. Health is measured by responses to the following question: How serious a problem would you say poor health is for you personally these days? Changes are tracked for four cohorts: 18-29, 30-39, 40-49, 50+ in 1974 and 44-55, 56-65, 66-75, and 76+ in 2000. RESULTS: For poor health as a very serious problem personally, small increases occur between 1974 and 2000 for the three youngest cohorts, but a decrease is evident for the oldest cohort. Using a more expansive definition (poor health as a very plus somewhat serious problem) substantial increases are found for the three youngest cohorts, but little change for the oldest cohort. Cohort changes for men and women, analyzed separately, parallel these overall trends. CONCLUSION: If poor health is a more prevalent accompaniment of aging, these findings suggest that the oldest cohort perceives poor health to have become less problematic than would be expected.

International Myths & Realities on Aging: A Five-Country Comparison

F. Forette (ILC-France, Paris, France), Y. Kudo (ILC-Japan, Tokyo, Japan), N. O'Bien (ILC-USA, New York, USA)

The PURPOSE of this paper is to report the results of a cross-cultural survey of public attitudes, perceptions and experiences related to aging and longevity in five countries; the Dominican Republic, France, Japan, the United Kingdom, and the United States. In each country, an omnibus survey METHOD was used to interview a nationally representative sample of people aged 18 or older. This survey was conducted by telephone in France, Japan, the United Kingdom and the United States, and in person in the Dominican Republic. While there are many similarities across the RESULTS of the research in the five countries, the differences are very substantial and indicate that experiences of aging, attitudes toward aging, and perceptions of old age vary markedly among the countries. A major CONCLUSION drawn from this study is the necessity of measuring and comparing attitudes in older countries vs. developing countries in building a base of knowledge for cross-cultural comparisons of aging policies and programs.

Predictors of Vital Aging: Factors that Compensate For Less Health and Wealth

N. Whitelaw and N. Cutler (National Council on the Aging, Washington, DC)

PURPOSE: This research explores the degree to which factors other than health and wealth promote vital aging as a social-psychological construct encompassing such personal attitudes as looking forward to living to age 75 and beyond, feeling in control of one's life, believing that life in general is working out better than expected. METHOD: The analysis is based on the American Perceptions of Aging in the 21st Century survey (January 2000, n=3000) conducted for the National Council on the Aging. The sample design includes a substantial over-sample of older adults. RESULTS: Not surprisingly, health and income are positively correlated with indicators of vital aging. Beyond such descriptive analysis, however, from the dual perspectives of personal well-being and social policy it is more important to empirically discover the how and why of higher levels of vital aging for those older men and women whose health and financial status would predict lower levels. Consequently, further analysis demonstrates the degree to which such factors as interaction with family and friends, community involvements, financial and health literacy, and perceived access to health care serve as compensatory factors that promote vital aging. CONCLUSIONS: Along with other recent studies this research documents that vital aging is not a simple reflection of personal health or wealth, but is responsive to continued interaction with family, friends, and community. Additionally, for middle-aged and older persons more generally, vital aging is enhanced by higher levels of health and financial literacy and efficacy.

SESSION 197

A longitudinal study of the relationships among passionate activities, affect, and psychological adjustment among seniors.

François L. Rousseau & Robert J. Vallerand (Laboratoire de Recherche sur le Comportement Social, Department of Psychology, Université du Québec à Montréal)

Although the benefits of activity engagement for seniors are well-documented, little is known about the psychological processes underlying those benefits. Vallerand et al. (2000) recently proposed a concept of passionate activities that may help explaining how activity engagement influences seniors' psychological adjustment. Vallerand et al. define passion as an activity that one finds interesting, important, and invests time in. Vallerand et al. proposed that there are two types of passion: harmonious and obsessive. Harmonious passion is in harmony with other activities in an individual's life and generally leads to positive consequences. Obsessive passion, on the other hand, tends to be in conflict with other activities in an individual's life and generally leads to negative consequences. In the present study, the relationships among passion, affect, and psychological adjustment were examined among 177 community-dwelling adults 50 to 91 years of age. Participants completed a first questionnaire (T1), followed by a second questionnaire three months later (T2). Results from hierarchical regression analyses showed that harmonious passion at T1 led to an increase in positive affect experienced during the practice of a passionate activity at T2, while obsessive passion at T1 led to an increase in negative affect at T2. In return, positive affect led to improved psychological adjustment while negative affect led to decreased psychological adjustment. These results suggest that harmonious passion, through its influence on positive affect, can lead to better psychological adjustment among seniors, and may therefore play a key-role in successful aging.

Affective Adaptation in the Context of Cataract Surgery: Does Experience Make a Difference?

N. Knoll, N. Rieckmann, & R. Schwarzer (Department of Health Psychology, Free University Berlin, Germany)

The goal of the present study was to investigate affective adaptation to a moderately stressful medical procedure, cataract surgery, in elderly persons. The sample consisted of 80 elderly inpatients at a Berlin eye-clinic (mean age = 71,79) who underwent cataract surgery. Central outcome variables were positive and negative affect assessed at two points in time pre-surgery (day of admission, day of surgery) and two time points post-surgery (day after surgery, six weeks after surgery). Main predictor variables were a total of fourteen coping strategies assessed on the day of admission to the hospital as well as first or second eye surgery. Results indicate different changes in positive and negative affect for first- and second-eye patients pre- and post-surgery. Moreover, coping strategies predicted positive and negative affect pre- and post-surgery as well as pre-surgical change of affect. Differential results suggest use of different coping strategies in both patient groups. Also, coping strategies were differentially related to outcome criteria depending on whether patients were operated on for the first or the second time. In terms of affect change and employment of coping strategies, prior experience with the stressor seems to make a difference for cataract patients.

Clinical Implications of Social Gerontology's Continuity Theory

L. MacBeath, (Psychiatrist, Private Practice, Vancouver, BC) R.C. Atchley, (Chair, Dept of Gerontology, Naropa University, Boulder, CO, USA) R.J. Mewhort, (Nurse Specialist, Geriatric Psychiatry, Galiano Island, BC)

PURPOSE: To determine if findings from Atchley's 20-year longitudinal study can be applied as a psychotherapy intervention in clinical settings with elderly patients having difficulties coping with aging changes. Atchley's Continuity Theory identifies how people can adapt to even unexpected and challenging changes by maintaining and adapting their successful life patterns in new circumstances. METHOD: Cognitively intact patients, aged 62 to 90, identified by their Family Physicians as not adapting well to aging changes, were referred to the study. Physical and psychiatric assessments, and an ADL check-list, were completed. A problem list was developed for each patient. Structured psychiatric interviews, which included review of life values, goals, expectations, and personality style, were then conducted by either the psychiatrist or the nurse specialist. Continuity strategies of each patient were listed, and patient implementation of these strategies was monitored over time. RESULTS: Profiles were developed comparing patients who were most successful and least successful at reconnecting with previous life patterns to help them cope with current problems. Patients who benefited usually reuired only one or two clinical sessions. CONCLUSION: Continuity strategies were effective for the majority of patients. Implications for health promotion training in younger years was primarily derived by studying those unable to identify previous strategies that were currently effective.

Death Anxiety and Death Denial: Nigerian Older People

Bolanle Elizabeth Adetoun CESDEG PO Box 2192 Garki-Abuja FCT Nigeria

Ninety-two Nigerian men and 120 Nigerian women older adults completed Templer's (1970) Death Anxiety Scale (DAS) and Feifel and Nagy's (1981) death fantasy measure of positive and negative death metaphors. They were each also asked to write his or her own metaphor of personal death. Results of the DAS showed that the two groups did not differ significantly on the level of conscious death anxiety, but men scores were significantly higher on both positive and negative personal death metaphors scales. Also, significantly more Nigerian men wrote personal metaphors of their own and more often used a neutral metaphor to describe their personal death. Nigerian women more often used a positive or a negative metaphor. The men thus evidenced less death denical than the Nigerian women did.Implication for health and human rights are briefly discussed.

Death Anxiety, Health Control Orientation, and Psychological Adjustment of Chinese Elderly with Chronic Illness

C. Tang, A. Wu (Department of Psychology, Chinese University of Hong Kong) T. Kwok (Department of Medicine, Chinese University of Hong Kong)

This study examines the associations among self-efficacy, life satisfaction, death anxiety, health locus of control, and psychological adjustment of Chinese elderly who had chronic illness. A total of 237 Chinese elderly aged 60 or above and resided in Hong Kong were individually interviewed. Results showed that Chinese elderly were not extremely fearful and anxious of death, and their level of death anxiety was related to low levels of self-efficacy and life satisfaction. Negative psychological adjustment was related to death anxiety and external health control orientation. Psychological distress of Chinese elderly could be mitigated by high levels of slef-efficacy, life satisfaction, and internal health locus of control. Chinese cultural beliefs about death-related and health control issues were discussed with regard to how they affect Chinese elderly's adjustment to chronic illness as well as the planning of social and medical services and policies for the elderly.

Death Anxiety, Health Control Orientation, and Psychological Adjustment of Chinese Elderly with Chronic Illness

C. Tang, A. Wu (Department of Psychology, Chinese University of Hong Kong) T. Kwok (Department of Psychology, Chinese University of Hong Kong)

This study examines the associations among self-efficacy, life satisfaction, death anxiety, health locus of control, and psychological adjustment of Chinese elderly who had chronic illness. A total of 237 Chinese elderly aged 60 or above and resided in Hong Kong were individually interviewed. Results showed that Chinese elderly were not extremely fearful and anxious of death, and their level of death anxieety was related to low levels of self- efficacy and life satisfaction. Negative psychological adjustment was related to death anxiety and external health control orientation. Psychological distress of Chinese elderly could be mitigated by high levels of self-efficacy, life satisfaction, and internal health locus of control. Chinese cultural beliefs about death-related and health control issues were discussed with regard to how they affect Chinese elderly's adjustment fo chronic illness as well as the planning of social and medical services and policies for the elderly.

Elderly facing physical limitations after a fracture: the impact of learning resources on performance in occupations

BROUSSEAU, Martine (Ph. D, student in Education, UQTR, Trois-Rivières, Qc, Canada) DENIS, Marie-Claude (, UQTR, Trois-Rivières, Qc, Canada GAGNON, Gaetan (, UQTR, Trois-Rivières, QC, Canada DUSSAULT, Marc (Ph. D, UQTR, Trois-Rivières, Qc, Canada

PURPOSE: The purpose of the study is to test the effect of two learning resources (Bandura's self-efficacy and Sternberg's, Audy et al.'s cognitive efficiency) on performance in occupations for 60 elderly facing physical limitations after a fracture. METHOD: The study used face-to-face interviews with structured questionnaires (SEFA, OEFA, COPM, PPT, PES) and was conducted in the community one month after the participants were back to their home. RESULTS: Multiple stepwise regression show that the 2 learning resources explains 43 0f the variance of performance on occupations. Moreover, one self-efficacy variable (self-efficacy belief) has a moderator effect on performance explaining 4 % more variance and showing that when self-efficacy beliefs are low, performance in occupations becomes better with the use of strategies as measured with the cognitive efficiency instrument (PES). CONCLUSION: In conclusion, the study brings insight into factors that affect performance in occupations and provide knowledge for educative-based program for elderly facing physical limitations.

Living with a Chronic Illness and Then Some: Data from the 1998 Ice Storm

M. A. M. Gignac (Arthritis Community Research & Evaluation Unit, The University Health Network & Department of Public Health Sciences, The University of Toronto, Toronto, ON, Canada), C. Cott (Arthritis Community Research & Evaluation Unit, The University Health Network & Department of Physical Therapy, The University of Toronto, Toronto, ON, Canada), & E. M. Badley (Arthritis Community Research & Evaluation Unit, The University Health Network & Department of Public Health Sciences, The University of Toronto, Toronto, ON, Canada).

This study had two goals. First, we examined the association of physical and psychological measures with older adults' reports of a traumatic stressor (the ice storm). Second, we examined whether the ice storm had any long-term physical or psychological impact on seniors with a chronic disabling illness. Respondents were 104 community-dwelling adults, aged ? 55 years with osteoarthritis (OA) and/or osteoporosis (OP), living in the Toronto or Kingston areas. All were administered a standardized questionnaire prior to the ice storm and approximately one year after the storm. Fifty nine Kingston area residents also completed a questionnaire about their ice storm experiences. Older adults who, prior to the ice storm, reported greater helplessness, depression, and dependence, subsequently reported that the ice storm had a greater subjective impact on them and greater ice storm stress and rumination. One year later, Kingston area residents who reported a high level of objective impact from the storm (e.g, displacement from home, loss of power, property damage) reported greater disability and pain, and less independence compared to Toronto respondents matched in terms of gender, age, and initial disability, and controlling for time 1 measures. Moreover, these findings were not moderated by the level of support participants received during the storm. The results suggest that traumatic stressors like the ice storm can have an impact on the physical health of individuals. Previous disaster research has focused mostly on the psychological consequences of major events.

Living with rheumatoid arthritis: The older adults' perceptions of stress, stress emotions and coping strategies

Patricia M. Melanson, MN, RN & Barbara Downe-Wamboldt, RN (Dalhousie University, School of Nursing, Halifax, Canada)

Purpose: The purpose of this longitudinal, descriptive and comparative study is to identify, describe and compare the illness-related stresses, stress emotions, and coping strategies of recently diagnosed elderly persons with rheumatoid arthritis (RA) with the illness-related stresses, stress emotions and coping strategies of elderly persons who have had RA since midlife. The Folkman and Lazarus transactional model of stress and coping guided this research. Method: This study included one semi-structured, audiotaped one-hour interview with each participant. The setting for the study was the homes of the participants living within a 100 kilometre radius of Halifax, St John and St John's metropolitan areas of Nova Scotia, New Brunswick and Newfoundland. Participants, aged 60 years and over, were asked to identify the most stressful situation related to RA that they had experienced in the past month, feelings related to the stressful situation and to describe what coping strategies they used to manage this situation. The sample included 16 recently diagnosed participants and 77 participants diagnosed since midlife. The data was transcribed and analyzed using content analysis. Results: The majority of the participants reported physical limitations to be their main illness-related stress. The participants most often reported the stress emotion of harm. Most of the participants dealt with their perceived illness-related stress by using confrontive coping strategies. Conclusion: Results of this study will add to the stress and coping literature by providing information on the stress of RA, stress emotions, and coping strategies of elderly persons with RA and changes in this appraisal over time.

SESSION 198

Biological Age for Assessing Efficacy of Health Strengthening Measures

N.Akhaladze (Institute of Gerontology Academy of Medical Sciences, Kiev, Ukraine)

Effects of health strengthening measure (cleaning up of body, periodic restriction of diet, physical exercise, psychophysical training) upon biological (BA) and cardiopulmonary (CPA) age were investigated in 18 men and 28 women aged 40-69 with multiple chronic pathology in history. METHOD: The individual biological age (BA) of every examined person was determined on the basis of a package of tests, developed by the Institute of Gerontology (Ukraine). Using special formula, BA and CPA indices were calculated for each person. These indices were calculated as difference between the BA and CPA and the chronological age of a given person. RESULTS: We found that both BA index and CPA index in both women and men were significantly lower than the population's standard. In general, women have benefited more than men from the complex of health promoting measures. Another important finding was that a duration of health promoting measures was an important factor. Indeed, after 10 to 15 yrs of practising health promoting measure, the BA of women was about 16 years lower than that of women of the same chronological age. CONCLUSION: Our findings strongly suggest that health promoting measures may have the so called geroprotecting effect. They significantly increase the quantity of health , as well as quality of life of people practicing such measures. We believe that our data shows that age-dependent pathological conditions are reversible.

Physical activity and functional capacity - a longitudinal follow-up from age 70 to 86

K Frandin, V Sundh (Department of Geriatric Medicine, Goteborg University, Goteborg, Sweden)

The aim was to study level of physical activity and functional performance from the age of 70 to 86 but also to compare previous activity patterns and performance in the subjects tested at age 86 with those who had died or otherwise dropped out. The 157 subjects, 96 women and 61 men, were born in 1911-12, and derive from a representative sample who have been followed since age 70. Variables like muscle strength, walking speed and balance were tested and an interview addressing walking habits, physical activity and self-rated fitness was performed. The results revealed a decline in all performance tests but the greatest decline was observed regarding balance function. The subjects tended to be less physically active and rated their physical fitness lower than before. However, more than half of the subjects still took a daily walk and subjects who had been most physically active before still belonged to the most active group. Between age 76 and 86 around 50% of the subjects had died. A significant difference between those who participated at age 86 and drop-outs (death or other reasons) could be demonstrated ten years earlier regarding daily walks, activity level, self-rated fitness, leg muscle strength and maximal walking speed. Simple tests could be used as predictors for severe decline in order to detect persons at risk in time. It is of great importance to stimulate people to be physically active as there is a clear relationship between physical activity level and performance even late in life.

The Effect of Counseling by Healthcare Professionals on Increasing Physical Activity in Older People

M. Hirvensalo, Department of Physical Education and The Finnish Centre for Interdisciplinary Gerontology, University of Jyväskylä, Finland/ E. Heikkinen , The Finnish Centre for Interdisciplinary Gerontology and Department of Health Sciences, University of Jyväskylä, Finland T. Lintunen, Department of Physical Education, University of Jyväskylä, Finland T.Rantanen, The Finnish Centre for Interdisciplinary Gerontology and Department of Health Sciences, University of Jyväskylä, Finland

Purpose: The aim was to study whether counseling by health care professionals is associated with increased exercise activity in older people. Methods: As part of the Evergreen study, data on physical activities were collected in 1988 and eight years later by structured interviews among 611 non-institutional people initially aged 65-84 years. Logistic regression analyses were used to study the association of recalling receipt of exercise counseling with increased activity. Those who remained sedentary were assigned as the reference groups. The models were adjusted for age, education, marital status and chronic conditions. Results: Altogether, 112 people of the 336 people who at baseline did not report home gymnastics became active over the follow-up. For participation in supervised exercise classes the numbers were 54 out of 548, respectively. Of all the subjects, 92% reported having been in contact with health care professionals during the follow-up, and 58% of them recalled on having been counseled on exercise issues. Those men and women who recalled having received counseling, started to participate in supervised exercise classes 5 to 6 times more often than those who did not recall being counselled (men OR 6.27 95%CI 1.19- 32.9), women OR 5.27 95%CI 1.97-14.1). For home gymnastics, the responding figure was 12.5 (95%CI 3.52-44.4) in men. Conclusion. We found a strong association between initiating new physical activities and recalling having received encouragement to exercise by health care professionals. Health care professionals should be encouraged to advise older patients about exercise issues.

The Program of Physical Rehabilitation

E. Mentheshashvili and O. Shoshitashvili

Moving activity have a special significance in aging among various factors and conditions. It's known that optimal muscular activity promote prolongation survival, wile hypokinesy about 4-6-fold decrease survival and especially among vice sportsmen. For amelioration and prolongation survival, Georgian wrestling Federation create special physical rehabilitation program tack account personal physiological peculiarities of aged people: moderate or low physical tolerance, low level reserve possibilities cardiovascular and respiratory systems. Our programs goal is elaboration a new respiratory and mobility stereotypes, adequate functional status and amelioration of cardiovascular and respiratory systems for physical tolerance. Our observation opposed on investigations of 60 persons (60-74 age) divided in two group (vicesportsmens and without sportive experiences). Program provides for volitional respiratory direction , general restorative training, gymnastic in piscine. We established indication and contraindications markers. The results show on the whole well subjective transference of procedures, amelioration of working and psychical status, stability or positive dynamics of outer respiratory indices. There was existed difference effect of program as among as well between groups. But long (6 month) duration program decrease deferens between groups and reassure that moving activity develop new horizons also in one's declining youthfulness.

The Role of Tai Chi in Healthy Aging: A Review of the Literature

Maria C. Tan (University of Alberta, Edmonton, Canada)

Tai Chi is a Chinese martial art involving patterns of smooth movements and body weight shifts that integrate mental concentration, meditative breathing, and purposeful body movement. Taught as an activity to improve flexibility, balance, and relaxation, Tai Chi is practiced chiefly by middle-aged and older adults; it can be modified to accommodate various physical ability levels and health conditions. Purpose: To highlight findings from a literature review on the health promotion aspects of Tai Chi. Method: English language scientific journal articles, books, and instructional videocassettes on Tai Chi were reviewed. Results: Clinical research on Tai Chi is relatively recent. Findings support Tai Chi's contribution to fall prevention/balance improvement, cardiorespiratory maintenance and rehabilitation, and the maintenance of joint range of motion. In addition, a growing body of anecdotal evidence suggests that Tai Chi has health-enhancing effects on physical and mental well-being, self-awareness, and cognitive function. Conclusions: Tai Chi uses a holistic approach of addressing the physical, mental, and spiritual facets of well-being, and complements other treatment interventions and healthy lifestyle behaviours. It contributes to healthy aging in terms of preventive care, health maintenance, and rehabilitation. While objective, physiological benefits of Tai Chi have been studied, gaps exist in research examining its affective, cognitive, and functional effects. Further research in these areas, while needed, will nonetheless face the challenges of longitudinal designs, measurement issues, and sampling bias due to self-selection. Qualitative approaches may be better suited to exploring the various ways Tai Chi affects individuals.

Walking speed and functional independence in later life

S. Shinkai, S. Watanabe, S. Kumagai, Y. Fujiwara, Y. Yoshida, Y. Aoyagi, T. Suzuki (Tokyo Metropolitan Institute of Gerontology, Tokyo, Japan), H. Shibata (Obirin University, Tokyo, Japan)

We investigated the association between physical performance measures and functional independence in later life. Out of the population aged 65 years or over living in Nangai (n=940), Japan, in 1992, we measured hand grip-strength, one-leg standing, finger-tapping, and walking speeds in 731 and 601 subjects who had no initial disability in the five basic activities of daily living (BADL) and the five instrumental activities of daily living (IADL), respectively. Their functional status was assessed each year for the subsequent 6 years. The outcome event was the onset of BADL disability, defined as a new disability in one or more of the five BADL, or death of a subject who had shown no disability at the previous follow-up, or the onset of IADL disability, defined as a new disability in one or more of the five IADL prior to BADL disability. Even after controlling for age, sex, and a number of chronic medical conditions with the Cox proportional hazard model, lower scores on each baseline performance measure showed increased risk for the onset of BADL and IADL disabilities. Among four measures, walking speed was highly and most sensitive in predicting future BADL and IADL disabilities. In conclusion, walking ability as measured by walking speed is a crucial physical performance for functional independence in later life.

SESSION 200

[1] "Me mother would have curled up and died" : older women talking about sex

Rebecca L. Jones (The Open University, Milton Keynes, UK)

The purpose of this research is to explore some of the ways in which older women manage talk about sex. A considerable body of research demonstrates that many retired-age people continue to be sexually active or interested. Nevertheless, the idea that older people are asexual still exists as a hegemonic discourse, as does the idea that older people have difficulty speaking about sex. Older people's awareness of these discourses may create tensions when they talk about sex. Two main data collection methods were used: small group workshop sessions and interviews. A small data set was used which is analysed in depth. The research analyses both the content of the accounts generated and the ways in which those accounts are produced. Drawing on feminist theory and aspects of discourse analysis (especially 'positioning' and 'interpretative repertoires'), the research considers the ways in which speakers both perpetuate and resist ideas of older people as asexual. Speakers position themselves in many different ways: as not an older person themselves; as an older person, but not a typical one; as a purveyor of wisdom; as a professional. Respondents draw on a range of interpretative repertoires which include: sex is natural within marriage, whatever your age; marriage is of overriding importance; male sexual desire in uncontrollable; a decline in attractiveness is inevitable as you age; sexual practices have changed significantly. The research suggests that speaking about sex as an older woman is neither as impossible nor as straightforward as has sometimes been assumed.

[2] Sexuality of women from 60 to 74 years of age in the city of Recife

S. G. Kitover (Unicap for the Third Age, PROCOM, Universidade Católica de Pernambuco, Recife, Brazil)

Sexuality in elderly women is a theme not yet very much researched in national literature. The aim of this paper was to study the sexuality of women from 60 to 74 years of age in Recife-Pernambuco, Northeast of Brazil, having as subjects 30 women, 10 from each social-economic class, with different degrees of education - in three age groups: 60-64, 65-69 and 70-74, considered in this research as social-economic classes: low, middle and high. Masturbation, menarche, sexual initiation with a partner, experiences of old age, perception of their own bodies, menopause, and other aspects were investigated. Myths, taboos and prejudices were considered. It began with a psycho-social-historic perspective, since the Creation, in a Judeo-Christian tradition. The answers to the questionnaire with 36 open questions were analyzed according to quantity and quality, completed by interviews and histories of life. Among the results in all classes and age groups that women pretend to have an orgasm during their entire sexual life was predominant. In higher social-economic class, the incidence of practice of masturbation and sex without love were increased. Dialogue with partners was unanimously avoided. One of the 30 women, would like to have a new marital relationship. Menarche and menopause were the events that caused the greatest impacts related to femininity, with less effect for women of middle class. In conclusion, there were no relevant differences in sexual experiences in function of social classes, although the expression is not the same.

[3] Strengthen exchanges in moral problems with the elderly to promote both physical and moral health

He Defang (Bureau for Retired Cadres with or without Special Treatment,Ministry of Labour and Social security p.r.c.)

In general, the elderly, after retirement, and especially those in towns and cities, face adaptation to their new role in society. Their financial income is reduced, their old ideas confront with the new, their physical health is gradually reducing, etc. While guaranteeing their material needs in daily life, a problem worth our studies is their needs in moral life so as to help them safely lead their twilight years. The crux of the matter is to strengthen exchanges with them in moral problems as a principal means in satisfying their needs in moral life. 1. The whole society should pay considerable attention to contacting the elderly government administering and servicing organs are entrusted with important responsibilities in providing a healthy life in their twilight years, and particularly in establishing exchanges with them. The family is still the main support for the elderly in our country. So it is necessary to underline the importance of contacts at this level, and increase family relations and harmony. The young should look upon today's elderly as their tomorrow. They should multiply their contacts, try to understand, respect and love the elderly. The elderly have similar life experience and thinking, and find it easier to exchange and communicate, and are willing to enjoy among themselves. 2. Wide exchanges and correct guidance Exchanges can be conducted among the elderly on state matters, family matters and all other problems of interest to them. However, it is necessary to provide correct guidance, so that they learn more, have healthy mentality, take correct attitudes, and benefit from the contacts. 3. Provide conditions for the contacts. One should create a kind of good habit of respecting the elderly, understanding them, loving them and protecting them. It is necessary to develop services for the elderly, ensuring them the possibility of further studies and enjoyment.

[4] Welcome the second spring of human being in the 21st century

Xing-hua Wang (China Gerontology committee Heilongjiang Hearbin China)

There is only one spring in human life, but there is another spring in human's mind - the second spring. For creating energetic, valuable and happy second spring the only way is to live in reasonable and healthy life. For every individual, a reasonable attitude to ageing must be without superstition and old age sadness. If he did so he can create two second spring gardens in his life, one is in the family and the other is in the society. The family is where the love exited and the society is an open world for happiness. Having three factors, such as happy daily life, high spirit and scientific knowledge, it is easy to create the second spring of human life in relationship, generation-gap relationship and national relationship. Our society should be full of true concern to aged poverty and spread scientific knowledge, despising the attitude to sickness and no discrimination to old people. The whole society should care about aged people and help them to create the second spring of human life. May the age people live in a happy and healthy life in the 21st century.

[5] Relationship between QOL and Activity of Daily Living, Blood Test among nonagenarians in Japan: Report of Kakegawa Population Study

Suzuki M, Kanamori M. (School of Medicine Hamamatsu University, Hamamatsu, Japan) Shiraki M. (University of Shizuoka, Hamamatsu College, Hamamatsu, Japan) Yamazaki S, Sato H, Ito S (Kakegawa Tokuiku Health Center, Kakegawa, Japan) Kobashi G.(Department of Public Health, Hokkaido University School of Medicine, Sapporo, Japan) Hirose N. (Department of Geriatric Medicine, Keio University School of Medicine, Tokyo, Japan)

PURPOSE: Japanese life expectancy is one of the longest in the world, resulting in the rapid increase of the old generations, especially that of the oldest old. Recently, promotion of quality of life (QOL) in a late stage of life is considered to be important. However, studies of QOL in the oldest old are not sufficient. This study was conducted to know the level of QOL and what factors affect the QOL in the oldest old in Japan. METHODS: Subjects of this study were nonagenarians living at home in rural area (Kakegawa, Shizuoka, Japan). After the informed consent was obtained from participants or their proxy, life satisfaction index (LSI), activity of daily living (ADL) was obtained using the questionnaire. Blood was collected, and then biochemical markers and peripheral blood count were measured. RESULTS: Forty two nonagenarians (14 men and 28 women) were enrolled into this study. The mean of LSI point in all subjects was 9.30 (±3.79); 9.08 (±3.32) in men and 9.47 (±4.08) in women. Nonagenarians were divided into 2 groups according to the level of LSI; high LSI group (HLSI) and low LSI group (LLSI). The level of ADL and parameters of blood test was compared between 2 groups. ADL level in HLSI was higher than that in LLSI. However, ADL level in women was lower than that in men. The level of High-density lipoprotein cholesterol (HDL-C) was high and HbA1C level was low in HLSI, compared to that in LLSI. In women, the ratio of body fat was high and the level of triglyceride, total cholesterol was low in HLSI, compared to that in LLSI. The level of bone density was lower in HLSI women. CONCLUSION: Nonagenarians in HLSI have high ADL level and have healthy profiles of blood test. This suggests that QOL in the oldest old is associated with physical health.

[6] SOJO Model for Healthy Aging. Part-I: Concepts and Procedures

A. M. M. Kamal, T. Iwanaga, T. Ohida (Dept. of Public Health Administration, National Institute of Public Health, Tokyo, Japan.)

PURPOSE: SOJO (System Oriented Joyful Operation) is a community based process model which has been being implemented at various community settings through out Japan for many years aiming health promotion among the elderly people. The objective of the presentation under Part-I is to introduce SOJO model specially its concept and procedures. METHOD: At the beginning of the model, participants from the locality have a joyful workshop where they share views among themselves to establish a healthy community. During the workshop, they set their ideal goal as an image of healthy life and make a master plan based on the required conditions to realize the goal. In the course of implementation, participants get together monthly to evaluate activities and make new action plan based on the evaluation report. RESULTS: The unique characteristics of the model are that regardless of age, education and economic background of the participants, and with a nominal cooperation from the professional and administration, participants, working through this model, learn how to make a role in planning, decision making and implementation of their own issue, health for example. After implementation of SOJO model at different settings of elderly people in Japan, developments such as participation, empowerment and personal skills among the elderly people have been documented. Specific out comes reflecting such development have been described under application of the model in part-II. CONCLUSIONS: SOJO model's proven capability to develop participation, empowerment and personal skills among the elderly people has special implication for health promotion resulting in healthy aging.

[7] The Effect of a Structured Life Review Process for the Homebound Elderly in Yamagata, Japan

H. Imuta (Yamagata Univ, Yamagata, Japan) , S. Yasumura (Fukushima Medical Univ, Fukushima, Japan) , T. Ahiko (Murayama Public Health Center, Yamagata, Japan), A. Fukao (Yamagata Univ, Yamagata, Japan)

PURPOSE: This study examined the therapeutic effect of life review process to improve physical and psychosocial function in Japanese homebound elderly. METHOD: Forty-six eligible homebound participants, aged 68 years and over and living in Yamagata Prefecture, were randomly allocated to an intervention group or a control group. The subjects in an intervention group were asked to participate in the life review process at least twice a month for three months. Each session started with giving a health information and followed by the life review process which taking an hour to finish. All subjects of two groups were measured dependent variables at the beginning and end of three months period (pretest and posttest). Dependent variables consisted of physical (Activities of Daily Living, Visual Deficit, and so on), psychological (Subjective Well-being, Life Satisfaction, and so on), and social variables (Functional Ability, Frequency of getting out of house within a week, and so on). The control group conducted only pretest and posttest. RESULT: Pretest and posttest scores in all physical, psychological, and social variables didn't significantly change in both groups. CONCLUSION: Unfortunately, our result reveals little positive effects on the physical, psychological, and social variables. There may be some limitations; 1) a half of sample of homebound elderly subjects with dementia was selected, 2) this intervention was short-term design, and so on. However, a life review process had no negative effects for Japanese homebound elderly sample.

[8] Quality of Life of Indian Elderly: A Factor Analytic Approach

N.K.Chadha(University of Delhi,India),M.Easwaramoorthy(DIPR,Delhi,India),Priya Bir(Aditi Mahavidhalaya,Delhi,India)

The concept of quality of life has gained significance in aging due to the need for integrated approach towards understanding the aged and requirement for an outcome measure for health care and welfare policies. There are economic, physical, psychological and social dimensions acting on an aging individual, variables related to these dimensions are interactive and interdependent and can be best understood in the light of a multidimensional approach. For this purpose, 580 elderly from Tamil Nadu state were interviewed. Four dimensions of quality of life were assessed, namely- economic well-nbeing, physical well-being, psychological well-being and social well-being by administering various psychological tools. The data were subjected to centroid method of factor analysis with orthogonal rotation. Results indicate five factors: (1) perceived psycho-social wellness, (2) physical wellness, (3) awareness and activities, (4) adequacy of financial status, and (5) adequacy of family and social support. These results provide a comprehensive understanding of elderly and carries various implications for research and policy making.

[9] Is aging associated to decreased quality of life?: the doctor and the patient impressions

Matheus Roriz Silva Cruz, Elisabete Michelon (Instituto de Geriatria e Gerontologia - PUCRS, Porto Alegre, Brazil)

PURPOSE: Study the physician evaluation of patient´s quality of life (QOL) and patient´s self perceived QOL and their relation to patient´s age. METHOD Following a routine medical visit, seventy-two outpatients and inpatients were interviewed by the attending physician using a questionnaire that included questions related to each domain of QOL based on the WHO-QOL (QOL-100) instrument and referred here as the Geriatric Global Impression method (GGI). After the interview, the physician rated the overall patient´s QOL on a scale from zero to 10 being zero the worst and 10 the best QOL. The patient was then asked to rate his/her self perceived QOL using a numeric scale. The age of the individuals were considered according to official records. The statistical analysis used the Spearman's correlation test. RESULTS: The study included 72 patients being 47% inpatients and 68% were women.. Mean age was 75 (s.d.=8) years; minimum age was 61 years and maximum age was 100 years. Twenty three percent of patients rated their QOL between 0 and 5; 17% between 5.1 and 7.5; and 60% between 7.6 and 10. The association between age and the patient´s self-perceived QOL was significantly positive ($r=0.251$; $p=0.038$). The physician evaluation of patient´s QOL was not associated to patient´s age. CONCLUSIONS: The majority of the elderly patients studied (77%) rated their QOL above 5. The patient´s self perceived QOL was positively associated to increasing age. No significantly correlation was found between the physician´s evaluation of patient´s QOL and patient´s age.

[10] The Geriatric Global Impression (GGI) method in the assessment of Quality of Life

Matheus Roriz Silva Cruz, Elisaabete Michelon (Instituto de Geriatria e Gerontologia - PUCRS, Porto Alegre, Brazil)

PURPOSE: Study the association between the physician's evaluation of patient's quality of life (QOL) and the patient's self perceived QOL using the Geriatric Global Impression (GGI) method. METHOD: Following a routine medical visit, seventy-two outpatients and inpatients were interviewed by the attending physician using a questionnaire that included questions related to each domain of QOL based on the WHO-QOL (QOL-100) instrument and referred here as the Geriatric Global Impression method (GGI). After the interview the physician rated the overall patient's QOL on a scale from zero to 10 being zero the worst and 10 the best QOL. The patient was then asked to rate his/her self perceived QOL using a numeric scale, a categorical scale and a scale of facial expression. The statistical analysis used the Spearman's correlation test. RESULTS: We studied 72 patients, 47% were inpatients and 68% were women. The average time used in the interview was 15 minutes. There was a statistically significant association between the physician evaluation of patient's QOL and all the instruments used for the evaluation of patient's self-perceived QOL. ($p<0.001$) CONCLUSIONS: The GGI method used by the physician in this study was able to significantly correlate to patient's self-perceived QOL. After undergoing validation studies this method can be used by the clinician to effectively evaluate patients QOL.

[11] Spirituality and health risks and behaviors among African American Elderly

Gregory A. Bechtel, (College of Arts and Sciences Cleveland State University 1860 East 22nd Street Cleveland, OH 44115)

PURPOSE: To determine the relationship of spirituality and health risk/ behavior patterns among 33 African American elderly residing in a rural southern community in the United States. METHODS: Triangulation methodology using structured interviews, a Health Risk Appraisal and the Spirituality and Well-being scale were used to assess the relationship between spirituality and health risks and behaviors among a group of well seniors participating in a community-based senior citizen center. RESULTS: Using both qualitative and quantitative analysis, no relationship was found between health risk or health behaviors and perception of spirituality. However, spirituality was strongly linked to social support networks that may influence risk behaviors and patterns of health behavior. While the degree of spirituality was not related to Appraised Age or Achievable Age using psychometric instruments, the majority of participants strongly linked the concept of spirituality and health risk/ behaviors during structured interviews. CONCLUSIONS: The findings from this study suggest that health care providers should realize that while spirituality and health outcomes might not be directly linked, clients in this study tended to conceptualize the two concepts as interacting. While the participants in this study could not clearly differentiate how spirituality affected health risk and behaviors, this may have been due to the inadequacies of the instruments or in differences between perception and data-based evidence. Thus, health providers who treat African American elderly must recognize the importance of perceived spirituality in care when providing holistic care.

[12] Images Toward Aging

M. Iwai (Department of Health Services Administration, Nippon Medical School, 1-2-5 Sendagi, Bunkyo-ku, Tokyo, 113-8602 JAPAN)

PURPOSE: The purpose of this qualitative study was to examine Japanese attitudes toward aging. Of particular interest was to discern if there are age differences in self-perceptions regarding the positive and negative aspects of the process of growing old. METHODS: The data were collected via a written questionnaire that included eight open-ended questions, such as "In your opinion, when does a person become old?" and "What comes to mind as you think about the positive/negative aspects of aging?" Questionnaires were distributed one week prior to the Gerontological Psychology lecture and were collected during the lecture. 215 people representing different age groups completed the questionnaire. RESULTS: The findings suggest that most respondents anticipate negative aspects of growing old themselves (e.g. lack of physical energy and mental deterioration). Also, most subjects held strong negative images toward aging. Even younger subjects expressed negative feelings. Reasons for negative attitudes toward aging included the perception that many older adults with whom respondents were acquainted did not seem happy. The stigma of death associated with old age also contributed to a negative view of aging. Positive descriptors of aging included such things as wisdom, rich life experiences, being kind and gentle, having communication skills, being patient, and knowing the meaning of life. Younger respondents believed that the aged have extra time for hobbies, such as traveling. CONCLUSION: Younger respondents viewed aging more seriously while people over age 50 viewed aging as a more "natural" phenomenon and tried to spend their lives more fully.

[13] Attitudes toward old age, educational motives, and subjective well-being among old people attending university

Pereira da Silva, Flavia (Universidade Federal de Pernambuco, Brazil) Liberalesso Neri, Anita (State University of Campinas, Brazil)

OBJECTIVES: Educational programs addressed to old age contribute to successful aging by their positive effects on cognition, self-development and subjective well-being of participants, and on individual and social attitudes toward aging. This investigation was aimed to analyse attitudes concerning old age, educational motives and subjective well-being of people aged 60 and more. METHOD: Subjects were 100 students of an Open University of Third Age (86% women; 70% aged 60 to 69; 43% widowed; 27% married; 83% with more than 8 years of school. Instrumentation involved: a 30 item Differential Semantic scale of attitudes toward aging (domains: cognition, agency, social relations and personal; a single item scale of satisfaction with life; eight item domain referenced scale of satisfaction (physical and mental health and social involvement) and a five item scale of motives to attend the program. RESULTS: Statistical analysis showed high overall and domain referenced satisfaction, mostly when the subjects compared themselves with others of the same age. Women, the oldest and those with lower level of scholarity were the most satisfied. Positive attitudes toward aging were correlated with life satisfaction and with satisfaction of motives to attend University. Higher but moderately negative scores toward old age occurred in agency and cognition. There were associations between the motives knowledge improvement and self-development, and between investment in social contact and useful occupation of free time. CONCLUSION: Results confirm the positive effects of education on adaptation of old people and suggest that gerontological education can contribute to their empowerment, either as individuals, or as an age group.

[14] Effects of emotional interaction with pets on well-being among the Japanese elderly

T. Ando (Yokohama National University, Yokohama, Japan), Y. Kodama (Kyoritsu Women's Junior College, Tokyo Japan), H. Osada (Tokyo Metropolitan University of Health Sciences, Tokyo Japan)

Importance of pets in old age has been gradually acknowledged. However, a few studies focusing on this issue have been conducted in Japan. The purpose of this study was to examine the effects of emotional interaction with pets on well-being among the Japanese elderly. Subjects were pet owners (dog and/or cat), ranging in age from 60 to 74 years, living in Metropolitan area. Mail surveys were carried out in 1999 and completed for 552 persons. The response rate was 92.0%. The demographics of pet ownership and quality of emotional interaction with pets (Animal-Human Bonding Scale) were inquired. Well-being was measured by the Japanese version of Geriatric Depression Scale and AOK Loneliness Scale. Multiple regression analyses showed the emotionally close relationships with pets had significant negative effects on depressive states and loneliness when the effects of socio-demographic variables, health status, and social support network were controlled. The results suggested the importance of emotionally close relationships with pets for quality of life in old age.

[15] Kansas ElderCount County Chart Book

Mercedes Bern-Klug (University of Kansas Medical Center, Center on Aging Kansas City)

Purpose: Describe the planning and process of producing Kansas ElderCount Chart Book. Method: This poster will contain a time frame for the planning of Kansas ElderCount; a listing of the advantages and drawbacks to attempting to plan and produce Kansas ElderCount; and future plans for the continuation of Kansas ElderCount. Results: This poster will contain pages from the Kansas ElderCount Chart Book. Each of the 105 Kansas counties will have their own page listing 30 key variables describing the well-being of older adults in that county. The poster will also contain information about the cost of producing Kansas ElderCount, how outside funding was secured, and plans for distributing the chart book. Conclusions: Building consensus from 40 aging specialists throughout the state as to the most important demographic indicators of older adult well-being can be challenging, but the final product justifies the effort. Being able to compare key demographic data among counties and among congressional districts is an important step toward gauging the well-being of older adults over time.

[16] Wellness as a Lifelong Pursuit

A. Segall, D. Bailis, B. Payne, N. Dunn, (University of Manitoba, Winnipeg, Manitoba, Canada)

PURPOSE: The purpose of this study was to examine the health status, health beliefs and wellness-oriented lifestyle behaviour of older adults. METHOD: Study participants were part of a larger research program. Two subsamples of older adults (65 years and over) were compared: members of a wellness facility (n=268); and a matched sample of community residents (n=316). Beliefs about health consciousness and a range of personal health practices were compared between samples and across age groups (65-69, 70-74, 75+). RESULTS: The subsamples are similar in their age distribution, gender split, marital and employment status. In contrast, Wellness Institute (WI) Sample members have higher levels of formal education and household income, than Community Comparison (CC) Sample members. All study participants rated their health in positive terms. WI Sample members were much more likely, however, to rate their current health as better than it was two years ago, compared to the CC Sample (p<.001). Both groups were found to be quite health conscious and the vast majority (90%) believe that they are doing a good job of looking after their health. Despite common beliefs, WI and CC Sample members differ in terms of several personal health practices. WI Sample members are more likely to engage in preventive medical care (such as a flu shot), to be non-smokers, and to be more physically active (p<.001). CONCLUSION: The findings suggest that older adults recognize that regular physical activity contributes to improvements in health. The concluding discussion focuses on the health benefits of active living in later life and wellness as a lifelong pursuit.

[17] Impact of objective health on well-being among the very old

P. Hillerås(123). H, Agüero-Eklund(23), A. F. Jorm(4), K. Ericsson(123), B. Winblad(23). 1) H.M. Queen Sophia University College and Nursing, Stockholm, 2)Stockholm Gerontology Research Center, Stockholm, 3) Karolinska Institutet, Department of Clinical Neuroscience, Occupational Therapy and Elderly Care Research, Division of Geriatric Medicine, Huddinge University Hospital, Huddinge, Sweden, 4)and Deputy Director at Psychiatric Epidemiology Research Centre, The Australian National University, Canberra, Australia.

Although the literature on studies of well-being in elderly samples is quite extensive nowadays, no research has been done on the impact of specific medical disorders on very old people. The aim of this study was to assess whether there is an association between objective health, measured as clinical medical diagnoses, and well-being among the very old. The study involved 105 people, 90 years or above, who were not cognitively impaired, living in the inner parts of Stockholm. Subjects were given a medical examination covering eye diseases, osteoarticular diseases, cancer, cerebrovascular diseases, bronchopulmonary diseases, heart diseases, and endocrine diseases. Well-being was assessed with the Positive and Negative Affect Schedule and the Life Satisfaction Index-Z. The data suggested there is no association of physical diagnoses with well-being, despite the fact that a self-rated health measure was found to be associated with life-satisfaction. There are, however, some limitations of this study such as the small sample size and diagnoses that were not covered. The present study concludes that relatives and health care providers should be aware that well-being in very old people may be more closely related to how they look upon the disease than the disease itself.

[18] Successful Aging and Control Perceptions

J. G. Chipperfield, L. P. Chuchmach, V. H. Menec & B. Havens (Health, Leisure & Human Performance Research Institute & Department of Community Health Sciences, University of Manitoba, Winnipeg, MB, CANADA)

PURPOSE: Our study identified individuals who have aged "successfully," comparing them on a variety of characteristics. The focus was on perceptions, including perceptions of control, which are regarded as a key component of successful aging. METHOD: Participants of the Aging in Manitoba Project were interviewed to assess their status in three domains that we used to define successful aging: physical, cognitive, and social (Schulz & Heckhausen, 1996). Successful agers (n = 210) were compared to their counterparts (n = 1156) on their perceptions of control over four domains (health, feelings, leisure, task achievement) and a variety of other perceptions including concern for and importance of health. RESULTS: Successful aging correlated significantly with older age and higher education; thus, subsequent ANCOVAs included these variables as covariates. Compared to their counterparts, successful agers had higher internality on health locus of control ($F = 3.19$, $p < .05$) and reported significantly stronger control perceptions over health ($F = 11.88$, $p < .001$), feelings/thoughts ($F = 3.14$, $p < .05$), leisure ($F = 16.58$, $p < .001$), and task achievement ($F = 29.60$, $p < .0001$). In contrast, they did not differ on other perceptions, such as the value for ($t = -1.29$) and importance of ($t = -1.54$) health. CONCLUSIONS: Given that successful agers, who reported higher internality and perceived control across several domains, did not differ from their counterparts in other perceptions (e.g, value for health), the stronger control perceptions may not simply reflect a tendency by successful agers to positively value or perceive the world around them. Rather, as suggested by other researchers, the stronger control perceptions may be central to successful aging.

[19] A Lifespan Analysis of Perceived Control and Well-Being

J. G. Chipperfield, A. Segall, D. S. Bailis & R. P. Perry (Health, Leisure & Human Performance Research Institute & Department of Psychology, University of Manitoba, Winnipeg, MB, CANADA)

PURPOSE: Our study examined perceived control (PC) and well-being (WB) over the adult lifespan. METHOD: Participants (n = 3930) were interviewed to assess four domains of PC (physical health, fitness, comfort, and emotions) and three indexes of WB (self-rated, physical, and mental health). Correlations between PC and WB were examined within age groups (<25, 25-34, 35-44, 45-54, 55-64, 65-74, 75+ years), and differences between correlations were tested across ages. RESULTS: The strength of the PC-WB associations varied across age groups. A linear pattern emerged for mental health, the correlations being significantly stronger for the oldest relative to younger groups for PC over physical health ($z = -2.89$), fitness ($z = -2.92$), comfort ($z = -1.65$), and emotions ($z = -3.42$). For self-rated health, age differences emerged for PC over physical health and comfort: The magnitude of the PC-WB associations increased over age, peaking at 55 to 64 years and then declining. For physical health, age differences in the PC-WB association were restricted to PC over physical health, the association peaking at 45-54 years and subsequently declining significantly ($z = -3.60$). CONCLUSIONS: The magnitude of the PC-WB relationship differed by age group, peaking at different ages depending on the measure of WB and/or the domain of PC. These findings provide direction on the potential role of control-enhancing interventions during the lifespan. For example, they may suggest that control-enhancing interventions would have the most powerful effect on physical and self-rated health in mid-life and on mental health in later life.

[20] Social Comparison, Marital Aggrandizement, and Marital Satisfaction among Older Adults

N. O'Rourke, P. Cappeliez (School of Psychology, University of Ottawa, Ottawa, Canada)

Marital aggrandizement is defined as the propensity to negate the occurrence of negative experience over the course of ones marital history (e.g.I have never regretted my marriage, not even for a moment. If my spouse has any faults, I am not aware of them). This construct has been identified as significantly associated with marital and life satisfaction among older adults. The current study examines the contribution of both marital satisfaction and relative relationship quality (i.e, compared to other couples) as predictors of marital aggrandizement. An international sample of older married adults completed the Marital Aggrandizement Scale (MAS; O'Rourke, 2000) as well as ratings of marital satisfaction and the perceived quality of their relationship relative to other couples (N = 551). A hierarchical regression equation was computed with the MAS as the dependent measure. Marital satisfaction ($F[2,548] = 8.40$, $p < .01$) and relationship quality compared to others ($F[2,548] = 46.05$, $p < .01$) were entered as a first step (R2 = .30, $p < .01$). The product of these independent variables was next entered resulting in a significant increase in prediction of MAS scores (change R2 = .08, $p < .01$). The interaction between these two variables is significantly associated with observed variance of the MAS. It would appear that ones level of marital satisfaction and the perceived quality of others marriages are associated with marital aggrandizement among older adults. Furthermore, the additive effect of perceiving oneself as happily married, more so than others, is significantly associated with marital aggrandizement. Further study is required to determine the direction of relationship among these variables.

[21] Secondary Control and Psychological Well-Being in Older Adults

A. Swift, J. G. Chipperfield, L. P. Chuchmach & R. P. Perry (Health, Leisure & Human Performance Research Institute & Department of Psychology, University of Manitoba, Winnipeg, MB, CANADA)

PURPOSE: Our study examined the relationships between Rothbaum et al.'s (1982) four types of secondary-control and psychological well-being. It was expected that secondary-control would significantly predict negative/positive affect and life satisfaction. METHOD: Intercorrelations assessed the relationships between the four types of secondary-control, and multiple linear regression was used to examine whether secondary-control strategies would predict negative and positive emotion as well as life satisfaction. Data collected from the 1996 Study of Adaptive Strategies (n = 353) was used to carry out these analyses. RESULTS: Correlational analyses revealed positive significant relationships between all four of the secondary-control measures. For the analyses of negative affect and life satisfaction, interpretive control emerged as the strongest predictor; higher levels of interpretive control predicted less negative emotions (B = -.28***, p = .000), and higher levels of life satisfaction (B = .28***, p = .000). Illusory control was the only secondary-control measure that predicted an increase in positive emotions (B = .14***, p <= .05). Vicarious control also emerged as a significant predictor of negative emotions and life satisfaction. CONCLUSIONS: Our findings suggest that, of the four types of secondary control, interpretive control has the most powerful implications for the psychological well-being of older adults. Specifically, having increased levels of interpretive control appears to predict less negative affect and higher levels of life satisfaction. This finding suggests that secondary-control must be taken into account when examining the psychological health of older adults. Other relevant findings related to vicarious and illusory control will also be discussed.

[22] Using Time-Linked Word Cues to Elicit Autobiographical Memories in Older Adults

M. L. Norman and J. L. Harris (The University of Memphis, Memphis, TN, USA)

This study investigated the effect of time-linked word cues on the distribution of autobiographical memories in younger and older adults. Twenty healthy, English-speaking participants in two age groups (younger: 25-40 and older: 70-85) provided personal memories in response to a series of word cues. The word cues included 150 inanimate object nouns categorized as either general or time-linked words. General words entered the English lexicon before the 19th century and are in current use. Time-linked words were further classified as either dated or contemporary. Dated words entered the lexicon over 50 years ago and have fallen out of use, whereas contemporary words entered the lexicon after 1960. Supporting previous research, general, but not time-linked, words prompted a characteristic reminiscence bump among older adults. Dated words prompted the recall of events from earlier years, whereas contemporary words prompted the recall of more recent events. Conversely, among younger adults, the word cues' temporal characteristics did not influence memory distribution. The results of this study suggest that time-linked word-cues may alter the temporal distribution of autobiographical memories among older adults, indicating the need to consider the temporal characteristics of lexical cues in future reminiscence research.

[23] Ranking elderly according to their well-being, assessed by ordinal indicators

V. Horstmann (Gerontology Research Centre, Lund Sweden)

PURPOSE: In studies of elderly the focus is often on constructs like well-being, loneliness, and health, concepts that are often assessed by a number of manifest variables. It is common to base inference on factor analysis or structural equation modelling, relying on an assumption of normality. In a study of well-being in 84-year old people, the three measurable indicators, life satisfaction, general adjustment, and depression, were all categorical, ordinal. The aim of the study was to test for differences in well-being between individuals with varying degrees of sleeping problems. For that purpose, we suggest to use, without requiring normality, an alternative way of combining evidence simultaneously from the ordinal indicators. METHOD: The main idea in the presented technique is the construction of a set of ranks for all individuals, based on the relevant indicators simultaneously; the ranks can then be used in the succeeding test situation. The procedure is an extension of the technique in the widely used Mann-Whitney test. RESULT: The ranking of the 84-year old people according to their well-being corresponds closely to the values of each of the three indicators. The power of tests that are based on our procedure is high compared to some other simpler techniques. CONCLUSION: When the outcome of a study is considered as a composite of several manifest variables, that cannot be regarded as normally distributed, the method suggested here provides a useful tool for testing hypotheses of differences between groups.

[24] Health Behaviour in Aging People

Vladislav Bezrukov, Alexander Polukhov, Vera Chaykovskaya, Georgiy Korobeynikov

PURPOSE: The aim of investigation was to use subjective estimation of sense of coherence and wellbeing life-satisfaction as criteria of health behavioral in aging people. Human behavioral reactions are complex and many-sided. Psychic activity provokes emotional states, which change the objective parameters. METOD: This presentation is a small part of pilot studying of the European survey on aging protocol (the supervisor of National project Prof. Vladislav Bezrukov, 1998). The life-satisfaction and well being were studied (Lykken & Tellegen, 1966). The Ukrainian version of the Sense of Coherence Questionnaire (Antonovsky, 1983, adapted Bezrukov, 1998) was examined. Cognitive functional state: memory and speed were studied (Wechsler, 1955). Two groups: 43 town people aged 35-82 and 31 village people aged 32-85 was examined. RESULTS: The results are showed that differences between town and village people are not reliable. At the same time average age in town group is higher than in village group. This circumstance indicates bigger functional conservation of cognitive functions among town people than among village people. Apart from this it can be supposed that subjective well-being estimations among town group are higher than among corresponding village group. This fact can characterize higher probability of low health behavioral among village people than among town people. CONCLUSION: According to analysis result the subjective estimation of well being is connected with sense of coherence, especially with manageability. The inter relation among well-being estimation and cognitive functions shows that cognitive functions among town people group is more functionally conserved than among village people group.

[25] School reminiscences among older women

Annika Toivoniemi University of Lapland Faculty of Art and Design Rovaniemi, Finland

PURPOSE: This study approaches the reminiscences of school from the perspective of speech and interaction. The main objective of the study is to clarify how, in social situations, aged women reminisce about their school days. In my study, the question is therefore about the individual relationship to personal memories and, on the wider level, to the reminiscences of other group members. The point of departure for the study is, on the one hand, to examine how language is used for socialising and, on the other hand, to study the social aspect of language. METHODS:The material for this study in the Elvi project includes the discussions of five women of over 65 years of age from the lake village area of Sodankylä. These women were in a workgroup that reminisced about school. Discourse analysis is adapted to interpret their school reminiscences. The purpose of the analysis is to perceive the full range of their reminiscences contained within the discourse in detail. RESULTS AND CONCLUSIONS: The study indicates how the narration of reminiscences by aged women takes shape and the significance given to it by the social group in great detail. Women consider the possibility for new points of view and interpretations as one of the greatest benefits in reminiscing. The results of the study also indicate that reminiscing is not chaotic and neither is mutual understanding among the speakers based on chance; rather, interaction in reminiscing is, along with its details, an organised function. The significance of reminiscence is ultimately created by the listener's reasoning process and from the interaction of expression and context.

[26] Religion across the life-span: social and family influences on religious beliefs among elderly women

Susan Fletcher [Cleveland State University, Cleveland, USA]

Religion is known to be an important means of negotiating life meaning and purpose among the elderly. The purpose of this study is to investigate how social and/or family differences during childhood impact the ability to sustain religious beliefs during the final stages of life. Fifteen women, who resided at various assisted-living facilities, participated in qualitative interviews about their current and past religious beliefs. They were distributed among fundamental Christian, Catholic, liberal Protestant, and Jewish faiths. Those women arriving at religious beliefs independent of their original family maintained consistent beliefs throughout their lives and relied on their beliefs to generate meaning in later life. The majority of women, regardless of childhood influences, expressed an increased need for religion during the second half of life. The women cited a growing awareness of human frailty for their increasing dependence on religion. The study suggests that the role of family support in develping religious beliefs during childhood greatly influences the role such beliefs play during the later years of life. It also reinforces previous findings indicating that the role of religion increases with age.

[27] Changes in Health-Related Quality of Life among older Coronary Heart Disease Patients

C.H.M. van Jaarsveld, R. Sanderman, I. Miedema, A.V. Ranchor (Northern Centre for Healthcare Research, University of Groningen, The Netherlands), G.I.J.M. Kempen (Dept. of Health Care studies, Section Medical Sociology, Maastricht University, The Netherlands).

PURPOSE: The objective was to study changes in Health-Related Quality of Life (HR-QL) following Acute Myocardial Infarction (AMI) or Congestive Heart Failure (CHF) in elderly people (>57 yr). METHOD: HR-QL was conceptualized and measured by physical, psychological (depressive symptoms/anxiety), and social (and role) functioning. Pre-morbid data (T0) were available from a community-based survey in 1993. Incident AMI and CHF cases, developed after 1993, are prospectively followed. Assessments were done at 6 weeks (T1), 6 (T2) and 12 months (T3) after diagnosis. RESULTS: Analysis include 89 AMI patients (mean age=69.5 yr) and 119 CHF patients (mean age=74.5 yr). At the pre-morbid assessment, AMI patients did not significantly differ on HR-QL compared to a reference group of elderly people. While CHF patients were on average older, and had worse HR-QL. At T1, all HR-QL measures (including anxiety) showed worse functioning compared to T0, except for depressive symptoms which presented later (at T2). Effect on physical functioning was largest. Effects on psychological and social functioning were less pronounced, but still significant. Effects maintained during the 12 months follow-up. CONCLUSION: The negative consequences on HR-QL among AMI and CHF patients are not temporarily. No recovery of functioning was seen in both groups, while functioning of CHF patients even continue to decline.

[28] On the life quantity of the old

Zen Zuo Wu, Qin Rui Liang (The Old Aging Committee of Linfen Prefecture, Shanxi Province, China)

The goal to improve the life quantity of the old is to keep health, to prolong the progress of getting old. This is not only for the life quantity of the old, but also for the social and self-value of the old. It is a systematic engineering, which is very important and complicated. Everyone and all society should pay great attention to it. A good atmosphere and environment should be established. The basic method to improve the life quantity of the old is mainly to exploit the resource of the old, to develop widely the education of the old, to raise the ability of the old, and to realize the social and self value of the old.

[29] Transitions, adaptation, and coping skills indicated by the Self-Discovery Tapestry life-review instrument

Phyllis J. Meltzer, [Gerontology Research Center, California State University, Fullerton, Fullerton, California, USA]

Abstact The Self-Discovery Tapestry form encourages individuals to analyze their adaptive skills following transitional events. It is utilized as an assessment and counseling instrument. This life-review instrument was developed to imitate the weaving of a tapestry as individuals, using colored pens, indicate their life histories—continuous elements, transitional events, and future goals. Life-span theories support the Tapestry form's development. The research, conducted in conjunction with and subsequent to doctoral dissertation research, presents evidence of several types of adaptive behaviors being recognized by the individuals completing the Tapestry form. Transitional events as well as adaptive and coping skills of more than 400 mature North American individuals were recorded, classified, and analyzed. The types of events differed according to cohort. Among the results: older adults frequently indicated financial events, normative personal transitions, and exhibited greater continuity; younger adults generally indicated greater numbers of geographical moves, deaths of persons or pets, and brief spans of continuity. There is, however, considerable overlap of types of transitional events and adaptive behaviors. Most individuals are able to analyze their own transitional and coping styles as they adapted to new circumstances and regarded their completed Self-Discovery Tapestry forms as an affirmation of their meaningful productivity. Life-span theories were supported by the research results. The Self-Discovery Tapestry proved to be an effective instrument that encouraged mature individuals to recall transitional events and analyze their adaptive coping styles. Many individuals from varying backgrounds and ages utilized transitional events to develop adaptive strategies.

[30] Quality of Life in Older Adults

*Gandelli M, Muzzoni B, Gornati R, Segù F, Antoniello N. (*II.AA.RR, RSA "F. Pertusati" Pavia), Perotta D, Magri F, Ferrari E. (Department of Internal Medicine and Medical Therapy, Chair of Geriatrics, University of Pavia, Italy)*

The assessment of the Quality of life is a crucial aspect of the management of elderly subjects. Thus we studied 24 healthy old subjects without cognitive impairment (64-92 years; MMSE >21) resident in a Senior Home. In this homogeneous group we evaluated the relationship between self perceived measures of physical and psychological health status (Sickness Impact Profile- SIP-and Short form Health Survey- SF-36) from one hand and cognitive (MMSE), affective (GDS), nutritional (MNA) and objective physical performance test (Walking test), from the other. The evaluation of the quality of life by the SIP was significantly related to the IADL score and the Walking test. However, some dimensions namely psychosocial and particularly the physical one, seems to be better related to cognitive (MMSE), functional (ADL and IADL), nutritional (MNA) and physical (Walking test) performances. By considering the SF-36, the eight SF-36 measures showed a good correlation coefficient with all the parameters evaluated. In conclusion, in this population the QoL seems to be mainly dependent on the functional status rather than on comorbility and disease severity; furthermore the QoL, evaluated by a simple and low cost questionnaire, may give useful information for the management of elderly subjects.

[31] Relationship of volunteering and self-esteem among the older adults in Korea

Joohyun Kim, Gyounghae Han(Department of Child Development and Family Studies, Seoul National University, Korea)

There has been recent increase of the participation in volunteering activities of the elders in Korea. However, little empirical studies were done to examine the relationship between the volunteering and the well-being of the elderly. The purpose of this study is to examine the effects of the participation in volunteering activities on the self-esteem of the elders. Main research questions of the study were : 1) Is there a significant differences between volunteering and non-volunteering elders in terms of socio-demographic characteristics and the self-esteem. 2) What are the perceived rewards of the volunteering and how supportive are the family members for the elder's participation? 3) Do the perceived rewards and family support affect the level of self-esteem of the volunteering elders? In order to explore these questions, data were gathered from 152 elderly volunteers and 143 non-volunteers in Korea, through the structured questionnaire. The statistical methods used for the data analysis were discriptive statistics, t-test, and multiple regression. Results showed that volunteering elders were younger, healthier, and economically better-off than non-volunteering elders. The proportion of the women and retired were higher among volunteers than non-volunteers. Participation in the volunteering activities was a significant variable predicting the level of self-esteem. Perceived rewards of volunteering has a significant positive effect on the self-esteem of the elders while family support showed no significant effect. The results confirm the notion that participation in volunteering activities is one of the ways to the successful aging.

[32] Medical and psychological factors related to the maintenance of independent living in old age

W. D. Oswald, B. Hagen, R. Rupprecht (Institute for Psychogerontolgy, University of Erlangen-Nuremberg, Germany)

In 1991 the longitudinal study Maintaining and Supporting Independent Living in Old Age (SIMA) was started. One major study aim was to analyse the possible loss of independent living and the development for need of care in a sample of former healthy and independent living subjects aged 75 years and older. Mean age of subjects in 1991 was 79.5 (+- 3.5) years. Data from 340 participants (63.5 % women) was available for multivariate Cox regression analyses adjusted for basic demographic parameters. Loss of independent living was defined by living in a care facility, keeping the own household not alone, need for long-term care insurance support, need for assistance or suffering from a kind of dementia. According to one of these criteria after seven years 161 subjects (47.4 %) had lost their ability of living independently. Analyses revealed the following main risk factors (Hazard ratios are given in brackets, for each of them $p <= 0.003$): passive personality (2.3), apoplexy (2.1), few everyday activities (1.9), inferior psychopathological status, low fluid intelligence performance (1.8 each), poor well-being, poor health status (1.7 each), high degree of multimorbidity, depression, and vision impairment (1.6 each). These results clearly contradict to the widespread gerontological opinion that one medical factor alone, i. e. apoplexy, is responsible for the loss of independent living in old age. Results indicate that maintaining independent living in old age is influenced significantly by several medical as well as psychological factors.

[33] Healthful Feeding Workshop for Successful Aging at Altitudes

Germán MONTEVILLA-VARGAS Plinio Rogelio Vergara Serrano Ruben Otto Streuli (Gobierno Municipal de La Paz and Adventist Development Relief Agency) (La Paz - Bolivia.)

PURPOSE:The Quinua, Cañagua and Tarwi are exotic foods in Andean regions at 3500-4300m above sea level. The purpose of this paper is to present and study that early eating such foods compound with dark green and orange vegetables and fruits we can get successful aging. METHOD:The workshop was planed by Municipal Government of La Paz City (GMLP) and Adventist Development Relief Agency (ADRA-Bolivia) in the winter of 2000. The research design was made as a pilot experience in Kupini Village Center. La Paz have 7 major city districs, this Village was selected randomly. The sample of 123 families showed us that migrants from mountain area were 60%, Valleys 28% and from flat lands (less than 300m above sea level) 12%. Our work consisted in 6 training courses to 47 family groups focussing on intergenerational relationships with multidisciplinary team. At the same time, we made medical check ups to 156 elderly persons with Nuestra Señora de La Paz University's medical students.The major problem was the time scheduling wetween formal and informal workers. RESULTS: For family groups from Valleys and flat lands the Quinua, Cañagua and Tarwi were unknown. However, through the training they were more interested about these teaching materials and changing in their food intake patterns introduced along the educational workshops. From 156 elderly people (60 and over), 36% were in transit from rural to rural areas; among them only 8% had disability problems. In the past, when the Kupini Village neighbors were living in rural areas, the Incas' food (Quinua,Cañagua and Tarwi)were well known; nevertheless, in their actual lifes they forgot it and their elderly members have more health problems. CONCLUSION: Around the Andean Mountains the people produce extraneous foods which seems to have powerful effects on the aging process. However, the migration from rural to urban areas is changing the ethnic food intake patterns. The teaching objective was reached successfuly and had been created expectancy for the following actions. In our opinion, the protein, vitamins, minerals and other nutrient contents of the Quinua, Cañagua and Tarwi should be explored.

[34] Studying successful aging in a culturally-relevant way: the relationship between value orientations and understandings of successful aging

Sandra Torres (Dept. of Sociology, Uppsala University, Uppsala, Sweden)

The field of cross-cultural gerontology has been deemed to be atheoretical by virtue of its failure to generate theoretical frameworks of its own. In order to contribute to the rectification of cross-cultural gerontology,a culturally-relevant theoretical framework for the study of understandings of successful aging (SA) has been proposed. This framework assumes that value orientations concerning human nature, man-nature, time, activity and relationships shape the manner in which successful aging is understood. This study aims to shed preliminary empirical light the framework in question. In order to test the proposed relationship between value orientations and understandings of SA, the anthropological instrument designed by Kluckhohn and Strodtbeck has been conducted. This adaptation entails the design of new vignettes that tap into the understandings of SA that are assumed to follow from these value orientations. Qualitative interviews with 30 Iranian immigrants to Sweden have been conducted using these vignettes. The results confirm the hypothesis — they attest to congruence between value orientations and understandings of SA. Thus, it is argued that they therefore pave the way for a theoretically sound approach to the study of individual, generational as well as cross-cultural understandings of SA. Last but not least it must be mentioned that a variety of understandings of SA were found. This variety suggests that there are other ways of understanding the concept in question besides the master nature, future, productivity and individuality oriented ones that characterize the gerontological literature.

[35] Decision-Making Style and Life Satisfaction among the Elderly of Japan

S. Okada, H. Lim (Graduate School of Human Life Science, Osaka City University, Osaka, Japan), M. Okada (College of Social Sciences, Ritsumeikan University, Kyoto, Japan)

PURPOSE: The aim of this presentation is to examine how decision-making style of the elderly of Japan is associated with life satisfaction. METHOD: Participants in Old Adult Day Care were recruited from four Day Care Centers. We conducted face-to-face interviews with 75 participants using the structured questionnaire. The questionnaire included several measures concerning decision-making style, ADL, and life satisfaction as well as several demographics. In this study, we used standardized measures for ADL and life satisfaction. RESULTS: 76.0% of the participants were female, and 38.7% lived alone. The average age of the participants was 79.7 years (SD = 8.1). The data indicated that the decision-making style measure was reliable as evidence by the moderate internal consistency. The alpha coefficient for the measure was 0.69. Principal component analysis was conducted in order to confirm the constructs of the measure. As a result, all items (7 items) loaded onto the two factors (active and passive decision-making styles: ADM and PDM) hypothesized by us. Results of multiple regression analysis indicated that ADM had a significant effect on life satisfaction after controlling for several demographics. On the other hand, PDM had no effect on life satisfaction. CONCLUSION: The study suggested that the active decision-making style of old persons positively influenced life satisfaction and that, as previously pointed out by many professionals, decisional autonomy of the elderly had a significant impact on the quality of life.

[36] Subjective Life Expectancy and the Accumulation of Assets among Elderly Japanese People

T.Nakata (Hokusei Gakuen University, Sapporo, JAPAN)

The aim of this study is to clarify the relationship between subjective life expectancy and the accumulation of assets among elderly Japanese people. Advance researches suggest that people can forecast their longevity and subjective life expectancy has an effect on their economic behavior. It is well known that Japanese have a high saving rate. A relevant factor of that may be anxiety for their future life. In that context, we can imagine that the longer people feel their life, the more they build up their assets. However it holds true that the other factors, for example income that people can get from their job etc, affect the accumulation of the assets. So I will examine what contributes to the accumulation of assets among elderly Japanese people. Analyses are based on data obtained from the Sapporo 1999 Study, a cross-sectional study of a random sample of 488 men who were 60 and older in 1999. And I use the self-rated life expectancy as endogenous variables and satisfaction rating for health, marital status, the number of cohabitants, and job prestige score (present jobs or jobs before respondents retire) as exogenous variables. Results of path analysis don't offer any support for the hypotheses. The accumulation of assets isn't associated with subjective life expectancy, but is influenced by the job prestige score. I conclude that subjective life expectancy has no effect on economic behavior like building up assets and is demonstrated by the high status of social stratification.

[37] The well-being of Chinese octogenarians in rural Hubei province: A qualitative investigation.

Zeng Erkang, Wu Zhien (Department of Gerontology, Tongji Medical College, Huazhong University of Science and Technology, Wuhan, China) James T. Sykes (Institute of Aging, University of Wisconsin, Madison, USA) Cheng Zhongwen (Institute of Aging, Zhongxiang, Hubei, China)

The 10.5 million persons aged 80 and above in China account for 16% of the world's octogenarians. More than 80% of these old persons live in the countryside. Findings from this investigation into the psychological health of octogenarians are important to improve the quality of rural elders and to inform government aging policies. From four rural towns in the Zhong-Xiang region 632 non-institutionalized octogenarians were identified. 136 elders were randomly selected. The interview instrument focused on the subject's personal assessment of well-being. Of 682 key words identified from interview records, 24 frequently occurring words were selected for analyses. Software: STATA 5.0 was used for statistical analysis. Fifty-three subjects were male, 83 female. 103 were illiterate. 104 were widowed. 116 were peasants. 34 reported they lived comfortably; 89 lived without worrying about food and clothes. 115 subjects relied on support from their children. 113 reported good health and ability to care for themselves. The core questions were: What brings you happiness? What causes you to worry? and To what are you looking forward? In rank order, subjects reported expectations of a good old age, filial piety, and independence brought them happiness. Sources of anxiety included poor health, worry about their children and poverty. An overwhelming numbers of subjects were looking forward to good health, good economic status, filial piety and comfortable lives. Our findings leave unanswered questions about how support systems for rural octogenarians can be strengthened and, for those without family support, how the community should provide care.

[38] Perceived Experiences of Well Senior Women Engaged in Occupational Lifestyle Redesign

Elysa G. Lipschutz, OTR/L [Nova Southeastern University, Fort Lauderdale, FL, USA]

Purpose: Demographic trends warrant exploration of interventions to maximize the well-being of older adults. This qualitative study explored the experiences of well senior women engaged in an occupational lifestyle redesign program in order to explain how participants' perceived the functions of this intervention and its influences on their well-being. Occupational lifestyle redesign enables participants to develop and enact a customized array of health promoting occupations. Methods:Grounded theory procedures were used to construct a conceptual model of the perceived experiences of six, well women, aged 58 to 80, engaged in the eight, 2-hour, weekly sessions of the Lifestyle Redesign Program at Nova Southeastern University (NSU). Results: Results illustrated how the women first experienced an opportunity to share themselves and build connections with one another while learning of the role of occupation in their lives. The women then became more self-aware and generated and realized occupational options for enhanced well-being. In turn, the women identified goals and enacted changes related to their occupational selves. The women subsequently revealed how the experience of these functions of occupational lifestyle redesign influenced their perceived well-being by facilitating: (a) their sense of connection, (b) new perspectives about themselves and occupation and

(c) their incentive to act to maximize their lifestyles. Conclusion: Results of this study: (a) inform programming aimed at promoting the well-being of well elderly through the use of occupational lifestyle redesign, (b) support the belief in occupational therapy that occupation influences health and (c) demonstrate the value of studying and explaining a phenomenon from the participants' perspectives.

[39] Predicting Adult Adaptation from Questionnaire and Narrative Assessments of Generativity; A Longitudinal Study.

Stephanie Kuiack, Joan E. Norris (University of Guelph, Guelph Ontario) and Michael W. Pratt (Wilfrid Laurier University, Waterloo Ontario)

Abstract: Erikson's construct of generativity refers to one's concerns with the care for future generations as a legacy of the self. The present research examines the longitudinal prediction from questionnaire and narrative measures of generativity to life satisfaction and social adaptation among adults four years later. The study involves a standard questionnaire as well as a narrative component. 55 adults from three age groups (<30, 30-50, 60+) were asked to complete the Loyola Generativity Scale (LGS) and tell stories about past learning experiences. Stories were scored for the presence of redemptive patterns which refer to the tendency to transform bad experiences into good (McAdams et al, 1997). These same participants completed a similar questionnaire and interview four years later. Generativity on the LGS showed stability over the four years (r=0.75). High generative concerns on the LGS as well as narratives scored high in redemptive structure at Time 1 were both related to a greater sense of importance of sharing one's life experience with others, greater perceived social support, availability of social support, greater life satisfaction and higher self esteem four years later (p<.05). This study supports the notion that generative concerns on the LGS questionnaire are enduring and predict to a range of positive life outcomes for adults across the lifespan four years later including those over age 60. Furthermore, narrative structure was shown to be a useful tool in assessing components of generativity and provided parallel insights into the subsequent adaptation and satisfaction of these adults.

[40] Spirituality in nursing homes: Is it happening?

Terry Tirrito, College of Social Work, University of South Carolina,Columbia, SC. 29208

The purpose of this study was to investigate the religious services offered to nursing home residents. The literature indicates that prayer and religion positively affect the health of older persons (Koenig, 1997). Building on research evidence, this study examines the services offered to residents in nursing homes. While there is renewed interest in the importance of religion in the live of older persons in gerontological literature, there is little study of religion in nursing homes. In practice religion and spirituality are marginally addressed. Current reimbursement and regulation policies in nursing homes focus on medical and psychiatric treatment but little attention is given to spiritual care. The Internet was used to contact nursing homes regarding religious services offered by the facility. The results found that beyond meeting requirements of regulatory agencies few non traditional (prayer groups, family prayers, outside visits to churches) services are offered. Although there is evidence that religion is essential to the well being of nursing home residents this information is not incorporated into daily services offered to residents in nursing homes.

[41] Response of Target Population to a Physical Intervention Program Promoted by Health Care Sectors.

S. Vestergaard(1), G. Dalsgaard (2), L. Puggaard(1) (1. Institute of Sports Science and Clinical Biomechanics, University of Southern Denmark, Odense University Ageing Research Center, Denmark. 2. The Health Services, Frederiksborg County, Denmark)

PURPOSE: Possibilities to participate in physical activity for the more frail elderly people, falling in the gap between existing activity offers and rehabilitation, are lacking. Therefore, Strengthen Your Body, a county-municipal training intervention program was initiated targeting this population. As such this study evaluates the level of functional ability (FA) of participants in this community exercise intervention program and possible intervention effects on FA. Furthermore, it examines correlation between ascend-descend stair test (ADST) and conventional measures of FA. METHOD: Community-dwelling participants (n=230) enrolled after receiving information about the weekly class-based exercise program from e.g. the public assigned home help. Information about subjective (activity of daily living-questionnaire, ADL) and objective (physical performance test, PPT) FA was obtained and participants performed a timed ADST. Paired t-test analyses the intervention effect. Pearson test analyses the association: age vs. FA and ADST vs. subjective and objective measures. RESULTS: Preliminary results indicate that age and FA were positively correlated. The FA of the enrollees is only slightly different from the FA in the respective age group in a comparison with large population studies in Denmark. Evaluation of post-exercise FA is ongoing. ADST correlated with both ADL-mobility and PPT. CONCLUSION: Level of FA of the participants suggests that the target population did not enroll and that further focus on reaching the more frail elderly people is important. Furthermore, it seems that ADST can be used as an indicator of FA.

[42] Physical capacity and activities among the oldest old: the Umea 90+ study

von Heideken P, Gustavsson J, Kallin K, Lundin-Olsson L, Nygren B, Lundman B*, Norberg A*, Gustafson Y. (Department of Community Medicine and Rehabilitation, Geriatric Medicine, Umeå, Sweden *Department of Caring Sciences, Umeå, Sweden)*

PURPOSE: To study physical capacity, activities, falls and fractures among the oldest old. METHOD: A population based study was performed in the municipality of Umeå, where all persons born before 1906 (n=86) and in 1910 (n=115) were asked to participate. The data collection consisted of structured interviews and assessments in the person's home. Data was also collected from medical charts, relatives and caregivers. Physical capacity was examined with Studentski's mobility screen and Berg's Balance Scale. Fear of falling was investigated with Falls Efficacy Scale, FES. ADL was measured with Barthels ADL-index and the ADL staircase. RESULTS: One hundred sixty-five persons (82%) agreed to participate while 25 persons (12%) refused and 11 (6%) died before inclusion. Seventy-nine percent were women, 42% lived in their own homes while 58% lived in institutions. Ten percent were independent in their ADL, 34% needed assistance only with their IADL and mean of Barthels ADL-index was 13.3 (SD 7.0). Eightyfour percent were able to walk and 79% of them had some kind of walking aid. Fiftythree percent had sustained a fall the previous year, 26% had the previous five years had a hip fracture and 18% a radial shaft fracture. Thiryfour percent were afraid of falling indoors and 43% outdoors, mean of FES was 87.0 (SD 37.2). Bergs Balance Scale was practicable in 82 persons (50%), mean 37.9 (SD 14.7). CONCLUSIONS: The majority of the oldest old are dependent in their IADL and 79% had walking aids. Fear of falling, falls and fractures are major health problems among the oldest old.

[43] Physician Physical Activity and Risk for Osteoporosis?

A. C. A. Souza, R. H. Schneider, Y. Moriguchi (Laboratory of Osteoporosis and Bone Metabolism on Geriatric and Gerontology Institute PUCRS, Porto Alegre, Brazil)

The health of the bone has been related with physical activity and sedentarism with osteopenia or osteoporosis. Physicians maybe at risk for bone resorption due to their sedentary activity. We have studied a group of medical doctors and compared this group with a normal population. We studied the bone density of 59 healthy physicians (32 males and 27 females), with a mean age, respectively, of 38 ± 7.06 and 34 ± 2.06 years. The bone densitometry was performed in the Lumbar Spine and proximal right femur regions. We calculated the vertebral density of L1-L4 individually. The values were compared with of the American standard population, respectively for males and females. We observed in the male group that L3 and L4 had significantly lower density (p<0.002) than the normal male population. Males doctors also presented lower density ($p<0.005$) in the hip, trochanter ($p<0.005$) and Ward's Triangle ($p<0.001$). However, in the female group only the Ward's Triangle showed a lower density ($p<0.009$). The mean density values L3-L4 is lower in the male group compared with the female group. These preliminary results showed that sedentarism of the medical professionals have a negative influence in femoral bone density and lower lumbar vertebrae for both sexes. In females we observed the same tendency, but without statistic significance, except the Ward's Triangle.

[44] Field Evaluation of Cycled Coupled Movements of Hand and Foot in Older Subjects

Capranica Laura, Olivieri Berardo (IUSM of Rome, Italy)

The aim of the present study was to verify by means of a field test: 1) age-related differences in rhythmic flexion-extensions of ipsilateral hand and foot, either in-phase and anti-phase associations; 2) differences between preferred and non-preferred limbs in older subjects. The subjects, seated in a chair that allowed independent motion of the hand and lower limb in the sagittal plane, had to perform flexion and extension movements around the elbow and knee joints with a 1:1 frequency ratio. Two homolateral (right upper and lower limbs; left upper and lower limbs) conditions were tested in two coordination modes: in phase (isodirectional) and anti-phase (nonisodirectional). Each test condition, which lasted 60 s maximum, was performed at three velocities (80, 120, and 180 beat.min-1) by older (10 females and 9 males: age 54-87 yrs.), adults (8 females and 8 males: age 18-28 yrs.), and children (12 females and 13 males: age 10 yrs.) subjects. Statistically significant differences ($p<0.01$) were found for age, phases, velocities, and age x phase x and velocity interaction. Older subjects always showed lowest values and, within the first 10 s, tended to end both all the anti-phase conditions (95 0.000000e+00rror), and the 180 beat/min in-phase condition (100 0.000000e+00rror). No statistically significant difference was found between preferred and non-preferred limbs. This test represents a useful tool to investigate the quantification of cyclic coupled movements of hand and foot allowing, with an inexpensive apparatus and simple measurements, to evaluate the age-related changes in older subjects' interlimb coordination.

[45] Training-related enhancement in muscle power production in sedentary elderly subjects

P. Caserotti (1), P. Aagaard (2) E. B. Simonsen (3), L.Puggaard (1), (1) Institute of Sports Science and Clinical Biomechanics, University of Southern Denmark, Odense University, Odense Denmark; 2) Team Denmark Test Center Bispebjerg Hospital Sports Medicine Research Unit, University of Copenhagen, Copenhagen, Denmark and 3) Institute of Medical Anatomy Dept C, Panum Institute)

PURPOSE: The ability of the muscle system to generate mechanical power (product of force of contraction and velocity of movement) deteriorates with increasing age with special emphasis on the velocity determinant. This may result in a greater difficulty in demanding tasks where rapid execution and intense muscle force are required (e.g. when trying to reverse a forward fall). The aim of this study was to elucidate the effects of physical training on the determinants of muscle power, force and velocity in 75-year old men. METHODS: 37 community-dwelling healthy elderly men were divided into a training group (TG) and a control group (CG). TG performed 8 months of all-round physical training, 75 minutes twice a week. Muscle power was assessed by two jumps (counter movement, CMJ, and squatting jump, SQJ), performed on a force platform. Jump height (JH), peak power (Wpeak/kg-1), velocity at Wpeak (Vwpeak) and force at Wpeak (Fwpeak/kg) were determined. Maximal vertical force (Fmax/kg-1) was also determined for the CMJ as an indicator of the eccentric muscle capability. RESULTS: After training, Wpeak assessed during the CMJ increased for the TG ($P<0.05$) and decreased in the CG ($P<0.05$). Significant changes in Vwpeak ($P<0.05$) were the main contributors to these changes in both groups. Not significant but similar tendency was observed for the SQJ. Fmax/kg-1 in the CMJ did not increase in TG after training but a larger increase in Wpeak was observed for CMJ versus SQJ. CONCLUSION: All-round physical training increased significantly the ability to perform the movement at higher speed and contrasted the decline observed in the CG during CMJ. Only a tendency was observed for the SQJ. Adaptive neural mechanisms (e.g. reduction of inhibitory mechanisms following eccentric contraction) may explain the differences between the two jumps after the training. The velocity component seemed to be the critical determinant for muscle power production both for the increase in TG and decrease in CG.

[46] Influence of preparatory set on anticipatory muscle activation in older adults

S.G. Brauer, Y. Burns (Department of Physiotherapy, University of Queensland, St Lucia, Australia)

PURPOSE: Changing the preparatory set for a task changes the complexity of the programming required prior to a movement. While young adults show a delay in anticipatory muscle activity when poorly prepared for a movement, the effect in older adults is unknown. Older adults show a delay in anticipatory muscle activity in comparison to young adults and a delay with complex tasks. Delayed postural muscle activity when poorly prepared to move could result in an ineffective movement and lead to a fall. The purpose of this study was to determine whether the timing of hip muscle activity was influenced by age and whether older adults were influenced more by a low preparatory set than younger adults. METHOD: Twenty young (21±3 years) and twenty-five elderly (71±5 years) females performed a rapid, reaction-time step task at high, neutral and low levels of preparatory set. Surface electromyography was recorded from the stance-limb gluteus medius, tensor fascia latae, and from the step-limb hip adductors. Group, preparation and group x preparation effects were determined with multivariate ANOVA. RESULTS: Postural muscle activity of older females was delayed in comparison to younger females across all preparation conditions ($p = 0.002$). In all subjects, muscle activity was delayed to a similar extent in both the neutral and low-preparation condition in comparison to the high-preparation condition ($p < 0.020$). CONCLUSION: Older females exhibit delayed postural muscle activity with rapid stepping in comparison to young. The influence of a low preparatory set was similar in both groups.

[47] Influence of muscle strength, body weight and composition on regional bone mineral density in healthy postmenopausal women

Blain H1, Vuillemin A2,3, Teissier A4, Guillemin F2, Durant R1, Jeandel C1 (1 Antonin Balmès Gerontology Center, Montpellier, France; 2 Faculty of Sport, Nancy, France ; 3 School of Public Health, UPRES EA 1124, Faculty of Medecine, Nancy, France; 4 Centre de Rééducation Jacques Parisot, Bainville-sur-Madon, France

PURPOSE : The study's aim was to investigate the relationship between body weight and composition and quadriceps strength on femoral neck and lumbar spine bone mineral density (BMD) in healthy postmenopausal women. METHOD: The relationship between isokinetic quadriceps strength, measured by Biodex, and BMD, measured by dual energy x-ray absorptiometry, was studied in multiple regression models controlling for age, body composition and menopausal treatment in 56 women aged 60 to 81 (70.5 ± 6.2 years). RESULTS: Weight and age were associated with femoral neck BMD (33% and 100f variance explained, respectively) and lumbar spine BMD (23% and 80f its variance). When body weight and quadriceps strength were excluded from the model, lean mass and age were associated with femoral neck BMD (29% and 140f variance explained, respectively) and lumbar spine BMD (28% and 110f variance explained, respectively). When quadriceps strength was added to the model, it was strongly associated with femoral neck BMD (300f variance explained), independently of lean mass (9%) and age (7%), whereas it was not found to be significantly associated with lumbar spine BMD. CONCLUSION: Lean mass explained a great part of the strong association between body weight and femoral neck and lumbar spine

BMD. Quadriceps strength explained a great part of the association between lean mass and BMD at the femoral neck but not at the lumbar spine site, suggesting a site-specific effect of muscular strength on bone and the possible association of age-related decline of muscle strength with age-related bone loss.

[48] Study of the Effects of Group Exercise Sessions on Frail Elderly in Long- term Care Facility

Elizabeth Baum, David Jarjoura, David Faur, Ann Polen, Gregory Rutecki, [Northeastern Ohio Universities College of Medicine, Affiliated Hospitals at Canton, Ohio and Northwestern University Medical School, Chicago, Illinois, U.S.A.]

Purpose: To determine if routine exercise sessions in frail nursing home and assisted living residents result in improved physical and/or psychological function. Methods: Twenty residents at a long-term care facility (LTC) were randomized to a strength training exercise group or an art therapy group (control) for 6 months. At 6 months the control group crossed over to the exercise group and both groups were followed for an additional 6 months. Objective measures of physical and psychologic function were obtained at baseline, 3, 6, 9 and 12 months using the timed get-up-and-go test, Berg Balance Scale, Physical Performance Test (PPT) and Mini-Mental Status Exam (MMSE). The exercise session, conducted by an exercise physiologist, included strength and flexibility training using therabands, balls and soft weights for 1 hour 3 times per week. Results: With measures at baseline there was a significant overall impact on the four measures of the exercise intervention (p=.013). Exercise benefit as measured by effect sizes (in standard deviation units), was positive for each measure (timed get up and go .5, PPT .40, Berg .32, and MMSE .54), and except for the Berg, 90% confidence intervals were above zero. Conclusion: Frail elderly in a LTC facility were able to routinely participate and benefit from a strength-training program. This program can be delivered with low cost equipment by staff and volunteers with minimal training. The advantage of such a program is that it provides not only recreational, but also therapeutic benefits.

[49] Physical Activity: A way to prevent aging in 2000 A.D.

J. Alice, V.H. Barraza, A. del C. Ontivero (Geriatric's Consulting-Rooms, Rosario, Santa Fe, Argentina)

PURPOSE: To demonstrate that physical activity improves both objectively and subjectively the quality of life of Aged Adults, preventing disabilities through revitalization (i.e. the whole of actions tending to retain functionality, especially in the locomotor and cardiorespiratory systems) and rehabilitation (i.e. the recovering of the psychic and physical potentiality lost because of definite pathologies like diabetes, cardiovascular disease, muscular diseases, etc.). METHOD: Non institutionalized men and women older than 65, regardless of previous pathologies. Evaluation of previous individual condition with regard to the practice of sports or physical activities. Variables: 1- Subjective perception of one's own quality of life. 2- Previous diseases, paying special attention to: a) diabetes; b) cardiovascular illness; c) muscular disease; d) pulmonary disease. Re-evaluation after 1 year practicing physical activities. Variables: a) Subjectively: improvements of quality of life and sleep. b) Objectively: improvements in the clinical parameters and biochemical standards specific to each pathology listed above. RESULTS: Physical level: prevention of obesity, decalcification and loss of muscular mass; improvement of strength, elasticity, agility and general physical condition; increase in respiratory capacity and articulator mobility; strengthening of cardiac contraction connected to effort - fatigue. Psychic level: sense of well-being; increase of optimism and intellectual activity; better intercourse with people; decrease in perceptions of loneliness and isolation. CONCLUSION: Physical activity gives longer life to elderly people, improves quality of life, stimulates social intercourse, and improves creativity as well as the linking among individuals and social capabilities as a whole.

[50] The role of mobility in the pathogenesis of disorders in the healthy elderly people

Bashkaeva M. S, L.B. Lazebnik (Russian Medical Academy of Post-Graduate Education, Department of Gerontology and geriatrics)

The goal : to estimate the mobility status - the capability of movement in the lonely elderly people. Methods. Specialized questionnaire was suggested to 1147 lonely people elder then 60 in the out-hospital department of Moscow. The estimation of data of demographical, medico-social and function status of each person was carried out. Results. Forced immobilization is the pathologic reason for the mobility limitation of the elderly. The main reasons are the loco-motor organ diseases (35% of all examined cases); central nervous system disorders (25%); eye diseases (10,6%); coronary artery disease (9%); malignancy (4%); comorbidity (16%). We suggested 5-staged quality classification for the elderly according to their mobility. I) The person could move outside his home (76,8% of studied population); II) The mobility is limited by the yard borders (4,5%); III) The mobility is limited by the borders of the home (14,4%); IV) The mobility is only within the room limits prisoner of the room (2,2%); V) Chained to bed (2,1%). In conclusion the complex analysis of the parameters and stages of immobilization and functional capability of the elderly let to put out main clinic-functional groups that are the basis of the rationale choice for treatment in geriatric practice and for making correct therapeutic decisions.

[51] A new method for determining exercise intensity based on the walking velocity of the elderly

Yukitoshi Aoyagi, Taketo Furuna, Satoshi Nishizawa, Miho Sugiura (Department of Kinesiology, Division of Human Science Research, Tokyo Metropolitan Institute of Gerontology, Itabashi, Tokyo, Japan), Fumiharu Togo, Shujiro Sugita (Department of Kinesiology, Division of Human Science Research, Tokyo Metropolitan Institute of Gerontology, Itabashi, Tokyo, Japan and Japan Science and Technology Corporation, Kawaguchi, Saitama, Japan), Shigemura Matsuki, Yasuhito Kumazaki, Mamiko Naka, Shigeru Inoue, Tomoko Takamiya, Fumiko Ono, Yumi Uchida, Chiyo Inokuchi (Tokyo Metropolitan Health Promotion Center, Shinjuku, Tokyo, Japan)

This study examined interrelationships between preferred and maximal walking velocities, maximal oxygen uptake (VO2max), and knee extension torque in 10 healthy male and 13 healthy female volunteers, aged 65-74 years. Furthermore, it determined the percentages of oxygen uptake reserve (02reserve) and heart rate reserve (%HRreserve) when exercising at 30-70% of the maximal walking velocity. The two walking velocities were calculated from the time taken to walk a 5 m distance (from the 3 m to 8 m mark) of an 11 m, straight, flat walkway. There was a significant correlation between the preferred and the maximal walking velocities ($p < 0.05$), the former corresponding to 53-54% of the latter, irrespective of the sex. The maximal (or preferred) walking velocity significantly correlated not only to the knee extension torque but also to the VO2max in both men and women ($p < 0.05$). As a result, a linear and regular relationship was found of 02reserve and %HRreserve to various submaximal walking velocities within a given range. For both men and women, 40-60%of the maximal walking velocity corresponded to 30-50% of VO2reserve and HRreserve. Thus, it appears that 60% of the maximal walking velocity (110-115% of the preferred walking velocity) could represent moderate exercise for the elderly. This new method of using walking velocity for determining exercise intensity would make it possible for the elderly to exercise simply, safely, and effectively.

[52] Effects of physical training on psychosocial functional ability in 75-year old men and women

Kurt Lüders, Lis Puggaard, Kirsten Schroll Bjørnsboe (Institute of Sports Science and Clinical Biomechanics, University of Southern Denmark, Odense University, Denmark).

Purpose: The purpose of the study was to evaluate the effect of physical training on psychosocial functional ability in 75-year old men and women. Methods: The subjects were 91 75-year old men and women. The group was divided into three groups (training-, social- and a control group). The training group participated in physical class-based exercise during ten months with two session of 90 minutes per week. The exercises consisted of various activities involving muscle strength, endurance and flexibility exercises. Psychosocial functional ability was measured, before and after the training, by means of general health questionnaires and psychometric scales. The psychometric scales included: 1. Profile of Mood State (POMS), 2. Pain and soreness in the musculoskeletal system (Lundgren et al, 1990), 3. Self-esteem Scale (Kjørmo, 1987), 4. Depression Scale (CES-D Scale) and 5. Cognitive functions (MMSE). The answers given in the questionnaires were followed by in-depth interviews with the training group. Results: All groups felt very good/good health before and after the training. The training group felt significant better fitness after the training. The same tendencies were found in feeling of stress, problems with insomnia, experiences of mood and depression. In feeling of loneliness and satisfaction with life there was a tendency to feel better in the training group and the social group. Conclusion: The training group felt significant better fitness and lower degree of depression after the training. In most others psychosocial parameters there were found minor positive, but not significant, changes in the training and the social groups.

[53] Study on the improving function of old people's health by China's community development

Ke-jian Tan (Shanxi Academy of Social Sciences Taiyuan Shanxi china)

The construction of China's community is having a rapid development in recent years. It is not only due to the government's improvement of community administrative structure and system, but also due to the formation of non-government pattern. These two community development patterns play the following important roles in improving the health of Chinese old people: 1) to provide assistance to the daily life of the old people; 2) to enrich the spiritual life of the old people; 3) to provide opportunity and help for the redevelopment of old people; 4) to help old people who remain single to solve their marriage problem; 5) to assist old people in settling the family problem.

[54] Meta-analysis: Self-efficacy for exercise in older adults

J. Kruger (University of Illinois at Chicago, Chicago, IL, US)

Health promotion interventions that encourage physical activity adoption are viewed as an important public policy issue. Identifying key relationships is foundational to tailoring exercise interventions that can result in changing habits to produce health benefits for the elderly. The purpose of this study was to summarize the literature and evaluate the effects of physical activity interventions on self-efficacy in older adults. A meta-analysis was used to integrate study findings and allows results to be combined statistically to determine the overall effects in diverse populations and study conditions using decision rules to distinguish systematic patterns. An effect size for individual studies was calculated using formulae recommended from Hedges and Olkin (1985). The population consisted of 251 studies, published between the years of 1967-2000 that focused upon: adults 60 years of age and older, engaged in physical activity interventions and use of the SCT framework to encourage behavior change. Of the population of 251 articles, 52 were used in the analysis, yielding a 21% inclusion rate. Statistically significant beneficial effects were found across all studies for self-efficacy with an overall moderate effect (d =+.55). Thus, a significant impact through physical activity interventions was found, suggesting the involvement in regular physical activity can move the typical inactive person from the 50th to 70th percentile using the standard normal curve, demonstrating a success rate gain by 20% which has considerable public health benefits for older adults. The use of the self-efficacy framework has implications for designing and implementing health promotion programs for older adults.

[55] Assessing long-term benefits of exercise: Focus group results

J. Kruger (University of Illinois at Chicago, Chicago, IL, US) Y. Aoyagi, S. Nishizawa, M. Sugiura (Tokyo Metropolitan Institute of Gerontology, Tokyo, Japan)

The purpose of this study was to examine the effects of physical activity among Japanese older adults. When considering the number of older adults will reach over 70 million by the year 2030, integration of strategies and skills associated with the long-term adoption of physical activity are needed. Older Japanese adults may be more physically active than other populations; although little is known about the types of activities in which they participate. In addition, little is known about the long-term benefits of exercise from the older adults' perspective. In developing appropriate measurement instruments, we conducted focus groups with men and women aged 60+ to determine: types of activities performed and perceptions about exercise. Subjects participated in two focus groups, which were transcribed and coded to identify major themes. Results indicated that women primarily participated in activities related to activities of daily living, occupational activities and intermittent recreational activities. Men on the other hand were more likely to engage in more structured and vigorous activities such as softball and mountain climbing. Determinants of long-term physical activity suggest that for the benefits to be realized, the behavior must be enjoyed and performed regularly. Our data suggest that in a relatively fit population, social relationships and diversity in activities may be necessary to maintain regular participation older adult population. Future investigation of the long-term benefits of physical activity are needed to encourage exercise maintenance until the social, psychological, and physical natural reinforces of exercise can be experienced as consequences of exercise behavior.

[56] Relationships of physical fitness with leisure time physical activity and exercise experiences among Japanese elderly

R. Kozakai (Graduate School of Medicine, Nagoya University, Nagoya, Japan and the National Institute for Longevity Sciences: NILS, Obu, Japan), W. Doyo (NILS, Obu, Japan), S. Tsuzuku (NILS, Obu, Japan), K. Yabe (Reseach Center of Health, Physical Fitness & Sports Nagoya University, Nagoya, Japan.) F. Ando (NILS, Obu, Japan), N. Niino (NILS, Obu, Japan), H. Shimokata (NILS, Obu, Japan),

PURPOSE: To assess the relationships of physical fitness components and performance with leisure time physical activity (LTPA) and exercise experiences (EE) in the elderly Japanese. METHODS: Subjects were 565 males and 561 females aged 60 to 79 years participating in the National Institute Longevity Sciences - Longitudinal Study of Aging. They were interviewed about LTPA and EE in earlier period (13-20 years). Flexibility, grip and knee extensor strength, leg extensor power, sit up, reaction time (RT) and balance were measured as physical fitness components. As physical performance, comfortable and maximum gait velocities were measured. Measurements at the initial visit were compared between the subjects who were engaged in LTPA (LTPA(+)) and those who were not (LTPA(-)), and between subjects who had exercise experiences (EE(+)) and those who did not (EE(-)). RESULTS: The proportion of LTPA(+) was 78.6 0n males and 69.2 0n females. EE(+) was 51.3% and 26.2%. Compared with LTPA(-), LTPA(+) showed higher ability at physical fitness. Significant differences were found in RT, balance and both gait velocities among males. Significant differences in both gait velocities were found in females. EE(+) also associated with higher physical fitness. Between EE(+) and EE(-), there were significant differences in grip and knee extensor strength, leg extensor power, sit up, RT and both gait velocities among both genders. Significant difference in balance was found only in females. CONCLUSION: There were significant effects of EE on both physical fitness components and performance, but the effects of LTPA on physical fitness components were relatively small.

[57] Motor Ability and Bone Mineral Density of Community Dwelling Elderly in Okinawa, Japan

Yoshihiko Ojiri, Seizo Sakihara*, Kiyomi Tome*, Masafumi Akisaka**, Hideyo Yoshida***, Tatsuro Ishizaki*** and Takao Suzuki***. (*School of Health Sciences, Faculty of Medicine, University of the Ryukyus, Okinawa, Japan. **Faculty of Health Education, Ibaraki University, Ibaraki, Japan. ***Tokyo Metoropolitan Institute of Gerontology, Tokyo, Japan.)*

PURPOSE: This study examined the relationships between motor ability and bone mineral density (BMD) of elderly men and women in a rural community of Okinawa, Japan. METHOD: Among 796 men and 1182 women aged 65 years and older who have no disability in the activities of daily living and non-institutionalized, 316 men (39.7%) and 713 women (60.3%) participated and completed the motor ability test. The test included an assessment of grip strength, one-leg standing with eyes open, 10 meters walking at preferred and maximum speed. BMD of a heel was measured by ultrasound bone-densitometer (CUBA Clinical, McCue). RESULTS: All motor performances decreased significantly with age in both elderly men and women. The decrease in motor performance at age 85-89 years relative to the level at age 65-69 years in men and women were 23% and 31% of grip strength, 16% and 28% at preferred speed, 12% and 29% at maximum speed for walking velocity, respectively. BMD decreased significantly with age in both elderly men and women. These tendencies had surpassed in the women (30%) compared to the men (13%). Significant correlation between motor ability and BMD was observed for women (r = 0.285 ~ 0.312), but not for men (r = 0.019 ~ 0.094). CONCLUSION: These results indicate that maintenance of higher motor performance by physically active lifestyle may prevent the decrease of BMD with aging, and consequently may contribute to reduce the risk of becoming bed-ridden in elderly people.

[58] New Cardiorespiratory Endurance Index and Standards for Assessing Age-related Fitness Decline in Japanese

T. Yoshioka (Department of Health and Behavioural Science, Kobe City College of Nursing, Kobe, Japan), T. Shiraishi (Department of Practical Science of School Education, Osaka Kyoiku University, Osaka, Japan), S. Fujimoto (Institute of Health Science and Physical Education, Osaka City University, Osaka, Japan)

PURPOSE: Cardiorespiratory endurance is a major health-related fitness indicator. We have developed a new cost-effective assessment tool that predicts cardiorespiratory endurance with simple parameters and minimal error. In this study, we epidemiologically clarified age-related fitness decline and standards of the assessment index for Japanese men and women. METHOD: The assessment tool uses a simple index with an age-predicted maximal heart rate: the slope of the modified relative heart rate (%HR) on work rate (WR) during submaximal incremental exercise on a cycle ergometer (%HR-WR-Slope). The %HR-WR-Slope was measured in 8863 Japanese (3077 men and 5786 women) aged 13 to 72 years. The subjects were divided into 20 age-groups in units of 3 years for each sex. We calculated mean and standard deviation (SD) of the measured values of the %HR-WR-Slope in each group. RESULTS: A linear regressive relationship between the mean value of %HR-WR-Slope and age was observed after 20 years of age in both men and women. The regression lines of men and women ran almost parallel, with a superior level for men. The slope of the regression line of %HR-WR-Slope on age was gentle (7% or less per decade) for each sex. We developed Japanese standards of the %HR-WR-Slope that referred to age and sex by using the regression equation of the mean value and the SD. CONCLUSION: The results based on a large population are considered reliable and useful standards that refer to age and sex assessment of cardiorespiratory endurance by %HR-WR-Slope.

[59] The Impact of Jubilation in the Old Man

Adán D. Pérez Cascante, Antonia Lavanderos Vélez

The classification for ages highlights the interest of the society, while the functional age underlines the direct facts about the individual. Ideally, both types of consideration should be taken intc account. The problems arise when one doesn't give a person the opportunity to work, according to their capacity, because of environmental restrictions that frequently are not but simple matters of the social control. A bigger conscience of these different reference squares would allow us to develop flexible trajectories along the life. The necessity that presents the society of having people " beginner " and veteran it could be respected, but with smaller pressure on people, for not forcing them to assume a premature responsibility or the jubilation, or you would deprive of the opportunities that are qualified to take advantage.

[60] Gait characteristics in healthy middle-aged and elderly adults

W. Doyo (National Institute for Longevity Sciences: NILS, Obu, Japan), R. Kozakai (NILS, Obu, Japan), S.Tsuzuku (NILS, Obu, Japan), N. Niino (NILS, Obu, Japan), F. Ando (NILS, Obu, Japan) and H. Shimokata (NILS, Obu, Japan)

PURPOSE: Along with a reduction in motor and sensory functions, the natural history of aging causes a shift in the locus of function in motor performance like walking (DeVita P and Hortobagyi T, 2000). We aimed to describe gait characteristics during walking at freely chosen speed in healthy middle-aged and elderly adults. METHOD: Subjects were 24 males aged 40-79yrs who were participated in Longevity Sciences of Aging at National Institute for Longevity Sciences in Japan. We divided the subjects into two groups according to each age; 40-59yrs (middle-aged) and 60-79yrs (elderly) groups. The subjects walked over force platforms while being videotaped (60Hz). Linear velocity of center of mass, step length and range of motion and joint torque in ankle were calculated. All variables were analyzed with a Student t-test comparing middle-aged and elderly. RESULTS: Linear velocities of center of mass during stance phase were 1.47±0.13 and 1.26±0.20 m/sec in middle-aged and elderly, respectively. Step lengths were 0.70±0.04 and 0.64±0.09 m/steps. Range of motions in ankle were 34.8±3.8 and 35.7±5.5 degrees. Joint torques in ankle were 1.47±0.13 and 1.26±0.20 Nm/kg. There were significant differences in the linear velocity and the joint torque between the groups, whereas no significant differences were observed in the step length and the range of motion. CONCLUSION: Elderly adults had a decline in the linear velocity of center of mass and the ankle peak torque when walking at freely chosen speed.

[61] Individual vs group exercise programs in frail elderly: effects on muscle strength and physical performance.

C. Martinelli, F. Schena, (Centre for Research on Bioengineering and Motor Science, Rovereto, Italy), G. Noro (Geriatric Unit, St. Chiara Hospital, Trento, Italy)

The aim of this study was to determine the feasibility and the effects on muscle strength and physical ability of exercise programs alternatively based on group or on individual physical activity performed by frail elderly living in nursing facilities. 27 older subjects (5 men and 22 females, mean age 81.22.3y) were divided in 3 groups respectively assigned to individual training (Gr.IT) using isotonic machines, group training (Gr.GT) using gym exercises and elastic bands and control group which continued the programmed activities of the facility. 36 exercise sessions (50 min duration) in 3 months were scheduled for the two training groups. Basal (B), after training (T) and 4 months follow up (F) assessments were performed by each subject to determine anthropometric values (BMI), functional (PPT, Up&Go, Tinetti test, POMA, 15 mt walking) and physiological evaluation (leg and arm max isometric strength). Compliance to exercise programs was very high (>90%) in both the groups. A highly significant improvement in motor performance and in muscle strength was measured in T (ranging from +23% to +65%) and it was larger in Gr.IT than in gr.GT with the relevant exceptions of Up&Go and stairs climbing tests. No changes were determined in control group. In F the values were reduced from T but still enhanced in respect to B in 7 of 11 tests. These data demonstrate that also frail elderly can improve their physical functions and strength through individual training using fitness apparatus. However some daily activities respond better to specific training on skills.

[62] The contribution of physical activities in quality of life in the third age

Auristela Duarte Moser [PUCPR Curitiba - Brasil] Ana Lúcia Bonifácio [PUCPR Curitiba - Brasil] Ana Maria Moser [PUCPR / UNIVALI / USP Curitiba - Brasil] Elisângela Perségona. [PUCPR Curitiba - Brasil]

Introduction: Each day more studies highlight physical activities as an important resource to minimize the degeneration due to aging process, making possible to aged people to keep a satisfactory life's quality. Since physical activities have potential to stimulate many organism's essential functions, it does not show itself just as supporting in the chronic degenerative's treatment and control, (diabetes, hypertension and osteoporosis), it's also essential at keeping the locomotion skills, main subject responsible for the aged's autonomy. Methodology: In this research 28 aged people took part, being 27 women at the average age of 67, attending a parish in Curitiba. At first, postural and flexibility evaluations were made to elaborate an exercise's program to fit the group's physical requests. The activities were developed twice a week, for forty minutes each, where breathing and aerobics exercises were accomplished, rhythm activities and senior dance (dances that were developed specially for aged people), in addition to relaxing exercises to motor control and global coordination. The equipment used were balls,sticks, chairs and a stereo. Results: After one year of activities, it was possible to check, in a second evaluation, that all the participants showed an expressive improvement in the aspects related to pains, active mobility coordination and static and dynamic balance. It was also observed a bigger awareness about one's own body potential, and that through these groups activities there was an improve of self esteem, of self confidence, of the social relations and personal well being, according to verbalization of the participants. The conclusion was that physical activities, besides the physical benefits, also contributes to the life's quality improvement at the third age.

[63] Prevalence of Gambling and Problem Gambling among Older Adults in Manitoba

J.Wiebe, (Addictions Foundation of Manitoba, Winnipeg, Canada), D. Kostyk, (Addictions Foundation of Manitoba, Winnipeg, Canada), G. Kolesar, (Addictions Foundation of Manitoba, Winnipeg, Canada), D. Kennedy (Addictions Foundation of Manitoba), J. Borody (Addictions Foundation of Manitoba, Winnipeg, Canada)

The purpose of the study was to improve understanding of the extent and nature of gambling among the older adult population in Manitoba. In phase 1 of the research process, 1000 older adults 60 years of age and older were randomly selected and were interviewed by telephone. In phase 2, in-depth telephone interviews were conducted with 61 older persons identified in phase 1 as experiencing gambling-related problems and also with 22 older persons who were experiencing problems from someone else's gambling. The results showed gambling to be a fairly common activity among this population in Manitoba. Of those who do gamble, most are not having any problems related to their gambling, as measured by the South Oaks Gambling Screen Revised. Of the total sample, 2.8% reported experiencing problems as a result of their gambling. Differences between non-problem gamblers and problem gamblers have been identified. Of the total sample, 5% reported being negatively affected by someone else's gambling. These individuals gave assistance to the gamblers and identified how they were negatively affected. In conclusion, most older adults gamble. Most do not experience problems from their gambling. An important issue identified is the negative affect of other's gambling on older adults.

[64] Elders, Crime, & the Criminal Justice System: Myth, Perceptions, & Reality in the 21st Century

Max B. Rothman (SE Florida Center on Aging, Florida International University, North Miami, Florida, USA Burton D. Dunlop (SE Florida Center on Aging, Florida International University, North Miami, Florida, USA

The abstract must not exceed 1,600 characters (250) words.... Gerontologists routinely examine the implications of an aging society on issues of long term care, housing, education, politics, religion, the labor market, and the economy. They rarely focus on how aging impacts the criminal justice system. This presentation will document current facts about the nature and extent of older people's involvement with crime and criminal justice. It will provide a gerontological framework for interpreting facts and for separating fact from myth, as well as identify salient policy, research, and ethical issues that emerge from a frequent disjuncture of popular stereotypes of aging with reality. The presentation is based on a newly-published book which includes contributions by gerontologists, criminologists, psychologists, sociologists, and lawyers. It also includes current data concerning the relationship between alcohol use and criminal activity by older people. The presentation will review various roles older people carry out at all levels of the criminal justice system, including victims, prisoners, offenders, jurors, witnesses, judges, and lawyers. There will be a specific emphasis on unique issues related to elder criminality and older prisoners. Using a gerontological framework, the presentation examines how stereotypes that contradict the heterogeneity have been broadly applied in the formation of practices and public policy regarding older adults involved in the system. Specific issues from four other countries, besides the United States, will be included. The presentation raises critical policy and ethical questions for the future concerning how prevailing perceptions of "old age" exert both positive and negative effects on older people.

[65] Psychosocial aspect releated with people between 55-75 and their future challenges

JOSE JAVIER YANGUAS LEZAUN, (Research and New Proyects Development´s Director. Matia Foundation. San Sebastian. SPAIN.) FRANCISCO JAVIER LETURIA ARRAZOLA. Technical Social Services Director. Matia Foundation. San Sebastian. SPAIN.

Purpose: To know the social relationships from the sample; to study the self-perception; to describe the mood related with retirement; to observe how do they spend their freetime and the cultural services of their interest; to calibrate the disposition to take part in volunteers activities. Method: Sample of 1007 older adults from a total of 150.470 people aged 55-75 years in Gipuzkoa (Spain). An estratified sampling in different stages was designed with a selection of the sample units by the method of randomed paths and a final selection by the Kish´s method. The stratification attended to criteria like age, gender, county and town of residence. Being the test in their houses. $p<.05$ Results: *Differences in gender in: relationship with relatives($p=.038$) and friends($p=.000$), studies($p=.000$), outside home activities($p=.000$), reading($p=.003$), sports($p=.002$), to provide informal careinformal care($p=.003$), volunteers activities($p=.047$). *Differences in aged: relationship with sons($p=.000$) and grandsons($p=.000$), healthy activities($p=.000$), cultural activities($p=.008$), sports($p=.000$), to provide informal care($p=.000$). *Differences in marital status: freetime activities($p=.000$), provide informal care($p=.000$). *Differences in cultural level: healthy activities($p=.000$), sports($p=.001$), to provide informal care($p=.001$), cultural activities($p=.000$). Conclusion: Differences have been shown specially in aged, gender and cultural level in the sampple. The future old will be different from the current one. In addition, it makes necessary a change in the services available today and specially in the concept to provide this services.

[66] Psychophysiological Mechanisms of Health in Elderly Workers

Georgiy Korobeynikov, Galina Fedko

PURPOSE: Modern research of aging dynamics for human professional activity shows, that 25 year old working men have a primarily decline of work-related health, increasing of fatigue, deterioration of memory vision and reaction (Arlinger S, 1989; Monk T.H, 1990). However, the compensation of negative influence of work environment on human health is used as professional adaptation. All of these factors allow to work productively without decreasing of reliability on aging worker. METOD: 60 men and 90 women, mental workers in four ages group: 20-29, 30-39, 40-49 and 50-60 were examined. The persons were requested to perform a special computer test with working algorithm changes. The psychophysiological mechanisms of occupational stress were studied by informative mathematical methods with entropy parameters (Shannon C.E, 1948) and measure of system organization (Glushkov V, 1974). RESULTS: The results showed that in young age group the informational processing realization by self-finishing quest responses in work condition. The strength of determinism of psychophysiological organization under work environment influence was observed in age group 30-39. The informational processing realization by exhaustive quest responses in this age group. Aging decline of perception and processing of information provokes the compensation of psychophysiological mechanisms of adaptation. One of the main mechanisms is increase of psychophysiological organization stochastic. At the same time type of informational processing changes to a self-finishing quest response. CONCLUSION: Thus, within the aging reduction of perception, processing and speed of reaction increases the tension from work environment to elder worker.

[67] Retirement Intentions of Same-Sex Couples

Steven E. Mock (Graduate Student, Department of Human Development, Cornell University, Pre-Doctoral Fellow, Cornell Employment and Family Careers Institute, Ithaca, NY, U.S.A.)

PURPOSE: The retirement intentions of same-sex couples are examined. METHOD: A mixed methods approach is employed, drawing on survey data and in-depth interviews of same-sex couples who participated in the Cornell Couples and Careers Study (1998, Phyllis Moen, Principal Investigator, Alfred P. Sloan Foundation Grant # Sloan FDN 96-6-9). Forty women and thirty men comprise the same-sex couples in this study. The average age of the women is 38, and 45 for the men. The average individual income for women is $48,000 and for the men is $50,000. For the basis of comparison, fifteen cohabiting opposite-sex couples and fifteen married couples from the Couples Study are matched with the same-sex couples. RESULTS: The hypothesis that retirement age and degree of retirement preparation will be delayed by "coming out" in adulthood and interruptions in the career path (such as childbearing or adoption) is not borne out in the results. Consistent with a rational choice perspective, on a within couple basis, retirement plans are influenced more by the partner with higher income and the greater age difference. Concordant with gender socialization theory, men in same-sex relationships tend to plan independently from their partners and report more financial planning, while female same-sex couples report greater interdependence with their partners' retirement plans and less financial planning. CONCLUSION: These results have practical applications for workplace policies and pension plans, Social Security legislation in the U.S. which does not recognize same-sex partners as surviving spouses, and financial planning services attuned to the needs gays and lesbians.

[68] Self-rated Health: The Role of Ethnic Background

V. Menec (Department of Community Health Sciences, University of Manitoba, Winnipeg, Canada)

PURPOSE: Self-rated health is a variable that has been gaining increasing interest in the research literature. Studies show, for example, that it is related to successful aging, as defined in terms of mortality or functional status, even when more "objective" health measures are controlled (e.g, Mossey & Shapiro, 1982). This study examined whether cultural differences exist in ratings of health. METHOD: Participants were drawn from the Aging in Manitoba study. Eight ethnic backgrounds were examined: British, Dutch/Belgian, French, German, Polish, Russian/Ukranian, Canadian, and "other". "British" served as reference group. Analyses were conducted for self-rated health, morbidity, functional status, and mortality. Age, gender and education, as well as self-rated health, morbidity and functional status (when not used as outcome variables) were controlled. RESULTS: Seniors of Russian/Ukrainian origin rated their health as poorer than those of British background ($\beta = -.19$, $p < .0001$). Similarly, individuals with a German ethnic background rated their health less positively than their British counterparts ($\beta = -.15$, $p < .01$). No differences emerged between these ethnic groups for morbidity and functional status. However, seniors of Russian/Ukrainian and German background were less likely to have died six years later than individuals of British origin (AOR = .71 and .70, respectively, $p < .05$). CONCLUSION: The finding that self-rated health, but not morbidity and functional status differed across ethnic groups suggests that subjective perceptions of health are culturally bound, with some ethnic groups systematically responding more pessimistically than others. This "pessimism", however, did not translate into greater mortality.

[69] Needs And Attention Expectations In Health Of The Old Users.

M.J. Arias Merino, A. Martínez Ramírez (Instituto Mexicano del Seguro Social IMSS, Jalisco, Mex.), I. Orozco Mares, and E.D. Arias Merino. (Universidad de Guadalajara) M.J. Arias Merino

PURPOSE: To identify from the perspective of the old users of the IMSS their needs and attention expectations in health. METHOD: A qualitative study was undertaken in old user groups that were living in the influence area of two Family Medicine Units (FMU). From a thematic guide on needs and attention expectations to the health, mainly those related with the accessibility and availability of the services, were performed interviews to depth in the address of the elders, recorded, transcribed to a word processor and subsequently analyzed. The data were categorized by content analysis. RESULTS: The perceptions of the elders with respect to their needs of attention in health were: deficient organization of the health services; the inconvenient dealing of the health personnel in the medical care, the acquisition and utilization of the medicines, need of information and/or support on their illness and the related to the physical structure of the FMU. Their expectations were: they would like that the physicians put more interest in their illness, overcoat to recover part of their functionality, to reduce the waiting time for their consultation. They use other alternative resources for their health care (homeopathy, shaman, herbolary, self-prescription) CONCLUSION: The needs of attention of the old users are linked to their condition of being old, to their life process of aging, to the presence of pathologies and to the social-cultural context, it is clear that their expectations are directed to maintain their functionality. The IMSS requires to reinforce the health services directed to this population.

[70] Workshop in health self care for Elders

N. Kunakov (Clínica Indisa, Santiago de Chile)

Purpose: To enhance the elder's quality of life through the capacitating of health's monitors in the community. Method: We invited 30 elders that were leaders and trained them in Self Care, Oral Health, Cancer Prevention, Nutrition, Sexuality and Depression. In each class we did a test about the past class, soon we explained the problems and later we made them work in little groups to search the problems and the solutions for each theme. One year later, we phoned each person and asked them about this workshop and their experience. Results: Assisted 24 persons, between 60 and 70 years old, 50% was men. All are leaders in retirement associations. The initial test was right in 80%. At first it was very difficult for them to work in groups, but it became easier after the third class. The conclusions in each group were very similar. One year more later all the people remember the workshop, they say that was interesting and the themes most remembered are Oral Health, Cancer and Sexuality. All people helped other persons in individual form, like a friend, but nobody worked with elders groups in their community. Conclusions: It is possible to teach the elders about health, they are very espectative about this because the health is a important worry for them. They know a lot about the correct health, but it is important to organize this knowledge. At the end I think that elder people in my country still need to be encouraged to do some activities.

[71] Self-Perceived health status and mortality in the Mexican Elderly Population

J.C. García, J.L. Torres, L.M. Gutiérrez, S. Villa. (Geriatrics Clinic, National Institute of Medical Sciences and Nutrition, Mexico City)

PURPOSE. Elucidate if the self-perceived health status can predict mortality in the Mexican elderly population. METHOD. Retrospective cohort from January 1994 to July 1999 in the outpatient and inpatient setting of a tertiary care center in Mexico City. The question was: With relation to people of your same age how would you say is your health at this moment? Excellent, very good, good, bad or very bad. We document survival through the charts. We made survival analysis before constructing proportional hazard models with Cox regression using demographic variables, functional information and associated diseases. RESULTS. 2277 patients were included. 844(37.1%) were male and 1433(62.9%) female patients, 802(35.2%) from the outpatient and 1475(64.8%) from the inpatient setting. Mean age 76.11 years, 1232(54.1%) older than 75 years. There were 293(12.9%) patients with excellent-very good self-perceived health (median survival 63.6 months), 881(38.7%) with good self-perceived health (median survival 56.8 months) and 1103(48.4%) in the bad-very bad group (median survival 38.7 months). In the proportional hazard models the self-perceived health status 1.21(CI 1.1-1.33), being older than 75 years 1.18(CI 1.04-1.34), to stay in the inpatient setting 1.72(CI 1.48-1.99), the score in Katz 1.13(CI 1.03-1.25), Lawton 1.24(CI 1.13-1.35), MMSE 1.31(CI 1.20-1.43), and the following diseases: ischaemic heart disease 1.33(CI 1.16-1.51), cancer 2.56(CI 2.25-2.91), pneumonia 1.39(CI 1.13-1.70), liver disease 1.60(CI 1.34-1.93), undernutrition 1.30(CI 1.06-1.60), and nephropaties 1.18 (CI 1.00-1.40) were significant for mortality. CONCLUSION. The self-perceived health status maintains a significant relationship with the mortality risk even after adjusting for demographic, functional and basal medical status.

[72] The Relationship Among Health Status, Life Style and Perceived Aging of the Elderly in City

Cho, Yoo-Hyang. (Department of Nursing, ChoDang University, SungNamRi #469, MuAnEup, MuAnGun, 534-800, KOREA.)

Purpose : This study was descriptive correlation study, tried to the relationship among health status, life style, and perceived aging of the elderly in small city area. Health status means that subjective health status and disease status of chronic and acute. Life style means that health maintenance method, smoking and drinking status. And instruments of aging factors are divided that psychological part and physical disable part. Method : The survey was conducted through the home-visit interview during half month at February, 1999 by the students of nursing department who were previously trained. The survey targeted the elderly aged 65 years or more living at home and in elderly homes in urban area. Results : When asked what they thought of their health, 45.1% replied that they were healthy. There was a significant difference between male and female elderly about their own health, disease and health maintenance methods. The degree of perceived aging factors were 77.2%, that was a significant between smoking habit and health maintenance habits. Perceived aging of the elderly is found to be lower than that they have good life style. Conclusion : These results indicate that should be to provide health promotion program of the elderly and development of medical services. And it is very important that changed life styles of the elderly.

[73] Self-perceived Health Status and its Related Factors Among the Elderly

Yih-Jing Tang1, Meng-Chih Lee2, Yuh-Shyun Wang1, Lifen Wu3, Hsiao-Chiang Huang1, Liang-Jen Chuo4 and Chorng-Song Chou4 (Departments of Family Medicine1, Nursing3, Psychiatry4 and rehabilitation5, Taichung Veterans General Hospital; 2Department of Family Medicine, Chung Shan Medicine and Dental College Hospital, Taichung. Taiwan)

PURPOSE: To determine senior residents' self-perceived health status and the related factors including demographics, physical conditions, mental and psychological status, living independence and health services utilization. METHOD: A total of 472 cases were sampled from 54,219 senior residents registered in Taichung City by a stratified systematic random sampling. Personal interview using questionnaires, scale tests and blood examinations was performed. Of them, 20 cases died, 6 cases couldn't complete, and 446 subjects completed the questionnaire. RESULTS: A majority of the elderly (78.3%) had good or excellent perceived health status, while 21.7% of the elderly had poor self-perceived health status. Univariate analysis indicated the poorer self-perceived health status was associated with female subjects, single, less education, lower income, poor visual activity, poor mobility, poor sleep, no exercise, no smoking , no drinking, fall and pain history, having depression and other psychological disorder, higher numbers of chronic diseases and medications, more physician visits, impaired blood urea nitrogen and creatinine level and higher scores of ADLs and IADLs. However, multiple logistic regression analysis revealed that only the following variables were associated independently with poorer self-perceived health: depression, suffering from heart disease or diabetes, physical pain, taking analgesics, more physician visits, impaired ADLs, no exercise, lower income, and no smoking. CONCLUSION: The self-perceived health status in the elderly was related with bio-psycho-social factors as well as functional disability. The further efforts to improve health status in the elderly should focus on the intervention of these factors.

SESSION 202

Home Care Research: International Comparisons

R. Bernabei (Centro Medicina dell'Invecchiamento, Rome, Italy) Home Care and Comprehensive Geriatric Assessment: International Perspectives. L. Branch (Centre for Studies of Aging and Human Development, Duke University, Durham, NC, USA) Understanding Home Care in the United States. M. Hollander (Hollander Analytical Services Ltd, Victoria, BC, Canada) Home Care in Canada. S. Gui (Shanghai Research Centre on Aging, East China Normal University, Shanghai, China) The Need for Family Care for Seniors in Shanghai in the 21st Century. I. Chi (Department of Social Work and Social Administration, University of Hong Kong, Hong Kong) Home Care Services in Hong Kong.

With concerns about escalating health care costs, reform in the 1990s has seen a philosophical shift throughout the world in favour of enhanced home care. Community care is embraced both as less expensive than medical and hospital care, as well as more appropriate for an aging population. This symposium with five speakers from five different countries (Italy, the United States, Canada, Hong Kong and Mainland China) examines recent developments at the policy and implementation levels in different countries. The first paper will provide international comparative data of home care users collected using the MDS-HC Minimum Data Set for Home Care. Data are presented from Canada, Italy, Japan, and the United States. The second paper by Dr. Branch from the United States reviews the variety of home care programs available in the United States and assesses their effectiveness. The third paper by Dr. Hollander discusses the organization, management and financing of home care services in Canada, providing an overview of the more common approaches to funding and emerging trends. The next paper by Dr. Gui, presents data on the current and projected needs of the elderly in Shanghai in order to assess their needs for home care. The last paper by Dr. Chi follows from a review of community services for the elderly in Hong Kong and presents recommendations for the integration of nursing, social, and health care services for the elderly. It is evident from these papers that the collection of similar data allows for comparisons of policies and their effectiveness cross nationally. Worldwide interest in expanding and reforming community services means countries can learn from one another in search of a common goal - more appropriate services for seniors in the community that allow them to age in place.

Home Care and Comprehensive Geriatric Assessment: International Perspectives

R. Bernabei (Centro Medicina dell'Invecchiamento, Rome, Italy)

In reviewing the literature, the differences in the characteristics of the population studied and the types of intervention make it difficult to draw definitive conclusions about the efficacy and cost-effectiveness of home care programs. One of the most significant drawbacks in trying to "learn from each other" is that no international comparisons have been possible because patient-level data have been obtained with different assessment instruments. Such comparisons have been made possible since the MDS-HC (Minimum Data Set for Home Care) was made available in the late nineties. The lecture will describe the principal functional and clinical characteristics of home care patients in four different countries, Canada (654 pts)-Italy (3506 pts)-Japan (1779 pts) and USA (14361 pts). This presentation will lay down the groundwork for the design of national effective home care policies. These data highlight the potential benefits of establishing an international database on home care patients. Such an effort would allow us to investigate and compare the characteristics of this population, both today and in the future, as well as to evaluate changes in policy from nation to nation affected by the availability of services and the introduction of new innovative medical or social programs. Such comparisons have not been possible to date. By way of example, the Italian population in the home setting is more severely cognitively and functionally impaired as compared with the home care patients enrolled in Michigan and Georgia (USA), and Ontario (Canada). These differences can be explained because of the different availability of community and institutional services in the four nations and the different social environment of home care patients in the three countries.

Home Care in Canada2

M. Hollander (Hollander Analytical Services Ltd, Victoria, BC, Canada)

This presentation will focus on the organization, management and financing of home care services in Canada. It will touch briefly on the extent to which people who need care actually receive it. The organization of home care services across Canada will be discussed, as will the place of home care in the broader health context. The presentation will also provide an overview of "best practices" for organizing a broader system of care for the elderly, called continuing care, which includes home care. The presentation will address the way home care services are financed in Canada. It will also provide an overview of the more common approaches to funding, and of emerging trends in funding such as tendering. The presentation will close with a discussion of the cost-effectiveness of home care in the Canadian context.

Home Care Services in Hong Kong

I. Chi (Department of Social Work & Social Administration, University of Hong Kong, Hong Kong)

HKSAR Government commissioned a consultant project of "Review of Care Services for Elderly Living in the Community" in March, 1998. Outcome of the review is expected to lead to substantial improvement in the organization, coordination and delivery of comprehensive in-home service. A long-term care system and enhanced home care program is proposed for Hong Kong that provides or arranges to provide a coordinated continuum of services to a defined population and is willing to be held clinically and fiscally responsible for the outcome of the health status (quality of life) of the population served. This paper will focus on reporting the recommendations made on the integration of nursing, social and health care for the elderly living in the community.

Understanding Home Care in the United States

Laurence G. Branch (Duke University Center on Aging and Human Development, Durham, NC, USA)

As in other countries, home care is an important component to the continuum of care of frail older people in the U.S. But "home care" can mean a variety of things, often depending on who is paying for the service and who is monitoring its quality. The home and community based services that are funded by the Title XX amendment to the Social Security Act are typically social services and often include housekeeping, grocery shopping, food preparation, and assistance paying bills, taking medications, and using the telephone. At the other extreme are the home care services provided under the Medicare program (Title XVIII of the Social Security Act). This home care benefit is typically triggered by a hospital discharge and emphasizes medical rehabilitation services such as skilled nursing care, physical therapy, occupational therapy, and speech therapy for homebound recipients. If such skilled medical rehabilitation services are necessary, some ancillary housekeeping assistance may also be provided. Conceptually, between the social home care of Title XX and the medical home care of Medicare, are the home and community services offered as an alternative to institutional care funded by the Medicaid program. The recipients of Medicaid's home care are typically certified as nursing home eligible in the state in which they reside, and the array of services is often a complete blend of the medical home care of Medicare and the social home care of Title XX. The Veterans Health Administration also operates a home care program for frail veterans that blends both medical and social home care services. Each of these four federal funding sources for home care impose their own guidelines and regulations over such things as eligibility (as discussed), duration, intensity, and qualifications of the providers. In addition to these major federal home care programs, there are also a large number of state programs. The research on the effectiveness of home care programs such as these has been summarized by Weissert. When targeted rigorously, home care in the U.S. can be a cost effective alternative to institutional care.

SESSION 203

Social Policy and Social Ethics

A. Jamieson (Birkbeck College, University of London, UK) Older People and Ethical Issues in Social Policy: The Case of Inter-generational Equity. T. Anme (National Rehabilitation Research Institute, Tokorozawa, Japan) To Use or not to Use: The Ethical Dilemma of Public Long-Term Care Insurance. D.A. Wolf (Center for Policy Research, Syracuse University, New York, USA) Private Actions, Public Values: Towards a Social 'Balance Sheet'. G. Naegele (Institute of Gerontology, University of Dortmund, Dortmund, Germany) The Generational Contract in Germany Under Pressure.

Changes in the population balance, and the trend towards increasing individualism, are challenging the social contract between generations. Equity considerations are among the central issues in this process, where the interests of the younger generations are contrasted to those of the older. While the challenge is more or less common to all modern countries, there is substantial variation in how different countries are responding, in part due to path dependency on already instituted social policies and practices. Variation in responses is also related to the balance of priority given to past contributions, present needs, or future utility in the distribution of scarce resources. The latter tends to favor the younger, the former tends to favor the older. The symposium is highlighting not only the dilemmas associated with inter-generational equity, but also issues of intra-generational equity in a life span context, more specifically between the childless and those with children from an American setting, and between elders from different social classes, or more specifically elders from the former East and West Germany. Other issues are the ethical dilemmas of a public long term care insurance program in a traditional collectivistic culture (Japan), and a comparative analysis of the extent to which the presentation of a dilemma as ethical or moral simply serve to hide the harsh economic reality behind it in a political climate that does not favor solidary social policies.

Older people and ethical issues in social policy: the case of inter-generational equity

A. Jamieson (Birkbeck College, University of London, UK)

In social policy, questions about equity are among the core ethical issues. Answers to questions of what is 'right' and 'wrong' are not given, but based on first principles, whether explicit or not. They can derive from a specific philosophical or religious system, from tradition and practice, or from self-interest. The ethical dimension of decisions made by policy makers or practitioners is not always recognised. On the other hand, arguments sometimes purport to be based on moral values, where in fact the exhortation of 'morals' merely serves as a political instrument. This paper will consider some examples of policy issues affecting older people, and examine the underlying ethical questions. It will also explore, through cross-national comparative analysis of different welfare systems, whether politics or ethics are at the root of some of the differences found in welfare systems. It will focus on some of the major issues associated with resource allocation, i.e. pensions and health & social services. Much of the gerontological literature on the topic of ethics or values in social policy is argued within a framework of inter-generational equity, i.e. in terms of distribution of resources between generations. The paper will analyse some of these arguments in the light of policy debates and trends in different countries. It will be argued that the key issues in social policy affecting older people are less to do with inter-generational equity, and more to do with distribution of resources between different social groups across societies as a whole. —

Private actions, public values: towards a social 'balance sheet'

D.A. Wolf (Center for Policy Research, Syracuse University, New York, USA)

A recent book (The baby boom: How family-friendly America cheats the childless, by Elinor Burkett) argues that tax, spending, and regulatory policies are biased in favor of parents (especially mothers), and against the childless, creating an inequitable situation. In stark contrast, analysts such as Nancy Folbre and others have argued that society fails to recognize (and to compensate) the social contributions made by under- or uncompensated childrearers (especially mothers), an equally inequitable situation. Similarly, my 1999 paper (The family as provider of long-term care: Efficiency, equity, and externalities) argues that the social value of informal care provided by family members justifies differential tax treatment of parents and nonparents. These diametrically opposing views can only be resolved through the computation of the net value, over the lifetime, of contributions to collective well-being through taxes, receipt of transfers and services, and private actions that have public - that is 'external' - value. This paper addresses the question of identifying, and measuring, to the extent possible, the flows of tangible and intangible, priced and unpriced, 'goods' between two distinct segments of society: parents and the childless. I pay particular attention to the role of informal elder care in these flows. Many studies of informal care have noted both the large but hidden 'costs' associated with elder care, and the strongly gender-biased nature of those costs. However, there has been little attempt to embed issues raised by informal elder care in either a lifetime or a broader social context. This paper will focus on difficulties, and logical conundrums, that arise in any attempt to draw up a comprehensive social 'balance sheet'.

The generational contract in Germany under pressure

G. Naegele (Institute of Gerontology, University of Dortmund, Dortmund, Germany)

Currently, the generational contract in Germany is under pressure. However, this pressure is not only due to financial reasons but also to societal challenges in terms of the well-known demographic and labor market trends and the less known differences in economic welfare within the German population. One prominent starting point are the demographic and labor market related challenges by which the public social security systems are confronted for years. In Germany, social security is mainly based on the Bismarck model and the pay-as-you-go-principle. At the same time, social security is built upon the generational contract, e.g. the active generation finances via contributions the benefits for the passive generation. Against the background of the challenges mentioned a new/modern conseptionalisation of the generational contract is required. Additionally, despite the growing economic welfare of seniors there are still substantial financial inequalities within the older German population. Apart from the 'classical' reasons linked with inequality earlier in the life course, they mirror gender differences, cohort-effects, long-term effects of migration and the economic differences between East- and West-Germany. Consequently, it is increasingly required to interlink the question how to conceptualize a new/modern generational contract with the dimension of intra-generational solidarity. Moreover, the growing 'richness' among seniors has become an issue among German social gerontologists, and have by some been contrasted to the poor financial status and the tight time budget of the young, in particular in the case of unemployment. In a growing number of publications the question is raised how, and to which extent, the elderly might 'pay back' parts of the goods the society is 'donating' (financing) for it's seniors. The paper will describe the different starting points of rediscussing the generational contract and will draw attention to current answers on both the political and socio-gerontological level.

To use or not to use: the ethical dilemma of public long-term care insurance

T. Anme (National Rehabilitation Research Institute, Tokorozawa, Japan)

Choices in public long-term care insurance appear to be not so much hindered by a lack of insight into how choices should be made in theory, as uncertainty as to how choices could be made in practice. Changing social values 'from family care to community care', expedite both requirement of social care and disclosure hidden problems such as elder abuse. The paper examines how policy-makers have dealt with the priority issue in long-term care over the past decades by means of social norm with ethical dilemma under a collectivistic culture. In many Asian countries, family care has dominated and often the eldest sons' spouse, as daughter-in-laws, are expected to take the responsibility for elder care. Social pressure is so strong that they are often forced to take elder care against their will. Such situation itself, in some meaning, could be named 'caregiver abuse'. Our study shows it is difficult to decide immediately which is abuser or abused in many cases of suspected elder abuse. Looking at the increasing requirements of social care, the broad accessibility and the good overall quality of long-term care, it may be concluded that the issue of choice has not come off badly under this system. The degree to which the system can respond adequately to likely developments, such as changing social norms and growing waiting lists, rests on the further empowerment of consumers, and the community and market enrolled in long-term care.

SESSION 205

Nutritional Assessment and Treatment

P. Senet (Service de gerontologie L'Orbe, Ivry sur Seine, France. Nutritional status in elderly patients with chronic leg ulcers); H. Heseker (Department of Nutrition and Health, University Paderborn, Germany. Risk factors of nutrition related problems among elderly people in a German community.). E.M. Simonsick (National Institute on Aging, Bathesda, USA. Association of weight and weight change with change in walking endurance over 1 year); H. Payette, (Research Centre in Gerontology and Geriatrics, Sherbrooke Geriatric University Institute, Faculty of

Medicine, University of Sherbrooke, Québec, Canada. Benefits of Nutritional Supplementation in The Free-Living Frail Undernourished Elderly.); Wija A van Staveren (Wageningen Agricultural University, Wageningen, The Netherlands. The SENECA study: the importance of diet and other lifestyle factors for survival and quality of life ten years later.)

Issue: This symposium will explore the interrelationships of malnutrition in the elderly and poor subjective, clinical, and functional health. It will include discussion of risk factor identification, as well as examination of the impact of nutritional interventions. Structure: The symposium will consist of 5 presentations of 15 minutes each, followed by a question period. Content: P. Senet will begin the symposium with an examination of the prevalence of malnutrition indicators among elderly clinical patients presenting with leg ulcerations. H. Heseker will then describe risk factors associated with eating difficulties and poor appetite identified in a large cohort of free-living elderly. This will include the association between high risk for malnutrition and other health risks. The consequences of overnutrition for mobility loss in older adults will then be the topic of the presentation by E. Simonsick. In this unique study, both body weight and weight gain will be examined as potential challenges to the wellbeing of older adults. Functional status is also a theme in H. Payette's report, in which she will describe the outcome of nutrition intervention with frail community-living adults. The intervention's impact on older participants' perceived wellness will also be discussed. In concluding this symposium, Way van Staveren will outline how nutrition and other lifestyle factors are associated with both survival and quality of life among older European participants in the 10- year follow-up of the SENECA study. Conclusions: Understanding risk factors associated with poor nutritional status and ultimately compromised wellbeing of older adults will assist in the development of successful intervention strategies.

Association of weight and weight change with change in walking endurance over 1 year

E.M. Simonsick, T. Harris (National Institute on Aging, USA), A. Newman (Univ. of Pittsburgh, USA), M. Visser (Vrije Univesiteit, the Netherlands), S. Kritchevsky (Univ. of Tennessee - Memphis, USA), M. Nevitt (Univ. of California at San Francisco, USA)

Overweight and obesity are highly prevalent among older Americans; yet, few studies have investigated the consequences of overweight for mobility loss in old age. Using data from the Health, Aging, and Body Composition (Health ABC) study, we examined the cross-sectional and longitudinal relationship of body weight to performance on a test of walking endurance, the Long Distance Corridor Walk (LDCW). The population consisted of 2,103 initially well-functioning men and women aged 70-79 who completed the LDCW in Year 1 and had a clinic visit in Year 2. At baseline, time to walk 400 meters was 3.3 seconds slower (p=.0001) for each additional 3 kg of body weight over 60 kg, independent of race, sex, age, site (Memphis or Pittsburgh), height, and walking behavior. In Year 2, 21% did not complete the LDCW. Risk of non-performance increased by 6.1% (p=.0002) for each additional 3 kg of baseline body weight, independent of race, sex, age, site, height and weight change. When baseline 400 meter time and walking behavior were included, risk declined to 3.2%, but remained significant (p=.0356). Weight gain >1.5 kg over the year increased risk of non-performance by an additional 32% (p=.0426). Among those completing the 400 meter walk in Year 2, times were .54 seconds slower (p=.0306) for each additional 3 kg of body weight, independent of all other factors. Excess weight is associated with poorer walking endurance in initially well-functioning 70 year-olds and contributes to a steeper rate of decline in walking ability over time.

Nutritional status in elderly patients with chronic leg ulcers

P. Senet [Service de gerontologie L'Orbe, Hopital Charles Foix, Ivry sur Seine, France], M.E. Sireix [Service de Reducation vasculaire, Hopital Europeen Georges Pompidou, Paris, France], P. Rumeau[Service de gerontologie L'Orbe, Hopital Charles Foix, Ivry sur Seine, France], D. Lecoz [Service de Reducation vasculaire, Hopital Europeen Georges Pompidou, Paris, France], C. Debure [Service de Reducation vasculaire, Hopital Europeen Georges Pompidou, Paris, France], S. Meaume [Service de gerontologie L'Orbe, Hopital Charles Foix, Ivry sur Seine, France].

Purpose Unlike in patients with pressure sores, little is known on the nutritional status of patients with chronic leg ulcers. Method We have studied, one week after admitting, the medical records of inpatients over 70, with leg ulcers, lasting for more than 3 months. Ulcers were both venous and arterial. We collected age, sex, duration of ulcers, brachial circumference (BC) and Body Mass Index (BMI), blood albumin and prealbumin. Our anthropometric and laboratory values were tested against norms obtained in community dwelling people aged over 70, living in the same area. We used a non parametric univariate test for our comparisons. Results: We have included 26 patients, aged 82 ± 6.9 years, one man for two women. 45% of our patients had had their ulcers for more than a year. There was no significant difference in our population with the norms for average BMI, BC, and blood albumin. Prealbumin was significantly lower in women (194.3 ± 42.8 Vs 270 ± 5 mg/l) but not in men. 8 patients had a blood albumin or prealbumin below the norm, of which 3 had an albumin under 30 g/l or a prealbumin under 140 mg/l, none had decreased BC or BMI. Conclusion : We had a 30.7% prevalence of undernutrition, with 11% serious denutrition. Measuring blood albumin and prealbumin looks relevant in looking for denutrition in elderly patients with chronic leg ulcers. Improving the patient's nutritional status could, then, prove to speed up the healing of leg ulcers.

Risk factors of nutrition related problems among elderly people in a German community.

H. Heseker, A.C. Schmid (Department of Nutrition and Health), M. Weiss (Institute of Sports Medicine, University Paderborn, Germany)

Purpose: The prevalence of nutrition problems increases with aging. Malnutrition is often not recognized and therefore the magnitude of the problem is often underestimated and preventive measures are introduced lately and are often less effective. Involuntary weight loss may cause an increased risk for the need of assistance in performing the basic activities of daily living. Therefore risk factors were identified and the outcome of nutrition related problems was studied. Method: We studied the nutrition and health situation as well as physical activities in a random sample of the non-institutionalized or institutionalized elderly German population. 490 persons (268 male and 222 female) in the age of 65 to 100 years participated in this questionnaire-based examination, including the pre-test of the MNA. Results: In our study low physical activity, chewing or swallowing difficulties, gastrointestinal diseases, multiple intake of prescription drugs were associated with low or reduced appetite. Besides dysphagia was correlated with a low intake of fruits and vegetables. Low appetite and subsequently low food intake were associated with weight loss, lower BMI and a higher susceptibility to infections. Additionally elderly people with a high risk of malnutrition - determined by MNA - and physical inactive people reported a higher number of falls in the year before the examination. A substantial proportion of elderly people with chewing and swallowing difficulties or gastrointestinal diseases didn't receive adequate nutritional support. Conclusions: Multiple-risk-factor intervention strategies have to be developed and evaluated to reduce the risk of malnutrition, underweight, immune deficiency and falls among elderly persons in the community.

Benefits of Nutritional Supplementation in The Free-Living Frail Undernourished Elderly.

H. Payette, V. Boutier, C. Coulombe (Research Centre in Gerontology and Geriatrics, Sherbrooke Geriatric University Institute, Faculty of Medicine, University of Sherbrooke, Québec, Canada), K. Gray-Donald (School of Dietetics and Human Nutrition, Macdonald Campus, of McGill University)

Purpose: To evaluate the impact of nutritional supplementation on nutritional status, muscle strength, perceived health and functional status in a community-living frail undernourished elderly population. Methods: Eighty-three adults aged 80±7 years receiving community home-care services and at high risk of undernutrition were enrolled in a 16-week intervention study in which they were randomized to either an experimental (addition of a nutrient dense protein-energy liquid supplement to increase total energy and nutrient intake) or a control group, and visited in their home on a monthly basis. Outcome variables measured at the start and end of the study at subjects' homes by a dietitian blinded to treatment assignment included anthropometric indices, handgrip strength, isometric elbow flexion and leg extension strength, lower extremity function, perceived health and quality of life. Study groups were compared on an "intention to treat" basis using ANOVA for repeated measures, unpaired and paired t-tests and their non-parametric equivalents where appropriate. Results: Total energy, nutrient intakes, and weight increased significantly in the supplemented group ($p<.001$). No significant changes were observed with respect to other anthropometric indices, muscle strength or functional variables. However, beneficial effects were observed in the experimental subjects with respect to perceived vitality, fatigue and weakness ($p<.01$). Conclusions: Nutrition intervention is feasible in the free-living frail and undernourished elderly and results in significant improvement of nutritional status with respect to energy and nutrient intake and weight gain. Weight loss is reversible, however increased physical activity may also be required to improve health and functional status.

The SENECA study: the importance of diet and other lifestyle factors for survival and quality of life ten years later.

Wija A van Staveren, Lisette CPMG de Groot, Annemien Haveman-Nies (Department of Human Nutrition, Wageningen University, Wageningen, The Netherlands)

Purpose: In 1988 a European multi center study, named SENECA (Survey in Europe on Nutrition and the Elderly, a Concerted Action), was initiated in elderly people born between 1913 and 1918. Nine of the original 19 participating towns in 12 European countries decided to continue the longitudinal study by conducting a second survey in 1993 and a Finale in 1999. The aim of SENECA's Finale was to identify dietary and lifestyle factors important for survival and the maintenance of health of SENECA participants since 1988. Method: In the latter study vital status was known for 1251 subjects (98% of the original baseline population) and from this group 307 men and 472 women survived. For the dietary factors data were collected in the baseline and in 1993 with an adapted dietary history method. Anthropometry and blood chemistry was used to obtain information about nutritional status and health. Data on other lifestyle factors and health were collected by standardized questionnaires. We used the data collected at baseline to examine the relationship with survival and quality of life in 1999. Results: The results indicated that single modifiable factors as dietary quality, smoking and physical activity are related to 10 year mortality. The mortality risk for men was 1.3 (95% CI 1.0-1.8) for a low quality diet; 1.4 for inactivity (95% CI 1.1-1.8) and 1.5 for smoking (95%CI 1.2-1.8). For women these risks were slightly higher. Conclusion: We concluded that even at ages 70-75 diet and lifestyle still matter for survival 10 years later.

SESSION 206

Cytamin Correction of Premature and Accelerated Aging among Lorry-Drivers

A. S. Bashkireva, V. Kh. Khavinson (St. Petersburg Institute of Bioregulation and Gerontology, St. Petersburg, Russia), V. G. Artamonova (I. I. Mechnikov St. Petersburg State Medical Academy, St. Petersburg, Russia)

Enhancement of the organism adaptation and functional reserves and reduction of regulatory mechanism tension caused by adverse environmental impacts allows to prevent premature and accelerated aging (PAA). Principal role is allocated to studying various PAA factors entailing decreased physical and mental work capacity (PWC and MWC, correspondingly) and, thus, disturbing adaptation to occupational requirements. To raise prenosological diagnosis reliability both the organism individual aging rate (by indices of individual biological age (BA) compared to the population standard) and adaptation capacity (by indicators of the total organism adaptation reactions) shall be assessed. Efficacy of cytamin-based modern gerotechnologies in assessing, preventing and correcting PAA, occupational, age- and work-related diseases at motor transport enterprises was estimated. Biological age was defined by PWC and MWC data and their totality in 150 lorry-drivers (aged 30-59) divided into 5 equal groups. Group 1 received Cerebramin(r), 2 - Vasalamin(r), 3 - Cerebramin(r) + Vasalamin(r), 4 placebo and 5 - no preparations. Predicted biological age (PBA) and aging rate index (BA - PBA) were also calculated. Applied multiple-regression BA model appeared adequate in estimating occupational hazards impact on a driver s organism. This enables to timely reveal individuals predisposed to pathology, disability, PAA and mortality and monitor examinations to correct the current functional state and aging rates with optimal adaptogens and geroprotectors. Cerebramin and Vasalamin regulated and restored PWC, MWC, and organism defense forces, raises resistance to occupational hazards. Investigations proved cytamins interpolymer complexes of tissue-specific proteins and nucleic acids to be effective agents of preventing PAA among lorry-drivers.

Dehydroepiandrosterone associated to low density lipoproteins reduces their increased susceptibility with ageing to lipid peroxidation

A. Khalil, J.-P. Fortin, J.-G. Lehoux and T. Fülöp Jr, Inst. Univ. Gériatr, Lab. Biogérontol, *Dept. Biochim, Fac. Méd, Univ. Sherbrooke, Sherbrooke, Qc, Canada*

Purpose: The incidence of atherosclerosis and its related diseases increase with aging. The aging process may enhance lipoprotein modification, which leads to the increase in the susceptibility of LDL and HDL to oxidation. DHEA the most abundant steroid hormone in humans was shown to have antiatherogenic effects and this hormone is decreasing dramatically with aging. Method: In this study we determined the presence of DHEA/DHEAS and the evolution of their contents in HDL and LDL with aging. Moreover, we studied the susceptibility of LDL to oxidation with age in the presence or absence of vitamin E or DHEA. Results: We demonstrated that vitamin E is unable to restore the decreased resistance to oxidation of LDL from elderly subjects to the level of LDL obtained from young subjects. Furthermore, our results provide evidence that DHEA is integrative part of LDL and HDL and disappear to almost non-detectable levels with aging. DHEA incorporated in the LDL from elderly subjects increased their resistance to oxidation in a concentration dependent manner, by increasing significantly the lag-phase and decreasing the plateau of conjugated diene, hydroperoxide and TBARS formations. The increased resistance provided by DHEA was higher than that with vitamin E. DHEA seems to act either by protecting Vitamin E from disappearance from LDL under oxidation or to scavenge directly the free radicals produced during the oxidative process. Conclusion: Our results suggest that DHEA exerts an antioxidative effect on LDL, which could have antiatherogenic consequences

Dehydroepiandrosterone (DHEA), DHEA sulfate, and aging. Contribution of the DHEAge study to a sociobiomedical issue

S. Legrain (Department of geriatrics, CHU Bichat, University of Paris 7, France), N. Lahlou, M. Roger (Hospital Saint Vincent de Paul) G. Thomas (Inserm 444), JC Souberbielle (Hospital Necker), J. Raison (Hospital Broussais), O. de la Charrière, S. Nouveau (l'Oréal), B. Rakoto Arison (Institut de sexologie, V. Faucounau (Fondation Nationale de Gérontologie), F. Forette (Hospital Broca), EE Baulieu (Inserm U 448 and College de France) on behalf of the DHEAge trial investigators.

The secretion and blood levels of DHEA and its sulfate (DHEAS) decrease profoundly with age. The question is posed whether administration of the steroid to compensate for the decline counteracts defects associated with aging. To assess this issue, 280 healthy individuals (women and men 60 79 years old) were given 50 mg DHEA or placebo, daily for a year, in a double blind placebo controlled study. Numerous measures were performed to assess the efficacy and the safety of DHEA administration. This paper presents the results on bone, libido and skin. Besides the reestablisment of a " young " concentration of DHEAS, a small increase of testosterone and oestradiol was noted, particularly in women, and may be involved in the significantly demonstrated physiological clinical manifestations reported. Bone turnover improved selectively in women >70 years old, as assessed by dual-energy x-ray absorptiometry (DEXA) technique and the decrease of osteoclastic activity. A significant increase in most libido parameters was also found in these older women. Improvement of the skin status was observed, particularly in women, in terms of hydration, epidermal thickness, sebum production and pigmentation. These encouraging results must lead to further controlled studies for a longer period. They do not support the hypothesis of DHEA creating " supermen / women " (doping).

Effect of Oxidative Stress on some Drug Metabolizing Enzymes Expression in Rat Astrocytes

D. Gradinaru ("Ana Aslan" National Institute of Gerontology and Geriatrics, Bucharest, Romania), J.M. Heydel, H. Goudonnet, Y. Artur (Unité de Biochimie Pharmacologique, Faculté de Pharmacie, Dijon, France), J. Magdalou, A. Minn (UMR CNRS/ UHP-7561, Faculté de Médecine, Vandœuvre-lès-Nancy, France)

Reactive oxygen species (ROS) produced during the normal metabolism and under conditions of oxidative stress, are thought to be implicated in the aetiology or progression of several neurodegenerative pathologies and in the normal brain aging. However, recent studies pointed out that ROS could initiate complex intracellular redox modulatory systems that regulate gene transcription and translation of many phase I and II drug metabolizing enzymes. By the use of primary cultures of rat astrocytes, this study aimed at following up the effects of an induced oxidative stress caused by the exposure to redox-cycling xenobiotics, on some oxidoreductases and conjugation enzymes expression, such as: NADPH-cytochrome P450 reductase (P450-red), NAD(P)H:quinone oxidoreductase (QR), nitric oxide synthase (NOS) and UDP-glucuronosyl transferases (UGT). Using quantitative RT-PCR assays, we showed that after a 48-hours treatment with moderate concentrations of menadione, paraquat, or the lipophilic iron donor ferric complexed to 8-hydroxyquinoline (FeHQ), QR and UGT expression was significantly increased. By contrast, we could report significant higher mRNA levels for P450-red only after paraquat exposure. As regards the astrocyte iNOS expression, results clearly show that quinones and bipyridinium compounds had different effects on this NOS isoform induction, being detected only for paraquat-treated cells. In the presence of the antioxidant melatonin in the culture medium, or the cycloheximide- an inhibitor of protein synthesis, the upregulation of these detoxification enzymes was suppressed. Results suggest that the regulation of these genes could be mediated through common electrophile/ antioxidant-responsive elements (EpRE/ARE), enhancing the further development of protective agents for aging and disease progression.

Effects of Pineal Peptides on Free Radical Processes in Ageing

A. V. Arutjunyan, V. Kh. Khavinson (St. Petersburg Institute of Bioregulation and Gerontology, St. Petersburg, Russia)

The pineal gland plays an important role in the regulation of various physiological functions of the organism. Melatonin (N-acetyl-5-methoxytriptamine), which is an indole hormone produced mainly in the pineal gland, possesses protective activity against the damage caused by reactive oxygen species (ROS). Our recent data show that beside melatonin the pineal gland contains peptides possessing antioxidative activity (AOA) that is especially revealed in ageing. The antioxidative effect of pineal gland peptide Epithalamin is mediated by an increase in endogenous AOA including antioxidative enzymes (Cu,Zn-superoxide dismutase, glutathione peroxidase) and ceruloplasmin. Synthetic pineal tetrapeptide Epitalon (Ala-Glu-Asp-Gly) - regarded as one of the active fragments of Epithalamin - suppresses ROS production and lipid peroxidation processes in the brain, liver and blood of experimental animals (aged LIO rats and CBA mice). Our clinical investigations confirm a significant age-related decrease in antioxidative defence indices in humans. Administration of Epithalamin to patients with age-related pathology (10 mg of the drug injected intramuscularly, daily for 10 days) eliminates imbalance in pro- and antioxidation systems. Study of free radical oxidation processes provides indication of validity of various approaches to the antioxidation state maintenance including antioxidant therapy of age-related pathologic processes predominantly with natural antioxidants. The presented results and data on the ability of the pineal peptides to extent longevity in rodents and protect them from carcinogenesis demonstrate that the described peptides can be employed as such compounds. Our data on the clinical application of Epithalamin as a geroprotector confirms this concept.

Factors Affecting Longevity

K.K. Reddy, A. Papa Rao, T.P.K. Reddy (Department of Physical Anthropology, School of Biological & Earth Sciences, Sri Venkateswara University, Tirupati - 517 502. Andhra Pradesh. India)

A high prevalence of coronary heart disease (CHD) in parallel with economic development among South Asian countries is observed. In India, studies suggest the prevalence of CHD to be about 10% - a figure about four times the prevalence of CHD in USA. South India shows still higher rates of CHD prevalence. In view of the fact that low high-density lipoprotein cholesterol (HDLC) and/or hypertriglyceridemia (in the presence of normal cholesterol with elevated central obesity) have been implicated as a cause for high rate of CHD in South Asians, especially among Indian origin. It is interesting to note that the Kurichias of Kerala (a tribal population) in India are enjoying longevity relatively free from age associated chronic problems. The CHD prevalence rates (Obesity:2.87; Central Obesity:3.71; Hypertension:2.70; Hypercholesterolemia:0.71; Hypertriglyceridemia:2.60 and low HDLC:1.24) among Kurichias is lower when compared to other Asian populations and Western countries. The low prevalence of CHD risk factors in the Kurichias provide some evidence that supports not only low fat intake and stress free economic activities but also other factors, including genetic make up and increased intake of foods rich in antioxidants, play a key role in their health and longevity.

Glutathione peroxidase under oxidative stress in aging

A. Valuch, S. Opris, C. Rusu, R.Nita (Nat. Inst. Gerontol.Geriatics, Bucharest, Romania)

PURPOSE: We studied influence of hiperglicemie from noninsulino dependent diabetus mellitus (NIDDM) in human aging. METHOD: Glucose is analysed enzimatic with Cormay kit no 2203. Glutathione peroxidase is determinated on erythrocytes with Ransel kit RS506. Hb is determinated by Drabkin method. RESULTS: Erythrocyte glutathione peroxidase presents an unsignificant statistically negative variation with aging (25 - 66 years); for woman ($r = -0.199$, $p = 0.268$, $n = 33$) and men ($r = -0.209$, $p = 0.174$, $n = 25$), where r is correlation coefficient, p probability coefficient and n number of cases. Under oxidative stress (NIDDM) both groups women ($r = 0.046$, $p = 0.888$, $n = 11$) and men ($r = 0.092$, $p = 0.726$, $n = 17$) presents a positive unsignificant statistically variation. CONCLUSIONS. Human erythrocyte glutathione peroxidase is unchanged both in normal aging and that accompanied by oxidative stress (NIDDM).

Radioisotope Uptake Studies of Atherogenic Potential of

Serum from Elderly Patients with CHD

F. Revnic ("Ana Aslan" N.I.G.G, Bucharest, Romania) C.R.Revnic (U.M.F. "Carol Davila", Bucharest, Romania)

Heart disease is the most common and costly of the ultimately complications of atherosclerosis(angina pectoris and myocardial lesions).The aim of our study was to investigate the atherogenic potential of serum from patients with CHD associated with major risk factors for atherosclerosis upon vascular endothelium permeability,upon 3H Cholesterol uptake and upon vascular proliferation.Material and methods.16 patients aged between 45-78 years old frm 2nd Medical Clinique of University Hospital admited for IHD(with angor of effort,spontaneously angor or heart stroke in their hystory) have been selected for our study.Only patients with normal blood glucose and without hypolemiant medication.patients have been divided in 4 groups of 4 patients each:1)Control with intact coronary arteries2).Patients with CHD without major risk,3)Patients with arterial hypertension as major risk factor,4).patients with CHD and associated risk factors:cigarette smoking and alcahol intake. Experimental studies have been performed on aortic rings incubated with serum from patients belonging to the 4 groups of patients, separately in order to find out any modifications in endothelial permeability(using 45Ca as well as to study 3H Cholesterol incorporation within endothelial membrane and the uptake of 3H Leucine to study the atherogenic potential of serum upon protein synthesis.The radioactive uptake has been performed according with the published method(F.Revnic,Rom.J.Geront.&Geriatrics10,3,1987) using a Beta Berthold Scintilation Counter.There is a positive corelation between advanced age in group 2 patients with cholesterol,total lipids and Tg level($p<0.01$) versus patients<50 years old from the same group.In group 2patients with cholesterol,lipids and Tg level($p<0.01$) versus patients<50 years old from the same group.In group3,both <50>patients the levels of cholesterol,total lipids and Tg are elevated In group 4 in both<50>patients the levels of cholesterol,lipids and Tg are above normal,but with a significant increase in patients over 50.Our data have pointed out an increase in 45Ca uptake when aortic rings have been incubated with serum from group 2 patients accaunting for a modification in permeability of endothelial wall.Concerning 3H Cholesterol and 3H Leu uptake by the aortic rings incubated with serum from patients of group 4, a significant increase in 3H Cholesterol and 3H Leu uptake has been recorded accaunting for the atherogenic potential of serum from CHD patients.

Skin effects of oral DHEA supplementation in the DHEAge Study

O. de Lacharrière, S. Nouveau*, P. Bastien*, V. Faucounau**, EE Baulieu***, F. Forette** (*Prospective Clinical Research, L Oréal Research, Clichy, 92110, France, ** Hôpital Broca, Fondation Nationale de Gérontologie, Paris, 75013, France ***INSERM, U488, Le Kremlin Bicêtre, 94276, France)*

The effects of a one year daily oral DHEA supplementation (50 mg/d) on skin were examined in the DHEAge study conducted in healthy volunteers (140 men and 140 women, 50% aged 60 to 69 years ; 50%, 70 to 79 years).Sebum production was measured by using specific tapes (Sebutape, CuDerm, Dallas) applied on defatted forehead skin. Absorbed lipids gave spots (one spot=one active sebaceous glands) then quantified by image analysis. Skin pigmentation was determined by chromametry (Minolta CR200, Chromameter) according to a three-dimensional L,a,b reference CIE standard system. Skin surface hydration evaluated by the measurement of electrical conductance of high-frequency electric current (10MHz, Dermodiag, L'Oréal). Epidermal thickness was determined by skin echography (25 MHz probe) on the back of the hand. Sebum production was significantly increased by DHEA on the whole population. This change was mostly related to the effect occurring in women, particularly those>70 physiologically hyposeborrheic. A significant decrease of the facial pigmentation (b value i.e. yellowness) at M12 for the whole DHEA-treated population was observed. This decrease was more pronounced in women>70. Suface skin hydratation was significantly increased for the whole DHEA-treated population at M12. In the population with the lower DHEAS blood concentration at M0, the DHEA supplementation had reduced significantly the epidermal atrophy observed in controls during the one year-period of the trial. In conclusion,oral administration of DHEA induces a measurable improvement of the skin.The effects of DHEA are mainly observed in subjects with the lowest level of DHEAS blood concentration at entry.

The State of Microcirculation and Some Connective Tissue Microstructures in Aging and Atherosclerosis

N.Kakauridze, N.Kipshidze Research Institutute of Therapy. 4 Ljubliana st, Tbilisi. 380059 Georgia

The aim of the work is to study the alterations of skin several microstructurs in atherosclerosis and proceeding from this to estimate aorta damages in early (preclinical) stage. The following indices and morphological microstructures were studied: -the specific share of capillaries (SSC) the specific share(SS) and ultrastructure of elastic fibers (EF) in derma papillary layer; and wall ultrastructure (US). We examined 103 patients (males) with atherosclerosis and 50 men withouth them.35 male cadavers were examined too. The patients and sectional material (with atherosclerosis and controls) were divided into three age subgroups. For the morphological examination in the skin bioptats were studied: by method Verhoeff was used to reveal EF which that of Gomori was used to examen capillaries .The SSEF and SSC was determined by mean of system automatic analysis of the images..Ultrastructure of cells and EF were examined under electron microscope. The connective tissue consisting elements is changed in skin during atherosclerosis: elastic fiber and SSEF in papillary layer is reduced, Thin EF disappear and fibrils are thickened, they undergo elastolisis and sometimes turn into a structurless mass.The SSC of capillaries in the papillary layer is reduced, capillary wall undergo ultrastructural alterations , atherosclerotic microangiopathy develops. The existing metabolic and anoxic state papillary derma in atherosclerosis form the condition for changment of structural -functional changes of Fibroblasts. Fibroblasts become secretorless. These suggestion is confirmed by sectional material, that reveals a close correlation between aorta atherosclerosis and wall -connective tissue element -elastic lamellae changes and alteration of derma connective tissue. The above mentioned alterations in atherosclerosis develops from a young ages and intensify at the adult and elderly as well as in connection with the gravty of atherosclerosis.

SESSION 207

Assessing Life Expectancies of Institutionalized Older Persons in Hong Kong

Eric Wong (Center for Clinical Trials and Epidemiological Research, The Chinese University of Hong Kong, Hong Kong), Elsie Hui, (Medical and Geriatric Unit, Shatin Hospital, New Territories, Hong Kong), Jean Woo (Department of Medicine and Therapeutics, The Chinese University of Hong Kong, Hong Kong)

PURPOSE: To predict life expectancies of institutionalized older Chinese persons aged 65 years and above METHOD: A 18-month prospective cohort study of survival in 590 residents of five nursing homes from October 1995. Information on demographics, the Abbreviated Mental Test (AMT), medical diagnoses, falls and hospitalizations were documented. Disability in activity of daily living was assessed with the Patient Assessment Instrument (PAI), which is total score of 4 for the best and 20 for the worst. Weibull accelerated failure time model was used to derive a mathematical model to predict the life expectancies. RESULTS: Of the 590 elderly enrolled in the study, 54 (9.15%) were excluded from the analysis due to lost to follow-up. Of the remaining 539 samples (median age 80 years; 70 0.000000emale; 57.5% AMT 6 and below; median length of stay 33 months) 18 months survival rate was 86.4%. Weibull model identified that decreased survival was significantly associated with, male, cancer, CAMC, increased age and PAI. There was a significant interaction between PAI and male. The goodness of fit of the model was satisfactory. CONCLUSION: It is forecasted that there will be 11.3% (868,300) of population in Hong Kong are aged 65 years and above by the year 2010, and consequently long-term care services such as nursing homes particularly will be in greater demand. The survival model we derived would be helpful for health care administrators to plan the future policies and demand for nursing home services.

Demand for formal long-term care services by the Dutch elderly

F. Portrait (department of Economics, Free University Amsterdam, Amsterdam, The Netherlands) D. Deeg (department of Social Gerontology, Free University Amsterdam, Amsterdam, The Netherlands) M. Lindeboom (department of Economics, Free University Amsterdam, Amsterdam, The Netherlands)

Markets for care services in most OECD countries face severe supply constraints and as a result observed utilisation differs from actual demand. Most studies on care try however to identify demand parameters using information on actual use. Strong assumptions are required to justify this. This paper takes a different approach. In the Netherlands, state committees (RIO) assess the demand of care applicants. Their decision is exclusively based on the current situation of the elderly and is not affected by supply conditions. Consequently, the care services recommended by the expert reflect the true individual demand of the elderly. We have access to an unique dataset from one of the RIO's that provide extensive information on the care applicants and the outcome of the intake procedure. This enables us to characterise the allocation mechanism conditional on application for care. The selection process preceding the application is characterised using information from a random sample of the Dutch elderly (LASA data set). Evidence suggests that the decision of state experts is only based on health status and on availability of informal and private care. On the other hand, additional factors - like loneliness and income - affect the decision to apply for care. Consistency of assessment among state experts is rejected by our model. Calculations based on our estimates show that for instance, 230f the men aged 75 apply for care and about 50f them are rejected by the committees. For men aged 75, the corresponding statistics equal 11% and 12% respectively.

Factors Affecting the Unmet Long-Term Care Need of Elderly in Korea

Jaeil Kim (Department of Public Administration, Dankook University, Seoul, Korea)

The only way to meet the long-term care need without a structured formal home care policy may be to live with certain types of informal caregivers. This study explores factors affecting the unmet long-term care need of elderly persons in Korea. In particular, it examines the effect of the presence of children in the home, as well as the effect that formal home care has on the reported unmet needs of the population. Data from the 1998 Elderly Living Condition Survey (ELCS) is used to analyze the Korean model. The unmet need is defined as the gap between the amount of long term care need, as assessed by an individual, and the actual resources the individual has at his/her disposal to meet that need. Predictors for unmet need model for the survey shows that high levels of functional difficulties and being in advanced age group are factors that are related to unmet need. Especially, living with a child is the most influential predictor in the model. The Living with a Child model presents that physical limitations are not significant predictors in the model. Also, having a son is the most influential predictor for the model. The finding indicates that Korean elderly living with a child is a matter of fact rather than a health related decision. Further examination of the relationship between unmet need and different types of living arrangements, number of children and household members, found high fluctuation in the unmet need rate depending on the living and the family situation. This finding suggests that the Korean elderly have to live in certain types of living arrangements in order to meet the needed care. This could be the result of Korea not having structured formal home care, where the only way to meet the need is to live with certain types of informal caregivers. Comparing above results to a previous research about the elderly in U.S. supports the findings. The U.S. case shows that: ´. physical limitations are significant predictors, 2. having a daughter is the most influential predictor, 3. the unmet need rate is consistent regardless of living arrangement factors. Thus, the impact and the need of formal home care can be seen from the differences shown in these studies of two countries.

Fitness and fatness as predictors of institutionalization and survival in elderly people

E.Heikkinen, T. Törmäkangas (The Finnish Centre for Interdisciplinary Gerontology and Department of Health Sciences, University of Jyväskylä, Finland)

Purpose: To examine the relative roles of physical fitness and body mass index as predictors of need for institutionalized care and survival among elderly people. Method: As part of a larger multidisciplinary longitudinal study of the elderly residents of the City of Jyväskylä, Central Finland, all the 75-year-old people (N=380) were invited to comprehensive examinations in 1989. During the subsequent 10 years information concerning the need for institutionalized care was collected from the elderly care centers and dates of deaths were obtained from the official register of the province of Central Finland. Maximal walking speed in a distance of 10 meters and maximal isometric knee extension strength were used as indicators of physical fitness. BMI was used to describe anthropometric properties. On the basis of the baseline information the participants were divided into BMI tertiles and into two physical fitness categories (<mean). Results: In relation to physical fitness the elderly people belonging to the above mean-value group had a lower need for institutionalized care and better survival irrespective of BMI. The need for institutionalized care was highest among those belonging to the heaviest BMI tertile and had their physical fitness value below the mean, whereas the worst survival was among those whose physical fitness value was below the mean and who belonged to the lowest BMI tertile. Conclusion: Among elderly people physical fitness seems to be a more important predictor of both the need for institutionalized care and survival than fatness alone. The results emphasize the importance of physical activity for elderly people.

Risk factors associated with future institutionalization

M. P. Beaudet (Health Statistics Division, Statistics Canada, Ottawa, Ontario, Canada)

This study examined health and socio-demographic factors that have been shown to be associated with institutionalization among older persons. The National Population Health Survey (NPHS) is a longitudinal survey designed to study health and its determinants. Data from the NPHS were used to examine the relationship between selected risk factors in 1994/95 and entry into a long-term care facility in the following four years among respondents 65 or older. An estimated 124,000 older Canadians (5 %) entered a long-term care facility in the years 1995 through 1999. Results from a multivariate logistic regression indicate that women had close to three times the odds of entering a long-term care facility (OR= 2.6; 95% CI=1.1, 5.9). As expected, persons 80 or older had higher odds of being institutionalized (OR=10.9; 95% CI=5.5, 21.6). Being in a low income category and having received publicly funded home care services in the year prior to the interview were also significant predictors of institutionalization (OR =2.1; 95% CI=1.1, 4.4 and OR=2.6; 95% CI=1.2, 5.7, respectively). Surprisingly, none of the health, social support and medication use variables that have been shown to be associated with institutionalization were predictive of entry into a long-term care facility. The results of this analysis illustrate the importance of longitudinal analysis in examining factors associated with institutionalization.

The Determinants of Retirement Homes in Taiwan

Shu-Chuan Jennifer Yeh (National Sun Yat-Sen University Kaohsiung, Taiwan, R.O.C.)

PURPOSE: The purpose of this study is to examine factors that influence retirement home selection. METHOD: A pre-tested closed structured questionnaire was distributed to 500 potential retirement home residents. Total 314 were returned for a response rate of 62.8%. The respondents were at least 50 years old and working full-time at the three private companies that were located in a major metropolitan area. Stratified random sampling was used to conduct this research based on the organizational size, total employee numbers. The questionnaire consisted of 34 questions using Likert-type scales with responses ranging from most to least important factors in making a retirement home selection. Eight background questions were asked to provide limited demographic information. Multiple regression analysis was used to analyze this research. Stepwise regression was used to analyze partition variation of each variable. RESULTS: After controlling several background variables, the following variables showed positively associated with entering a retirement community home ($p<0.05$): respondents with higher income, and showing higher agreement on the idea of retirement homes. Regarding to facilities-related determinants, greater number of amenities, nature and extent of the therapeutic services, as well as internal and external appearance showed statistically significant ($p<0.05$). On the other hand, the percentage of male children, owing a house, and frequencies of contacting with friends and families were negatively associated with entering a retirement community home ($p<0.05$). CONCLUSION: The concept of living in a retirement home is still new for most people in Taiwan. Culture is the most important determinant in this study. Higher income group and less social activities persons might be more willing to stay in a retirement home after they retire.

The Relationship between Regulatory Status, Quality of Care and 3-year Mortality in Residential Care Facilities

G. Bravo, M.F. Dubois, P. De Wals, R. Hébert (Research Center, Sherbrooke University Geriatric Institute, Sherbrooke, Canada)

PURPOSE : To determine whether the regulatory status of a long-term care (LTC) facility and the quality of the care it provides affect the risk of death among dependent older residents. METHOD: The study involved 299 older adults from 88 LTC facilities who were chosen randomly and followed for 3 years. At baseline, subjects were assessed in their living environment with respect to their functional autonomy, cognitive abilities and quality of their care. The exact date of death for the 143 residents who died during the follow-up period was retrieved from their medical files. Medical records were also used to collect disease-related information suspected of altering the risk of mortality. The effect of regulatory status and care quality on length of survival was investigated by means of a Cox's proportional hazards model. RESULTS: Controlling for age, comorbidity, and baseline functional abilities, the length of survival of a resident is not significantly influenced by the regulatory status of the facility in which he/she lived at baseline (HR = 1.09; 95% CI: 0.55 to 2.18). However, residents with poor quality ratings at baseline had shorter survival times than those provided with good care (HR = 1.73; 95% CI: 1.27 to 2.18). Median survival was 28 months among residents classified as receiving inadequate care compared to 41 months for those adequately cared for ($p = 0.002$). CONCLUSION: Quality of care has a much stronger influence on residents outcome than regulation per se. This finding underscores the relevance of testing innovative interventions aimed at improving the quality of care provided in LTC facilities, regardless of their regulatory status. Study funded by Health Canada, Grant #6605-05-1998/2590036.

SESSION 208

Canada takes action towards healthy active living for older adults

Bruce Taylor (Health Canada, Ottawa, Canada) 'Federal Active Aging Initiatives'. Diana Dampier (Active Living Coalition for Older Adults (ALCOA), Toronto, Canada) 'ALCOA, a Coalition Approach to Promoting Active Aging'. Margaret Horn (National Indian and Inuit Community Health Representatives Organization (NIICHRO), Kahnawake, Canada) 'Spirit in Motion: Active Living and Aging'. Jack Brownell (Canadian Seniors Games Association, Rothesay, Canada) 'Seniors Games in Canada'. Robert Petrella (College of Family Physicians of Canada, Mississauga, Canada) 'Physical Activity Strategy of the College of Family Physicians of Canada'.Nancy Ecclestone (Canadian Centre for Activity and Aging, London, Canada) 'National Leadership Training Initiatives'.

This roundtable will present the physical inactivity issue and its impact on the health and well being of older Canadians. National initiatives developed to address the issue through the promotion and support of an active lifestyle will be highlighted. Member organizations of ALCOA will present how they address physical inactivity among seniors and how they contribute to the implementation of the Blueprint for Action. A discussion period to answer questions, raise further issues and discuss the applicability of programs to other countries will follow. Health Canada - Federal Active Aging Initiatives An overview of the development and implementation of the Blueprint for Action will be provided. Included are the extensive community based consultation used in its development and the goals and objectives. The presentation will also describe other initiatives at the federal level to promote active living for older Canadians. ALCOA - A Coalition approach to Promoting Active Aging The Active Living Coalition for Older Adults (ALCOA) is a national organization comprising 23 national and provincial member organizations involved with health, aging, physical activity and creating healthy environments. This presentation will describe how ALCOA functions as a coalition and national initiatives underway to promote healthy aging. Spirit in Motion: Active Living and Aging The National Indian and Inuit Community Health Representatives Organization (NIICHRO) developed culturally relevant training tools and trained 300 Community Health Representatives across Canada to promote active living among seniors in Aboriginal communities. NIICHRO's approach emphasizes motivating elder Aboriginal people to become more active and encouraging activities that include traditional lifestyles. Senior Games in Canada The Canadian Seniors Games Association will describe their program providing opportunities for enrichment, fulfillment and improved quality of life and health provided through participation in a variety of recreation, sport and organized games activities. It will outline how games held at the local, regional, provincial and national levels lead to approximately 100,000 older adults participating in active living and will describe the short and long term benefits of participation reported by the seniors themselves. Physical Activity Strategy of the College of Family Physicians. This presentation will describe initiatives to improve the delivery of physical activity to those at risk of a sedentary lifestyle. The results of the activities to date will be identified including the publication of resource materials, workshops and links to allied groups enabling family physicians to improve the delivery of physical activity. Canadian Initiatives Promoting Active Living: From Research to Action Nancy Ecclestone of the Canadian Centre for Activity and Aging will outline two national strategies that translate evidence-based research into strategies leading to appropriate resources for those delivering physical activity programming for older adults. The first is the recent National Leadership Training Initiatives project and the second is the ALCOA research newsletter for practitioners of programs for older adults. ANTICPATED OUTCOMES: An increased awareness of participants of the importance of physical activity and an understanding of initiatives that have been developed in Canada to promote active living that may be applicable in other countries. Resources developed will be distributed.

ALCOA - A Coalition Approach to Promoting Active Aging

D. Dampier (Active Living Coalition for Older Adults, Toronto, Canada)

The Active Living Coalition for Older Adults (ALCOA) is a national non-profit organization supported by Health Canada. ALCOA's purposes and initiatives are to promote a culture and environment that supports and motivates older Canadians to include physical activity as an essential part of daily living. ALCOA has attracted 24 national and provincial organizations involved with health, aging, physical activity and creating healthy environments. Bringing together individual strengths and a common interest in healthy aging, members have forged a collaborative partnership that is continually expanding its efforts to promote active living for all older adults. The presentation will introduce the unique structure and function of the Coalition and will provide an overview of its strategy to implement the Blueprint for Action. The strategy includes working with our partners in the areas of Marketing and Communications, Influencing Policy, Communicating Research in Clear Language, Leadership and Coordination and Collaboration. It will also describe the evaluation plan for the Blueprint. Benchmarks achieved to date towards the implementation of the Blueprint will be highlighted followed by future plans and challenges. Physical inactivity is an important health issue that must be addressed by government, seniors' organizations, health providers and service deliverers. The coalition approach is one method that has been successful in bringing together multi-disciplinary stakeholders to address a common cause.

Physical Activity Strategy for Family Physicians

Robert Petrella (College of Family Physicians of Canada, London, Canada)

The College of Family Physicians of Canada is the national medical association that supports family physicians in providing high quality health care to their patients. In addition to training and Annual Scientific Assemblies, the College is active in continuing medical education and produces a number of publications. The College's monthly clinical journal has a circulation of almost 30,000.This presentation will identify the results of the Physical Activity Strategy Committee of the College of Family Physicians of Canada to improve the delivery of physical activity to those at risk of a sedentary lifestyle. The presentation will highlight the following initiatives specific to older adults: 1) The endorsement, distribution and promotion of Canada's Physical Activity Guide to Healthy Active Living for Older Adults; 2) The Problem Based Small Group Learning (PBSGL) module for physical activity and older adults that awards medical education credits for completion of modules; 3) A Production Video in which a family physician discusses the importance of counselling older patients on the benefits of a physically active lifestyle and older adults demonstrate activities. 4) PACE-CAN and STEP projects endorsed by the Committee tosupport family physicians in counselling and encouraging their older patients to be active and 5) peer reviewed publications. This presentation will highlight what the Physical Activity Strategy has accomplished and will identify the priorities for the future.

Seniors Games in Canada

Jack Brownell (Canadian Seniors Games Association, Rothesay, Canada)

The Canadian Seniors Games Association (CSGA) believes that every Canadian age 55 years and over has the fundamental right to opportunities for enrichment, fulfillment and improved quality of life and health provided through participation in a broad variety of recreation, sport and organized games activities. A number of activities have been adopted ranging from active sports such as swimming, golf, track and softball to more passive pursuits such as floor curling, bridge and billiards. It is the duty and responsibility of the CSGA to promote the ongoing operation of Seniors Games at the national level. The Association believes this can be accomplished most effectively through the development of provincial programs, which have existed for 25 years in Canada. Provincial Games organizations are encouraged to begin competitions at the local / community level, then the district and regional levels and end with provincial competitions. No matter what the level of competition reached by the seniors, the process of participation strengthens attitudes and forms sound habits with regard to mental and physical health. Indeed the social aspects of the games are just as important as the performance of the physical activity. Many seniors have stated that their daily practice for the predicted timed swim, or walk has developed into a daily exercise program long after the competition has passed. Due to provincially operated Seniors Games, approximately 100,000 older adults 55 yrs+ took part in organized activities this year. The direct benefits are increased levels of mental and physical health and social interaction.

Spirit in Motion: Active Living and Aging

Margaret Horn (National Indian and Inuit Community Health Representatives Organization (NIICHRO), Kahnawake, Canada).

The National Indian and Inuit Community Health Representatives Organization (NIICHRO) is a national non-profit organization formed to strengthen and enhance existing health education programs and other activities carried out in Indian and Inuit Communities. NIICHRO's goal is to improve the quality of health care services offered to Indian and Inuit people through the work of the community health representative. NIICHRO works in the areas of environmental health, health delivery, medical administration, counselling, home visits, education, community development and mental health. NIICHRO has direct contact with front line workers through their magazine 'In-Touch'. Through the 'Spirit in Motion' project supported by Health Canada, NIICHRO developed culturally relevant training tools (exercise video and training manual) and trained 300 Community Health Representatives and other health professionals across Canada to promote active living among senior population in Aboriginal communities. \ NIICHRO's approach emphasizes motivating elder Aboriginal people to become more active and encouraging activities that include traditional lifestyles. The training approach utilizes a 'train the trainer' model where a core group of representatives are trained and they in turn train a larger number of community health representatives. This model has been adapted by other national organizations.

Two Canadian Initiatives Promoting Active Living: From Research to Action

Nancy A. Ecclestone (Canadian Centre for Activity and Aging (CCAA), The University of Western Ontario, London, Canada)

The Canadian Centre for Activity and Aging (CCAA) is a research and educational institute that translates research into strategies promoting the independence of older adults. This session will describe a recent CCAA National Leadership Training Initiatives project (2000-2003) that is supported by Health Canada. It will involve stakeholders across Canada in developing guidelines for practitioners and strategies for implementation of education and leadership training courses targeting older adults living in the community and those living in long-term care facilities (nursing homes) or living in a homebound environment. Also, Nancy Ecclestone, co-chair of the ALCOA research committee, will outline a new initiative of ALCOA to produce a research newsletter in plain language for practitioners of programs for older adults. Thus, this session outlines two national strategies that translate evidence-based research into strategies leading to appropriate resources for those delivering physical activity programming for older adults.

SESSION 209

Comparison of Parkinsonian patients developing Dementia Vs Dementia patients developing Parkinsonism.

Vaneet KHANNA MD FRCP, North Manchester General Hospital, UK

Response to treatment in Parkinsonian patients who then go on to develop Dementia varies from Dementia patients who later go on to develop Parkinsonism. Data was collected from the Medical records of 50 patients attending the Movement Disorder Clinic at North Manchester General Hospital. Data Consisted of MiniMental state Examination at the time of Diagnosis of Parkinsonism and Dementia and finally during the study period in May 2000.Response to Treatment was assessed and graded as significant improvement, partial improvement and poor responders. Webster rating scales for functional assessment at the time of diagnosis as well at the time of review. 41 patients were selected and divided into 2 groups. Group A consisted of 19 patients who had Dementia and after a mean period of 8 years developed Parkinsonian disorder as well. Group B comprised of 22 patients who had Parkinsonian disorder who after a mean period of 9 years went on to develop Dementia. In group A (Dementia + PD) there were no patients who showed significant improvement with Rx. 56% continued to show partial response to Rx, 44% were poor responders to Rx. In the Group B (Parkinson's + Dementia) 32% continued to show significant improvement despite development of dementia, 47% managed to have partial improvement on RX while 21% were poor responders to Rx. This study suggests that majority of Parkinsonian patients who in later life go on to develop Dementia continue to respond to pharmacological manipulation. Unfortunately majority of Dementia patients who go on to develop Parkinsonian disorder are resistant to anti-parkinsonian pharmacological manipulation.

How Well Does the Levodopa Challenge Test Predict Dopamingergic Responsiveness in Parkinson's Disease?

PK Sarkar, S Walsh, and AES Ritch (City Hospital, Birmingham, UK), P Nightingale (Queen Elizabeth Hospital, Birmingham, UK)

The clinical diagnosis of idiopathic Parkinson's Disease (PD) remains more difficult in older individuals and drug therapy is less effective.. The value of the levodopa challenge test in predicting dopaminergic responsiveness was assessed. 44 patients fulfilling the PD Society Brain Bank criteria and 54 controls were assessed by the tap test (number of taps on 2 plates 20cm apart over 15 seconds) and walk test (time in seconds to walk 6m and return). These were repeated for patients 1 and 2 hours after an oral dose of Cocareldopa 100/25 and 1 month after chronic dosing with levodopa. Barthel index was completed at baseline and after 3 months treatment. 39 (88.6%) of patients (mean age 79 years) had a positive result to challenge (>20% improvement in either test) and 41 (93.2%) at 1 month, predictive value 85%, sensitivity 95%, specificity 100%. Percentage improvements were greater for responders at 1 month for tap test ($p<0.001$), walk test ($p<0.05$) and at 3 months for Barthel score ($p<0.001$). Median tap and walk scores in controls (mean age 79 years) and in patients were 49.5v35.5 ($p<0.001$) and 14v20sec($p<0.001$), improving to 48 and 54 ($p<0.001$) and 12.5 and 12sec($p<0.001$) for patients initially and at 1 month. Median Barthel scores were 13 at baseline and 18 at 3 months ($p<0.001$). There was a linear relationship between percentage improvement in tap ($r=0.86, p<0.001$) and walk ($r=0.87, p<0.001$) scores initially and at 1 month. The levodopa challenge test can predict the degree of improvement to be gained on longterm therapy.

Managing a Progressive Illness in Old Age:Parkinson's disease and the older person and carer

M.Lloyd (Department of Sociological Studies, University of Shefield,UK), M.Gonsalkorale (Salford Royal Hospitals NHS TRust, UK)

The authors are a social reseracher and consultant geriatrican concerned with the managment of Parkinson's disease in the community. This paper will present the combined findings of a survey of community care for PD people and their carers(342 postal questionaire returns and 26 case studies) and a multidisciplinary intervention in geriatric medicine (EPICS) initiated through a 12 month pilot project. The average age of PD respondents in the community care survey was 70 years and 470f carers were aged over65. Numbers of community care assessments and services provided were low overall and showed no significant increase with age or length of illness (110f over 65s had had a community care assessment). Weaknesses at the health and social care interface and communication problems between professionals were limitig the effectiveness of care management. The EPICS project introduced a single assessment process and the use of service user-held records. Front-line professionals incorporated standardised measures (BARTHEL Index, AMTS and HADS) into their assessments and jointly agreed (client and professional)goals. The project demonstrated that more people were enabled to stay at home without institutionlisation and there was high service user satisfaction with their participation in assessment and service delivery processes. A community care follow-up project(which will report in June 2001) is refining the cmbioned use of localised service information packs with a care pathway folder which is carried and coordinated by the service user/carer themselves.

SESSION 210

Age differences in health and lifestyle after acute myocardial infarction

Dee Jones, Robert West (University Of Wales College Of Medicine, Cardiff, UK)

Purpose: Studies of rehabilitation following acute myocardial infarction (MI) provide little information on age differences. Most previous studies have focused on younger people particularly younger men, although a significant and increasing proportion of MI patients are aged over 65 years. A multicentre trial of rehabilitation following MI (n=2287) included 948 older people. Data were collected on admission from clinical records, following discharge by structured interview using standard measures in patients' own homes, at six months by second interview using the same standard measures and at 12 months clinical examination in outpatients. We report here an analysis of the controls. Results: Comparisons showed many highly significant age differences in health status, 'natural history' of rehabilitation and lifestyle changes following MI. At discharge clinically significant anxiety was identified in 23% of older people compared with 36% of younger people ($p<0.001$), depression in 16% v 21% ($p<0.001$) and severe disability in 27% v 18% ($p<0.001$). At six-month follow up these differences persisted but there was little difference in medication (32% v 31% received five or more prescribed medications per day) or readmissions to hospital (24% v 27%). More older people undertook no physical exercise (31% v 20%, $p<0.001$). Conclusion: This study shows major differences between young and older patients in a number of domains of health and lifestyle, both early after MI and six months later. These findings have implications for the management and aftercare of older people following MI, Programmes should be designed with sufficient flexibility to respond to the specific needs of older people so that they do not continue to feel excluded from services currently available.

Aortic Pulsewave Velocity as an Independent Predictor of Cardiovascular Mortality over 70 Years Old Subjects

S. Meaume, A. Rudnichi, A. Lynch, C. Bussy, C. Sebban, A. Benetos, ME Safar, Geriatric departments (SM, AL, CB) Charles Foix Hospital, Ivry sur Seine, France Department of Internal Medicine (MES) and INSERM 337 (AB), Broussais Hospital, Paris France Covance (AR), Rueil-Malmaison, France

PURPOSE : Aortic pulse wave velocity (PWV) is a significant and independent predictor of cardiovascular mortality in hypertensive subjects and in patients with end-stage renal disease, but its contribution to cardiovascular risk in subjects above 70-100 years old has never been tested. METHOD : A cohort of 141 subjects (mean age : 87+/- 7 years) was studied in two geriatric Departments in Paris suburb.Together with sphygmomanometric blood pressure measurements, aortic PWV was measured using a validated automatic device. RESULTS : Blood pressure, heart rate, gender, the presence of dementia, but no age, explained 34% of the PWV variability in this cohort. In addition to low plasma albumin, PWV was the major predicting factor of cardiovascular, but not global, death. The adjusted odds ratio was 1,16 (95% confidence intervals : 1.00-1.35). antihypertensive drug therapy and blood pressure level, including pulse pressure, had no additive role. CONCLUSION : In subjects 7O-100 years old, aortic PWV is a strong independent predictor of cardiovascular death, a finding that remains to be confirmed by an intervention study.

Cardiovascular morbidity among Danish centenarians

K. Andersen-Ranberg (Geriatric Dept. Odense University Hospital and Aging Research Center, Institute of Public Health, University of Southern Denmark, Odense, Denmark), M. Schroll (Geriatric Dept. Bispebjerg Hospital, Copenhagen University, Copenhagen, Denmark) and B. Jeune (Aging Research Center, Institute of Public Health, University of Southern Denmark, Odense, Denmark).

Purpose: This study is focusing on the presence of cardiovascular disease in Danish centenarians in order to assess the morbidity and mortality risk in a group of extremely old subjects, who have survived most of their fellow birth cohort members. Methods: A population-based study of all Danes celebrating their 100th birthday from 1 April 1995 to 31 May 1996, a total of 276 persons. All participants were visited at their domicile for an interview (incl. proxies) and a clinical examination (incl. BP, ECG and blood-test). Further health information was retrieved from GPs, and the national discharge register. Results: In all, 75% (N=207, M:F=1:3.6) of eligible subjects participated in the study. Based on the clinical examination and medical files a cardiovascular disease incl. hypertension (>160/>100) was present in 149 (72%) subjects. Twenty-seven percent had suffered from myocardial infarction. Hypertension defined according to WHO was present in 52% (>140/>90), and moderate hypertension (>160/>100) in 31%. Atrial fibrillation was diagnosed in 17%, while 7 subjects had a pacemaker. Chronic heart failure was found to be present in 32%, but is believed to be higher. Data on natriuretic peptides will be presented. Conclusion: Danish centenarians have survived to extreme ages in spite of a high prevalence of cardiovascular diseases. Not only improvement in life style, but also better knowledge of treatment indications, together with more effective therapies, including secondary prevention, may explain the increasing number of centenarians by improving the survival of 80+year-olds.

Morphologic and Functional Characteristics of the Heart in Longevivals

D. State, G.I. Prada, M. Georgescu, S. Galaftion (Ana Aslan National Institute of Gerontology and Geriatrics, Bucharest, Romania)

The purpose of the study was to identify the specific functional and structural changes in the heart of longevals. 61 longevals beyond the age of 90 (range 90-105) have been studied. 42 were women (mean age 93.8 years) and 19 men (mean age 92.7 years). We investigated echocardiographic changes at the level of valvular apparatus (mitral, aorta, pulmonary, tricuspid), thickness of the ventricular wall and interventricular septum, left ventricular mass, changes in the ventricular kinetics (hypokinezia, akinezia, diskinezia), resting systolic function (FE and FS) and the assessment of the diastolic ventricular performance. We used an ultrasound machine with a color Doppler facility (Apogee 150). The following echocardiographic changes were found: degenerative stenotic valvular lesions in 260f the longevivals; aortic atheromatosis with a transaortic gradient lower than 20 mmHg in 78.3%; calcification of the mitral ring in 60.6% and septum sigmoidum in 390f longevivals. Resting systolic function (FE and FS) was below 50 0n 690f longevivals. Ventricular diastolic function was decreased in all longevivals, mainly due to the disorder of ventricular relaxation (E wave < A wave, E/A ratio lower than 1) and to a lesser extent due to restrictive diastolic dysfunction. Conclusions: most prevalent lesions in longevivals are atheromatous lesions, wide valvular stenosis, and calcification of the mitral ring (60.6%); septum sigmoidum without any sign of obstruction of the ejection chamber of the left ventricle has been found in one third of the longevivals; decreased systolic function at rest and ventricular diastolic relaxation predominantly affected.

Personal, Chronological and Environmental Factors Contributing to Cardiopulmonary Arrest during Bathing in Japan

R. Takahashi, S. Watanabe, S. Matsushita (Tokyo Metropolitan Institute of Gerontology, Tokyo, Japan), S. Hori (Keio University School of Medicine, Tokyo, Japan), A. Hamamatsu (Tokyo Medical Examiner's Office, Tokyo, Japan), Y. Asakawa, F. Endo (Gumma University School of Medicine, Maebashi, Japan)

Incidence of cardiopulmonary arrest (CPA) during bathing is on the rise in Japan and is likely to persist as a public health problem because it most often occurs in the rapidly increasing population of elders. This study was conducted to assess personal, chronological and environmental factors contributing to the risk of CPA in Japanese elders. From October 1, 1999 to March 31, 2000, ambulance emergency call data from over 95% of the total population in Tokyo were collected. There were 1087 total emergency calls during bathing (accidents occurring in a bathroom or in a bathtub); 574 calls reported CPA. Incidence of the calls was the highest in December and January and between 8p.m. and 24p.m.. Twenty-nine percent (311) of the calls were made for persons who were aged 80 to 89 years old; 56%(610) were made for males. Logistic regression analysis indicated that CPA was associated with increasing age [odds ratio (OR)=1.3/10 yr.; 95% confidence interval (CI): 1.2, 1.4] and female gender (OR=1.4; 95% CI: 1.1, 1.8). Lower atmospheric temperature, but not atmospheric pressure, was significantly associated with increased risk of CPA during bathing (OR=1.4/10C decrease; 95% CI: 1.0, 1.9). The incidence of CPA was the lowest between 4p.m. and 8p.m.(OR=0.6 95%; CI: 0.4, 0.8) and the highest between 4a.m. and 8a.m. (P=0.08; OR=1.8; 95% CI: 0.9, 3.7). Bathing time and environment are important factors contributing to CPA in Japanese elders, especially women. Choosing bathing time and controlling temperature in the preparation and bathing environment may decrease risk of CPA during bathing among elderly Japanese.

Physical activity of old individuals with high risk for atherosclerotic cardiovascular disease

E. L. Klein, Y.M. Garcia, L. M. R. Hartmann, E. T. Carvalho Filho, L, W Jacob Filho (Disciplina de Geriatria Δ Medical School of São Paulo University, São Paulo, Brazil).

PURPOSE:Elderly out-patients of a Geriatric Health Care unit, considered at high risk for cardiovascular disease had their present and past standard of physical activity compared to their clinical manifestations of atherosclerosis. METHOD: Patients were assigned to a group of follow-up if they had at least three risk factors and/or clinical manifestation of atherosclerotic cardiovascular disease. At first consultation in this group they were asked about their present and past pattern of physical activity and this information was compared to their clinical manifestations of atherosclerosis. RESULTS: 181 patients were seen, 64.1% females. Mean age was 76.0. 30.4% had physical activity at present, and 39.3% in the past. The most frequent present activities were walking (70.4%), gymnastics (11.1%), and physiotherapy (7.4%). Most frequent past activities were walking (34.6%), soccer (17.3%) and swimming (7.7%). 24.9% had risk factors but not clinical atherosclerosis; 22.2% had physical activity at present and 26.7% in the past. Among patients with atherosclerotic lesions, 33.1% had physical activity at present and 30.1% in the past. Lesions were on central nervous system (CNS) (27.2%), coronaries (51.5%), peripheral artheries (2.9%), and more than one territory (18.4%). Present activity was less frequent for patients with CNS lesions (p=0.0275). There was no difference for past activity. CONCLUSIONS: practice of physical activity decreased with time in these elderly; one third of them have some kind of physical activity at present; walking was the most frequent activity described; atherosclerotic lesions showed no relationship with past activity, but CNS lesions correlated negatively with present activity.

Respiratory symptoms and body mass index in a group of elderly subjects

M H Shamssain (The Institute of Pharmacy, Chemistry & Biomedical Sciences, School of Sciences, University of

Sunderland, Sunderland, United Kingdom)

PURPOSE: To investigate the association between body mass index (BMI) and respiratory symptoms in elderly subjects. METHODS: We studied 2000 elderly subjects from the north east of England. We used St. Georges Respiratory Questionnaire to assess the prevalence and severity of respiratory symptoms. We used SPSS to analyse data. RESULTS: Mean (SD) age, height, weight and BMI were 76.9 (8.3) y, 160.8 (10.9) cm, 62.4 (11.8) kg, and 24.1 (4.2) kg/m2, respectively. Cough most days a week, cough several days a week, and cough few days a months were high at low BMI, low at medium BMI, and high again at High BMI. The prevalence rates of shortness of breath (SOB) and wheeze followed the same pattern. CONCLUSION: The present study illustrates that there is a U-shape relationship between the prevalence rates of respiratory symptoms and BMI in elderly subjects. These results will help to design follow-up studies to implement strategies for intervention research in elderly subjects. in elderly subjects.

Risk factors for symptomatic venous thrombosis in geriatric patients. A multicentric hospital-based case-control study.

Sebastien Weill-Engerer (hopital Rothschild, Paris, France), Sylvie Meaume (hopital Charles Foix, Ivry-sur-Seine, France), Amina Lahlou (hopital Charles Foix, Ivry-sur-Seine, France), François Piette (hopital Charles Foix, Ivry-sur-Seine, France), Olivier Saint-Jean (hopital Charles Foix, Ivry-sur-Seine, France), Annick Sachet (hopital Charles Foix, Ivry-sur-Seine, France), Jean-Yves Beinis (hopital Charles Foix, Ivry-sur-Seine, France), Claude Gallinari (hopital Charles Foix, Ivry-sur-Seine, France), Anne-Sophie Grancher (hopital Charles Richet, Villiers-le-Bel, France), Jean-Pierre Vincent (hopital Emile Roux, Limeil Brevannes, France), Henri Naga (hopital Emile Roux, Limeil Brevannes, France), Joel Belmin (hopital Rene Muret, Sevran, France), Rosella Salvatore (hopital Charles Foix, Ivry-sur-Seine, France), Marie Kazes (hopital Bicêtre, Le Kremlin Bicêtre, France), Eric Pautas (hopital Charles Foix, Ivry-sur-Seine, France), Andre Boiffin (hopital Charles Foix, Ivry-sur-Seine, France), Jean-Bernard Piera (hopital Charles Foix, Ivry-sur-Seine, France), Monique Duviquet (hopital Charles Richet, Villiers-le-Bel, France), David Knafo (hopital Georges Clemenceau, Champcueil, France), Andree Piau (hopital Bichat-Claude Bernard, Paris, France), Dragoslav Miric (hopital Rene Muret, Sevran, France), Alain Jean (hopital La Rochefoucauld, Paris, France), Valerie Bellamy (hopital Rothschild, Paris, France), Olivier Tissandier (hopital Rothschild, Paris, France), Alain-Ferdinand Le Blanche (hopital Charles Foix, Ivry-sur-Seine, France)

Purpose : although venous thrombosis is frequent among elderly, especially when hospitalized, little is known about the relevance of clinical risk factors when they occur simulteaneously. The objective of this study was to identify independent risk factors of symptomatic venous thrombosis or pulmonary embolism in geriatric patients. Method : all patients of 18 geriatric departments where submitted to clinical surveillance over a period of 16 months. Potential clinical risk factors for patients presenting a clinical suspicion of venous thrombosis or pulmonary embolism were determined prospectively before performing confirmation complementary investigations. Patients were therefore classified in two groups: confirmation of pulmonary embolism or venous thrombosis, and negative examination. The relevance of potential clinical risk factors was calculated by logistic regression. Results : out of 1,063 examinations evaluated, 374 confirmed the suspected diagnostic while 689 did not. Seven factors were identified to be independently related to the development of venous thrombosis or pulmonary embolism: age over 74 (OR=2.6), hospitalization in an intermediate-stay or long-stay unit (OR=1.8), obesity (OR=4.6), history of deep vein thrombosis or pulmonary embolism (OR=1.7), absence of oral anticoagulant therapy (OR=2.2), treatment with heparin at a dosage greater than 3000 anti Xa IU/day (OR=1.8), wearing of elastic stockings (OR=1.6). A risk score for symptomatic deep vein thrombosis or pulmonary embolism applicable to geriatrics was elaborated. Conclusions : This study identified a number of independent medical risk factors for symptomatic venous thrombosis or pulmonary embolism in geriatric patients. Systematic screening of asymptomatic geriatric patients presenting several of these risk factors should be considered.

The impact of lifestyle advice on the cardiovascular risk factors of Japanese immigrants in Brazil

Y. Moriguchi, E.H. Moriguchi, P. Ishikawa (Institute of Geriatrics & Gerontology, PUCRS University, Porto Alegre, RS, Brazil), Y. Yamori, (WHO Collaborating Center, Kyoto University, Kyoto, Japan)

PURPOSE: To evaluate the impact of healthy lifestyle advise on the cardiovascular risk factors (RF) profile of Japanese immigrants living in the southern Brazil. METHOD: The subjects of the study were Japanese immigrants living in the two states located in the most south part of Brazil, age range 45-59 years, that were followed from 1970 to 1999 in regular health examinations. All of them received a systematic healthy lifestyle advise that consisted in the education on: (a) diet: salt restriction (<6g/day), animal fat restriction, (b) normalization of body weight, (c) rest: 8 hr sleep every night and 30 min. siesta after lunch, (d) exercise: 60 min. walk every day, (e) quit smoking. The non-compliant group (NC) consisted of 160 participants that did not follow any of the given advises. The compliant group (C) consisted of 107 participants that followed at least three of the five given advises. The comparison of the prevalence (%) of the RF was done using chi-square test. RESULTS: There were no differences in the baseline RF prevalence. The differences in the main measured cardiovascular RF are as follow (in %): Overweight (BMI>25): 54.1% male, 49.5% female in NC vs. 32.0% male, 22.2% female in C, $p<0.05$. Hypertension (BP>140/90): 32.8% male, 36.4% female in NC vs. 7.5% male, 9.2% female in C, $p<0.05$. ECG ST-T changes: 9.0% in NC vs. 0.9% in C, $p<0.01$. CONCLUSION: The long term compliance with healthy lifestyle advice is fundamental to keep the prevalence of cardiovascular RF lowered.

SESSION 211

Balancing Work and Family Responsibilities in an Aging Society: International Perspectives

M. Evandrou, K. Glaser and U. Henz (Age Concern Institute of Gerontology, King's College London, London, England) Balancing work and family life: multiple role occupancy in mid-life and quality of life. J. Mears and E. Watson (University of Western Sydney Campbelltown, Australia) 'I go to work for a holiday': Paid Work and Care, the Australian Experience. M. Reichert (Institute of Gerontology at the University of Dortmund, Germany) Combining Work and Eldercare in Germany: Does the Long Term Care Insurance make a difference? J. Phillips, M. Bernard and M. Chittenden (Centre for Social Gerontology, University of Keele, Keele, England) Evaluating the effectiveness of support for working carers.

Abstract This symposium addresses issues of balancing work and family responsibilities, which have become the focus of policy and practice debates in the last decade. Our convenor and Chair, Anne Martin - Matthews will open the symposium by highlighting the key issues in work-family life research drawing on key findings of national Canadian research on work-family life balance, conducted in the 1990s by CARNET: The Canadian Aging Research Network. Four papers will be presented drawing specifically on empirically based research in the UK, Germany and Australia. The first of two papers from the UK will highlight the multiple roles of mid-life individuals and the impact of this on quality of life and well-being. The degree of variation in patterns of multiple role occupancy by socio-economic group, ethnic origin, education and health and material resources is examined. Women who play a central role in balancing work and family life provide the focus for the second paper from Australia, which argues that the current definitions of care fail to identify the size and value of the enterprise and its impact on work opportunities. Recent data from Germany in the third paper will address the question of whether long-term care insurance has made a difference to the possibility of combining work and eldercare. The fourth paper, again from the UK, will focus on what workplace-based support is considered effective by working carers and their managers in public sector organisations. All the papers will addresses methods and implications of work-life balance for carers, older people, their families and communities. In conclusion, our discussant, Margaret Neal will draw together the implications of this research for developing policies and practices to support carers balance work and family commitments and make comparisons between the symposium findings and the well-established literature in the US.

Balancing work and family life: multiple role occupancy in mid-life and quality of life

M. Evandrou, K. Glaser and U. Henz (Age Concern Institute of Gerontology, King's College London, London, Great Britain)

Individuals undertake a variety of roles within work and family life. Balancing various responsibilities among those in middle and later adulthood is of particular interest given socio-economic and demographic changes, such as rising female labour force participation, increases in longevity, and rises in the age which children leave home, which are likely to create additional roles. This paper investigates the complex inter-relationships between the multiple roles of mid-life individuals, focussing on work and family commitments. The extent to which men and women in mid-life undertake a multiplicity of roles is explored using a series of typologies. The degree of variation in patterns of multiple role occupancy by socio-economic group, ethnic origin, education, health and material resources is also examined. The project also investigates the likely effects of multiple work and family responsibilities in mid-life on measures of quality of life and well-being in later life (health, financial resources and social activities). The research is based upon secondary analysis of longitudinal data containing paid work and caring histories (Family and Working Lives Survey, and the Retirement and Retirement Plans Survey). Initial results indicate that although the proportion of mid-lifers occupying multiple roles at one point in time is low, this proportion rises to 24% when we examine occupancy over the lifecourse. There is an association between paid work and caring, which has implications for the accumulation of future pension entitlements and health status. The findings will inform debate on how policy can best aid those endeavouring to balance paid work, family life and caring responsibilities.

Combining Work and Eldercare in Germany: Does the Long Term Care Insurance make a difference?

Monika Reichert (Institute of Gerontology at the University of Dortmund, Germany)

Balancing work and family life, particularly in relation to the care of older people, is increasingly an issue in Germany, given socio-economic and demographic changes. In the context of combing work and eldercare, special emphasis is put on the question whether and to what extent the long-term care insurance (LTCI, Pflegeversicherung) changed the situation of working carers. The LTCI, which was introduced in 1995, provides benefits, which have -it is assumed - the potential to either facilitate or inhibit a combination of work and care. For example, the possibility that older people in need of care choose benefits in kind (additional support by professional helpers) instead of benefits in cash might enable carers to stay in the workforce or work longer hours. To examine the consequences the LTCI has on working carers, data from two representative cross-sectional surveys of care giving households, which were carried out before (1992) and after (1998) the LTCI came into force, are compared. Both data sets provide information on the number and socio-demographic characteristics of working carers as well as on relevant employment related aspects so that differences between "before" and "after" can be highlighted and interpreted. In addition, the implications of the findings for working carers, older people and the LTCI will be discussed.

Evaluating the effectiveness of workplace based support for Carers.

J. Phillips, M. Bernard and M. Chittenden (Centre for Social Gerontology, University of Keele, Keele, Staffordshire, England)

Employers are increasingly under pressure, both from within organisations and from recent government legislation and policy in the UK, to develop family-friendly policies to support informal carers in the workplace. Traditionally policy has been focused on childcare and to date, there has been little review and evaluation of what formal workplace schemes exist to assist working carers of disabled and older adults. There is also little information about the kinds of strategies carers informally use to help them remain in employment. The paper will explore the use, relevance and effectiveness of a range of workplace policies and practices from the perspective of working carers. It will highlight whether existing family-friendly policies and programmes are the kinds of services carers want or need to assist them in balancing work and care. The research on which this paper is based was conducted using firstly, an initial self-completion questionnaire survey of employees in two large public sector organisations, and secondly, a longer questionnaire to 359 carers of older adults. Third, in-depth interviews were conducted with a small sample of working carers and senior managers. These interviews assisted us in identifying what opportunities and barriers existed for working carers. Preliminary findings suggest that informal support is vital within the workplace. The findings will be discussed with relevance to how workplace based support should develop to help carers of older adults. Alongside this comparisons will be made with US and Canadian studies.

'I go to work for a holiday': Paid Work and Care, the Australian Experience.

J. Mears and E. A. Watson (University of Western Sydney, Sydney, Australia)

Our research set out to explore the experience of working carers - women who were both working full time and carrying a major responsibility for care of an elderly relative. The data comprised interviews with forty women. In the symposium paper we examine how our participants balanced the demands of caring and paid work, how caring shaped and constrained the other areas of their lives, and the implications of this in the present and for the future. We also examine the nature of the support, both informal, from family and friends, and formal, from community services and within the workplace. We make use of a broad definition of 'a major caring responsibility'. The study found that, for these women, continuing in paid employment was of central importance, for financial security (immediate and longer term) and because work was personally rewarding. While few women had reduced their hours of work as a result of caring responsibilities, nearly all had accepted restrictions and forgone opportunities for advancement, e.g, postponing or abandoning education and not seeking promotion. Workplaces were, in general, unresponsive to the problems these women confronted. Because they had paid work, they were often seen to be a lower priority by hard-pressed community services. We argue that current narrow definitions of care in policy fail to identify either the size of the caring enterprise or its value. Support for carers is not 'welfare' but astute and compassionate investment, an arena of productive work that is of value for all.

SESSION 212

Alzheimer's Type Dementia (AD) and Caregiver Stress

Massaia M, Ferrario E, Pallavicino di Ceva A, Cappa G, Bo M, Molaschi M, Fabris F (Institute of Gerontology. University of Torino. Corso Bramante 88, 10126 Torino. Italy)

PURPOSE: aim of the study was the identification of the patient's and caregiver's features associated with an high level of stress in the latter. METHOD: a cross-sectional multicentric analytic study was performed in a sample selected from caregivers enrolled in 12 sections of the AIMA, an Italian Alzheimer's Disease Association. The Greene Relative's Stress Scale (RSS) was utilised as outcome measure. The predictive variables were included in two protocols. The caregiver's protocol was focusing on degree of depression (Hamilton Depression Scale), caregiving burden and charges; in the patient's protocol were inserted the Global Deterioration Scale (Reisberg), Katz's ADL and Blessed Dementia Scale. The linear correlation coefficient R, multiple regression stepwise method and ANOVA were used in the statistical analysis. RESULTS: The sample (mean age 57.8±13.8) was composed by 423 caregivers. They take care of 423 AD patients (mean age 73.3 ± 8.9). A mean of 12.8 ± 8.8 hour a day was spent to look after or to support the patient. This large employment of time was considered from 61.40f the subjects the main problem influencing their social (51%) and daily (55.7%) living. The increasing mean of the hours spent in caregiving shows a positive correlation with the RSS score ($F= 9.68$, $p<0.001$). Caregivers stress also is positively correlated with age ($p<0.01$), degree of depression ($p<0.001$), monthly charges for the assistance ($p<0.001$) and the number of lost functions in the ADL ($p<0.001$); not correlation with GDS and Blessed. CONCLUSION: lost functions in the ADL ($p<0.0002$), behavioural disturbances ($p<0.0001$), psychotropic drugs use ($p<0.02$) are the main features that influence the caregiver's stress level, independently from the degree of cognitive deterioration (GDS and Blessed).

Caregiving Burden: A Comparison of Blood-Related Caregivers and Non-Blood-Related Caregivers in Korea

Hyunsook Yoon (Graduate School of Social Welfare, Hallym University, Kangwondo, Korea)

This study examines the different impact of caring - caregiving burden - for an impaired elderly in two types of adult-child caregivers: (1) blood-related caregivers (sons and daughters) and (2) non-blood-related caregivers (daughters-in law and sons-in law). The sample consisted of 264 adult-child caregivers who were providing care to elderly with functional and/or cognitive impairment. 65.50f adult-child caregivers were non-blood-related and most of them (97.1%) were daughters-in law. The results of this study indicate that caregiving experience is different according to the blood relationship of the caregiver to the elder. Specifically, non-blood-related caregivers report higher level of social burden ($t=-2.153$, $p<.032$). Caregiver's age and elder's level of cognitive impairement are important variables explaining the different level of social burden in two types of adult-child caregivers. The family cooperation is a significant predictor of the lessening four dimensions of caregiving burden (financial burden, physical burden, social burden, and emotional burden) of the non-blood-related caregivers' perception of their caregiving. The results have important implications for intervention models aimed to lessen the caregiving burden for adult-child caregivers.

Factors influencing caregiver's psychological morbidity among primary caregivers of CVA and DM discharged inpatient elders

Roger L. Amidon (Department of Health Administration School of Public Health University of South Carolina; USA) Cheng-Chieh Lin, Ming-May Lai (Department of Family Medicine, Center of Community Medicine, China Medical College Hospital, Taichung, R.O.C.), Tsai-Chung Li (Department of Medical Research, China Medical College Hospital, Taichung, R.O.C.)

In traditional society of Taiwan, taking care of elderly family members is the responsibility of younger family members. Therefore, it is important to examine the psychological morbidity of primary caregivers of elders. The study sample consisted of 121 primary caregivers of consecutive CVA or DM discharged inpatient elders in China Medical College Hospital from July, 1998 to April, 1999. Face-to-face interviews with trained interviewers were conducted to collect information about sociodemographic factors, psychological morbidity, perceive social life, and so on. The statistical analyses were mean, standard deviation, proportion, t-test, and Chi-square test. Most of them are less than 44 years old (60.0%). Forty-nine (40.5%) are male. The prevalence of psychological morbidity in this sample is 24.3%. Primary caregivers without psychological morbidity have a lower proportion of living with inpatients than those with psychological morbidity ($p<0.05$). Primary caregivers without psychological morbidity have a lower proportion of who are informal than those with psychological morbidity ($p<0.05$). Primary caregivers with psychological morbidity reported significant higher scores of perceived affected social life than those without psychological morbidity ($p<0.05$). There is a score reduction in life satisfaction among caregivers with PMPM ($p<0.001$). A significant longer duration of care is psychological morbidity ($p<0.05$). Our study identifies living with inpatients, type of caregiver, duration of care, perceived affected social life, depression, and life satisfaction are associated with psychological morbidity of primary caregivers for CVA and DM discharged inpatient elders.

Factors related to the outcome of caregiving of the impaired elderly: A longitudinal study in rural Japan.

Y. Arai (National Institute for Longevity Sciences (NILS), Japan), S. Zarit (Penn State University), M. Sugiura, M. Washio, H. Miura, K. Kudo (NILS, Japan)

This longitudinal study investigates the experiences among Japanese caregivers who provide informal care at home to the impaired elderly over 1 year. The objectives of the study are to determine if changes suggest wear and tear, adaptation, or a trait model of caregiving, and to identify factors associated with successful and unsuccessful adaptation over time. Between 1998-1999, 47 pairs of the impaired elderly and their caregivers were followed in Matsuyama Town in a rural area of northern Japan. Caregivers were interviewed initially and then again 12 months later. Findings indicated that the mean score of the Zarit Burden Interview at T2 was significantly lower than that of T1, suggesting that caregivers adapted to their role over time. Outcomes were categorized as successful and unsuccessful, depending on the pattern of change over the year's period of time. Two factors were found to be related to the outcome in univariate analyses: Caring someone with dementia, and caregiver being a spouse. Logistic regression demonstrated that caring someone with dementia was five times more likely to belong to the unsuccessful outcome while spouse caregivers were five times more likely belong to successful outcome. There was also a trend for a daughter-in-law to be more likely to have unsuccessful outcomes. The present study suggests that 1) changes in burden among caregivers in Japan are similar to those observed in most studies in the West 2), and that care of the demented elderly is particularly stressful for family members.

Social network, perceived social support and feeling of burden in family caregivers.

Acrich - Gutmann Luisa, Seidmann Susana, Stefani Dorina School of Psychology Research Department - University of Buenos Aires - Argentina

The purpose of this paper is: 1) to analyze in a critical-comparative way the differences between two groups of women family caregivers of chronically ill patients - mothers who take care of chronically ill children, and daughters who take care of chronically ill elderly parents 2) to study in each group of women caregivers the influence of the size of the network of relatives, the perceived social support and the satisfaction with that support with the feeling of burden. Different test of univariate and multivariate statistical significance were performed, such as tests of percentage differences and arithmetic mean for independent samples, ANOVA and two-factor ANOVA. Mothers differ significantly from daughters in the strong and moderate degrees of perceived social support and in the feeling of burden. Mothers show, in a higher percentage than daughters, that the responsibilities implied in the caregiving of a chronically ill child almost never negatively affect their health, their personal and social lives, their finances and their psychological well-being; while daughters show in a higher percentage than mothers that caregiving a chronically ill parent frequently affects them in a negative way. The expectations and prescriptions of the role of mother can partially explain the differences found. Mothers who are satisfied with their social support obtain significantly lower marks in the Feeling of Burden Questionnaire than those who say they are not satisfied. Satisfaction with positive emotional bonds with the members of the network would partially explain the moderating role it has when facing the caregiving of a chronically ill child.

The assessment of quality of life in primary caregivers of CVA and DM hospitalized elders

Cheng-Chieh Lin (Department of Family Medicine, Center of Community Medicine, China Medical College Hospital, Taichung, R.O.C.), Tsai-Chung Li (Department of Medical Research, China Medical College Hospital, Taichung, R.O.C.), Chia-Ing Li (Center of Community Medicine, China Medical College Hospital, China Medical College Hospital, Taichung, R.O.C.)

The aims of this study are to measure the extent to which there is a decrease in quality of life measured by Short-form 36 among primary caregivers of CVA and DM hospitalized elders and to identify the predictors that explain the variation of their reduced quality of life. The study sample consisted of 187 primary caregivers of consecutive CVA or DM hospitalized elders in China Medical College Hospital from July, 1998 to April, 2000. Face-to-face interviews with trained interviewers were conducted to collect information. The statistical analyses were t-test and multiple linear regression. The mean age of these inpatients is 46.9 years old. Sixty (32.1%) are male. Regression models estimated the reduced quality of life among their primary caregivers by comparing them to the normal population of Taiwan. After controlling for age and gender, the estimated effect of caregiving on General Health, Vitality, Role-emotional, and Mental Health scales was significantly negative, as much as a 3-10 point reduction on this 100-point scale. The estimated effect on Physical Functioning and Bodily Pain scales was significantly positive, as much as around 5 points higher. Worsened Bodily Pain of caregivers is correlated with reduced ADL and IADL in inpatients. The degree of care demand for daily living is negatively correlated with Bodily Pain, Vitality, Social Functioning, Mental Health scales. The life satisfaction is positively correlated with Vitality and Mental Health scales. Our study demonstrates that primary caregivers of hospitalized DM and CVA elders have better status of Physical Functioning and Bodily Pain and diminished quality of life in General Health, Vitality, Role-Emotional and Mental Health. The declines in quality of life could be linked to care-receivers' physical status and workload of caring.

The burden of informal care of the elderly in Hong Kong

Liu CP, Leung AC, Tsui LL, Tang WY, Li SY (Aged Care Research & Development Unit, Haven of Hope Christian Service, Haven of Hope Hospital, 8 Haven of Hope Road, Tseung Kwan O, Hong Kong)

This is to evaluate burden of informal care to community-dwelling frail elderly in Hong Kong; to identify risk factors contributing to caregiving stress; and to make recommendations for lessening the stress. This randomised controlled trial was implemented in July 2000 and 130 community-dwelling older persons age 65 and over plus their informal carers were recruited to experimental and control group respectively. Minimum Data Set- Home Care is used to examine elderly subjects¡≈ health risks, while the Cost of Care Index was to assess carers¡≈stress. Mean age of overall elderly respondents was 74.9 (SD=7.2, range=60-96), 54.6% of them were male, and 12% of them did not have carers. 145 carers were successfully interviewed, 51% of carers were spouses of care-recipients, and 44.9% were children of child-in-law. 50.4% of carers claimed that caring for the elderly has made them anxious, 48.3% felt physically fatigue, and 16.5% of carers¡≈ appetite was negatively affected. 40.7% of them perceived their care-recipients as a demanding person to care for, and 33.3% of them complained their care-recipients of trying to manipulate them. 38.6% reported that caregiving caused them to dig into savings. Logistic regression analysis reveals that care-recipients¡≈ manipulative character (OR=9.2, 95%CI=2.7-31.3), and disruption of routine in home (OR=3.4, 95%CI=1.1-10.1) attributed to carers¡≈ poor appetite. In conclusion, Informal support from family members is still an important means of care for the elderly in Hong Kong. Yet, the burden of care adversely affects caregivers and care-recipients relationship. More education and understanding of the caregiving process plus better community services support to informal carers are required to sustain this virtue.

SESSION 213

Opportunities for Learning and Healing through Art in Later Life

Frank Campbell (Instructional Media, Simon Fraser University, Vancouver, British Columbia, Canada) Rebuilding Family History with Images. Sarah Dobbs (Visual Arts Burnaby) and Cheryl Wanamaker (Burnaby Hospital, Canada) "Ribbons Of Life": An Intergenerational Visual Arts Project. Chris Mulat (Zion Park Manor, Surrey, British Columbia, Canada) Creating "Walls of Healing" in a Long Term Care Facility. Colleen Hussey (Behavior Stabilization Unit, Memorial Pavilion, Royal Jubilee Hospital, Victoria, British Columbia, Canada) Adapting Visual Arts Approaches for People with Dementia.

This symposium will demonstrate the importance and value of providing people with innovative techniques for creative expression, which are appropriate to their needs and level of ability. Each of the four presentations offers a distinctive process for involving people in exploring their own creativity. The first presenter describes his use of family photographs, stories, 8mm films, and slides to weave a visual collage that has personal meaning to the client and his family. This presentation will demystify some of the techniques used in the making of such an unusual family document and describe the healing qualities of such a project. The second presentation describes a community initiative designed to make a connection between residents of a care facility and students of the neighbourhood school. Artists worked with the students to share a variety of printmaking techniques and then, each student worked with a senior to create a work of art. The outcome of this intergenerational project is that each piece created was an expression of the resident's life, past and/or present. The next presentation details the development of a project that involved everyone associated with a long term care facility including residents, family members, staff and friends. The original idea was to decorate the interior walls of the facility in a way that was meaningful to the people who lived there. Residents' stories beginning with "I remember when" became the theme for the project. Everyone collected articles such as photographs, antiques, toys, and tools for visual displays that were created and hung throughout the facility. Each display presents a snapshot of a moment, event or activity in someone's life that everyone can share and enjoy. People with a dementing illness have special needs and considerations, which must be assessed and accommodated when designing successful art activities. This final presentation describes a series of techniques which take into account the strengths and challenges of this unique population. Assessment criteria as well as ideas for specific projects and activities will be discussed.

Adapting Visual Arts Approaches for People with Dementia

Colleen Hussey (Behavior Stabilization Unit, Memorial Pavilion, Royal Jubilee Hospital, Victoria, British Columbia, Canada)

This presentation will explore how the visual arts can be adapted when working with people with dementia. Due to the cognitive, sensory and physical deficits associated with a dementing illness, the approach to art when working with people with dementia should recognize the interests, strengths and limitations of each individual. Thus programming is often 1:1 or organized within small groups. Assessment of individual interests may consider past experiences, learning orientations (visual, etc.), and reaction to color and environment. Assessment should also include consideration of physical tolerance, verbal ability, hearing, vision and motivation. Criteria used to assess limitations may include initiation deficits, sensory and comprehension deficits, restlessness, distractibility, mood fluctuations and safety issues. Projects can then be designed with the client, allowing as much personal choice and involvement as possible. Slides will be shown of works by people with dementia clients that have enhanced or assisted as aids in their environment, or have been created for relaxation and enjoyment, or as an opportunity to give to others and receive recognition.

Creating "Walls of Healing" in a Long Term Care Facility

Chris Mulat (Zion Park Manor, Surrey, British Columbia, Canada)

Walls often conjure up images of confinement, barriers and isolation, but not the walls at Zion Park Manor, a long term care facility in Cloverdale, British Columbia. At this facility, walls are canvasses of self-expression. Upon completion of a building expansion, there were walls that were completely empty. It was decided that we would undertake a project that would help to make the environment a reflection of the residents who live there. As with any artwork, the project began with an inspiration, a myriad of thoughts. An incubation period followed, as ideas formed and developed. It was planned that the walls would come alive with theme displays, as a gallery of resident histories and life experiences. This led to months of collecting items and stories which would be used in the displays. Contributors had a sense of fulfillment and purpose as they realized that they were creating "walls of history" in their home. They were also sharing in a healing process. Many of the residents would forget about their illnesses and pain, and become lost in a discussion beginning with "I remember when". The walls of history and healing have promoted friendships and relationships as common interests are identified. In the special care unit, residents can remove articles from the display and carry them around. This ongoing project means that all residents can be involved in self-expression. Together, they are creating walls of history, by sharing their life memories with those around them. By doing this they are also sharing an healing experience.

Rebuilding Family History with Images

Frank Campbell (Instructional Media, Simon Fraser University, Vancouver, British Columbia, Canada)

When my father passed away ten years ago, I felt a need to capture images of his life for our family. It felt important to develop a sense of his life through photographic images, and be able to share his photos with his brothers and sisters in Great Britain. Given this, I developed a technique that allows people to share their stories and family memories through video art documentation. As an example of this process, a retired gentleman wanted to create a video piece that illustrated his life as a drama teacher. He contributed all his photos, 8mm film and his slides of his theatre life for the production. These various media were then transformed into one document. This proved to be very beneficial for the younger family members to learn about and come to appreciate the interesting life he had led. This presentation will demonstrate a variety of methods for capturing images such as narrating over the images, or filming in situ. The use of video for documenting family history provides an innovative and effective way for seniors to connect with family members, share their stories, and enrich relationships across the generations

"Ribbons of Life": An intergenerational visual arts project

Sarah Dobbs (Visual Arts Burnaby/Cultural Services, Burnaby, British Columbia, Canada); Cheryl Wanamaker (Burnaby Hospital, Burnaby, British Columbia, Canada)

Many seniors are institutionalized in environments that offer little visual stimulation. "Ribbons of Life" was a curatorial initiative designed to facilitate the involvement of seniors within the community in an art program that culminated in a touring exhibition. "Ribbons of Life" are works of art created by seniors and students that explore the individual history of the seniors who participated in the project. The project began in January of 2000. Four artists visited schools within Burnaby in a series of outreach programs that allowed each artist to share their techniques with the students. Some of the students were then selected to go with each artist to Burnaby Hospital's long term care facility, Cascade Residence, and meet with the seniors. Using a variety of techniques such as water-based monotype printmaking, painting and collage, the residents were then guided by artists and assisted by students in creating works of art that represented their history. Works of art were created as was a building of community and intergenerational relationships. Students and the public have been exposed to the lives of seniors-in-care and the important contributions this group has made to community. The intergenerational aspect of this project has played a key role to its success. The act of making art works increased not only the dexterity of the seniors, but also their emotional well-being by helping to alleviate the three plagues of seniors-in-care: loneliness, helplessness and boredom (Dr. Thomas' Eden Alternative). Through this initiative the public's awareness of the arts and the contribution made to the community by seniors has also increased.

SESSION 214

Diet, Oxidative Stress, Antioxidants and Aging

Alberto Boveris (Universidad de Buenos Aires, Buenos Aires, Argentina) Biology of Aging and Neurodegenerative Diseases. The Mitochondrial Theory. Virginia Junqueira (Escola Paulista de Medicina, UNIFESP, Sao Paulo, Brazil) (Dietary versus Supplemental Antioxidants in the Elderly: Why and When) Federico Leighton (Universidad Catolica de Chile, Santiago, Chile) (Effect of Vegetarian, Occidental and Mediterranean Diets, and Wine Consumption, on Oxidative DNA Damage.) Richard Weindruch (University of Wisconsin, Madison, WI, USA) (Caloric Intake, Oxidative Stress and Aging.)

This symposium presents and discusses the modulation of oxidative stress by diet, specific dietary components and antioxidant supplementation, in relationship to aging or aging related biochemical markers and chronic diseases. The mechanisms of free radical generation in mitochondria and particularly the role of NO and the gene expression profile response to oxidative stress and its response to caloric restriction will be examined as novel areas with high impact potential. Structure: The session will start with a review of the oxidative stress mitochondrial theory of aging, followed by caloric restriction, its relationship to mitochondrial function and its consequences on gene expression; DNA damage as a consequence of oxidative stress and its modification with diets and wine; and antioxidant defenses in elderly patients and its response to supplementation will close the presentations. Content: The subject will be introduced reviewing the role of mitochondria in reactive oxygen and nitrogen species generation (RO/NS) and the evidences supporting their role in aging and in the pathogenesis of neurodegenerative diseases. Then caloric restriction, capable of retarding the aging process, will be considered with special focus on gene expression changes in rat tissues, detected with oligonucleotide microarray technology. The effect in humans of several different diets, with widely different content of prooxidant and antioxidant components, will be reviewed focusing on DNA oxidative damage as a marker of oxidative stress. Finally, the reduced antioxidant mechanisms in elderly persons and their response to antioxidant supplementation will be considered. Conclusion/Anticipated Outcomes: The symposium focuses on oxidative stress and new insights on its mechanism and effects on gene expression. It is apparent that oxidative stress can be partially controlled by reduction of free radical generation (caloric restriction and diet) and by improved defenses (diet and antioxidant supplementation). DNA damage would play a key role in aging and chronic diseases and appears as a valid marker for oxidative stress. General conclusions from the data to be discussed is that the key role of mitochondria in oxidative stress is confirmed, that the aging process and the pathogenesis of chronic diseases are markedly influenced by oxidative stress and that this is a process clearly susceptible of exogenous regulation.

Biology of Aging and Neurodegenerative Diseases: The Mitochondrial Theory

A. Boveris, L. B. Valdez, S. Lores Arnaiz, S.Alvarez and L. E. Costa (Laboratory of Free Radical Biology, School of Pharmacy and Biochemistry, University of Buenos Aires, Buenos Aires, Argentina.)

The concept that mitochondria are involved in aging derives from the views of Gerschman et al. (1954) and Harman (1956) linking senescence to the injurious effects of the free radicals produced in the univalent reduction of oxygen in cell and tissues. This hypothesis is more attractive when applied to mitochondria than to cells and tissues after considering that: (a) mitochondria are the more important subcellular site of free radical production, especially considering O2- and NO; (b) O2- steady-state concentration in the mitochondrial matrix is about 5 to 10 times higher than in the cytosolic and nuclear spaces; (c) mtDNA is in close proximity to the sites of generation of the hydroxyl radical and peroxynitrite and is not protected by histones; (d) accumulation of faulty synthetized proteins might compromise energy transduction; and (e) dysfunctional mitochondria signal for lysosomal digestion and for apoptosis. During the last few years, experimental evidence has indicated that mitochondria evolve during aging to a state of oxidative stress and dysfunctionality. Mitochondrial aging by oxyradical and peroxynitrite induced damage occurs through mtDNA damage and relatively specific protein inactivation, such as adenine nucleotide translocase. This process leads to a state of dysfunctional mitochondria, which are not able to keep membrane potential and ATP synthesis. Dysfunctional mitochondria release O2-, Ca2+ and cytochrome c to the cytosol and signal for organelle digestion by primary lysosomes when the number of dysfunctional mitochondria in the cell is relatively small, or, for apoptosis, when the number of dysfunctional mitochondria in the cell is relatively large.

"Caloric Intake, Oxidative Stress and Aging"

Richard Weindruch, [University of Wisconsin, Madison, WI, USA]

PURPOSE: To discuss the relationship among caloric intake, oxidative stress and aging. METHOD: A 30-50% caloric restriction (CR) extends maximum life span and retards a broad array of pathophysiological changes in rodents. Currently, CR is being tested for its influences on the aging process in rhesus monkeys. RESULTS: In laboratory rodents, CR opposes the development of age-associated increases in oxidative stress and damage in postmitotic tissues such as skeletal muscle, heart and brain. Because these tissues are sites of prominent geriatric diseases and disorders, they likely represent critical targets for oxidative stress and damage. The recent use of oligonucleotide microarrays has provided information on the gene expression profile of aging skeletal muscle (Science 285:1390-3, 1999) and brain (Nat. Genet. 25:294-7, 2000) in mice and its alteration by CR. Aging resulted in a gene expression profile indicative of a marked stress response which was largely attenuated by CR. In rhesus monkeys, CR can be safely carried out and certain physiological effects of CR which occur in rodents (e.g, decreased blood glucose and insulin levels, improved insulin sensitivity, lowering of body temperature and oxidative damage), are also observed. There is also emerging epidemiological evidence linking lower caloric intakes to a reduced incidence of certain cancers and late-life neurodegenerative diseases. CONCLUSION: Studies in rodents are providing an improved understanding of how CR retards the aging process. The experiments in rhesus monkeys and epidemiological data are supporting the notion that CR would have similar actions in people.

Dietary vs. Supplemental Antioxidants in the Elderly: Why and When

VBC Junqueira [UNIFESP, São Paulo, Brazil], CM Almada Filho [UNIFESP, São Paulo, Brazil], M Najas [UNIFESP, São Paulo, Brazil], SC Poppe [USP, São Paulo, Brazil] and LR Ramos [UNIFESP, São Paulo, Brazil].

The purpose of this paper was to investigate the oxidative stress status in elderly people and the relation between these parameters and the dietary intake of antioxidant vitamins. Elderly subjects (90; age: 78±7) were selected by chance from the EPIDOSO population and evaluated for plasma levels of vitamin E (VTE), b-carotene (bC), vitamin C (VTC), lipid oxidation products (LPO), antioxidant enzymes, polymorphonuclear (PMNs) cells activity, and daily dietary intake of the above-mentioned vitamins. They were randomly divided (45/group) into placebo (P) and vitamin (V) group, both receiving daily, for 100 days, placebo or 800mg VTE, 2g VTC, 15mg bC, and 100mg Se. Basal levels of VTE (21.5mM), bC (0.9mM), and VTC (38mM) were found to be much lower than those of younger subjects, while the activity of glutathione peroxidase (GPx; 20.2U/gHb) and catalase (CAT; 201U/mgHb); the levels of LPO (2.74hmol/ml plasma), and PMNs oxidative burst (3.38mV/min/102cells) were found to be higher than in younger subjects. The differences found in plasma levels of vitamins couldn't be attributed to their low intake, as this population had a satisfactory intake of them. Supplementation increased the plasma levels of VTE, bC, and VTC, leading to a decrease in the activity of the measured enzymes, LPO, and PMNs oxidative burst. Data presented here are indicative of a lower absorption of the studied micronutrients, together with an adaptative increase in the measured enzymes. Supplementation restores antioxidant status, decreasing levels of lipid oxidation, and PMNs reactive species production. Financial support: FAPESP and CNPq

Effect of Vegetarian, Occidental and Mediterranean Diets, and Wine Consumption, on Oxidative DNA Damage

F. Leighton, R. Foncea, M. Espinoza, P. Strobel, D.D. Perez, O. Castillo, A. Cuevas, J. Rozowski (Molecular Basis of Chronic Diseases Program, P. Universidad Catolica de Chile, Santiago, Chile)

PURPOSE: Diet is a source of antioxidants and also of prooxidant nutrients. Markers of oxidative damage are employed to measure indirectly the intensity of the oxidative stress. Among DNA oxidation markers, 8-oxo-2'-deoxyguanosine (8-oxodG) is frequently employed. This communication presents and discuss our measurements of oxidative DNA damage in healthy volunteers receiving various diets, and the additional effect of wine supplementation. METHOD: Six groups of volunteers, n=20 each approximately, vegetarians and matched omnivorous controls plus intervention groups receiving occidental diet (high-fat), mediterranean diet, and high fat diets rich in either monounsaturated or polyunsaturated fatty acids. Intervention groups (12 weeks) were temporarily (3-4 weeks) supplemented with 240 ml/day red wine or white wine. Measurements of 8-oxodG were performed in leukocyte DNA, employing HPLC with electrochemical detection. Results are expressed as 8-oxodG/10(5)dG. Parallel measurements of plasma antioxidants and antioxidant capacity were performed. RESULTS: The average values obtained for each group varied from 4 to 18 8-oxodG per 10(5) deoxyguanosine. In summary, in addition to correlations with plasma antioxidant status, the 8-oxodG measurements show marked changes, statistically significant, as follows: Vegetarian Diet < Omnivorous Controls; Mediterranean Diet < Basal Diet <Occidental Diet; All Intervention Diets + Red Wine <<the corresponding diet; White Wine supplementation showed a small, statistically significant, reduction. CONCLUSIONS: The level of oxidative DNA damage is markedly influenced by the diet. High-fat diets increase, and mediterranean diets decrease DNA damage relative to usual diet values. Red wine supplementation decreases DNA damage values to the lowest levels observed among various dietary groups. Financial support PUC-PBMEC 1998-1999.

SESSION 215

Cerebrospinal Fluid Tau Phosphorylated At Threonne 231 is an Early Biological Marker for Alzheimers Disease and Shows Improved Disease Discrimination Over Total Tau

Raymond P. Zinkowski, Katharina Buerger, John F. DeBernardis, Daniel J. Kerkman, Cheryl B. Miller, Russel E. Kohnken, Stefan J. Teipel, Tero Tapiola4, Hiroyuki Arai, Kaj Blennow, Stanley I. Rapoport, Peter Davies, and Harald Hampel

Tau protein phosphorylation and accumulation in the form of paired helical filaments is a common pathological feature found in Alzheimer's disease (AD) brain. Total tau protein (t-tau) in cerebrospinal fluid has been reported to be elevated in AD, however its levels are also elevated in other neurodegenerative diseases as well. Hence, construction of new assays was initiated to improve the diagnostic power of tau as an AD biomarker in CSF. We have developed a new sandwich ELISA assay that detects phosphotau in CSF. In this assay, tau is captured with two backbone-directed antibodies, tau-1 and CP-27. The captured tau is detected by CP9, which is specific for tau phosphorylated at threonine 231. We have compared the diagnostic accuracy of measuring phospho-tau (p-tau231) and total tau (t-tau) in CSF obtained from AD patients, healthy controls, other neurological disorders, frontotemporal dementia, vascular dementia, Lewy Body dementia, and other dementias. For p-tau231 and t-tau, sensitivity and specificity levels were determined using Receiver Operating Characteristic (ROC) curve analysis. From sensitivity and specificity levels, the per-cent of correctly allocated cases (% assay accuracy) was calculated. CSF phospho-tau231 % Accuracy Total Tau % Accuracy AD vs. Healthy Controls AD vs. Other Dementias AD vs. Frontotemporal Dementia AD vs. Vascular Dementia AD vs. Lewy Body Dementia AD vs. Other Neurological Disorders 98.1% 80.7% 90.7% 87.3% 76.8% 94.4% 83.2% 71.1% 66.0% 84.8% 81.4% 89.9% Longitudinal studies have demonstrated a linear decrease in p-tau231 levels during the course of AD progression. T-tau was not altered over time. Preliminary data also suggests that p-tau231 may be a useful marker to detect incipient AD in patients with mild cognitive impairment. Collectively, the data suggests that CSF p-tau231 represents an AD biomarker that can be utilized to differentiate AD patients from healthy controls and other forms of dementia and has the potential to track disease progression.

Combined use of cerebrospinal fluid biomarkers in the differential and early diagnosis of dementia

E.Vanmechelen, H.Vanderstichele (Innogenetics, Ghent, Belgium), K. Blennow (University of Göteborg, Göteborg, Sweden)

Using several phospho-tau-specific antibodies in cerebrospinal fluid (CSF) studies it has been suggested that increased phosphorylated tau is a more specific marker for Alzheimer's disease (AD) than total tau. Therefore we evaluated CSF-phospho (181P) -tau and CSF-total tau (Innogenetics) with CSF-ß-amyloid (1-42) (Innogenetics) in several non-AD dementia and stroke patients with increased CSF-total tau levels. In 92 longitudinal CSF samples from 23 stroke patients, a marked increase is observed in CSF-total tau between day 2 and week 3, while CSF-phospho-tau is not significantly altered. Improved diagnostic performance of CSF-phospho-tau compared to CSF-total tau is demonstrated in comparing 80 AD patients with 69 frontotemporal dementia or 43 patients with dementia with Lewy bodies. Thus, elevated CSF-total tau is accompanied with increased CSF-phospho-tau predominantly in AD patients. The use of CSF-ß-amyloid(1-42) adds a key additional element to the differential diagnosis of dementia. Significantly decreased levels of CSF-ß-amyloid (1-42) are observed in AD (n=80) and DLB (n=43) compared to controls (n=40), while in 69 patients with FTD (median Mini-Mental State Examination score of 22), CSF-ß-amyloid (1-42) is not significantly altered. Furthermore, in a longitudinal follow-up study of 15 patients with mild cognitive impairment (early AD) who at follow-up progressed to AD with dementia, 8 of the 15 had high CSF-total tau, 6 had increased CSF-phospho-tau levels, while 14/15 showed low CSF-ß-amyloid(1-42) levels. This suggests that combining CSF-phospho-tau and CSF-total tau with CSF-ß-amyloid (1-42) is not only valuable for differential diagnosis of dementia, but could further improve the diagnosis of AD in its very early stages.

Phosphorylated tau in human cerebrospinal fluid is a diagnostic marker for Alzheimer's disease

K. Ishiguro (Mitsubishi Kasei Institute of Life Sciences, Machida, Japan), H. Ohno (Mitsubishi Chemical Corporation, Tokyo, Japan), N. Itoh (Mie University School of Medicine, Tsu, Japan), K. Urakami (Tottori University, Yonago, Japan), H. Arai (Tohoku University School of Medicine, Sendai, Japan)

Microtubule-associated protein tau in cerebrospinal fluid (CSF) has been proposed as a diagnostic marker for Alzheimer's disease (AD). However, there is overlap between AD patients and non-AD controls, and the level of total tau in CSF (CSF-total tau) is elevated not only in AD but also in certain acute neurological conditions. To improve the diagnostic accuracy, we measured phosphorylated tau in CSF (CSF-p-tau), because phosphorylated tau accumulates as pathological paired helical filaments in neurons of the AD brain. Immunoblot showed that CSF contained a 32 kDa N-terminal fragment of tau partially phosphorylated on Ser199, Thr231 and Ser235 of the human tau containing 441 amino acid residues. Based on the results, we developed a sandwich ELISA for detecting CSF-p-tau. To quantify levels of CSF-tau phosphorylated at Ser199 (CSF-p-tau199) by the sandwich ELISA, we surveyed a total of 537 CSF samples from AD (n=236), non-AD demented and non-demented diseases (n=206) and normal controls (n=95). The CSF-p-tau199 levels in the AD group were significantly elevated ($p<0.0001$) compared to those in all the other non-AD groups including acute neurological conditions such as Creutzfeldt-Jacob disease and meningoencephalitis. Receiver operating characteristics (ROC) curves demonstrated a sensitivity of 85.2% and a specificity of 85% for the CSF-p-tau199, whereas a sensitivity of 77.1% and a specificity of 77.6% for the CSF-total-tau. The elevated CSF-p-tau199 in the AD group was noted irrespective of age, severity of AD and number of ApoE4 alleles. These data indicate that the elevated CSF-p-tau level is a more specific diagnostic marker for AD.

What We Can Learn About Aging from Human Cell Cultures

Vincent J. Cristofalo (President, Lankenau Institute for Medical Research, Wynnewood, Pa. and Thomas Jefferson University, Philadelphia, Pa)

Normal fibroblast cultures derived from human tissues have a finite replicative capacity, which has been interpreted as a manifestation of cellular aging in vivo. There are a number of parallels between the phenotypes of aging cells in vivo and in vitro. In addition several studies have shown an inverse correlation between replicative life span and donor age. In all cases, however, the correlation was weak and in most, the health status of the donors was unknown. We have determined the replicative life spans of 124 fibroblast cell cultures, established from donors of different ages, who were subjects in the Baltimore longitudinal study on aging. All were healthy, according to the standards of the study, when the biopsies were taken. We found no significant correlation between replicative life span and donor age. Unfortunately, many have interpreted this finding as indicating that cell culture aging has no relevance to human aging. This is not correct on several counts. First of all, absence of evidence is not evidence of absence. It could be that we were simply unable to resolve a relationship because of the intrinsic variation. The most probable explanation of the failure to detect significant differences, however, is the result of the selection that takes place for the most vigorously growing cells during the process of establishing the culture. Thus the cells that grow to establish the culture are those with the greatest replicative potential. Our data do not preclude the existence of senescent fibroblasts in vivo. Presumably proliferating cells in vivo exist as a mosaic of cells with different replicative histories. What remains unclear is whether the process and pathway of the senescence in vitro duplicates the process in vivo. But it is not necessary that a one-to-one relationship exist between the model and the in vivo counterpart it is proposed to model for the model to be informative. We use cell culture as a heuristic model, which permits the manipulation of cellular processes which have an indisputable role in human aging. These studies allow us to understand underlying mechanisms. Several examples of studies using human cell culture in this way will be presented

SESSION 216

International Perspectives on the Meaning of Place

G. Rowles (University of Kentucky, Lexington, KY, USA) and R. Rubinstein (University of Maryland Baltimore County, Baltimore, USA) Rural-Urban Contrasts in the Meaning of Place in the Context of American Culture. M. Cattell (The Field Museum of Natural History, Chicago, IL, USA) Landscapes of People: The Meaning of Place Among the Abaluyia of Western Kenya. H. Ravdal (University of Kentucky, Lexington, KY, USA) Perspectives on the Meaning of Place in Norway. F. Oswald and H.-W. Wahl (The German Centre for Research on Ageing at the University of Heidelberg, Heidelberg, Germany) Place Attachment and the Meaning of Home in Older Adults in Germany.

Increasing concern with understanding the relationship between the meaning of place and the experience of aging has resulted in a growing literature focused on: the emotional significance of home, neighborhood and community; attachment to possessions as markers of place; the role of life experience and affinity with place; vicarious involvement in environments displaced in time and space; cosmologies of environments as sacred and spiritual spaces; and explorations of the relationship between place affiliation and well-being. This symposium explores the universality of such themes. The session is organized around four papers representing contrasting cultural perspectives from three continents. An opening presentation on the meaning of place to elders in the United States, compares findings from two decades of ethnographic research conducted independently in rural Appalachia and urban Philadelphia. The paper reveals sub-cultural diversity in expressions of place meaning within American environments. There follows a report on the meaning of place among Abaluyia farmers in Kenya. Here, the focus turns to cosmologies of place in which environments are inhabited by spirits and viewed as sacred. Land and place are imbued with prescriptive meanings related to home, ethnic identity, kinship, gender and the continuity of generations. Building on the work of architect and philosopher Christian Norberg-Schulz, a third paper considers the role of stability and permanence as distinctive elements of the contemporary cultural meaning of place to elders in Norway. A central theme is that the transformations of life (including aging) must be anchored in the durable and meaningful and that place provides a source of such anchoring. The final contribution provides a more focused perspective on a theme permeating all of the presentationsthe meaning of home and its relationship to well-being. An empirical comparative study identifies themes of physical, behavioral, cognitive, emotional and social bonding as central features of the meaning of place to elders in both eastern and western Germany. Significant time will be allocated for discussion of similarities and differences among the focal themes of the four papers. It is anticipated that one outcome of the session will be confirmation of some universal themes in the meaning of place to elders as well as identification of characteristics of place affiliation that are unique to individual cultures. While specific manifestations of the meaning of place to elders differ considerably among the four cultures considered, it is clear that place is a critical component in identity in old age, is closely linked to well-being, and deserves to be a focus of attention for policy-makers in all cultures. It is hoped that the session will provide a catalyst to further internationally comparative research in this domain.

Landscapes of People: The Meaning of Place among Abaluyia of Western Kenya

Maria G. Cattell (The Field Museum of Natural History, Chicago, US)

This paper examines the meaning of place among Abaluyia peasant farmers of western Kenya. It is based upon ongoing anthropological research begun in 1982. Data are from participant observation, field-designed formal instruments, and numerous informal and in-depth interviews. In indigenous Abaluyia cosmology, natural features of the landhills and plains, plants, trees, rocks, rivers and "the lake" (Lake Victoria)are inhabited by spirits. Certain trees, in particular, are regarded as sacred. Human features in the landscape include houses dotted over the hills and valleys, among cultivated fields and fruit trees. Land has primary utilitarian value as the chief productive resource for house-building materials, farming and animal husbandry. The land puts food on the table and cash in the pocket. Above all, land is invested with meanings related to home, ethnic identity, kinship, gender, land rights and the continuity of generations. For example, relations among husbands and wives, parents and sons, and brothers are expressed in the deployment of houses and fields in family homesteads. Home is the place where ancestors are buried, where sons inherit land from fathers and women have the right to cultivate and be buried in their husband's land. At home a person is identified by clan or other local categories; "abroad" (outside Luyialand), the same person's identity shifts to the ethnic group category of Luyia. Such complex, multivalent meanings of place figure significantly in Luyia individuals' personal and social identities and in their ties to each other and to the land.

Perspectives on the meaning of place in Norway

H. Ravdal (Sanders-Brown Center on Aging. Program in Gerontology, University of Kentucky, Lexington, KY, USA)

The purpose of this paper is to explore the meaning of place and the essence of place experiences to older persons in Norway. Architect and philosopher Christian Norberg-Schulz maintained that transformations of life must be anchored in something durable to be meaningful, and that place best represents this notion of stability and permanence. Since aging is by definition a series of transformations, and the culmination of a life of change and transition, the significance of place to older individuals has particular implications for gerontology. The paper will consider important influences on place experience such as climate, nature, traditional and regional lifeways, history, and more recent cultural influences of modernity and post-modernity. Assuming a life course approach, and centering on a discussion of pervasive values and metaphors in Norwegian life, the paper will engage the work of architect and historian Christian Norberg-Schulz and other Norwegian contemporary place-philosophers, as well as survey information provided through statistical population research (Statistics Norway). It will further incorporate life histories of older Norwegians to qualitatively illustrate how these values and metaphors affect the experience of place and expression of place meaning in late life. The selective emphasis on preservation of environment and place in present day Norwegian culture is, despite rapid change, a reflection of a national recognition of the importance of maintaining a sense of permanence and stability in the natural and built landscape. This is consequential in environmental planning pertaining to the needs of the older population today and in the future.

Place Attachment and the Meaning of Home in Older Adults in Germany

F. Oswald, H.-W. Wahl (The German Centre for Research on Ageing at the University of Heidelberg, Heidelberg, Germany)

Gerontology often focuses on objective housing conditions, intending to keep older adults independent as long as possible. Less attention has been paid to subjective experiences of home or to place attachment and its impact on autonomy and well-being. Purpose of this contribution is to present empirical data on the meaning of home among community-dwelling older adults. Subject groups included: (a) persons with versus persons without competence loss; and (b) persons living in eastern versus persons living in western Germany, i.e, exposure to different levels of home modification after reunification in 1990. Data was drawn from two studies, one with N = 126 older adults, aged 61-92 years (M = 76.4); 42 participants were in good health, 42 suffered from severe mobility impairment, and 42 were blind. A sample from another study consisted of N = 227 highly competent elders of the birth cohort 1930-1932 (66-69 years old) from a longitudinal study on adult development, half from eastern, the other half from western Germany. To empirically address the meaning of home, semi-structured in-depth interviews were conducted and transcribed. The variety of meanings ascribed to the home could be reduced to 13 detailed categories or five global categories respectively, focusing on physical, behavioural, cognitive, emotional, and social bonding. Whereas healthy participants were more appreciative of the physical aspects of the home and impaired participants emphasised the cognitive and biographical significance of the home, no differences were found regarding emotional bonding. Concerning regional differences, those who had experienced recent objective environmental change were also more attached to physical aspects of the home. Differences and similarities in the meaning of home are discussed in terms of possible adaptive mechanisms, such as coping with personal or environmental stress. Results may contribute to our understanding of how people create their everyday life at home and why they want to stay put.

Rural-Urban Contrasts in the Meaning of Place in the Context of American Culture

G. Rowles (University of Kentucky, Lexington, KY, USA) and R. Rubinstein (University of Maryland Baltimore County, Baltimore, USA)

This presentation melds insights from two independently conducted research programs, each spanning more than two decades, on the meaning of place to elders in the United States. Findings from research in small rural communities in Appalachia are compared and contrasted with insights from a similar series of studies conducted in metropolitan Philadelphiawith the objective of identifying environmentally and culturally related variations between the two settings. Both research programs employed an ethnographic approach using a variety of qualitative methods (participant observation, in-depth interviews, case studies, and indicators of place affiliation) to identify experiential components of place meaning, reveal the phenomenological meaning of specific environments to elders (e.g. home, neighborhood and community), describe processes through which places become imbued with meaning through habitation, trace the manner in which the meaning of place evolves with advancing age, explore the role of personal possessions and environmental cues in sustaining place affinity, and chart the relationship between place meaning and well-being together with the implications of such a relationship for policy and practice. Comparison of findings reveals commonality in the processes of establishing and maintaining place meaning and in the relationship of a sense of place to personal identity. However, contrasts in specific manifestations and expression of these processes are revealed between the rural and urban setting. These contrasts are shown to be a function of differing environmental and social characteristics of the two settings as well as location- and cohort-related variations in the culture of aging.

SESSION 217

Lessons from the Front Lines in Dementia Care

Nancy Gnaedinger (Consultant in Gerontology, Victoria, Canada)

The purpose of the study was to learn about the experiences and assessments of front line workers providing "client-centred care" to elderly people with dementia, in residential care facilities in British Columbia. Methods included in-depth one-to-one interviews with practice leaders in dementia care in B.C, observation of residential care facilities, and focus groups with front line workers including Care Aides, Activation Aides, Housekeepers and others. It was learned that the philosophy of client-centred care is embraced by front line workers, but the model is difficult to implement without increases in staff-to-resident ratios, some rotation of front line staff, formal involvement of front line staff in decision-making, more education in dementia and training in dementia care for all levels of staff, better leadership among both nurses and front line workers, changes in some operational realities such as the use of casual labour, and changes in the design of the built environment.

Strategies of remembering among relatives of Alzheimer Patients.

Author's name: Yair Goldberg, Social Anthropologist, Israel (from Tel Aviv University on March 1998).

Abstract: Purpose: why and how the damage (caused by Alzheimer disease) on patients' Remembering, also changes the relatives' recollections of both the Patients' image and their own. Method: Participant observation for approximately nine years. For Seven of these nine years, it also included activity in a self-help Organization established by the relatives of Alzheimer's patients. Throughout the nine years, participant observation also was employed during interviews of relatives. Results: The uncertainty generated by the damage caused by Alzheimer's disease to the memory and, hence, remembering of the patient, reveals the importance of remembering for social-negotiation processes and the influence on them in social constructions of images of patients and their relatives. Alzheimer's disease also demonstrate the reciprocal dependence between remembering and forgetting, indicating that forgetting is one of the strategies of the remembering function. Remembering and forgetting can appear dialectically. Remembering and forgetting can be dynamic: they can change because of the influences of circumstances on them. Relatives tend to forget the image of the patient, while continuing to remember themselves and their social goals. This helps in their efforts to minimize the uncertainty caused because of the damage to the patient's remembering. Conclusion: relatives of Alzheimer's patients deal with the disease. They see themselves as being harmed by the disease, even though they themselves are not ill. This linkage between uncertainty and the social construction of memory is an additional channel for building the body of Anthropological knowledge with respect to environmental- adaptation mechanisms for managing conditions of crisis and transitions.

The Social Construction of Caregiving

Joanie Sims Gould (The University of British Columbia, Vancouver, Canada) Charles Barbour (The University of British Columbia, Vancouver, Canada)

As Canada's population ages the role of the family in care of older Canadians is increasingly critical. However, to date, definitions of caregiving have had significant discrepancies, gaps and overlaps. Caregiving, although an important concept in an aging population, has no one clear definition, but multiple definitions that often fall under the general label of caregiving. Employing a critical perspective, this investigation highlights how caregiving as a socially constructed concept in gerontological literature has been defined. Using two methodologies: genealogy and discourse analysis, this investigation critiqued current gerontological research on caregiving. Two prominent themes emerged which included: 1) the medicalization of aging and age-related concepts, and 2) the concept of burden. This presentation, adopting a postmodernist theoretical orientation, will include a discussion and analysis of the social construction of caregiving with respect to the emergent themes. An alternative model of caregiving emphasizing individuality and plurality will be presented. Implications of this new model for caregivers, care receivers, policy makers and researchers will also be addressed

The social construction of caregiving in Denmark

M. Lewinter (Dept. of Sociology, U. of Copenhagen, Copenhagen Denmark)

In doing a literature review for a project on caregiving in Denmark, I found that the majority of studies in international journals dealt with informal care, while studies in Scandinavian countries dealt overwhelmingly with formal care. The analysis which will be presented at the conference argues that development of caregiving research is anchored in the nature of the welfare state of respective countries, and will examine the Danish construction of caregiving. Denmark has a liberal system of public income transfers and services that seek to support individual independence and to intervene before family resources are exhausted. Hence the development of formal care which is needs assessed and allotted across social groups. Elder care has come to mean formal care, and hence research focus on home help and nursing homes. However this focus has masked the extensive role of family members in caregiving (and their problems), which has become a serious problem as public budgets become tighter. The paper will conclude with reflections on some deleterious consequences of this social construction, for instance unjust cost transfers, increasing burden on family caregivers and conflict with some citizens' view of caregiving.

SESSION 218

A comparison of leisure constraints between Hispanic and White older adults

Richard Gitelson (Arizona State University West, Phoenix, USA) Fran Bernat (Arizona State University West, Phoenix, USA) Sara Aleman (Norhtern Arizona University, Flagstaff, USA)

Much has been written about the importance of how we approach our growing old and the implications our choices have on our mental and physical health and the quality of our lives (Rowe & Kahn, 1999). But what if the resources and opportunities are not equal. The objective of this paper was to compare two ethnic groups living in separate communities which share a common border, in terms of the following, 1) resources, 2) the types of recreation activities that the two communities of elders pursue, and 3) the constraints that impact on their recreation choices. Older adults, defined as 55 years or age or older, were sampled in three communities in Arizona. Two of the communities are age-restricted and the populations are nearly 100% white. The neighboring community is not age restricted, and although mixed in terms of ethnicity, nearly all the older individuals are of Mexican descent. The individuals in the study were asked what they did that they enjoyed and what were the constraints to participation in these activities. The results showed statistically significant differences between the two groups in terms of participation in several broad categories of leisure and the constraints they faced in engaging in these activities. The results appear to support marginality theory and the differential access model. This latter model, similar to marginality theory, posits that inequalities arise because of ... systematic, institutionalized historical and contemporary discriminatory practices based on factors such as racial characteristics, ethnic origins, social class background and gender (Taylor, 1992, p. 15-16).

Aging and Old Age; An Interdisciplinary Perspective

Elisa Dulcey-Ruiz, Graciela Mantilla, Guillermo Zapata, Myrta Muñoz, María Eugenia Gómez, Silvio Velásquez y Martha Inés Franco

A question is posed on the status of Gerontology as the study of aging and old age, around which the debate related to multi- and inter-disciplinarity turns as a mega-tendency. This point of view is illustrated with the launching of a project under the lifespan perspective, constituted by three specific lines of analysis: (1) perceptions of aging and old age, (2) conditions, styles and quality of life and (3) analysis of situations of marginalization, such as the forced movement of old people in Colombia. Studies on the perception of aging and old age carried out in Colombia from the seventies to the late nineties are analyzed. Similarly, studies on the conditions, styles and quality of life are reviewed, from the biological and psycho-social standpoints. Finally, situations of marginalization under conditions of social crisis such as the forced movement of the population being experienced in Colombia (almost two million people in the year 2000 - 5% of these being persons over 60 years old) are taken into consideration. As a conclusion it is stated that in spite of persistent marginalization situations both perception of aging and the conditions, styles and quality of life have suffered important modifications in a positive sense. The above tallies with a higher emphasis on research and on the culture of aging, which is consistent with the present accelerated aging of the Colombian population.

Cohort Changes in U.S. Racial Attitudes: 1972-1998

S. J. Cutler, N. L. Danigelis (Dept. of Sociology, University of Vermont, Burlington, VT, USA)

Using attitudes from the domain of race relations as a case study, this research examines whether sociopolitical attitudes become more conservative or rigid with aging. Data are drawn from 22 nationally representative surveys of the adult population of the United States (the National Opinion Research Center's General Social Surveys) conducted between 1972 and 1998 (N=38,116). The attitudes of four cohorts on 10 dimensions of race relations are modeled over periods ranging from 21 to 26 years using GLM with appropriate controls for composition effects. For the four cohorts as a whole, significant trends over time in a liberal direction were found on eight of the attitudinal dimensions, one trend was nonsignificant, and one was significant in a conservative direction. Year by cohort (Y x C) interaction effects were nonsignificant on seven of the eight liberal trends, indicating that attitude change occurred in a liberal direction and to approximately the same degree for each of the four cohorts. The one significant Y x C interaction effect in the presence of the overall liberal trend was due to the oldest cohort becoming more liberal at a faster rate than the youngest cohort. The significant Y x C interaction effect for the one conservative trend stemmed from the youngest cohort becoming more conservative at a faster rate than the two oldest cohorts. These findings demonstrate that attitude change with aging is prevalent among older cohorts and neither necessarily in a conservative direction nor at a slower rate than among younger cohorts.

Elder Women's Position and Demographic Change: Hypotheses on Gender and Aging in Transitional Settings

Kathryn M. Yount [Emory University, Atlanta, Georgia, USA] Harris S. Solomon [Emory University, Atlanta, Georgia, USA]

Progression of the demographic transition in less developed countries (LDCs) has triggered unprecedented population aging, with higher life expectancies of women compared to men contributing to the feminization of aging in these settings. These shifts in population structure create a practical imperative to understand the position of macro-social change on their means of social support. Unfortunately, social theories have tended to conceptualize gender and aging as separate domains or dimensions of social inequality, and have failed to integrate notions of structure, agency, and temporality into explanatory models of human behavior at the later stages of life. Attempts to develop more integrated macro-micro models of the gendered process of aging have given little heed to their application in less developed settings. This paper makes use of empirical qualitative and quantitative data from the Middle East to establish the historical bases of elder women's position in the family and their customary claims to familial support. Then, after describing the effects of specific macro-social and demographic changes on these claims, a set of hypotheses are proposed, which consider the forms of resistance and adaptation that elder women adopt to secure support during periods of physical and mental decline.

The Domestic Unit as the Key Building Block for an Aging Society

Otto von Mering (University of Florida, USA)

In the USA, the past three decades witnessed the rise of alternative, single- and multiperson living arrangements, encompassing one-to-four generations. This change is co-eval with the relative decline of the atomistic American parent-child 'household,' or so-called normative biological 'family.' Instead of this terminology, the concept of 'domestic unit' is proposed as the key behavioral building block for doing systematic and holistic research in a particular technological service industry-oriented culture. Just like a pluripotent stemcell, it captures the change-making behavioral capacity of people who, facing ordinary and exceptional life-transitions, create different structures to provide essential support, care and resource management suitable for any intentional residential life-space of kin and unrelated persons. The concept is instrumental for analyzing how domestic life ways evolve in response to the impact of current socio-political forces, particularly in "medically and socially underserved" inner city and rural areas: (1) significantly extended longevity and chronic illness; (2) notable changes in marriage, divorce and parenting patterns; (3) a growing part-time, and temporary agency-contingent workforce without permanent employer ties; (4) rapid expansion of third- and fourth-generation elders performing voluntary or low-pay shadow work and bartered services; (5) declining affordable public, employer-funded and private health and long-term care insurance. Fieldwork in Florida, together with information from the Census and CDC, NGO's like the Children's Defense Fund, OWL, Urban Institute, Fellowship for Intentional Community and National Gay and Lesbian Taskforce, document the scientific utility of the 'domestic unit' as the uniform entity for the comparative study of human living arrangements anywhere.

The Transfer of Decision Making Across the Ages

Sandra Loucks Campbell (Sheridan College, Oakville, Ontario, Canada)

There have been few studies of the power held by older adults, although authors have written about disempowerment. This initial finding gave the impetus to seek a beginning understanding of the place power plays in the lives of older adults. Based in grounded theory, non-structured interviews were conducted with a small number of individuals. Data analysis of these taped interviews resulted in the development of a game metaphor of the transfer of decision making that occurs from older to younger individuals. The study concluded with the evolution of three constructs. First, we bring expectations based on our own upbringing as children and based on our own context and reality to both our own aging process and to our relationships with others. Second, an older person gains or loses autonomy according to the amount of resources they have, the positive or negative state of their health, whether they are isolated from or integrated into society, and whether they are dependent on another for care. The individual's emotional state and fears of aging will also have an impact on the loss or gain they experience. Finally, a cross generational power struggle occurs as elders and younger people try to determine who will make the decisions about the older person's life. The conclusions of this study have led to the implementation of a comprehensive study of decision making in long term care that is currently underway.

Triple Power Blocks: Construction of Powerlessness Among Older People in Hong Kong

P.K. Kam (Department of Applied Social Studies, City University of Hong Kong, Hong Kong)

This paper presents a sociological study of the issue of powerlessness in old age. It analyses the social processes involved in the reproduction of old age powerlessness in the Chinese context. The analyses are based on the data collected from in-depth qualitative interviews with 54 Chinese older people. This study reported that a low self-image, a sense of uselessness and a lack of control over future life and a pessimistic view towards old age prevailed among older people in Hong Kong. It found that the powerlessness problem was not a natural result of old age. Three power blocks were identified as the social factors that structured the reproduction of the problem. The first one was the structural deficiencies, which were concerned with how the economic, social and political structures interplayed to condition the powerlessness situations in old age. The second one was related to the impact of the changes of Chinese culture in contemporary society, which had affected the position, status and power among older people in both family and society. The Chinese welfare ideology also had a role in sustaining or producing the powerlessness problem. The third power block was concerned with the daily interaction and power relationship between older people and socials service professionals. Disempowering professional practice was found to have a significant effect on inducing, sustaining or reinforcing the powerlessness problem. This paper also discusses the implications of the findings for policy and practice responses to address the issue of powerlessness in old age.

SESSION 219

Aging and Its Policy Implication in China

Xiaochun Qiao, Ph.D (Carolina Population Center University of North Carolina at Chapel Hill University Square, CB#8120 123 West Franklin Street Chapel Hill, North Carolina 27516-3997 USA)

Abstract: Purpose: Exploring the aging process and corresponding serious social issues in the first half of 21th century in China Method: Population projection method was used to predict the population aging in the first half of the coming century. Series of population indicators was calculated in combination with social indicators. Results: That problems of aging confronted by Chinese people in the early of 21st century will be affected by both sharp transitions of age structure and the reform of economic institution. The combination of this two part, plus the biggest magnitude of elderly population, will make the problems of aging in China more serious than any countries else where the transitions of age structure have happened. The seriousness of the problems of aging is caused by the speed and the level of aging, the change of family structure, the adaptability of traditional convention and social institution, and the power of economy of the country. The severity of the problems of aging in the new century in China will be elicited by the shrink of family scale, lack of social security and the low level of economic development. Due to the large proportion of one-child family, the traditional virtue, i.e. support and care of the elderly by family, will automatically disappear. Through the analysis of the determinant factors, we also explored the implication of the policy toward to resolving the problems, and raised that early constructing the systems of social security in both urban and rural areas are necessary and urgent. And setting up the system of social care, promoting the nursing home and reinforcing the health service are alternative means. Conclusion: The problems of aging in the new century are not only the problem of the elderly, but also the problem of the young people, and the problems of the socioeconomic development of China in the new century. This means that if the problems could not be early and sufficiently settled, it would severely affect the development of young and mid-aged people as, well as the sustainable development of China.

Declining Family Support for Older People in Ghana: Nature and Causes of Shifts in Support

I.Aboderin (International Institute on Health and Ageing, University of Bristol)

Abstract PURPOSE: Family support for older people in Ghana is declining, exposing increasing numbers of elderly to destitution and poverty. Explanations of the decline in the literature - blaming, on the one hand, modernisation and weakening norms and on the other, worsening economic strain - are conceptually and epistemologically limited, failing to provide a solid understanding of nature and causes of the decline. This study aimed to develop a fuller, interpretively grounded, understanding of the decline that illuminates the interrelationships between normative and material changes in briging it about. METHOD: In-depth interviews were used to explore three generations' experiences and attitudes regarding old age support, and their own interpretations of the current problems. The respondent sample (N=51) was selected to include older parent-adult child dyads, where possible triads with the grandchild, and a spectrum of gender, socio-economic-, and ethnic groups.RESULTS: The decline in family support was found to be underpinned by two major shifts. First, a decreasing capacity of the young to provide for the old, coupled with a fundamental priority of the needs of the young in resource allocation decisions. Second, a shift in the basis of filial support towards greater dependence on parents' past conduct and affective relationship with their children. CONCLUSION: Ultimately, these shifts and the decline are the result of a complex interaction between economic strain and modernisation. Whilst the effects of the economic crisis - some hitherto unexplored,have been the dominant force, the role of modernisation has mainly been to exacerbate their impact, in ways not so far addressed in the literature.

Filial Piety of Young and Middle-Aged Couples

Myung Cha Kim (Dept. of Home Management, Sookmyung Women's University, Seoul, Korea), Seon Young Ahn (Dept. of Home management, Sookmyung Women's university, Seoul, Korea)

The purpose of this research was to compare the filial piety between young and middle-aged couples. The sample was composed of 207 young couples who under age 35,and 196 middle-aged couples who were 40-55 years old. They had at last one parent and lived in Seoul, Korea. The main methods chosen for analyzing the data were factor analysis, paired t-test, t-test and regression analysis. The major findings were as follows: 1.The filial piety was composed of obedience, emotional support, economic support, service care, rising in the world and gaining fame, ancestor worship, maintaining one's physical health, and repaying parents according to one's circumstances. 2.The fiflial piety of the young and middle-aged husbands was significantly higher than their wives. 3.The filial piety of the middle-aged husbands and wives was significantly higher than young husbands and wives. 4.As for the regression analyssis, caregiving rewards from parents, mother's(mother's-in-law)health, father's(father's-in law)health, proximity of residence,father's age, and income were significant predictors of filial piety totally in four groups. Especially caregiving rewards was the strongest predictor commonly in four groups. So, reciprocal relationship between elderly parents and their adult childre is highly recommended. In conclusion, Korean families have maintanind filial piety still, but there differences of filial piety according to age and sex. It means that even nowadays Koreans have patriarchal familism.

Illness and weakening of friendship ties in later life

Peeter Tammeveski (Pennsylvania State University, University Park, USA)

This ethnographic study investigated changes in ethnic friendship ties upon the onset of illness induced frailty among community dwelling elderly. The participants of the study were 45 ethnic Estonians ages 75-92 who had resettled in the US as World War II refugees. The data were collected through interviews and participant observations. The results indicated that ethnic friendship ties attenuated considerably when the elderly experienced long lasting illness induced frailty. Such weakening of ethnic friendships, however, contrasted starkly to the strong ethnic community ties prior to illness. This change was linked to the concepts of nationalism, selfhood, and public/private that the elderly held. For the participants of the study, an ideal Estonian was a self- sufficient person who contributed to the ethnic group. Illness diminished one's ability to be self- sufficient and, hence, complicated the relationship of the individual with the national community. The frail Estonians were no longer able to participate in the community activities with full vigor and were reluctant to ask for assistance from their ethnic friends. The healthy, however, were cautious in offering companionship or assistance to a sick friend because illness was seen as a private matter which was not readily accessible to an outsider. The author of the study argues that the potential positive contribution of lasting friendship ties to illness experience is undermined by the existing ideologies moral self, illness, and national order.

Influence of Time on Social Preferences: Testing Socioemotional Selectivity Theory among Taiwanese and Mainland Chinese

Helene Fung (University of Alberta, Edmonton, Alberta, Canada) Phillina Lai & Rita Ng (Stanford University, Stanford, California, USA)

PURPOSE: Socioemotional selectivity theory holds that as people recognize the inevitable constraint of time imposed by mortality, their social goals change, motivating them to limit social contacts to those with whom they are emotionally close. This theory was tested among Taiwanese and Mainland Chinese. METHOD: Younger (18-35 years old) adults and older (65 years old or older) adults in Taiwan and Mainland China were asked to choose from among emotionally close and peripheral social partners in different experimentally manipulated time contexts. In addition, time perspective was measured by Carstensen and Lang (1995)’s Future Time Perspective Scale. RESULTS: As predicted, older adults in both cultures were more likely to prefer emotionally close social partners than were younger adults. Mainland Chinese, who as a group have shorter actuarial life expectancy, were more likely to prefer emotionally close social partners than were Taiwanese. These age and cultural differences were eliminated when differences in perceived time were statistically controlled for. CONCLUSION: Findings suggest that time perspective plays a role in both age and cultural differences in social preferences.

Solace to Bereaved

K.Balakrishna Moorthy (People's Action for Social Service, Tirupati, INDIA)

To provide emotional and psychological support through respite services to the Elderly People who are bereaved by the sudden death of close kith or most lovable member of the family. Gathering information about Elderly individuals who are affected by the sudden death of their close kith or most lovable family member, through a network of Volunteers established by the voluntary organsiation - People's Action Social Service (PASS), Andhra Pradesh, INDIA. The individuals will be approached by the team of organisation consisting of counsellors, psychiatrist's, and social workers. The team will approach the family members of the affected Elderly individual and counsel with the same. Efforts will be made to identify the next most approachable member of the family to maintain a sustained , affectionate relationship with the affected individual. Routine follow-up would be organized, So as to enable the affected individuals maintain a balanced psychological state. An achievement of 60% to 700ositive results were obtained through the respite services. The family is the best institution that can rehabilitate the affected older persons psychologically. And to achieve this the organsiation strives various strategies to identify and link other family members to the affected elderly individual.

The era evolution of Chinese filial piety's culture and its gerontology meaning

Wang Di ('Institute of Population Research, Hangzhou Teachers College, Hangzhou Zhejiang China) Zhou Shaoxiong (Institute of Area Culture Research, Hangzhou Teachers College, Hangzhou Wang Di)

The filial culture is one of the important contents of Chinese family ethical culture. It is said: "The monarch is courtesy and his subjects are loyal, the father is kind and the children are filial." From managing a household to managing a country, the filial culture has further influence on the stability and development of Chinese families and society. The content of Chinese filial culture develops with the era evolution. The ancient said, "Being not filial has three, without children is first." The multiplying of the family is the main assignment of filiation at that time. It shows the ancient Chinese population reproduction thoughts' characteristic. In the modem times, the family will provide for the aged because of the poor material conditions and the low social insurance. The traditional standpoint of filiation is that people bear children to prevent from the aged. It shows the cultural quality that Chinese people love the aged and provide for the aged. In the 21st century, especially in the comparatively well-off society, the filial culture has its new character. The content of the filial culture rises from the material demand to the spiritual demand. It means the aged will demand firmly the family feelings and the children comfort. The era evolution of Chinese filial culture is the adjustment and construction of the Chinese family ethical thoughts. For Gerontology, it means we will set up the new generation relationship which coordinates the aged society to ensure that the aged gains the happy family life and develops healthily.

SESSION 220

Support of older people and their family carers by using information and communication technology

M. Nolan (University College of Borås, Borås, Sweden) The EU funded ACTION project (Assisting Carers using Telematic Interventions to meet Older persons' Needs). E. Hanson (University of Sheffield, Sheffield, England), H. Berthold and B. Andersson, (University College of Borås, Borås, Sweden) Development of multimedia caring programmes. E. Hanson (University of Sheffield, Sheffield, England) User focused research methodology in R & D work. L. Magnusson (University College of Borås, Borås, Sweden), Quality of Life and information and communication technology. L. Magnusson (University College of Borås, Borås, Sweden) Critical issues regarding commercialisation.

ISSUE: The following key issues will be addressed with reference to the EU funded project, ACTION (Assisting Carers using Telematics Interventions to meet Older persons' Needs): areas of further research and development work to explore the role of ICT to enhance the quality of life and care for older people and their family carers; ways of working in partnership with frail older people and their families; development of an international collaborative network. The overall aim of the ACTION project was to enhance the independence, autonomy and quality of life of frail older people and their family carers by offering information, education and support via information and communication technology. The partner countries consisted of England, Northern Ireland, the Republic of Ireland, Portugal and Sweden. STRUCTURE AND CONTENT A. Five short presentations, as an introduction to the discussion: The EU funded ACTION project, development of multimedia caring programmes, user focused research methodology in R & D work, quality of life and information and communication technology, critical issues regarding commercialisation B. Discussion around the following topics: areas of further research and development work in the area of health and social telecare, user involvement, a way forward to meet the researcher's ethical responsibilities, taking key research outcomes to the market. CONCLUSIONS/ANTICIPATED OUTCOMES: recommendations for further research and development work in the field, innovative models for working with users, a multidisciplinary and user-focused international network to develop and support further research, development and commercialisation in the field.

Critical issues regarding commercialisation

L. Magnusson (University College of Borås, Borås, Sweden)

PURPOSE: To discuss the importance of an awareness of commercialisation as an integral part of research dissemination activities. METHOD: To present experiences from the commercialisation of products and services developed within the ACTION project (Assisting Carers using Telematics Interventions to meet Older persons' Needs). RESULTS: The following areas will be addressed during the presentation: key ethical issues such as the potential risk of conflict between the two goals, quality of life and cost effectiveness; the use of a consortium agreement as the basis for a successful co-operation; an awareness of the meaning of intellectual property rights and commercial property rights; the importance of developing a business plan at an early stage that is handled as a living document; the benefits and difficulties surrounding co-operation and collaboration with commercial partner/s or companies; the University's role and responsibilities in the commercialisation process; ICT and the health care market. CONCLUSION: Based on the experiences of the commercialisation of the ACTION project, the importance of an early awarenes of the critical issues with regard to commercialisation, including the ethical responsibilities surrounding the exploitation of the results of the project, will be emphasised.

Development of multimedia caring programmes

E. Hanson (University of Sheffield, Sheffield, England), H. Berthold and B. Andersson (University College of Borås, Borås, Sweden)

PURPOSE: The purpose of the multimedia caring programmes developed in the ACTION project (Assisting Carers using Telematics Interventions to meet Older persons' Needs) is to provide education, information and support to frail older people and their family carers in the following areas: caring in daily life, respite care services, financial information and economic support, and planning ahead. METHOD: A user-focused iterative approach was adopted to develop and test the multimedia programmes. This involved close collaboration with older people, family carers and professional carers using a variety of research methods such as interviews, focus groups, questionnaires and user trials. The development phase involved gaining detailed feedback over a period of time to develop and review the structure and content of the programmes. These were then tested in a number of care settings across the partner countries, including family carers own homes. RESULTS: Results highlight that older people and family carers found the multimedia programmes easy to learn, easy to use, informative with regard to their caring situation and enjoyable due to their multimedia format. Professional carers found the programmes highly informative with regard to local service provision and claims and benefits in their particular health care context. They also highly rated the educational content of the caring in daily life programmes due to their clear, accurate and culturally-specific material. CONCLUSION: The ACTION multimedia programmes demonstrate that older people and use of new technology sit well together if they are designed from the outset with a user perspective.

Quality of Life and information and communication technology

L. Magnusson (University College of Borås,Borås, Sweden) and E. Hanson (University of Sheffield, Sheffield, England)

PURPOSE: To explore the impact of the ACTION services on the quality of life of frail older people and their family carers. METHOD: Qualitative semi-structured interviews were carried out with frail older people and their family carers before and after the field study period. Interview data were content analyzed according to the key areas of the interview schedule. Emerging themes that highlighted core similarities and differences across the partner countries formed the focus of the analysis. RESULTS The themes were as follows: Competence Family carers explained that ACTION had helped to improve their knowledge and skills such that they were able to care more effectively for their relative; Support Participants considered that ACTION helped to reduce a sense of isolation, created a sense of presence and provided easier access to care professionals; Older people and ICT. Despite initial reservations that they would damage the system, participants' overall views after using the system were that they found it useful, simple to use and it directly benefited them in their caring situation. Early introduction to benefit novice carers. The importance of introducing ACTION early on in the caring trajectory was highlighted by novice and experienced family carers. Creating an optimal environment. Participants deemed the location of the system itself important and the most suitable location was dependent on each individual family's needs. CONCLUSIONS The results highlight the potential of user-friendly ICT to enhance the quality of everyday life of frail older people and their family carers.

The EU funded ACTION project (Assisting Carers using Telematic Interventions to meet Older persons' Needs)

M. Nolan, L. Magnusson (University College of Borås, Borås, Sweden)

PURPOSE: To provide an overview of the EU-funded project, ACTION (Assisting Carers using Telematic Interventions to meet Older persons' Needs). METHOD: In accordance with EU-funded projects, the work of ACTION was divided into five phases. During the first phase, the users' needs were identified across the partner countries. Based on these results, phase two involved developing the services i.e. programmes, video phone service and adaptation of technology, in close co-operation with the users. During phase three, the services were tested and evaluated in twenty homes, four nursing/residential homes, hospitals and health care centres. These results formed the basis for the prototype version of the ACTION services. This prototype was evaluated in phase four. The multimedia caring programmes were evaluated by 1,802 users across the project partner countries and the full services were field tested and evaluated in 39 homes and 25 professional sites, including nursing/ residential homes, hospitals and health care centres. During the final and current phase, the services are being presented and results have been disseminated in the partner countries, across Europe, North America, Australia and New Zealand. A company has been established to commercialise the services. RESULTS: This presentation will consist of showing an 11 minute video to provide an overview of the project including the ACTION services and its key benefits for users. CONCLUSIONS: The project results highlight the potential of using information and communication technology in home care. The findings also demonstrate the importance of involving users at all stages of research and development projects.

User focused research methodology in R & D work

E. Hanson (University of Sheffield, Sheffield, England)

PURPOSE The purpose of the user focused research methodology employed in the ACTION project was to ensure that the ACTION services were user friendly and acceptable for frail older people, their family carers and professional carers across the partner countries. METHOD The methodology consisted of the following: - development of local user groups in each of the partner countries and an international user advisory board to advise the research teams about the ACTION services throughout the project, - questionnaires, focus groups and interviews with users to develop the structure and content of the ACTION services, - user trials with family carers and professional carers to provide detailed feedback regarding the ACTION services, - usability and user acceptance testing of the ACTION services in the field, i.e. in a variety of care settings including family carers, own homes across the partner countries. RESULTS The ACTION services demonstrated high levels of usability and user acceptance amongst frail older people, their family carers and professional carers in each of the partner countries. Key considerations arising from the research teams experiences of working in partnership with users include: - the education and training of participants, - reciprocity with participants, including practical considerations, - positive aspects of peer support - barriers to involvement. CONCLUSION The outcome of this approach has been the development of an expert user panel consisting of older people and family carer participants from the ACTION project to provide advice and support regarding dissemination activities for further work in the field and models of commercialisation.

SESSION 221

The International Network for the Prevention of Elder Abuse (INPEA): Promoting Global Communication and Collaboration

Elizabeth Podnieks (Ryerson Polytechnic University, Toronto, Canada) Strategies to Address Elder Abuse in North America; Bridget Penhale (University of Hull, Hull, UK) Elder Abuse in Europe; Toshio Tatara (Shukutoku University, Chiba, Japan) Status of Efforts to Combat Elder Abuse in Asian Countries: An Interim Report; Lia Daichman (University of Belgrano, Buenos Aires, Argentina) International Network for the Prevention of Elder Abuse (INPEA): GENESIS; Linda Mello Machado (Candido Mendes University, Rio de Janeiro, Brazil) Elder Abuse in the Latin American Region

Since first identified as a social problem more than twenty years ago, elder abuse has become an issue of world-wide concern. The United Nations and World Health Organizations have both placed elder abuse on their agendas. At the World Congress of Gerontology (Australia 1997), the International Network for the Prevention of Elder Abuse (INPEA) was established to create a global network of national and regional organizations on elder abuse. The primary goal of INPEA is to increase society's ability, through international collaboration, to recognize and respond to the mistreatment of older people in whatever settings it occurs, so that each individual can achieve an optimal quality of life in keeping with his or her cultural values and traditions. INPEA provides a means of promoting awareness and acknowledge of the problem, dissemination of information, education and training, advocacy, research, and assistance to individual countries. With Regional Representatives on six continents, a web site and newsletter, INPEA has undertaken a program to facilitate the sharing of information on elder abuse between developed and developing countries and to promote international collaboration on elder abuse projects. The represented regions include North America, Latin America (including Mexico, Central America and the Caribbean), Europe (including the Middle East), Asia, Africa and Oceania. In 2001, the identification and development of National Representatives, whose work will be coordinated by the Regional Representatives, will be promoted. This Round Table with INPEA members, including Regional Representatives and Executives, provides an opportunity to discuss current INPEA initiatives in the development of the web site, the six regions and National Representatives. Brief presentations will be made by or on behalf of each Regional Representative and by an Executive member. Initiatives in countries and regions throughout the world, which could be replicated in other developed and developing countries, will be discussed. The interchange will draw attention to the continuum that exists from countries that have little or no awareness of elder abuse to those countries where there is active concern and involvement in relation to the abuse and neglect of older people. The group discussion will also highlight the benefits of the national and international networking that INPEA facilitates. Participants will be invited to share their vision of how elder abuse can be prevented through research, advocacy and education while working together to effect a positive change for the collective.

Elder Abuse in Europe

Bridget Penhale (University of Hull, Hull, UK)

This presentation will provide an overview concerning elder abuse in Europe. The issues and developments in relation to the European Region concerning elder abuse that have taken place in recent years will be explored. This will draw attention to the continuum that exists from countries that have little or no awareness of elder abuse to those countries where there is active concern and involvement in relation to the abuse and neglect of older people. The development of a regional network, in the face of such a diverse spectrum, will be examined. Attention will be given to a specific project that was undertaken during 2000 concerning the development of a European network as part of the organization, INPEA. The outcome of the project, and possible future developments, will be explored.

Elder Abuse in the Latin American Region

Laura Mello Machado (Candido Mendes University, Rio de Janeiro, Brazil)

By 2020, seven of the ten largest elderly populations will be living in developing countries. In Latin American countries, the elder is mainly cared for by his family. However, the government should provide social and medical support for the family to properly fulfill this role. The implementation of day-care centers, day-care hospitals, quality long-term care facilities and legislation that protects the elderly is fundamental to decrease the burden on the family. Reports from Adult Protective Services and from Public and Social Health Services lead us to assume that there is a high prevalence of elder abuse in Latin American countries; however, very little research is being carried out. The purpose of this presentation is to show research data and actions being taken throughout Latin America, in order to identify, prevent and treat elder abuse and neglect. The Latin American INPEA Regional Representative promotes the collaboration of all countries of the region in the development of creative strategies to prevent elder abuse. The planning of efficient community-based programs that help to combat elder abuse must be culturally sensitive and embrace the ethnic diversity of the region.

International Network for the Prevention of Elder Abuse (INPEA): GENESIS

Lia Daichman (University of Belgrano, Buenos Aires, Argentina)

Since first identified as a social problem more than twenty years ago, elder abuse has become a world-wide phenomenon. The 1997 World Congress of Gerontology, held in Adelaide, gave us the opportunity to highlight the issue of elder abuse. One of the Round Table sessions established the first International Network for the Prevention of Elder Abuse (INPEA). INPEA provides a means of promoting awareness and knowledge of the problem, disseminating the information, educating and training, and promoting research and assistance to individual countries. The main goal of INPEA is to increase society's ability, through international collaboration, to recognize and respond to the mistreatment of older people in whatever settings it occurs, so that each individual can achieve an optimal quality of life in keeping with his or her cultural values and traditions. Links between national findings and experiences, similarities, and differences are discussed, and possible ways to move forward will be covered. It is our commitment as gerontologists to go on working in this field, combining our efforts with other international groups that share similar interests, in the belief that this work will be an important factor to better the quality of life of the world's aging population.

Status of Efforts to Combat Elder Abuse in Asian Countries: An Interim Report

Toshio Tatara (Shukutoku University, Chiba, Japan)

The purpose of the study is to find out the nature and extent of efforts to combat elder abuse in Asian countries. A mail survey of several countries is being conducted, and additional information is being gathered through e-mail, as well. The preliminary findings show that very little has been done to address elder abuse problems in Asian countries. Many of these countries do not have definitions of elder abuse and their citizens have not yet recognized what elder abuse is and whether it is a serious social problem.

Strategies to Address Elder Abuse in North America

Elizabeth Podnieks (Ryerson Polytechnic University, Toronto, Canada)

It has been estimated that four to ten percent of seniors in North America will experience one or more forms of abuse or neglect at some point in their later years. The North America Region of the International Network for the Prevention of Elder Abuse (INPEA) has focused on the dissemination of information about abuse, effective treatment approaches and program development. The membership has worked collaboratively to understand the nature and scope of elder mistreatment, develop models of intervention, increase public awareness, educate the public and government and train professionals. Much has been accomplished through local, regional, national and international conferences and through professional meetings and publication. This presentation will address current initiatives in Canada and the United States, which could be replicated in other developed and developing countries. Participants will be invited to share their vision of how elder abuse can be prevented through research, advocacy and education while working together to effect a change for the collective.

SESSION 222

Strategies To Meet Emerging Demands for Eldercare in Developing and Developed Countries

Phoebe S. Liebig, (Gerontology and Public Administration, Leonard Davis School of Gerontology ,University of Southern California, Andrus Gerontology Center, Los Angeles, California 90089-0191 USA). U.S. Strategies for Elder Care. D. Jamuna, (Asst. Centre for Research on Ageing, Dept. of Psychology, Sri Venkateswara University, TIRUPATI-517 502 A.P) Strategies to Meet the Caregiving Needs of the Elderly in India. Sung Jae Choi (Seoul National University, Department of Social Welfare, Seoul, 151-742, South Korea). Elder Care issues in Korea. Monica Fereira, (HSRC / UCT Centre for Gerontology, University of Cape town, Cape Town, Observatory 7925, SOUTH AFRICA.). African-grown elder care strategies in a changing South Africa. Sujatha Ramamurti (Division of Nutrition & Dietetics, Dept. of Home science, Sri Venkateswara University, TIRUPATI - 517 502. India.) Strategies to Meet the Nutritional Needs of the Elderly in India. R.M. Gutmann, Strategies to Meet Emerging Demands for Eldercare in Argentina.

The world is greying, but more so Asia and other developing countries where the bulk of the elderly are going to be in the coming decades. Demographic and epidemiologic transitions are pushing up the life expectation (at birth) of individuals leading to the prolongation of the older years. While the developed countries on the one hand (where this process has already taken place) are facing one type of problems eg, high cost of social security and inadequate social and familial supports, the developing countries on the other hand are confronting another type of problem eg, absence of adequate provisions of social security by the State. In view of their own national priorities, the developing countries, with their formidable (and yet growing) numbers of the elderly needing assistance, can ill afford to finance a State owned social security system (as it would take a lions share of the national budget). The joint/extended family, the traditional care provider for the elderly in most developing countries, is being torn asunder by the ravages of modernisation, urbanisation and migration, gradually shifting the responsibility of elder care to oneself/spouse or the State. Thus, many traditional cultures are facing the dilemma of whether to revive and refurbish the family (parent-adult married children conglomerate) as primary care providers or in the alternative to allow the caregiving go the way of the developed west that emphasizes self / spouse care and state care (instead of care by adult married children). May be, the developing countries could take a lesson or two from the experience of the developed countries to fashion their own policy. Not of less importance in this context is the objective of promoting a healthy, disability free longevity, which would reduce the burden of intensive elder care by the family or the State. Otherwise, it would become a stupendous task for the populous developing countries steeped in poverty and poor hygiene. The foregoing are issues that would need to be urgently addressed at some length in the context of changing socio-economic and cultural milieu of the countries concerned. In the light of these considerations, the expected outcomes of this symposium are: 1. To highlight the implications of the demographic and epidemiological transitions in the developing and developed countries for elder care. 2. To appreciate the commonalties and differences among the experiences of the developed and developing countries in the context of existing policies on elder care. 3. To consider possible strategic interventions to improve the overall quality of life of the elderly within the constraints of the culture of the countries concerned.

African-grown elder-care strategies in a changing South Africa

M. Ferreira (Institute of Ageing in Africa, University of Cape Town, CT, South Africa)

South Africa's older population (60+ years) of 2.7 million is projected to more than triple by 2050. The effects of demographic and epidemiological transitions, specifically the consequences of urbanisation and the HIV/AIDS epidemic, increasingly impact older South Africans, resulting in a growing demand for health and social care for this population. Despite these imperatives, older persons have been marginalised in policies of the new African National Congress-led government, in favour of children and youth. The government's health and social welfare policy response systems, as well as the roles and capacity of non-governmental organisations and African families to provide elder care in the future are examined. Selected traditional, or non-formal best practices are reviewed, as feasible, African-grown solutions to the care needs of increasingly vulnerable numbers of older persons, within a context of deepening poverty, dwindling resources and competing demands, normative in developing and thus African countries.

Strategies To Meet Emerging Demands for Eldercare in Argentina

GUTMANN, Ramon M. - Secretariat for Social Promotion - Government of the City of Buenos Aires

The purpose of this presentation is to show the achievements as well as the permanent difficulties in planning and delivering programs devoted to the care and protection of the elderly in Argentina. This is a result of the complex situation that puts Argentina in a special position within Latin America. It is necessary to discriminate the social variables that make this country a heterogeneous one with both rich and very poor regions. The federal and the local political authorities sometimes maintain strong controversies. As a result there is a deterioration in the situation of the elderly population. The conclusion is that taking into account a) the general conditions of globalization in the region b) the permanent controversies and the lack of continuity in policies for the elderly c) the diminishing number of adult children taking care of an increasing number of older adult parents d) the insufficient budget the federal and some local governments dedicate to programs for the elderly, the general situation of the elderly is likely to become worse. The empowerment of the Seniors' Organizations may guarantee to some extent a limited number of changes in this field.

Strategies to Meet the Care giving Needs of the Elderly in India

D. Jamuna (Centre for Research on Ageing, Dept. of Psychology, S.V. University, Tirupati Δ 517 502, INDIA.)

This presentation focuses on the status of care giving in India with an objective to suggest some strategies to meet the emerging demands of elder care. As a result of the impact of socio-cultural and technological changes and in view of demographic and epidemiological transition, the elder care scenario is fast dwindling. In the absence of formal care services and in view of poor social security measures, the elder care needs are not being met adequately. On the basis of various surveys conducted on a sample of 1,480 adult carers and elderly men and women, it was found that there is a shift in stance in the attitude towards elder care. A majority perceived care giving as burdensome and pointed out the need for alternative care services, especially respite care and home help services. Keeping the findings in view strategies on elder care suitable to the context are suggested.

U.S. Strategies for Elder Care

P.S. Liebig (Andrus Gerontology Center, University of Southern California, Los Angeles, USA)

U.S. eldercare strategies are shaped by the demographics of aging, especially of the "baby boomers," and by social and political values: individualism, self-reliance and reluctant welfare statism. Non-governmental solutions, with a heavy reliance on for-profits, are preferred, as is devolution to state and local governments. Evolving from this context, aging policies have been designed primarily to foster the independence of elders via social insurance (e.g. Social Security), limited social services (meals), means-tested/income-tested programs for income, health and housing, and tax credits to induce retirement savings, homeownership, long-term care insurance purchase, etc.—unique among developed nations. Self-care, until the aged can no longer fend for themselves, and then institutionalization, has been the dominant paradigm. Thus, despite a growing recognition over the past two decades of the vital roles played by informal caregivers, U.S. policies and programs have seldom focused on sustaining elders within the family context or supporting family caregivers financially or practically. Some (e.g, local zoning against granny flats) have actually been "anti-family" or resulted in age-segregation (e.g, senior housing). However, in the past decade, a new four-pronged strategy has emerged: 1) a greater willingness to pay family givers (although generally not spouses); 2) tax credits for family caregivers; 3) enhanced development of home- and community-based services to help elders and their families; and 4) this past year (2000) the enactment of a $125 million national caregiver initiative that will provide direct services (e.g, respite, counseling) to family caregivers. While these changes mean U.S. aging policies have become more family-centered, the value of independence remains key. This contrasts with aging policies and programs in Asian nations that enhance family caregiving roles, e.g, co-residence housing incentives, day care, so that age-segregation and social isolation are avoided. Mutual lessons to be learned are emphasized.

SESSION 223

An Experimental Study on a Care-Management Hospital Discharge Pattern

ML.Perälä,T.Hammar,A.Noro,P.Pöyry,P.Rissanen,J.Teperi (National Research and Development Centre for Welfare and Health, STAKES)

PURPOSE: The focus of this study is patients hospital discharge practices, seamless co-operation between home services and hospitals and between primary health care and social services. A new working pattern for patient discharge from hospital was developed as a part of the research project Integrated Services in the Practice of Discharge to eliminate the shortcomings in patient transitions and home care services. The aim of this study is to evaluate the impact of the working pattern from patients informal caregivers and staffs points of view. METHOD:The new working pattern will be implemented in the home help and home nursing by action research. Its impact will be evaluated in a controlled study, which involves 22 elected pair of municipality-hospital randomly assigned between experiment and comparison group. The patients will be selected using inclusion and exclusion criteria. The data will be gathered through interviews with patients, questionnaires sent to informal caregivers and staff, and documents. Evaluation elements are connected with patients managing at home and the quality of life, informal caregivers care burden and staff job satisfaction, and quality, accessibility and costs of services. The baseline measurement will be carried out in the beginning of 2000, after which the implementation of the new working pattern will be started in the experiment group. When the new working pattern is established (1 year) the follow-up measurements for the patients will be started in 2002.

Falling short of the mark: Tales of life after hospital discharge

LeClerc, Chantale Marie, RN, (St. Michael's Hospital, Toronto,

Ontario, Canada) Wells, Donna L, RN, (University of Toronto, Toronto, Ontario, Canada) Craig, Dorothy, RN, (University of Toronto, Toronto, Ontario, Canada) Wilson, Jean L, RN, (St. Michael's Hospital, Toronto, Ontario, Canada) Holmes, Carol, RN, GNC(C) (Toronto Rehabilitation Institute, Toronto, Ontario, Canada) Waldburger, Beth, RN, BScN (Toronto Community Care Access Centre, Toronto, Ontario, Canada)

PURPOSE: The purpose of this qualitative, descriptive study was to explore the every day issues, challenges, struggles and needs of elderly, community-dwelling women in the first weeks post hospital discharge. METHODS: Over the course of 11 months, 14 elderly women were recruited into the study from an acute-care hospital and a Community Care Access Centre in Metropolitan Toronto. After having signed a written consent, the women were interviewed in their homes 6 to 8 weeks following hospital discharge. In addition, using a method based on photo novella or photovoice, 4 of the women took photographs of their every day lives. These photos were used as triggers during the interviews. The interviews were content analyzed to identify the themes and patterns of the women's experiences. RESULTS: The overarching theme was that formal hospital discharge plans Fall Short of the Mark because they failed to reflect the complexity of the post-hospitalization experience by focusing primarily on very basic physical and medically related needs. However, life post-discharge was characterized by intense physical and emotional struggles. Furthermore, plans were reductionistic because hospital professionals framed the plans in the context of the acute illness and not the reality of the women's post-discharge recovery. CONCLUSIONS: The results of this study highlight the needs to improve hospital discharge planning and to rethink the nature of home care services. However, recommendations will not impact on the situation unless we also begin valuing our elders by engaging in discourse with them around their needs, wants, struggles and challenges.

Implications of the Transfer of Specialized Care to Patients and Caregivers after Hospital Discharge in Quebec

N. Guberman, E, Gagnon (Direction de la santé publique, Québec), D. Côté (Université du Québec à Hull, Québec), C. Gilbert (Université du Québec à Chicoutimi), N. Thivièrge (Université du Québec à Rimouski), M. Tremblay (Université du Québec à Chicoutimi).

The transfer of specialized care to the home following hospital release is an integral part of the restructuring of health services in most Western countries. A Quebec study of patients from five sectors with reduced hospital stay: antibiotherapy by intravenous, hip fractures, pulmonary disease, strokes and palliative care, examined the division of responsibilities for this care between patients, caregivers and home care professionals, and the rational underlying this division, from the perspectives of both patients and professionals. Based on 120 qualitative interviews with patients and/or caregivers (majority over 65) and 15 focus groups with home care and hospital professionals in five regions of Quebec, this study reveals that many specialized professional acts are being transferred to patients and caregivers from a perspective of promoting self-care and patient autonomy. If for some patients the opportunity to assume these activities is seen as a gain in independence, others consider it an obligation for which they are ill-prepared and incompetent, leading to feelings of anxiety and insecurity. These are reinforced by a perception of insufficient supervision and emergency services. As well, lack of consideration in the transfer process of the specific context and conditions of the home as a place of care reinforces these negative experiences. This suggests that more attention be given to patient/caregiver preparation for the realities of care in the home environment before and after hospital discharge, and to reviewing current supervisory and emergency measures. To achieve this, hospital and home care professionals need to better understand the self-care experience from the patients' perspective.

Older people as partners in research

J Reed (Centre for Care of Older People, University of Northumbria, UK)

The purpose of the study was to investigate discharge from hospital, and identify potential startegies for improvement. Method - Appreciative Inquiry interviews were carried out by a group of 37 professionals and older people with different organisations to find out what their experiences of good practice were. The interviewers participated in a training programme, and were supported and advised throughout by the project team. Results, several key factors in good discharge practice were identified, including the need for inter-agency communication, and the interviewers developed action plans to take these forward. Conclusion The inclusion of older people as research partners enhanced the study, but also required support and planning from the project team. This will be further discussed.

SYSTEMATIC REVIEW OF DISCHARGE ARRANGEMENTS FOR OLDER PEOPLE: INTERVENTION CHARACTERISTICS AND EFFECTS

S G PARKER (University of Sheffield, Sheffield, UK) S M PEET, A MCPHERSON, A M CANNABY R BAKER, A WILSON, J LINDESAY, G PARKER, K ABRAMS, D R JONES (University of Leicester, Leicester, UK)

PURPOSE We performed a systematic review of randomised controlled trials (RCTs) to test the hypothesis that the outcome of hospital discharge procedures for older people can be improved by intervention. METHODS A systematic literature review and meta-analysis was performed using standard methods (NHS Centre for Reviews and Dissemination CRD Report No.4 1996.) including dual independent appraisal and data extraction. The search strategy was designed to provide a comprehensive retrieval of RCTs of interventions to improve the discharge from hospital of older people. RESULTS Final synthesis used data from 56 RCTs in which a total of 16985 subjects had been randomised to a discharge arrangement (8621) or control (8364). Overall no significant effect on was seen on mortality at 3, 6 or 12 months or length of stay. Risk of readmission to hospital was significantly reduced by intervention with a relative risk reduction of 17.5% ($p=0.001$). This effect was observed in interventions provided by a single professional or a team and was most apparent in interventions provided both in hospital and in the patients home (20.5%, $p=0.02$). However, analysis by specific service types (discharge planning, comprehensive geriatric assessment or discharge support arrangements) did not show this effect. CONCLUSION The evidence from these trials does not suggest that discharge arrangements have effects on mortality or length of hospital stay, but supports the concept that arrangements for discharging older people from hospital can have beneficial effects on subsequent readmission rates. The review does not support the choice of a specific service model.

Uniform data sets and co-morbidity analysis in post acute care

S. Arino, F. Martinez, E. Valles, and A.Salva.

Outcomes assessment becomes paramount in any evidence based health care system and systematic analysis from high quality uniform data set, based on comprehensive geriatric assessment, could contribute to do so. Accurate identification of co morbid conditions and its relative importance on medical outcomes are essential in assessing patient's health status and quantifying risk of adverse results. PURPOSE: The aim of this work is to explore the behaviour of co morbidity in the post acute care setting assessed with a crosswalk Charlson index developed from the Resident Assessment Instrument's Minimum Data Set. METHOD: Patients admitted to all Public Geriatric Post Acute Care Units in Catalunya (Spain) during January 1999 - September 1999 were studied using and adapted version of the RAI v1 and RUG III instrument. RESULTS: A total of 2691 assessments were analysed. Sixty three percent were female patients, mean age 77 ± 10.8. Main diagnosis on admission was fracture of femur (22% cases) followed by CVA (18.2% cases). Mean MDS-Charlson index 5.6 ± 2.2, being cardiovascular co morbidity the most common . Baseline characteristics RUGIII-ADL index on admission 9±4.8. Cognitive Performance Scale 1.8±2, mean length of stay 49±43.3 and in-hospital mortality 8%. CONCLUSION: Dependency on activities of daily living, poor cognitive performance scale, higher resource consumption and in-hospital mortality were associated with higher MDS-Charlson index. Co morbidity accounts to explain variation across the above outcome variables, therefore control for various levels of co morbid illness in post acute care will be needed.

SESSION 224

A criticism of Wood schedule: a gerontologic reasoning

Marie-Pierre LABERNADIE, Bertrand PLACINES, Pierre DUBOE (Centre de Gérontologie de Pontacq-Nay , 64800 Nay , France)

Is the Wood schedule applicable in geriatry? The wood schedule associates to the deficiency of an organ a functional inability , wich generated a handicap in the social life . This reasoning is interesting in rehabilitation notably when only one causal factor is in reason and internes . On the other hand , the geriatrics is characterized by a polypathology and this schedule presents some limits . It is possible to propose the following reasoning: the polypathology , generating has loss of autonomy wich product of the dependence schedule . The polypathology can be landed by the theory of J.P.Bouchon wich associates 3 propositions: first , the ageing altered not the working of an organ but his functional reserves; second, the decompensation of an organ reaches his own functional reserves; third , the decompensation of one organ decompensated others organs . The autonomy maybe appreciated by the theories of self-organizing system and notably the on F.Varela with 2 notions: the physical autonomy with the enactive function and the psychic autonomy understood like being the decisional capacity of the subject to interact in this environment . The dependence is defined by the theory of A.Memmi , like a restricting relation accepted or not with the being , an object , a group , a real or ideal institution which are a matter for the need satisfaction . This proposition of reasoning geriatric permits to fear the set of the intervening factors in gerontology . Some decisional processes can be elaborated from this modelling.

A multimedia computer program for measuring functional ability in the elderly.

James C. Wall (University of South Alabama, Mobile, U.S.A.)

PURPOSE: The purpose was to develop a tool that therapists could use to measure functional abilities in elderly subjects. A computer program was written to collect data (using the mouse button for input), calculate and store the results. The program will also graph the results alongside data obtained from non-impaired subjects. The program includes multimedia instructions on data collection and analysis. METHOD: The timed up and go test, which was developed to assess fall risk in the elderly, requires the subject to rise from a sitting position, walk three meters, turn around and return to their original sitting position. This test is included in the program together with an expanded version that allows the individual tasks within the test to be timed. The modified test has the patient walk in one direction at a comfortable speed while returning at a fast walking speed. During these walks stride times and walking speeds are measured. Step times while turning are also measured. If the test is videotaped then the program may also be used to determine the durations of foot/floor contact. All of these measurements have been shown to be useful in determining those at risk of falling. RESULTS: A study of non-impaired young and elderly subjects, has produced reliable and valid results that have been incorporated into the program as baseline data. CONCLUSION: The program allows therapists to objectively measure functional abilities in an economical way. The approach may also be used to measure other functional tasks such as ascending and descending stairs or other activities of daily living.

Coping with activities of daily living in different care settings in Finland

Laukkanen (Health Centre of the City of Jyväskylä); Karppi, P,M.D.(Head of Geriatric UnitCentral Finland Health Care District); Heikkinen, E,M.D (Department of Health Sciences and The Finnish Centre for Interdisciplinary Gerontology); Kauppinen, M, (Statistician The Finnish Centre for Interdisciplinary Gerontology)

PURPOSE: To measure the functional capacity of elderly people cared for in different health and welfare care settings in Fin and, with functional capacity defined in terms of coping with activities of daily living. METHOD: Subjects were all elderly (65 or over) cl ents (N=5652) of health centre hospitals, nursing homes, and home nursing and home help services in Central Finland. Coping with activities of daily living (ADL) was measured with the Evergreen ADL index, which comprises nine physical activities of daily living (PADL) and nine instrumental activities of daily living (IADL). Results: Assessments of functional capacity were obtained for virtually all subjects: only 33 (0.6%) forms were returned with incomplete data. The mean ADL sum score (range 0-54) was lowest for women receiving home nursing (17.3), and highest for women in long term care at health centre hospitals (48.4). Age showed no association with the mean ADL sum score in any of the care settings. Conclusion: The Evergreen ADL index was easy to use and successfully distinguished between clients in different care settings. It seems that policies of assigning clients to different settings are sound and sensible because the main defining criterion was their level of functional capacity rather than their age.

Functional Autonomy Measurement System: Developement of a social subscale

Pinsonnault, Eugenie (Gerontology and geriatrics research centre, Sherbrooke Geriatric University Institute, Sherbrooke, Quebec, Canada). Desrosiers, Johanne (Gerontology and geriatrics research centre, Sherbrooke Geriatric University Institute, Sherbrooke, Quebec, Canada). Kalfat, Hadj (Association Audoise Sociale et Médicale, Limoux, France). Dubuc, Nicole (Gerontology and geriatrics research centre, Sherbrooke Geriatric University Institute, Sherbrooke, Quebec, Canada). Delli-Colli, Nathalie (Sherbrooke Geriatric University Institute, Sherbrooke, Quebec, Canada) Colvez, Alain (INSERM unité 500, Montpellier, France)

PURPOSE: Aging is accompanied by psychological, sociological and biological vulnerability which can result in the loss of functional autonomy. To plan the best care, it is important to assess the level of functional autonomy. The Functional Autonomy Measurement System (SMAF) was developed to measure functional ability through five subscales (ADL, mobility, communication, mental functions and IADL); however, it does not assess social functioning. This presentation will describe the procedures followed to develop a social subscale of the SMAF and verify its interrater reliability. METHOD: The social functioning subscale was developed from the input of a panel of experts in Quebec and France, through focus groups and nominal groups. The interrater reliability study was also carried out in Quebec and France. Seventy-eight older people presenting a decrease in functiona autonomy were assessed twice by a nurse and a graduate student. RESULTS: With the data from the panel, the experts were able to clarify the definition of social functioning and the factors involved. From the nominal groups’ results, six social items were constructed (activities, relationship, resources, respect for others, roles and self-expression). The results of the interrater reliability study showed a percentage agreement of 60 0.000000or the subscale and between 47% (social activities) and 81% (respect for others) for the individual items. An intraclass correlation coefficient of 0.70 was obtained. After this first study, the new scale was modified to improve and clarify the wording for each item. The reliability of this modified scale is presently under study. CONCLUSION: The new scale will contribute to a more comprehensive evaluation of functional independence in older people. *Supported by the FRSQ France-Quebec co-operation program on aging

Measuring physical function in frail older people: self report versus physical performance measures

Caroline Stretton (Clinical Trials Research Unit, University of Auckland, Auckland, New Zealand), Nancy Latham (Clinical Trials Research Unit, University of Auckland, Auckland, New Zealand), Arier Lee (Clinical Trials Research Unit, University of Auckland, Auckland, New Zealand), Anne Moseley (Rehabilitation Studies Unit, University of Sydney, Sydney, Australia), Ian Cameron (Rehabilitation Studies Unit, University of Sydney, Sydney, Australia), Craig Anderson (Clinical Trials Research Unit, University of Auckland, Auckland, New Zealand)

PURPOSE: To compare two approaches to assessing physical function in older people: motor performance measures and self-reported health-related quality of life. Both approaches measure physical function along an activity continuum, but the relationship between the two has not been well established. METHOD: As part of a large pragmatic, multicentre, randomised controlled trial of strength training and vitamin D supplementation to improve physical disability in older people, we assessed the relationship between direct physical performance and health-related quality of life in the first 60 randomised subjects. Physical function was assessed at baseline, and at 3 and 6 months post-randomisation and included four motor performance measures (isometric quadriceps strength, timed Up-and-Go, gait speed and the Berg Balance Scale) and a variety of self-report measures, including the Physical Component Summary measure (PCS) and the Physical Functioning sub-scale (PF) of the SF-36. RESULTS: As assessed by Spearman's rank correlation coefficients, there was a weakly significant association of motor performance to the PCS. However, motor performance, cognition and self-efficacy predicted only 400f the total variability of the PCS in a multivariate regression model. In contrast, motor performance was strongly correlated with the PF of the SF-36, and the same covariates predicted about 700f variability of PF. CONCLUSION: Motor performance and self-report measures assess related dimensions of physical health. Psychosocial factors including patient self-efficacy and cognition are important additional determinants of health-related quality of life in older people.

Self-Reported Health Status of Older Adults at Risk for Functional Decline

M.Whitridge, Homecare (Calgary Regional Health Authority, Alberta, Canada), E.Valge (Valge Health Management Consulting, Alberta, Canada)

PURPOSE: Self-reported health is a determinant of survival and predictor of use of health services. The purpose of this study was to a) examine what self-rated health means to older adults at risk of functional decline and b) explore the relationships between an objective measure of health and health risk, (i.e. Risk Indicator Tool (RIT)) and self-reported ratings of health. METHOD: Participants (N=14, mean age= 75) were community dwelling, cognitively intact seniors on Home Care, at risk of functional decline. Qualitative interviews were completed within seven days of their RIT assessment. Audiotaped transcripts were thematically analyzed using qualitative software (NUD*ist(c)). RESULTS: Self-reported health was comparable to objective ratings assessed with the RIT. However some aspects of emotional and physical health were not accounted for on the RIT. Participants described their health in relation to themselves not to their cohorts. Many described health as taken for granted or as expected for their age. Emotional aspects of health included the importance of a positive attitude, supportive social interactions and functional independence in their chosen environments. The meaningfulness of the terms health and health risk were challenging for participants and they found it difficult to put a numerical value on their status of health and health risk. CONCLUSIONS: Our findings are consistent with the self-rated health literature. Responses of participants confirmed the multidimensional nature of health and the importance of context in narrative discussions about health and health risk, particularly with older adults. Respondents in our study may have been affected by ill health, functional consequences and experience with health care providers

Using Life-Space to Assess Mobility

P.S. Baker, E. V. Bodner, R. M. Allman. (Center for Aging, University of Alabama at Birmingham and the VA Medical Center, Birmingham, AL, USA)

PURPOSE: Life-space, a spatial measure of mobility, is the area through which persons routinely and purposely move. The UAB Study of Aging Life-Space Assessment incorporates frequency, extent, and independence of movement. The correlation of seven scoring methods with self-reported function and observed physical performance and one-week test/retest reliability of the Life-Space Assessment is evaluated. METHODS: Medicare beneficiaries from 5 central Alabama counties were interviewed in their homes in 1999-00. Functional measures included LS, ranging from 0 (room-bound) to 5 (unlimited movement), a composite physical performance measure (PPM), the physical component score of the SF12 (PCS), ADLs, and IADLs. Telephone interviews were made 1-2 weeks after the baseline interview. RESULTS: The sample (N=321; mean age 75.1, SD=1.5) was 46% rural, 42% African American, 47% male; 25% had incomes <\$8000/yr.; 18% reported education < 6th grade. For all scoring methods, baseline and 1-2 week follow-up LS correlations >0.9 (p<.01). Maximal LS, distance attained with assistance, correlated only with PPM (.2). All other measures of LS significantly correlated with PPM (range 0.5-0.6); PCS (range 0.3-0.5); ADLs (-0.3-.4); IADLs (-0.3-0.4) (p<.001 for all). Highest correlations were for the LS measure incorporating all attributes of mobility, and measures of LS level attained without assistance. CONCLUSIONS: Life-space correlates with self reported function and observed physical performance. It is stable over a one week period. A simple dichotomous measure of independent life-space may be as useful as the most complex for baseline assessments. Longitudinal assessments will establish the best scoring method to detect change in mobility.

SESSION 226

Mental Health Disorders of the Elderly in India

Bela Shah and Ravinder Singh (Indian Council of Medical Research, New Delhi, India)

Ageing as a phenomenon, and its accompanied changes in the mental status of the aged has been traditionally well recognized in India. However, it is only in the last two decades that focused research on mental health disorders of the elderly has been undertaken. This paper presents the observations made in some landmark studies on the mental health status of the elderly in India, and describes in details the research undertaken by the Indian Council of Medical Research on the psychiatric disorders of the elderly. In one of the earliest Indian studies, the prevalence of mental illness in outpatients aged fifty and above was reported to be 50 per1000. In another study conducted amongst the rural population in South India the prevalence rate of mental morbidity was observed to be 89 per1000 amongst the aged. In one of the first major studies by the Indian Council of Medical Research (ICMR) on "Problems of aged seeking psychiatric help, it was observed that 43% of the hospital based study group suffered from depressive illness. The prevalence rate of mental morbidity observed was 59 per 1000. Depression was twice as frequent as mania. -Based on ICMR's "Severe Mental Morbidity Survey", it was estimated (1996) that 1.2 million of elderly in a rural population were suffering from mental illnesses. In a study on "Gero-Psychiatric Morbidity" conducted by ICMR in Uttar Pradesh, psychiatric morbidity was found to be 42.2% in geriatric group as compared to 3.97% in non geriatric group. Psychiatric illness in the elderly above 80 years was twice as much as in those aged 60-80 years. In hospital based screening programmes conducted at New Delhi, approximately 13.5% of elderly attending Geriatric Clinic at a tertiary hospital were reported to be suffering from mental problems, depression being major problem. As is evident from the various studies conducted all over India, mental health service delivery needs to be strengthened and streamlined. Future research should include this as a priority.

Mental Health Issues Among Residents of the Homes for the Elderly in Jakarta

Tony Setiabudhi PhD. (Trisakti Medical School/ Indonesian Society of Gerontology Jakarta/ Indonesia)

During the preparation on celebrating the International Year of Older Persons/ IYOP 1999); several activities were carried out in Indonesia e.g. Setting up the Collaboration of Homes of the Elderly/ Association of the Homes of the Elderly in Jakarta. This momentum was initiated by a join cooperation between Jakarta Communication Forum of the Elderly and HelpAge Indonesia (Yayasan Emong Lansia). This event was exposed in 1998 and Mr. Wahyudi Nugroho was elected as their first chairman and soon after this election : many positive activities were already done. Mental Health Issues is one of their concern; and within this year when they are administering some surveys in relationship with DEMENTIA some Mental Disorders are also found and detected. This paper tries to give a rough picture on this matter since we do not have an accurate data on it yet. We are sure that this preliminary report will stimulate other researcher to continue. We hope that in the near future the Psycho-Geriatrics community in our country are able to coordinate a better program.

Older adults showing neglect: access to and evaluation of public (outreaching) health care

F. de Boer, C. Smits, and J. de Lange (Netherlands Institute of Mental Health and Addiction)

The purpose of the present study was to develop a manual for public health care staff to improve the care of older clients with mental health problems showing neglect. Two studies provided data for this manual: an access study focused on the referrals of these elderly to public health care, and a qualitative study on the evaluation of this care. In two cities in the Netherlands we asked all institutions who may have been in touch (in 2000) with older persons with mental health problems showing neglect of themselves or of their homes to report these cases . In in-depth interviews 14 older persons, a personal network member, and the staff involved evaluated the provided public health care. The analyses of the access study are ongoing. The majority of the interviewed elderly received unasked-for help. The help consisted of house-cleaning and calling in home care and often agreed with clients' wishes. Hoarding clients whose houses were cleared or who were evicted were dissatisfied. Public health care workers were seen as "traitors"; clearing workers were accused of theft. Some staff members were also dissatisfied, in other cases they were, contrary to their clients, satisfied. Although public health care services aim to provide client oriented care, they often fail to do so, due to organizational, communication, co-operation and attitude shortcomings. The manual informs public health workers of these shortcomings and of ways to overcome them.

Principles, Treatment and Philosophy of Psychiatric Rehabilitation of elderly patients in Africa

Debo Akande (Potche University, Vanderbijlparke, South Africa)

Research has shown that mental health professionals can be guided in their attempts to improve existing rehabilitation efforts by becoming more aware of the current body of rehabilitation research and conceptual knowledge and integrating that knowledge into their repertoires of therapeutic techniques and principles. Mental health professionals must also learn as Anthony, Cohen and Cohen (1983) suggested that the rehabilitation of the psychiatrically disabled elderly patient is not simply a matter of organizing environment resources so that there is a place in the community to refer the client. The most salient variable determining rehabilitation outcome is the degree to which a particular elderly client experiences a psychiatric rehabilitation approach within that community milieu.

The RAI-Mental Health (RAI-MH): A New Assessment Instrument for Geriatric Psychiatry

John P. Hirdes (University of Waterloo and Providence Centre, Toronto Canada), Brant E. Fries (University of Michigan and Ann Arbor VA Medical Center, Ann Arbor USA), John N. Morris (Hebrew Rehabilitation Center for the Aged Boston USA) Terry Rabinowitz (Fletcher Allen Health Care Burlington USA)

Purpose: This presentation provides and overview of the development and applications of the RAI-Mental Health (RAI-MH), a new comprehensive assessment instrument for use w th geriatric, acute, long stay and forensic psychiatric patients. This study will emphasize findings on elderly psychiatric patients. Method: The original RAI-MH development effort was a 6-country initiative lead by interRAI (a 20-country research network) and the Ontario Joint Policy and Planning Committee (JPPC). More recently, over 5,000 psychiatric patients in 34 hospitals in 3 Canadian provinces were assessed with the instrument and their resource use was track over a 24 hour period on the nursing unit and for 7 days for other costs. Results: The RAI-MH can be used to do cross-sectoral comparisons of the care of elderly persons with mental health needs. For example, patients in geriatric psychiatry units had comparable levels of cognitive impairment as noted in long term care facilities, but showed substantially higher rates of behaviour disturbance. In addition, rates of restraint use and psychotropic medication use were substantially higher in psychiatric settings compared with long term care. Conclusions: The RAI-MH provides new opportunities to evaluate and improve the care of older adults with mental health needs. In addition, it can be used to develop person specific care plans, support equitable funding, track outcomes and bench mark the quality of mental health services.

SESSION 227

A Comparison of the Quality Assurance of Elderly Services in Hong Kong and Canada

Kam-Tong CHAN, PhD

Quality Assurance in human services is becoming a world-wide trend in ensuring the standards of care render to people in care. For Hong Kong, the government has introduced a new quality assurance system, namely Service Performance Monitoring System (SPMS) in April 1999. The SPMS is consisted of three components, namely Funding and Service Agreement; the Service Quality Standards and External Assessment. Such system is also applied to services for the elderly people. Concerning the quality assurance system for the elderly people in Canada, the care providers would apply accreditation from the Canadian Council for Health Services Accreditation (CCHSA). The major objective of this paper is to compare the quality assurance system for the elderly people in Hong Kong and Canada. A framework consisted of 6 major elements is constructed for the comparison. These 6 elements, the scope of quality assessment, focus of assessment, mechanism, levels of assessment, process and outcome will be discussed.

Demonstrating Quality Outcomes in Residential Aged Care Through the Government Accreditation Process

Jill Pretty (Aged Services Association NSW & ACT. Sydney Australia)

This research sought to identify areas of commendable practice from the Commonwealth Government's accreditation process that impacted on the quality of care and lifestyle for frail older people in residential care. A survey of the Church and Charitable Aged Care facilities was conducted in New South Wales. Each facility was asked to complete a two page questionnaire following their accreditation visit. One of the questions requested facilities to give details of any commendable ratings they achieved. These results were collated and commendable practices contributing to quality of care and lifestyle were identified. 1000 questionnaires were distributed and 25% were returned. 38% achieved a commendable rating. The most common areas of commendable practices were Staff Development and Education and Leisure Activities for residents. Staff development highlighted that competency based training for all care staff had been provided to meet the National Competency Standards Certificate III Level. Comprehensive staff performance systems enabled staff to identify their educational and personal development goals. These needs analysis were used to develop further educational program. The second commendable outcome focussed on the social needs of residents. Innovative programs had been developed for residents who were suffering from the advanced stages of dementia. These programs showed how residents were able to maintain a degree of social independence both within the facility and in the community. The findings of the survey showed that the educational needs of staff and social independence of residents with dementia have been highlighted as key areas for maintaining quality outcomes for residents.

Development of Regional Clinical Practice Guidelines for Residential Care

Anne Earthy (Continuing Care, Simon Fraser Health Region, New Westminster, British Columbia, Canada)

The development of regional clinical practice guidelines (CPG's) for the frail elderly contributes to evidence based, consistent, cost effective and meaningful care. Before and after data was collected to demonstrate that CPG's can improve resident outcomes. Two years ago this health region's Residential Clinical Practice Council identified pertinent foci of care for this population and prioritized the development of CPG's. These included: Maintaining Healthy Skin, Managing Pressure Ulcers, Lower Extremity Ulcers, Dysphagia, Bowel Care, Maintaining Continence, Chronic Pain, Agitation and Excessive Behaviours, Assisting Persons with Feeding Tubes, and Managing Persons at High Risk for Falls. Most of these CPG's have been implemented in 5 care agencies and information has been shared within the region. The implementation process included benchmarking data, education, application to individual residents with follow up and data collection processes to illustrate compliance with care standards. The results have shown improved resident outcomes; decreased bowel and skin prescribed medications, briefs and linens, increased toileting of residents, decrease of serious injuries related to falls, increased fluid intake. By working together within the region interdisciplinary guidelines have contributed to improved resident care and consistent care between agencies.

Implementing the New National Accreditation System for Aged Care Facilities in Australia: a Process Evaluation

D.P. Boldy and L.Grenade (Department of Health Policy and Management, Curtin University of Technology, Perth, Western Australia)

Australia has recently introduced a new accreditation system, which includes the establishment of an independent Aged Care Standards and Accreditation Agency. This represents a major philosophical shift, with a particular emphasis on 'continuous quality improvement'. More specifically, the new accreditation process focuses on examining the management systems that facilities have in place to ensure that quality care is being provided. The objectives of this study are to: assess the extent to which service providers support the new accreditation system; identify the ways in which the process has been implemented; assess the extent to which service providers regard particular aged care standards and requirements as appropriate; and identify strengths and weaknesses, and any areas for change or improvement. A retrospective descriptive study design has been adopted, involving in-depth interviews with key personnel in 16 aged care facilities in the Perth metropolitan area that had recently been accredited (i.e. within the previous 3-6 months). A range of facilities are being included, taking into account criteria such as size and level of care provided Interviewing is not due to be completed until early 2001. However, findings to date indicate broad support for the principles and philosophy of the new system, although a number of concerns have also been identified. One of these is the perceived inadequate funding environment within which aged care facilities are operating, this being regarded as a key reason why some facilities may find difficulty in meeting particular standards, especially those related to management systems.

Monitoring quality of long-term institutional care and benchmarking

Noro Anja (Stakes, Helsinki, Finland), Finne-Soveri Harriet (Stakes/Kustaankartano, Helsinki, Finland), Björkgren Magnus (Chydenius-Institute, Kokkola, Finland), Pia Vähäkangas (Chydenius-Institute, Kokkola, Finland), Häkkinen Unto (Stakes, Helsinki, Finland), Laine Juha (Stakes, Helsinki, Finland)

PURPOSE: To implement the resident assessment instrument (RAI) in long-term care facilities to monitor quality of care, productivity, and costs of care and use the data in care planning and monitoring of outcomes of care and benchmarking of the best practices. METHOD: Project began in 2000 in which RAI (Resident Assessment Instrument) was implemented in three municipalities, and about 2200 residents in 80 wards were twice assessed with RAI in residential homes and health centre hospitals. The first data assessment was conducted in April, and the second assessment in October. In benchmarking meetings results were discussed with participants and results were disseminated by an Internet feedback database to participants. Four elderly care organisations were involved in this project. A computerised data collection system has been developed based on RAI system. RESULTS: Results of quality issues, case-mix including resource utilisation groups, dementia, depression in units and the benchmarking figures have been discussed and results disseminated to participants. Also the productivity figures among units have been calculated and staffing ratios discussed. Longitudinal results will be presented including productivity figures among units, and quality indicators. The variation in productivity figures, as well as in quality indicators, were quite high between units. A clear difference in case-mix was found between residential homes and health centre hospitals indicating need for separate benchmarking indicators and quality thresholds for both types of institutional long-term care. CONCLUSION: The experience from the first year have been promising, and all those who started with the project will carry on.

Quality Care for Australian Nursing Home Residents: Development of Clinical Indicators of Care.

L. Spencer (School of Health, University of New England, Australia), M. Courtney (Centre for Nursing Research, Queensland University of Technology, Australia)

PURPOSE: This study aimed to develop indicators of clinical care designed specifically for residents with high level needs in Australian nursing homes. METHOD: This study was conducted over three phases - an exploratory phase to compile 10 case studies of best practice, a national randomized survey and a trial of the clinical evaluation. RESULTS: During Phase 1 and 2 a series of 18 clinical indicators of quality care were identified and assigned to one of four care domains: resident health, personal care, resident lifestyle and the care environment. These were subsequently complied into an Australian Quality Matrix (AQM) of clinical care. In Phase 3, the draft AQM was trialed and revised in a 60 bed high level stand-alone metropolitan facility. During the trial period the prevalence and/or incidence rates of eight indicators were noted to improve, four deteriorated and six remained relatively static. The definitive version of the AQM and the 18 clinical indicators identified will be presented in this paper. CONCLUSION: The study concluded that the Australian Quality Matrix should be the subject of a multi-centre trial to confirm its validity and reliability. It further recommended that future research address the differences between urban and rural outcomes detected during the project.

Rolling Out Best Practices in a Continuing Care Setting - Becoming a Learning Organization

Debra F. Elm (The Good Samaritan Society, Edmonton, Canada)

Upon recognition of the need to put research practices in place, The Good Samaritan Society, a multi-site continuing care service provider, developed a best practice process and restructured the organization accordingly. The process was developed based on the CURN model and Peter Senge's writing on the "Learning Organization". Six steps are involved in the process: 1. The identified need; 2. Literature Search and Bench marking; 3. Developing processes and protocol; 4. Developing the roll out a plan; 5. Implementation; 6. Evaluation. Five Best Practice Specialists were hired, each with an area of expertise. The specialists are responsible for gathering information, developing the processes and evaluation. A Best Practice Council which includes the leaders of the organization and representatives of all disciplines, was formed and is responsible for reviewing and approving the process. The presentation and discussion of information at the council meetings are done in a way which facilitates learning and coming to a consensus or shared vision. Once a consensus has been reached, commitments are made by all to be stewards of that vision. This process has been in place for three years and best practices have been developed for wound care, pressure relief, transferring residents, infection control, environmental standards, dementia care, diabetes care, venous stasis care, admission process, dysphagia care and restraint reduction. An evaluation of the best practice process itself is done annually where barriers to the implementation of the best practice process are identified and recommendations are made to overcome them.

SESSION 228

A Study on Resource Based Relative Values for Home Care Nursing Services

Yasuko Ogata (University of Tokyo, Tokyo, Japan), Yasuki Kobayashi, (University of Tokyo, Tokyo, Japan), Takashi Fukuda (University of Tokyo, Tokyo, Japan), Katsumi Mori (University of Tokyo, Tokyo, Japan), Michio Hashimoto (Yokohama City University Hospital, Kanagawa, Japan), Kayo Otosaka (Kohoku Home-visit Nursing Care Station, Kanagawa, Japan)

Purpose: The purpose of this study was to investigate the resource based relative values of actual visiting nursing services for the aged, and to analyze the relationships between the relative values and the 3 dimensions of nursing service (time, mental effort and physical effort). Method: Nurses at 3 home-visit nursing care stations (HVNCS) in the Metropolitan area answered questions on relative values of Total Work (TW) and relative weight for the 3 dimensions of actual nursing services. TW was defined as comprehensive evaluation of nursing services in terms of both work intensity and time. With TW as the dependent variable and the 3 dimensions as independent variables, multiple regression analyses were carried out. Degrees of influence on TW by service type and individual respondent were examined. The validity of the results was reconfirmed by comparing the measured time with the answered time. Results: 32 respondents at 3 HVNCSs were all female and their average age was 35.6 years old. They had HVNCS experience of 2.4 years. They visited 240 aged persons homes and provided a total of 99 kinds of nursing services. Services provided more than 20 times were analyzed. TW and 3 dimensions scores were standardized using common logarithms. The 3 dimensions explained 76% of TW in the multiple regression analysis. Service type and individual respondent characteristics explained little of TW. Answered time and measured time were not significantly different by nursing service. Conclusion: Most of the variation of TW was explained by the 3 dimensions.

Assessing Older Peoples' Need for Nursing - the contribution of the RCN's Nursing Older People Assessment Tool

Pauline Ford, (Royal College of Nursing, London, England.) Brendan Mc Cormack, (University of Ulster/Royal Group of Hospitals, Belfast, Northern Ireland)

This paper presents an overview of the work of the Royal College of Nursing (RCN) in developing an assessment tool to determine the need for registered nursing by older people in continu ng care. In the past, health care has been provided free and social care 'means-tested'. The erosion of the UK National Health Service's responsibility for continuing care provision through the development of eligibility criteria has resulted in the majority of older people having their care services means-tested, including their nursing care. The RCN has argued that older people have interrelated health and social care needs, that nursing care is an integral component of health care provision and that therefore older people should not have to pay for nursing care. This paper describes the work undertaken by the RCN to develop a tool for use in assessing older people's need for registered nursing - "The RCN Nursing Older People Assessment Tool". The underpinning theoretical framework, derived from theories of personhood articulated by Seedhouse (1997) and Kitwood (1997) and informed by Agich (1993) will be outlined. Examples of how the use of this tool has influenced practice will be drawn from the results of two research studies (Ford & McCormack, 1999; Ford et al, 2000). Issues of determining the validity of the tool and the challenges in doing this will also be addressed (Ford et al, 2000). The presentation will conclude with an agenda for the development of person-centred approaches to assessment with older people.

Changes of Images toward Elders and Demented Elders after Practicum among Nursing Students

Jung Hee Kim (Inha University, Inchon Korea)

Caregiverspositive attitudes toward elders are crucial in ensuring quality of care. Effects of practice on images toward demented elders and elders in general were examined. Thirty six senior nursing students were assigned to day care centers for demented elders (Group 1) and for elders with CVA (Group 2) for 1 week. The students images were obtained right before and immediately after the practicum using self-reported questionnaire. The images toward elders were measured with 50 items of semantic differential scale, from which 4 factors were identified in a previous study such as vitality, mildness, cooperativeness, and prudence. Data were analyzed with paired t-test. The image of vitality toward both demented and general elders was changed toward positive direction in both groups. The image of mildness changed toward negative direction for the demented in both groups, while the change for general elders was observed in Group 2 only. In Group 2, the image of mildness for general elders was negative compared to that for demented elders in the pre-test. As for cooperativeness, Group 2 showed changes toward positive direction. The image of prudence was changed toward positive direction for demented elders in Group 1 and to negative direction for general elders in Group 2. According to the pre-test, the image of prudence was negative for demented elders in Group 1 and positive for general elders in Group 2, compared to their respective counterparts. The images toward demented elders and elders in general came to be more similar after practicum.

Effects of a critical pathway of PLF for lumbar spinal stenosis

Hae-Ok Park, (Inha Univ. Hospital, Inchon, Korea) Kyu Jung Cho, (Inha University, Medical School, Inchon, Korea) Sr. You-Ja Ro, (Catholic University, School of Nursing, Seoul, Korea)

(The abstract is the following:) PURPOSE : The aims of this study were to determine whether a critical pathway(CP) for patients with spinal fusion would have effects on the quality of care and cost-effectiveness, and whether nurses using the CP would be more satisfied with their job. METHOD : Data from 25 females aged 59.2 +7.2 years underwent the CP were compared with those from a control group. Measures included the quality of nursing care, patient satisfaction at discharge, the length of stay, and the medical charge. Nurses' job satisfaction before and after the application of CP were compared with those from another ward. RESULTS

: The CP group showed higher scores in total and every item of quality of nursing care and more satisfied with discharge care (P<.05) than the control group, although it showed no difference in patients' satisfaction about the general nursing care between groups. The mean length of stay of the CP group was shorter than that of the control group without statistical significance. The charge of medication and treatment of the CP group were smaller than that of the control group (P<.05). Nurses of the CP ward showed higher job satisfaction after the CP application (P<.05). On the contrary, nurses on a different floor showed no change in job satisfaction at the same period of time. CONCLUSION : The results of the study support that the CP enables to improve the quality of care and job satisfaction, to reduce the medical charge, and consequently to increase patient satisfaction with care.

Improvement of a Tool as an Incentive to Improve Quality of Care in Physiotherapy

J. DANZIGER, (CHIEF PHYSIOTHERAPIST, MINISTRY OF HEALTH, JERUSALEM, ISRAEL).

Improve quality of care in physiotherapy in Nursing Homes. The Ministry of Health in Israel controls the hospitalization of nursing patients and maintains the quality of care given to these patients in government, public and private institutions. Professionals have established a system to examine the care given in these institutions by allotting scores in different areas of care, using a specially designed scoring method. The tool examines if the work is carried out according to the compendium of regulations issued by the Ministry of Health. At the beginning of the year 1999, the tool was changed. The tools are basically the same but they differ in the level of specification . The new tool is more detailed and specific. Changing of the tool caused lowering of the scores in physiotherapy. Methods: Both tools were used to mark the scores in physiotherapy care in 50 Nursing Homes. Results: In 45 our of 50 Nursing Homes the scores in physiotherapy care were lower when using the new tool. Conclusions: The new tool is a much more sensitive tool and points out more clearly areas in the physiotherapy service that need improvement. Steps were taken by the Physiotherapy unit in the Ministry of Health to improve the quality of the services in Nursing Homes. The steps included study days and workshops on quality care.

SESSION 230

The Role of Vitamin K in Bone Metabolism

Hajime Orimo

Osteoporosis is defined as a systemic bone disease characterized by low bone mass and deterioration of microstructure which make the bone susceptible to fractures. It is a metabolic bone disease caused by the imbalance between bone resorption and bone formation. Among various fractures related to osteoporosis, hip fracture is the most serious one, because it causes the disability and impairs the quality of life of the elderly. Therefore, the prevention and management of hip fractures are issues of great importance in geriatric practice. Hip fracture occurs exclusively in the elderly and its incidence is increasing all over the world, particularly in Asian countries, and it is now being recognized as a global burden. Serum level of vitamin K, was lower and that of undercarboxylated osteocalcin was higher in the patients with hip fractures than in the controls. Furthermore, increased serum level of undercarboxylated osteocalcin was shown to be a predictor of hip fracture. Oral administration of vitamin K2 was proved to be effective in increasing bone mineral density in the patients with osteoporosis. Vitamin K2 was shown to stimulate the calcification in vitro of osteoblast and to induce apoptosis in vitro of osteoclast. In this symposium, various topics on these issues will be discussed.

Dietary Vitamin K Intakes and Hip Fracture Risk

S.L. Booth (USDA Human Nutrition Research Center on Aging at Tufts University, Boston, USA)

Vitamin K is a potentially modifiable dietary factor in the risk for hip fracture. Three vitamin K-dependent proteins have been identified in bone and cartilage, and it is assumed that any role of dietary vitamin K is mediated through the gamma-carboxylation of these proteins. The predominant dietary source of vitamin K in North America is phylloquinone (vitamin K-1). Average dietary intakes of phylloquinone among adults are below recommended dietary intakes. Several epidemiologic studies suggest that low reported dietary intakes of phylloquinone are associated with an increased risk of hip fracture in men and women. In contrast, the associations between dietary phylloquinone and bone mineral density (BMD) are inconsistent among studies. A gene-nutrient interaction between apolipoprotein (apo) E genotype and dietary intakes of phylloquinone in the risk for hip fracture has also been suggested. Fasting plasma phylloquinone concentrations may be influenced by polymorphisms of apo E. Individuals with the E4 allele may have a greater risk for hip fractures and lower BMD than for individuals without the E4 allele. However, there are currently no epidemiologic studies that report significant interactions between the E4 allele and phylloquinone intakes and BMD or hip fracture risk. A criticism of these epidemiologic studies has been the overall confounding effect of poor nutrition. Furthermore, the putative mechanisms of vitamin K action on bone are not well understood, which limits the interpretation of existing studies. To define the potential dietary role of phylloquinone in age-related bone loss, phylloquinone supplementation trials are required.

Effect of vitamin K on bone fracture with special reference to Natto intake in Japan

Masao Kaneki

Purpose: The increasing evidence indicate a significant role for vitamin K in osteoporosis. However, the knowledge on vitamin K status in humansis limited. Therefore, we investigated the impact of fermented soybean food, natto intake to vitamin K status and bone health. Method: Serum vitamin K was measured in three groups of postmenopausal women living in Tokyo, Hiroshima and United Kingdom. Results: We found a large geographical difference in serum vitamin K2 (menaquinone-7) level in postmenopausal women. Serum menaquinone-7 concentration was 5.26 + 6.13 ng/ml (mean + S.D.) in Japanese women in Tokyo, 1.22 +1.85 in Hiroshima, 0.37 + 0.20 in British women, respectively. Natto contains a huge amount of menaquinone-7 and is eaten frequently in eastern (Tokyo), but scarcely in western (Hiroshima) Japan. Serum concentration of menaquinone-7 was remarkably higher in frequent natto eaters, and natto intake resulted in a marked, sustained increase in serum menaquinone-7 concentration. As the lower hip fracture incidence in eastern than western Japan was shown previously, we analyzed the relationship between the regional difference in natto intake and regional fracture incidence. The statistically significant inverse correlation was found between the female hip fracture incidence and natto consumption in each prefecture throughout Japan. Conclusion: These findings indicate that the large geographical difference in menaquinone-7 level may be ascribed, at least in part, to natto intake, and suggest the possibility that higher menaquinone-7 level resulting from natto intake may contribute to the relatively lower fracture risk in Japanese women.

The EPIDOS study : undercarboxylated osteocalcin measured with a specific immunoassay predicts hip fracture in elderly women.

P. Szulc (INSERM Research Unit 403, Lyon, France)

Vitamin K plays an important role in bone metabolism. Its high levels were found in bone tissue. Vitamin K stimulates the formation of gammacarboxyglutamic acid (GLA) which is present in three proteins of bone matrix: osteocalcin (OC), Matrix GLA Protein, protein S. Vitamin K stimulates differentiation and metabolic activity of osteoblasts as well as inhibits osteoclasts activity and bone resorption. Vitamin K concentration is decreased in patients with hip fracture. Patients treated with vitamin K antagonists had a decreased bone mineral density (BMD). OC contains three GLA residues. Its level is positively correlated with histomorphometric parameters of bone formation. Some fraction of circulating OC is not fully gammacarboxylated and its affinity for hydroxyapatite is decreased. This fraction called undercarboxylated osteocalcin (ucOC) can be a marker of vitamin K status. EPIDOS is a prospective population-based study on osteoporotic fractures in elderly women. To determine the value of serum ucOC to prospectively predict the risk of hip fracture, ucOC was measured using a direct and specific enzyme-linked immunosorbent assay. Women with the baseline concentration of ucOC in the highest quartile had an increased risk of hip fracture (O.R. = 2.0, $p<0.01$) also after adjustment for femoral neck BMD. Women who had both low femoral neck BMD and increased ucOC had an elevated risk of hip fracture (O.R. = 5.5, $p<0.001$). Total OC was not predictive of hip fracture. This direct immunoassay for ucOC is rapid, specific and has a negligible cross-reactivity with total OC. In elderly women, ucOC predicts hip fracture risk independently of bone mass.

SESSION 231

Aging in Israel - An Overview of a Few Sociological Aspects

Nurit Sharlin, Director, Center for Environmental Studies, Western Galilee College, Israel and Shlomo Sharlin, Director, Center for Research & Study of the Family, University of Haifa, Israel; Head, Dept. of Social Work, Judea & Samaria College, Israel. Community based project: Prevention and intervention for improvement of environmental quality conducted by veterans Dan Soen, Head, Dept. of Sociology & Anthropology, Judea & Samaria College, Israel; Social Sciences Dept, Ha'Kibbutzim College, Tel-Aviv. Project renewal - Age and Content in Israel's Distress Neighbourhoods Shlomo Sharlin and Ester Eshel, Director, Dept. of Social Services, Or-Yehuda, Israel; Dept. of Social Work, Judea & Samaria College, Israel The unavoidable obligation: The influence of the inter-generation caring on the "sandwich" generation's marital quality Ahuva Even-Zohar, Dept. of Social Work, Judea & Samaria College Elderly parent placement reflected in family structure: Adaptation and cohesion

The paper will discuss the results of the research, that seemed to support the underlying hypothesis. A strong connection has been indeed found between the coefficients of cohesion and adaptability on one hand and the decision to place the elderly parents in a Home on the other hand. Israeli society is unique in its aging pattern owing to its particular history. From an unusually young society in its pre-State days (prior to 1948) it turned in the wake of the ongoing mass migration and the natural process into an aging society. While in 1955 elderly people (aged 65+) constituted a mere 4.7% of the population (85,200 in all), in 1998 their weight reached 11.6% (!) of the population (700,800 altogether) - an 8.2 fold growth over a period of less than 45 years. Life expectancy at birth arose among males from 64.9 in 1949 to 75.3 in 1990; among women - from 67.6 in 1949 to 78.9 in 1990. The symposium tries to touch upon some of the outcomes of this dynamic social change. On the one hand, the Panel will deal with the overall satisfaction of the elderly with their communities, as well as with their active involvement in community projects, all of which attest to their social integration. On the other hand the Panel will explore the plight of middle-aged families as they try to deal with their responsibility to their aged members. Dr. Nurit Sharlin and Prof. Shlomo Sharlin: Community based project: Prevention and intervention for improvement of environmental quality conducted by veterans. In recent years many distressed neighbourhoods confront vandalism and physical deterioration of housing and public sites. Shortly after urban renewal intervention, physical negligence and environmental nuisances tend to occur once again. This paper will present an effort to overcome such a problem by involving volunteers living in these areas. The project involves volunteers recruited from among the aged population, senior high-school students, representatives of various business and industrial councils, jointly with representatives of the municipality and other social organizations in the community, who go through workshops and training to become environmental trustees. The paper will discuss the organization and training of the project program. A model for intervention will be presented and discussed. Among the program goals are": · Development of an action model according to community characteristics; · Developing a program for the identification of needs, on-going stable activities, responsibility and collaboration with the local authorities; · Providing tools for the improvement of environmental quality for the residents by themselves. A follow-up study of the results and evaluation of the training and implementation of specific projects will be presented and discussed. Participants will be able to discuss with the presenters implementing such a project. 2) Prof. Dan Soen: Age and content in Israel's distress neighbourhoods The Abstract has already been forwarded earlier and confirmed by your committee !!! 3) Prof. Shlomo Sharlin and Ms. Ester Eshel: The unavoidable obligation: The influence of the inter-generation caring on the "sandwich" generation's marital quality The aged population continues to rise all over the world due to the rise of life expectancy and decrease of childbirth. It is expected that the percentage of the aged among the general population will double by the year 2025, while the group of 85+ will quadruple and become 12.8 of all aged. It is expected that both the health and functioning of the aged will deteriorate and some might reach complete dependency. There are two aspects in treating the aged: (1) Social aspect - the resposibility of the government to its citizens, and (2) Family aspect - the responsibility of the familty to their aged. At the threshold of the 21st century, there might be an obligation of the aged offspring for more responsibility of care taking, which might be hard, long and exhausting. There will be a rise of roles, - 3 - mental and familial distress will become vigorous. These offspring are defined as the Sandwich Generation: Parents who are taking care of their elderly parents while simultaneously also tending to their own offspring. The paper will present the meaning of role changing and its influence on the marital quality of the sandwich generation in Israel. Resuts of a study of 100 such families will be presented and discussed. An effort will be made to identify why some families succeed in this onerous task while other fail in providing care and maintaining healthy marital relationships. 4) Ms. Ahuva Even Zohar: Elderly Parent Placement Reflected in Family Structure: Adaptation and Cohesion This inquiry focuses on the decision of placement of an elderly parent in light of family structure. Our hypothesis suggest that: where the coefficients of cohesion and adaptability are high, there will be a tendency to care for the aged parent in the home of the adult offspring. Conversely, where the coefficients of cohesion and adaptability are low there will be a propensity to place the parent in residential care. In addition we hypothesize that when the coefficients of cohesion and adaptability are midrange, the probability of taking the elderly parent into the offspring's home are higher than when the coefficients are low. The theoretical base for this study derives from the classic work of family theory, and more particularly - the intergenerational dimensions of these theories. Structural, systemic and cotextual approaches are examined. The key concept of Olson's circumplex model is introduced, utilizing the major variables of cohesion and adaptability. This model projects sixteen categories that classify family functioning centered on two major concepts of cohesion and adaptability. The research discussed in the paper was based on 152 offspring of elderly parents acting as caregivers. The distribution was as follows: · 77 offspring whose parents live with them, as a two-generational family, so to speak; · 75 offspring whose parents live in the home for the aged. The study was based on two questionnaires: · A demographic questionnaire intended to depict the parents and their offspring; · A self-report measure - FACES 3, meant to reflect family adaptability and cohesion (Olson, 1985).

Project Renewal: Age and Content in Israel's Distress Neighbourhoods

Dan SOEN (Dept. of Sociology & Anthropology, College os Judea & Samaria, Israel; Dept. of Social Sciences, Ha'Kibbutzim College of Education, Tel-Aviv).

About 12% out of a total budget of US$ 1.5 billion spent over 18 years on Israel's PROJECT RENEWAL have been allocated to improving the condition of the elderly residing in distressed neighborhoods. The purpose of the presented study has been to find out to what extent has the target population benefited from these inputs. The study is based on a survey carried out on a national sample of the neighborhoods financed by the PROJECT. Based on the finding of the study it is maintained that in as much the elderly population of the relevant neighborhoods is concerned the budget was well invested. Analysis of the questionnaires shows the elderly population to be well integrated socially. A check of improvement of the housing conditions of the elderly reveals that what with the inputs of the PROJECT their housing condition compares favorably with the other sectors of the population. Their content with the situation is remarkable. Analysis of the utilization of the socio-cultural amenities and public services made available to the elderly in their neighborhoods reveals that only a relatively small group takes advantage of the new opportunities offered by the community. And yet, the survey indicated that the mere availability of these amenities and services contributed to a high satisfaction coefficient among the elderly. The Paper goes on to analyze the assessment made by the elderly of the changes affected in the neighborhoods through the PROJECT. It draws attention to the fact that the opinion of this age-group is not different from that of the population as a whole. Last but not least, the data assembled in the survey shows that the elderly are by far the most satisfied segment of the population residing in the distressed neighborhoods. Since this segment is considered the weakest, their content is a clear evidence that decision-making and priorities set by the planning teams have been in the correct direction

SESSION 232

Eldercare by Eldercarers: Rethinking Community Care

Deborah A. Sears (Carewest Day Hospital, Calgary, Canada) Elizabeth A. Gislason (Carewest Day Hospital, Calgary, Canada) Marlene A. Smart (Carewest Day Hospital and Mental Health Consulting Services Calgary Regional Health Authority, Calgary, Canada) Diana Didrickson (Carewest Neuro Rehabilitation Program, Calgary, Canada) Discussant Joan Buhr (Community Care, Calgary, Canada) Discussant.

Issue: The movement from institutional care for the frail elderly to community care has alerted the above discussants of an emerging pattern of eldercare. Our observations from our work in community geriatric rehabilitation, suggest that eldercare is often managed on behalf of the frail elderly by an eldercarer who may also be in need of eldercare. Structure: The convenor will introduce the issue and each discussant representing geriatric psychiatry, psychology, social work, occupational therapy and speech pathology will present their observations, case examples, and research relevant to the issue. The attendees will be encouraged to discuss the issues related to "Eldercare by Eldercarers" and to further provide anecdotal findings and research results. Content: Issues related to "Eldercare by Eldercarers" raised for discussion. Anticipated Outcome: If the discussants and the attendees conclude that the issue of "Eldercare by Eldercarers" warrants further investigations and researches, an international network will be formed to address the topic.

Eldercare by Eldercarers: A Psychiatrist's Perspective

Marlene A. Smart (Mental Health Consulting Services, Calgary Regional Health Authority, Calgary, Canada).

Issue: As the population ages we are seeing an increasing number of elderly caregivers providing support to their loved ones. Because of their advanced age, these eldercarers are at significant risk for physical and emotional/mental health concerns. As a result of their concern for their loved ones, they are often reluctant to seek the care they need for themselves. Observations from clinical practice will be included in the discussions.

Eldercare by Eldercarers: A Psychologist's Perspective

Deborah A. Sears (Carewest Day Hospital, Calgary, Canada).

This is a call for health service professionals to share with others their experience and observations regarding the real health costs of eldercare by eldercarers. The assumption is made by health policy makers and financial planners that the elderly can be adequately cared for in their homes with external supports such as bathing assistance, meal preparation, and medication monitoring; while all other care needs such as personal hygiene, transfers, and safety monitoring can be met by other members of the household, most often the spouse. It is our observation that this assumption is not always met. It is most questionable when the carer is the spouse. Case examples will be provided for discussion with the attendees.

Eldercare by Eldercarers: An Occupational Therapist's Perspective

Elizabeth A. Gislason (Carewest Day Hospital, Calgary, Canada).

Issue: A number of cases will be discussed which highlight the problems that arise when eldercarer's who themselves may have undiagnosed functional deficits, are expected by the health system to care for spouses with a variety of medical problems. Some of the cases will speak directly to the issues related to the care of spouse's with Alzheimer's or other dementias.

SESSION 233

Slowing the Brain Drain — Games for Residents with Mild Cognitive Impairment

Kathy Laurenhue (Mather Institute on Aging, Evanson, IL, USA) (Slowing the Brain Drain — Games for Residents with Mild Cognitive Impairment) Carly Hellen ("Alzheimer's Disease-Activity Focused Care") Jitka Zgola ("Care that Works", "Doing Things")

Issue: Anecdotal evidence suggests that keeping the mind stimulated slows the progress of mild cognitive impairment. At the very least, engaging residents in satisfying activities improves their sense of well-being. However, many people don't know how to get beyond crossword puzzles to individualize brain games for residents. Nor do they understand how to adapt the activities for varying degrees of impairment. Structure: Over the course of the 1.5 hours, participants can be confident that whether they stay the whole time or circulate to other tables, they will receive creative ideas for stimulating activities to serve a broad range of interests and abilities. Content: This round table will give participants hands-on experience with a variety of exercises which they can take back and use. Outcomes: Participants will receive training in a variety of exercises provided as handouts. Handouts will also include brain stimulation theory that can't be easily taught in this format. Participants will also receive a resource list for creative product companies and useful publications.

Alzheimer's Disease: Activity Focused Care

Carly Heller

The success of an activity is not a magnificently produced product, nor an outcome that meets the needs or specifications of the caregiver. Success is calling forth the person with dementia's best in his or her relationship to self and others. Therefore, success is spelled: S = sensitivity U = understanding C = creativity C = connectedness E = enabling S = safety S = satisfaction

Understanding the qualities of a successful activity includes knowing how to relate an activity analysis to a specific activity in relationship to the resident. An activity analysis is a process by which an activity is clearly understood so it can be selected or rejected as a meaningful engagement for a resident. There are three basic components of an activity analysis:

1. Understanding the selected activity's effects on A. the cognitive, physical and psychosocial abilities of the resident B. the cognitive, physical and psychosocial risks to the resident

2. Adaption qualities of the activity to A. be implemented one to one with the resident B. be implemented in a small group (3 - 6) residents C. be implemented to a large group of residents (6 or more)

3. Modification qualities of the activity to A. be meaningful for residents with mild dementia B. be meaningful for residents with moderate dementia C. be meaningful for residents with severe/terminal dementia

Therefore, any activity can be considered by using the three basic activity analysis components. The analysis will be demonstrated and explained. The conference participants will then be invited to look in their pockets, purses, etc, select an item and create an analysis that reflects its appropriateness and inappropriateness as a therapeutic activity: benefits, risks number of residents and level of abilities/inabilities.

Slowing the Brain Drain - - Meaningful Activity for Residents with Mild Cognitive Impairment

Jitka Zgola (Giverny Consultants Ltd, Wreck Cove, Nova Scotia, Canada)

Issue: The key to providing satisfying activities to persons with cognitive impairment is identifying activities that comply with the individual's interests and abilities and presenting them in a manner that compensates for the challenges that person faces. Structure: This presentation will invite participants to identify activities that would be truly meaningful to them, associate criteria for identifying meaningful activity and then see how these activities can be presented to cognitively impaired persons so that success is ensured. Content: The principle concepts presented here will be, the range of activities that contributes to a satisfying lifestyle, the criteria for individually meaningful activity, how such activities can be identified for the individual and method of presentation that accommodates the most common difficulties experienced by persons with dementia. Outcomes: Participants will come away with a practical method of finding an optimum fit between activities offered and the needs, interests, abilities of their clients.

SESSION 234

Behavioral presentation of older Hong Kong Chinese people with dementia and the impact of dementia on family caregivers

Jenny Chung (The Hong Kong Polytechnic University, Hong Kong, SAR, China), Behavioral and activity profiles of nursing home residents with dementia. Claudia Lai (The Hong Kong Polytechnic University), Agitated behaviors in older people with dementia in Hong Kong. Gemma Wong (The University of Hong Kong, Hong Kong, SAR, China), Working with family caregivers to understand behavioral problems in the demented elderly. Teresa Tsien (The Hong Kong Polytechnic University), Care for family caregivers: An evaluation of a pilot social intervention project.

This symposium reports the behavioral presentation of people with dementia in Hong Kong and its impact on family caregivers. It also addresses, in part, how problematic behaviors could be managed in the Hong Kong context. The symposium consists of four papers from four different researchers. The convenor will introduce the contents and summarize the conclusion of the symposium. Each presentation will last 15 minutes and there will be a 30-minute open discussion after the four presentations. An overview of dementia services in Hong Kong will be given should time permits. In the literature, there s little information concerning cultural differences in terms of behavioral presentation and management in dementia care. This symposium addresses this particular aspect by studying people with dementia in Hong Kong, which is a fairly homogeneous society. In the first paper, Chung investigates the activities and behavioral profiles of individuals with dementia in nursing homes. An observation tool, the Dementia Care Mapping developed by Kitwood & Bredin (1997), was used to assess the activities and behavioral patterns of subjects. Subjects were found to be largely passive, with little stimulation in their life in the home. Mismatch of activity with residents' functional and cognitive abilities, and the home's care culture, contributed to a non-stimulating care environment. Lai reports findings from both nursing homes and community samples in her study. Using a validated Chinese version of the Cohen-Mansfield Agitation Inventory (Cohen-Mansfield & Billig, 1986), subjects were noted to have relatively lower agitation scores. Moreover, reported agitated behaviors in the subjects were more benign in nature - mainly belonging to the categories of verbally and physically non-aggressive behaviors. In this study, the community subsample showed a somewhat higher score than the nursing home subsample. In the l iterature, studies have consistently reported that caregiver stress is significantly associated with problematic behaviors in people with dementia. Using the Chinese versions of a multidimensional burden inventory and the Caregiving Hassle Scale, Wong studies the type and the frequency of problematic behaviors that occur in community subjects, and its relationship to the caregiver burden. The result shows a significant association between the level of burden and the frequency of behavioral isturbance. Wong concludes that the provision of adequate social support and psychoeducation for the caregivers would enhance their coping skills and help to reduce the frequency of problematic behaviors. Tsien's report is about outcomes of a pilot Social Intervention Project that aimed at the reduction of stress for family caregivers and improvement of the physical and mental abilities of older people with dementia. Programs in the project included center-based respite, home-based respite and individual care management. The preliminary result showed that center-based respite was more effective in reducing stress for family caregivers than the other two programs. However, the programs did not help in improving the physical or mental abilities of older people with dementia. To conclude, this symposium addresses the interesting topic of behavioral presentation in people with dementia, and the impact of dementia on family caregivers. It will also discuss how behavioral problems are managed. There is a lack of systemic review of cultural differences in terms of behavioral presentation and management in the literature. This symposium, therefore, will be a timely presentation addressing this topic.

Agitated behaviors in older people with dementia in Hong Kong

Claudia K Y Lai (The Hong Kong Polytechnic University, Hong Kong)

When validating the Cohen-Mansfield Agitation Inventory (CMAI, a tool for the assessment of agitated behaviors in older persons) in a sample of older people with dementia in Hong Kong (n=164: nursing homes subsample: n=24; community subsample: n=39), only slight differences could be found in the range of agitated behaviors observed as compared with reports from overseas. However, more prominent differences are observed with regard to the intensity of agitated behaviors. Local subjects with dementia had relatively lower total scores. This finding is corroborated by results of studies by other local researchers (Chan, 2000). Moreover, agitated behaviors in subjects were noted to be more benign in nature - mainly belonging to categories of verbally non-aggressive behaviors such as repeatedly asking questions, and physically non-aggressive behaviors such as handling things inappropriately. Verbally and physically aggressive behaviors against others were not very common. Two observations that are similar to reports from advanced countries include the relatively low occurrence of inappropriate sexual expression and use of dangerous objects to harm self or others. Inappropriate sexual expression occurred in 5 - 13 % of subjects, as compared to the 2-14 % reported in the Western literature. Only 4% of local subjects had reportedly attempted to harm others or themselves with dangerous objects, while "bearing or using a weapon" was not observed at all in a study by Souder and associates (1999). The findings point to an interesting area of cross-cultural comparisons in behavioral presentation. To conclude, the range of behavioral presentation of agitated behaviors was more benign and its presentation less intense in Hong Kong Chinese. Working with family caregivers to understand behavioral problems in elderly people with dementia.

Behavioral and activity profiles of nursing home residents with dementia. J.C.C. Chung (The Hong Kong Polytechnic University, Hong Kong)

J.C.C. ChungDepartment of Rehabilitation Sciences, The Hong Kong Polytechnic University, Hung Hom, Hong Kong.

The literature has shown that persons with dementia residing in long-term care facilities are largely passive and engaged only minimally in meaningful activities (Bowie & Mountain, 1993; Perrin (1997). Mayer and Griffin (1990) reported that persons with dementia engaged in stimulus-seeking behaviors, despite their impaired cognitive functions. The development of dementia-related services in Hong Kong is largely drawn upon the insights and experiences of overseas empirical studies. Little is known about the perceptions of its service-users in local care contexts. This explorative study examines the behavior manifestation and activity profiles of 32 nursing home residents with dementia. By means of an observational tool, "Dementia Care Mapping" (Kitwood & Bredin, 1997), each subject was mapped for an average of six hours. Preliminary data analysis indicated that most subjects engaged in apathetic and withdrawn behaviors such as dozing (15%) and the passive observation of their surroundings (28%). Some used pacing and repetitive actions as a form of self-stimulation. Aggressive behaviors, both verbal and physical, were less frequently observed. Subjects with better cognitive functions generally had better engagement in functional and recreational activities, such as eating, self-care, and physical activities. Results suggested that patterned care of nursing homes, mismatch of activity with residents' functional and cognitive abilities, and care culture contribute to a non-stimulating care environment, which deprives residents with dementia of an appropriate level of participation in meaningful activities. This study uncovers some limitations of Hong Kong residential services for persons with dementia, which need to be addressed in order to promote quality dementia care. Agitated behaviors in older people with dementia in Hong Kong

Care for Family Caregivers: An Evaluation of a Pilot Day Respite Care Project

Teresa Tsien (The Hong Kong Polytechnic University, Hong Kong, SAR, China)

In Hong Kong, minimal resources and services were allocated to support family caregivers in their caring process. From the findings of the author's study on the impact of caregiving and needs of demented elderly caregivers, the majority of the respondents suffered from physical and mental aspects of health and social life. The two critical factors that disabled caregivers from the continued care, were deterioration in their own health and the inability to manage difficult behaviors of the demented elderly. Respite care was one of the most needed programs (Tsien & Cheng 1997). Adequate social support and planned intervention helped to reduce the frequency of undesirable behavior presented by elderly with dementia (Cohen et al, 1997) and the stress of caregivers (Zarit et al, 1980). A pilot day respite care project that aimed to reduce stress for family caregivers and improve the physical and mental abilities of elderly individuals with dementia was conducted. A total of 18 families had participated in the center-based and home-based respite care. The evaluation results evidenced the satisfaction rate of the caregivers to center-based and home-based respite care were 90% and 60% respectively. Moreover, center-based respite care was found to be more effective in reducing the stress for family caregivers than home-based respite care because center-based respite care offered a longer break for the caregivers. These findings were consistent with the Western results. However, both types of the day respite care did not help in improving the physical or mental abilities of elderly with dementia.

Working with family caregivers to understand behavioral problems in elderly people with dementia

G.K.C. Wong (The University of Hong Kong)

Behavioral disturbance is a common feature of dementia and causes the most hassle for the caregiver in caring for the demented elderly person at home. Consistent findings reveal that caregivers' burden is significantly associated with behavioral disturbance, rather than with cognitive or functional disabilities (Cohen et al, 1997). Therefore, identification of the type and frequency of the behavior presentation through a standardized assessment tool could help to provide appropriate management strategies in order to reduce the caregiving stress. The participants were a group of family caregivers (N=73) caring for their demented older relatives at home. A multidimensional burden inventory - Chinese version - and the caregiving hassle scale - Chinese version - were adopted to measure the level of burden amongst the Chinese family caregivers, as well as the type and frequency of daily hassles presented by the demented elderly at home. The identified behavior hassles were mainly wandering, restlessness, agitation, emotional outburst, lack of cooperation, waking at night and occasional aggression. The result illustrates that there is a significant association between the level of burden and the frequency of behavioral disturbance ($r = .756$, $p<0.000$). It was further supported by their verbal report that they had no problem taking care of their confused older relatives at home. It was only when there was an outburst of disruptive behavior that they felt stressed and hassled. Therefore, intervention in terms of a psychoeducation model and adequate social support would enhance caregivers' coping skills and help to reduce the frequency of the undesirable behavior presented by elderly persons with dementia (Cohen et al, 1997)

SESSION 235

The English National Plan for the Health and Social Care of Older People: Part I

Ian Philp (National Director Older People's Services) Department of Health, London, UKJune Crown (Chairman)Age Concern England, London, UK

1. How and why a national plan for health and social care for older people was developed. 2. What are the roles of government and non-government organisations in the implementation of a national plan. 3. What lessons are there from other countries for helping to implement the English National Plan? 4. What lessons are there for other countries from the English national plan? Structure: (i) 25 minute presentation by Professor Philp about the development and content of the English National Plan for modernising health and social care of older people. (ii) Modernising health and social care for older people 5 minute response by Dr Crown about the role of an NGO in shaping and implementing the national plan. (iii) 3x 10 minute responses from international authorities on health/social care policy for older people (Robert Kane, Alex Kalache, A.N. other - all to be confirmed) on advice on implementation and lessons to be drawn for other countries. (iv) hour for audience questions and comments and panel responses (chaired by June Crown) Content: The National Service Framework reflects the issues that are of prime importance to older people in relation to their health. They wish to remain healthy and independent as long as possible. If they need acute care, they, like the rest of the population, want it within reasonable time, of high quality, with easy access, and they want to be assured that they are not discriminated against merely on the basis of chronological age. If

they need continuing care they want services to be integrated, accessible and provided in an environment that is both professional and dignified. The voluntary sector has a significant role to play in this interesting new approach to policy making at the national level. Policy development - The voluntary sector has access to a wide range of information about older people, their needs and their priorities, as well as about many of the practical problems with existing services. It can therefore collaborate with professionals and Government officials in the development of the strategy, to ensure that it is appropriate and realistic. This approach improves the chances of the strategy being welcomed by key stakeholders when published and assists in generating political commitment to the main proposals. Policy Implementation - The successful implementation of a policy for older people needs the participation of many agencies in the public, private and voluntary sectors. The voluntary sector is experienced in working across these sectors and so can play a valuable part in bringing together implementation groups at national and local levels that will be able to achieve change. Monitoring - It is essential that a major new initiative such as the National Service Framework is monitored so that progress can be recognised, problems identified at an early stage, and lessons learned that may benefit future work. The voluntary sector is also well placed, because of its experience of working with older people and providing services to them, to help to develop suitable monitoring systems and to analyse the findings. Advocacy - Age Concern England seeks to work constructively with Government and other bodies concerned with the welfare of older people. It is, however, independent of such bodies, so has an important role in advocacy that is not always open to statutory agencies. This is important in keeping issues on the agenda that might otherwise be overlooked and could be of assistance in ensuring that the exciting ambitions of this National Service Framework are realised. Anticipated Outcomes: This will be the first presentation outside of the UK of a much anticipated and hugely ambitious policy development from England. It will describe a vision for health and social care of older people and generate debate about how to develop and implement advanced models of health and social care for older people. It is likely to generate considerable interest from social and clinical gerontologists, practitioners, policy-makers and all those working to improve the care of older people. Discussion will inform the implementation of the national plan in England, and stimulate similar initiatives appropriate for the culture and systems of care in other countries.

The English National Plan for the Health and Social Care of Older People: Part II

Ian Philp

The English national plan consists of six inter-related programmes of activitiy : a National Service Framework for health & social care of older people providing :- · Care closer to home- Intermediate Care · Improved access to services- Care Direct · Integrating health & social care services- Care Trusts · Promoting health in the elderly- Health Promotion · Funding and Quality in Long Term Care The plan is led by a National Director (an older person's "Czar"). There are also underpinning programmes for research, human resources and information systems development with £1.4 billion ($2billion) p.a. additional investment in older people's services as part of the Government's modernisation agenda for health and social care services. National and Regional Task Forces have also been established to support the older people's programme. The centre-piece programme, the National Service Framework will be published early in 2001. It has two central principles: · Eliminating age discrimination · Delivering Person Centred Care It will promote a "whole systems" approach with a specific focus in four areas: · Promoting health and independence · Improving general hospital care · Developing Intermediate care · Ensuring older people receive a high quality of care and palliative care. It gives detailed attention to the care of older people with · Stroke · Dementia · Falls · Old age depression

SESSION 236

Characteristics of a Sample of Community-Dwelling Older Adults Related to Driving Status

R.V. Sims, R.M. Allman, P.B. Baker, E.V. Bodner (The Center for Aging of the University of Alabama at Birmingham and the Birmingham Veterans’ Affairs Medical Center, Birmingham, AL, USA)

We performed a cross-sectional analysis of data from the UAB Study on Aging to examine associations between demographic and health variables and driving status among a sample of older community-dwelling adults. Medicare beneficiaries from 5 central Alabama counties were interviewed in their homes in 1999-00. Functional measures included a composite physical performance measure (PPM), the Mini-Mental State Examination (MMSE) and questionnaires on Activities of Daily Living. The sample (N=321; mean age 75.1, SD=1.5) was 46% rural, 42% African American, 47% male, 25% with incomes <$8000 (US)/yr and 18% reported education < 6th grade. Subjects were stratified by unlimited (N=160), short distances only (N=64), stopped (N=61) and never (N=40) driving. Across more restricted driving strata (i.e, from unlimited to stopped), participants became increasingly older, female and unmarried, less educated and white and demonstrated progressively higher Geriatric Depression Scale scores. Worsening self-reported health, MMSE scores and PPM’s and fewer blocks walked seemed to parallel this progression. All p values for differences across driving strata were < 0.0001. The 40 participants, who reported never driving, had better self-reported health, were more fit and less depressed than former drivers. Demographic, health and functional variables were related to driving status in older community-residing seniors.

Injurious Crash Risk and Medical Conditions and Medication Use among Elderly Drivers

Xinjie Cui (Alberta Health and Wellness; University of Alberta, Edmonton, Canada); Donald P. Schopflocher (Alberta Health and Wellness; University of Alberta, Edmonton, Canada); Allen R. Dobbs (DriveABLE; University of Alberta, Edmonton, Canada) and Stephan Gabos (Alberta Health and Wellness, Edmonton, Canada)

Purpose: Identify medical factors (diseases and drugs) associated with injurious crash risk among elderly drivers. Methods: Population-based case-control study. Cases included elderly (=65.5) drivers who had emergency room visits due to injuries related to motor vehicle crashes (n=915). Control/case ratio was 10:1 and total sample size was 10,065. Data on medical diagnosis and prescription drug use from government administrative databases were modeled against injurious crash using multivariate logistic regression modeling techniques where driver characteristics, comorbid conditions and co-medications were statistically controlled for. Results: Use of benzodiazepines, non-tricyclic antidepressants, ophthalmic solutions, antibiotics, or topical antifungal medications was associated with an increased risk of injurious crash. Adjusted odds ratios (OR) for these medications ranged from 1.17 to 1.80. The relationship between diseases and injurious crash risk was complex and often involved interactions with comorbid conditions and medications. For example, diabetic drivers who also had disorders of joints/spine but were not on diuretic medications had an increased injurious crash risk (adjusted OR, 2.36). Female drivers with sleep disorders who were free from acute pulmonary infection had a 3-time increase in injurious crash risk (adjusted OR, 2.98) compared to healthy male drivers. Also, both intestinal diseases and a history of injury were associated with an increase in injurious crash risk, with an adjusted OR of 1.27 and 1.51, respectively. Conclusions: Certain medical diagnoses and prescription medications are associated with injurious crash and some interact with one another to affect crash risk.

The Effects of a Simulated Cellular Phone Conversation on Visual Search for Traffic Signs

Lisa McPhee, Geoffrey Ho, Wanda Dennis, Charles Scialfa & Jeff Caird [Department of Psychology, University of Calgary, Calgary,

Alberta CANADA]

PURPOSE: Younger and older drivers searched for traffic signs in digitized images of traffic scenes. The intent of the study was to determine the impact of a simulated cell phone task on age differences in search performance. METHOD: There were 16 younger (Mage = 22 yrs) and 16 older (Mage = 64 yrs) adult drivers were involved. Everyone was in good health and normal for their age with respect to visual function. The search task required that observers determine whether warning and regulatory signs were embedded in traffic scenes. Participants searched for these signs when that was the only task to perform and also while listening and responding to the logical memory (LM) test of the Wechsler Memory Scale. RESULTS: People were less accurate, slower, made more eye movements and fixated objects for longer durations when engaged in the simulated cell phone task. They also judged search to be more difficult under the cell phone condition. Content of the cell phone conversation was remembered less well in the dual-task condition. Older adults were slower and less accurate on all tasks but this did not interact with either clutter or cell phone use. Age differences in memory for content were greater in the cell phone condition. CONCLUSION: Cell phone use had a deleterious impact on search performance but did not interact with age. However, the main effects imply that in driving conditions where dual tasks like cell phone usage compromise search, older adults will be at greater risk.

SESSION 237

Films and Videos on Art and Elderhood: Focus on Poetry and Visual Arts

James Vanden Bosch (Terra Nova Films, Inc, Chicago, Illinois USA)

Writing in the Upward Years: May Sarton (30 minutes, released in 1991) - this video focuses on the role of aging in the creative process and how it has affected Sarton's life. It features scenes of the poet reading selected works in which she has charted the waters of her own aging. Augmented by archival photographs, the dramatic reading and candid interviews provide a rare and intimate portrait of a journey into older age. // The Traveling Brushes (29 minutes, released in 1999) - Narrated by Julie Harris, the documentary profiles the lives of five mid-life and older women. All artists, they joined together on the Eastern Shore of Maryland more than 15 years ago to take trips so they could paint landscapes. Despite their personal challenges of widowhood, or life as a caregiver, these women exemplify what it means to live life with meaning, passion and fulfillment. // Something Else (19 minutes, released in 1989) - Psychotherapist Emily Atwater is hired to determine eccentric Arthur Munson's mental competency. The problem? He's covered his house with 50,000 beer cans. Is Arthur Munson a folk artist or certifiable? The filmmaker was inspired by the lifework of John Milkovich, who, with his wife's blessing, transformed their simple home into a neighborhood treasure or an eyesore, based on differing opinions. // Why? (12 minutes, released in 1994) - When 60-year-old art student Carol Halstead was repeatedly asked what she was doing in school at such an age, she offered this mesmerizing fusion of photographs, drawings, paintings, cartoons, and computer graphics as her response

SESSION 238

Arterial hypertension control in elderly - could we do any better?

M. Dubrava, M. Figurova, Z. Mikes, J. Janosiova, S. Krcmery (Geriatric Department, School of Medicine, Comenius University, Bratislava, Slovakia)

PURPOSE: Nowadays it is no doubt, that arterial hypertension (AH) should be treated effectively also in elderly patients (pts). Scientific evidence for well-known therapeutic guidelines in AH is impressive. Unfortunately, there is little known about results, achieved in everyday clinical practice in elderly. METHOD: Retrospective study in a setting of an university acute geriatric department. Medical records of all pts with AH older than 64 years (yrs) hospitalised in 1998 were analysed (n = 469, average age 76.6 yrs, 25 % older than 80 yrs). 39 parameters were monitored in each patient, including blood pressure (BP) values at admission and during the last three days of hospitalisation, presence of polymorbidity and AH treatment. RESULTS: At admission, 70% pts who were not hospitalised because of AH, had systolic blood pressure >140 mm Hg and 18% of them were taking no antihypertensive drug. During hospitalisation the average BP was reduced from 163/91 to 144/80 mm Hg (average decline 39/23 mm Hg in patients admitted because of AH, 22/13 mm in others). Polymorbidity concerning diseases with potential interference with treatment of AH was frequent: three and more out of 21 monitored diseases were present in 85% of patients. The most preferred antihypertensive agents were ACE inhibitors and diuretics (at admission/discharge 37/59% and 41/57%). CONCLUSION: The AH control in elderly outpatients is not completely adequate. Our results achieved in BP control during hospitalisation in elderly are not completely in accordance with guidelines. The debate continues whether guidelines are entirely applicable for this age group.

EFFECT OF A DIETARY INTERVENTION ON HYPERTENSION IN THE ELDERLY

Sujatha Ramamurti & M. Saimala, (Dept. of Home Science, S. V. UNIVERSITY TIRUPATI-517 502 A.P India)

The objective of the study was to assess the effect of dietary intervention on hypertension in a co-morbidity free sample of (N=225) community dwelling hypertensive elderly in the age group 60-80. The subjects were randomly assigned to five age matched treatments and one control group. The treatment groups received independent supplements of (a) Safflower biscuits (b) Ascorbic acid 500 mg (c) Potassium chloride 600 mg (d) Potassium chloride 1200 mg (e) high fibre supplement respectively, while the control group received a placebo for a period of sixty days. Pre and post-tests of Blood Pressure were conducted to assess effects of the supplements. Biochemical analysis included assessment of lipid profiles, serum ascorbic acid levels, sodium and potassium levels in urine, serum and erythrocytes. Fibre supplementation and potassium supplementation significantly lowered blood pressure and certain lipid fraction levels. Implications for a pure dietary as well as drug cum dietary interventions are considered.

Hypertension and Cognitive Dysfunction in the Elderly: Correlation with Age and Anti-Hypertensive Treatment

L. T. Cavalini, D. Chor (Epidemiology and Quantitative Methods in Health, National School of Public Health, Oswaldo Cruz Foundation, Rio de Janeiro, Brazil)

Both hypertension and cognitive dysfunction are highly prevalent conditions among the elderly population, and have a direct influence on quality of life. For this reason, it is the interest of public health to identify associations between these disorders. We have performed a case-control study, with 99 cases and 208 controls, to study the association between arterial hypertension and cognitive deficit in a group of individuals at least 65 years old. Cognitive function was evaluated by the Mini-Mental State Examination (MMSE), which identified cases and controls. Interview and review of medical records allowed subjects classification by exposure status (hypertension). A strong inverse association was found between hypertension and cognitive dysfunction, in elderly people, only in their 80s and over (OR = 0.13; CI 95% = 0.03 0.54). This association was significant only among those diagnosed as hypertensives for at least five years. There was no association between hypertension and cognitive dysfunction in the 65 to 79 year-olds. The anti-hypertensive treatment categories (regular, irregular, not-treated) had less chances of cognitive dysfunction (respectively, 64%, 58% e 44%) than the not hypertensive group, although in the not-treated hypertensive group, with no statistical significance. The inverse association between hypertension and cognitive deficit among the most elderly confirms the hypothesis of other authors that in this age bracket, a certain level of arterial pressure is needed to maintain cognitive function, and our findings suggest that only in treated hypertensive subjects this effect is obtained.<?xml:namespace prefix = o ns = "urn:schemas-microsoft-com:office:office" />

Management of Arterial Hypertension in Old and Senile Patients

N.N.Kipshidze; T.G.Zubiashvili; Research Institute of Experimental and clinical Therapy, Tbilisi, Georgia.

The aim of the present work was to study the efficiency of combined hypotensive therapy at arterial hypertension (AH) in old and senile age. 182 patients with AH old (60-74y) an senile (75-89y) whis revealed LVH were examined. All patients underwent clinical, electrocardiographic and echocardiographic investigations before and after a long-term hypotensive therapy (12 months). Combined using of drugs with different mechanisms of action (selective beta-adrenoblocator athenolol, calcium antagonist - corinfar and inhibitor angiotensintransforming captopril ferment) allows to carry out long-term treatment, using a small therapeutic doses that levels side effects of drugs. On the basis of long-term combined hypotensive therapy (corinfar+ athenolol, corinfar+captopril, captopril+ athenolol) regression of LVH was achieved in 62-770f cases, with less mass of LV miocard in 10-12% and with stable normalisation of AH in 95.90f cases. Improvement of systolic, diastolic functions, normalisation of bioelectrical activation of LV miocard were observed.

The role of ACE-Inhibitors in the treatment of hypertensive elderly patients

Gosch M. (Landeskrankenhaus Hochzirl Hochzirl 1 6170 Zirl Austria)

Purpose: What is the role of ACE-Inhibitors in the treatment of hypertensive elderly patients Method: Research in the literature on this topic Results and Conclusion: Hypertension has a high prevalence among elderly patients. Randomised trials have already demonstrated that treating healthy older persons with hypertension is highly efficacious. Nevertheless some questions are coming up. On one hand the generalisation of these trial results, particulary for older persons with serious medical comorbidities and poor functional status, is not clear. On the other hand different antihypertensive drugs have shown to be effective. Which drug for which patient? Even data from randomised intervention trials showing that the treatment affects cardiovascular morbidity and mortality, were missing, ACE-inhibitors have been used for more than a decade to treat high blood pressure. For a younger population the captopril prevention project showed no differences between ACE-inhibitors and conventional antihypertensive treatment (diuretics, beta-blocker) concerning the primary endpoints (myocardial infarction, stroke and other cardiovascular death). The STOP-2-study confirmed these results also for elderly patients. Treating elderly patients we must be aware of physiological changes with age and the comorbidities. Of significance among this patient is the declining renal function. Admissions for uraemia that are related to the use of ACE-inhibitors are still commonplace, even many cases are preventable by monitoring the renal function, but guidelines are still missing . Concerning the comorbidities ACE-inhibitors have benefits compared to other antihypertensive drugs, especially in cases of heart failure, diabetes and coronary heart disease.

SESSION 239

Atrial fibrillation and cognitive function: A Slovak study

Stefan Krajcik (Slovak Postgraduate Academy of Medicine, Bratislava, Slovakia Peter Mikus (National Institute of TB and Respriatory Diseases, Bratislava, Slovakia) Andrea Sobolova (National Institute of TB and Respiratory Diasease, Bratislava, Slovakia) Vladimira Pipiskova (National Institute of TB and Respiratory Diseases, Bratislava, Slovakia) et alt.

Purpose: Relation of atrial fibrillation (AF) and cognitive function. Method: MMSE questionnaire administrated at 210 patients with AFand 253 controls over 60 years of age, both inpatients og geriatric or long term care departments. Results: The study group had significantly lower MMSE score than the control group (19.36 vs. 20.6), This difference persisted after exclusion of hypertonics and diabetics (17.2 vs.18.7). Deleterious effect of risk factors was summed up. The poorest score was found in patients with combination of AF, DM a hypertension (17.2), then in those without AF having combination of DM and hypertension (18.7). The best was in patients without risk factors (20.86). The stroke incidence was higher in the study group (21.4% vs 15.38%). The deleterious effect of AF was more pronounced than that of stroke (20.18 after stroke without AF, 19.43 with AF without stroke). The most pronounced decline of cognitive function was found early in the course of AF (MMSE score: 23.05 in those with duration maxim. 1 year an 16.3 in those with max. 3 years) Conclusion: AF is significant independent risk factor of vascular dementia.

Atrial fibrillation and cognitive impairment in elderly patients

Gosch M, Talasz H, Benvenuti-Falger U, Rhomberg H.P. (Landeskrankenhaus Hochzirl Hochzirl 1 6170 AUSTRIA)

Purpose: to determine differences in the cognitive status of elderly patients with sinus rhythm and atrial fibrillation Method: The design of our study was prospective and descirptive. We included 717 pateints aged over 70, who came to our geriatric assessment ward. The mean age was 81.3. Two of three patients were female. Patients with a stroke in their history were excluded. The cognitive function was measured by the Mini-Mental-State examination and the Clock Completion. Furthermore we checked the activities of daily living by the ADL-Score of Barthel. By doing an ECG we divided the patients into two goups, one with sinus rhythm and the other with atrial fibrillation. 623 patients, mean age of 81.1, had sinus rhythm, 93 patients, mean age 82.3, had atrial fibrillation. Results: The MMSE score was significant lower in the group of patients with atrial fibrillation. The mean MMSE was 21.6 in patients with atrial fibrillation, 23.6 in patients with sinus rhythm. By using the Mann-Whitney-test we find a high significance ($p<0,001$). In the Clock Completion we found nearly the same result. The mean score in patients with sinus rhythm was lower, exactly 3.3, compared to 4.1 in patients with atrial fibrillation. Also this result was statistically significant by using the Mann-Whitney test ($p<0.05$). We observed a lower ADL-score in patients with atrial fibrillation, but the difference was not significant. Conclusion: Atrial fibrillation is associated with lower levels of cognitive function in elderly patients, even though they have not had a stroke in their history.

Nonvalvular atrial fibrillation (NVAF) and stroke prevention in old patients in long term care units

A. Gentric - J.J. Chever - J. Jouquan

The prevalence of NVAF increases with age (>10 % in persons older than 80 years). The risk of stroke is five fold increased in patients with NVAF, particularly when other risk factors are present : âge (>75 years), hypertension, cardiac failure, prior stroke. In both primary and secondary stroke prevention in NVAF patients, it has been shown that the risk of stroke was significantly reduced by Warfarine (68%) and to a lesser extent by Aspirin (28 %). The aim of our study was to determine the proportion of old patients hospitalized in the 7 long term care units of our district who were receiving an antithrombolic treatment. Of the 1790 patients hospitalized, 138 patients (7.75 %) had a NVAF (101 females, 37 males, mean age 82.1 years) , 62 patients were demented (DSM IV criteria). Of the 138 patients with NVAF, 9 (6,5 %) received Warfarine (INR : 2-3), 2 (1.4 %) were treated with Aspirin (325 mg per day), 55 patients received 75 to

160 mg of Aspirin per day (ineffective or non evaluated dosage in NVAF). Of the 129 patients who didn't receive Warfarine, only 29 (21.7 %) had a validated contraindication. Only 6,5 % of long term care units patients with NVAF received Warfarine. Comparable studies were undertook in the USA or the UK with a proportion of 30 % of patients treated. Contraindication to Warfarine account for a quarter of non prescription thus other reasons should be identified to improve stroke prevention in the elderly.

Usefulness of prophylatic measures in the Korean elderly with atrial fibrillation

S.Y. Choi, M.D, C. H. Kim, M.D.(Department of Internal Medicine, Seoul National University College of Medicine. Seoul, Korea)

The purpose of this study was to assess the prevalence of atrial fibrillation, and the incidence of new thromboembolism, in elderly Korean patients with atrial fibrillation. Among the elderly (65yr) patients exhibited atrial fibrillation without valvular heart disease, 156 patients that did not exhibit contraindication against anticoagulation therapy were enrolled for a review of associated diseases, risk factors of thromboembolism, medication for anticoagulation therapy, and new thromboembolism. The average length of follow up was 42months. The prevalence of atrial fibrillation was 6.2% with the condition increasing with age. Among 156 patients, thirty-one patients (19.9%) received anticoagulation therapy with warfarin (Group 3). Fifty-three patients (34.0%) received aspirin (Group 2). Seventy-two patients (46.1%) were under observation without any specific medication (Group 1). The frequencies of patients with previous evidence of thromboembolism were 9.7% in Group 1, 22.6% in Group 2, 67.7% in Group 3 (p<0001). The rate of new thromboembolisms was 4.5%/patient-year for all patients, 7.1%/patient-year in Group 1, and 2.7%/patient-year in Group 2, 0%/patient-year in Group 3. The rate of new thromboembolisms in the patients with histories of thromboembolism was 36.0%/patient-year in Group 1, 3.8%/patient-year in Group 2, and 0%/patient-year in Group 3. The cumulative rate of new thromboembolisms was significantly different in the three groups, in the total number of patients, and the patients with histories of thromboembolism (Group 1 vs. Group, 2 p=0.014; Group 1 vs. Group 3, p=0.001; and Group 2 vs. Group 3, p=0.12 using the Kaplan-Meier method and log-rank test), but not in the patients without previous thromboembolism. Warfarin and aspirin are highly efficacious in the treatment of thromboembolism in elderly Koreans with nonvalvular atrial fibrillation and evidence of previous thromboembolism.

SESSION 240

Complaints Management: It Is Worth the Hassle

Netha Dyck and Wendy Whalley (Winnipeg Regional Health Authority, Winnipeg, Manitoba, Canada)

The purpose of this presentation is to highlight the goals, objectives, policies and implementation strategies that were used to develop the complaints management program, as well as the outcomes and quality initiatives that have resulted. The challenges and opportunities encountered will also be discussed. The Winnipeg Regional Health Authority (WRHA) encourages and fosters the philosophy that every complaint is an opportunity for quality improvement. Based on a strong commitment to continuous improvement, the WRHA has developed and implemented an innovative regional approach to complaint management that is used in both acute and continuing care sectors. Through the regional statistical analysis, quality performance issues were identified and quality improvement initiatives were developed. The outcome achieved through the program is a consistent client-focused approach to complaint management that assists in satisfactory resolution.

Developing care planning in residential care home services - potentials and problems

David STANLEY (Centre for Care of Older People, University of Northumbria, Newcastle upon Tyne, England)

The purpose of the programme was to improve the care of older people in residential care homes by working with agency staff to develop and evaluate existing care planning and practices. Action research methodology was used, employing a cycle of enquiry, intervention and evaluation. The action elements were informed by a best practice review and the baseline of existing practice in the two study sites was identified. Practitioners and managers collaborated with researchers in working towards shared goals that could promote improvements in services. A workshop enabled care staff to recognise what providing better care involved, and managers to recognise what care staff required in order to provide better care. Best practice approaches (key working, life story maps, work with carers / families) were introduced and evaluated. Results indicated that all stakeholders gained. Residents benefited from enhanced care, care staff were enthusiastic to develop new practice skills and managers were keen to promote and support the project. However, conflicting interests also emerged during the course of the study, centring on the differential treatment of participating residents, others perceptions of the beacon role of participating care staff, and the resource implications. The study concluded that baseline care provision could be improved through the approaches adopted, but also recognised that there were powerful inhibitors to the improvement process. This presentation will focus on the interplay between these two sets of competing dynamics.

Modeling Information Systems for Planning, Management, and Evaluation in Elderly Care: A Business Process Analysis Approach

Richard Pieper, Gerhard Nunner (University of Bamberg, Bamberg, Germany)

The productivity, effectiveness, and efficiency in elderly care systems has to be enhanced in aging societies by information technologies. The introduction of IT implies not only the application of readymade IT from other fields. The availability of reusable IT components and of higher level programming languages supports the design of information systems by social planners (end user programming) in cooperation with information technologists. For the modeling of information systems new procedures and tools have to be developed which are adapted to the problem situations of social care and support the cooperation between social care experts and IT experts. The approach of object-oriented business process modeling is introduced as a framework to specify the interface of management and work processes in social care and information system design and to structure development processes. Using the case of strategic planning for elderly care, special aspects of modeling social care systems are identified and strategies, concepts and tools introduced for - description, analysis, and modeling of care planning and care provision - specification of user requirements and system requirements, and - cooperation in development and implementation between social care experts and information technologists. The framework utilizes the experience of an EU-research project developing a PC program for strategic planning in elderly care and the results of a pilot study on the usability of the framework with social care practitioners. Both indicate the need for a methodology adapted to this specific field for IT applications.

Needs-management in care institutions: Perspectives from organization-theory

Elisabeth Reitinger (Institute of Organization and Supply management, Vienna University of Economics and Business Administration, Vienna, Austria)

Purpose: The research interest of the ongoing study stems from the every-day-challenge in the work of care institutions: How to organize basic provisions for elderly in a needs-oriented way? In addition to improving knowledge in care, medicine and gerontology, it will be argued that organization-theory contributes fundamentally to understanding this complex problem. Methods: A theoretical framework based on systems-theory will be elaborated. Needs-management in care institutions will be interpreted within this theoretical frame. Case studies conducted in the City of Vienna will offer empirical evidence. Results According to systems-theory, organizations consist of communication, rather than people, buildings, rules or a combination of these. It differentiates between social systems (organizations) and psychic systems (e.g. the elderly). The core function of needs-management is to design an interface between both systems in such a way that individual needs become relevant to organizational communication. Organizations reproduce themselves recoursively (autopoiesis) through communication inside the organization and through interactions with their environment. The selection of themes that become part of communication is crucial for organizational responsiveness to the needs of the elderly. Needs-management has to open opportunities influencing these selections and communications. Conclusions: Because care institutions are made up of communication, only those themes and needs of elderly people will be taken into account, that become part of this specific communication. Therefore, the management of spaces, where such communication is given room, is essential. Needs-management has to create awareness of the communications behind the communications and to allow and initiate reflections about them.

Supporting clinical and program decision-making in the community: The role of a best practice resource centre

Kevin Brazil (Department of Clinical Epidemiology and Biostatistics, McMaster University, Hamilton) Larry Chambers (Department of Clinical Epidemiology and Biostatistics, McMaster University, Hamilton) Joan Royle (School of Nursing, McMaster University) Maureen Montemuro R. (Samuel McLaughlin Centre for Research and Education in Aging and Health, McMaster University)

This report will provide an overview on the development of a Long Term Care Best Practice Resource Centre. The results of both a feasibility study and the outcomes of a one year pilot will be presented. The pilot project involved a hospital as the information service provider and two demonstration sites a Community Care Access Centre and a nursing home who used the the services of the Centre. The presentation will include: a review of information needs of providers in the participating sites; how the service was used during the trial; and, how a Resource Centre can be most responsive to staff needs and concerns. The audience will also receive an update on current activities to establish a Resource Centre to serve Central South Ontario.

SESSION 241

Constructing dementia and dementia care in daily practices

Jonathan Parker (University of Hull, UK)

Purpose: This paper describes some of the ways in which the daily practices of social care staff add to the construction of dementia and dementia care in those settings. It explores the concept of daily practices and its development within family theory in the context of dementia care. Method:The model of daily practices is applied to a small study of a day care setting for people with dementia. The data for this study are taken from observations of the daily practices of, and interviews with, social care staff working with people with dementia in a local authority day centre in the UK. The data is analysed by reference to the concept of practices across a range of constructive levels and domains deriving from the data. A process of axial and selective coding was used to make connections between observed practices, perceptions of care and dementia care. Results: A number of levels of practice and construction were identified from the observations made and interviews undertaken. These concerned the physical environment, a cognitive and intellectual level and an emotional/personal level. At each level of practice and construction, a number of constructive domains were noted. These overlapped across levels. The domains included 'holding and homogenising', 'demarcating and distancing' and 'care-giving and control'. Conclusion: The construction and reconstruction of practices is multidirectional and influence at each level can produce effects at other levels - including policy, procedure and practice. It is especially important to attend to the personal biographies of staff to provide a supportive environment that encourages reflection on practice and the development of approaches that take cognisance of the individual needs of the person with dementia.

Spouses of Persons with Dementia: Self Expression and Intervention

R. Ingebretsen (NOVA - Norwegian Social Research, Oslo, Norway) and P. E. Solem (NOVA - Norwegian Social Research, Oslo, Norway)

PURPOSE: To study 1) how spouses of persons with dementia cope with losses and care-giving tasks, 2) how this is affected by former and present spousal contracts and attachment patterns, 3) influences the life space and self expression of the care-giving spouse, and 4) how these factors have to be considered by intervention. METHOD: Twenty-eight spouses (9 males and 19 females) of persons with dementia were interviewed at an early stage of dementia and then four times over period of five years. The interview was semi-structured and covered a process of increasing need for help and support. The subjects were 60-87 years at the baseline. RESULTS: The study has developed a model to understand the consequences of changes in relationship contracts and attachments patterns on the self-expression of the care-giving spouse. Three patterns of consequences are found; restricted spontaneity, increased independence, and released potentials for care giving and closeness. The latter is more typical of male care-givers. Intervention strategies discussed are to bring in alternative interpretations of the situation, alternative ways of relating to the spouse with dementia, and ways to develop and sustain other social relationships. Interventions offering practical help, respite or institutional placement has to be adapted to the individual needs of the care-giver, the often-implicit relationship contract, attachment patterns and the balance between closeness and distance in the relationship. CONCLUSION: Effects of dementia care-giving like restricted spontaneity, increased independence, and released care potentials and closeness requires differential intervention strategies. —

________________ Per Erik Solem NOVA Pb 3223 Elisenberg N-0208 Oslo Phone: +47 22 54 12 67 Facs: +47 22 54 12 01

The meaning of caring for a demented relative

Calda, Celia (Third Age Open University, UNATI, Rio de Janeiro State University, UERJ, Rio de Janeiro, Brazil)

This study focuses on the meaning of being-there as defined by the situation of being a caregiver of an elderly relative undergoing a demential process. Understanding such a meaning is seen as essential for the improvement and broadening of traditional approaches concerning dementia and support of caregivers. The theoretical and methodological framework is based upon Martin Heidegger's approach to phenomenology. Data were collected by means of interviews carried out with main caregivers of elderly relatives undergoing demential process being counseled at the UNATI/UERJ out-patient facilities. The speech of interviewees was analysed according to the Heideggerian phenomenological method at two distinct moments: the first one when, through the caregivers' vague and median understanding, the set of units of meaning were obtained; at the second moment, the understanding interpretation was carried out. Meanings revealed were: caregivers are tied to a time that is past (temporality); they are caregivers because there is no other way (factuality); caregivers are occupied rather than preoccupied (occupation vs. preoccupation); caregivers provide care patiently (tolerance). The conclusion highlights the importance of discussing time and caregiving in relation to health care. Regarding time, caregivers may be ready to adjust their daily life according to professional orientation without denial of their own expectations. Concerning caregiving, it is essential to be aware that, at first, caregivers are likely to follow orientation provided by health workers. However, as the routine of caring for a relative is incorporated to daily life, caregivers are bound to make decisions independently from health workers.

The Nature of Caring for Dementia in Thailand

S. Sasat (The Royal Thai Army Nursing College, Bangkok, Thailand), R.M. Bryar, (School of Nursing, University of Hull, UK), and A.J. Newens (School of Nursing, University of Hull, UK)

To explore the nature of caring for elderly demented relatives living at home in Thailand. Structure and semi-structure interviews were carried out with 44 pairs of known cases of demented patients and their principle carers. Significant correlations were found between levels of strain in carers and the cognitive impairment and physical dependence of subject. Spouse carers experienced significantly less strain, but reported more stress and physical strain and a poorer current relationship than younger relative carers. 94% of subjects and 57% of carers had a small support network. 75% of carers needed information about dementia illness and how to provide care at home and 60% felt the elderly relative should receive financial support. The primary motivation to care was derived from a strong filial obligation based on the Buddhist belief of 'reciprocity.' Policy recommendations include providing health education, financial support, and carers support groups.

SESSION 242

Chiropractic care of the older person: An evidence-based approach

Gleberzon, B.J. (Canadian Memorial Chiropractic College, Toronto, Ont.)

This article is an attempt to develop an evidentiary basis for chiropractic care for older persons. A qualitative review of the literature was conducted, with synthesis and interpretation by the author. Fifty nine articles were found within the search parameters. These were in areas of chiropractic geriatric education (N=3), demographics/epidemiology (N=9), case studies (N=25), clinical trials (N=4), and clinical guidelines (N=18). The literature indicates the utilization of chiropractic services is very common among older adults, particularly for spinal pain, headaches, and strain and sprain injuries, and that the medical community is becoming more accepting of this treatment approach. Chiropractors also emphasis the importance of health promotion and prevention, often recommending healthful lifestyle choices. Older patients report they believe chiropractic care is important to their health. The evidence suggests spinal manipulative therapy (SMT) is effective for the treatment of acute and chronic low back and neck pain, and certain types of headaches. Extrapolating these findings to older patients must be done with caution; nevertheless, it is reasonable to predict that older adults respond as well as younger adults to the use of SMT for spinal pain. Although not without risk, SMT is a very safe treatment, especially when compared to analgesic therapy. The evidence supporting the benefits of chiropractic care for non-neuromusculoskeletal conditions is less robust. In summary, utilization rates of chiropractic services is increasing, and the evidence supports the effectiveness and safety of chiropractic care, especially for neuromusculoskeletal conditions, and older patients believe chiropractic care is important for their overall health.

Complimentary Therapies in a Rural Aged Care Setting

Lyn Reid (Hepburn Health Service, Daylesford, Victoria, Australia)

The use of complimentary therapies at Hepburn Health Service have become a valuable addition to the quality of care of the aged residents. Over the past 7 years complimentary therapy has expanded to encompass all 92 beds of the service and is conducted 5 days per week. The purpose of complimentary therapy is to enhance the residents quality of life by providing therapies which assist the resident to relax, calm down, decrease pain and assist with their overall well-being naturally, rather than using medical interventions. Therapies include massage, foot spas, spa baths and aromatherapy. These therapies are used for a variety of ailments, such as pain, stiffness, rashes, wound care and used to assist with residents' anxiety, stress and fear levels. Results from treatment have been difficult to measure; however, anecdotal evidence supports current research findings into the use of complimentary therapies in aged care. Hepburn Health Service has found complimentary therapy to be an important and integral part of the care delivered in the aged care units. By providing this therapy the service is assisting with providing holistic care to residents in a natural way.

Factors associated with registered massage therapy utilization among chronically ill seniors in Toronto Canada.

K. Willison (Institute for Human Development, Life Course and Aging, University of Toronto, Toronto, Canada)

Purpose: To identify social psychological and socioeconomic factors associated with the utilization of registered massage therapy (MT) by an urban chronically ill elderly population. Method: This descriptive, multi-site, exploratory, cross-sectional study makes use of questionnaires (n=90) as well as in-depth interviews (n=20). Toronto-area respondents are derived by the help of randomized registered massage therapists (practicing in Toronto Canada) to obtain a convenience sample of the population under study. To meet the study's objective, the "Behavioral Model of Health Services Use" developed by Andersen & Newman (1973) is used to operationalize Max Weber's notion of Life Chances. Predisposing, enabling as well as perceived need characteristics are then considered. Results: Findings to date mirrors existing research concerning the characteristics of those who commonly seek out complementary/alternative health care services. Data collection for this on-going study will be completed by late April with bivariate and descriptive analysis scheduled for completion by mid-June (2001). Pre-testing of the questionnaire has yielded a sample of n=31. Final target group sample size is set at n=90. Conclusion: Preliminary results support Max Weber's concept of life chances as a suitable determining indicator of MT utilization. This original contribution to the social gerontological literature is the first study of its kind in Canada to primarily focus on the use and non-use of registered massage therapy by seniors (aged 60+). Increasing usage of complementary/alternative medicine (CAM) such as massage therapy, combined with a rising number of seniors who may potentially use CAM, makes this a timely topic.

Herbal Product Use Among Western Kansas Elderly

Mary Morgan Liane Connelly RN, CNAA, Glen McNeil MS, RD/LD [Fort Hays State University, Hays. USA]

Purpose: This presentation will describe an ongoing study that describes herbal product use among the older adult population in Western Kansas. Indications for use, frequency of use, and expenditures on herbal products by the older adult will be discussed. Implications for practice in rural areas will be provided. Method: A survey design was used in this study for the purpose of describing the actual use of herbal products by this group. Forty-four percent of the 1070 surveys mailed were returned. Results: Of the 44% that were returned, forty-two percent (42%) of the sample reported use of herbal products. The average cost per month was 1-25 dollars. The majority of the respondents obtained herbal product information from advertising, TV and health food stores. Conclusions: Herbal product use is on the rise among older adults. Health care practitioners must become more prepared in the area of herbal products and their use in order to adequately serve the older adult population.

Herbal Remedies as a Self-Care Practice for Older Adults with Chronic Illness

Kristine Votova (Simon Fraser University, Vancouver, Canada)

Chronic illness is a reality for many older adults. Another reality is that more and more adults are using alternative therapies as self-care in response to chronic illness. In fact, use of herbal remedies, a popular aspect of alternative therapies, is widespread among all age groups (Drew & Myers, 1997). Is herbal remedy use dependent upon the adult's ability to cope with the disease and the perceived severity of disease (i.e, specific subjective factors)? Or do objective factors such as the type and duration of illness and exposure to the medical community impact herbal remedy use? Furthermore, are pain and the severity of pain important determinants of herbal remedy usage? Responses from Wave III (N=879) of an extensive panel study, the North Shore Self-Care Study, were analyzed to address these queries. Descriptive analysis revealed that about half of the older adults described arthritis as their primary chronic condition (48.8%) with high blood pressure (26.2%) and heart disease (25%) following. Logistic regression revealed that being female and having arthritis increased the likelihood of using herbal remedies (p>001). Lower income and reporting moderate levels of pain also impacted herbal remedy usage for older adults with chronic illness, only the association was not as strong. For older adults who use herbal remedies in addition to prescribed medications, a greater understanding of the interaction between the two is necessary to ensure that adverse drug reactions are prevented. Furthermore, awareness of an older adult's coping abilities will assist in understanding herbal remedy usage and the importance of herbals for the community dwelling older adult.

Medicinal herb products and medication use in elderly Canadians

C. I. Neutel (University of Ottawa Institute of Health of the Elderly, Ottawa, Canada), W.Walop (Health Canada, Ottawa, Canada)

Canadians have shown an increasing interest in medicinal herbs (MH) over the past decade. The objective of this study is to determine whether people use medicinal herbs and conventional medicine simultaneously. Data collected on 16,260 randomly selected Canadians over 60 in 1996-7 for the National Population Health Survey, included demographic variables, chronic conditions and drug and other health product use in the last two days before the interview. It was found that 5.9% of the population used MH, the most frequently used being garlic, ginseng and echinacea. MH were used more often by women (6.5%) then by men and was especially high for persons with self-reported depression and stress. Use of MH increased with use of conventional medication: from 3.4%MH use for those with no medications, 8.3%MH for one medication and 10.0%MH for 5+ medications. Especially vitamin use correlated highly with MH use: 2.7%MH use for those with no vitamins, 9.2%MH for one vitamin and 30% MH for 4+ vitamins. MH use also increased with number of chronic conditions reported but to a lesser degree. Of persons using any type of MH, 90.2% also used either vitamins or conventional medication in addition. We conclude that physicians need to be aware that many of their patients who take conventional medication, may also be taking MH, not always prescribed by their physician; and that the likelihood of MH use increases with the number of conventional medications.

SESSION 243

Health Habits, Self-efficacy, and Health Locus of Control among Chinese Elderly with Diabetes Mellitus

A. M. S. Wu, C. S. K. Tang (Department of Psychology, Chinese University of Hong Kong, HKSAR, China), T. C. T. Kwok (Department of Medicine, Chinese University of Hong Kong, HKSAR, China)

The psychological factors contributing to elderly patients’ decision to implement healthy habits, that in turn significantly determine their health status, are essential for the planning of social and medical services and policies for the elderly. The aim of this study is to examine the association of health habits with self-efficacy, health locus of control (HLC), and health value among those Chinese elderly with diabetes mellitus (DM). One hundred and ninety-four (119 males and 75 females) Chinese participants with DM who were 60 years old or above and attended an outpatient clinic for DM were individually interviewed. Correlation analysis results showed that age, educational level, DM duration and years of follow-up by DM nurse were all not associated with health habits practice of Chinese elderly (p>.05). On the other hand, their healthy habits were significantly correlated with their health value (r = .495), self-efficacy (r = .499), internal health locus of control (r = .384), as well as external – doctor health locus of control (r = .343) (p<.00). In other word, Chinese elderly with DM who value their health, are confident of their ability to practice various health habits, and view their illness as controllable by both doctor and themselves are more likely to engage in healthy habits. Health-promotion programmes for Chinese elderly should incorporate these results to enhance their efficiency.

Health information needs among English and Chinese speaking community-dwelling older adults in a Canadian metropolitan city

R.Y.M. Wong (University of British Columbia, Vancouver, Canada), L. Constable (Vancouver/Richmond Health Board, Vancouver, Canada), B.L. Beattie (University of British Columbia, Vancouver, Canada), P. Semeniuk (Vancouver Hospital and Health Sciences Centre, Vancouver, Canada)

To identify the self-perceived health information needs among English and Chinese speaking older adults in a major Canadian city, we conducted a cross-sectional survey of 442 community-dwelling individuals who attended public health forums, adult day centre programmes and other seniors groups from February to June 2000. All participants received a 2-page telephone contact list of commonly used community services printed in their native language before completing a self-administered questionnaire. Most respondents (38.2%) were between 65 and 74 years old, and 71.5% were females. Thirty-six percent completed the English survey, with the rest completing the Chinese version. Most respondents described their understanding of health concerns as about average or better. Women who were 75 years or older and English speaking tended to report poor understanding of their health concerns. Most respondents (94.3%) indicated that they would keep the community contact telephone list for future use. The most frequently selected services included support services (24.8%), personal emergency response systems (16.9%), and special services and programs (13.8%). Regardless of age, gender or language spoken, the most commonly selected source of health information was the family physician (51.1%). Television was identified as the most popular media (31.3%) for obtaining health information, while use of the Internet was scant (1.5%), particularly among older respondents. We concluded that a printed telephone list of community contacts was useful in addressing the health information needs of older adults, especially when printed in their native language. The family physician and television were important channels for disseminating health information.

Helping Patients Over the Barriers to Healthy Aging

Lyn MacBeath, FRCP(C), (Psychiatrist, Private Practice, Vancouver, BC)

PURPOSE: Medical care cannot substitute for healthful habits and life-enhancing living. How can we help our patients to effectively apply the findings of relevant healthcare research in making healthful lifestyle changes? With the demographic pressure of our aging population, new strategies are required in clinical practice for optimization of health outcomes with age and effective use of healthcare resources. METHOD: A physician-run pilot program of 8 to 12 weeks duration entitled Healthy Aging was developed for patient groups of variable sizes. The program has combined functions of both education and support group. Participants, and non-participant age-matched controls, were given questionnaires for identifying up to three lifestyle changes they wished to make and their readiness to change each one using Prochaska's Stages of

Change Measurement Scale. Follow-up questionnaires were distributed at the end of the course, and one year later, to monitor progress of the two groups and their use of healthcare resources. RESULTS: Usual barriers to making change were identified by the participant group and processed. Topics found to be most helpful included Communication Skills and Writing a Living Will. Over time the participant group identified various strategies and resources for making the changes they desired. CONCLUSION: Acknowledging barriers to change, and applying psychological insights and psychiatric expertise to move beyond them, were essential steps for most participants in making real change. Group work was supportive and motivating. The non-participant group was less effective at maintaining change over time.

Physical Activity, Health and Aging: Perceptions of Elderly Women of Portuguese Origin.

Josianne Roma (University of Ottawa, Ottawa, Canada) Geneviève Rail (University of Ottawa, Ottawa, Canada) Hélène Dallaire (University of Ottawa, Ottawa, Canada) Suzanne Laberge (Université de Montréal, Montréal, Canada) Philippe Voyer (Université Laval, Québec, Canada)

The purpose of this presentation is to identify the perceptions of physical activity, health and aging and their link to the health promotion strategies of economically disadvantaged elderly women of Portuguese origin. The methodology borrows from ethnography and favours, as a starting point, the meanings which elderly women ascribe to their successful aging strategies as well as their perceptions of physical activity and health. In-depth, semi-structured interviews taking the form of informal conversations were conducted with 10 women between 65 and 75 years of age from the Ottawa region. Conversations were recorded, transcribed, and then analysed using the NVivo qualitative content analysis software. The participants' perceptions of physical activity, health and aging are discussed in the results. In brief, these women, five who engage in some forms of physical activity (mostly walking) and five, who are inactive, perceive physical activity as an important strategy to improve their health and see it as a means to maintain and create social links. The participants have various definitions of health, which are often associated to a certain degree of autonomy. They also identify ways in which they can prevent sickness or illness, and mostly mention good nutrition and exercising. All the participants have a positive outlook on the future and many have projects they are planning on undertaking. With regards to aging, all the women indicate feeling good at their age and all are very positive about their life. The study indicates that regular physical activity is part of the successful aging strategies of the active participants and can become one of the successful aging strategies of those who are inactive, since they are aware of the benefits that physical activity can have on their health, well-being and future.

Sources of efficacy for Walking and Climbing Stairs among Older Adults

Sandra O'Brien Cousins, M.P.E, Ed.D, (University of Alberta, Edmonton, Canada) Maria C. Tan, BScOT (University of Alberta, Edmonton, Canada)

The sources of personal confidence for active living in late life are largely unknown. The purpose of this study was to identify the main contextual and cognitive determinants of beliefs about being able to walk blocks and climb flights of stairs among older adults. In addition, we were interested to find out if work-time physical activity (WTPA) interferes with leisure-time physical activity (LTPA). The specific goals of this study were to 1) clarify which contextual variables (demographic, lifestyle, health) influence self-efficacy for distance walking and stair-climbing; 2) explore which self-referent beliefs predict efficacy for walking and climbing stairs; and 3) examine the relationship of WTPA and LTPA. In total, 389 adults over age 50 successfully completed surveys gathering information on: i) 6 demographic characteristics of age, gender, health, education, cultural background, and lifelong physical activity; ii) self-referent beliefs such as exercise efficacy, support, health value, motivation, exertion, enjoyment and risk; and, iii) seven day recall inventories of WTPA and LTPA. Linear regressions predicting efficacy for flights of stairs one could climb showed that the significant demographic predictors were: being born outside Canada, healthier, younger, habitually active, and male. For blocks walked, being healthier and male were significant. The only significant cognitive predictor for stairs was perceived exertion, while, for walking efficacy, only the belief about enjoying exercise in a variety of settings was predictive. There was no relationship between WTPA and LTPA suggesting that energy spent at work tasks does not necessarily interfere with an active leisure lifestyle.

SESSION 244

Cultural Issues in the Recruitment, Assessment, and Treatment of Ethnically Diverse Caregiver Populations

V. Mitrani [University of Miami School of Medicine, Miami, USA] Measuring Family Interactions in Dementia Caregiver Families: Comparisson of Cuban American and European American Families. S. Argüelles [University of Miami School of Medicine, Miami, USA] On-The-Phone Discussion Groups in An Ethnically Diverse Sample of Caregivers of Alzheimer's Individuals. D. Loewenstein [University of Miami School of Medicine, Miami, USA] Sensitivity and Specificity of a New Semantic Interference Test for Ethnically Diverse Alzheimer's Disease Patients. T. Argüelles [University of Miami School of Medicine, Miami, USA] Practical and Theoretical Apects of Recruitment and Retention of Hispanic Caregivers of Alzheimer's Disease Patients. M. Pelaez [Family Health and Population Programs, PAHO, Washington, D.C. USA] -discussant. C. Eisdorfer [University of Miami School of Medicine, Miami, USA] -co-discussant.

This symposium addresses research on the importance/impact of culturally appropriate methods when working with ethnically-diverse Alzheimer's (AD) individuals and their caregivers. The focus of this session is on the recruitment/retention, assessment, and treatment of AD patients and their caregivers. The session proposes a culturally-specific framework for the recruitment and retention of ethnically diverse caregivers into clinical trials. This method highlights the importance of the recruiters' characteristics and it transcends the subjects' ethnic barriers. Addressing the ethnic differences is crucial in the assessing of family interactional patterns which will assist in the implementation of culturally-appropriate interventions such as the on-the-phone caregiver discussion groups. The assessment of the AD individuals' memory using a culturally sensitive and specific instrument concludes this session. Overall, this symposium provides descriptive information, data, and suggestions on how to work with a group of AD patients and caregivers who are ethnically diverse.

Measuring Family Interactions in Dementia Caregiver Families: Comparison of Cuban American and European American Families

Victoria B. Mitrani [University of Miami School of Medicine, Miami, United States]

The assessment of family interaction patterns among dementia caregivers is a valuable tool for developing and implementing family-based interventions, providing a road map for identifying maladaptive interactional patterns to be targeted in treatment. These maladaptive patterns, which are interdependent and repetitive, block the ability of the caregiver to receive support from family members, and the ability of family members to offer relief to the caregiver. This presentation will focus on the adaptation of the Structural Family Systems Ratings (SFSR) for assessing interactions among caregiver families. The SFSR is a family observational coding system that assesses family interactions along five dimensions of family functioning: Structure (family roles and alliances), Developmental Stage (adjustment to live-cycle changes), Resonance (interpersonal boundaries), Identified Patienthood (the family's perception of the locus of the problem), and Conflict Resolution (the manner in which the family manages problems and disagreements). The SFSR has been adapted for caregiver families using data collected within a large-scale (224 families) longitudinal (four time points) randomized family intervention trial to prevent and alleviate distress in European American and Cuban American dementia caregivers. At each assessment, families enact a set of three family exercises which are videotaped and coded using the SFSR. Culture plays an important role in shaping family interactions. Attention to ethnic differences is crucial for the development of culturally-congruent interventions. Clinical experience with the REACH families indicates that differences between Cuban American and European American families is most pronounced in the dimensions of Structure, Resonance and Conflict Resolution.

On-The-Phone Discussion Groups in an Ethnically Diverse Sample of Caregivers of Alzheimer's Individuals

Soledad Argüelles [University of Miami School of Medicine, Miami, USA], Sara Czaja [University of Miami School of Medicine, Miami, USA], Mark Rubert [University of Miami School of Medicine, Miami, USA], Carl Eisdorfer [University of Miami School of Medicine, Miami, USA]

The demands of caring for a family member with Alzheimer's disease can often times prevent caregivers to attend community support groups. An attempt to provide caregivers with the emotional/social assistance that support groups provide is the Computer Telephone Integration System (CTIS) Discussion Groups. This presentation will provide an overview of the CTIS, and it will specifically describe the on-the-phone Discussion Group experience in caregivers who participated in a caregiver project (Resources for Enhancing Alzheimer Disease Caregivers Health-REACH). A brief description of the technical aspects of the on-the-phone Discussion Groups will preamble the discussion, especially in light of the caregivers' diverse ethnic background. A total of 51 caregivers (25 white non-Hispanic and 26 Cuban-American) participated in 6 Discussion Groups (3 in English and 3 in Spanish). Participants of both ethnic groups discussed a wide array of caregiving topics including: behavioral management techniques for patients' problematic behaviors, access of community and family resources, and time allocation for leisure activities. Most participants viewed their Discussion Groups experience as positive. They enjoyed and benefited from both the practical and emotional support provided. Some viewed group participation as respite time, while others began attending community support groups and socializing with group members outside the group experience. Overall, this descriptive presentation depicts an alternative/innovative way of conducting support groups with ethnically diverse caregivers of Alzheimer's patients.

Practical and Theoretical Aspects of Recruitment and Retention of Hispanic Caregivers of Alzheimer's Disease Patients

Trinidad Argüelles [University of Miami School of Medicine, Miami, USA]

>Generally the literature suggests that recruitment of minority >participants for intervention studies is somewhat challenging. This paper >will discuss a model of recruitment that was developed on the basis of >recruitment and retention strategies used with caregivers of Alzheimer's >disease (AD) patients in two research studies: 1) The Resources for >Enhancing Alzheimer's Caregiver Health (REACH) program, a caregiver >intervention project and 2) A project concerned with assessing the >functional status of AD patients. The first project included Cuban-American >and White-American caregivers, while the second project included Hispanic >-American caregivers of diverse backgrounds as well as White-American >caregivers. This presentation will provide an overview of the recruitment >model and a summary of the recruitment results obtained in both studies. In >addition, data regarding participant retention will be presented. Generally >the data indicate that the effectiveness of recruitment strategies vary as a >function of ethnicity. The results also indicate that participate retention >varies as a function of the patient's level of functioning, and that such >retention decreases as level of functioning declines. These data and the >model of recruitment and retention will be discussed in terms of guiding >recruitment strategies for caregivers with diverse ethnic backgrounds.

Sensitivity and Specificity of a New Semantic Interference Test for Ethnically Diverse Alzheimer's Disease Patients

David Loewenstein [University of Miami School of Medicine, Miami, USA], Amarilis Acevedo [Mount Sinai Medical Center, Miami Beach, USA],Lynn Schram [Mount Sinai Medical Center, Miami Beach, USA],Raymond Ownby [University of Miami School of Medicine, Miami, USA]

Disruption of semantic networks required for information processing is one of the earliest deficits observed in Alzheimer's Disease (AD). We have developed a semantic interference task which involves a three trial learning paradigm for ten common household objects borrowing from the paradigm developed by Fuld and Colleagues (1981). Another semantically related ten common household objects are then presented and recall for this second list of items is then assessed. Recall for the first group of target objects are assessed immediately after the recall of the second group of objects and after a 20-minute delay. This allows for an assessment of both proactive and retroactive interference for semantically similar targets. This new test demonstrates excellent interrater reliabilities and concurrent validity when compared to standard memory measures. High discriminative validity is also demonstrated in that 34 of the most mildly impaired Alzheimer's patients (mean MMSE score =24.89 (3.0) could be discriminated from normal elderly controls with 96.9 sensitivity and 80.5 specificity. Further, analyses suggest that this measure retains high sensitivity/specificity for Spanish-speaking elderly, suggesting that this object memory test may be more culturally fair with diverse cultural/ language groups. These findings suggest that use of a simple object memory test which assesses proactive and retroactive interference may be particularly sensitive to disruption in semantic networks secondary in both English-speaking and Spanish-speaking patients early AD. Further, they may be superior to standard measures of delayed recall and rate of forgetting in the early identification of the disorder.

SESSION 245

A Tribute to the late Dr. Tom Kitwood: Enhancing Personhood Well-Being in Contexts of Dementia/Chronic Illness

C. LeNavenec (Faculty of Nursing, University of Calgary, Calgary, Canada). An overview of Kitwood's Personhood Concept and Indicators of Personhood Well-Being: The Interpersonal Context. M. Downs (Bradford Dementia Group, University of Bradford. Bradford, UK). The role of the cultural context in the lived experience of dementia. O. von Mering (University of Florida, Gainesville, FL, USA) . Informal Caring Practices in the American Culture of Managed Care. D. McCulloch (School of Public Policy, Economics & Law, University of Ulster at Jordanstown, Newtonabbey, Co. Antrim, UK). Approaches for Estimating Costs and Benefits of Medical and Social Interventions for People with Dementia and their Families.

This purpose of this symposium is to revisit the research done by the late Dr. Tom Kitwood at the University of Bradford in the UK regarding the interdependence of contextual factors and personhood well-being of older people with dementia or chronic illness and their families. The focus of this session is the implications of this theoretical model for clinical practice, program development and policy, and research pertaining to cost and related types of outcome indicators.

Approaches for Estimating Costs and Benefits of Social and

Medical Interventions: The Economic Context

D. McCulloch (School of Public Policy, Economics & Law, University of Ulster at Jordanstown

Degenerative diseases like Alzheimer's or Motor-Neuron Disease, and chronic conditions (stroke), disable a patient, and burden a carer, permanently. Their costs, in terms of resources and opportunities forgone, are significant, and the best use of the resources applied to these patients is therefore an important problem. The usual technique applied to the health sector, cost-effectiveness analysis (CEA), has tended to rely on the comparison of tightly-defined interventions in contexts where differences in costs and/or outcomes can be clearly identified, for example, on the basis of evidence from Randomised Controlled Trials. This approach is problematic for the diseases and conditions of interest, that is, when there is no cure, when care takes place in context which are (scientifically) uncontrollable, and when the science behind the disease or condition is not well understood. Using the example of Alzheimer's Disease, this paper explains why a programmed-budgeting and marginal analysis (PBMA) approach, incorporating quality of life measures for patients and their carers, might permit a clear description of existing outcomes and their resource costs, as a preliminary to an improvement in the allocation of resources.

Informal Caring Practices in the American Culture of Managed Care

Otto von Mering (University of Florida, Gainesville, Florida, USA), Nannette Hoffman, M.D. (VA Medical Center, Gainesville, Florida, USA)

The rise of managed care and decline of Social Security, Medicare, Medicaid, child- and long- term care benefits burden more families and communities whose needs outstrip conventional resources. The purpose of this presentation is to discuss how they abatted the impact by having related and unrelated elders and young reconstitute themselves into variable domestic units, (re)inventing mutual caring practices, and altered resource management, autonomous income generation, volunteer 'shadow work', bartered services and habitat selection. Increasingly, as informal case managers of body and mind, elders become co-equal stakeholders in weighing the financial and ethical place of clinical evidence in care decisions. They promise to become the key public persuaders that medical science does not exist to create the deathless life on earth.

The role of the cultural context in the lived experience of dementia

M. Downs (Bradford Dementia Group, University of Bradford, UK)

The social psychology of dementia was introduced to the field of dementia studies in England by Kitwood. His work cogently argued the critical importance of the social environment to the well-being of people with dementia. This interest in the social world of people with dementia can also be expanded to include the cultural and economic realities in which people with dementia live. The aim of my presentation is to present an overview of the role of the social and cultural context in the lives of people with dementia and their families. This discussion will focus on three inter-related areas: (1) the meanings attributed to dementia-like symptoms over time and cultures; (2) families' response to their relative with dementia across time and cultures will be explored with reference to the amount of care provided by families and the 'burden' experienced in this caring; and (3) the government's response across time and culture to the needs of people with dementia and their families. The author's conclusion will emphasize that the experience of dementia is as much a function of the cultural context as it is of the degree and extent of one's neurological impairment.

SESSION 246

Emerging Careers: Creating Student Opportunities

Pat Spadafora (Sheridan College, Oakville, Canada) Helen Hamlin (United Nations)New York, USA

Purpose: Professionals in the field of gerontology are well versed in the shifting demographics in Canada. They are equally well aware of the challenges inherent in attracting students to careers in this emerging field. There is a need to respond to commonly held stereotypes and ageist attitudes. We must address perceptions of elders and the opportunities for working with elders if we hope to shape career choices. This round table will encourage discussion about two specific issues: 1. Attracting students to careers in the "helping" professions - (i.e. gerontological social work, nursing, physiotherapy, occupational therapy, geriatric medecine, recreation/activity therapists) 2. Sensitizing students in other disciplines about the impact of an aging population on their respective disciplines. Structure: The cohosts, representing a faculty and an adminstrative perspective in a community college, will present the issues and opportunities as they perceive them. The intent is to engage the session participants in thoughtful reflection, interactive brainstorming and solution focused problem solving. Content: The hosts will descibe current gerontology programming at Sheridan College. Further, they will outline the Sheridan Elder Research Centre (SERC), an innovative facility which will open on campus in September, 2003. This initiative is multidisciplinary and builds on the unique program strengths at Sheridan. Although the physical structure will not open for some time, there is considerable activity taking place in the interim period. One of these activities is a proposal for a post graduate progam in Aging and Design, which brings together faculty and students fron both the Interior Design Program and the Social Service Worker-Gerontology Program. For this session, the proposed program will be one of the exapmles used to describe issue number two, sensitizing other professions to the realities of an aging population. We will also present and facilitate discussion about the broader issues in attracting students to this field and will propose ideas to respond to the concern. Using a collaborative approach, we will build on ideas generated from the audience. Anticipated Outcomes: It is our expectation that, at the end of this session, we will have these 'products': 1. Clarification of the issues, as perceived by session participants. 2. An articulated strategy to address these issues. 3. Identification of collaborative opportunities and partnerships as a follow up after the conference

SESSION 247

Continuity and change: long term marriage relationships in the context of chronic illness and disability

Mo Ray (Keele University, Keele, Staffs, UK)

Despite an enormous literature about informal caring and a significant body of research exploring long-term marriage, few studies have specifically examined the impact of chronic illness on long established marriage relationships. This research discusses an in-depth qualitative study with 13 long married couples. Using semi-structured interviews, participants were interviewed jointly and singly. Couples were interviewed again approximately 6 months after initial contact. Interview transcripts were analysed using grounded theory. The concept of reorganisation is a term used to conceptualise the active attempts couples engaged with to manage change and uncertainty. Reorganisation had as its goal a need to stabilise and ultimately assimilate new modes of behaviour or role responsibility when change disrupted the usual routines and divisions of labour in the marriage. Couples often made use of their perceptions of long-standing continuities and marital identity themes when they talked about their strategies for managing change. In conclusion, the importance of long-standing relationship continuities is highlighted as an important means of managing change and uncertainty. Comment is made about the importance of formal services and practitioners recognising and working with relationship continuities and the active attempts couples make to manage change.

Does recency of widowhood affect health among older people?

J.K. Kim, E.M. Crimmins (Andrus Gerontology Center, University of Southern California, Los Angeles, California, USA)

This study examines whether recency of widowhood is related to health status among older persons. Using the data from multiple studies (Health and Retirement Survey (HRS), Asset and Health Dynamics among the Oldest Old (AHEAD), MacArthur Research Network on Successful Aging Community Study (MacArthur)), health status of the married is compared to that of the recently widowed and the long-term widowed (N=3,589 in HRS, N=2796 in AHEAD, N=518 in MacArthur) to examine the effect of widowhood and the recency of widowhood on health outcomes. The study investigates a variety of mechanisms through which widowhood and health are related. Regression results showed that longer-term widowhood was associated with a higher probability of acquiring some conditions. Recent widowhood was related to a higher likelihood of developing depression while longer-term widowhood was not. The study findings suggest that longer-term adverse effect of widowhood on health should not be neglected. The increased likelihood of getting depression among the recently widowed and high prevalence of depression among longer-term widowed imply that treatment or prevention of depression would be appropriate for the recently widowed who are at high risk of getting depression and the longer-term widowed who suffer from chronic depression.

Informal Social Support Among Institutionalized Elderly with Schizophrenia

T.F.Smith (Health Studies & Gerontology, University of Waterloo, Waterloo, Ontario), J.P. Hirdes (Health Studies & Gerontology, University of Waterloo, Waterloo, Ontario)

PURPOSE: These analyses report upon the supportive needs of three patient groups residing in psychogeriatric settings. METHOD: The study sample (N=129), based upon existing data from three Canadian facilities, was composed of 57% males and the mean age was 77 years old. Analyses were restricted to patients with a primary diagnosis of either organic disorder (52%), schizophrenia (26%), or mood disorder (22%). Data collection was based upon the Resident Assessment Instrument-Mental Health (RAI-MH). RESULTS: Patients with a primary diagnosis of schizophrenia were associated with lower levels of informal support resources and lower levels of received support compared to patients with a primary diagnosis of either organic or mood disorder. Patients with schizophrenia were more likely to be never married (59%) with only 5% being currently married. Research subjects with a diagnosis of either organic or mood disorder were more likely to be currently married (37% and 21% respectively). Approximately 38% of patients with an organic diagnosis were in contact with family and/or friends over the last 7 days while 35% had contact within the last 30 days. Of those with a mood disorder, over 50% had contact with informal supports within the last 7 days. Of those diagnosed with schizophrenia, only 12% had contact with the last 7 days. Over 70% of the patients diagnosed with schizophrenia were coded as not receiving any emotional support from informal sources over the prior 30-day period. CONCLUSIONS: These findings demonstrate the paucity of informal supports for those older patients with long-term schizophrenia.

Synergism of Frail Rural Elderly Couples Sustains Their Independence

Fran Racher RN, BScN, (Community Health) (Brandon University, Brandon MB, Canada, R7A 6A9

In this phenomenological study, a purposive sample of 19 frail rural elderly couples were interviewed as dyads to identify programs, services and relationships perceived by the couples as beneficial to their ability to continue to live independently in the community. Communication between the partners, as well as roles and relationships were observed and discussed. Findings showed that mutually supportive dyads generated a synergism or energy that acted as a vital resource to couples. Research results led to the development of a continuum of spousal relationships and a trajectory of couple communication. Support to the couple as a unit, to the couple relationship and to address the couple's needs may be important strategic directions for future policy development and resource planning.

SESSION 254

[1] Barriers to Accessing the Internet for Older People with a Communication Disability

L.E. Worrall, J. Egan, D. Schmidt (Communication Disability in Ageing Research Unit, The University of Queensland, Brisbane, Australia)

This study examined the barriers in accessing the Internet for older people with communication disabilities. Most people in the community learn the Internet by reading (a barrier for people with communication disability) or by attending classes where good comprehension skills are necessary. This project enlisted the help of volunteers who used a specially modified training manual to train 20 people with aphasia and 5 people with Parkinson's Disease to use the Internet. This study reports on the barriers to training older people with communication disabilities in an Australian context. Baseline observed Internet usage and baseline interview results of participants will be reported. Barriers included local access to Internet linked computers, recruitment of suitable volunteers, variations in Web browsers and access to specialized computer hardware. Reading comprehension difficulties of on-line material were an anticipated barrier but were not found to be a particular problem for participants. While the results of the full training program will determine the success of an Internet Training Program for people with communication disabilities, this study has identified that many of the barriers are not specific to the communication disability.

[2] Risk of development of functional disability in elderly Hong Kong Chinese: Longitudinal and cross-sectional analysis

S.C. Ho, Y.M. Lam, J. Woo (Centre of Gerontology & Geriatrics, The Chinese University of Hong Kong, Hong Kong; Department of Community Health & Epidemiology, Queens University, Canada)

PURPOSE: To determine social, psychological, lifestyle and health factors influencing functional disability in Hong Kong Chinese aged 70 years and over METHOD: We conducted a three-year longitudinal follow-up study on a cohort of 2030 subjects aged 70 years and over selected by stratified disproportional random sampling. Baseline information regarding social, psychological, lifestyle and health factors was obtained through structured face-to-face interview. The data collection was repeated at 18 months through telephone, and at three-years through face-to-face interviews. We applied the multiple logistic regression method to simultaneously model the cross-sectional (baseline) and longitudinal information using the overall activity of daily living score (ADL) from the modified Barthel Index, collected at baseline and in the two followup interviews, as the outcome variable. We applied the generalized estimation equation method to estimate the regression coefficients taking into account the intra-subject correlation. An individual will be classified as having functional disability if the ADL score is below 20. RESULTS: After adjusting for age and sex, factors that increased the risk of functional disability include an increase in baseline and followup episodes of hospitalization (longitudinal OR=1.175, 95%CI 1.055-1.310; cross-sectional OR=1.217, 95%CI 1.104-1.340); falls during the prior 12 months (longitudinal OR=2.054, 95%CI 1.622-2.602; cross-sectional OR=1.862, 95%CI 1.459-2.377); and an increase in depression score (longitudinal OR=1.127, 95% 1.083-1.173; cross-sectional OR=1.108, 95%CI 1.073-1.142). The lack of practice of exercise (longitudinal OR=1.579, 95%CI 1.232-2.024; cross-section OR=1.587, 95%CI 1.294-1.948), better mental score at baseline and its positive changes were associated with a decreased risk of functional disability. CONCLUSION: Among the modifiable factors, the prevention of falls, the preservation and promotion of mental health, and the practice of exercise are important factors for the preservation of functional ability in the older Chinese population.

[3] Outcome After Amputation For Limb Arteriopathy In The Elderly

C Le Du1, C Cattenoz1, S Brenugat2, P Jouanny1, Y Kerdilès2. Departement of Geriatric Medicine and 2 Vascular Surgery, University Hospital Rennes, France

PURPOSE: The prevalence of limb arteriopathy is more than 5 0n the elderly. Critical ischaemia occurs in 200f the patients, and 25% will have amputation after one year follow-up. The aim of this study is to analyze the factors that influence outcome and autonomy after amputation in old patients. METHOD: Between 1993 and 1998, 80 patients aged over 65 years (48 male and 32 female, mean age 78.4 years [65 to 94 years]) were amputed for critical limb ischaemia (stages III or IV) after unsuccessfull or unpossible vascular reconstruction. : 48 transfemoral and 38 transtibial amputations. Outcome was analyzed in univariate (Kaplan-Meier) and multivariate (Cox). Surgical related mortality was 5% (4 octogenarians with major amputations). In the patients with below-knee amputation, 12.5% had a major amputation of the same limb in the first month. 7.9% had major amputation of the other limb. RESULTS: Mean survey was 35 months [1.5 to 84 months]. Survival after 1, 3 and 6 years-follow-up were respectively 76.2, 54.2 and 22%. In univariate analysis, age over 80 years, nursing home living, neuropsychological disease and unpossible prosthetic rehabilitation, badly inlfluenced long-term mortality. In multivariate analysis, nursing home living and prior smoking, badly influenced but successfull prosthetic rehabilitation was protective. Quality of life : 63.5% had prosthetic rehabilitation, in which 67.5eeded help for moving. 79.40f private home patients returned back home, in which 76eeded help for some activity of day-living. 87.50resented with disability before amputation and 55.5% after. CONCLUSION: Rehabilitation after amputation in old patients is often difficult due to frequent related loss of autonomy. Regular follow-up of prosthetis and/or rolling chair is necessary for better psychological acceptation of amputation.

[4] Disabilities in ADL and IADL of patients with Alzheimer's disease leading to death and institutionalization

Ankri J (RFR12, Université Paris5, Paris France) Cerase V (RFR12, Université Paris5, Paris France) Harboun M (RFR12, Université Paris5, Paris France) deStampa M (RFR12, Université Paris5, Paris France) Schwald N (RFR12, Université Paris5, Paris France)

Purpose : To document the role of patient characteristics (specially disabilities in ADL and IADL and comorbidity) in determining wether a patient will need institutionalization, we undertook an analysis of outcome of primary degenerative dementia visiting ou Day Hospital. Method :The first hundred elderly persons living at home referred for dementia and related disorders to our day hospital and followed during one year formed the study group for this report. The diagnosis of probable AD was made on the basis of the NINCDS-ADRDA and DDSM IV criteria All patients underwent a general medical examination, CT sacn, screening blood tests, chest RX, EKG, and psychometrics tests including MMS of Folstein. Depression was evaluated by a psychologist. For all patients, a primary caregiver accompanied the patient to the initial visit and was interviewed by a trained social worker about ADL and IADL. Patients were seen every six month, where a standardized evaluation based on the RAI instrument was performed. Results :Death rate at one year of follow up appears low and linked to comorbidity. For those still living preliminary results on ADL and IADL's evolution of this prospective cohort will be presented here. Especially the main characteristics which lead them to institutionalization versus those who remain at home. Conclusion Longitudinal study of demented people appears indispensible for better understanding ADL and IADL's evolution and the factors leading to death and institutionalization.

[5] Life Satisfaction and Functional Capability in Elderly People Submitted to Amputation of Lower Limbs

Maria José D'Elboux Diogo {Nursing Department, Medical Science Faculty, State University of Campinas, Campinas, São Paulo, Brazil}

Evaluate the current level of independence for daily activities and the global life satisfaction of the elderly people submitted to amputation of lower limbs; to evaluate, both individually and comparatively, the level of life satisfaction in different realms; to identify the relation between satisfaction and life with a basis on the physical capability/independence domain and Barthel's index. METHOD: Forty elderly people (30 men and 10 women), aged 60 years old or above, who had been submitted to amputation above the malleoli were interviewed. The instrument used to gather data including the evaluation of the functional capability in accordance with Barthel's Index, the global evaluation of life satisfaction (adapted from Cantrill's model) and the evaluation of life satisfaction concerning the health sphere, physical capability/independence, mental capability and social interaction/involvement, both at personal level and in comparison to other elderly people. RESULTS: In general, the elderly in this study presented a high level of functional independence. As to the evaluation of global life satisfaction, the elderly presented medium values. People with higher Barthel's index values showed average-to-high life satisfaction at the time of the interview. Life satisfaction concerning the investigated realms was found to be high both individually and comparatively. CONCLUSION: Results showed that independently from Barthel's scale, the elderly see themselves as satisfied, that is, the subjective evaluation was seen as positive.

[6] Attitudes of physically disabled persons toward the aged, own aging, and physically disabled people

Resende, Marineia Crosara de (State University of Campinas, Brazil) Liberalesso Neri, Anita (State University of Campinas, Brazil)

OBJECTIVES: Being old and being physically disabled mean to be challenged by physical and social barriers, since human environments are not programmed to support the needs of these less independent and active minorities. As attitudes are regulators of self and behavior, knowing them is useful to the management of behavior of special populations like these. This investigation was aimed to describe and compare attitudes of adults with physical disability toward aged people and own age, and toward persons with physical disability (PPD). METHOD: Subjects were 242 adults (65.3% women) aged 24 to 39, members of an association of paraplegics. Instrumentation comprised: a 30 item DS Scale covering the domains cognition, agency, social relations, and persona, assessing the concepts " An aged person is", "When I will be old I will be", "A physically disabled person is"; the Barthel Index, and a personal information questionnaire. RESULTS showed small variability and predominance of positive attitudes toward the oldest and PPD. Independently of their attitudes concerning PPD, subjects showed higher and more positive attitudes toward own old age than to the aged. There were found positive correlations between attitudes toward old age and toward PPD. To all the concepts the most negative scores occurred in the domains persona and agency. CONCLUSION: Results reply others found in literature about the higher value attributed to ideal objects, indicate a tendency of adaptation deriving of social comparison, and suggest awareness of the limits to social image imposed by both conditions.

[7] Biomarkers as predictors of disability over a 24-year period in a Swedish sample.

Kozma Ahacic, (Department of Social Work, Stockholm University, Stockholm, Sweden) Marti G Parker (Department of Social Work, Stockholm University, Stockholm, Sweden) Mats Thorslund, (Department of Social Work, Stockholm University, Stockholm, Sweden)

Biomarkers as predictors of disability over a 24-year period in a Swedish sample. PURPOSE: It is plausible that the same general aging process gives rise to early recognizable signs of aging, so-called biomarkers, and later disability. If impairments in mobility, hearing, vision, and dental health are signs of early aging, they should also predict later disability. METHOD: In 1991/92 a nationally representative sample of the adult Swedish population was interviewed. Persons aged 76+ who had also been interviewed in 1968 (n=497, response rate 92.6%) were the basis for correlation estimates. Dichotomized variables were used in complimentary logistic regression analyses. RESULTS: Mobility limitations, hearing and vision problems, and poor dental health showed a steep increase after age 40. Among the oldest, a majority had these problems. Correlation analyses showed that mobility explained nearly half the variance in ADL and IADL disability. Hearing, vision and dental health explained a few percent. People with disabilities in 1992 had about twice the odds to have had mobility limitations, hearing and vision problems, or poor dental health in 1968. While mobility and dental health were also significant correlates and predictors of cognitive disability, vision and hearing were not. CONCLUSION: While hearing, vision and dental health were independent areas of impairment only weakly connected with mobility and disability, their predictive ability supports their use as biomarkers. The hypothetical relation between sensory deficits and cognitive disability, an association most likely to be connected to biological aging, was not found. This could suggest that biomarkers reflect an aging due to environmental influences rather than biological determinants.

[8] To promote the research on the disabled elderly

Ding Qiwen (China Federation of the Disabled Beijing China)

The paper will discuss the status and development of the disabled elderly in China. It would discuss the importance of developing the research on the disabled elderly in order to promote the quality of life of those elderly disabled. Lastly the author would make recommendations concerning the promotion of research in this field.

[9] Health and Quality of Life

Vicente Spinola Dias Neto; Giselle H. de P. Rodrigues; Juliana P. Magnatti (Pontifícia Universidade Católica de São Paulo Sorocaba Brazil).

PURPOSE: To determine the relation between the quantity of pathologies presented by a population over than 60 years old, their autonomy in activities of daily living (ADL), instrumental activities of daily living (IADL), and the consequences on their quality of life. METHOD: Interviews, based on a standard questionnaire, have been done with all of the older people (n=409) from two city districts of Sorocaba, SP, Brazil. The software EPI-INFO 5.0 has been used to compute the results. RESULTS: Among those who had total autonomy, in ADL, 52.3% was 60-69, and only 9.75%, 80-99. Those who had difficulty to do four or more, 20% was 60-69 and 53.3%, 80-99. In IADL, those who presented total autonomy, 55.3% was 60-69 and 4.56% was 80-99. Those who needed help in four or more IADL, 31.34% was between 60-69 and 80-99. The autonomy is influenced by the number of pathologies too. Those who had difficulty to do one to three ADL, 1.26% had no pathologies and 40.5% of them had four or more. Those who needed help to do one to three IADL, 5.98% had no pathologies and 26.49% had four or more. Among those who had difficulty in four or more ADL, 33.3% had four or more pathologies, and to do four or more IADL, 1.49% had no pathologies and 34.32% had four or more. Patients that didn't have any pathology: 43.7% was 60-69; 37.5%, 70-79; and 18.75%, 80-99. Among those who had four or more pathologies: 47.12% was 60-69; 40.22%, 70-79; and 12.64%, 80-99. CONCLUSION: The decrease of autonomy occurs proportionately of an increase of pathologies. This decrease is also seen with the increase of age. But, differently of expected, older patients have less pathologies than younger ones. So, if the rate of decrease is bigger when related to the quantity of pathologies, we conclude that the autonomy, and consequently the quality of life, are directly influenced by the number of pathologies, more than by the age of the patients.

[10] UNKNOW ISCHEMIC OPTIC NEUROPATHY IN ELDERLY PEOPLE

Serrano MP(1), Ramírez JM.(2), Triviño A.(2), Tena-Dávila MC.(1) (1)Unidad Geriátrica Municipal. Área de Sanidad. Ayuntamiento de Madrid. SPAIN (2)Instituto de Investigaciones Oftalmológicas Ramón Castroviejo. Universidad Complutense de Madrid. SPAIN

PURPOSE: To identify visual field abnormalities connected with nerve fibre defects occurring in a population aged over 65, and how these abnormalities relate to vascular pathology at other levels. METHOD: Clinical history and complete eye examination including computerized perimetry (Humphrey 2.4.6 and 30.2) of 49 individuals (22 male, 27 female, with an average age of 70,4) with no know ocular pathology. The statistical analysis was performed using SPSS. RESULTS: 54 abnormal field were detected and related to ischemic optic neuropathy in association with systemic vascular pathology ($p<0,05$) at a risk level of 1,5 versus 0,5. CONCLUSIONS: Among apparently healthy persons there are a great many visual field defects, and these may indicate vascular pathology at other levels

[11] Drug toxicity in 90-year-old and over patients

L. Merle, T. Dantoine, Y. Nouaille, F. Bouthier, J.P. Charmes

As part of a survey among 2018 elderlies aged 70 or over consecutively admitted to an acute care geriatric unit aimed at studying the relation between clinical status and treatment given prior to admission, late old (LO) patients (567 = 28.1 %) aged 90 or over (92.9 ± 2.7 years) were compared with early old (EO) patients (1451=71.9 %) aged 70 to 89 (82.3 ± 5.1). Adverse drug effects were divided into definite, probable, nil and impossible to identify. LO patients were mostly women (76.6 %). Ageing was associated with a weight loss ($p<0.0001$) both in women (EO/LO : 56.0 ± 13.1 / 51.8 ± 11.5 kg) and in men (65.4 ± 13.5 / 59.0 ± 10.8) and a decrease of total proteins concentration in women only (65.6 ± 7.0 / 63.3 ± 6.9 g/L ; $p<0.01$). The number of drugs given on admission (NDA) was not different both in EO and LO women (6.3 ± 3.0 / 6.0 ± 2.9) and in EO and LO men (6.4 ± 3.3 / 5.9 ± 3.1). However the NDA was higher in patients admitted with an adverse drug effect than in those without both in EO (7.4 ± 3.1 / 5.6 ± 3.1 ; $p<0.0001$) and in LO patients (7.0 ± 2.7 / 5.2 ± 2.9 ; $p<0.0001$). The frequency of adverse drug effect occurrence was stable with ageing (definite adverse drug effect : 19.2 % in EO and 18.9 % in LO patients) which suggests that besides the number of drugs given the general condition of the elderly, specially in women, is a main factor of medication induced problem ; undernutrition, together with the well known renal function deterioration might be added risk factors, whatever the age.

[12] You and your sensory environment a life long learning experience

Bev O'Sullivan, Pender Island, BC, Canada Klari Varallyai, Campbell RiverPhysiotherapy Clinic, Campbell River, BC, Canada

The discussion will heighten the participant's awareness of the sensory environment around the seminar. The focus of this session is on the importance of sensory motor learning towards improving safety, independence, and interdependence between seniors and their environment. Practical application utilizing a variety of sensory feedback to maximize participant's own sensory awareness or lack of it towards independent living, mobility and self care. Sensory awareness of one's environment can be called a form of education or as frequently happens, due to decreased awareness- "a re-education process". In the last twenty years before the millennium and for years to come, a greater number of people retire at an earlier age than 65. The aging population lives healthier therefore longer than previous generations. Their common wish is to remain independent for as long as it is feasible. To ensure retiring and aging population that they can and are able to remain independent and self sufficient they need to have the following: · functional skills (including sensory/motor) · to be physically mobility and relatively pain free · to be mentally functional · to be somewhat stable emotionally As a lifelong educational program in sensory awareness of our environment is a must,as well as the sensory motor learning to maintain and improve wherever possible and to be able to re-learn sensory awareness in case of some loss of the sensory appreciation of both the in and outdoor world. Often due to gradual loss of sensory experience, individuals involved may not even realize the decreased ability to read and process sensory clues, let alone to act upon sensory stimulation. It is well known that as the aging population's mobility and over all social interaction decreases, the day to day functional skills are known to slow down and in certain cases disappear all together. Often an unfortunate accident- ie a fractured hip - brings it to everyone's awareness around injured seniors the decreased sensory awareness - "a presumably forgotten experience" now present and therefore needs to be improved. The importance of our sensory awareness of the environment around us for us to function safely and efficiently cannot be emphasized often enough. To re-discover and re-educate our senses, we need to be extra sensitive how and when we approach our family members or friends, and our clients (if one is a health professional). The importance of a specific therapy needs to be equally sensitive to the unique anatomy, physiology and sociology and cultural and spiritual background of the aging individual. We keep in touch with our sensory environment through our basic senses which are: touch - skin vision - eyes hearing - ears taste - mouth smell - nose The following diagram (*Adaptation of Human Performance Model from R.G. Marteniuk, Information Processing in Motor Skills, New York: Holt, Rinehart & Winston, 1976), is an adaptation which shows the relationship that exists between a sensory stimuli and the resultant motor process. Input — Information — Information — Perception — Information — Performance Reception Transmission Decision Transmission Action Visual — Eyes ——— Nervous ——— Brain ——————— Nervous —— Movement Stimuli System System In the daily life of a senior information processing of a sensory stimuli decoded in the following way: 1. receive information from the external or internal environment (internal ie. digestive system urinary system) 2. the process and the action upon receiving information takes place 3. end result depending which sensory organ stimulated, a motor response During this conference we heard a great deal of new research and I'm happy to say we also received positive feedback that many of the earlier findings and practical experiences (from the field) are as true today as they were at the time they were first documented. In conclusion, the intent of this paper (round-table presentation) is to heighten the awareness of the challenges, the sensory environment brings into our life, whatever age we may be. As Aging Is Everybody's Future, we would like to finish our round-table discussion with a short practical presentation to share a few of the activities we utilize to maintain and improve sensory experiences some of us may have forgotten or lost or just needs to be brought into our awareness. (The practical part will include short sensory journey through our five basic senses) We welcome you all to join and have fun with us.

[13] The Self-perceived Handicap by a Geriatric Institutionalized Population with Hearing Loss

K.M.M. Silveira, - Phonoaudiology Dept. Alfenas University - Minas Gerais - Brazil I.C.P. Russo, - Titularof Catholic University - São Paulo - Brazil J.D. Soares, M.D, - Gerontology Research Centre and Program, Unifenas - Alfenas University - Minas Gerais - Brazil

Abstract This study aimed to evaluate the self-perceived handicap of 50 hearing impaired residents and nurses from three nursing homes that shelter senior citizens in the city of Franca, São Paulo, and Alfenas, Minas Gerais in Brazil, through the application of the Nursing Home Hearing Handicap Index - NHHI, created by Schow & Nerbonne (1977). Fifty hearing impaired residents, 25 males and 25 females, ranged from 60 to 90 years old, with sensorineural hearing losses of different degrees and their respective nurses, were the subjects of this research. The results showed 82% of the residents with some degree of self-perceived hearing handicap, females (92%) showing statistically significant higher perception than males (72%) $p<0.05$ t-Student. The comparative answers given by the residents and their nurses revealed a higher degree of perceived hearing handicap for the nurses. The NHHI showed to be an effective tool in the hearing handicap assessment of elderly citizens, living in nursing homes, playing an important role in the audiologic rehabilitation of this population.

[14] Vitamin intake and transparency of human lens in middle-aged and elderly Japanese

H.Nomura (Chubu National Hospital,Obu,Japan), T.Imai(National Institute for Longevity Sciences,Obu,Japan:NILS), F.Ando(NILS), N.Niino(NILS), H.Shimokata(NILS), Y.Miyake(Nagoya University School of Medicine,Nagoya,Japan)

PURPOSE: Cataracts are the most common cause of age-related vision loss and are one of the structural markers of aging. The relationship between the dietary vitamin intake and the transparency of human lens was investigated. METHOD: Subjects comprised 1988 Japanese (987 male and 1001 female), who participated in the longitudinal study of aging at the center of National Institute for Longevity Sciences (NILS-LSA) from 1997 to 2000. Participants aged from 40 to 79 were selected by random sampling from the local community. According to the 3-days dietary records, the daily average intake of carotene, vitamin C (VC), and vitamin E (VE) was calculated for each subject. The light scattering intensity, as an indicator of lens transparency, was measured at anterior cortex (AC) and anterior nucleus (AN) on the Scheimpflug lens image using an anterior eye segment analysis system. The relationships between the vitamin intake and the light scattering intensity of lens were assessed using correlation analysis. RESULTS: In cross-section analysis, carotene intake was negatively correlated to the scattering intensity at AN in male ($p<0.05$) and female ($p<0.01$). VC intake was negatively correlated to the scattering intensity at AN in females only ($p<0.05$). VE intake was negatively correlated to the scattering intensity at AN in males only ($p<0.05$). There was no significant association between the scattering intensity at AC and the intake of carotene, VC, and VE. CONCLUSION: The antioxidants intake, such as carotene, VC, and VE, may protect NILS-LSA participants from decreasing the transparency at anterior nucleus of lens.

[15] Aging and Vision Loss - Implications for service providers and CNIB's Seniors Program.

Leona Burkey & Cathie Dallas (Seniors Program Coordinators, Canadian National Institute for the Blind, Edmonton & Calgary AB, Canada)

PURPOSE: The CNIB's Seniors and Vision Loss Program helps visually impaired seniors sustain their independence through community-based support and education. METHOD: CNIB staff help coordinate a network of peer support groups and provide education to seniors' groups and service providers. A successful training module was created specific to the needs of blind and visually impaired seniors in order to train facilitators to deliver support at the community level. RESULTS: This program is a qualified success - to date, thousands of seniors have been educated about aging and vision loss and thousands of visually impaired seniors have received support through the network in their own communities. The training module inspires dedication by providing essential education to facilitators who work at the community level. A large network is coordinated by only two CNIB staff - the program is unique and highly effective. CONCLUSION: It is estimated that 3 out of 4 people over the age of 75 are affected by significant vision loss. This alarming statistic raises the importance of education for service providers about the realities and implications of aging and vision loss today. As the only provider of extensive services for people experiencing vision loss in Canada, the CNIB will continue with programs and education for older adults. (This poster presentation will include literature and practical information and suggestions for service-providers.)

[16] Back to hearing: Rehabilitation in presbyacusis

GOTTSCHALK, Mónica (HOGAR ADOLFO HIRSCH, San Miguel, Buenos Aires, Argentina)

PURPOSE: To regain, as much as possible, the ability to hear and listen, to provide the optimum basis for minimizing the handicap. METHOD:

Acoustic stimulation in sound qualities. Concrete sound experience: a series of different sounds, individual instruments, more than one instrument, series of popular music, series of sounds-noises from everyday life, series of words, sentences, short poems. Listen carefully in order to recognize from sounds (daylife, familiar, street, music) to language (words, sentences) RESULTS: Stimulation-training of: audiosensorial memory, timber gestalt, concentration, attention, discrimination, time-spatial-sequential sound location. CONCLUSION: Overcoming of communicative fences.

[17] Exercise limitation in elderly: Is cardiopulmonary exercise testing clinically useful

CM Chu, CY Yung, VL Chan, GCY Wong, EMF Leung (Department of Medicine& Geriatrics, United Christian Hospital, Kwun Tong, Hong Kong, China)

PURPOSE: To study the use of cardiopulmonary exercise testing (CPEXT) in elderly Chinese patients with exercise limitation METHOD: Over a period of 12 months, subjects of age 65 or above seen in medical clinics of a district hospital were arranged to have CPEXT if they had: (1) more than one medical diagnosis which might cause exertional dyspnoea, but the key limiting disorder was not definite; (2) the degree of dysnoea felt to be disproportionate to baseline investigation findings or (3) exertional dyspnoea was thought to be unexplained from primary diagnosis, lung function tests and echocardiogram. The subjects underwent incremental maximal exercise testing on a treadmill with a modified Harbor protocol. The results were interpreted using diagnostic algorithm compared to expected responses during exercise. Correlations were made between primary diagnosis and key pathophysiological mechanisms limiting exercise. RESULTS: A total of 18 subjects were recruited (3 males) with mean age of 69 (SD 4.6). The key pathophysiological mechanisms limiting exercise as delineated by the CPEXT included: cardiac pump (27.8%), cardiac ischaemia (5.6%), ventilatory limitation (22.2%), pulmonary vascular (5.6%), pacemaker malfunction (5.6%), deconditioning (22.2%) and normal in 11.1%. In the remaining 72.2%, CPEXT results showed that the pathophysiological mechanisms limiting exercise were heterogeneous and not entirely predictable. Only 27.8% had a mechanism of exercise limitation that was obvious from the primary diagnosis and correctly predicted by the physician. CPEXT is useful to delineate the underlying pathophysiological mechanism. CONCLUSION: Our study suggested that maximal CPEXT is useful in selected elderly patients with unexplained exercise limitation.

[18] Concept of Instincts and Age-Related Pathology Prevention Based on the Advances of Traditional Oriental Medicine

Yu. R. Roumyantsev (St. Petersburg Institute of Bioregulation and Gerontology, St. Petersburg, Russia)

The work bases the theory of instincts distinguishing 7 primary human instincts self-preservation, birth giving, altruism, investigation, domineering, freedom and dignity preservation. In every individual, certain instinct domineers determining the personality type. Masculine or feminine instinct orientation underlies formation of masculine or feminine types of personality. This research has been designed to reveal the correlation between instincts and certain intrinsic organs and systems of organs. Impact of such individual data as year, month, date and time of birth associated in traditional oriental medicine with activity of certain organs and their role in constitutional individual passport formation are the focus of this work. The domineering instinct is a constant acquiring additional peculiarity in various life periods under the influence of changing activity of other instincts or their combination, as well as by constitutional expressiveness of certain instincts. This periodicity constitutes 10-12 years since the birth date and embraces intermediate periods of 3-4 years. Each intermediate period is marked by the activity of certain organs and systems of organs determining the individual background , against which various diseases occur and progress. Role of masculinity and femininity in etiopathogenesis of psychosomatic diseases and neuroses is important. Long-term experimental and clinical trials on peptide tissue-specific bioregulators cytomedins enables conducting preventive therapy since early childhood with respect to the life period and individual constitutional peculiarities. In this context, development of chronotherapy principles in restoring biorhythmic disorders of the organism neuroendocrine functions with cytomedins appears to have a significant preventive potentiality.

[19] Homebound Level and Mortality among the Community-dwelling Elderly

S. Yasumura (Fukushima Med. Univ, Fukushima, Japan), H. Imuta, A. Fukao (Yamagata Univ, Yamagata, Japan), T. Ahiko (Yamagata Public Health Center, Yamagata, Japan)

PURPOSE: The aim of the present study is to examine the relationship between homebound level and mortality among the community-dwelling elderly. METHOD: Of the 2310 eligible subjects aged 65 years and over of Yamagata in Japan, 2217 subjects responded to the baseline interview survey in September 1997. The questionnaire consisted of age, gender, frequency of outdoors within a week as level of homebound, ADLs, functional status, physical, psychological and social variables. All subjects were followed up until 1 December 1999. Cox proportional hazard model was used to analyze the relationship between homebound level and mortality. RESULTS: During the follow-up period, one hundred and thirty three subjects died. The subjects with less frequent outdoors had a significantly higher mortality controlling for age, gender, and functional status ($p < .01$). The subjects who never or almost never go out of their own room had about twice high mortality compared to those who go out of their house at least once a week. CONCLUSION: Our findings suggest that level of homebound measured as frequency of outdoors within a week is significantly related to mortality among the community-dwelling elderly. Information on the frequency of outdoors within a week is important to select persons with high risk for mortality among the elderly.

[20] Is lifestyle important for health outcomes in elderly Hong Kong Chinese?

J. Woo, S.C. Ho (Centre of Gerontology & Geriatrics, The Chinese University of Hong Kong, H.K.)

PURPOSE: To determine if physical activity, dietary habit, smoking and alcohol intake in Hong Kong Chinese aged 70 years and over affected mortality, morbidity, self-perceived, health, mental health and use of health and social services. METHOD: A 3 year longitudinal follow-up of a cohort of 2030 (559 M; 612 F) subjects selected by stratified disproportional random sampling. Baseline information regarding physical and psychological health, and lifestyle factors, was obtained, and repeated after three years. Multiple logistic regression was used to examine the effect of lifestyle factors on each of the following outcomes: mortality, development of new disease, falls, self perceived health, depression (GDS >= 8), and use of health and social services. RESULTS: Being a current smoker increased mortality (OR 1.34; 95%CI 1.0-1.8). Factors reducing risk include physical activity >= 20 min/day (OR 0.46; 95%CI 0.36-0.57); occasional alcohol intake (OR 0.64; 95%CI 0.43-0.97); and daily fish consumption (OR 0.60; 95%CI 0.41-0.86). Factors inversely associated with depression include physical activity >= 20 min/day (OR 0.69; 95%CI 0.52-0.93); occasional alcohol intake (OR 0.58; 95%CI 0.35-0.94); while occasional vegetable intake 2-3 times per week appear to increase the risk (OR 2.67; 95% CI 1.06-6.72). Physical activity >= 20 min/day also reduced hospitalization (OR 0.7; 95%CI 0.53-0.92). Good self perceived health was associated with occasional alcohol intake (OR 1.77; 95%CI 1.18-2.65) and inversely associated with smoking (OR 0.56; 95%CI 0.39-0.80) CONCLUSION: Even among with a mean age of 80 years, lifestyle factors are important in achieving better health outcomes.

[21] Predictors of women's intention to use dual energy x-ray: Testing the theory of planned behavior

P. Werner (Department of Gerontology, University of Haifa, Israel), I. Vered (Institute of Endocrinology, Sheba Medical Center, Israel), Y. Shatz (School of Social Work, University of Haifa, Israel)

PURPOSE: To examine women's intentions to use dual energy x-ray (DXA) for bone density screening of osteoporosis using the Theory of Planned Behavior. METHOD: One hundred and fifty-one women (mean age = 57.34, range 45 - 71) completed a questionnaire including questions based on the Theory of Planned Behavior (attitudes, subjective norm, perceived behavioral control, past behavior and knowledge about osteoporosis) to predict their intention to use DXA. Six hypothetical scenarios varying by age (45, 50 and 60 years old) and family history, were presented. RESULTS: Factor analyses of the scenarios revealed two factors: one for scenarios describing a 45-year woman (regardless of family history) and a second factor for scenarios describing 50 and 60-year old women (regardless of family history). Stepwise regression analyses showed that women's attitudes, perceived behavioral control, past behavior and knowledge were significant predictors of intention to use DXA in the factor describing women aged 50+ ($R2 = 0.52$). Only attitudes and past behavior, were significant predictors of intention in the factor describing women aged 45 ($R2 = 0.14$). Subjective norm did not significantly predict intention. Attitude provided the best explanation of intention (Beta = .40 in the 50+ factor and Beta = .28 in the young one). The external variables of age and education had indirect effects on intention. CONCLUSION: In predicting women's intention to use DXA, their attitudes, their degree of confidence in their ability to carry out the behavior (i.e, perceive behavioral control), their knowledge and past behavior are important considerations.

[22] A short instrument to assess risk of functional impairment in the elderly at community setting

J Silva (National Institute of Geriatrics, Santiago, Chile), C Albala (Nutrition and Food Technology Institute, Santiago, Chile), J Jerez (National Institute of Geriatrics, Santiago, Chile), Villalobos A (MINSAL, Santiago, Chile), Barros C (Catholic University, Santiago, Chile), Escobar MC (MINSAL, Santiago, Chile), McDowell I (Dep Epidemiology University of Ottawa, Ottawa Canada)

Purpose: To develop an instrument to predict risk of functional impairment in the elderly. Methods: Cross sectional study in a community sample of 780 people aged 60 y and over. All the subjects were interviewed collecting data on self-assessment of health, physical and mental impairments, history of chronic diseases, geriatric syndromes, socioeconomic conditions and lifestyles. A subsample of 267 subjects underwent a standardized clinical evaluation acting as gold standard, performed by 3 geriatricians trained and standardized (Kappa index=0.62). Subjects were classified in non healthy, healthy on risk of functional impairment and healthy without impairment risk. Statistical analysis performed with SAS, included comparison of means, simple regressions, multiple regressions and factor analysis. Results: 62 variables identified having significant differences between outcomes, were run in a factor analysis. Five new variables explained 35.6% of the total variability. A summary of stepwise selection for each factor is shown. Factor 1: Taking bath or shower, Managing one's own money, Dressing and undressing, Cooking, Taking one's own medications, Factor 2: Feeling depressed, Yesavage short version, Memory self-assessment, Feeling distress, Income Factor 3: Taking object from floor, Physical self-assessment, Climbing stairs, Taking one's own medications, Cutting one's own toe nails. Factor 4: Education, MMSE short version, To read newspapers, To dress and undress, Eating fruits Factor 5: Blood pressure seated, Walking parks, Blood pressure standing, Hypertension history, income Conclusion: The most important variables to predict functional impairment were IADL, followed by mood disturbances, physical fitness and blood pressure. Factors 4 and 5 also included education, reading and healthy eating patterns.

[23] Profile of a Brazilian Population

Vicente Spinola Dias Neto; Giselle H. de P. Rodrigues; Juliana P. Magnatti (Pontifícia Universidade Católica de São Paulo Sorocaba Brazil).

PURPOSE: This study shows the prevalence of pathologies and the quantity of medication used among patients over 60 years old. METHOD: Interviews, based on a standard questionnaire, have been done with all of the older people (n=409) from two city districts of Sorocaba city, São Paulo, Brazil. The questionnaire wanted to define the social profile, pathologies, medications used and the autonomy of this population. The software EPI-INFO 5.0 has been used to compute the results. RESULTS: 95.8% had some pathology. Of these, 21% had one; 27% had two; 25.2%, three; and 22.9% had four or more pathologies. These people had diseases like: cardiovascular (54.9%), musculoskeletal (35.43%); neuropsychiatric (21.5%) and 35.95% of the population had no diagnostic for their diseases. These older people used drugs like: antihypertensives (46.5%); nonsteroidal anti-inflammatory agents (23.88%); sedatives (22.3%); oral antidiabetic drugs (12.9%). We noticed that 19.4% of them used one kind of drug; 20.2%, two kinds; 18.1%, three kinds and 21% used four or more. Between 80 to 99 years old (13.29%), 4.19% didn't use drugs; 3.14% used only one kind; 1.58%, two kinds; 2.88%, three kinds and 1.50%, four or more. CONCLUSION: The importance of showing the total population of two city districts is to determine what's happening with this people and, as soon as possible, to improve a kind of preventive health program. So, with this study, we could show that the patients have been using a lot of drugs, maybe unnecessarily. Differently of expected, patients over than 80 years use fewer drugs than the others. And some of them are without adequate treatment for their diseases or without diagnosis.

[24] The living conditions of the elderly with chronic renal failure under hemodialysis treatment

Rita de Cássia Helú Mendonça Ribeiro (University of São José do Rio Preto at College Nursing São José do Rio Preto, São Paulo, Brazil) Rosalina Aparecida Partezani Rodrigues (University of São Paulo at Ribeirão Preto College Nursing, Ribeirão Preto, São Paulo, Brazil)

The purposes of this study were to characterize elderly people with chronic renal failure under hemodialysis treatment and to outline their living conditions. Such a group was assisted at a university hospital in the interior of São Paulo state, consisting of eight subjects aged from 65 to 72 years old who were under hemodialysis treatment and lived in São José do Rio Preto - SP and neighboring towns. The theoretical and methodological framework was based on Meihy's thematic oral history and on Bardin's suggestions for data analysis. This analysis was classified into two categories: the elderly's living conditions before the hemodialysis treatment and the elderly's living conditions during it. From those categories, subcategories were classified: food and hydration; physical disorders; daily-life activities (DLA) and health/disease process. These categories showed some changes in the elderly's living conditions before and after the hemodialysis treatment, which can be understood as biopsychosocial alterations affecting the elderly's living conditions with emphasis on the health-disease and treatment process.

[25] The Elderly Health Attention Group (GRASI): Report of experience in an university hospital

M.J.D.Diogo, M.F.Ceolim, F.A.Cintra (Nursing Department, Faculty of Medical Science, State University of Campinas, São Paulo, Brazil)

This study aims to report the experience of implantation of the Elderly Health Attention Group (GRASI) in the outpatient's medical clinic of a University Hospital (Hospital de Clínicas - Universidade Estadual de Campinas), the core of which was the elaboration and development of an educative program designed to this age group and their relatives. The program included topics requested by the clients, such as increased risk for falls, changes in memory, sleep and vision, as well as issues considered important by the researchers, such as self-care, emotional aspects, senescence and senility. The experience was evaluated as a significant contribution for their daily life as well as a good opportunity for acquiring new knowledge and new friendships.

[26] Plasma brain natriuretic peptides (BNP) level in community-dwelling elderly is associated with the functional impairment

Masanori Nishinaga, Tomio Hamada, Takayuki Fukui, Kiyohito Okumiya, Yukari Morita, Daisuke Kuzume, Yoshinori Doi(Kochi medical School, Kochi, Japan) and Kozo Matsubayashi(Kyoto university, Kyoto, Japan)

PURPOSE: To elucidate the relation between the plasma BNP level and neurobehavioral function in community-dwelling elderly people. METHOD: We studied 315 eligible elderly people aged over 65 years; mean age 79 years (range 65 to 93years in the town of Kahoku, Kochi. We measured LV end-diastolic diameter (Dd), fractional shortening and the ratio of peak early filling velocity to peak atrial systolic velocity (E/A) and left ventricular mass Index (LVMI) by echocardiography. The plasma samples were analyzed for BNP. To evaluate of cognitive and neurobehavioral functions, we used 1) Mini-mental State Examination (MMS) 2) Hasegawa Dementia Scale Revised (HDSR), 3) Timed Up & Go test, assessing gait/balance and 4) Button score, assessing manual dexterity, both are useful and easy-to-administer predictors of declines in basic activities and instrumental activities of daily living. RESULTS: Elderly were classified into 3 groups based on plasma BNP concentration (Normal: < 18.5 pg/ml, Moderate: 18.5-100 pg/ml, High: 100pg/ml<) . (1) Normal group was 13%, Moderate :70% and High was 17% of all eligible elderly. (2) High group was older than the other groups (82.8, 78.9, 76.2 years, respectively, ANOVA p<0.001). (3) Among the 3 groups, there were no differences in sex, Dd, E/A, LVMI and systolic/diastolic blood pressure. (4) MMS and HDSR scores of High were lower than the other (ANOVA p<0.05). The times of Up & Go and Button test of High were longer (ANOVA , p<0.05). (5) Multivariate logistic regression analysis identified age, plasma concentration of BNP as independent factors of the cognitive impairment. CONCLUSION: The high plasma concentration of BNP is associated with cognitive impairment and functional decline in community-dwelling older peoples. Thus blood plasma BNP level in the community-dwelling elderly people may be one of the indexes of frailty.

[27] Attitudes of Geriatric Patients towards Adult Immunization

T. S. Narayanan, M.D. Shobhana Chaudhari, M.D. Francis Rice, RNP Ana Miller, RN (New York Medical College/ Metropolitan Hospital Center, New York City, NY 10029, USA

PURPOSE: Prophylactic vaccination of all Geriatric patients (influenza Vaccine) decreases the mean number of hospital admissions for respiratory infections (71%), congestive heart failure (27%) , and over all mortality by 50%. Latest CDC 2000 guidelines recommend the mean age of routine flu vaccinations to 50 years with a goal of vaccinating 900f population at risk by 2010.This project was undertaken to study the attitudes of elderly patients towards adult immunizations. METHODS: In a city hospital serving ethnically diverse and under served populations, we prospectively evaluated patients attending geriatric clinic from October to December 2000 by a questionnaire. Results were analyzed to know the differences between those who took the vaccination and refused the vaccination. RESULTS: Out of 209 patients who were eligible, 23 (11%) refused the vaccine. Mean age of both groups were (Mean +2SD) 74 +_7.8,74 +_ 8 respectively (p=0.96). Racial distribution was similar between both. Afro-American were 34.8%, 39%, (p=0.67), while Hispanic constituted 60%, 47.6% (p=0.25) respectively. Out of those refused, 11 patients (47%) felt they are not at risk, 10 (43%)were afraid of side effects, 2 (8.6%) felt that the vaccine does not work and 2 (8.6%) felt more than 2 factors.none felt further need of advice or receiving at other time or place. CONCLUSIONS: Inspite of persistent and extensive health care efforts, significant number of patients (11%) refused vaccination , possibly due to lack of knowledge of immunizations indicating the need of active physician participation, in order to achieve the goal as above.

[28] Educative Action of Multidisciplinary Team in a Secondary Prevention Program in Coronary Artery Disease

S. L. Medeiros, (Instituto Dante Pazzanese de Cardiologia de São Paulo. São Paulo, Brazil); C. M. Bogus, (Instituto de Saúde . São Paulo, Brazil)

Purpose: Evaluation of education strategies of the multidisciplinary team in the Program Heart Care Network in the Institute "Dante Pazzanese" of Cardiology Method: During 2 years (1999-2000) the multidisciplinary team (MT) selected 200 old patients (among 4000 registered in Heart Care Network Program) to participate in the Educative Program (EP) to be orientated about the risk factors for Coronary Artery Disease (CAD), to facilitate the understanding of the disease and reinforce the treatment adherence. The goal was to discuss the self-created risk factors and training abilities for healthy habits adoption substituting compartmental bad patterns. The MT used different pedagogic methods as: expositive classes , dynamic group, dialog exposition and shared experiences. The evaluation about knowledge gains was obtained through formularies with objective questions. Indirect evaluations were obtained through graphic representations and dynamic group. Results: The disease knowledgement and therapeutic procedures increased from 79% in the beginning tests to 91% after the participation in the EP. The understanding about risk factors was demonstrated by 84% of the patients that changed some eating habits (63%) other habits (20%). Conclusion: The quantitative and qualitative data showed some MTs appropriate strategies to reach the principal goal that is to control CAD . Investments must be done to valorize the educational actions to promote health; to better prepare MT to collect and evaluate the behavioral changing process and in the communication among the team also with the patients and motivational strategies, especially with oldest ones.

[29] The Seniors Health Resource Team: A Demonstration Model - Clinic on Wheels

S. Lundstrom, E. Stelmack, A. Moore (Winnipeg Regional Health Authority - Long Term Care Community Services, Winnipeg, Canada)

The Seniors Health Resource Team consists of a registered nurse and occupational therapist who provide direct service, health promotion, injury and illness prevention and chronic disease management to a target population of 1500 seniors living in congregate housing. The Team will share how they have mobilized existing services and agencies to provide health care education, primary health care, resources and research to individuals, families, groups and the community. By providing pertinent information to the family doctor, home care, hospitals or other services, this team develops care plans that allow clients to receive the care they need where and when they need it. This team approach has prevented crisis management for those with long term illness. The team provides monthly clinics, group education, home and site visits. Focus groups and surveys identified varied needs and this resulted in implementing walking groups, fall prevention activities, caregiver and diabetes management support groups. Community organizers are involved in planning and designing gardening projects, street and building modifications, and the Friendly Watch. The Team has facilitated agencies to reach seniors with their services and resources making them more accessible. Summary findings indicate that community development and advocacy make the community a place that addresses the determinants of health. The team has successfully reached isolated and vulnerable seniors and early results show a reduction in medication misuse, prevention of falls and injuries, and management of chronic diseases.

[30] Nurse led clinic for high risk older patients

Tak-yin Lau (United Christian Hospital, Hospital Authority, Hong Kong S.A.R. China)

This paper discusses the contribution of a nurse led secondary prevention clinic as a better model to bridge the gap between acute hospital care and home for high risk older patients. Data on hospital readmissions, A & E department visits, length of stay, compliance to treatment plan and treatment regime, satisfaction of patients and care givers were collected after the patients joined the clinic. Data analysis during the clinic's first three months revealed that frail elderly patients and patients requiring continuous nursing care needs, such as patients with chronic wound ulcers and patients who had percutaneous endoscopic gastrostomy performed, seemed to benefit most from participation in the clinic. Results shown that if a healthcare provider is available to manage early signs and symptoms of deterioration of general health status of patients, hospital readmissions may be decreased and patient's outcomes may be improved. The provision of health education and counseling and the nurse specialist as the first point of contact for patients and caregivers encourages the families to take care of the elderly patients thus further improve the quality of life of these patients.

[31] Evaluation of Handwashing Practice in the Prevention of Nosocomial Infections in the Elderly

L.Fustier (Centre Gérontologique Départemental, Marseille, France), E.Grandini (InterClin-Noso 13,Marseille,France), N.de Rekeneire (National Institute on Aging, Bethesda, USA)

Nosocomial infections are a big public health problem and handling transmission is the principal cause . We conducted a study based on an audit on the handwashing practice in a geriatric hospital. 141 persons were observed, including 28 nurses, 64 nursing auxiliaries (47 %) , 28 housekeepers, 4 doctors, 2 nurse's chiefs and 6 students . In 78,7% of cases, the observations were realized during the day . The recommendations about the staff clothes are largely followed but the wearing of a wedding ring in 22,7% of cases is not correct . The mean time of the handwashing is 68,17 seconds . The time spent to soap the hands is 39,25 seconds and the time of rinsing is 28,92 seconds . This time differs according to the units . The handwashing duration is better in nurses and nursing auxiliaries.In the equipment preparation, 33% are not adapted: empty distributors...The opening dates are not noted on the bottles in 73,7% of cases . The rising time is not tidy in 54,6% . 23,4% of the persons dry one's hands by rubbing which is not correct . A risk of contamination is shown in 22,7% of people at the end of the practice . This evaluation shows that the staff really knows our protocol . The actions to start are to inform about the respect of the duration especially in rinsing . This audit permitted us to quantify the equipment and to improve it . Then, we rewrote our protocol regarding the results insistent on the time, the rinsing and drying . This audit only studied the quality of the handwashing, we plan to analyse in a second time the observance of this practice .

[32] Developing an Injury Prevention Program - A Minimal Lift Policy

Debra F. Elm (The Good Samaritan Society, Edmonton, Canada)

Staff injury from lifting and transferring residents are very costly and put the residents at risk for falls and injury. The Good Samaritan Society (GSS), a multi-site continuing care service provider, implemented a "Minimal Lift Policy". The objective of this policy is to prevent injury of both staff and residents while allowing the resident to use as much of their own ability as possible. A literature search was done to determine the risks and causes of injury while lifting and transferring. Each cause was evaluated and strategies were put into place. Transfer decision trees were developed to determine the appropriate transfer method for each resident. The number of residents that require each transfer type was determined using the decision tree to ascertain the number of mechanical lifts required. Lifts were then purchased. Education modules were developed which are mandatory for all staff to complete after which both knowledge and practice competencies must be demonstrated. Unit teams were formed to teach staff the transfer methods and to be consulted in unique situations. To evaluate the injury prevention program the residents were surveyed to determine their feelings of safety with the lifting before and after the program was implemented. A staff survey was completed to determine staff knowledge and the level of risk for injury. Injury rates and the costs of those injuries to the organization were compiled prior to implementation. The staff survey will be again completed and injury rates and costs will be again reviewed in three months time. The results will be available for the presentation.

[33] Psychosocial Variables in a Screening Study of Older Adults: Scale Development and Construct Validity

S. Koffman, G. Hicks, K. Arnette, P. Watkins, Lily Sizemore, Joan Lawrence, Mike Johnson, Jessica Gallion (Department of Psychology, Eastern Washington University, WA, USA), N. Jackson, R. Browers (Department of Counseling, Educational and Developmental Psychology , Eastern Washington University, WA, USA), L. Bennett, P. Hastings (Department of Counselor Education, Gonzaga University, WA, USA)

The screening study, which demographically and clinically defines the population, is an essential step in developing ethical methodology and adequate sampling procedures for ongoing research in geropsychology, as well as being integral in grant writing, program planning and service provision. Clarity of construct definition and increased validity in the variables of interest to the geropsychologist is accomplished through refinement of instrumentation. The present study addressed both of these needs. We assessed a variety of psychosocial variables across an eastern Washington State population of older persons (N= 500, mean age = 72) in both institutionalized and independent living conditions, in urban and rural settings, of diverse SES, race and ethnicity, and with a range of medical and psychiatric diagnoses. The variables included in the screening study were factor analyzed. They are: a demographics questionnaire, the Mental Status Exam, Instrumental Activities of Daily Living, Symptom CheckList- Revised (SCL 90-R), Subjective Quality of Life (SF-36), Geriatric Depression Scale (GDS), Life Satisfaction Inventory-A (LSIA), Irrational Beliefs Test (IBT), Ego Integrity Scale (EIS), and the GRAT, (a subjective experience of gratitude scale which is still in development). The descriptive statistics of the screening study variables and population norms will be presented. Further research will be suggested.

[34] Prevention of aging dependence to 2006

Ricardo Moragas Moragas (Gie, Pcb,Universitat De Barcelona, Barcelona, Spain) Nuria Rodriguez Avila (Gie, Pcb, Universitat De Barcelona, Barcelona, Spain) Ramon Cristofol Allue (Gie, Barcelona Science Park)

Purpose: The main objective is to analyze the demand dependan persons of Sanitary and Social Services up to the 2006 in Spain. Method: Estimate of the quantitative demand in cost of services for ages and sexes and qualitative for causes of the dependence through direct survery and demographic models based on current and future pathologies whose incidence will increase: Alzheimer's, Parkinson's, neurological, skeletal sclerosis, endocrine, etc. Valuation of innovations in prevention, cure and rehabilitation of the dependence that can reduce the demand of sanitary and social services. Results: Costs of dependence by personal services, medication and technical aids in each of 12 types of systems and pathologies. Conclusions: cost of dependence is increasing in most pathologies but growth is different and way slow in some pathologies. The spanish health and social services wil have to redesign its structure financially and service wise to cope with the increased demand.

[35] Obstacles to Mammography Compliance Among Low-Income Middle-Aged Women in Puerto Rico

M. Sánchez-Ayéndez, C. M. Nazario, A.L. Dávila, M. Bustillo, M.C. Larriuz, G. Martínez, N. Figueroa (Graduate School of Public Health, University of Puerto Rico Medical Sciences Campus, San Juan, Puerto Rico)

Despite evidence in favor of breast cancer screening with mammograms and that screening has increased in the last years, mammogram compliance among low-income, minority and women over 50 years of age has been slow. This poster presents the first stage of a three-year project that contemplates a study of low-income middle-aged women in Puerto Rico in regard to compliance with 1997 U.S.A. National Institutes of Health (NIH) screening mammogram guidelines. This first-stage centered on focus groups conducted to obtain qualitative data to develop instruments to be administered to women who will participate in a survey. Women from different geographic regions in Puerto Rico who attend community health centers participated in the sessions. Focus groups results indicate that women view cancer as a cell disorder and that breast pain or discomfort is a factor associated to the disease. The women have knowledge of breast self-exam, clinical breast-exam, and mammogram as early detection tests as well as of the usefulness of mammograms over other methods. They indicated no clear knowledge of 1997 NIH guidelines. Apprehensions about the discomfort caused by the mammography procedure and fear of a cancer diagnostic were the most prevalent personal barriers for mammogram compliance. Other factors were: cost, lack of transportation, patient-physician-relationship, and conflicts with child-care-provider role. The focus groups served to incorporate pertinent issues to mammography compliance and vocabulary for the development of a questionnaire that will be applied to 200 women in 2001.

[36] Healthy Brain Program: Novel Approach to Healthy Aging Promotion

Stephen J. Kiraly (UBC, Vancouver, Canada) Stephen G. Holliday, (VMDA, Vancouver, Canada) Brenda Bray, (VCMHS, Vancouver Canada) Rebekah Kiraly (Trent U, Peterborough, Canada)

Purpose: To acquaint the participant to the brain as an organ which requires care and maintenance. Specifically, we expose inconclusive material, isolated reports and fads which may prove to be worthless or dangerous. We strive for evidence based facts which will clarify the confusing and often contradictory information from the marketplace. Method: A didactic and cognitively oriented approach is used. The program is modeled after healthy heart programs which abound. Additional features are developed specifically for brain health. A core lecture outline and eight workshop outlines, each corresponding to one of the Eight Pillars of Longevity, will be presented in a pictorial and text format. The Eight Pillars are: Safety, Nutrition, Physical Exercise, Cognitive Exercise, Sleep, Stress Management, Hormone Replacement and Treatment of Existing Disease. The information in each of the workshops is based on analysis of many studies and reports. References are provided. Results: Participants have been very enthusiastic, attendance has been excellent and they given very positive feedback. Most are eager to return for more presentations and workshops. Conclusion: The Healthy Brain Program has excellent audience participant acceptance and it appears to be a worthwhile effort. It may have efficacy similar to the already proven healthy heart programs. Systematized research is needed to evaluate effects of consistent participation in various groups. The program may have great preventive potential. If followed, it may greatly improve quality and length of life and it would reduce health costs.

[37] Colon hydrotherapy in treatment of chronic constipation

Sylvester Yong (Dotolo Research - Asia Singapore)

Purpose: To assess the effectiveness of colon hydrotherapy in the treatment of chronic constipation in the elderly. Common factors causing constipation in elderly include dehydration, poor diet, dental problems, side effects of medication, lack of exercise and immobility. The use of laxatives and enema offers some degree of relief but the sufferings and problem tend to persist. Colon hydrotherapy offers an added option to therapy by facilitating the removal of faecal wastes from the entire length of the colon, providing immediate relief as well a long term improvement in the patients. Method: Colon hydrotherapy is carried out using the Toxygen Model BSC UV colon hydrotherapy instrument. It is designed to introduced water into the colon gently and safely. Water is introduced to flush the entire length of the colon. Flushing action is facilitated by gentle abdominal massage to loosen stagnated waste which is then carried out of the colon (solids and gas) with the discharging water. A series of 22 elderly patients with a history of chronic constipation (without organic causes) were treated with colon hydrotherapy. Their response were evaluated at the end of a series of colon hydrotherapy sessions ranging from between 4 to 10 sessions over a period of 4 weeks. Results: In the majority of patients, there was significant improvement in symptoms, reduced level discomfort, reduced use of laxatives and need for enema, and improved feeling of relief.

[38] Hospital Admissions for Influenza-like Illness: Who is at Risk?

V. Menec (Department of Community Health Sciences, University of Manitoba, Winnipeg, Canada)

PURPOSE: Influenza-like illnesses place considerable pressure on the hospital system during the winter months (Menec et al, 1998). This study examined characteristics of patients hospitalized for influenza-like illnesses. METHOD: Administrative data were used to identify admissions to all Winnipeg acute care hospitals during the winter months of 1995- 96 to 1998-99. Influenza-like illnesses (ILI) were defined based on ICD-9-CM codes as influenza, pneumonia, and acute and chronic respiratory diseases, such as chronic bronchitis and asthma. RESULTS: Seniors aged 65+ constituted the majority of adult admissions for ILI in all four study years (69.9% to 75.5%). The percentage of 75+ year olds was particularly large and increased steadily over the four years (42.6% to 52.8% of all adult admissions). In comparison, the percentage of 65+ year olds admitted for reasons other than ILI ranged from 55% to 55.5%, with the percentage of 75+ year olds remaining relatively constant over the four years (32.8% to 35.5%). Further analysis indicated that among individuals aged 65+ years old, admission rates for ILI (age and sex standardized) were considerably higher for seniors living in senior apartments than their counterparts living at home. Compared to individuals in senior apartments, admission rates were only slightly higher among personal care home residents in 1997-98 and 1998-99 and, indeed, were lower in 1995-96 and 1996-97. CONCLUSION: Given that influenza vaccination is effective in decreasing hospitalization for influenza-like illnesses among seniors, influenza vaccination programs should be further expanded. Particular emphasis should be placed on targeting individuals living in senior apartments.

[39] Serum albumin and outcomes in patients with fractures on a geriatric rehabilitation unit (GRU)

Serrano MP, Tena-Dávila MC. Unidad Geriátrica Municipal. Área de Sanidad. Ayuntamiento de Madrid. SPAIN

PURPOSE: To analyse predictive value of serum albumin in patients admitted to the GRU with fractures, and the influence of that parameter on the results. METHOD: The study covered 265 patients, 42 male and 223 female, with an average age of 81.38. Serum albumin was determined at admission and related to physical and mental disabilities recorded previously, on admission and on release, measured by Barthel and the Red Cross scale. They were also related to the average stay and complications that required transfer to the hospital for acute patients. The statistical analysis was performed using SPSS RESULTS: Mean albumin was 3.43 mg/dl, 148 (55.8%) patients had albumin level lower than 3.5 mg/dl and albumin was associated with other variables: People transferred to the acute patients hospital (average 3.1, $p=0.008$), Functional failures (average 3.27) vs Good functional outcome (average 3.47)($p=0.003$). The average stay was related with albumin level ($r=-0.212$, $p=0.002$). CONCLUSIONS: In patients where albumin levels were low more time was required to achieve functional recuperation and there were more instances of transfer for intercurrent disorders.

[40] Intensive Geriatric Rehabilitation in Demented Pattients with Hip Fracture: Functional Outcomes and Length of Stay

Ranieri P, Guerini F, Pea S, Gatti S, Franzoni S, Rozzini, R, Trabucchi M. GERU, H. P. Richiedei, Gussago, (and Geriatric Research Group, via Romanino 1, 25121 Brescia.)

Aims: To evaluate the effect of intensive geriatric rehabilitation on functional recovery and length of stay (LOS) in demented patients with hip fracture. Subjects: 70 hip fractured elderly patients (mean age 81.7±7.8 years, 88 0.000000emale, 8.30f all new admission) consecutively admitted to Geriatric Evaluation and Rehabilitation Unit over a period of one year. Twenty-six (37.7%) patients had severe cognitive impairment

(MMSE<18). Methods: Three days after admission a multidimensional evaluation was performed including information on demographics, cognitive status (MMSE), physical health, functional disability (BADL, IADL, Tinetti scale), and nutritional status (PNI). Patients received five daily sessions per week of 30-45 minutes each. Patients were discharged when the rehabilitation team judged that the maximal effect of rehabilitation has been reached. The efficacy of the rehabilitative treatment was estimated by the difference between Tinetti score at discharge and on admission. We defined motor independence and safe gait by Tinetti score >18. Results: The endpoint of motor independence and safe gait was reached by 28 patients and was found to be less likely in patients with poorer functional status on admission, very old age, and malnutrition. The mean LOS was 42.2±21.9 days. Conclusions: Data suggest that demented patients with hip fracture can benefit from geriatric assessment and intensive rehabilitation. In hip fractured patients dementia is not associated with lower likelihood of reaching the rehabilitative endpoint. Length of stay is not different between demented and non demented patients.

[41] Aged and Rehabilitation

L. Vértes (chief physician, President of Gerontological Section at Hungarian Association of Rehabilitation, Budapest, Hungary)

The author, based upon the literary data and his own cases as well as 347 of his old (average 74,5 years) patients getting into multimorbidity the significance of the rehabilitation, what in addition refers of the dialectic relationship of the prevention, the therapy and the rehabilitation. That means, that the rehabilitation may be successful only in the case, if it asserts itself in all somatic, psychic and social fields. The expectans and the results of the rehabilitation are determined not only by the diagnosis, but individual conditions of the patients. The complexity of the questions reflects firmly the heterogenity what generally characterizes the elderly people living in the involution. It is obvious out of these that the rehabilitation in itself is an abstract idea, and doesn't give proper help for recognising the concrete and real state. Our tasks is always to determine the functional capacity of the old person. We have to save the senior citizens from segregation. That is we have to insure their social integration in the rehabilitation.

[42] MusicTherapy in the Elderly

L. Vértes (Chief physician, General Secretary of the Hungarian Association of Gerontology, General Secretary of Music Therapy Association in Hungary, Budapest, Hungary)

The relaxing, anxiety relieving, euforiant, tranquillizer effect of music has been examined in the elderly. The author tried to induce associations with positive aestetic, affective and emotional content. Due to the different musical educations and taste of patients they played easily understandable pieces of music within the frames of a lecture held on different topics which they propagated under titles arousing interest. The number of participiants was 4025.On the basis of the results of randomized tests it has been concluded that adequately chosen music has a definitive favourable subjective relaxing, tranquillizer psychich effect. Listening to music collectively influences beneficially especially those aged patients who had lived in isolation at home. The most favoured were the compositions of romantic, viennese classic and baroque periods and hungarian folk song. This latter was especially popular among aged patients. The author based the concept on the observations that musical talent is one of the gifts evinced at the earliest age which lasts the longest.

[43] An Empirical Review of Mindfulness Meditation with Applications to Older Adults

A. Schultz (Arizona State University, Tempe, USA)

Mindfulness meditation, in the form of mindfulness-based stress-reduction and relaxation programs, has spread across the United States within the last 20 years. Currently over 240 such programs are in operation (Salmon, Santorelli, & Kabat-Zinn, 1998), with a number of them based in Veterans Administration Medical Centers. The empirical literature on mindfulness meditation was reviewed in order to evaluate its impact on both self-regulatory (e.g, pain, anxiety, health care utilization) and phenomenological (e.g, control beliefs, spirituality) outcomes, with a focus on applying mindfulness to older adults. Psychinfo, Medline, and Dissertation Abstract databases were searched for mindfulness meditation terms. After obtaining empirical articles, relevant empirical citations from the articles were also gathered. Study components including sample size, control groups, randomization, follow-up data collection, and relative quality of MM interventions were uniformly addressed for all quantitative studies. Studies were also examined for use with older adult populations and/or special applicability to older adults. The empirical literature on mindfulness meditation was found to be in an early stage of development. Nonetheless, preliminary support was found for the positive effects of mindfulness meditation on a wide array of outcomes. While few studies have directly assessed the utility of mindfulness meditation with older adults, theory integrating salient characteristics of many older adults with the mindfulness literature suggests that mindfulness may have important implications for health and quality of life in aged populations. Target variables relevant to older adults such as temporal focus, control beliefs, and active acceptance were expanded upon.

[44] Ergonomics a catalyst for change for retirement and the ageing role of physiotherapists in the change.

Bev O'Sullivan, Pender Island, BC, Canada Klari Varallyai, A.L.L. Ergonomic International Ltd, Campbell River Physiotherapy Clinic, Campbell River, BC, Canada

The aim of ergonomics is to help the retiring and ageing population to remain independent and self sufficient. The understanding of Ergonomic principles and solutions will enable seniors to put ergonomic strategies into practice. The practical application will help seniors to remain relatively independent and to experience a high quality of life experience in their golden years. The growing number of senior citizens in the 1990's and year 2001 is a well known fact worldwide. Increased ability to maintain independence is a fact of life shared by all of us. Ergonomic experience from industry enables physiotherapists to be the "catalyst for change." The increased awareness of the environmental factors influencing the musculo-skeletal system, therefore independent living, such as light, sound, temperature, clothing, furniture, tools, etc. are being recognized and evaluated to maximize senior's abilities and to minimize the loss of functional skills. Educational programs to promote independence in the homes and at large are introduced to the public via preventative health education programs. These programs include practical sessions about self- care, safety in the home, and activities such as gardening, walking, etc. This information is especially important for the senior citizens in their daily tasks to remain independent as well and interdependent. Their wealth of knowledge of the past and present is vitally important to plan for the future. The utilization of ergonomic principles creates an increased user friendly environment and safer surroundings both at home and in the community. Ergonomic knowledge helps to promote A Quality of Life.

[45] Functional Recovery in Very Old Subjects with Femoral Fractures: A Case Report in Centenarians

Muzzoni B, Casarotti D, Cravello L, Albertelli N, Pelanconi L, Carbone P, Magri F, Ferrari E. (Department of Internal Medicine and Medical Therapy, Chair of Geriatrics, University of Pavia, Italy)

Aging is associated with an impairment of bone mass and an increase of the falls incidence. Therefore also a light trauma may expose old subjects to fractures. The femoral fractures are the most important causes of functional inability, loss of autonomy and worsening life quality in elderly people, and the rehabilitation represents a crucial moment for elderly subjects. Two centenarians women (100 and 103 ys) underwent a femoral fracture because of an accidental fall and were submitted to surgical osteosynthesis. Before this event they were in good physical and mental conditions, according to ADL, IADL and CIRS score. Longitudinal observation showed a good recovery of the functional autonomy independently from the fracture s site (subtrochanteric versus subcapital), the kind of surgical operation (gamma nail or endoprothesis) as well as the rehabilitative context (rehabilitation in clinical structure or at home). At the time of our observation one of them was able to walk by cane and the other by sustaining help. Our data show that the age alone was not an absolutely negative risk factor, but it may acquire unfavourable prognostic significance where is coupled to a bad health status and to poor performances in ADL and IADL.

[46] Reality Orientation in aged women home residents in Curitiba making use of activities with music

Ana Maria Moser (PUCPR / UNIVALI / USP Curitba Brasil) Maria Regina de Souza Godeli (USP São Paulo Brasil) Andressa Mores (PUCPR Curitiba Brasil) Carolina Esmanhoto Bertol (PUCPR Curitiba Brasil) Fernanda do Vale (PUCPR Curitiba Brasil) Leticia Barreto (PUCPR Curitiba Brasil)

The present research had as its purpose to work with old ladies the orientation to the reality, through the music, aimed at optimizing life quality. There were eight ladies, who were between 60 and 101 years old, living in an private asylum (which fare is around US $250.00). There were several diseases diagnosed such as Alzheimer's Disease, Parkinson's Disease and others. The procedure consisted of the application of a previous and post test and nine meetings with 40 minutes each. These meetings were composed by warming exercises and a main activity, always utilizing music as facilitator to develop the activities. The main results in the post test were: increase of verbalizing among the aged women, increase of the behavior frequency in the activity, helping behavior among them and concluding the exercises. Through the meetings we observed that they frequently cared more of each other and even signs of affectivity in relation to themselves and to the applicators. As well as verbalizations represent self-corporal awareness (I cannot get any lower) and willing (I do not want to pee in my diaper). Concluding that, these kinds of musical activities should be utilized to motivate elder people with some kind of deficiency to develop activities once these activities are adjusted to their difficulties and also the staff works its own difficulties.

[47] Formation of little musical band with aged carriers of AVC

Ana Maria Moser [PUCPR / UNIVALI / USP Curitiba - Brasil] Ana Carolina Carvalho [PUCPR Curitiba - Brasil] Andréa Ferrari [PUCPR Curitiba - Brasil] Daniele de Sá [PUCPR Curitiba - Brasil] Flávia Muniz [PUCPR Curitiba - Brasil] Franciele Tozo [PUCPR Curitiba - Brasil] Jordana Scheuer [PUCPR Curitiba - Brasil] Eliane Vendramin [PUCPR Curitiba - Brasil] Maria Regina de Souza Godeli [USP São Paulo - Brasil]

The objective of the present research was to use music to facilitate the development of motor and social abilities in aged residents in an home for elderly in the city of São José dos Pinhais Pr. Seven people (4 women and 3 men), who were between 55 and 78 years old, participated, and the majority (71%) carrying of Cerebral Vascular Accident with sequels. The procedure consisted of the application of a previous and post test (for verification of the interpersonal relationship) and of nine sessions with average duration of thirty minutes, twice a week. In each session three dynamics were accomplished by music, and in the third and fourth session, the aged themselves confectioned the musical instruments correspondent to rattle, triangle and bumbo. From the fifth session was trained a little band with the music chosen by the aged themselves. The main results indicate a bigger easiness in the manage of the musical instruments and an accompaniment of the rhythm of the music, beside a bigger integration of the aged, perceived through the increase of the frequency of verbalizing and the compliments among them, and even the beginning of a courtship. The interpretation of the results evaluated the importance of the music utilization in the rescue of abilities in aged, providing an optimization of the life quality. Moreover it was also considered that in activities with aged it must be emphasized the adaptation of the applicators in relation to the difficulties presented by the aged and also the necessity of co-responsibility of the institutional team.

[48] Rehabilitation Program for Aging Chernobyl Disaster Survivors

Georgiy Korobeynikov, Galina Fedko

PURPOSE: There are many medical consequences obtained before accident on of Chernobyl Nuclear Power Plant. The purpose of the study approbation of the prevention lifestyle program for Chernobyl disaster survivors. METOD: Sixty persons, disaster survivors and workers of Chernobyl Nuclear Power Plant station aged 32-56 have rehabilitation during 21 days. The used of complex of training prevention programs as lifestyle change intervention. The study of the effect of preventive lifestyle program for Chernobyl disaster survivors. The functional age and tempo of aging as criterion of health status were studied. RESULTS: The results showed the increasing of the functional age (71,7+5,62) and tempo of aging (1,58+0,09) for comparative of calendar age (48,81+1,91) in patients in the moment of start of the prevention course. This associated with the acceleration type of aging and decline of health of Chernobyl disaster survivors. After preventive course program, the average parameters of functional age in-patients decrease (66,76+4,31). But, the tempos of aging in-patients after preventive course remains accelerate (1,36+0,06). The decrease of arterial blood pressure, heart rate in rest and after physical load, increase of vital capacity of lungs and static balance are showed about health promotion in Chernobyl disaster survivors during the preventive course. CONCLUSION: According to data the subjective estimation of self-sense, activity and mood in Chernobyl disaster survivors improve during preventive course. This fact indicated the promotion of psychological health of Chernobyl disaster survivors during lifestyle change intervention

[49] Differences in response to rehabilitation in elderly population in community hospital

A. Krajewski, L. Lowe, J. Vidi, B. Park, A. Lochurst Humber River Regional Hospital, Downsview, Ontario, Canada

Elderly patients often experience a decline in physical functioning during the course of acute illness requiring hospitalization. This decline leads to prolonged hospital stay, nursing home placement and mortality This study evaluates the relationship between early reactivation and change in functional status for patients admitted to community hospital acute care for elderly unit. The study population included 118 patients(52 with stroke at age 67.8 +13.5 , 34 hip fractures - 81.3+ 9.2 and 32 frail elderly - 83.5+9 years) consecutively referred for rehabilitation services over a 6 month period. The Modified Barthel index (MBI) was administered by physiotherapy and occupational therapy staff on admission and discharge. MBI measures functional independence in personal care and mobility. The hip fractures had the lowest total score at admission 13.5 points and improved to 40 points. The stroke group gained form 35.4 to 63.9 points. The frail elderly improved form 23 to 42.3 points. The lowest improvement in the later group was seen in terms of personal hygiene like bladder control. Nine of 32 frail elderly went to long term facilities, the rest went home. The was not significant difference in total length of stay between groups (16.2 days for frail elderly, 15.5 stroke and hip fracture 12 days). In summary we believe that rehabilitation should be continued for frail elderly. MBI can be used as the standard tool in the geriatric population undergoing reactivation . It became an invaluable instrument to assess ability of patient to care for themselves, to assess progress, to predict outcome and to help with discharge planing issues.

[50] Older patients need more information and active rehabilitation after an acute myocardial infarction.

I.Grumme-Rönnquist, I.Odén (Danderyd Geriatric Clinic, Danderyd, Sweden), T.Kahan (Karolinska Institutet, Danderyd

Hospital, Division of Internal Medicine, Danderyd, Sweden). Par 3 I.Odén

Purpose: Cardiac rehabilitation(CR) after an acute myocardial infarction(AMI) improves prognosis and well-being also in older people. This study aimed to examine age or gender differences in attending a CR program after an AMI, compliance in attending, need for further information and need of acute care after an AMI. Method: A questionnaire was mailed 6 months after discharge to all patients hospitalised in our hospital for an AMI during 01.05.97 through 30.04.98. Results: 391 questionnaires were sent out and 313 answers were received. Mean age was 71.105 were women. 204 patients were offered CR. 117 attended. Reasons for not attending were other diseases, problems with transportation and costs for the patient. 196 patients did not attend and 109 were not offered CR, 40/105 women vs 69/208 men. Patients over 65 attended to lesser extent than younger, and older women attended more seldom than older men. 52% of the patients over 80 wanted more information regarding their disease. 40% of the patients paid an unscheduled visit to the emergency ward or primary care unit due to heart problems and 22% were re-hospitalised. Conclusions: There is a need for more patient information and CR to older patients after an AMI. This would best be met through co-operation between cardiologists, geriatricians and primary-care physicians in creating suitable CR programs. A reduction of re-hospitalisations and unscheduled visits could be expected.

[51] Chiropractic Care of the Elderly

Terry J. Gromala (Health Services Research & Policy, University of Minnesota, Minneapolis, MN, USA)

Over 6,000 elderly (65+ years) chiropractic patients in Minnesota are described in this retrospective study. This secondary database analysis used 1999 and 2000 data from the American Chiropractic Network, which provides professional management services for many health plans in Minnesota. We examined patients' chief complaints, primary diagnoses, severity, procedures, episode of care or treatment, patient satisfaction reports and outcomes of care compared to baseline functional and pain assessments. Finally, we compared elderly patients' outcomes between two chiropractic groups, who participate in ACN's quality improvement program. Findings demonstrate that most chief complaints of elderly patients are of neuromusculoskeletal origin and have chronic histories. Regional low back pain and neck pain were most common. The majority of procedures include chiropractic adjustments and manipulation, followed by specific supportive therapies and education. Controlling for similar conditions, the length of care resulted in a slightly longer, but not significant, length of care than for patients from 40 to 64 years of age. Elderly patients reported very high patient satisfaction, compared to young ages (18-39) and middle-aged (40-64) patients. Improved function and reduced pain were found for the primary diagnoses of elderly patients. Finally, elderly patients who saw providers participating in the quality improvement program reported better outcomes and patient satisfaction compared to providers not in the program. This study provides descriptive data and preliminary norms for elderly chiropractic patients. Elderly patients seen by providers in quality improvement programs had better outcomes and were more satisfied with their care.

[52] Electrical Stimulation of Quadriceps During Rehabilitation Following Proximal Femoral Fracture

Mark Barber (Academic Section of Geriatric Medicine, Glasgow Royal Infirmary, UK), Virginia Braid (Academic Section of Geriatric Medicine, Glasgow Royal Infirmary, UK), Sarah Mitchell(Academic Section of Geriatric Medicine, Glasgow Royal Infirmary, UK), Brendan Martin (Department of Medicine for the Elderly, Hairmyres Hospital, East Kilbride, UK), Stan Grant(Institute of Biomedical and Life Sciences, University of Glasgow, UK), Malcolm Granat (Department of Bioengineering, Strathclyde University, Glasgow, UK) and David Stott (Academic Section of Geriatric Medicine, Glasgow Royal Infirmary, UK)

PURPOSE: Proximal femoral fracture (PFF) is associated with high levels of disability and dependency. Quadriceps weakness may be an important factor in poor outcome. We hypothesised that electrical stimulation (ES) to quadriceps increases leg extensor power (LEP) and decreases disability following PFF. METHOD: A Case control study of elderly post-surgical PFF patients, comparing the addition of 6 weeks of ES (10 patients, mean age 79.0 years) to standard physiotherapy alone (19 patients, mean age 78.4). ES consisted of 7 seconds of stimulation of quadriceps followed by 23 seconds of relaxation for 36 repetitions. This was delivered daily as an in-patient and twice weekly once discharged. Our outcome measures were LEP (Nottingham Power Rig), functional mobility (Elderly Mobility Scale), disability (Barthel Index) and quality of life (Nottingham Health Profile) and were measured at baseline, after 6 weeks (the end of the intervention) and at 16 weeks. RESULTS: A median of 12.5 (range 4-20) sessions of ES were given to those who reached the 6-week assessment. LEP increased significantly in the ES group (fractured leg mean improvement at 6 weeks 307% (standard error 110), non-fractured leg 164% (72)) compared to the control group (51% (14) and 30% (11) respectively), Mann-Whitney U tests both $p<0.02$ for between group comparisons. There were non-significant trends towards greater improvements in EMS and Barthel scores in the treatment group. CONCLUSIONS: ES of quadriceps was associated with increased LEP and a tendency for reduced disability following PFF. A randomised controlled trial is warranted.

[53] Electrochemical-activated solutions (ECAS) influence on enzymes of antiradical protection

A. Podkolzin, A.Megreladze, O.Mrikaeva, E.Zukova (National Gerontology Center, Moscow, Russia)

Purpose: The influence of electrochemical-activated solutions (ECAS) with various redox potential on activity of main enzymes of antiradical protection of an organism - catalase (Ct), peroxydase (Pr) and SOD was researched. Material and methods: It was researched the ability of lysed erythrocytes of the rabbit to inactivate a peroxide of hydrogenium at the presence of ECAS various concentrations, obtained with usage of the water electrochemical clearing apparatus "Izumrud"(Russia). We have utillized also SOD of high clearing (93 % of cleanness) from erythrocytes. Results: It was shown, that ECAS in concentration 1-20 % and time 1-20-minute exposition has effected to influence activity of all 3 enzymes of antiradical protection of an organism. The effect of ECAS was dose-dependent and time-depend also. The double effect of ECAS was shown: the activation (on 85-130 %) at small concentrations and small exposure time and moderate suppression at high concentrations and long-lived period of an incubation with enzymes. The ECAS effect also directly and proportionally depend on the value of negative redox potential of ECAS and was maximum for fresh-prepared ECAS. Conclusion: The usage of electrochemical-activated water by usual apparatus of electrochemical clearing of water allows to influence enzymes of antiradical- protection of an organism, which add now important value in connection withprobable involvement of free radicals during ageing processes.

[54] Measuring Client Satisfaction in Geriatric Rehabilitation

P. Stolee, J. Esbaugh, J. Wagg, M.J. Borrie, M. Vickers (Southwestern Ontario Regional Geriatric Program, London, Canada), M.G. Woodbury (St. Joseph's Health Care London, Canada)

Client-centred care is frequently identified as an important component of the quality of clinical interventions. We sought to enhance client-centred care in geriatric rehabilitation, and to evaluate the effectiveness of these strategies using a client satisfaction measure. Admission, discharge and follow-up data were collected on patients admitted to a geriatric rehabilitation program consisting of 10 beds for short-term musculoskeletal rehabilitation and 26 beds for interdisciplinary assessment and rehabilitation of clients with complex physical and psychosocial problems [N=168, mean (SD) age: 79.7 (7.1) years, 124 females, mean (SD) days stay 37.6 (18.3)]. Strategies to enhance client-centred care included increased client/family involvement, individualized goal-setting and enhanced clinical coordination. The client satisfaction questionnaire developed for the study included three global questions [two 10-point scales and a 100 mm visual analogue scale (VAS)] and specific questions intended to measure important aspects of client-centred care (such as involvement in care planning). Mean overall satisfaction was high (>8.5/10, >80/100 on the VAS) throughout the study but not affected by introduction of client-centred strategies, nor by reductions in mean length of stay. Client satisfaction did not correlate with improvements in functioning and quality of life assessed using instruments such as the Functional Independence Measure (r<.05). Similar ratings were obtained at discharge and at the 6 week follow-up. Although the global measures produced similar overall results, their inter-correlations were only moderate (r~.50). The use of client satisfaction information to improve and evaluate the quality of care in geriatric rehabilitation may require more in-depth exploration of variations in responses.

[55] Maintenance of Functional and Quality of Life Outcomes in Geriatric Rehabilitation

P. Stolee, M.J. Borrie, J. Esbaugh, J. Wagg (Southwestern Ontario Regional Geriatric Program, London, Canada), M.G. Woodbury, R.J. Petrella (St. Joseph's Health Care London, Canada), I.A. Connidis (University of Western Ontario)

We aimed to determine if functional and quality of life gains achieved during inpatient geriatric rehabilitation were maintained after discharge. Admission, discharge and post-discharge follow-up data were collected on 78 frail older patients [mean (SD) age: 80.6 (6.7) years, 74.4% female, mean (SD) days stay: 37.4 (15.9)] admitted to a geriatric rehabilitation program consisting of 10 beds for short-term musculoskeletal rehabilitation and 26 beds for interdisciplinary assessment and rehabilitation of patients with complex physical and psychosocial problems. Outcome measures included self-rated health and quality of life (5-point scales), the Functional Independence Measure (FIM), the Spitzer Quality of Life Index (QLI), and Goal Attainment Scaling (GAS, an individualized measure). Follow-up data collection included telephone follow-up at 6 weeks and 3 months post-discharge, and home visits at 3 months for a random sample (n=35). The majority (84.9%) of patients were discharged to the community; 75.7% received formal community services. At three months, a total of 10 patients had died; another 10 could not be located or refused follow-up assessment. For those patients with whom follow-up was possible (N=58), we found that significant gains (p<.001) were achieved during inpatient stay [Mean (SD) improvement: self-rated health: 0.7 (1.2); self-rated quality of life: 1.0 (1.1); FIM: 14.5 (17.7); QLI: 1.5 (1.9); GAS: 17.0 (11.1)], and that these gains were maintained at three months. Follow-up GAS scores indicated that further improvement on individual goals occurred after discharge. Inpatient geriatric rehabilitation can achieve durable improvements in function and quality of life for frail older patients.

SESSION 255

International Perspectives on Knowledge Transfer: Working Together to Enhance Evidence-based Policy and Services for Seniors.

Carol McWilliam (University of Western Ontario, London, Canada) Canada's National Consensus Process to Create Evidence-based Redress of Seniors' Issues. Andrew Dillon (National Institute for Clinical Excellence, London, England) National Institute for Clinical Excellence. Penelope Hawe (University of Calgary, Calgary, Canada) Working Invisibly: A Model for Knowledge and Skill Transfer in Health Promotion Practice in Australia. Johnathan Lomas (Executive Director, Canadian Health Services Research Institute, Ottawa, Canada) The Challenges and Opportunities for Progress in Knowledge Transfer.

ISSUE: Despite advancements in information technology and high emphasis on research dissemination, knowledge transfer from research to the policy, programming and practice arenas continues to present a tremendous challenge. Limited success has left researchers, policy makers, and service providers frustrated, consumers disillusioned, and seniors all over the world underserved by evidence-based policy and service evolution. Given our aging populations, it is both time and timely to critically examine the strategies currently being put to the test by international leaders in knowledge transfer, with a view to extrapolating from pooled international expertise ideas for refining future efforts. This symposium will explore three models of knowledge transfer: Canada's National Consensus Process for Creating Evidence-based Consensus on Issues of Seniors' Independence; Great Britain's National Health Service permanent infrastructure for professional knowledge transfer, the National Institute for Clinical Excellence; and Australia's capacity development approach to knowledge transfer at the grassroots level of service delivery. Dr. Jonathan Lomas, internationally renowned expert in knowledge transfer, will fulfill the role of discussant, comparing and contrasting the utility, the strengths and the limitations of each model. Symposium participants will have an opportunity to ask questions, to raise issues and concerns, and to contribute their creative ideas as they and the panel of experts work with Dr. Lomas to refine knowledge transfer in a changing world, for the benefit of our aging global population. STRUCTURE: The Canadian, British, and Australian models of knowledge transfer, together with an evaluation of their effectiveness, will be presented by their respective spokespersons in sequential, 15-minute overviews. Dr. Jonathan Lomas will then discuss the key elements contributing to the strengths and limitations of each model. The symposium convenor will then facilitate discussion by the audience. In a 15-minute closure, Dr. Lomas will summarize recommendations for trans-jurisdictional international refinement of knowledge transfer, with due consideration of its applicability to facilitating policy, program and service evolution for an aging population. CONTENT: Dr. C. McWilliam will present a brief overview of the structure and process of Canada's National Consensus Process, together with evaluative data on the nature, scope and extent of knowledge transfer that resulted. Dr. A. Dillon's presentation will include an overview of the organization and operating methodologies of the National Institute for Clinical Excellence, and results of formal research on the implementation and impact of this knowledge transfer endeavor. Dr. P. Hawe will present an Australian approach to knowledge transfer at the grassroots level in a national health promotion endeavor, including the strategy for planning and evaluating this capacity-building approach to knowledge transfer. Dr. J. Lomas will elaborate the strengths and limitations of each model and, following consultation with the audience, will present new ideas for knowledge transfer arising from this international exchange of experience. CONCLUSIONS: This symposium will create an international understanding of the state of the art of knowledge transfer, capitalize on the synergy of sharing international expertise to develop refined strategies for future endeavors, and stimulate international collaboration to enhance knowledge transfer on behalf of an aging global population.

Canada's National Consensus Process to Create Evidence-based Redress of Seniors' Issues.

C. McWilliam (University of Western Ontario, London, Canada), G. Gutman (Simon Fraser University, Vancouver, Canada), M. Penning (University of Victoria, Victoria, Canada), M. Stewart (University of Alberta, Edmonton, Canada), and R. Tamblyn (McGill University, Montreal, Canada).

Abstract PURPOSE: The purpose of this three-year National Consensus Process was to promote knowledge transfer from research on seniors' issues to policy, programming and practice arenas. METHOD: The National Consensus Process was designed to combine the strengths identified in many previously tried dissemination strategies with policy issue filtration and consensus-building strategies. Research evidence from a $7.5 million investment by the Federal Government in research on seniors' issues, combined with data from related international research from a total of 783 studies selected for their scientific rigor was condensed through systematic literature review and syntheses, and disseminated in policy fact sheets, other print materials, an interactive website, and both formal and informal discussion groups. Facilitated by a National Consensus Committee that developed unique opinion leader strategies and consensus building activities, participants representing over 500,000 Canadians, including academics, policy makers, program planning personnel, service providers and individual citizens (25% of them seniors themselves) identified key messages from the research, prioritized the issues, discussed and prioritized potential action strategies, and implemented follow-up actions. RESULTS: Sixteen municipal, provincial, and federal policy branches, 67 health planning authorities, 56 educational institutions, 7 professional associations, 12 seniors' advocacy groups and other community organizations with a vested interest in seniors' issues, participated. The scope and depth of this project presented many challenges and opportunities. Evaluative results suggest limited knowledge transfer. CONCLUSION: Knowledge transfer is an ongoing, long-term endeavor, and both the strategies and their evaluation need to be evolved with this in mind.

National Institute for Clinical Excellence

A. Dillon (National Institute for Clinical Excellence, London, England)

Abstract: PURPOSE: The purpose of the National Institute for Clinical Excellence, established in April 1999, is to provide guidance to health professionals in the National Health Service (NHS) in England and Wales on the management of disease and conditions, on the organization of care and on the use of specific new and existing health technologies. METHOD: The Institute provides guidance appropriate for both patients and carers. The organisation and operating methodologies are designed to achieve this aim with the range of guidance being produced. The 'virtual' nature of the Institute is an important aspect of the knowledge transfer strategy. RESULTS: There are many advantages of an inclusive approach and involving partnerships with public and private sector organisations. Several challenges and advantages are associated with considerable operating transparency. The significance of involving stakeholders in topic selection and in the formulation and interpretation of evidence is especially noteworthy. CONCLUSION: The Institute's approach to dissemination, including its relationship with the media, its alliances with conventional and web-based medical publishers and the use of its own web site contain several valuable lessons. The Institute's involvement in the implementation is important, particularly with reference to the role of other national agencies. The style of presentation of guidance is in keeping with the Institute's ambition to ensure that its work is accessible to all health professionals. The formal research, commissioned by the Institute, to examine the implementation and impact of its guidance affords insights for future knowledge transfer endeavors.

Working Invisibly: A Model for Knowledge and Skill Transfer in Health Promotion Practice in Australia.

P. Hawe (University of Calgary, Calgary, Canada), L. King (New South Wales Cancer Council, Australia), M. Noort (Nepean Health Services, Australia), B. Lloyd (University of Sydney, Australia).

Abstract: PURPOSE: The purpose of this four-year Australian knowledge and skill transfer project was to build capacity in health promotion practice through application of unique capacity-building strategies. METHOD: Informal learning theory suggests that the one of the most powerful opportunities for cultural change, values reorientation and system change comes from workplace situations which are not always fully exploited for their learning potential. Using these insights, change agents in the health promotion workplace crafted occasions for "accidental learning" among colleagues by creating more "accidents" demanding specific skills and insights. Change agents also encouraged colleagues to become more engaged in workplace learning by encouraging proactivity, creativity and reflectivity. A series of checklists were developed to plan and evaluate capacity-building endeavours by health promotion workers. Funding was subsequently made available for a round of research-to-practice grants, encouraging health promotion workers to use the checklists and report on their usefulness in capacity-building in hospitals and community health services. RESULTS: The strength of this model is that learning happens without it being labeled as such. This suits health care settings, where many professionals might feel that they have nothing to learn, or no time to learn. CONCLUSIONS: Sometimes the best route to organisational change is the slow one. While the focus of our work has been in health promotion, the model has applicability to those attempting to foster evidence-based practice in other fields, including gerontology.

SESSION 257

Systems of Coordination and Integration of Care of the Frail Elderly

Howard Bergman (Division of Geriatric Medicine, McGill University, Montreal, Canada) Dennis Kodner (Metropolitan Jewish Health Systems, New York, USA) Roberto Bernabei (Università Cattolica Sacro Cuore, Istituto di Clinica Medica, Rome, Italy) Darryl Wieland (Division of Geriatrics, University of South Carolina, Columbia, USA)

Proposals for Integrated Health and Social Care Systems (IHSCS) for frail elderly have been developed in Canada, the European Union, United States, and in other countries around the world. The goals of these systems are to meet, comprehensively, appropriately and with effectiveness, the complex social and health care needs of frail elderly persons. They are defined along five dimensions: 1) extent of health and social care offered; 2) responsibility for enrolled persons or for catchments' area population; 3) case management; 4) some form of financial responsibility; 5) public/private funding and/or ownership. Demonstration and established programs combined these dimensions in a variety of ways, adapting features of IHSCS to local, regional, and national characteristics of their respective health and social care systems. This diversity suggests that there are more than one ways to reach the goals of integration. Also, within countries, IHSCS have been and still are implemented on a trial basis, though some of them have been implemented in more extensively and in a variety of settings, while some are now, after evaluation, permanent providers of care in their respective regions or countries. The objective of this invited symposium is to discuss the programs, the evaluation designs used in these trials, the results obtained, and implementation issues. Experiments and programs from Italy (Rovereto's program, and implementation of an integrated program in 25 Health Agencies), Canada (the SIPA project) and the United States (PACE, S/HMO, HomeFirst programs) are presented. They will be discussed in terms of: 1) Program description: clinical, financing, organizational models, and the target population; 2) Evaluation design: location characteristics, number of sites, sample size, sample design (experimental, quasi-experimental, etc.), statistical procedure, data collection and sources; 3) Results: structural features of the program, process of care, health services uses and costs, quality of care, and health outcome; 4) Discussion of the results: internal validity, difference between expected results and observed results; 5) Generalisability issues: external validity of the study, extension of the program to milieus others than the experimental sites.

Fully Integrated Care Systems for the Frail Elderly: Two American Models

Dennis L. Kodner, Corinne Kay Kyriacou, (Metropolitan Jewish Health System and Institute for Applied Gerontology, Brooklyn, USA)

The frail elderly have complex medical problems and physical disabilities. Yet, the delivery of health and social services are often fragmented and uncoordinated, and no single organization or system exists level at the community level with clinical and financial accountability for the care of these at-risk individuals. This situation usually results in unmet needs, and also contributes to inappropriate hospitalization and institutionalization, as well as poorly controlled costs. Despite global differences in the funding and organization of elder care, countries nonetheless share a common interest in better models of coordinating and integrating care. The United States, despite its lack of a universal health care system, has led in experimentation with so-called fully integrated (or managed care) models for the frail elderly for over 15 years. This paper will examine two such American models: the Social Health Maintenance Organization (Social HMO), which has been in operation since 1985; and, HomeFirst, a new home-based managed long term care program that was launched in July 2000. The discussion will focus on key program characteristics; evaluation design; evaluation results; and, generalizability issues.

How did I implement an integrated home care coordinated by case-management in Italy

Roberto Bernabei, MD

Home care was poorly developed in Italy up to the late nineties and is now rapidly increasing in terms of agencies and patients. The Italian Research Council (CNR) promoted research to find the best home care model to be implemented in the country in the early nineties and our group was in charge of that grant. We tested with a randomised clinical trial a new model of home care based on case-management and services integration versus a traditional not integrated model . The results showed a better function and a lower institutionalisation in the treated group after one year. This new model of care was provided of a new assessment system, the MDS-HC, and, by means of a CNR-Pfizer grant, was made available to the interested Health Care Agencies of the National Health Service. 25 of the 250 Health Agencies in which the country is divided adopted the same care model case-management based and the same assessment instrument. A database was created and patients characteristics and quality of care comparisons between the participating home care agencies are presented.

The Program of All-Inclusive Care for the Elderly (PACE) in the United States

D. Wieland (Palmetto Richland Memorial Hospital, Columbia, South Carolina, USA), G.P. Eleazer (Division of Geriatrics, University of South Carolina School of Medicine, Columbia)

PACE is a prepaid, capitated program of comprehensive primary, long-term, and acute care delivered by non-profit or public providers. PACE is intended for frail, disabled elderly persons certified by the states as eligible for nursing-home care. Acting as insurer, each PACE site pools payments from Medicare (the universal federal health insurance program for seniors) and Medicaid (the means-tested state program) or alternative payers. Assuming full financial risk, PACE provides a comprehensive array of services determined as necessary and appropriate by an interdisciplinary evaluation and management team. Since its beginnings as a national demonstration program based on the On Lok program in San Francisco, 25 PACE sites have been established in 13 states, with additional sites in development, serving nearly 7,000 participants. We provide an overview of evaluative and comparative research concerning the PACE model, its outcomes and costs, identifying remaining and emergent research and policy issues. The review includes studies contracted by the U.S. Health Care Financing Administration [HCFA], and the National PACE Association, as well as independent research. Using a quasi-experimental design, the HCFA evaluation found numerous differences in the pattern of service delivery, most notably, significant reductions in Hospitalizations and nursing-home use among PACE participants. These changes were accompanied by improved survival, health-related quality of life, functional status, and participant satisfaction. Evaluation of first-year costs suggests that combined Medicare-Medicaid expenses would have been 4-6 0gher than the total PACE capitation. While the evidence suggests PACE is cost-effective, challenges to its expansion are addressed in new research.

The SIPA project in Montreal, Quebec, Canada

Howard Bergman, François Béland, Paule Lebel, MD (McGill/ Université de Montréal Research Group on Integrated Services for the Elderly, Montreal, Canada)

The SIPA (Système de soins intégrés pour personnes âgées) project is a community based demonstration project which simulates capitation and is clinically and financially responsible for providing through consolidated case management the full range of complex health and social care (HSC) to frail elderly persons living in two neighbourhoods in Montréal, Canada. Reductions in in-patient care, emergency rooms use, and institutionalisation were expected. 1254 elderly persons agreed to participate and were randomly allocated to the SIPA or control group. The control group received usual health and social care available to frail elderly in Montréal. Utilisation of HSC was assessed with data from administrative files, from hospitals, nursing homes, SIPA and other agencies records. Elderly persons in both groups have a high number of medical problems and a high level of disability. They are high users of medical, emergency room, acute hospital and nursing home services. No differences were found between experimental and control groups in emergency room use but there was a 20% reduction in the length of stay (LOS) in the SIPA group. There was no difference in hospitalisation rates and LOS. Use of physician services and of prescribed drugs was comparable. However, in the SIPA group, there was a three-fold reduction in acute care hospital patients who became bed blockers and a two-fold reduction in institutionalisation rates.

SESSION 258

Cross-National Comparison of Social Isolation and Loneliness

J. de Jong Gierveld (NIAS, Wassenaar, The Netherlands), Conceptual Development, Definitions and Measurement of Loneliness; V. Burholt (University of Wales, Bangor, Wales), Changes in Levels of Loneliness and Social Isolation among Older People in Rural Wales; B. Havens (University of Manitoba, Winnipeg, Canada), Social Isolation, Geographic Isolation, Ethnocultural Background and Social Loneliness among Aging in Manitoba Respondents; P. Dykstra, (NIDI, Den Haag, The Netherlands), Gender Differences in Dutch Older Adult Loneliness; M. Jylha (University of Tampere, Finland), Loneliness in Old Age: Cross-national and Longitudinal Analyses; T. van Tilburg (Vrije Universiteit, Amsterdam, The Netherlands), Loneliness among older adults in Canada, Italy and the Netherlands: A multi-facet comparison; Proposed Discussant: D. Perlman (University of British Columbia, Vancouver, Canada)

ISSUE: Loneliness is frequently posited as a universal experience among older persons, especially among the very old and oldest-old. Loneliness has two diverse conceptual roots, one in psychology where it is related to depression and the other in social science where it is related to the subjective experience of isolation. If loneliness is truly a universal experience, the results of research into these phenomena should be, similar if not, the same among diverse cultures and societies. In addition, the impact of geographic isolation should also be minimal. Should the research not confirm universality, the effects attributed to loneliness may derive from other factors or may be mutable. STRUCTURE: The symposium will begin with an introductory presentation that sets out parameters of social loneliness among older persons. Three additional presentations identify aspects of loneliness in three diverse settings. Two presentations compare social loneliness measured cross-nationally with the same instruments. The discussant will address the issues as a social psychologist. CONTENT: Careful conceptualization and operationalization of loneliness is an important sine qua non for empirical research. The interrelationship of loneliness with characteristics of the life course of older persons are affected by the measuring instruments of loneliness that are used. In rural Wales, some longitudinal study respondents maintained consistently low levels of loneliness and social isolation throughout the study, while others showed changes in levels. Both quantitative and qualitative data from the study identify factors associated with increases and decreases in loneliness and social isolation. Descriptive and predictive analyses of determinants of geographic location, gender, ethnocultural background, previous health status and the consequences of use of health services and death as related to social isolation and loneliness are reported from the 1996 Aging in Manitoba (AIM) study. Based on data from two Dutch studies little gender difference was found in loneliness among those in first marriages, however, gender differences emerge among those in second and third partnerships. Gender differences are also observed among the non-married. Using the ELSA data for cross-national comparisons, a gradient of higher percentages of loneliness was found from northern European cites to rural southern Europe and loneliness was more frequent in the oldest age groups. However, longitudinal analyses in the TamELSA sample showed both increasing and decreasing loneliness with age, where loneliness was related to poor health and closeness to death rather than to age per se. Another cross-national study using an eleven-item scale, developed in the Netherlands examines differences in loneliness among older adults living independently in Canada, Italy and the Netherlands according to the level of loneliness, its determinants and its measurement. CONCLUSION/ANTICIPATED OUTCOMES: The opportunity to discuss the determinants and consequences of social loneliness in diverse settings and cultures from a cross-national perspective is expected to further our understanding about the degree to which loneliness is a universal experience of older persons. The policy and program implications of demonstrating that loneliness is not universal may lead to developing policies and programs that can be expected to redress social loneliness among older persons.

Changes in Levels of Loneliness and Social Isolation among Older People in Rural Wales

G. Clare Wenger and Vanessa Burholt (University of Wales Bangor, Bangor, Wales)

PURPOSE: The Bangor Longitudinal Study of Ageing, which was conducted in rural Wales from 1979 to 1999 followed a cohort of survivors from more than 500 people over 20 years. Using both quantitative and qualitative data from the study, the factors associated with increases and decreases in loneliness and social isolation are identified. METHOD: The study was based on a population sample and survivors were followed up every four years. From 1983 to 1987 an intensive study of 30 people aged 75+ in 1979 were studied intensively. Customary measures of loneliness were used, as well as an aggregate measure devised by the research team. Social isolation was similarly measured using an aggregate measure. Respondents were classed as demonstrating low, moderate or high loneliness or isolation. Subsequently, models of loneliness, social and isolaltion and morale were refined using statistical modelling. RESULTS: Some respondents maintained consistently low levels of loneliness and social isolation as long as they remained in the study. Others showed changes in levels. In this paper, both quantitative and qualitative data from the study are explored seeking factors associated with increases and decreases in loneliness and social isolation. CONCLUSION: Outcome measures of these two variables of interest are compared with items from the aggregate measures and other identifiable intervening variables. The paper discusses which change variables contribute most to levels of loneliness and isolation and which of these produce long-term as opposed to short-term effects.

Conceptual development, definitions and measurement of loneliness

J. Gierveld (Netherlands Institute for Advanced Study in the Humanities and Social Sciences, NIAS, Wassenaar, the Netherlands & Vrije Universiteit, Amsterdam, the Netherlands).

PURPOSE: to provide an overview of the conceptualization, definitions and most important measuring instruments of loneliness as used to empirically investigate different subtypes of loneliness via survey research. METHOD: the literature about the concept of loneliness, especially about loneliness among older persons, will be dealt with as well as the results of empirical research investigating the determinants and consequences of loneliness.RESULTS: Most scholars agree about the central facets of the concept of loneliness. However, some researchers opt for a unidimensional operationalization of the concept, others make a plea for a multidimensional perspective. Some researchers opt for measuring instruments including the word loneliness, others refrain from using the word loneliness. Some developed their measuring instruments in laboratory situations, others in student populations and still others with a broad in vivo set of respondents. These decisions have direct consequences for the outcomes of the research. CONCLUSION: A careful conceptualization and operationalization of loneliness is an important sine qua non for empirical research in the social field. The interrelationship of loneliness with characteristics of the life course of older persons, such as marital and partner history, with current household composition, with indicators of the size and composition of the social network, and with gender, and health status are - to a certain extent - affected by the measuring instruments of loneliness that are used. Research clearly points out that some measuring instruments are more useful for research among young adults and other instruments are reliable and valid for use in a broader set of age categories

Gender differences in Dutch older adult loneliness

P.A. Dykstra (NIDI, The Hague, The Netherlands).J. de Jong Gierveld (NIAS, Wassenaar, The Netherlands),

PURPOSE: To identify gender differences in loneliness by looking at social skills, relationship expectations, and sources of support outside the partner.METHOD: The analyses are based on the Dutch Living arrangements and Social Networks of older adults survey (NESTOR-LSN), and the Longitudinal Aging Study of Amsterdam (LASA) data sets, which are supplemented with data from in-depth interviews with selected respondents. RESULTS: Previous research has indicated that gender differences in loneliness vary by marital history. There generally is little difference in loneliness among men and women in first marriages. However, gender differences emerge among those in second and third partnerships, where women tend to be more lonely than men. Gender differences are also observed among the non-married: single men tend to be more lonely than their female counterparts. Conclusions: We explore and report on a set of hypotheses aimed at uncovering gender differences in loneliness, looking at (a) social skills, (b) relationship expectations, and (c) sources of support outside the partner.

Loneliness among older adults in Canada, Italy and the Netherlands: A multi-facet comparison

T. van Tilburg (Dept. of Sociology and Social Gerontology, Vrije Universiteit, Amsterdam, The Netherlands), B. Havens (University of Manitoba, Canada), J. de Jong Gierveld (NIAS, Wassenaar, The Netherlands), P.A. Dykstra (NIDI, The Hague, The Netherlands)

PURPOSE: To examine differences in loneliness among older adults living independently in Canada, Italy and the Netherlands according to the level of loneliness, its determinants and its measurement. METHOD: Loneliness has been measured with an 11-item scale, developed in the Netherlands and used in Canada and Italy as well as in the Netherlands. Analyses were performed to assess cross-cultural differences. Attention was paid to three aspects: (1) the intensity of feelings of loneliness, (2) determinants of loneliness such as differences in household composition, health and (support exchanged within) personal relationships, and consequences of loneliness such as mortality. Special attention was paid to (3) the measurement of loneliness; in particular whether insufficient scale homogeneity and differential item functioning suggest cross-national differences in the meaning of loneliness. RESULTS: Previous research has revealed that loneliness is a pervasive social problem and is experienced in many cultures. To date, cross- cultural studies have rarely taken into account more than one of these aspects. Furthermore, cross-Atlantic differences in loneliness among older adults have rarely been studied. CONCLUSION: The present study describes differences in loneliness among older adults Canada, Italy and the Netherlands based on the level of loneliness, its determinants and its measurement. That the experience of loneliness is universal can be concluded only if the examination of all three aspects results in absence of cross-cultural differences.

Loneliness in Old Age: Cross-national and Longitudinal Analyses

M. Jylhä (School of Public Health, University of Tampere, Tampere, Finland)

PURPOSE: We used data from six areas in the European Longitudinal Study on Ageing (ELSA) and the three waves from the Finnish ELSA study sample (TamELSA) to examine the cross- national and longitudinal patterns of loneliness in old age. METHOD: At the baseline of the ELSA project, representative population samples aged 60 to 89 stratified by gender and 5-year age group were interviewed in Tampere (Finland), Berlin (Germany), Florence (Italy), Belgrade (Yugoslavia), Amiata (Italy), and rural regions of Greece, using a standardized structured questionnaire. In Tampere, a ten-year follow-up was conducted in 1989: 84% of the survivors (435 persons) and 395 persons from new cohorts aged 60-69 years were interviewed. In a 20-year follow-up 398 person (93% of the survivors, followed in the National Population Registry) were interviewed. The respondents were asked, "Do you feel lonely?" The preset alternatives were 'often', 'sometimes', 'never', and 'cannot say'. RESULTS: In cross-national comparisons, we found a gradient of higher per cent of loneliness from cities in northern Europe to the rural areas in southern Europe. Feelings of loneliness were more frequent in the oldest than in the youngest age groups. However, longitudinal analyses in the TamELSA sample showed both increasing and decreasing feelings of loneliness with age on an individual level. Loneliness was related to poor health and closeness of death rather than to increasing age, per se. CONCLUSION: To better understand the association between aging and loneliness, we need approaches that are sensitive to cultural contexts and individual meanings attached to social interaction.

Social Isolation, Geographic Isolation, Ethnocultural Background and Social Loneliness among Aging in Manitoba Respondents

Betty Havens and Madelyn Hall (University of Manitoba, Winnipeg, Canada)

PURPOSE: To identify the relationships among social and geographic isolation, ethnocultural background, gender and health status and the expression of social loneliness within a longitudinal panel of very old adults. METHOD: Descriptive followed by predictive analyses of the determinants and consequences of social isolation and social loneliness from the 1996 Aging in Manitoba (AIM) respondents (N=1868). Among the determinants are geographic location (urban to remote), gender, ethnocultural background (ethnic descent, language spoken, immigration) and previous health status. Among the consequences are use of health services (physician visits, hospitalization, pharmacare, home care, nursing home) and death. RESULTS: In previous AIM research, we found a modest similarity among determinants and consequences between gender and social isolation, but not social loneliness. This research carries these analyses further. CONCLUSION: If social loneliness is the subjective expression of isolation, then the determinants of both measures will be the same, as will the consequences, whether considering gender, ethnocultural background or previous health status. Social loneliness is usually considered to be a universal experience among older people. If social loneliness is a universal phenomenon, then older people with similar health and social cultural characteristics, especially those living in the same location, should experience the same intensities of social isolation and social loneliness and the latter two attributes should have the same impact on typical consequences. Further understanding of these relationships not only increases our understanding of very old people, but also contributes to our understanding of social loneliness as potentially less universal than previously believed.

SESSION 259

Ethnicity and End-of-life Decisions in Multicultural Populations - An Overview

Reva N. Adler (University of British Columbia, Vancouver, BC, CANADA. OLDER ADULTS, ETHNICITY AND HEALTH DECISIONS: AN OVERVIEW OF THE LITERATURE) Sharon Brangman, (Associateand Head,Division of Geriatrics, Upstate Medical University, Syracuse, NY, USA - END-OF-LIFE DECISIONS AND OLDER AFRICAN AMERICANS: APPROACHES TO MULTI-CULTURAL CARE) Susan Feldman, (Director, Alma Unit for Research on Ageing, Victoria University, Melbourne, Victoria, Australia - Ethnicity and End-of Life-Decisions in Multicultural Populations: Vietnamese Women Show Us How it is)

Issues: By the end of the year 2000, 20% of the U.S. population will be comprised of individuals of African, Hispanic, Native American or Asian-Pacific descent. As industrialised societies become more culturally diverse, health care professionals face the growing challenge of meeting the needs of older adults from numerous ethnic backgrounds. In this setting, an understanding of the influence of ethnicity on health decisions and the decision-making process is critical to the preservation of clinical efficacy and patient dignity. Investigators have identified significant differences in attitudes toward truth telling, perceptions of debilitated health states, treatment limitation, personal autonomy, and completion of advance directives between cultural groups. This symposium will address the current state of scholarship in these areas, focusing on practical considerations in clinical settings. Structure: This symposium will be comprised of three presentations, each addressing a specific aspect of the interface between ethnicity, ageing and health behaviour. A discussion period, inviting audience participation, will follow the presentations. Content: Dr. Adler will provide an overview of the recent health services literature addressing ethnicity, ageing and health decision-making. In particular, she will focus on data addressing the impact of culture on attitudes toward clinical disclosure, decision making structures and perception of illness, suffering and quality of life. Dr. Brangman will discuss an approach to working with older African Americans around their end-of-life decisions, based on the current state of scholarship in the field. She will concentrate on the process utilised in developing this approach, and will provide suggestions for use of these methods in working with other cultural groups. Dr. Feldman will discuss the findings from a longitudinal study of Older Australian Vietnamese women, making particular reference to the everyday decisions that have direct impact on their quality of life. She will discuss how these older women chose to represent themselves in research about their lives, the issues that they selected when talking about the final stage of life and specifically, the relationship of spirituality, community and family to their health and well-being. Anticipated Outcomes: At the conclusion of this symposium, the participants will be familiar with the current state of scholarship regarding the interface between ethnicity, ageing and health decisions in three industrial, multicultural societies. The symposium will provide data relating to decision-making in two distinct ethnic groups. Approaches to working with other cultural groups around end-of-life decisions will be discussed.

Ethnicity and End-of Life-Decisions in Multicultural Populations: Vietnamese Women Show Us How it is

Feldman, S, (Victoria University, Melbourne, Australia) Kamler, B (Deakin University, Melbourne Australia) Threadgold, T (Cardiff University, Cardiff, Wales)

A large Australian research grant project entitled 'Stories of Ageing: A Longitudinal Study of Older Women's Self-Representation' provided an opportunity to explore and gain a broader understanding of the health and end-of-life decision making of women as they age. This large study also aimed to challenge stereotypes about ageing and included approximately 40 women living in their own communities, outside of institutional care. The women worked in small groups to write and film stories of their lives. This study included a sample of women from Vietnamese backgrounds. Eleven Australian/Vietnamese women aged between 55-74 met regularly over a period of two years in two-three hour workshop settings to record video diaries. These workshops were conducted with the assistance of an interpreter. In this setting the women were taught video techniques and to think of the video camera as a visual aid for the telling of their stories and the representation of the elements that they considered overall as important in their lives. Analysis of the video footage produced by these women also assisted the researchers to gain a more comprehensive understanding about the everyday decisions that have direct impact on the quality of life for older Australian/ Vietnamese women. Each woman produced a video that provided the researchers with visual access to their lives, revealing just how these older Australian/Vietnamese women chose to represent themselves. Analysis of the videos and the translated talk of the women from the face-to-face workshops, provided the researchers with insights into the complexity of the issues that these women selected as impacting on the final stage of their life. The video representation of the final stage of life revealed the centrality of spirituality, community and family in relation to the maintenance of their ongoing health and well-being. This study confirmed that end-of life decision making for older Australia/ Vietnamese women stretches beyond a narrow definition, and their key concerns commonly extended into more practical and social arenas. The findings of this longitudinal study have broad implications for Older Australian/Vietnamese women in both the public and private domains of their lives. It also has implications for researchers who undertake projects in collaboration with older women from multicultural backgrounds and for the development of the health services and supports that ethnic women rely upon as they grow older.

Ethnicity and End-of-Life Decisions in Multi-cultural Populations

Reva N. Adler (Division of Geriatric Medicine, University of British Columbia)

Developing a conversant understanding the influence of ethnicity on health decisions and the decision-making process is critical to the preservation of clinical efficacy and patient dignity in multicultural societies. This presentation will examine the North American data comparing health behaviour and attitudes across a range of cultural groups. Specifically, significant differences in attitudes toward truth telling, perceptions of debilitated health states, treatment limitation, personal autonomy, and completion of advance directives will be examined. Areas of concentration will include scholarship addressing health behaviour and beliefs within communities of African, Latino, Asian and European descent. Focus will be placed on enhancing cultural sensitivity while at the same time avoiding the use damaging stereotypes in clinical practice with individual patients.

SESSION 260.

Physical Activity and Aging: International Initiatives

Donald H. Paterson (Canadian Centre for Activity and Aging (CCAA), The University of Western Ontario, London, Canada) (The Importance of Cardiorespiratory and Muscle Fitness in Older Adult Programs) Nancy A. Ecclestone (Canadian Centre for Activity and Aging (CCAA), London, Canada) (Canadian Initiatives Promoting Healthy Active Aging for Older Adults) Federico F. Schena (Center for Research and Bioengineering and Motor Science, Rovereto, Italy) ("The Health in the Movement": A Project for Health Promotion through Physical Activity in Elderly) Wojtek J. Chodzko-Zajko (University of Illinois at Urbana-Champaign, Urbana IL, USA) (The ACSM Active Aging Partnership: A National Initiative for the Promotion of Healthy Aging in the United States of America)

This symposium describes the development of program strategies in Canada, Italy and the United States of America with the goal of improving fitness and function of older adults. The research basis of the benefits of physical activity in the elderly and the development of program activities in each of three countries will be addressed. Canadian initiatives include national physical activity promotion (Canada's Physical Activity Guide to Healthy Active Living for Older Adults and A Blueprint for Action for Active Living and Older Adults). As well, progress with programs of the Canadian Centre for Activity and Aging (CCAA) will be outlined. The latter have been developed and tested and are applicable for national distribution. From Italy, results of the impact of a regional project on changes in lifestyle in the elderly population will be presented. The United States of America initiative, Active Aging Partnership (AAP), a national initiative of the American College of Sports Medicine, will address projects in the areas of education, research and practice. This session will inform and generate ideas regarding different methods of addressing the physical activity needs of the aging population in three countries.

Canadian Initiatives Promoting Healthy Active Aging for Older Adults

Nancy A. Ecclestone (Canadian Centre for Activity and Aging (CCAA), London, ON, Canada)

Strategies have been initiated to promote physical activity for older adults in Canada. Round Table of Leaders in Physical Activity and Aging, hosted by Canadian Centre for Activity and Aging (CCAA). Canada's Physical Activity Guide to Healthy Active Living for Older Adults (1999). A Blueprint for Action for Active Living and Older Adults: Moving Through the Years -a national framework of action. ALCOA National Forum on Older Adults and Active Living, hosted by CCAA. CCAA National Leadership Training Initiatives Project, supported by Health Canada (1999-2002). Researchers, program deliverers, organizations and individuals have participated in consultations and forums on active living and older adults - facilitated by Health Canada, CCAA, ALCOA, La Fondation en adaptation motrice (FAM) and Canadian Society for Exercise Physiology (CSEP). Priority goals and recommendations regarding the active living needs of older Canadians were outlined in: Proceedings of the Round Table of Leaders in Physical Activity and Aging (1998), A Blueprint for Action for Active Living and Older Adults (1999), Proceedings of the ALCOA National Forum on Older Adults and Active Living (1999). A comprehensive plan, involving specific actions and programs, is being developed to address these goals and recommendations. The CCAA is playing a role, particularly in the areas of research and leadership training. The leadership training programs of the CCAA available for national distribution include: Community (Seniors' Fitness Instructors Course), Home Care (Home Support Exercise Program),Long-term Care (nursing homes), Residential and Day Care (Restorative Care and Functional Fitness in Long-Term Care), Active Living Community Development Program.

The ACSM Active Aging Partnership: A National Initiative for the Promotion of Healthy Aging in the United States of America

Wojtek J. Chodzko-Zajko, (University of Illinois at Urbana-Champaign, Urbana IL, USA)

The ACSM Active Aging Partnership: A National Initiative for the Promotion of Healthy Aging in the United States of America In the fall of 2000 the American College of Sports Medicine (ACSM) launched a major new programming initiative - The Active Aging Partnership (AAP). This initiative is designed to spearhead US national initiatives for the dissemination of information about research, clinical practice, and educational opportunities in the area of active aging. In this presentation, the Chair of the AAP will summarize the scope and content of this new program. The AAP is designed to be a coalition of national organizations who come together to share resources and ideas in the area of aging and physical activity. In addition to ACSM, partners include the National Institute on Aging, the American Geriatrics Society, the American Association of Retired Persons, the Centers for Disease Control and Prevention, and several other organizations. The partnership is developing joint initiatives in the following areas; Education: 1. Public/ consumer education initiatives 2. Professional/Continuing education projects: Research: 1. Funding investigators to evaluate successful physical activity programs 2. Identifying research gaps through joint roundtable conferences Practice: i. Identifying model programs ii. Develop referral network/national clearing house The partnership will sponsor symposia and colloquia at national meetings, it will ally with industry and foundation partners, and will reach out to similar organizations in other countries with the goal of increasing the effectiveness of communication in this area. Chodzko-Zajko will summarize the status of current projects and discuss future developments. Particular attention will be placed on the need to interface with similar groups from other countries in order to move toward an integrated global strategy for active and successful aging.

"The Health in the Movement": A project for health promotion through physical activity in elderly.

F. Schena (Center for Research on Bioengineering and Motor Science, Rovereto, Italy)

The project "The Health in the Movement" began 12 years ago in the city of Verona and it is actually utilized in many cities of Italy with particular extension in the provinces of Verona and Trento, actually engaging more than ten thousand people. The Civic Administration, the local office of Preventive Health and the University Centre for Motor Science cooperate in the development of a series of initiatives aimed at inducing in the elderly an active style of life. The structure of the project is mainly focused on the organization of physical activity (PA) classes for people aged from 55y to 75y living in the community. Each class is formed of about 20 subjects, recruited in a determined area, matched for health status and functioning ability, which was previously determined through a specific medical and physical evaluation. Group exercises are proposed and supervised by a physical education teacher with specific expertise in PA for aged people. Physicians, physiologists and teachers work in a very close way to elaborate and to upgrade PA programs. Several different courses are available: gymnastic, swimming, aquagym, resistance training, walking groups, all normally lasting 6 months. In addition special courses are offered to subjects living in nursing houses or to people with chronic diseases (diabetes, CHD, BPCO, osteoporosis).The project is completed by conferences, targeted to the elderly, on the different topics of PA and ageing and by a detailed program of scientific research in biologic and social fields to analyse the effects observed in the participants to the projects and upgrade protocols and programs.

The Importance of Cardiorespiratory and Muscle Fitness in Older Adult Programs

D.H. Paterson (Canadian Centre for Activity and Aging (CCAA), The University of Western Ontario, London, Canada)

Aging is characterized by a loss in function. Cardiorespiratory fitness (VO2max) and muscle strength decline to threshold levels for maintenance of independent living. Cross-sectional studies have reported that different aspects of fitness were independently associated with functional limitations. The present study reports data from a longitudinal follow-up of a random survey of 441 independently living men and women, initially aged 55 to 85 years. In the eight-year follow-up 10% of the sample had become dependent. From the host of initial measures, multiple logistic regression revealed that cardiorespiratory fitness and muscle strength were determinants or explanatory variables of dependence at ages 63 to 93 years. Amount of daily physical activity was not related to maintenance of independence. Rather, in older age cardiorespiratory fitness and strength may drop below needs for activities of daily living, and older adults, to remain independent, require physical activity of a type and intensity to impact on fitness.

SESSION 261

Comparative Case Studies of Older Workers in the United Kingdom and Australia

P. Taylor, (Open University, U.K), L. Brooke (Lincoln Gerontology Centre, La Trobe University, Melbourne, Australia), L. Rolland (JobsEast, Area Consultative Committee, Melbourne, Australia)

PURPOSE: This paper reports on the first stage of a longitudinal research study based on case studies of the constraints and opportunities faced by older workers within a range of private, not-for-profit and public organisations in Australia and the United Kingdom. The purposes of this paper are, firstly, to examine current age management practices within organisational case studies in the United Kingdom and Australia; secondly, to develop emerging themes from the analyses of these case studies; and thirdly, to comparatively analyse individual, business and social policy perspectives within the national contexts of these case studies. METHOD: The methods utilised in this longitudinal case study approach are primarily based on qualitative data collected through semi-structured interviews and focus groups. Demographic data which provides background contextual data was also analysed. RESULTS: The comparative analysis of case studies in the United Kingdom and Australia found that there are common issues affecting how older workers are utilised and valued in their organisations. Some of the common issues which arose in both countries concerned responses to technological change, labour force shortages and skills of the older workforce. Differences between the findings were related to broader social policies and cultural influences which affected age management practices and also potential areas for change. CONCLUSION: These comparative analyses show key factors which benefit or constrain older workers based in individual, business and social policy perspectives. The paper indicates directions for all three stakeholder sectors which can support enhanced employment outcomes for older workers.

Investigating the learning styles of older women employees in low skilled jobs

A.Withnall (University of Warwick, Coventry, UK)

The learning styles of older women workers (aged 45+) were investigated as part of an international EU-funded project into the training of older workers in small and medium sized enterprises. 26 older women employed in low-skilled jobs in took part in a series of workshops designed to help them identify their learning histories and/or completed a newly designed Learning Style Inventory (Building Excellence). Evaluation of reactions to the workshops and Inventory showed that the women did not perceive learning or training to be relevant to their lives and that this Inventory, in its present form, was not appropriate to their situations. It was concluded that (i) some older employees might need to be helped to understand the role that training might play in improving their working lives before any programmes are devised (ii) the BE Inventory should be revised to make it more user-friendly for low-skilled workers

Managing Flexible Employment in Later Life: A Case Study of the UK Media Industry

Kerry Platman (Open University, England, UK)

Purpose: Organisational change, downsizing and early retirement programmes have led to a decline in secure, full-time employment for older workers. Meanwhile, portfolio working, or freelancing, has been presented as an ideal option for professionals wishing to remain in paid work in later life. This research examines the mythology and the reality of such flexible jobs in the years preceding and following statutory retirement age. Method: This is a case study of the UK's media industry, an expanding sector with an established freelance workforce. In-depth interviews were conducted with 50 people who were able to offer experiences and insights into the practicalities of freelancing. These included older and younger freelances, recruitment agents, union officials and employers. Results: The study found that older freelances displayed both ingenuity and endurance in retaining a labour market foothold beyond the age of 50 years. However, freelancing was far from being an ideal employment state. Older freelances faced cumulative insecurities due to the lack of labour market protection, the rapid turnover of staff who commissioned freelance work, and the pressure to deliver cutting edge services at low cost. Conclusions: This case study of freelancing in the media industry focused on a group of highly trained and experienced professionals who, it could be argued, were well-placed to take advantage of flexible employment opportunities in later life. The findings challenge the assumption that portfolio working, or freelancing, is a liberating state in which individuals gain control over the timing and nature of their exit from the labour market.

Re-employment Success of Older Displaced Workers

J. Bowman, R. Eisenstadt, G. Thomas (Institute of >Gerontology, University of Louisiana, Monroe, >Louisiana, U.S.A.)

PURPOSE: Each year millions of Americans experience job displacement. Because older workers often experience job losses during their peak earning years, the consequences for these individuals can be troublesome. Therefore, we examine factors that affect duration of unemployment and re-employment success of older displaced workers. METHOD: Data is from the 1998 Current Population Survey, Displaced Worker Supplement. The sample consisted of displaced workers 20 years of age and older (n = 5,838). Comparisons were made with sub-samples of displaced workers younger than 40 and 40 years of age and older (n = 2,634). Descriptive and regression analyses were performed on each sample. RESULTS: As displaced workers age, so does their duration of unemployment. For example, the younger sub-sample experienced 9 weeks and the older group, 14 weeks. Eighteen percent of the younger workers received unemployment insurance (UI), while 27% of older workers received UI. Forty-three percent of the sample exhausted their retirement benefits, even more disturbing, however, were the 47% of older workers who exhausted pension funds. Regression results indicate that older displaced workers who experienced longer periods of unemployment, and who had exhausted retirement benefits, experienced wage losses. Moreover, once re-employed, older displaced workers tend to experience earning losses at an increasing rate. While having a college education decreases duration of unemployment, one's occupation may have more to with one's re-employment success. CONCLUSIONS: Implications include programs and policies that increase financial management, job search and readiness skills across the life course.

SESSION 262

Master Plan for the Third Age Habitat I

Eduardo Frank, Arch. (Centro EA/3E - Estudio de Arquitectura por la Tercera Edad - Buenos Aires, Argentina) Susana Koham, Arch. (Centro EA/3E - Estudio de Arquitectura por la Tercera Edad - Buenos Aires, Argentina) Norma Sharovsky, Arch. (Centro EA/3E - Estudio de Arquitectura por la Tercera Edad - Buenos Aires, Argentina)

Third age architecture is much more than a habitat without barriers. It is not the result of applying an exhaustive catalogue of forms and recipes. It is not a question of designing orthopaedic spaces which finally reinforce the exclusion models. Rather, it generates the need for thinking again the architect's role, as a pedagogic one, as well as the need to place oneself in the place of the other within a universal habitat system criterion, as the environment receipting the ageing, and to design new alternatives to the institutionalisation model. The extension of life in one's own house in addition to the protected dwellings and new models for elderly people's homes must be a response to the new needs. Institutional architecture, which even today is articulated on the basis of closure, authority and control models designed in accordance with the industrialism's rhythms and efficiency parameters, and considering the architecture as an orthopaedic operator, reveals the society's opinion on old age. This situation generates the need to raise again the question of the architect's role and his responsibility as an operator for the rationalization of human, physical and financial resources in order to optimise the equation.

Master Plan for the Third Age Habitat II

Irene Susana Koham (Centro EA/3E - Estudio de Arquitectura por la Tercera Edad, Buenos Aires, Argentina) Master Plan for the Third Age Habitat. Norma Sharovsky (Centro EA/3E - Estudio de Arquitectura por la Tercer Edad, Buenos Aires, Argentina) Master Plan for the Third Age Habitat. Eduardo Frank (Centro EA/3E - Estudio de Arquitectura por la Tercera Edad, Buenos Aires, Argentina) Master Plan for the Third Age Habitat. Patricia Guido (A.G.E.B.A - Asociación Gerontologica de Buenos Aires, Buenos Aires, Argentina)

An impassable city, an institution with barriers, a dwelling with physical or spiritual obstacles, even in different degrees, are similar forms of exclusion. Our analytical position in front of the design for the old age implies a practice which infers the necessity of a Third Age Master Plan, by the development of a physical resources infrastructure tending to unify the actions in course and to incorporate answers to the new demands by means of architectural responses.

Master Plan for the Third Age Habitat III

Susana Koham, Arch. (Centro EA/3E - Estudio de Arquitectura por la Tercera Edad - Buenos Aires, Argentina) Norma Sharovsky, Arch. (Centro EA/3E - Estudio de Arquitectura por la Tercera Edad - Buenos Aires, Argentina) Eduardo Frank, Arch. (Centro EA/3E - Estudio de Arquitectura por la Tercera Edad - Buenos Aires, Argentina)

The increase in the old age population over the number of births is causing a change in social structure and, consequently, new needs in the areas of health, housing and education. Planning is a necessary tool for each area, especially architecture, in order to establish new programmes and projects in accordance with the existing demand and its future projection which, on the basis of scientific and technological improvements, may give an adequate response by means of architectural actions. In order to improve third age life quality through the Habitat, we must design a Third Age Habitat Integral Programme by developing research work and an adequate methodology. Tasks: a) To map out the actual demand and existing offer, in order to establish whether the old age population needs are fulfilled; b) To elaborate Contrast Models of Architectural Typologies which may operate as a Target-Image for the existing typologies. Methodology to be implemented intends to open a clear breach between the Contrast Model and the existing ones. During the analysis stage, this will be useful to measure the distance between the present situation and this ideal Model.

Master Plan for the Third Age Habitat IV

Norma Sharovsky, Arch. (Centro EA/3E - Estudio de Arquitectura por la Tercera Edad - Buenos Aires, Argentina) Susana Koham, Arch. (Centro EA/3E - Estudio de Arquitectura por la Tercera Edad - Buenos Aires, Argentina) Eduardo Frank, Arch. (Centro EA/3E - Estudio de Arquitectura por la Tercera Edad - Buenos Aires, Argentina)

Cities can no longer ignore the breach between the reality and the ideal model to fulfill the third age habitat, and it is imperative for those planning cities to think about the old age problem and to propose the development of an infrastructure offering responses to it. In this regard, governments cannot work isolated in their planning departments desks. They must arrive at a solution after an evaluation of their possibilities, always respecting the population's needs. This combination results in a strategy to be followed and stimulates the citizen to take part in it. The master plan will be a first experience of research work to be developed on physical resources, aimed at the definition of strategies firmly based on reality, tending to dignify the human subject, and stimulating social participation in programs contemplating the functional differences and optimizing the economic equation. Our position as architects is that the results of these works must go beyond the field of the academic discussions and materialize in facts to be incorporated by our society in order to improve our life quality.

SESSION 263

Effects of Dispositional Coping on Subjective Well-Being and Everyday Activities in Cataract Patients Undergoing Surgery

N. Rieckmann, N. Knoll, R. Schwarzer (Free University Berlin, Germany)

The model of assimilative and accomodative coping (Brandtstädter, 1999) proposes that there are stable interindividual differences in the tendency to adhere to or disengage from blocked goals. Also, it is assumed that, in dealing with age-related losses, flexible adjustment of one's goals by means of reappraisal and orientation towards new goals (accomodative coping) is crucial for successful adaptation. The present study examines how this theoretical framework applies to the situation of elderly people undergoing cataract surgery as a sample case for both age-related resource loss (vision impairment) and resource gain (improvement of vision after successful surgery). Data from 150 cataract patients (age 42 - 92) were collected using questionnaires at three measurement points in time (one week pre- and both one and six weeks post-surgery). Two scales were used at baseline to assess dispositional coping styles: Tenacious Goal Pursuit (TGP) and Flexible Goal Adjustment (FGA). Outcomes were measured at all three occasions and include emotional and cognitive facets of subjective well-being (SWB) as well as indicators of behavioral adaptation in everyday life. Results indicate that the coping styles are differentially related to outcomes: FGA is positively associated with SWB at all occassions, whereas TGP goes along with a larger range of activities. Moreover, FGA serves a buffering function in that its relation to SWB is stronger in patients with high multimorbidity. Overall, findings underscore that accomodative coping with losses is adaptive and show that this may - at least temporarily - also be the case for situations that offer new opportunities.

Factors associated with progression and regression through states of disability in elderly people

Pascale BARBERGER-GATEAU Catherine VERRET Karine PERES Ahmadou ALIOUM (all from Université Victor segalen Bordeaux2, Bordeaux, France)

PURPOSE : to identify factors of progression and regression through increasing grades of disability and towards death. METHOD: PAQUID is a prospective cohort study of cerebral and functional ageing in south-western France. A random sample of 3777 community dwellers aged 65 and over was followed for 8 years. Three grades of increasing disability were identified, based on a combination of items of mobility, Instrumental Activities of Daily Living and Activities of Daily Living. A five-state Markov model was used to estimate transition intensities between autonomy, the three disability states and death, and the impact of risk factors. RESULTS: age was associated with an increased risk of disability progression and limited the probability of regression. Female sex increased the risk of disability progression between the first two stages and decreased the risk of mortality, whatever the disability level. A low educational level was associated was an increased risk of disability progression. Subjects living in rural areas had a lower risk of mortality. When adjusting for these sociodemographic factors, a depressive symptomatology, and lower cognitive performances increased the risk of disability progression but also mortality, and depression was associated with a lower probability of recovery. In multivariate models, physical factors associated with disability progression were dyspnoea, cardiovascular disease, hypertension and stroke. Most of these factors were also associated with a lower probability of recovery and increased the risk of death. CONCLUSION: pathologies that are not directly involved in the genesis of disability such as

Older Women's Experiences with Chronic Pain: Physical, Psychological and Social Challenges

K. A. Roberto (Center for Gerontology, Virginia Polytechnic Institute and State University, Blacksburg, VA, USA)

Chronic pain frequently accompanies many non-fatal diseases common in old age. Women, given their longer life expectancy and greater likelihood of having multiple disabling health problems, are more likely than their male counterparts to suffer from chronic pain. Little is known, however, about the personal experiences of older women living with chronic pain. The purpose of this qualitative investigation was to identify the challenges older women face in their everyday lives as a result of their pain and explore how they cope with and manage their pain. Twenty older women, who engaged in focus groups, discussed the influence of chronic pain on their daily lives. Eight of these women also participated in in-depth individual interviews. The women described their pain in many different ways, indicative of the subjective nature of the pain experience. Managing pain forced many of the women to withdraw from social activities that they valued and interfered with sleep patterns, household tasks, and recreational activities. Varied acceptance by social network members added to the challenge of adjusting to complications associated with pain. Self-care practices that supported independence contributed to women's perceived success in daily functioning. Listening to the voices of older women living with chronic pain provided insight into the psychosocial issues of the pain experience. Acknowledging older women's experiences with pain enhances our understanding of the complex interweaving of personal and social factors involved in the everyday management of chronic pain in later life.

Perceived Independence as Handicap in Older Adults with Musculoskeletal Disability

Cheryl A. Cott, Monique A.M. Gignac, Elizabeth M.Badley (Arthritis Community Research and Evaluation Unit, University Health Network/ University of Toronto, Toronto, Canada)

Abstract: PURPOSE: To examine the relationship between disability and perceived handicap in older adults with musculoskeletal disability. The relationship between disability and handicap is an important issue in the rehabilitation and disability literature. Conceptual models of disablement such as the ICIDH increasingly emphasize that the relationship between disability and handicap is not a direct one, but is modified by external factors such as the physical environment, the social situation and the resources available to the individual. Handicap is conceptualized as being experienced in a number of dimensions with the dimension of interest in this research being perceived physical independence. We hypothesized that perceived physical independence would be related to level of physical disability, as well as contextual factors such as the use of assistive devices, modification of the performance of activities and receipt of assistance, and psychological resources such as helplessness, mastery and appraisals of lost capacity. METHOD: Face to face structured interviews were conducted with 286 community dwelling seniors with chronic musculoskeletal disability. Separate hierarchical regressions were conducted for domain-specific measures of physical independence across five domains of disability. RESULTS: Domain-specific physical independence was consistently related to disability and perceptions of helplessness. Other factors such as age, gender, education, use of assistive devices, size of helping network and perceptions of lost capacity also contributed to perceived physical independence but their contribution varied by domain. CONCLUSION: These findings support the argument that the social situation and resources available to the individual have an impact on perceived handicap in older adults over and above that of disability.

The Influence of Sociocultural Risk Factors on the Disablement Process among Older Mexican Americans

M. Kristen Peek [UTMB, Galveston TX]; Kenneth J. Ottenbacher [UTMB, Galveston, TX]; Kyriakos S. Markides [UTMB, Galveston, TX[]

The process of becoming disabled and recovery from disability has largely been overlooked in research focusing on older Hispanic adults. Moreover, the role that sociocultural risk factors may play in the disablement process has not been examined among the older Hispanic population. We examine the influence that degree of acculturation, nativity, and migration experience have on the disablement process in older Mexican American adults. Using two waves of data from the Hispanic Established Populations for the Epidemiologic Study of the Elderly (n = 2439), the hypothesis that sociocultural risk factors have a role in the disablement process is tested using structural equation models (LISREL 8.30). Results indicate that both nativity (being US born) and acculturation (interview given in Spanish) are directly associated with lower levels of disability (beta = -.07, p < .01; beta = -.07, p < .01). Moreover, acculturation is associated with increased levels of functional limitations, while nativity is associated with decreased levels of limitations. In conclusion, sociocultural risk factors appear to have differential effects on the disablement process. Sociocultural factors should be accounted for in theories and models focusing on health and disability among older Hispanic adults.

SESSION 264

Understanding Health, Illness and Aging within Canada's Baby Boom Population Presenters Details:

Leigh Turner [McGill University, Montreal, Canada. Individualistic and Communal Values: Examining Assumptions about self-fulfillment in the lives of Baby Boomers] Daryl Pullman [Memorial University of Newfoundland, St John's, Canada. The Normative Force of Appeals to Human Dignity in the Context of Elder Care] Miss. Ayumi Goto [Memorial University, St John's, Canada. Perceptions of Dignity in the Transition Stories of Adult Children of Seniors] Darrin Hodgetts [Memorial University, St John's, Canada. The Imperative to Provide Senior Care: Psychological, Physical, Relational and Societal Consequences]

Canada's baby boom population is aging. As this cohort enters their senior years, it can be expected that they will continue to shape social policy in general and that related to healthcare in particular. Yet aside from some general demographic trends, few specifics are known about the perceived needs and expectations of this group. What values are most important to Baby Boomers in Canada? What stories do Canadian Baby Boomers tell about family obligations, understandings of the public good, and encounters with local health care systems? How do Baby Boomers experience and understand their responsibilities toward parents, children, spouses or partners, extended families, communities, and careers? What values and narratives inform the understanding of Canadian Boomers as they live through profound changes to family structures, social support systems, spiritual and religious life, technological systems, and the workplace? The Norms and Narratives project (funded by the Social Sciences and Humanities Research Council of Canada) explores this rich and complex moral topography. This national project includes researchers from five Canadian Universities and numerous government and community partners including Health Canada, the Catholic Health Care Association, the Canadian Policy Research Network and the Canadian College of Health Service Executives. The project was developed to investigate the views of people in Canada aged between 45 and 55 years regarding the delivery of health care, the type of health services available, and their own perceived health care needs as they enter their senior years. Participants from a range of social backgrounds are being recruited from various health care and community organizations from across Canada. Using research materials drawn from focus groups, popular media sources, interviews, and scholarly literature the "Norms and Narratives" project is tracing the intellectual, emotional, and experiential contours of Boomer lifeworlds. While exploring differences in understanding connected to class, religion, culture, socioeconomic status, and gender, the multi-disciplinary team also searches for commonalities in attitudes and experiences shared by members of the Boomer generation. The symposium consists of a number of theoretical and empirical papers that set the context for the project and provide initial findings. Dr. Leigh Turner (Religious Studies) explores the dynamic tension between individualistic and communal values as expressed in the everyday experiences of baby boomers. Dr. Daryl Pullman (Bio-Ethics) reviews theoretical issues pertaining to the manner in which appeals to dignity inform understandings of aging and elder care. Ms Ayumi Goto (Community Health) explores the question of what constitutes dignity for both adult children and their aging parents as they experience various life transitions. Dr. Darrin Hodgetts (Health Psychology) examines several of the theoretical issues raised in the earlier papers through an analysis of participants talk regarding the consequences of caring.

Individualistic and Communal Values: Examining Assumptions about self-fulfillment in the lives of baby boomers

Turner, L, Hodgetts, D, Pullman, D, Murray, M.

The Norms and Narratives research group is finding that some of the more all-encompassing claims about "modernity" and "post modernity" do not seem to capture the moral imagination of Canadian Boomers. Specifically, while Boomers have concerns about careers and personal fulfillment, Boomers simultaneously experience obligations towards family members, communities, and social institutions. Though Boomers sometimes make reference to self-fulfillment, self-interest, and narrow personal interests, they are not overwhelmingly captivated by "the culture of narcissism," the "triumph of the therapeutic," or the language of "expressive individualism." Rather, Boomer morality is multifaceted, and mingles personal concerns with a sense of obligation to many parties. Furthermore, few Boomers express a "protean sense of self"-the postmodern, fluid, constantly changing selves traced by psychiatrist Robert Lifton. Buffeted by change and societal turbulence, Boomers also experience continuities in self-understanding, conceptions of family life, and understandings of key social institutions. This project is challenging some prominent social narratives about moral life in "late modernity" or "post modernity." Talking with Boomers reveals hints of a moral imagination richer, more complex, more variegated, and-perhaps-more fundamentally decent and caring, than is captured in many of the dominant social science characterizations of contemporary moral life in Canada and the United States

Perceptions of Dignity in the Transition Stories of Adult Children of Seniors

Goto, A, Pullman, D, Hodgetts, D.

As their relationships to their aging parents change, adult children of seniors must often manage a variety of transitions in their personal and social life stories. Their parents' loss of independence will often mark a diminution in their own independence as they face the challenge of caring for those who once cared for them. How do adult children understand "dignity" as it relates to their aging parents, and what constitutes "dignity" for them as caregivers? Are there universal themes about dignity that emerge from these transition stories, or are the stories so diverse that "dignity" becomes a highly particularized notion? The question of what constitutes dignity and how adult children perceive of it for both themselves and their aging parents is one avenue of exploration pursued in the "Norms and Narratives Project". Dignity, it turns out, is a dynamic concept. While perceptions of dignity inform the manner in which children respond to their aged parents, how they respond in turn impacts how they perceive the dignity of their parents, even as it affects their sense of their own personal dignity. This paper examines some of the transition stories told by adult children of aging parents with a view to understanding how considerations of dignity inform their capacity to negotiate these transitions.

The Imperative to Provide Senior Care: Psychological, Physical, Relational and Societal Consequences for Caregivers

Hodgetts, D. J, Flynn, B-J, Goto, A. Pullman, D, Murray, M.

Within contemporary society, both formal and informal approaches to caring for seniors have been subject to increased social and financial pressures. Although quantitative information on the level of resourcing for institutional and home care services is readily available, less is known about the qualitative experience of caring for seniors. This paper explores the way people describe the impact on themselves and on their families of providing senior care. It draws upon accounts presented by research participants in focus group discussions and individual interviews, which were conducted as part of the "Norms and Narratives" project. In making sense of their own situation and that of those receiving care, participants repeatedly refer to various restraints on their ability to provide quality senior care. In doing so, they highlight the psychological, relational and physical health consequences of attempting to provide such care in a period of healthcare restructuring and changing family structures. Shared explanations are used to invoke the consequences of care are explored as a strategy for preserving one's sense of identity as a worthy member of society.

The Normative Force of Appeals to Human Dignity in the Context of Elder Care

Pullman, D, Goto, A. Hodgetts, D.

Appeals to human dignity are common in moral discourse, and are especially prevalent in the literature on aging. We are told to treat people with dignity and to respect the dignity of others. Some talk about the need to live with dignity, while others express a desire to die with dignity. For all the talk about dignity, however, there is little discussion about the content of this notion. What do we mean by "human dignity"? How does one acquire it in the first place, and in what sense can one's dignity be lost or taken away? If we are to preserve and enhance the dignity of elders and of those who provide their care, some attempt must be made to answer such fundamental questions. This paper begins to unpack the rich and complex notion of human dignity. It reviews a number of ways in which considerations of dignity are invoked in the health care literature in general, and by those involved in various aspects of elder care. While some appeals to dignity carry universal normative force (i.e. they apply to everyone, everywhere), others are more culturally and individually referenced. Implications of this analysis for social and health care policies that aim to preserve and enhance the dignity of elders and their care-givers will be discussed.

SESSION 265

Decisions made by persons with dementia

Bonnie Dobbs (University of Alberta, Edmonton, Alberta, Canada), Penny MacCourt (University of Victoria, Victoria, B.C, Canada), Kate Oakley (University of Ottawa, Institute on Health of the Elderly, Ottawa, Ontario, Canada), Holly Tuokko (University of Victoria, Victoria, B.C, Canada)

The ability to make decisions regarding the care of self and property is fundamental to the concepts of competence, autonomy, and independence. Decision-making is multi-factorial, complex, influenced by a myriad of factors (e.g, specific cognitive abilities, attitudes, beliefs, environmental milieu) and domain-specific. There are a number of situations where decision-making capability may be questioned. This symposium will address issues relevant to decision-making for persons with dementia. Decision-making in persons with dementia has a role to play from the diagnosis through to care planning and ongoing care management. There is evidence to suggest that decision-making indices may be useful in the early detection of dementia. This research also suggests that decision-making, within specific domains, may be impaired early in the course of a dementia prompting the need for assistance with decision-making. This raises important issues about when and how assistance with decision-making can be provided and the impact this loss of autonomy may have on the individual with dementia, their family, and other care providers. Each of the four presentations in this symposium will address specific aspects of these issues. Dr. Oakley will describe the use of a decision-making task in the early detection of cognitive decline. Dr. Dobbs will discuss factors affecting the decision to stop driving. Ms. MacCourt will describe the values that underlay health care decision-making and describe similarities and differences between choices made by elderly persons and health care providers. Dr. Tuokko will discuss decision-making in the context of financial management. This symposium will highlight the variety of ways dementia may affect decision-making, factors that affect decision-making in the context of dementia and provide directions for future research in this area.

Awareness of financial skills

H. Tuokko and K. Cramer (University of Victoria, Victoria, B.C, Canada)

It is known that persons with dementia may have difficulty making decisions on their own behalf. In certain situations, such as those involving financial matters, it may become necessary for a legal determination of incapability to make specific decisions. Central to making such a determination is whether people are aware of problems they may be experiencing in handling financial issues. A three-part measure of awareness of financial skills was developed to examine the extent to which people with dementia are aware of their limitations in this area: Part 1 - self-report of financial functioning; Part 2 - informant report of financial functioning parallel to Part 1; Part 3 - performance measure assessing a subset of tasks from Part 1. Awareness was examined as the congruence between self-report, informant report, and performance tasks. The measure was found to be reliable (internal consistency of .92 and .97, respectively, for Parts 1 and 2; inter-rater reliability of .995 for Part 3) and valid (content, convergent and discriminant validity were examined). The awareness measure and measures of memory and executive functioning were administered to 25 persons with dementia. The preliminary findings suggest that both executive and memory functions were related to awareness of financial skills. The construct of awareness and its relation to cognitive impairment are important to the incapability assessment process and within the broader context of decision-making.

Decision-making and driving in persons with dementia

Bonnie M. Dobbs (University of Alberta, Edmonton, Alberta, Canada)

Voluntary driving cessation is often advocated as a means of reducing older driver crash rates. This approach is based on the presumption that the amount and type of self-regulation is commensurate with objective ability change. The assumption that driving will be appropriately adjusted to accommodate ability declines presumes that the individual will have insight into those declines. It seems reasonable to presume that healthy older drivers might have insight into ability declines relevant to driving and restrict their driving accordingly. However, it is equally reasonable to presume this same relationship would not hold if the individual's insight was impaired. However, when insight is impaired, as is often the case with a dementing illness, ability declines may not be recognized. Reported self-regulation and actual driving performance were examined in a sample of healthy older drivers (n = 64) and older drivers with clinically significant cognitive impairment (n = 218). An examination of video taped serious driving errors committed during the on-road assessment most often showed either no evidence of awareness of the driving error or a reaction that was incongruent with the seriousness of the driving error for those individuals with cognitive impairment. Not surprisingly, measures of self-perceptions of driving competency were found to be unrelated to on-road performance for the cognitively impaired sample, even in the early stages of the illness. These findings underscore driving as an area of decision making for which external interventions are appropriate when insight is impaired because of the potential for serious consequences for personal and public safety.

The Use of Support Groups to Help Older Adults Dealing With Substance Abuse Problems

D. Bradshaw (Seniors Well Aware Program, Vancouver, B.C, Canada). C. Spencer, Gerontology Research Centre, Simon Fraser University, Vancouver, B.C.

Peer support and self help groups have been well recognized in the gerontological field as means to help older adults deal with life changes and stresses such as retirement, loss of a spouse, or major changes in health. Clinical practice is beginning to demonstrate that similar kinds of support are also an extremely important aid when seniors are experiencing substance abuse problems. These can operate an adjunct to outreach counselling and as additional support for relapse prevention. However, there is still surprisingly little gerontological or addictions' literature addressing when and how these groups work. Based on research of the experience of older clients and staff in a British Columbia seniors addiction program, this presentation describes who benefits and why, as well as the systemic challenges that exist in establishing and maintaining these types of support groups for seniors. For older adults in British Columbia, these groups are not limited to abstinence models or information-giving by group coordinators. Results show that they take on far more diverse forms and goals with seniors often taking on a lead role in the structure and functioning of the group. The groups often focus on sharing life experiences, rebuilding socialization skills and a sense of fun and purpose in life, normalizing daily activities, and reducing harms of drinking.

Values and care decisions of elderly persons and health care professionals

Penny MacCourt (University of Victoria, Victoria, B.C, Canada)

Health care professionals often make long-term care decisions about marginally incompetent elderly people, particularly when they appear to be living alone at risk. Without standardized objective criteria for assessing either risk or capability to live alone, the decisions are value-laden. We would expect that age-cohort differences and the adoption of professional and organizational values would lead to different values between health care professionals from elderly persons. A between-groups design was used to examine whether elderly persons and professionals would: (1) make different long-tem care decisions for a hypothetical marginally incompetent elderly person, and (2) whether their decisions would reflect differences in under-lying values between the two groups. Data was gathered from 86 professionals and 81 elderly persons using a scenario about an elderly woman (Mrs. Smith) living alone at risk. Respondents were asked to choose between community and institutional care based on their appraisal of the situation and on information provided about local resources. Questions were asked about their decisions to reveal underlying values, and to explore the circumstances (e.g, perceived risks, burden on children)under which respondents alter their original decision. Elderly people rated the risks to Mrs Smith living alone higher, and chose institutional care for her more frequently than did professionals. Elderly persons were more influenced by the burden on family that living at risk caused, than were professionals. Elderly persons' decisions were more reflective of the values of beneficence and family interdependence, than were those of professionals, whose decisions reflected of the value of autonomy.

What's in a decision?

Kate Oakley (University of Ottawa, Institute on Health of the Elderly, Ottawa, Ontario, Canada)

A deficit in judgement and decision-making ability is typically listed as one of the symptoms of Alzheimer's disease. Yet evidence to support this belief is based primarily on anecdotal reporting by physicians. Given the extent of the belief, the current study sought to verify whether the above assumption could be generalized across individuals with dementia and to determine whether any deterioration is domain-specific or domain-general. In addition, this research investigated whether any breakdown in decision-making ability occurred at each stage of the decisional process. Based on psychophysics subjective probability methodology, young adults, 'normal' seniors, and individuals diagnosed with possible or probable dementia made 2-AFC decisions in both memory and perceptual domains and indicated their choice on a response-panel. The difficulty of the decision as well as the age of the decision-maker influenced results. That is, individuals were less accurate, more over-confident (or less under-confident), and less well calibrated and resolved when the decision was difficult compared to easy decisions. This effect was exacerbated with increased age, as well as cognitive loss associated with dementia. Interestingly, the results further support the position that a deficit in decision-making ability does not necessarily arise from a failure to make accurate judgements. Instead, results demonstrate that some specific aspects of the decision-making process are sensitive to the effects of age and others to pathology associated with dementia. Judgement and decision-making is particularly useful in the early detection of cognitive loss associate with dementia. This research is funded by the Alzheimer's Association, US

SESSION 266

Problems of elderly workers

Victor W. MARSHALL (Institute on Aging, University of North Carolina, Chapel Hill NC, USA) Canadian research on older workers Masaharu KUMASHIRO (Department of Ergonomics, Institute of Industrial,Ecological Sciences, University of Occupational and Environmental Health, Fukuoka, Japan) Occupational ergonomists ready for an increasingly aging workforce: solution- oriented strategies for effective use of aging workers Sol ENCEL (Social Policy Research center, University of New South Wales, Sidney / Australia) Mature workers in Australia recent developments Johannes DOLL (Institute of Psychology, University of Porto Alegre/ Brazil) The situation of elderly workers in Brazil Jose Luis VEGA-VEGA (Faculty of Psychology, University of Salamanca / Spain) Stereotype formation on older workers. The role of implicit theories Gabriele MAIER (Institute of Gerontology, University of Heidelberg / Germany) Older workers a new target group for human resource management: empirical findings.

Labour force participation of aged people 55-65 has declined during the last decades in most of the countries. The image of the elderly worker very often is a rather negative one: Older workers sometimes are perceived as being slower, less motivated, less creative, less flexible, less competent. As far as research is valuable, it points to a greater degree of competence. We need much more research on the special abilities of elderly workers. - The demographic change in most of the countries of the world leads to an elderly work force. What can be done for achieving productive aging? Measures of special training- and placements-programms for elderly employees will be discussed

Canadian research on older workers

Victor W. Marshall (Institute on Aging, University of North Carolina, Chapel Hill NC, USA)

PURPOSE: This paper reviews Canadian research on older workers, identifying major projects, themes, and gaps. METHOD: Literature review RESULTS: Canadian research on older workers is quite recent and not plentiful. Government research conducted in house relies primarily on nationally representative surveys and this supports a general overview of working patterns by age, with limited opportunity to portray longitudinal patterns. Government-supported research and other research by academics includes secondary analyses of national data files but also includes firm- and industry-based studies. With an institutionalized retirement age of 65, Canada's actual average retirement age is 52. Labour force participation of males aged 55-64, and 65+ has generally declined but is sensitive to demand characteristics. CONCLUSION: Older persons appear to face greater labour force instability than younger persons but this inference requires further research. Work and retirement patterns are shaped by a mix of public and corporate policies, economic swings, demographic patterns and technology.

Mature Age Workers in Australia: Recent Developments

S. Encel, Social Policy Research Centre, University of New South Wales, Sydney, Australia

In Australia, as in other industrialised countries, there has been a steady fall in the labour force participation rate among older men (i.e. over 50) since the 1970s. The decline is related to a continuing rise in unemployment, especially long-term unemployment, among men in these age groups. Three State governments in Australia have introduced programs to assist the older unemployed (two of them in 1999), but the Federal government has refrained from following suit. The issue has now been examined in an extensive review by a committee of the Federal parliament. The committee's report strongly recommends the introduction of measures to assist older workers, including special training and placement programs and incentives for employers.

Occupational Ergonomists Ready for an Increasingly Aging Workforce : Solution-Oriented Strategies for Effective Use of Aging Workers

Masaharu KUMASHIRO,(Department of Ergonomics, Institute of Industrial Ecological Sciences, University of Occupational and Environmental Health , Japan)

The aging of Japan's labor population is proceeding at a pace not seen anywhere else in the world. As measures to cope with this rapid aging of Japan's workforce, the Ministry of Labor proposed in its 1997 White Paper on Labor, three tasks to expedite the utilization of Japan's elderly work force: (1) consideration of health issues, (2) review of wage systems and retirement pay, (3) and reevaluation of job content and the workplace environment. To satisfy those three conditions, tools for work ability assessment must be developed. The author has developed a method for work ability diagnosis and evaluation as one step towards the ERGOMA strategy and actions for achieving productive aging (Kumashiro, 1999). The essence of this method is the formula $P = f(W, A, C, M)$ where P is the value of labor performed by aging workers, with a substantial economic effect; W is the work conditions and environment (including a database of success stories); A is the capacity for duties (skill plus knowledge plus experience); C is the ability to adapt to work (one's functional age); and M is the worker's motivation (desire to perform work). This report discusses the development of practical ergonomics interventions aiming for the effective use of aging workers, involving three areas of concern: the three major issues addressed by Japan's Ministry of Labor, the author's strategy and actions for each of these.

Kumashiro, M. (1999) : Strategy and actions for achieving productive aging in Japan, Experimental Aging Research, 25, 461-470.

Older workers - a new target group for human resource management: empirical findings

Gabriele Maier (Institute of Gerontology, Ruprecht-Karls-University, Heidelberg, Germany)

Current demographic trends in industrialized countries indicate an increase in average age within the workforce. Ususally older workers (typically over 45 years) are regarded as a homogenous group, are often stereotypied as less competent, less motivated, and therefore debared from programs of Human Resource Management. This junior-staff-directed perspective of companies obviously no longer fits when the number of older workers increase. Analyzing the research on older workers leads to the conclusion that there is an abundance of scientific evidence to show that older workers are no less effective than younger ones but on the other hand there is a lack of human resource strategies in managing age at the workplace. Hence this study particularly focuses the subjective view of older workers, their bosses, and the perspective of the personnel departments regarding the development and implementation of models of HR strategies to integrate older workers and combat age barriers in employment (i. e. training, development, promotion and job design). Data collection is based on semi-structured interviews with 140 men 45 to 60 years old) working in various companies of chemical industries in Germany. Results show that their is a different attitude towards HR strategies: whereas most of the older workers prefer skill- and job-orientated, non-age specific programs, their bosses and representatives of personnel departments mostly still opt for an early exit or age-specific strategies. These findings point to the need of a holistic approach and company specific, flexible implementation when developing HR strategies encompassing not only the commitment of older workers, but changing attitudes within organizations especially by using senior managers as consultants to establish a change.

Stereotype formation on older workers: The role of implicit theories

José Luis Vega Vega (Department of Developmental and Educational Psychology, University of Salamanca, Spain), Belén Bueno Martínez (Department of Developmental and Educational Psychology, University of Salamanca, Spain) and Carmen Tabernero Urbieta (Department of Social Psychology, University of Salamanca, Spain)

People may vary in the degree to which they are engaged in the processes that are implicated in stereotypical judgments. Older workers are sometimes perceived as being slower, less creative, less flexible, more resistant to change, disinterested on training, and prone to illness in accidents. We hypothesized these beliefs and attitudes are generated on the base of implicit theories about the fixedness versus malleability of human attributes (entity versus incremental theories). Data have been collected from two samples of workers, under and over 40 years of age. Participants have been selected form two contexts: workers from elderly institutions and workers from other institutions. A total of 200 workers have been tested on auto and hetero-perception of worker characteristics, attributions of feilure and implicit theories of personality. The results from correlational analyses focus on how implicit theories can explain the stereotype about older workers, but also how these implicit theories are installed on older worker and predict differences in perceptions of groups. The present study presents data to understand the cognitive processes involved in the formation, use, and maintenance of stereotypes on older workers. Data will be presented as well about the context of the older worker situation in spanish population. Therefore changing the attitudes, prejudice or stereotype of staff towards older workers and the own old workers may be a vital prerequisite to the development of good practice for older workers. These attitudes and beliefs are of critical importance for the quality of work life.

The elderly worker in Brazil

Johannes Doll (Federal University of Rio Grande do Sul, Porto Alegre, Brazil)

In order to understand the situation of elderly workers in Brazil, we first have to consider the general employment situation and the historic moment of the Brazilian economy, which is marked by a great number of informal work (Cardoso et al. 1997), by extreme differences between the regions of Brazil, by great differences between industrial and country workers and by a tendency of modernization and reengineering which brings up, upon other consequences, the decrease of employment and the coexistence of brand new and archaic kinds of production (Jornada et al, 1999). The situation of elderly workers is marked too by a retirement system, which still allows retiring after 30 (women) and 35 (men) working years and which leads to the fact that, although a lot of people get retired, they continue working. The general situation for regularly employed elderly workers is not as difficult as generally assumed. In comparison to the younger workers, the percentage of unemployment is lower and, in the enterprises, they get higher salaries. Nevertheless, a restart after having lost employment is much more difficult for them. The study examines the image that personal managers, younger and elderly male workers have of the abilities and restrictions of elderly workers by interviews in 20 enterprises. The study shows that the images of the three groups (personal manager, younger worker, elderly worker) correspond in some characteristic aspects, while in others they differ strongly.

SESSION 267

Diverse Solutions to Helping Older Persons with Addiction Problems

E. McKee (COPA, Toronto ON M6R 3B2 Canada), Addictions and Older Persons. An Overview; J. Barr (Centre for Addictions and Mental Health, Peterborough ON K9J 2V4 Canada) Older Adults with Substance Misuse Problems: Mobilizing our Community Resources to Help; C. Spencer (Gerontology Research Centre, Simon Fraser University, Vancouver B.C. Canada) The Use of Support Groups to Help Older Adults Dealing With Substance Abuse Problems.

Approximately 6-100f older adults have an addiction to alcohol or other drugs. Increasingly, it is being recognized that older adults needs in this area are often different than younger adults and a range of approaches is being offered to help. In this roundtable, four presenters will discuss solutions that have been developed in cities and small communities in Canada and the United States. The content will cover: a brief overview of addictions and older persons; a home-visiting model of treatment that incorporates 'best practices'; innovative application of a 'home visiting' service to detoxification; community development of appropriate addiction resources for older persons with addictions living in small towns; the effective use of different type of support groups; and overcoming challenges/opposition to a harm reduction public health model in a 12-Step community. An example of cross-border consultation will be given. Organized to encourage audience participation, the session will include a discussion of the barriers to treatment, including ageism and negative attitudes towards addiction problems, and several strategies to address these barriers. The expected outcome of the session is an increased awareness of addictions and older persons, and more specifically, of interventions shown to work well with older adults. The need for an interdisciplinary and intersectoral approach to dealing with this issue is highlighted.

Older Adults with Substance Misuse Problems: Mobilizing our Community Resources to Help

J. Barr (Centre for Addiction and Mental Health, Peterborough, ON, Canada)

Based on prevalence data it is estimated that in Peterborough County, Ontario, Canada there may be as many as 3,300 individuals over the age of 55 suffering from alcohol and/or other substance abuse problems, most of whom are unidentified, and not receiving treatment. This presentation will discuss a project aimed to improve awareness, identification, and support of older adults experiencing substance misuse problems in Peterborough County by primary and secondary care providers. A Working Group, comprised of four organizations in Peterborough was convened to improve case consultation and coordination within the community of health care workers, and increase referrals between the addictions and gerontology fields. Elements of successful treatment from the COPA and LESA programs (home visiting and harm reduction) and an educational workshop aimed to improve service providers' awareness, knowledge and skills in the identification and support of older adults with substance misuse problems, was provided. The clinical and training results, as well as the collaboration required, may be applicable to other small urban and rural areas in Ontario and in other jurisdictions.

Older Persons and Addictions: Development of Home Visiting Addiction Treatment and Detoxification

E. McKee (Community Outreach Programs in Addictions (COPA), Toronto ON Canada)

Approximately 6-100f older Canadians have an addiction to alcohol or other drug. Addictions among older persons is not a well understood or well researched issue. As a result, they often do not receive appropriate treatment. The Community Outreach Programs in Addictions (COPA) program in south west Toronto, Ontario, Canada has been assisting older persons with addictions problem since 1983. It is only one of eight senior-specific addiction programs across Canada. This presentation provides an overview of the harm reduction and home visiting model used by COPA with older persons who may not otherwise qualify for addiction treatment. In the past two years, COPA has added a home detoxification component, which a recent evaluation shows is proving to be helpful in stabilizing and improving older persons life situations. This model of treatment has served to inform other communities of responses to addiction treatment and older persons.

SESSION 268

Arts Across America: The National Center For Creative Aging

Susan Perlstein (National Center for Creative Aging/ Elders Share the Arts (ESTA), Brooklyn, New York, USA)

With the aging of America comes the search for meaningful engagement, lifelong learning, and community involvement. Interest in arts and aging is drawing a new and broad audience. Prevailing myths and misconceptions about aging and creativity influence research, practice and policies. Many believe that arts are for only the talented and privileged rather than a creative process available to all people to express themselves, to heal, to find meaning, to celebrate and to connect to community. The National Center for Creative Aging is leading a creative arts and aging movement across America. The purpose of this center is to support the exchange of information, resources, research, and policy development and provide technical assistance. This presentation will demonstrate the importance of sustaining quality creative arts programming for the well-being of older people. In this session, we will review recent research and practice in aging and creativity in the United States; and consider the impact of policy. "Best practices" from each of four regional centers will be highlighted.

The Artworks Studio Program: New learning for veterans in a continuing care environment

Marilyn Magid (George Derby Centre, Burnaby, British Columbia, Canada)

In recent years, there has been increasing interest in creativity among health professionals who work with the elderly. In fact, the study of aging is increasingly showing that later life can be an especially creative age, and that the introduction of creative arts in clinical care settings can profoundly influence health and well-being. Developing new skills adds to one's ability to adapt to aging, thereby promoting maintenance of independent functioning, an increased sense of accomplishment, and personal satisfaction. Since 1946, Veteran's Affairs Canada has provided support for creative arts departments in hospital environments across Canada, presenting a wide range of creative activities, including painting, drawing, weaving and pottery. This presentation will describe the Artworks Studio program that is offered at George Derby Centre, an intermediate care facility in Burnaby, and at Brock Fahrni Pavilion, an extended care facility in Vancouver. By using adaptation tools and techniques participants who wish to engage in creative pursuits may do so, despite physical or cognitive challenges they may face. A description of the program philosophy, processes and procedures will be presented with emphasis given to the range of possibilities for residents exploring their own creativity, in many cases, for the very first time. Perspectives of clients and other health professionals on the value of a creative arts program in continuing care will be shared. It is hoped that this type of program will be reproduced or adapted to meet the needs of different client groups in other community and residential environments.

SESSION 269

Programmed Cell death

Rita B. Effros (UCLA School of Medicine, Los Angeles, USA) Apoptosis resistance of T cells during aging: impact on immune function. Katsuiku Hirokawa (Department of Pathology and Immunology, Tokyo Medical & Dental University Graduate School, Tokyo, Japan) Age-related increase of apoptosis in the human thymus, bone marrow and gastrointestinal cancer. Yoshio Hayashi (Department of Pathology, Tokushima University School of Dentistry) Acceleration of Autoimmune Exocrinopathy with Aging in Murine Sjogren's Syndrome through Fas-mediated Apoptosis. Tamas Fulop (Institut Universitaire de Gériatrie, Sherbrooke, Qc, Canada) Changes in the apoptosis of polymorphonuclear granulocytes with aging: implication of signal transduction pathways and mitochondria.Junda D. Liu (Beijing Hospital, Institute of Geriatrics, Beijing, China) Modulatory Effect of Chinese Herbs on Apoptosis of Lymphocytes in the Elderly. Mark A. Smith (Case Western Reserve University, Cleveland, Ohio USA) Abortive apoptotic signaling in Alzheimer disease: a last gasp or a survival mechanism? Shun Shimohama (Department of Neurology, Graduate School of Medicine, Kyoto University, Kyoto, Japan) Apoptosis in Alzheimer's disease: Comparison with development and aging.

Issue: This invited symposium will address the problem of programmed cell death (or apoptosis) in relation to aging and related diseases. Apoptosis is an essential physiological phenomenon occurring throughout life. However, a dysregulation of apoptosis might occur with aging and could increase the susceptibility to diseases which are more frequently associated with aging such as cancer, neurodegenerative diseases and infections. The modulation of the apoptotic process could provide powerful tools to influence the physiological and pathological aging. Structure: The Symposium will be composed of six oral presentations over-viewing various aspects of apoptosis in relation to physiological and pathological aging. Content: The first part will be devoted to the role of apoptosis in the dysregulation of the immune system with aging and the potential interventions for modulating it. Dr. R. Effros will discuss the research that has been conducted on the influence of the resistance of T cell apoptosis on the immune functions changes with aging in mice and humans. The role of the caloric restriction as a mean to restore normal T cell apoptosis will be shown. Dr. T. Fulop will discuss the role of the decreased modulation of neutrophil apoptosis in the altered immune response with aging. The intracellular signal transduction pathways and the mitochondrial alterations leading to apoptosis will be reviewed. Dr. K. Hirokawa will continue by discussing how the increase of apoptosis in the human thymus, bone marrow and gastrointestinal cancer influences the immune function and the progression of cancer with aging. Dr. J. Liu will discuss how the alterations of apoptosis in T cells with aging could affect the immune response, but can be favourably influenced by Chinese herbs. Finally, Dr. Y. Hayashi will discuss the role of apoptosis in various T cell subsets in relation to autoimmune diseases in murine model with possible implications to humans. The second part will be devoted to the apoptosis in the nervous system with aging mainly in relation to its role in neurodegenerative diseases. Dr. M. Smith will discuss the role of apoptosis in the nervous system with aging and in Alzheimer's disease. The new concept of apoptotic avoidance, termed abortive apoptosis in Alzheimer's disease will be discussed. Dr. S. Shimohama will discuss the apoptosis in the pathology of AD in comparison with development and aging of the brain with the implication for possible future treatments. Conclusions: There are marked differences in apoptosis with aging depending on the cells studied which might be explained by the differential dysregulation of the molecular pathways involved. The further understanding of the apoptotic process with aging mainly in the immune and nervous systems will help to design powerful interventions to decrease age-related diseases such as cancer, neurodegenerative diseases for a better quality of life of elderly persons.

Abortive apoptotic signaling in Alzheimer disease: a last gasp or a survival mechanism?

Arun K. Raina1, Ayala Hochman2, Akihiko Nunomura3, Shun Shimohama4, Atsushi Takeda5, George Perry1 and Mark A. Smith1 [1Case Western Reserve University, Cleveland, Ohio USA; 2George S. Wise Faculty of Life Sciences, Tel Aviv University, Tel Aviv, Israel; 3Asahikawa Medical College, Asahikawa, Japan; 4Kyoto University Graduate School of Medicine, Kyoto, Japan; and 5Tohoku University School of Medicine, Sendai, Japan]

PURPOSE: Several lines of evidence implicate an apoptotic mechanism in the selective neuronal death that characterizes Alzheimer disease (AD). However, somewhat paradoxically, the terminal phases of apoptosis, such as chromatin condensation, and apoptotic bodies, are rarely/never seen. To further resolve this issue, in this study, we investigated caspase activation as a biochemical index of apoptosis to determine the extent of the apoptotic cascade in AD. METHOD: Antisera against major upstream (8, 9) and downstream (3, 7) caspases were used for immunocytochemical and immunoblot analyses of AD (n = 10) and control (n = 10) cases. RESULTS: Upstream (8, 9) but not downstream (3, 7) caspases were selectively increased in AD compared to controls cases, especially in association with neurofibrillary tangles in hippocampal and cortical pyramidal neurons. CONCLUSION: Given that execution of apoptosis requires amplification of the caspase-mediated apoptotic signal, our results indicate that in AD there is a lack of effective apoptotic signal propagation to downstream caspase effectors. Therefore, it appears that, although initiated, apoptotic signals in AD do not progress through to cell death. This novel phenomenon of apoptotic avoidance, which we term abortive apoptosis, or abortosis, may represent an exit from the caspase-induced apoptotic program that leads to neuronal survival in AD

Acceleration of Autoimmune Exocrinopathy with Aging in Murine Sjogren's Syndrome through Fas-mediated Apoptosis

Yoshio Hayashi (Department of Pathology, Tokushima University School of Dentistry)

Purpose: To evaluate the age-associated changes in autoimmune exocrinopathy, we analyzed a NFS/sld murine model for Sjogren's syndrome. Methods: Apoptotic cells were detected by flow cytometry. Autoantigen cleavage was analyzed by immunoblotting. Serum autoantibodies were detected by ELISA. Results: Severe autoimmune lesions developed in the aged mice. A higer proportion of mouse salivary gland cells bearing Fas was found in the aged, whereas no significant changes were seen on infiltrating CD4+FasL+ T cells. We detected an increased cleavage product of autoantigen, and an increase in serum autoantibody production in the aged. Fas expression was decreased on splenic CD4+ T cells, and anti-Fas mAb-stimulated apoptosis was downregulated on CD4+ T cells. Conclusion: Age-associated dysregulation of CD4+ T cells may play a crucial role on acceleration of autoimmune exocrinopathy through Fas-mediated apoptosis.

Age-related increase of apoptosis in the human thymus, bone marrow and gastrointestinal cancer.

Katsuiku Hirokawa (Department of Pathology and Immunology, Tokyo Medical & Dental University Graduate School)

Purpose: The cell number in most organs are known to decrease with age and this is presumed to be due to apoptosis increasing with age. In fact, many of the age-linked physiological dysfunction could be ascribed to a dysregulation of apoptotic process. Thus, it is important to know the age-related change of apoptosis in organs/tissues in normal and diseased conditions. Results: The thymus starts to involute in the early phase of the life as early as the 1st decade. The adult thymic tissue is disrupted into small fragments due to marked infiltration of fatty tissue. Most of these fragments contain lymphoid tissue, where a detectable amount of thymopoiesis is observed even in the elderly people. However, proliferative activity of thymocytes in adult thymic tissue significantly decreases with a concomitant increase of apoptosis. This cellular equilibrium in favor of apoptosis is one of underlying causes of age-related thymic involution. Bone marrow is also known to decrease in total volume with age, especially prominent in long bones such as femur. Cellular marrow in the sternum is relatively well maintained until the 8th decade and decreases at the 9th decade. Proliferative activity of hemopoietic cells is significantly higher in the subjects of the 6th decade than those of the 3rd decade, but decreases in those over 9th decade. Apoptosis, however, increases gradually with advance of age. Myelodysplastic syndrome (MDS) is a common disease in the elderly, where an abnormally enhanced cell proliferation occurs together with a marked increase of apoptosis. The enhanced apoptosis is caused by increased expression of growth factor, FAS, FAS-L, and I-NOS in different type of cells. Development of tumor cells is also based partly on the imbalance between cell proliferation and apoptosis. But this imbalance appears to change with age. When the incidence of apoptosis is compared between cancer cells of different age, it increases with age. The fact may explain why cancers in the elderly often show relatively benign behavior as compared to those in the younger people. Conclusions: Thus, it is of importance to examine genetic background how apoptosis changes with age.

Apoptosis in Alzheimer's disease: Comparison with development and aging

Shun Shimohama, M.D, Sadaki Fujimoto, Yoshihisa Kitamura, and Takashi Taniguchi*, (Department of Neurology, Graduate School of Medicine, Kyoto University, Sakyoku, Kyoto 606, Departments of Environmental Biochemistry and Neurobiology*, Kyoto Pharmaceutical University, Kyoto 607, Japan)*

Purpose: Alzheimer's disease is the most common human neurodegenerative disorder characterized by the progressive deterioration of cognition and memory associated with the presence of senile plaques, neurofibrillary tangles, and massive loss of neurons. It is now generally recognized that massive neuronal death due to apoptosis is a common characteristic in the brains of patients suffering from neurodegenerative diseases, and apoptotic cell death has been found in neurons and glial cells in AD. Results: The current findings regarding the evidence for apoptosis in AD and the possible involvement of apoptosis-regulating factors, Bcl-2 and caspase families, are discussed in the pathology of AD in comparison with development and aging of the brain. Conclusion: Modification of the apoptotic cascade could be considered as a therapeutic strategy for the diseases.

Apoptosis resistance of T cells during aging: impact on immune function

Rita B. Effros, Carolyn C Spaulding, UCLA School of Medicine, California (Los Angeles, USA)

PURPOSE: Appropriately timed programmed cell death is a critical component of normal immune function. Since the immune system of aged mice and humans shows a progressive accumulation of poorly functional T cells, we sought to determine if senescent T cells were altered in their capacity to undergo apoptosis. METHOD: The effect of aging and caloric restriction on T cell apoptosis was examined in mice. Splenic T cells were evaluated for apoptosis induced by heat shock, irradiation, staurosporine, galectin-1, or antibodies to Fas and CD3. In other experiments, human T cells were repeatedly stimulated to proliferate using antigen and IL-2 until they reached replicative senescence. Induced apoptosis was compared in T cells from early passage and senescent cultures. ELISA, Annexin V staining, and morphologic criteria were used to evaluate apoptosis. RESULTS: Aging in mice is associated with increased numbers of splenic lymphocytes and T cells and a marked resistance of T cells to apoptosis, changes that were totally reversed by caloric restriction. Similarly, human T cells that had been "aged" in cell culture and had characteristics identical to expanded T cell populations in the elderly (e.g,short telomeres, non-proliferative, no CD28 expression), were resistant to apoptosis and showed increased bcl2 expression. CONCLUSIONS: Aging in both humans in mice is associated with reduced T cell apoptosis, providing a possible explanation for the age-related increased proportions of non-proliferative, senescent T cells. Caloric restriction, which retards aging and extends maximum lifespan, is associated with reversal of this effect, suggesting that ongoing appropriate T cell apoptosis may be health-enhancing.

Changes in the apoptosis of polymorphonuclear granulocytes with aging: implication of signal transduction pathways and mitochondria

T. Fülöp Jr, A.C. Goulet, S. Desgeorges, N. Douziech and G. Dupuis Inst. Univ. Gériatr, Lab. Biogérontol, *Dept. Biochim, Fac. Méd, Univ. Sherbrooke, Sherbrooke, Qc, Canada*

Purpose: Apoptosis is playing an important role in several pathologies such as cancer, neurodegenerative and immune diseases. Our aim was to study the apoptosis of polymorphonuclear granulocytes (PMNLs) in aging under several stimulation. Method: PMNLs of healthy young (20-25 yrs) and elderly (65-x yrs) subjects were studied for apoptosis after 18 hours of culture without or with stimulation. The agents used were: PMA, H_2O_2, FMLP, G-CSF, GM-CSF, GSH, oxLDL, LPS, IL-2, DHEA, Vitamin C, N-acetyl-cystein (NAC). The apoptosis was assessed by DNA ladder, Giemsa staining and flow cytometric expression of Annexin V/PI. Results: It was found that without stimulation the susceptibility of PMNLs to apoptosis was slightly increased with aging. Under stimulation such as PMA, H_2O_2 the apoptosis was almost 100%, FMLP increased it also, while the other stimulants could prevent to different extent the apoptosis. Marked age-related changes were observed in the extent of apoptosis under stimulation with LPS, GM-CSF and IL2 known to rescue PMNLs apoptosis. GM-CSF was not able to rescue PMNLs of elderly from apoptosis. This seems to be related to the altered signal transduction pathway elicited by GM-CSF (Jak2 and STAT 5, MAP kinases) in PMNLs of elderly. The activation and the activity of CASPASE 1, 8 and 3 could not be modulated by GM-CSF in PMNLs of elderly subjects. The mitochondrial permeability was also altered with aging. However, caspase 9 was not activated. Thus, we demonstrated that the Jak2/STAT pathway is participating to the survival of PMNLs under GM-CSF stimulation. Moreover, this and the MAP kinase pathways are altered during healthy aging. The mitochondrial apoptotic pathway did not seem to be directly involved in the neutrophil apoptosis. Conclusion: These changes in apoptosis of PMNLs with ageing could play a role in the altered immune response with aging leading to infections, cancer and degenerative diseases

Modulatory effect of Chinese herbs on apoptosis of lymphocytes in the elderly

J.D. Liu (Beijing Hospital, Institute of Geriatrics, Beijing, China)

Purpose: To study the modulatory effect of Chinese herbs on proliferative responses and apoptosis of lymphocytes in the elderly. The lymphocytes had been co-cultured in RPMI 1640 media with extracted or synthetic effective substances of Chinese herbs for 72h. The proliferative response was measured by the MTT method. Apoptosis of lymphocytes was determined by CD95 (Fas antigen) phenotype assay, Hoechst 33342 and Propidium Iodide (PI) staining procedure, Flow Cytometry, DNA fragment analysis. It was found that Rg1 (from Ginseng) BP5 (from Pollen) and 4W (from Caterpillar Fungus) revealed significantly modulatory effect on apoptosis of lymphocytes in the elderly. Those results implicated the possibility of developing a novel antiaging immunomodulators at molecular level of immune function of lymphocytes.

SESSION 272

Comparative Care Provision Time Study of Dementia Sufferers Versus Non-dementia Sufferers

Jo Hardy (Mary Ogilvy Homes Society; Hobart, Australia); Jo Jones (Vaucluse Lodge Nursing Home, Hobart, Australia); Carolyn Wallace (Southern Cross Homes Rosary Gardens, Hobart, Australia).

Purpose: To explore the hypothesis that providing nursing care interventions within a residential care setting for dementia sufferers is more time consuming than for non-dementia sufferers. This study will attempt to quantify the actual time taken to meet care needs, thus providing firm data on which to plan for improved care delivery. Method: Participating residents were randomly selected using a primary diagnosis of dementia as the determining criteria for group A and the absence of this diagnosis for group B. Care interventions measured were those described in the Australian Department of Health and Aged Care Resident Classification Scale. Measurable care interventions were defined and passive observers recorded the time taken to deliver these over three consecutive 24-hour periods. Results: Preliminary results from this study indicate that there is a significant time differential in care provision between group A and group B. This data gives valuable evidence to improve planning for dementia care for the future given the anticipated increase in the "old old". Conclusion: This study provides firm data on which to base policy directions for both short and medium term in dementia care provision. The results have significant ramifications for issues such as carer stress, integrated or segregated care models, funding mechanisms, capital funding requirements, targeted staff education and community awareness.

Patients with Alzheimer's disease living at home: costs and consequences of the disease

C Bayle (Hopital Broca, 54 rue Pascal, 75013 Paris, France), A.S Rigaud (Hopital Broca, 54 rue Pascal, 75013 Paris, France), F Fagnani (CEMKA, 43 Boulevard du Marechal Joffre, 92340 Bourg-la-Reine, France), L Traykov (Unite INSERM 324, 2ter rue d'Alesia, 75014 Paris, France), M.L. Seux (Hôpital Broca, 54 rue Pascal, 75013 Paris, France) , O. Hanon F(Hopital Broca, 54 rue Pascal, 75013 Paris, France), F. Forette (Hopital Broca, 54 rue Pascal, 75013 Paris, France)

The objective of this retrospective longitudinal study was to assess the total costs of caring for home-based patients with mild to moderate Alzheimerss disease (AD). The study included a stratified sample of untreated AD patients (n=50). Outcome measures included the MMSE, the Katz Activities of Daily Living (ADL) scale, the Lawton Instrumental ADL (IADL) scale, the NeuroPsychiatric Inventory (NPI), the General Health Questionnaire and Zarit scale to assess caregiver burden. Sociodemographic data were recorded from structured interviews of both patients and caregivers. The Broca model contained the following parameters: patient distribution according to both age and location of care and MMSE score, mortality rate, progression of MMSE score and unit costs for accommodation and resource use as a function of MMSE score. Net costs of caring for AD patients at home were defined as additional costs incurred for AD patients compared with those of a non-AD reference elderly population living at home. There was a rapid increase in net costs associated with increasing severity of cognitive deficit. The Broca model also showed that unpaid assistance is the most costly component of the total cost of care. MMSE scores correlated strongly with functional status. Indeed, the IADL emerged as a robust indicator of the overall magnitude of behavioural, cognitive and dependence problems of the patient. Thus, these results suggest that the Broca model provides a satisfactory link between costs incurred in caring for an AD patient at home and disease severity.

Primary Care Expenditures for Newly Diagnosed Alzheimer's Disease

SM Albert, S Glied, H Andrews, R Mayeux, Y Stern (Columbia University, New York, USA)

PURPOSE: Prior research is inconsistent on whether people with Alzheimer's disease (AD) use primary care services to a greater extent than elders who do not have AD. METHOD: We investigated this question in a population-based study of Medicare enrollees in New York City, concentrating on outpatient and ambulatory care in newly identified AD cases. Medical service expenditures were identified using person-level Medicare (1996) and Medicaid (1996-98) claims. RESULTS: Compared to non-demented elders, elders diagnosed with AD for the first time were nearly three times as likely to have primary care costs in the top quartile of Medicare reimbursement (odds ratio, 2.8, 95) CONCLUSION: In this NYC sample, incident AD was associated with increased primary care needs.

The Pathos Model For Evaluation of the Level of Medical and Technical Care

Vetel Jm Ch Le Mans France Prevost P Ersm Cnam France Ducoudray Jm Probtp France Leroux R Ch Vierzon France

The PATHOS model is an information system on the care requirements necessary to ensure treatment of pathological conditions that was compiled in liaison between the French National Association and the medical department of the French National Health Insurance Organization (CNAM). It forms a complement to AGGIR The system enables : - indentification, on a pre-compiled list, of 50 « pathological conditions best summarizing the set of disease entities with which the patient presents on the day of the survey. - completion of the clinical status description by a « care requirement profile » selected from 12 possible profiles which indicates the gravity . Each pathological condition previously identified is associated with corresponding care profile, - determination of an indicator expressing the global care level for a patient to be implemented for the 8 types of identified actor of care: geriatrician, psychiatrist, nurse, physiotherapist, psychologist, biology, other examinations,.medications The data processing algorithm is complex and necessitates computerized processing. THE PATHOS INDICATOR BOARD : definition and interpretation. Comparison of these 8 indicators in two facilities makes it possible to measure the difference between the population (concerning the medico technical care and not the loss of autonomy) of each facility. In the same department, these indicators, constituted at different times, show the evaluation and evolution of the required resources as these are affected by the course of patients’ pathologies. At a later stage, studies should be undertaken with a view to standardizing the means allocated as a function of the indicators. the presentation will describe the tool and present examples.

Utilization of the Pathos Model

PREVOST P (ERSM. RENNES. FRANCE) VETEL JM (CH du MANS. LE MANS FRANCE) DUCOUDRAY JM PROBTP PARIS FRANCE LEROUX R CH de VIERZON. VIERZON FRANCE

The Pathos Model evaluates the level of medical and technical care necessary to manage the polypathologies of an elderly at a said time, at home or in institution. The Model describes a clinical situation and measures 8 indicators giving useful data for individual or group. 1- Individual level : As the AGGIR Model, Pathos is only one element of the information necessary for individual health care. It is a tool to synthetise the sanitary state of a person. 2- Collective level : As AGGIR, in its medical and technical specific domain, PATHOS is a comparison tool used for units or populations. it allows : - to help the management of units or services by describing the patients according to the evaluation of the accurate medical needs in 8 domains by comparing the resources with the national average of the National Health Department data bank for similar structures. - to allocate financial support to the structures not yet covered by satisfying medicalised information system, whether they belong to the heterogenous geriatric medical or medico social field. the Model evaluating the required care can be confronted with interest with those measuring the actual distributed care. - To elaborate the Regional Sanitary Scheme : the model provides information useful to analyse the functioning of hospital and community network, and is essential for sanitary planning in the gerontologic field. The report will describe the different level of concern of Pathos, with examples from the national data bank of the National French Health Department.

SESSION 273

Culturally Inclusive Aged Care: Features of Good Practice for Health Personnel

David Brous, (Impact Consulting Group, Melbourne, Victoria, Australia)

PURPOSE: Australian aged residential services may be inappropriate for older Australians from culturally and linguistically diverse backgrounds. By 2001, this cohort will represent 25% of the population aged 70+ years. To achieve equity, at least 22% of beds/places in the residential aged care sector should be accessed by ethnic older persons. In recent years, the formal aged care system has provided care which is consumer-focused, addressing clearly identified quality standards. Achieving these outcomes requires approaches and competencies in health personnel which move outside conceptual boundaries defining mainstream aged care. METHOD: Qualitative research was undertaken for the Australian Government's Department of Health and Aged Care to develop case studies of best practice between ethnic communities and residential care providers and to prepare a practical guide for facilities to provide culturally appropriate care to ethnic aged residents. RESULTS: Best Practice is the delivery of high quality services which effectively accounts for linguistic, cultural and religious differences and meets the needs of ethnic older people to achieve outcomes in tune with preferences and expectations. Best practice requires commitment to access, equity, and user rights strategies. These form the basis of indicators on best practice in ethnic aged care, covering planning and needs analysis, accessibility, communication, cultural relevance, individual client assessment, service coordination, cost effectiveness, participation, consultation, education, quality assurance, continuous improvement, commitment to best practice, and accountability. CONCLUSION: The paper assesses forms of best practice that should be adopted by health personnel in the provision of residential care services to aged persons from diverse cultural and linguistic backgrounds.

Improving Quality through the Peer Review Process

Netha Dyck and Wendy Whalley (Winnipeg Regional Health Authority, Winnipeg, Manitoba Canada)

The purpose of this presentation is to describe the outcomes of the Peer Review process and to present the current statistical analysis in relation to compliance with the new draft Personal Care Home (PCH) standards. The presentation will also highlight the challenges and opportunities the team encountered during development, implementation and evaluation of the Peer Review Program. The Winnipeg Regional Health Authority (WRHA) has demonstrated leadership in the development and implementation of a regional quality monitoring and improvement program for PCH services in Winnipeg. In collaboration with Manitoba Health, the WRHA has incorporated the draft provincial PCH Program standards and the CCHSA AIM standards into the quality monitoring program. The outcome data obtained from the Peer Review validates client-centred best practices and improved quality organizational performance. The Peer Review process has resulted in a strong commitment to innovation and client-centred continuous improvement.

Managing Scarcity: Case talk and decision making in multi-professional meetings

Pirjo Nikander (University of TampereDept. of Sociology and Social PsychologyTampere, Finland)

Pirjo NikanderUniversity of TampereDept. of Sociology and Social PsychologyFIN-33014 University of TampereTampereFinlandManaging Scarcity: Case talk and decision making in multi-professional meetings This paper focuses on the analysis of interactional decision making in multi-professional meetings. Using video-taped data gathered in the project: 'CONSTRUCTING AGE, HEALTH, AND COMPETENCE: Argumentation and Rhetoric in Institutional and Personal Discourse', the paper seeks to demonstrate how 'well-informed' and 'rational' professional decisions over questions of the health care of elderly clients are reached, and how issues of well-informed-ness and rationality are negotiated in everyday institutional talk.Multi-professional teamwork in the decision-making concerning the elderly is, in Finland seen as a tool for rational and well-judged administration. Meetings where decisions about a) home health-care benefits of elderly clients and b) about elderly clients' placement in nursing homes were videotaped. The analysis is based on a detailed, discursive reading of transcribed data. The analytic focus is on the multi-professional naming, sorting, and organising practices through which elderly clients are placed or declined membership in specific categories of care-recipiency. Analysing institutional discourse affords detailed understanding of how professionals accomplish their demanding work of communicating, decision-making, and reasoning. It also shows how professionals in multi-disciplinary meetings manage conflicting demands: between social and professional priorities and codes dictated mainly by economic scarcity and bureaucratic rationality, on the one hand, and notions of the client's best interest, on the other.

Team climate and organizational justice as predictors of quality of care in long-term care

Timo Sinervo (STAKES, National Research and Development Centre for Welfare and Health, Helsinki, Finland) Marko Elovainio (STAKES, National Research and Development Centre for Welfare and Health, Helsinki, Finland) Marja-Leena Perälä (STAKES, National Research and Development Centre for Welfare and Health, Helsinki, Finland)

PURPOSE: The aim of the study is to explore whether climate of work unit and organizational justice in leadership are related to quality of care in long-term care of elderly patients. Previous studies in social and health care have shown that fair treatment of employees is related to job satisfaction, turnover, job involvement and health. Furthermore, team or organizational climate has been related to organizational commitment, innovation at work and work stress. Job performance and quality of care have been associated with job involvement, organizational commitment, job satisfaction, stress and leadership. METHOD. The random sample of this study consists of the employees in 192 Finnish long-term care institutions (residential homes, health center hospitals and intensive service housing). The data were collected using two questionnaire surveys, which were linked together. The participants were head nurses, registered nurses, practical nurses and other employees of the institutions (N=1912), who were asked to evaluate their work, organization and quality of care. The data were analyzed using multi-level modelling, in order to take into account the variation between work units. RESULTS.

Preliminary results showed that both organizational justice and team climate were related to quality of care at the work unit -level. Ouality of care, team climate and organizational justice were perceived being better in smaller units. Further analyzes will be completed in spring 2001.

The Quality of Long-term Institutional Care

M.Vaarama, S.Kainulainen, M-L Perälä, T. Sinervó (Stakes, National Research and Development Center for Welfare and Health, Helsinki, Finland)

Purpose: To examine the interaction between material and non-material resources, quality of the care and client and personnel satisfaction in the long-term institutional care Method:192 public and private institutions were selected by stratified random sample. A range of quality measures were used that enable comparisons between the opinions of personnel and relatives. The data was obtained from self-completed questionnares: directors (192), chief nurses (315), care personnel (2998) and relatives of the residents (2445) of these institutions. The data was analysed in multidiciplinary design. This paper summarises the results of other designs in the production of welfare design. The main statistical method is linear regression analysis. Results: Public institutions had lower material resources than private ones. Still, they cared for most dependent clients. The majority (70 %) of institutions provided high quality care, but a third - mainly public institutions - faced problems in interaction with the elderly residents, client empowerment and inclusion of the relatives. Some evidence of low professional and ethical quality was also found. The clients, relatives and personnel were most satisfied with service housing, either public or private. Lowest quality was found in public hospital bedwards Δ even they most often had some quality assurance procedures in use. Privacy and homeliness were important for the client satisfaction, small care units for personnel. Both appreciated high professional quality, peaceful atmosphere and friendly interaction with low time pressure. Conclusion: Sufficient material resources, qualified staff and well employed non-material resources are keys to a good quality, satisfactory long term care.

SESSION 274

Comparison of Public Long term care insurance in Germany and Japan

B. Reisach,N (c) (University Witten/Herdecke, Institut of nursing science, Witten, Germany)

The Japanese long term care insurance was introduced in April 2000, five years after Germany did so. It is modelled closely after the German long term care insurance (LTCI) with some importent differences. Literature review was undertaken, five weeks research period in Japan at the women's univerity in Kochi and discussions with Japanese and German policy experts. The German LTCI compared with the Japanese differs in administration, individuals who are covered, the assessment instrument, the benefits: range, levels, amount and eligible; also in financing and premium amount. The two insurance systems have a number of things in common as well as many different features. Both countries have introduced compulsory basic coverage in view of the rising importance of long term care insurance against the backdrop of demographic developments. However the Japanese system is much more sophisticated within the classification of claims. That might be the real relief for family care givers and caretakers. In the German system dementia is not a stand alone benefit trigger, whereas in Japan dementia alone can trigger benefits. In Germany the individual must suffer from functional inability to perform the Activities of Daily Living. The entitlement to benefits generally arises in Germany later. Research is needed to clarify the question how many people become dependent of care because of this late access to benefits.

Direct Care Resource Use and Reimbursement for Cognitively Impaired Nursing Home Residents

G. Arling (Cookingham Institute, University of Missouri at Kansas City, Missouri, USA)

PURPOSE: Measure direct care resource use among cognitively impaired nursing home residents on conventional and Alzheimer's special care units in order to develop a more effective payment system through the state Medicaid program. METHOD: Resident-specific time study involving direct care staff from 54 nursing units in 26 facilities in the state of Indiana. The sample consisted of 1507 cognitively impaired and cognitively intact residents on conventional and special care units. Direct care time (minutes/day) was collected by staff type and adjusted for salary differentials between staff. Health and functional data were collected with the MDS assessment instrument. RESULTS: After adjusting statistically for resident case mix (RUG-III), there was no significant difference in direct care resource use between cognitively impaired and intact residents on conventional units. However, residents on Alzheimer's special care units had significantly greater resource use than residents on conventional units. Special care units had higher staffing, particularly nursing assistants, in relation to their resident case mix. Also, effects of cognitive impairment appeared to have been mediated by ADL limitations and medical conditions. CONCLUSION: The study raises important issues about reimbursement policy and service delivery for dementia residents. Should cognitively impaired and intact residents with similar health and functional conditions receive the same reimbursement? And, should care for dementia residents be subject to a double standard according to unit type (conventional or special care), or should services be integrated into one system of care for all dementia residents?

Interplay of Different Forces: LTC Insurance in Preparing for Retirement Years

Hyojin Kang (Cornell University, Ithaca, U.S.A.)

This study tries to analyze a planning process rather than an isolated outcome of purchase/non-purchase of long-term care (LTC) insurance to characterize multiple aspects of LTC. The purpose of this study is to compare factors related to obtaining LTC insurance with those linked to overall LTC planning for retirement years using bivariate probit model. The data is the 1st wave (1995) of Cornell Retirement and Well-being Study (grant #IT50 AG11711, Phyllis Moen). Both perceived likelihood of purchasing LTC insurance (1=100%, 0=otherwise) in retirement years and overall LTC planning for retirement years (1=plan a lot if any of three categories, 1) prepare financially 2) learn about retirement or health insurance options 3) consider different housing arrangements, 0=otherwise) are used as dependent variables. Respondent's caregiving experience explains both dependent variables significantly though whether a respondent has provided care is negatively related to overall planning unlike in the case of LTC insurance. In contrast, whether a respondent is currently providing care is positively related to overall planning only. Other characteristics like age, health status, residence area, type of residence, and income explained either LTC insurance or overall planning significantly. Results of this study suggest that there exist more aspects to consider other than coverage against costs in planning how to finance LTC in retirement years. In particular, family structure in the context of caregiving status seems to play an important role. Developing alternatives to LTC insurance is recommended to recognize overall LTC planning as well as outcome of LTC insurance.

Technically Immature and Inappropriate Assessment to Classify the Benefits of Japanese Long-Term Care Insurance

H. Sumii (Hiroshima Prefectural College of Health and Welfare), S. Hashimoto (Hokumo Clinic), K. Miyake, M. Hidaka, S. Kasahara, M. Kunisada, M.Oba, T. Arimura, H. Hashizume (Japan Kaigo Research)

Japanese long-term care insurance system since April 2000 determined the level of insurance benefits. The insured person must be assessed and classified into six stages (from I to VI), before provided them. This study checked the reliability of the determination system. Method: With 60 model samples from public recognition guideline, the similarity, discretion and the influence of their stages examined by the judgment software program (http://www3.wind.ne.jp/hassii/kaigo/win32/josyu32.lzh) with A.I.mode. Similar models revealed the combination of matching (>80%), distance (<30), and the difference of middle evaluation score (<40). The number of reverse-correlation models, which are changed their stages with the two items alteration of 73 questions were checked. Results: The models of similar stages existed together in view of matching, the distances, and the difference, especially among from I to III or from V to VI stages. The discretion of the stages from I to III is especially uncertain. The reverse-worse phenomenon that as the disability get better, as the stages get worse at V stage (one item change:8 cases, two item change: 636 cases) next at IV stage(one : 3 cases, two : 99 cases), and the reverse-better phenomenon that as the disability get worse, as the stages get better at II stage (one : 49 cases, two : 4290 cases) next at VI stage (one:12 cases, two:721 cases) were detected. The alteration with positive-worse at I stage (28767 cases), next II stage (9059 cases), and the alteration with negative-better at VI stage (2994 cases), next V stage (2816 cases) were recognized. Conclusion: This study revealed that the recognition system would be technically immature and inappropriate to classify the risk of the long-term care. The main failures were caused by the reasons that the inappropriate nursing times were calculated through statistical tree analysis by 73 investigation questions, which are only based on their physical and mental conditions, in addition neither the family situation nor their need of the long-term care services were reviewed for this assessment system.

The effect of public long-term care insurance plan on care management and care planning

Joji Onishi, Yuichiro Masuda, Masafumi Kuzuya, Kazumasa Uemura1), and Akihisa Iguchi Department of Geriatrics and 1; Third Department of Internal Medicine, Nagoya University Graduate School of Medicine Nagoya, Japan

Purpose: The purpose of this study was to examine the change in knowledgeability on the side of managers of Japanese geriatric hospitals regarding 1) the concept of care-management as the methodology to supply care services to the elderly smoothly, and 2) comprehensive assessment for the elders as the technical skill in the process of materializing care-management. Method: (Design) Subjects were interviewed and inquired over telephone according to structural questionnaire. (Subjects) Managers (directors and office managers) of geriatric hospitals in 1996 and 1999. Results: In 1996, the rate of knowledgeability for care-management on the side of managers of geriatric hospitals was 70.0%(28/40) as a whole. It increased to be 97.3%(71/73) in 1999. With regard to MDS-RAPs, knowledgeability rate increased from 57.5%(23/40) of 1996 to 95.9%(70/73) of 1999. However, regarding care-planning, almost all of the hospitals which performed care-planning were those in the category required to submit care plans to the municipal government. At geriatric hospitals which were not required to submit such plans, they did not perform such planning neither in 1996 nor 1999. Conclusions: It can be concluded that the decision to introduce long-term care insurance system in Japan led to deeper understanding for methodology of care-management and comprehensive assessment on the side of managers of geriatric hospitals.

SESSION 275

Adherence to Nasal Continuous Positive Airway Pressure (nCPAP) in Geriatric Patients with Obstructive Sleep Apnea (OSA)

Helmut Frohnhofen, Bernhard J. Hoeltmann** (* Department of Geriatric Medicine, Prosper Hospital, Recklinghausen, Germany ** Department of Geriatric Medicine, General Hospital, Grevenbroich, Germany)*

Introduction: Only a minority of geriatric patients with symptomatic obstructive sleep apnea (OSA) accept nCPAP therapy. As the adherence to this expensive therapy in geriatric pateints is unknown, we investigated prospectively therapy adherence in geriatric patients with initial acceptance of nCPAP and compared it with the adherence of consecutive non geriatric OSA patients admitted to our sleep laboratory for treatment of OSA. Methodes and Results: We included 26 geriatric pateints (69±9y) and 59 sleep lab patients (56±9y, p<0,01). Both groups did not differ in OSA severity (Respiratory Disturbance Index RDI 41±13/h vs. 43±21/h), Sleepiness (Epworth Sleepiness Scale ESS 11±3 vs. 11±4) or initial nCPAP preassure necessary (10±3 mbar vs. 9± 2 mbar). After 30±25 weeks 13 (54%) of the geriatric patients and 29 (45%) of the sleep lab patients were found to be compliant Δ characterized by use of the device every night for more than 4 h per night. The daily use of nCPAP was sig. correlated to the difference in the hypersomnia score (ESS) in sleep lab patients and showed a trend in geriatric patients (p< 0,03; r= 0,29 vs. P< 0,06; r= 0,42). There were no correlations between daily use of nCPAP and other variables in both groups. Conclusions: Adherence to therapy with nCPAP in geriatric patients is comparable with the adherence to nCPAP therapy in sleep lab patients. The improvement of sleepiness seems to be the most important predictor of therapy adherence in both patient groups.

Age-related differences of serum melatonin in men age from 31 to 95 years old.

*Zi-Yan Zhao, Yue-Rong Fu, Yi Xie, Yu-Yang Li, Xin-Hua Li, Jian-Ping Liu, Fang-Hong Lu and Yvan Touitou (Shandong Academy of Medical Sciences, Jinan, P.R. China and * Faculty of Medicine Pitie-Salpetriere, Paris, France)*

It has been documented that night plasma melatonin secretion declined with age. However, there were results recently that did not support this point. In this present study, we examined serum melatonin in 88 men aged from 31 to 95 years old. METHOD: in 25 healthy men aged 30s, 40s, 50s and 60s year old, blood samples were drawn for a 24-h period at 2-h intervals from 8:00 to 22:00 and hourly from 22:00 to 8:00; and in 63 men, both healthy and patients, aged from 60 to 95 years old, samples were drawn at 08:00 and 02:00. RESULTS: Circadian pattern of serum melatonin was similar in the four healthy age groups (30s, 40s, 50s and 60s), with a peak at midnight and very low level during daytime. There was no significant difference among these groups. The 02:00 serum melatonin levels showed significant decline with age (P < 0.01), especially in men >70 years old, while there were no significant differences when comparing healthy persons with patients suffering mainly from hypertension, ischemic coronary heart diseases or the two diseases combined. The 08:00 serum melatonin levels showed no difference with aging and diseases. CONCLUSION: our results confirmed circadian melatonin rhythm, and the decline of night melatonin levels with aging, whereas it failed to show any significant influence of hypertension and ischemic heart diseases on night melatonin levels.

Beneficial Effect of Controlled Release Melatonin on Sleep Quality and Hemoglobin A1C in Type 2 Diabetic Patients

*D. Garfinkel , J. Wainstein, A. Halabe, Z. Matas (*Department of Medicine Diabetic Unit and ^Biochemistry Laboratory, The E. Wolfson Medical Center, Holon 58100), M. Laudon (Neurim Pharmaceuticals Ltd, Tel Aviv), N. Zisapel (Department of Neurobiology, Tel Aviv University, Tel Aviv) (Israel)*

PURPOSE: To evaluate the effect of Controlled Release Melatonin (CRM) on sleep quality, and on glucose and lipid metabolism in Type 2 diabetics. METHODS: In a randomized, double-blind crossover basis, 38 Type 2 diabetics (11 men, 27 women, age 46-77 years) who complained of insomnia, were given either 2mg of CRM (CIRCADIN,Neurim Pharmaceuticals,Tel-Aviv, Israel) or a placebo for 3 weeks. Following one week of placebo to all subjects (wash out), patients who had received CRM were given placebo and vise versa for another 3 weeks. Quality of sleep was assessed by wrist-actigraphy for 3 consecutive nights at the end of each 3 week treament period. At baseline and at the end of each treatment period, we assessed fasting glucose, fructosamine, insulin, C-peptide, triglycerides, cholesterol (total, HDL and LDL) as well as some antioxidants (malone dialdehyde, conjugated diens, catalase, gluthatione peroxidase and reductase). The long term effect on Hemoglobin A1C (HbA1C), was evaluated by measuring HbA1C levels before and after 6 months of 2mg CRM treatment; these latter tests were performed in another group of 34 type 2 diabetics. RESULTS: CRM induced a significant improvement in sleep efficiency (a 3.6% increase, $F(1,21) = 4.53$, $p<.05$), a 38.6% decrease in wakes after sleep onset ($F(1,21) = 9.32$, $p<.01$), and a 33.3% decrease in the number of awakenings ($F(1,21) = 10.7$, $p<.01$). CRM had no significant effect on the laboratory tests including serum glucose, fructosamine, insulin, C-peptide, or antioxidant levels. However, following 6 months of 2mg CRM, a decrease was observed in HbA1C concentrations ($p=0.04$), the effect being even more significant ($p=0.01$) in diabetics who had HbA1C levels above the median. CONCLUSION: Controlled release melatonin 2mg improves sleep quality in type 2 diabetic insomniacs and also has a beneficial effect on HbA1C, particularly in patients with unsatisfactory diabetes control.

Melatonin Effectively Facilitates Benzodiazepine Discontinuation in Patients with Sleep Disturbances

N. Zisapel (Department of Neurobiochemistry, Tel Aviv University,Tel Aviv), J.Wainstein (Diabetes Unit, The Wolfson Medical Center, Holon), M. Laudon (Neurim Pharmaceuticals Ltd. Tel Aviv), D. Garfinkel (Aging Research and Department of Internal Medicine E, The Wolfson Medical Center, Holon and Maccabi Healthcare Services) Israel.iv), Israel.

BACKGROUND and PURPOSE: Benzodiazepine (BZD) users frequently develop dependency and may experience rebound insomnia when trying to discontinue the drug. Paradoxxically, though BZD are widely prescribed for insomnia, they were found to suppress nocturnal production of melatonin. This pineal-product is involved in the regulation of the sleep/wake cycle and in the promotion of good sleep. We have previously found that in elderly insomniacs including those treated with BZD, melatonin replacement therapy significantly imprroves sleep quality. We assessed whether melatonin administration could facilitate BZD discontinuation in patients suffering from insomnia. METHODS: In a double blind design, 34 BZD users received either 2 mg of Controlled - Release Melatonin (CRM - CircadinTM, Neurim Pharmaceuticals, Israel) or a placebo, nightly for six weeks. Patients were encouraged to reduce their usual BZD dose by 50% on week 2, to 25% for weeks 3 & 4 and discontinue the BZD completely for weeks 5 & 6. . Later, CRM was administered for another 6 weeks to all subjects and BZD discontinuation attempts resumed. BZD consumption and the subjective sleep quality scores were reported daily and all patients were all allowed to continue taking CRM. RESULTS: By the sixth week 14/18 subjects receiving CRM discontinued BZD use, as compared to only 4/16 in the placebo group ($p = .006$). Furthermore, in spite of the higher rate of BZD discontinuation, sleep quality scores were higher in those receiving CRM as compared to the placebo group ($p=0.04$). Following another 6 weeks on CRM, six additional subjects of the placebo group discontinued BZD. After more than one year of follow-up, almost 80% of the patients who had stopped taking BZD using CRM, continue to do so while maintaining a good quality of sleep. CONCLUSION: Controlled-Release Melatonin may effectively facilitate discontinuation of benzodiazepines while maintaining good quality of sleep. .

Palliative Oxygen Therapy and Cognitive Functions in Elderly Patients with Stroke and Obstructive Sleep Apnea

Bernhard J. Hoeltmann, Helmut Frohnhofen** (* Department of Geriatric Medicine, General Hospital, Grevenbroich, Germany **Department of Geriatric Medicine, Prosper Hospital, Recklinghausen, Germany)*

Introduction: Obstructive sleep apnea (OSA) and cognitive impairment are frequent in elderly stroke survivors. Treatment of OSA with nasal continuous positive airway preassure breathing (nCPAP) is refused by the majority of elderly patients. We studied the impact of palliative noctural oxigen therapy on cognitve function in elderly patients with recent stroke and OSA who refused nCPAP. Methodes: 29 concious stroke patients with proven OSA (polysomnography) and moderate handycap (Barthel Index >50) were randomly assigned to receive 3l/min (group 1, n=15, 72±8y) or 0.5l/min (group 2, n=14, 69±6y) nocturnal oxigen by a face mask. LPS50+ and AKT two validated German tests for multiple cognitive functions were performend at the beginning of the study and after one week of treatment. Results: Patients of group 1 improved significantly in 5 of 12 subtests (visual cognitive functions, word fluency, spatial recognition) and in the mean total score of LPS50+ and in perceptual speed of the AKT. Patients of group 2 improved in one subtest of LPS50+. Conclusion: Our results confirm a causal relationship between nocturnal hypoxemia and daytime cognitive function in elderly patients with OSA and ischemic stroke. Further studies are warrented to clarify the benefits of longterm oxigen therapy in these patients.

SESSION 277

Disability in Asian Developing Countries

S. Ebrahim (Department of Social Medicine, University of Bristol, UK) Disability, health and social policy in south-east Asia, P. Srinivas (Gleneagles Medical Centre, Penang, Malaysia) Appropriate services for Asian developing countries: community and hospital models of geriatric care, S. Ebrahim (Department of Social Medicine, University of Bristol, UK) Demographic trends and medical training, S. Jitapunkul (Faculty of Medicine, Chulalongkorn University, Bangkok, Thailand) Appropriate research on disability for Asian developing countries.

This symposium adresses the situation and strategic actions toward disability among the elderly population in Asian developing countries with particular emphasis on Southeast Asian countries. The focus of this session is the prevalence, type and burden or impact of disbility; appropriate health and social policy; appropriate models of community and hospital services for geriatric care; need of medical training; and research which is essential and appropriate for developing countries. Content: Worldwide, the proportion of people aged 60 years and over is growing faster than any other age group. Global aging will put increased economic and social demands on all countries. Most of these old people live in developing countries and their numbers will continue to rise at a far more rapid rate than in developed contries. In terms of regions, the majority of the world's older people live in Asia. The rapid speed of population aging in developing countries has not allowed socioeconomic development to keep pace. Meeting the challenges of population aging will require innovative planning and substantive policy reforms in developing countries, most of which do not yet have comprehensive policies on aging. As nations industrialize, their economic progress is inevitably accompanied by a shift from communicable to noncommunicable diseases. Chronic diseases not only kill; they are significant and costly causes of disability and reduced quality of life. The likelihood of experiencing major disabilities dramatically increases in very old age. But disabilities associated with aging can be prevented or delayed. Policy makers and doners must act now by putting policies, programmes and intersectoral partnerships into place that can help to halt the massive expansion of chronic noncommunicable diseases. National policy has to be comprehensive and relevant to this situation and should aim toward security in old age, promoting good health and independence of the elderly population, and maintaining an attitude in society of family support for the elderly and non-formal care. Asian developing countries must concentrate on the development of effective models integrating social and medical interventions with various dimensions of care. Appropriate medical services for geriatric patients both in communities and institutions are essential. These services have to comply with the cultural and socioeconomic status of each country, which may be different from those existing in developed countries. Thus, education and training for health and social personnel are also required. Due to resource scarcity, it is essential for Asian developing countries to conduct research which will mostly benefit their own people. Disease-by-disease biomedical research should not be emphasized. Research which concentrates on independence maintainance and disability prevention must be of central interest. Conclusion: In the 21th century, population aging is one of the biggest challenges facing Asian developing countries, where rapid aging is accompanied by rapid changes in socioeconomic circumstances and disease patterns. There is an urgent need for these countries to have comprehensive policy, innovative planning and collaborative actions to meet these challenges.

Appropriate research on disability for Asian developing countries

S. Jitapunkul (Faculty of Medicine, Chulalongkorn University, Bangkok, Thailand)

Asian developing countries are in a transitional period of being an aging society. Although their people live longer, it seems that the extension of life is in bad rather than good health. Because of resource scarcity, it is essential for Asian developing countries to conduct research which will mostly benefit their own people. Disease-by-disease biomedical research should not be emphasized. Research concentrating on independence maintainance and disability prevention must be of central interest. Disability researchs in the elderly population should cover the following areas: 1. Natural course of functional capacity 2. Type, size, trends and consequences/burden of disability 3. Causes and risk factors of disability especially those that are preventable or modificable 4. How to maintain or slow declining of functional capacity 5. How to prolong contribution to the society by the elderly population 6. Implications of public policy. All of the above aim to help the elderly to remain healthy and independent and continue to play an active role in their society. That is the ultimate goal - "SUCCESSFUL AGING"

Appropriate services for Asian developing countries: Community and hospital models of geriatric care

P. Srinivas (Gleneagles Medical Centre, Penang, Malaysia)

The purpose of the presentation is to review the geriatric services in a developing Asian country-Malaysia. Rapid socioeconomic development in Malaysia has brought improvements in life expectancy with declining mortality rates leading to an ageing population. In 2000 the proportion of the older persons aged 65 years and above is 4.2% of the total population but by 2020, the aged above 65 years will comprise 6.1% of the total projected population of 33.7 million. The Ist phase of the National Health Programme for Older Persons was implemented from 1997 till 2000. Pilot projects on community based care of the elderly have been successfully launched in the districts of Bentong, Karak, Kuala Keda and Kubang Pasu. An acute Geriatric Assessment unit (30 bedded) with a adjoining rehabilitation ward has been established at the University Malaya Medical Centre, Kuala Lumpur. A 12 bedded Geriatric Unit with a day care centre is functioning at the Seremban General Hospital. Improvement of existing links between hospital and community services is being achieved. Conclusion: The Health Programme for older persons in Malaysia has a strong disease prevention and health promotion component with considerable community and NGO participation. Programme implementation has been rapid and now emphasis is on a phase of consolidation where programme evaluation and a review of important interventions needed is ongoing. The increasing aged dependency ratio in Malaysia will maintain the impetus for further development of appropriate services for the elderly.

Demographic trends and medical training

S. Ebrahim (Department of Social Medicine, University of Bristol, UK)

Background The demographic trends in most countries of the world are raising concerns about how best to train doctors for the future. In developing countries, many doctors and nurses will find better job opportunities overseas. This raises questions about the relevance of "needs-related" medical curricula in an increasingly global market for health professionals. The following points will be discussed: - Increasing sub-specialisation in medicine produces doctors who are unable to deal with the complexity of multiple pathology found in most older people. - Undergraduate medical education reforms are forcing specific training in geriatric medicine out of the curriculum. - Postgraduate education requires reorganisation - including mandatory attachments in geriatric medicine - to ensure that all doctors are capable of managing elderly patients appropriately. - Globalisation of employment for doctors and nurses means that curricula in developing countries may not meet the needs of those who practice in post-industrialised countries. - Traditional medical careers are changing so that many doctors will need to gain new skills and consider career changes over the course of their lives.

Disability, health and social policy in south-east Asia

S. Ebrahim (Department of Social Medicine, University of Bristol, UK)

Background. In south-east Asia demographic trends are advanced, resulting in an ageing population which raises many questions. What impact will this have on disability levels? How will health and social services cope? Will the family continue to look after elderly people? How can affordable care to alleviate disability and suffering among frail elderly people best be organised? Methods Appointed country experts in ageing and health care for elderly people were appointed by ASEAN and a regional advisor performed a series of visits to each country to assess the situtation of frail elderly people. Demographic data were complied from United Nations Year Books and additional information was obtained from reports of ad hoc studies and published work. Results The family was regarded as the major foundation of support for frail elderly people in all ASEAN countries. It was frequently stated that the family role should not be supplanted by community-based services, but that existing traditions of filial respect and social integration of elderly people should be built upon. Relevant social policies that would aid family support are: pensions, housing for extended families, caring and disability allowances, disability-friendly public transport, respite care and organisations for elderly people. In addition to these, health policies that might be helpful include free primary health care for frail elderly people and their carers, specialist geriatric medicine and psychogeriatric services, community rehabilitation programmes, nursing homes and training for family care-givers. Few of these policies have been adopted universally be all ASEAN countries, reflecting their diversity. The more developed countries of the region (Brunei, Malaysia, Philippines, Singapore, Thailand) were more likely to have implemented policies on tax relief for carers, caring allowances, subsided travel, and respite care. These countries were also more likely to have geriatric and/or psychogeriatric services. Conclusions ASEAN now comprises countries as diverse as the Union of Myanmar, the Peoples Republic of Laos and Singapore, so no one "formula" for family support and community care will be found. However, it is clear that many of the policies currently in place do not support familes and run counter to caring for frail elderly people at home. More attention should be given to policy analysis for its impact on family support in countries undergoing rapid social and demongraphic transitions. Investments in training, research, information exchange, service development and expansion, and new legislation will all be required to support families and meet the challenges of ASEAN's ageing population.

SESSION 278

Association between Nutritional Risk and Falls among Frail Older Adults

C. Shanthi Johnson (School of Nutrition and Food Science, Acadia University, Wolfville, Nova Scotia & Canadian Centre for Activity and Aging, London, Ontario, Canada).

PURPOSE: The purpose was to examine the association between the level of nutritional risk and falls among frail older adults. METHOD: This retrospective study involved 96 frail older adults with a mean age of 82 years. Nutritional risk was measured using the Nutrition Screening Initiative's Determine Checklist. For this study, falls was defined as ending up on the floor or ground unintentionally. The incidence of falls in the last four months along with the frequencies and nature of falls were recorded. Other factors related to falls such as age, gender, health problems, medication use were assessed using a series of questions. RESULTS: The results showed that 26 percent of older adults had suffered falls. Both fallers and non-fallers were similar in terms of age, prevalence of self-reported health problems and medications use (p>0.05). However, the level of nutritional risk among fallers was higher compared to non-fallers (score = 5.7 vs 4.8; p<0.05). Regression analysis showed that the level of nutritional risk predicted falls among the frail elderly (p<0.05). CONCLUSION: The findings suggest that the level of nutritional risk is a risk factor for falls among frail older adults. However, falls prevention initiatives seldom include nutritional strategies. The results of the present study provide impetus to address nutrition and dietary issues in falls prevention interventions and strategies.

Evaluation of the Home Falls and Accidents Screening Tool (HOME FAST)

L.Mackenzie, J.Byles, N.Higginbotham (Centre for Clinical Epidemiology and Biostatistics, University of Newcastle, Newcastle, NSW, Australia)

PURPOSE: To describe the development and evaluation of a concise home safety screening tool designed to detect older people at high risk of falls, trips and accidents. METHOD: A review of published home safety tools, field-testing of pooled items and an expert panel selected the items for the HOME FAST. Content and construct validity were appraised using expert opinion from 142 health professionals. An inter-rater reliability study (n=40 raters) was conducted. A prospective study (n=129) was used to establish the predictive validity of the HOME FAST using sensitivity data and ROC curves. RESULTS: 25 items were associated with the falls history of the field-test participants. Using a version of Thurstone scaling, all items were considered to be contributors to increased risk of falls by experts. Factor analysis of the scores allocated for each HOME FAST item revealed the factors of function and physical environment underpinned expert perceptions of the dimension of home safety. Inter-rater reliability kappa scores were acceptable (item kappa scores .40-.80). ROC curves indicated that the HOME FAST was better than chance in predicting those at risk of falls (area under curve = 0.67). Use of a weighted hazard score or a hazard count yielded similar results. CONCLUSION: The HOME FAST has been evaluated as a screening tool for falls. As home hazards are only one aspect of the multi-factorial nature of falls in older people, further work needs to be done to investigate the predictive validity of the HOME FAST in combination with other important risk factors.

Falls and Visual Function among Community-dwelling Elderly People

N. Niino, H. Nomura, R. Kozakai, Y. Fukukawa, F. Ando, H. Shimokata (National Institute for Longevity Sciences, Aichi, Japan), H. Sugimori (St.Mrianna Univ, Kanagawa, Japan), S. Yasumura (Fukushima Med Univ, Fukushima, Japan), H. Haga (Tohoku Bunka Gakuen Univ, Miyagi, Japan), N. Nishihara (Hamamatsu Health Care Center, Shizuoka, Japan)

Purpose: Falls are one of the major health problems among the elderly because of the frequency and the physical, psychological and social consequences. The purpose of the present study was to investigate the relationship of visual function to the incidence of falls among community-dwelling elderly people. Method: Four hundred and seventeen people living in Hamamatsu City of Shizuoka Prefecture in Japan participated in this study. They consisted of 160 males and 257 females; the mean ages were 73.4 and 73.8 years. At the beginning of the study (August 1999), visual function including near vision, distant vision, kinetic vision, and stereoscopic vision was measured. Information on age, gender, physical and mental health status were also obtained. In August 2000, a survey on falls was conducted. The association between visual function and falls was analyzed using chi-square test and multiple logistic regression analysis. Results: During the 1-year study period, 87 people (20.9%) experienced at least one fall. The proportion of fallers was significantly higher among females (24.1%) than males (15.6%). Out of four types of visual function, low distant vision (<0.3) was significantly associated with falling by chi-square test (p<0.05). After adjusting for age, gender, physical and mental health, low distant vision remained a significant predictor of falls (p<0.05). Conclusion: Low distant vision was a significant and independent predictor of falls among community-dwelling elderly people.

Falls in elderly: An investigation into contributing factors

Yun, Hong (Department of Occupational Therapy, Tan Tock Seng Hospital, Singapore), Lynette, Soo Ping, Sim (Department of Rehabilitation Services, Changi General Hospital, Singapore)

The elderly population has recently been the focus of increased attention in the local healthcare arena. However, research into falls remain in its infancy. With their specialized skills and holistic philosophy, occupational therapists can play an invaluable role in establishing the knowledge base of this emerging health problem. The literature indicates there existed a wide array of factors contributing to falls in older persons. Furthermore, a majority of studies into falls in elderly had reported dire consequences following a fall, including a fear of falling and self-imposed immobility. A descriptive cross-sectional study was undertaken to determine the circumstances of falls in elderly people in Singapore, the consequences of the fall as well as feelings towards the falling episode. Participants were a convenience sample of elderly people who were admitted to a community hospital following a fall in the past year. Self-report data of the falling episode as well as other relevant information were obtained using a semi-structured interview questionnaire that comprised of open and closed questions. Data were analyzed and summarized using descriptive statistics and content analysis. The results indicated that the participants possessed certain risk factors associated with falling. The findings also suggested that falls were related to the dynamic interaction between personal, environmental and situational factors. This thus supported the emerging view that falls are complex events with multifactorial antecedents. Besides injuries, psychological and functional consequences were also prevalent. Other important areas of concern included views on home modification and mobility aids.

Musculoskeletal pain and falls in older women

SG Leveille (Hebrew Rehabilitation Center for Aged, Boston, MA) J Bean (Hebrew Rehabilitation Center for Aged, Boston, MA) JM Guralnik (National Institute on Aging, Bethesda, MD)

Many older women have pain in multiple musculoskeletal regions. It is unknown whether musculoskeletal pain and, specifically, widespread pain, places elders at risk for falls and fall-related fractures. To examine the risk for falls due to musculoskeletal pain, we studied 1002 women aged 65 and older living in the East Baltimore area. Participants in the Women's Health and Aging Study, representing the one-third of women living at home with disabilities, were followed semi-annually for 3 years beginning in 1991. Of the 935 women who participated in at least one follow-up examination and had complete information, 39 0.000000ell in first year, 36 0n year 2, and 39 0n year 3. After adjusting for several major risk factors for falls, women with widespread pain had an increased likelihood of falling during follow-up (adjusted OR = 1.60, 95%C.I. 1.21, 2.13) compared to those with none or mild pain in only 1 musculoskeletal site. Women who had moderate to severe lower extremity pain but not widespread pain also had an increased risk of falls (adjusted OR=1.39, 95%C.I. 1.07-1.81). Among women with musculoskeletal pain, risk for falls was lower in those who used daily analgesic medication. Risks for recurrent falls and fractures due to falls were also elevated in women with musculoskeletal pain, and most consistently among women with widespread pain. Musculoskeletal pain, particularly widespread pain, in older women is a substantial risk factor for falls and requires further attention by researchers and clinicians.

Prediction of recurrent falls in vertebral osteoporotic women: a cohort study

T.Masud, R.O.Morris, R.Baker, E.J.Bassey (Clinical Gerontology Research Unit, City Hospital, Nottingham, UK)

Vertebral osteoporosis subjects have an increased risk of peripheral fractures, particularly if they are recurrent fallers. Identification of fall risk is important allowing targeted intervention. This study aimed to identify simple clinical tests, which can predict recurrent fallers. Women with at least one vertebral fracture were studied prospectively. The following tests were performed at baseline and 12 months: Geriatric Depression Score (GDS), Abbreviated Mental Test Score (AMTS), postural sway, ability to rise from a chair without using arms, "get up and go test' (GUAGT), tandem walk, time to walk 10 metres, number of steps to turn 180 degrees (STEPTURN), leg extensor power and blood pressure drop on standing. Demographic details and fall history were recorded. Telephone interviews were conducted at intervals to record fall episodes. 104 women, mean age 78±7, range 63-91 years were studied. 86 (82.7%) completed follow up. 18 of 86 (20.9%) reported 2 or more falls during follow-up. Logistic regression analysis showed that a history of recurrent falls (/2 falls) in the preceding year (r=0.30, p=0.002), GUAGT (r=0.27, p=0.035), STEPTURN (r=0.23, p=0.011), timed 10m walk (r=0.2, p=0.019), sway (r=0.15, p=0.035) and the AMTS (r=-1.16, p=0.037) were significantly associated with recurrent falls. The GUAGT and a history of recurrent falls in the preceding year remained significantly associated with recurrent falls in multivariate analysis. In conclusion, the "get up and go test" in combination with a history of recurrent falling may prove useful as simple clinical predictors of recurrent falling amongst elderly women with vertebral osteoporosis.

The heterogeneous nature of falls among older adults: Identifying the need for differing intervention strategies

P.Raina (University of British Columbia, Vancouver, BC Canada T. Lipskie (Health Canada, Ottawa, ON Canada) K. Turcotte (University of British Columbia, Vancouver, BC Canada)

Abstract Purpose: The reasons for heterogeneity of injuries resulting from falls among older adults must be understood to inform prevention. The circumstances, nature and the severity of fall related injuries seen in emergency department were examined to understand the heterogeneity among adults 45 years or older.Methods: Data were extracted from the Canadian Hospitals Injury Reporting and Prevention Program (CHIRPP) database for falls (slip/trip/fall) related injuries and if the person was 45 years or older. The sample was divided into two age groups, older adults (45-64; n=1454) and seniors (65+; n=1396). Analyses were done to describe the falls related injuries between and within these age groups.Results: Falls, as a proportion of all CHIRPP injuries, increased steadily with advancing age. The most common location was "home (37.6% for 45-64; 44.3% for seniors), second being "road/ground" (9.5%) for older adults and "nursing homes" (11.3%) for seniors. "Body movements" was the most common activity when falls occurred for two groups (45.1% for older adults and 51.8% for seniors), followed by "occupation" (13.5%) for older adults and "household activities" (8.0%) for seniors. The top three for older adults were "ice/snow" (22.4%), "stairs" (14.3%), and "fell off something" (12.2%). The top three for seniors were "walking" (15.0%), "stairs" (13.0%), and "ice/snow" (10.9%). The number of "injuries" was similar between two groups, however severity of injury varied between the groups with 17.7% older adults and 35.6% seniors being admitted to hospital. Conclusions: Heterogeneity in the circumstances and outcomes related to falls suggest targeted approach to prevention.

SESSION 280

A Day In The Life Of A Healthy 92 Year Old Man

J. Strenger, J. Hanczik, Hungarian Association of Gerontology; Budapest, Hungary Retina Workshop;Szigetvár, Hungary

- Brief description of content: We want to show the epigenetic aspect of our case. I.N, a 92 year old man who is in exceptional physical and mental health. He gave his conscent to video presentation. He was followed through an out patients appointment and is annual check-up. He also completed a questionnare. In this film he is captured performing his daily routine of living in his 4 room flat in Pécs, Hungary. And lot of his daytime activities . He lives alone and is completely independent and talks freely about the wide range of his life experiencies. He was born into a good family the youngest of 8. During World War I. the family was ruined. When he was 12 he witnessed his father committing suicide. He had to work hard every day as a Jack-of-all-trades. Also during this time the young István become a diving and gymnastics champion, much admired by the young ladies as an Adonis. In 1943 he suffered a gangrenous perforated appendicitis, and spent 1.5 years in hospital, in the meantime he tried to help save the life of one of his sisters husband. He become a portrait sculptor and presented one to Pope John Paul II. He then became the fine arts advisor to the University of Pécs. And finally in August 2000. received a Knighthood from the Order of Saint István. In the near future we would like to test his anti-oxidative status and molecular genetic structure.

Bernice

Terry Coles, (Maple Lake Releasing, Winnipeg, Manitoba, Canada)

A psychological portrait of the choices women face as they age. Bernice has two role-models, her embittered Aunt and a client who embraces age. Bernice has lessons to learn from both of them.

The Other Side

Terry Coles, (Maple Lake Releasing, Winnipeg, Manitoba, Canada)

Four families share initimate stories of becoming caregivers. The Other Side is a twenty minute video examining the issues that people face when someone close to them has had a stroke. After teaching art for many years to a stroke recovery group at Central Neighbourhood House in Toronto, Laurel Angeloff was moved to make a film about the caregivers of her students. Five different caregivers talk candidly about the issues and emotional decisions they had to make, their struggles and triumphs. This short but intimate film strikes a chord with anyone who has faced this challenge

The Research Program on the Phenomena of Longevity and Georgian Longevities

Simon Dalakishvili(Academy of Sciences of Georgia, Tbilisi,CIS Georgia)

The video describes the history of study of the phenomena of longevity by the Problem Council of Gerontology and Geriatrics at the Presidium of Georgian Academy of Sciences and the experimental teamwork carried out with the scientific centers of the U.S.A, England, Czechoslovakia and Japan. It considers the role of medical, biological, economical, social and psychological factors in the formation of the phenomena of longevity. It represents the ideas of individuals aged 100 and more concerning the issues of reaching the longevity.

SESSION 281

Changing Demography, Faster Ageing and Economic Shifts in South-Asian Region: Are they Mutually Supportive?

Moneer ALAM (Institute of Economic Growth, Delhi, India)

Abstract: Not so uniformly, but most of South Asia is transitioning - both economically and demographically. In many ways, however, these transitions and their emanating changes may not be mutually compatible. To specify, while demographically mediated changes in the region would accelerate ageing and adulthood, liberalization and market driven shifts may cause them to suffer from expenditure compressions, labour market issues, rising age dependencies, old age poverty, inadequate social securities, etc. This study addresses to some of these issues with a focus on ageing and its ramifications for India and its neighborhood. This articulation, inter alia, postulates:· declining non-adult, rapid ageing, growing "old old", · low income levels and restricted familial abilities for elderly support,· bulging of labour market, · low health standards, · missing old age security, etc. Drawing upon the trends in macro parameters and other analytical evidences, we observe that changes in age composition remain a dormant issue in most ongoing economic formulations in the region. An illustration may be the deceleration in (quality) employment followed by unceasing trade and financial liberalization. Informalisation and insecurity of labour are other critical issues. Arguably, this phenomenon lacks conformity with the region's bulging population in working ages. Loss of conformity may further be noted from the neglect for rampant ageing and its ramifications - particularly for impoverished, low-income households. Given these, the study concludes by stressing the need to recognize the risks of economic-demographic incompatibilities in the region. It also attempts to identify options for mobilizing resources to finance social and health security for the aged.

Developing Master plan for Korean Elderly's Wellbeing through Construction of Welfare Infrastructure in 21th Century

Mee-Hye Kim (Department of Social Welfare, Ewha Womans University, Seoul, Korea)

The major purposes of this study are 1) to conceptualize the welfare infrastructure for Korean elderly; 2) to develop a research framework for the analysis of the welfare infrastructure; 3) to analyze the existing welfare infrastructure; and 4) to suggest the future direction for the development of a master plan designed to promote Korean elderly's quality of life in 21th Century. This research is based on literature review and analyses of secondary data on the policies and programs for Korean elderly. In this study, the concept of the welfare infrastructure is defined as the foundation of welfare, based upon which policies and programs can be effectively implemented and the benefits from those can be distributed equitably. Five areas as of the welfare infrastructure as well as variables affecting each of these areas are identified on the base of demographic characteristics, needs and problems of Korean elderly. The areas are economy, health, housing, social activity and leisure, and long- term care. The economic area functions as the primary basis which other areas depend on. This study finds that the welfare infrastructure is insufficient across the five areas. The area of social activity and leisure is the least sufficient. Therefore, new programs need to be developed and more resources should be invested in this area. Long-term care is another area which needs updating physical facilities as well as community programs. However, five areas interact to affect Korean elderly's wellbeing. The future direction for development of the master plan is suggested to begin with balanced construction of welfare infrastructure and then, undertake the investment of resources into the prioritized areas.

Financing Problems in Old Age's Health: A Discrimination Paradigm?

A. Herrera (HOSPITAL CLINICO UNIVERSIDAD DE CHILE.)

Old age's health problems exist in public and private systems. It's a hard solution problem and it doesn't visualize appropriate manners to face it. In 1981, this problem had the most relevance when the Chilean provisional system was modified from a "delivery system to a system of capitalization", drastically decreasing the sources of salaries of old people. Actually, 73 % are retired from the public system and 11% from the private one, representing 38% of the fiscal presupposed cost. 79.6% is beneficiary of the healthy public system and 8.9% the private one. The individual expenditure and annual in old people's health is 3.4% and 2.3% times higher than the people between 18 and 44 years old, and the cost of the project increases between 2.5 and 6 times more than the people among 18 and 44 years old. Solutions proposed by some authors: Solutions in a short period of time (old age people, actual population): 1) "direct subsidy", 2) financing with nation's funds. Solutions in a long period of time (future old people): 1) "voluntary individual save" being necessary 2) the economical increased sustained. Conclusion: When they retired, the current price decrease, forcing old people to leave the private system, therefore, it would be discriminating against the old people who cotised. Immediate Needs: To reform the previsional system and health system; "new health model", fair collective, solidarity. Local subsidy for the homeless old age people. Gratefully, Adela Herrera Geriatrics

Social-Policy for the Elderly in Albania: A Necessity for the Future

Luan Shahollari (Center for Economic and Social Studies, Tirana - ALBANIA)

Changes in the social sphere ocurred later than in that political and one in Albania, as in the other former -communist of CEECs. As the beginning of the transition it has been operated learning by doing hastily, but later, the legal framework became much more qualified, as a result, actually are fixed some pickets of the social protection on the whole. The analysis of results, problems and suggestions for the future are the purpose of this study. The main of description is the using of empirical and statistical as well as of some questionaries data that are made recent times. The full paper includes tables, as well as, some compared data of Ballkan's countries. The results of work done shows that Albania has not yet a special social policy for the elderly. During the last three years some improvements have been achieved in the macroeconomic framework. For this reason, there is a future need to build a special strategy and social policy for edlery, as a legal packet, possible to be approved by Parlament. Second to carry out with caution all legal acts with the intention to improve the economic status of retired pensions, avoiding the tendency to increase the number of premature pensions, generated from different political parties. Third, paying pensions system must go together with voluntary insurance. It's time to make the necessary amendaments in the laws to brake the existed mistrust in establishing a Private Insurance Institute. Four, to have to implement coherent measures in the medical system, for subvention of drugs, curative places, asylums, urban and interurban transportation etc. At last but not least, it is necessary to raise the level of pensions payment on the whole, of rural areas especially, because they are lower than pensions of urban zones.

Tradeoffs between Public and Private Economic Support of the Elderly: A Natural Experiment in Taiwan

A.E. Biddlecom, A.I. Hermalin, M.B. Ofstedal [Population Studies Center, University of Michigan, Michigan, USA]

The purpose of this study is to examine how public money transfers affect private money transfers, a relationship that is at the core of questions about the effectiveness of public redistribution programs. We take advantage of a "natural" experiment that occurred in Taiwan to examine this link. Beginning in July 1994, elderly subsidy programs were implemented in 8 hsiens (counties) and cities, while in the other 15 hsiens no such subsidy was provided. We use nationally representative, longitudinal data from 1989-1996 on approximately 4,000 older persons to examine three research questions: 1) Over time, how do private transfer monies vary with receipt of (public) pension monies? 2) Whether and to what degree do private transfers respond to amounts received in the state-sponsored subsidy scheme? 3) How well did the state-sponsored subsidy scheme "protect" the economic well-being of older persons? Preliminary results indicate that of older persons who were receiving primary financial support from children in 1989, only 54% continued to receive their primary support from children in 1996 and nearly one-third had shifted to pension or retirement funds as their major source of income. The results suggest that the 1994 subsidy scheme may have had a significant impact on the distribution of support for older adults. The results are valuable not only for Taiwan, as policymakers formulate a public pension system for the nation, but also for other countries that are either contemplating such systems or need to make changes in existing systems.

SESSION 282

European Union initiatives for specialized healthcare for older people I

D O'Neill (Trinity College Dublin, Dublin, Ireland

The European Union contains one of the greatest concentrations of older people within a single geo-political entity. The challenge of ensuring the maximum support to facilitate successful ageing has provoked a number of Europe-wide initiatives. For example, the most recent Bio-Sciences research strategy has dedicated a significant proportion of its budget to ageing issues. This symposium will outline the origins and proposed course of these projects. A Stuckelberger (CH) will present the genesis and evolution of research strategies specifically targetted at the ageing process. The Fifth Framework of the EU research has dedicated a significant resource to research into ageing. Roger Smith (UK) will present on the development of the Geriatric Medicine Section of the European Union of Medical Specialists. This was founded in 1997, following recognition of geriatric medicine by at least 8 of the member states of the European Union. Although there are over 10,000 geriatricians in the EU, development has occurred at different rates and in different ways in the member countries. The Geriatric Medicine Section of the EUMS has produced a consensus document on the minimum training standards for the recognition of geriatricians in Europe. Desmond O'Neill (IRL) will present on the European Union Geriatric Medical Society, the nucleus of which formed in 1999. There will be an inaugural meeting in August 2001 in Paris. The society is complementary to the Clinical Section of the European Region of the IAG and will promote research and academic excellence in geriatric medicine in the European Union The Public Health Section of the European Commission has funded the planning of a European Master's Course in Gerontology in response to the need to prepare health and social systems to support successful ageing in a focussed and co-ordinated way. Anders Vidiik (DK) will present the origins and development of what has the potential to be a very important academic focus for gerontology and the health and social sciences in Europe in the future.

European Union initiatives for specialized healthcare for older people II

D O'Neill (Trinity College Dublin, Dublin, Ireland

Although specialized healthcare for older people has been proven to be effective, there has been an unmet need to provide an academic focus for the estimated 10,000 geriatricians in the European Union. The European Union Geriatric Medical Society, uniting societies for geriatric medicine in member states will be launched at an inaugural scientific meeting in August 2001 in Paris. The mission of the society is to develop geriatric medicine in the member states of the European Union as an independent specialty caring for all older people with age-related disease, to support that these services become available to all citizens of the European Union, to promote education and continuing professional development, and in particular an annual scientific meeting. It is envisaged that in conjunction with the Section of Geriatric Medicine of the EUMS, to promote geriatric medicine to the European Commission and Parliament. to promote evidence-based guidelines for the most efficacious preventive and treatment strategies for older people in the European Union and to liaise with other European bodies promoting the specialty in Europe, such as the Section of Geriatric Medicine of the EUMS, the clinical section of the International Association of Gerontology (European Region) and the European Academy of Medicine and Ageing. Further details are also available on http://www.eugms.org

Building Ageing into the EU Framework Programmes: Lessons and Challenges

Astrid Stuckelberger (Swiss Research Programme on Ageing, Genève, Switzerland)

Europe has the world's oldest popualtion structure. All of the countries of Europe are ageing, as reflected in the growing numbers and proportion of older persons (65+), and the increasing median age of the total population. The aged population, itself, also has been ageing, with growing numbers of persons at the oldest old ages, 85+, representing slightly over 20% of the total aged population in the region. Adding to the picture, rates of fertility and mortality have fallen from high to low. If current trends in fertility and mortality persist, the balance between active and non-active working force will be threatened creating an economic turmoil: the labour force is ageing, along with the population of voting age, while the school-age population is shrinking. The situation has been underlined by a UN report in 2000, with significant numbers of immigrants needed to replace the retirees. After prioritizing assistive technologies and telematics for the Integration of Disabled and Elderly People (TIDE), the European Commission has launched the 5th Framework Programme (FP5) of Research and technological development (RTD) for the period 1999-2002. It includes four thematic programes, of which "Quality of Life and Mangement of Living Resources " (QoL) addresses RTD in the life sciences. The QoL programme includes 6 problem-oriented Key Actions, each addressing a common European challenge, including "The Ageing Population and Disabilities". Today bringing diversity together in Europe, has underlined the need to integrate and unify standards, definitions, research tools as well as to strenghten collaboration and networking. Thus FP5 offers the opportunity to build a true European team working and addressing key issues in ageing, not only through research and collaboration, but more so through cross-dissemination, inter-action and teaching exchange. Considering the challenge ahead, considering the diversity of situations (North-South and East-West), the multiculturality and multi-ageing processes, Europe is only a microcosm of a larger world and could certainly serve as a model for global scales. A brief presentation of the socio-demographic situation in Europe today within the context of the EU Framework Programmes will be presented and discussed.

European Master in Gerontology

A. Viidik (University of Aarhus, Aarhus, Denmark)

There is a need for professionals trained in gerontology to meet the challenges of the ageing of the societies in Western Europe. This need arises from the lack of comprehensive, multidisciplinary academic training programs in gerontology (from the social sciences and social work to demography, psychology, healthcare and biology) on the same level as the well established Master in Public Health programs. The objective was to develop a European Master in Gerontology Study Program and offer it to interested consortia of European universities for implementation. A flexible structure with respect to acceptability in different countries was ascertained. It offers a European dimension in the curriculum and enables students to take different parts of the study in different European countries and thus attain a first-hand experience of different European settings in the field of gerontology. This two-year study program is a part time study programme calculated on the European Credit Transfer System; 90 credits (2400 hours) equally spread over two academic years. There are full weeks (30-40 hours) residential study at a university in the beginning of each module followed by home study. The first study year contains the core modules: introductory module (including biology of ageing) followed by modules for psycho-gerontology, social-gerontology and, health-gerontology. A methodology module (qualitative and quantitative research in gerontology) runs in parallel with the other modules and/or is integrated into them. The first year concludes with an integrative module and summer school, in which multidisciplinarity is emphasised. The second study year consists of elective modules and the completion of a dissertation. The elective modules are selected by the students to meet their professional needs. The dissertation is introduced at the beginning of the year and its theme is developed gradually in collaboration with a supervisor. Three months at the end of the second year is devoted to the dissertation. This programme will thus enable the study of gerontology to the level of a Masterfis degree in more than one European country. Further, it will promote language skills and ability to work in different European countries as well as enhance professional gerontological skills and expertise. Since this programme is issue-orientated, it offers an opportunity for individual specialisation according to professional needs. It offers key qualifications and skills that are necessary for thinking and working productively and successfully in multidisciplinary environments. It was developed under European Commission DG V contract No.: SOC 98 200505 05F03. A full programme description is available at http://www.scw.vu.nl/master/emg

Training in Geriatric Medicine in the European Union (EU)

Roger Smith (University of Edinburgh, Scotland)

Geriatric Medicine was officially recognized as a specialty by the European Union in 1997. One of the most major initiatives of the new Geriatric Medicine Section of the European Union of Medical Specialists (EUMS) was to formulate the training requirements for the specialty of Geriatric Medicine as laid down in chapter 6 of the Charter on Training of Medical Specialists in the European Union. It will also cover the general aspects of training in geriatric medicine, the requirements for training institutions, teachers and trainees. It will discuss obtaining competency and will describe the recommended curriculum for training in geriatric medicine. The responsibilities of National Authorities take into account national rules, EU legislation and recommendations from the Geriatric Medicine Section of the (UEMS). They are also responsible for quality assurance of training programmes, training institutions and teachers. It is recommended that there is a common 2 year period of training in general internal medicine followed by a minimum of 4 years of specialist training in geriatric medicine. The opportunity to train in recognised programmes in other EU counties should be available. The requirements for training institutions, trainers (teachers) and trainees will be discussed. Competency reqires knowledge, objectives and skill objectives whish include communicative, diagnostic, therapeutic, rehabilitative, academic, teaching, research, and administrative skills. It is hoped that the aims of the Geriatric Medicine Section of UEMS which are harmonisation of specialty between member countries, promotion of quality of services, development of guidelines for specialist training and stimulation for continuing professional development will be enhanced. In the symposium it is hoped to help other countries to develop their training guidelines and to learn from others where training has already been established.

SESSION 283

Attitudes of elderly towards death and Illness

Manish Gera, T. S. Narayanan, Hemangi sane, A. Ashutosh, Manish Chopra, Shobhana Chaudhari, Francis Rice, (New York Medical College/ Metropolitan Hospital Center, New York City, NY, USA

PURPOSE: With rapid growth in number and increasing life expectancy, geriatric population is becoming more ethnically diverse. Provision of high quality of care to elderly requires a special set of knowledge, skills and attitudes. This study is undertaken to know the attitudes of elderly population with different ethnic background towards their illness and death METHOD: We prospectively evaluated 3 major ethnic groups of elderly from different continents. Questionnaire was distributed in these populations and their responses were evaluated. Student t test was used for statistical analysis. RESULTS: There are 3 groups of population; USA (n-46), Africa (n-49), India (n-51) Sex distribution: Males: USA 32, Africa 20, India 41 Following were the answers to the questionnaire: Want aggressive treatment: USA 26, Africa 11, India 41 Want CPR even if futile: USA 26, Africa 20, India 36 Want to fight with disease: USA 44, Africa 11, India 47 Believe in rebirth: USA 20, Africa 15, India 40 Wish predicted death: USA 9, India 4, Africa- unknown. Want to die in the hospital: USA 27, Africa 15, India 4 Religious belief helps to cope up with illness: USA 27, Africa 11, India 32 Preoccupied with illness USA 4, Africa 10, India 25 CONCLUSION: There are significant differences in attitude in various ethnic groups, which may influence the approach of the health care professionals while dealing with geriatric population in view of changing ethnic structure of the American population.

Doctors' Attitudes Towards Euthanasia in Hong Kong

Alice Ming-lin Chong (Department of Applied Social Studies, City University of Hong Kong, Hong Kong), S.Y. Fok (Division of Applied Social Studies, City University of Hong Kong, Hong Kong).

In recent years, there have been ardent debates on the legalization of euthanasia in many countries. Hong Kong seems to be an exception, until very recently. The present research is the first in any Chinese societies that explores the doctors' attitudes towards euthanasia and to find out factors affecting such attitudes. Besides euthanasia in general (GE), three different types of euthanasia were also examined, including active (AE), passive (PE) and non-voluntary (NVE). Two-third of doctors in Hong Kong were randomly selected as the sample. Three waves of self-stamped questionnaires and reminding postcards were sent from July to August 1998. 1,188 were finally received, making a response rate of 25%. In average, the participants tended to support euthanasia in general, they agreed with passive euthanasia, but were against active euthanasia. No significant trend was found in non-voluntary euthanasia. Multiple regression models found that those who found their religious belief to be important, and those who always treated terminal-ill patients, were less likely to support euthanasia. Male and Buddhist respondents tended to be more supportive except for non-voluntary euthanasia. Those respondents with poor health status, and those who reported "always" in receiving request to withdraw/withhold treatment for terminal-ill patients were also more supportive of euthanasia except for active euthanasia. In conclusion, this study shows a certain degree of acceptance of euthanasia among the doctors. However, different doctors tend to define passive euthanasia differently. Therefore more discourse on euthanasia is recommended.

Technology and natural death: a study of older people

Merryn Gott, Sheffield Institute for Studies on Ageing, University of Sheffield, Sheffield, UK. Jane Seymour, Sheffield Palliative Care Studies Group, Sheffield, University of Sheffield, UK.David Clark, Sheffield Palliative Care Studies Group, University of Sheffield, Sheffield, UK.Sam Ahmedzai, Sheffield Palliative Care Studies Group, University of Sheffield, Sheffield, UK.

PURPOSE: There is evidence that older people fear euthanasia ‘by the back door’, while also worrying about practices which may prolong dying. This presentation reports work in progress exploring older people’s beliefs and risk assessments regarding the use of innovative health technologies in end-of-life care. METHOD: A two-phase study design has been adopted. Firstly, focus groups have been held involving participants from voluntary groups representing older people in Sheffield, UK. These considered: 1) concerns older people are likely to have about innovative health technologies at the end of life; 2) how a ‘vignette’ could be drafted to explore these concerns during individual interviews; and 3) how an advisory steering group could be organised. Phase II will involve interviewing a systematically selected sample of older people living in 3 contrasting localities within Sheffield using these vignette scenarios. RESULTS: Data from the focus groups conducted during Phase I will be available to present and will include: 1) older peoples’ anticipated concerns about the use of innovative health technologies during end of life care; 2) participants’ experiences of situations where such technologies have been used; 3) participants ideas about ‘natural death’ in relation to distinctions they may draw between ‘natural’ and ‘unnatural’ technologies. CONCLUSION: Care of older people at the end of life in the UK is poorly informed by systematic inquiry into beliefs, understandings and preferences. This study will aid the ongoing development of guidelines for clinical practice and form a basis for information packages for older people and their family carers.

Treatment Choices in Life-Threatening Illness: Attitudes and Preferences of Elderly Australian Veterans and War Widows

Felicity Barr, Anthony Ireland et al, (Department of Veterans' Affairs; Sydney, Australia)

BACKGROUND: Rates of undesirable outcomes - death, institutional placement or complications - reach 50 percent for selected hospital interventions in veterans and war widows aged 85 years or more. PURPOSE: To identify the attitudes and choices of elderly veterans and war widows in respect to complex hospital interventions for elderly persons with severe illness. To assess the impact of recent personal experiences and selected social factors upon these attitudes and choices. METHODOLOGY: A population of veterans and war widows aged between 75 and 89 years was selected and informed consent obtained. Persons who had suffered bereavement in the past six months were excluded. Five clinical scenarios of elderly hospital patients with potentially life-threatening illnesses were presented to small groups of participants. After semi-structured discussion, participants registered their individual responses to nominated treatment interventions in respect of each patient. Participants were also asked whether they possessed any form of Forward Directive for their own future healthcare or whether they believed that their next of kin fully understood their preferences in these matters. RESULTS: Collective attitudes toward specific interventions and towards an aggressive or conservative philosophy of care are described. The impacts of age, gender, spouse/carer status, recent hospital experiences and self-appraised health status upon individual responses are also assessed. CONCLUSION: Veterans and war widows were selective and critical regarding healthcare interventions for their peer group. Drastic measures to preserve life were not universally welcomed.

Who Cares for the Dying

Karen Henderson (How to Care, Toronto, Canada)

Death: we don't talk about it, we don't prepare for it, we don't learn from it. We waste precious time at the end of life being frightened by it. Canadians are not dying well. According to the June 2000 Senate Subcommittee Report: Quality End-of-Life care: The Right of Every Canadian we face a possible crisis in end-of-life care. The report states: <sum>Over 220,000 Canadians die each year <sum>750f all deaths occur in people over 65 years of age <sum>750f deaths take place in hospitals and long term care facilities <sum>each death potentially affects the well being of an average of five other people <sum>an estimated 50f dying Canadians receive integrated and interdisciplinary palliative care How did we get like this? With candor and insight gained from 14 years of caregiving and the recent death of her cognitively impaired father in a long term care facility, Karen Henderson, founder of Caregiver Network and How to Care.com examines her experience with death. She will present ways that both formal and informal caregivers can help each other learn to cope with death in a way that helps all of us regain the lost art of dying. Program Description A frank overview of death in long term care with discussion on such issues as the dying process, medical interventions, staff attitudes and family involvement,

SESSION 284

Acute care of Frail Older Persons

Duncan Robertsonof Nedicine (GEriatric Medicine) Department of Medicine Univertsity of Alberta Edmonton,AB. Canada

ISSUE: In most parts of the world,older persons constitute the highest per capita users of acute care services. Yet hospitals and the care they provide to seniors, especially to frail older persons,often fails to meet their special needs. While some innovative practices and service delivery models have been developed and evaluated they are not widely implemented. STRUCTURE: This round table discussion provides an opportunity for health care professionals and others interested in the topic to learn about innovations in acute care of older persons in various parts of the world. CONTENT: A brief history of specialized institutional and community-based services for frail older persons will be followed by an examination of issues and challenges in acute elder care in 2001. Innovative models of care delivery, outcomes of evaluative studies and strategies to overcome institutional and system barriers to application will be discussed. ANTICIPATED OUTCOMES: In keeping with the 2001 World Congress theme of Working together in a changing world participants will share information and learn strategies for improving acute elder care.

SESSION 285

Cognitive activity in aging and Alzheimer's disease.

N.Yu. Bachinskaya (Institute of Gerontology, Kyiv, Ukraine)

Study on the higher nervous activity in aging and at mild stages of Alzheimer's disease (AD) was undertaken in 300 apparently healthy subjects of different ages and in 60 AD patients. Methods used: MMSE, WAIS, CAMCOG, intellectual working ability during fulfillment of an experimental-psychological task, memory on 10 words and 8 figures, EEG, neurological status, global clinical investigation. Age changes of the integrative activity of the brain involve such processes as perception, processing and analysis of incoming information. Functional systems responsible for spatial transformation and operative forms of information processing undergo greatest changes with age. Comprehensive mechanisms and the ability of categorical generalization mainly provide the intellectual maintenance at late stages of ontogenesis. It is noteworthy that the indices characterizing the intellectual-mnestic activity of elderly subjects have a wide range of individual differences. They depend on the constitutional personality stamp, education, profession, lifestyle and many other factors. The most important among them are the cerebrovascular disturbances and neurodegenerative processes. Gradual onset and slow but irreversible progression of the dementia are typical for AD. The expression of cognitive deficits in AD patients are characterized by early appearance of dysphasia, agnosia or some form of apraxia. By enhancing cognition and memory, effective therapies should therefore have beneficial effects on the functional performence of patients. Donepezil hydrochloride (Aricept) is in clinical use for the symptomatic treatment of AD. The results of 12-weeks studies demonstrate that Donepezil treatment has beneficial effects on patients' cognitive functions and daily living activity as well as on caregiver's burden.

DHEAS, Cortisol Serum Levels, and DHEAS/Cortisol Ratio in Alzheimer's Type Dementia

Massaia M, Ferrario E, Pallavicino di Ceva A, Zannella P, Cappa G, Bo M, Molaschi M, Fabris F (Institute of Gerontology. University of Torino. Corso Bramante 88, 10126 Torino. Italy)

PORPOSE: elevated cortisol concentrations damage the brain, and in particular the hyppocampus; therefore a relation between dementia of Alzheimer type (AD) and decreased DHEAS serum levels could be hypothesised. Our research has been performed to evaluate DHEAS and cortisol serum concentration differences and their ratio in an AD patients group and in a cognitively healthy control group. METHOD: In our case-control study entered 158 subjects (mean age 75.7 ± 7.2) affected by AD according to DSM IV and the NINCDS ADRDA Work Group criteria; controls were 180 cognitively normal individuals (mean age 76.5 ± 8.7). The sample was enrolled among 426 subjects consecutively afferred to our Geriatric Institute in 1997. Exclusion criteria were vascular dementia, insulin dependent diabetes, neoplasm, hyperlipidemia, CHD, previous

MI, stroke, severe liver/renal failure. Linear correlation coefficient R, two sample t-test and ANOVA were used in the statistical analysis. RESULTS: The total sample mean age was 76.2 ± 8.0 yrs, without any significant difference between AD and controls (t= -0.98, NS). DHEAS serum levels show a negative correlation with age in the total sample ($p< 0.001$) and in AD and controls ($p<0.001$). Cortisol levels didn't show any correlation with age and with diagnosis; DHEAS/cortisol ratio shows a negative correlation with age ($p=0.001$) both in the total sample and the two groups ($p=0.001$). The ANOVA on six age cohorts didn't show any statistically significant differences of DHEAS and cortisol mean levels and DHEAS/cortisol ratio between AD and normal controls. CONCLUSION: DHEAS and cortisol levels don't seem to be correlated with AD.

MRI correlates of normal brain ageing in an elderly Australian sample

T.C. Lye, D.A. Grayson, H.P. Bennett, H. Creasey, O. Piguet (Centre for Education and Research on Ageing, University of Sydney, Sydney, Australia), & G.A. Broe (Prince of Wales Medical Institute, Sydney, Australia).

The aim of this study was to define MRI correlates of normal brain ageing, with the specific purpose of investigating whether volumes of the hippocampus are selectively correlated with age-related memory performance. MRI-based volumetry was employed to measure hippocampal volumes in 102 community-dwelling individuals aged between 81 and 94 years (mean age=85). Participants were assessed on a variety of clinical and experimental instruments, including a comprehensive neuropsychological test battery. All participants underwent neurological examination, and an extensive medical history was obtained from an informant to confirm details of each participant's functional ability. Three measures of the hippocampus were compared to determine which measures were predictive of memory functioning: (1) hippocampal volumes adjusted by whole brain volumes; (2) hippocampal volumes adjusted by total intracranial volume; and (3) visual ratings of the hippocampus. All hippocampal measures were found to be significant predictors of delayed recall of short stories, although whole brain adjusted hippocampal volumes and visual ratings of the hippocampus were the best predictors of memory functioning in this group. Hippocampal measures were generally not associated with performance in other cognitive domains. When the sample was reduced to include the most cognitively healthy participants, in 57 individuals rated by an informant as showing no evidence of dementia (Clinical Dementia Rating = 0) the left hippocampal volume (whole brain adjusted) remained a significant predictor of long-term retention of short stories. These findings suggest that hippocampal volumes are selectively correlated with memory functioning in healthy individuals in their ninth and tenth decade of life.

Slow waves in Alzheimer s Disease: a preliminar study with Magnetoencephalography

A.Garnica, P.López-Riquelme, P. Gil Gregorio and J.M. Ribera Casado (Servicio de Geriatria,Hospital Clinico San Carlos,Madrid,Spain). A. Fernández-Lucas, C. Amo-Usanos, F. Maestú-Unturbe, Tomás Ortiz-Alonso (Centro MEG Complutense, Madrid,Spain)

PURPOSE: to assess the relationship between patterns of ALFMA (Abnormal Low Frequency Magnetic Activity) and the clinical and neuropsychological diagnosis of Alzheimer´s disease (AD). METHOD:a 148-channel MEG using a whole-head magnetometer (MAGNES 2500WH, 4D-Neuroimaging, San Diego, USA) was recorded during a 10-min resting period in 26 subjects (17 patients with probable AD according to NINCDS-ADRDA criteria and 9 age-matched controls). The MEG was recorded with a 678.17 Hz sampling rate, using a band-pass filter of 0.1-100 Hz. For statiscal analysis (following the Dipole Density Method) the total brain volume was divided into ten regions and the number of succesful dipole fits was determined for each of these regions representing temporal, frontal, prefrontal, parietal and occipital left and right hemispheres; both for delta (1.5-4.0Hz) and theta (4.0-8.0) bands. Neuropsychological variables measured were: CAMCOG and MMSE. Subjects were classified in stages by Functional assessment stages scale (FAST). RESULTS:Two kinds of statistical analysis were carried out, a T-Student-mean comparison for independent samples, showing a significant higher density of delta activity over the left temporal area ($T= 2,135$; $p< 0.05$) in the AD group. On the other hand a discriminant analysis was performed both for MEG and Neuropsychological variables. In this case a combination of left temporal and parietal delta activity, right prefrontal and parietal theta activity, and the MMSE and Recent memory (CAMCOG) scores could classificate accurately the 100 0f the subjects. CONCLUSION:The combination of magnetoencephalography and clinical and neuropsychological variables could be a powerful parameter for the diagnosis of AD.

SESSION 286

[1] Functional adaptation after congestive heart failure and acute myocardial infarction. A prospective study

G.I.J.M. Kempen, C.H.M. van Jaarsveld, R. Sanderman (Department of Health Care Studies, Section of Medical Sociology, Maastricht University, The Netherlands)

PURPOSE: to study the impact of 3 pre-morbidly assessed psychological resources (i.e. neuroticism, mastery and self-efficacy expectancies) on functional adaptation after congestive heart failure (CHF) and acute myocardial infarction (AMI) in late middle-aged and older persons. METHOD: patients with new episodes of either CHF (N=134) or AMI (N=79) were included. Due to the prospective design of the study initial baseline levels of functional disability and chronic medical morbidity could be adjusted, next to age, gender and the severity of either CHF or AMI. Functional decline (outcome measure) was defined as change in functional status between baseline and 8 weeks after the diagnosis of either CHF or AMI. Data were analyzed with multiple regression analysis. RESULTS: baseline, pre-morbid levels of functional disability were significantly higher for CHF patients compared to AMI patients. Functional disability increased substantially and significantly in both groups of patients. Significant unique contributions of self-efficacy expectancies were found for functional adaptation after CHF, while mastery significantly contributes to functional adaptation after AMI. Neuroticism was not related to functional decline after either CHF or AMI. CONCLUSION: pre-morbidly assessed levels of psychological resources influence functional decline after cardiac disease substantially in late middle-aged and older persons, but the impact of specific resources can be considered differential for CHF and AMI.

[2] Comparison between echocardiographs finds differences with aging for left ventricular hypertrophy

Vicente Spinola Dias Neto, Giselle Helena de Paula Rodrigues, Pierre, H. (Pontifícia Universidade Católica de São Paulo, Department of Geriatrics Medicine)

PURPOSE: To set up a relationship between electrocardiography (ECG) and echocardiography (ECO), for left ventricular hypertrophy (LVH), among old people (>65 years) and younger adults (25 to 50 years), women and men. METHOD: The medical registrations of 218 patients, normal and with cardiopathies, have been analyzed. From the ECG, have been observed the Sokolow-Lyon rate (S-L rate), left atrium anomaly and the points score of Romhilt-Estes. And from the ECO, the left ventricle masses rate. Have been used: G test of Cochran to compare the positives percentages, MC Nemar test to compare LVH on the ECO with the ECG variables in each studied group, the Qui-square test to compare the sex in each etary group and the etary group in each sex. RESULTS: Among men (25-50 years), haven't been observed difference between the criterions, and the points score showed bigger positive percentage (31.2%). Men (>65 years) presented S-L rate with a positive percentage smaller (10.8%) than the positiveness of the ECO for LVH (37.3%); the same occurring for the women: older ones with 7.6% for the S-L rate, and 40% for the ECO; and younger ones with 9% and 50%, respectively. The concordances study showed concordance percentage bigger, for left atrium anomaly and LVH on the ECO, among men (69.2%), than women (43.8%). In etary group, the concordance between ECO and the electrocardiographics criterions was bigger for the women >65 years. CONCLUSION: The S-L rate is more specific among men (25-50 years) than the sensibility of the left atrium anomaly and the Romhilt-Estes points score. The S-L rate has lower sensibility among older men and 25 to 50 years old women. The elderly degenerative processes have stronger influence on the women for the LVH diagnostic.

[3] Analysis of association between apolipoprotein E polymorphism and cardiovascular risk factors among oldest-old.

Carla Schwanke, Ivana Da Cruz, Yukio Moriguchi, Rosane Scheibe, Ney Leal, Emilio Moriguchi (Institute of Geriatrics and Gerontology of PUCRS University, Porto Alegre, RS, Brazil.

PURPOSE: to establish the gene frequencies of Apolipoprotein E and to analyze the association of cardiovascular risk factors with the Apo-E gene polymorphism in 80 years old or older. METHOD: 70 subjects of the Veranópolis Project, were studied. The technique of identification of the APOE genotypes used PCR-RFLP and Hha I as restriction enzyme to observe the alleles E2, E3 and E4 whereas the genotopic frequency were: E3E3 (0.70), E3E4 (0.22), E2E3 (0.06), E2E2 (0.02). The most frequent genotypes were compared regarding to their association with biological variables and cardiovascular risk factors. RESULTS: The frequencies of E2, E3 and E4 alleles were 0.05, 0.84 and 0.11 respectively. The evaluation showed that E3E4 subjects presented a mean age significantly greater than observed in individuals with the E3E3. Individuals carrying E3E3 showed mean levels greater of diastolic arterial pressure and body mass index than E3E4. The levels of uric acid were highest in E3E3. These findings were not reported in the previously in literature reviewed. Individuals with the E3E4 genotype showed significantly higher LDL-cholesterol and fibrinogen plasmatic levels than E3E3 ones. The results suggested that E4E4 could be associated with early mortality as describe in literature. A balance between the factors considered neutral or protective and the cardiovascular risk ones could be occurring among the genotypes, masking or reducing the negative effects of the E4 allele.

[4] Altered paraoxonase activity and increased HDL susceptibility to oxidation with aging

I. Seres, G. Paragh, T. Fulop Jr, A. Khalil*. University of Debrecen, Medical and Health Science Center, First Department of Medicine, POB 19, Debrecen, H-4012, Hungary. *Inst. Univ. Gériatr, Lab. Biogérontol, *Dept. Biochim, Fac. Méd, Univ. Sherbrooke, Sherbrooke, Qc, Canada*

Purpose: Paraoxonase (PON) is associated in human serum with high density lipoprotein (HDL) and its arylesterase/paraoxonase activities are reduced in hypercholesterolemia, diabetes and vascular cardiac diseases explaining the reduced antiatherogenic activities of HDL. The incidence of atherosclerosis and its related diseases increase with aging. The aging process may enhance lipoprotein modification, which leads to the increase in the susceptibility of LDL and HDL to oxidation. The aim of our study was to determine the PON activity in healthy elderly and correlate it to the susceptibility of HDL to oxidation. Method: Lipid parameters and the PON activity was measured in the sera of 128 healthy individuals of various ages (y=18-34 years, n=27; middle-aged = 35-64 years, n=61, elderly = 65 x years, n=40). The HDL oxidation was done by -radiolysis of water and lipid peroxidation parameters measured (TBARS, conjugated dienes and vitamin E). Results: The lipid parameters showed a significant increase of total cholesterol with aging, however neither the HDL nor the Apo A1 levels did not change with aging. The PON activity significantly decreased with aging ($p<0.0001$) and a strong negative correlation was found with aging ($r = -.3824$, $p<0.001$). The correlation was even stronger when the PON activity was correlated to HDL ($r = -.4489$, p<001). There was an increased HDL susceptibility to peroxidation with healthy aging. The peroxidative parameters (TBARS and conjugated dienes) increased and the antioxidants (Vitamin E) decreased. Conclusion: the decreased PON activity and vitamin E levels contribute to the increased susceptibility of HDL to oxidation with aging explaining at least partly the increased incidence of atherosclerosis leading to cardiovascular diseases with aging.

[5] Relationship of hypertension between age-related and artery sizes of aneurysm and dissection in ageing

Liu Zhenan, Director/MD (Department of Gerontology, Liu Hua Qiao Hospital,Guang Zhou,CN), Ou Shanxing ,Vicer Director/ MD(Department of Radiology, Liu Hua Qiao Hospital,Guangzhou,CN)

PURPOSE: The object of this prospective study was to determine both the sizes of the aortic aneurysm and dissection in relation to hypertension and age. METHOD: The study group comprised 32 subjects (30 males and 2 females, mean age of 72 years) was divided into 2 groups by age (in decades).The classifications of dissection: DeBakey type I 11 cases, DeBakey type II + IIIa 5 cases, DeBakey type IIIb 4 cases ,and aneurysms 12 cases were performed. Images with diagnostic quality were obtained by the three-dimensional CT angiography and CT virtual endoscopy (3D-CTA/CT-VE) . Among sizes ,types of aortic aneurysm and dissection were evaluated by CTA/CT-VE or MRI, then the linear regression models were analyzed to data. RESULTS: The mean size of the aortic diameter involved in part was about 4.8cm (range 3.5-7.2cm). The Sizes of the aneurysm and dissection in men were showed significant difference with increasing hypertension and age ($p < 0.01$) and positive relative($r=0.90$),and none of these values were significantly different in control. CONCLUSION: The results in sizes of aortic dissection were showed positive relative with increasing hypertension and age in pronounced older men. CTA and CT-VE provide us with an important noninvasive imaging of the aneurysm of aorta, dissection and their branches in relevant to diagnosis and therapy.

[6] The correlation between the plasma t-PA, PAI level and allele genotype of APOE among 1058 elderly in Shanghai, China

Ma Yong-Xing, Wang Chuan-Fu, Lu Pei-Fang (Department of Aging, Antiaging and Cognitive Function, Shanghai Institute of Gerontology and Geriatrics, Huadong Hospital,Shanghai,China)

The allele genotype of APOE and Plasma t-PA, PAI level of 1058 elderly (65-85 years old) in Shanghai were determined in order to evaluate if there was any correlation between genotype of APOE and fibrinolytic activity. The level (IU/ml) of t-PA, PAI in various allele genotype of APOE were as follows: (1) APOE 3/3 (803 persons): t-PA 0.44±0.15, PAI 0.72±0.15 (2) APOE 2/3 (101 person): t-PA 0.44±0.14, PAI 0.73±0.15 (3) APOE 3/4(133 persons): t-PA 0.44±0.13, PAI 0.73±0.15 (4) APOE 2/4 (15 persons): t-PA 0.43±0.11, PAI 0.6±0.14 (5) APOE 2/2 (2 persons): 0.46±0.74, PAI 0.51±0.13 (6) APOE 4/4 (4 persons): t- PA 0.4±0.20, PAI 0.85±0.07. No significant difference of the levels of t-PA (F value =0.135) and PAI (F value =1.628) in various APOE allele phenotypes were found. It is suggested that the effect of APOE4 as a risk factor of cerebro-cardiac vascular disease and dementia (VD, AD) in the aged may be mediated by certain mechanisms other than fibrinolytic activity changes.

[7] Circulating cell adhesion molecules in dependence on aging

V. Richter, F. Rassoul, K. Purschwitz, M. Wittek, G. Vierig (Department of Clinical Chemistry and Pathobiochemistry, University of Leipzig, Germany), Th. Kuntze (Heart Center, Clinic of Heart Surgery, University of Leipzig, Germany), B. Hentschel (Institute of Medical Informatics, Statistics and Epidemiology, University of Leipzig, Germany), W. Reuter (Clinic of Internal Medicine IV, University of Leipzig, Germany)

Binding and recruitment of monocytes to vascular endothelial cells and further subendothelial migration are early steps in the development of atherosclerosis and are mediated through cellular adhesion molecules (CAMs). CAMs are also found in soluble forms in the circulation, and several data indicate that their increased plasma levels may be related to risk factors for atherosclerosis and to underlying atherosclerosis. The aim of the present study was to assess in subjects with different cardiovascular risk profile the levels of circulating CAMs (cCAMs) in dependence on age. The following groups of subjects (18-82 years old) were included: 179 male and female control subjects, 80 vegetarians (subjects with favourable risk profile), 70 patients with angiographically proved coronary artery disease, and 112 patients with peripheral arterial disease. Serum levels of intercellular cell adhesion molecule-1 (cICAM-1), vascular cell adhesion molecule-1 (cVCAM-1), and endothelial-leukocyte adhesion molecule (E-selectin) were determined by the use of monoclonal antibody-based ELISA assays (R&D Systems, Europe Ltd.). Patients with cardiovascular diseases showed a tendency of elevated cVCAM-1 levels in comparison with control subjects. However, an age-dependent increase of cVCAM-1 levels was found in all groups of subjects with different cardiovascular risk included in the study. In contrast, cICAM-1 and cE-selectin levels were not correlated with age. These data indicate that cVCAM-1 may be a marker for biological aging independent of cardiovascular risk profile.

[8] Long term antihypertensive treatment did not reduce activity and cognitive function in the very old

H.Yu, A.Moriguchi, H.Matsushita, S.Nakamura, Y.Nakamoto (Hanwa 2nd Senboku Hospital, Sakai, JAPAN), T.Ogihara (Osaka University Dept. of Geriatic Medicine, Suita, JAPAN)

Abstract: Efficacy of medical treatment for very old hypertensive patients is not established. We evaluated the effect of anti-hypertensive agents for long term on the activity of daily life (ADL) or degree of dementia in hospitalized very old hypertensives. We employed 37 hospitalized hypertensives with medication and 74 patients without hypertension as control. Brain magnetic resonance imaging, electrocardiogram and measurements of serum creatinine were performed. Blood pressure (BP) was also evaluated at admission and 6 months after admission. The degree of ADL or dementia was graded into 8 or 5 stages, respectively. Patients with stroke, myocardial infarction, renal failure or obvious diabetes mellitus were excluded. Both systolic and diastolic BP at admission was higher in patients under medication compared with control (154/81 vs. 136/73 mmHg, $p<0.05$, respectively). At 6 months after admission, while systolic BP in hypertensive patients was higher than that of control (134 vs. 122 mmHg, $p<0.05$, respectively) diastolic BP was not different. The frequency in complication of hypertension such as lacunar infarction, left ventricular hypertrophy, renal insufficiency was not different between these two groups. The degree of either ADL or dementia was not different between hypertensive patients and control. There was no significant correlation between BP level and degree of ADL or dementia. Active treatment using anti-hypertensive agents for very old hypertensives did not affect on their degree of either ADL or dementia. Medical treatment might be necessary even in very old because their activity or cognitive function was maintained.

[9] Carotid Arteries Structural Changes and Stroke in the Elderly

G.I. Prada, D. State, M. Georgescu, A.M. Georgescu (Ana Aslan National Institute of Gerontology and Geriatrics, Bucharest, Romania)

Our objective was to identify the influence of structural changes in carotid arteries in the elderly upon the occurrence of ischemic stroke. A study has been carried out on 871 consecutive patients referred for ultrasound vascular investigation for various reasons (dizziness, occlusive peripheral arterial disease, sequelae of stroke). The age range was 60 to 105 years (mean 82.4 years). Prevalence of stroke among these patients was 15%, and gender distribution in stroke patients was: 43% women and 57% men. The patients were investigated by both Doppler ultrasound technique and echotomography. Nearly all elderly patients (99%) demonstrated a certain structural modification at the level of common carotid artery and/or internal carotid artery. This change did not necessarily correlated with the presence of stroke in the past history of these patients. The number and dimensions of atherosclerotic plaques demonstrated in the carotid tree did not correlate with the presence of stroke unless some other risk factors were concomitantly encountered, such as: smoking and diabetes mellitus. Especially when smoking was present in the past medical history of the patient, the number, localization and size of atheroma correlated very strongly with the coexistence of stroke, irrespective of the age of the subjects ($p<0.001$). Moreover, the severity of stroke was not influence by the mere number of atherosclerotic plaques. Instead, their localization and structure (mainly the calcium content) were more important. In conclusion, Doppler and echotomographic techniques need to be corroborated with other clinical information in order to increase their capacity to predict the risk of stroke in elderly patients.

[10] Peripheral Obliterating Atherosclerosis and N-3 Fatty Acids in Elderly Patients.

NL Terra, AJG. Bos, RO Ehlers, JC Lehmkuhl, RS da Cunha, EH Moriguchi, Y Moriguchi(Institute of Geriatrics and Gerontology of Pontifical Catholic University of Rio Grande do Sul. Porto Alegre. RS. Brazil)

PURPOSE: To observe the efficacy and tolerability of N-3 fatty acids on the treatment of peripheral atherosclerosis in elderly people. METHOD: Seventeen patients (9 men and 8 women) took part in this study, they average on age 67 years-old. All subjects had atherosclerosis on their lower extremities with intermittent claudication and were on treatment with vasodilators and platelet aggregation inhibitors. The length of walk up to the start of the symptoms were graded in all participants before and after the treatment period. All the patients were submitted to a full physical examination, analysis of the total Cholesterol, HDL-c, LDL-c, Triglycerides, platelet aggregation, and Doppler echography of the lower extremities, at the beginning and immediately after the end of the treatment. During five months the volunteers had added up to their current treatment, six capsules of n-3 fatty acids 3 times daily, taken immediately after meals. The capsules contained 300 mg of the ethyl ester of eicosapentaenoic acid of high purity. They were questioned about the appearance of any side effects. RESULTS: At the end of treatment, a clinical improvement was observed in all patients. The distance covered until the appearance of the pain increased, there was an improvement on the blood flow and improvement of the serum lipids. CONCLUSION: Based on the obtained results, observed tolerability and presence of minimal side effects, we conclude that oral n-3 fatty acids are useful on the treatment of peripheral atherosclerosis.

[11] The dispersion of QT-interval in the ECG of the elderly

A. E. Tàmmaro, P.Tarlarini (Geriatric Institute PAT, Milano, Italy)

PURPOSE: To assess 1) the feasibility of the determination of QT-interval dispersion (QT-D) in the elderly, and 2) if such parameter is influenced by some demographic, clinical, pharmacological, and ECG variables. METHOD: QT-D and QTc-D (i.e. the dispersion of rate-corrected QT-interval) were calculated from the difference between the longest and shortest of the intervals measured on the 6 standard precordial leads of 500 pts aged between 65 and 102 yrs consecutively admitted to our institute. A comparison was then made between the mean values of QT-D and QTc-D in groups of pts selected on the basis of presence-absence or of the value of the above variables. RESULTS: QT-D measurement resulted feasible in a high percentage (83.8%) of the studied population. Significantly higher values of QT-D and QTc-D were found among pts with ischemic heart disease, ECG signs of myocardial ischemia, under digitalis treatment, and with high maximum values of QT, QTc, and JT (QT QRS) intervals. Pts aged 85 yrs and over showed higher qt-D and QTc-D values, but only for the former the difference resulted statistically significant. CONCLUSIONS: The high grade of feasibility of QT-D measurement and the association between QT-D and QTc-D and some variables resulting from the study of an older population suggest the necessity of larger, prospective studies. These could be of aid in the debate about the actual value of QT-D as a marker of serious arrhythmogrenicity and risk of sudden death.

[12] Effect of beta-blockers on cardiac events in the elderly patients with healed myocardial infarction

Norihiro Takeda,Akio Kimura,Hiroki Furuta,Akiko Ikeda,Hikaru Ino,Takaaki Taniwa,Katsuhiko Katayama,Toshihiko Takenaka,Takahiro Hayashi,Ken Kanamasa,Kinji Ishikawa

Purpose: It has been already proved that beta-blockers are effective to reduce the cardiac events in healed myocardial infarction (MI) but less used in the elderly patients (pts). We analyzed to compare the effect of beta-blockers in the elderly and younger pts to find the rational of encouraging more use in the elderly pts. Method: Among all consecutive 6602 pts (age 58.5±10.4 years) from 1986 to 1999 with healed MI, the incidence of cardiac events were studied retrospectively. 4017 of them were treated with beta-blockers and 2585 were without beta-blockers. The mean observation period was 12.3±16.3 months, cardiac events were defined as fatal and nonfatal recurrent MIs, sudden death and death by congestive heart failure. Results: There were 94 cardiac events among 2585 pts (3.6%) who were not on beta-blockers, while there were 101 among 4017 pts (2.5%) with beta-blockers ($p<0.01$). In pts less than 60 years, the incidence of cardiac events were 42 among 1253 pts (3.4%) without beta-blockers, 56 cardiac events among 2268 pts (2.5%) with beta-blockers. In pts from 60 years to 69 years, 22 cardiac events among 737 pts (3.0%) without beta-blockers, 30 cardiac events among 1207 pts (2.5%) with beta-blockers. In pts older than 69 years there were 32 cardiac events among 518 pts (6.2%) treated without beta-blockers, there were 16 cardiac events among 550 pts with beta-blockers (2.90<0.01). Conclusion: This observational study demonstrates a benefit of beta-blockers use on long-term prognosis after MI in the elderly pts.

[13] Prevention of and Treatment for Genetically Determined Age-Related Cardiovascular Pathology

D. L. Strekalov, D. V. Solovieva (St. Petersburg Institute of Bioregulation and Gerontology, St. Petersburg, Russia)

This study was designed to develop an approach to the treatment-and-prevention measures by molecular genetic and clinical data of age-related cardiovascular pathology. Enrolled patients (mean age 51.2 y. o.) were subject to standard clinical laboratory and molecular genetic investigations. Genes responsible for the following factors were studied: lipid metabolism - Apo E (Cys112Arg, Arg158Cys), Apo CIII (C/G, position 5163), PON (Gln192Arg); vascular constriction activity and the left ventricular hypertrophy factor ACE (I/D, intron 16); coagulation function prothrombin (G/A, position 20210), V factor (Arg506Gln), PAI-1 (4G/5G promoter, position -323), vessel wall condition MTHFR (C/T, position 677). We used genomic DNA of venous lymphocytes. DNA was amplified by polymerase chain reaction. In the patients of the studied age group arterial hypertension (50% of the cases), ischemic heart disease (16% of the cases) and functional apoplexy (8% of the cases) were diagnosed. Hereditary predisposition to arterial hypertension a risk factor for ischemic heart disease and functional apoplexy was revealed in 28 % of the patients. We devised 2 levels of recommendations regarding the revealed unfavorable gene allelic polymorphism. Level 1 was preclinical and implied risk factors estimation, life style modifications and diet restrictions. Level 2 was supplemented by prescription of pathogenetically based treatment-and-prevention measures. In both cases long-term measures of medical observation and diagnosis were required. Clinical recommendations to the treatment and prevention in case of hereditary predisposition to age-related pathology were formalized as a conclusion form of molecular genetic analysis according to the genotyping

[14] Asymmetry of common carotid artery velocity is a marker for cardiovascular disease in elderly patients

Kyoji Okazaki, Hiroshi Nakano, Tatsuya Suzuki, Kenzo Oba (Division of Geriatric medicine, Nippon Medical School, Tokyo, Japan)

PURPOSE : The aim of this study is to clarify the clinical usefulness of the high to low velocity ratio between the two carotids (velocity ratio), measured by ultrasonic quantitative flow measurement system in elderly patients. METHOD : We studied 230 aged 60 to 91 years (average 65.1 +/- 10.8 years). Carotid blood velocity was measured using QFM-1100 ultrasonic blood flow meter. We divided the subjects into two groups depending on the velocity ratio; high (H) group (>or = 1.4; n=91) and low (L) group (<1.3; n=139). The end point of the study was the occurrence of angina pectoris, nonfatal myocardial infarction, or death from coronary heart disease. The average follow-up period was 3.0 +/- 1.2 years. RESULTS : The incidence of the ischemic heart disease (IHD; myocardial infarction or angina pectoris) was significantly higher in H group than L group (19.4 vs 35.2%; P=0.009). On multiple logistic analyses, only H-group (OR=1.96: p=0.037) was significant predictor for IHD. There were 5 angina pectoris, 17 nonfatal myocardial infarction, and 1 death from coronary heart disease during follow-up period. The risk of the end point of defined events was significantly higher in H group than G group (18.7 vs 4.3 %; p=0.0004 by log-rank test). Uric Acid (RR=1.34; p=0.013) and H-group (RR=4.78: p=0.002) were significant predictors with the Cox proportional-hazard model. CONCLUSION : The high to low velocity ratio between the two carotids, measured by QFM, is a useful clinical marker for cardiovascular disease in elderly patients.

[15] Hypertension in the elderly with salty taste disturbance and Angiotensin II type 2 receptor gene polymorphism.

Shoroku Sakurai, Kohya Okaishi, Masashi Okuro,Miyuki Onishi, Akiko Matsuo, Noriko Fujiwara, Shigeto Morimoto,Toshio Ogihara

Purpose: Hypertension in the elderly is highly dependent on excess intake of sodium, at least partially based on salty taste disturbance, little is known about association of gene polymorphisms with hypertension in the elderly with salty taste disturbance. Method: To clarify the role of gene polymorphisms in this mechanism, 202 elderly subjects were enrolled (mean age + SD; 81 + 7 years) for determination of magnitudes of NaCl (1.25%, 2.5%, 5%, 10% and 20%) in aqueous solution. Thresholds for salty taste were divided into six grades. We analyzed A1166C polymorphism of human AT1 receptor gene, C3123A polymorphism of AT2 receptor gene mapped on human X chromosome, angiotensinogen M235T polymorphism, and angiotensin-I converting enzyme gene I/D polymorphism. Results: There was a significant (p=0.013) association of salty taste threshold with the AT2 receptor gene polymorphism, but not with other polymorphisms. Thus the female elderly subject with AA genotype of the AT2 receptor gene required about 2.5 times higher concentration of NaCl solution to detect salty taste compared to those with CC genotype. On the other hand, there was significant (p=0.0003) correlation between the salty taste threshold and decrease in diastolic blood pressure from the value at ambulatory measurement to that after restriction of salt intake for 4 weeks. Conclusions: These observations indicate participation of AT2 receptor gene polymorphism in salty taste disturbance and in salt-sensitive increase in blood pressure in elderly patients with hypertension.

[16] Aortic calcification as a marker for arteriosclerosis obliterans of lower extremities in the elderly

Masashi Okuro, Yoshichika Baba, Miyuki Onishi, Kohya Okaishi, Shoroku Sakurai,Noriko Fujiwara, Jin Yang, Ryuichi Morishita, Shigeto Morimoto, Toshio Ogihara

Arteriosclerosis obliterans (ASO) is one of the major health problems in the elderly, since this disease causes decreased ADL and QOL. In this study, we examined clinical significance of aortic calcification in ASO in the young and the elderly after adjustment of known risk factors for ASO. Method: The subjects were young [65-75 years] ASO patients (n=34) and control subjects (n=60), and elderly ASO patients (n=33) and control subjects (n=82). ASO was defined as those with ankle-brachial pressure index (ABI)<0.2, and controls were those with ABI>0.9. We classified calcification of aortic arch on the chest X-ray into 4 groups as no (grade 0), speckled (grade 1), linear (grade 2) and circular (grade 3) calcification. Result: The distribution of grades of the calcification (0 to 3) were 47%, 29%, 24%, 0% in young ASO patients, and 80%, 17%, 3%, 0% in the young controls (ANOVA p<0.001), and 9%, 24%, 46%, 21% in elderly ASO patients, and 22%, 42%, 31%, 6% in elderly controls (ANOVA p=0.013), respectively. Logistic regression analysis using diabetes mellitus, hypertension, hypercholesterolemia and high serum Lp(a) as confounding factors revealed that the aortic calcification is the highest risk factor among these confounding factors both in the young group and elderly group. Discussion: ASO is known to occur in iliac and femoral arteries which comparatively locate near to the aorta. In consequence, our results indicate that calcification of aortic arch is a predictor for ASO both in young and elderly subjects.

[17] Initiation of warfarin therapy in old old inpatients: a new loading dose protocol

V. Siguret, E. Pautas, M. Debray, S. Moulias, I. Gouin (Hôpital Charles Foix, Ivry-sur-Seine, France)

Purpose: Under warfarin therapy, risk of major bleeding increases after the age of 80. Elderly patients require a lower dose of warfarin than youngers to obtain the same desired anticoagulant effect. However, most of the age adjusted warfarin protocols propose a starting dose 6 mg or over, often leading to overanticoagulation in very elderly patients. We propose a new warfarin loading dose protocol derived from Fennerty's, in order to reach an International Normalised Ratio (INR) between 2.0 and 3.0. Method: The maintenance daily dose of warfarin is predicted after three intakes of 4 mg of warfarin on days 0, 1 and 2 (6 p.m.), using a simplified algorithm based on INR testing on day 3 (10 a.m.). Results: This protocol was validated in 28 inpatients (6 men, 22 women), mean age 84 (range 71-97), needing a recommended target INR of 2.5. The maintenance dose was defined as the actual warfarin dose required to obtain two successive INRs between 2.0. an 3.0 within 72 hours. INR was performed using Neoplastin CI (Diagnostica Stago). There was a strong correlation between the predicted daily warfarin dose on day 3 and the actual daily maintenance dose (y = 0.94x + 0.27, R◊ = 0.84). The mean actual maintenance warfarin dose was 3.1 mg vs 3.0 mg for the predicted one. The mean time to reach a stable INR was 10 days. Conclusion: this warfarin loading protocol is reliable in old old in-patients. A larger study is in progress to strengthen its validation.

[18] Cytokine and Natriuretic Peptides in Aged Patients with Acute Congestive Heart Failure

M. Sakai, T. Taniguchi, T. Imai (Division of Cardiology, Tokyo Metropolitan Geriatric Hospital, Tokyo, Japan)

We investigated the pathophysiological role of inflammatory cytokine, interleukin-6 (IL-6), and atrial natriuretic peptide (ANP) and brain natriuretic peptide (BNP) in aged patients with acute congestive heart failure (CHF). The subjects included 30 patients (mean age 82 years) with CHF and 5 control patients (mean age 85 years) without CHF. In the severity of acute CHF on admission, 5 patients were classified according to the Killip class as class 1 (no CHF), 15 patients as class 2 (mild to moderate CHF), 13 patients as class 3 (severe CHF) and 2 patients as class 4 (shock). A comparison was made of plasma levels of IL-6, ANP, BNP and cGMP among 3 groups of class 1,2 and 3+4. Plasma ANP and cGMP levels showed no significant differences among 3 groups. Plasma BNP and IL-6 levels increased significantly in the groups with CHF compared with the control group (BNP: class 1 89±32, class 2 828±572, class 3+4 742±452pg/ml; IL-6: class 1 4.0±2.7, class 2 9.9±48.7, class 3+4 38.1±61.2pg/ml). However, plasma BNP and IL-6 levels showed no significant differences between the groups of class 2 and class 3+4. Plasma BNP levels showed no significant correlation with plasma IL-6 levels. Thus, IL-6 suggests an important role in the pathophysiology of CHF even in the elderly, independent of the secretion of BNP.

[19] Prevalence of Urinary Incontinence after stroke

M.Song (College of Nursing, Seoul national University, Seoul, Korea), S. Ryu, M. Kim (Graduate school of Seoul National University, Seoul, Korea)

PURPOSE To investigate the prevalence and the types of urinary incontinence and symptoms, the management strategies, and the impact of urinary symptoms among stroke survivors. METHOD One hundred and ninety-eight stroke patients(113 men, 76 women, mean age 65.5years, mean stroke period 46.57 months)were recruited from two university hospital inpatients units and outpatient clinic, and a rehabilitation hospital. Data were collected by interview utilizing survey questionnaire and chart review. RESULTS The results were as follows: The prevalence of urinary incontinence after stroke was 47%. Urge, functional, stress, overflow urinary incontinence were present in 95.5%, 44.9%, 43.8%, 20.20f patients respectively. Prominent Urinary symptoms were weak stream(49.2%), urgency(46.0%), feeling of incomplete voiding(36.5%), hesitancy(33.4%), intermittent stream(22.2%), straining(19.6%), burning sensation(6.7%), and pain(4.8%). Reported management strategies were fluid restriction in 25.8%, frequent toileting in 15.7%, use of diaper in 5.6%, scheduled voiding in 5.6%, and catheterization in 5.60f patients, and 75.30f incontinent patients didn’t treat their urinary continence. Prescribed medical treatment consisted with pharmacological therapy(11.2%), pelvic muscle exercise(3.4%), others(10.1%). Subjective quality of life of incontinent group was significantly lower than those of continent group(t = -7.309, p = .000). CONCLUSION The prevalence of urinary incontinence among stroke survivors was 47%. But most of incontinence after stroke were not given management or treatment. Therefore the development of the management program for poststroke UI patients is recommended.

[20] Clinical usefulness of evaluation of pulse wave velocity on stroke incidence

Hiroshi Nakano, Kyoji Okazaki, Tatsuya Suzuki, Kenzo Oba (Division of Geriatric medicine, Nippon Medical School, Tokyo, Japan)

PURPOSE : The aim of this study is to clarify the clinical usefulness of carotid to femoral pulse wave velocity (PWV), as an index of cerebral infarction (CI), in cross-sectional and longitudinal follow-up studies. METHOD : We studied 260 outpatient (134 males and 126 females), aged 25 to 91 years (average 67.6 +/- 11.0 years). PWV was measured using PWV-200 (Fukuda Denki Co, Ltd.) aortic pulse wave velocity meter. We divided the subjects into two groups depending on the PWV; high (H) group (>or =10 m/sec; n=89) and low (L) group (<10.0 m/sec; n=171). The end point of the longitudinal study was the occurrence of CI events. The average follow-up period was 3.1 +/- 1.6 years. RESULTS : In the cross-sectional study at baseline, the mean age, uric acid, mean systolic blood pressure in H group were significantly higher than in L group. The incidence of lacunar infarction in H group was significantly higher than in L group. However, on multiple logic analysis, age was only significant predictor of CI. The five-year incidence rates of new CI in H group (7.87%) was significantly higher than in L group (1.17%) (p=0.012; Log Rank test). H-group was only significant predictor for CI (RR-15.1; p=0.015) with the Cox proportional-hazard model. CONCLUSION : These results suggest the importance of the assessment of PWV for predicting the existence of cerebral infarction in patients with stroke risk.

[21] Relation of serum lipoprotein (LP)(a) concentration to atherosclerotic disease and severity of atherosclerotic change of major arteries

Ken-ichi Nakahara, Satoru Matsushita

PURPOSE: LP(a) is a genetically determined multi-isoformic lipid-containing particle that has been found in atherosclerotic plaque. The role of LP(a) in atherosclerotic disease remains controversial. We investigated the role of LP(a) as a risk factor for atherosclerotic disease and contribution to the development of atherosclerotic change in major arteries in autopsy patients. METHODS: Serum LP(a) concentration of 581 consecutive autopsy patients was measured within two weeks before death. The history of the patients was retrospectively surveyed from patient records. The atherosclerotic changes of major arteries were scored into 0 to 4 by macroscopic examination. Coronary arteries were cut every 5 mm and scored for their stenosis. RESULTS: The LP(a) concentration was significantly elevated in patients with myocardial infarction(p<0.0001), arteriosclerosis obliterance(p=0.0058), and hypertension(p=0.0271), but was not in patients with cerebral infarction and angina pectoris. LP(a) concentration revealed significant relation to the atherosclerotic change in aorta (p=0.0013), carotid artery (p=0.0037), subclavian artery (p<0.0001), coronary artery (p=0.0004), common iliac artery (p=0.0036). By multi-regression analysis, LP(a) was an independent risk factor for atherosclerotic change in carotid artery, subclavian artery, and common iliac artery, but not in mid cerebral artery, basilar artery, aorta, coronary artery, and mesenteric artery. CONCLUSIONS: Elevation of serum LP(a) concentration was an independent risk factor of atherosclerotic progression of middle sized arteries, but was not of coronary arteries. This fact suggests that there may be another additional mechanism between LP(a) concentration and pathogenesis of myocardial infarction.

[22] Role of Endothelium-Dependent Flow-Mediated Dilatation of the Brachial Artery in Predicting Coronary Events

K. Iijima, M. Hashimoto, J. Ako, M. Eto, S. Kim, Y. Ohike, T. Watanabe, M. Yoshizumi, Y. Ouchi (University of Tokyo, Tokyo, Japan)(Kobe University, Kobe, Japan) M. Akishita, N. Sudoh, K. Toba (Kyorin University, Tokyo, Japan)*

PURPOSE: Impaired endothelial function is thought to be the initial step in atherosclerosis. Flow-mediated vasodilation (MD) of the brachial artery has been used to measure clinical endothelial function, however, its relation to coronary events has not been explored. This study was undertaken to elucidate whether MD of the brachial artery predicts coronary events. METHOD: Three hundred and eighteen subjects 18 to 87 years of age who were examined MD were enrolled. MD was measured using high-resolution brachial artery ultrasonography. After MD measurement, the incidence of coronary events (angina pectoris, non-fatal acute myocardial infarction, cardiac death and coronary artery revascularization) were documented. Average follow-up period were 44 months (max 67 months). RESULTS: A total of 22 events was documented in the 304 subjects during the observation period. According to the MD, we classified the subjects into 3 groups (less than 3.5% 3.5-7.0%, more than 7.0%). Of the 22 events, 13 occurred in subjects with lower endothelial function, compared to 4 events in the subjects with higher endothelial function. By Cox regression analysis, MD showed significantly negative association with future coronary events. CONCLUSION: Impaired flow-mediated vasodilatation of the brachial artery may predict future coronary events.

[23] Autonomic nervous activity and QT dispersion during ERCP

Satofumi Morishita [Second Department of Internal Medicine, University of Tokushima,2-50 Kuramoto-cho, Tokushima, Japan 770-8503

PURPOSE: Cause of cardiac accidents during endoscopic retrograde cholangiopancreaticography (ERCP) was examined from the view points of QTc dispersion, spectral analysis of heart rate variability and serum catecholamine level. METHOD: Twenty-three patients undergone ERCP (ERCP group) and 15 patients premedicated scopolamine butylbromide and diazepam (C group) were studied. Electrocardiographic data during ERCP procedure was analyzed using the QT analysis software (Fukuda Denshi). The changes of QTc dispersion, autonomic nervous parameter from spectral analysis of heart rate variability (LF, HF, LF/HF) and serum catecholamine levels were analyzed (before endoscope insertion, at insertion, stomach passage, duodenum achievement of endoscopy, canulation of Vater papilla, during cholangiopancreaticography and immediately after pulling out endoscopy. RESULT: QTc dispersion was significantly increased during all phase of ERCP procedure, especially during cholangiopancreaticography. Moreover, catecholamines (Ad,NA, DA) at this phase were significantly increased in comparison with the C group. The HF power during ERCP procedure was decreased and decreasing ratio of HF power showed significant inverse correlation with the change of QTc dispersion (r=-0.54, P<0.05). However, there was no correlation in increasing ratio of catecholamine and LF/HF indicating that LF/HF could not become an index of sympathetic nervous activity. CONCLUSION: These results suggest that ERCP procedure gives rise to increase QTc dispersion and decreasing HF power, and arrythmogenic condition might occur.

[24] The Causal Diseases and Duration of Bedridden State of Elderly Subjects in a Care Hospital

Akiko Mastuo, Kohya Okaishi, Miyuki onishi, Noriko Fujiwara, Yang Jin, Masashi Okuro, Shouroku Sakurai, Shigeto Morimoto, Toshio Onishi, and Toshio Ogihara

PURPOSE: Bedridden state in the elderly is one of the most serious problems in Japan. We investigated the cause and duration of bedridden state of Japanese elderly subjects. METHODS: Subjects studied were 211 elderlies with completely bedridden state (35 males and 176 females, mean (+SD) age: 82+9 years). Causal diseases and onset of bedridden state were examined in 1998, and two-year mortality in 2000. RESULTS: Apoplexy (cerebral infarction or cerebral bleeding) was the most prominent cause [n=96, 46%, male/ female ratio: 14/82], followed by dementia [n=49, 23%, 7/42], bone disease [n=30, 14%, 4/27], diseases of internal medicine (include heart failure, pneumonia, asthma, etc.) [n=19, 8%, 5/12], and parkinsonism [n=11,5%, 2/9]. The duration (months) of bedridden state was longer in the following order; cerebral bleeding (60+44), cerebral infarction (57+48), dementia (49+37), hip fracture (45+38), diseases of internal medicine (31+26), and parkinsonism (2+23). The mean age (years) was higher in the following order; hip fracture (89+3), dementia (84+8), cerebral infarction (82+8), parkinsonism(82+4), diseases of internal medicine

[25] Is it possible to improve treatment of severe hypertension? An experience of group assistance.

R.D. Miranda, K.E.C.S. Moreira, A.M.Z. Gagliardi, A.P. Guarnieri, L.R. Ramos. (Federal University of Sao Paulo, Geriatric Division, Sao Paulo, Brazil)

Purpose: Due to the huge number of patients in our ambulatory clinic, geriatric consultation (generally long and complex) in less than 3 or 4 months is quite rare. Thus, one of our greatest challenge is controlling elderly patients with severe hypertension. Objective: Evaluate the effectiveness of a new model of assistance, which we call the quick return method. Methods: The method consists in assisting a group of 3 persons simultaneously, focusing on the blood pressure measurement (seated and upright positions), stimulation of adherence, and adjustment of antihypertensive medication. A simple but specific chart was created allowing us to easily view the evolution. When blood pressure is normalized or have a significant improvement, patient returns to the regular assistance, following the treatment of the other problems. Patients come to ambulatory each 2 to 4 weeks. We analyzed data of 100 consecutive patients enrolled in the quick return. Results: Medium Age= 77.4 years old; Male=29%; average number of visits= 4 (2 11); Systolic blood pressure initial= 184.6 and final=147.5; Initial diastolic= 103.8 and final= 83.2. Conclusion: We concluded that this is a very simple model, easy to implement, and a relatively small number of visits could contribute a lot to a better control of hypertensive elderly patients, specially in clinics limited by a high volume of patients. We believe that the quick return assistance, with a more often contact with the nurse and physician, can improve adherence to medical treatment.

[26] Circadian Variation of Blood Pressure and Catecholamines in Natural Longevous Subjects

H. Mitsubayashi, H. Kawamura (Dept. of Med. Nippon Dental

Univ. Sch. of Dentistry,Tokyo, Japan), M.Jumabay, Y.Izumi, Y.Ozawa(2nd Dept. of Med. Nihon Univ. Sch. of Med,Tokyo, Japan), D.Rehemudura, M.Mahmut, Y. Mu, A. Zu Heng, S. Zhen Wang(Dept. of Med. Xinjiang Medical Univ, Xinjiang, China)

PURPOSE: The purpose of this study was to clarify the relationship between blood pressure variation and urinary catecholamines in longevous people. METHOD: A cross-sectional observational study was conducted on 260 elderly subjects in Xinjiang, China. All of subjects were divided into three groups. 1. Longevous Uygur group: (103 subjects, age >=90 years); 2. Elderly Uygur group: (107 subjects, aged 65-70 years); 3. Elderly Han group: (50 subjects aged 65-70 years). Blood pressure (BP) and pulse rate (PR) were monitored every 30min for more than 26 hours using ambulatory blood pressure monitors (ABPM). Office and mean 24-hr BP and PR were analyzed in each group with conventional statistics. Urinary catecholamines were measured HPLC-DPE methods. RESULTS: 1. ABPM has shown that the prevalence of hypertension is lower in longevous group than other elderly groups ($P > 0.001$). 2. White coat effect is common in longevous groups. 3. The ratio of dipper type were 52 0n longevous Uygur group, 51 0n elderly Uygur group and 45 0n elderly Han group. 4. Urinary norepinephrine (NE) and dopamine(DA) concentrations were not different among three groups. However, urinary epinephrine (E) concentrations in elderly Han group was higher than other groups (Elderly Han group 6.8±7.8g /day, Longevous Uygur group 4.2±2.7g/day, Elderly Uygur group 3.8±2.0 g/day, $p<0.05$). CONCLUSION: Dipper type variation of normotentive blood pressure and lower urinary epinephrine concentration may be one of the important factors in longevity.

[27] Human lipid peroxidation and blood pressure changes in normotensive and hypertensive patients crenotherapy-treated with sulphured mineral water and peloids

Hernández-Torres A.; Ramón-Giménez J.R.; Cuenca-Giralde E.; Márquez-Montes J. (Agency of Health Technology Assessment of National Health Institute "Carlos III". Universitary Hospital "Clínica Puerta de Hierro". ASEPEYO. Madrid. SPAIN)

PURPOSE: The absorption of sulphur, in a topical way, mainly in the form of hydrogen sulphide, contained in the sulphured mineral-medicinal water and peloids, could act as a precursor of GSH, increasing SH radicals present in the cysteine of the glutathione tripeptide and acting as an antioxidant and free radical scavenger. METHODS: Prospective clinical study in human beings, in a Spanish spa of sulphured mineral waters and peloids, evaluated the change obtained in human oxidative balance and blood pressure (BP) before and after crenotherapy administration with the mentioned waters in groups of patients classified according to their BP. The sulphured mineral water crenotherapy influences TBARS elimination in hypertension volunteers and its effect on BP. 110 volunteers of a Spanish spa, were studied. 49 normotensive (NBP) and 61 hypertensive (HBP), this last one treated either with pharmacological BP drugs (HBPD) or not (HBPnD). The group made up of dependent paired samples of the same size. 55 men and 55 women, (mean age: 68.5), were included in our study. There was no statistically significant differences (ssd) between the age of both groups. The levels of urinary production of TBARS obtained in relationship to the groups of volunteers classified according to their BP were analysed, and habits, medical conditions, solar radiations received during treatment, administration approach, diet, sex, smoking, etc. and we studied especially the influence on hypertension. The treatments were baths: 37.5-39°C, 15 minutes, jets, peloid application, and inhalatory therapies, followed by 30-45 minutes rest, to improve the organic reaction. We studied BP changes in relation to: crenotherapy, age, administration approach and urinary elimination of Malondialdehyde (MDA). In the statistical analysis performed, the means were compared using Student's "t" Test and ANOVA and a multiple linear correlation to weight (Stepwise backwards), in elderly population samples, in the final results. RESULTS: There was no ssd in the urinary elimination of TBARS on arrival at the spa between normotensive and hypertensive subjects and neither were there differences after the treatment. Hypertensive women showed a greater decrease of urinary TBARS elimination. Among hypertensive patients we found a more important decrease of urinary production of MDA when compared to the normotensive ones. Therefore hypertensive patients showed less aging. BP did not condition TBARS elimination since there were no ssd between urinary TBARS elimination from hypertensive and normotensive patients. The decrease in urinary TBARS elimination was observed, as long as the treatment was administered topically. The systolic and diastolic blood pressure (SBP/DBP) in normoten-sive volunteers decreased in 7 and 4 mm Hg. respectively. The patients with HBPD in 10 and 6.5 mmHg. and the HBPnD in 11 and 12 mm.Hg, obtaining three groups with ssd ($p<0.01$). The patients who received more benefits from crenotherapy were the hypertensive ones, since their BP decreased between 5.5 and 10.2%, being the hypertensive women those presenting the most important decrease in BP. CONCLUSIONS: There was no correlation between BP and TBARS no matter the sex, as the TBARS elimination decreased in both cases. There were not any relationship between BP and urinary TBARS elimination. The decrease in urinary elimination of TBARS in hypertensive patients showed ssd, which were more significant in women. At the end of the treatment, systolic and diastolic pressure decreased in both men and women. Crenotherapy decreased BP in both normotensive volunteers and those with high BP, treated or not. This effect was more noticeable among hypertensive patients without pharmacological treatment although there is also a decrease in normotensive volunteers, being more important in hypertensive women than in men ($p<0.01$). SBP and DBP values decreased after crenotherapy with sulphured mineral waters. The BP reduction was independent of age and sex. The topical treatment with sulphured mineral-medicinal water and peloids, relaxation, moderate physical exercise and the spa atmosphere decreased the BP values, avoiding HBP. The first of these measures could be the most important in avoiding HBP due to its possible vasodilator action .

[28] Determination of Aspirin Resistance in High-Risk Carciovascular Patients

R. Lenzen, D. Poser (Protest. Geriatric Center Berlin, FRG), A. Loew, H.Riess (Dep. of Medicine, Div. of Hematology, Charité Campus Virchow Clinics, Berlin, FRG), E. Steinhagen-Thiessen (Protest. Geriatric Center Berlin, FRG)

Although Aspirin(ASA) reduces major cardiovascular or cerebrovascular events by 23%, recurrent stroke or myocardial infarction(MI) still occur in patients receiving ASA. Purpose: Identification of patients(pats) after recurrent stroke or MI with insufficient inhibition of platelet function(PF) by ASA, i. e. ASA-resistance. Methods: Determination of PF by the PF-Analyzer 100 (in-vitro-bleeding-time, iv-BT) and by flow cytometry(FC) (CD42b, CD41, CD62P, Fibrinogen, PAC-1). Study populations: 11 healthy volunteers receiving ASA 300 mg/d for 5 days. PF determination before and after the 5 day period. 70 inpatients (mean age 75 years) with recurrent stroke or MI, daily receiving ASA 100mg (n=14), ASA 300mg (n=44), ticlopidine (n=3), clopidogrel (n=9). Results: Controls: iv-BT was significantly extended by 300mg ASA form 95+/-13 sec to 163+/-38 sec ($p<0.0001$), and platelet activation was reduced from 7.4+/-4.5% to 4.0+/-1.5% ($p<0.011$). Determination of the 95% confidence interval revealed 86 sec as maximum limit for iv-BT, and 5% activation for FC. 22 pats(50%) of the 300-ASA-group had an iv-BT of >138sec and 30 pats (63%) a <5% platelet activation, indicating an effective ASA response. However, 6 pats (18%) of the 300-ASA-group revealed an iv-BT of <86sec and 14 pats (32%) still showed platelet activation of >5% by FC. 4 pats (9%) exhibited both parameters of ASA-resistance. Effects of ticlopidine and clopidogrel on PF could be detected by FC, but not by iv-BT. Conclusion: ASA-resistance represents an important risk factor in patients with recurrent stroke or MI, which can easily be detected by iv-BT, pointing towards a different regimen of PF inhibition, if necessary.

[29] Comparison of the risk factors of aortic sclerosis between Korean and Japanese community-dwelling groups

Tomio Hamada, M. Nishinaga, T. Fukui, Y. Morita, K . Okumiya, Y. Doi, T. Ozawa (Kochi Medical School, Kochi, Japan), K. Mtsubayashi(Kyoto University)

PURPOSE: We studied whether there was the life-style difference in risk factors of aortic sclerosis. METHODS: We investigated the severity of aortic sclerosis and the risk factors of aortic sclerosis between Korean (K group: n=77) and Japanese (J group: n=120) men of community dwelling over 65 years old. We measured pulse wave velocity (PWV), ankle-brachial index (ABI) to evaluate the severity of aortic sclerosis. Blood pressure, body mass index (BMI) and the blood samples (total cholesterol, HDL-cholesterol, total protein, etc.) were examined. RESULTS: (1) we could not find significant difference of the PWV between J and K groups. However, the incidence of ABI<0.9 in K group was higher than that of J group (p<0.05). (2) The K group was younger than J group (75 vs. 79, p<0.01). Blood pressure and BMI of K group were higher than those of J group (148/88 v.s.139/78mmHg, p<0.01, 23.5 v.s.22.3kg/m2, p<0.05). (3) The total cholesterol, HDL-cholesterol and serum albumin of J group were higher than those of K group. CONCLUSION: Though K group was younger than J group, the aortic sclerosis of the K group was same as or more severe than J group. These findings suggested there is the life-style difference in risk factors of aortic sclerosis.

[30] Determination of the Dosage of Fluindione Needed for Anticoagulation in the Elderly

L. LECHOWSKI (Hopital Sainte Perine, Paris, France), D. TORTRAT (Association Claude Bernard, Paris), M. HARBOURN, B. FORETTE (Hopital Sainte Perine, Paris, France)

PURPOSE: In the elderly patient, it is difficult to determine the dosage of antivitamin K (AVK) needed to obtain a steady state for INR between 2 and 3. The aim of this study was to set up a method for rapidly knowing the dosage of fluindione to reach that goal.METHOD: Thirty patients aged over 70 years (mean: 86, range: 71 - 96), who were receiving heparin and who needed an oral anticoagulation, were given fluindione (10 mg daily) during 3 days. We measured the INR 38 and 62 hours after the start of treatment. We then adapted the dosage of fluindione (+ 2.5 mg) to obtain a stable INR between 2 and 3.RESULTS: We were able to determine a function predicting the dosage of fluindione (+ 5 mg) that maintained a steady state INR value between 2 and 3.CONCLUSION: This method could be very useful in geriatric practice to shorten the duration of heparin treatment and to reduce the risks of AVK adaptation.

[31] The factor in stroke onset after cardiac surgery

Daisuke Kuzume, Kiyohito Okumiya, Masanori Nishinaga, Yukari Morita, Yoshinori Doi, Shiro Sasaguri(Kochi Medical School, Kochi, Japan), Kozo Matsubayashi(Kyoto University, Kyoto, Japan)

PURPOSE: We evaluated the factor in the onset of stroke after cardiac surgery. METHODS The subjects operated on cardiac surgery were 105 (mean age; 65.3 years, men; 76, women; 29). We studied the association between postoperative stroke onset and many factors, i.e. diabetes, hyperlipidemia, smoking, hypertension, atrial fibrillation, cardiac systolic function, heart diseases, use of heart-lung machine, and so on). RESULTS: Three subjects had postoperative stroke. The association between postoperative stroke onset and atrial fibrillation was shown significantly (E'square test, p=0.02). Twenty-two (31%) of 72 subjects had new onset of atrial fibrillation. Two of three patients of stroke had new onset of postoperative atrial fibrillation and one patient had been having atrial fibrillation ever since preoperation. CONCLUSION: New onset of postoperative atrial fibrillation were shown frequently and there were significant association between stroke onset after cardiac surgery and atrial fibrillation. We should manage postoperative atrial fibrillation carefully to prevent the onset of stroke after cardiac surgery.

[32] End-stage Heart Failure Patient and Outpatient Inotropic Therapy

A. G. Kocheril, J.K. Dave (University of Illinois College of Medicine, Urbana-Champaign, USA)

PURPOSE Geriatric patients with decompensated end stage heart failure have poor quality of life and frequent hospitalizations. While the effectiveness of outpatient intravenous inotropic therapy is debated, it is acceptable in selected patients. There is concern regarding increased mortality with inotropic therapy that has not been consistently shown with low dose intermittent therapy used in newer protocols. Patients with end stage heart failure patients prefer symptom control and better quality of life as the main goal of therapy, even with some increase in mortality. METHODS 83-year-old female with end stage (New York Heart Association Class IV) heart failure due to ischemic cardiomyopathy and severe mitral regurgitation was presented for exacerbation of heart failure. She had had nine hospitalizations for heart failure exacerbations during the previous 15 months Her medications included lisinopril 20 mg daily, bumetanide 2.5 mg daily, digoxin 0.25 mg daily, spironolactone 25 mg daily, and warfarin 5 mg daily. The patient was considered high-risk for mitral vale replacement due to severely reduced LV function (Ejection fraction 10%). Examination was remarkable for blood pressure 90/50 mm of Hg, pulse 100 per minute, weight 114 lbs, bibasilar crackles and severe edema of both legs to the knees. In the outpatient setting, dobutamine was infused at 2.5 mcg/kg/min for 6 hours twice a week. RESULTS During the next 15 months, she had only one hospitalization for exacerbation for heart failure. blood pressure improved from 90/50 to 112/70, weight dropped from 52 Kg to 46 Kg and functional status improved from NYHA class IV to class II. CONCLUSION Outpatient dobutamine therapy is an alternative therapy for heart failure what may improve symptoms and reduce the number of hospitalizations for carefully selected patients with advanced heart failure refractory to optimal oral heart failure agents. Further investigation is needed to assess effectiveness of outpatient inotropic therapy compared to established therapy protocols.

[33] Protocol Design for Switching RV to LV Pacing in End-Stage Heart Failure Patients: The SWRLE Study

A.G. Kocheril and J.K. Dave(University of Illinois College of Medicine, Urbana-Champaign, US)

PURPOSE Pacing in congestive heart failure is one of the most promising therapies of the new millennium. Preliminary studies showed benefits of biventricular and left ventricular pacing in advanced heart failure patients, including symptomatic improvement, increased in cardiac output, and improved quality of life. While controlled trials are in progress, these do not include patients with existing pacemakers or defibrillators. The effects of left ventricular pacing in heart failure patients with existing pacemakers has not been extensively studied. We hope to clarify the effects of left ventricular pacing in patients with advanced heart failure and existing pacemakers. METHODS SWRLE studies the effects of left ventricular pacing by switching from a right ventricular to left ventricular pacemaker lead in advanced heart failure patients with existing pacemakers or defibrillators, aiming to resynchronize the contraction and relaxation sequence of both ventricles and to optimize left ventricular activation pattern. Patients older than 18 years of age with class III or IV heart failure and an existing dual chamber pacemaker or defibrillator will be enrolled by April 1, 2001 in this prospective observational study. The Medtronic 2188 coronary sinus lead will be used to pace the left ventricle. The hypothesis is that SWRLE will result in an improvement in exercise tolerance and quality of life. All patients will be followed up at 3 months. Inclusion started on October1st 2000 and is to be completed by April 1st 2001. Measurement will include functional status, cardiac output, quality of life, and brain naturetic peptide levels. CONCLUSION The hypothesis is LV pacing improves cardiac function by effects on atrio-ventricular delay, AV synchrony, bi-ventricular synchrony, left ventricular activation pattern and left bundle branch block in advanced heart failure patients. If this hypothesis is confirmed, then patients with advanced heart failure might be treated by right atrial- left ventricular pacing rather than the current practice of right atrial - right ventricular pacing.

[34] Time of stroke onset is crucial

Abhaya Gupta [Department of Medicine, University Hospital, Cardiff, UK] Peter Thomas [Department of Medicine, Prince Philip Hospital, Llanelli]

PURPOSE : Information on the time of stroke onset is important. This information can help the stroke service providers in organisation of early rapid stroke treatments. There is a paucity of literature on time of stroke onset in relation to 24 hour clock. We sought to determine the time of onset of focal neurological deficit amongst hospitalised stroke patients. METHOD : Consecutive elderly patients admitted with a diagnosis of acute stroke from January 2000 were included. A structured questionnaire sought to determine the time of stroke onset symptoms. Information was obtained from the patient, carer or general practitioner. RESULTS :Out of 53 patients included, age range was 65 to 104 years, male:female 57:43. 86% had ischemic stroke, 10 0.000000e+00morrhagic stroke, 4 0id not have CT brain. 18(34%)woke up with stroke. 21(40%) had symptom onset between midnight and midday. 14(26%) had stroke onset between midday upto midnight. CONCLUSIONS : A large number of stroke patients had stroke onset in morning hours and 'woke up' with stroke. This subgroup may delay seeking emergency help and thus miss the potential benefits of acute stroke treatments. Further studies into the reasons for early morning strokes are needed.

[35] The Impact of Age on the Functional Recovery from Stroke

J. Kovanen, A. Lukinmaa, H. Takkunen (The Rehabilitation Unit of the Health Department of the City of Helsinki, Helsinki, Finland)

There are opinions, that the rehabilitation of elderly patients may not be as effective as that of younger patients. The aims of this study were to clarify the effect of age on the functional recovery and outcome of stroke patients. The new stroke patients in Helsinki, who are considered to benefit of intensive rehabilitation come after an acute treatment in the Helsinki University Central Hospital to the rehabilitation wards of the Koskela Hospital. The material consisted of 500 consecutive patients admitted to the rehabilitation unit during 1998-2000. The patients were classified according to their median age, 73 years, to the younger group of 250 patients (median age 64 years) and the older group of 250 patients (median age 79 years). The rehabilitation is based on comprehensive, multidisciplinary and function-oriented treatment. The assessment instrument is the FIM, Functional Independence Measure (The Uniform Data System for Medical Rehabilitation). The range of the FIM score is 18-126, the higher the better. The rehabilitation period was usually 2-3 months before the discharge home or to institutional care. The median FIM score of the younger group was on admission 80 (18-125) and at discharge 106 (20-126). The respective figures of the older group were 75 (19-120) on admission and 104 (18-126) at discharge. After the ward rehabilitation period 19% of the younger group needed long-term care. The respective figure of the older was 33%. The main reason for this statistically significant difference was the frequent need of nursing home care in the older group. The social network as well as the social and health services were of crucial importance. As a conclusion, the functional recovery was equal between the groups. Subsequently the age should not be used as a criterion to choose stroke patients for rehabilitation.

[36] The clinical significance of determination of plasma D-dimer in highly aged patients with unstable angina pectoris.

LS Gong, B Zhang et al (Beijing 306th Hospital, Beijing P.R. China).

OBJECTIVE: To investigate the clinical significance of plasma D-dimer level in highly aged patients with unstable angina (UA, mean age 80.75+/- 3.81). METHODS: The plasma levels of D-dimer in 50 cases of angina pectoris, UA group 28, SA (stable angina) group 22, and 16 healthy volunteers were determined and analyzed by half-quantity latex method. The serum levels of firbrin degradation products (FDP), fibrinogen (FIG) were detected simultaneously. RESULTS: The plasma D-dimer levels in the UA group were much higher than those in the SA group and healthy volunteer groups ($p<0.001$). The quantity of FDP in the UA group was also higher than that in the healthy volunteer group ($p<0.05$), but it was not related to the quantity of D-dimer ($r=0.11$, $p>0.05$). CONCLUSIONS: The plasma D-dimer level was higher markedly in highly aged patients with UA, which may reflect the activities of coagulase and fibrinolysin. Detection of plasma D-dimer may be helpful in investigating the pathogenesis of UA, estimating the prognosis of the disease and guiding the clinical treatment

[37] Ultrasonographic study on carotid arteriomegaly specific for aortic aneurysm

K. Kin, T. Iwamoto, T. Sugiyama, M. Takasaki (Department of Geriatric Medicine, Tokyo Medical University, Japan), S. Ishimaru (the 2nd Division of Cardiovascular Surgery, Tokyo Medical University, Japan)

Aortic aneurysm (AA), usually asymptomatic until rupture, is found out incidentally in the elderly, while carotid ultrasonography is widely used to evaluate atherosclerosis. Then, to clarify whether ultrasonographic findings of the diffusely dilated carotid artery is useful for screening AA, 953 consecutive patients with a variety of diseases were enrolled. They were all men. Using B-mode ultrasonography, the carotid diameter from the interface between the adventitia and media of the proximal wall to the interface between the media and adventitia of the distal wall was determined on the bilateral common carotid arteries, and a dilated carotid artery was considered present when the sum of the bilateral carotid diameters was 22 mm or more. The presence of AA was also evaluated by chest X-ray film and abdominal ultrasonography, and, if it was suspected, computed tomography or angiography, or both were carried out. Patients with dilated carotid artery, namely carotid arteriomegaly, were seen in 66 (the dilated group), and the mean age was 71.8. In the dilated group, there were 53 patients with AA and 5 patients with dissecting aneurysm. In the non-dilated group (n=887), there were 192 patients, diagnosed to have AA. These data indicated the sensitivity of carotid arteriomegaly for AA was 0.22, while the specificity of carotid arteriomegaly for AA was 0.98. In conclusion, ultrasonographic findings of carotid arteriomegaly could strongly suggested the possibility of AA, although findings of a non-dilated carotid artery could not rule out the possibility of AA.

[38] Preoperative dobutamine stress echocardiography for evaluation of cardiovascular risk in elderly

Ch. Klimczak, C.Sebban, F.Piette (Service d'Explorations Fonctionnelles, Département de Médecine Interne Gérontologie ; Hôpital Charles Foix, Ivry-sur-Seine, France) E. Coignard, J. Evans (Service de Cardiologie, Hôpital Pitié-Salpêtrière, Paris, France)

Over 4% of patients undergoing general surgery have known ischaemic heart disease; 10 to 15% have multiple cardiovascular risk factors and 15% are over 65 years of age. Perioperative cardiac morbidity and mortality is observed mainly in these cases. Clinical evaluation of cardiovascular risk (myocardial infarction, cardiac failure, sudden death..) is difficult in the elderly. Limited physical capacity makes exercise stress testing or stress myocardial scintigraphy difficult. Stress echocardiography using dobutamine provides a solution to this problem. From the authors experience and published data, stress echo has an excellent negative predictive value (about 94%) which means that a negative test is a very good predictor of a low risk of cardiac events during the perioperative period. On the other hand, a positive test identifies a sub-group of patients with high cardiovascular risk. These patients require special attention both in the perioperative period and thereafter.

[39] The influence of sex gender on secondary prevention in elderly patient with healed myocardial infarction

Akio Kimura, Norihiro Takeda, Hiroki Furuta, Toru Watanabe, Hikaru Ino, Takaaki Taniwa, Toshihiko Takenaka, Takahiro Hayashi, Ken Kanamasa, Kinji Ishikawa The First Department of Internal Medicine Kinki Univ. School of Medicine Osakasayama, Osaka, Japan

PURPOSE: Recently, cardiac events were markedly reduced in elderly patients with myocardial infarction(MI). The purpose of this study is to investigate the better therapeutic strategies considering of sex gender for elderly patients with in elderly patients with healed MI. METHOD: A total of 6290 patients with MI was studied retrospectively from 1986 to 1999. We analyzed the incidence of the cardiac events in the 1069 elderly patients (>= 70 years old) after MI depending of the sex gender. Cardiac events were defined, fatal and nonfatal recurrent MIs, sudden death and death by congestive heart failure (CHF). The patients background such as, risk factors, combined medications, thrombolysis and interventional therapies were analyzed in relation to cardiac events. The single and multivariate analysis (Cox-Hazard model) were performed. RESULTS: The total incidence of cardiac events was 4.8% (51 events/1069 patients) in elderly patients, whereas 2.8% (143/5221, p<0.01) in younger patients. Among elderly patients, beta blockers was the only effective drug for male patients by the multivariate analysis(p<0.05). While, antiplatelet agents was the only effective drug for elderly female patients, (p<0.05). CONCLUSION: In the elderly patients, the effective drugs for secondary prevention after MI were different by sex gender. It may be needed the different therapeutic strategies for elderly patients with MI by sex gender.

[40] Improvement of long-term prognosis after myocardial infarction on the elderly patients in these 14 years

Akio Kimura, Norihiro Takeda, Hiroki Furuta, Toru Watanabe, Hikaru Ino, Takaaki Taniwa, Toshihiko Takenaka, Takahiro Hayashi, Ken Kanamasa, Kinji Ishikawa The First Department of Internal Medicine Kinki University School of Medicine Osakasayama, Osaka, Japan

PURPOSE: The purpose of this study is to clarify the recent changes in long-term prognosis of the elderly patients with myocardial infarction (MI). METHOD: We studied the incidence of the cardiac events after MI, depending of the observation years. A total of 6290 patients with MI from 1986 to 1999 at southern Osaka was registered and studied retrospectively. We divided 3 groups depending of the year observation (Early=1986-1989, Mid=1990-1994, Latest=1995-1999). Patients were divided into 2 groups ; <70 and 70<= years old. Cardiac events were defined, fatal and nonfatal recurrent MIs, sudden death and death by congestive heart failure (CHF). The patients background such as, risk factors, combined medications, thrombolysis and interventional therapies were analyzed in relation to cardiac events. RESULTS: Baseline characteristics showed no differences among the observation periods. The total incidence of cardiac events among the elderly patients were significantly higher than younger patients (25.0 vs 52.4 /1000 person-year, retrospectively, p<0.01). Among the younger patients, the cardiac events depending of the year observation were 35.6 (Early), 20.8 (Mid) and 18.2 (Latest), showing a marked reduction from Early to Mid. Among elderly patients, however, these were 59.5 (Early), 56.2 (Mid) and 33.9(Latest), showing a marked reduction from Mid to Latest. At the latest period, the prognosis of the elderly patients was improved and sudden death and death by CHF were significantly diminished (p<0.01). There was a significant increase in the application of revascularization therapy in the latest in the elderly patients. CONCLUSION: Cardiac events of the elderly patients was markedly reduced at the latest 5 years within these 14 years. This change may be explained by the improvement of therapeutic strategies of elderly patients with MI.

[41] Characteristics of the Cardiovascular Diseases in the Context of Polypathology in the Eldery

M. Georgescu, A.M. Georgescu, G.I.Prada, D.State (Ana Aslan National Institute of Gerontology and Geriatrics, Bucharest, Romania)

The authors followed the analysis of data regarding the characteristics of cardiovascular diseases during the evaluation of the health status in a population group represented by patients admitted to a clinic specialized in delivering medical services for elderly. They investigated 400 patients admitted to the Ana Aslan National Institute of Gerontology and Geriatrics, and used SF-36 questionnaire containing 36 questions grouped into 8 scales that describe health status. For the population 50 - 86 years, the scores for the 8 dimensions of health status were around 50 percent which means a reduction to half of the health status in this age group. Our sample was close to the general structure of the population in Romania. Physical functioning, emotional role, functional role and social functioning are small as compared to the general population, and general health, vitality and body pains have higher scores than general population, The last aspects seem to be explained by the fact that these patients perceive themselves as protected and cared for in the Clinic.

[42] Pulse pressure and cardiovascular risk in the elderly

Denisa Chirita, Gabriel Ioan Prada (National Institute of Geriatrics and Gerontology ANA ASLAN, Bucharest, Romania)

The purpose of this investigation was to evaluate the independent role of pulse pressure as a determinant for cardiovascular prognosis in older patients. A retrospective study was carried out on 3187 patients admitted to Ana Aslan NIGG in 1999. 173 patients were included, age range 65 - 87 years of age. Each had more than 2 major cardiovascular risk factors (hypertension, hypercholesterolemia, low high-density lipoprotein, cigarette smoking, diabetes mellitus) and were diagnosed, for at least 5 years, with ischemic heart disease and/or chronic heart failure and/or hypertension. All patients received standard medical treatment for their medical condition. We considered the following major cardiovascular events for the last 5 years: myocardial infarction, stroke, need for revascularization, number of emergency hospitalizations for unstable angina or aggravated heart failure. We divided the patients into two groups: group A- with a pulse pressure higher than 60 mm Hg (51 patients), and group B-pulse pressure lower than 50 mm Hg (79 patients). Group A had 2.5 times more major cardiovascular events/patient when compared to group B. When analyzed separately for hypertensive patients, group A had 2.7 times more major cardiovascular events/ patient. In conclusion, in older patients the pulse pressure is a major determinant of cardiovascular risk, especially in hypertensives. Pulse pressure can be an independent determinant of cardiovascular prognosis. Implications can be further evaluated in accordance with the principles of evidence-based medicine.

[43] Association of the ACE Gene Polymorphism with Hypertension and Blood Pressure in Men but Not Women

YH Choi, WH Lee, SW Park, HC Gwon, JW Kim, JS Kim, DK Kim, SH Lee, KP Hong, JE Park, JD Seo, WR Lee (Samsung Medical Center, Sungkyunkwan University School of Medicine, Seoul, Korea)

PURPOSE: Controversy exists as to whether the angiotensin-converting enzyme deletion-insertion (ACE D/I) polymorphism is associated with hypertension and blood pressure. METHOD: We used data from a large population-based sample of 4100 men and 3132 women who attended health screening examinations. The ACE genotypes were determined by using a polymerase chain reaction assay. RESULTS: The overall frequencies of the genotypes DD, DI, and II were 14.4, 49.1, and 36.5, respectively in the entire sample. In men, mean systolic/diastolic blood pressure (SBP/DBP) was 125.1/84.9, 123.5/83.7, and 124.2/84.0 mm Hg for DD, DI, and II genotypes, respectively (ANOVA, P=0.08). In women, mean SBP/DBP was 122.2/80.2, 122.1/79.0, and 123.0/79.6 mm Hg respectively (P>0.05). In men of age 45 and above (N=2564), mean SBP and DBP were 128.1 (SE 0.8) and 87.2 (0.5) mm Hg for DD genotype, and 126.0 (0.3) and 85.1 (0.2) mm Hg for DI+II genotype (P=0.03 and 0.001 for SBP and DBP respectively). The prevalences of hypertension were 156/372 (41.9%) and 786/2192 (35.9%) among DD and DI+II genotypes respectively. The odds ratio for hypertension among men (age >45) for the DD genotype was 1.29 (95CONCLUSION: In our large, population-based sample, there is an association of the ACE gene with hypertension and with blood pressure level in Korean men but not women. The result suggests that ACE gene is a candidate gene for hypertension and influences blood pressure in a sex-specific manner.

[44] Orthostatic Hypotension and Non-Invasive Continuous Finger Blood Pressure Measurement in the Elderly

Emmanuel Bulckaen ; Hélène Bulckaen ; François Puisieux ; Philippe Dewailly (Hôpital Gériatrique Les Bâteliers, Chru Lille, France)

PURPOSE: To examine the influence of orthostatism on postural blood pressure (BP) changes with non invasive continuous finger blood pressure measurement (finapres method) in older adults. METHOD: In geriatric short-stay department, 11 inpatients (6 women and 5 men; mean age: 79+/-7) were included in the study. The set of BP was obtained for each subject by one examiner using finapres method during 20 minutes between 2:00 p.m and 6:00 p.m (10 minutes of supine rest, the getting up and 10 minutes after the patient stood). Orthostatic hypotension (OH) was defined as a systolic blood pressure decline/20 mm Hg or a diastolic blood pressure/15 within 2 minutes of standing up. RESULTS: All patients had a drop in BP in the first minute but no had symptomatic drop in BP. Six participants (54%) experienced significant orthostatic BP decline. Among them, 4 (67%) had systolic OH and 2 (33%) had systolo-diastolic OH. Two of three patients with falls, had OH. OH appeared 19.5+/-4.5 secondes (range 12 to 26 secondes). CONCLUSION: OH is responsible many unexplained falls in the elderly. The standard method can not detect a early drop in BP. The finapres method seems to be a good method to detect OH in the elderly. Obviously, further studies are needed to confirm such assertion.

[45] Correlation Between Fibrinogen and Aortic Valve Sclerosis Assessed by Echocardiography in the Community Dwelling Elderly

T.Fukui (Department of Medicine and Geriatrics, Kochi Medical School, Kochi, Japan), M.Nishinaga, T.Hamada, Y.Morita, F.Yamasaki, A.Ishimoto, K.Okumiya, K.Matsubayashi, Y.Doi

Purpose : Plasma fibrinogen levels are known to be an independent risk factor for cardiovascular events. Although arotic valve sclerosis (AV sclerosis) is speculated to be associated with cardiovascular mortality, the underlying mechanisms are poorly understood. In addition, few studies have evaluated the association between AV sclerosis and plasma fibrinogen levels. Methods : We assessed echocardiograms from a total of 123 men and women of 65 years of age or older (mean age 78.0 years) resident in a rural village in Japan. AV sclerosis was defined by focal areas of increased echogenicity and thickening of the aortic valve leaflets without restriction of leaflet motion. Levels of plasma fibrinogen, lipids, Lp(a) lipoprotein, blood sugar, atrial natriuretic peptide (ANP), brain natriuretic peptide (BNP), left ventricular (LV) mass, and aortic pulse-wave velosity were measured. Results : AV sclerosis was present in 39 of the 123 subjects (32%). The subjects with AV sclerosis were older than those without (80.3 vs. 77.8 years ; p=0.01). Plasma fibrinogen levels were signficantly higher in subjects with AV sclerosis than in those without (320 vs. 284 mg/dl ; p=0.009). The prevalence of AV sclerosis did not significantoy differ for sex, blood pressure, level of plasma lipids, Lp(a) lipoprotein, blood sugar, ANP, BNP, LV mass, or aortic pulse-wave velosity. Multiple logistic regression analysis identified only the plasma fibrinogen level (p<0.05) and age (p<0.05) to be independent predictors of AV sclerosis. Conclusion : We conclude that increased serum levels of fibrinogen, as well as advanced age, are closely correlated to AV sclerosis in the community dwelling elderly.

[46] Pulse Pressure in the Elderly

YC Chia (Department of Primary Care Medicine, Faculty of Medicine, University of Malaya, Kuala Lumpur, Malaysia), CT Chua (Department of Medicine, Faculty of Medicine, University of Malaya, Kuala Lumpur, Malaysia)

Pulse pressure in the Elderly YC Chia, CT ChuaAimPulse pressure is being recognised more and more as a predictor of cardiovascular mortality and morbidity. We examined the pulse pressure of a group of elderly patients attending outpatient services.MethodAll patients aged 60 years and above, attending the primary care outpatients services in 1998 were recruited into the study. History of known hypertension, diabetes mellitus and antihypertensive therapy were obtained. Blood pressures(BP) weight and height were measured in all subjects. Conventional hypertension was defined as BP >and equal to 140/90 , and isolated systolic hypertension (ISH) as systolic >and equal to 140 and diastolic less than 90 mm HgResultsA total of 1429 were screened. Their mean age, systolic, diastolic and pulse pressure of the group was 67.6 years, 137, 79 and 58 mm Hg respectively. The pulse pressure correlated significanlty with age and BMI. There was a significant difference between the mean pulse pressure of the normotensive, isolated systolic hypertension (ISH) and conventional hypertensive group (49, 71 and 61 respectively p< 0.005) There was also a significant difference between the mean pulse pressures of men and women, those on and not on antihypertensive therapy and known and non hypertensives, diabetics and hypercholesterolnaemics respectively.There was however no significant difference between the mean pulse pressure of those treated with diuretics, beta-blockers,calcium channel blockers, ACE-inhibitors or alpha-blockers as monotherapy.ConclusionWider pulse pressures are seen in the elderly, hypertensives, diabetes, hypercholesterolnaemics and those with a bigger BMI. Such subjects already carry greater cardiovascular risks. Hence greater efforts should be made to narrow the pulse pressure, particularly in these groups of patients.

[47] Hypertension in the old olds: Prevalence and Treatment in Comparative Urban/Rural Survey.

B. Bien, J. Wilmanska, B.Z. Wojszel (Department of Clinical and Social Gerontology, Medical University of Bialystok, Poland)

PURPOSE: The aim of the study was to estimate the prevalence of hypertension, their probable underdiagnosis and efficacy of antihypertensive treatment in the rural and urban community dwelling elderly in advanced old age. METHOD: The survey was carried out, as a screening, in systematically sampled 463 people 75 and over year old, coming from area served by primary health units (230 in urban Δ Bialystok and 233 in rural area - Sokolka). Single measure of Blood Pressure (BP) was made in probant's home by visiting gp or community nurse. Medical anamnaesis concerning earlier diagnoses and pharmacological treatment was carried out. The diagnosis of hypertension (H) was established according to the WHO-ISH criteria. RESULTS: Almost the same percentage of people (42,1% in urban and 40,3% in rural area) declared known hypertension. 16,2% of the elderly in urban and 30,5% in rural area had underdiagnosed hypertension (persons without antihypertensive treatment, but with elevated BP and unaware of hypertension). In general, 49,1% of the elderly in urban and 70,4% in rural area had elevated systolic or/and diastolic BP, independently on antihypertensive medication. 31,7% of the elderly in Bialystok and 22,3% in Sokolka had normal BP without antihypertensive treatment ('healthy'), successfully medicated were respectively 19,1% and 7,3%,. Unsuccessfully medicated were 28,3% in Bialystok city and 32,2% in Sokolka and 20,9% persons in urban and 38,2% in rural area had elevated BP without any antihypertensive treatment. CONCLUSIONS: The results of the study confirm the high prevalence of hypertension in advanced old age population, higher in rural than urban area, and low efficacy of antihypertensive treatment. The differences between urban and rural samples can be partly explained by socio-demographic characteristics of the two studied populations.

[48] Research on the characteristics and diagnosis of left ventricular dysfunction (LVD) from COPD associated with respiratory failure in elderly persons

Zhu Benhong, Wu Jingchuan (et al. Department of Respiratory Medicine, Xinhua Hospital, Shanghai Second Medical University, China PR)

The Left Ventricular Dysfunction(LVD) resulting from the COPD associated with respiratory failure in the elderly persons, similar to the clinical variance of COPD, is very hard to detect. To improve the early diagnosis of LVD resulting from the COPD associated with respiratory failure in the elderly persons, we assess the statistics obtained from multigated radionuclide ventriculography (MUGA) and clinical analysis of 25 patients suffering from COPD. The statistics are then divided into two groups according to the regional ejection fraction of left ventricular septum

(LVEFs): NLLV group (LVEFs>40%) and LVD group (LVEFs<40%). The latter occupied 64 per cent of the total population. The LVEFs values of the two groups (NLLV and LVD) are 60+6% and 36+7% respectively (p<0.01). The group, whose LVEF is less than 40 per cent, accounted for 20 per cent of the total population. This group (LVEF<40%) is subsumed in the group whose LYEFs is less than 40 per cent. Those whose LVEF is more than 40 per cent and those whose LVEF is less than 40 per cent have LVEFs values of 47+8% and 26+12% respectively (p<0.05). There is also a certain degree of correlation between LVEF and LVEFs Values (r=0.81 p<0.05). The traditional method of judging the clinical variance, chest radiograph and pulmonary function is not able to identify the existence of LVD when diagnosing COPD. The results of this research show the validity of the early diagnosis of the LVD resulting from the COPD associated with respiratory failure in elderly persons by setting the LVEFs value below 40 per cent using MUGA. The cause of LVD includes the overload of the heart due to ventricle mutual dependence, hypoxaemia, hypercapnia, respiratory failure, cor pulmonale and the degree of functional declining of the heart. The left ventricular dysfunction thus caused has the characteristics of left ventricle change succeeding right ventricle overload, the functional damage of left ventricle systole proceeding the diastole, and poor synchronization and coordination of left-right ventricle systole and diastole.

[49] Management of congestive heart failure in geriatric out-patient clinics: a Canadian survey

Nahid Azad (Regional Geriatric Assessment Program, The Ottawa Hospital Civic Campus, Ottawa Canada), Pierre-Marc Legault (University of Ottawa, Ottawa, Canada, Anna Byszewski (Regional Geriatric Assessment Program, The Ottawa Hospital Civic Campus, Ottawa, Canada), Frank Molnar (Regional Geriatric Assessment Program, The Ottawa Hospital Civic Campus, Ottawa, Canada), Barbara Power (Regional Geriatric Assessment Program, The Ottawa Hospital Civic Campus, Ottawa, Canada)

Background: The incidence and prevalence of heart failure increases with age and CHF is one of the most common causes for admission of seniors to hospital. Systematic review of 116 RCTs of outpatient management enhancing programs has demonstrated that such programs improve patients' outcomes. Purpose: To describe the approaches employed in Canadian CHF clinics and to determine the degree to which management enhancing strategies are incorporated. Method: Survey of 11 Canadian CHF clinics to determine program structure and outcome measures employed. Results: 10 out of 11 clinics responded. Formal clinical pathways were employed in only 4, Cardiologists were present in all 10 but were only routinely used in 4. Nurses saw all patients in all 10. Other disciplines were mainly involved on a PRN basis ; Physiotherapists in 6, Pharmacist in 8, Social Worker in 8, Dietician in 7, and Occupational Therapists in 5 clinics. Teaching (one-on-one and handouts) was provided in 10 clinics while 7 employed videos, 6 tele-teaching and 4 classroom teaching. Clinic availability 1 to 5 times a week. Home Care routinely used in 8 clinics. Phone follow-up may happen up to 6 months. In terms of outcome measures; quality of life measured in 4, dyspnea in 3, and mood in only 1clinic. Conclusion: Complex geriatric patients with CHF are a considerable challenge to health care system. The current composition of CHF clinics does not take advantage of structured interdisciplinary management. An enhanced multi-disciplinary approach, use of clinical pathways and improved measurement of outcomes merit further investigation.

[50] Blood Pressure Changes of Elderly People during Japanese Style Bathing

Y. Asakawa (Gunma University School of Health Sciences, Maebashi, Japan) R.Takahashi (Tokyo Metropolitan Institute of Gerontology, Tokyo, Japan) F.Endo (Gunma University School of Health Sciences, Maebashi, Japan)

Purpose: Changes in blood pressure in Japanese style bathing, whole-body soaking in rather hot water, have been suspected one of the inducing factors for bathing accidents: cardio-pulmonary arrest and fall. This study examined blood pressure changes during Japanese style bathing and its effecting factors. Method: Blood pressure changes of 30 male who are aged 65 and over were measured during 5 minutes bathing at 42 centigrade. Blood pressure was taken every 2 minutes during the bathing process from undressing, soaking in a tub to getting out of the bath. The variables to see blood pressure change, coefficient of variation and the difference of maximum and minimum value of each blood pressure measurement were calculated. The relationships between blood pressure change variables and age, presence of cardio-pulmonary disease and of hypertension (140/90mmHg and higher) were examined. Result: Age was significantly correlated with coefficient of variation of systolic blood pressure, diastolic blood pressure, and of mean blood pressure(r=0.42,r=0.37,r=0.37;P<0.05). The difference of maximum and minimum value of measured systolic blood pressure was also found to be significantly correlated with age(r=0.38,P<0.05). 81-year old person, whose coefficient of variation was the highest of all subjects, showed the largest maximum-minimum difference of 89mmHg, with no subjective symptoms of dizziness or instability. Conclusion: Changes of blood pressure are bigger in older persons during bathing, which may result in serious accident by blood pressure drop without any predisposing symptoms.

[51] Postural Hypertension and its association with Nocturnal Blood Pressure changes

Kannayiram Alagiakrishnan,(University of Alberta, Edmonton, Canada) Kamal Masaki, (University of Hawaii,Honolulu, U.S.A) Irwin Schatz, (University of Hawaii,Honolulu, U.S.A) Patricia Blanchette, (University of Hawaii, Honolulu, U.S.A)

Aim of study: To study the relationship between postural hypertension(rise of 10 mm of Hg or more of SBP or DBP on standing for 3 minutes) and its association with nocturnal changes in blood pressure. Methodology: This is a cross sectional study. 62 community dwelling elderly aged 65-94 years were recruited for the study. Patients screened for the presence of postural hypertension using standard sphygmomanometer, by checking their blood pressure in the supine position and after standing for 3 minutes. 31 patients with postural hypertension and 31 controls with no rise of 10 mm HG or more of SBP or DBP on standing for 3 minutes. 24 hour BP monitoring done in all patients and nocturnal blood pressure patterns noted. Results: 42 elderly women and 20 elderly men participated in the study. The median age was 74.5 years. There were 25 Caucasians, 11 Chinese, 22 Japanese and 4 Mixed Ethnicity. Postural hypertension was associated with 21 (65.6%) Dippers , 10 (31.2%) Non Dippers and 1 (3.2%) Extreme Dippers. Postural Normotension was associated with 20 (66.6%) Dippers, 10 (33.4%) Non dippers and 0 (0%) Extreme Dippers. Conclusion: Our study shows postural hypertension is associated with all types of nocturnal blood pressure patterns. In our study,there was no significant association between postural hypertension and extreme dippers as cited in the literature. This investigation was supported by a research center in minority institution award, P 20 RR/ AI 11091, from the national center for research resources, National Institute of Health.

[52] Propophol anaesthesia at the patients elder than 60 years

N.S. Davydova (Ural Medical Academy; Ekaterinburg; Russia) , N.V. Yegorova (Sverdlovsk regional clinical wars veterans hospital ; Ekaterinburg; Russia) M.V. Chuguyevsky (Sverdlovsk regional clinical wars veterans hospital ; Ekaterinburg; Russia) K.Y. Repin (Sverdlovsk regional clinical wars veterans hospital ; Ekaterinburg; Russia) O.G. Malkova (Ural Medical Academy; Ekaterinburg; Russia

Propophol anaesthesia at the patients elder than 60 years Sverdlovsk regional clinical wars veterans hospital N.S. Davydova, N.V. Yegorova, M.V. Chuguyevsky, K.Y. Repin, O.G. Malkova Purpose of research: to estimate the cerebral, reactivity and central haemodynamics at elderly patients group under propophol anaesthesia. Research carried out at the patients of wars veterans hospital operated in ophthalmologic (38 patients) and urologic (18) departments. Induction and maintenance of anaethesia was effectuated with propophol (4,5 - 5 mg/kg/h), 0,1 mg phentanil injected at the induction and if necessary 0,05 - 0,1 mg every 30 minutes. Cerebral bloodflow investigated by transcranial doppler with hyper- and hypocapnic tests. Realization of intravenous anaesthesia by propophol produced at the elderly and senile patients the expressed vasoconstricting effect on main cerebral vessels and the authentic decrease of cerebral bloodflow speed parameters for 34%. The diffusing reduction of vasomotoric reactivity index due to significant restriction of the constriction reserve on a background of normalization of a dilatation reserve. The prevalence of compensating dilatation reactivity pial vessels according to reduction of main bloodflow parameters is established. The more importent index of central haemodynamics is the reduction of cardiac one by 32 %. Other parameters authentically did not change. Thus indirect vasoconsticing action of propophol on main cerebral vessels accompanied by compensating peripheric vasodilatation protecting the brain from ischaemia.

[53] Observation of Therapeutic Effects of Multiple Drugs on CoronaryHeart Disease

DUAN DONGMEI, SUN SHULING

Nitroglycerin, polarized light, energy, compound and svate were used in turn to treat angina pectoris and myocardial infarction in 40 cases at our hospital. In another 20 cases, svate was used alone as the control group. The clinical symptoms and signs, EKG, heart monitor, blood rehology, and cardiac function were observed and tested to evaluate the therapeutic effects of multiple drugs. Materials and Methods: In the first 10 days, nitroglycerin 5-10 mg, KCt lg, Insuling 8 u, and ATP 40 nag were dissolved in 500 mi of 10 glucose solution with 200 u of CoA added into the Murphy's lagena every day. The speed of the intravenous drip of nictroglycerin was 30 ug/min. In the succeeding 10 days, 1 u of svate and 40 rag of ATP were dissolved in 250 ml of 5 glucose solution with 200 u of CoA added into the Murphy's lagena every day. The Control Group: 2 u of svate was dissolved in 250 ml of 5 glucose solution. The intravenous drip was done for 14 days as a course of treatment. After 7-14 days rest, the next courese of treatment would be carried out. Results: In the 40 cases of multiple drug group, 23 cases showed a significant reduction in angina pectoris, 16 cases were effective but 1 case failed to respond to treatment. The total effective rate was 97.5%. In teh 20 cases of control group, 10 cases showed a significan reduction of angina pectoris, 3 cases were effective, and 7 cases were not effective. The total effective rate was 65%. Conclusion: The multiple drug group had good therapeutic effects on various kinds of angina pectoris and AMI. It had cooperative effects to dilate the coronary artery, strengthen the heart, remove fibrin, resist coagulation, reduce the blood viscosity and resist embolism. The treatment of multiple drugs had rapid effects on angina pectoris and AMI. It is convenient to use. It is safe, nontoxic and worthy of clinically popularizing.

[54] Health Conditions of Older Family Caregivers of Stroke Patients

M, Yuki (Miyagi University, Miyagi, JAPAN)

Stroke is the third leading cause of death and the leading cause of adult disability in Japan. In addition, stroke also frequently causes victims to become secluded or remain bed ridden. At present, the presence of a family member care provider is an essential condition for enabling stroke patients, who have some sequela but have been discharged from the hospital and are residing at home, to continue leading their lives in their own homes. The purpose of this study was to investigate health conditions of older family caregiver (OC)(65 years and over) for stroke patient compared with younger caregiver (YC)(64 years and less). Subjects were 302 family caregiver for stroke patients at home , discharged from A hospital (long-term care wards) in Japan 1994-1998. The Care Burden Scale by Zarit is used for caregiving burden measurement, 23 items of health conditions questionnaires for caregiver health, and Tokyo Metropolitan Institute of Gerontology Index for patient ADL. Ninety-nine family caregiver, OC:N=44, YC:N=54, was analyzed with t-test and O square test. The results shows that there were no significant differences on number of family, ADL of patient, caregiving length, caregiving hours, and level of caregiving burden between OC and YC. OC had significantly higher percentage of stomach disorder than YC.

[55] The prognostic significance of 99mTC-MIBI cardiac imaging in elderly patients with CHD

Huang Cuiyao, Jiang Yawen (Gao Ruzhen Liuhuaqiao Hospital, Guangzhou, China)

Purpose: To realize the prognostic value of 99MTC-MIBI cardiac imaging for cardiac events. Methods: 420 CHD inpatients diagnosed by WHO criteria of CHD, aged from 61 to 83, and excluding congenital, rheumatic and other kind of heart disease at the beginning of the study. During the following period, they accepted serumologic check and EKG every six months. Cardiac arrest history was also recorded. Myocardial infarction and cardiac death, as the most important event, were observed intensively. The patients were defined as normal (group A) or abnormal (group B) according to the result of 99MTC-MIBI cardiac imaging. Group A, with 102 males and no females, and group B, with 315 males and 5 females, were followed-up from January 1988 to December 1999, with an average span of 9.8 years. Results: 75 cardiac events occurred among all patients with the frequency of 17.3%. 3 happened in group A, whose occurrence of total cardiac events is 22.6% (72/320) (1.9% per year). The discrepancy between the two groups had statistical significance. 96% (72/75) of cardiac events presented abnormal cardiac imaging, 21.7% abnormal EKG examined at the same time, 52.1% abnormal Holter EKG. In this study, 16 patients underwent coronary angiography, and discovered serious occlusion in 1 to 3 coronary branches, all of them abnormal in cardiac imaging. Conclusion: These suggest that 99MTC-MIBI cardiac imaging demonstrated high sensitivity and specificity in diagnosis for heart ischemia, and was also quite valuable for its diagnose in the early time, estimation of its severity, and judgement of its prognosis, and especially to forecast for cardiac event.

[56] Predictors of Survival Among Elders Suffering Strokes in Taiwan: Observation From a Nationally Representative Sample

Shu-Li Wang, Wen-Harn Pan, Meng-Chih Lee, Shu-Ping Cheng, Ming-Cheng Chang (Departments of Public Health and Family Medicine, Chung Shan Dental and Medical College, Taichung, Taiwan)

PURPOSE: In Taiwan deaths due to stroke now rank second only to cancer, with more deaths resulting from strokes than from any other single pathology. It is important to understand stroke prognosis among elderly stroke survivors, with respect to survival and attendant predictive factors, because aged population in Taiwan is growing rapidly. The aim of the present study was to discern factors affecting survival in stroke patients from a nationally representative elderly sample. METHOD: A total of 99 stroke survivors, from a representative national sample of elders aged e 65 years on December 31, 1988, whose strokes occurred in the period 1989-1993,were followed for mortality until July 1, 1995. Personal data were gathered through home interviews conducted by well-trained community nurses, and mortality data were obtained from the national census office by using identification card numbers. Cox proportional hazards regression analysis and the stepwise technique were used to search for important prognostic factors of survival. RESULTS: Women experienced a higher mortality rate (139.8 per 1000 person-years) than men (126.4 per 1000 person-years). Stroke patients who received continuous treatment for diabetes experienced mortality risk similar to those of patients without diabetes and much lower risk than those with discontinuous diabetes treatment. Cognitive impairment was also independent predictor of survival (relative risk 2.69, $P<0.05$). In addition, patients with both cognitive and mobility impairment had a 2-to 3-fold greater risk of mortality than those with only a single abnormality. CONCLUSION: This first report on the various prognostic factors related to survival of elderly stroke patients in Taiwan's Chinese population emphasized the benefit of continuous diabetes treatment in improving survival chances. These stroke patients should also be monitored for cognitive and mobility impairments and undergo rehabilitation.

[57] Comparison of ADA Diagnostic Criteria with WHO Criteria for Diagnosis of Diabetes Mellitus in Elderly.

M. Staszwewska, S. Lambru, A. Dontas, (Research Center of Studies of Age related Changes in Man, Athens, Greece).

PURPOSE: The aim of the study was to compare the criteria of ADA for the diagnosis of Diabetes Mellitus (DM) and Impaired Glucose Tolerance (IGT) with those of WHO in ambulatory elderly people living in a resident home. METHOD : Fasting Plasma Glucose (FPG) was examined according to ADA criteria and Oral Glucose Tolerance Test (OGTT) according to WHO method in persons without known DM. Body Mass Index (BMI) and Waist Hip Ratio (WHR) was carried out too. 303 elderly subjects aged >70 years (mean age 83.1 + 6.6) were examined: 212 women (70%) and 91 men (30%). RESULTS : According to WHO criteria, 18.1% suffered from DM (women 19.7%, men 12.1%) with mean value of BMI 25.9 and WHR 0.90. Although, 30.4% had IGT (women 28.8%, men 34.1%), with BMI 25.5 and WHR 0.90. According to ADA criteria, 3.6% suffered from DM (women 3.8%, men 3.3%) with BMI 28.2 and WHR 0.91. Although, 6.4% had IFG (women 6.2%, men 6.6%) with BMI 28.5 and WHR 0.94. Sensitivity and specifisity of ADA method comparing to WHO criteria was respectively 15.4% and 100%. The cross results showed that subjects with DM according to ADA criteria, had 27% IGT and 73% DM according to WHO criteria. In opposite, subjects with DM according to WHO criteria had only 23.6% IFG and 14.5% DM according to ADA criteria. CONCLUSION: Suggesting by ADA criteria, seems are not sensitive enough for the diagnosis of Diabetes Mellitus and using them in screening could lead to significant devaluation rate of the prevalence in elderly, higher than in younger age group has already been proven.

[58] Apolipoprotein(a) phenotype and retinopathy in elderly diabetics-prospective study

T.SUZUKI, K.OKAZAKI, H.NAKANO, K.OBA (Division of Geriatric Medicine,Nippon Medical School, Tokyo, Japan

The aim of this study was to clarify the relationship between apolipoprotein(a) phenotype and diabetic retinopathy in elderly patients on the basis of a prospective study. Serum Lp(a) concentration and apolipoprotein(a) phenotype were analysed in 250 diabetic patients . Apolipoprotein(a) phenotypes were classified into 7 subtypes (F,B,S1,S2,S3,S4,O(Null)) by the method SDS electrophoresis with Western blotting. Patients were defined as the high molecular group with S3, S4, O (Null) and as the low molecular group with F, B, S1, S2 . Diabetic retinopathy is classified to 4 groups non-retinopathy group (R0), simple retinopathy group (R1), pre-proliferative retinopathy group (R2), proliferative retinopathy group (R3). The distribution of the diabetic retinopathy in the high molecular group was changed for 4 years as follows: R0 73.2%;57.6%,R1 5.4%13.7%, R2 14.6 %;18.0%, R3 6.8%;10.7. That in the low molecular group was changed for 4 years as follows: R0 62.3%4;45.8%,R1 13.3%8.9%, R2 13.3;20.9%, R3 11.124.4%. The frequency of diabetic retinopathy in low molecular group was significantly higher than that of diabetic retinopathy in high molecular group on the 4 years follow-up period. On multiple logistic regression analysis, low molecular group is an independent risk factors for diabetic retinopathy by follow-up investigations. These results provide a significant evidence of a contribution of low molecular Lp(a) to the increased risk for the diabetic retinopathy on the prospective study.

[59] Study of hypertension and diabetes in the elderly population in Pernambuco, Brasil, 2000

Margarida Santos, Maria do Carmo Araujo (Public Staf of Health in Recife Pernambuco Brasil)

In Brazil, diabetes reached 7.6% of the population among 30 to 60 years and 20% of the population above 70. It is the 4th basic cause of death and responsible for 30% of the inabilities in those older than 60 years. The hypertension answers for the 3rd death cause. Pernambuco state of the Brazilian federation, with population of 7,399,131 of the which 7.9% are more than 60 years. Rising accomplished in 5 hospitals of the Public System of Health in this state, verified that 43% of the hospital internment of this age group are due to complications of hypertension and diabetes. Not existing rule of the actions of health regarding these pathologies. Objective: To accomplish rising of the prevalence and hypertension complications and diabetes in the 60 year-old larger population in the state of Pernambuco with the purpose of subsidizing the implantation of a politics of health gone back to these pathologies Method: Rising marries the house accomplished through the community agents of health by means of filling of questionnaire before tested. Results: 1) number of people disabled above the expected living in home, without its relatives know as maintaining them appropriately clean and alimentados, 2) diversity in the treatment forms, 3) lack of clinical accompaniment and medicaments in the identified cases. Conclusion: project to gather scientific community and professionals of health with the purpose to define norms for control of these pathologies.

[60] Prevalence of Diabetes Mellitus and Impaired Glucose Tolerance in Elderly

S. Lambru, M. Staszwewska, A. Dontas, (Research Center of Studies of Age related Changes in Man, Athens, Greece).

PURPOSE: The aim of this study was to determine the prevalence of Diabetes Mellitus (DM) and of Impaired Glucose Tolerance (IGT) in subjects with good functional abilities residing in a retirement home. METHOD : Known DM was deduced from detailed medical history of the examined subjects. Unknown DM and IGT were diagnosed by the two hours oral glucose tolerance test (OGTT) according to WHO criteria, which was carried out if the person did not report known DM. All subjects were examined for Body Mass Index (BMI) and Waist Hip Ratio (WHR). 566 subjects aged >70 years (mean age 82.7 + 6.6) : 389 women (68.7%) and 177 men (31.3%) were examined. RESULTS : Prevalence of known DM was18.2% (women 17%. men 20.9% =NS) with a mean value of BMI 26.9% + 4.7 (women 26.8, men 26.9) and WHR 0.91 + 0.08 (women 0.90, men 0.93). According to the OGTT 18.2% subjects were classified as suffering from undiagnosed DM (women 20.8%, men 12.1% = NS) with a mean value of BMI 26 + 4.6 (women 26.4, men 24.6) and WHR 0.90 + 0.08 (women 0.89, men 0.92 0. In addition, 30.4% of the examined subjects presented an IGT (women 28.8%, men 34.1% = NS) with a mean BMI 25.3 + 4.7 (women 26.1, men 23.9) and WHR 0.90 + 0.08 (women 0.89, men 0.92). Persons with normal glucose metabolism had a BMI 25.5 + 4.1 (women 25.7, men 25.0) and WHR 0.89 + 0.11 (women 0.88, men 0.92). CONCLUSION: Total prevalence of DM (known and discovered by OGTT) at this age group, was high (36.4%). IGT was present in 30.4%. Thus, only 33.2% of the examined elderly subjects had a normal glucose metabolism. BMI is increased in persons with impaired glucose metabolism, specially those with previously known DM.

[61] Influence of hypertension on incidence of chronic complication in diabetic patients

Y. M. Li, J. D. Liu (Beijing Hospital, Institute of Geriatrics, Beijing, China)

160 cases of NIDDM were studied during past 10 years. The diagnosis and type of diseases were met with the criteria designed by WHO for hypertension and diabetes. Of these patients, 42 cases were preliminary hypertension (26.2%). The research data were obtained from comparison between hypertension (H) group and patients with normal (N) blood pressure. The results showed that no differences were found in age, period of disease, serum level of cholesterol and triglyceride, in two groups. But, the serum level of insulin in H group (143.6 ± 87.2 pmol/L) were significantly higher than that of N group (104.0 ± 61.7 pmol/L), $p<0.05$. The incidence of nephritic diseases, proliferative retinal lesion, stroke and coronary heart diseases in H group were remarkably increased than N group respectively ($p<0.05$ and $p<0.01$). In the 42 cases of NIDDM

with hypertension, 12 cases suffered from hypertension earlier than NIDDM, 18 cases were diagnosed NIDDM first. The period of NIDDM last longer in latter group (9.3 ± 6.3 years) than former group (4.1 ± 4.0 years), $p<0.05$. In contrast, the period of hypertension last longer in former group (20.7 ± 7.8 years) than latter group (5.4 ± 4.7 years) $p<0.01$. It was concluded that hypertension is an important factor on incidence of complication of diabetic patients.

[62] Glucoregulation and Autonomic Nervous System Function Following Ethanol Administration in Older Patients with Diabetes Mellitus

J.L. Gilden, T.Hassan, A. Akbar, S.P. Singh (Finch University of Health Sciences/The Chicago Medical School and VA Medical Center, North Chicago, IL, USA)

Alcoholism is a widespread social problem. Long term abuse is known to be associated with autonomic dysfunction as well as hypoglycemia. Acute alcohol (ETOH) administration to normal subjects produces selective alterations of regional cerebral blood flow (CBF)and changes in glucoregulation. . In addition, the autonomic nervous system (ANF) plays a role in normal glucoregulation. However, the effects of 2-3 drinks of alcohol on glucose regulation in older diabetic patients and its relationship to changes in ANF has not been well studied. Ethanol (ETOH= 0.4 gm/Kg) was administered orally to 10 non-alcoholic male diabetic patients [(mean age=67 yrs; range=54-77) (3 Type 1 DM: 7 Type 2 DM) (glycosylated hemoglobin= 6.6 to 9.8%) (EKG expiratory:inspiratory RR ratios= 1.0-1.22)]. ANF (hemodynamic response to upright posture for systolic (SBP), diastolic (DBP), and pulse pressure (PP) (mmHg), heart rate (HR), and CBF by Transcranial Doppler for end diastolic velocity (EDV), as well as glucose (BG) and endogenous insulin levels (C-peptide) were evaluated before and 1 hour after ETOH administration. Following ETOH, BG decreased significantly from average of 217 to 159 mg% ($p<.02$) without changes in C-peptide levels. Greater decreases in response to upright posture occurred for both DBP ($p<.02$) and PP ($p<.01$), with increases in HR ($p<.05$). Decrease of orthostatic SBP correlated with ETOH levels achieved ($R= -.7$; $p<.05$). Patients with more ANF dysfunction had greater DBP decreases ($R=.8$; $p<.02$). The chchchchchangeschanges changes in orthostatic hemodynamic parameters (HR and PP), as well as the BG decreases correlated with the decrease in CBF ($R=.9$; $p<.05$; $R= -.7$; $p<.05$). In conclusion, acute administration of 2-3 drinks of ETOH to diabetic patients can adversely affect both ANF and BG. These hypoglycemic and hypotensive effects are also associated with decreased cerebral blood flow and are greater in older diabetic patients with more autonomic dysfunction.

[63] Prevalence of diabetes mellitus and glucose intolerance among the elderly in the Canary Islands (Spain)

P.L. de Pablos, B.J. Anía (Hospital Doctor Negrín and Universidad de Las Palmas de Gran Canaria, Spain), F. Rodríguez-Pérez, F.J. Martínez-Martín (Hospital Doctor Negrín, Spain).

PURPOSE: To estimate the prevalence of diabetes mellitus and impaired glucose tolerance among the elderly living in the community in the Canary Islands (Spain). METHOD: We studied 243 subjects aged 65 or older randomly sampled from the municipal roster of a mid-size town having 12381 inhabitants of whom 1745 (14%) were 65 or older. An oral glucose tolerance test was performed in the fasting state in all subjects except those already diagnosed with diabetes. The 1985 World Health Organization (WHO) and 1997 American Diabetes Association (ADA) criteria for the diagnosis of diabetes and glucose intolerance were both applied. RESULTS: The prevalence of diabetes mellitus according to WHO was 32.1% (23.6% for men, 41.4% for women) and did not increase with age. The diagnosis of diabetes was already known by 68% of diabetics. Prevalences of impaired glucose tolerance (WHO) and impaired fasting glucose (ADA) were 24.0% and 12.1% respectively. CONCLUSION: In this population one third of the elderly is diabetic, and more than half has either diabetes mellitus or glucose intolerance according to WHO criteria.

[64] Treatment of lower respiratory infections with Meropenem of elderly

Yinan Zhou (Department of Respiratory Tract Disease, HuaDong Hospital, ShangHai, China) Huili Zhu (Department of Respiratory Tract Disease, HuaDong Hospital, ShangHai, China) Jin Gong (Department of Respiratory Tract Disease, HuaDong Hospital, ShangHai, China)

Purpose: To evaluate the effectiveness of Meropenem therapy for lower respiratory infections in the elderly (average 83.5 years old). Method: 31 cases of inpatients from April 2000 December 2000 were treated. The dosages of Meropenem used were 0.5g every 8-12 hours by vein for average 10 14 days. The analysis was done according to the improvement of clinical symptoms, the clearance rate of bacteria in sputum and the results of lab. Results: Clinical efficacy was 80.64%. The clearance rate of bacteria in sputum was 84.37%. There was no damage of renal or hepatic function. Conclusion: Meropenem can be considered as an effective and safe agent in treatment of serious lower respiratory infections in the elderly, especially for infections within hospital.

[65] Acute infective exacerbation of elderly COPD relation between bacteriologic etiology and lung function

Zhang Yueli, Pang Zhonghua (Respiratory Department of Huadong Hospital, Shanghai 200040 PRC China)

The aim of this study was to evaluate the relationship between decrease of lung function and the sputum culture in acute exacerbation of elderly COPD. Sixty-seven elderly patients admitted to our hospital with an acute infective exacerbation of COPD were investigated with the clinical data, chest film, lung function tests and sputum bacteria culture. The patients were categorized according to the lung function test. Lung function tests revealed an FEV1 of 50% to 75% of the predicted value in 35 patients (group C), an FEV1 of 35% to 49% of the predicted value in 19 patients (group B), and an FEV1 of <or =35 of the predicted value in 13 patients (group A). The sputum cultures were positive in 48 of 67 cases. The results of cultures in discovering microorganisms were about 71.6% . For all patients together, the most frequently isolated bacteria were Gram-negative bacillus (65.8%), followed by Candida albicans (20.6%), and Gram-positive cocci (13.6%). In group A patients, 10 of 13 had bacteria. In group B patients, 14 of 19 showed bacteria. In group C patients, 24 of 35 had bacteria. The average number of bacteria per patient from group A, group B and group C was 9.46, 6.53 and 3.23, respectively ($P<0.001$). There is a correlation between deterioration of lung function and the bacteria isolated from patients with acute infective exacerbation of COPD. The more the impairment of lung function, the more the chance of bacteria infection, the more the positive rate of sputum cultures.

[66] The Effect of Pulmonary Rehabilitation on Physiological function in Patients with COPD

Kwua-Yun Wang National Defense Medical Center; Taipei, Taiwan, ROC Chi-Hue Chiang Tri-Service General Hospital, National Defense Medical Center; Taipei, Taiwan, ROC Wen-Yi Shau Graduate Institute of Clinical Medicine, College of Medicine, National Taiwan University; Taipei, Taiwan, ROC

PURPOSE: The purpose of this study is to investigate the effect of pulmonary rehabilitation (PR) on physiological function in patients with COPD. METHOD: We take a convenience sample (n=28) from a teaching hospital. Eighteen patients are to be the study group and 10 patients are to be the control group. The study group divided into bicycle with education program (group 1; n=9), education program (group 2; n=6), and walking with education program (group 3; n=3). Pulmonary function, SaO2, and related questionnaires data were collected. Means and their 95 for the control group were decreasing (-0.0311/week, $P=0.002$). For the study groups, the slowly decreasing FVC were not significant. The change trends of FEV1 for group 1 and 3 were lower than that of control group ($P=0.025$ and 0.009). CONCLUSION: The exercise with education program has the beneficial in the elderly with COPD.

[67] Clinical effect of Aztreonam in the treatment of elderly with lower respiratory tract infection

Zhong-Hua Pang, Hui-Li Zhu (Division of Respiratory tract disease, Hua-Dong Hospital, Shanghai, the People's Republic of China)

PURPOSE: To study the clinical effect and safety of Aztreonam in the treatment of elderly with lower respiratory tract infection. METHOD: 80 cases with lower respiratory tract infection were consecutively admitted to our hospital from 1995 to 2000 and their clinical data were retrospectively reviewed. The dosage of Aztreonam was 1 gram/each time, every 8 to 12 hours for intravenous injection or 2 gram/each time, every 12 hours. Their clinical symptoms, signs, and the dynamic changes of the laboratory data and bacterial spectrum were monitored before and after treatment with Aztreonam. The side-effects were carefully recorded. According to the guiding principles of the antibiotic investigation issued by the ministry of health in 1993, 4 grades were subclassified. The complete recovery and significant effect were considered as efficiency. RESULTS: It showed that the effect of Aztreonam on the patients with the lower respiratory tract infection caused by Gram's negative bacilli was much better with total efficiency rate of 78.7% and 76% of the clearance rate of bacteria. Its side-effects were rare with no otic and renal toxicity observed. CONCLUSION: The effect of Aztreonam in the treatment of patients with Gram's negative bacilli infection was satisfactory, good and safe. Its side-effect was rare with no otic and renal toxicity. So, it's especially suitable for the elderly and patients with renal insufficiency.

[68] Impact of COPD in the Elderly

F. Halici, G.I. Prada (Ana Aslan National Institute of Gerontology and Geriatrics, Bucharest, Romania)

Chronic obstructive pulmonary disease (COPD) is a major cause of disability and death. It is thought that its true mortality exceeds that of pulmonary neoplasm. It is estimated that COPD affects 150f older men. This study attempts to reveal the importance of COPD in the elderly. We analyzed 2400 patients admitted to Ana Aslan National Institute of Gerontology and Geriatrics between January 2000 and December 2000. We found 53 patients diagnosed with chronic obstructive pulmonary disease (COPD), 39 of them (73,4%) had a predominance of emphysema, 10 of them (19%) had a combination of chronic bronchitis and emphysema and 4 of them (7,6%) had a combination of chronic bronchitis and asthma. The age range was 63-91 years (mean 71 years). Age distribution was: 60-69 years - 17 patients (32%), 70-79 years - 22 patients (41,5%), 80-89 years - 9 patients (17%), >90 years - 5 patients (9,5%). Gender distribution was: men 77,36% and women 22,6%. All of the patients with COPD founded by us, represented only 2,080f the total number of patients admitted to our clinic during one year. This is much lower than the figures given by other studies, perhaps due to patients’ less industrialized areas of origin and lower rates of cigarette smoking. Another reason could be the fact that it is most of the time undetected clinically (maybe due to decreased mobility and reduced expectation on the part of physician and patient). There was a significant difference between men and women with COPD; it was more prevalent in men (77,36%), p< 0,05. Prevalence was higher in the age group 60-79 years, especially heavy smokers (20 cigarettes * 20 years). The prevalence of patients with COPD is decreasing sharply in older age, after 80 years and is more prominent as emphysematous type (type A) disease. These findings suggest that either the COPD is underdiagnosed in older age or the patients died earlier from different complications and associated diseases. The impact on elderly patients quality of life seems to be influenced mainly by emotional reactions to their condition, therefore therapy aimed at developing strategies for coping with daily living might have greatest effect.

[69] Should we offer non-invasive ventilation to elderly COPD patients who declined intubation in acute exacerbation?

PT Lam, CM Chu, WM Lam, MF Leung (Department of Medicine & Geriatrics, United Christian Hospital ,Hong Kong)

Purpose: To estimate the survival of severely ill COPD elderly patients and to identify possible predictors so as to help prioritize patient for non-invasive ventilation (NIPPV) . Method: A retrospective study was done in this group of patients who were admitted with acute respiratory failure, who declined intubation in case of respiratory arrest, but agreed to a trial of NIPPV , between 1.10.1999 to 30.4. 2000. Their baseline, outcome and survival data were recorded. Kaplan-Meier plot was used to examine survival. Comparisons between groups were performed with log-rank test. Results: A total of 15 cases were included in analysis, with 14 males and 1 female, at mean age 74.8 (SD 6.6) years. The median survival after NIPPV was 18 days (range 2-302 days). There were 8 deaths within 18 days. Those (7, 46.7%) survived could all be weaned off from NIPPV and survived for ?6 months. Baseline variables were tested as predictors of survival for ?180-days and none was statistically significant . However, those with low Katz's ADL score or high pre-NIPPV CO2 showed trends towards worse prognosis. Conclusion: The survival appeared to have a bimodal distribution. A significant proportion (46.7%) did benefit from NIPPV and survived for >6 months even though they declined intubation. A prospective study with larger sample size is underway to study survival and to identify predictors, so that this group can be better identified. Meanwhile, prior to the identification, NIPPV should be given a trial for all this group of seniors.

[70] Nocturnal Oxigen Desaturation in the Elderly (70+): A Population Based Study

Bernhard J. Hoeltmann Helmut Frohnhofen**,Carsten Neifer* (*Department of Geriatric Medicine, Grevenbroich General Hospital, Germany ** Department of Geriatric Medicine ,Prosper-Hospital Recklinghausen, Germany)*

Finger-pulse-oximetry provides a simple method for screening of severe apneas, that is well accepted by elderly people. The lack data about NOD in the elderly led us to perform sleep study in 100 randomly selected people out of a total of 5105 inhabitants aged 70+ living in the rural city of Grevenbroich. 61 persons agreed, 39 refused to be studied. Refusers were older (80 vs. 77y) and showed a lower Berthel´s Index (77 vs. 96) than participants. The Results for Oxigen desaturations Index 4% (ODI4%) are shown below: Measure ———Total———Male———Female n-particip.—n=61(100%)—23(38%)——38(62%) Age(y)————77±5—— ——76±5———77±5 BMI————————27±7————26±3————28±4 ODI4% <5 /h————27(44%)——11(48%)——16(42%) 5-9/h———— 17(28%)————6(26%)——11(29%) 10-19/h————11(18%)————6(26%)—— 5(13%) 20->——————6 (10%)————0(0)————6(16%) The results of our study confirm, that elderly people have a very high prevalence of frequent nocturnal oxigen desaturations. Although the recovery rate of our study was exeptional for this age the data may de biased, since elder and more handicapped people refused to participate. The prevalences may be underestimated.

[71] The clinical significance of the surveillance of SIL-2R, IL-4 & IL-5 in elderly persons with lower respiratory infection

Zhu Benhong, Shen Xia, Shen Zheng, Zhu Weiqi, Xu Xianghui, Yang Tianyun, (Department of Respiratory Medicine, Xinhua Hospital, Shanghai Second Medical University, Shanghai, China PR)

AIM: To explore the clinical significance of the participation of SIL-2R, IL-4 and IL-5 in the course of infection on the elderly persons with lower respiratory infection. METHOD: To employ ELISA, by means of Reader Organon Technique to detect SIL-2R, IL-4 and IL-5 on the 25 cases of elderly persons with lower respiratory infection and 30 cases of the normal elderly persons during the period from July 1996 to June 1997. RESULT: The result on the basis of statistics shows that SIL-2R 6104+1980 pg/ml, and IL-5 26+17 pg/ml of the elderly persons with lower respiratory infection are obviously higher than those of the normal (p<0.05), while IL-4 3+5 pg/ml is lower. CONCLUSION: SIL-2R and IL-5 on the elderly persons with the lower respiratory infection participate in the course of inflammation and they are the efficiency index of the infectiousness and immunity.

[72] The clinical characteristics and risk factors of multi-organ failure (MOF) from COR

Zhu Benhong (et al. Department of Respiratory Medicine,Xinhua Hospital Attached to Shanghai Second Medical University,China PR)

To inquire into the unique nature of MOFE, the clinical features and the key to the treatment, we examined 60 cases who died during 1992 to 1994 according to the standard of the diagnosis of COPD, cor pulmonale and MOFE. The elderly patients with cor pulmonale induced by COPD who die of MOFE amount to 91.6 per cent of the total population. The rates of failure of the lung and heart are among the highest: 100%and 84% respectively. The failure of 4 organs makes up 49%,and the failure of 5 organs 31%. Among the most common risk factors, pulmonary infection tops all, which takes up 100%; hypoxaemia accounts for 100%, hypochloremia 84%, hyponatremia 69%, acidosis 73%. MOFE resulting from cor pulmonale induced by COPD in the elderly persons has the characteristics of insidious development, dull reaction, multi-organ influence, little chance of recovery, and a high death rate. The lung and the heart, whose failures occur in a very early stage, are the two most important organs which invite good attention in the early treatment of MOFE. The control of infection and the remedy of hypoxaemia and derangement of the internal environment are the important measures of the treatment.

[73] Prethrombogenesis state and therapeutic effect of Dan Shen during acute exacerbation of chronic COPD

Zhu Benhong (Department of Respiratory Medicine,Xinhua Hospital,Shanghai Second Medical University,Shanghai PR. China)

Abstract: The acute exacerbations of COPD are often associated with prethrombogenesis state in elderly persons. The prethrombogenic state and therapeutic effect of Dan Shen have not been assessed during acute exacerbation of COPD in elderly persons. These 22 patients had serial measurements of VIIIR:Ag, AT-III:Ag, Fg,and blood viscosity with clinical evidence of exacerbation (Pa02 7.69±1.41 Kpa). VIII R:Ag was elevated (>126%) in 15 patients, AT-III:Ag was decreased (<0.23 g/L) in 13 patients, Fg was elevated (>4 g/L) in 13 patients, blood viscosity (H.C.) was elevated (>7.28) in 12 patients, blood viscosity (L.C.) was elevated (>9.87) in 19 patients, and plasma viscosity was elevated (>1.84) in 17 patients.The values of blood viscosity (H.C.) were 8.7±2.0 and 6.4±0.8 respectively in patients with elevated level and normal level of VIII R:Ag (P<0.01). VIII: R:Ag was elevated in all patients in whom blood viscosity (H.C.) was elevated. There was a significant correlation between the values of VIII R:Ag and blood viscosity (H.C.) (r =0.51 P<0.05). Blood viscosity (L.C.) was elevated in all patients in whom blood viscosity (H.C.) was elevated. Plasma viscosity was elevated in all patients in whom Fg was elevated.There was a significant correlation between the values of Fg and plasma viscosity (r=0.52 P<0.05). Blood viscosity (H.C.) and blood viscosity (L.C.) were significantly decreased with major effect of Dan Shen (P<0.05). It is thus concluded that during acute exacerbation of COPD in elderly persons,VIII R:Ag is a more sensitive indicator in hypercoagulability state, AT-III: Ag is an objective indicator in anticoagulant change, Fg is a principal indicator relative to plasma viscosity, and comprehensive therapy with Dan Shen has clinical significance against prethrombogenesic state. Key words: chronic obstructive pulmonary disease factor VIII related antigen (VIII R:Ag) antithrombin III blood viscosity.

[74] Clinical analysis of Klebsiella pneumoniae and Escherichia coil producing ESBLs in patients with respiratory tract infection

Hui-Li Zhu, Zhong-Hua Pang (Division of Respiratory tract disease, Hua-Dong Hospital, Shanghai, the People's Republic of China)

PURPOSE: To investigate the antibiotic resistance of strains producing ESBLs among Klebsiella pneumoniae and Escherichia coil in elderly with respiratory tract infection, and the prognosis of these patients. METHOD: We analysed 92 strains of Klebsiella pneumoniae and Escherichia coil in 78 elderly with respiratory tract infection. 16 strains of ESBLs producing E. Coli and 28 strains of ESBLs-producing K. Pneumoniae were determined by a double-disk synergy test and antibiotic susceptibility test by Kirby-Bauer test. We evaluated the prognosis and relationship between antibiotics used and ESBLs producing. RESULTS: The prevalence of ESBLs in isolates of 59 K. Pneumoniae was 47.5%, E. Coli was 48.5%. ESBLs producing strains had higher resistance rate to aminoglycosides (except amikacin), quinolones , the second and third-generation cephalosporins and ampicillin, but few of which was resistant to imipenem and amikacin. The susceptibility rate of these strains to sulfonamides and cefoxitin was about 37.5%~50%. The mortality of patients with infection of ESBLs-producing strain was higher than that of patients with respiratory tract infection of non ESBLsproducing strains, and antibiotics used were higher frequency. CONCLUSION: The results indicated that such antibiotics as imipenem, amikacin, sulfonamides, cefoxitin and others which are susceptive to ESBLs-producing strain can be used. The prognosis of patients with respiratory tract infection of ESBLs-producing strain was poor. The unreasonable using of antibiotics may result in appearance of ESBLs-producing strain.

[75] Urinary tract infection caused by extended spectrum-lactamase producing organisms in a geriatric practice

CY Yung, A Lau, CM Chu, EMF Leung (Department of Medicine & Geriatrics, United Christian Hospital, Hong Kong, China)

PURPOSE: To study the urinary tract infection (UTI) caused by extended-spectrum b-lactamase (ESBL) producing organisms in a geriatric practice in Hong Kong METHOD: Patients in acute geriatric wards of a district hospital were recruited if they had features of urinary tract infection and urine cultures growing extended spectrum-lactamase producing organisms were studied. RESULTS: 69 patients (47 female) were recruited. 41 lived in nursing homes and 59 in the community. Common presenting features included fever (73%), failure to thrive (38%) and symptoms of lower UTI (33%). Only 3% had symptoms of upper UTI. Common comorbidities were: cerebrovascular disease (58%), diabetes mellitus (39%), uremia (29%), previous hip fractures (15%) and dementia (7%). Multiple comorbidities were common with Charlsons score ranging from 0-7 (mean: 2.5, S.D.: 1.8). 28% had long-term (>2 weeks) bladder catheterization and 19% had recent bladder catheterization. 35% were double incontinent. 56 needed diapers. Using Subjective Global Assessment, malnutrition was detected in 67%. Urine dipstick tests were performed in 61 patients: positive white cell esterase in 89% and nitrite in 83%. Peripheral white cell counts ranged from 3.3 to 28.3 (mean: 11.5, SD: 5.6). Urea ranged from 1.3 mmol/l to 91 mmol/l (mean: 12; S.D.: 14.9). Bacteremia was found in only 9%. Empirical choice of antibiotics included: cefuroxime (54%), amoxycillin-clavulanate (17%) and sultamicillin (8.7%). 58% required subsequent change in the antibiotic therapy. CONCLUSION: Typical urinary symptoms were not common. Urine dipstick was useful to predict the presence of bacteriuria. The choice empirical treatment for these patients can be difficult.

[76] Pneumonia Mortality Trends in Elderly Spanish during the period 1975 - 1995

C. Trescoli (Internal Medecine Department, Hospital de la Ribera, Alzira, Valencia, Spain)

Pneumonia is one of the most important causes of death in the Spanish Elderly population. Purpose: Identify changes in pneumonia mortality rates in the elderly Spanish population (>65 years) from 1975 to 1995. Method: The Spanish National Institute of Statistics registers all deaths by its primary cause using the ICD-8 code (Institute Classification of Diseases). We collected pneumonia mortality rate data (per 100000 inhabitants) by sex and 5-year age groups using the ICD-8 code: 480-486 (pneumonia all causes with or without microorganism) from 1975 to 1995 in Spain. A regression equation on the natural logarithm of mortality rates was used to calculate the mean annual percentage of variation. Results: Pneumonia mortality rates for the elderly for both sexes was 240.6 in 1975 and 107.4 in 1995. Mean annual mortality rates were significantly higher for men, 177.5 than women, 132.9 during that period of time. There was a 44% total reduction in mortality rates during that period with an annual decrease 4.3% (95%CI: -4.8 to -3.8) for both sexes. This reduction in pneumonia mortality did affect both sexes (annual decrease in men: 4.0% and women: 4.6) and all 5 year age groups, especially young elderly (annual decrease in 65 to 75: 8.5% and >85 years: 4.3%). Summary: Pneumonia mortality rates were higher in men than women during the 1975 - 1995 period. There is a gradual reduction in annual pneumonia mortality for both sexes and all 5-year age groups, specially the young elderly.

[77] Prospective study on the relationship between nosocomial infections and natural killer cell activity and serum immunoglobulin in the elderly

Lu Pei-Fang, Ma Yong-Xing, Yu Xiao-Feng (Department of Aging, Antiaging and Cognitive Function, Shanghai Institute of Gerontology and Geriatrics, Department of Geriatrics of Huadong Hospital,Shanghai,China)

Objective: Prospective study on the relationship between nosocomial infections and natural killer cell activity and serum immunoglobulin in the elderly. Methods: Prospective follow-up of elderly (>60 years) patients for nosocomial infections in geriatric ward from Jan. 1996 to Dec. 1997 after assay of nature killer cell activity and serum globulin in 1995 in the healthy inspection of the aged in O.P.D. Results The relative morbidity of nosocomial infections in the elderly with nature killer cell 20% is significantly higher (77/101=76.24%) than that with nature killer cell 20% (24/101=23.76%). No significant correlation of nosocomial infections and serum Immunoglobulin was found. Conclusions: The elderly with lower nature killer cell activity is rather easily complicated with nosocomial infections. Nature killer cell activity may be one of the important causes of nosocomial infections in the elderly. It is suggested that routine examination of nature killer cell activity is very important for prophylaxis of nosocomial infections in the elderly.

[78] Comparative study on serum antibody titers for JC and BK virus

Masako Tajima (Teikyo University, Tokyo, Japan), Mayumi Mori (Tokyo Metropolitan Geriatric Hospital, Tokyo, Japan), Kenzo Kato (National Institute of Health Japan, Tokyo, Japan), Hisamasa Akabane (Yokosuka Kyosai Hospital, Yokosuka, Japan), Naoto Aoki (Tokyo Metropolitan Laboratory of Public Health, Tokyo, Japan), Hiroyuki Shimada (International University of Health and Welfare, Ohtawara, Japan)

Purpose: We previously reported the difference between anti-JCV and anti-herpesviridae titer in elderly patients. Using newly developed hemagglutinin (HA) particles produced by recombinant baculovirus, we conducted a survey on antibody titers in Japanese patients to delineate differences between closely related human polyomaviruses, JCV and BKV, in elderly patients. Method: Sera (606 samples, age; 0-89 years) were collected between 1999 through 2000, and examined for anti-JCV and anti-BKV antibody titers by hemagglutination-inhibition (HI) test. Specificity of purified HA antigen made by baculovirus was confirmed by HI test and western blotting. Sera with 8-fold or more increase in HI titers were judged as positive. Results: Average antibody titer for JCV was higher than BKV, in neonate-1 years old (yo) patients. In 2-9 yo patients, BKV titer was higher than JCV. In 10-39 yo patients, no apparent difference was noted. However, in 40-89 yo patients, JCV titer was significantly higher than BKV titer, where BKV titer decreased age-dependently. Percentage of patients with high antibody titers (512-fold or more), in 50 yo or older patients, was 5.1% for BKV and 19.2% for JCV. In patients between 20-89 yo, anti-BKV positive rate was around 70% while anti-JCV positive rate increased age-dependently, up to 100% on 80-89 yo patients. Conclusion: In the patients 40 yo or older, average BKV antibody titer decreased age-dependently while JCV antibody titer increased. Although, replication of JCV and BKV has been known to be enhanced by the presence of immuno-suppression, JCV replication may be enhanced by mechanisms associated with aging, also.

[79] Prospective survey of nosocomial infections (N.I.) in 1840 geriatric ward elderly patients

Lu Pei-Fang, Yu Zhi-Zheng, Zhao Shang-Min (Department of Aging, Antiaging and Cognitive Function, Shanghai Institute of Gerontology and Geriatrics, Department of Geriatrics of Huadong Hospital,Shanghai,China)

Objective: To find the general rules of N.I. in geriatric ward, and the prophylactic measures. Methods: By prospective follow-up of 1840 elderly patients in the geriatric ward from Jan 1996 to Dec. 1997. Results: 18.12% (333 case-times/1840) of nosocomial infections with mortality 14.4% were found. The N.I. occurred chiefly in the patients with malignancy, renal failure, stroke, diabetes mellitus and those long term keep beds. The incidence of N.I. were highly correlated with age, period of hospitalization and invasive diagnostic-therapeutic procedure. The prognosis of N.I. was closely related to the severity of the original diseases. 79% of the N.I. were pulmonary infections and 9% urinary tract infections. 67.9% of positive sputum culture were Gram-negative bacilli. The incidence of nosocomial infections is significantly correlated with old age, period of hospitalization, long term keep the beds, invasive diagnostic-therapeutic procedures, functional declining of vital organs and decreased immunological function.

[80] Morbidity and Clinical Risk Factors for Post-influenza Pneumonia in the Elderly in Japan

Miyuki Onishi, Shigeto Morimoto, Toshio Onishi, and Toshio Ogihara(Department of Geriatric Medicine, Osaka University Medical School, Osaka, Japan.)

Post-influenza pneumonia is one of the biggest health problems in the elderly, since it is the main cause of excess death in winter season. We investigated morbidity and the clinical risk factors for post-influenza pneumonia in the elderly. Methods: Subjects studied were 1087 elderly inpatients (mean age: 83years, 99 with and 988 without influenza vaccination) in a long-term care hospital with a follow-up period from December 1, 1998 to March 31, 1999. The items investigated were: 1. the morbidity of post-influenza pneumonia in the 988 non-vaccinated and 99 vaccinated elderly subjects, 2. clinical risk factors for post-influenza pneumonia in the 988 non-vaccinated elderly subjects, identified by multiple logistic analysis among the following covariates: age, gender, cerebrovascular disease, ischemic heart disease, heart failure, past history of lung disease, asthma, renal failure, diabetes, dementia, hypoalbuminemia and bed-ridden state. Results: The numbers of the subjects who suffered from the influenza itself were 349 (35%) in the non-vaccinated group and 14 (14%) in vaccinated group. The morbidity rates of post-influenza pneumonia in the influenza patients among these groups were 27% (95 subjects) without and 14% (2 subjects) with vaccination. The independent risk factors for post-influenza pneumonia in non-vaccinated subjects were past history of lung disease (p=0.001, relative risk; 2.47) and hypoalbuminemia (p=0.001, 2.50). Conclusion: Vaccination for influenza significantly decreased the morbidity of influenza itself and tended to decrease that of post-influenza pneumonia. Past history of lung disease and hypoalbuminemia were significant clinical risk factors for the post-influenza pneumonia among non-vaccinated elderly subjects.

[81] Investigation of Pathogens of Sputum of Bacterial Pneumonia in Bedridden Inpatients

Kohya Okaishi, Shigeto Morimoto, Toshio Onishi, and Tishio Ogihara (Department of Geriatric Medicine, Osaka University Medical School, Osaka, Japan).

PURPOSE: Elderly inpatients are susceptible to suffer from pneumonia. Particularly, pneumonia constitutes the leading cause of death in the elderly. In the present study, we investigated major pathogens of pneumonia from a specimen of sputum in elderly subjects with completely bedridden state. METHOD: The subjects studied were 110 elderly people aged 65 years and older (82 females, 28 males, mean age : 81.1 years) who were admitted in the ward of the Department of Internal Medicine of a hospital for the elderly, serving as a hospital and a long-term care facility for the elderly. They were diagnosed as having bacterial pneumonia from the Center for Disease Control and Prevention (CDC) definition. A follow-up study was performed from 1997 to 1998. RESULTS: The causal bacteria for pneumonia in the elderly were more often identified as follow: Streptococcus agalactiae (GroupB) (34.5%), MRSA(methicillin resistant Staphylococcus aureus) (28.2%), Streptococcus pneumoniae (8.2%), Klebsiella Pneumoniae (7.3%), MSSA (methicillin sensitive Staphilococcus aureus (5.5%) and Pseudomonas aeruginosa. (3.6%). CONCLUSION: From these results, special attention should be focused that MRSA was highly identified as a major pathogen of pneumonia in bedridden inpatients.

[82] Asymptomatic bacteriuria in elderly diabetic women

K. Oba, H Nakano, K Okazaki, T Suzuki (Division of Geriatric Medicine, Nippon Medical School , Tokyo, Japan)

The aim of the present study was to determine the prevalence of and the risk factors for asyptomatic bacteriuria ASB in elderly women (65 years) with type 2 diabetes. The present study included 99 type 2 out-patient diabetic women 88 and consecutive 299 non-diabetic women attending the outpatient in 1996. Patients with known urinary tract abnormalities, symptoms of a urinary tract infection or the use of antimicrobial drugs during the previous a month were excluded. ASB was defined as the presence of more than 5 leukocytes /high-power field (HPF) in a random urine sample. Diabetic women more often had ASB than non-diabetic women (54.5 vs. 27.1%) (P<0.01). Duration of diabetes was significantly higher in diabetic women with ASB than in diabetic women without ASB (13.8 vs. 9.0 years). The prevalence of ASB was significantly increased in patients with a duration of diabetes exceeding 15 years (0-4 years; 50.0%, 5-9 years; 36.8%, 10-14 years; 45%,15 years; 80.8%). However, no differences were evident in HbA1C (7.8 vs. 7.3%) and BMI (24.1 vs. 23.4kg/m2). Diabetic women with ASB more often had diabetic retinopathy, diabetic neuropathy and cerebrovascular disease than those without ASB. However, no statistically significant differences were evident in prevalence of diabetic nephropathy, hypertension, hyperlipidemia, constipation, ischemic heart disease and dementia. The prevalence of ASB was increased in elderly women with diabetes and increased with longer duration of diabetes but was not affected by measures of glucose control.

[83] Silent cerebral infarction: A potential risk for pneumonia in the elderly

H Sasaki, T Nakagawa, K Nakajoh, N Okamura, T Matsui, H Arai.

Objective: To determine whether patients who have silent cerebral infarction are more likely to develop pneumonia than are controls without silent cerebral infarction. Methods: We examined 269 community-residing participants of the senior day-care center without history of previous stroke, and then followed them over a two-year period to assess pneumonia. On the basis of computerized tomography scans, they were divided into two groups; no infarction (n=102) and cerebral hemispheric infarction (n=167). Cerebral infarcts were further divided into deep and superficial infarcts. Results: The incidence of pneumonia was significantly higher in subjects with silent cerebral infarction (19.8%) than in controls (4.9%) (odds ratio, 4.67 [95% CI, 1.87-11.67]; P<0.01). Deep infarcts were more closely associated with the incidence of pneumonia (29.1%) than superficial infarcts (7.6%) (odds ratio, 5.00 [CL, 1.91-13.08]; P<0.01). Conclusions: Amongst hemispheric silent cerebral infarcts, those located in the deep brain structures may be an important predictor of the development of pneumonia.

[84] Complicated Urinary Tract Infection and Asymptomatic Bacteriuria - The effective Approach

J.D. Soares (Gerontology Research Centre and Program, Unifenas - Alfenas University - Alfenas - MG - Brazil) B.C. Gomes (Unifenas - Alfenas University)

Diagnosis and treatment of complicated Urinary Tract Infection (UTI) in older persons in the Log-Term Care (LTC) setting presents practitioners with special clinical challenges and is a more complex proposition than management of UTIs that arise in younger persons. Key decision points should be routinely addressed: 1. Is a culture needed? 2. Which drugs should be used? 3. How long they should be used? In old patients with complicated UTIs the spectrum of infecting pathogens is much broader, and a urine culture should be routinely performed. In our series of 120 patients a small percentage of cultures showed E.coli, whereas most indicated various species of gram negative bacilli, such as Proteus sp, Klebsiella, Enterobacter, Serratia, Pseudomonas sp, Enterococcus faecalis, Staphylococcus aureus. When the cause was E.coli in a complicated UTI in old population a multiple - antibiotic - resistant strain is more likely to be present. As many as 50% of all LTC elders have asymptomatic bacteriuria, without symptoms (frequency, urgency, dysuria, etc.) and they showed evidence of pyuria in sedimentoscopy (Addis - count). Routine follow-up cultures induce a high prevalence of asymptomatic bacteriuria and over diagnosis of UTI and unnecessary antibiotic therapy. The presence of UTI - like symptoms in older persons does not always indicate infection. Symptoms such as incontinence, urgency and nocturia are common in older men and women without UTI and can coexist with asymptomatic bacteriuria. In older patients, pyuria is not necessarily a dependable marker of UTI. Urinalysis cannot be relied upon to distinguish an urinary tract colonization from infection. The Follow-through can be problematic for several reasons: 1. Uncontaminated specimen may be difficult. 2. 52% of all LTC patients had asymptomatic bacteriuria. The asymptomatic bacteriuria is common in a chronically ill and debilitated patient, but is a benign condition and is not known to contribute to morbidity or mortality. The treatment of asymptomatic bacteriuria is not clinically beneficial nor cost effective.

[85] Performances of 5 Tests for Diagnostic of Helicobacter Pylori Infection in the Elderly

N. Salles-Montaudon (Hôpital Xavier Arnozan, Pessac, France), N. Broutet (Hôpital Pellegrin, Bordeaux, France), L. Monteiro (Hôpital Pellegrin, Bordeaux, France), N. Gras (Hôpital Pellegrin, Bordeaux, France), A. de Mascarel (Hôpital du Haut-Lévêque, Pessac, France), J.P. Emeriau (Hôpital Xavier Arnozan, Pessac, France), F. Megraud (Hôpital Pellegrin, Bordeaux, France).

Purpose : The diagnostic of Helicobacter pylori (Hp) infection is difficult to determine in the elderly because of the high frequency of atrophic gastritis and drug intake (antibiotics or antisecretory drugs). The aim of this study was to evaluate the diagnostic performances of 5 tests in the elderly. Methods : We evaluated the diagnostic performance of 5 tests : culture and histology of biopsy specimens, serology (ELISA), urea breath test (13C-UBT), and detection of Hp antigens in stool samples (HpSA). Patients were considered Hp + when the result for culture was positive or when 2 of the other tests performed were positive. Results : 167 patients were included in this study [55 men, 112 women; mean age : 85.6 +/- 5.1 years, 86 (51.5 %) patients were undernourished, and 89 (53.3 %) took drugs at the time of inclusion]. Hp infection was found in 38 (22.8 %) patients. Performances estimated for each test were as follow : Performances (%) Culture Histology Serology 13C UBT HpSA Sensitivity 86.9 77.8 90.9 74.3 74.1 Specificity 100 95.4 88.8 79.5 98.7 Performances of culture, histology and 13C UBT were lower in the 85-100 years age group, in the undernourished group and in the chronic atrophic gastritis group. Only the performances of the 13C UBT were significantly lower in the treated group (p < 10-6). Conclusion : Patients over 90, undernourished, with drugs consumption, or chronic atrophic gastritis may decrease tests performances by producing an unfavorable environment for Hp overgrowth.

[86] CMV antibodies in long term care geriatric wards.

S. Moulias, R. Salvatore, S. Meaume (Long term units, Hôpital Charles-Foix, Ivry/Seine, France), A. Devillechabrolle, R. Moulias

(Laboratory Biology of Aging, Faculté Pitié-Salpétrière, Paris, France).

Nosocomial infection risk may concern also latent viral infection as Herpes family virus. Method: we have compared 97 elderly patients in long term units, 72 healthy elderly living at home, 100 healthy blood donors and 60 AIDS and ARC patients for CMV IgG antibodies (passive hemagglutination). Results: high concentrations (>2560) of anti-CMV IgG showed no significant discrepancy between long stay elderly patients (73 %) and AIDS patients (65 %). These concentrations in both pathological groups were higher than those observed in healthy elderly (29 %, p<10-5) and blood donors (29 %, p<10-5). These results were not due to an elevation of IgG concentrations in elderly patients, at the opposite a reverse correlation (r=0.38) was observed between anti-CMV IgG and total IgG (p<0.01). Conclusion: high antibody response towards CMV in elderly long term care patients may be due either to exogenous nosocomial infection, or to endogenous reinfestation, due to a lowered immune status. Correlation with morbidity and mortality deserves further studies.

[87] Urinary Tract Infections in Nursing Home Residents in Hong Kong

Kwok-fai Hui, Kwok-yiu Sha, Man-fuk Leung (Department of Medicine and Geriatrics, United Christian Hospital, Hong Kong)

Purpose: To study the commonest bacteriological causes of urinary tract infections in nursing home residents in Hong Kong, and to review their sensitivity patterns to the common antibiotics being used. Method: All patients coming from nursing homes covered by a regional hospital with urinary tract infections (positive culture with a significant bacterial count) admitted to the geriatric wards would be reviewed, during a 6 month period from 1/1/2000 to 30/6/2000. Results: 51 episodes of urinary tract infections were identified. Mean age of the patients was 84.0 (range 68 to 100). 80.40atients were in groups 4 and 5 in Rankin Scale. Escherichia coli was the commonest organism isolated from the urine (47.2%), followed by Proteus (18.9%) and Pseudomonas (13.2 %). 39 episodes (76.5%) were non-catheter related, whereas 12 episodes (23.5%) were catheter related. In the latter group, the most common organism isolated was Escherichia coli (50%), followed by Proteus (28.6%). The traditional drugs, including ampicillin and cotrimoxazole, were not useful as they had a high resistance rate. Beta-lactam/beta-lactamase inhibitor and second-generation cephalosporin still had a resonable sensitivity pattern among the commonest organisms isolated (greater than 68%). However, the sensitivity pattern of quinolones was fair, with only 440f Escherichia coli sensitive to quinolones. The catheter related infections had a higher prevalence of resistant organisms. Conclusion: The commonest bacteriological cause of urinary tract infections is Escherichia coli in nursing home residents in Hong Kong. Beta-lactam/beta-lactamase inhibitors and second-generation cephalosporins are still reasonably sensitive to the organisms isolated.

[88] The Effect of Age on the Presentation and Outcome of Tuberculosis

G.Kaltenbach (Center of Gerontology, University Hospital of Strasbourg, France), F.Grunenberger (Department of Internal Medicine and Nutrition, University Hospital of Strasbourg, France), T.Vogel, D.Heitz, C.Martin-Hunyadi, M.Kiesmann, M.Berthel (Center of Gerontology, University Hospital of Strasbourg, France), J.L.Schlienger (Department of Internal Medicine and Nutrition, University Hospital of Strasbourg, France), F.Kuntzmann (Center of Gerontology, University Hospital of Strasbourg, France)

Purpose : Comparison of clinical and radiological features of tuberculosis in two groups of patients, under and over the age of 65 years. Method : Between 1980 and 1997, 83 patients diagnosed as having tuberculosis were treated in two departments of Internal Medicine and Geriatrics. They were divided into young (< 65 years) and elderly (>65 years) patients and differences in presentation between the two groups were analysed. Results : 41 elderly (mean age 80 years) and 42 young (mean age 40 years) patients were studied. A past history of tuberculosis was found in 18% of elderly and in 10% of young patients (p=0.43). Cancer was more often associated with tuberculosis in elderly patients (15% vs 2%, p=0.09). The sites of disease were similar in both groups with 2/3 of pulmonary infection. Comparison of the presenting symptoms showed no significant difference for weight loss (66% vs 52%, p=0.31), fever (56% vs 52%, p=0.90) and cough (32% vs 33%, p=1). The skin testing was positive for the majority of the young adults (84% vs 58%, p=0.11). The commonly observed biochemical abnormalities in elderly patients were lymphocytopenia (p<0,01) and increased erythrocyte sedimentation rate (p=0.03). There was no significant difference in radiologic findings between both groups with miliary tuberculosis in about 10% of patients. The mortality was high (22%) for the frail elderly patients with associated diseases. Conclusion : Except slight differences in biochemical features, the clinical and radiological presentation of tuberculosis was similar in young and elderly patients.

[89] Predictors of Mortality in Old Patients with Nosocomial Bacteremia: What About Functional Status

G. GAVAZZI, [Department de medecine interne et gériatrie, Centre Hospitalier Universitaire,Grenoble, France] P. ESCOBAR, [Department de medecine interne et gériatrie, Centre Hospitalier Universitaire,Grenoble, France] P.COUTURIER, [Department de medecine interne et gériatrie, Centre Hospitalier Universitaire,Grenoble, France] A. FRANCO. [Department de medecine interne et gériatrie, Centre Hospitalier Universitaire,Grenoble, France]

Purpose : Bloodstream infections (BI) are associated with a higher mortality rate in elderly patients In overall population nosocomial acquired bloodstream infections (NBI) are associated with a higher mortality rate. To détermine specific pronostics factors in elderly patients with NBI, we analysed retrospectively the charateristics of 62 NBI. Methods : It's a retrospective study concerning 62 NBI diagnosed between 04/96 and 09/99 in 3 differents units of gériatric's département (acute care, readaptation care and long term care). BI, polymicrobial BI, nosocomial BI are defined according CDC definitions. Epidemiological characteristics (demographic data, immunosuppresive treatment, duration of hospitalisation), underlying disorders (active malignancy, dementia, stroke, prior colonisation with MRSA, recent surgery or invasive interventions, tube feeding, bladder or intreveinous catheter), clinical findings (detailed activity daily life (ADL) before NBI, delirium, thrill, hypothermia <36°C or hyperthermia >38.5°C, shock) biological findings (neutrophiles count, lymphocyte count, albuminemia) were collected for each patient. Type of microorganism , and source of BI were also collected for each episode. Results : Of 62 patients Mean age was 83.9 (SD 1). Female account for 66%. Cocci gram negative bacteria were more frequent acounted for 630f all BI. Escherichia coli was the most frequent microorganism (44%), and Staphyloccocus aureus the second (18%). Source of BI were respectively, Urinary tract infection (41.9%), undeterminate source (35.5%),skin and soft tissue (4.8%), digestive (4.8%), post-surgical(3.2%) and pulmonary (1.6%). Statistical analysis showed that mortality was significantly correlated with age >85 ans, ADL score <2, incapacity to walk from bed to toilet, incapacity to wash himself, hypothermia, hypoalbuminemia (<25g/l), Bladder catheter, Cocci gram positive bacteremia. Conclusions : This study find the pronostic factors already found in previous studies ; it shows also that the incapacities to activities of daily living, particularly to walking and to wash himself are important indepedant factors for the outcome of very old patients with nosocomial BI.

[90] Deaths By Pneumonia in Elderly of the Southeast Area of Santiago of Chile

E Gallegos C, M Grosman C, VH Carrasco M. (Geriatrics Service Centro de Rehabilitación CAPREDENA. Santiago de Chile y Servicio de Geriatría Hospital Universitario de Getafe. Madrid,*

España)

Purpose: In the winter the Health Ministry accomplishes a campaign that provides extra resources to the health care system. Pneumonia is the third cause of death and explains 11% of the mortality. To determine the epidemiological characteristics and associated diseases. METHOD: The present study, of descriptive type, is based on the analysis of the whole the death certificates with diagnosis of pneumonia as cause of death, issued in the south-east area of Santiago of Chile, in greater of 65 years, in 1999. RESULTS: 520 deaths for pneumonia are registered, rate of 39.8 deaths by 100,000 inhabitants. 53% women. 72% occurs in >75 years, 47% dies in their houses and 46% dies in the months of May -June - July (Autumn - winter). In these months dies 45.2% of the cases of the year and a 54.5% expire in a hospital. The prevailing associated disease is the Dementia (21%), COPD (18%), Cancer (13%), ICTUS (12%) and Cardiac diseases (10%). 61.4% of the patients with dementia die in their houses; 60.8% of the patients with ICTUS die in a hospital; 52.3% of the patients with cancer die in their domicile. 53.2% of the patients with COPD expire in the months of May - June - July, as opposed to patients with cancer, since in this era only expires a 35.5%. CONCLUSION: 1- The deaths by pneumonia occurred are concentrated in the months of autumn - winter and exists greater quantity of deaths income. 2- The observed results of greater mortality in ages more extreme and the pathologies associated with event of the death.

[91] A Clinical Report of Spondylodiscitis

P. Gareri, G. Ruotolo, F. Talarico, S. Giancotti, G. De Sarro*, D. Galasso Medicine II Unit, "Pugliese- Ciaccio" Hospital, Catanzaro; *Chair of Pharmacology, Department of Experimental and Clinical Medicine "G. Salvatore", Policlinico Materdomini, University of Catanzaro.*

A 71-year old woman was hospitalized for the onset of a continuous-remitting fever since a week. It reached peaks up to 39 °C, accompanied by a macular papular exanthema from upper extremities to the palm of the hands and by headache, sweating, myalgia, anorexia, photophobia, torpidity of sensory. Fever had been preceded by a "tache- noir" to left leg. On her hospitalization she appeared to be dehydrated, tetraplegic and with urinary incontinence. Physical examination showed an hepatosplenomegaly, right inguinal and armpit mesoadenitis. Hematochemical exams, Weil-Felix test and a cervical Nuclear Magnetic Resonance (NMR) were performed. Weil-Felix test was positive for proteus- OX19, suggesting the diagnosis of Rickettsiosis. Cervical NMR showed a wide change in the intensity of the signal of vertebral bodies C5- C6 and in particular of intervertebralis disk, with erosions of vertebral tabular and a prevertebral and posterior abscess. Therefore, diagnosis of spondylodiscitis with an abscessual anterior epidural collection was made. Antibiotic treatment was performed at first with minocycline 200 mg/day orally for 40 days and continued with teichoplanin 400 mg/day i.v. and sulfametoxazole 800 mg trimethoprim 160 mg twice daily orally for a total period of sixty days. Two months later a full recovery of upper limbs motor activity was obtained and a good recovery of lower limbs too, with a persisting steppage gait at the left lower limb requiring the use of a stick. A control cervical NMR suggested the reduction in prevertebral and anterior epidural abscesses and in the hyperintensity of disk signal. Furthermore, a decrease in the width of spinal canal was shown. Brain NMR showed an altered signal in periventricular white matter and anterior horn..

[92] Internal stool bag for bed bound elderly patients with decubitus

M. Fujii and H. Sasaki

For the purpose of the prevention from stool contamination, we have developed a new type of medical instrument for bed bound elderly patients with decubitus. In cooperation with Terumo company, Japan, we have recently produced an Internal stool bag (IASB) for protection against such things as urinary tract and decubitus infection of these patients. IASB consists of two parts. One is the attachment apparatus on the patient's perianus and the other is the bag apparatus for defecated stool. Each part is made from soft and water-proof latex, and the inside of the bag is coated with jelly. The method of IASB use is as follows. First, IASB is genty fixed on the patient's perianus by the attachment apparatus. Next, the bag apparatus is inserted into the rectum in a way similar to digital examination. After the patient's defecation, the bag including stool is pushed out from patient's anus. We twist it, and take it off from the patient's buttock tenderly. During this process there are few bad smells, and clean up one's anus can be done quickly. So that, we can manage patient's decubitus and urinary tract clear from stool contamination. It is a very useful method of defecation care for bed ridden elderly patients, especially those who have infectious decubitus, not only at nursing units and hospitals but also at home.

[93] A hospital study of community acquired pneumonia in the elderly : microbiology and prognosis factors

AL Fauchais MD (1), F Puisieux MD (1), O Leroy MD (2), T Vrielinck MD (3), H Bulckaen (1), N Asseray (1), G Ferard (1), P Dewailly (1) (1) Geriatric department (2) Infectious disease department University hospital of Lille France (3) Geriatric department CH Somain France

Purpose : to better known bacteriological features and prognosis factors of elderly (>65 years old) exchibiting community acquired pneumonia (CAP) in France Method : prospective multicentric study Results : We studied 215 patients (110 wemen, mean age 83 yr.) admitted in our units between May 1997 and Marsh 1999 with CAP. Pneumonia was nursing-home acquired in 41 cases. The main associated diseases were neurological disorders (n=64), denutrition (n = 59). A microbiological diagnosis was assigned in 125 patients. main organisms werre S pneumoniae (21%), Staphylococcus spp (22%), H influenzae (33%), Klebsiella-Enterobacter-Serratia spp (29%). During hospital stay, 73 patients exhibited CAP related complications. Finally 44 patients died. multivariate analysis identified 5 independant predictos of mortality : age >88 years, mental confusion, severe underlying conditions, occurrence of CAP related complications and lack of improvment with initial AMT. Conclusion: We proposed a simplified prognosis index taking into account only tree factors (age >88, mental confusion and weight loss). The 30 days mortality among the 27 patients with the two former conditions was above 50% while mortality among the 98 < 88 and without mental confusion was 7%.

[94] Silent Peptic Ulcer Disease in the Elderly Patients

Abbasi J. Akhtar (Charles R. Drew University of Medicine and Science, Los Angeles, California, USA)

PURPOSE: Precise pathogenesis of pain in peptic ulcer disease (PUD) is incompletely understood. Sometimes the first manifestation of PUD may be one of its complications, such as bleeding or perforation. This study was conducted, to determine the frequency of painless PUD in the elderly population and its comparison with the younger age group. METHOD: Records of 390 patients, 29 to 95 years of age with endoscopic and/or radiological diagnosis of PUD were reviewed retrospectively. Presence or absence of pain, and use of non-steroidal anti-inflammatory drugs (NSAIDs) were recorded. Patients were stratified according to the age group and sex: 29-65 yrs (Group I), 168 patients (98 males, 70 females), 66-80 yrs (Group II) 130 patients (70 males, 60 females) and 80-95 yrs (Group III) 92 patients (47 males, 45 females). Fequency of pain in PUD was determined and the data were analyzed. RESULTS: Endoscopy was performed in 360 patients (92%). In 30 patients (8%), the diagnosis was made by upper gastrointestinal barium studies. Patient characteristics, regarding absence of pain are shown in Table 1. CONCLUSION: Our study confirms earlier observations that painless PUD is common in the elderly, its incidence increases with aging in both sexes, more so in women. NSAIDs consumption significantly increases the incidence of painless PUD. Table 1 Group I Group II Group III Male 16 (10%) 26 (20%) 23 (25%) Female 12 (7%) 31 (24%) 28 (30%) NSAID User 15 (9%) 35 (27%) 39 (42%)

[95] Aging with the stigma of AIDS: A man of the cloth shares his personal story.

Pamela S. Tyler, MGS, LNHA, LSW student in Gerontology (University of Kentucky, Lexington, KY, USA)

AIDS is an issue of concern for older adults especially in countries where the aged population is growing exponentially. Scant research on the topic has established that older adults are the least likely of at risk age groups to use condoms, to consider themselves vulnerable for infection, to be targeted for prevention messages via the media or AIDS organizations, to be HIV tested/diagnosed in the early stages of the disease, and to receive specialized support services once diagnosis is made. One factor contributing to these findings is likely to be the stigma associated with being older and participating in the behaviors associated with HIV/AIDS transmission. The purpose of this poster presentation is to offer a personal account of how the stigma of being diagnosed with the HIV virus impacted the life of an older male member of the clergy. His story is one of strength and courage as he not only has to admit to his congregation that he is HIV+ but also chooses to come out by disclosing his homosexuality. His story is explored through a narrative methodological approach during a series of personal interviews. The findings illustrate how stigma associated with HIV/AIDS diagnosis can dramatically influence the social network of older adults. While case studies cannot be generalized to entire populations, particularly in a group as diverse as older adults with HIV/AIDS, this chronicle can provide researchers, healthcare providers, and caregivers insight into the powerful impact of the stigma associated with this disease.

[96] Analysis of abnormal serum alanine aminotrasferase (ALT) level in the elderly

Xi Zhong-hua (Department of Geriatrics of Hua Dong Hospital . Shanghai. China)

As more people live longer than ever before, the incidence of various diseases resulting from senile degenerative changes and impaired immune system has increased. As a result, more and more cases of drug-induced liver damage occurred during the pharmaceutical treatment. The increased incidence of senile hepatitis and liver tumor has also induced more cases of liver function abnormality. In this article, we analyzed three major causes responsible for abnormal serum alanine aminotransferase (ALT) level in the elderly. First, in most senile patients, abnormal serum ALT level is drug induced. These drugs include antihyperlipidaemic agents, hypoglycaemic agents, antituberculous agents, antineoplastic agents and agents used for prostate diseases. Second, the increased ALT level accompanied by higher serum AFP level usually indicates the possibility of liver cancer. Finally, in some senile cases, the increased ALT level is caused by viral hepatitis. So according to these causes, certain measures should be taken in the elderly to prevent liver damage, to prolong their lifetime and to improve their quality of life.

[97] Safety and efficacy of TTS-Fentanyl compared with sustained release morphine in patients with cancer pain

Ute Richarz-Barthauer on behalf of the study group (Janssen–Cilag, Baar, Switzerland)

Purpose: Continuous pain affects millions of elderly individuals worldwide and remains poorly addressed in terms of both treatment and effective management. Sensitivity to the side effects of pharmacological intervention is an important aspect when considering effective pain relief in the elderly. This study compared the safety and efficacy of TTS-fentanyl with sustained release morphine (SRM) in elderly patients with chronic cancer-related pain. Method: Pooled analysis based upon two open, randomized, parallel 4-week studies. Safety assessments were conducted throughout the studies; efficacy parameters included pain control, drowsiness and sleep quality. Patients randomized to TTS Fentanyl were prescribed the lowest dose, 25g/h patch every 72 hours, with incremental titration of 25g/h to achieve adequate pain control. Patients randomized to SRM started on 30 mg SRM 12 hourly. Results: Preliminary analysis suggested that while TTS-fentanyl and SRM were similar in terms of efficacy parameters, patients rated TTS-fentanyl above SRM in terms of side effects. A scheduled analysis of the pooled data from these studies is planned for January 2001. Conclusions: TTS-fentanyl is equally as effective as, although better tolerated than SRM in strong-opioid-naïve elderly patients with cancer pain. The results from the pooled analysis are awaited with interest.

[98] Estrogen binding in liver cancer

J. Vrioni (New York Med college), T. Theodoropoulos (Univ. of S. Florida Tampa, USA)

Hormonal infuences such as sex hormones and growth factors may have a role in the pathogenesis of liver tumors and hepatocellular carcinoma.We recently reported on the binding of gonadotropin releasing hormone (GnRH) to this tumor (Vrioni et al, GSA, 1999). Now we report on the binding of Estradiol 17- (E2) to plasma membranes obtained from liver cancer in old humans. The membranes were obtained by differential centrifugation on discontinious sucrose gradients. 125I- E2 binding was studied following incubation in Tris-HCL buffer, pH 7.4, at 37C, for 30-60 min at the 10-11 to 10-10 M concentration range. The calculated binding capacity to tumor membranes was 0.06 0.009 fmol/ g protein, whereas for normal aged liver membranes it was 0.02 0.004. Comparatively, the binding capacity of E2 to normal aged pituitary membranes was 0.18 0.02 fmol/ g protein. Analysis of the binding kinetics suggested the presence of more than one binding sites. In conclusion, the E2 receptors present in this tumor are structurally or functionally incomplete. Their siginficance in terms of the pathogensis of these liver tumors or some of their feminizing signs is presently unclear.

[99] Lung Cancer Mortality in Elderly Spanish during the period 1975 - 1995

C. Trescoli (Internal Medecine Department, Hospital de la Ribera, Alzira, Valencia, Spain)

There is a close correlation between lung cancer incidence and mortality in the patients older than 65 years. Purpose: Changes in lung cancer mortality rates in the elderly population (>65 years) from 1975 to 1995 by sex. Method: The Spanish National Institute of Statistics registers all deaths by its primary cause using the ICD-8 code (Institute Classification of Diseases). We collected lung cancer mortality data (per 100000 inhabitants) by sex and 5-year age groups using the ICD-8 code: 162(tracheal, bronchial and lung malignant tumour) from 1975 to 1995 in Spain. A regression equation on the natural logarithm of mortality rates was used to calculate the mean annual percentage of variation. Results: Lung cancer mortality rates in men was 51.5 (40 - 64 age group) and 233.3 (>65 year group) in 1975 and 94.3 and 386.8 respectively in 1995. For women was 7.5 (40 - 64 age group) and 31.2 (>65years) in 1975 and 7.4 and 31.6 respectively in 1995 There was a 2.9% (95%CI: 2.7 - 3.1) mean annual lung cancer mortality rate increase in elderly men during this period, speciallly the very elderly (5.3% in >85, 95% CI: 4.4 - 6.2). Women had a 0.0% (95% CI: -0.2 - 0.4) mean annual lung cancer mortality rate increase. Conclusion: Lung cancer mortality rates are tenfold times higher in elderly men than women during the 1975 - 1995 period and there is a mean annual lung cancer mortality increase in elderly men that is not seen in elderly women.

[100] A New Technique of Stenting for Elder Patients with Inoperable Pyloric or Antral Malignant Stenosis

H. TOKUMO, H. KOMATSU, M. NAKAO, K. KUNIHIRO, and K. ISHIDA (Department of Gastroenterology, Hiroshima General Hospital, Hiroshima, JAPAN)

PURPOSE: The self-expandable metal stent (EMS) for a malignant pyloric or antral stenosis may be considered as one of the best treatments for keeping the elder patients' quality of life (QOL). In this paper, we introduce a new technique with which gastrostomy is utilized as an access point to induce the EMS to the pylorus or the antrum. SUBJECTS and METHOD: Twelve patients with inoperable malignant pyloric or antral stenosis were included in this study. In the initial 4 cases, Z stent or Wallstent designed for the esophageal stenosis was selected, and introduced orally. In the remaining 8 cases, gastrostomy was utilized as an inducing route. Concretely, after suturing the abdominal wall and gastric wall in the opposite position to the stenosis, puncture with a needle was followed. A guide-wire passed inside the needle was introduced to the stenosis by manual operation and then it was passed though the stenosis. A hand-made covered Z stent was introduced to the position of the stenosis over the placed guide-wire and then it was released. RESULTS: In all cases, the EMS was successfully positioned and the stenosis was relieved. The mean survival time after stenting was 2.5 months. The mean operation time for each technique was 63.5 minutes via oral route and 39.5 minutes via gastrostomic route, respectively. CONCLUSION: The EMS for elder patients with inoperable pyloric or antral stenosis would contribute to improve their QOL. To apply the EMS for such patients, the gastrostomic access technique would be most useful.

[101] Compassionate use of TTS-fentanyl in elderly patients with cancer-related pain

J. Menten (University Hospital Gasthuisberg, Leuven, Belgium); M. Desmedt (Cliniques Universitaires Saint Luc, Brussels, Belgium); D. Lossignol (Institut Jules Bordet, Brussels, Belgium); A. Mullie (Algemeen Ziekenhuis St Jan, Bruges, Belgium)

Purpose: Misconceptions about pain sensitivity, pain tolerance, and ability to use opioids often result in the undertreatment of cancer pain, especially in elderly patients. Regardless of the patients age, pain requires aggressive assessment and management. Controlled-release formulations, such as TTS-fentanyl, offer potential benefits over conventional formulations for elderly patients, e.g. longer dosing intervals. This study examined the compassionate use of TTS-fentanyl in patients with cancer-related pain. Methods: Patients were stabilized on oral morphine before being switched to TTS-fentanyl. The initial TTS-fentanyl dose was calculated using standard conversion tables; opioid-naive patients received the lowest strength patch (25 mcg/h). Dose titration was permitted in 25 mcg/h increments/decrements and oral morphine was provided as rescue medication. Pain relief, ease of use, presence of constipation, and laxative use were assessed periodically. Results: Six hundred and sixty-six patients were enrolled into the study; 181 (26%) were between 60 and 70 years old, and 140 (21%) were above the age of 70 years. In the total population, the total daily oral morphine dose dropped rapidly following the switch to TTS-fentanyl and 60 - 65% of patients rated TTS-fentanyl as good to excellent. TTS-fentanyl was well tolerated with a low incidence of treatment-related adverse events. Constipation was recorded as mild to moderate by 38% of patients while 43% used laxatives. A formal scheduled analysis is planned for the elderly population in March 2001. Conclusions: In the total population, TTS-fentanyl was effective and well tolerated; the formal results for the sub-analysis of the elderly population are awaited with interest.

[102] The Role of the Geriatric Nurse Practitioner in an Oncology Emergency Center

Vi Ho RN, MSN, GNP, Eva Lu Lee RN, MSN, ANP, Neomi Badrina RN, MSN, Sally Fernandez RN, MSN, ANP (MD Anderson Cancer Center, Houston, Texas, USA)

PURPOSE: To identify and develop innovative measures in effectively caring for the elderly cancer patients in despite of the increase of acuity and census in the emergency center. METHOD: Data were gathered and reviewed to identify the major chief complaints, age, length of stay (LOS) in the Emergency Center (EC), its peak hour, and measures to improve the flow of the EC. The result of a 3 months pilot study was evaluated and compared with previous existing data. RESULTS: About 270f the patients visiting the EC are gereiatric oncology patients (65 years and older). Their medical needs could be classified as urgent (66%), emergent (1%), or non-emergent (33%). Their common complaints were fever (33%), pain (15%), respiratory problems (10%), fluid and electrolytes imbalance (10%), weakness (7%), bowel/bladder problems (4%) and other such as cardio/ vascular related complaints (13%). The results of the pilot study, utilizing a Geriatric/Adult Nurse Practitioner to evaluate those patients, indicated the patient's LOS had decreased by 46 munutes. Satisfaction surveys were done. The Nurse Practitioner was viewed as a valuable provider. The over all satisfaction had increased with results of 66 0ood and 33 0.000000e+00xcellent. Since then the EC had created a fast-track programs utilizing the nurse practitioners. CONCLUSION: Geriatric oncology patients have many needs. Innovative measures can help in decreasing the length of stay and increasing patient's satisfaction during their visit in the EC. Since the utilization of Nurse Practitioner in our oncology EC is a success, we would recommend this system to others.

[103] Clinical aspects and clinical outcome of very old patients with colorectal cancer

Y.martin, V. Abitbol , C.bussy, P.chaibi, A.lahlou, W.ourad, F.piette (Hôpital Charles Foix, Ivry Sur Seine, France).

Purpose : to describe clinical aspects of colorectal cancer in very old patients and to assess their clinical outcome under care of geriatricians or gastroenterologists. Method : We retrospectively reviewed all medical files of patients older than 75 years hospitalised in a geriatric hospital between april 1995 and april 1999 with newly diagnosed colorectal cancer. Clinical presentation, comorbid conditions, complementary explorations and clinical outcome were described and compared with matched patients from an universitary gastroenterology unit. Results : We found 18 patients older than 75 years (mean age 85.3 years, range 75 - 94) with newly diagnosed colorectal cancer in our institution. Atypical onset symptomatology, including falls, was common. Ten of the 18 patients had severe comorbidity. Nevertheless, 13 patients underwent curative surgery and 6 patients survived more than one year (frequently at home). Those patients were matched ,according to age, sex and tumor location, with 18 patients from gastroenterology unit, including only 4 patients with severe comorbidity. Fourteen matched patients underwent curative surgery and 6 survived more than one year. Preoperative evaluation of preexisting comorbid conditions and of nutritional status appeared to be insufficient in the 2 groups. Medical specific treatment of colorectal cancer was underused in the 2 groups. Conclusion : Very elderly patients with newly diagnosed colorectal cancer and severe comorbid conditions may survive longer than one year in good condition after undergoing curative surgery. Attention should be raised on better preoperative evaluation and on medical specific management by geriatricians as well as by gastroenterologists.

[104] The prevalence of cancer in an acute geriatric unit

JM Jiménez P, VH Carrasco M, F Guerrero F, MJ Salcedo C, F Guillén L. Servicio de Geriatría Hospital Universitario de Getafe, Madrid Spain

Purpose: To determine the prevalence, different types and frequency of cancer in the elderly patient. To analyse the tumors with a new diagnosis, their form of presentation and the extension studies. Methods: A one year retrospective analysis of the records of our AGU (Acute Geriatric Unity) was carried out to identify patients who went into the hospital with the final diagnosis of tumors. The patients were studied by a protocol previously done which included 52 variables. The records were performed on file maker 4.0 and statistical analysis on Epi info. Results: 132 patients underwent into the AGU (76 women, 56 males); the mean age was 83.4 years, the mean stay was 11.2 days, and a mean 2-3 functional state according to the Red Cross Scale (RCE) score. Overall, 42 (31.8%) were a new diagnosis, 32 of them underwent into an extension study with the next results: 6 (18.78%) carcinoma in situ, 5 (15.62%) extension to the adjacent organs, 3 (9.37%) regional metastases. The most common fatal malignances neoplasm were: Colorectal (22.72%), Gynecologycal (16.66%), Prostate (15.15%) carcinoma. The most frequent cause for income to the AGU was respiratory infection (28.78%) follow by functional impairment (21.96%) and constitutional syndrome (16.66%). Conclutions: A total of 11.22% of the income to the AGU were neoplasms. 31.8% were unknown cancer, and 76.9% of them underwent through an extension study. The most common fatal malignances were 1) Colorectal 2) Gynecologycal, 3) Prostate neoplasms. Our data are similar to the describe on the major publications.

[105] Lung cancer. Comparison between adult and elderly in a Hospital area of Madrid.

L.C. Arranz S, V.H. Carrasco M*, M. Montes L*, M. Muro D**, A. Esteban P**, J.M. Jiménez P*, F. Guillén L*, D. Gómez S**. (Geriatric Department*. Radiology Department**. Universitary Hospital of Getafe. Madrid-Spain)*

PURPOSE: To establish the prevalence of Lung Cancer on the population related to a public hospital in one area of Madrid. To compare and analyze clinic variables between adults (<65 years) and elders (>65 years). METHOD: A one year (1999) retrospective analysis of the records of our hospital (influence area of 250.000 inhabitants) was carried out on the patients with lung cancer. The patients were studied by a protocol previously done. Statistic analysis in Epi Info 6. RESULTS: 72 patients (37 adult and 35 elderly, 89% and 91% male respectively). History of smoker habit: 97% and 94% respectively. The principal means of diagnosis were bronchoscopy (49 0n adults and 63 0n elders ($p<0,05$))and fine-needle aspirates (49% and 29% respectively ($p<0,05$)).The histological types were: Adenocarcinoma: 35% and 37% ($p>0,05$); Squamous cell: 30% and 51% ($p<0,05$); Small cell: 24% and 9% ($p<0,05$); Large cell: 8% and 17% ($p<0,05$); Bronchoalveolar: 5% and 9% ($p>0,05$). The use of therapies was significantly greater in the adult group: Surgery (30% vs. 17%), Chemical therapy (62% vs. 38%)and Radiotherapy (22% vs. 11%). The survival to 6 months was 81% vs. 55%, and per year were 49% vs. 36%. CONCLUSION: The estimate prevalence was 28 over 100.000. The diagnostic technique more used was fine-needle aspirates in adult and bronchoscopy in elderly. The prevailing type in elderly was squamous cell carcinoma and Adenocarcinoma was in adult. The adult group were more treated. The survival was smaller in aged people both in six month and one year period.

[106] Myelodysplasia in the elderly : clinical features and comments about 16 aged inpatients

JF Desson, (Department of Geriatric Medicine, Cote de Nacre Hospital, Caen, FRANCE), F Vabret, A Davy (Department of General Medicine, Clemenceau Hospital, Caen, FRANCE), M Macro, S Cheze, O Reman (Department of haematology, Clemenceau Hospital, Caen, FRANCE)

Because of the population aging, the frequency of myelodysplastic syndrome (MDS) is increasing after the age of 75. The propensity of MDS to transform to acute myeloid leukemia (AML) leads in some cases to active chemotherapy, according to health status, FAB classification, age itself being considered as an essential prognosis factor. Most of the time, only blood support is proposed for the elderly. 16 old patients (median age = 80.6 y) with MDS were followed in our department, between 1996 and 2000. 13 patient died, 11 of them at hospital. 11 patients had pancytopenia. Bone marrow examination was performed in 13 cases. Cytogenetic analysis was abnormal in 2 cases. Infectious or haemorrhagic complications and AML occured in 10 and 7 patients respectively. Chemotherapy was attempted in 4 cases and transiently effective in only one. In our study, altered health status and chronic diseases associated with MDS prevented us to initiate chemotherapy. Blood support and complications required many hospitalizations. Most of the time, death occured at hospital, in opposition to the patient and family wishes. Chemotherapy agents are generally proposed for high-risk MDS, but its toxicity is very important in the elderly. The use of growth factors has to be evaluated in this population. Improvement of prognosis criteria needs validated data, creating new scoring systems for elderly people who can possibly benefit by new chemotherapy agents. Quality of life has also to be evaluated in the aged MDS patients, with geriatric scales according to the frequent misinterpretation of the self-evaluation in the elderly. At last, psychologic and socioeconomic considerations, as well as cognitive impaiment, are essential for treatment decision.

SESSION 287

Canada-Mexico Working Together on the Continuum of Care for Seniors

N. Garrard (Division of Aging and Seniors, Health Canada) Developing a Policy Framework on the Continuum of Care for Seniors: the Canada_Mexico Experience. A. Lara Esqueda (Programa de Adultos Mayores, Secretaria de Salud, México) Developing a Policy Framework on the Continuum of Care for Seniors: the benefits for Mexico.

Canada and Mexico have undertaken a process that will lead to the creation of a policy framework that outlines the necessary key elements in the continuum of care for seniors. This roundtable will include presentations from Health Canada, Secretaríat de Salud de México and the Pan-American Health Organization (PAHO), as well as concluding remarks from a discussant, Dr. Enrique Vega from Cuba. As part of the Canada-Mexico Memorandum of Understanding on Health Matters, Health Canada and the Secretaríat de Salud de México have undertaken a three-year plan of action on healthy aging issues. The purpose of the collaboration is to address health issues of importance to both countries in responding to the health and well-being of seniors. One of the main priorities of the plan of action is to develop a policy framework that outlines the necessary key elements in the continuum of care for seniors. The intent of this tool is to guide policy and program decision-making with respect to the health and well-being of seniors. The two countries will share their experience in developing and consult on a preliminary draft a joint policy framework. The session will build on the theme of the Congress by highlighting the collaborative process developed to undertake this initiative. Health Canada and the Secretaríat de Salud de México will render presentations on the overall process and method established to develop the joint policy framework and how the results of the collaboration (i.e, the policy framework) will be used or beneficial in Mexico. PAHO will demonstrate the value of this experience within the overall philosophy of technical cooperation between pan-American countries. Finally, the discussant will initiate the roundtable by providing some remarks on the benefits of the collaboration and comments on the draft policy framework. * Please note that if our proposed roundtable is approved by the Congress, we will take the initiative of inviting participants from Latin-American countries to participate in our discussion.

Developing a Joint Policy Framework on the Continuum of Care for Seniors: the benefits for Mexico.

O. Velazquez, A. Lara Esqueda , F. Martínez Abaunza, R. Mena Lopez (Programa de Adultos Mayores, Secretaria de Salud, México)

Similar to the Canadian experience in the last decades, aging in Mexico is also influenced by life conditions and other factors. Mexicans aged 60 years old and over represent approximately 7% of the current total population; this cohort is expected to increase to 13% over the next 25 years. In Canada, this cohort represents currently around 17% of its total population. This would mean that Canada has close to 25 additional years of experience than Mexico in developing policies, programs and services for the care of seniors. In order to improve the development of programs for the care of seniors, it is of the utmost importance for México to learn from the Canadian experience in developing an integral continuum of care for seniors. The Canada-Mexico Memorandum of Understanding on Health Matters is facilitating this learning experience. Mexico will make good use of its experience in developing a joint policy framework with Canada which will identify the successes and challenges in developing the necessary continuum of care for seniors and an aging population. With this information, Mexico will use the most effective best practices and avoid or enhance the practices which provided some challenges to establish policies, objectives and plan of action . For Canada, this joint initiative provides an opportunity to assess the

Canadian models of care for seniors and, therefore, strengthen its policies and programs for seniors. It will also expand its capacity and experience of providing technical expertise in the area of aging to other countries of the region.

Developing a Policy Framework on the Continuum of Care for Seniors: the Canada-Mexico Experience

N. Garrad, N. Levesque, S. Carbone (Division of Aging and Seniors, Health Canada, Ottawa, Canada)

This first section of the roundtable will provide a brief overview of the Canada-Mexico Plan of Action on Healthy Aging Issues. The method to create a joint policy framework to guide policy and program decision-making on the continuum of care for an aging population will then be defined. The main activities of the working group, consisting of representatives from Canada, Mexico, and PAHO, will be presented. These activities include: 1) an environmental scan to develop common knowledge about the meaning of continuum of care for seniors and the environment in which it exists in each country; 2) the creation a common conceptual framework; and, 3) focus testing the draft framework with key stakeholders in both countries. Finally, the major considerations, such as clear communication and sound project coordination, in developing a collaborative process among two different cultures and languages will then be discussed. This presentation will demonstrate that collaboration among two countries must be primarily based on a flexible developmental process and a solid understanding of each other realities. It will also establish the value of sharing experience and policy development expertise on the continuum of care for seniors among pan-American countries.

The Benefits of Collaboration on Aging Issues among PAHO countries.

Martha Pelaez, Regional Advisor on Ageing, Pan-American Health Organization

This presentation will position the Canada-Mexico collaboration on healthy aging issues within the context of the philosophy of technical cooperation between countries and the spirit of PAHO/WHO. As the population of the PAHO countries ages, building on and sharing expertise on aging issues is becoming increasingly important. By working collaboratively on the policy framework, Canada and Mexico are building on their experiences to develop a useful tool to assist Latin-American countries plan, and developed countries assess, the necessary continuum of care for their aging population. The speaker will discuss the benefits of working together to identify common solutions for an aging population in PAHO countries.

SESSION 289

Longitudinal Studies - Multidisciplinary Aspects

K. W. Schaie (Gerontology Center, Pennsylvania State University, University park, PA, USA) Interdisciplinary Aspects of the Seattle Longitudinal Study. R.A. Dixon (Psychology, University of Victoria, Victoria, BC, Canada) The Victoria Longitudinal Study: Research on Change with Aging. J. Smith (Max Planck Institute for Human Development, Berlin, Germany) Age Trajectories from 70 to 100+: Longitudinal Findings from the Berlin Aging Study. M. Martin (DZFA, University of Heidelberg, Germany) Psychological resources, health behavior, and health in middle and old age: The ILSE study. B. Hagberg (Gerontology Research Center, Lund, Sweden) Multidisciplinary predictors of survival after age 80 years of age: The Lund 80+ study.

This symposium will address issues of change and prediction of change and survival based on results from five renowned longitudinal studies that are all multidisciplinary in character. The presentations from the studies will cover several aspects related to aging and changes in old age as well as methodological intricacies that are encountered when conducting multidisciplinary longitudinal research. From the Seattle Longitudinal Study cognitive development will be discussed in relation to, among other things, behavior genetic factors, micro-environments and chronic diseases. Longitudinal change patterns concerning neuropsychological profiles, health and personality will be presented from the Victoria Longitudinal Study. In the Berlin Aging Study the focus will be on age- and death-related trajectories from age 70 to 100+ in different areas of psychological functioning. Changes in health, health behavior and psychological resources in two cohorts will be discussed based on data from the ILSE study. Finally the presentation from the Lund 80+ study will discuss the differences in prediction of survival from age 80 to 90 when variables from single disciplines are considered separately as contrasted to when they are analyzed simultaneously. The symposium provides opportunities to reflect on and discuss the merits of multidisciplinary longitudinal research both from empirical and methodological points of view.

Age Trajectories from 70 to 100+: Longitudinal Findings from the Berlin Aging Study

J. Smith (Max Planck Institute for Human Development, Berlin, Germany)

Initial data in the multidisciplinary Berlin Aging Study (BASE: Baltes & Mayer, 1999) were collected in 1990-1993 from a representative, age by sex stratified sample (N = 516). Four longitudinal follow-ups of the survivors have since been completed at approximately two-yearly intervals (1993-1994, 1995-1996, 1997-1998, and 2000). In addition, we also follow the mortality of BASE This presentation will focus on age- and death-related trajectories (70 to 100+) found in three aspects of psychological functioning (cognitive ability, personality, and social relationships). In general, BASE findings suggest that the amount, onset time, and rate of age-related change differs across psychological dimensions. In the area of intelligence and cognitive functioning, negative age differences between 70 and 100+ years were substantial and were closely associated with indicators of biological deterioration. In contrast, age-related changes in personality, self-related beliefs, and social relationships were smaller and located primarily in the 80s decade. Interindividual differences in level of functioning and onset of decline were substantial in all areas of functioning, reflecting the combined influences of biogenetic factors and life history experiences. BASE findings also indicate that many of the oldest-old (over 85 years) show decline or dysfunction in multiple areas of psychological functioning and that this decline profile is death- related.

Interdisciplinary Aspects of the Seattle Longitudinal Study

K.W. Schaie, S.L. Willis (Gerontology Center, Pennsylvania State University, University Park, PA, USA)

The primary focus of the Seattle Longitudinal Study (SLS) has always been the monitoring of age changes and generational differences in adult cognitive development. However, we have progressively added other domains as independent variables in order to understand individual and group difference patterns in cognitive development. These domains include studying the influence of chronic diseases and use of prescription medication, the careful description of family environments in the family of origin and the current family to consider behavior genetic factors, the description of participants micro-environments, and the assessment of ApoE genotypes and neuro psychological status in our older study participants. We will discuss the inter disciplinary implications of these expansions of our study design.

Multidisciplinary predictors of survival after 80 years of age: The Lund 80+ Study.

B. Hagberg, O. Dehlin, G. Samuelsson, T. Svensson (Gerontology

Research Center, Lund, Sweden)

In Lund 80+ the subjects are examined at baseline with medical, psychological and social measurements. All domains contain important information predicting future survival. Objective and subjective health, lifestyle and habits, mental status, cognitive performance level, memory and learning, coping style, locus of control, life satisfaction, social network with structure and support, socio-economic status, education and occupation are assessed for each gender separately. Bivariate and multivariate analyses of variables predicting survival from medical, psychological and social disciplines separately are compared to multidisciplinary survival analyses, utilizing information from all domains simultaneously. The relative importance of the variables from the different domains, is found to differ as the models are expanded to all domains. The significance of survival prediction from different contexts will be discussed.

Psychological resources, health behaviors, and health in middle and old age: The ILSE

M. Martin & D. Zimprich (German Centre for Research on Ageing, & Institute of Gerontology, Heidelberg, Germany)

PURPOSE: The goal of the current study was to examine the interrelations between age-related differences and 4-year changes in psychological resources, health behaviors, and health in two cohorts born 1930/32 and 1950/52. METHOD: Data from the Interdisciplinary Longitudinal Study on Adult Development and Ageing (ILSE) are used to examine the level differences and structural relations between latent change constructs of psychological resources, e.g, cognition and social support, health behaviors, e.g, exercising, and well-being and physical health in two age-groups. The influence of individual biographies of stressful life events on health and health behavior changes is controlled. RESULTS: For all constructs and both age groups used in this study, there were interindividual differences in the amount and direction of intraindividual change over time. There were age differences in the type and number of stressful life events and relatively small changes over time. Results from Structural Equation Models focusing on latent difference constructs suggest direct and indirect influences of psychological resources on health and well-being. CONCLUSION: Our findings suggest age differences in the level of stressful life events, psychological resources, health behaviors, and health. However, the structural relations between latent differences in these constructs were comparable and support the assumption of self-regulatory processes for the maintainance or improvement of health and well-being in middle-aged and young-old adults.

The Victoria Longitudinal Study: Research on Change with Aging

R. A. Dixon, D. F. Hultsch (Department of Psychology, University of Victoria, Victoria, BC, Canada)

The Victoria Longitudinal Study (VLS) is a large-scale investigation of multiple aspects and processes of human aging. Three independent samples (originally aged 55-85 years) are tested at 3-year intervals. Each occasion of measurement involves about 10 hours of testing, with measures tapping such domains as cognitive speed and resources, memory and knowledge, metacognition and awareness, neuropsychological profiles, health and medications, sensory and physiological status, background and current lifestyle, and personality-affect. Research has focused on longitudinal change patterns, as well as individual differences in variability and predictors of change. We provide an overview of the VLS and illustrative research results.

SESSION 291

The Institute of Healthy Aging of the Canadian Health Research Institutes (CIHR)

Réjean Hébert, Scientific Director

The Canadian Institutes of Health Research (CIHR) is a new funding agency launched in June 2000. It replaces the Medical Research Council and integrates the National Health Research and Development Program (NHRDP). Its objective is to "to excel, according to internationally accepted standards of scientific excellence in the creation of new knowledge and its translation into improved health for Canadians, more effective health services and products and a strengthened Canadian health care system". CIHR is a new structure for funding research based upon virtual institutes and a multidisciplinary approach. The scope of research it covers is broadened since it encompasses not only the biomedical and clinical research but also the research on health services, health of populations, societal and cultural dimensions of health, and environmental influences on health. The Institute of Healthy Aging (IHA) is one of the 13 CIHR institutes. Each Institute is directed by a scientific director who is supported by an Institute Advisory Board including representatives from the research community, the public, voluntary and private stakeholders and by the general public. The Institutes are not involved in the usual investigator-initiated core programs of CIHR and these proposals continue to be peer-reviewed by committees. The Institutes are involved in the development of strategic initiatives targeted to important health problems. Specific competitions based on request for application will be put forward by the Institutes and a peer-review process will ensure that funding is allocated to the most excellent proposals. These strategic initiatives has to be developed with partners in order to increase the budget available for funding and use the institute budget as a lever. A support development grant (400 thousand dollars per year) allows the Institutes to fund networking activities (workshops) and dissemination and transfert activities. The primary focus of the IHA will be to increase the research capacity in aging by training awards and infrastructure support (team, group, center) for new investigators. A consultation process is actually underway to identify the problems that should be prioritised by the institute.

SESSION 292

National Efforts to Promote Healthy Lifestyles: Multiple Strategies to Increase Physical Activity in Older Persons

Marcia G. Ory (National Institute on Aging, Bethesda, Maryland, USA) Symposium overview. Robin Mockenhaupt (Robert Wood Johnson Foundation, Princeton, New Jersey, USA) Building Organizational Capacity to Increase Physical Activity Among Adults Aged 50 and Older. David Buchner (Centers for Disease Control and Prevention, Atlanta, Georgia, USA) National Initiative on Activity Friendly Environments. Katie Sloan (AARP, Washington, D.C, USA) AARP's National Health and Fitness for the Fifty Plus Population. Wjotek Chodzko-Zajko, (University of Illinois at Urbana-Champaign and American College of Sports Medicine, Indianapolis, Indiana, USA) National Initiatives for Public and Professional Education in the Area of Aging and Physical Activity.

ISSUE: Although the benefits of increased physical activity and exercise are well known, the majority of older Americans are not meeting recommended levels of physical activity. A variety of individual, organizational and environmental barriers to initiating and maintaining a healthier lifestyle have been identified. While individual organizations have been addressing these barriers for the past decade, only recently has there been a coming together of different national organizations to provide a coordinated research, practice and education base for designing programs and policies to increase physical activity in older American populations. STRUCTURE: This symposium is organized around different national efforts reflecting a range of public-private approaches for increasing physical activity in different types of older populations (i.e, from healthy but sedentary adults to frail elders with many functional limitations) and in different settings (e.g, home/community; medical settings; workplace). After national efforts are highlighted, two discussants from outside of the United States will be invited to respond from their country perspective regarding lessons learned from other countries. CONTENT: After a brief symposium overview and comments about efforts at the National Institute on Aging, the first presentation will describe the Robert Wood Johnson Foundation's sponsorship of a National Blueprint for encouraging organizational capacity building in this area as well as their new initiative on replicating and expanding evidenced based programs. The second presentation will describe the Center for Disease Control and Prevention initiative on activity friendly environments addressing how community environments can facilitate or impede walking. The third presentation will address efforts by AARP to promote health and fitness of adults fifty and older by the use of social marketing strategies combined with other media, partnership, policy initiative and volunteerism activities. The fourth presentation will describe the American College of Sports Medicine's active aging partnership and their efforts to promote public and professional education. CONCLUSIONS/ANTICIPATED OUTCOMES: This invited symposium will highlight some of the major national efforts for increasing physical activity, demonstrating the benefit of public-private partnerships that can address many of the known barriers to initiating and maintaining healthier lifestyles.

AARP's Health and Fitness Programs for the Fifty Plus Population

Katrinka Smith Sloan, MA (AARP, Washington, D.C, USA)

PURPOSE: AARP—the largest membership organization focused on the concerns of older Americans— is embarking on a research and demonstration effort to better understand how to increase the physical activity of people age 50 and older in the United States. By addressing this issue within its wellness priority, AARP is carrying out its mission to serve the needs of people age 50 and older through information, advocacy and community service. METHOD: AARP is employing media, policy initiatives, partnerships, and volunteerism, to build on evidence-based programs that have demonstrated success in increasing physical activity. It will employ the discipline of social marketing to assure that its program will be well aligned with the motivations and interests of mid-life and older adults. Social marketing uses commercial marketing methods to create behavior change for the benefit of individuals and society. RESULTS: Results, to date, of qualitative and quantitative physical activity research with mid-life and older adults, will be shared, as well as a discussion of how AARP is using social marketing methods to apply what it has learned to physical activity programming. CONCLUSIONS: AARP seeks to contribute to the physical, psychological, and social well being of mid-life and older adults in the United States. This presentation will demonstrate how a national membership organization can use its resources to improve the health and fitness of older adults through its focus on increasing physical activity.

Building Organizational Capacity to Increase Physical Activity Among Adults Aged 50 and Older

Robin E. Mockenhaupt, (Senior Program Officer, Robert Wood Johnson Foundation, Princeton, NJ, USA)

Purpose: The National Blueprint: Increasing Physical Activity Among Adults Age 50 and Older outlined a comprehensive approach to increasing physical activity among mid-life and older adults in the US through development of a national plan. Method: The project brought together key organizations to develop and implement the plan. A Steering Committee of six organizations collaborated to initiate and implement the process of development. These organizations include AARP (formerly the American Association of Retired Persons), the American College of Sports Medicine, the American Geriatrics Society, the Centers for Disease Control and Prevention, the National Institute on Aging, and the Robert Wood Johnson Foundation. The plan was developed with input from over 45 organizations with expertise in related fields to physical activity and aging. Results: The document was released and disseminated to multiple organizations and agencies throughout the US. It serves as a guide to inform and support the planning work of these groups related to increasing physical activity among America's aging population. Conclusions: A broad-based, national effort to create a national plan can serve as a framework for collaborative engagement of organizations and agencies in achieving mutual goals and improved health outcomes for 50+ adults. This can provide a stimulus for future program and policy development for organizations and agencies, and for the field as a whole.

CDC's National Initiative on Activity Friendly Environments

David M. Buchner, M.D, M.P.H, Centers for Disease Control and Prevention, Atlanta

Purpose: This paper will review aspects of the CDC "ACEs" inititiative that relate to older adults. Method: Literature review and program analysis. Results: CDC surveillance data show that older adults are the least physically active age group, and that activity levels in older adults have not changed over the past decade. National strategies to increase activity in older adults emphasize walking, and walking is by far the most common physical activity of older adults. CDC is addressing promotion of walking in older adults as part of its Active Community Environments (ACEs) initiative. This initiative is investigating how physical activity levels of a community are affected by features of the environment, such as sidewalks, bikeways, trails, parks, and recreational facilities. Some data suggest our environments are less conducive to walking than in the past. For example, walking as a form of transportation is declining. Neighborhood safety is correlated with amount of walking in older adults. Unconnected neighborhood designs, such as cul-de-sacs, are associated with less walking. Ultimately, the initiative should lead to an ability to design communities in a way that promotes physical activity, including walking. Conclusions: The presentation will review some of the existing literature on environmental determinants of behavior, and discuss components and future directions of the ACEs initiative.

National Initiatives for Public and Professional Education in the Area of Aging and Physical Activity

Wojtek J. Chodzko-Zajko, (University of Illinois at Urbana-Champaign, Urbana IL, USA)

Purpose: This paper will review national initiatives on public and professional education in the area of aging and physical activity sponsored by the Active Aging Partnership, a US coalition of organizations including the National Institute on Aging (NIA), the Centers for Disease Control and Prevention (CDC), the American College of Sports Medicine (ACSM) , the American Geriatrics Society (AGS), the Robert Wood Johnson Foundation (RWJ), and the American Association of Retired Persons (AARP). Method: Recent initiatives designed to educate health professionals and members of the general public about the health benefits of physical activity will be reviewed. Results: In recent years ACSM has identified the dissemination of information about healthy aging as a central component of its organizational mission. In the area of public information, numerous initiatives have been developed, some examples include; (1) ACSM active aging pages have been developed for distribution to the general public; (2) a media campaign has prepared content for press, magazines, www sites etc.; (3) the College has published "Current Comments" in response to topical issues and news items. The College has also developed a number of initiatives in the area of Professional Education, for example: (1) ACSM has sponsored numerous research symposia on topics germane to physical activity and aging, (2) in October 2000, the ACSM organized a Special Conference on physical activity and aging; (3) a course leading to an advanced certificate of clinical competence has been developed and implemented in multiple sites around the country; (4) a comprehensive slide set has been developed for professional education and dissemination. Conclusions: Chodzko-Zajko will discuss future plans of the partnership to impact knowledge and information in the area of physical activity and aging, and to translate this information into clinical practice

SESSION 293

High-Risk Patient Intervention Program Evaluation

Patrick McGowan, (Institute of Health Promotion Research, UBC, Vancouver, BC, Canada); B. Lynn Beattie, (Division of Geriatric Medicine, UBC, Vancouver, BC, Canada); Neena Chappell, (Centre on Aging, U of Victoria, Victoria, BC, Canada); Heather Clarke, (Research and Evaluation Consulting, Vancouver, BC, Canada); David Gayton, (Peace Arch Hospital, White Rock, BC, Canada); Lawrence Green, (Centers for Disease Control, Atlanta, Georgia); Malcolm Maclure, (BC Pharmacare, Victoria, BC, Canada)..

This study is a randomized control trial to test whether a pharmacist and nurse home-care team can reduce hospital re-admissions of seniors discharged from hospital on 6 or more medications. After being discharged from the hospital, seniors were visited in their homes by a research assistant who administered four functional ability tests: Modified Mini-Mental State Examination; ADL portion of the Older Americans Resource and Services Multidimensional Functional Questionnaire; Timed Up and Go Test; and Center for Epidemiologic Studies Depression (CES-D) Scale. When the tests were completed and consent forms signed, seniors were randomly assigned to either the Experimental or Control Group. In total, 283 seniors were admitted into the study. Of these, 174 seniors were placed in the Experimental Group and 109 seniors in the Control Group. There were 161 female participants and 122 male participants, and the mean age was 78.13 (SD 6.88). To test the effectiveness of the randomization process in recruitment, a series of statistical tests were conducted. Results showed the Experimental and Control groups were similar with respect to age, gender, number of prescription, over-the-counter and herbal medications, as well as with mean scores on the four functional ability tests. Outcome measures include: number of times hospitalized; number of emergency room visits; number of physician visits; number of prescription medications; whether seniors started to receive home care services; and whether senior was admitted to institutional care. The outcome measures are being examined for each senior for the one-year period prior to being admitted to the study, and for a one-year period following discharge from the program.

Home Follow up of High Risk Hospitalized Elders

Bernard KONG, Jimmy WONG, Shirley WONG (WONG CHUK HANG HOSPITAL, HONG KONG)

PURPOSE: Study the effectiveness of home follow up intervention by a geriatric nurse fully supported by geriatrician SUBJECTS & METHODS : Since May 1999, 100 frail elders discharged back to home were randomly assigned to study and control group. Study group receive a total of 4 scheduled visits by a geriatric nurse within 6 months while control group only received four phone consultations with no direct assess to specialty nursing service. In the study group, elders or carers could contact the nurse directly via mobile phone daily from 9am to 8pm for medical consultation and the nurse had full support from the geriatrician. Both groups were comparable in age, sex, physical function, mental ability and activities of daily living upon discharged. The number of emergency services attendance were the same in both groups prior to admission. RESULTS: Majorities of the calls were related to medical and drugs inquiry. Top three problems were risk of fall, inadequate medical knowledge and drug compliance. Out of 50 elders in the study group, 10 had emergency admissions, 4 dead, 2 admitted to nursing home, one refused service and one moved to China. There was a significant reduction of readmission < 28 days (7 Vs 15, P < 0.041), acute and emergency attendance (22 Vs 61, P < 0.001) and acute hospital admission (16 Vs 50, P < 0.003). Although there is a trend of increasing clinical admission (16 Vs 10). Statistically this is not significant. CONCLUSION: High Risk Elders required special medical attention especially after they were discharged. This study showed that home intervention program delivered by geriatric nurse supported by geriatrician reduced unnecessary acute health service utilization and decreased the cost of health care. Both elders and carers appreciated the program.

Hospital-Based Geriatric Home Care in Very Dependent Elderly People

Viloria A, Mora J, Mesa C, Alonso P, Pastor E, Torrijos M, Ribera JM (Servicio de Geriatria, Hospital Clinico San Carlos, Madrid, Spain)

AIM: To describe the functional, medical and social parameters related to a poor prognosis in a geriatric population included in a hospital-based home care program (HCP). METHOD: Data were collected from patients included in the HCP in the last ten years. Demographic, social, medical and functional parameters are assessed in the first visit and when discharged. Data on mortality, rate of hospitalisation and institutionalisation were considered. A multivariate analysis was applied (logistic or linear regression as indicated) to know the main factors related to these parameters, confidence interval 95%, p < 0.05. SPSS. RESULTS: n = 1310, women 62.4%, mean age 83.5 +/- 7.4 y.o. (50-102). Most of them (72.3%) were referred from Hospital Services (HS) and the rest from Primary Care (PC). These patients had 4.9 chronic conditions in average, dementia 44.9%, pressure ulcers 36.2% and presence of catheters 25.9%. Main caregiver data: female 84.3%, mean age 64.0 +/- 14.0 y.o. Functional assessment: 76.3 0ependence for more than 3 activities of daily living (ADL), 53.1% very bad mobility. Mortality during the permanence in the HCP 46.3%, more than a half being at home. Those who died were less independent in ADL (4.9 vs. 4.3 lost activities), had a worse mobility, and came more probably from HS (49.6% vs. 38.0%) than the other patients (p < 0.001). These patients always had more proportion of pressure ulcers or catheters. Logistic regression confirmed these results and remarks the dependence for eating as a valid prognostic factor. Institutionalisation and use of hospital resources: Need of a social intervention was identified in 25.8% of the cases, and 11.5% were sent to a long-term care facility during their follow-up. Those placed in an institution were more dependent, having an older main caregiver (67.0 vs. 63.3 y.o), and needing more hospital resources (39.0 vs. 16.0% admissions) than the others (p < 0.01). Conversely, the rate of hospital admission was more related to medical conditions and the presence of a male caregiver. Follow-up: Average time of follow-up was 199.9 days. This was associated with more use of hospital resources (mainly readmission of those coming from HS), more pressure ulcers, higher mortality and/or necessity of social intervention. CONCLUSIONS: 1) Physical status (e.g. ADL, mobility) is the main factor to explain mortality and admission in an institution in our HCP. 2) Caregiver conditions secondarily may explain the institutionalisation and use of hospital resources in these patients. 3) Medical conditions and the presence of pressure ulcers and/or catheters are related to hospitalisation and more time of permanence in the HCP.

The In-Home Care Experience of Patients Following Total Hip or Knee Replacement

Maureen Loft, RN,N (cand), St. Joseph's Health Care London, London, Canada Carol McWilliam, RN, University of Western of Ontario, London, Canada Catherine Ward-Griffin, RN, University of Western, Ontario, London, Canada

Purpose: The purpose of this research was to gain an enhanced understanding of the in-home care experience in relationships with care providers, following discharge from hospital, of patients who had undergone total hip or knee replacement. METHOD: The research methodology of phenomenology was utilized to discover and interpret the experiences as expressed by the participants. Narrative data were collected using in-depth interviews of a purposeful maximally varied sample of nine patients over 65 years of age, audio-taped following informed consent. Interpretive analysis using immersion and crystallization techniques was conducted to illuminate the essences and themes of the participants' experiences. RESULTS: Findings illuminate themes and patterns revealing the limited empowerment of older persons receiving in-home care following joint replacement.

CONCLUSIONS: Insights gained from the participants will be used to enable health care providers to consider the participants' perceptions of their knowledge, status, and authority in their care relationships after discharge from hospital to in-home care. This understanding may, in turn, be used to refine and develop educational programs aimed at enhancing the empowerment of the patients undergoing total hip or knee replacement.

SESSION 294

An Ounce of Prevention: Community and Institutional Education Strategies to Help Prevent Abuse of Older Persons

C. Ward-Hall (B.C. Coalition to Eliminate Abuse of Seniors, New Westminster, B.C, Canada) Educating Seniors and Others About Abuse: A Decade of Experience from a Provincial Organization; C. Spencer (Gerontology Research Centre, Simon Fraser University, Vancouver B.C. Canada) Respecting Residents Rights: Preventing Institutional Abuse Through Resident and Family Education.

Between 4 and 10 per cent of adults in Canada will experience abuse or neglect in later life from someone they know and trust. It is well recognized that it is far more advantageous to prevent elder abuse from occurring than to have to deal with its aftermath. Yet there can be important barriers to successfully educating seniors and others in a way that leads to change. In this roundtable, three presenters will describe education approaches that have developed in two Canadian provinces, followed by audience discussion on approaches being used in their own communities, looking at some of the continuing challenges and successes. In Elder Abuse- Not Me: Personal Empowerment and Prevention, B. Gleason focuses on education as an essential element in abuse prevention. Given that there are significant literacy and educational barriers to reaching seniors, is our prevention education being heard by seniors? Are we educating in a way that seniors and professionals understand? How can you tell if you are reaching seniors? What prevents them from hearing you? How do you avoid that? In Educating Seniors and Others About Abuse: A Decade of Experience from a Provincial Organization, C. Ward-Hall describes the different prevention education approaches that have been used by the B.C. Coalition to Eliminate Abuse of Seniors to reach specific target audiences (e.g. seniors renting and building managers; seniors in the Iranian community; the financial and legal communities serving seniors) and the lessons that have been learned along the way. In Respecting Residents Rights: Preventing Institutional Abuse Through Resident and Family Education, C. Spencer describes the need for and development of plain language information for British Columbian seniors in care and their families and how these materials can also serve as a staff training tool. The expected outcome of the session is an increased awareness of effective educational strategies for reaching seniors and others on this issue.

Educating Seniors and Others About Abuse: A Decade of Experience from a Provincial Organization

C. Ward-Hall (B.C. Coalition to Eliminate Abuse of Seniors, New Westminster, British Columbia, Canada)

The B.C. Coalition to Eliminate Abuse of Seniors has been providing seniors, service providers, industry, and the public with information and education materials on abuse and neglect issues affecting seniors for over ten years. This presentation describes the different prevention education approaches used by the provincial organization during three projects to reach specific target audiences (e.g. seniors renting and building managers; seniors in the Iranian community; the financial and legal communities serving seniors) and the lessons that have been learned along the way. Successful strategies include involvement of the target audience from the beginning; identifying their specific needs and typical means of receiving information; fitting the information into their personal or business realities; reviewing of draft materials by the target audience and formal evaluation/feedback. Staff in private industry such as banks often have only a narrow window of opportunity (10 minutes before work) to receive information of any kind (whether that is client relations, or improving awareness of financial abuse). Those working in rental housing often work in isolation with few opportunities to upgrade their skills in dealing with and helping older tenants. Both situations can make it challenging to get abuse prevention information to the places where it may be much needed

Respecting Residents Rights: Preventing Institutional Abuse Through Resident and Family Education

C. Spencer (Gerontology Research Centre, Simon Fraser University, Vancouver, Canada)

Prevention of abuse and neglect of older residents in institutional care has typically focussed on staff education and training. However, abuse can occur when residents and their families lack information on what their rights and the responsibilities of the facility staff are. As a result, many seniors feel they are leaving their rights at the door when they live in a care facility. This presentation describes a project funded by the Law Foundation of British Columbia to help address this knowledge gap by providing plain language rights information to seniors in care and their families. The process begins by identifying common issues and questions regarding rights through focus groups with (a) seniors and family caregivers; (b) staff and administration. There can be both simple misunderstanding and different values operating. We combine those identified issues with peoples legal rights as identified in the provincial statutes and regulations governing these facilities, as well as Canadian common law, translating the concepts and ideas into everyday examples more useful to the end users. This process has been successfully used in one other Canadian province, as both a resident and staff training tool. Additional considerations for the project from the outset have been: (a) recognizing the challenges of protecting cognitively impaired seniors; and (b) the best means and best time to provide the information (e.g, how soon before or after going into care, providing it through long term care or seniors agencies).

SESSION 295

Quality of Life: Concept, Measurement, and Research

Elisa Dulcey-Ruiz (Centro Psicologia Gerontologica, Bogota Colombia) ("Evaluation Methods of Quality of Life Measures: Colombian Findings) Gema Quintero (Southeast Florida Center on Aging, Florida International University, Miami Florida, USA) ("The Nonspecific Concept of Quality of Life, Development and Implementation of a Quality of Life Instrument in Cuba") Anita L. Neri (Cidade Universitaria Campinas, Campinas San Paulo, Brazil) ("Quality of Life Research")

Issue: This session focuses on the conceptual frame work, methods, and findings for quality of life measures. We also analyzed instruments measuring quality of life in three different Latin American Countries: Colombia, Brazil and Cuba. Structure: Because quality of life is an unspecific over utilized concept, we begin with the development of a conceptual framework for quality of life measures. Different methodology and assessment instruments will be presented. Their administration and results will be discussed. A brief examination of quality of life measures in Latin American countries: Colombia, Brazil and Cuba and their implementation with older adult populations will be presented. Content: Many instruments have been developed to measure quality of life. Those instruments have utilized physical limitations, symptoms, emotional and intellectual performance, and even health services provision measures to quantify quality of life. The concept is rich and nonspecific. It requires multidimensional evaluation with its corresponding indicators. This table examines the methodology of instrument selection, sources of information and data collection used in the measurement for quality of life measures. The presentation begins with the standardization analysis of quality of life instruments focusing on physical health and psycho-social well-being. It concludes with stressing the importance of examining the parameters on which they are based, searching for greater integration and co adherence. Also discussed are the subjective and objective views on quality of life taking into account the dimensions of time: past, present and future, in the interrelationship between the individual and their environment. The implementation of quality of life instruments in three Latin American countries showed cultural similarities and differences. Conclusions: The concepts, methods and evaluation of quality of life measures must be consistently and rigorously revised. Analysis of quality of life measures in different countries can contribute to the establishment of more enriching criteria for its conceptualization and application.

Evaluation Methods of Quality of Life Measures: Columbian findings

Elisa Dulcey-Ruiz (Centro Psicologia Gerontologica, Bogota Colombia)

This presentation examines instrument selection, sources of information and data collection used in the measurement for quality of life. Two investigations will be described. The first addressing the standardization and utilization of an instrument with an emphasis on physical and psychological health. The second investigation analyzed two instruments with a psychosocial focus. It concludes by stressing the importance of examining the parameters and searching for greater integration and co-adherence.

Quality of Life Research

Anita L. Neri, (Cidade Universitaria Campinas, Campinas San Paulo, Brazil)

This presentation discusses the subjective and objective views on quality of life taking into account the dimensions of time: past, present and future, and the interrelationship between the individual and their environment. Methodological and controversial complexities in the measurement of subjective and objective quality of life are identified. It concludes with methodological aspects in the quantification of quality of life. Yes, "Quality of Life..." E.D. Rui

The Nonspecific Concept of Quality of Life. Development and Implementation of a Quality of Life Instrument in Cuba.

Gema Quintero, M.P.H. (Southeast Florida Center on Aging, Florida International University, Miami Florida, USA)

This presentation begins by examining the nonspecific and over utilized concept of quality of life. A survey instrument was developed in Cuba to measure quality of life. It's conceptual framework was based on three fundamental dimensions: functional level, socioeconomic status, and life satisfaction. It's administration and results concluded emotional issues had the greatest impact on quality of life. Quality of life requires multidimensional evaluation with its corresponding indicators.

SESSION 296

Caregiving issues and service models for elders with disabilities

Barbara M. Silverstone (Lighthouse International, New York, New York, USA), Amy Horowitz (Lighthouse International, New York, New York, USA), Cynthia Stuen (Lighthouse International, New York, New York, USA)

Issues: A substantial body of research has consistently documented the importance of family members in providing emotional and instrumental support to older relatives, as well as the stresses experienced by the family as a consequence of caregiving. Most of this research has focused on caregiving to elders with dementia and to a lesser extent on those with physical disabilities. Although there are few comparative studies, the literature suggests that there are differences in family caregiving behavior and outcomes as a function of the kin relationship of caregiver and care receiver, the type and stage of the disability as well as cultural influences. In addition, much less is known about the role families play in the rehabilitation of older persons with a disability and the extent to which families influence both short and long-term functional and psychosocial outcomes for the elder. Research addressing the latter requires a conceptual and methodological shift from a primarily caregiving perspective (i.e, what family members do for the disabled elder), to one that addresses the family as partner in the rehabilitation process and their potential to facilitate and/or hinder the elder's maintenance and/or recovery of function. Further, service models and interventions will differ depending upon all the factors discussed above. Structure of session: Presentations will be made by the three participants addressing patterns of caregiving and family support among older persons with disabling conditions, followed by an interactive question and answer discussion among all attendees. Content summary of presentations: Drawing upon current research and program models, presenters address how key family characteristics (e.g. perceptions of the disability, attitudes towards independence and autonomy, understanding of the rehabilitation process and goals, as well as the elder's perception of family support) influence the well-being of all members in the family system. Dr. Silverstone focuses on theoretical issues related to traditional, but various, caregiving patterns. Dr. Horowitz discusses a broader conceptualization of caregiving as it applies to families of elders with physical disabilities in the context of rehabilitation, and draws on the evaluation findings of a demonstration project to involve families in the rehabilitation of their disabled relatives. Drawing on the latter as well as other programs, Dr. Stuen addresses some of the practical models of interventions, ranging from formal services to families to support groups for spouses and partners, that have been successfully implemented. Methods for facilitating the involvement of families as active members of the rehabilitation team for elders with disabilities are also discussed. Conclusion/outcome: Evidence from the research literature and clinical/service demonstrations support the need for involvement of the family network of older persons with disabilities in order to enhance the quality of life of both the elder and the family. Attendees will have a more comprehensive understanding of the different types of family support needs depending on both type and stage of elder disability, the type of kin relationship of the caregiver and carereciever, as well as cultural influences. Attendees will be given case examples illustrating the critical importance of appropriately timing the intervention in order to successfully address the various stresses experienced by family members of elders with disabilities over time.

A Family-Based Model of Rehabilitation: Evaluation findings and methodological issues

Amy Horowitz (Lighthouse International, New York, USA)

Although family caregiving to the elderly has been the topic of extensive research, there is substantially less known about the influence of the family in the context of geriatric rehabilitation. Yet it has been suggested that the attitudes and behaviors of social supports can significantly influence both functional and psychosocial outcomes for the elder. At the same time, family members may experience specific stresses associated with their relative's disability which may be addressed through direct involvement in the elder's rehabilitation program. Recent research findings related to these issues are reviewed, with a particular focus on the evaluation findings of a recent research/demonstration project in family-based rehabilitation funded by the AARP Andrus Foundation. The project goal was to maximize functional outcomes for the elder and enhance both the elders' and families' psychosocial adaptation to the disability. The research plan incorporated both pre and 2-month post service in-depth interviews with both the visually impaired elder and his/

her closest relative/friend. Hierarchical regression analyses were conducted for both elder and family outcomes variables to identify the independent influence of greater family participation in services. The fact that both positive (e.g, increase in family life satisfaction) and negative (e.g, increase in elder depression) findings emerged suggests that elder and family interests may not always coincide. Also discussed are the methodological problems that can arise and influence findings and their interpretation. (e.g, timing of the evaluation vis-à-vis service development; ceiling effects resulting from open, rather than targeted, services).

A New Family-based Model of Rehabilitation: From Theory to Practice

Cynthia Stuen (Lighthouse International, New York, USA)

Among the general population, there is little awareness or understanding of vision rehabilitation. When lack of awareness is combined with ageism, older people are even less likely to receive family support for vision rehabilitation. Involvement of families in the vision rehabilitation process has, until very recently, been relatively obscure. However, overall adjustment of older visually impaired persons has been found to be significantly associated with attitudes, behaviors and perceptions of family members. Extrapolating from general theories of caregiving and rehabilitation processes, a new model of family-based rehabilitation was constructed and demonstrated. Practice case examples document that vision loss can create pain for family members and manifest itself as guilt and resentment. Helping families deal with the pain is the first step in helping older people get the positive reinforcement and support they need to adjust to vision impairment. In constructing a new family based model, it is critical to determine how, when, and to what extent to involve the family so as not to diminish the autonomy of the older person. Various strategies involve staff training, new application and assessment processes, and utilization of peers to help coach and/or share their experiences. Other interventions focus specifically on just the partner/spouse relationship. Successful practice-based interventions for adopting a family-oriented model of rehabilitation for older persons will be shared.

Towards a Unifying Theory of Family Caregiving Patterns

Barbara M. Silverstone (Lighthouse International, New York, New York, USA

To date, the prototypical family caregiving arrangement as regards older people in need of support has been a single relative (usually a female spouse or daughter caring for a very frail and impaired individual (usually with dementia). It has become increasingly apparent that other types of caregiving arrangements vital to the well being of older persons exist which have required fresh approaches both in terms of research and practice. This presentation examines the premises and assumptions underlying family caregiving research and practice and offers a theoretical model which reflects the diversity among elderly care receivers, their caregivers, and the disabling conditions leading to the need for care. Research and service models reported in the literature over the past 20 years will be summarized and analyzed. Put forth will be a more encompassing theoretical framework that can lead to a fuller understanding of caregiver behavior and point to appropriate interventions.

SESSION 297

Dementia and Personhood: Matters of the Heart and Mind

K. McGilton and D. Pringle (University of Toronto, Toronto, Canada) Relationships between residents and providers in long-term care: What matters and how do we encourage relationships that matter? B. Dobbs and N. Keating (University of Alberta, Edmonton, Alberta, Canada) Dementia and Driving Cessation: More than Loss of Mobility. H. Tuokko (University of Victoria, Victoria, B.C, Canada) and P. MacCourt(Seniors Outreach Team, Nanaimo, BC, Canada) The process(es) of decision-making by and for persons with dementia. A. Smith and K. Kobayashi (University of British Columbia, Vancouver, Canada) Making sense of dementia in an intergenerational context: The case of a Japanese Canadian family. P. Stephenson (University of Victoria, Victoria, Canada) and C. Russell (University of Sydney, Sydney, Australia). Isolated elderly men and dementia: reflections on a new research agenda. J. Graham, for the UBC Dementia and Personhood Collaborative Research Group: A. Carswell, J. Graham, A. Martin-Matthews, D. O'Connor, J. Perry, B. Purves, (University of British Columbia, Vancouver, Canada), N. Keating (University of Alberta, Edmonton, Canada)

ISSUE: This is the first of a two-part symposium and roundtable presentation that will extend the conceptual and methodological issues addressed during a recent Canadian Institutes of Health Research Tri-Council Workshop. Bringing together an international roster of researchers and health professionals interested in aging, dementia, personhood, identity, and dignity, these papers address the wider cultural matrix which embodies the familial, social and political ecologies and representations through which the progress of neurodegeneration is experienced. STRUCTURE: The five papers present approaches which focus on the meanings of cognitive decline and qualities of life from the point of view of the sufferers affected, while heuristically working towards a model which allows for the development of evidence-based therapeutic strategies of maintaining dignity and personhood in the presence of decline. The functional and cognitive changes that have been the markers of a clinical phenomenology of dementia are explored in respect to how the dementing experience is associated with inter-individual, cultural and wider contextual determinants which address intention, communication, interaction, and performance of those experiencing dementia. These invited papers examine how the essential value of experiential knowledge attends to the cultural complexity, pluralism and boundaries of contemporary experience of frail elderly Canadians. They portray the transformative nature of multidisciplinary, cohesive and collaborative research frameworks which guide the pluralistic examination of personhood and dignity in dementia in Canada presented here and will be taken up in the roundtable session to follow. CONTENT: The symposium opens with McGilton & Pringle examining quality relationships between residents and heath care providers in long-term care facilities. Dobbs & Keating take us out to the community, where the forfeiture of driving privileges is associated with losses in identity and self-esteem. Tuokko & McCourt follow this up with recent research findings on value-laden factors related to care decisions made by and for older persons. Smith & Kobayashi then localize these values to the specific case of intergenerational negotiation in Japanese-Canadian nisei-headed families. Finally, by turning our attention to problems experienced by isolated elderly men in Australia and Canada, focusing on issues of class, poverty, and indigenous status, Stephenson & Russell push us to re-examine the medicalization of dementia when it is encountered on the street, and the prescribed societal values that constrain our constructs. ANTICIPATED OUTCOMES: Although we are entering an era of pharmaceutical treatments for dementia, the hope and expectations resting on these treatments have unfortunately overshadowed the experiences and needs of the people living with these conditions. This symposium-roundtable presents the findings of an interdisciplinary research project to advance a conceptual framework for research strategies (e.g. a series of stepped and concurrent methodological approaches) that accommodate a national, and perhaps international, interdisciplinary dementia research agenda focusing on personhood and dignity. By integrating clinical and critical interpretive frameworks, the papers in this symposium and roundtable presentation articulate individualized (identified through qualitative techniques) and standardized indicators (outcomes) to guide the design and evaluation of interventions across cultural, personal, functional and clinical domains that enable individuals with dementia to maintain identity and dignity.

Dementia and driving cessation: More than the loss of mobility

B. Dobbs and N. Keating, (University of Alberta, Edmonton, Alberta, Canada)

For many individuals with a dementia, the forfeiture of driving privileges is a major loss. Within the research community, this loss has been framed almost exclusively in terms of loss of mobility. Thus, researchers have focused on the negative outcomes of driving cessation such as increased dependence and social isolation, with an emphasis from program developers and policymakers on the provision of alternate means of transportation for those who no longer are able to drive. The loss of driving privileges, however, can have consequences that go beyond affecting the mobility of the individual. In this presentation, we argue that the primary consequence of license forfeiture as a transportation issue obscures the associated losses to identity and self-esteem. In North American culture, the prerogative to drive is synonymous with competence, self-regard, and social membership, with loss of driving privileges associated with feelings of diminished self-worth, reductions in self-esteem, and a loss of identity. A reconceptualization and exploration of the centrality of driving to sense of self will advance our understanding of the psychological impact of driving cessation. This information is basic to the development of programs aimed at preserving dignity and self-esteem of individuals with dementia experiencing forfeiture of driving privileges.

Isolated elderly men and dementia: reflections on a new research agenda

P. Stephenson, (Centre on Aging, University of Victoria, Victoria, B.C.) & C. Russell (School of Behavioural and Community Health Sciences, University of Sydney, Lidcombe, Australia)

In response to an earlier 'masculinist' bias in social gerontology, the past twenty years have yielded a tremendous increase into research on the the lives of older women and claims that the issues associated with aging are predominantly 'women's issues' have become relatively commonplace. Unfortunately our view of elderly men has remained largely frozen in time and the problems experienced by isolated elderly men remain largely unanalysed today. This paper focuses on the issues of class, poverty, isolation, and especially indigenous status as they are reflected in compromised health among isolated elderly men in Australia and Canada. We are particularly concerned with the development of dementia as experienced by men living on the streets, or intermittently in poor housing. The paper concludes with a discussion of adjusting research agendas to reflect the need for policy relevant information.

Making sense of dementia in an intergenerational context

A. Smith (Department of Anthropology & Sociology, University of British Columbia, Vancouver, Canada) and K. Kobayashi (School of Social Work & Family Studies, University of British Columbia, Vancouver, Canada)

This study focuses on intergenerational negotiations between parents and adult children in a nisei (second generation) Δ headed Japanese Canadian family during the clinical evaluation of a parent for dementia. Intergenerational negotiations are explored according to parent's and children's: (1) adherence to traditional issei (first generation) values; (2) roles and responsibilities within the family; (3) perceptions of mental illness; (4) and understandings of dementia. The case study is selected from a larger qualitative investigation of 16 families where a relative was evaluated at an outpatient dementia clinic. Data collection methods include participant observation of the clinical evaluation and in-depth interviews with family members. Results indicate that adult children play a key role in negotiating the referral of the affected parent to the clinic and in diffusing the stigma associated with being evaluated for a psychiatric condition. This case also reveals how adult children interpret the disclosure of ambiguous diagnostic information by clinicians as confirming the presence of Alzheimer disease in a more definitive way than is warranted by evaluation results. This interpretation appears to be an effort to resolve distressing uncertainty about the nature of memory and behavioural problems in the affected parent. This case study underscores the influence of cultural values on the familial management of the clinical evaluation. Specifically, it suggests that in Japanese Canadian nisei-headed families, a primary consideration is family members' concern around having an elder diagnosed with a condition that potentially could diminish not only the individual's but the family's dignity and status within the community.

Relationships between nursing staff and residents: professional, friend, family, companion, or?

K. McGilton and D.Pringle (Faculty of Nursing, University of Toronto, Toronto, Canada)

The quality of life of residents of long-term care facilities is of concern to providers and of interest to academic researchers. Both research findings and experience in working with residents have demonstrated that the type of relationships these residents have with their direct care providers, who for the most part are not professional workers but rather are health care aides, can help them to take pleasure in their daily lives or can leave them feeling isolated and lonely. Unfortunately, we know little about the types or characteristics of relationships that benefit residents and the nature of long-term care creates challenges and opportunities quite different from the "professional" or "therapeutic" relationships characteristic of acute care. Furthermore, since the majority of residents have some degree of cognitive impairment, it is difficult to determine if they are part of the relationships that they take pleasure in. There are few theories providing guidance as to the nature of the relationships that should be encouraged; and it is still unclear whether health care aides can be taught how to develop these relationships or whether this capacity is innate and therefore must be part of what aides bring to their jobs. In this session, we will examine the research on relationships between residents and health care aides, explore a range of theories that provide guidance for relationship development particularly involving cognitively impaired residents, propose a typology of relationships that may be appropriate in long term care and discuss how research in this area might be developed.

The process(es) of decision-making by and for persons with dementia

H. Tuokko (Centre on Aging, University of Victoria, Victoria, B.C, Canada) and P. MacCourt (Seniors Outreach Team, Nanaimo, BC, Canada).

The role of the person with dementia in the process of health care decision making, in any setting, from the diagnostic level through to care planning, has emerged as an area of great importance and concern. Of particular concern are procedures for determining decision-making incompetency or incapacity. Under what circumstances is a person's right to autonomous decision-making questioned? If a health care professional, or any other individual or group of individuals, is involved in making a decision on behalf of an elderly person, what are the factors that need to be considered? We will describe current work on factors related to care decisions made by and for older persons. In so doing, we acknowledged that these decisions are not purely technical judgments but are value-laden and that values operate at the personal, professional, institutional, and societal levels. Those circumstances where the decisions made by older persons and others (e.g, health care professionals, family) may appear in conflict will be highlighted for discussion. Finding ways to assist persons in communicating their health care preferences (e.g, extending autonomy) seems to be of particular relevance to maintaining the personhood and dignity of those with dementia.

SESSION 298

Caffeine reduces cerebral blood flow in patients recovering from an ischaemic stroke

S Ragab, M Lunt, T Birch, DF Jenkinson (Royal Bournemouth Hospital, Bournemouth, England, UK)

PURPOSE: Caffeine causes a reduction in cerebral blood flow (CBF) in healthy individuals. The purpose of this study was to investigate if a similar reduction in blood flow occurs in stroke patients. METHOD: The study used a randomized, double blind, cross over design. Eighteen patients recovering from an ischaemic stroke in the middle cerebral artery (MCA) territory 2-10 weeks previously, attended two sessions having abstained from caffeine for 48 hours. At each session, CBF was measured 4 times using xenon clearance, twice before the oral administration of 250mg caffeine or matched placebo, and twice after. Three MCA velocity readings (Vmca) using transcranial doppler were made prior to administration and four after. RESULTS: Ingestion of 250mg caffeine resulted in a significant fall in CBF and Vmca compared to placebo. On the affected side, caffeine caused an average decrease in CBF of 10ml/100g/min from a baseline of 43ml/100g/min (-24% [95% Confidence Interval -17% to -31%] p<0.00001). On the unaffected side, CBF decreased by an average of 10ml/100g/min from a baseline of 43ml/100g/min (-24% [95% CI -18% to -30%], p<0.000001). Vmca on the affected side decreased by 15% ([95% CI -8% to -22%],p<0.001) and on the unaffected side decreased by 15% ([95% CI -10% to -19%], p<0.0001). CONCLUSION: This study demonstrates that caffeine reduces CBF and Vmca in both the affected and unaffected hemisphere. Since caffeine is widely consumed by stroke patients this effect could have adverse clinical consequences through exacerbation of existing cerebral ischaemia.

Effect of Fancia on improving microcirculation disturbance

Mao Weng, Zhu Hanming, Zhen Zhixue (HuaDong Hospital, Shanghai Institute of Gerontology and Geriatrics, Shanghai, China)

Objective: To study the immediate effect and co-effect of Fancia (inhalant) on improving microcirculation disturbance and criteria for evaluation of the therapy. Methods: 60 patients with cardio-cerebro-vascular diseases divided into four groups were observed by microcirculation of nailfold (MN) before and after treatment with Fancia using Tian Niu's Test Multiple Quantitative Evaluation Method (MQEM) as an evaluation index. Results: After treatment with Fancia, the score value of morphology, hemodynamics and the nailfold microcirculation as a whole were significantly decreased (0.8967±0.7195, 0.7517±0.7041, 0.5867±0.3842, 0.4567±0.7817, 2.4933±2.2846, 1.8533±1.0817, P<0.001), especially the capillary loop diameter, the capillary density, the velocity of blood flow and RBC aggregation remarkably improved. There was no significant difference between the pure-Fancia treatment group and co-Fancia treatment group or simple hypertension group and the hypertension with coronary disease group or the cerebro-cardio-vascular disease group and non-cerebro-cardio-vascular disease group before and after treatment . Conclusion: It is suggested that Fancia (inhalant) has a distinct and immediate effect on improving microcirculation, but its effect is not specific - Fancia may be used as a symptomatic therapy for cardiovascular disease and an aid for non-cardio-vascular disease.

Endogenous Dehydroepiandrosterone (DHEA) and DHEA Sulfate (DHEA-S) in Ischemic Stroke: Effects on Outcome

L. Denti, G. Valenti, M. Maggio, A. Cecchetti, S. Perelli Ercolini, M.F. Merli, A. Giordano, F. Ablondi and G.P. Ceda. (Chair of Gerontology and Geriatrics, University of Parma, Parma, Italy)

Dehydroepiandrosterone (DHEA) and DHEA sulfate may function as neuroprotective or neurotrophic factors to protect central nervous system against a variety of insults. To date, no data are available on the potential role of endogenous DHEA and DHEAS in neurological and functional outcome of patients with ischemic stroke, especially in the very old. We evaluated the relationship between hormonal concentrations determined within 24 hours of stroke onset and clinical outcome, in 74 patients, aged 82.9+/-7.4, consecutively admitted to a Geriatric Ward. DHEA, DHEAS and cortisol serum levels were related by logistic regression to neurological evolution, assessed by NIHSS at 1 week and at 1 month or discharge, as well as to poor outcome, defined as severe disability (Barthel index < 60/100) or death, at 1 month or discharge and at 3 months. A significant association with neurological improvement at 1 week was found for DHEA-S (positive) and cortisol/DHEA-S molar ratio (negative), independent of age and admission NIHSS score. However, disability or death (poor outcome), at 1 month (or discharge) and at 3 months, were correlated only to cortisol levels at multiple logistic analysis adjusting for admission NIHSS score, neurological complication, therapy and pre-morbid functional status. In conclusion, our data support a neuroprotective effect of endogenous DHEAS, at least in the short-term. However, no predictive value was apparent for functional outcome or death, which turned out to be related to cortisol and other clinical covariates. Work partially supported by Grant n 9906153187-010 from MURST- Rome

Influence of the magnetotherapeutic pillow on microcirculation of nail-fold of patients with cervical spondylosis disease

Mao Weng, Zhu Hanming, Zhu Yongfen (Huadong Hospital, Shanghai Institute of Gerontology and Geriatrics, Shanghai, China)

Objective: To observe the adjunctive efficacy of magnetotherapeutic pillow with a shape of cervical spine curve in patients with cervical spondylosis disease . Methods: 15 patients sleep with their heads on the magnetotherapeutic pillow for two months and the examination of microcirculation of nailfold and their clinical symptoms and signs were taken before and after treatment, and the combination of the two parameters was used as criteria to test the efficacy. Results: The score value of morphology hemodynamics and the nailfold microcirculation as a whole post-treatment were significantly decreased with an average of 0.88 low (0.78±0.60, 0.33±0.39, 0.63±0.39, 0.42±0.24, 2.19±1.21, 1.49±0.88, P<0.05~0.01), and especially the capillary loop diameter and velocity of blood flow improved remarkably. The clinical symptoms were improved also: 3 cases were remarkably improved (20%), 8 cases were improved (53%), the remarked effective rate, the effective rate and total effective rate of the therapy were 20%, 66% and 86%. Conclusions: The magnetotherapeutic pillow aids improvements of patients' microcirculation and the relief of their clinical symptoms. It is helpful to the prophylaxis and therapy of cervical spondylosis disease.

Subarachnoid Hemorrhage in the Elderly : Management Outcome in the Endovascular Era

S. Navarro, B. Jarraya, N. Taright, A. Srour, J.-P. Sichez, A. Biondi-Dormont, R. van Effenterre, Ph. Cornu(Salpetriere Hospital, Paris, France)

PURPOSE: The number of aged patients referred for aneurysmal subarachnoid hemorrhage (SAH) has increased. The purpose of this study is to answer the following questions : What is the outcome of these patients ? What are the significant prognosis factors ? Is there a place for a neurosurgical treatment in this period of life ? METHOD : We retrospectively analysed the data of fifty patients with aneurysmal SAH , over 70 years old, who were consecutively admitted from March 1996 to March 2000. All were admitted in the neurosurgical care intensive unit. All were considered for neurosurgical treatment whenever possible, regardless of their age. This included either open microsurgery or endovascular surgery. RESULTS : At admission, 800f the patients had an American Society of Anesthesiology score < 3. Fifteen patients were treated by open surgery, seventeen by endovascular surgery, eighteen were not treated. Overall outcome (Glasgow Outcome Scale and Modified Rankin Scale) revealed 34% with good recovery, 6% with severe disability, 60 0ead, and no vegetative state. Fourteen patients (28%) experienced an acceptable Quality of Life state (return to home with no or only moderate disability). Low level of consciousness, World Federation of Neurological Surgeons grade >= 3 and existence of blood clots on CT-scan at admission were correlated with poor outcome. No significant outcome difference was noted between open surgery group and endovascular surgery group. CONCLUSION: At admission, the patient prognosis may be estimated by clinical and neuroradiological data. Endovascular surgery may be a promising minimally invasive treatment.

SESSION 299

Community Hospitals for Elderly in Singapore - A Model

David Yong (Ang Mo Kio Community HospitalSingapore)

PURPOSE: To describe our experience with community hospital care for elderly in Singapore METHOD: A descriptive study RESULTS: Singapore has one of the fastest ageing populations in the world. Recent initiatives by government have targeted an integration and expansion of health care resources for the elderly. Since 1993 Ang Mo Kio community hospital provides subacute, rehabilitation , day hospital-type and respite care services for the elderly. These services help the older person to regain functional independence and the family cope with those with disabilities in the community. The staff comprise aged care trained community physicians, nurses, therapists and social workers, supported by other specialists who are visiting or through referrals. The main conditions are strokes, falls and fractures, recent acute illness or surgery with deconditioning and amputees. The team also provides services to nursing homes and day centres in the vicinity, and participates in community health promotion projects. It is also a training centre for aged care. There is a pharmacy, Xrays and laboratory, renal dialysis centre, an acupuncture clinic, an equipment shop and the Singapore Diabetic Society co-located here to provide related services. The community hospital is integrated vertically 'upstream' to the acute referring hospital and horizontally to other community hospitals. Furthermore community hospital provides a leadership and support role to the other community aged care services 'downstream'. Recently there are trends towards quality assurance and audit in these facilities. CONCLUSION: Community hospital is poised to play a bigger role in providing services for older people in transition back into and in the community in Singapore.

Economic evaluation of a geriatric day hospital: Cost-benefit analysis based on functional autonomy changes

M. Tousignant, PT, (University of Ottawa and Gerontology and Geriatrics Research Center, Sherbrooke Geriatric University Institute, Sherbrooke, Canada) R. Hébert, MPHIL (Gerontology and Geriatrics Research Center, Sherbrooke Geriatric University Institute, Sherbrooke, Canada) J. Desrosiers, ERG, (Gerontology and Geriatrics Research Center, Sherbrooke Geriatric University Institute, Sherbrooke, Canada)

PURPOSE - The purpose of this study was to investigate whether the benefits related to a geriatric day hospital (GDH) program exceeded the costs using a cost-benefit analysis based on functional autonomy changes. METHOD - Sample. The sample was composed of 151 patients admitted to the GDH program at the Sherbrooke Geriatric University Institute (SGUI) in the Province of Quebec, Canada. Data from a previous longitudinal study tracking autonomy changes in 554 olders over 75 years of age living at home were used to create a comparison sample. Clinical data collection. After admission to (T0) and at discharge (T1) from the GDH program, functional autonomy was assessed by a trained nurse using the Système de Mesure de l'Autonomie Fonctionnelle (SMAF). Cost estimation. Based on financial reports, costs associated with resources consumed by the GDH program were established. Benefit estimation. Benefit in dollars per day was estimated through regression equations based on functional autonomy changes T1-T0 related to the GDH program. Two scenarios for spreading the benefit per day were used: 1) time to go back to the pre-admission SMAF level; and 2) median time from survival analysis to institutionalization or death from the comparison sample. RESULTS - The results show that for every dollar invested in the GDH program, the benefit for the health system was $1.63 based on the time to go back to the pre-admission SMAF level as the spreading period of the benefit ($p=0.047$), and $2.07 for the survival analysis scenario ($p=0.001$). CONCLUSION - Based on our convenience sample of SGUI patients, the benefit related to the GDH program seems to exceed the costs. Other studies are required to replicate our results and to compare costs and benefits for other types of care.

Impact of the Day Hospital program at the Sherbrooke Geriatric University Institute

Johanne Desrosiers (Centre de recherche en gérontologie et gériatrie, Institut universitaire de gériatrie de Sherbrooke et Université de Sherbrooke) Réjean Hébert (Centre de recherche en gérontologie et gériatrie, Institut universitaire de gériatrie de Sherbrooke et Université de Sherbrooke) Hélène Payette (Centre de recherche en gérontologie et gériatrie, Institut universitaire de gériatrie de Sherbrooke et Université de Sherbrooke) Sylvie Côté (Centre de recherche en gérontologie et gériatrie, Institut universitaire de gériatrie de Sherbrooke) Pierre-Michel Roy (Institut universitaire de gériatrie de Sherbrooke et Université de Sherbrooke) Lise Trottier ((Centre de recherche en gérontologie et gériatrie, Institut universitaire de gériatrie de Sherbrooke)

PURPOSE: The Day Hospital at the Sherbrooke Geriatric University Institute is a specialised geriatric outpatient service for people aged 65 and older referred for one or more physical, psychological or social problems. The purpose of this study was to: 1) evaluate the effect of the program on the nutritional risk, pain, functional autonomy, balance and walking, grip strength, well-being, psychiatric profile, perceived social support and leisure satisfaction of the clients in the program and on the caregivers' burden; 2) compare the effects of the program according to the diagnoses of the participants; and 3) evaluate whether improvements were maintained three months after the program. METHOD: A pre-experimental longitudinal design was used. Each Day Hospital client was evaluated in person using reliable, valid tools on three occasions: 1) at admission (T1); 2) at termination (T2); and 3) three months later (T3). RESULTS: A total of 151 people participated in the T1 and T2 measures. Significant improvements were observed for all the participants on all the variables studied except for nutritional risk, perceived social support and the caregivers' feeling of burden. The effects of the program on the Stroke / Neurological diseases and Locomotive disorders / Amputations diagnosis groups were more marked. For the subjects presenting the Gait disorders and falls diagnosis, only the total score on the functional autonomy scale improved. The greatest improvement in their feeling of well-being occurred in the Cognitive function disorders / Psychopathologies diagnosis groups, and a reduction in the feeling of burden among their caregivers was also observed. All the gains observed were still present three months after the program (T3; n=126), with the exception of leisure satisfaction. CONCLUSION: Despite the limitations inherent in the research design, the results suggest that the Day Hospital program improves the functioning of its clientele and maintains it for at least three months.

Seven-year experience of elderly care in a Geriatric Day Hospital

G. Sergio, G. Capobianco, P. Monini, A. Tognetti, S. Baglio, R. Cinque and L. Bartorelli (UOC Geriatria, Dipartimento Tutela Salute dell'Anziano, ASL Roma C, Roma, Italia)

The Authors present a seven-year activity program of geriatric multidisciplinary evaluation and intervention in Day Hospital. 24 elderly patients on average/daily; Jan 1994 - Dec 2000 (N=4483, 2690 women, 1793 men, mean age 74; 30100 daily presence registrations): 2466 (55%) patients received mainly diagnostic and medical assistance; 1493 patients (74%) were mainly physically rehabilitated, 524 patients (26%) mainly neuropsychologically rehabilitated (Alzheimer or vascular type dementia patients). Physical Rehabilitation (PR) consisted of group exercise according to the method "body/conscience" (45 min at a time, 3 days a week for 4-6 weeks) and individual treatment: 10% of all patients performed 2 rehabilitation cycles a year. Neuropsychological Rehabilitation (NR) consisted of: 1) "formal" Reality Orientation Therapy (ROT) to a group of 5 patients (45 min at a time, 4 days a week, for 4 weeks, 2 twice a year); 40% of the patients have been partecipating this treatment for at least 3 years; 2) individual cognitive rehabilitation with computerized memory training utilizing programs of different levels of difficulty (30 min a session, either 2-3 days a week, 4 weeks, 2 periods a year or see ROT frequency); 3) occupational therapy (2 hrs a time, see above) by group and individual standard procedures. PR/3 yrs (N=60) vs Controls/3yrs (N=51) showed a significant positive effect (one way analysis of variance) on the Tinetti scale (balance) ($F = 81.6$, $p<0.001$), the BADL ($F=155.4$; $p<0.001$) and the IADL scale ($F=201.4$; $p<0.001$). NR/3yrs (N=27) vs Controls/3 yrs (N=16) showed a similar trend upon the MMSE score ($F=40.8$; $p<0.001$).

The Essentials of Program Evaluation at a Geriatric Day Hospital

Tanya Dutton (McGill University, Montreal, Canada) Diane Podsiadlo (Royal Victoria Hospital, Montreal, Canada) Nancy Mayo (McGill University, Montreal, Canada)

Purpose: The main purpose of this project was to determine the extent to which the goals and objectives of a Geriatric Day Hospital were comprehensive, meaningful, and met as a form of program evaluation. Methods: The program's goals and objectives were first refined for the purposes of program evaluation. Goals were then selected based on their relevance to the program purpose and client outcomes. Objectives were operationalized with each goal. The objectives were evaluated against a standard criteria selected to indicate clinically meaningful change. Client data (n=130) was obtained to help determine whether the goal, decrease disability was met. Four parameters were established and were used to judge whether the goal had been met by means, 95 (6-Minute Walk). The proportion of individuals who met at least one disability objective was 72%, which suggests that the Geriatric Day Hospital did indeed meet their goal of reducing disability. Conclusions: The Geriatric Day Hospital did meet their goal of reducing disability in their population. The program is still advised to review the strengths of their interventions, targeting of clientele, and what is considered meaningful change for this population of frail elderly.

SESSION 300

Bodies In Space: Creative movement for the older adult

Dean Fogal (TooBa Physical Theatre Centre, Vancouver, British Columbia, Canada)

This workshop encourages the older adult to explore moving the body through space. Conference participants may watch or join in with the gentle exercises which stimulate non-verbal storytelling through the body. This work deepens creativity and allows for a wonderful release of emotion in a completely non-threatening environment. Participants are encouraged to explore the movement of their bodies through the use of gesture and simple self-generated choreography. An increased physical efficiency and appreciation of the beauty of one's own body is fostered by this work which has its roots in Corporeal Mime. The workshop will also address how the exercises taught can be adapted to all levels of physical ability

SESSION 301

Early Assessment, Treatment, and Rehabilitation of Osteoarthritis

J. Guralnik (National Institute on Aging, Betheseda, USA)The Occurrence and Functional Impact of Osteoarthritis in Older Person. M.A.Acanfora (COMLAT-IAG Rehabilitation Committee, Buenos Aires, Argentina) Could Drugs Therapy Reduce Pain and Modulate Osteoarthritis Evolution? C.L. Catalán (Dept. Rehabilitation and Physical Therapy, Hogar Frances, Buenos Aires, Argentina) Management of Osteoarthritis with Physical Therapy. M. Barbagallo (Institute of Internal Medicine and Geriatrics, University of Palermo, Italy) Generalised Osteoarthritis and Bone Mineral Density in the Elderly. S.Yamamoto (Tokyo Metropolitan Geriatric Hospital, Dept. of Orthopedic Surgery) Treatment of Osteoarthritis of the Knee in Japan

Osteoarthritis is one of the most important causes of immobility and disability in the elderly. This disease is usually found among the elderly and although it is one of the most frequent causes of morbidity and medical consultation, it is frequently not considered because it is so common and is sometimes considered to be an elderly ailment. The mistake in regarding this situation as normal, delays not only the assessment but also the right treatment resulting in immobility, serious disabilities and increasing health expenses. An early assessment, treatment, and rehabilitation program must be carried out in order to avoid the above mentioned problems. The purpose of this Symposium is to provide an overview of the main issues related to Osteoarthritis and its influence on health status and mobility or disability of older people. The session will begin with an epidemiological review of this pathology and its impact on functional status, pain and quality of life. The benefit of an early diagnostic and medical treatment could offer modulation in the evolution of this disease and pain management. Physical Therapy provided with sense and in time would manage pain and encourage patients to begin with early physical activation to prevent atrophy and improve muscular strength. The presence of osteoporosis and its correlation with osteoarthritis, both very common in older people, will be presented and discussed. The experience in Japan for treatment of knee joint osteoarthritis to maintain functionality will be presented.

Could Drug Therapy Reduce Pain and Modulate Osteoarthritis Evolution?

Miguel Angel Acanfora (COMLAT Δ IAG Latin American Rehabilitation Committee)

This paper is an update on management of Osteoarthritis with conventional and new drugs to control or reduce pain, as well as a revision of some drugs that seem to modulate the Osteoarthritis evolution in addition to potentially delaying disability. International trials were studied and updated and compared with our experience to find the real outcomes and benefits in the use of NSAIDs (non- steroidal anti-inflammatory drugs) and Sy-SADOA (Symptomatic slow-acting drugs for osteoarthritis) given orally or percutaneously. The gastrointestinal and adverse side-effects were pointed out and summarized, and iatrogenic effects specific to patients with multiple pathologies in the daily use of therapy were focused on. Administration of drugs and Physical Therapy and its interrelations and convenience were detailed. The outcomes and utility of treatment and the way they could help patients and physicians to manage Osteoarthritis pain and delay its evolution were shown and compared. Conclusions: The prescription of drugs by physicians to reduce pain and inflammation, and the rationed use by patients could offer relief of symptomatology. More trials and studies must be encouraged regarding disease evolution.

Generalized osteoarthritis and bone mineral density in the elderly

M. Barbagallo, LJ Dominguez, R. Ruggero, MA Alessi, L.Granvillano, D. La Milia (Institute of Internal Medicine and Geriatrics, University of Palermo, Italy)

PURPOSE: Osteoarthritis and osteoporosis are both extremely common diseases in the elderly. Aim of the present study was to study the relationship between osteoarthritis and bone mineral density (BMD) in the elderly. METHODS:120 women older than 65 yrs were studied. 60 women with generalized osteoarthritis (OA) and 60 controls (NL) of the same age, sex, anthropometric characteristic and working activity. In all subjects, BMD was measured at vertebral and femoral sites using dual energy X-ray absorptiometry (DEXA; DPX-100 Lunar). RESULTS: Mean age and BMI were respectively 69.1±0.92yrs and 28.6±0.52 in the OA group vs 68.9±0.91yrs and 27.5±0.33 in NL group (p=NS). Only 11/60 subjects with osteoarthritis (18.3%) have a reduced BMD in one of the sites examined. When compared to normal controls, OA subjects had increased BMD at all the sites examined: spine 1.026±0.178 vs 0.964±0.051 g/cm2 (p=0.011); femoral neck 0.81±0.116 vs 0.777±0.057 g/cm2 (p=0.019); Wards Triangle 0.690±0.140 vs 0.640 vs 0.066 g/cm2 (p=0.032); throchanter 0.724±0.100 vs 0.686±0.048 g/cm2 (p=0.010). A significant positive relationship was present between the severity of ostearthritis of the spine (measured by Kelgreen scale) and the BMD of femur and other sites not clinically and/ or radiologically involved by the disease. CONCLUSIONS: Our present results suggest that the presence of ostearthritis may protect from postmenopausal bone loss and the occurrence of osteoporosis. Further studies are needed to elucidate the mechanism(s) and to confirm the hypothesis that a reduction of bone turnover and/or an increased production of bone growth factors (non measured here) may be involved.

Management of Osteoarthritis with Physical Therapy

Carmen Luz Catalán (Dept. of Rehabilitation and Physical Therapy, Hogar Frances, Buenos Aires, Argentina)

The usual role of Physical Therapy in the treatment of Osteoarthritis is for instilled disability. Serious joint damage may prevent patients from having good mobility and good quality of life. Early diagnosis, global assessment, and referral to Physical Therapy could offer an excellent way to reduce the disease's impact and to provide advice to patients for future management in their daily activities, thereby improving mobility and preventing further injuries. The convenience of physiotherapy prescription and a suitable exercise program for each patient should be specified. The adverse effects of a massive way of working, especially with elder patients who suffer multiple pathologies, will be demonstrated. The large number of modalities that physiotherapists may employ in the treatment of their patients as well as our experience in the matter will be presented. Conclusions: The role of Physical Therapy and Physiotherapy in treatment of Osteoarthritis may offer pain control as well as reduce and rationalise the use of drugs. This is a good modality of treatment to improve muscular strength, to promote mobility, and to delay disability, ultimately reducing social and health cost of Osteoarthritis.

The Occurrence and Functional Impact of Osteoarthritis in Older Persons

J. Guralnik (National Institute on Aging, Bethesda, USA)

PURPOSE: This presentation will be an introduction for the symposium, reviewing the epidemiology of osteoarthritis and research evaluating the impact of osteoarthritis on functional status, pain, and quality of life in older persons. METHOD: Pertinent literature that focuses on osteoarthritis in older persons will be reviewed. Emphasis will be on prevalence and incidence of osteoarthritis and the impact of osteoarthritis on a number of relevant outcomes. Large intervention trials aimed at preventing the functional consequences of osteoarthritis will also be assessed. RESULTS: Osteoarthritis is one of the most common chronic conditions that affects older persons, with increasing prevalence at higher ages. In persons over 75 years old over 80% have some symptoms of osteoarthritis. Although a number of risk factors for osteoarthritis have been identified in epidemiological research, no marker of early disease that will allow for early intervention is available. Pain and decreased range of motion that result from osteoarthritis have an important impact on functional ability, and arthritis is the most common condition that older persons ascribe their disability to. Exercise has been found to be a valuable adjunct to symptomatic treatment for osteoarthritis. CONCLUSION: With the aging of the population, osteoarthritis will become increasingly more important as a cause of decreased functioning and greater health care expenditures.

Treatment of osteoarthritis of the knee in Japan

Seizo Yamamoto (Tokyo Metropolitan Geriatric Hospital, Dept.of Orthopedic Surgery)

Prevalence of primary osteoarthritis of the knee in Japanese women is expected to be 10 Δ 50%. Almost over 90% of osteoarthritis is varus angulation type. And valgus angulation is few. Conservative treatments are including use of patient education, weight loss(if overweight), physical therapy (range of motion exercise, quadriceps exercise, use of a cane, shoe inserts to correct abnormal biomechanics due to angular deformities), intra-articular (IA) hyaluronic acid (HA),nonsteroidal anti-inflammatory drugs (NSAIDs). Arthroscopic lavage with debridement is useful in patients with concomitant meniscus disease or symptoms of locking of the knee. Severe symptomatic patients with OA knee who have pain that has failed to respond to medical therapy and progress limitation in ADLs are considered osteotomy or total joint arthroplasty. Long term result of the total knee arthroplasty is excellent.

SESSION 302

Functional Immunity in Aging: Implications to Infections

R. B. Effros (UCLA School of Medicine, Los Angeles, California USA) (Memory T cells in the elderly: Lessons from HIV infection) G. Butenko (Institute of Gerontology, Kiev, Ukraine) (Primary and secondary immune responses in aging) R. Solana (Department of Immunology, "Reina Sofiacute; " University Hospital, acute; rdoba, Spain) (NK cells and T cells expressing NK cell differentiation antigens in the elderly) A. Ben-Yehuda (Geriatric Unit, Hadassah University Hospital, Jerusalem, Israel) (Influenza vaccination for the elderly: Current status and novel approaches)

ISSUE: According to the classical view of immunity in aging the response to incognate antigens declines while immunological memory is maintained. However, more recent detailed studies indicate that although the frequency of memory type cells increases they may not necessarily represent a consequence of immunological memory accumulation throughout the life span. The symposium is designed to elucidate the source and nature of the "memory type" lymphocytes in aging, along with a better understanding of the innate immunity in old age, and to examine novel approaches for efficient vaccinations of the elderly. STRUCTURE: The symposium will start with a brief introduction (by A. Globerson), and be followed by talks of R.B. Effros, G.M. Butenko, R. Solana and A. Ben-Yehuda, presenting the state of their art from studies in their laboratories. CONTENT: The introduction will focus on the state of the art on the immune system in aging. It will emphasize the point that the immune system does not just undergo a unidirectional decline, but is characterized by cellular shifts from primary to "memory type" lymphocytes and from Th1 to Th2 cytokine networks. It will call attention to the possible impact of these dynamic changes on immunity and infection in old age. The first speaker (R.B. Effros) will then present data on the fate of T lymphocytes that are subject to chronic antigen stimulation and the implications to long-term immunological memory in old age. These studies are based on the in vitro model of lymphocyte replicative senescence and the in vivo relevance is viewed through analyses of cells from HIV infected subjects. The results indicate that "memory type" lymphocytes may eventually senesce. The second speaker (G.M. Butenko) will discuss the question of whether the "memory type" lymphocytes in aging represent a consequence of immunological memory accumulation throughout the life span. His results indicate that newly generated T lymphocytes in aging may have a priori properties of "memory type" cells. These presentations will be followed by an updated insight into the nature of cells involved in innate immunity in aging. This issue will be discussed by focusing on the natural killer (NK) lymphocyte compartment. The studies presented (by R. Solana) indicate phenotypic and functional changes in this immune cell compartment, that result in a shift from mature T lymphocytes to mature NK and NK/T cells and senscent/effector T lymphocytes. The last speaker (A.Ben-Yehda) reports on novel approaches for Influenza vaccination to the elderly. It takes in account the reduced production of Th1 cytokine (IL-2) in the aged and thus provides this cytokine along with the vaccine incorporated in liposomes. This strategy may offer an efficient vaccine to combat influenza and possibly other infections in the elderly. CONCLUSIONS AND ANTICIPATED OUTCOME: The symposium introduces a new overall view of the immune system in aging, showing its functional status. It may thus lead to novel practical approaches for vaccinations and protection against infection in the elderly.

Influenza vaccination for the elderly: Current status and novel approaches

Arie Ben Yehuda, Gideon Friedman, Yecheskel Barenholz and Eli Kedar, (Hadassah University Hospital and the Hebrew University Medical School, Jerusalem, Israel)

PURPOSE: To establish a useful protective vaccine to influenza in the elderly INTRODUCTION: Influenza has been one of the commonest causes for morbidity and mortality among the elderly during the winter season. Each winter brings an increased influenza-related mortality rate, most of which occurs among elderly persons. The increased rate of the disease and its poor outcome have been attributed to a decline in lymphocyte function that occurs with age. Specifically, memory T cells that have lost their ability to be co-stimulated to produce IL-2 accumulate with age, thus leading to an abortive immune response to the virus and to the vaccines that have been developed against it. The World Health Organization recommends yearly vaccination of elderly persons and about 40-60% of the vaccinees develop protective immunity. Despite the limited efficacy vaccinated subjects have lower frequencies of hospitalization for respiratory diseases, congestive heart failure and death from any cause compared to unvaccinated subjects. An enhanced immune response may further reduce the morbidity and mortality from influenza, and this presentation will describe some strategies to develop novel more effective vaccines. METHOD: One such strategy uses liposome-mediated immunization. .Liposomes are phospholipid particles that have been shown to act as a delivery system to antigen presenting cells. RESULTS: We found that young adult mice and humans who were immunized with the hemagglutinin antigen that had been entraped in liposomes containing IL2 developed a higher titer of protecting antybodies than did those immunized with the free antigen or with the liposomal antigen without IL-2. Other approaches include intranasal preparations, using cold adapted live attenuated viruses or various vehicles. CONCLUSIONS: Newer vaccines may encompass better clinical efficacy and prove to be cost-saving.

Memory T cells in the elderly: lessons from HIV infection

Rita B. Effros and Mirabelle Dagarag, UCLA School of Medicine, California (Los Angeles, USA)

PURPOSE: To analyze the cellular and genetic basis for reduced T cell function in the elderly, particularly within the memory pool. METHOD: We have reported that the proportion of CD28-negative T cells increases progressively with age in humans, with the most dramatic change observed within the CD8+ T cell memory subset. A putative scenario for the generation of such cells is the process of replicative senescence, which we have modeled in cell culture. The experimental system involves establishing T cell cultures from peripheral blood of normal healthy adults donors by stimulation with an irradated allogeneic B cell line in the presence of IL-2. The cultures are restimulated every 3-4 weeks and subcultivated until they reach irreversible cell cycle arrest. The cells are characterized throughout the long-term culture for surface phenotype, telomere length, telomerase activity, CTL function, cytokine production, and apoptosis. RESULTS: In response to repeated antigenic stimulation and exposure to IL-2, naïve CD8+ T cells eventually reach an end-stage memory/effector phenotype that is characterized by an irreversible cell cycle arrest, loss of CD28 expression, telomeres in the 5-7 kb range, potent antigen-specific CTL function, altered cytokine profiles, and apoptosis resistance. Cells with this same phenotype are dramatically increased during HIV infection, with the progressive accumulation of CD28-negative T cells over time in individual donors correlating with disease progression. Ongoing experiments on peptide-specific CD8+ T cell clones established from HIV-infected donors are in progress to further characterize the functional and effector characteristics of this end-stage memory cell. CONCLUSIONS: The final differentiative state of chronically stimulated CD8+T cells is an end-stage memory cell that has unique phenotypic, genetic and functional characteristics. The demonstration that chronic HIV infection leads to the accelerated generation of such cells provides unique insights into its possible etiology in the context of aging. (supported by NIH AI 47665, AG10415, and AG05920)

NK cells and T cells expressing NK cell differentiation antigens in the elderly

Olga DelaRosa, Raquel Tarazona, Javier G. Casado, Ester Peralbo, Julia Carracedo, Rafael Ramirez, Corona Alonso, and Rafael Solana (Department of Immunology, Faculty of Medicine, "Reina Sofía" University Hospital, and Research Unit, "Reina Sofía" University Hospital, Córdoba, Spain)

NK cells play a significant role in the defense against infections as a consequence of both their cytotoxic capacity and the cytokines produced. Age-associated alterations have been demonstrated in NK cells. Although NK cell cytotoxicity is well preserved in healthy elderly people other NK cell characteristics such as proliferation, expression of different NK markers, or response to IL-2, are decreased in aging, indicating that senescence is associated to a defective functional capacity of NK cells, that is partially compensated by an increased number of mature NK cells. The clinical relevance of the altered NK cell function in aging is shown in studies that demonstrate that low NK cell number or function associate to infections and increased mortality risk. We have also observed an increase in the percentage of T cells co-expressing NK cell markers (CD56, CD94, CD16, CD161) in aging. Analysis of these cells according to the CD28 phenotype demonstrate that the expression of CD16, CD94 and CD56 is increased in CD8+CD28- cells from elderly individuals. The study of telomere length in these subsets using the Flow-FISH technique show that CD3+CD28- T cells have shorter telomeres than CD3+CD28+ cells. These T cells do not correspond to an expansion of the classical Va24+ NK/T cells that represent only a minor subset (<1%) of T lymphocytes. Phenotypic differences were also observed in Va24+ NK/T cells from young and elderly individuals. Taken together these results support a shift in lymphocytes from ab T lymphocytes to mature NK, NK/T cells and senescent/effector T lymphocytes.

Primary and secondary immune responses in aging

G.M. Butenko (Institute of Gerontology, Vyshgorodskaya st. 67, 04114 Kiev, Ukraine)

The primary and secondary immune responses are both impaired in aging. This holds true of the primary response to a greater degree, although the secondary (anamnestic) immune reactions are affected as well. In our experiments on the CBA mice we have shown that in old animals after antigen priming the immune cell expansion was less pronounced and proportion of cells shared between antibody producing and memory cells shifted to the latter however did not reach the young organism's level. In the case that a second antigen administration was made in a 2 days interval after the first one, the level of antibody producing cells became equal to the young one. At the same time proportion of cells with memory cell markers increased in old organism 3-4-fold. This is assumed to be the consequence of immunological memory accumulation through life span. Although in heterochronic bone marrow radiation chimeras the previously existing immune memory dramatically decreased or vanished, the proportion of cells with naive/memory phenotypes maintained at a level, which is characteristic of the host organism. So, despite the replacement of bone marrow cells and their progeny by the cells of opposite ages the features of mature immunocompetent cells are dependent on the regulatory signals of recipient not on the simply "immunological experience". All these events should be considered in infection immunology.

SESSION 303

Environmental Gerontology at the Beginning of the New Millennium

H.-W. Wahl (The German Centre for Research on Ageing at the University of Heidelberg, Heidelberg, Germany) and G. D. Weisman (University of Wisconsin, Milwaukee, U.S.) Environmental Gerontology at the Beginning of the New Millennium: Major Achievements and Some Concerns. S. M. Golant (University of Florida, Gainesville, U.S.) Theory in Environmental Gerontology: Challenges and Promising New Pathways. L. N. Gitlin (Thomas Jefferson University, Philadelphia, U.S.) Methods in Home Environmental Research: Lessons Learned and New Directions. T. Toyama (University of Kyoto, Kyoto, Japan) Holistic Approaches to Dementia Design. Y. A. W. Slangen-de-Kort (Eindhoven University of Technology, Eindhoven, Netherlands) Where Is the Person in Environmental Gerontology? H. Kendig (University of Sydney, Sydney, Australia) Discussant

The goal of this symposium is to critically and constructively review the state of the art of environmental gerontology at the beginning of the new millennium. First Hans-Werner Wahl and Gerald Weisman will provide their evaluation of the major achievements of the ecological perspective for gerontology, the lives of older persons, and for society as a whole, along with the challenges confronting the field. Steven Golant will then consider the latest theoretical developments in environmental gerontology, offering a framework to assess the heuristic value of old and new ideas with particular emphasis on temporal change in person-environment relations in later life. Third, Laura Gitlin, focusing on the domain of home modification, will elaborate on new research directions and corresponding methods. Todashi Toyama will specifically address the challenges which dementia presents for environmental gerontology, emphasizing the value of post-occupancy evaluations of group living environments. Fifth, Yvonne Slangen-de Kort focuses on critical linkages between environmental gerontology and personality research, taking the position that the study of aging and environment should be transformed to the study of aging with environments. Finally, Hal Kendig will consider and further integrate the substance of these papers.

Environmental Gerontology at the Beginning of the New Millennium: Major Achievements and Some Concerns

H.-W. Wahl (The German Centre for Research on Ageing at the University of Heidelberg, Heidelberg, Germany) and G. D. Weisman (University of Wisconsin, Milwaukee, U.S.)

This introduction to the symposium begins with the observation that environmental gerontology has revealed many faces in terms of theory, methods, results, values and application since in emergence almost 50 years ago. Review of these multiple facets of the field provides a broad and useful perspective for this symposium. While classical theories, such as those of Carp, Kahana, and Lawton, have been widely recognized in gerontology, theoretical development in the 1990's has slowed and diversified into multiple mini-theories. Philosophical and methodological tensions between interactional and transactional approaches continue; the field does not yet possess an armementariium of data collection strategies of repeatedly proven quality. Despite these limitations, there are substantial empirical findings within the environmental gerontology paradigm [see recent summaries of Day et al, Gitlin, Wahl, and Weisman et al.]. This literature provides a major contribution to our understanding and ability to optimize both normal and pathological [particularly dementia] aging; this research base enhances the ability of environmental gerontology to contribute to the ability of care providers and society as a whole to meet the needs and expectations of elders. Among the major challenges for the future are more focused efforts in the realms of theory and methods, progress in the selection and/or integration of individual, group, organization, or place as the unit of analysis, and clearer consideration of the environmental needs of forthcoming cohorts of elders.

Holistic Approaches to Dementia Design

Tadashi Toyama (University of Kyoto, Japan)

Today it is estimated that there are over 1.6 million persons with dementia in Japan. Of this population one third receive care in traditional institutions, such as hospitals, extended care facilities, and nursing homes. In Japan the philosophy of care for persons with dementia is undergoing change. Since around 1990 a new form of care has been introduced. This alternative is called "group living" and a number of these new facilities have been built in Japan. The author has been intensely involved in the process of evolving these alternative "group living" facilities both in terms of designing the structures and then through extensive evaluation. At the beginning of this process the knowledge gained by in-depth post occupancy evaluations of existing group living facilities and the activity patterns of the residents the author identified cultural elements believed to be helpful to person's with dementia. From these studies, designs which were culturally specific to Japanese traditional homes were developed. As each new "group living" facility has been established they have been evaluated. The evaluations have been repeated at three-monthly intervals and this process has continued for a period of 3 years in some instances. Two case studies of these evaluations will be presented in order to describe the data collected. The method of these evaluations included interviews with staff members and activity tracking maps of each identified resident made every 10 minutes to record their activities. The results show that "group living" facilities have brought about increased resident activity and involvement, and has improved their well-being. The process the author describes demonstrates the value of behavioral research in creating new forms of architecture and care for persons with dementia in Japan.

Methods in Home Environmental Research: Lessons Learned and New Directions for Research

Laura N. Gitlin, (Thomas Jefferson University, Philadelphia, PA, USA)

Most older people live at home and express the desire to age in place. Little research examines however the role of home environments in supporting this goal and promoting life quality. This is due to the methodological challenges in examining person-environmental transactions in the home. This paper identifies new directions in home enviornmental research by first examining current knowledge and methodologies in use. Two streams of research, falls and home modification studies, contribute to our current knowledge of the role of home environments in supporting elders. In this research, the environment is treated primarily as an independent variable in which its relative contribution to positive (safety) and negative (injury from falls) outcomes is examined. Self-report or direct observation of discrete environmental features is the principle methodology used. Recent efforts, however, attempt to link characteristics of persons and environments by examining discrete functional actions (toileting) in relationship to particular environmental set ups (toilet height). Chief among the challenges in person-environment research is developing conceptual and operational definitions for measurement. Only select dimensions important to home life (safety, security, and accessibility) have thus far been examined. Environmental attributes contributing to higher order functioning (engagement, stimulation, satisfaction, novelty, comfort, personal control) remain relatively unexplored. A related issue is whether relevant dimensions of home environments differ by impairment-type (cognitive vs. physical). Finally, home environments are not static, standard or uniform. Applying a reliable and valid metric is important but remains difficult. Of most importance is developing methodologies by which to examine the dynamic, transactional nature of person-environment fit and conceptualizing and operationalizing change. Frame-by-frame videotape analyses or use of microchip processors that detect movement provide micro-perspectives of environmental contexts of self-care practices. These approaches offer promising new approaches to the study of complex interactions.

Theory in Environmental Gerontology: Challenges and Promising New Pathways

S. M. Golant (University of Florida, Gainesville, Florida, USA)

Several generalizations characterize past environmental gerontology theories explaining the appropriateness of residential and/or care settings and how they impact the lives of their elderly occupants. First, they have generally failed to conceptualize how changes in either the attributes of older individuals or their environmental preferences influence their responses to currently occupied shelter and care settings. Second, except in the instance of extreme environmental changes (e.g, moves from conventional residences to nursing homes), theoretical efforts have assessed the shelter and care setting occupied by the older person as a momentary situation. Third, theoretical treatments have emphasized the effects of environmental content (e.g, dwelling attributes or characteristics of social relationships) as opposed to the influence of the individual's behavior circuits or activities within their environments. Fourth, most theoretical models have failed to specify how individual variations in the assessed salience of environmental content and behavior circuits explain environment-behavior relationships. Fifth, theorists have displayed little consistency in how they have defined constructs to specify individual or environmental outcomes. Sixth, the complexity of construct specifications and interrelationships has made most theoretical models impractical to operationalize in empirical research. New theoretical efforts by the author attempt to alleviate several of these weaknesses by defining environmental change as a central construct, conceptualizing temporal assessments of both environmental content and individual's behavior circuits, and conceptualizing outcomes as an individual's set of multidimensional emotional responses. This formulation is mindful of the practical difficulties researchers confront when operationalizing complex theoretical models.

Where is the person in environmental gerontology?

Y. A. W. Slangen - de Kort (Eindhoven University of Technology, Netherlands)

The purpose of this presentation is to argue that after years of studying aging and environment, one of the major research challenges today is to study ageing with environments. In the past we have seen numerous studies investigating characteristics of housing and other environments and their appropriateness for elderly users. Other studies have focused on characteristics of ageing individuals that are good indicators (determinants) of successful aging. More recent studies, adopting the ideas of person-environment fit, have been focusing on optimal combinations of the two: what environmental characteristics are beneficial for which elderly users. However, in our view, we have fallen in the same loophole as the earliest architectural psychologists in regarding elderly users as passive entities who accept their environments as stable and unadjustable artifacts. This view proven unacceptable in environmental psychology in general and is likely to fall short as well in environmental gerontology. The author will argue that it is interesting and enlightening to study what older individuals actually do with, or rather to their environments and discuss ways of studying this behavior. Some exploratory studies indicate that this behavior is highly dependent on the very specific spatial, financial, stuctural, personal and social characteristics of the person and situation. This will pose serious challenges to generalizability and validity of the research and calls for new methods and techniques for studying 'aging in place'. However, we would like to argue that this will be way towards understanding environmental competence and proactivity with regard to aging with environments

SESSION 304

A Service Provision Model for Rehabilitation of Visually Impaired Older Persons in Quebec

Baignée, Diane (Institute Nazareth and Louis-Braille, Montreal, Canada) Couturier, Julie-Anne (The School of Optometry of the University of Montreal).

The population of older people experiencing age-related vision loss is increasing dramatically as the older population is growing and should even double by the year 2030. Although vision impairment is not life threatening like many age-related health conditions, it has a significant impact on the quality of life and independent living for older persons. Isolation and fear of nursing home placement are common difficulties experienced, along with significant depressive disorders developed following the onset of vision loss. On the basis that older visually impaired persons need to have access to services that will help them continue living as independently and productively as possible in their own home and community, professionals in the aging network need to develop collaborative partnership in delivering services. The Institute Nazareth and Louis-Braille, a rehabilitation agency for the blind and visually-impaired population, provides services through the medicare system to 4000 persons aged 65 and older. Home and community-based services, such as low vision, orientation and mobility, activities of daily living, communication, and psychosocial support are offered by a multidisciplinary team. Considering their positive influence, peer support groups have been implemented as part of the programming. The rehabilitation process has a strong impact on self esteem and integration into community activity. A partnership is also established with the University of Montreal School of Optometry to enhance quality of training for first-line service care optometrists and a collaborative project is at its initial stage of development with an ophtalmology care unit for a better service continuum

Coping with and adapting to age-related vision loss

David Kolker (University of Toronto, Toronto, Canada)

The purpose of this cross-sectional exploratory study is to: - Examine the various emotions that the individual encounters when first diagnosed with the eye disorder; - Look at what strategies and technical devices they utilize in order to adapt to daily life; - Examine what impact the family has on the visually-impaired elder; - Investigate what services the visually challenged senior uses; Method: A self-administered questionnaire was distributed to three CNIB peer support groups. Study participants had a choice of completing a large print questionnaire, or flistening to it on tape and then writing their answers on a piece of paper. A convenience sample was utilized that included 22 study participants. Results: Visually-impaired elders express negative emotions, especially for the most part depression and anger, in the period of six months after being first diagnosed. Later on the individual acquires a more positive outlook due to using different strategies, and accessing services and devices. Some of these strategies elders utilize to cope with the handicap may be techniques that they have used all of their life or it could be something new that they have developed. For the most part elders presently utilize low-tech devices. Most study participants discussed how family makes a difference in adjusting to a visual impairment. Conclusion: This study indicates that diagnosis is only the first step in coping and adapting with a visual impairment and not the last one. Coping and adapting with a visual handicap is a socially constructed process, which depends on society, family, and the elder. Furthermore, health care professionals can help facilitate this process.

Effect of Retinalamin and Cortexin on the Development of Age-Related Macular Degeneration

S. V. Trofimova, V. Kh. Khavinson (St. Petersburg Institute of Bioregulation and Gerontology, St. Petersburg, Russia)

Retinal degeneration is of high incidence in the elderly and aged patients being the 3rd most frequent cause of blindness. It is entailed by metabolic disorders complicated by generalized atherosclerosis manifestations often occurring at this age. This is the main cause of involution-associated chronic degeneration in the retinal macular region and subsequent central sight loss. Methods of treatment applied in today s ophthalmology cannot stop this pathology being purely symptomatic. Our investigations were designed to estimate the effect of Retinalamin(r) and Cortexin(r) on development of age-related macular degeneration in 64 patients (127 eyes) aged 61-82. Retinalamin is a polypeptide complex isolated from calf retina. It normalizes metabolic processes in the retinal membrane, improves the functional interaction of pigmented epithelium and external segments of photoreceptors. Cortexin is a polypeptide complex isolated from calf cerebral cortex normalizing metabolism in the central nervous system and optic nerve fiber. After treatment, ophthalmoscopic picture of the eyegrounds improved in 71.1 % of the cases: hemorrhages resolved, macular edema diminished. The drugs increased the retinal functional activity and improved retinal blood flow in 85.8 % of the cases, thus not only stopping the pathology progress but also increasing visual functions. Visual acuity raised in 79.5 % of the cases (in 46.4 % - by 0.2-0.4), number of central scotoma significantly reduced in 77.9 %. Consequently, regular application of Retinalamin and Cortexin (2-3 times a year) facilitates stabilization of the pathologic process evidencing the prevalence of bioregulation therapy over the conventional methods of

Old, Deaf and Dumb ? No way! Communicating with the Hard of Hearing.

J.P. W. Tremblay, Christine Cabedoce (Programme Aînés, Institut Raymond-Dewar, Montréal, Canada).

Thirty to eighty percent of the aged present a hearing problem from mild to total deafness. Althought the lost of hearing is not life threatening, nor is it physically obvious, it will limit ones autonomy, increase social isolation as well as increase the occurence of depression and anxiety. Although hearing aids do exist, they do not correct ones hearing as a pair of glasses can correct myopia. It is an understatement to say that most professionnals do not grasp the debilitating reality of the condition. It is often misunderstood the serious consequences on their practice from their evaluations of the patient, as well as the intense mental suffering. Yet, simple strategies do help the aged to better understand. The author, a clinical psychologist, will present an ongoing clinical program that helps the Hard of Hearing to better cope with this condition and will demonstrate a series of simple stategies that can facilitate communication with the aged. The coordinator of the program will present the specific services developed, community based as well as institutionnal, for the aged who are Hard of Hearing. Participants will be exposed to the actual sound that Hard of Hearing do hear. The participants will find it much less stressful to communicate with the Hard of Hearing and should be able to make a more accurate cognitive assessment of these patients.

Outcomes of Hearing Aid Fitting for Older Adults

L. Hickson, P. Stanz (Communication Disability in Ageing Research Unit, Department of Speech Pathology and Audiology, The University of Queensland, Brisbane, Australia).

Hearing impairment is highly prevalent in older people, occurring in approximately 60% of the population over 60 years of age. Clinical intervention for older people with hearing impairment in Australia has a predominantly technological focus with hearing aids being the most common form of treatment. The purpose of the present study was to investigate the outcomes of hearing aid fitting for a sample of 755 older Australians. The majority of participants had mild to moderate hearing impairment and were fitted with in-the-ear hearing aids. Outcomes were measured via a postal questionnaire distributed three months post aid fitting. Results were generally positive with 65% of participants reporting using their aid(s) five or more hours per day; 91% were either very satisfied or satisfied with their aid(s); and participants, on average, considered that their aid(s) provided between a lot and a moderate amount of benefit across different listening situations. A high percentage of participants did report some problems with their aid(s) however, with the most frequent problems being the quality of the participant's own voice (55%) and aid whistling (51%). Although the outcomes of aid fitting in terms of use, benefit and satisfaction were very good, the high prevalence of reported problems is a concern. These problems may detrimentally affect outcomes in the long term. The results of the study suggest that further research into the prevention of problems with hearing aids is necessary, and long-term follow up is recommended.

Senile local eye amyloidosis in age related macular degeneration

Victor V.Ermilov MISR University for Science and Technology, College of Medicine,Department of Pathology,6th of October City,Egypt

Age related macular degeneration(AMD) is now the leading cause of blindness in developed countries.The role of amyloidosis in the mechanism of accelerated aging of the ocular fundic tissues has not yet been investigated.With the help of selective methods of revealing amyloid and by performing electron microscopy,we investigated 111 enucleated eyes of people over 60 years age.We found morphologic signs of AMD.100 eyes were included into group I. It was the atrophic type of AMD(geographic atrophy of the retinal pigment epithelium).11 eyes made up group II with exudative ("wet")AMD.Amyloid was found in 47 eyes.Both in the atrophic and exudative forms of AMD in the eyes with amyloidosis,morphologic changes in the form of drusen combined with changes in the retinal pigment epithelium cells prevailed.In group I amyloidosis was found in 39%,in group II-in 80%.As well as in other forms of senile local amyloidosis the amyloid found in AMD was resistant to potassium permanganatis and alkaline guanidine hydrochloride which was applied for 2 hours.Ultrastructural investigation showed that amyloid fibrillae are localized on the inner collagen surface of Bruch's membrane in the subretinal space.Our investigation has shown that the transformation from the atrophic type to exudative("wet")form of AMD in the injured ocular fundic tissues,the frequency of amyloidosis is doubled.Senile local amyloidosis is an important component of Bruch's membrane change when aging

The Evaluation of the Risk Factors and of the Diagnosis Proceeding in Presbycusis

C. Ciucurel (Ana Aslan National Institute of Gerontology and Geriatrics, Bucharest, Romania)

Presbycusis must be considered a consequence of the senescence of the auditory system on which different external and internal factors can graft, but these ones must be seen only as risk factors and not etiological agents. The purpose of this paper is to identify the risk factors associated to the presbycusis. The research represents an analytical inquest of observation (case-witness) with a transversal character. The subjects of the study (N=120) can be divided into five age categories (subjects aged 50 years and over), 65 men and 55 women. Among them 43 were found with presbycusis, using the Hearing Handicap Inventory for Elderly - Screening Version, physical tests, audiometry, auditory brainstem responses. The distribution of the presbycusis on the age categories had a progressive evolution from 12.5% (50-55 years old) to 50% (76-80 years old). The evaluated risk factors were: extracranial vascular modifications, EEG modifications, EKG modifications, diabetes mellitus, obesity, the plasmatic lipids modifications, hypertension and smoking. A significant association ($p < 0,01$) of presbycusis and the following risk factors has been established: extracranial vascular modifications to both sexes, women EEG modifications, men EKG modifications, diabetes mellitus under 65 years for both sexes, obesity at women, hypercholesterolemia to both sexes, the hypo-HDLcholesterolemia at women, hypertension at women, smoking at women. As a conclusion a special attention must be paid to the association of presbycusis to metabolic and cardio-vascular disorders which can produce physiopathological modifications at different levels of the auditory system. Sex and age adjust the action of these risk factors.

Visual Problems in Latino American Rural Elderly

Fernando Gómez, Carmen Lucía Curcio, Marcela Villa. [Geriatric and Gerontological Research Group, Caldas University, Manizales, Colombia]

Objective: To evaluate self-reported visual disability and to screen of visual function in rural Colombian elderly to determine the prevalence of visual problems and describe their characteristics in this group. Design: Descriptive epidemiology and cross-sectional study. Setting: Two rural coffee grower areas in Colombian Andes mountains. Subjects: Of a total of 381 inhabitants of two rural communities with a mean age of 68.3 (SD 7.4) were screened 280 (73%) Measurements: A personal interview assessing demographic information, functional ability, falls was obtained. The Geriatric Depression Scale (GDS) was used. Self-reported visual problems were obtained, visual acuity and screening of and fundoscopy were assessed. Results: 780f the elderly people informed visual problems compared with 63% with objective problems found by examination: 73.4% refractive problems (especially presbicia), 15.8Conclusions: Self-reported visual problems were correlated with objective visual problem assessment in rural elderly. The prevalence of visual problems in rural areas in developing countries is higher than in developed countries, especially refractive problems. Moreover, rural elderly with visual problems have higher dependence in ADL and depression rates than general elderly population.

SESSION 305

Experiences with External Hip Protectors in Aged People in Institutions and Home.

R. Heikinheimo, P. Jäntti (Hospital of Oulu Health Center, Finland), A. Jalonen-Männikkö (Health Center of Tampere,Finland).

The first study of the use of Finnish external hip protectors,"Safety Pants" in homes for the aged showed, that whereas among the controls here occurred seven fractures in the hip region, only one occurred among the users of Safety Pants. In another study it was found that instead of six expected fractures there occurred only one. In an inquiry among 71 homes for the aged three hip fractures occurred with the Safety Pants on and in 22 homes at least one certain hip fracture had been avoided. The 716 Safety Pants used in the latter study cost altogether about US $20 000. When in this way 27 hip fractures were avoided and the cost of the treatment of these is about $10 000, each and altogether more than 200 000, these savings were thus achieved with 10% investments. In the Central District of Tampere Health Center Safety Pants were distributed to the circulating nurses in the autumn 1998 -1999 to be given to the aged of their area who in their opinion most needed them. Problems : 1. Can the nurses estimate the possible fallers and bone breakers? 2. Can they persuade them to use Safety Pants? 3. Can this reduce the number of hip fractures? and 4. Is the use of Safety Pants economical also among the home dwelling aged? The preliminary results are promising: In control areas the number of hip fractures increased by 14 (49 - 63), but in the Central District diminished by 4 (43 - 39). Using the Safety Pants was also economical: The 150 Safety Pants cost only 36 000 - FIM (US $ 5 000), less than the cost of the treatment of one hip fracture 70 000 - FIM (US $ 10 000).

Hip Protectors in Elderly Orthopedic Patients: A Prospective Case Cohort Study

Klaus Hindso & Jes Bruun Lauritzen, (Department of Orthopedic Surgery, Hvidovre Hospital, Bispebjerg Hospital, University of Copenhagen, Denmark)

PURPOSE: To evaluate the effect of hip protectors on risk of subsequent hip fracture among elderly orthopedic patients admitted with fall and/or fracture. METHOD: Open prospective case cohort study among 1,170 elderly orthopedic patients more than 74 years of age admitted to orthopedics with fall or fracture. A total of 711 patients at Hvidovre Hospital were offered three sets of hip protectors (SAFEHIP) and 459 patients at Bispebjerg Hospital were controls. Home-dwellers accounted for 90.9% and nursing homes residents 9.1%. Patients were followed from 1 to 1 year. RESULTS The annual rate of subsequent hip fracture in the control group was 5.4%. Primary acceptance of hip protectors was 60%. Based on intention to treat analysis the adjusted relative risk (RR) was 0.89 (0.52-1.5, 95%CL). Based on continued use referred to as still possessing hip protectors including seldom use to every day use (n 256) the adjusted RR was 0.71, (0.37-1.4). For those who used hip protectors often or every day the non-adjusted RR was 0.43, $p<0.05$ (n 131). 143 falls on the protector were reported with no hip fracture. CONCLUSION: Hip protectors demonstrated a significant 57% risk reduction for subsequent hip fracture among the subgroup of subjects who wore hip protectors on a regular basis. Based on intention to treat the risk was reduced by 11% and for those who were registered as having and still possessed hip protectors the RR for a new hip fracture was reduced by 29%, but these reductions were not statistically significant.

Intervention programme to increase adherence to the use of hip protectors

Meyer G (University of Hamburg, Hamburg, Germany) Warnke A (University of Hamburg, Hamburg, Germany) Bender R (University of Bielefeld, Bielefeld, Germany) Muehlhauser I (University of Hamburg, Hamburg, Germany)

PURPOSE: The risk of hip fractures can be reduced by hip protectors. But, compliance to wear the protector is poor. We studied the effects of an intervention programme to increase adherence and reduce hip fractures in a 18-months randomized-controlled-trial. METHOD: After baseline assessment of 942 high risk subjects in 49 nursing homes the institutions were cluster-randomized (computer-generated, concealed) to the intervention group (IG, n=25) or to standard care (control group, CG, n=24). Intervention comprised an education programme and providing 3 hip protectors (Safehip) for each participant. The education programme addresses staff and residents targeting relevant aspects known to interfere with the use of the hip protector and uses modern concepts of adult education. Standard care consisted of brief information about and demonstration of the hip protector to the staff. Compliance was analysed for the first 6-months. RESULTS: Baseline risk for falling was comparable between groups. For 60 (IG) and 88 (CG) subjects the study was terminated because of death (87%) or moving to another institution. Of the total of 459 IG residents 37% experienced 484 falls; of the 483 CG residents 42% had 705 falls. The hip protector was worn in 74% versus 130f falls. There were 8 hip fractures in the IG and 16 in the CG. CONCLUSION: Implementing the hip protector in nursing homes by following a structured approach consisting of an education programme and providing the hip protectors increases adherence to the use of the hip protector.

Short term acceptance of semi-rigid hip protectors in elderly inpatients.

P. Rumeau [service de gérontologie L'Orbe, Hôpital Charles Foix, Ivry sur Seine, France], G. Lefranc [service de gérontologie L'Orbe, Hôpital Charles Foix, Ivry sur Seine, France], J.B. Piera [service de médecine physique et de réadaptation, Hôpital Charles Foix, Ivry sur Seine, France], F. Piette [service de gérontologie La Triade, Hôpital Charles Foix, Ivry sur Seine, France].

Abstract Purpose: Hip protectors are efficient against hip fractures but their acceptance is said to be low. We tried to assess acceptability of an hip protector in our gerontology ward . Method: Voluntary at risk patients received, according to availability, an Hips(r) (Qvortrup Medical, Denmark) protector. We didn't ask them to wear it at night. Wearing was assessed by four preplanned controls over 15 days. No notice of the controls was given to the nurses nor the patients, and the controller didn't incite the patients to wear the device. Patients could quit whenever they wanted. Patients were considered wearing the protector if they were actually wearing it on two controls, and were still wearing it at the end of the fortnight. Medical records were not collected until the end of the study to avoid a bias in selecting the patients. Results: We included 30 patients over 7 months, aged 86 ± 6, with MMS = 12.5 ± 9, only 2 eligible patients declined taking part. 27 had previously fallen, 17 had one or more fractures related to osteoporosis, 16 had a neurologic condition, 19 a dementia. 18 patients were wearing the protector at the end of the study, 5 from the 15 first and 13 of the last 15. There was no significant difference in age and MMS both between wearers and not wearers, and the first and last 15 patients included. Conclusion: Hips(r) hip protectors has a good short term acceptance in elderly inpatients, what ever their mental status. Acceptance improves with use.

SESSION 306

Advances in Psychotherapy for the elderly

Joel Sadavoy (Mount Sinai Hospital/university of Toronto, Toronto Canada Laura Machado (institue of gerontology of Candido Mendez University, Rio de Janeiro, Brazil Molyn Leszcz (Mount Sinai Hospital and University of TOronto, Toronto Canada Patricia Guido (Sociedad Argentina de Gerontologia y geriatria, Buenos Aries Argentina

The psychotherapies have been adapted to treating the elderly and have shown effectiveness for this group as they have for younger patients. This symposium examines the application of psychotherapy in four domains emphasizing the demonstrated utility in each area and the modifications and techniques particularly useful for the elderly. The session is organized into four sections: Dementia, depression, personality disorders, and group therapy with complex disorders The Dementia section analyses the most effective types of psychotherapeutic interventions for patients and their families, emphasizing the utility in stress reduction of caregivers, reduction of the risk of family abuse, delaying admission to a facility, relieving patient suffering, and improving quality of life for patient and family. Psychotherapy of depression is addressed from a psychodynamic perspective, examinig indications contraindications and utility of this form of intervention. Special emphasis is placed on models of understanding transference and countertransference. The group therapy technique is examined in detail emphasizing the integrated use of interpersonal, self psychology and cognitive behavioural techniques with patients who present with complex comorbid clinical pictures. Similarly, individual dynamic psychotherapeutic techniques for challenging and perplexing behaviours associated with personality disorders will be presented in detail. with emphasis on practical management of the therapists counterreactions. Psychotherapies are effective but complex interventions. This session will provide participants with a guide to the utlity, indications, and practical applications of various techniques to the most most common clinical problems of the elderly

Group Psychotherapy for the elderly

Molyn Leszcz (Mount Sinai Hospital and Universityof Toronto, Toronto, Canada)

Abstract Purpose: to present integrated approaches to group therapy of the elderly. Method: The data derive from detailed clinical records of ongoing multidisciplinary group therapy of geriatric patients in a specialized psychiatric day hospital. Patients are admitted primarily for treatment of depression. This group includes patients with comorbid mild cognitive impairment, and frequent histories of massive psychic trauma suffered in the Holocaust. Methods of treatment include integrated application of self psychology theory, cognitive and behavioural interventions and interpersonal psychotherpay techniques. Conclusion: Integrated Group psychotherapy techniques have proven highly effective as determined by overall clinical outcome and patient satisfaction

How effective are psychotherapeutic approaches for patients with dementia and their families?

Laura Machado (Institute of Gerontology of Candido Mendes University, Rio de Janeiro, Brazil)

It is known that dementia causes suffering not only for the patient himself, but foremost for his family. Until recently, however, research has focused primarily to the pharmacological treatment of dementia, targeting cognitive and behavioral symptom control; very little has been done concerning non-pharmacological interventions, that address psychological and relational aspects of the patient, as well as qualifying members of the family to properly look after the sick person. The purpose of this paper is to analyse the most effective types of psychotherapeutical interventions to manage dementia patients, as well as interventions with the family, for these reduce the stress from caregiving, reduce the risk of family abuse, delay patient admission to a facility, relief patient suffering, thus significantly improving the patient and the family quality of life.

Individual dynamic psychotherapy for personality disordered elderly

Joel Sadavoy (Mount SDInai Hospital and the university of Toronto, Toronto Canada)

Personality disorders persist into old age and often create major therapeutic challenges. This presentation demonstrates that dynamic understanding and psychotherapy remains one of the pillars of therapy for this group of patients. Method: Using clinical material, the presentation applies psychodynamic principles in therapy as a robust method for both understanding and intervening especially when combined with other methods in an integrated fashion. In this presentation the theoretical basis for framing understanding of PD in old age will be presented including psychodynamic formulation techniques for age specific stressors and presentations of PD symptoms, approaches to organizing therapy and practical interventions. Results and conclusions: The clinical cases clearly reveal the effectiveness of these clinical interventions as a model for both understanding the clinical pictures and helping therapists deal with their own complex feelings during therapy.

Psychotherapy of Depression in the Elderly

Patricia Guido (Sociedad Argentina de Gerontología y Geriatría, Buenos Aires, Argentina)

Depression is not only one of the most frequent pathologies in aging, but is also one of the most frequent consulting reasons in elderly psychotherapy. During the last few years the theoretical developments of elderly psychotherapy and its efficacy were on the increase. There is no contraindication for psychotherapy in the elderly, except with psychotic patients, schizophrenia or patients with moderate or serious dementia disorders. Psychoanalytical psychotherapy as antidepressive therapy is based on the technical and theoretical principles of psychoanalysis with some technical variations. Psychotherapy in the depressed elderly, as in other age groups, requires a permanent analysis of transference and countertransference as they allow the therapist to conduct the therapeutical process. Although prejudice in society and in some professions towards this kind of treatment exists, the clinical experience shows that the elderly improve their symptoms and display their possibilities from psychotherapy, sometimes faster than younger adults. Psychotherapy can diminished the dose of psychopharmacological drugs. It is necessary to go on working on theoretical developments and psychotherapy research, as an effective way of treating depressed elderly.

SESSION 307

A Survey of Residential Care Facilities in Ottawa-Carleton Region: Care Needs and Health Service Provision

F. Aminzadeh, (Regional Geriatric Assessment Program of Ottawa Carleton, Canada) WB. Dalziel, FRCP (C) (RGAP of Ottawa-Carleton, Canada) S. Amos, (RGAP of Ottawa-Carleton, Canada) C. Martell, (RGAP of Ottawa-Carleton, Canada)

PURPOSE: Demographic changes characterized by a rapid growth of the older population coupled with the inadequate funding of community care and long term care sectors have led to a proliferation of unlicenced residential care facilities as an alternative living arrangement for frail older adults. However, there is a lack of systematic research on residents' care needs, service provision, and the potential role of specialized comprehensive geriatric assessment programs (CGA) in the care of at risk residents. This study is part of a larger research initiative examining the above issues. METHOD: A survey of senior administrators of all residential care facilities in the Ottawa-Carleton Region. RESULTS: Preliminary results reveal considerable variability among facilities with regard to resident profile, availability of nursing and social services, staff ratio and professional training, access to a dedicated facility physician, use of specialized CGA programs and other available community services, cost, and membership status with the Ontario Residential Care Association. Overall, respondents' comments point to a progressive increase in age and complexity of care needs of residents, limited staff ratio and training, inadequate case finding and underutilization of CGA program. The findings identify the priority services and educational needs in this setting. CONCLUSION: The results highlight the need for more anticipatory and systematic approaches to better targeting of at risk residents and meet the staff educational needs.

Innovative Approaches to Knowledge Creation: Merging Technology and Talent for Senior's Health

Shirlee Sharkey (Saint Elizabeth Health Care, Markham, Canada)

PURPOSE: The purpose of our Fostering Real Time Talent Initiative is to combine information and communication technologies with knowledge and experience, to transform caring and health services delivery to seniors. As a non-profit organization providing community-based health care to over 100,000 seniors in Ontario each year, Saint Elizabeth Health Care has created a continuous knowledge exchange process that supports and enhances the cross-functions of a diverse and highly mobile workforce. METHOD: The organization applied creative approaches to traditional educational and professional development building strategies, using technology as a facilitator. Drawing on innovation research and best practice models, Saint Elizabeth Health Care developed a comprehensive framework for knowledge creation, exchange and transfer. RESULTS: Emerging from this technology-enabled Talent Initiative is a more competent and skilled employee base. Clinicians with varied backgrounds and areas of specialization access state-of-the-art, real time information. The end result is the fostering and development of highly skilled, mobile, knowledge clinicians of today and tomorrow. CONCLUSION: In a world experiencing global aging, there exists the need within the health care system to do things differently. Our Fostering Real Time Talent Initiative and its ongoing expansion brings together a tradition of caring, talent, and technology in a whole new way.

Telemedical consultations to a geriatric nursing home

PO Sandman (Dept of Advanced Nursing, Umeå, Sweden) Stefan Sävenstedt (Dept of Advanced Nursing, Umeå, Sweden. Gustaf Bucht (Dept of Geriatric Medicine, Umeå, Sweden) Lennart Norberg (Dept of Geriatric Medicine, Umeå, Sweden)

Purpose: To investigate the possibilities and limitations of using remote medical consultations with videoconference technique by specialist in Geriatric Medicine to nursing home. Method: Two wards in a nursing home were given medical support from a specialist in geriatric medicine using a videoconference. Data was collected from, videotaped telemedical sessions with a systematic registration of tasks dealt with and assessment of the interactions between doctor and nurse, systematic registration of consultations that took place outside telemedical sessions and tape-recorded interviews of the participants. Data were analyzed using booth quantitative and qualitative methods. Results: There was an average of 13.1 problems tasks dealt with per ward per week and 69% of them could be dealt with using distance consultations. The most common way of presenting problems/tasks by nurses was both to give an opinion and a suggestion of what to do with an aim to get this sanctioned by the doctor. The most common response from the doctor was to sanction the nurses suggestions. The experience of telemedicin rounds was that they needed more preparation and were better structured than ordinary rounds. Mutual trust between doctor and nurses was important and the role as link between patient and doctor was emphasized.

Visioconferencing between remote hospitals for the professionals of gerontology

A. Franco, P. Couturier, C. Montani, G. Gavazzi, S. Moine, M. Debray (Gérontologie, CHU, Grenoble, France), C. Hohn, P. Basset, A. Sagnier (CH, Chambéry, France), F. Picot, L. Mackern, B. Bahmane (CH, Annecy, France) F. Tarpin-Lyonnet (CH, Crest, France), J. Tyrrell, S. Banerjee, R. Culet, M. Frossard (Lab.Gérontologie, UJF; UPMF, Grenoble, France)

PURPOSE : Analysis of visioconferencing (VC) between geriatricians of remote french hospitals used to communicate and share continuing education and information. METHOD : As a tool of telemedicine (Télémédecine en Gérontologie, Franco, Frossard, Montani, Serdi Ed, Paris, 2000), VC is used every Monday from 2 to 3 PM between gerontologists of the Academic Hospital of Grenoble and colleagues from 3 General Hospitals (Chambéry since 1995, Annecy 1998, Crest 2000) of the Alpine Region of France. Commercial VC devices (Picturetel and Sony Trinicom 5000) with a mobile camera use 128 Kb RNIS telephone lines. For more than two sites a telecom bridge is scheduled with the provider. Technics and coordination are leaded by Grenoble’s site. RESULTS : Participants are mainly senior and junior geriatricians, psychologists, physiotherapists. Nurses miss the VC for timeless reasons. Contents are : a) analysis of papers (neurologic, Alzheimers’ and cardiovascular diseases, falls, incontinence, rehabilitation; b) internal and general medicine ; c) congress informations; d) clinical discussion about cases and numerical images; e) gerontology internet sites review. Cost is weekly $15 by site with an additive $ 20 for the bridge. A writen summary of the VC (Petit Bulletin du Gériatre) is sent to participants by e-mail and located on a website (www.gerontonline.com). CONCLUSION : After an experimental phase VC appears to be an organizer of a geriatric web. All participants wish to maintain it as a routine tool and new sites are candidates, thus leading to consider a new technical and coordinating organization.

SESSION 308

The Consumer Directed Care/Payment for Care Movement Worldwide

Robyn Stone (Institute for the Future of Aging Services, AAHSA, Washington, DC) ("Consumer-Directed Care: A Global Perspective") Jane Tilly (Urban Institute, Washington, DC) ("Consumer Direction of the Netherlands and France: A Tale of Two Countries") Yoko Crume (North Carolina Department of Health and Human Services, Division on Aging, Raleigh, NC) ("Why Consumer-Direction is Not an Option in Japan") Anna Howe (Consultant Gerontologist, Melbourne, Australia) ("Back to the Future: Lessons from an Early Australian Initiative with a Cash Alternative to Nursing Home Care") Janice Keefe (Mount Saint Vincent University, Halifax, Canada) ("Money or Services: Giving Canadian Caregivers These Options")

Programs which provide a direct payment to persons with disabilities have received increasing attention as a way in which dual objectives can be met; one of increasing consumer empowerment and control and the other of providing adequate services in a cost effective manner. Financial compensation directed at informal caregivers is another program approach that has been developed in many countries throughout the world. This symposium will emphasis the policy issues and ethical concerns which emerge within specific programs that are described as "consumer-directed or payment for care". The session will begin with an overview of the types of program that exist world wide. Findings from a study of the Netherlands and French long-term care systems, including the role of consumer-direction will be reviewed by Jane Tiley. Dr. Crume will discuss the new Japanese LTC program, and will explain why, in contrast to the German system, consumer-direction was not included as an option in Japan. A well established Australian policy of paying family caregivers to care for someone who would otherwise have been in a nursing home will be reviewed by Anna Howe. Dr. Howe will analyze why consumer direction has not progressed beyond the disability community and discuss its potential for expansion into aging services. Professor Clare Ungerson, will use empirical evidence drawn from recent published work in the USA and Europe, plus data from an ongoing cross national study of consumer directed care systems in five European countries, to discuss the ways in which consumer directed care is likely to affect the care relationship and the social and economic position of care givers and care users. Janice Keefe will use Canadian data to describe what informal caregivers in Canada identify as important programs and analyze the policy implications of introducing such programs. This final paper will highlight key ethical issues and dilemmas that arise in consumer-direction programs and provide a cautionary reflection of the underlying implications of introducing these policies through the world. Participants of the symposium will gain knowledge of the scope of existing programs and the problems that emerge out of research studies in this area.

Back to the Future: Lessons From an Early Australian Initiative With a Cash Alternative to Nursing Home Care.

Anna Howe, Consultant Gerontologist, Melbourne, Australia

In 1972 the Australian Federal Government introduced a Domiciliary Nursing Care Benefit which was paid to family caregivers caring for someone who would otherwise have been in a nursing home. The DNCB was paid at 50% of the cost of nursing home care. Although a pioneer cash alternative to services, the DNCB was never widely taken up. This paper begins with an account of the early implementation of the DNCB and then explains its marginalization, due to a lack of indexation to nursing home care benefits and a significant decline in relative value. It then reviews options for reviving the DNCB that were considered in 1991 as part of a major review of aged care programs in Australia, and why little action was taken. The place of the DNCB in repackaging of several caregiver support programs in the late 1990s is then discussed. The paper concludes with an assessment of the lessons learned from this experience with reference to current policy debate about consumer directed care, and of the prospects for renewed interest in cash benefits instead of services on the part of government, older clients and family caregivers in Australia.

Consumer Direction in the Netherlands and France: A Tale of Two Countries

Jane A. Tilly and Joshua Wiener of The Urban Institute, Washington, DC, USA.

This study assesses policy implications for long- term care for older people of consumer-directed home and community services programs. Government officials and key stakeholders, representing the views of consumers, workers, and provider agencies, were interviewed in France and the Netherlands; government documents were analyzed; and published quantitative research was reviewed. Quantitative studies and interview data indicate that a subset of older beneficiaries want to and can manage their services. While quality of care for consumer directed services has been a contentious issue, available evidence suggests that consumer-directed care is at least no worse than agency-directed services and may provide significant benefits related to quality of life. For workers, consumer-directed care has some disadvantages, including fewer fringe benefits. Governmental programs in France and the Netherlands have not provided extensive consumer or worker support and have not aggressively regulated quality of care. Policymakers should consider consumer-directed home and community services as part of long-term care reform for older people.

Consumer-Directed Care: A Global Perspective

Robyn Stone DrPH (Institute for the Future of Aging Services, AAHSA, Washington, DC)

Policies on Consumer direction and payment for care are developing across the globe in an attempt to meet the needs of the aging and disabled population and increase the role of the consumer in their care plans. This paper will provide a framework for the symposium discussion by highlighting the differences and similarities in policies focused on consumer direction and those more specifically described as payment for care options. Attention will be given to identify how the focus of these policies differ by whether they are advocated by the independent living or the seniors movement. By providing definitions of key concepts in this area, identifying global trends in policy develop and highlighting key issues affecting all countries, this paper will be a solid foundation upon which the papers more specific to individual countries and comparison among countries will be centered.

Consumer-Direction Without Cash Payment Option in Japan

Yoko S. Crume (North Carolina Department of Health and Human Services, Raleigh, USA)

The public long-term care insurance program for older adults started in Japan in April, 2000. Prior to launching the program, the Japanese policy makers extensively reviewed a similar program in Germany. Both the Japanese and German programs are unique in the world in that they represent the public insurance approach to long-term care with comprehensive service coverage. However, the Japanese program differs from the German model in several key areas including its decision not to provide cash payment option for family caregivers. In this presentation, the issues of consumer-direction in the new Japanese long-term care insurance program will be explored including a discussion of why Japan decided to forgo the cash payment option. A case study will be utilized to illustrate how a service recipient and her family interact with her care-manager.

Money or services: What are the policy implications of giving Canadian caregivers these options.

JaniceM. Keefe and Pamela Fancey (Mount Saint Vincent University, Halifax, Canada)

This presentation will discuss policy implications of introducing various models for supporting informal caregivers in Canada. Data from the 1996 General Social Survey indicate that an equal proportion of caregivers chose financial compensation compared to community supports to assist them to continue their caregiving role although caregivers who were younger, male and from "have-not" provinces were more likely to choose financial compensation. Models of financial compensation and direct services to support caregiving are briefly described and Canadian examples are presented. We conclude that models of financial compensation and service availability should be viewed as complementary; that both the persons in need of care and their family caregiver should be considered clients and that the philosophy of consumer-directed care should be adopted in order to recognize the centrality of both these individuals in the assessment process. We acknowledge that the consequences of each approach vary significantly depending upon the stakeholders involved. These consequences include justice, ethical and programmatic issues. Particular attention is given to the impact of these consequences for consumers and, where appropriate, family caregivers.

SESSION 309

Aging Well in Rural Areas

Hana M. Hermanova, Director (Center on Aging, West Virginia University, Morgantown, WV, USA)

ISSUE 70% of populations in developing countries live in rural areas as compared to 25% in developed countries; in general, the majority of the world's 60+ populations are rural. The symposium Aging Well in Rural Areas sets a framework for understanding the multiple challenges of aging in rural/remote areas. It is generally accepted that rural aging is characterized by: · The exodus of young generations, thus eroding the existing networks · Inequities in access to existing education, jobs, health and social infrastructures · Socioeconomic and environmental hardships and challenges Efficient information systems and research collecting reliable data, are essential for addressing the changes and challenges in rural aging at the beginning of the 21st century, even in remote and deprived rural areas. Knowledge of migration patterns, changes in intergenerational relations, health and functional limitations, availability and affordability of services, access, rural aging and development of society are key issues to set out a coherent framework for rural aging policies at the local, regional, national and international levels. STRUCTURE The session based on paper presentations will - introduce the policy framework for aging well in rural areas, - address areas critical for creating realistic rural aging policies in the 21st century, among them - the epidemiology of rural aging as source of essential information - Minimal data sets on rural aging as prerequisits for creating realistic Rural Aging Policies at different levels. - Case studies addressing the multidimensional issues of rural aging in a developing country. - A coherent framework for rural aging policies at different levels and the critical need - implementation, i.e. ensuring that policies are put into effect and outcomes are monitored, measured and evaluated, will be presented. CONTENT The symposium will provide an updated information on rural aging and its main challenges in the 21st Century. - The policy recommendations developed by the 2000 Forum on Rural Aging (part of the first International Conference on Rural Aging, Charleston, WV, July 2000) will be presented as basis for developing a Plan of action in Rural Aging in 21st Century. - Epidemiology of rural aging addressing health and function, lifestyles and their anticipated changes, living arrangements, use of services and socioeconomic status of rural elderly as source of policy related important information for rural aging . - Sub-saharan Africa example of Minimal data sets on aging in countries lacking data as basis for planning. - India case study, illustrating the enormous differences and diversity existing in rural aging within one country . - Primary health care delivery in rural areas illustrated by examples of dental care and community based rehabilitation. - Identification of issues important for the Plan of Action in Rural Aging in 21st Century. CONCLUSIONS/ANTICIPATED OUTCOMES Dissemination of knowledge in "Aging Well in Rural Areas" Identification of knowledge gaps Recommendations concerning policy oriented research and rural policy development and implementation Considering a "Plan of Action in Rural Aging in the 21st Century"

Aging in Villages in India

Vinod Kumar, (St.Stephen's Hospital, Delhi, India)

75% of India's eighty million elderly live in villages in diverse cultural traditions. Majority are poor illiterate without access to services. Female elderly are more vulnerable. Traditionally, joint families, social interactions and spiritual practices contribute to active aging. However, youth migration to cities for opportunities is unfavourably influencing family structure and care of elderly. Weather extremes, insanitation, unsafe drinking water and indoor pollution also marginalise rural elderly. Studies (1995-1996) by country's National Sample Survey Organisation (NSSO) show 75-80% of elderly as actively involved with life and only 5% live alone. However, when compared to urban counterparts, rural elderly had higher dependency ratio (9.2%), physical disabilities (40%), work participation (38.6%), economic dependence (70%) and non-receipt of retirement benefits (65%). Urban rates were 7.4%, 35%, 21.4%, 68% and 21% respectively. Comparing with earlier NSSO study (1986-87) with similar methodology, overtime trends indicated that economic condition and property holding of only rural elderly had declined. Policy framework on rural aging need cost effective culturally adjusted strategies to enable communities, families and individuals to ensure quality life in later years. Research to assess healthy aging determinants, intergenerational relationships, support networks and extent/type of older persons' contribution is important. Based on age integrated society inclusive of elderly, rural development programmes slow down out-migration, strengthen family structure, and improve generational relationships. An accessible primary care system with trained staff should provide health promotion. Gender sensitive programmes, NGO participation, health insurance and indigenous medical systems should also be components of policy formulations

An Epidemiological Perspective on Aging Well in Rural Areas

Gary R. Andrews (Centre for Ageing Studies, Flinders University, Australia

PURPOSE: This paper reports global findings related to the epidemiology of aging in rural locations in developed and developing countries. METHOD: The paper reviews findings from current sources and draws policy implications for future action. RESULTS: Rural populations tend to have higher levels of very old persons and a greater proportion of men. Problems experienced compared with urban counterparts include: lower incomes resulting in reduced self-sufficiency and impeded social participation; less infrastructure and services; problems of access to services and health; difficulties with intra-regional and inter-regional transport; gender inequalities, including the changing role of rural and farm women in terms of family care for older generations; loss of family and community networks as younger generations move to the cities, and lack of mental health care. An additional consideration is the issues associated with aging of native indigenous populations in many countries, many of whom tend to live in rural and remote areas. Such groups as a rule have shorter life expectancy, suffer higher levels of morbidity and have even poorer access to health and care services than the rest of the population. CONCLUSION: More data on health of older persons in rural areas is vital for informed policy formulation and creation of programs that can effectively improve health and well being of rural dwelling older people in the developing and developed worlds. Action is needed now for rural development policies to take account of population ageing and the needs of older persons, improved coordination and integration of public health and care services in rural areas, support for NGO and community group efforts, and greater use of new technologies for communication.

Community Based Rehabilitation of Rural Elderly

Rueben Eldar (Fleischman Unit for the Study of Disability, Loewenstein Hospital, Raanana, Israel)

Older adults following a disabling event could be rehabilitated in rural areas on community level by primary care teams, assisted by family; they could be provided with appropriate assistive technology and their immediate environments could be adapted to changed needs, and they could be taught to practice self-rehabilitation. This would enable them to continue living in own homes, at least partially independently, and would allow them to age relatively well in spite of chronic disease and disability.

Creating a Minimum Data Set on Ageing and Older Person in

Africa

P.R. Kowal, J.E. Dowd, R.de Graft Agyarko (Evidence and Information for Policy, World Health Organization, Switzerland), N.A. Apt (Centre for Policy Studies, University of Ghana, Ghana), M. Ferreira (Institute on Ageing in Africa, University of Cape Town, South Africa), C.P.B. Mkai (Bureau of Statistics, United Republic of Tanzania), N. Madzingira (Institute for Development Studies, University of Zimbabwe, Zimbabwe), K. Peachey (Regional Development Office, HelpAge International, Kenya).

As most of the older population in Africa is living in a rural setting, combined with the increasing migration of younger generations to urban settings with many then returning home when old, ill or dying, information about the situation of older persons will be of increasing importance. The importance of this population is not only a public policy issue (i.e. health care planning and costs) but importance social insurance as younger generations are relying more on this older cohort for support. The goal of this project is to develop the evidence-base to inform policy for older persons in sub-Saharan Africa. Four countries, Ghana, South Africa, the United Republic of Tanzania and Zimbabwe, have begun work in three main areas: 1) creating a Directory of Ageing Research and Information on Older Persons in Africa; 2) creating a Minimum Data Set (MDS) with a sustainable data management system; and in countries that request assistance, 3) developing and implementing a comprehensive ageing survey on the health, mental, social and economic well-being of older persons in Africa. Available data sources, and methods and strategies to obtain data for the MDS are being evaluated. The core MDS Indicators and available data elements will be presented as they relate to the ageing policy recommendations from the Organization for African Unity. The possibilities of applying this methodology to other sub-Saharan African countries, Latin America and the Caribbean as well as Asia is being explored.

Enhancing Global Geriatric Oral Health Outcomes

D. Berkey (University of North Carolina at Chapel Hill, NC, USA), R. Berg (University of Colorado, CO, USA), R. Meckstroth (University of West Virginia, WV, USA)

Meeting the substantial dental needs of rural elderly requires recognizing significant barriers and then formulating efficient and effective strategies to address these challenges. Internationalizing this discussion can bring new insights, establish key collaborations, and promote enhanced outcomes. The convening of the First International Conference on Rural Aging (ICRA) in Charleston, WV during June of 2000 provided an opportunity for a global oral health promotion effort. This presentation will summarize 10 country/region specific barriers and recommendations regarding better education, research, policy, and financing of oral health care, analyze the similiarities and differences of issues by country/region (e.g, prevalence and incidence of oral disease, workforce availability, etc), and portray resultant ongoing or planned international collaborations by experts from Japan, China, India, Africa, Australia, Spain, Germany, UK, Uruguay, and USA. The ICRA meeting has provided an impetus for global geriatric oral health promotion efforts.

SESSION 310

Aged Care for a Traditional Aboriginal Population in Remote Central Australia

M. Arch, M. Paddy, (Nganampa Health Council, Alice Springs, Australia)

Nganampa Health Council is an Anangu (Aboriginal) controlled community health organization providing health services to people living on the Anangu Pitjantjatjara (AP) Lands in remote Central Australia. These lands cover some 103,000 square kilometers and the Pitjantjatjara people have freehold title to this area. There are 3,000 people of whom 326 Anangu are aged 50 or older on the AP Lands. Nganampa Health Council has recently been funded to begin an Aged and Disability Care Program which is still in its developmental stage. The program aims to develop and maintain services which are affordable, sustainable, appropriate, and responsive to the needs of older and disabled Anangu and their carers, and which will enable older and disabled Anangu to remain on the AP Lands. We describe the process of developing this program. The key components of the program, its strengths and limitations, and the desired future directions are discussed.

Ethnology on widowhood rituals in the "bembe" land (Congo)

Martin YABA MAMBOU (Congolese Society of Gerontololy-Brazzaville)

Summary translation (into English); the enclosed text The "Bembés", a linguistic entity belonging to the "Kongo" group located in southern Congo have developed with the passing days socio-cultural representation systems linked to mourning usual rituals. The latter as far as widowhood is concerned are dependant on proper beliefs, habits and customs, animism practices. In the "Bembe" mentality aged women are considered guardians of cultural survivals and real-living libraries. This work aim comes within the research framework carried out in anthropology, ethnology, psychology and sociology on ageing with the viewpoint of enhancing cultural patrimony in identity crisis. Our matter is based on the socio-cultural representations developed around mouring rituals for aged widows on the Bembe land. So this study is aiming at an analysis of the cultural foundation of rituals to evaluate their impact on the aged women's real-life experience. To lead this, we proceeded through a methodological approach focused on anthropological talks, field surveys, testimonies, biographical accounts and oral sources method. It appears that the Bembe group has acceptance patterns concerning aged widows that take into account the socio-cultural realities peculiar to it. The rituals revolve round sexual taboos, symbols, cultural prohibitions, social and food habits, magico-religious beliefs. Two essential function characterize mourning rituals: firstly, the social regulation of attitudes, habits and behaviours between social institutions and the dead; secondly the function based on moral, physical, psychological and socio-material ill-treatments, the victims being once more the aged widows. Eventually, the cultural foundation of mourning rituals based on customary laws in the Bembe mind not only works as a social regulation, but also makes the rituals be undermining those widows' corporal integrity.

Health Problems in Aged Australian Indigenous Community

PJ Rudolph (Bega Garnbirringu Health Service, Kalgoorlie, Western Australia)

Persons aged over 65 years make up only 2.6% of the Australian Indigenous population compared with 13% for the population in general, and little is written about this group of people. Minority Indigenous populations in other countries are in a similar situation. The medical problems of Aborigines aged 70 years and older in contact with the Aboriginal Medical Service in central Western Australia (living both in the community and in residential care) were reviewed with the aim of 1) advancing the knowledge of health needs for this unique group of Australians and 2) improving understanding as to why so few Aboriginal people live to old age. Of the 49 people identified, the most common medical diagnoses are hypertension (39%), diabetes (33%) and cataracts or retinopathy (30%). The main reasons for admission to a nursing home were dementia (53%) and stroke (29%). Geographical, cultural and language isolation exists, with 53% of those living outside of residential care continuing to live in small Indigenous communities. There is an apparent reduction in the prevalence of diabetes in the group aged 70 plus from as high as 75% of those aged 50 to 65, and alcohol abuse was not identified in the group studied but is as high as 38% in those aged 30 to 60. Treatment of cardiovascular disease and diabetes needs to be emphasised as does accessibility to ophthalmological services. Providing culturally appropriate care in the appropriate geographical location for older people who are disabled with many conditions, particularly dementia or stroke, remains a challenge. The contribution of diabetes and alcohol abuse toward premature death cannot be underestimated.

Service Needs and Preferences of Urban Aboriginal Seniors: A Key Informant Case Study

Sid Frankel (Faculty of Social Work, University of Manitoba, Winnipeg, Canada)Sharon Taylor-Henley (Faculty of Social Work, University of Manitoba, Winnipeg, Canada)Anne Charter (Faculty of Social Work, University of Manitoba, Winnipeg, Canada) John O'Neil (Department of Community Health Sciences, Faculty of Medicine, University of Manitoba, Winnipeg, Canada)

The overall purpose of this study is to provide decision support for comprehensive program development for Aboriginal seniors in an urban context. Method: Findings are based on data from key informant interviews with Aboriginal senior service providers, supplemented by analysis of available socio-demographic data and review of the professional, academic and "gray literature." Results: Findings include the following: Culturally appropriate and accessible services for Aboriginal seniors are extremely limited in the case study area, despite the fact that it constitutes the urban area with the highest proportion of Aboriginal population in Canada. Respecting the elderly is a primary value of Aboriginal peoples. It is important to maintain older persons as an active part of the family. Caring for the elderly is a communal, rather than exclusively filial or familial, responsibility. A holistic healing model should be incorporated into any program seeking to address the needs of Aboriginal seniors in order to adhere to Aboriginal cultural imperatives. The presence of Aboriginal health care providers in a program or facility and Aboriginal governance of the entity are defined as essential ingredients of cultural appropriateness. Transportation, subsidized cultural food, interpretation and translation services for several language groups are required to enhance accessibility due to the presence of both resource limitations and linguistic barriers. Aboriginal-specific information, outreach and advocacy are required to assist Aboriginal seniors in accessing services because of their limited bureaucratic skill and isolation from mainstream service systems. Conclusion: Specialized Aboriginal-governed services are required throughout the continuum of care.

Traditional or Western Health Care Decisions in American Indian Elders

Margaret P. Moss, DSN (University of Minnesota, Minneapolis, Minnesota, USA)

Purpose: The full study was engaged to understand the beliefs and behaviors of aging in the Zuni Indians of New Mexico from their own perspectives. Methods: Classical ethnographic methods were used including participant observation, interviews, photography, and videography. The time in the field included over 1800 hrs from entree and data gathering, through verification and exiting, and lasted from August of 1998 through April of 2000. Results: The findings to be discussed in this presentation revolve around the hierarchy of decision-making by elders regarding accessing either traditional or western medicine for health problems. After the PI made several site-visits it was clear that there is a general course followed by the elders. There are specific times one seeks care by the Indian Health Service (western)and specific reasons one would seek out a medicine man, bone presser, or stomach massager. The elder is particularly likely to seek out traditional modes of care whether used in conjunction with western medicine or alone. There is also, in many cases, a specific order for seeking these provider and to stray from the order is to confound the outcome. Conclusion: Health care providers and provider systems need to be aware that it may be necessary,in the eyes of the American Indian elder, to take in the information they are given and then based on that information and their own beliefs and practices choose who, how, and in what order to carry out their care.

SESSION 312

IBYCUS: A Poem by John Heath-Stubbs,

Terry Coles, (Maple Lake Releasing, Winnipeg, Manitoba, Canada)

A stunning look into the human condition through a vision of the interior world of the British poet John-Heath Stubbs. Performance meets documentary in this study of poetry, life and film. John Heath-Stubbs is one of the most celebrated poets of his generation. His vivid poems have been bring to mind landscapes of the past. These have been created while Heath-Stubbs as lost his sight to a progressive disorder.

The Age Old Question:Defining Old Age

Sandra Kerr, Program Director, Continuing Education, and Elaine Vayda,Emeritus in Social Work and with Act II Studio (Ryerson Polytechnic University, Toronto, Ontario, Canada)

Act II Studio, a theatre school for older adults in Continuing Education at Ryerson Polytechnic University partnered with the ONtario Coalition of Senior Citizens' ORganisation to create a presentation dealing with the realities of ageism and ageing at the beginning of the 21st Century. We started with the premise that in the 20th century, better nutrition, improved public health measures, emphasis on preventive medicine, modern dentistry, and social insurance and income supports have made aging a gradual process that can last 30 years or more beyond age 65. However, stereotypes based on a more rapid decline into obsolescence still persists and inform attitudes and social policy regarding seniors. To test this premise, eigth focus groups of seniors were held throughout the province, seeking to get a cross section of authentic experiences, ideas and attitudes toward growing old. The script was developed through improvisations using transcripts of these groups. The play, If not know, when? has been performed six times throughout ONtario and more performances are planned in 2001. The play is appropriate for trained professionals, caregivers of seniors and the elderly and intergenerational audiences from adolescents to seniors. It raises awareness that older persons are not a category, but are individuals coping with aging with varying levels of success. They bring unique reactions to the inevitable losses and to the physical, emotional, social and financial consequences of aging.

SESSION 313

"Care-cultural" Orientation and Social Milieu

Baldo Blinkert (University of Freiburg, Germany), Thomas Klie (Protestant University of Applied Sciences, Freiburg, Germany)

The study was guided with two intentions: we liked to get information about the mentalities of the potential care-givers in the future and we intended to develope an instrument for regional and local social planning for the elderly in case of care-needing. In 1998, 400 citizens aged between 40 and 60 years living in a south German city have been interviewed in an oral standard interview. The important results: the "care-cultural" orientation compared to todays care-givers will be in a big change: only 13 % will be willing to give care to close relatives, 38 % prefer nursing homes in each casethe moral orientation is a decreasing factor for the decision to be willing to become a care-giver for close relatives: much more important are "cost to benefits"-weighing upsthere is a significant relationship between the social milieu and the "care-cultural" orientation: in the lower class, many more people are willing to become a care-giver for parents and partners, in the higher classes the number of citizens, who are willing to give care to their parents and partners is much lower. For the future, we expect in Germany a decreasing of the number of members of the lower classes. The results of the study show, that in the near future we will have a big change in the care-cultural orientation; the number of care-needing people given to a nursing home will rapidly increase, if new concepts and forms of share-responsibility in case of care-needing in the community will not be developed.

From Good Intentions to Good Practice. Do Goals and Principles of Medical Care Help?

Duncan Robertson B Lynn Beattie Division of Geriatric Medicine, University of British Columbia, Vancouver, BC. Canada and Geriatrics and Palliative Care Committee of the British Columbia Medical Association, BC , Canada

The British Columbia Medical Association - the professional association for physicians in the Canadian Province of British Columbia - has, for many years, had a Council on Health Promotion that makes recommendations to improve the heath and well-being of British Colombians. PURPOSE: In anticipation of 1999, the International Year of the Older Person, the Geriatrics and Palliative Care Committee, one of the subcommittees of the Council, initiated a collaborative process to develop provincial goals and principles for medical care of older persons. METHOD: This paper describes the process of development and the subsequent use of the principles by the Canadian Medical Association as a basis for developing a national Policy Statement. The BCMA Committee began a process for developing principles for medical care of the elderly that reflected best practice based on health care research and, where that was not available, on expert opinion. The committee consulted widely with individual physicians and physician groups, with the Provincial Chief Medical Officer and with the Seniors’ Advisory Council of BC. The document, when approved by the BCMA , was subsequently reviewed by the Canadian Medical Association and a consultation process with relevant national associations was initiated. This resulted in certain changes reflective of a broader consensus. RESULTS: The Goals and Principles approved by the Board of the BCMA in 1999 may be viewed at http://bcma.bc.ca/AboutBCMA/Commitees/StandingCommittees/CoHPCommitees/Goals&Principles.htm The Principles approved by the Board of the CMA in 2000 may be viewed at. http://cma.ca/inside/policybase/2000/03 005.htm CONCLUSION/OUTCOMES: The authors seek wide distribution of these Goals and Principles, and informed discussion and debate on their application. Does a clear statement of goals and principles that we believe should underpin policies, programs and practices related to care of older persons translate into improved care and better outcomes for seniors, particularly frail older persons?

Preparing for an Aging Population in an Israeli HMO

Yosef Bregman, John Lemberger (Maccabi Healthcare Services, Tel Aviv, ISRAEL)

Purpose: To describe service provision in an aging HMO population Method: Maccabi Healthcare Services is Israel's second largest HMO(in Israeli parlance sick fund) with 60f its members aged 65+. In preparation for the doubling of this population in the next eight years, Maccabi's directors prpeared a master plan for providing health services for its elderly members. Although considered a young HMO, the changing demographics of the members, including a large percentage of elderly new immigrants, especially from the former Soviet Union, presage a need to prpeare for the immediate future. Results: The following elements are in different stages of implementation: 1. Additional geriatric services by recruiting geriatricians, 2. Raising the awareness, understanding and knowledge of staff at all levels of the organization, but most significantly among family physicians, 3. Health promotion and prevention programs targeted to the elderly, as well as efforts intended to insure that middle-aged members age more successfully than today's aging population, 4. Establishing multi-disciplinary comprehensive geriatric assessment units at the regional level, and 5. Reviewing and reconstituting the home care system to reflect the needs of an aging, frail population. Conclusion: Management commitment and leadership can bring about a radical change in health care delivery for aging members of an HMO, and change the way the organization views its elderly members.

Promoting Health in Aged Care

Sharon Smart (University of Ballarat Ballart, Victoria AUSTRALIA)

The world's population is ageing and it is prudent to investigate means to reduce the demands on health and welfare services. One example is in the provision of preventive services and programs that meet the needs of the elderly community which will be more economically viable than current treatment methods. During the 1990s rapid policy change occurred in Australia, particularly within residential aged care. Doctoral research to investigate the Ottawa Charter and its application was conducted in a retirement village in Victoria, Australia, that offered a continuum of residential aged care. Using constant comparative analysis, interviews were conducted with retirement village residents and staff and the results indicate that residents had positive attitudes regarding their own current lifestyle. They also reported that there was minimal community involvement and expressed concern for the welfare of staff faced with administrative change. Staff stated that they experienced a feeling of being overwhelmed by changes in legislature and the associated accreditation process. This had increased their administrative work leading to stress, and reduced care time with residents. In an effort to create an environment which promotes health and well-being of residents, their relatives and staff rather than one that merely maintains essential services and care, it is argued that the concepts of the Ottawa Charter can be used as a model for future directions in the care of our elderly. The adoption of a health promoting environment which fosters a focus on health improvement, rather than illness management alone, will improve the health care delivery to the aged.

Putting the Person at the Centre

Brendan Mc Cormack, (University of Ulster/Royal Group of Hospitals, Belfast, Northern Ireland) Pauline Ford, (Royal College of Nursing, London, England.)

Person-centred care is a phrase commonly used in contemporary health care practice (Fulford et al, 1996). The philosophy extends humanistic theory and aims to create services and practices that are responsive to the individual needs of people. It is argued (McCormack, 1998) that at the core of person centredness is the concept of authenticity. This concept reflects an individual's life values and the manifestation of these values in care decisions. Maintaining an individual's authenticity is a complex activity and this paper will explore the factors that challenge such a philosophy in practice - organisational factors, individual attitudes and care approaches. The paper will explore common principles of person centredness that underpin a number of research and development activities in contemporary gerontological nursing. Research perspectives drawn upon will include - an understanding of the concept of autonomy from a person centred perspective; person-centred assessment approaches; 'conversations with people with dementia' and development work that actively involves older people with dementia. Examples of these areas of work by staff of the Royal College of Nursing's Gerontological Nursing Programme and the University of Ulster will be drawn upon to illustrate the challenges to being person-centred and factors that can lead to success. It will be argued that paying attention to the values of both the older person and the care workers is crucial to success. Approaches to doing this in practice will be presented.

SESSION 315

An Approach to the Suffering of the End Stage Dementia Patient Para 2 B.Z. Aminoff (Geriatric Department and Memory Clinic, Sheba Medical Center, Israel)

B.Z. Aminoff

Dementia patients suffer profoundly until death. It is impossible to alter the cognitive and functional status of a dementia patient by means of medication, rehabilitation or by any other means. Medical ethics or religious practices do not permit either passive or active euthanasia. Thus the only way in which to treat a dementia patient is by careful and accurate diagnosis to diminish and prevent suffering. The suffering of an end stage dementia patient is not only a function of the basic progress of the disease, but is mainly a function of the quality of medical and nursing care. No patient, at any stage of the disease deserves to suffer. On the contrary, at every stage of the disease suffering can be treated and prevented. Physicians, nurses, relatives and society all accept the suffering in the end stage dementia patient as a natural process of the disease, and are usually not aware of the fact that a great deal of suffering is caused by incorrect medical and nursing care, that may be inadequate, unsuccessful or negligent. No objective methods for the evaluation of the suffering of end stage dementia are known to exist. The Mini Suffering State Examination (B.Z. Aminoff, 1999 Berlin, 4th European Congress of Gerontology) for the first time presented a method for the diagnosis and evaluation of the level of suffering of an end stage dementia patient which could enable suitable treatment .

Biographical Pain at the End of Life

M.L. Johnson (International Institute on Health and Aging, University of Bristol, United Kingdom)

Purpose: To provide a constructive critique of the concepts of pain which have become prominent in the literature, particularly the ideas projected within the hospice, palliative care and bereavement fields. To argue that two principal contentions (1) That all pain can be alleviated, and (2) That non-physical pain is best described and understood as spiritual pain, are unsubstantiated claims which do not accord either with the evidence of the lived experience of large sectors of the populations of developed societies. Method: The analysis will subject the literature in these areas to careful scrutiny, in order to expose the sets of assumptions and ideologies which have produced a way of categorising extreme pain and its management. The focus will be on the profound anguish which frequently manifests itself as finitude is reached. Of those who by reason of great age or life threatening illness, face iminent death there is a subset of individuals fro whom life review produces unbearable, often deep, burried recollections of situations which are now beyond reclification. In a world where both spiritual literacy and the facilities of confession and forgiveness, the options are severly restricted. The pain experienced is not spiritual, nor is it amenable to drug or counselling therapies. It is argued that in order to address this pain which arises out of biographical experience, we need to reconceptualize and to conduct more empirical enquiry. Conclusion: There is a need to create a new way of understanding profound and irresolvable pain. The concept 'biographical pain' is offered as a framework for clearer thinking which recognises the changing cosmologies of secular societies.

Dying in Hospital: Issues for Older Peopel

Margaret Brown (Hawke Institute, University of South Australia, Adelaide, Australia)

Purpose: This paper will present the findings of research that examined the care of 20 dying patients in two acute hospitals in South Australia. The findings of this research raises question about the care of elderly people dying in the acute hospital setting. The research was funded by the National Health and Medical Research Council of Australia

Method: Both quantitative and qualitative methods were used. The study was conducted in two stages, the first involved collecting data from the death registers from the two hospitals. The second stage involved non-participant observation of the care provided to patients who were dying and interviews with selected staff involved in the care of these patients. Criteria for selecting patients included; over the age of 18, a terminal prognosis and an estimated six days to live. Intensive Care and Palliative Care wards were excluded.

Results: Retrospective data from the hospital death registers guided the selection of wards for the non-participant observations. The mean age of the patients was 76 years. The data indicated that the majority of care was associated with routine and technological care. There was little care that emphasized the patient as a person. Some of the care observed could be described as best practice, however the data also revealed that some care could be considered to be unacceptable according to the current standards of palliative care. The presence or absence of family members had the greatest positive impact on the care these patients received.

Conclusion: This research revealed that there does not appear to be a 'culture of care' for dying patients in the acute hospitals. Recommendations have been made for strategies and procedural policies to be reviewed so that a palliative care approach can coexist with acute care in hospitals.

End-of-Life Care in Canada: National and Administrative Data to Identify and Demystify Trends

D.M. Wilson (University of Alberta, Edmonton, Canada); and C. Truman (Sherwood Park, AB)

The purpose of two conjoint investigations was to: (a) identify Canadian trends in location of death for 1950 through 1997, and (b) explore hospital utilization by terminally ill and dying persons. Both investigations involved quantitative analysis of population databases. The first investigation identified a continuing hospitalization-of-death trend, with hospital deaths peaking in 1994 at 77.3%. Following 1994, an ongoing decline in hospital deaths occurred (72 0n 1997). The second investigation involved Alberta hospital inpatient utilization data, seeking to explore hospital utilization both during the hospital stay which ended in death (N=38,468 in the years 1992/93 through 1996/97) and over a five year period for all individuals (N=7,429) who died in hospital during the 1996/97 year. The last hospital stay was infrequently resource intensive; 51.80f all inpatients had no diagnostic or treatment procedures performed. Procedures averaged 1.7 (0 to 10 range) and the cost weight averaged 14.6 (0.5 to 316 range), with both distributions positively skewed. Hospital utilization over a five year period similarly varied. Admissions ranged from 1 to 50 (4.5 mean, positively skewed distribution). Similarly, total days in hospital ranged from 1 to 4,963 days (54.9 mean, positively skewed distribution). Procedures averaged 6.2 (0 to 92 range, positively skewed distribution). The cost weight of care averaged 42.1 (0.8 to 462.6 range, positively skewed distribution. In conclusion: Hospitals across Canada are extensively used for end-of-life care purposes, but it also appears that a shift away from hospital death and dying is occurring. Furthermore, half of all persons who died in hospital received nursing care alone. This information belies the myth of extensive utilization of hospital resources by terminally ill and dying persons.

End-of-Life Care in Rural Canada

Michael MacLean (Faculty of Social Work, University of Regina, Regina, Saskatchewan, Canada

While there are many initiatives in palliative care taking place in rural areas of Canada, there has not been much published research on this topic. The purpose of this presentation is to give information on the components of a rural palliative care model based on the experiences of formal caregivers in rural areas who are working in this area of social services and health care. Focus groups were held with social and health care providers in six regions of Canada to get the views of these practitioners on how to provide excellent end-of-life care to people who are dying and to their family members. Based on these focus groups, a model of palliative care in rural Canada is presented that includes components of definitions, integrity of the rural communities, accessibility of services, teamwork, palliative care consultants, flexibility in the provision of services, education for the health care and social service provider, social support for the family and the formal caregivers and cultural awareness. This model of end-of-life care will be discussed.

Ethnicity, Aging and Care: End of Life Issues for Ethnic Seniors and Their Families

Noreen M. Lerch, MSN (Student, University of Victoria, School of Nursing, Victoria, British Columbia, Canada).

Ethnicity is an important variable in gerontology services and influences the way that elders are perceived and treated within their community, the rates and distribution of illness, the ways people identify health problems, the informal networks used for assistance and the usage patterns for biomedical health care. There is a dearth of relevant research about end of life issues for ethnic seniors but we know that language and culture are formidable barriers facing older immigrants who have migrated later in life. They are faced with aging in a foreign culture surrounded by a language and people they do not understand. In this paper the issues facing ethnic seniors and their families are examined through a review of the literature, demographics and issues and implications for health care policy. Canadian perspectives are reflected and examples from the Indo-Canadian group of migrants are used to illustrate some issues and how they are experienced. It was concluded that ethnicity and race do make a difference to the experience of aging, whether this is in connection with preferred lifestyles and expectations of old age, roles in the family and residence patterns, gender and independence, culture-specific needs for care or to problems of racism and stereotyping. In the coming years, when the aging baby boom cohort reaches 65 and older, the population will be more racially and ethnically diverse. Health care policy will need to address these differences.

Ontario's Advance Directives on Care Choices Initiative: Supporting Seniors' Expression of their Wishes for Future Care

Wendy Hulko (Ontario Seniors' Secretariat, Toronto, Canada)

CONTEXT: One of 10 initiatives under Ontario's Strategy for Alzheimer Disease and Related Dementias announced September 10, 1999. PURPOSE: To enhance and protect seniors' rights, to enable seniors to make informed choices and to not leave seniors vulnerable to the wishes of others. METHOD: Education and training strategies to increase awareness of the process of advance care planning among seniors in Ontario and to ensure that providers have the information and skills to support seniors with this process. Dissemination of educational materials to ensure the appropriate training of providers, such as allied health professionals and physicians. RESULTS: In this presentation, the speaker will provide an overview of the development of the advance directives action plan, which supports elements of this initiative, the implementation process and the status of this initiative. CONCLUSION: This initiative incorporates ideas and suggestions arising from stakeholders, in particular many dedicated and interested consumer and provider groups. The advance directives on care choices initiative is a critical step towards enhancing and protecting seniors’ rights in Ontario.

SESSION 317

A Community Based Interdisciplinary Dementia Assessment and Management Program- Experience from the Victoria Geriatric CARE Program

Ted Rosenberg, June Swanson , Jan Broome BOT, Bonnie Davoren , Jocelyn Carter, BPT, Blanche Black and David Brook MDDept of Geriatric Services, Capital Health Region, Victoria Canada

Purpose- Dementia is associated with dependency, a higher risk of depression for patients and caregivers, and premature nursing home placement. As the population ages, the personal, social and public health burden from dementia will increase substantially. Care and services are often fragmented amongst specialists, primary care physicians, case managers and community agencies leading to poor acceptance by patients and families. The purpose of this program was to develop a program which integrates specialized individual geriatric assessment with group education and long term individual follow-up. Methods All consecutive patients and caregivers referred for geriatric assessment were enrolled in our program. Demographics and Caregiver satisfaction were measured. Outcomes including the Care Giver Stress, Quality of Life and Depression are measured Results The average age and MMSE of patients was 80.6 and 20.4. Alzheimer's Disease was the most common diagnosis (62%). Most patients lived with their caregiver (78%) and were unknown to the home care program (71%). 410f caregivers were spouses and their average Zarit score was 34.2. There was a very high level of satisfaction in the program. Data from SF-36, depression scales and caregiver reaction scales will be presented. Conclusions A Dementia CARE Program which integrates assessment, education support and long term follow up appears to be highly regarded by caregivers and may improve long term outcomes.

Case report : 30 year old patient suffering from severe prefrontal dementia

Jean-Claude LENERS / Long Term Care (Centre Hospitalier Neuro-Psychiatrique Ettelbruck-Luxembourg)

In our neuro-psychiatric long term unit, we have a young man in our care who is 30 years old. It has been more than a year since he was first admitted to our nursing home. The whole history started about four years ago and for more than three years the assessment was always quite difficult, suggestive of a more degenerative dementia or a more psychotic disease. His stereo-tactical biopsy done more than half a year ago suspected a motoneurone disease inclusion dementia. Also genetic testing was done to look for mutations in his chromosomes, all results were negative. We would like to discuss the possibility of taking care of such a young man in a ward of mainly other younger people but suffering from quite different diagnoses (mentally ill people). A complete report will be made on the assessment tools and diagnostic investigations done over the past 3-4 years and we will insist on his behaviour symptoms and how to manage these in a typical neuro-psychiatric long term care.

Cognitive Heterogeneity in Colombian patients with Alzheimer's Disease: Suggesting other analysis in oral tradition cultures

D.Matallana, C.Cano, P.Montanes, M.I. Garcia, S. Plata, R. Garcia, O. Pedraza, M. Montalvo, L. Morelo, M. Jimenez (Aging Institute, Memory Clinic, Javeriana University, San Ignacio Hospital, Bogota, Colombia)

Even though progressive cognitive deficits are the hallmark of Alzheimer's disease(AD), over the last ten years, a frequent neuropsychological, among others, deviation from the classical progression has been reported. Cognitive outcome, in 90 AD patients (mean age= 74.83; 58F; 32M) and 150 Normal subjects (mean age= 67.78; 85F; 65M) was the aim of the present research. Discriminative analysis (descriptivly) was performed to establish (1) a frontier between groups in terms of its homogeneity (AD versus Control group, where results showed a 1000rediction in terms of sensitivity and specificity of the diagnostic procedure) and (2) heterogeneity in cognitive functioning (by clustering subjects distances regarding its functioning on his/her cognitive domains). Throughout a factorial analysis, clusters of patients and normal controls were achieved, on each cognitive domain, where, for all subjects, a tendency of dispersion on praxic and executive domains were observed. Though, AD patients had a greater dispersion, functional heterogeneity was present in both groups. Nonetheless, (accounting that longitudinal report has to be done in terms of the progression of such profiles) whereas different clustering of AD patients expresses itself heterogeneously, analyzing outstanding cases of the normal control group (with no cognitive impairment) doubts regarding instruments used to assess the cognitive domains, referred previously, lead us to a different type of assessment on oral tradition cultures. In conclusion, an alternative procedure of testing attention and executive functions is suggested, where such evaluation is based on language content.

Complex Medical Comorbidity and Neuropsychological Decline in Geriatric Rehabilitation Patients

Louise Patrick, C. Psych, Peter Gaskovski, & Daniel Rexroth, Psy. D. (SCO Health Service, Ottawa, Ontario)

PURPOSE: The etiology of cognitive dysfunction in geriatric rehabilitation patients is not well understood. The extent to which medical comorbidity, within a context of advanced age and depressive symptomatology, is associated with patterns of intellectual deficits has received little empirical attention. The purpose of this study was thus to investigate the relationships among age, complex medical comorbidity, depressive symptomatology and performance on neuropsychological measures in frail geriatric patients undergoing physical rehabilitation treatment. METHOD: Data was gathered from patients consecutively admitted to the Geriatric Rehabilitation unit of the SCO Health Service in Ottawa, and referred for neuropsychological evaluation, over a one year period. Prevalence and severity of illness across 13 organ group dimensions (based on the Cumulative Illness Rating Scale) were studied in relation to patterns of cognitive decline across various aspects of intellectual functioning. RESULTS: Findings revealed that medical comorbidity significantly predicted cognitive decline in frail elderly patients beyond effects attributable to age, depressive symptomatology, and neurological and psychiatric impairment. Even mild illness, when cumulative across several organ group dimension, was associated with cognitive deficits. The presentation further outlines illness in which organ group was associated with diffuse cognitive impairment and which cognitive function is most frequently declined in relation to physical illness. CONCLUSION: The clinical implications of findings, in terms of diagnoses and prognoses of cognitive dysfunction in the frail elderly, are discussed.

Do residents in long-term institutional care with severe cognitive impairment lack a diagnosis of dementia?

Noro Anja (Stakes, Helsinki, Finland), Finne-Soveri Harriet (Stakes/Kustaankartano, Helsinki, Finland), Björkgren Magnus (Chydenius-Institute, Kokkola, Finland)

PURPOSE: To assess relation between severe cognitive impairment and explaining diagnoses in the long-term institutional care (LTIC). METHOD: The subjects were drawn from database including 2400 RAI (Resident Assessment Instrument) assessments of elderly residents in (LTIC) long-term institutional care. The data was collected during April to September in 2000. Logistic regression was used as the analysis method. Cognitive skills were graded by using Cognitive Performance Scale (CPS) included in the RAI-system. The scale ranges from 0-6, where 4 to 6 represents severe cognitive impairment. The dependent variable was classified as 0 if CPS was 0-3 and 1 if CPS was 4-6. As predictors were used gender, age, length of stay (LOS), previous history of mental diseases, diagnosis of any form of dementia, stroke, aphasia, hemiplegia, depression and hallucinations, in addition to type of institution. RESULTS: Of the residents 43.5% were assessed to have severe cognitive impairment, 74% were women and average age was 82 years, average LOS 2,4 years, and 15% had earlier diagnoses mental disorder. In logistic model subjects with longer LOS had severe cognitive impairment. From the diagnoses Alzheimer disease (OR=10.8), aphasia (OR=2.8), other dementia (OR=5.3) and hallucinations (OR=1.79) were connected to severe cognitive loss. Depression (OR=0.64) and delusions (OR=0.52) together with pain had a significant negative association with severe cognitive loss. CONCLUSION: Assessment of cognition was in accordance with given diagnoses of dementia, and diagnoses of mental disorders do not interfere. In addition, assessing depression in severely demented individuals is unstructured and unreliable.

The Neuropsychological Profile of Mild Cognitive Impairment

L Traykov (Unite INSERM 324, Paris, France), A.S. Rigaud (Hopital Broca, Paris, France), F Latour (Hopital Broca, Paris, France), N. Raoux (Unite INSERM 324, Paris, France), F. Boller (Unite INSERM 324, Paris, France), F. Forette (Hopital Broca, Paris, France)

The recent developments in drug treatments for Alzheimer's disease (AD) have highlighted the importance of early diagnosis and the need to characterise the cognitive profile of the earliest stages of the disease. Recent study suggested that onset of AD is commonly preceded by an interim phase known as mild cognitive impairment (MCI) (Petersen 1999). Persons who experience this condition are at increased risk for the development of AD. The objective was to examine the pattern of neuropsychological impairment in patients with MCI. We investigated 15 MCI subjects (MMSE=29.1±0.9) and 15 normal controls (NC) (MMSE=29.5±0.5). All subjects were assessed with detailed neuropsychological battery designed to measure memory, language, visuospatial functions, praxis and attention/executive functions. MCI patients had a significantly worse scores on Story Recall ($p< 0.001$) and on all measures of the Free and Cued Selective Reminding Test ($p < 0.05$ to 0.01) than NC. Furthermore MCI had greater number of perseverations ($p < 0.02$) on Modified Card Sorting Test and lowest performance on Stroop ($p < 0.02$) and graphic sequences ($p < 0.03$) tests. Despite the similar degree of overall cognitive deterioration, the findings show more impaired episodic memory in MCI than in NC. Moreover, the data suggest that MCI subjects had particular problems with response inhibition and speed of attentional switching. As preventive strategies are developed and new cognitive enhancing therapies emerge, these results may help us to define which domains are expected to improve in MCI populations.

The use of an inhouse psychological assessment tool in a psychiatric ward for older adults suffering form dementia

Z. Guernina (Thames Valley University)

The purpose of this study is to use an easy, friendly tool to facilitate further in depth assessment by assisting in the choice of the most appropriate psychometric test after outlining the patient's cognitive functioning. The psychological package (PAP) has been piloted and ward staff have been involved in the process of evaluation through different stages. The results show that after audit, the psychological tool proved useful and invaluable in a multidisciplinary team.

SESSION 318

Anemia in the Elderly: Clinical Impact and Practical Diagnosis

L. Balducci, W Ershler, D. Lipschitz, B. Robinson, G. Rothstein, H. Cohen (Discussant)

This symposium is supported by an educational grant from Amgen Inc. and aims to be a highly educational meeting, with CME accreditation. This satellite symposium aims to illustrate the clinical impact of anemia in the elderly and to presents a cost effective, convenient and exhaustive work-up of anemia in the elderly. The presentations will review old and new management opportunities for anemia in the elderly and lay the biological basis to understand anemia in the elderly. 1. Introduction and overview of the symposium. L Balducci, M.D, H Cohen, M.D. 2. Epidemiology of anemia in the aged (with information on diagnostic work- up). L Balducci, M.D. The objective of this presentation is to provide the attendee with current knowledge of the prevalence and incidence of anemia, its demography, risk factors, pathophysiology and etiology. This information will constitute the scientific basis for designing an effective diagnostic work-up for anemia in the elderly, which will be presented to the audience. 3. Biological interactions of aging and anemia a focus on cytokines. W. Ershler, M.D. Inflammatory cytokines and their elevation in aging have been implicated in various age-related aspects, and correlations have been found between inflammatory cytokines and anemia. This presentation will focus on available information on cytokines and their production in aging, and identify possible biochemical effects of these cytokines on mechanisms leading to anemia in the elderly. 4. Medical and functional consequences of anemia in the elderly. D. Lipschitz, M.D. This presentation will focus on clinical consequences of anemia in the elderly, and potential clinical complications of non-treatment of this condition. The topics presented will include: anemia as independent risk factor of death, impact of anemia on cardiovascular and cerebrovascular conditions, and impact of anemia on functional dependence and on pharmacological complications. 5. Cost of anemia in the elderly. (Speaker to be confirmed). The objective of this presentation is to estimate the costs of anemia in the elderly. These costs include direct and indirect costs, as well as mounting intangible costs. Cost minimization is essential for the management of anemia. The speaker will provide : · An estimate of the total cost of anemia · An estimate of the pure medical cost of anemia · An exam of different strategies of cost minimization for the management of anemia in the older person. 6. Qualitative disorders of hemopoiesis in the aged a focus on myelodysplasia. G Rothstein, M.D. With aging, quantitative as well as qualitative changes occur in hemopoiesis. The qualitative changes include proliferative senescence, resistance to apoptosis, increased concentration of cytokines in the hemopoietic stroma. These changes may lead to myelodysplasia and eventually to AML. A new series of interventions, from use of hemopoietic growth factors to use of anti-cytokine antibodies may reverse these changes and reverse, or ameliorate, the risk of myelodysplasia and aplastic anemia in the elderly. The goals include: 1. A practical approach to the diagnosis and the management of anemia in the older person 2. Timely recognition and prevention of the complications of anemia in the elderly (delirium, congestive heart failure, functional dependence) 3. Appreciation of the cost of anemia in the aged At the end of the conference the attendee should be able to: 1. Initiate an exhaustive work up of anemia in the elderly 2. Institute proper and timely treatment of anemia 3. Prevent the complications of anemia in the older person 4. Defend the investment in the management of anemia in a forum of public health, health care delivery study, hospital, clinic and pharmacy administration.

SESSION 322

[1] Early and late menopause: delayed hormonal and metabolic effects.

L.Berstein, V.Gamajunova, E.Tsyrlina, I.Kovalenko, Ju.Kvatchevskaja (Petrov Research Institute of Oncology, St.Petersburg, Russia)

Timing of menopause is very important for the course of aging (successful or unfavourable) and depends on complex of genetic, anthropometric, behavioral and endocrine factors. Early menopause is associated with a higher risk of cardiovascular disease and osteoporosis and delayed menopause may increase the risk of breast and especially endometrial cancer. As one can understand, the optimal time of the onset of menopause lays between these two extremities. To know better the hormonal and metabolic consequences of early and late menopause we studied a total 118 postmenopausal females at mean age of 61.9 and the age of onset of 49.9 yrs. Anthropometry, fat topography, glucose tolerance, basal and reactive insulinemia, lipid fractions, FSH, LH, estradiol, testosterone and SHBG levels were evaluated. Notwithstanding of similar mean age and body mass (Quetelet) index females with menopause onset >52 yrs (LMP, average age at menopause 53.7 yrs, n=47) were characterized by higher blood cholesterol and insulin (120 min) concentrations than females with menopause onset < 52 yrs (n=71) or < 48 yrs (n=38). In LMP group some studied hormonal and metabolic parameters (f.e. fasting glucose or waist/thigh ratio) correlated primarily with age at menopause while in females reporting about earlier menopause with its duration. Strength of correlation in the pair blood FSH/blood LH was weaker in LMP group. Therefore, postmenopausal females of the same age and weight who differ by the timing of menopause belong to the groups with different hormonal status which might be important for their health and deserves further studies.

[2] Effect of Dietary Restriction from Old on the Carbonylated Albumin Contents in Plasma and Urine

R. Takahashi, K. Nishizawa, S. Goto (Department of Biochemistry, School of Pharmaceutical Sciences, Toho University, Chiba, Japan)

We previously found that the content of oxidatively modified proteins, measured as protein carbonyls, increased in the kidney but not in other tissues (brain, liver, lung and heart) of old rat (F344). In the kidney, serum albumin was one of highly carbonylated proteins. In order to better understand the mechanism of accumulation of carbonylated albumin in the kidney of rats with age, we further examined whether the contents of carbonylated albumin in plasma and urine are altered with age and dietary restriction for 3.5 months initiated from early senescence (26.5 month-old). Regardless of age, the protein carbonyl contents of albumin was higher in urine than in plasma. There was no significant difference in the content of carbonylated albumin in urine between young and old rats but the amount of urinary proteins, mostly albumin, increased with age, and dietary restriction reduced the amount of urinary proteins. Although no significant difference was observed in the protein carbonyl contents of albumin in plasma between young and old rats, the amount of carbonylated albumin remarkably decreased by dietary restriction.

[3] The effect of peptides on generation of reactive oxygen species in mitochondria.

S. V. Mylnikov (Department of genetics, St.-Petersburg State University, St.-Petersburg, Russia), T. I. Oparina (D. O. Ott Institute of obstetrics and gynecology, St.-Petersburg, Russia), V. Kh. Khavinson (St.-Petersburg Institute of bioregulation and gerontology North-Western branch of Russian academy of medical sciences, St.-Petersburg, Russia

In our previous works we investigated antioxidant and geroprotective effects of synthetic peptides synthesized in the St.-Petersburg institute of bioregulation and gerontology. It was established, that the introduction of epithalon (Ala-Glu-Asp-Gly), and vilon (Lys-Glu) in a nutritious medium increased activity of antioxidant enzymes in Drosophila melanogaster. One of the reasons of such effect can be magnification of generation of reactive oxygen species (RAS) in mitochondria. In this case activation of enzymes is compensatory induced reaction. The goal of the present work was comparative study of effects of vilon and eptithalon on the contents of RAS in mitochondria and soluble cellular fraction (SCF), and also on common antiradical activity of SCF in D. melanogaster. The object was inbred line, selected for high fitness. Epithalamin and vilon were added to nutrition medium as 0.000010f medium weight. Concentration of RAS was detected in mitochondrial and SCF in 10 and 25 days old flies using chemiluminescent method. The reduction of RAS contents in mitochondria was achieved in females after feeding on vilon. The effect expressed in 1.7 fold reduction of the RAS contents in mitochondria of young females, in 1.5 fold at mature ones and the contents of RAS in SCF of mature females was increased in 1.4 fold. Possible mechanism of vilon action seems to be as follows. Vilon interacts with mitochondrial membrane and release penetration of RAS to SCF with its strong antioxidant systems. Removal of RAS from mitochondria prevents injury of mtDNA and matrics. The latter retard aging.

[4] Responsiveness of P21WAF1 to EGF decreased in old cells

TJ Tong, DL Yang, XD Peng, ZY Zhang (Dept of Biochem & Mol Biol, Peking University, Health Science Center Beijing, China)

One aspect of senescence may be a loss in the ability of cells to respond to mitogenic signals, such as epidermal growth factor (EGF). Cellular senescence is always associated high expression of p21 WAF1 gene. In order to understand the responsiveness of p21WAF1 to EGF during cell aging, the expression of p21WAF1 was examined in human diploid fibroblasts by Northern blotting after EGF stimulation. The results show that p21WAF1 was over-expressed in senescent fibroblasts (55~65PD), and induced by EGF obviously in young cells (23~29 PD). The peak of the induction appeared around 3 h after the stimulation. After 3-6h the expression declined gradually. At 12 h later the expression level of p21WAF1 was even lower than that one before stimulation. These effects are more obvious in young ones than in old ones. The EGF-responding region of p21 WAF1 in young cells was between C1620bp and C800bp upstream of TATA box as shown by green fluorescence protein reporter gene. Neither binding sites of STAT1, nor that of p53 exists in this fragment. It is concluded that EGF has dual effects on expression of p21WAF1 in 2BS (i.e. after transient induction of p21WAF1, the repressing effects appear and the responsiveness of p21WAF1 to EGF in old cells was decreased. The related regulatory region of p21WAF1 may be p53 and STAT1 independent. (Supported by the National Natural Science Foundation of China, Grant No.39930170 and Major State Basic Research Program of P.R. China, Grant No. G2000057001)

[5] Differential gene expression profiles in liver and kidney from aging rats.

L. Teillet (Hôpital Sainte-Périne, AP-HP, Paris, France and Service de Biologie Cellulaire, CEA Saclay, Gif-sur-Yvette, France), P. Ribière (Service de Biologie Cellulaire, CEA Saclay, Gif-sur-Yvette, France) and B. Corman. (Service de Biologie Cellulaire, CEA Saclay, Gif-sur-Yvette, France).

Purpose. Determination of gene expression profiles using cDNA arrays is now used to elucidate the mechanisms of aging. In the present study, we address the question of tissue specificity of these changes in genes expression in both kidney and liver. Method. Liver and kidneys were removed from 10 and 30 mo-old female WAG/Rij rats. Total RNA were extracted and transcripted into cDNA in the presence of 32P dATP. These labelled cDNA were hybridized with rat Atlas cDNA expression array from Clontech. The resulting hybridizations were quantified with a phosphorimager and analyzed with the Atlas Image software. Results. From the 1176 cDNA probes present on the Clontech membranes, 300 to 400 were detectable in kidney or liver. The experimental variability in gene expression was assessed by comparing hybridization profiles in different 10 mo-old rat livers. From this experiment, it was considered that changes in gene expression would be confident when the ratios between two conditions were lower than 0.5 or larger than 2. According to these criteria, 7 genes in liver and 8 genes in kidney were down-regulated (ratios ranging from 0.5 to 0.4) and 8 genes in both organs were up-regulated (ratios ranging from 2 to 4). These up- or down-regulated genes were all different in the two considered tissues.

[6] Effects of Weight-lifting or Running Exercises on Bone Aging in Male Rats

Maria do Carmo Sitta, M.D. Wilson Jacob Filho, phD. José Maria Santarem, M.D. Vanda Jorgetti, M.D. Institution: Department of Gerontology - University of São Paulo - Brazil

Seventy-one male Wistar rats submitted to different types of physical activity (sedentary control, aerobic and anaerobic training) were employed to study bone mineral density (BMD), biomechanical properties, biometrics indices and cortical thickness. The animals were sacrificed with 3, 8 and 18 months of age. The specific training began at 3 months of age after the femur was resected from the initial control. The aerobic exercise was performed on a treadmill running, three times a week, for 60 minutes a day, at 16 meters per minute. The anaerobic exercise was performed three times a week on an effort board specially designed in our laboratory with a slope at 18 degrees with weight progressively bigger during the whole experiment. The BMD was measured using a dual-energy X-ray absorptiometry and the biomechanical properties were measured using universal test equipment. The total BMD and stiffness were bigger in the running with 8 months of age when compared to the control and anaerobic groups. With 18 months the total BMD, the strength and cortical thickness were bigger in the weight-lifting group. The running group had the same tendency of the control group but with values significantly higher of stiffness and bone density with 8 months of age. The weight-lifting group had the highest density, cortical thickness and strength with 18 months of age. The physical activities, specially the weight-lifting exercise, delayed the bone loss and modified the natural tendency of bone aging, improving the bone quality.

[7] Deletion polymorphism of the angiotensin-converting enzyme (ACE) and HindIII polymorphism in the lipoprotein lipase gene (LPL) are associated with myocardial infarction (MI) and longevity

L. D. Serova, N. A. Malygina, I. V. Kostomarova, R. T. Sajgitov (Russian Research Institute of Gerontology, Moscow, Russia), A. S. Melentjev, I. A. Melentjev (Russian State Medical University)

Cardiovascular diseases (CAD) are the leading cause of death in Russia. Suggesting that old age individual is somewhat protected from the propensity to die. It is possible that certain alleles of CAD genes exert a beneficial influence at an advanced age, as alternative certain mutations exert a negative effects. The purpose is to investigate associations between myocardial infarction (MI), longevite and alleles of candidate of CAD (deletion polymorphism of angiotensin converting enzyme (ACE) and Hind III polymorphism in the lipoprotein lipase gene (LPL). MATERIAL and METHODS: Polymorphism of genes was studied by the method polymerase chain reaction in 90 patients with angina on exertion (average age 72,2+6), in 58 patients with MI, in 34 subjects age over 90 years (average age 93,O+2,8). For the control group we have chosen 66 healthy donors (mean age 56,1+5,2). RESULTS: The D allele frequency of gene ACE was decreased in cohort of patients age over 90 years as compared in patients with MI (0,47 versus 0,74, p< 0,01). The H+ allele frequency of gene LPL was decreased in cohort of patients age over 90 years as compared in control and in patients with MI (O,47 versus 0, 66 and 0,81, p<0.0001). It may be due to negative selection H+H+ genotype. The H+H+ genotype frequency was decreased in subjects age over 90 years as in patients with MI (0,11 versus 0.69) and the frequency of heterozygotes was increased (0.71 versus 0.24). Conclusion: Thus the deletion allele of ACE and the H+ allele of LPL gene appear to be risk factors for MI. The deletion allele of polymorphism ACE gene and HindIII polymorphism of LPL gene are associated with MI and longevite.

[8] Association of Genetic Variants of Angiotensin Converting Enzyme to Bedridden Elderly Inpatients with Stroke

Noriko Fujiwara, Shigeto Morimoto, Kohya Okaishi, Yang Jin, Miyuki Onishi, Masashi Okuro, Shoroku Sakurai, Akiko Matsuo, Toshio Onishi, and Toshio Ogihara (Department of Geriatric Medicine,Osaka University Medical School, Osaka, Japan)

Bedridden state is one of the most important target states to be prevented in the elderly. On the other hand, genetic variants of angiotensin-I converting enzyme (ACE) has been known to associate with several diseases related to bedridden state. In the present study, we investigated possible association of the genetic variants of ACE gene with bedridden state itself and to the clinical factors in elderly subjects. We identified 278 elderly subjects in completely bedfast state [83±8 (SD) years], and a random sample of non-bedfast control subjects (n=289) [82±10 (SD) years] admitted to the same long-term care hospital for the elderly. We evaluated duration of bedridden state and the following clinical factors as confounding factors in 1998 and 2000; age, sex, dementia (Mini-mental state examination<23), cerebrovascular accident (CT examination), stroke (MRI, CT), hypoalbuminemia (<3.0 g/dl), and renal dysfunction (Cr>2.0 mg/dl). ACE gene I/D polymorphism significantly associated with bedridden state (p=0.00001, ANOVA). ACE gene DD type was 4 times more in patients with bedridden state caused by stroke than in non-bedridden patients with stroke. In addition, the mean bedridden period was significantly less in those with DD genotype compared to those with ID and II genotypes in stroke patients with bedridden state. Our observation suggests that ACE gene I/D polymorphism is a genetic factor associated with occurrence and duration of bedridden state caused by stroke in the elderly.

[9] Effects of caloric restriction and insulin on Na,K-ATPase

activity in old rats

O. V. Sokolova (Institute of Gerontology, Kiev, Ukraine)

In previous works it was shown that the regulation of Na,K-ATPase activity was mediated by low molecular weight proteins (invertors) which appeared in cells of insulin treated adult rats. This mechanism changed in old rats for the reason of the insufficient production of invertors. We supposed that the caloric restriction could restore the invertor mechanism of hormone regulation of Na,K-ATPase activity in old rats. Purpose: to investigate the influence of insulin and calorie restricted diet on the Na,K-ATPase activity in hepatocytes of old rats. We used Wistar female rats (25 mo). From age 18 to 25 months rats were fed with 50 % restriction of the diet (CRD-rats). As a control were used the old rats fed ad libitum. Na,K-ATPase activity was measured as the difference between total and magnesium ATPase activities. Na,K-ATPase activity of CRD-rats did not differ from the enzyme activity of control rats. The insulin (1.6 U/kg, i.p.), 40 min after injection to CRD-rats provoked the activation of Na,K-ATPase in the liver. The hepatocyte cytosol and blood plasma of CRD-rats injected by insulin activated Na,K-ATPase in the fraction of isolated hepatocyte plasma membranes of CRD-rats. Cell cytosol and blood plasma of insulin-injected rats fed ad libitum as well as insulin itself in vitro did not induce the increase of Na,K-ATPase activity. It could be supposed that there was Na,K-ATPase activating factor in the cells and blood of insulin-treated CRD-rats. Therefore, caloric restriction favoured the prolonged maintenance of the invertor mechanism in old rats and it regained hepatocyte capacity to respond to insulin action similarly to adult animals.

[10] The influence of thyrosine on the glucocorticoid function of old rats under conditions of chronic stress

Gorban E.N, Topolnikova N.V, Bobrovnitsky J.A. (Institute of Gerontology Acad. Med. Sci. Ukraine, Kiev, Ukraine)

PURPOSE: To study the influence of introduction of catecholamins' precursor thyrosine on the glucocorticoid function of adrenal glands (AG) under conditions of chronic stress. METHOD: Experiments have been conducted on Wister male rats aged 7 to 27 month. The situation stress was modeled by changing regimens of feeding, drinking, lighting during 1,5 month. The rats were fed with thyrosine (625 mg/ rats x day 5 times) a week. The glucocorticoid function of AG was estimated at the intensity of 11-OCS secretion by the isolated AG. The concentration of 11-OCS in the medium was measured by fluorometric method. Behavioral reactions were determined by the spontaneous motor activity, which was assessed by the distance traveled by a rat within the fist two minutes of test. RESULT: The intensity of 11-OCS secretion by the isolated AG of the old rats has grown twice, that according to our previous studied influences negatively upon the adaptive potentialities of rats: the behavioral indices were worsened. According to modern concepts, the stress-caused increase of glucocorticoid secretion contributes to the depression of an excessive reaction of the organism to the stress. Oral introduction of 11-OCS precursor thyrosine to the old rats, which were influenced by chronic stress, prevented the rise of 11-OCS secretion that could be positive. Introduction of thyrosine to the control rats didn't cause changes of the 11-OCS secretion. CONCLUSION: Oral introduction of 11-OCS precursor thyrosine to the old rats leads to the inhibition of glucocorticoid function of AG during the stress that quite possibly contributes to the rise of adaptive possibilities under those conditions.

[11] Immune parameters in a non-hospitalized elderly group

Lázaro M, Pallardo B, Fernández C, Figueredo MA, Ribera JM (Geriatric and Immunology departments. Hospital Clínico San Carlos 28040-MADRID SPAIN)

AIMS: To know basal values of different immune parameters in a group of elderly people living in the community. To assess differences according to gender. SUBJECTS AND METHODS: 249 voluntary retired workers from our hospital (59% women). Age: 67.0+4.2 y. We assess the complement components (C-3, C-4), rheumatoid factor (RF), immunoglobulins (IgA, IgG, IgM), total leucocytes and lymphocytes, lymphocytes B (BL), lymphocytes subpopulation (CD4, CD8, CD4/CD8 ratio), natural killer (NK), cutaneous retarded hypersensitivity (score), and the most common haematological and biochemical parameters. Technics: Standard laboratory test, Flow cytometry (EPICS Profile II) with monoclonal antibodies Cytostat B4-B11; T4, T8 HNK1 (Coulter Clone) and multitest IMC (Bio-Merieux). RESULTS: men women p — Leuc 6699.4+1615.2 6105.4+1470.5 ns Lymph 2100.7+ 671.8 2105.1+ 656.8 ns BL(%) 9.4+ 5.0 11.3+ 4.1 <.01 IgG 1155.7+ 320.0 1116.1+ 253.8 ns IgM 112.7+ 69.3 136.8+ 85.6 <.01 IgA 276.1+ 114.0 254.1+ 122.0 ns RF 18.5+ 6.6 20.9+ 18.8 ns CD4 (%) 42.2+ 9.7 47.3+ 9.1 <.001 CD8 (%) 30.3+ 10.8 25.0+ 10.2 <.001 CD4/CD8 1.6+ 1.0 2.2+ 1.3 <.001 NK (%) 12.8+ 10.5 9.8+ 5.8 <.05 Score 13.2+ 7.4 10.0+ 7.2 <.01 C3 118.5+ 29.7 121.1+ 25.2 ns C4 26.4+ 9.0 26.8+ 8.5 ns Hemoglob, haematocr, platelets, monocytes, creatinine and GPT showed significant higher values in men than in women. There were not significant gender differences in leucocytes, neutrophiles, glucemia, total cholesterol, total proteins, and TSH values. CONCLUSION: There are important gender differences among the most common inmune parmeters in elderly people living in community.

[12] Immune parameters in elderly people: A 5-year longitudinal follow-up

Lázaro M, Pallardo B, Fernández C, Figueredo MA, Ribera JM (Geriatric and Inmunology departaments. Hospital Clínico San Carlos. 28040-MADRID SPAIN).

AIMS: To know the eventual changes in basal immune patterns after a 5 years follow-up in a group of elders, according with gender. SUBJECTS AND METHODS: 112 voluntary retired workers from our hospital (60.6% women). Age at the initial study: 67.0+4.2 y. Complement components (C-3, C-4), rheumatoid factor (RF), immunoglobulins (IgA, IgG, IgM), total leucocytes and lymphocytes, lymphocytes B (BL), lymphocytes subpopulation (CD4, CD8, CD4/CD8 ratio), natural killer (NK), cutaneous retarded hypersensitivity (score) were evaluated at the begining and 5 years later. Technics: Standard laboratory test, Flow cytometry (EPICS Profile II) with monoclonal antibodies Cytostat B4-B11; T4, T8 HNK1 (Coulter Clone) and multitest IMC (Bio-Merieux). RESULTS: basal 5 years later Leuc 6229.4+1453.2 6082.4+1429.0 ns Lymph 2153.9+ 644.9 2012.5+ 650.4 ns BL(%) 10.6+ 4.1 10.6+ 4.1 ns IgG 1135.6+ 253.2 1097.6+ 268.8 ns IgM 129.8+ 82.0 122.0+ 75.0 ns IgA 271.0+ 118.9 281.1+ 151.0 ns RF 19.4+ 6.8 20.5+ 23.1 ns CD4 (%) 44.5+ 8.2 44.7+ 8.6 ns CD8 (%) 27.8+ 10.5 25.5+ 8.8 < .01 CD4/CD8 1.8+ 0.8 2.0+ 0.9 < .01 NK (%) 10.2+ 5.3 14.5+ 7.3 < .001 Score 11.6+ 6.9 12.6+ 7.0 ns C3 116.1+ 25.7 127.3+ 34.2 < .001 C4 27.0+ 9.9 28.4+ 13.3 ns According to sex we found lower basal significant values of BL, IgM, CD4, CD4/CD8, and C3 in men, with higher CD8, NK and Score values. All these differences were maintained 5 years later. CONCLUSION: Results show a significant increase in NK and CD4/CD8 ratio due to a decrease in CD8 values. The relevant differences found according to gender are maintained after five years.

[13] Lymphocytes subpopulation in elderly people: Influence of alcohol, tobacco and drugs

Lázaro M, Fabre C, Fernández C, Figueredo MA, Ribera JM (Geriatric and Immunology Departments. Hospital Clínico San Carlos 28040-MADRID SPAIN).

AIMS: To know the influence of toxic habits and polipharmacy on lymphocyte subpopulation in a group of retired workers. SUBJECTS AND METHODS: 225 voluntary retired workers from our hospital (59% women). Age: 66.9+4.6 y. Complement components (C-3, C-4), lymphocytes B (BL), lymphocytes subpopulation (CD4, CD8, CD4/CD8 ratio), natural killer (NK), cutaneous retarded hypersensitivity (score) were determined. Technics: Standard laboratory test, Flow cytometry (EPICS Profile II) with monoclonal antibodies Cytostat B4-B11; T4, T8 HNK1 (Coulter Clone) and multitest IMC (Bio-Merieux). Drinkers (>8gr alcohol/d), Smokers (yes or not), Polypharmacy (3 or more drugs/d). RESULTS: DRINKERS SMOKERS yes (26) not (199) yes (39) not (186) — BL (%) 8.7+ 2.5 10.8+ 4.7* 8.8+ 3.9 10.9+ 4.7 CD4 (%) 43.1+11.9 45.5+ 9.3 43.5+ 9.6 45.6+ 9.6 CD8 (%) 28.9+ 9.5 27.0+10.9 31.8+13.2 26.2+ 9.9* CD4/CD8 2.0+ 2.1 2.0+ 1.1 1.6+ 0.9 2.0+ 1.3* NK (%) 12.2+ 4.5 10.9+ 8.5 7.1+ 1.1 8.3+ 0.6 Score 16.9+ 6.7

10.7+ 4.3 14.3+ 6.8 10.8+ 7.5* C3 116.1+23.8 120.5+27.6 121.4+29.2 119.8+26.7 C4 28.7+12.6 26.3+ 8.0 28.7+12.5 26.2+ 7.7 TBC 9.8+ 4.8 6.5+ 4.3* — * p<0.05 There were not statistical differences referred to the polypharmacy. CONCLUSION: 1) CD4/CD8 ratio is reduced in smokers probably due to the increase in CD8 values, 2) Global and TBC score values are increased in drinkers, c) Polypharmacy do not introduce significant changes in this population.

[14] Immune parameters in elderly people: Influence of chronic diseases

Lázaro M, Pallardo B, Fernández C, Figueredo MA, Ribera, JM (Geriatric and Immunology Departments. Hospital Clínico San Carlos 28040-MADRID SPAIN)

AIMS: To assess the influence of some common chronic diseases on immune parameters in an elderly population. SUBJECTS AND METHODS: 249 voluntary retired workers from our hospital (61% women). Age: 67.7+4.6 years. Complement components (C-3, C-4), rheumatoid factor (RF), immunoglobulins (IgA, IgG, IgM), total leucocytes and lymphocytes, lymphocytes B (BL), lymphocytes subpopulation (CD4, CD8, CD4/CD8 ratio), natural killer cells (NK), cutaneous retarded hypersensitivity (score) were determined. Technics: Standard laboratory test, Flow cytometry (EPICS Profile II) with monoclonal antibodies Cytostat B4-B11; T4, T8 HNK1 (Coulter Clone) and multitest IMC (Bio-Merieux). We compare subjects with or without Diabetes Mellitus (DM), thyroid disease (TD), chronic obstructive pulmonary disease (COPD), and previous history of tuberculosis (TBC), repeated bacterial infection (BI), allergy (A) or dermatological diseases (CD). RESULTS: patients with DM (10.4%) had higher CD4 values (<.05) and CD4/CD8 ratio (<.01). Patients with COPD (7.2%) had higher CD8 values (.05) and a lower CD4/CD8 ratio (<.05). In TBC patients (5.2%) NK and score values were increased (<.001). Score values and IgM were also higher (.002 and .05 respectivly) in TD patients (6.8%). No differences were found related with BI (16.3%), A (4.4%) or CD (6%). CONCLUSION: Different chronic common disorders may contribute to alter normal immune parameter values in the elderly.

[15] Relationship between loss of CD 95- and increase of CD28- T cells in aging.

P. Sansoni, R. Vescovini, F. Fagnoni, G. Passeri, G. Bologna, M. Pedrazzoni, G. Lavagetto, M. Passeri (Dpt. of Internal Medicine and Biomedical Sciences, University of Parma, Italy, C. Franceschi (Dpt. of Experimental Pathology, University of Bologna, Italy),

PURPOSE: Elderly people are particularly prone to severe infections induced by novel pathogens. Since primary immune responses relie on the availability of naive T cells, we evaluated the T cell reservoir throughout the life span. METHODS: 120 healthy subjects from 18-105 years were studied. Peripheral blood mononuclear cells (PBMC) were obtained by Ficoll density centrifugation. Phenotype analysis was performed with a Facscan cytofluorimeter by using whole blood stained with a wide panel of monoclonal antibodies. T cells and purified CD95- cells were stimulated with immobilized anti-CD3 alone or plus anti-CD28. RESULTS: We identified "naive" T cells as CD95- T lymphocytes that require a costimulatory signal in order to proliferate. A progressive age-dependent reduction of "naive" T CD95- cells both in percentage and absolute number was found. The reduction of CD95- cells was accompanied by an increase of CD28- T cells and this phenomenon was particularly evident within CD8+ cells. A multiple linear regression analysis showed that CD95- reduction was significantly related to the aging process while the expansion of CD28- cells may represent a compensatory mechanism for the loss of CD95- cells. CONCLUSION: The absence of CD95 antigen can define putative "naive" T cells previously identified by a double-staining with CD45RA and CD62L; moreover, these cells show activation requirments typical of "naive " T cells. The exaustion of naive CD8+ reservoir, in advanced aging, suggest that this T cell pool is a major target of the aging process and may define a parameter possibly related to the human life span

[16] Towards a new immunological theory of aging

S. Meaume, R. Moulias (Hôpital Charles Foix 94200 IVRY - FRANCE)

Immunosenescence is observed mainly in the sick or the frail elderly. • Analysis of experimental and clinical data showed direct links between immune stimulation, cytokines production and aging like manifestations as sarcopenia, hypercatabolism, lowered renal and hepatic clearances, hypercoagulability, arteriosclerosis, osteoporosis, APP formation, skin atrophy, cardiac wall dysfunction, etc.. • Aging is associated with factors for permanent immunostimulation (AGE antigenes, cells suffer), or transitory immune stimulation (ischemia, infection, trauma) • Cytokines production leads the elderly to a chronical low grade inflammatory syndrome associated with frailty, cardiovascular risk, multi organ dysfunction, multi organ failure if acute worsening. • In this situation TH1 lowered function and TH2 switch of imune response and IL6 increased gene expression could be understood as adaptative mechanisms to lower acute destructive cell mediated immune response. The down regulation of somatotropic axis and lowered IGF1 production permited also to lower T cell answers . Conclusion. The classical manichean view of aging mechanisms have to be criticized. A large part of biological "abnormalities" of aging are likely adaptative mechanisms.

[17] Age-specific Effects of Tryptophane and Nicotinic Acid Combination on Blood Lipoproteid Spectrum under Stress Conditions.

A. P. Yastrebov, S.I. Spektor, V. N. Meshchaninov, D. L. Shcherbakov, V. V. Emelyanov, A. G. Solodovnikov (Ural State Medical Academy, Yekaterinburg, Russia).

PURPOSE: Dyslipidemia accompanies development of stress syndrome (Shcherbakov D.L, 1999). Nicotinic acid can be used as hypolipemic drug (Klimov A.N, Nikul'cheva A.G, 1972). Nicotinic acid metabolism is linked with metabolism of essential amino acid - tryptophane (Rodwell V, 1993). We investigated the effect of tryptophane and nicotinic acid combination on blood lipoproteid spectrum in middle-aged and elderly under stress. METHODS: Study was performed on male 80 rats: 40 middle-aged (10-12 months) and 40 old (22-24 months). Both groups were divided into 3 parts: 1) underwent immobilization stress, 2) were given tryptophane (TRP) (60 mg/kg) and nicotinic acid (NA) (30 mg/kg) combination, 3) underwent both procedures. Stress reactions were controlled by morphological and biochemical analysis of epinephros. High density, low density and very low density lipoproteins (HDL, LDL, VLDL) were detected in blood serum, and atherogenity coefficient (AC) was calculated by Klimov method (Klimov A.N,1977). RESULTS: Immobilization induced blood proatherogenic lipoproteid spectrum shifts in both groups. AC in old increased from 1.63±0.27 to 2.58±0.41 (p<0.05), in middle-aged - from 1.23±0.15 to 1.56±0.26 (p<0.05). Preliminary injection of TRP and NA combination prevented such shifts in old (AC - 1.65±0.20, p>0.05, compared with control), due to increase HDL by 31%, but enhanced them in middle-aged (AC - 1.65±0.20, p<0.05, compared with control) due to increase of LDL by 24% and VLDL by 28%. CONCLUSION: Administration of TRP and NA combination prevents proatherogenic stress-specific shifts in lipoproteid metabolism only in old. Presence of link between this phenomenon with lipid peroxydation level in this group will be further investigated.

[18] Towards Novel Fullerene-Based Pharmaceuticals for Anti-Aging Medicine

V. K. Koltover (Institute of Problems of Chemical Physics, RAS, Russia), E. N. Gorban (Institute of Gerontology, NAMS, Ukraine)

The goal of this study was to demonstrate the prospects of applications of the novel carbon-based pharmaceuticals - enterosorbents, fullerenes and endometallofullerenes. The dietary enterosorbent, SKN non-coated nitrogen-containing carbon, was found to increase the mean value of Wistar rats' life-span by 43% that is comparable with the life- span prolongation effects of the calorie-restricted diets (Frolkis et al, 1989). The discovery of fullerenes (Kroto et al, 1985) has furthered our searching of novel carbon-based drugs. Endohedral metallofullerenes (M@C2n) are carbon clusters that contain metal atoms trapped within a fullerene cage. Recently we have developed a simple extraction scheme that first afforded to produce M@C2n in the large preparative amounts (Laukhina et al, 1998; Koltover et al, 2000). M@C82 are easily modified into novel powerful enterosorbents as well as into water-soluble antioxidants. In addition, M@C2n with the appropriate particle-emitting radionuclides inside, among them - beta- emitting 89Sr, 90Y, 47Sc, 64Cu, 149Pr, 153Sm, 166Ho, and 177Lu can be synthesized while technological advances in the molecular biotechnology provide targeting vectors to deliver therapeutic doses of ionizing radiation with high specificity for the treatments of primary or metastasis cancer tumor cells. In conclusion, fullerenes and endohedral metallofullerenes, due to their unique physical and chemical properties, provide obvious prospects for designing the targeted NMR relaxants and novel therapeutic pharmaceuticals in the coming millennium.

[19] Changes with Age in Heart Structure and Function in Dietarily Restricted Rats

Y. Ito, H.Tauchi, T.Sato (Institute for Medical Science of Aging, Aichi Medical University, Aichi, JAPAN), E.A.Jeckel-Neto (Institute of Geriatrics and Gerontology, Pontifical Catholic University of Rio Grande do Sul, RS, Burazil)

PURPOSE: We investigated the effects of dietary restriction on the heart, a major organ necessary for the maintenance of life, from the viewpoints of structure and function. METHODS: Male rats were divided into two groups, one given food ad libitum (AL) and the other with a dietary restriction (DR). The DR group rats were limited to 60% of the food consumed by the AL group. The rats were killed at regular intervals and the hearts were examined in terms of weight, thickness of the ventricle walls, diameter of the cardiac muscle fibers, and sign of the onset of cardiomyopathy, as well as heart rate and blood pressure. RESULTS: Heart weight gradually increased with age. In measurements of wall thickness, there was no marked change with age in both groups in the right ventricle. In the left ventricle, there was a peak at 18 months in the AL group, after which it became thinner, whereas in the DR group it grew thicker after the 24th month. No marked change was seen in cardiac muscle fiber diameter in either the right or left ventricle in the AL group, but in the DR there was an increase with age in both ventricles. This was particularly marked in the left ventricle. No significant difference was seen between the two groups in maximum and minimum blood pressure at any time and in cardiomyopathy. CONCLUSION: The hypertrophy of cardiac muscle and increase in heart weight with age continued with time, even in the DR group, and a uniform blood pressure was maintained, so the role of the heart in maintaining life is thought to be mainly its action as a mechanical pump.

[20] Over-expression of glucagon receptors in hepatocytes of aging rats is prevented by food restriction.

L. Teillet (Hôpital Sainte-Périne, AP-HP, Paris, France and Service de Biologie Cellulaire, CEA Saclay, Gif-sur-Yvette, France), S. Gouraud (Service de Biologie Cellulaire, CEA Saclay, Gif-sur-Yvette, France), H. Bakala (Université PARIS VII, Paris, France) and B. Corman (Service de Biologie Cellulaire, CEA Saclay, Gif-sur-Yvette, France)

Purpose. Glucose homeostasis is currently impaired with age, resulting in tissue accumulation of advanced glycation endproducts (AGEs). This age-related reduction in glucose tolerance may be due to insulin resistance, but also to a rise in glucagon receptor activity. To test this hypothesis, the relationship between AGE accumulation and glucagon receptor expression was investigated in rat liver. Method. Female WAG/Rij rats were fed ad libitum or food restricted by 30 0.000000rom 10 to 30 months. Receptor density was measured in binding experiments on isolated hepatocytes. Intracellular cAMP and AGEs were determined by ELISA with specific antibodies. Results. The density of glucagon receptors increased from 58823 ± 8775 to 109184 ± 7574 sites per cell between 10 and 30 months in animals fed ad libitum. Food restriction prevented this over-expression of glucagon receptors (47108 ± 6585 sites per cell in restricted 30 mo-old rats). Intracellular cAMP accumulation induced by maximal concentration of glucagon was 35% larger in 30 that in 10 mo-old animals (341 ± 28 versus 249 ± 10 pmol/4min/106 cells respectively), and similar in 10 mo-old and restricted 30 mo-old animals. AGE content in collagen isolated from liver was threefold larger in senescent than in adult rats. Food restriction prevented this AGE accumulation. Conclusion. Increase expression in liver glucagon receptors and intracellular cAMP content may contribute to the age-related reduction in glucose tolerance. Chronic food restriction from 10 to 30 months in rats prevented this over-expression of glucagon receptors as the collagen-associated AGEs accumulation.

[21] Effects of caloric restriction on the hypothalamus-pituitary-testicular axis functions during aging in NIDDM rats

Tadashi Shinkai , Kyoko Miyasaka, Minoru Ohta, (Tokyo Metropolitan Institute of Gerontology Tokyo, Japan), Akihiro Funakoshi (National Kyushu Cancer Center, Fukuoka Japan) and Akinori Hattori (Tokyo Metropolitan Geriatric Hospital, Tokyo , Japan)

A strain of non-insulin dependent diabetes mellitus (NIDDM) rats has been discovered and named Otsuka Long-Evans Tokushima Fatty (OLETF). They have developed mild obesity during aging. It has been reported that testosterone plays a role in the development of obesity. We examined that the relationship between obesity and the hypothalamus-pituitary-testicular axis dysfunction and that effects of caloric restriction (60% and 80% of the amount of food consumed by an ad libitum group) on the dysfunction using 7, 15 and 25 weeks old male OLETF and non-diabetes mellitus (control) rats. Body weights were higher in OLETF rats than in controls, whereas testis weights were lower in OLETF rats than in controls. Plasma testosterone levels significantly decreased at 25 weeks of age in OLETF rats. Plasma luteinizing hormone (LH) levels were higher in OLETF rats than in controls at 7, 15 and 25 weeks of age. Moreover, hypertrophic LH-producing cells (signet-ring cells) were observed in OLETF rat pituitaries. Plasma leptin levels markedly increased in OLETF rats. Caloric restriction suppressed the weight gain of OLETF rats and decreased plasma leptin levels. Plasma testosterone levels of the 80% group recovered to half of controls at 25 weeks of age in OLETF rats. On the other hand, testosterone levels did not increase in the 60% group. These results indicate that obesity atrophies testes and decreases testosterone synthesis and secretion and that the appropriate caloric restriction can improve the testicular dysfunction in male obesity.

[22] Sodium Overload During Aging did not Change ACE Activity and Blood Pressure in Wistar Rats

C.P. Almeida, T. Rodrigues, A. Futerlieb (Dept. of Physiology, UFRGS University, Porto Alegre, Brazil) E.A. Jeckel-Neto (Institute of Geriatrics and Gerontology, PUCRS University, Porto Alegre, Brazil) E. Oliveira; M.C. Irigoyen (Heart Institute, INCOR, USP University, São Paulo, Brazil).

This paper aims at: showing the relationship between Angiotensin-Converting Enzyme (ACE) and blood pressure; comparing animals submitted to a normal diet and animals submitted to a salty diet; comparing the altering in different ages. METHOD: 73 Wistar males rats have been used, aged 3, 6, 9 and 12 months and divided into 2 groups. One group received water with 1% NaCl from weanling and the other group received plain water. In conscious animals, intra-arterial blood pressure was measured by a data acquisition system (CODAS 1kHs). After death the lungs were homogenized in sodium borate buffer (50 mM) with sucrose (0.34 M). The supernatant was incubated with Hip-His-Leu. The total protein was measured by Bradford method. RESULTS: The ACE in the control group (from 11.14±1.5 to 9.22±2.36 nmol/min per milligram protein) has significantly decreased and the blood pressure got higher in the 12-month-group (from 99.13±5.41 to 109.67±4.45 mmHg). However, the other age groups have not had these changes. The groups which had a salty diet have not had any changes at any age. CONCLUSION: The decrease of the ACE activity at the older age (12 mo) in the intact rats seems to be associated with the higher values of blood pressure found in this group. Sodium overload did not change blood pressure and ACE activity, that remained inhibited. The data suggest that alteration in blood pressure during the aging process depends on association changes of renin-angiotensin system.

[23] A "new" tool for an old problem: Brain volume, aging and dementia

R. Verduga, D. Crespo (Department of Anatomy and Cell Biology, Cantabria University, Cantabria, Spain), C. Fernandez-Viadero, (Nursing Home for the Aged, Health & Social Welfare Service. and Department of Anatomy and Cell Biology, Cantabria University, Cantabria, Spain)

PURPOSE: Aplication of Cavalieri stereological method on brain neuroimaging for brain volume quantification. METHOD: Images from computerized axial tomography of 16 elders with normal aging (NA) and 26 elders with senile dementia of Alzheimer type according to DSM-IV criteria. Cognitive evaluation was performed with CAMCOG and MMSE. Brain volume parameters in cm3 (cerebral volume CV, Cerebral volume/ cranial volume CVCV and ventricular volume VV) was calculated by the unbiased method of Cavalieri. RESULTS:The population has a mean age average of 86.7+6.8 years, without differences by sex. Of the 26 patients with dementia 2 have minimum (MD), 6 have mild (MID), 8 have moderate (MOD) and 10 have severe dementia (SD). CONCLUSION: The Cavalieri method is an easy, fast and unbiased method for the analysis of very irregular and complex human structures like the brain. With this method we obtain significant differences on any morphometric parameters between normal aging and dementia. Supported by Grant of Fundacion Valdecilla 12/98.

[24] Neuropathology of a community sample of elderly demented and non-demented individuals.

MRC CFAS Neuropathology group (Margaret M Esiri, Radcliffe Infirmary, Oxford, UK; Fiona E Matthews, MRC Biostatistics Unit, Cambridge UK; Carol Brayne, Institute of Public Health, Cambridge UK; Paul G Ince, Institute for the Health of the Elderly, Newcastle-upon-tyne, UK, John Xuereb, Cambridge Brain Bank Laboratory, Cambridge, UK; John Broome, The Walton Centre for Neurology and Neurosurgery, Liverpool, UK; James McKenzie, The Walton Centre for Neurology and Neurosurgery, Liverpool UK , Marco Rossi, The Walton Centre for Neurology and Neurosurgery, Liverpool, UK; Ian McKeith, Institute for the Health of the Elderly, Newcastle-upon-tyne, UK; Jim Lowe; University of Nottingham, Nottingham UK, James H Morris, Radcliffe Infirmary, Oxford, UK)

PURPOSE: To test the assumption that dementing disorders, as defined by diagnostic protocols used in specialist practice and research, underlie the dementia syndrome encountered in the community. METHOD: Neuropathology was performed on 209 deceased individuals who participated in the MRC cognitive function and ageing study (MRC CFAS). The study is a prospective population based sample of elderly people from five UK centres. Risk factor information, cognitive function data and dementia status, diagnosed using the AGECAT algorithm, were collected longitudinally. Neuropathology was standardised using the CERAD protocol to assess Alzheimer’s-type pathology (ATP), vascular lesions and other causes of dementia. RESULTS: Vascular pathology (78%) and ATP (70%) were frequent. Dementia was present in 47%, of whom 64% had ATP indicating probable or definite Alzheimer’s disease. However, 330f non-demented individuals had equivalent densities of ATP. 600f demented people and 35on-demented had neocortical neurofibrillary pathology. Among the latter 10% had moderate or severe neocortical tangles. Vascular lesions were equally frequent in both groups although multiple vascular pathology was increased in the demented group (47% vs. 32% respectively; p=0.04; Odds ratio 1.9, 95% CI 1.04-3.4). CONCLUSION: ATP and vascular pathology were the major pathologies most strongly related to cognitive decline in this elderly sample, but most individuals had mixed disease. There were no clear thresholds of these pathologies which predicted dementia status. The findings challenge conventional diagnostic criteria for dementia in this setting. Additional factors must determine what burden of ATP and vascular pathology are associated with cognitive failure in an individual.

[25] Presenile Dementia and Cerebral Hemorrhage within a Large French Pedigree

DRODE M (Medecine interne et geriatrie CHG Pau - France) , de la FOURNIERE F (Medecine interne et geriatrie CHG Pau - France), VITAL A (Anatomopathologie CHR Bordeaux - France), KERVINIO C (Medecine interne et geriatrie CHG Pau - France), SAUVANIER M, (Medecine interne et geriatrie CHG Pau - France), REVEL V (Medecine interne et geriatrie CHG Pau - France), ALBERT D (Medecine interne et geriatrie CHG Pau - France), VITAL C (Anatomopathologie CHR Bordeaux - France)

PURPOSE : A large pedigree 5 subjects with presenile dementia (mean age of onset : 48 + 2 years) and one subject with stroke was identified. METHOD : All demented subjects fulfilled the NINCDS-ADRA clinical criteria for probable Alzheimer's disease (AD) Seizures and myoclonus were found in 3 AD patients. RESULTS : The neuropathological examination of the brain of two AD patient showed numerous neuritic plaques and a large amount of amyloid deposits within the blood vessels (congophile angiopathy). The pattern of inheritance of the dementia/ stroke syndrome within this family is compatible with autosomal dominant inheritance. CONCLUSION :The clinical and neuropathological protein displayed by affected individuals within this family does not concern chromosome 1, 14, 19 or 21. Locus of chromosome 17 is under study for identification.

[26] Oxidative Stress and Relationship with Dopatherapy in Parkinson's Disease: A Case Control Study

SAUVANIER M (Medecine Interne et Geriatrie - CHG Pau - France), REVEL V (Medecine Interne et Geriatrie - CHG Pau - France), BONNABAU H (Faculte de Biochimie Universite de Pau et des Pays de l'Adour - Pau - France), DRODE M (Medecine Interne et Geriatrie - CHG Pau - France), KERVINIO C (Medecine Interne et Geriatrie - CHG Pau - France), de la FOURNIERE F (Medecine Interne et Geriatrie - CHG Pau - France), ALBERT D (Medecine Interne et Geriatrie - CHG Pau - France), PLACINES B (Medecine Interne et Geriatrie - CHG Pau - France), DEHORNE M (Laboratoire Dehorne 59 Boulevard Lelasseur 44000 Nantes - France)

PURPOSE : A preliminary study enabled to establish a significant reduction of glutathione peroxidase in platelets (GPXp) in Parkinsonian patients versus younger or elder control individuals (*). To better understand this relationship, we have carried out a new survey which encompasses other variables and particularly the level of circulating dopamine. METHOD : 50 Parkinsonian patients and 100 control individuals were included. We investigated the following variables : age, sex, GPXp levels, superoxide dismutase in erythrocytes (SODe), glutamate, cysteine and circulating dopamine. These variables were compared with chi2 square tests and student tests, followed by a multivarious analysis. RESULTS : GPXp level was significantly reduced in Parkinsons disease patients in comparison with control individuals, irrespective of age and sex. On the other hand, we did not find a significant relationship between GPXp and circulating dopamine levels. The other dosages were not different between both groups. CONCLUSION : These results confirm the relationship between Parkinsons disease and oxidative stress, independently of potential confusion factors. On the other hand, the hypothesis that there is a link with the dopamine level has not been demonstrated. Further investigations are required to determine whether dopatherapy has a deleterious effect with regard to oxidative stress in Parkinsonian patients.
(*) de la FOURNIERE F et al. Decreasing activity of the platelet

glutathione peroxydase in aged patients with parkinsons disease. La revue de geriatrie 2000, 25(7) : 457-462.

[27] Effect of age and gender on the endothelium-dependent vasodilatation in human mesenteric microvessels

S. Vallejo; A. Sánchez-Ferrer; MG. Giorgi; P. López-Dóriga; J. Solís. R.Petidier, N. Martínez-Velilla (Research Unit and Service of Geriatrics, Hospital Universitario de Getafe, Getafe, Madrid, Spain), C. Peiró; CF. Sánchez-Ferrer. (Deparment of Pharmacology, Faculty of Medicine, Universidad Autónoma de Madrid, Madrid, Spain).L. Rodríguez-Mañas. (Research Unit and Service of Geriatrics, Hospital Universitario de Getafe, Getafe, Madrid, Spain).

Purpose: To analyze the effect of age and gender on endothelium-dependent responses in human vessels. Methods: Branches of human mesenteric arteries were obtained from abdominal fat of 88 patients suffering surgical procedures (45 women), free of known vascular disease. Mean age was 43.5 ± 1.9 years (range: 18-91). Microvesseles were mounted in a myograph to analyze their reactivity. Endothelium-dependent responses to bradykinin (BK; 0.01-3 µM) were tested in vessels precontracted with KCl 35-50 mM. Results are expressed as the means of the pD2 values (Log of the effective dose, number of moles, required to produce half the maximum effect) of the vascular segments from every patient. Simple regression analyses (age v pD2) were performed, trying to find the best fitted model. Results: There was a weak lineal relationship between age and endothelium-dependent vasodilatation (r^2= .04; p= .07). When the data were analyzed by gender, no changes were observed for men, but in women the best fitted, most explicative model was a polynomial one (r^2= .20; p= .01). The NO-dependent component of the response (i.e, vessels preincubated with indomethacin) showed the strongest lineal relationship with age (r^2= .21; p= .01), without differences by gender (r^2= .37; p= .01 for women and r^2= .36; p= .02). Conclusions: Several components of the endothelium-dependent responses show separate and different relationships with age and gender.

[28] Components of the aging-associated endothelial dysfunction in human mesenteric microvessels

S. Vallejo; A. Sánchez-Ferrer; MG. Giorgi; P. López-Dóriga; J. Solís. (Research Unit and Service of Geriatrics, Hospital Universitario de Getafe, Getafe, Madrid, Spain). C. Peiró; CF. Sánchez-Ferrer. (Deparment of Pharmacology, Faculty of Medicine, Universidad Autónoma de Madrid, Madrid, Spain).L. Rodríguez-Mañas. (Research Unit and Service of Geriatrics, Hospital Universitario de Getafe, Getafe, Madrid, Spain).

Purpose: To analyze the mechanisms contributing to the age-associated endothelial dysfunction. Methods: Branches of human mesenteric arteries were obtained from abdominal fat of 70 patients suffering surgical procedures (39 women), free of known vascular disease. Mean age was 46.5 ± 2.3 years (range: 18-91). Microvessels were mounted in a myograph to analyze their reactivity. Endothelium-dependent responses to bradykinin (BK; 0.01-3 µM) were tested in vessels precontracted with KCl 35-50 mM. Results are expressed as the means ± SEM of the pD2 values (Log of the effective dose, number of moles, required to produced half the maximum effect) and compared by t test or two-way ANOVA, as required. Results: pD2 for BK were 7.712 ± 0.035 in vessels (n=73) from >65 years and 7.250 ± 0.038 (n=21) from < 65 years (p< 0.001). To abolish the BK-induced vasodilation preincubation with L-NAME (100 µM) plus indomethacin (10 µM) was needed in < 65 yr, but only L-NAME (100 µM) in >65yr. Pretreatment with SOD (100 U/ml) or indomethacin (10 µM) increased the vasodilator responses to BK in >65 years group. The preincubation with both Indomethacin plus SOD restored the endothelial function in this group. In <65 years group, these pretreatments did not modify the responses to BK. Conclusions: Endothelial dysfunction associated to aging embraces three separate mechanisms: lost of a cyclooxygenase-derived vasodilator, interference with NO by an increased generation of superoxide anions and the release of a cyclooxygenase-derived vasoconstrictor substance.

[29] Telomere Shortening with Aging in Human Thyroid and Parathyroid Tissue

Makoto Kammori1,2, Ken-Ichi Nakamura2, Hajime Kanauchi1, Masaki Kawahara1, Yoshikazu Mimura1, Michio Kaminishi1, Kaiyo Takubo2 1 Endocrine & Metabolic Unit, Department of Surgery, The University of Tokyo, Tokyo, Japan, 2 Department of Clinical Pathology, Tokyo Metropolitan Institute of Gerontology, Tokyo, Japan.

PURPOSE & METHOD: Progressive telomere shortening with aging was studied using normal thyroid tissue specimens from 44 human subjects aged between 0 and 98 years (yrs) and normal parathyroid tissue specimens from 19 human subjects aged between 0 and 83 yrs. RESULT: There has hitherto been no information documented about telomere length in such thyroid and parathyroid tissues and age-related shortening at rates of 90 and 94 base pairs (bp) per year, respectively, were observed. Telomere lengths of normal thyroid tissues were 16.1±1.43 (mean±SE), 14.8±1.04, 13.65±0.87, 10.47±0.77 and 8.73±1.08 kilobase pairs (kbp) for age groups less than 2 yrs, 21-40 yrs, 41-60 yrs, 61-80 and 81-98 yrs, and parathyroid tissues were15.58±2.04, 16.68±0.86, 13.77±0.85 and 9.66±0.51 kbp for the first few of these. Significant shortening thus did not occur in the young generations, with substantial decrease in both thyroid and parathyroid tissues only after 60 yrs of age. CONCLUSION: These findings are consistent with the idea that thyrocytes and parathyrocytes have a mechanism to lengthen telomeres.

[30] Why is the Proportion of Centenarians Increasing Today? Is it Possible that Centenarians Originate from a Frail Part of a Generation?

S.V. Ukraintseva, A. I. Yashin (Max Planck Institute for Demographic Research, Rostock, Germany)

In our century there are observed two important processes in human populations, which go in parallel: 1) The increase of survival and proportion of frail individuals over time. 2) The increase of the proportion of centenarians over time. We suggest here a hypothesis on relation between these two processes. The main point of this hypothesis is that some of centenarians may originate from initially frail part of a generation, and then change from relative frailty to relative robustness later in life. Hence the increase of survival and proportion of initially frail individuals in human populations over time may promote the increase of centenarians proportion in the populations. We suggest empirical evidences supporting this hypothesis got from human and animal studies of aging. We show that the antagonistic change in relative frailty during an individual life was observed in many experimental researches. We discuss possible biological mechanisms which may explain initial frailty of some centenarians: (i) antagonistic gene action in different ages; (ii) deviation from optimal health parameters as a possible consequence of slower aging; (iii) antagonistic change in the resistance to stress during an individual life.

[31] Criteria of Normal Aging

Ma. Magdalena Ionescu (Geriatric Clinic, MéxicoCity, México), M. Dumitru (Geriatric Clinic, Mexico City).

The normal age related changes of the organism are essentially characterized by a linear regression in the number of units. The regression of the active cellular mass is asymmetric and asynchronous with different organs or even within the organ. The present paper presents our conclusions determining the essential peculiarities of the biochemical, hydroelectrolitical and hemostaseological framework in the progressive physiological aging. A 10 to 50% regression was estimated in the metabolically active cellular mass in parallel to the decrease in the water amount of the organism, and to increase in total lipid. The hydroelectrolytic changes are determined by the condensation of the proteic molecules which lead to deep modifications in the cellular features. Our studies converged to a hyperlipoproteinemia in the elderly. The immunologic unbalancing in the elderly has some aspects pleading for the fact that its functions are secondarily disturbed by many other changes occurring both in the normal aging or following chronic pathology. As regards the hemostaseologic changes in normal aging, we consider that the structural and metabolic changes lead to hyperhemostasia or thrombogenic status under the name of "thrombophilic status".

[32] Aging dynamics of body mass and longevity of human

I. G. Gerasimov, D. Y. Ignatov (Scientific Research Institute of Medical Problems of Family, Donetsk Medical Government University named after M. Gorky)

The body mass (M) of males and females (age 0 - 90 years) were analyzed. The age dynamics of M is described by function (FM) of periodic extinguishing oscillations: M = A*[exp(-Tt)*cos(wt) + 1], there A - amplitude, T - increment of extinguishing, t - age, w - frequency of oscillations. On the basis of FM analysis common regularity of age alterations for M, entropic equivivalent (EE) equivalented to thermodynamics entropy, and intensity of mortality (IM) are fo- und out. Age indices of first three extremums coincide with such in extremums and/or bend points (first derivative equals zero) of EE and IM age dependence. Thus both M and EE are an characte- ristic of thermodynamic state of biosystem. The period of oscil- lations is approximately 35 years and equilibrium index of M is approximately equal 60 kg. While, second, third and fourth ext- remums of FM is correspond to middle (70-75 years), maximal (100-110 years) and maximal known (140-150 years) longevity. It is significant that after 40 years entropy reflected by EE increases and aspires to limiting index compatible with existence of biosystem. The extrapolation of M on the age after 90 years demonstrates, that amplitude of oscillations FM equals zero epproximatly by 145 years. As existence of biological systems condition on presence of oscillation processes so absence of last, evidently, signify destruction of system as a biological one. In this case, age 140-150 years really appears limiting for human, as species. In conclusion, the age dynamics of human M is well described by function of periodic extinguishing oscillations. Aging alterations of M, EE and IM have common regularitys, and the body mass, as EE, is thermodynamic characteristic of biological system. FM extremums correspond to extreme ages of human life and a biosystem existence ceases in the absence of mass oscillations.

[33} Effect of new preparation made of deer antlers on the level of the blood testosterone and reproductive capacity of rats with accelerated aging

V. Frolkis, V. Bezrukov, B. Pugach (Institute of Gerontology AMS Ukraine, Kyiv, Ukraine) S. Komissarenko, Z. Datsenko (Institute of Biochemistry NAS Ukraine, Kyiv, Ukraine)

The purpose - to investigate the effects of new preparation made of deer antlers upon the level of testosterone and reproductive capacity of rats at physiological and accelerated aging. Studies were performed on 44 male and 88 female Wistar rats aged 17 months and 10 months, respectively. A single X-ray irradiation (400 R) of male rats served as a model of accelerated aging. New preparation from fraction separated from deer antler extract (1 % solution in ethanol) was administered per os with drinking water (10mg/kg b.w.) daily during 30 days. Control rats were given ethanol solution. Blood plasma testosterone was determined radioimmunologically. The results of first series of experiments revealed that the preparation increased 2-fold blood testosterone in 17-mo. rats. Blood testosterone concentration in control rats did not change. Preliminary irradiation resulted in a significant decrease of blood testosterone. However, testosterone concentration in the irradiated rats, which were given preparation, was three times higher than in control animals. The second series of experiments dealt with reproductive capacity of male rats. They were taken to females, creating "families" (1 male +2 female). In the "families" of rats which received the preparation all females had offspring, whereas in the control ethanol-treated animals only 50 % of females had offspring. The number of newborns in the experimental "families" was 7.5±0.8 vs. 4.6±1.2 in control "families" ($p<0.05$). In the "families" of irradiated males, which received preparation and of control, which received ethanol, an equal number of females had offspring (33.3 %) and number of newborns. New preparation can be used as gero- and radioprotector.

[34] The Effects of Aging on Autonomic Parameters Associated to Valsalva´s Maneuver in Normal Individuals.

J.D.Soares (Gerontology Research Center and Program, Unifenas - Alfenas University - Alfenas - MG - Brazil)

One group of 50 healthy normal subjects, age range (20-85 years old) was used to study the changing in Autonomic Function (AF) during the aging process by Valsalva´s maneuver. Each individual performed each maneuver 2 to 4 times. Autonomic Functions was evaluated based on RR interval variations indices, Valsalva´s ratio, and barorreflex sensitivity (Barorreceptor Sensitivity Δ BRSI). There is a linear and negative correlation between the BRSI and aging (Y=9.45-0.078X R=-0.494, $p<0.01$). Relative Bradycardia, Relative Tachycardia, Total Bradycardia Time and Velocity were progressively altered during aging process. The author showed different statistical models to correlate the RR interval variations indices during the aging process. The Barorreceptor reflex obtained by the phenilephrine test decreased progressively after 40 years old (R = 0..58, $p<0.01$) and more intensely after 50 years old (R=0.57, p <0.01) comparatively with younger ages. These data confirmed the fact that autonomic cardiovascular function decreases progressively with the aging process in normal individuals.

[35] The effect of aging on autonomic cardiovascular control during head-up tilt.

P.J. Pretorius, J. Carter, A.P. Blaber (School of Kinesiology, Simon Fraser University, Burnaby, BC, Canada)

The purpose of the study was to investigate the effect of aging on autonomic nervous control of the cardiovascular system during orthostatic stress. Methods: A 70-degree head-up tilt (HUT) test was used with recreationally active subjects in three age ranges (19-21y, N=12; 40-45y, N=12; 57-67y, N=8) of equal gender mix. Continuous beat-by-beat non-invasive blood pressure (BP) and heartbeat R-to-R interval (RRI) were recorded before and during HUT. Coarse graining spectral analysis was used on the BP and RRI time series to investigate age-related changes in cardiovascular orthostatic control mechanisms. Results and Discussion: Supine BP was not different between age groups; however, with HUT systolic BP decreased 7 0n the 19-21y group, did not change in the 40-45y group and increased 14 0n the 57-67y group. This may reflect a decrease in arteriolar elasticity with aging. Across all age groups, systolic BP total harmonic and low frequency spectral power increased and percent fractal power decreased with HUT indicating increased sympathetic activation. RRI decreased 15 0.000000rom supine to HUT regardless of age group, but mean RRI was 13horter in the 19-21y and 57-67y groups compared to 40-45y. RRI high frequency and total harmonic spectral power decreased with HUT in the 19-21y group and also decreased with age. The parasympathetic (PNS) indicator decreased with HUT and age with similar PNS values during HUT. Conclusions: With aging the autonomic sympathetic/parasympathetic nervous systems undergo shifts which may not be reflected in resting RRI or BP. Support: Heart and Stroke Foundation of B.C. & Yukon

[36] A comparative pharmaco-clinic study of ceftriaxone after subcutaneous and intravenous administration in the elderly.

Y. GRUMBACH, L. HARY** , F. MELIN-COVIAUX** , M. ANDREJAK** (*Gerontology Unit, **Pharmacology Unit, University Hospital Center, Amiens, France)*

The incidence and severity of lower respiratory-tract infections in the elderly hospitalized in a long-term care unit require a first line empirical antibacterial therapy with a third-generation cephalosporin. This randomised, open-label study was designed in order to assess comparatively the efficacy, safety and pharmacokinetics of ceftriaxone when administered either subcutaneously or intravenously at a daily dose of 1 g over a 7-day period in this indication. The results on 27 patients, mean age 82 years hospitalized in a long-term care unit, confirmed the clinical and biological efficacy of ceftriaxone. A bitherapy was only used in 2 patients. Ceftriaxone was clinically and biologically well tolerated whatever the route used, and the local tolerance was excellent when using the subcutaneous route. With regard to pharmacokinetics, the halt-life of ceftriaxone (15.1 (0.9 hours with the subcutaneous route and 13.8 (1.1 hours with the intravenous route), the plasmatic clearance (0.656 (0.032 l/h and 0,702 (0.059 l/h respectively) were not statistically different between the two routes. As the mean of the total area under the curve for drug concentrations (1574 (74 mg.h/l and 1500 (103 mg.h/l respectively) were statistically equivalent, it could be concluded that the intravenous route and the subcutaneous route are bioequivalent. These results demontrated that ceftriaxone by subcutaneous route could be alternative to the intravenous in the elderly

[37] Age-related peculiarities of radioprotector effect of Spirulina platensis on glucocorticoid function of adrenal glands

Gorban E.N, Topolnikova N.V. (Institute of Gerontology Acad. Med. Sci. Ukraine, Kiev, Ukraine)

PURPOSE: To study the radioprotector effect of extractum of blue-green seaweed Spirulina platensis (SP) on glucocorticoid function of adrenal glands (AG) and lipid peroxidation (LP)in hepar of adult and old rats. METHOD: Experiments have been conducted on Wistar rats aged 6 and 28 month. After single roentgen irradiation (X-irradiation) in dose 2 Gy the rats were fed during 1 month by extractum SP in dose 500 mg/kg body weight daily. It was determined intensity 11-oxycorticosteroids (11-OCS) basal secretion by isolated AG, reactivity of isolated AG on ACTH. To study LP it was measured in hepar levels of malonic dialdehyde (MDA), catalase (Cat), superoxyddismutase (SOD)activities. RESULT: X-irradiation didn t change basal secretion of 11-OCS isolated AG, increase of MDA level and decrease of SOD and Cat activity in hepar of adult and old rats, and decrease the reactivity of AG on ACTH in adult ones. Feeding by SP in adult animals decrease of basal secretion of 11-OCS by isolated AG and SOD activity, didn t change reactivity of AG on ACTH, level of MDA and Cat activity. In old animals fed by SP indices of AG glucocorticoid function and LP in hepar didn t change against control. In group of irradiated animals fed by SP reactivity of isolated AG of adult animals on ACTH and MDA level and SOD activity restored to control level. CONCLUSION: The result demonstrated an efficiency of the use of extractum of SP to correct radiation impairment of AG glucocorticoid function and LP in hepar adult animals. 13. PURPOSE: To study the radioprotector effect of preparation of blue-green seaweed Spirulina platensis on the glucocorticoid function of adrenal glands (AG) and the POL system in hepar of adult and old rats. METHOD: Experiments have been conducted on Wistar male rats aged 8 and 26 month. After single irradiation (2 Gy) the rats were fed during 30 days with spirulina 500 mg/kg body weight daily. It was determined 11-OCS level in plasma, intensity of 11-OCS basal secretion by isolated AG, reactivity of isolated AG on ACTH. The levels of malondialdehyde (MDA), catalase (Cat), superoxyddismutase (SOD)were measured in hepar. RESULT: 1 month later of irradiation did not change 11-OCS in plasma and basal secretion of 11-OCS in adult and old rats. In adult rats unlike in old ones irradiation activated the POL processes in hepar and lowered the reactivity of AG on ACTH. Spirulina feeding in adult rats led to the lowering of basal secretion of 11-OCS by isolated AG and activity of SOD, did not change reactivity of isolated AG on ACTH, the level of MDA and the activity of Cat. Spirulina feeding prevented of decrease the reaction of isolated AG on ACTH, levels of MDA and SOD activity in adult irradiation rats unlike in old ones. CONCLUSION: The preparation of spirulina has radioprotector effect on the glucocorticoid function of AG and on the hepater POL system in adult rats unlike in old ones in the remote terms after single irradiation.

[38] Microelements and the chronic pathology in the elderly.

Manuela Udrea MD St.Luca Chronic Diseases and Geriatrics Hospital,Bucharest Speranta Babeanu,Centre of Diagnosis and Therapy Bucharest, Livia BrazdesNatl.Inst.of Gerontology and Geriatrics Anna Aslan,Bucharest

Purpose:Studying a possible correlation among some microelements and the aged people with chronic pathology. Method:The study included 48 subjects with chronic non inflammatory pathology aged from 47 to 91 years old, mostly women. The laboratory tests comprised the blood level of Zn,Cu and Cd by Xray induced emission by accelerated heavy particles. Selenium could not be evaluated that element being under detectable blood level. Results. The range of values of the 3 studied microelements was ver large. The ;abortaory performing these analysis claims the values were normal. It seems the data do not confirm the literature regarding the Zn decrease with age and that Cd was not increased. Conclusion: It is a preliminary study, however we could conclude that the 3 microelements studied in elederly with chronic pathology had normal values. The failure of evaluating Se blood level suggests its supplemental administration. On the other hand such a large variation of the serum concentrations requires a reevaluation.

[39] Age and Oncological Burdening in Families of Breast Cancer in Ukraine

Ganina K, Boroday N, Nosa P, Glushchenko N, Dobryden L, Slyusar N. R.E.Kavetsky Institute of Experimental Pathology, Oncology and Radiobiology, National Academy of Science of UkraineInstitution of Oncology, Medical Acad. of Science of Ukraine, Kyiv, Ukraine.

From 1977 breast cancer (BC) occupies the first place in Ukraine among women population and with each year it increases. Hereditary factor puts together 55,68±2,44% with environmental factors 44,32±3,89%. The aim is to define age peculiarities in BC women with different burdening degree on cancerous pathology. Methods. The epidemiological, medico-geographic diffusion analysis of BC in Ukraine, clinic-genealogical and cytospectrophotometrical methods were used in this investigation. Results. Medico-geographic analysis showed a tie of harmful environmental factors in making BC, the most morbidity chronicled in industrial regions, Odessa regions, Crimea and Kiev. An age comparison on the fifth anniversaries in women with burdening on cancerous pathology (174 women) and without burdening (73 women) exposed more young age in ◊ group with two lances before menopausal and postmenopausal periods. Correlation between these groups puts together 43,9 and 17,4% in groups with burdening and without burdening on cancerous pathology. Like so in families with overburdened heredity arose an accumulation neoplasm in more early age, that showed the typical hormonal disturbances. The patients from the families without accumulation neoplasms had the presence of disturbances in more elderly age. Cytospectrophotometrical analysis of DNA content in buccal epithelium exposed considerable augmentation on BC women on comparison with healthy women and women with benign proliferation processes. Maintenance of DNA content can be a marker of malignancy in organism.

[40] Influence of Cortex Spreading Depression and Transcranial Anode Polarization on Limbico-Neocortical Mechanisms of Emotional Behaviour in Aged Rats

V. M. Sheverova (Research Institute of Biology of Kharkov National University, Kharkov, Ukraine).

The problem of cortex-subcortex interrelations and working out non-medicines methods for correction of disturbances that is arising in the psychoemotional sphere with age are very actual. Experiments carried out on 44 aged Wistar rats (24 month-old). The electrodes were implantated into neocortex, hippocampus, hypothalamus and reticular formation. It was used such methods: self-stimulation behaviour, anconditioned reflex avoidence reaction and EEG registration. Functional reversible turning-off of cortex was obtained by Leao method. Polarizing electrodes were located in the region of frontal bone. Strength of direct current -5-20-25 mkA. It was shown the cortex spreading depression provocted the decreasing of electric activity and displacement of biopotentials into diapason of slow waves in subcortex structures. Such changes on EEG correlated with inhibition of self-stimulation and the increasing in the thresholds of arising of active avoidence reaction at 20-th-30-th min. of experiment. Polarization decreased a guota of slow activity and increased an amplitude of main rythms in rats with low type of background EEG, provoked displasement of biopotentials into diapason of alfa-freguencies and increased alfa-indexes. In 1,5-2 hours after beginning of seance and for the space of 13-14 seances polarization increased frequency of self-stimulation and the thresholds of evoidance reactions, transformed "neutral" zones hypothalamus into reward ones. So functional decortication provocted development of inhibition processes in limbico-reticular structures and suppressed of emotional activity of rats. Polarization increased the level of total physiological activity in old animals, exert activating influence on cerebral mechanisms of positive emotional behaviour.

[41] L-Carnitine Counteracts the Age-related Decline in T-maze Learning Ability in Rats.

Sandra Lohninger, Alois Strasser, Hermann Bubna-Littitz (Institute of Physiology, VMU Vienna, Vienna, Austria)

L-Carnitine is of particular interest because of its reported capacity to influence several brain aging processes. However, data on T-maze learning ability are inconsistant. Thus, we examined the effect of L-carnitine on the learning ability of old rats. 100 mg/kg/bw/d L-carnitine was administered orally to 12 old (21 months) male Spraque Dawley rats for a period of 2 months. 12 old (21 months) and 12 young (7 months) control animals received tap water exclusively. The performance of old rats treated with carnitine and old control rats was compared to that of young animals in a multiple T-maze. The mean run time values were significantly lower in the group of old rats treated with carnitine in comparison to old controls (288 209 vs. 471 170 s; p = 0.01), and similar to the mean run time values of the group of young rats (293 209 s). Also for the T-maze parameter mean correct responses we were able to demonstrate that L-carnitine treated old rats made significantly less errors (p = 0.03), and significantly more animals reached the T-maze goal in comparison to old control animals (p = 0.01), whereas no significant differences were observed between old carnitine treated rats and young controls. Thus, the results of our study clearly demonstrate that carnitine treatment improves the learning ability of old rats and seems to be able to reduce the loss of cognitive functions that occurs with aging.

[42] Involvement of P21WAF1 in apoptosis of normal human fibroblast during cell aging

Z-Y Zhang, Y Huang, L Yang, X-D Peng, T-J Tong (Dept. of Biochem & Mol Biol, Peking University, Health Science Center Beijing, China)

Senescent human fibroblasts are more resistant to apoptosis than young ones. Cellular senescence is always associated high expression of p21 AF1gene.To understand if p21 WAF1 was involved in the regulation of senescent cell apoptosis, we constructed p21 WAF1 antisense retroviral recombinant vectors, and transfected it into human diploid fibroblasts (2BS). The results showed that apoptosis was accelerated and senescence process was delayed in antisense p21WAF1 stable transfected cells, in which over-expression of antisense p21WAF1 leads to repression of the endogenous p21WAF1 expression. We have also shown that phosphorylation level of retinoblastoma protein (pRb) increased in senescent 2BS cells over-expressing antisense p21WAF1. The phosphorylation level of pRb was accumulated further in response to sodium butyrate induced apoptosis. Taken together, our results suggest that down-regulation of p21WAF1 in senescent 2BS cells promotes apoptosis through pathways of delaying cell senescence process and increasing retinoblastoma protein phosphorylation. (Supported by the National Natural Science Foundation of China, Grant No.39930170 and Major State Basic Research Program of P. R. China, Grant No. G2000057001)

[43] Geriatric autopsy database and its application to genomic research

Motoji Sawabe, Tomio Arai, Ken-ichi Nakahara, Takayuki Hosoi, Hajime Orimo (Departments of Pathology and Internal Medicine, Tokyo Metropolitan Geriatric Hospital, Tokyo, Japan)

Purpose: Human genome project has completed the entire draft sequencing of human genome, identifying thousands of genes of unknown function. To study the correlation between genetic data and human diseases, exact clinical and pathological information are required. We have developed a complete geriatric database designed for genetic research based on autopsy cases. Methods and Materials: Recent consecutive autopsy cases for six years have been registered to the database. Clinical and pathological data were saved on a PC server. DNA have been extracted from frozen autopsy kidneys with each ID, being encrypted. Written informed consents were taken from the bereaved family and this project was admitted by the ethical committee. Results: More than 1,200 cases were registered in the database. The male:female ratio was 1.1:1 and the average age was 72 years. Fifty-three cases more than 95 years of age were included. The clinical diagnoses and pathological data were coded according to ICD-10. Using our materials, a molecular study on ApoE genotype has already been published. Conclusion: We have developed a geriatric autopsy database which is a powerful resource for genomic research, especially for the SNPs of the candidate genes of the geriatric diseases.

[44] Retinal damages in the non-arteritic ischemic optic neuropathy

Ramírez JM, Salazar JJ, Ramírez AI, De Hoz R, Rojas B, Triviño A. Instituto de Investigaciones Oftalmológicas Ramón Castroviejo. Universidad Compluntense de Madrid. Spain.

PURPOSE: To study the different types of cellular death (necrosis and apoptosis) in the non-arteritic ischemic optic neuropathy. METHOD: Transmission electron microscopy was used to study human retinas with non-arteritic ischemic optic neuropathy. RESULTS: The damages were located in the ganglion cell layer (GCL), inner nuclear layer (INL), and outer nuclear layer (ONL). Apoptosis was observed at the photoreceptor level, where was also death by heterophagy, although this was less frequent. In the INL apoptosis alternated with necrosis in all of the cell types existing in this layer and in the GCL there was a large number of apoptotic ganglion cells. CONCLUSION: The apoptosis is alternated with the necrosis in the nuclear layers. Thus the behaviour of the non-arteritic ischemic optic neuropathy in human is similar to that found in animal models.

[45] Astroglia and age-related macular degeneration

Ramírez JM, Ramírez AI, Salazar JJ, De Hoz R, Rojas B, Triviño A. Instituto de Investigaciones Oftalmológicas Ramón Castroviejo. Universidad Compluntense de Madrid. Spain.

PURPOSE: To study the morphological changes of the astroglia in relation to the Age-related Macular Degeneration (AMD). METHOD: Electron microscopy and immunohistochemical techniques (anti-GFAP) were used to examine the changes in retinal astroglia in normal (young and older) and pathological (AMD) human retinas. RESULTS: There were large numbers of hypertrophy and reactive astrocytes in the AMD group. In this group trunk-shaped astroglial protrusions with high GFAP reactivity passed trough the internal limiting membrane (IML) and formed a glial membrane in the vitreous humour. The astrocytes of the glial membrane had a large number of cellular organelles and glial filaments, numerous microvilli and gap junctions. The AMD group showed an increase in the thickness of the ILM and in the basal membrane of the capillaries. Additionally, a larger number of acellular capillaries were found. CONCLUSION: The loss of astroglial cells accompanying normal aging together with the extensive retinal ischaemia could cause the astrocytes to migrate to vitreous where there was a metabolic reserve. These cells could protect to the ganglion cells from oxidative damage.

[46] Age-related change of the DNA binding activity and the expression of the glucocorticoid receptor in rat liver

Ryoichi Abe and Sataro Goto (Department of Biochemistry, School of Pharmaceutical Sciences, Toho University, Funabashi, Chiba, JAPAN)

Purpose: The ability to maintain homeostasis decreases in older ages. Glucocorticoid (GC) is a hormone released from the adrenal cortex in response to stress to cope with deleterious changes. It is conceivable that reduced GC action is a mechanism of the age-related decrease in the stress response. GC binds to its receptor (GR) in the cytoplasm and the complex translocates to the nucleus and acts as a transcription factor of various target genes. In the present work we studied whether expression of the GR gene and properties of GR change with age. Method: Male F344 rats were used. The DNA binding activity of transcription factors in the liver whole tissue extracts was studied by electrophoretic mobility shift assay (EMSA). The GR mRNA and the protein were estimated by RT-PCR and Western blot, respectively. Results: The DNA binding activity of GR from old rats (28-33 month-old) was 64% of that of young rats (8-11 month-old). No age-related change was observed in the binding activity for NF1. The activity for Sp1 was decreased to 78% of that of young counterparts with no statistical significance. The RT-PCR and Western blot analysis revealed that quantity of GR mRNA of old rat livers was 56% of that of young ones, while the amount of GR protein did not change with age. Conclusion: These findings suggest that not only the mRNA level for GR but also the quality of GR protein decrease with age, providing one of possible mechanisms of reduced stress resistance in old age.

[47] Sex differences in antioxidant system in Drosophila melanogaster.

T. I. Oparina (D. O. Ott Institute of obstetrics and gynecology, St.-Petersburg, Russia), S. V. Mylnikov (Department of genetics, St.-Petersburg State University, St.-Petersburg, Russia),

The goal of the present work was to analyze the level of free radicals and activity of antioxidant enzymes in Drosophila melanogaster. The objects were set of wild type and congeneric inbred lines of Drosophila melanogaster pre-selected for reproductive traits. We analyze the level of lipid peroxidation products (conjugated hydroperoxides and Shiff's bases), generation of reactive oxygen species, antiradical activity, SOD and catalase activity in extracts of flies tissues. In all lines production of reactive oxygen species was 1.2 fold higher in males as compared with females. At the same time, catalase and total antiradical activity was always 25-60 0gher in males in all lines. We did not observe sex differences in SOD activity. The level of lipid peroxidation also has demonstrated sex differences, but its direction was depended from concrete line. High level of antioxidant enzymes activity in males seemed to be compensatory reaction for increased level of reactive oxygen species and products of lipid peroxidation. Because of this, mortality rate and longevity in both sexes in analyzed lines were comparable on magnitude.

[48] RAGE and Cellular Pertubation in Alzheimer's Disease

A.R. Stern (Great Neck South High School, Great Neck, NY, USA)

Receptor for Advanced Glycation Endproducts (RAGE) is a member of the immunoglobulin superfamily of cell surface molecules which has been shown to interact with amyloid fibrils in vitro and in vivo. In view of the increased expression of RAGE in neurons in the brains of patients with Alzheimer's disease (AD), a murine model was developed to test whether RAGE amplifies cell stress induced by the amyloid-beta peptide (A-beta). Transgenic mice with targeted overexpression of RAGE in neurons were crossed with other transgenic mice overexpressing a mutant form of amyloid precursor protein which results in increased levels of A-beta in the brain. At 3-5 months of age, double transgenic mice displayed evidence of cell stress, as manifested by expression of inflammatory mediators (Interlukin 6 and macrophage-colony stimulating factor) and activation of the transcription factor NF-kB compared with single transgenics and notransgenic control animals. Furthermore, cell stress in double transgenic mice was associated with decreased synaptophysin and microtubule-associated protein 2 immunoreactivity, consistent with accelerated neurotoxicity. In vitro studies with neurons from transgenic mice overexpressing RAGE showed increased susceptibility to NF-Kb activation over several hours followed by increased caspase 3 activity at longer times. Taken together, these data suggest that neuronal RAGE can function as a cofactor promoting A-beta-induced cell stress, and that this may result in exaggerated cytotoxicity. Finalist, Gerontology category, 2001 Intel International Science and Engineering Fair.

[49] Immunocytocheminal Study on the Changes of Cell-Death Controlling Factors in the Hippocampal Formation of the Aged Rats

S. J. Shin(Department of Psychiatry, Chook Ryoung Evangelical Hospital, Namyangju, Korea), H. W. Woo(Ewha Medical Research Center, Division of Neuroscience, Ewha Womans University, Seoul, Korea)

PURPOSE : Hippocampal formation and entorhinal cortex play a part in learning and memory. This study sought to investigate the change of cell-death controlling factors in the hippocampal formation and entorhinal cortex of aged rats. METHOD : Ten aged rats and ten controls were studied. We performed immunocytochemical method using antibodies against NOS, VIP, c-fos, bcl-2, bax and p53 and insitu hybridization. RESULTS : 1) The number of nNOS-immunoreactive(IR) neurons in the entorhinal cortex was significantly decreased in the aged rats(>30%). Morphologically, the number of dendritic branches seemed to be decreased and the length of dendrites showed a tendency to shorten in the aged group. A major loss of nNOS mRNA positive neurons was observed in the hippocampal formation of the aged rats(>30%) . 2) VIP-IR cells were mildly decreased in the hippocampus and subiculum(<15%), and moderately decreased in the dentate gyrus and entorhinal cortex of the aged rats(15-30%). 3) c-Fos-IR nuclei were moderately decreased in the hippocampus(15-30%), and severely decreased in the dentate gyrus,subiculum and entorhinal cortex of the aged rats(>30%). 4) Bcl-2 mRNA positive neurons were moderately decreased in the hippocampus, subiculum and entorhinal cortex(15-30%), and severely decreased in dentate gyrus of the aged rats(>30%). 5) Bax-IR neurons were similarly distributed between the control and the aged rats. 6) P53-IR neurons were only observed in hippocampal CA1 region of the aged rats. CONCLUSION : These results indicate the involvement of neuronal system containing NOS, VIP, c-fos, bcl-2 and p53 in the brain aging process, and provide the morphological evidence for the changes in immunoreactivity fo cell-death controlling factors in the hippocampal formation and entorhinal cortex of aged rats.

[50] Program of Age-Related Pathology Prevention and Professional Longevity Extension among "Gazprom" Personnel

R. I. Vyakhirev, N. N. Gouslisty, S. V. Okhotnikov (OAO "Gazprom", Russia), V. Kh. Khavinson (St. Petersburg Institute of Bioregulation and Gerontology, Russia)

Professional activity at "Gazprom" - the largest Russian enterprise - is associated with the impacts of extreme natural, environmental, social and psychological factors, which entail a decrease in the organism adaptation abilities, premature aging and early development of diseases. The main risk group embraces gas-extraction and gas-transportation personnel working in the North and Western Siberia. Increased incidence of chronic diseases, augmented premature mortality rate and complete invalidity in this group cause a significant economical damage to the company and decrease the working potentiality of its staff. Declined economical and demographic situation in the country, persisting natural processes of the staff aging, increased negative psychological and informational loads, higher pathology incidence among the company workers necessitated the development of the "Program of Active Professional Longevity Extension and Age-Related Pathology Prevention among "Gazprom" Personnel". This program was devised to prevent age-related pathology, inhibit the processes of aging, restore and maintain the main functions of organs and tissues in "Gazprom" staff by means of bioregulators. Bioregulators are nucleoprotein complexes or peptides applied in the form of tablets or solutions for intramuscular injections. The technology of active professional longevity extension, health and working ability preservation and age-related pathology prevention was integrated with over 12 000 "Gazprom" workers in the period of 1995-2000. Result of the technology application facilitated a significant extension in the working life, decreased losses by work, lowered biological age and raised quality of life among the company personnel.

[51] Loss of Functional Caveolae During Senescence of Human Fibroblasts

Keith Wheaton, Kari Sampsel, Francois-Michel Boisvert, Alice Davy, Stephen Robbins and Karl Riabowol (Department of Biochemistry and Molecular Biology, Southern Alberta Cancer Centre, University of Calgary, Heritage Medical Research Building, Calgary Alberta.)

Purpose: Primary human fibroblasts have a finite replicative lifespan in culture that culminates in a unique state of growth arrest, termed senescence that is accompanied by distinct morphological and biochemical alterations. Senescent cell responses to extracellular stimuli are believed to be altered at a point after receptors are bound by ligand, leading to improper integration of the signals

[52] Age changes of functions correlations and a problem of biological age assessment

T. Smirnova, V. Kroutko, V. Dontsov, A. Mamay (National Gerontology Center, Moscow, Russia)

PURPOSE: Comparative analysis of correlations between biological age biomarkers (BAB) in different age groups was the aim of research. METHOD: 13 parameters used as BAB in the "Kiev test" of biological age (BA) definition (Voitenko V.P, Tokhar A.V, Polyuhov A.M, 1984) for 159 essentially healthy women in the age of 25 - 69 years were determined. The women inspected were parted into 3 age groups: 25 - 39 years (young age); 40 - 54 years (average age) and 55 - 69 years (elderly age). Significance of correlations between continuous parameters was estimated by t-test, and significance of contingency between discrete BAB - by chi-square test. RESULTS: the authentic relation between age and the number of significant correlations within BAT was detected. In the average group increase of number of correlation as compared to the young group was stated. In the elderly age group the number of authentic correlations was minimum. Age dynamics of interlinks between the biomarkers allow to make definite conclusions concerning age features of an organism homeostasis maintenance. For example, the nature of correlations of exhalation delay with other biomarkers demonstrates, that the capabilities of the gas-transporting system in the young age are limited by the main anatomic features, in the average - by system resources of blood circulation, and in the elderly - are strictly connected with lung function. CONCLUSION: the age changes of correlation links connections between BAT reflect modification of regulatory links and depend on increase of organs and systems operation tension for the average age and with disturbance of different systems operation conformity in the elderly age. The methods of BA definition should take into consideration the age dynamics of system organization of functions of an organism.

[53] The aging retarding effect of Ge-132

Xie Shu-Zhen, Ma Yong-Xing, Chen Shu-Ying (Department of Aging, Antiaging and Cognitive Function, Shanghai Institute of Gerontology and Geriatrics, Huadong Hospital, Shanghai, China)

1. Ge-132 oral liquid composed of Carboxyethyl Germanium Sesquioxide (Ge-132). 2. After 40-60 mg for 2 months in 75 persons of the aged, the mean value of NK activity (19.9±7.3%, 22.9±6.4%, P<0.01), SOD (449±25, 1±28g/gHb, P<0.01), Catalase (15.3±3.2, 17.2±1.4U/mgHb, P<0.001), GSH (2.3±0.3, 2.5±0.3mg/gHb, P<0.01), MQ (97±16, 105±19, P<0.01) and CO, CI, SV, SI, LVET, LVETI and arterial compliance were significantly increased, but the LPO (4.50±0.97, 4.16±0. 70nM/ml), and the simple light reaction time (red: 401±112, 335±66ms, P<0.05; green, 361±63, 328±64ms, P<0.01) significantly decreased. There were no apparent changes in the control group. 3. The mean life span of the male fruit fly was significantly increased in the middle and high concentration of Ge-132 oral liquid treated group than that in the control group (56±10, 63±12; 62±11 days, P<0.05~0.01). 4. It is suggested that Ge-132 has an age-retarding and geroprotective effect.

[54] Hutchinson-Gilford Progeria Syndrome

Vicente Spinola Dias Neto; Giselle H. de Paula Rodrigues; Izilda das Eiras Tâmega (Pontifícia Universidade Católica de São Paulo Sorocaba Brazil).

The Hutchinson-Gilford progeria syndrome is a very rare, but well-known inherited condition of uncertain etiology in which features of premature and accelerated aging are mixed with those of delayed maturity and immaturity. The incidence of progeria has been estimated to be 1 per 8 million births. And, until 1990, only 76 cases had been found worldwide in the literature. Appearance at birth and birth weight are usually normal but growth typically starts to become retarded after one year. All organ systems undergo degeneration to such an extent that the patient resembles a little old man or woman. The syndrome is characterized by short stature, micrognathia, alopecia, sculptured nose, prominent scalp veins, loss of subcutaneous fat, prominent joints, skeletal hypoplasia and dysplasia, persistent open fontanelles, pathological fractures, hyperlipidemia and early arteriosclerosis. Generalized osteoporosis and osteolysis can occur. There are no intellectual disturbs in patients with this syndrome, intellectual disturbs in patients with the age. The life span in progeria is shortened by early arteriosclerosis, and death usually occurs in the second or third decade of life and usually results from cardiac or cerebrovascular complication. We report a case of an eight years-old girl, which was admitted, in our hospital, with short stature and loss of hair. On examination, the child was short for her age and bald. She has too: appearance of three years old, despite her old aspect; dry and wrinkled skin; prominent scalp veins; craniofacial disproportion; short and sculptured nose; delayed dentition; arms and legs symmetrics and hypoplasics; normal intelligence, although her conduct is like an adult. There isn' t another case like that in her family. With all of those characteristics, we conclude that is a case of Hutchinson-Gilford progeria syndrome.

[55] Prevention of ageing as a new area of gerontology

V. Kroutko (National Gerontology Center, Moscow, Russia)

A really new scientific area should have a unique subject, method and concept of true, distinguishing it from other areas of science. A process of natural ageing of a living organism is the basic subject and the point of effort application of ageing preventive measures. The method of this science is a combination of unique preventive techniques for retardation of natural ageing. Concept of true is a set of natural ageing retarding effects established with the help of special evidential base, which includes unique experimental procedures, grounded on the analysis of survival curves, and special mathematical methods of the analysis and forecast. The biological age is the base concept for this study. At a population level the above mentioned effects have an integral expression in an increase of an average species life span (ASLS). At a personal level - in an increase of an expected life span (ELS). In the National Gerontology Center the development of complex Aging Prevention Technology is conducted. The Technology includes: computer-controlled procedures for speed definition of natural ageing of a human organism as a whole and of its separate subsystems; estimation of risk factors; definition of Expected Life Span (ELS) on this basis; choice of personal age retardation measures set and help in putting these means into daily practice. The principal novelty of the Ageing Prevention Technology lies in the fact that it is oriented to diagnostic and correction of inner processes of wearing and exhaustion of reserves even in an absolutely healthy organism during its normal functioning, instead of dealing with particular diseases. The Technology surpasses the available foreign techniques for solution of the given problem. Five features may be pointed out. First, it exceeds them in the general methodology, offering an author's development of the system theory of ageing. Second, the advantage is embodied in the algorithm of diagnostics, as it gives capability of definition of both integral biological age, and partial ages of separate systems of an organism and it helps to calculate an expected life span as well. Third, the Technology comprises a developed computer system for optimization of personal diets enabling to retard the process of ageing. Forth, the advantage of the Technology is in its methodology of selection and applying of age retarding means, as it employs an integral method of simultaneous impact on basic processes of ageing of different levels. Fifth, it uses original ageing constraining means.

[56] Action of free radicals oxidation in the development of endothelial dysfunction in elderly people.

O.Korkushko (Institute of gerontology AMS of Ukraine, Kiev, Ukraine), V.Lishnevskaya (Institute of gerontology AMS of Ukraine, Kiev, Ukraine), G.Dugak (Institute of gerontology AMS of Ukraine, Kiev, Ukraine),

PURPOSE. Investigation of the relationship between free radicals oxidation system, antioxidant defense, and the functional state of the endothelium in elderly people.METHOD. Thirty healthy subjects (age range, 60 - 79 years) were examined and 20 healthy others (age range, 20-29 years) served as control.Their action was assigned by the content of malondialdehyde (MDA), lipid hydroperoxides (LHP), erythrocyte superoxide dismutase (SOD), plasma, erythrocyte catalase, and reduced glutathione.The endothelium was studied by measurement of the volume velocity of skin blood flow using laser doppler flowmetry (Transonik - USA), the quantity of nitrogen oxide metabolite NO2 (Griss reagent), the level of plasma endotelin (Endothelin - 1 ELISA, AMERSHAM FARMACIA BIOTECH - England).RESULTS. In elderly people, the levels of MDA, LHP exceeded the values of young while the levels of SOD, catalase, reduced glutathione were decreased. The functional state of endothelium revealed lower increment of skin blood flow velocity compared to the young in response to hyperaemia, pronounced spastic reaction after the subcutaneous injection of adrenalin, a decreased of plasma NO and an increased of endotelin. CONCLUSION. The mathematical processing of the data obtained revealed the existence of relationship between the degree of endothelial dysfunction and the action of FRO in elderly people.

[57] Coal-Workers: immune system, hormonal status and efficiency

Olga A. Trunova, Grigory S. Peredery, Valentina M. Kulyas, Yelena A. Aslanova (State enterprise Research Institute for medical-ecological problems of Donbass and coal industry, Donetsk, Ukraine)

Purpose: prognosis for labour factors influence upon health and occupational efficiency of coalminers on the basis of physiological and biochemical indices study. Method: 271 coalminers aged 20-29, 30-39, 40-49 years examined during their working activity. Control group consisted of 30 donors - non coalminers aged 20-29 years. RIA concentrations of ACTH, follicule stimulating hormone, thyroxin, cortizol, aldosterone and testosteron, phagocytosis activity of neutrophils, the spontaneous and induced NBT-test indices, the lysozyme level and immunoglobulin (IG) A, G, M, E in the serum blood were studied. The following physiological indices were measured: arterial pressure, pulse, muscle strength and endurance, top speed of air current at the expiration, vital lung capacity, minute respiratory volume, latent period of visual-motor reaction, vegetative tone (by cardiorhythm indices) and physical efficiency were measured. Results: High concentration of hormones of hypophysial adrenal system (ACTH and cortizol) and thyroxin at the age of 30-39 years reflects the state of hightened activity of adaptation mechanisms. Against this background prenosologic indications of failures of harmonious correlarions between the activity of hypophisial and gonadotropic hormones appeare. Adaptation out of strain gradually passes to the cachexia. The same changes of hypophysial and gonadal system in workers of the other occupations develop as a rule two ten-years later at the age of 50-59 years. Chronic industrial stress causes of premature coalminers occupational ageing and development of pathologic changes of the body in young and middle working age. Emaciation of phagocytic function of neutrophiles against a background of hyperimmunoglobulinemia A in middle aged coalminers probably is connected with hightened demands to the respiratory organs profection under intensive dust load. Sensitized influence of mine environment causes significant increase IGE concentration. Necessity of neutralization and extraction of tissue decay products from the body is closely connected with the results of sensitized influence. It is followed by hightened activity of autoimmune processes. Development of the identical immune hormonal changes under such different states of the body as occupational stress, normal ageing, etc. Is generally known fact. Under working activity age changes in the body cause narrowing of activation range for physiologic and psychologic functions; as a result of it the level of vegetative protection of the activity decreases up to 10-15 b/min. It is achieved by its strategy change. Workers with large length of service decrease work rate 20% and change its content which is directed to the limitation of behavioural activity and displayed by the shortening of work operations on 40-60 min under simultaneous increase (1.6-1.7) of break length in the work. As a result of such changes index of effective use of working hours decreases from 82 to 69%; decrease of efficiency reaches 30%. Results of coalminers hormone status estimation display the dinamics of body adaptation to the factors of industrial environment and working activity. Deficiency of adaptative resources and development of stress-syndrome in coalminers of coal mines is observed after 5-7 years of work at the age of 30-39 years. As a rule stress-age-syndrom is followed by the development not only destructive but protective mechanisms. The last ones are displayed at the behavioural and homeostatic levels as efficiency decrease and functional strain with preservation of occupational activity reliability. Conclusions: A presence of the definite accordance of the calendar age and activation energetic components of the responding, the immune and hormonal changes of the regulation allow to connect the health peculiarities and the activity strategy, used by coalminers, with the occupational ageing.

[58] Immunogenetic HLA peculiarities in patients with ischaemic heart disease in different age periods.

L.D.Serova, T.V. Karpova, N.V.Khrabrova,L.P.Minashkina (The Institute of Gerontology, Moscow, Russia)

PURPOSE: to study association between HLA immunogenetic system and the origin of ischaemic heart disease (IHD) in old people. METHODS: HLA distribution was studied in 163 IHD patients in five age groups: I 36-46 years, II 47-60 years, III 61-70 years, IV 71-90 years, V >90 years. Control group consisted of 507 practically healthy people. We identified 52 HLA I classes by means of a double-step microlymphocytotoxic method. HLA frequecy was determined, relative risk (RR), ethiology fraction (EF). RESULTS: The frequency of certain HLA allels in IHD patients differed from their frequency in practically healthy people (Table). Occurrence peculiarities of HLA system antigens in patient with IHD in different age period. HLA Frequency (%) I II III IV V Control n=42 n=54 n=31 n=17 n=19 n=507 RR/EF RR/EF RR/EF RR/EF RR/EF RR/EF A10 28,6 2,4/0,17 31,3 2,7/0,12 31,8 2,8/0,2 29,4 2,7/0,2 10,5 0,8/-0,25 14,5 B21 9,5 3,2/0,06 4,2 1,5/0,01 9,1 3,4/0,06 10,0 4,4/0,07 5,3 2,3/0,03 3,3 B22 7,1 2,0/0,04 8,2 2,3/0,05 9,1 2,8/0,06 11,7 3,4/0,07 5,3 1,9/0,03 4,1 A9 23,1 1,1/0,02 25,9 1,2/0,04 23,1 1,1/0,02 23,5 1,1/0,02 42,1 2,5/0,25 22,7 B5 10,2 0,8/-0,02 22,0 1,9/0,11 18,2 1,5/0,06 30,0 2,9/0,19 42,1 4,7/0,33 13,6 CONCLUSION: Occurrence of HLA alleles in IHD patient over 90 years is significantly different from that in more younger patients. At that maximum difference was observed when compared patients over 90 with 36-45 age group. These observations make it possible to suppose that the mechanism of IHD development in the older age group is different from the same mechanism in younger age groups. Most probably IHD in old people is not determined genetically but is due to additional aggravating factors that appear in the process of aging, such as metabolism disturbances that cause atherosclerosis and IHD.

[59] Antibody Titer for Influenza Vaccination in Octogenarians in a Nursing Hospital in Japan.

S. Saeki, T. Onishi (Hanwa Daiiti Senboku Hospital, Osaka, Japan), M. Onishi, S. Morimoto*, T. Ogihara* (*Department of Geriatric Medicine, Osaka University Medical School, Osaka, Japan)*

Purpose: Many elderly people suffer from influenza every year and their mortality is high. On the other hand, vaccination rate for influenza was very low in Japan compared to those in European countries and U.S.A. We examined the effects of influenza vaccination on the antibody titers for AH1, AH3 and B in old-old elderly patients aged 80 years or more (range 80-95 years) (n=87) compared to those young-old subjects aged 65 to 79 years (n=58) in a nursing hospital for two influenza seasons (1997/98, 1998/99). Method: Elderly subjects had 0.5 ml of influenza vaccine (Biken HA vaccine) subcutaneously in November. Serum antibody titers for AH1, AH3 and B were measured by hemagglutination method before and one and two months after the vaccination. Results: Antibody titer was elevated sufficiently from before to one and two months after vaccination not only in young old subjects but also in old-old subjects. There was no significant difference in the mean values in each antibody titer before and one and two months after the vaccination between the old-old subjects (being AH1: 5.7, 25.0, 13.4, AH3: 20.5, 164, 129, and B: 7.9, 20.2, 17.0) and the young-old subjects (being AH1: 6.8, 36.8, 15.5, AH3: 20.7, 196, 118, and B: 6.9, 22.8, 17.0). Conclusion: Influenza vaccination seems to be effective in not only young-old subjects but also in octogenarians and nonagenarians.

[60] Effect of lipoproteins on NK cell activity

Tomiya Yasumasu, Kazuo Takahara, Kazuhiko Isozumi¶, Takao Sadayasu†, Ryouji Kouzuma and Yasuhide Nakashima‡ [*Department of Medical Technology I, School of Health Sciences, and ‡the Second Department of Internal Medicine, University of Occupational and Environmental Health, 1-1 Iseigaoka, Yahatanishi, Kitakyushu, Japan ¶Ashiya Central Hospital, Onga, Fukuoka-prefecture, Japan †Seiwakai Clinic, Onga, Fukuoka-prefecture, Japan]*

PURPOSE: It is unknown that whether hypercholesterolemia should be considered a risk factor for diminished immunity in old age. To evaluate the role of plasma lipoproteins in the physiological relevance of their immunoregulatory properties, we investigated the relationship between plasma lipoprotein levels and natural killer (NK) cell activity in elderly subjects. METHOD: The association between NK cell activity and lipoprotein levels was examined cross-sectionally in 41 samples of elderly male (mean age ± SD, 66.8 ± 1.7 years) who lived in the same community and underwent a medical check. NK cell activity was assayed by release of 51Cr from K562 target cells. Total cholesterol and high density lipoprotein (HDL) were measured by enzymatic techniques. Triglyceride was measured by H_2O_2 colorimetric assay after elimination of free glycerol. Low-density lipoprotein (LDL) was calculated using the Friedewald equation. Apolipoproteins were measured by immunoturbidimetric method. RESULTS: Simple regression analyses revealed direct relations between NK cell activity and HDL ($r = 0.42$, $p < 0.01$), Apo A-1 ($r = 0.48$, $p < 0.005$) and Apo A-2 ($r = 0.34$, $p < 0.05$). Multiple regression analyses showed independent direct relation between NK cell activity and Apo A-1 ($b = 0.36 \pm 0.11$, $b = 0.48$). CONCLUSION: It is concluded that NK cell activity is related directly to plasma Apo A-1 level in elderly subjects. The mechanisms of this association are unknown, but Apo A-1 is contributed to the composition of the anti-atherogenic fraction of HDL and could also potentiate the NK cell activity.

[61] Evaluation of Thyroid Function and Autoimmunity in Elderly Patients in an Acute Geriatric Unit

A.Lemma,E.Gvozdenovich,O.Levalle,G.Maccallini,A.Tropea,C.Aranda(Unidad de Geriatria,Division Endocrinologia,Hospital General de Agudos Carlos G.Durand,Buenos Aires,Argentina)

PURPOSES:To assess thyroid function in a group of elderly hospitalized patients and to compare it with a group of independent elders. To assess the incidence of thyroid autoimmunity measuring thyroid peroxidase antibodies (aTPO) and of elevated TSH levels in hospitalized patients. To find an association between thyroid function and illness degree. METHOD: Subjects:A:327 hospitalized patients, aged 60-101,201 women,126 men who were divided in two groups (1) those whose clinical condition allowed their treatment in the gerontology unit and (2) those who required an intensive care unit. Blood samples were taken on their first day of admission. B: 35 independent elders who live in their own home, 27women, 8 men, aged 63-90. Measurements:TSH, T4, FT4, T3 and aTPO. RESULTS: Thyroid function results expressed as median and range: n TSH UI/ml FT4 ng/ml WOMEN 201 1.50 (0.01-28) a 1.15 (0.2-5) d MEN 126 1.73 (0.04-57) b 1.15 (0.2-5.8) e GROUP B 35 2.50 (0.51-8.24) c 1.15 (0.71-2.15) f a and b vs c; d and e vs f :p ns. The presence of aTPO is expressed as positivity index (PI), and aTPO serum level greater than 1UI/ml was considered a positive result. PI = 37% in women; PI = 18.2% in men. Elevated TSH levels were present in 13% of women and in 15% of men, with 46% and 37% positive aTPO respectively; showing that 5.8% of all patients had both elevated TSH and aTPO. Neither TSH nor FT4 or T3 proved any significant difference between subgroups (1) and (2). CONCLUSIONS: No significant changes were found in the biochemical thyroid evaluation between hospitalized and outdoor patients. We found a high prevalence of thyroid autoimmunity and a 2:1 women:men ratio by measuring aTPO.

[62] Autologous transfusion in the elderly in Japan

T. Kumakawa, M. Teratani, N. Takahashi, H. Sekiguchi, K. Inaba. (Department of Blood Transfusion, Tokyo Metropolitan Geriatrics Hospital, Tokyo , Japan.)

Transfusion of autologous blood averts some of the problems encountered with heterologous transfusion such as febrile and allergic reactions, immunological incompatibility, immunization, immunosuppression, and the transmission of infections such as viral hepatitis and HIV. With the recognition that HIV can be transmitted by blood transfusion, the practice of autologous transfusion has grown considerably in recent years. While each country's population is aging very quickly in the world, the age of patients for autologous transfusion is increasing. We discuss here 103 cases of autologous transfusion in elderly J patients (18 male and 85 female, and their average age was 73.2 years old. Average volume of autologous blood collected pre-operatively was 800ml. Recombinant erythropoietin and oral iron have been tried in all cases. There were no untoward effects in any of these cases. In conclusion, autologous transfusion is possible and safe for the elderly in Japan.

[63] Hypogammaglobulinemia in the Elderly

Hélène BULCKAEN ; Emmanuel BULCKAEN ; François PUISIEUX ; Philippe DEWAILLY (hôpital Gériatrique les Bâteliers, CHRU Lille, France)

Purpose : Althrough fortuitous discovery of hypogammaglobulinemia (hg) is frequent in the elderly, very few studies have focused on diagnosis and prognosis of this biological disorder. The aim of this study was to determine prevalence and etiologies of hg in elderly inpatients. Method : a prospective study was carried out during nine months in our geriatric unit. At the admission, all inpatients had blood protein electrophoresis. When gammaglobulins were found under 6.6g/l, immunological, nutritional and viral makers were achieved. Control patients, matched for age and sex were recruited simultaneously from our department. Patients and controls were followed up during a mean period of 9±3 months. Results : 37 (6.8%) patients aged over 65 years exhibited hg during period of the study. 33 patients, 11 men and 22 women (mean age 82.7±7 yr) were involved in this study. 4 patients declined to participate. We discovered a classical etiology only in 12 patients. The gammaglobulins level was 5.7±0.9g/l (range 3.2 to 6.6 g/l) in the group of 21 inpatients without etiology of hypogammaglobulinemia (hg group) versus 10±2.7g/l in the control group (p<0.0001). Positive correlations were found in hg group between gammaglobulins level and mininutritional assessment (MNA) (p=0.01) and between gammaglobulins level and the body mass index (p=0.01). The MNA was significantly different between the 2 groups. During the following period, infectious occured 4/17 patients and 1/21 control. Comments : hg is frequent in the elderly but etiology remained undetermned in 650f hg despite large investigations. Our study suggest that this hg 1) may result from nutritional causes, in particular a deficiency in micronutrients, 2) may be a maker of undernutrition to correct to decrease the risk of infectious disease.

[64] Primary Sjogren's syndrome in the elderly: clinical and immunological characteristics

AL Fauchais MD(1), PY Hatron MD(1), H Bulckaen MD(2), U Pasturel MD(1), F Puisieux MD(2), E Hachulla MD(1), B Devulder PhMD(1) 1 Internal medicine department 2 Geriatric department University hospital of Lille, 59000 France

Purpose : the objective of the study was to determine clinical and immunological characteristics of primary Sjogren's syndrome (pSS) in patients with an older onset of the disease Method : retrospective study Results : we included 153 patients (142 female) that were retrospectively studied in our unit. All patients fulfilled four or more of European Community Criteria proposed in 1996 for the diagnosis of pSS. In 28 patients, the onset of the disease occured after the age of 65 years, and they represent the elderly group described in this report. Of the 28 (18%) patients with elderly onset of pSS, 25 were female and 3 male and the disease onset occured between 65 and 82 years (mean 70+/- 4). Parotid swelling were more commun in yong group; althouth Raynaud's phenomena and intertitial pulmonar involvement were higher in young group, prevalence of hematologic manifestations was higher in elderly group. The immunological features were similar in the two groups, except for SSb, more commun in young onset group. Conclusion: pSS is not uncommun in elderly and should be carrefully diagnose in this age group characterised by frequent idiopathic sicca syndrome.

[65] T-lymphocytes-regulators of somatic cells growth deficient as aging mechanism

V. Dontsov (National Gerontology Center, Moscow, Russia)

Purpose: Purpose: The analysis of series of experimental facts indicates on ability of T-lymphocytes to regulate the growth, regeneration and self-renovation of nonimmune - somatic cells of any tissues of organism. These facts requires the close theoretical and experimental study this problem. Material and methods: Both the theoretical computer models of interaction of several proliferated cells in evolution aspects, and experimental models on mice were used: the lymphocytes regulation of: liver regeneration; mice and rat submandibular salivary glands hyperplasia on isoproterenol injection (Seljefenomenon) and tumour growth and the immune reaction as these processes interferention. Results: Isolated T-lymphocytes were investigated by methods of cell and molecular biology and immunology. The review of references and our researches has shown, that specific T-lymphocytes subpopulations are able to stimulate and suppress the growth of somatic cells of different tissues types by somaticcells regulating growth factors secretion. Specific effects (specific regeneration memory etc.) and non-specific effects (different types cells growth interaction etc.) has been shown. These cells may be isolated by various methods and in detail to characterize. The influences of some immunopharmacology agents on these cells permit to influence the somaticcells growth processes. The decrease of such T-cells function with age can be important for ageing processes, especially for sel-renovated tissue consisted of proliferated somatic cells. Conclusion: It permits to think about the existence of specific, separate from immune, system in organisms. The main purpose of this system existence, represented by some T-lymphocytes subpopulation, is to regulate cell-to-cell interaction during different types cell proliferation and tissue growth. The decrease of function of these cells with age to determine the decrease of cell self-renovation and growth potention decrease in old organism.

[66] Gastroduodenal tuberculosis : unusual presentations in the elderly - report of two cases

JF Desson, A Vandevoir, M Benoist, M Alix (Department of Geriatric Medicine, Cote de Nacre Hospital, Caen, FRANCE), F Vabret, A Davy (Department of General Medicine, Clemenceau Hospital, Caen, FRANCE)

Case 1 : A 72-old male patient, treated for chronic lymphoid leukemia, had mild and sustained fever and loss of weight. Clinical examination, laboratory data and chest radiography were normal. Gastric endoscopy revealed an ulcer of the antrum, with histological evidence of tuberculous lesions. Stomach fluid analysis was positive for Mycobacterium tuberculosis (MT). Antituberculous agents were given and progressively effective in a few months. Case 2 : Loss of weight and weakness occured, for a few weeks, by a 65-old male, paraplegic patient, associated with diarrhea. Microbiological samples for MT were negative. Systematic biopsies were performed, despite normal macroscopic aspect of the duodenum and revealed typical tuberculous lesions without villous atrophy. Antituberculous treatment was initiated and proved to be effective. Gastroduodenal tuberculosis is uncommon in developped countries and especially affects the immunocompromised patients. Diagnosis is difficult when only digestive tract is affected. Mycobacterium tuberculosis is isolated in only 50 percent of the cases. Dramatical outbreak of MT favours unusual presentations of tuberculosis. In our experience, systematic investigations for gastroduodenal tuberculosis seems to be justified in case of impaired healthy state in the immunocompromised elderly people

[67] The Clinical Analysis of 150 Cases of Brain Infarction

Sun Shuling, Duan Dongmei

We use svate, weinaolutong, tanshin, ligustrazine and CoA Synthetically to treat 150 cases of patients with brain infarction of pre-senile and senile period.

[68] Copper requirements estimated from serum copper levels in female elderly inpatients

N.Saito, S.Ootani, H.Kushihashi, H.Nagatomo, S.Saito, I.Nakajima, T.Murata, M.Kawahara and K.Uchino (Miyazaki Aiwa Hospital, Miyazaki City, Japan)

Purpose: Inpatients with long-term tube nutrition were often accompanied with hypocupremia, because of a few copper (Cu) contents. Therefore, Cu-rich liquid foods such as milk cocoa or Ensure liquid were supplemented to tube nutrition in ones with hypocupremia. When serum Cu was improved to near normal range (70 to 132 ug/dl), total Cu intakes were estimated as the requirement volumes. Method: Six female elderly inpatients with hypocupremia were recruited, who were aged 78.+/-9.9 years (M+/-SD). Milk cocoa and Ensure liquid were supplemented to tube nutrition. Fasting blood sample was obtained early in the morning for measuring serum Cu using colorimetry. These inpatients were suffered from cerebrovascular lesions and dysphagia, resulting in disturbed physical movement. Results: Serum Cu changes were investigated in 6 cases. Case 1 : 85 years old(yo), serum Cu increased from 15 ug/dl to 74 ug/dl by total 0.298/day of Cu intake in period of 4 months(M). Case 2 : 71 yo, from 15 ug/dl to 91 ug/dl by 0.298 in 4M. Case 3 : 88 yo, from 18 ug/dl to 76 ug/dl by 0.37 in 2.5M. Case 4 : 87 yo, from 34 ug/dl to 77 ug/dl by 0.299 in 2M. Case 5 : 64 yo, from 31 ug/dl to 110 ug/dl by 0.247 in 5M. Case 6 : 74 yo, from 18 ug/dl to 68 ug/dl by 0.279 in 2M. As the summary serum Cu increased from 21.8+/-8.4 ug/dl to 82.7+/-15.4 ug/dl by 0.299+/-0.04?/may in 3.3+/-1.2M. The average value was estimated as average requirement. By addition of the two SD to the mean volume, the recommended allowance was calculated to be 0.38 mg/day of Cu intake. Conclusion: The recommended allowance of Cu intake was estimated to be 0.38 mg/day in female elderly inpatients with tube nutrition, showing a low volume of Cu intake.

{69} Effect of Melatonin on the Life Span and Biological Age Markers in CBA Mice

N.Yu. Zavarzina, I.G. Poplovich, A.V. Shtylik, M.A. Zabezhinski, O.A. Zimina, V.N. Anisimov (Petrov Research Institute of Oncology, St. Petersburg, Russia)

Method: 100 female CBA mice were randomly subdivided into 2 groups (50 mice per group) and starting at the age of 6 months, one of the group were exposed to melatonin with drinking water (20 mg/l) during night time 5 consecutive days monthly until the their natural death. Body weight and temperature, food consumption, estrus function, locomotor activity, physical strenght, survival and tumore pathology have been monitored during all periods of observation. Results: It was shown that body weight gain and food consumption were similar in the control and melationin mice. As compared with the control group, the body weight of mice treated with melatonin was increased at the age of 15, 18, and 21 months. Melatonin did not change the muscle strenght evaluated in wire hang test. The rectal body temperature did not change with age in the control mice, whereas significantly decreased in the melatonin-treated mice. The treatment with melatonin resulted in the decrease in locomotor activity of animals at the age of 6 and 9 months as compared with the controls. The administration of melatonin slowed down the aging of the estrus function. The survival dynamics were similar in the control and melatonin mice from 6th to 23rd months of their life and then was reduced in the melatonin-treated group. The maximum life span was increased by 2 months in the mice treated with melatonin as compared with the control. The treatment with melatonin was followed by an increase in the incidence of lymphomas and lung adenocarcinomas. Conclusion: Our data suggest that melatonin should not be recommended as a potent geroprotector.

SESSION 323

Creating the National Framework on Aging

Dave Arsenault (Director, Seniors Policy and Programs, Community Development, Government of Alberta)

The development of the National Framework on Aging, under the direction of the Federal/Provincial/Territorial Ministers Responsible for Seniors, was developed to respond to the needs of an aging population. This presentation will outline how the NFA was developed and how it has evolved over the last few years into a tool for the design and development of programs and services that meet seniors needs.

National Framework on Aging: The Canadian Experience

Dave Arsenault (Director, Seniors Policy and Programs, Community Development, Government of Alberta) Creating the National Framework on Aging; Ann-Marie Julien (Division of Aging and Seniors, Health Canada) The Seniors Policies and Programs Database; Provincial representative (not yet identified) The NFA in Action: Making a difference in policy and program development

ISSUE: The National Framework on Aging is a tool to assist in the development of programs and policies that are responsive to seniors and an aging population. STRUCTURE: Conduct a session on the National Framework on Aging, highlighting the potential use of the framework and the Database in the development of responsive policies and programs. CONTENT: The National Framework on Aging is a voluntary framework to assist in guiding current and future policy development related to seniors and aging issues. The Federal/Provincial/Territorial Ministers Responsible for Seniors requested the development of the Framework to assist them in responding to the needs of an aging population. The Framework includes a vision statement and five principles developed in consultation with Canadian seniors and approved by Ministers. A Policy Guide has been developed to support these principles. The newest component of the National Framework on Aging is the Seniors Policies and Programs Database which is an innovative, fully bilingual Database providing current information on a wide range of Federal/ Provincial/Territorial policies, programs, and services designed for seniors, in areas such as health, housing and income support. The Database allows individual policy analysts, program developers and researchers in every jurisdiction access to a resource that can help them review and develop policies and programs for seniors. This workshop session will be a mechanism for providing a progress report on the development of the NFA, including its key elements: the Policy Guide and the Database. This session will explore how the tools of the National Framework on Aging can and have been used, from the perspectives of different jurisdictions, to move towards its vision "Canada, a society for all ages, promotes the well-being and contribution of older people in all aspects of life". CONCLUSIONS: Better understanding of how Canada is contributing to the health and well-being of older Canadians by incorporating a broad based, voluntary approach to meeting seniors needs.

The National Framework on Aging in Action

Provincial Representative from the Committee of Officials (Seniors)

This workshop presentation will explore how the tools of the National Framework on Aging can and have been used, from the perspectives of different jurisdictions, to move towards its vision "Canada, a society for all ages, promotes the well-being and contribution of older people in all aspects of life".

The Seniors Policies and Programs Database

Ann-Marie Julien (Division of Aging and Seniors, Health Canada)

The newest component of the National Framework on Aging is the Seniors Policies and Programs Database which is an innovative, fully bilingual Database providing current information on a wide range of Federal/ Provincial/Territorial policies, programs, and services designed for seniors, in areas such as health, housing and income support. The Database allows individual policy analysts, program developers and researchers in every jurisdiction access to a resource that can help them review and develop policies and programs for seniors.

SESSION 324

Pushing back the limits of early diagnosis of Alzheimer's Disease

Karen Ritchie (INSERM, Montpelier, France) "What is Mild Cognitive Impairment", David Bennett (Rush Presbyterian St. Luke's Medical Center, Chicago, U.S.A.) "Clinical and Pathological Features of older persons with Mild Cognitive Impairment", Hyman Schipper (McGill University, Montreal, Canada) " Heme Oxygenase-1: A Novel Biomarker of Early Sporadic AD" Gary Small (University of California, Los Angeles, U.S.A.) "Using Brain Imaging for Preclinical Detection of Alzheimer's Disease." Howard Chertkow (McGill University, Montreal, Canada) "Low and High Tech Approaches to the early diagnosis of Alzheimer's Disease". Organized by Howard Chertkow

Issue: More than a dozen agents are currently under development for preventative treatment of Alzheimer' s disease (AD). The critical time to initiate such therapy is at the earliest stages of AD, but exactly when can AD be accurately detected? In this symposium, we will focus on the stage of Mild Cognitive Impairment that in many cases precedes AD, and on our increasing ability to reliably diagnose future AD even before clinical dementia is clearly present. Structure: Five speakers from North America and Europe will present various aspects of mild Alzheimer's Disease, Mild Cognitive Impairment (MCI) and preclinical diagnosis, focussing on the natural history of mild memory loss in the elderly and diagnostic markers that can be used to predictu which MCI individuals will progress to AD. Content: Karen Ritchie will describe studies in France to delineate subgroups of MCI, with differing prognoses. The opposing view that all subjects with MCI will progress to AD will also be presented. David Bennet will focus on clinical/pathological correlation studies carried out in MCI individuals who were part of the Religious Orders Study in Chicago. Participants in this study underwent longitudinal cognitive assessment and post-mortem examination. Results suggest that MCI is an intermediate stage between normal and AD in terms of the course of cognitive decline and the severity of brain pathology encountered. Hyman Schipper will discuss his own work with heme oxygenase 1 (HO-1), a serum marker for early AD, along with other blood, urine, and CSF biomarkers of promise. HO-1 may provide a sensitive marker even at the MCI stage. Gary Small will review novel imaging studies of non-demented elderly subjects which, when combined with APO-E genotype, offer the possibility of pre-clinical detection of early AD. Howard Chertkow will review the possibility that in the future, complementary use will be made of low tech markers (clinical, cognitive, and neuropsychological) along with high tech markers (anatomic and functional imaging, neuroendocrine cortisol measures, smell detection, and spectroscopy) in order to stratify risk of progression in MCI individuals.. Conclusions: It is hoped that the audience will come away with a better understanding of the "pre- Alzheimer's state" of mild memory loss and its current taxonomic uncertainties. Attendees will be presented with the current landscape in terms of promising experimental approaches to diagnosing AD at the preclinical and MCI state.

Classification of Mild cognitive impairment, and how this determines the significance of this entity

Karen Ritchie (INSERM, Montpelier, France) "What is Mild Cognitive Impairment",

PURPOSE: This presentation will discuss the taxonomy of Mild Cognitive Impairment (MCI). MCI has been proposed as a nosologic entity referring to elderly persons with subclinical cognitive deficits due to incipient dementia. Classification criteria, which have been derived from small, selected clinical groups, are currently disputed, and have not yet been assessed within the general population. METHOD: Subjects meeting current criteria for MCI and also age-associated cognitive decline (AACD a similar concept that is assumed to be related to normal cognitive aging processes rather than incipient dementia) were identified within each of three waves of a longitudinal population study, which included a standardized neurologic examination. RESULTS: In the general population, the prevalence of MCI was estimated to be 3.2% and AACD 19.3%. MCI was a poor predictor of dementia within a 3-year period, with an 11.1% conversion rate. Subjects with MCI also constituted an unstable group, with almost all subjects changing category each year. Discriminant function analysis failed to isolate a homogeneous clinical group. Subjects classified as AACD, contrary to the theoretical assumptions underlying the disorder, represented a more stable group, with a 28.6% conversion rate to dementia over 3 years (relative risk = 21.2). CONCLUSIONS: MCI criteria perform poorly when applied to a representative population sample. Modifications to current diagnostic criteria are proposed to increase their capacity to detect incipient dementia

Clinical and Pathological Features of older persons with Mild Cognitive Impairment

David Bennett (Rush Presbyterian St. Luke's Medical Center, Chicago, U.S.A.)

PURPOSE: Older persons display a spectrum of cognitive abilities ranging from normal, to Mild Cognitive Impairment, to dementia. The extent to which Mild Cognitive Impairment represents the earliest manifestations of the pathology of Alzheimer's disease is unknown. METHOD: More than 850 older nuns, priests, and brothers participating in the Religious Orders Study underwent annual evaluation for an average of more than 5 years. Cognitive performance tests were summarized to yield a composite measure of episodic memory and a global measure of other cognitive abilities. Starting levels and rates of cognitive decline were estimated with repeated measures random effects models. Cox proportional hazards models were used to compare risk of developing Alzheimer's disease among those with mild cognitive impairment to those without cognitive impairment. Post-mortem data were analyzed from 100 persons. The neuropathologic indices of Alzheimer's disease were summarized to yield a composite measure of Alzheimer's disease pathology. Linear regression was used to examine the relation of Alzheimer's disease pathology to diagnostic group, to level of cognitive function proximate to death, and to the slope of cognitive decline prior to death. RESULTS: The starting levels and slopes of decline in episodic memory and global cognition among persons with mild cognitive impairment were intermediate to that of persons with Alzheimer's disease and no cognitive impairment, with the latter group not showing significant decline. Overall, persons with mild cognitive impairment were more than 4 times as likely to develop Alzheimer's disease than persons without cognitive impairment. Persons with mild cognitive impairment had levels of pathology similar to those persons with Alzheimer's disease. The relation of Alzheimer's disease pathology to level and rate of decline of episodic memory was stronger than its relation to level and rate of decline global cognition. CONCLUSIONS: Loss of cognitive function, especially episodic memory, is often due to the pathology of Alzheimer's disease, even among persons without clinically diagnosed dementia. These data suggest that the public health importance of Alzheimer's disease is much larger than currently recognized. Supported by the National Institute on Aging, RO1AG15819, P30AG10161, PO1AG14449.

Heme Oxygenase-1: A Novel Biomarker of Early Sporadic AD

Hyman Schipper (McGill University, Montreal, Canada) ,

PURPOSE: Developing biomarkers that can aid in the diagnosis of early Alzheimer's Disease, even at the stage of Mild Cognitive Impairment, represent a current challenge to neuroscientists. This presentation will review the current experimental status of CSF, blood, and urine biomarkers, focussing on our recent work with Heme oxygenase-1 (HO-1). HO-1 is a 32 kDa stress protein that catalyzes the degradation of heme to biliverdin in brain and other tissues. METHOD: Immunostaining techniques were applied to human brain tissue from AD individuals subjects and compared to normal control specimens matched for age and post-mortem interval. Subsequently, blood lymphocyte HO-1 mRNA levels were measured in subjects with AD, normal elderly, MCI, and a variety of neurological and medical disorders. RESULTS: We demonstrated increased HO-1 immunoreactivity in neurons and astrocytes of post-mortem hippocampus and temporal cortex derived from AD subjects. Furthermore, we have demonstrated colocalization of HO-1 protein to neurofibrillary tangles and senile plaques in AD specimen. In contrast to the over-expression of HO-1 in AD brain, we observed that blood lymphocyte HO-1 mRNA levels are significantly suppressed in subjects with probable sporadic AD relative to normal elderly controls (NEC) and patients with other neurological and medical conditions. Furthermore, lymphocyte HO-1 mRNA levels in individuals with mild cognitive impairment (MCI) were intermediate between those of the AD and NEC subjects. CONCLUSIONS: Our findings indicate that peripheral HO-1 gene suppression is a very early event in the natural history of sporadic AD and a potentially useful biological marker of this condition.

Low and High Tech Approaches to the early diagnosis of Alzheimer's Disease

Howard Chertkow (McGill University, Montreal, Canada)

PURPOSE: The natural history of Mild Cognitive Impairment , and in particular, the chances of developing dementia over longitudinal follow-up remains unclear. There are few reliable predictors for the chances of developing dementia over longitudinal follow-up in MCI. METHOD: We followed 90 elderly subjects over a mean follow-up period of 38 months. All received detailed clinical, neuropsychological, genetic, and imaging assessments. This included a detailed evaluation of time of onset of symptoms. A large battery of cognitive reaction time markers, along with MRI volumetric measurements of hippocampal volume and atrophy were carried out as well . RESULTS: At end of follow-up period, 51 subjects had deteriorated to dementia, and 39 had not. Kaplan-Meier curve analysis indicated a decline to dementia rate initially of about 15% of the subjects per year, but also indicated that even 10 years after onset of symptoms, 30% of the cohort would remain non-demented. Presence or absence of Apo-E4 genotype, a risk factor for Alzheimer's Disease, had no significant bearing on decline to dementia over follow-up. It was found that an algorithm with seven cut-off scores accurately stratified risk of progression. Critical factors were Age, MMSE, logical memory 1 and 2, lexical decision reaction time, trigram recall on the Brown Peterson task of working memory, and an atrophy ratio measure from the MRI results. Subjects who exceeded none of the cutoff score had 0% chance of progression to dementia (ie, AD) while those exceeding three cut-off scores had a 100% chance of progressing. CONCLUSIONS: There appears to be a subgroup (about 1/4 of MCI subjects) who will not deteriorate to dementia over long-term follow-up of up to 10 years from onset of symptoms. It appears feasible to design an initial practical "low tech" approach for physicians to use with MCI patients to stratify risk of progression, along with a complimentary "high tech" assessment valid for stratifying "uncertain" cases. This will allow physicians to better select elderly individuals for future preventative therapies for AD. Supported by the FRSQ, the Alzheimer's Society of Canada, and the CIHR (Canadian Institutes of Health Research).

Using Brain Imaging for Preclinical Detection of Alzheimer's Disease

Gary Small (University of California, Los Angeles, U.S.A.)

PURPOSE: This presentation describes three novel brain imaging strategies for preclinical Alzheimer's disease (AD) detection. METHOD: (1) Measures of relative cerebral blood flow (rCBF) were obtained using functional magnetic resonance imaging (fMRI) while older non-demented subjects memorized and retrieved unrelated word pairs. (2) Cerebral metabolic rates using positron emission tomography (PET) were measured during mental rest in non-demented older persons. (3) A novel radiofluorinated derivative of 1,1-dicyano-2-[6-(dimethylamino)-naphthalen-2-yl] propene (FDDNP) was utilized to visualize neurofibrillary tangle and senile plaque in AD brain. The genetic profile of apolipoprotein E (APOE-4) was also assessed in each individual. RESULTS: Subjects with the apolipoprotein E-4 (APOE-4) genetic risk for AD showed significantly greater rCBF during memory retrieval in regions affected by AD. (2) APOE-4 was associated with lowered inferior parietal, lateral temporal, and posterior cingulate cortical metabolism, which predicted cognitive and metabolic decline two years later. (3) FDDNP provided excellent neurofibrillary tangle and senile plaque visualization in AD brain, matching thioflavin results from the same specimens. Areas of low glucose metabolism (FDG-PET) matched areas of high FDDNP activity retention (particularly entorhinal, medial temporal regions) in AD. CONCLUSIONS: Functional brain imaging has the capacity to aid in preclinical detection of AD.

SESSION 325

Reconsidering the Roles of the State and Family in Providing Care for the Frail Elderly

Betty Havens (University of Manitoba, Winnipeg, Canada)("Policies That Have Positive or Negative Impacts on Informal Care in Canada") Taewha Lee (College of Nursing, Yonsei University, Seoul, Korea) ("Caregiving for the Frail Elderly in Korea: Who Provides the Care, How Much Care and Cost of Care") Katie Maslow (Alzheimer's Association, Washington D.C, USA) ("Respective Roles of Families and Government in Care of People with Dementia in the US") Brenda Morginstin (National Insurance Institute, Jerusalem, Israel) ("Emerging Issues in the Development of Family-Supported Long-Term Care") Judith Phillips (Centre for Social Gerontology, University of Keele, Keele, England) ("The Shifting Balance of Responsibility for Older People and Carers in Britain")

Issue: Changes in family structure, the increasing proportion of women in the labor market, and the declining ratio between those needing care and potential caregivers are raising questions about the family's ability to care for the elderly and disabled. However, it is most likely that the informal network, which supplies the bulk of input in the elderly care sector, will continue to be an essential component of the system of care. Therefore, just as it is important to address the needs of the elderly, it is also essential to address the needs of family caregivers. The support for informal carers is a necessary prerequisite to motivate people to go on caring for their elderly family members and to contribute to the "normalization" of their lives. Structure: Presentations will focus on different approaches taken by five countries with different cultural and socio-political backgrounds (USA, Korea, England, Canada and Israel) and will discuss the dilemmas confronting their systems of formal and informal care of the elderly Summary: Major changes in Korean society call for new policies that expand the role of the sate in the care of vulnerable populations such as the disabled elderly. New governmental endeavors will be discussed. Of major concern in the USA is the growth in the numbers of people with dementia. The development of governmental programs to pay for home and community-based care has been hindered by the unsubstantiated fear of substitution of government-funded services for unpaid family care. One major issue, discussed from the British perspective, is the balance between family and work responsibilities. Developing flexible family and workplace support is crucial for enabling families to continue to provide support for the frail elderly while enabling caregivers to fulfill work obligations and careers. Supportive services, such as home care for the frail and disabled are relatively well developed in Canada. However, much variation exists among the Canadian Provinces, which have significant implications for the informal system of care. The importance of the development of national policies will be discussed. In Israel, the Community Long-Term Care Insurance Law represented a change in the perception with regard to the responsibility of care, now viewed more as a shared responsibility between the family and the State. However, future developments will need to consider more profoundly the changing needs of the family and consider different directions to reinforce the family such as providing more choice and flexibility. Conclusion: The emerging issues related to family care of the elderly include the overriding needs of family caregivers for training and information, as well as the need for supportive services such as respite care, consumer directed care, and balance between family and work obligations. Some countries are more advanced than others in recognizing and addressing family needs. These countries may offer ideas and policies that could assist policy makers and service providers to strengthen the informal system of care and find a more appropriate balance between family and state responsibility for the care of frail elderly.

Caregiving for the Frail Elderly in Korea: Who Provides the Care, How Much Care and Cost

Taewha Lee (College of Nursing, Yoinsei University, Seoul, Korea)

Korea is undergoing changes such as globalization, the onset of the information age, a trend toward decentralization, and the possible reunification of the Korean peninsula. Traditional family ties and mutual cooperation in communities have diminished. The changing family structure, and the growing trend toward nuclear families, call for national policies dealing with these social changes. Many of the welfare functions once carried out under the extended family system have now fallen upon the government and local communities. The social insurance system, which substitutes for the weakened private support system, has begun moving in a more desirable direction. The Korean government has established the Elderly Health and Welfare Policy Committee in which many experts of private and public institutions have been developing policies to improve the quality of life of the elderly by expanding health service coverage and home help services. The following issues will be explored: who requires care, who are the formal and informal caregivers, who pays for the care, what are the direct and indirect costs and benefits of family caregiving in Korea. Korean government health care policies that deal with and protect frail elderly from economic destruction and other disadvantages are not fully established. These problems are a major obstacle to securing long-term balanced development and social integration. In the 21st century, the creation of a new paradigm is required, which is capable of harmonizing government and family roles in caring for the elderly, and building a safety net for this vulnerable population.

Emerging Issues in the Development of Family-Supported Long-Term Care

Brenda Morginstin (National Insurance Institute, Jerusalem, Israel) Jenny Brodsky (JDC-Brookdale Institute, Jerusalem, Israel)

The overwhelming majority of Israel's elderly reside at home with family network providing the backbone of care. Israel's Community Long-Term Care Insurance Law (CLTCI), providing home care for some 12% of the elderly, has changed perceptions with regard to the responsibility of care, now viewed as a shared responsibility between the family and the State. In planning future developments the long-term care system will need to recognize the evolving needs andexpectations of family caregivers in order to encourage continued family support. Some of the current issues include: - Services in kind or cash: Although the CLTCI program provides in-kind services, the question of whether cash benefits would be more effective in meeting the needs, continues to be a subject ofdebate. Current research, comparing similar elderly groups, who either receive cash benefits under Disability Insurance, or in-kind services under CLTCI, will provide new insights as to differential preferences, patterns of service acquisition, and degree of family involvement for these two groups. - Contracting agencies quality of care and choice:Services are provided by for-profit and non-profit agencies (65% and 35% respectively). What is the role of the State in assuring quality of care? To what degree do families and elderly wish to exercise autonomy in choosing care provider agencies, as opposed to the more paternalistic model under which social workers assign the care agency? Recent research findings will be discussed. - Models of care for supporting family caregivers: Neighborhood support services, is an innovative model being developed in Israel. Possibilities of expanding this model, which seems to offer more flexibility in enhancing the partnership between formal and informal care, will be explored.

Policies That Have Positive or Negative Impacts on Informal Care in Canada

Betty Havens (University of Manitoba, Winnipeg, CANADA), Carol Donovan (Health Canada, Ottawa, CANADA) and Marcus Hollander, (Hollander Analytical Services Ltd, Victoria, CANADA)

PURPOSE: To describe some of the public policies that relate to providing care to frail elderly Canadians with specific reference to their impacts on family and other informal caregivers. Variations among Canadian Provinces are highlighted in these descriptions that relate primarily to provision of home care and to a lesser extent to long-term residential care across Canada. METHOD: An environmental scan of relevant policy statements and reports of informal caregivers across Canada was undertaken to identify similarities and differences that occur among provinces. RESULTS: The differences among provinces were greater than the similarities as the provincial jurisdiction over formal long-term care has led to unique responses to formal care provision and these variations have had differing impacts on family and other informal caregivers. CONCLUSION: Advantages and disadvantage of various provincial policies to providing care to frail elderly Canadians will be described in view of a grassroots movement to establish a national Canadian policy on long-term care, especially home care

Respective Roles of Families and Government in Care of People with Dementia in the U.S.

Katie Maslow (Alzheimer's Association, Washington)

In the United States, federal and state government programs pay for more than half of all medical care and nursing home care for people with Alzheimer's disease and other dementias (or elderly people and people with Alzheimer's disease and other dementias). Some in-home and community-based services are also paid for by government programs, but families provide most of this care, with huge expenditures of time and other resources. Awareness of the burden of caregiving has increased considerably in the U.S. in the past five years, but concerns about costs and unsubstantiated fears about possible substitution of government funded services for unpaid family care continue to hinder the development of government programs to pay for home and community-based care

The shifting balance of responsibility for older people and carers in Britain: the role of state, family and employers.

Judith Phillips (Centre for Social Gerontology, University of Keele)

In the promotion of community care, a specific policy objective in the UK is the empowerment of caregivers of frail older people. Traditionally the majority of formal provision to assist frail older people and family carers has come from the public sector. However, the state has had an ambiguous relationship with caregivers and contributed little specifically to maintaining carers in employment. There are increasing developments by employers themselves, which indicate a commitment to supporting carers in the workplace. If families are to continue to take on the primary care giving role then both state and employer support will be vital in helping them balancing work and family commitments. The paper is based on a review of the literature on the respective roles of working carers and their families, employers and the state in meeting the care needs of frail older people. Additionally the paper will draw on findings from a large-scale survey and in depth interviews with employees and managers in two large public sector organisations. Preliminary findings indicate the increasing importance of developing flexible family and workplace support. The findings will inform debate on the relative contribution of state, family and employer in supporting older people given demographic trends, workplace factors and social policy.

SESSION 327

A Comparison in Social Welfare Planning of the Newly Industrialized Countries and Australia

Yusnani Mohd Yusof (Department of Geographical Sciences and Planning, The University of Queensland, Brisbane, Australia)

PURPOSE: This paper discusses social welfare planning for the elderly in the newly industrialized countries, compares it to an industrialized country like Australia, and examines the differences that exist between them. METHOD: The social welfare policy matrix identifies gaps in the provision of health, social welfare, income security, housing and the environment in the newly industrialized countries. The focus of the finding is management-driven and is a definitive source for analyzing the extent of welfare for the elderly or its likely future. RESULTS: There exists a substantial difference between countries like Malaysia, Japan, Singapore and Australia. In Japan, the elderly enjoy comprehensive lifelong health lifestyles under the 'New Golden Plan', and in Malaysia 'Long Term Care Insurance' provides the elderly access to public health care but does not have mandatory care insurance. Welfare through income supports to individuals is available in Australia, while in Malaysia income supports are disbursed to the needy. CONCLUSION: Conceptualizing policy responses to the present and future social welfare needs of the elderly in the newly industrializing countries does not necessarily mirror those of the developed countries. However the gaps essentially provide a possible benchmark to support the formulation of new policies or the adjustments that are needed to ensure that the elderly population in newly industrialized countries live well into their old age.

'Can we grow older comfortably?, the case of the Netherlands'

Jan B. Kune

Purpose: to find out the economic and welfare implications of ageing in the Netherlands in the coming decades. Method: a simple economic model confronting future production capacity and national consumption expenditures. Findings: aging in the Netherlands will result in a smaller proportion of the population being employed in the decades after 2010/2020. Also the volume of pension savings will decrease. Under the plausible assumption that 2 percent yearly growth in per worker production can be realized in the coming two decades and 1 percent in the years after 2020, it is demonstrated that per capita consumption of the working population increases from 1995 to 2020 by 80.6 percent and that of the 65+ population by 125 percent. Only with a zero growth rate of labour productivity all the time average welfare will decrease by about 8 percent, whereas a minor 0.4 percent productivity growth with unchanged labour participation rate suffices to maintain welfare at its present level. More detailed findings are given in the paper. Conclusion: the Dutch society can adapt its economy succesfully and grow older comfortably in the 21th century.

From Public to Private? Recent developments in financing and service delivery in Sweden

Lennarth Johansson(National Bord of Health and Welfare, Stockholm, Sweden)

Until the 1990s, services and care for the elderly were predominantly financed and provided by the public in Sweden. However, due to a combination of reasons, i.e. the economic recession and attached cost containment, a liberal-right wing political shift in power, increased focus on users' empowerment and freedoom of choice implied a breakthrough in private alternatives of service delivery and a successive shift of costs over to the user. During the last decade, private run elder care has expanded steadily. From a one-percentage proportion of elder care in 1990 to roughly 7-8 percent of elder care in 2000. The services are contracted out to private (for-proffit) service providers. However eligibilty and access is still decided by the care manager in the municipality.One result of recent developments is that the competition has off course brougth an imperative to develope the services and care and issues such as targeting, service effectiveness and quality has been focused. On the other hand, recurrent shifts of providers has implied problems for both care personnel and care recipients. Increased fees for services has also forced some elderly to abstain from services do economic reasons. In conclusion: Recent developments of "privatization" of elder care seems to continue. New ideas of service delivery and financing are frequently discussed as well as the boundaries between public and private responsibilities for elder care. Issues regarding access, quality and costs for the user are increasingly beeing focused. The challenge for the future then, is whether one could strike a balance between the old and the new mixed model of elderly welfare in Sweden.

Social Policy Initiatives for an Aging Society: Implications for U.S. Fiscal Policy

James R. Storey (Congressional Research Service, Washington, DC, USA)

Official projections of U.S. Government finances indicate that short-term budget surpluses will give way to long-run deficits as population aging contributes to larger public benefit costs. Moreover, social problems associated with a rapidly aging population will generate pressure for benefit improvements over and above those associated with demographic trends. This paper analyzes the implications of these forces in terms of the likely size of budget resources that these social policy initiatives will require, the size of the budget shortfall under current law, and options for changing public policies to accommodate them. Attainment of desired social policy goals for the elderly in regard to retirement income, health care, housing, and long-term care will require some combination of a larger public sector relative to the national economy, strengthened private insurance markets, and increased saving for retirement.

The Canadian Report on Seniors: setting benchmarks for well-being

Patricia Raymaker, Chairperson, "National Advisory Council on Aging", Ottawa, Canada.

PURPOSE: Despite the availability of much information on seniors in Canada, there is a need to move a step beyond a description of indicators to monitoring and analyzing certain trends over time. The National Advisory Council on Aging has developed a bi-annual Report on Seniors to measure the status and progress of seniors' well-being in Canada through an analysis and comparison of key indicators over time from four major domains: health, wealth, social integration and living environment. The Report is intended to: · Monitor trends which are amenable to policy/program interventions. · Inform, support and evaluate policy and program development by identifying and anticipating emerging needs. · Advise and educate the public. · Create an advocacy tool and dispel myths. METHODS: A minimum set of indicators covering each policy domain for which regular, national-level data exist was determined in consultation with gerontologists and seniors' organizations. The data analysis and interpretative report were prepared by the Canadian Council for Social Development. Special attention was given to make the language and format accessible to a wide public. CONCLUSION: The report of seniors is expected to become an important tool for seniors advocates and policy-makers

The International Year of the Older Person in Israel: Did it Make an Impact?

Arnold Rosin (Chairman IYOP Committee, Ministry of Social Welfare, Jerusalem, Israel).

The United Nations declared 1999 as the International Year of the Older Person. Beyond the formal announcement, what was the practical aim, or the anticipated impact on society regarding the aged population? These questions will be examined in the light of the activities of the Year in Israel. The Minister of Labour and Social Affairs appointed a Public Committee comprising representatives from planning services, Ministries, academic institutions, NGO s and organizations working with aged. Sub-committees dealt with health, environmental issues, including dwellings, social and activity projects, and legal and economic aspects of aging in Israel. Ten local committees were organized throughout the country to plan and carry out events appropriate to the local population. The objectives were to give old people a platform for expressing their needs, demonstrate the creativity of older people, increase awareness of a positive image of the aged throughout the school system, draw attention of the legislature to economic issues in the field of housing, medications, long-term nursing care, and other social issues. Many of these objectives were achieved through joint planning such as with the Ministry of Education, interviewing Knesset (Parliamentary) Committees, publications and radio interviews. There were many special local events, such as conferences and workshops for the aged, public entertainments, often hosted by the mayors, exhibitions by schoolchildren and by adults of paintings or photographs on subjects of aged people, and an essay and poetry competition for the over-70 s on What is aging? This momentum has continued into the following years.

Who Benefits From Age Based Entitlement Programs?

John R. Gist [Public Policy Institute, AARP, Washington, DC]

ISSUE: Entitlement programs have become an ever-larger component of federal budget. Entitlement spending has been claimed to be skewed toward the affluent and blamed for the projected fiscal crisis occasioned by the retirement of the baby boomer cohorts. How real are the distributional claims and the concerns about the strains on the public budget? PURPOSE: To analyze the growth of different entitlement spending programs relative to growth in the economy, to identify the areas where growth is fastest, and to compare the distribution of entitlement spending benefits with the benefits from tax entitlements in recent years. RESULTS: The analysis shows that entitlement spending has not changed significantly as a percentage of GDP since the mid-1970s, despite rapid growth in health entitlements. The only real growth in entitlements as a percentage of GDP is in the area of health programs-Medicare and Medicaid. Social Security has remained at the same percentage of GDP for years, and other entitlement programs have grown slowly if at all. Although many entitlements are skewed toward the middle class, Social Security is almost as targeted on low-income people as are means-tested benefits. On the other hand, tax entitlement benefits are much more skewed toward the middle and upper classes than the largest spending entitlements. CONCLUSION: Entitlement spending shows no sign of overwhelming the ability of the economy to absorb the projected increased spending on baby boomers. While the retirement of the boomers will most certainly cause entitlement spending to increase, some estimates suggest that continued economic growth will allow us to absorb it without significant budgetary impacts.

SESSION 328

Multi-Nation Research on Ageing Well and Adult Well-Being: The Global Ageing Initiative

Barbara A. Hawkins (Center on Aging and Aged, Indiana University, Bloomington, USA) Round Table Convenor, Overview of Global Ageing Initiative and Ageing Well Research Project. Ingalill Rahm Hallberg (Department of Nursing, Lund University Sweden, Lund, Sweden) Findings from Sweden's Pilot Study of Ageing Well. Joseph Troisi (Institute of Gerontology and Geriatrics, University of Malta, Malta) Implications of UN Initiatives and Ageing Well Cross-Nation Research. Shashikant Karandikar (Centre for Gerontology and Elderly Medicine, Bharati Vidyapeeth Deemed University, Pune, India) Challenges of Ageing Well Research in Developing Countries - The India Experience. Vanessa Burholt (Centre for Social Policy Research and Development, University of Wales, Bangor, UK) The Challenges of EU Collaboration on Ageing Well Research. Carol Morse (Victoria University, School of Human Movement, Recreation and Performance, Melbourne, Australia) Funding Challenges for Australian Ageing Well Research. Barbara Masberg (Central Washington University, Ellensburg, USA) Discussant. Susan Feldman (Alma Unit for Research on Ageing, Victoria University, Melbourne, Australia) Discussant. Clare Wenger (Centre for Social Policy Research and Development, University of Wales, Bangor, UK) Discussant. Brian Winchester (Center for the Study of Global Change, Indiana University, Bloomington, USA) Discussant.

The Global Ageing Initiative is a collaborative international project involving more than 15 countries coordinated by a team at Indiana University. The Global Ageing Initiative research is responsive to the Ageing Well and Healthy Older People 21st Century Objectives as proposed by the United Nations. Through a coordinated program of social science research using an empirically-based model for ageing well our goal is to produce worldwide findings about the conditions that support healthy, productive, and active ageing. The ageing well model is based on the interactive processes between the environment (social, cultural, economic) and the individual (behavior and cognitive choices) as a means of measuring success and productivity in older adulthood. The contributions of five latent variables (physical health and functional status, cognitive efficacy, social support resources, life activity, and material security) on the outcome variable ageing well is under investigation within and across collaborating countries using cross-nation research methodology. The ultimate objective of this collaborative research is to apply the findings in policy analysis and community development that targets improvements in social context, economic circumstances, environmental conditions, available programs, public policies, and business practices that promote a positive, productive, and healthy ageing process. The focus of this Round Table is to present and discuss the possibilities, opportunities, challenges, and progress associated with doing a cross-nation study like the one undertaken by the Global Ageing Initiative. Presenters and discussants will report on the conceptual and methodological framework for the ageing well study, strategies and challenges associated with international collaborative research, findings from individual country pilot studies, and specific challenges in developing vs. developed countries. The Round Table will be structure as brief presentations by selected presenters (Hallberg, Troisi, Burholt, Morse, Karandikar, and Hawkins) enhanced by discussion from the discussants (Wenger, Masberg, Feldman, Winchester) and participants. Expected outcomes include (a) awareness of the Global Ageing Initiative and collaborating investigators; (b) information pertaining to the ageing well model; and (c) enhanced understanding of the challenges and advantages of cross-nation collaborative research that is aimed at producing findings to aid social gerontology theory development, practice enhancement, and policy analysis/development.

Challenges of Ageing Well Research in Developing Countries - The India Experience

Shashikant Karandikar (Centre for Gerontology and Elderly Medicine, Bharati Vidyapeeth Deemed University, Pune, India)

Dr. Karandikar will present an update on the progress and status of the ageing well research in India. He will interpret his findings within the challenges associated with collaborating on such research by developing countries. The presentation will include successful strategies and challenges for the future. Expected outcomes include (a) information associated with multi-nation research that involves more and less developed nations, (b) specific successes from the India partnership, and (c) challenges and recommendations for the future.

Funding Challenges for Australian Ageing Well Research

Carol Morse (Victoria University, School of Human Movement, Recreation and Performance, Melbourne, Australia)

Dr. Morse will describe the process of organizing the Australian collaborative team and the search for external funding to support the Australian study. She will provide case examples of how the Australian study utilized the cross-nation framework with embedded national initiatives and sub-study components to seek and obtain funding to support Australian research on adult well-being and the ageing well model. Expected outcomes from this presentation include (a) information on additional, country-specific sub-studies; (b) case examples of strategies for funding research that is part of a larger, worldwide initiative; and (c) insights on the challenges associated with funding the national component of an international project.

Implications of UN Initiatives and Ageing Well Cross-Nation Research

Joseph Troisi (Institute of Gerontology and Geriatrics, University of Malta, Malta)

Dr. Troisi will report on the progress of the Global Ageing Initiative's Ageing Well Research as it fits within the long range research plan of the

United Nations. He will discuss strategies for success, challenges to overcome, and recommendations for maximizing the impact of findings for world utilization and benefit. Outcomes from Dr. Troisi's presentation include (a) specific research questions from the Global Ageing Initiative's Ageing Well Research as matched with UN goals and objectives, (b) research methodology and procedures as developed by the Global Ageing Initiative Collaborating Investigators, and (c) specific examples of outcome findings as useful to UN planning and future initiatives.

Overview of the Global Ageing Initiative and Ageing Well Research Project

Barbara A. Hawkins (Center on Aging and Aged, Indiana University, Bloomington, USA)

Dr. Hawkins will open the Round Table with an overview of the development and overall design of the Global Ageing Initiative - Ageing Well Research Project. She will provide details on the theoretical framework and methodology guiding the research, as well as information pertaining to the collaborating nations and how the project evolved over the past three years. She will provide information on the study's instrumentation, data collection procedures, and outcomes from the first Working Conference of the Global Ageing Initiative held in June 2000. She will provide examples of project management strategies used by the cross-nation collaborative team of investigators that enhance overall project organization, ongoing communication, product development, and problem resolution. Outcomes from the presentation include (a) a general overview and orientation to the Global Ageing Initiative - Ageing Well Research Project; (b) introduction of the worldwide team of collaborating investigators; (c) encapsulation of progress, challenges, and future goals; and (d) methodological details pertaining to the multi-nation study.

Sweden's Pilot Study of Ageing Well

Ingalill Rahm Hallberg (Department of Nursing, Lund University Sweden, Lund, Sweden)

Dr. Hallberg will report findings from the Swedish pilot study pertaining to the Ageing Well Research project. The presentation will include information about survey instrument design and modifications, data collection training and procedures, preliminary results, recommendations for worldwide modifications to the multi-nation study, and strategies for enhancing cooperation and collaboration among collaborating nations. Outcomes from the presentations include (a) case example of pilot work and challenges associated with the multi-nation collaboration, (b) methodological challenges and issues confronting the multi-nation study, and (c) recommendations for world-wide cross-nation research on ageing and adult well-being.

The Challenges of EU Collaboration on Ageing Well Research

Vanessa Burholt (Centre for Social Policy Research and Development, University of Wales, Bangor, UK)

Dr. Burholt will chronicle and discuss the history of two years of working on building an EU collaboration in the Global Ageing Initiative - Ageing Well Research. She will outline the process and experiences with two EU applications, challenges associated with building EU multi-nation collaboration, and a report of the current status of the EU component of the world-wide project. Expected outcomes include (a) a case example of regional capacity building and collaboration from multi-nation research on ageing well, (b) recommendations for successful regional strategies, and (c) challenges for the future.

SESSION 329

Dynamic plantar pressure measurement as a new method for the remobilisation of elderly patients with partial weight-bearing on one lower limb

K.G. Gassmann, U. Runge (Department of Geriatric Medicine, Waldkrankenhaus St. Marien, Erlangen)

PURPOSE: In the aftercare of patients who underwent operations of the joints of the lower extremity a partial weight-bearing is often recommended for a period of several weeks. Due to various reasons many elderly patients can not appropriately apply partial weight-bearing on one limb only. This is a major cause for concern because the effects of full limb loading can lead to local complications. We studied for the first time whether dynamic insole plantar pressure measurement improves the compliance of postoperative patients with partial weight-bearing on one limb during ambulation. METHOD: Dynamic plantar pressure was measured in 15 geriatric patients (63 - 96 years). If the patient exceeds the preset weight limit (kp), an alarm will sound. Age, sex, weight, height, size, handgrip, MMS, acceptance of the method as well as compliance were recorded. RESULTS: The method is described. One third of the patients (n = 5) showed a good or very good compliance, 46% (n = 7) a moderate and 13% (n = 2) an unsatis- factory compliance with the required partial weight-bearing. A similar distribution of results was seen in the acceptance of the method. CONCLUSION: Dynamic in-shoe pressure measurement offers a new therapeutic option for the remobilisation of elderly patients who are not allowed to bear full weight on the operated limb. The majority of the patients accepts the new method and the compliance with the partial weight-bearing is improved.

Elderly Franco-Ontarians: Informed but Powerless With Regards to Physical Activity and Health

Hélène Dallaire (University of Ottawa, Ottawa, CANADA) Josianne Roma (University of Ottawa, Ottawa, CANADA) Geneviève Rail (University of Ottawa, Ottawa, CANADA) Suzanne Laberge (Université de Montréal, Montréal, CANADA) Philippe Voyer (Université Laval, Québec, CANADA)

This qualitative study was conducted with Francophone women aged 65 to 75 who were either physically active or inactive, and living in lower socio-economic conditions in the Ottawa-Carleton area. Data were gathered through individual interviews focussing on four main themes: the practice of physical activity, the perception of physical and human resources, the preferences with regards to physical activity, and the perceptions of physical activity, aging and health. Interview transcripts were content analysed using the NVivo software. The main results suggest that the participants know about the benefits of physical activity as it relates to health. For instance, they are aware that physical activity can slow down the aging process, diminish their sense of isolation and improve their self-esteem. However, the study also reveals a feeling of powerlessness among the participants when it comes to integrating physical activity in their daily lives. When they engage in physical activity, they do it out of a sense of obligation rather than for pleasure. Participants explain the various obstacles that contribute to their inactivity. The recommendations stemming from the study have been formulated with the intention of capitalizing on the participants knowledge of the benefits of physical activity. One of the main challenges resides in the formulation and implementation of novel solutions allowing elderly Francophone women to adopt physical activity as part of their lifestyle.

Mobility and Physical Activity as Predictors of Depressive Symptoms among Community-Dwelling Older Women

P. Lampinen, E. Heikkinen, R-L. Heikkinen (The Finnish Centre for Interdisciplinary Gerontology, and Department of Health Sciences, University of Jyväskylä, Jyväskylä, Finland)

PURPOSE: To examine associations of mobility status and physical activity with depressive symptoms among community-dwelling older women during an eight-year period. METHOD: As a part of the Evergreen project, two random samples each containing 800 community dwelling men and women aged 65-74 and 75-84 years were drawn from the local population register. At the baseline, in 1988, 78% (N=804) of the eligible women were interviewed. The follow-up interview was done in 1996 for 451 women representing 87% of those eligible in 1996. The 428 women who participated both at the baseline and in the follow-up interviews were selected for the analyses. Depressive symptoms were assessed using the modified Finnish version of Beck's 13-item depression scale. Physical activity was assessed on a seven-point scale ranging from the performance of necessary chores only to participation in competitive sports. Mobility status was operationalised as the ability to walk two kilometres and climb up a single flight of stairs. Participants were classified into four groups: 1. Mobile-Active, 2. Mobile-Sedentary, 3. Impaired-Active, and 4. Impaired-Sedentary. RESULTS: The women with impaired mobility had more depressive symptoms than those with intact mobility irrespective of the level of physical activity. Impaired mobility and physical inactivity, longstanding somatic illnesses and older age increased the risk of developing depressive symptoms during the follow-up period. The women with impaired mobility but active physical lifestyle had a lower risk for depressive symptoms compared to their more sedentary counterparts. CONCLUSION: Elderly women should be encouraged to prevent mobility problems through sufficient physical activity.

Physical Activity, Health Status and Depression among Older Adults in Canada

John Cairney (Brock University, St. Catharines, ON Canada) Brent E. Faught (Brock University, St. Catharines, ON Canada) John Hay (Brock University, St. Catharines, ON Canada) Robert Kerr (Brock University,St. Catharines, ON Canada)

PURPOSE: Epidemiological research suggests that physical activity may play an important role in the management of mild-to-moderate depression and anxiety. Studies of older adults with depression or anxiety have been limited, but physical activity appears beneficial to this population as well. The purpose of this study is to examine the relationship between physical activity and symptoms of psychological distress among a sample of adults aged 65 years and older. In particular, we are interested in whether or not the relationship between physical activity and symptoms of psychological distress remains statistically significant after adjusting for physical health status. METHODS: Secondary data analysis of the 1994 National Population Health Survey. We select a sub-sample of respondents aged 65 and older for the analysis (N=2393). RESULTS: Bivariate analyses reveals that physical activity is associated with lower psychological distress scores (r=-.174, p<.001). In multivariate analysis, after controlling for demographic factors and physical health status (chronic conditions and activities of daily living), physical activity remains significantly related to psychological distress. CONCLUSION: Among older adults, nearly 500f the relationship between physical activity and psychological distress is related to physical health status. In other words, individuals who are physically healthy tend to exercise more and have lower levels of psychological distress. However, even after adjusting for physical health, the relationship between physical activity and lower levels of distress remains significant supporting the proposition that physical activity is associated with better mental health among older adults. The implications of this study for further research and interventions are discussed.

Physical exercise and experienced bodily changes: The emergence of benefits and limits on benefits.

François L. Rousseau (Laboratoire de Recherche sur le Comportement Social, Department of Psychology, Université du Québec à Montréal), Brian P. O'Connor & Susan Anneli Maki (Department of Psychology, Lakehead University)

The objective physical benefits of exercise are well documented for individuals of all ages. In contrast, little is known about people's subjective experiences of the changes that take place in their bodies with age and physical exercise. This is unfortunate, because such information could result in more effective interventions aimed at increasing people's exercise levels. In the present study, levels of physical exercise, experienced bodily changes, and attitudinal and well-being variables were measured among 407 adults (aged 26 to 95 years). Cluster analyses of participants on exercise and experienced changes identified three groups at each of four age levels: (1) relatively sedentary people who experienced negative bodily changes; (2) moderate exercisers who reported the most positive bodily changes; and (3) high exercisers who reported only minimal bodily changes. At the low end of the physical exercise continuum, the subjective benefits of exercise appeared rapidly, with only minimal increases in exercise levels. However, attributions of negative bodily changes to aging, low levels of exercise motivation, self-efficacy, competence, and control, and negative exercise attitudes among sedentary people make the chances of small shifts in exercise behavior unlikely. The minority of high exercisers reported little or no positive bodily changes, yet they continued to score high on attitude and well-being variables. These results undercore (1) the complex relationships that exist among physical exercise, subjective experiences, attitudes, and well-being, and (2) the need for researchers to start considering both the objective benefits of physical exercise and the subjective experiences of individuals.

Walking ability and physical activity as predictors of mortality among old people over five years

M. Äijö, (Finnish Centre of Interdisciplinary of Gerontology, University of Jyväskylä), T. Rantanen (Finnish Centre of Interdisciplinary of Gerontology, University of Jyväskylä), M. Alén, (Department of Health Sciences, University of Jyväskylä), M. Kallinen (Central Hospital of Central Finland, Department of Physical Medicine and Rehabilitation)

PURPOSE: To investigate the simultaneous effects of walking ability and physical activity as predictors of mortality over five years in old people. METHODS: As part of the Evergreen Project altogether 200 people (65 men and 135 women) aged 80 or 85 years participated in a six-minute walk test to record walking distance. Level of physical activity was assessed in a interview. Using gender-specific cut-off values, people were categorized into good walkers and poor walkers and active and sedentary groups. These two characteristics were used to form four groups: active good walkers (n=74, reference), sedentary good walkers (n=31), active poor walkers (n=35) and sedentary poor walkers (n=60). RESULTS: 21 men and 20 women died during the follow-up. The mortality rates per 100 person-years were 2.1 for active good walkers, 1.3 for sedentary good walkers, 4.7 for active poor walkers, and 8.3 for sedentary poor walkers. The relative risks of death adjusted for gender and age were 3.4 (95% CI 1.5-7.6) among sedentary poor walkers and 2.6 (95% CI 1.0-6.7) among active poor walkers compared to active good walkers. The risk of sedentary good walkers did not differ from the reference group. After adjustment for coronary heart diseases, stroke and arthritis, the relative risks of mortality decreased somewhat in all groups. CONCLUSION: Poor walking ability was associated with increased risk of mortality. However, among people with poor ability to walk, physical activity was associated with lower mortality risk. Presence of chronic diseases probably explains only part of the effect observed here.

SESSION 330

Qualitative Analyses of Personal and Social Correlates of (Lifespan) Psychosocial Development

A. Clemente (University of Valencia, Valencia, Spain) Adult stages: Relations between the dimensions of personality and physical development. A. Gimeno (University of Valencia, Valencia, Spain) Sex differences in life events. A. Cordoba (University of Valencia, Valencia, Spain) Evaluation of life experiences across the lifespan. M. F. Domenech (University of Valencia, Valencia, Spain) Developmental analysis of perceptions of influence of relevant people on diverse life events. M. Albinana & E. Escolano

(University of Valencia, Valencia, Spain) The influence between personality and areas of development in different stages of adulthood. B. M. Gfellner (Brandon University, Brandon, Canada) Self conceptualization of older adults in three residential settings.

This symposium provides a lifespan perspective of personal and social factors that influence psychosocial development in relation to life events across various domains or areas of functioning. The studies reported in the symposium are based on research that combines the use of qualitative and quantitative methodologies. These feature the use of semi-structured interviews with open-ended questions that are typically followed up with the use of rating scales. The symposium includes six papers. The first five presentations are based on a data set of approximately 1300 subjects in Valencia, Spain who range from 14 to 92 years of age, partitioned into four age-groups including: adolescents, young adults, middle aged adults and older adults. This research program examined participants' self-descriptions of life events in six domains: work, economics, physical and health, personal, affective and social development. These life events were then rated in terms of the extent of positive and negative valence for the respondent. In addition, participants articulated personal self-descriptions and these were subsequently categorized according to the "Big Five" personality traits. Finally, participants generated a list of relevant network members and indicated the supportiveness or intrusiveness of each person in terms of achieving their own major developmental goals. In the first paper, Clemente, Albinana and Gimeno (Adult stages: Relations between the dimensions of personality and physical development) examine age and personality differences in relation to physical development and health. The second presentation (Clemente, Cordoba & Gimeno: Sex differences in life events) summarizes age and sex differences across six domains of life events including work, economics, physical, personal, affective and social. The third paper (Clemente, Cordoba & Gimeno: Evaluation of life experiences across the lifespan) focuses on age differences in the impact of normative and nonnormative life events across the six domains of development. In the fourth presentation, Clemente, Gimeno and Domenech (Developmental analysis of perceptions of influence of relevant people on diverse life events) examine age differences and the impact of positive and negative social network members in the six domains of development. The fifth paper (Clemente, Gimeno, Alninana & Escolano) considers age differences and the impact of personality in the areas of work and economics. In the final paper Gfellner examines spontaneous self-descriptions of older adults in three different residential settings (including personal care homes, elderly person's housing, and independent community homes) to elucidate the salient aspects of older adults' self-conceptualizations in relation to the environmental context. Taken together, the research findings discussed in this symposium extend our understanding of the issues and concerns relevant to older adults, and thereby offer directions for further research as well as policy and program development to improve the quality of life and promote optimal functioning for our aging populations.

Adult stages: Relations between the dimensions of personality and physical development

A. Clemente, M. Paz Albinana, & A. Gimeno (University of Valencia, Valencia, Spain)

The influence on personal development of life events, other people and reference groups and similarly, the dimensions of personality may depend on how they are perceived and the significance attributed to them in one's life. In the present work we analyzed the influence of personality dimensions on the area of physical development in a sample of 1300 subjects from 14 to 92 years of age. The instrument utilized was the Inventory of Personality with Life Events and Relevant Persons (Clemente & Gimeno, 1994). The independent variable was age group (adolescence, young adulthood, middle adulthood, older adulthood). The dependent variable was the self-descriptions of personality provided by subjects which subsequently, were categorized according to the Big Five Dimensions of Personality: Introversion/Extroversion; Agreeable/Disagreeable; Scrupulous/Unscrupulous; Stability/Instability; and Openness to Experience (Goldberg, 1989; John, 1989). Analyses of variance for the dimensions of personality by age group showed that introversion was the major influence in the area of physical development among older adults in comparison with younger age groups. Similarly, the dimensions of personality rated by subjects as positive had a greater influence on physical development for older adults than for those at younger ages. These results are consistent with Cohen and Syme (1986) and Taylor and Hoyt (2000) which suggest that in the later years of adulthood physical development and health play a crucial role in personality development.

Developmental analysis of perceptions of influence of relevant people on diverse life events

A. Clemente, A. Y. Gimeno & M. F. Domenech (University of Valencia, Valencia, Spain)

The social network of an individual is a most significant factor for one's development (Cochran & Niego, 1995; Berkman & Syme, 1979; Abramson, Metalsky & Alloy, 1989). The purpose of this work was to examine the role of individuals' social network members as currently reported over their lives. We used the instrument called "Influences on the Development of Life Events, Personality Characteristics and Relevant People (Clemente & Gimeno, 1994) in which respondents describe their own personal history in a semi-structured interview, and subsequently rate the importance of various events they have indicated. This instrument was administered to 1300 subjects between 14 to 92 years of age. The independent variables were age (categorized as adolescents, young adults, middle aged adults and older adults) and relevant persons rated as either admired (positive) or resisted (negative). These variables were considered in relation to the dependent variable: different areas of development (physical and health, economics, work, affective, personal and social). The findings showed that older adults reported a significantly greater positive influence of people in the physical and affective domains than the other age groups. For young and middle aged adults the influence of people considered relevant was significantly greater for the areas of economics and work in terms of both positive and negative factors. Finally, the influence of relevant people was similar in the personal and social domains for all age groups studied.

Evaluation of life experiences across the lifespan

A. Clemente, A. Cordoba, & A. Gimeno (University of Valencia, Valencia, Spain)

Life span psychology considers normative events to have a different impact than non-normative events due to the ability to predict them. In our work we examined this hypothesis utilizing a sample of 499 subjects between 14 to 65 years of age. Respondents wrote their own life history and subsequently selected the events they considered to have influenced their development. Then participants rated the influence in various life areas of development (including physical, economic, work, personal, affective and social) utilizing the Inventory of Interrelations of Personality with Life Events and Relevant Persons (Clemente & Gimeno, 1994). The results showed clear differences between the two types of events. Normative events had a significantly greater influence than non-normative events in the affective domain for all age groups as well as for events that happened in the past or in the past year. For the other areas and across age groups, respondents attributed greater influence to non-normative events in the economic, work, and social domains. These results contrast with the thesis that normative events are more predictable and with the importance of the affective impact (Thoits, 1983), and point to the interpretation that other characteristics of events (such as evaluation and social desirability) may be more important.

Self conceptualizationof older adults in three residential settings

B. M. Gfellner (Brandon University, Brandon, Canada)

Spontaneously produced components of self-conceptualization were investigated among elderly adults living in three residential settings:

personal care homes (PCHs), elderly persons' housing (EPHs), and their own homes. There were 151 participants: 50 in nursing homes (M = 80.8 years); 49 in seniors' housing (M = 75.3 years); and 52 in their own homes (M = 73.2 years). The sex ratio was 2:1 (100 women; 51 men). In comparison with community dwellers, those in PCHs were more likely to be older, women, widowed and to have a lower income although the groups did not differ in terms of self-rated health. Participants completed the Spontaneous Self-Concept Procedure (McGuire & Padawar-Singer, 1976) as part of a home interview. Verbatim self-descriptions were scored using a modification of Gordon's (1968) 30-category system with 90 0nter-rater agreement. Findings showed that older adults in the community (own home and EPHs) gave greater prominence to interpersonal factors and experiences than PCH residents. Seniors' housing (EPH) residents emphasized the importance of their physical environment and associated activities and interests while PCH residents focused on kinship and occupational roles. Similarities and differences between the groups are discussed in terms of distinctiveness differences among the environmental settings. Consideration is given to directions for further research in the area of policy development and housing options to maximize the quality of life among older adults in a variety of living environments.

Sex differences in life events

A. Clemente, A. Cordoba, & A. Gimeno (University of Valencia, Valencia, Spain)

Lifespan psychology focuses on the impact of life events on development in terms of the individual's experience and interpretation of them (Baltes, Reese & Lipsett, 1980; Pruchno et al, 1989). In the present work we analyzed how events considered relevant for each person influence his/ her development in various domains: physical, economic, work, personal, affective and social. These events were rated by respondents in terms of personal salience. Our objective was to assess possible differences in the six domains of functioning. The instrument utilized was the Inventory of Interrelations of Personality with Life Events and Relevant Persons (Clemente & Gimeno, 1994) in which participants reported their life stories. The sample included 499 subjects (182 men and 317 women) between the ages of 14 and 65 years. According to the results, men showed significantly higher ratings than women and across all age groups in reference to events in the areas of economics and work (whether these experiences were in the present or in the past). Women rated events as significantly higher in influence in the affective and social domains. These results are consistent with Kessler (1979), Elwell and Maltbie-Crannell, 1981, Conger et al. (1993) and Wethington et al. (1987).

The influence between personality and areas of development in different stages of adulthood

A. Clemente, A. Gimeno, M. Albinana, & E. Escolano (University of Valencia, Valencia, Spain)

Older adults experience a series of events that influence distinct areas of their development, especially in the field of work and economics. In large measure, these events are related to personality and coping styles (Kalish, 1983). In our work we attempted to clarify associations between self-perceptions of personality and coping styles in relation to two areas of development: work and economics. The sample included 1300 subjects between 14 and 92 years of age. We analyzed participants' life histories using the Inventory of Inter-relations in the Areas of Development (Clemente & Gimeno, 1994). The independent variables were: (1) age with four different age groups (adolescents, young adults, middles aged adults and older adults) and (2) self-descriptions of personality coded into ten categories with five considered positive and five negative following the work of Goldberg and John (introversion, extroversion, agreeable, disagreeable, scrupulous, unscrupulous, stable, unstable, open or closed to experience). The dependent variable was the developmental domain of work and economics as categorized in our inventory. Using analysis of variance we found significant effects for age and the dimensions of personality (both for positive and negative categories). Post hoc testing clarified our understanding of these effects and the subgroups in which these differences were relevant.

SESSION 332

Assessment of balance and mobility in frail elderly patients : validation of the Mini Motor Test.

Mourey F, Camus A, Mischis C, Pfitzenmeyer P. (Centre de Gérontologie de Champmaillot Dijon, France).

Purpose: Dimensions assessed by Mini Motor Test (MMT) include: mobility in lying position, balance in sitting position and transfer from sitting position to standing position, balance and postural adaptation in standing position and gait. The aim of this study was to establish the validity of the MMT. Method: The MMT has been tested in four populations from departments of geriatric medicine in Marseille, Saint-Etienne, Strasbourg and Dijon. The validation has been conducted in 101 patients (mean age: 83.93 ± 6.03 years). In these patients, all the causes of hospitalization were found but history of fall was noted in 65.34% of cases. This population showed a great diversity in independence level. To assess interrater reliability, the patients have been tested by two observers on the same day. The assessment included too the index of Katz ADL and the Mini-Mental State Examination of Folstein. Construct validity has been analyzed trough the comparison of scores obtained in the different items. Results: The interrater difference was not significant. The better correlation was found for standing position ability (97.03%) and the less one for reactive postural responses in standing position. A significant correlation has been observed between MMT score and Katz index score ($p<0.005$) while the correlation was not significant between MMT score and MMSE score. Conclusion: Our results showed that the MMT appear as an useful test in frail elderly. We think that a specific rehabilitation program could be elaborated from the results of MMT.

Balance function and fall-related efficacy in patients with newly operated hip fracture.

Annika Hellzén Ingemarsson (Department of Physiotherapy, Mölndal, Sahlgrenska University Hospital, and Department of Geriatric Medicine, Göteborg University) Kerstin Frändin (Department of Geriatric Medicine, Göteborg University) Karin Hellström (Department of Neuroscience, Rehabilitation Medicine, Uppsala University, Uppsala) and Åke Rundgren (Department of Geriatric Medicine, Göteborg University, Sweden)

PURPOSE: To investigate the relation between fall-related efficacy in daily-life activities and functional as well as instrumental tests of balance in patients with hip fracture. METHODS : Fifty-five elderly inpatients (mean age 82.3) with newly operated hip fracture were assessed during their the last week in hospital before discharge. Analysis of different aspects of balance using the Falls Efficacy Scale Swedish version FES(S), questions on fear of falling, Functional Reach (FR) and tests on a Balance platform (Chattanooga). RESULTS: The results showed a significant relationship between the subjective ability measured with the FES(S), and the objectively measured balance in the Functional Reach test as between fall-related efficacy measured with FES(S) and fear of falling. Very few significant correlations were found between the results from balance tests on the force platform and those obtained with FES(S) and FR. CONCLUSIONS: Both Falls Efficacy Scale, Swedish version and the Functional Reach have been shown to be useful in analysing balance function in elderly patients newly operated on for hip fracture. The Falls Efficacy Scale also indicates which of the daily activities the patient perceives as troublesome and thus require further training.

Benefit Of Balance-Training Program In Brittany

H Bastide1, N Loquen2, J Fonlupt2, J Lassale3, P Rochcongar4, P Jouanny1. 1Department of Geriatric Medicine, 4 Sport medicine, University hospital 2French Federation of Physical Education and

Volontary Gymnastic 3Brittany Health Insurance. Rennes, France

PURPOSE: Falls in elderly are a problem of public health due to high incidence and related morbidity/mortality rate. Prevention policy is necessary for reducing incidence. METHOD: We performed a balance stimulation program including 12 sessions of neurosensitive stimulation through various exercises for groups of 10 to 12 elderly volunteers. 96 older subjects were recruited (9 male and 87 female, mean age 70.0 +/- 7.9 years). 61 declared having fall and 34 in the past 6 months. Balance was appreciated with Tinetti test and monopodal standing test (MPST) mesured in seconds. RESULTS: Tinetti test was badly correlated with age (r=0.468; p<0.0001), medication number (r=0.266; p=0.010), male gender (p=0.044), past hip fracture (p<0.0001), hip prosthesis (p=0.0006) and declared difficulties for walking (p=0.0016) or standing (p=0.0009). MPST provided similary results. After the program balance was significantly improved (Tinetti 15.8 +/- 2.1 vs 17.1 +/- 2.8; p<0.0001 and MPST 17.8 +/- 8.4 vs 14.4 +/- 10.9; p=0.032). The most significantly improved items were monopodal standing (p<0.0001), balance vhen seated (p=0.011), standing up from a chair (p=0.032), standing with rotation or hyperextension of the head (p=0.032) and standing up (p=0.034). 83 0f the subjects declared having better balance and 73 % that they had more security in moving. 100 0eclared that they have made again past activities and 77 0erformed new activities. 69 % wanted to participate in a permanent program. CONCLUSION: This preliminary results showed that Brittany balance training program significantly improved balance perfomances in elderly volunteers, and that they secondarily improved their social activities due to greater moving security. These data support to promote public health intervention in elderly for improving balance and successfull aging.

Effects of a Rehabilitation Program in Elderly Fallers

N.de Rekeneire (National Institute of Aging, Bethesda, USA), J.Aiguier (Centre Gérontologique Départemental, Marseille, France), Ph.Sauvageon (Centre Gérontologique Départemental, Marseille, France), F.Mourey (CHU Dijon)

The aim of our study is the evolution of the rehabilitation technics on balance and gait in elderly fallers . 45 fallers hospitalized in an acute geriatric unit were evaluated .The objective evaluation of the balance and gait was realized by 2 clinical tests: the Tinetti scale(POMA)explores the balance and gait, and the AFAPA test (assessment of functional activities and postural abilities) includes an evaluation in bed, the sitting position, the standing posture and the gait . These tests were used before and after a rehabilitation program .45 fallers (75.6% women , mean age: 82.9 years oldand 24.4% men,mean age: 81 years old) were evaluated . 82% were living at home . At the admission, only 20% had no functional disability . Gait without help was possible for 42.2% of the fallers; 57% had a cognitive impairment.73.3% fell more than once.66.7% had a fear of falling, 28.9% presented a post fall syndrom . After 3 weeks of the rehabilitation program, the evaluation shows a significant improvement for 15.5% of patients in balance and 6.7 % in gait in the POMA. We see an improvement but not significant for 42.2 % in balance and gait .For the AFAPA,a significant improvement is shown in the mobility in bed for 28.9 %, the sitting position in 22.2% of the patients, the standing position in 22.2%, for the gait in 13.3%.The results are better in balance than in gait in the POMA, the improvement is higher in the AFAPA.The improvement is noted even in the older group and is better in patients without cognitive impairment . The results are worse in patients with a long length stay (frail population). Only 63.6% come back home .Our study shows the interest of the rehabilitation in fallers with a global improvement in balance and gait . It would have been interesting to explore the impact of our program in the secondary prevention of falls; the results of other studies are very cautious.

Impact of a Rehabilitation Program in Elderly Fallers

N.de Rekeneire (National Institute on Aging, Bethesda, USA), J.Aiguier (Centre Gérontologique Départemental, Marseille, France), Ph.Sauvageon (Centre Gérontologique Départemental, Marseille, France), F.Mourey (CHU Dijon, France)

This study explores the impact of selected rehabilitation techniques on measures of balance and gait in elderly fallers. 45 elderly fallers admitted to an acute geriatric unit were evaluated . Balance and gait were measured by 2 clinical tests conducted before and after the rehabilitation program: the Tinetti scale (POMA) for balance and gait, and the AFAPA test (assessment of functional activities and postural abilities) in bed, while sitting, while standing and gait. Subjects were 34 women (mean age: 82.9 years) and 11 men (mean age: 81 years); 82% lived in their own home. At admission, 20% had no functional disability. Unassisted gait was possible for 42.2% of the fallers; 57% had a cognitive impairment and 73.3% had more than one prior fall. 66.7% of the subjects had a fear of falling, and nearly one third evidenced a post fall syndrome. After 3 weeks exposure to the rehabilitation program, 15.5% of patients showed a significant improvement in balance and 6.7% improved their gait scores in the POMA. An improvement in balance and gait was noted for 42.2% of subjects but this was not significant . However, significant increases in functional and postural scores measured by the AFAPA were recorded for mobility in bed (28.9%), the sitting position (22.2%), the standing position (22.2%), and in gait (13.3%). Although the posttest results from the POMA are better for balance than gait, improvement in all categories is greater on the AFAPA measures. This improvement is noted even in the older group and is better in patients without cognitive impairment. Improvements are less frequent among patients with longer hospital stays(frail populations).63.6% returned home.Our study demonstrates an overall improvement in balance and gait from a short-term rehabilitation program, but it did not explore the impact on the secondary prevention of falls. The results of such studies on falls prevention appear inconclusive .

The mobility and balance performance of a group of elderly residents in Hong Kong

Yau Cheuk-ngok Daniel, Wu Yee-ming, Chiu Tak-yi, Chow Yuk-hing Ada, Liu Chi-pun, and Leung Chi-tat Antony (Aged Care Research & Development Unit, Haven of Hope Christian Service, Hong Kong, China)

PURPOSE: Published studies on mobility and balance performance of elderly people in Hong Kong are scarce. This study aims to describe the mobility and balance performance of a group of elderly people residing in residential care settings in Hong Kong. METHOD: A group of elderly residents (n=200) were recruited from four residential care facilities in the local district of Tseung Kwan O. Mobility and balance performance were measured by 3 functional tests including the 'Timed Up & Go Test'(UGT), 'Timed Sit-to-Stand Test'(SST), and the 'Timed Single-Leg-Standing Test'(SLT). History of falling and other relevant information were gathered by personal interview with a standardized questionnaire. RESULTS: Mean age of the subjects was 80.1 (SD7.2; range 62-96) and 61.50f the subjects were female. The prevalence of fall was 25.5%. Mean performance on the UGT, SST, and SLT for all subjects were 18.5 sec, 8.3 times, and 6.6 sec. respectively. High levels of reliability alphas were observed on the inter-rater and test-retest procedures. Bivariate analysis found significant difference between the faller and non-faller group on all of the 3 tests: UGT (p=0.02), SST (p=0.00), and SLT (p=0.00). Significant differences were also found between the outdoor-walker group and non-outdoor-walker group on the 3 tests (p=0.00). CONCLUSION: Mobility and balance performance of the elderly residents are important indicators for preventive measures. By using the functional tests of UGT, SST, and SLT, elderly residents who are at risk of falling and immobility can be identified and thus interventions can be provided promptly. The results of the study can also be used for comparisons and verifications of the mobility and balance performance status of elderly people in residential care settings.

SESSION 333

Music and Spirituality for Healing in Dementia and Palliative Care

Kevin Kirkland, MA, MTA (UBC Hospital, Vancouver, British Columbia, Canada), Howard McIlveen, MDiv (Richmond Hospital, Richmond, British Columbia, Canada) Then Sings My Soul: Spiritual therapy for people with dementia. Heather Mohan, MMT, MTA (North Shore Palliative Care program, Lion's Gate Hospital, North Vancouver, British Columbia, Canada) Meaningful Moments: Stories of music therapy in end-of-life care for persons with dementia.

These presentations will demonstrate the power of music and the combination of music therapy and spirituality as therapeutic, supportive interventions for persons with dementia in all stages of their lives, including palliative care. Outlining the foundation and implementation of a "spiritual therapy" program, the first presenters combine music therapy and pastoral care in a presentation of the importance of spirituality, religion and secular approaches for those with dementia. Through a case study and narrative inquiry, the second presenter explores the meaning in her music therapy practice in palliative care for persons with dementia and their family members. Persons with dementia have spiritual needs that are often difficult to address. "Spiritual therapy" for older adults with dementia offers a diverse approach to meeting spiritual needs. Although "spiritual therapy" is based on a Christian approach, it can be adapted for other spiritual faiths. Through lecture, experiential exercises and videotape, delegates will be introduced to an approach that goes beyond "activities" and addresses group process as well as an individual's spiritual path. Using a case study approach and narrative inquiry, the second presenter explores the meaning of her music therapy practice in palliative care for persons with dementia and their family members. The use of music therapy in palliative care is well documented. Music therapy can decrease pain and agitation and can promote relaxation. The shared experience of music and singing supports the expression of grief and can facilitate communication between family members and the person with dementia who is facing death. Music assists in the creation of meaningful moments between patients, family members and caregivers. Through case studies, stories, poetry and music, the power of music and spirituality for healing with persons with dementia will be demonstrated.

Meaningful Moments: Stories of music therapy in end-of-life care for persons with dementia

Heather Mohan (North Shore Palliative Care Program; Lion's Gate Hospital; North Vancouver, British Columbia, Canada)

This presentation will demonstrate the power of music as a therapeutic, supportive intervention for persons with dementia and their family members as they approach the end of their life's journey together. The presenter used a process of narrative inquiry and case study analysis to explore the meaning of her music therapy experiences in palliative care for persons with dementia and their family members. Feedback from caregivers and family members involved in these experiences was also considered. Music therapy was found to decrease pain perception, alleviate anxiety, promote relaxation, support the expression of grief and facilitate communication between family members and persons with dementia who are imminently facing death. In addition, music assisted in the creation of meaningful moments between patients, family members and caregivers. Case studies, stories, poetry, and live music will be used to demonstrate the scope of possible applications and power of music therapy with this population. Examples of clinical practice will be interwoven with personal reflections and theoretical contexts

Then Sings My Soul: Chaplaincy and Music Therapy in Group Dementia Care

Kevin Kirkland (UBC Hospital, Vancouver, British Columbia, Canada); Howard McIlveen (Richmond Hospital, Richmond, British Columbia, Canada)

This presentation will describe the foundation and implementation of a music-based spiritual therapy program for the elderly with all ranges of cognitive impairment. Participants will learn guiding principles for combining pastoral care with music therapy to meet the needs of body, mind and spirit. We will present on a model of spiritual therapy, described in our book "Full Circle: Spiritual Therapy for the Elderly," based on a combination of chaplaincy and music therapy. The program addresses dementia care with a traditional religious background, but participants will also learn about spirituality in a broader sense. Outcomes of participating in a group of this nature include grief resolution, accessing long-term memories, group cohesion, spiritual insights from the elderly, and enhanced verbal processing. Examples from practice will be given to demonstrate the potential and abilities of people with dementia. Music and spirituality provides an effective means for addressing the personhood of people with dementia in a program of care that honours the depth of responses and abilities within the population. Implications for further research will be noted.

SESSION 334

Nutrition and Immune/inflammatory Response

Katsuiki Hirokawa, [Tokyo Medical & Dental University Graduate School, Japan] : Differential effect of protein-free diet, oral antigen and VE in young and old animals. Philip C. Calder [University of Southampton, Southampton, United Kingdom] : Modulation of inflammatory responses by lipids - applications to ageing, Tamas Fulop [Université de Sherbrooke, Sherbrooke, Qc, canada] : Inflammation, atherosclerosis, nutrition and aging: is there any link?, Dayong Wu [Tufts University, Boston, USA] : Vitamin E and macrophage cyclooxygenase regulation in the aged, Bruno Lesourd [Université de Clermont-Ferrand, Clermont-Ferrand, France] : Influence of inflammatory process on Nutrition-Immune Response interelationships in healthy and diseased Elderly.

Abstract: Issue: Aging is associated with increased incidences of undernutrition, immunodeficiencies and inflammatory diseases. They are often associated in the Elderly: undernutrition leading to immunodeficiency and to chronic inflammation, immune deficiency to occurring diseases, then to inflammation and to undernutrition, inflammation to undernutrition and to immunodeficiency. Such association is always observed in elderly patients, being a component of the accelerated aging process linked to ongoing diseases. The same association is often seen in the frail Elderly, appearing to be part of the aging process. This symposium provides new insights in the recent knowledge of aging-related diseases and of aging-related cell metabolism. It mostly focus on inflammatory mechanisms. Structure : The symposium starts with the influence of energy and protein nutrition of immune responses (oral tolerance) in animals (Hirokawa). Then it focus (Calder). on the role of lipid nutrition (n-3/n-6 ratio) on inflammation and the consequences for age-related immune diseases. Then it focus on atherosclerosis (Fulop), a typical model of the aging process related to increased inflammation, bringing the importance of the oxydative process in such disease. Reduction of the oxydative process may be done through vitamin E therapy (Wu), to which particular attention is given to molecular mechanism activity. Finally, the important relationships of inflammation, immune responses and nutritional status in different categories of elderly is presented (Lesourd), with a particular on refeeding efficacy. Content : Aging is associated with decreased oral tolerance to protein antigen and to increased allergic reactions (Hirokawa). In experimental model antioxidant vitamin E treatment may not reduce the occurrence of allergic/auto-immune diseases. Pro/anti-inflammatory equilibriums change with aging leading to increased infections and chronic inflammatory diseases (Calder). Age-related changes may be reverse with fish oil consumption which increases the n-3/n-6 fatty acid ratio. Such treatment reduces the pro/anti-inflammatory ratios and induces amelioration of the symptoms of allergic and auto-immune diseases. Atherosclerosis, an auto-immune model of the aging process, is related to increased inflammation and decreased immune responses to oxidized LDL. The presence of carotis plaques is linked to the intensity of the inflammatory process (Fulop). In addition, undernutrition is associated to increased inflammatory processes and carotis plaques. Increased inflammation is associated with increased PGE2 production which leads to decreased immune responses (Wu). Such phenomenon may be reverse with vitamin E therapy, the molecular basis of such activity being presented. Finally a global view on the relationships between increased inflammation, decreased immune responses and decreased nutritional status is presented (Lesourd) through data in different groups of elderly. In addition the detrimental effect of the inflammatory process in refeeding efficacy of undernourished elderly is presented. Conclusion/ anticipated outcomes. The presented data show the importance of the inflammatory process on immune responses and the association between undernutrition and increased inflammation in aged persons. In addition the role of nutrition through some nutrients (protein, lipid, antioxidant vitamin E) to reduce the deleterious consequences of inflammation in aged persons is presented. The symposium brings new knowledge and new nutritional therapeutic possibilities to reduce the inflammatory process in the elderly, permitting perhaps in a near future to slow down the aging process

Differential effect of protein-free diet, oral antigen and VE in young and old animals.

Katsuiki Hirokawa, [Tokyo Medical & Dental University Graduate School, Japan]

Purpose: Protein is essential for development and maintenance of the immune system. Thus, protein free diet (PFD) containing satisfactory energy is detrimental to animals. Method : Regarding age difference, young immature rats are most susceptible to PFD and old rats are next in order. Young mature rats are relatively resistant to PFD. Diet containing well balanced nutrients and restricted calorie (60% of ad libitum) does not influence the immune functions of rats, regardless of age. Most contents of food act as antigens, but their antigenic capacity is suppressed by oral tolerance. Therefore, immune response usually does not occur to most food antigens. Results: Oral tolerance, however, is observed when new antigens are given orally in young animals but not in middle-aged or old animals. Thus, the young mice pretreated with oral administration of a new antigen do not respond to the same antigen administered intraperitoneally. However, the old mice pretreated with oral administration of a new antigen respond to the same antigen administered intraperitoneally. In the experiment of experimental allergic orchitis (EAO), oral administration of testicular antigens can prevent or ameliorate the extent of EAO in young mice. EAO can not be induced in old mice, but oral administration of testicular antigen promote the induction of EAO in old mice. Vitamin E is an anti-oxidant and known to be effective in reducing risk for various age-associated diseases and this effect is partly due to restoration of immune functions of aging subjects. In animal experiment using C57BL/6 mice, diet containing a high dose of vitamin E (VE) enhances the immune functions and promotes the recovery of immune functions after the stress. This beneficial effect of VE is observed in young C57BL/6 mice, but not in old ones. Conclusion: These results in animal experiments are helpful information for the health maintenance of human elderly. Namely, sufficient amount of protein intake is necessary for maintenance of immune system of the elderly. Oral administration of some specific antigen could enhance the immune response in the elderly. Individual variation is present in the effectiveness of vitamin E on the immune system of the elderly.

Inflammation, atherosclerosis, nutrition and aging: is there any link?

Tamas Fulop [Université de Sherbrooke, Sherbrooke, Qc, canada]

Abstract: Purpose: Atherosclerosis is the underlying cause of several cardiovascular diseases such as infarction, stroke. In recent years there have been shown that inflammation plays an important role in the pathogenesis of atherosclerosis. Activated T cells, macrophages and mast cells are present at all stages of the development of the atherosclerotic plaques. This means that this inflammatory response is immune mediated. It is well known that with aging there is an increase in the incidence of cardio-vascular diseases on the basis of the development of atherioslerosis. Moreover aging is associated with the increase of the inflammatory processes. Thus it is an important issue to study whether there is a relationship between aging, the development of atherioslerosis and inflammation and whether this can be modulated by nutrition. Method: oxidized LDL (OxLDL) obtained from individuals of various ages were studied in interaction with T lymphocytes in the presence or absence of monocytes to determine their response as to proliferate or die by apoptosis. An observational study was conducted with 120 subjects to determine their nutritional, inflammatory and atherosclerosis status. Results: One of the antigen playing a role in the immune response related inflammatory process is the OxLDL. The presence of monocytes will decide whether the lymphocytes will be activated (proliferate) or die by apoptosis. This important protective immune reaction become harmful if the immune response is dysregulated as it is occuring with aging. Here we demonstrate that the origin of lymphocytes (young versus aged) as well as that of oxLDL induce a differential response in regard to proliferation or apoptosis. We observed an increase in apoptosis and decrease of proliferation with aging suggesting that there is an acceleration of the development of the atherosclerotic process with aging. The signal transduction pathway differences elicited by OxLDL and AGE products on monocytes and lymphocytes in regard to aging and the atherosclerotic process will be also discussed. More the inflammatory response is increased more the level of acute phase proteins is increased. We were thus further interested to study the relationship between the markers of the inflammatory reaction (CRP, fibrinogen, TNF alpha and IL-6), the nutritional status (albumin, hemoglobin) and the presence of plaque (by B-mode ultrasonography anti-oxLDL antibodies) in healthy elderly and patients with stroke. Results suggest that malnutrition is related to an inflammatory process which is associated to the presence of carotis plaques. Conclusion: Thus the immune dysregulation with aging favour the development of an inflammatory process such as atherosclerosis and the nutritional status could further enhance this pathological process.

Influence of inflammatory process on Nutrition-Immune Response interelationships in healthy and diseased Elderly.

Bruno Lesourd#, Agathe Raynaud-Simon# [Université de Clermont-Ferrand, Clermont-Ferrand, France]*

Abstract: Purpose: Undernutrition leads to decreased Immune responses, mainly for Cell-Mediated Immunity (CMI). Such influence are more important at the extremes of life (Infancy and Elderly), the two ages where undernutrition is more prevalent. Undernutrition is often revealed in aged persons with occurring diseases, showing the importance of Inflammatory process in undernutrition occurrence. Methods: We explored immune responses in different groups of Elderly, well defined for Clinical and Inflammatory status to study the interrelationships of CMI and Nutrition. Very healthy, healthy, autonomous with chronic diseases, undernourished without and with inflammatory reaction Elderly groups were simultaneously investigated for nutrition and immune status. Monocyte (IL-1, IL-6) and lymphocyte (IL-2, IL-6) cytokine released were quantified in vivo, ex vivo and in vitro. We also quantified T-lymphocyte subsets and lymphocyte proliferation. Results: Very healthy Elderly have comparable lymphocyte responses (cytokine releases as well as lymphocyte proliferation) than young adults and even higher IL-6 in vitro monocyte releases. In contrast lymphocyte subsets reflect Immune Aging: decreased CD3+ and CD8+ subsets with parallel increases in CD2+CD3- and CD57+ subsets. There is a continuous decreases of CMI responses (monocyte as well as lymphocyte cytokine releases) from the healthiest to the more sick elderly groups. Such decreased CMI responses are strongly correlated to decreased nutritional status and to increased inflammatory process, both being interrelated. In addition we explored immune responses in profoundly undernourished Elderly (BMI < 18 kg/m2 , Albumine < 30 g/L), during protein-energy refeeding therapy. Undernourished Elderly who exhibits moderate inflammation (i.e. CRP $<$ 30 mg/L), rapidly improves their nutritional status and, in parallel, CMI responses. In contrast, undernourished Elderly with more important inflammatory process, had similar improvement of nutritional status and CMI responses but with delay. Both only starts to improve when inflammatory process have slown down. Conclusions: Inflammatory process seems of major importance in the Nutrition-Immunity relationships in Aged persons

Modulation of inflammatory responses by lipids - applications to ageing

Philip C. Calder [University of Southampton, Southampton, United Kingdom]

Abstract: The immune and inflammatory systems are self-regulated by a variety of balances, such as those between the Th1- and the Th2-type responses and between the pro- and anti-inflammatory cytokines. Ageing is associated with changes in immune cell function and in the production of inflammatory mediators and with a dysregulation of the various balances within the immune and inflammatory systems. These ageing-related changes are readily demonstrated in laboratory rodents, but they have also been observed in humans. Altered balances within the immune and inflammatory systems can lead to immunosuppression (which increases susceptibility to infection), to chronic inflammatory [autoimmune] diseases (which are driven by a dysregulated Th1 response and are characterised by the over production of the pro-inflammatory cytokines [TNF, IL-1, IL-6, IL-8]), or to allergic inflammation (which is driven by a dysregulated Th2 response). The key link between fatty acids and inflammation is the n-6 polyunsaturated fatty acid (PUFA) arachidonic acid (ARA; 20:4n-6). ARA is the precursor of prostaglandins, leukotrienes and related compounds which have important roles in inflammation and in the regulation of immunity. For example, prostaglandin E2 suppresses production of Th1-type cytokines by lymphocytes (so skewing the Th1/Th2 balance in favour of the Th2-type response). Most inflammatory cells contain a high proportion of ARA. However, the fatty acid composition of inflammatory cells is sensitive to change according to the fatty acid composition of the diet: the proportion of different types of PUFA in these cells is readily changed. Fish oil contains the n-3 PUFA eicosapentaenoic acid (EPA; 20:5n-3) and docosahexaenoic acid (DHA; 22:6n-3). Feeding fish oil results in partial replacement of ARA in cell membranes by EPA. This leads to decreased production of ARA-derived mediators. In addition, EPA is a substrate for cyclooxygenase and lipoxygenase and gives rise to mediators which often have different biological actions or potencies than those formed from ARA. Animal studies have shown that dietary fish oil decreases the production of the pro-inflammatory cytokines TNF-a, IL-1 and IL-6 and, in some circumstances, increases the production of the anti-inflammatory cytokine TGF-b. Supplementation of the diet of healthy human volunteers with fish oil-derived n-3 PUFA (1.2 to 14 g/day) results in decreased monocyte and neutrophil chemotaxis and decreases production of TNF, IL-1, and IL-6. Addition of fish oil to the diet of laboratory animals or healthy humans modulates adhesion molecule expression on the surface of monocytes and lymphocytes and alters the ability of such cells to bind to ligand-bearing cells. Taken together these observations indicate that n-3 PUFA possess anti-inflammatory properties, and so may be useful in the prevention of some age-related changes in the inflammatory system. Activated endothelial cells release adhesion molecules into the circulation and the concentration of these is increased in cardiovascular and inflammatory diseases. We have recently demonstrated that the concentration of soluble adhesion molecules increases with age in humans. Furthermore, providing fish oil to healthy elderly subjects resulted in a decreased concentration of some adhesion molecules, suggesting that fish oil decreases endothelial activation in vivo. Fish oil feeding has been shown to ameliorate the symptoms of some animal models of autoimmune disease. These changes are associated with abolition of pro-inflammatory cytokine production and the induction of anti-inflammatory cytokines and antioxidant enzymes. Clinical studies have reported that fish oil supplementation has beneficial effects in rheumatoid arthritis, supporting the idea that the n-3 PUFA in fish oil are anti-inflammatory and immunomodulatory.

Vitamin E and macrophage cyclooxygenase regulation in the aged

Dayong Wu, Simin Nikbin Meydani (Tufts University, Boston, USA)

Abstract: Aging is associated with increased incidence of immune and inflammatory diseases. Products of arachidonic acid metabolism, in particular prostaglandin (PGE2), play an important role in the regulation of immune and inflammatory response. We showed previously that the aged have higher macrophage PGE2 production compared with their young counterparts. This age-associated increase in PGE2 production is mainly a consequence of cyclooxygenase (COX) activity. We demonstrated further that increased COX activity in old mice is due to the increased expression of mRNA and protein for the inducible form of COX, COX-2. Vitamin E has been shown to reduce PGE2 production while improving the immune response in the aged. In aged mice, we showed that vitamin E-induced decrease in PGE2 production is due to decreased COX activity. However, vitamin E had no effect on COX mRNA and protein levels, indicating a post-translational regulation of COX by vitamin E. Further experiments indicated that vitamin E decreases COX activity through reducing formation of peroxynitrite, a hyperoxide shown increased to be involved in the activation of COX-2. Other homologues of tocopherols were also effective in inhibiting COX activity but their degree of inhibition varied. The varied potency to inhibit COX activity was not explained totally by differences in their antioxidant capacity. We have shown that vitamin E-induced inhibition of COX activity contributes to its improvement of T cell function in the aged. Further studies are needed to determine the effect of vitamin E on inflammatory diseases associated with aging.

SESSION 335

Altered composition of the AP-1 transcription factor during ageing of, and in immortalised, mammalian cells

A. Sheerin, M.H. Goyns (School of Sciences, University of Sunderland, Sunderland, UK), K.S.J. Thompson (BASF Pharma Research & Development, Nottingham, UK)

Changes in gene expression patterns are known to occur during ageing and to be susceptible to caloric restriction. It is unclear why a relatively small number, perhaps less than 1%, of active genes exhibit these changes, though the involvement of transcription factors is a possibility. We have used Western blotting to analyse the expression of the AP-1 transcription factor proteins in ageing (proliferating) cultures of human MRC5 fibroblasts and ageing (quiescent) rat liver, and compared these data to those of immortalised mouse 3T3 fibroblasts and rat hepatoma cell lines. As the MRC5 fibroblasts aged, the 46kd junB began to decline after 41 population doublings (pd) and was replaced by a 34kd species. The two junD species disappeared, and fra-1 began to decline, after 44pd. After 49 pd, fos and jun also decreased, but disproportionately, showing a decline in the fos/jun ratio. By contrast, there was little evidence of changes in AP-1 protein expression during ageing of the rat liver. However, analysis of fos and jun mRNA by fluorescent in-situ hybridization indicated a decline in the fos/jun ratio. When young proliferating MRC5 cells were compared to immortalised cells, several differences were observed. Both fos and jun expression appeared to be higher in the immortalised cells. The latter also exhibited expression of fra-2, expression of both the 46kd and 34kd junB species and a change in the relative levels of the two junD species with the larger species being more prominent. These data indicate that significant changes occur in AP-1 protein expression during ageing of mammalian cells and also indicate that immortalised cells are not simply cells in which the ageing process has been reversed or blocked, but rather exhibit additional characteristics.

Biological Age as a Biomarker in Geroprotectors Efficacy Assessment in Occupational Health

A. S. Bashkireva (St. Petersburg Institute of Bioregulation and

Gerontology, St. Petersburg, Russia)

Biological age by long-term work capacity examination for different professions allows to assess functional reserves and adaptation depletion stage and timely correct it with geroprotectors. Biologically active food additives cytamins interpolymer complexes of tissue-specific proteins and nucleic acids are effective agents of preventing premature and accelerated aging (PAA). Study was designed to apply biological age as a biomarker in cytamins efficacy assessment to prevent and correct PAA, occupational, age- and work-related diseases under adverse occupational conditions. 150 drivers (aged 30-59) divided into 5 equal groups were subject to physiological and psychophysiological examination. Group 1 received Cerebramin(r), 2 - Vasalamin(r), 3 - Cerebramin(r) + Vasalamin(r), 4 placebo and 5 - no preparations. Integral criteria of the elderly workers biological age and aging rates served as biomarkers. Biological age by long-term work capacity evaluation was proven adequate in prenosological diagnosis of occupational, age- and work-related diseases and in geroprotectors efficacy assessment for preventing and correcting PAA in elderly workers. Cerebramin and Vasalamin restored the organism defense forces, inhibited aging rates of separate functions and entire organism manifested in increased mental and physical work capacity as compared to the initial level. Application of a screening and monitoring system in main industrial occupations allows to timely diagnose aging processes, create and perform population gerontological data bases for various professions, estimate the efficacy of geroprotective multisystems. Thus, modern gerotechnologies employed to solve topical problems of occupational health promote work capacity increase, professional ability maintenance and professional longevity extension under adverse occupational conditions.

Cell Aging Studies at the Junction of Millennia: From "Correlative" to "Gist" Models

A. N. Khokhlov (Evolutionary Cytogerontology Sector, School of Biology, Moscow State University, Moscow, Russia)

Usually cytogerontological research reports are produced utilizing the "Hayflick's model". We already aware of the mechanisms of the aging in vitro phenomenon in contrast to the aging in vivo mechanisms. Perhaps, this is a consequence of the fact that Hayflick's model is CORRELATIVE, i.e. based on some detected correlations only. However, very frequently a good correlation does not have anything to do with the gist of the phenomenon. Thus, is evident the absence of CAUSE-EFFECT RELATIONSHIPS, which are totally indispensable for the GIST models. They are based on a definite CONCEPT of aging. In the case of Hayflick's model, such a concept is absent Δ we cannot explain, using "Hayflick's limit", why our organism ages. Therefore we consider as indispensable the elaboration of "gist" models of aging. We believe that one of such models could be our "stationary phase aging" model (Khokhlov, 1983, 1988, 2000), the basis of which is the assumption of the leading role that the cell proliferation restriction plays in the aging process. We assume that the accumulation of «senile» damage is caused by the restriction of cell proliferation either because of formation of differentiated cell populations during development (in vivo) or due to existence of saturation density phenomenon (in vitro). Cell proliferation changes lead to accumulation of macromolecular defects, which, in turn, generate deterioration of tissues, organs and eventually of the whole organism, increasing the probability of its death. We define cell aging as the accumulation in a cell population of various types of damage identical to the damage arising in a senescing multicellular organism. And, finally, we see as extremely important the determination how a cell is dying and what it is, in general, - the death of cell. The author's work is supported by Russian Foundation for Basic Research (grant 00-04-48049).

Cell Response to Stress as Aging Biomarker

Mariana Rachita, Nicolae Hanu ("Ana Aslan" National Instiute of Gerontology and Geriatrics)

Purpose: The paper proposes the accomplishment of a longitudinal cell culture study by means of an original procedure of "cell culture in homogenous sets" as well as an optometric method for cellular monolayer measuring. Materials and methods: Using the sugested method, you can act on the cells by a controlled induction of stress. The stress induction is made with the help of some factors wich can be physical, chemical, biological and/or taken all together. The reaction to stress consists in changes of the cell morphology that can be rendered evident by way of registration of the optical density variation in time, thus obtaining contraction curves. The analysis of contraction curve consists in electrocardiogram interpretation, that this way the contraction was called OPTOGRAM. The return to the cell state is ascertained by the relxation curves. Results: With the described method we rendered evident by longitudinal studies the differencies concerning the reaction to stress between young culture and the same cultures after they became older. The young cultures are different from the old ones in the aspect of relaxation curves. Thus, in young cultures these curves have a parabolic aspect, while in the old ones they have a characterstic close to linearity. Conclusions: Optogram can be considered as aging cellular biomarker. In the pharmacological and the cytotoxicity experiments, stress can be induced even by the substancies by the study.

Diagnostics of the prenosologic status and methods for its correction in gerontological patients.

Zakharchenro Mikhael Petrovich, Saint-Petersburg State medical academy, head of the department of human ecology, Saint-Petersburg, Russia. Khavinson Vladimir Khatskelevich, Saint-Petersburg institute of bioregulation and gerontology of NWD Russian academy of medical science, director, Saint-Petersburg, Russia.

Prenosologic states can be found in a considerable number of the so-called apparently healthy persons which are out of medical observation until they take medical advice in connection with some evident disease. These states differ from diseases in prevalence of non-specific changes over specific ones. Investigations convincingly show that the immune system is highly sensitive to the influence of the environmental factors, it is a critical target for considerable number of xenobiotics. This allows to use immunologic methods for diagnosing prenosologic status and prognosticating the consequences after the influence of environmental factors. Our studies show that the use of cytamines regulates and recovers the protective mechanisms of organism what allows to correct the prenosologic status, to prevent appearance in development of different diseases and pathological states and also to speed the rehabilitation of gerontological patients after diseases (illnesses of the immune, nervous, cardio-vascular, respiratory, urogenital, and other systems; surgical operations and traumas; acute and chronic infectious-inflammatory diseases; burns and frostbites; states after radiation and chemotherapy). Prescribing the cytamines may also be effective in the recovery period after different stress conditions. Different prenosologic states of organism, i.e. conditions between the health and disease are also the important aspect in use of cytamines. The uniquity of the new class of parapharmaceutical consists in the highly effective influence of these substances on cells in tissues and organs, at the same time they are not alien for the organism and do not have toxic and another side effects. So correction of the prenosologic status by cytamines provides the optimum state of the health of gerontological patients and increases their lifespan.

Possible Involvement of Superoxide Dismutase and Cytochrome C in ALS

Allan Davison, Amandio Vieira, Suiping Zhou, and Brian Bandy

On the one hand, fruit flies that over-express superoxide dismutase have increased life expectancy. On the other hand, elevated levels or side reactions of superoxide dismutase may be deleterious. Neuropathies like Down's syndrome or amyotrophic lateral sclerosis (ALS) can accompany overexpression or mutation of this ubiquitous enzyme. Peroxidatic activity has been suggested as a mechanism for the harmful effects. Cytochrome c, another superoxide scavenger that has well documented peroxidatic potential, can also kill cells. This paper compares peroxidatic activities of these two enzymes, and their potential for participation in age-related neurological disorders. We compared the abilities of superoxide dismutase and cytochrome c to exacerbate peroxidatic damage, using a synthetic target. We confirm that superoxide dismutase can sometimes accelerate peroxidatic damage. However, this peroxidatic activity is elusive, and when found requires very high concentrations of superoxide dismutase. Cytochrome c, in contrast, has uniformly high peroxidatic activity, which is dramatically increased by initial exposure to hydrogen peroxide. There is good reason to suspect that superoxide dismutase may bring both benefits and risks to the cell. Some have suggested that autocatalytic peroxidatic reactions involving superoxide dismutase could account for the long latent period and the sudden rapid onset of ALS. Nevertheless, experiments to date have largely ruled out a powerful and facile peroxidatic role for superoxide dismutase. There are peroxidatic mechanisms downstream in apoptosis, and there is at least the possibility that the peroxidatic properties of cytochrome c may act upstream also.

Study Regarding Lipids, Lipoproteins and Serum Antioxidant Status in Elderly Patients with Metabolic Syndrome

C. Rusu, C. Borsa, D. Gradinaru, C. Ionescu ("Ana Aslan" National Institute of Gerontology and Geriatrics, Bucharest, Romania)

Lipid, lipoprotein, apolipiprotein levels and antioxidant status represented by total serum antioxidant capacity (TAOC), the peroxidative susceptibility of serum low density lipoprotein (LDLox) and erythrocytes (ESP), were studied in 27 elderly patients (13 men and 14 women, mean age 61+12 years) with metabolic synrome and in 25 control patients (10 men and 15 women, mean age 60+9 years). Triglyceride (TG), fasting blood glucose and ESP levels in patients with metabolic syndrome were significantly higher than in control subjects (176+11 mg/dl vs. 140+36 mg/dl, p <0.001; 148+49 mg/dl vs. 93+7 mg/dl, p <0.001, and 1055+24 mmoles MDA/g Hb vs. 778+167mmoles MDA/g Hb, p<0.001, respectively). High density lipoprotein cholesterol (HDL-C) and TAOC were significantly lower in patients with metabolic syndrome than in the control patients (38+13 mg/dl vs. 58+15 mg/dl, p <0.001, and 64+11% vs 72+13%, p <0.05, respectively). No significant differences were found between groups in apolipoprotein AI and apo B, total cholesterol (TC) and LDL-C. Atherogenic index [Apo B x (TC - HDL-C)/ApoAI x HDL-C] in subjects with metabolic syndrome is positively correlated with TG (r=0.77, p <0.001), with LDL-C/HDL-C ratio (r=0.83, p <0.001) and negatively correlated with TAOC/LDLox ratio(r= -0.39, p <0.05), as an indicator of antioxidant status. In conclusion, this study suggests a link between hypertriglyceridemia, low HDL-C levels, glucose intolerance and serum antioxidant status in elderly patients with metabolic syndrome.

The protein-chaperon control of cellular senescence.

V.F. Semenkov, O.V. Artemieva, V.I. Karandashov, N.A. Gumilevskaya, L.D. Serova. (Research Institute of Gerontology, Moscow, Russia).

According theory of oxidative stress (D. Harman, 1956) senescence may be result of damage of membranes and DNA cells by active form of oxigen (AFO). We have studied possible influence of interaction of autologous serum (AS) of patients different age with the heat shock proteins or chaperons of peripheral blood leukocytes on oxidative metabolism or output AFO in induced luminol and lucigenin dependent chemiluminescence of cells (CLC). Synthesis of heat-shock proteins (p 65) by peripheral blood mononuclears and neutrophils after heating cells at 42C was determined in autoradiography with 35S-methionine labelled proteins. Alteration of proteins structure was obtained by heating on water bath or treatment ultraviolet rays (200-280 nanometers) AS before their interaction with of blood cells. Levels of immunoglobulins and acute-phase proteins in sera were measured by nephelometry analyzator (Beckman Instruments). The heating enhanced stimulatory activity of AS on CLC in 3 times in comparison with nonheating AS. Treatment AS by ultraviolet rays caused the same enhancing effect on CLC. Albumin and gamma-globulin of human serum activated CLC. Cohn II fraction of human gamma-globulin enhanced CLC only after heating. Strained through filter 0.2 micrometer heating AS lost the most parts of its stimulating property. AS reduced the suppressive influence of ATG (Fresenius), monoclonal antibodies CD8 or CD16 on CLC. Xenogenous rabbit and mouse sera and bovine albumin also increased CLC. Activation of heat shock genes in leucocytes by their heating at 42C reduced enhancing effect of AS on CLC. These data suggest the decrease of suppression of oxidative metabolism by proteins cells of the heat shock or chaperons type in consequence of their interaction with denatured or unfolded sera proteins and may be the important mechanism of aging.

The Time and Biological Age

L.M.Belozerova. Ontogenesis laboratory. Perm State Medical Academy

The time and ontogenesis is a most complex interdisciplinary problem to be studied in the joint of phylosophy, biology and psychology. The aim of the research is to study time binds to influence human being ontogenesis. Ontogenesis is the process to form an individual organism from the conception moment till the life end. It can be divided into 3 stages - development, maturity and aging. The leading factor of the organism changes in ontogenesis is physical time, attribute, general form of matter expessing genesis prolongation and subsequence of all material systems state changes and world processes. This time has one measure, one direction and it is uninverted, all system changes spring from the past to the future. Physical time may be called external by its attitude to the human organism. In the organism as in any other material system there is its own (inner) time resulted from changes tempi of matter, energy and information. The own time is in definite relations with inner time. Different relations types of both times are manifested in the biological age: 1) their coincidence shows that the tempo of age individual changes are appropriate to population age shifts tempo; 2) the external time forestalling in comparison with inner one demonstrates accelerated tempo of individual age changes; 3) lacking of inner time from external one indicates delayed tempo of individual age changes. There is another time type which brings its own contribution to complex age picture - it is subjective time. Together with the age increase subjective perception of external time is accelerated that may be explained probably by delayed physiological processes. The human being physical time is determined by the chronological age, the individual inner time measurement is the problem which has its future in gerontology. The type of their relations is being studied objectively by biological age determination.

SESSION 336

Gerotechnology - the European Perspective

J.A.M. Graafmans (CESAER, Leuven, Belgium) The Emerging Field of Gerontechnology. P. Topo, H. Hyppönen, O. Mäki, M. Rauhala (National Research and Development Centre for Welfare and Health, STAKES, Helsinki, Finland) Gerontechnology in Finland. F. Bouchayer (Ministry of Employment and Solidarity, Paris, France) Aging and Technology. Social Science Approaches in France. F. Marcellini (INRCA - Italian National Research Centre on Ageing, Ancona, Italy) The Situation of Gerontechnology in Italy. Z. Széman (Hungarian Academy of Sciences, Budapest, Hungary) A new Technology and its Ripple Effect in Hungary. H. Mollenkopf (The German Centre for Research on Ageing at the University of Heidelberg, Heidelberg, Germany) Gerotechnology - Challenges, Opportunities, and Concerns.

Given the increasing mechanisation of private and public settings, as well as the shift in the age structure of the population, technological appliances will have to be designed with the older user in mind (=>gerotechnology). The symposium aims to provide an overview on the efforts undertaken to face this challenge and the progress achieved in European countries with different levels of mechanisation and technical advancement. J. Graafmans reflects upon the major goals of the European Gerontechnology "movement" set up by The Netherlands and Scandinavian countries, and the milestones that have been reached in order to achieve those goals. Then P. Topo and associates will describe the situation in Finland, which has emerged as front runner in the field of gerotechnology; their contribution will address the challenges which sensory disabilities and dementia present for the development of technology and ethical concerns. Elderly people's coping with changes in their material environment are the focus of a comprehensive multi-disciplinary research programme being carried out in France. Results are presented by F. Bouchayer who stresses the importance of a social science approach in technology research and development. F. Marcellini addresses some major trends in the gradual diffusion of new technologies in Italy, a less industrialised European country where family ties and informal support networks are still strong. The situation is again different in Hungary, a Central European country at the threshold of becoming a member of the European Union. Focusing on the linkage of gerotechnologies to social services, Z. Széman uses the example of alarm systems to illustrate how a technical innovation combined with social innovation can benefit a whole society. Finally, H. Mollenkopf presents selected gerotechnology initiatives from Germany, a country which has achieved an intermediate level of mechanisation. She will conclude the session by reflecting on the major challenges, opportunities, and concerns arising from the papers presented in terms of future gerotechnology research and development.

A New Technology and its Ripple Effect in Hungary

Zsuzsa Széman (Institute of Sociology, Hungarian Academy of Sciences, Budapest, Hungary)

The paper shows what far-reaching changes, affecting even public administration units, can be achieved by a single civil organisation in the introduction of new technologies and their linkage to social services. The first attempt to improve the poor infrastructural situation of the elderly in their own home by introducing an alarm bell system was made in 1993. The model with units linked to a central computer and a 24-hour duty service was introduced in a district of Budapest with an ageing population. Parallel with the installation of the units, the civil organisation also undertook to provide care for these elderly persons in the frame of a contract. The model proved successful; it was developed between 1994 and 1998 in the capital. Then the civil organisation set it up also in smaller settlements. 150 settlements have so far been successfully provided with the technology which has been developed and adapted to local conditions and the Ministry of Family and Social Affairs would like to incorporate the system into the basic services. The paper presents data showing how a Western initiative which was first embraced by a civil organisation shifted to the competence of local authorities and how the civil organisation finally succeeded in having the technical innovation combined with social innovation of benefit for the whole society included in plans for the expansion of basic services for the elderly in Hungary.

Aging and Technology: Social Science Approaches in France

F. Bouchayer (Ministry of Employment and Solidarity, Department of Research MIRE-DREES, Paris, France)

How do elderly people, in their daily life, face changes concerning their material environment ? This is the central topic of a social science research programme carried out in France by MIRE and CNAV, from 1997 to 2000. 20 completed studies in sociology, anthropology, ergonomics, economy were realised, in the fields of housing, domestic and leisure appliances, transport, health, ICT, banking services, etc. Elderly people point of view were collected by qualitative interviews and in situ observations. Results reveals that: 1. To use, as well as not to use technological products participate in the process of identity adjustments and assertions linked to age an ageing. Then, to qualify as «reluctance» attitudes of people that prefer not to use technical goods can be a comprehension error. 2. An important part of the difficulties encountered by the elderly is due to unsuitable products. Products and services dedicated to the whole population are most frequently designed for young and every way able users. 3. The relationships between elderly persons and their relatives, friends, professional carers, play a central role. Departure of children, retirement, widowhood, demotorisation constitute transition periods that determine changes in the uses of technical devices. To conclude, we have to consider the risk of technological illiteracy in industrialised societies, where elderly people are mainly living in usual daily life environment. Products and services specifically dedicated to dependant and frail elderly are of course useful but they partly concern the field of elderly people and of ageing.

Gerontechnology in Finland

P. Topo, H. Hyppönen, O. Mäki, M. Rauhala (National Research and Development Centre for Welfare and Health, STAKES, Helsinki, Finland)

The first objective of the presentation is to give a short overview on the gerontechnological research in Finland. The second objective is to describe the results of two studies. The first study was made among deaf people, deaf blind people and people with aphasia on how their needs to gain access to email and virtual information have been met. The second study is the ongoing research project "Assessment of and ethical guidelines for welfare technology. Multimedia in dementia care and Internet-based shopping services as examples." The methods used in data gathering of the research projects were questionnaire surveys and letters, participatory observation and observation, semi-structured and structured interviews. The multimedia is assessed in a dementia care unit, shopping services in a home services office of a city of Helsinki, and the ethical issues are studied within two assistive technology development projects. The needs to use email and internet of deaf people, deaf blind people and people with aphasia have often not been met. According to the first findings of our projects it is necessary to involve the users - in our case ageing people and social and health care professionals - in the technology and service development in order to get sustainable solutions. For ageing deaf blind persons and persons with aphasia the access to the Internet and email is crucial. More attention should be paid to the value of access to virtual information and email of these user groups. The importance of user involvement in technology and service development should be emphasised more. Methods to encourage discussion on ethical issues in welfare technology development should be developed.

Gerotechnology - Challenges, Opportunities, and Concerns: The German Perspective

H. Mollenkopf (The German Centre for Research on Ageing at the University of Heidelberg, Heidelberg, Germany)

The first aim of this paper is to provide an overview of the main topics discussed in Germany in relation to gerotechnology: accessible technical devices for older people, tele-care and tele-rehabilitation, and seniors and the Internet. Prototypical research projects and initiatives are presented as examples from each domain: (1) the "Sentha" project ("Everyday technology for senior households") conducted by an interdisciplinary research group at the Technical University of Berlin; (2) the "TeleReha" study, conducted at the Berlin Geriatric Center, examining telematic applications in geriatric-rehabilitative contexts; and (3) the "Silvermedia" Computer & Internet Club for older adults run by the Berlin Institute for Social Research (BIS). The second aim of this paper is to draw conclusions from the results of the different European approaches to gerotechnology with regard to future research and development. The knowledge obtained using these different approaches should be used to maintain a high quality of autonomous living for older citizens and to prevent their exclusion from technological opportunities and advances.

The Emerging Field of Gerontechnology

J.A.M. Graafmans (CESAER, Leuven, Belgium)

Throughout history, many groups have applied their technology to specific problems of elderly people. This activity usually was performed in a crisis-driven mode dealing mainly with imminent problems related to the sickly aged. Solutions often came from medical or assistive technologies. To that respect, gerontechnology is unique by virtue of its deliberate comprehensiveness. The term gerontechnology was coined at Eindhoven University of Technology (Graafmans, 1989). This name supplemented an existing term 'Technology and Aging', which is still used and roughly parallel to gerontechnology. Bouma (1992), in an article in the first book devoted to this field provided the first publicised definition of gerontechnology as being 'the study of technology and aging for the improvement of the daily functioning of the elderly'. He pointed out that the terms 'Technology and Aging', in the context of ergonomics, then and still now, are intended as very encompassing designations including R&D, design, manufacture and marketing. Now a number of groups at universities, especially throughout Europe, North America and Japan, have formed under the rubric of gerontechnology. There are international conferences and governmental funding has been developed. COST-A5, a Europe-wide network for planning and investigating issues related to older people was established by European governments. Findings of this network indicated that specific training and education were needed to produce dedicated researchers and professionals. The full paper will elaborate on international developments in this field during the past decade and will briefly discuss how gerontechnology will unfold in the future.

The Situation of Gerontechnology in Italy

F. Marcellini (INRCA - Italian National Research Centre on Ageing, Ancona, Italy)

In recent years technological solutions have become more diffused in Italy and they are becoming important also for elderly people, even if they are not as widely used as in Northern European countries or in USA. The level of education plays an important role in the use and acceptance of technology: in Italy 75% of people aged 60 and over have 5 or less years of schooling, and also their income is often low. Nevertheless in the Centre and North of Italy, which are more industrialised than the South, it is possible to find innovative applications, even if some of them are in an initial or experimental phase. In the health system, there is a good diffusion of telecare and alarm systems; telemedicine is used for connecting hospitals with homes, rest houses or nursing homes. TED project is a recent example of technology for persons with dementia. But, as in Italy the family has still a strong role in caring for the older persons, probably the need of technological support is less felt. High technology is created by "research centres of excellence" (e.g. Scuola Superiore S. Anna, Pisa) for developing innovative products for living independently. In housing, only recently some public dwellings for elderly people have been built with IT domotic solutions. In conclusion gerontechnology is not widespread in Italy. Modern appliances are often a hindrance for elderly people, even if surfing Internet, Italian websites for older persons, and the use of cellular telephone are slowly becoming popular. It is thus necessary to improve the acceptance of technology.

SESSION 337

Health Status and Health Care of Indigenous Elders

P. McGowan (Institute of Health Promotion Research, University of British Columbia, BC, Canada) and M. Fitzgerald (Centre for Disease Control, Vancouver, BC, Canada) The Aboriginal Tuberculosis Program: A New Strategy To Deal With An Age-Old Problem. M. Arch, M. Paddy, (Nganampa Health Council, Alice Springs, Australia) Developing an Aged Care Program for a Traditional Aboriginal Population in Remote Central Australia. K. Braun, V.M. Tanji and R. Heck (University of Hawaii, Honolulu, HI, USA) Attitudes Toward Assisted Suicide and Planning for Death Among Indigenous, Immigrant, and Dominant Groups in Hawaii. R.T. Goins (West Virginia University, WV, USA), C.H. Hennessy, C. Denny (Centers for Disease Control and Prevention, Atlanta, GA, USA) and D. Buchwald (Department of Medicine, University of Washington, USA) Comorbidity and Health-Related Quality of Life Among Older American Indians. B. Finke (Indian Health Service, Zuni, NM, USA) and C.H. Hennessy (Centers for Disease Control and Prevention, Atlanta, GA, USA) Multiple Stakeholder Perspectives in Research on American Indian and Alaska Native Health and Aging.

Although specific demographic data on indigenous populations is often lacking, the size of the global indigenous population aged 60 years and over (8%) was estimated to be some 16 million at the beginning of the 1990's. Of these, an estimated 1.3 million indigenous elders live in industrialized countries where their situation parallels that of developing countries in a developed country context. In general, there is scant information on the situation on these growing populations of elders. This symposium will focus on issues related to the health status and health care of indigenous elders across diverse geographic and cultural settings including aboriginal Canada, Australia, the U.S. mainland, and Hawaii. Within these contexts, topics to be addressed cover disparities in health, well-being, and resource availability between indigenous elders and elders in the majority population, innovative programs and strategies to deliver health care to native elders, cultural orientations affecting health-related decision-making, and the process of involving relevant stakeholders in research on health and aging among indigenous groups. Similarities and differences in issues and strategies relevant to indigenous elders' health and the provision of services across these contexts will be explored, with an emphasis on the magnitude and growth of needs in these populations and related policy implications.

Attitudes Toward Assisted Suicide and Planning for Death among Indigenous, Immigrant, and Dominant Groups in Hawaii

K.L Braun, V.M. Tanji, R. Heck (University of Hawaii, Honolulu, HI, USA)

Several investigators have found that many U.S. minority groups feel and act differently than the dominant North American culture when it comes to end-of-life decision making. While there is clear proof of general ethnic-specific differences, empirical and everyday evidence acknowledge a range of within-group differences as well. This study presents a broader, empirical approach to the issue by trying to identify and measure attitudinal factors related to support of physician-assisted suicide (PAS) that may apply across ethnic groups. This study interviewed adults in five ethnic groups, used factor analysis to quantify attitudes toward planning for death, and used path analysis to test the relative influence of respondent characteristics, including ethnicity, and attitude factors (advocacy to discuss/document wishes, trust in family and physician to make decisions, reliance on religious guidance, fears and anxiety about life's end, and fatalism about the timing of death) on support for physician-assisted suicide (PAS). Findings verified that attitude factors had a direct effect on PAS support but that ethnicity had a direct effect as well, with significantly less support among Native Hawaiians. For Hawaii's indigenous people, lack of support is likely attributable to experience with discrimination, especially in health care access. Practitioners are encouraged to learn about the cultural traditions of the people they serve and to ask open-ended questions that will elicit underlying attitudes that influence end-of-life behavior.

Comorbidity and Health-Related Quality of Life Among Older American Indians

R.T. Goins (West Virginia University, Center on Aging, WV, USA), C.H. Hennessy, C. Denny (Centers for Disease Control and Prevention, Atlanta, GA, USA), D. Buchwald (Department of Medicine, University of Washington, USA)

The first two goals outlined in Healthy People 2010 are to increase quality and years of healthy life and to eliminate health disparities among different segments of the population. Since the association between physical health conditions and health-related quality of life (HR-QoL) may differ by race and ethnicity, our objective for this research was to compare older American Indian and Alaska Natives (AIANs) to their non-AIAN counterparts with respect to patterns of comorbidity and the relationship between comorbidity and HR-QoL. The data source for this analysis was the 1996-1998 Behavioral Risk Factor Surveillance System (BRFSS). We used data from the 50 states in the U.S. and the District of Columbia collected from AIANs and non-AIANs 50 years or older. Comorbidity consisted of 3 chronic conditions - diabetes, high blood pressure, and obesity. Distribution of each of these conditions and HR-QoL measures were examined. Odd ratios adjusted for age, sex, income, and marital status were calculated to assess the interrelationships of the individual chronic conditions with one another. Statistical testing and estimation of the association between the number of comorbid conditions and each HR-QoL measure were obtained by logistic regression and adjusted for age, sex, income, and marital status. Our study revealed that older AIANs more commonly reported diabetes and obesity but less often had hypertension than non-AIANs. Overall, we found that AIANs were more likely to have comorbid conditions than non-AIANs and these comorbid conditions had a significantly stronger negative impact on HR-QoL among AIANs than non-AIANs.

Developing an Aged Care Program for a Traditional Aboriginal Population in Remote Central Australia

M. Arch, M. Paddy, (Nganampa Health Council, Alice Springs, Australia)

In remote central Australia, 3,000 Pitjantjatjara people live a semi-traditional life style on 103,000 square kilometres of land to which they have freehold title, the Anangu Pitjantjatjara Lands. Pitjantjatjara people refer to themselves as Anangu. English is a second language on this land. Literacy levels are low for all age groups. Attendance at school is spasmodic. Employment opportunities are very limited. The cost of basic food is about twice that of Australian cities. Income levels are low with most people relying on social security payments. Few people have access to a private telephone or a private vehicle. There is no public transport and other infrastructure is limited. The average life is some 20 years less than the wider population. There is also a much higher level of morbidity in this population. Nganampa Health Council is an aboriginal community controlled organization which provides primary health services via clinics across the Lands. Until 1996, there were no specific services for aged Anangu on the Anangu Pitjantjatjara Lands. On the Anangu Pitjantjatjara Lands, there are 350 people aged over 50. They have limited access to housing, ablution facilities, laundry facilities, water, food and money. In 1995, Nganampa Health Council undertook a consultancy to ascertain what would be culturally appropriate, sustainable and affordable services to meet the most outstanding needs of senior Anangu. As a result, a program of basic community services and short-term residential care is being developed for senior Anangu.

Multiple Stakeholder Perspectives in Research on American Indian and Alaska Native Health and Aging

B. Finke (Indian Health Service, Zuni, NM, USA), C.H. Hennessy (Centers for Disease Control and Prevention, Atlanta, GA, USA)

The appropriate questions and methods for research on health and aging among American Indian and Alaska Native (AI/AN) populations cannot be determined by researchers alone. Multiple stakeholder perspectives are needed, including those of researchers, direct service providers to the elderly, AI/AN aging advocates, tribal and community leaders, and AI/AN elders themselves. A day-long symposium as part of the annual Indian Health Service Research Conference sought to identify key research issues in American Indian and Alaska Native aging by engaging the perspectives of representatives of all of the above constituent groups and developing a dialogue amongst them. The process by which this was attempted and the results of this effort will be presented.

The Aboriginal Tuberculosis Program: A New Strategy To Deal With An Age-Old Problem

P. McGowan (Institute of Health Promotion Research, University of British Columbia, BC, Canada), M. Fitzgerald (Centre for Disease Control, Vancouver, BC, Canada)

Tuberculosis (TB) remains the world's most important infectious cause of morbidity and mortality among adults. As well, the HIV pandemic has altered the global TB picture because HIV infection accelerates the progression from latent TB infection to active TB, while TB in turn accelerates the progression from HIV infection to AIDS. Canadian aboriginal people experience a disproportionately high rate of TB, especially in older persons. The purpose of this study was to develop and evaluate a lay-led education program. Two aboriginal communities were selected and community advisory committees were established. A TB awareness contest created interest and 200 subjects received honorariums to complete a TB questionnaire. Aboriginal newspapers/newsletters disseminated information about the contest, correct answers and a discussion. Advisory committees worked with the project researcher to develop a one-session, two and one-half hour lay-led program. The PRECEDE-PROCEED health promotion model was used in planning activities to change TB behaviors, such as getting a TB skin test, and accepting INH treatment. The program incorporated culturally appropriate processes along with effective theory and education practices. Lay leaders then piloted the program in seven communities to nearly 100 persons. Feedback from participants and leaders was used to modify the program. Fifty trained aboriginal leaders are now delivering the program to 500 persons. The primary hypothesis in this research is: "aboriginal persons living in communities receiving the education program who are offered chemoprophylaxis treatment will accept the treatment more than persons living in control communities not receiving the education program."

SESSION 338

An Elder Friendly Hospital: Creating a Cultural Shift to Realize a Preferred Future.

Belinda Parke (Capital Health Region, Victoria, Canada) Lesley Moss (Capital Health Region, Victoria, Canada) Tona Lundgren (Capital Health Region, Victoria, Canada)

PURPOSE: Present the "Elder Friendly Hospital" concept and explain the strategies taken by the Capital Health Region to improve outcomes for older hospitalized patients. Older Adults account for 62% of acute care medical and surgical hospital admissions in the Capital Health Region, Victoria, British Columbia. Evidence indicates that hospitals can unintentionally contribute to adverse clinical and social consequences in older adults. The significance of such consequences are observed in lasting functional disabilites. METHOD: System wide interdisciplinary working groups were established to create a network of organizational activity. Using a strategic planning process and incorporating population health data, research findings, critical incident case reviews, patient satisfaction surveys and utilization trends, a gap analysis was completed. The sum total of all activity was directed toward closing the gap and realizing a vision for the preferred future. RESULTS: The creation of a network of activity targeting care processes and services, hospital systems, policies and procedures and community relationships and partnerships. CONCLUSIONS: A gerontological developmental approach to hospital care that stretches from admission to discharge in multiple programs across an integrated health region that serves a population base of 340,000 residents.

Does patient age influence prostate cancer tumour severity at diagnosis?

S.M.H. Alibhai (University of Toronto, Toronto, Canada), M.D. Krahn (University of Toronto, Toronto, Canada), M.M. Cohen

(University of Toronto, Toronto, Canada), N.E. Fleshner (University of Toronto, Toronto, Canada), G. Naglie (University of Toronto, Toronto, Canada)

PURPOSE: Prostate cancer stage, grade, and prostate-specific antigen (PSA) level at the time of diagnosis influence cancer management and prognosis. While some studies suggest these tumour characteristics may change with age, data are conflicting. We investigated the impact of age upon these tumour characteristics. METHODS: Chart review of an age-stratified random sample of newly diagnosed, histologically confirmed prostate cancer in three cities in Ontario, Canada. Patients were identified by means of a comprehensive cancer registry. Comparisons were made across four age strata using chi-square analysis for stage and ANOVA for grade and PSA level. Natural logarithm-transformed PSA (lnPSA) levels were used because of skewness of the data. RESULTS: Three hundred and forty seven charts were reviewed. More men in the oldest age group (80 years or older) had American Urological Association stage A (impalpable) disease and stage D (metastatic) disease than younger men ($R2=0.029$, $p=0.017$). The proportion of patients with clinically localized disease (stages A and B) did not change with age ($p>0.10$). Tumour grade, as assessed by Gleason score, increased slightly with age ($R2=0.017$, $p=0.011$). lnPSA levels were also positively associated with increasing age ($R2=0.081$, $p<0.001$). Excluding patients diagnosed by transurethral prostatectomy attenuated only the relationship of stage with age. CONCLUSION: Aggressiveness of prostate cancer at diagnosis increases slightly with age. This is most likely due to decreased screening intensity and later diagnosis in older patients. Alternatively, prostate cancer biology may change with age.

Evaluation of Interventions to Improve Individualized Care and Information of Inpatients

I. Findl, E. Lehner, P. Benisch, H. Eichbauer, G. Fellinger, K. Klaushofer S. Kordasch, E. Melcher, R. Steinkellner, E. Zwettler, K. Koller (Hanusch-Hospital, Vienna, Austria)

The purpose of this analysis is to evaluate 3 different interventions at a geriatric department with regard to improving inpatient satisfaction: patient information booklet, pain management and conversation with the treating doctor at discharge. In the first part of the study, deficits in the organization of the department and in inpatient care were found via questionnaires of 94 inpatients and 28 staff members. As a consequence the above mentioned 3 interventions were implemented by an interdisciplinary team. In the second part of the study, under the use of the 3 interventions, the same questionnaire was applied to 90 patients and 27 staff members. The comparison of the satisfaction between the 1st and 2nd part of the study in the indicators which represent the interventions served as evaluation criterion. Statistical analysis included correlation analysis and factor analysis using SPSS. The patients and the staff members of the second part of the study assessed the information about organization and daily routine of the department, about pain management and about discharge management significantly better than those of the first series of interviews. In addition the staff members assessed the teamwork within and between the occupational teams better too. Summarizing, the interventions caused significantly higher satisfaction. Nevertheless, in some areas of patient information, eg. about the disease itself and the consequences for the patients' future, there was still a fair amount of dissatisfaction. Therefore, we plan to implement new interventions in the near future.

Factors Related to One Year Mortality After an Emergency Hospitalization of >75 Years Old

F Yvain, D Somme*, G. Magnier *, M. Gisselbrecht*, G. Potel**, O Saint-Jean*, *[Service de Gériatrie, Hôpital Européen Georges Pompidou, PARIS, France], **[Service de Médecine, Hôpital de Nantes, France].*

PURPOSE: >75 years old (y) patients (pts) are frequently hospitalized in emergency. However emergency hospitalization is a manifestation of frailty, and factors related to post-hospital discharge are important to asess for improvement of quality of care. METHOD: We prospectively studied consecutive >75 y pts hospitalized in emergency in an University Hospital in Nantes. Pts who died during the index hospitalization were excluded. We recorded for all pts, the following variables : age, sex, familial status (alone or not), admission motif (cardiovascular, infections, falls, iatrogenic, neurological, others), disorientation, discharge modality (home, nursing home, other institution), and early readmission (<90 days after discharge) (ER) to hospital. RESULT: 129 pts were studied and one-year follow-up was completed for 118 (91.5%). Age, sex, familial status, admission motif and discharge modality didn't differ significantly between pts died and pts alive one year after the hospitalization. In contrast, 51.40f pts disoriented during the hospitalization were dead at one year as compared with 24.10f pts not disoriented ($p=0.004$) and 48.40f pts ER to hospital were dead at one year as compared with 26.40f pts who were not ER ($p=0.03$). In multivariate analysis (logistic regression), with one-year mortality as dependant variable and all others variables independents, only ER and disorientation were significantly associated with one-year mortality ($p=0.048$ and 0.009, respectively). CONCLUSION: Our results suggest that disorientation during the first hospitalization and early readmission after an emergency hospitalization of a >75 y pts are associated with post hospital discharge mortality.

Geriatric Mobile Unit for managing frail elderly patients in an University hospital

P. Couturier, S. Fachler-Buatois, S.Moine, A.Franco (Unité Mobile de Gérontologie, Département de Médecine Communautaire, CHU Grenoble, 38043 GRENOBLE CEDEX 09.

Frail elderly patients constitute a significant proportion of all hospitalized patients. In many hospitals, admission in Geriatics department is not possible due to lack of bed. They are primarily managed within different specialities according to the main presenting problem. The management of such patients usually requires prolonged care in order to recover completely from the acute condition, to be followed by proper rehabilitation and biopsychosocial evaluation finally to be discharged at home or in different institutions. We reported a four year experience of a Geriatric Mobile Unit, presenting the needs of 28 non-geriatric units, based on the type of response obtained from 750 standardized geriatric evaluation at the patient's bedside. The results show that 80 % of patients, who require intervention of the GMU, are hospitalized through the emergency unit. Problems are usually complex including geriatric advice, geriatric orientation and more importantly placement within the community. The intervention on an average occurs 14 days after the admission, which suggests difficulties in the management of this population. The time necessary to evaluate them and to plan their management justify a team that includes at least a geriatrician, a geriatric nurse, and a social worker. The bedside evaluation is discussed in terms of feasibility and the level of satisfaction of hospital partners. Even if the satisfaction of the different specialists is high including opportunity and quality of the intervention, the results suggest that they expect a complete management of such patients with a quick redirection to the geriatric departement or different community services.

Outcomes of an Acute Care of the Elderly Unit with Defined Targeting Criteria

K. Hunter McIlveen, K. Lechelt, D. Wulf (Royal Alexandra Hospital, Edmonton, Alberta, Canada).

Research in progress. It has been suggested that more refined "targeting" might further improve outcomes for ACE (Acute Care of the Elderly) Units. In this study, targeting criteria of age and acute illness, as well as actual or potential risk of functional loss with hospitalization, are used in identification of patients who might benefit from the unit. Patients 65 and over admitted to medical units are screened by a Geriatric Assessment Nurse. Three groups of fifty patients meeting the unit criteria are being sought. These groups include patients admitted directly to the ACE unit, those admitted to another medical unit but transferred to the ACE unit when a bed becomes available, and patients admitted to another medical unit but not transferred. Assessment of

ADL/IADL function and mobility (Barthel Index, OARS) and cognitive function (MMSE, CAM) is completed at admission and discharge. The primary caregiver completes the Caregiver Burden Index. Demographic information, discharge location and length of stay are collected. Three months after discharge, a Research Assistant will repeat the functional assessment on a home visit. Statistical analysis will be used to examine for differences in the three groups. The effect of caregiver burden will be also be examined. Results of the hospital admission/discharge data will be completed in the Spring of 2001. Three month follow-up data will not be available at the time of the conference. Results of this study will provide information regarding the effects a specific targeting strategy for an ACE unit on outcomes for hospitalized older adults.

The Present Situation of Geriatric Hospital Care and New Concepts for it in Hungary

B. Boga, A. Császár, O. Regius, L.Vértes, J.Gabanyi (Hungarian Association of Gerontology, Budapest Hungary

In 2000 the Hungarian Association of Gerontology, conducted a survey to get an overwiev on the present status of hospital care for the elderly in Hungary. Our country will be a member of European Union in a few years, thus we should make our system comparable to the West European ones. We have received answer from 60% of the hospitals we asked. 40% of them have long-term departments. (dpts) Dpts. with nomination"geriatric" work only in 2 hospitals. Acute geriatric dpts do not exist. The acute elderly patients are treated in general dpts. Dpts for chronically ill are held as geriatric dpts though they provide patients without lower age limit and fulfill mainly nursing task. At the same time several elderly cared for there require broader medical provision. The head physicians are well-skilled in geriatrics but the dpts are understaffed. The infrastructure is insufficient. The dpts have mainly a supplement role for the acute dpts which work in a strict DRG system. Due to under-developed social care system the admission for social reason is frequent. The whole situation is amalgam of the residue of the previous era and the ill-transformed western system. It is needed a unified comprehensive concept for the geriatric hospital care. The board of the Hungarian Association of Gerontology elaborated a new concept for this with three basic purposes. According to these 3 sub-departments should work in the geriatric dpts: ambulatory assessment unit, acute care and functional-adaptive subdepartments.

SESSION 339

Chinese Immigrant Women Who Care for Aging Parents

Ho Hon Leung (McGill University, Montreal, Canada), and Lynn McDonald (University of Toronto, Canada)

According to governmental reports about 65% of immigrant seniors to Canada are mainly Chinese and South Asian. Under the existing immigration policy, most of these immigrant seniors are sponsored by their children and most are living with their children. For example, 65 percent of Chinese immigrant seniors compared to 18 percent of Canadian born seniors live with relatives (Government of Canada 1996). The purpose of this pilot study was to explore the experiences of a group of Chinese immigrant women who provided care to their parents and/or in-laws, and the experiences of their elderly relatives who received the care. Unlike the majority of caregiving studies, the focus of study was the dyad living in the same household. An ethnographic approach was used to explore the challenges of the caregivers such as time dependence, emotional, physical and social burden, and the well-being of the caregivers. The elderly parents/in-laws reported on their immigration experiences, how the care receiving experiences affected them socially and psychologically and their daily challenges. Both members of the dyad reported on their coping strategies for living together and the differences in their care experiences before and after their move to Canada. A purposive sample was recruited of 12 caregivers and 12 care recipients who are immigrants living in Toronto. The findings indicate that the dyads face unique caregiving issues attributable to cultural differences which are conditioned by the fact that older immigrants to Canada are not eligible for government transfer payments or welfare benefits for up to 10 years.

Late-in-life immigration as point of departure for elderly Iranian immigrant's explanatory models of illness

Azita Emami (Department of Caring Sciences, Mälardalen University, Eskilstuna, Sweden) Sandra Torres (Department of Sociology, Uppsala University, Uppsala, Sweden)

This study is based on the secondary analysis of data gathered in four studies that aimed at shedding light on the post-migration realities of elderly Iranian immigrants to Sweden. Inspired by the symbolic interationist perspective, this study aims to shed light on the variety of ways through which the process of late-in-life migration constitutes the point of reference for the explanatory models of illness that these elderly immigrants utilize. The results of the secondary analysis of data suggest that knowledge on the various strains associated with the process of late-in-life migration is needed if we are to understand how the elders in question make sense of the illnesses that afflict them.

Physical Health Status of Immigrant Seniors: Some Preliminary Findings

Anita Beltran Chen (Lakehead University, Thunder Bay, Ontario, Canada)

Given the multicultural nature of contemporary Canadian society, gerontologists are beginning to focus their research on the ethnic elderly. Ethnicity is thus used as a significant variable in analyzing gerontological issues. PURPOSES: This paper is a part of a larger study of Filipino seniors in Toronto. Its purposes are: to assess their physical health status based on their own subjective self-rating; to describe the nature of their health problems; to identify their primary caregiver and access to health care; and to describe their attitutde toward institutional care. METHOD: Data were obtained from structured interviews using a 22-page interview schedule with open and close ended questions. Field work was conducted in summer, 1998 using the snow-balling sampling design (N=41). RESULTS: A majority expressed their health to be "excellent" and "good" with arthritis and vision impairment as main problems. Daughters and spouses rank high as primary caregivers. Access to health care does not appear to be a problem. Negative attitude toward institutional care exits. CONCLUSION: The Filipino seniors in Toronto are in relatively good physical health. The relatively easy access to health care professionals is primarily due to their own family members, if not fellow ethnics, who are practicing health professionals themselves, such as nurses and doctors. Social dancing as a form of exercise is effective to relieve stiff joints, aches and pains. Among those without family members to count on as caregivers, reluctance to institutional care may constitute an impediment to adequate health care in old age.

SESSION 340

The Need for Theory: Critical Approaches to Social Gerontology for the 21st Century - Part 1

Simon Biggs (Haifa University, Israel), Carroll Estes (University of California, San Fransisco), Stephen Katz (Department of Sociology, Trent University, Peterborough, Ontario, Canada), Ruth Ray (Department of English, Wayne State University, Detroit USA), Jon Hendricks (University Honors College, Oregon State University, Corvallis, USA), Hans-Joachim von Kondratowitz (Deutsches Zentrum fur Altersfragen, Berling), Chris Phillipson (Centre for Social Gerontology, Keele University)

ISSUE: This double symposium raises the question: What sort of theoretical issues will be key in developing a critical social gerontology for the new millenium? The focus of each session will be the conceptual frameworks, determining issues and critical positions that will contribute to a radical interrogation of contemporary ageing and our personal and societal responses to it. It is hoped that such a possible geography for the study and experience of ageing may begin to emerge. STRUCTURE: Each session will consist of presentations by five leading speakers covering a key theoretical position or issue. Presentations will be followed by an opportunity for debate. CONTENT: In convening this double-symposium, we recognise the growth of dynamic and often challenging ideas that are emerging to develop a critical perspective on contemporary ageing. We also recognise the poverty of what could be thought of as the mainstream of gerontological thought. The scope of the issues to be addressed is formidable, including the place of feminist and political economic analysis, the role of identity formation and maintenance, the social construction of ageing, the effects of changing social institutions such as the family, critiques of power, marginalisation and globalisation, the relative merits of modern and post modern interpretations of contemporary ageing and beyond. An international grouping of speakers, who have been leading developmentin their particular fields, will expand upon key aspects of contemporary theory-building in social gerontology. Agreement is not expected. However, it is hoped that the symposia will work toward a more profound understanding of both the study and the experience of ageing as we move into a new millenium. OUTCOMES: A clearere understanding of the complex and contradictory nature of contemporary ageing. An exploration of the theoretical tools available to interrogate ageing as a field of study. The identification of core issues for a critical social gerontology in the 21st century.

Critical Configurations in Gerontological Theory: Multidisciplinarity or Nomadic Thinking?

S. Katz (Department of Sociology, Trent University, Peterborough, Canada)

In the past decade critical gerontologists have creatively borrowed ideas from political economy, feminism, the humanities and cultural studies to challenge and enhance the field of ageing studies. Contesting social gerontology's traditional focus on individual roles, masculinist lifecourse models, scientific standards and liberal political agendas, critical studies turn to macro-structural stratification models, constructivist and reflexive methodologies, and cross-cultural and interdisciplinary frameworks. Less attention has been given, however, to the discursive dynamics behind the new critical configurations. How are intellectual traditions such Marxism, feminism or poststructuralism fractured, diluted, transfigured and recombined in critical gerontology? What is the theoretical status of critical ideas in gerontology and how is it maintained? In addressing these questions this paper takes up the work of Pierre Bourdieu, Michel Foucault and Gilles Deleuze to suggest that critical thinking in gerontology is a Anomadic rather that A multidisciplinary enterprise. As such, critical gerontology has the potential to innovate theoretical responses to the problems and promises of our ageing society while shedding light on its own limitations as a sub-field of expertise.

Rethinking Family Development and Family Solidarity

A. Lowenstein (Centre for Research & Study of Ageing, University of Haifa, Israel)

The presentation will address two general questions. First, what have we learned about the social phenomenon of the family life course development and family solidarity over the past decade? Second, what do we need to know to improve the theory of family development and enrich the model of family intergenerational solidarity? The discussion will explore and critique issues of family trajectories and transitions that are today more age integrated, less disjunctive and more continuous and interdependent. The implications for the organisation of the family life course and the timing of various family transitions in light of the diversity and change that are today basic to these transitions will be analysed. The contingencies inherent in family relations, termed the latent kin matrix, will be discussed in light of the growing heterogeneity in intergenerational family relations. Conceptual and methodological issues related, for example, to level of analysis or to the concept of family life stage and timing will be explored. Findings regarding intergenerational family solidarity versus the emerging themes of family conflict and family ambivalence will be analysed. Finally, family identity will be presented as a concept that may serve as a paradigm to answer the above critique

Surface, Depth and Masquerade: An interrogation of the Personal and the Structural as factors influencing Age and Identity.

Simon Biggs (Centre for Social Gerontology, Keele University, U.K).

A key question for critical gerontology, as we enter a new millenium, will be how social theories can include personal and structural change without reducing one to the other. One way in which this problem has been conceived is in terms of surface and depth elements of identity. Surface privileges place and appearance. Depth refers to socio-historical embededdness and hidden motivation. In this paper I will explore the relationship between the hidden and appearance through the proposal that both are necessary to understand narratives of continuity and change in later life. Further, these narratives provide route-maps though which ageing identities can be negotiated. They result in strategies, actively adopted, to both protect and connect personal and the social will determine the degree to which strategies such as masquerade are used. Masquerade may be particularly important in understanding intergenerational exchanges and other forms of interaction where power and integrity are at stake. Three layers of analysis are proposed in order to make sense of this complex situation. The first of these include formal representations of social reality, the second refers to the experience of events and the third, to ageing in the imagination. These layers may be operationalised in order to interrogate surface and depth as aspects of an ageing identity.

The Perils and Possibilities of Critical Theory: Lessons from Feminist Criticism

R. Ray (Department of English, Wayne State University, Detroit, MI, USA)

Although "theory" (generalisable paradigms which explain and predict) has greatly influenced knowledge-making in gerontology, "critical theory" (perspectives which challenge and critique existing paradigms, methodologies, and knowledge-making itself) has had comparatively little influence on the field. Yet recent movement in the direction of feminist gerontology (Browne 1998; Calasanti, 1999, Garner, 1999; Ray, 1996, 2000) suggests that gerontology is now poised for a "critical turn." In this paper I offer some cautionary tales from feminist literary criticsm regarding the use of critical theory in the pursuit of knowledge and social change. Feminist criticism is an instructive case because it has undergone substantial internal critique but has endured long enough to produce three generations of feminist scholars. Drawing on lessons from feminist criticism, I argue that feminist gerontologists need to make their theory relevant to society at large and turn their critical energies toward activism.

Theoretical Perspectives on Old Age Policy: A Critique and A Proposal World Congress of Sociology, Vancouver BC, Canada, July, 2001

C.Estes (UCSF Institute for Health and Ageing, San Francisco, California, USA)

The last two decades have been characterised by an intensification of political struggles over the privatisation of the bedrock programs of old age policy in the US, Medicare and Social Security. This paper explores the theoretical strengths and weaknesses of current gerontological theorising for understanding and explaining old age policy in the context of the Ademographic imperative@ and attacks on entitlements for the elderly. Five major trends that frame and shape public policy for the elderly are examined in terms of the two dimensions of ideology and process: privatisation rationalisation, globalisation, medicalisation and informalisation. Political economy, feminist, critical and cultural theories are employed and revised in a multi-level analytical framework to understand the relationship between demography, capitalism, the state and old age policy.

SESSION 342

The Social and Political Context of the Elderly: The Argentine Case

GUTMANN, Ramon M. - Secretariat for Social Promotion - Government of the City of Buenos Aires.

The purpose of this presentation is to describe the situation of the elderly in Argentina from the beginning of the century until the present. This situation highly correlates with the functioning of the political power in office and the permanent controversies with other main political parties and movements (nation - provinces controversy). The outcome of these differences is the worsening conditions of the elderly population. Also taken into account is the perverse profile sustained by the previous military dictatorship (1976 - 1983). The figures used to describe this perspective are: health, education, housing, social security, social services and the role of the seniors' leadership in Argentina. The conclusion points out that the acceptance, rejections and demonstrations of solidarity to the elderly population became a mirror of the emerging values of these recent changing stages of the Argentinean society.

Ageing in the Indian Context

S.D.GOKHALE

In India, advances in medical sciences, Genetics and Bio & Information Technology, upgradation of the quality of life, declining death and birth rates, have cumulatively resulted in a rapid increase in the number of people in the age bracket of 60 plus. This has presented a number of challenges. The average life span has increased resulting in multi-generational families especially in rural areas. This has an impact on transmittal of values and familial relations. Women live longer than men. While, men can easily re-marry, widows may not because of cultural reasons. Since, the number of children has gone down the widowed mother may be compelled to stay with relations as a dependant. This leads to a feeling of loneliness; of being unwanted, increasing dependency ratio. For ages family is providing safety-net and takes care of ill, disabled or aged. Some believe that family as a social system may collapse before we know it. As a social scientist, my assumption is that the oriental family is only changing its face and form. Economic security is a concern emerging with demographic change. The government as well as society is looking at a number of options to provide income security to the elderly such as gratuity, provident fund and old age assistance. * The number of people above the age of 60 is increasing faster than the birth rate. * Dependency ratio is higher in widowed women. * Indian family is only changing its face and form and not withering away. * Multigenerational families are on an increase. * Longevity has upset the actuarial time table and made the pension calculation vulnerable.

SESSION 343

A simple set of Durkheimian nomie tools for elderly to master social activities

Bo G. Eriksson (Department of Sociology, Ubiversisty of Göteborg, Sweden)

Purpose: To reconsider the focus of the Durkheimian anomie analyses into a set of simple tools for persons, especially elderly, to form co-operative actions to pursue a self chosen life style. Method: First, an analysis of the Durkheimian anomie concept is transformed into a simple set of propositions suited for co-operative actions. Second, these propositions have been used as tools used by 70-years-olds in a longitudinal intervention study in a population in Göteborg, Sweden. Results: Co-operative activity successes, and failures, during a six years follow up, are presented. From these experiences, the potentials and limitations of these tools are discussed. Conclusion: This simple set of nomie tools are understood and mastered by elderly persons in their strive to perform a self chosen life style.

Elderly Suicide and the History of Modernisation

Karatu Kiemo (Sociology Department, Uppsala University, Uppsala, Sweden).

Purpose:The history of modernisation and the underlying demographic and socioeconomic changes has been theorised as being detrimental to the status, welfare and security of elders in the society (Cowgill, 1972). This study examines how such changes might impact on contemporary elders' risk for suicide. Method: In a cross-national comparative approach, a population study of 49 countries (WHO suicide data) has been undertaken. Countries are classified according to the magnitude of elders' suicide and the demographic and socioeconomic characteristics of such clusters assessed, as Corin (1996) recommends. Results: The findings demonstrate that low elders' risk for suicide is not typical of less modernised countries and high elders' risk for suicide is not common in more modernised countries (as it would be expected on the basis of modernisation theory). Our data show that high elders' risk for suicide is invariably found in countries that can be described as undergoing rapid demographic, socioeconomic and/or political changes. Conclusion: The modernization proposition regarding the decline of the status, welfare and security of elders in the course of modernisation can be queried for it is not supported by contemporary elders' suicide data. The data supports the view that modernisation is not necessarily averse to the welfare and security of elders (Palmore and Manton, 1974); that rapidity of social change may be problematic for elders (Hammarstrom, 1975); and that high levels of modernisation might augment elders' social integration (Cox, 1994) so as to occasion a low and/or a declining elders' risk for suicide in the more modernised countries.

Has loneliness amongst older people in Britain increased since 1945?

Christina R. Victor (Department of Public Health sciences, St George's Hospital Medical School, London, England), Sasha Scambler (Department of Public Health sciences, St George's Hospital Medical School, London, England).

Purpose: Loneliness has been consistently identified as one of the specific 'social problems' which accompanies old age and growing older. 90% of the general population of Britain feel that loneliness is a problem associated with old age. It is presumed that loneliness and isolation have become more prevalent in Britain the post-second World war period as a result of the decline of multi-generation households and changes in family structure. This paper examines the accuracy of this stereotype and considers if current cohorts of older people are more likely to report experiencing loneliness than previous generations of elders. Method: Analysis of historical and contemporary survey data. Historical data is provided by three 'classic' social surveys undertaken in England between 1945 and 1960 by Sheldon, Townsend and Tunstall with sample sizes ranging from 2-500. Contemporary data are provided by a survey of 245 people aged 65-74 living in South London undertaken in 1999. The questions used in all four surveys were highly comparable. Results: The prevalence of individuals reporting that they often experienced loneliness ranged from 5-9% and showed no evidence of increasing , nor did loneliness rates for specific age or gender specific sub-groups. Reported loneliness amongst those living alone had decreased from 32% in 1945 to 14% in 1999. Conclusion: The self- reported prevalence of loneliness suggests little variation between different cohorts of older people and offers little support for the assertion that changes in household and family circumstances have resulted in an increase in loneliness amongst older people.

Predictors of loneliness among community elders in Korea

Hye-Ryoung Kim (Department of Nursing, Inje University, Pusan, Korea)

The purpose of this study was to examine the predictive relationship between the predictors and loneliness among community elders in Korea. The subjects for this study were 531 elders who are 60 and over. They were living at the local area where the government has been supporting financially in Pusan, Korea. This is a descriptive study using cross-sectional design. Data collection was performed by 9 trained interviewers individually in subjects¡¯ house from April 3 to August 10, 2000. Loneliness using revised UCLA Loneliness scale, social network and perceived social support using NSSQ, Functional status using Instrumental Activities of Daily Living (IADL), and demographics such as age, gender and education were measured. Hierarchical multiple regression model was used to examine the relationship between loneliness and its¡¯ predictors. Demographics such as age, gender and education, and social factors such as social network, perceived social support and functional status significantly explained 26.9% of the total variance of loneliness (F=24.884, p=.000). Social network was the most significant predictor of loneliness (beta=-.331, p=.000). Perceived social support (beta=-.263, p=.000), functional status(beta=-.204, p=.000) and education (beta=-.147, p=.013) had effects on loneliness. The findings of this study will provide the grounds for assessment and intervention of loneliness of community elders in Korea.

Understanding the Experiences of Loneliness in Older People.

Sasha Scambler, Christina R Victor (St George's Hospital Medical School, London, UK)

PURPOSE: Loneliness and social isolation are indicators of both poor quality of life and poor self reported health status amongst older people, making this an important area for research and policy development. Despite the large body of literature there is no universal definition or understanding of the concept of loneliness and the many studies use differing and sometimes contradictory definitions. The aim of this study is to explore the possibilities of creating a sociological framework for the understanding of loneliness through the experiences and understanding of older people. METHOD: The results of a qualitative pilot study involving in-depth, semi-structured interviews with 15 adults between the ages of 66 and 88 are explored. RESULTS: Four themes central to developing an understanding of loneliness are reviewed. Key aspects of the experience of loneliness - including individual life choices, health status, financial independence and gender - are then developed into a model framework for understanding the concept and experience of loneliness in older people. The framework outline is presented and the first links between the individual and their perceptions on the importance of social contact, personality characteristics, lifestyle factors, material, social, physical and environmental resources and structural and causal mechanisms are presented. CONCLUSION: The model framework is presented as a useful tool in drawing links between the agentic powers of the individual and the structural mechanisms of social class, age, gender and race, reflecting individual experiences of loneliness in the social context.

SESSION 345

"The 3rd Life" - A Longitudinal Study of New Forms of Aging

Paul Schlecht (leading editor of Südwestrundfunk (SWR) Baden-Baden,Germany) Hermann Sturm (editor of Südwestrundfunk (SWR) Baden-Baden, Germany: "The 3rd Life": A Long-Term Project on Public Television) H. Strum (Sudwestrundfunk, Baden-Baden, Germany) P. Schlecht (Sudwestrundfunk, Baden-Baden, Germany) ("The Making of The 3rd Life") E. Olbrich (Department of Psychology, University of Erlangen, Germany) B. Fulgraff (Adult Educatin, University of Oldenburg, Germany) A. Kuhlmey (Health Sciences, Technical College, Braunschweig, Germany) ("An Aging "Pioneer-Generation": Styles of Life After Recruitment in Germany) B. Seidl (Sudwestrundfunk, Baden-Baden, Germany) ("Meaning in the Last Years of Life: A Pilot Film")

The Symposium will present the projekt "The 3rd Life", a longitudinal study of development after retirement, made by Südwestrundfunk (SWR), a German TV-Station, in collaboration with an interdisciplinary team of gerontologists. Starting with their transition from regular work to retirement in 1993. 30 women and men (born between 1926 and 1939) were interviewed every year, and systematic records of their everyday lives as well as of physical, social and psychological changes were assessed. Moreover, important live-events were recorded verbally and visually whenever they occurred. The project will run for two more years. It is intended to show the various forms of aging in our time. Modern societies do rarely offer meaningful tasks to persons after retirement; models of socially and psychologically productive styles of aging are seldom presented, and conceptualizations of good aging usually just demand "more of the old", i.e. performance and behavior of adulthood. This does not take into acount that men and women today can anticipate 20 to 30 years of life after their retirement, that many aging persons work actively in order to find new roles and to develop a new identity. Many of them claim that society should recognize and acknowledge their generative contributions. These themes have seldom been brought to the attention of the public, and they have not frequently been analyzed by social-gerontological research. The longitudinal study presented does describe "new" forms of life after retirment, using verbal communication and non-verbal (filmed) information. This refers to changes of physical and ecological conditions and of social contexts, it also encompasses new role-behavior in old age, and a continuing personal development. Since it is a historically new fact that whole generations can enter an extended period of retired life, a differentiated description of perceptions and experiences of "late freedom" is offered. Interindividual differences between goals and ways of their realization become evident as do (intraindividual) changes of commitments over time. In our analyses we have given special attention to potentials for development. After eight years we are able to identify different styles of living in old age, such as aging as a period of "increasing care for others", as a time of "strong relationships with one's family", or for other persons as a time of "calm disengagement". We could describe "curious" and "adventurous" forms of aging in a continuing situation of freedom, we could also recognize "denial" od "coping with restrictions" in our participants. The first presentation will deal with the scope, methods, and the organization of the study. The second will characterize the cohort from which our participants come and their specific situation. It will come to describe a "Pioneer-Generation". The third part of the symposium will present results. Our analyses strengthen positions of differential gerontology. They also demand the distinction between different pathways of aging.

An Aging "Pioneer-Generation": Styles of Life After Retirement in Germany

E. Olbrich (Department of Psychology, University of Erlangen, Germany), B. Fülgraff (Adult Education, University of Oldenburg, Germany) and A. Kuhlmey (Health Sciences, Technical College, Braunschweig, Germany)

Although models of socially and psychologically productive forms of aging are seldom presented in modern societies, many aging persons find new roles and develop a new identity in their later years. The study presented uses verbal and non-verbal (filmed) information. It differentially describes perceptions, experiences, and behaviour of participants in the longitudinal study "The 3rd Life". Interindividual differences between goals and ways of their realization in rather specific environments are described as forms or styles of aging. The social theme is prominent in these, although realizations differ. A commitment to active social participation, "new" relationships with children and grandchildren, changes in partnership, and "new" form of relationship to nature, sometimes also to god (religion), and others, will be described. Moreover, the experience of behavioural restrictions and of existential limitations will be adressed. Dealing with these cannot often be described in terms of coping. Rather, an acceptance of limitations begins to show.

Meaning in the Last Years of Life: A Pilot Film

B. Seidl (Südwestrundfunk (SWR) Baden-Baden, Germany)

One of the pilot-films produced by the author for Südwestrundfunk is presented. It shows two forms of finding menaning in the last years of life. Authentic statements of participants and film records are cautiously interpreted.

The 3rd Life: A Long-Term Project on Public Television

P. Schlecht (Südwestrundfunk, Baden-Baden, Germany) and H. Sturm (Südwestrundfunk, Baden-Baden, Germany)

In 1992, SWF SÜDWESTRUNDFUNK a public TV-Station in Germany, started a project intended to document differential forms of aging in a developed society. Starting at the time of their transition from work to retirement, 30 persons 17 men and 13 women from different occupations were selected, casted, and then followed over nine years. Assessments will end after ten years, i.e. in 2002. The project documents life after retirement as filmed by a professional camera team. In close cooperation with six gerontologists from the medical, the social-psychological, and the social-political sciences, additional data on physical, social, and psychological changes were collected, and careful theoretical interpretations on forms of coping with these changes were made. To our knowledge, "The 3rd Life" is unique in combining science, professional film-makers, and normally aging people from different social classes in an attemt to describe new concepts of aging on public TV.

The Making of The 3rd Life

H. Sturm (Südwestrundfunk, Baden-Baden, Germany) and P. Schlecht (Südwestrundfunk, Baden-Baden, Germany)

Regular interviews in front of a TV-camera, and the filming of important events whenever they occur not only demand a continuing motivation of participants. It must be paralleled by sensitivity, empathy and respect of interviewer plus camera team that come in addition to their professional skills. A demonstration of this work is presented. Forms of cooperation of the TV-crew with researchers and with aging participants in the study is described. Before all, the question is discussed, what influence participation I in a longitudinal study on aging, especially knowledge of one´s public presentation in films has on the development of participants, and how this can be controlled.

SESSION 346

Physical activity as a determinant of physical and cognitive functioning

V.S. Stel (EMGO Institute, Vrije Universiteit, Amsterdam), S.M.F. Pluym (EMGO Institute, Vrije Universiteit, Amsterdam), B.W.M. Schalk (EMGO Institute, Vrije Universiteit, Amsterdam), M. Visser (EMGO Institute, Vrije Universiteit, Amsterdam), M.G. Dik (EMGO Institute, Vrije Universiteit, Amsterdam)

ISSUE: Physical inactivity in old age is well known to increase the risk of morbidity and mortality. Physical activity may affect physical and cognitive functioning in old age through its effect on health status. However, a direct association between physical activity and functioning, independent of health status, can also be hypothesized. This hypothesis will be addressed using prospective data from the Longitudinal Aging Study Amsterdam (LASA). STRUCTURE: This symposium will start with a 5 minute introduction by the convener, introducing the topic of the symposium and describing the general characteristics of the LASA study. Five speakers will present their research during 10 minute presentations. After each speaker, 3 minutes are allowed for discussion/clarification. After the presentations, the discussant (E.M. Simonsick, National Institute on Aging, Bethesda MD, USA) will summarize the presented results (5 minutes) and will lead the general discussion with the audience (15 minutes). CONTENT: The potential influence of physical activity on functioning in old age is the central theme of this symposium. Several functioning outcomes will be presented, including falls, (mobility) performance, and cognitive functioning. Data from the Longitudinal Aging Study Amsterdam, a study among 3,107 elderly men and women aged 55 years and older (a representative sample of the Dutch elderly population) will be presented. This prospective study started in 1992 and participants are continued to be examined with 3-year time intervals. Only prospective data will be presented at this symposium. Speaker 1 will discuss different methods for assessing physical activity in the LASA cohort. Physical activity data obtained using an interviewer-administered questionnaire will be compared with 24-hour physical activity diaries and objective pedometer counts. Speaker 2 will discuss physical activity as a predictor of falls in older men and women. Information on falls was collected prospectively using fall calenders. High physical activity was associated with a 50% reduction in fall risk in both men and women. Speaker 3 will address whether sports activity and biological frailty markers (and their interaction) are determinants of decline in functional performance. Low cholesterol level was associated with an increased risk for performance decline in women. No interaction with sports activity was observed. Speaker 4 will address physical activity as a determinant of 3-year prospective change in mobility. Low overall inactivity and no participation in sports activities were important determinants of future mobility loss, independent of health status. Finally, speaker 5 will address life-time physical activity as a determinant of cognitive functioning in old age. Even after adjustment for current physical activity, regular exercise at young age (15-25 years of age) was an important determinant of information processing speed at old age. CONCLUSION: The results that will be presented during this symposium support the functional and cognitive benefits of physical activity in old age. The symposium will show that a variety of function dimensions are independently influenced by physical activity, including falls, mobility, functional performance, and cognition.

Albumin and cholesterol levels and decline of physical performance in the elderly.

B.W.M. Schalk, M. Visser, D.J.H. Deeg, L.M. Bouter (EMGO Institute, Vrije Universiteit, Amsterdam, The Netherlands)

PURPOSE: Previous studies have demonstrated a relationship of low albumin and low cholesterol levels with heart disease and mortality. Little is known on whether low levels of albumin and cholesterol are associated with physical functioning. The aim of our study is to investigate the association between cholesterol, albumin and future decline in physical performance. METHOD: We used data on 1042 men and women aged 55-84 years, participants of the Longitudinal Aging Study Amsterdam (LASA). Participants were classified into low (< 5.20 mMol/L) and normal total cholesterol and low (< 43 g/L) and normal albumin using baseline (1991/92) blood samples. Performance (6-meter walk, putting on a cardigan, repeated chair stands) was assessed at baseline and 3-year follow up. Decline was defined as a difference < -5 %. RESULTS: After adjusting for, age, performance score, body mass index, social economic status, exercise, smoking and chronic disease at baseline, women with low cholesterol levels had a odds ratio of 3.40 (95% CI: 1.43-8.08) for performance decline. In contrast, in men no relationship was observed (OR=1.33; 95% CI: 0.63-2.79). For both men and women, no significant association with albumin was found (p>0.2). Exercise was an important determinant of performance decline in men and women. However, no interaction between exercise and cholesterol levels was observed (p>0.2). CONCLUSION: Women with low serum cholesterol levels have a 3-fold increased risk for future decline in physical performance compared to those with normal cholesterol levels. In men no such relationship was observed.

Life-time exercise and cognition at old age

M.G. Dik, D.J.H. Deeg, M. Visser, L.M. Bouter, C. Jonker (Institute for Research in Extramural Medicine, Vrije Universiteit, Amsterdam, The Netherlands).

PURPOSE: Exercise intervention studies have shown positive effects of aerobic exercise on cognition, especially on information processing speed. To date, the association between life-time exercise and cognition has not been investigated. This study investigates the influence of life-time exercise on cognitive function at older age. METHOD: Study subjects, aged 55-85 years, were participants in the Longitudinal Aging Study Amsterdam (LASA), a longitudinal population-based study covering 6 years of follow-up, measured on three occasions. Respondents were retrospectively asked whether they had exercised earlier in life. We assessed cognition using the Mini-Mental State Examination (MMSE) and Coding Task (information processing speed). Data were analyzed with MANOVA for repeated measures, adjusted for sociodemographics (age, sex, education, socioeconomic status), health indicators (ApoE e4, chronic disease, depression) and health-related behavior (life-time work activity, current physical activity, smoking, alcohol, and body mass index). Complete data were available for 914 subjects. RESULTS: Overall, elderly who had exercised regularly during life had higher adjusted scores on information processing speed compared to elderly who had exercised never or sometimes (p=0.02). No significant differences between the exercise-groups were observed on MMSE (p=0.08). Analyses of separate age-periods during life revealed that elderly who had exercised regularly while they were 15-25 years had higher scores on information processing speed at older age (p=0.002) compared to elderly who had not exercised. Exercise during the other age-periods (26-35 years and 36-50 years) was not significantly associated with information processing speed. CONCLUSION: Our study suggests a beneficial effect of regular exercise early in life on information processing speed at older age. This effect could not be explained by current habitual exercise or other life-style factors.

Physical activity and the risk of falls in older men and women

S.M.F. Pluijm (EMGO Institute, Vrije Universiteit, Amsterdam), V.S. Stel (EMGO Institute, Vrije Universiteit, Amsterdam), M. Visser (EMGO Institute, Vrije Universiteit, Amsterdam), D.J.H. Deeg (EMGO Institute, Vrije Universiteit, Amsterdam), J.H. Smit (Department of Sociology and Social Gerontology, Vrije Universiteit, Amsterdam), P. Lips (Department of Endocrinology, VU-Hospital, Amsterdam)

PURPOSE: The role of physical activity in the prevention of falling remains controversial. In this prospective study, we examined the relationship between daily physical activity and falls in older men and women. METHOD: The study population consisted of 1383 participants (705 women and 678 men) of the Longitudinal Aging Study Amsterdam (LASA) who were 65 to 88 years old as of the first of January, 1996. The level of physical activity in the previous two weeks was estimated by means of a detailed, interviewer-administered questionnaire regarding walking, cycling, sports and household activities. During three years of follow-up, fall events were recorded with a 'fall calendar'. Data were analysed using Generalized Estimating Equation (GEE), adjusted for age, sex, chronic disease, urinary incontinence and cognition. RESULTS: Physical activity was non-linearly, inversely related to the risk of falls. As compared with people in the lowest quintile, people in the highest quintile of energy expenditure (expressed in kcal/d) had an adjusted relative risk for multiple falls of 0.76 (95% CI 0.59-0.97). Walking outside was also inversely associated with falls; people in the highest quintile, who walked at least 40 minutes per day, had a relative risk of 0.79 (95% CI: 0.61-1.00) as compared with women who never walked. Performing sports activities (yes/no) was not associated with multiple falls. However, when we distinguished between inside and outside falls, performing sports activities (yes/no) appeared to be protective against inside falls (RR: 0.69; 95% CI: 0.55-0.87), but modestly increased the risk of outside falls (RR: 1.19; 95% CI: 1.00-1.41). CONCLUSION: These prospective data indicate that a high level of total physical activity and walking activity protect against falls among older men and women.

Physical activity as a determinant of mobility loss

M. Visser (EMGO Institute, Vrije Universiteit, Amsterdam, The Netherlands), S.M.F. Pluym (EMGO Institute), R.J. Bosscher (Faculty of Movement Sciences, Vrije Universiteit, Amsterdam, The Netherlands), D.J.H. Deeg (EMGO Institute)

PURPOSE: The aim of this study was to investigate whether physical activity is a determinant of future change in objectively measured mobility performance. METHOD: Prospective data (3-year follow-up) on 2,109 men and women aged 55-85 years, participants of the Longitudinal Aging Study Amsterdam, were used. Physical activity of the past 2 weeks was assessed at baseline by questionnaire. Change in mobility performance was based on two performance tests (walking 6 m and 5 repeated chair stands) at baseline and follow-up. RESULTS: Mobility loss was observed among 45.6% of the respondents. Low physical activity was associated with a greater mobility loss and a threshold effect in the association was observed. After adjustment for baseline mobility function, health status, socio-demographic and lifestyle variables, persons in the lowest quintile of physical activity (<1h20min per day) experienced a greater mobility loss compared to those in the upper four quintiles (p=0.003). No participation in sports activities was also associated with a greater loss of mobility (p=0.009). The results were similar when a more stringent definition of mobility loss was used (mobility decline >1 SD, 11.8% of respondents) or when physical activity was expressed in kcal/day instead of min/day. When the population was stratified by health status (no chronic disease versus one or more chronic diseases), a similar association between physical inactivity and mobility loss was observed in both groups. CONCLUSION: Our results suggest that physical inactivity is an important determinant of future mobility decline.

Physical activity in older people measured by a questionnaire, a seven-day diary and a pedometer

V.S. Stel (EMGO Institute, Vrije Universiteit, The Netherlands), J.H. Smit (Department of Sociology, Vrije Universiteit, The Netherlands), S.M.F. Pluijm, (EMGO Institute, Vrije Universiteit, The Netherlands), P. Lips (Department of Endocrinology, VU Hospital, The Netherlands)

PURPOSE: Low physical activity is an important risk factor for falls. It is difficult, however, to assess precisely physical activity in an older population. In this study physical activity was assessed by three methods: a questionnaire, a diary and a pedometer. The aim of the study was to measure physical activity more precisely in older people and to validate the physical activity questionnaire by the diary and pedometer. METHOD: The study was performed in a subsample of men and women (n=439, age>65) of the Longitudinal Aging Study Amsterdam (LASA). During a home visit, an interviewer-administered questionnaire on physical activity of the last two weeks was completed. After the visit, respondents completed a diary and wore a pedometer, both for seven days. RESULTS: The mean physical activity by questionnaire was 150 minutes per day (median=133 [IQR: 81-206]), by diary 111 minutes per day (median=109 [IQR: 63-145]), and by pedometer 3358 steps (about 2,4 km) per day (median=3221 [IQR: 1702-4770]). Compared to the diary, both men and women scored significantly higher on the questionnaire (p<0.01). Agreement between the questionnaire and diary was higher in people with an average activity of <120 minutes per day (mean=11 [limits of agreement: -35, 56] compared to >=120 minutes per day (mean=62 [limits of agreement: -26, 151]. Spearman correlation's of .66 and .41 (p<0.01) were found between the questionnaire and the diary and pedometer, respectively. CONCLUSION: The questionnaire overestimates physical activities compared to the seven-day diary, but seems to be a useful instrument for classifying physical activity in older people.

SESSION 347

A City Transportation Service For Elderly Handicapped Persons In Rennes : A Nine-Year Experience

O. Michel, M. Michel, J-Y Housset, C. Cattenoz, P. Jouanny (Consultation of Gerontology, University Hospital, Rennes, France)

PURPOSE: Analysing the characteristics of an elderly population using a special transportation system for handicapped persons and the reasons for abandoning regular busses. METHODS: A special transportation service for handicapped persons, initially planned for people in wheel chairs, has been opened to elderly people with impaired mobility. The consultation of Gerontology has been choosen to appreciate the ability of the customers to use regular busses. A questionnaire was filled in this occasion. RESULTS: In a nine-year period (1992-2000), 852 elderly persons (mean age 80,5) who wanted to use this service were examined. The reasons for requesting the service were more focused on health-related needs (consultation with a paramedical worker or a specialist) than on social wishes (family, friends, hospital or cemetery visits, clubs) or shopping. All these people expressed difficulties with the regular busses : lack of benches at the bus stop, steps too high to go into or even more out of the bus, bus stops too shortly or too far from the pavement, trouble to manipulate the ticket, bus too jerky, impolite passengers or noisy children. 358 persons were admitted to the service, on various grounds: mobility disorders, cardiovasculars problems, sensory troubles, dementia. CONCLUSION: the fear of taking the bus, combined with the high cost of taxis severely increased the isolation of these elderly people. Solutions have been planned to facilitate the access and use of public transportation facilities.

Community Partnerships and Independent Living

A. Moore, M. Kohut, G. Kroeker (Winnipeg Regional Health Authority - Long Term Care Community Services, Winnipeg, Canada)

Support Services for Seniors is a unique, grant funded program in Canada between Winnipeg Regional Health Authority and its partners. It enhances the independence of older persons living in the community. A strength of Support Services is that communities are allowed to determine the needs of their seniors and tailor services to address those needs. The direction of the program comes from the citizens of the community rather than from government. These services empower people to improve their health. A range of services is coordinated, made accessible and affordable. They focus on promoting well-being, fostering and ensuring that social and physical environments meet the needs of seniors. There are 68 programs sponsored by 32 community agencies. In 2000 there were about 5,660 individuals using these services. Evaluations of the services indicate that socialization and service use was often noted in suggesting a lower incidence of depression and mental illness among seniors. It also indicates that the program directly reduces the amount of services provided by Home Care and delays premature Personal Care Home placement. The most direct and visible impact is with the congregate meals (270,000 meals served in 2000), daily hello and cleaning services. Support Services plays a complementary role with Home Care in health surveillance and monitoring. Support Services has resulted in more appropriate use of the formalized health care system and has facilitated a more integrated service delivery. The Support Services to Seniors program is viewed as a cost effective, quality service.

Developing an Agency and Consumers Network to Improve Communication and Policy Making for Aging Services

R. McCaslin (Department of Social Work, California State University, San Bernardino, USA), B. Bennett (San Bernardino County Department of Aging and Adult Services, USA)

A large and diverse county sought greater service efficiencies for elderly and disabled adults through a formal network of providers and consumer constituencies. This network would solicit ongoing input from the local level and channel that information to critical decision makers. Its philosophical orientation would encourage consumers to speak for themselves, with those groups unable to do so represented by advocates. Potential network members were involved in initial design through group discussions and written comments including rankings/ ratings of functions and membership of each key network component. Especially analyzed were differences among county regions and constituencies (e.g, providers versus consumers, aging versus disability services). The resulting San Bernardino County Aging and Adult Network (SB CAAN) channels direct knowledge of service problems to appropriate decision makers and requires response to those who initially raised the issues. SB CAAN consists of Provider and Consumer/Advocate Councils which convey input from member agencies and groups to a Service Management Team composed of staff from key county agencies. The Councils and the Service Management Team send representatives to a Policy Council of agency chief administrative officers who address policy changes involving agency/interagency contracts, initiate agency collaborations, and, with the County Board of Supervisors, address issues requiring legislative initiatives or new funding. An non-profit Aging and Adult Fund receives and distributes contributions on behalf of the elderly and disabled adults. Thus, reliable information on service issues is continuously routed to the decision making level best able to resolve the problem.

Geropsychology Roles and Service Delivery within a MultiCentre Facility: Change Agent, Support Provider, Assessor, Educator/Trainer

M. Gorman (Queen Elizabeth Health Sciences Centre, Halifax, NS, Canada)

This paper reviews delivery of psychology service over a 12-month period within a multi-centre health care facility, to serve as an important step towards ensuring quality service delivery and appropriate use of health care funding. This review can also inform both the public and professional colleagues (thus educating prospective customers) about the potential roles played by a psychologist in such a centre. These roles are carried out on an Outpatient, Inpatient, Day Hospital, and Long Term Care basis and with psychiatric, medical and geriatric populations. Community consultation and education/training responsibilities are also carried out in this position. This review includes comparisons with previous years' service delivery to model a database system that can monitor and reflect changes in "the system" and in the clientele/referral base, and subsequent program changes. The roles of change agent, support provided, assessor, and educator/trainer are discussed in terms of effectiveness, time (and stress) management and personal job satisfaction. Innovation is discussed in the context of career opportunities that can debilitate or enhance the role of psychology in the field of gerontology, with emphasis on the need to advance with these opportunities.

Multi Services make Elders active and Happy An Innovative and Successful Facility - Home Care Services

R Gangadharan, (Reddy's Heritage Foundation, Hyderabad, India)

Purpose: India is a country where elders used to spend most of their times in home without much of activity. With the longevity increasing, isolation without adequate physical and mental activity is not good for health and emotional well being. Therefore, Heritage started several programmes for the elderly. Method: Heritage Hospital India's premier healthcare institute for the elderly was started in October 1994. Several older adults feeling grateful, proposed setting up a programme for promoting health ageing. Therefore, Heritage Seniors Club was launched in January 1995. Several events were organised coinciding with World Elders Day, World Alzheimer's Day, World Diabetes Day, New Years Day, Festival Days and Moonlight days. These days are fun days for the members of Heritage Seniors Club, Caregivers Club, Diabetic Club, Dial a Driver Programme and Members of Alzheimer's Chapter and so on. Important and popular programmes include: · Asian Tour · Caregivers Club · Diabetic Club · Dial a Driver Club · Fashion Show · Golden Couple Contest · Heritage Show · Life Long Learning - Computer Course · Life Long Learning- Debates · Made for each Other Grand Parent - Grand Child Couple · Picnics · Seniors Club · Talk Shows Conclusion The events proved the point that several programmes have to be offered to the elderly to keep them active while giving them choices. The elders liked the opportunities given for attiring themselves well, appreciated efforts taken to offer services of various kinds and preferred interacting with people having similar interests and concerns. Having Fun was found to be the most preferred activity as could be seen from several accompanying photographs (to be shown at the conference!).

Social Mapping of Organisations Working for the Care of the Elderly: A Study in Mumbai

S. Siva Raju (Tata Institute of Social Sciences, Deonar, Mumbai, India)

Organisations working for the elderly are of recent origin in the developing societies like India. Most of these organisations are located in major cities like Mumbai and they may be categorised as Oldage Homes, Senior Citizens Clubs, Retired Persons Associations and Day Care Centres. Though these organisations/associations are catering to the needs of a particular section of the elderly, most of the activities of these organisations are carried out in isolation. In the process a considerable overlapping of the activities carried out by these organisations are noticed. To derive maximum benefit to the elderly in the society from these organisations, there is a strong need to provide a common platform for these organisations to come together and to share their common resources and experiences in their activities. In this regard, a project on social mapping of the organisations working for the care of the elderly in Mumbai is undertaken with a major objective to identify the strengths and inadequacy of these orgnisations and to assess their readiness and dilemmas to join in the networking of the organisations in the city. All together 150 such organisations were contacted and the data was collected from them with the help of an interview schedule. The findings revealed that most of the organisations especially senior citizens clubs have shown their readiness for networking. The study clearly revealed that given the clear cut activities as an important component in the networking, most of the organisations have favorable opinion to come forward and join in the networking process. Further the findings of the study revealed that there is a need to adopt a differential approach to these organisations for their inclusions in the networking process and also highlighted the need for adopting and alternative model for networking these organisations to expect them to play an effective role in improving the quality of life of the elderly in the society.

Venturing Out: The Challenge of Developing Community-Based Partnerships for Faith-Based Organizations Providing Senior Services

B. Lewis [University of Pennsylvania School of Social Work, Philadelphia, PA], B. Cohen [Center for the Study of Youth Policy, University of Pennsylvania School of Social Work, Philadelphia, PA], N. Morrow [University of Pennsylvania School of Social Work, Philadelphia, PA], T. Chuluun [University of Pennsylvania School of Social Work, Philadelphia, PA],

In what has been termed the "new partnership" between governmental and/or foundational-giving and the faith-based sector, religious organizations — previously accustomed to planning and providing community-based services in relative isolation — may find themselves thrust into a new arena of service delivery requiring skills in building and nurturing interorganizational ties. New efforts to reach out to the wider community of clients and service providers may involve consideration of the relative benefits to the organization of consolidating pastoral and social service functions in the delivery of services. The authors' work carrying out a senior center capacity-building project with the local division of a national faith-based organization provides an opportunity to examine a range of challenges for multi-service faith-based organizations in designing services for the low-income urban elderly population. The challenges include rethinking the mission of senior services, becoming more market oriented, and learning how to collaborate and share control. Data gathered from individual and focus group interviews were utilized as the basis for providing inter- and extra-organizational input to a newly-initiated advisory committee composed of pastoral and social service staff within the organization who have major responsibility for planning and delivering senior services. Implications of project findings for planning community-based senior services in faith-based organizations will be discussed.

SESSION 348

AGGIR French national tool for evaluation of the loss of autonomy and care level

VETEL JM CH LE MANS FRANCE DUCOUDRAY JM PROBTP FRANCE LEROUX R CH VIERZON FRANCE

The Autonomy-Gerontology Iso-Resources Group (A..G.G.I.R.) system comprises three components. 1/ 10 discriminant items scored on a 3-points scale, enable evaluation of the degree of gerontological autonomy of elderly subjects : these 10 discriminant and relevant items are those essential for evaluation of the loss of autonomy in the elderly. Each variable supposes 3 possible modalities : - A : Performs a function independently, completely, regularly and correctly - B : Performs a function independently but partially, or not regularly, or not correctly - C - does not perform or perform with help a function regularly correctly refers to time or refers to the usual environment, according to habits and customs 2/ The Iso-Resources Group computer program is a grouping program which enables each patient to be assigned to one of six groups that are iso-consumers of work load (time and penibility) in the context of geriatric dependence management. A table enables detection of the main signs characterizing each of the iso-resource groups but, in case-by-case routine practice, the computer program is essential to assigns the patients, immediately and precisely, to the correct groups. The Mean Ponderated Iso ressource Group is also calculated by the computer program, it indicates the mean loss of autonomy of a population 3/ 7 domestic and social items very usefull to establish the health care plan, but they are not taken in count to determine the Iso-Resource Group AGGIR : Where ? When ? How ? Why ? The AGGIR (autonomy gerontology Iso Resources Groups) system may be used with both outpatients and inpatients since it has been validated in the various health care structures. It is important to regularly update the data in order to have as clear a view as possible of the basic care workload of each unit and of the structure as a whole. Result presentation is essential in order to circulate information and promote use. The communication will present the system with examples.

Utilization of the AGGIR Model

PREVVOST P ERSM Rennes FRANCE VETEL JM CH Le MANS LE MANS FRANCE DUCOUDRAY JM PROBTP PARIS FRANCE LEROUX Robert VIERZON FRANCE

The AGGIR Model evaluates the activities actually performed by an elderly person and assigns each patient to an Iso Resource Group (G.I.R.). Each group is homogenous concerning the level of required basic care or nursing. The tool can be used for patients at home or in institution. The goals are different whether it focuses on an individual or a group. 1- Individual level : The AGGIR Model, as it describes the activities in various fields (physical, domestic, social) may contribute to the care management planning. At this level, the Iso Resource Group may be helpful to allocate individual financial help. 2- Collective level : the Iso Resource Group and the Mean Weighted Iso Resource Group (indicator of the mean level of basic care in a defined population) are excellent indicators to compare different units or populations. These indicators are completely relevant : - in the management of a unit or a service, to evaluate the real need of the concerned population for basic care and in comparing it to the Mean National Ratio measured from a national geriatric data bank. - in the setting up of a realistic and equitable financing system of the structures, based on the real needs of the elderly, according to the distribution of the Iso Resource Groups and especially on the Mean Weighted GIR of the structure. Our report will illustrate these different levels of utilisation of the AGGIR Model, with examples from the National data bank of the National French Health Department.

Developing an Information System for a Network of Specialized Geriatric Services

Marlene Awad Administrative Director Regional Geriatric Program of Toronto Sunnybrook & Women's College Health Sciences Centre

The Toronto RGP has been developing a computerized Information Network to enhance the coordination of our services to frail elders. The system, developed in conjunction with HealthLink Clinical Data Network will provide a central patient registry and database that can be shared across the RGP participating organizations. The information system is designed to meet the pressing information needs found throughout the health care system. Its design principles maximize interoperability in order to facilitate integration with other hospital and community information systems, security, and readiness for change. For our patients, the system will allow them to take information with them if they cross service areas and hospital boundaries and reduce information collection redundancy. For clinicians, it will provide patient information and reports quickly and easily, facilitate timely decision making and enhance case management wherever our patients make contact with our services. And, for managers it will readily provide such key information as patient volumes and demographics, waiting time, discharge and flow rates. This presentation will speak to the development of this project and provide a demonstration of the information system.

Geriatric Assessment: Lessons Learned

Ludomyr Mykyta (Western DomCare, Adelaide, Australia) Justin English (Western DomCare/University of South Australia, Adelaide, Australia)

Purpose: To develop best clinical practice initiatives for rural settings through the use of comprehensive assessment. Method: A comprehensive geriatric assessment tool was developed and administered over four rural regions in South Australia over a two year period. Data collected from subjects (n=480) included a combination of demographic and client characteristics as well as results from the utilisation of a number of standardised assessment instruments including IADL, ADL and dementia specific tools. Results: Quantitative data analysis has been incorporated to examine the data set. However, data analysis was not complete at the time of the abstract submission therefore results were not available. Conclusions: The paper provides important implications for clinical practice and policy development in rural settings.

Quality of care from the perspective of cataract patients; a new measuring instrument

H.J. Sixma (Netherlands institute for health services research, Utrecht, The Netherlands), M.D. Nijkamp (Eye Research Institute Maastricht, University Maastricht, The Netherlands), R.M.M.A. Nuijts (Eye Research Institute Maastricht, University Maastricht, The Netherlands)

PURPOSE. Patien views on quality of care are of paramount importance with respect to quality assurance (QA), quality improvement (QI) and the expected outcome of care. However, the relevance of patient satisfaction studies is often questioned because of conceptual and operational problems. The focus of this paper is on the development and assessment of a new measuring instrument for quality of care from the perspective of cataract patients: the QUOTE-cataract. METHOD. We developed the QUOTE-cataract questionnaire by using a combination of qualitative and quantitative methods. Expectations were derived from focus group discussions and concept mapping procedures. As part of a multi-center study, empirical data were obtained on the opinions and experiences of 300 patients who experienced cataract surgery. The internal consistency of (sub)scales and the taxonomy and feasibility of the instrument were evaluated y using explorative and confirmative factor analyses and reliability analysis. RESULTS. The QUOTE-cataract instrument consists of general and cataract-specific quality aspects which relate to process, structure and outcome characteristics of the services that cataract patients received. Feasibility tests showed considerable differences between settings. Within settings, the new instrument was capable to select specific areas in which service quality was sub-optimal. CONCLUSION. The QUOTE-cataract is an assessment instrument for quality of care, tailored to the expressed needs of cataract patients. The instrument can be used in QA and QI studies. The conceptual framework underlying the instrument can also be applied in other groups of older people.

Should we consider frailty to improve DRG's case Mix for acute geriatric patients?

J.Petermans, S.Ceulemans*,J.P. Baeyens **I.Wauthy***, N.Swartenbroeckx***, M.C. Closon(*** * CHR de la Citadelle bd XII e de Ligne - 4000 Liège - Belgium ** AZ Sint Joseph - Nieuwpoortsesteenweg - Oostende - Belgium *** CIES - Ecole de Santé Publique - UCL - Clos Chapelle aux Champs - 1200 Bruxelles - Belgium)*

Diagnosis Related Groups (DRG's) are used for prospective payment in different countries, but DRG are poor predictors of cost or length of stay (LOS) in acute geriatric units. Frailty could have an impact on LOS, increasing risk for mortality or discharge to long term care facilities. Methods: Retrospective study based on 4432 acute geriatric admissions. Criteria for frailty were based on expert advice. Considered criteria for frailty were: age over 85, Katz score G or H, multiple pathology (>3 diagnosis), need for social support, pressure sore, NG tube feeding, geriatric assessment (falls, cognitive, continence). Each of the 7 criteria for frailty was balanced, maximum score for frailty was 10. The effect of frailty on mortality, risk for discharge to long term facilities and increased for LOS was considered within each DRG's group. Statistics: we used a distribution analysis to evaluated the effect of frailty score on mortality, risk for discharge to long term facilities and for increased LOS. Results: Analysis concerned a data collection of 4332 acute geriatric stays in 17 Belgian hospitals. Mean age was 81 years, sex ratio was 2.5 female for 1 male. 47 different DRG's groups were considered. Before admission, 70% of the patients were living home, 28.5 % were admitted from long term care facilities. In our population, mean score for frailty was 3.5 (q25=1.5 , P.50=3.4 , P.75 =5.1). 46% of the patient were home discharged. Frailty score is not related to an increasing risk for long term facilities discharge. Mortality was 13%. When frailty score was over 4, mortality risk was increased by two. Mean LOS was 21 days (q25: 12 days, Q75: 75 days). When frailty score was over 3.3, the probability of an increased LOS was 50%. Conclusion: Criteria for frailty were not exhaustive. We couldn't take into account items like poor nutrition and delirium. But geriatric frailty has probably an impact on LOS and on mortality risk in acute geriatric units.

Striving For Best Practice In Professional Assessment.

Justin English (Western DomCare/University of South Australia, Adelaide, Australia) Ludomyr Mykyta & Parasivam (Western DomCare, Adelaide, Australia)

Purpose: To develop a best practice model of professional assessment to ensure an efficient and effective delivery of home-based services to frail and disabled elders. Method: In 2000 an innovative model of professional assessment was introduced by one of Australia's largest providers of home-based care in order to reduce multiple assessments and to reduce the utilisation of assessment as a gate keeping tool for limiting access to services. Data was analysed from a random sample of 1500 clients drawn from a population of 5000 as well as through the use of a survey tool administered to the organisation's clinical staff. Results: Results revealed that, contrary to popular belief, carer advocacy plays a significant role in the professional assessment process to the point that clients with carers received significantly more services and service time than clients without such support. However, assessment, if not monitored, can also be utilised as a gate-keeping tool and as opposed to one that can provide significant benefits to the consumers through comprehensive need articulation. Conclusions: The authors argue that the professional approach does not preclude empowerment, and that assessment should not be utilised for gate-keeping of limited resources but instead for the benefits that it affords the consumer.

Use of a simple computerised clinical assessment in optimising the care of the elderly in Finland

T. Rajala, E.Vaissi (Health Office, City of Turku, Turku, Finland), Y. Lahtinen, P. Paunio (Assiciation of Municipalities in Finland, Helsinki, Finland)

During the years 1989 - 1994 a computerized database system DEP (Description, Evaluation and Placement) was developed for helping to arrange proper care for the elderly in the city of Turku. The DEP system contains information about ADL, memory and behavioral problems. From this information we developed the RaVa-index that measures the need of care in the frail elderly. The system has been used in practice in Turku since 1994. Follow up studies have been made from the material of all the elderly who get municipal support for their care (5000 persons). In 1998 ten biggest cities in Finland made a comparison of their care systems using the RaVa-index as a measure of the need of care (N=25114) and 11 biggest cities made the same study in the year 2000 (N=32588). In the follow up studies in Turku we have found out that the elderly who have normal memory sustain much more better their functionality in home care than in institutional care if their RaVa-index was at the starting point below 3. If the elderly had severe memory impairment, they sustained their functionality better in institutional care than in home care. In the study of the big cities in 1998 we found out that those cities that had the lowest costs of the care of the elderly had a well developed home care systems and they used less beds in long term institutional care than those who had high costs of the care of the elderly. In the study made in the year 2000 was noticed that many cities had improved their home care according to the results of the first study. The use of the same simple computerised assessment has shown its benefits both in the follow up studies and also in the comparison of different municipalities. The system is now used in about 100 municipalities in Finland. The Association of the Municipalities in Finland is coordinating the use of the system and an intranet version of the system has been developed.

SESSION 349

Cognitive impairment and dementia in the aged and preaged: Comprehensive mechanism and intervention

Ma Yong-Xing (Department of Aging, Antiaging and Cognitive Function, Shanghai Institute of Gerontology and Geriatrics, Huadong Hospital, Shanghai, China)

1. Prevalence rate of cognitive impairment in the aged (>60 yrs old): (1) age-associated memory impairment 15.27% (629/4120) with MQ (WMS)69. (2) 10.1% (475/4700) with HDS<30.5. (3) 4.1% (35/345) with IQ (WAIS)69. (4) Incidence of dementia and suspected dementia in 223 longevous 12% (27/223). 2. We found that cognitive impairment in the aged and preaged is intimately correlated with free radical metabolism, microcirculatory disturbance, arteriosclerosis, hypertension, coronary heart disease, diabetes mellitus, cerebrovascular disease, chronic bronchitis and emphysema, chronic renal failure and lower PaO2. 3. The frequency of APOE4 of AD (19.89%,37/93±2) is significantly higher than that of general aged population (6.22%, 213/1463±2) (P<0.001). The mean value of MMSE in APOE4 (16.6±10.96) is significantly lower than that without APOE4 (20.86±3.86) (P<0.05). 4. We have performed double blind trial on huperzine (742 cases), aniracetam (622 cases), Reinhardt and sea cucumber capsule. R.S.C. (sea products, 702 cases) and certain other traditional Chinese drugs to treat cognitive impairment including VD (MID), AD and VD+AD. Huperzine, aniracetam R.S.C. and were found to be effective to increase the MQ, MMSE and HDS-R score in memory impairment in the aged and preaged and mild or moderate dementia (VD, AD, VD+AD). 5. The mechanism of cognitive impairment in the aged is comprehensive and multifactorial. The measures for intervention of cognitive impairment in the aged must comprehensive too.

Effects of Psychomotor activation programmes for use in groups of cognitively impaired people

Patricia G.M. Staats, Marijke Hopman-Rock, Erwin C.P.M. Tak3 (TNO Prevention and Health,Leiden, The Netherlands) Rose-Marie Dröes (Vrije Universiteit Amsterdam, The Netherlands)

Purpose: To test the effects of the Psychomotor Activation Programme (PAP) on the behaviour and cognition of demented elderly people. Method: Randomized controlled trial with an experimental group and a control group. Post-test after 6 months. Setting. Group care projects for demented elderly people living in 11 different homes for the elderly in The Netherlands. One hundred and thirty-four subjects entered the study (72 in the experimental group and 62 in the control group), 42 of whom dropped out (27 in the experimental group and 15 in the control group). Individual behaviour and group behaviour were scored by using two Dutch scales (BIP and SIPO respectively) developed and validated for use in psychogeriatric populations. Cognition was measured with the short- and the long form of the Cognitive Screening Test (CST-14 and CST-20). Disability was measured with the Barthel Index. Medicine use, falls or other accidents, and life-events were registered. Results: Beneficial effects of the PAP were found on non-social behaviour (BIP, F=1.80, p<0.10, effect size 0.3) and on cognition (CST-14, F=2.63, P<0.05, effect size 0.4)(CST-20, F=3.77, p<0.05, effect-size=0.5). In participants with relatively mild cognitive problems, positive group behaviour increased (SIPO, F=4.46, p<0.05). Small increases in rebellious behaviour, restlessness, and negative group behaviour were found especially in the severely demented participants. Conclusions. The PAP has beneficial effects on behaviour and stabilizes cognitive performance. The PAP also seems to improve alertness.The findings were supported by a simultaneously conducted process evaluation.

Negative effect of ApoE4 on memory performance

Buxin Han (Institute of Psychology, Chinese Academy of Sciences, Beijing, China)

Purpose: Memory disorder is one of the typical clinical symptoms of Alzheimer's Disease (AD). Studies have confirmed apolipoprotein allele four (ApoE4) as a risk factor of AD (Matterson, 1997). Does ApoE4 correlate with memory performance? Method: Three studies on the relation between ApoE4 and cognitive (memory) aging were reviewed. Results: Kamigin (1997) did not observe the phenomenon that cognitive aging was interfered by education level among those participants with ApoE4. This indicated that ApoE4 can contract the effect of education on cognitive aging. Nilsson (1999) found that those who have ApoE4 showed significantly lower performance on memory tasks than those participants who did not have ApoE4. This memory disorder took place even five years ago. Raber et al (2000) recently found that mutant mice with ApoE4 showed significantly lower performance on Morris water maze than those mutant with ApoE3. Conclusion: The correlation between ApoE4 and memory performance has been proven from behavioral and genetic perspectives. Further questions: Is there a remedy for this negative effect? Do other genetic products (e.g, PS-1, PS-2) relating with AD have similar correlation with memory performance?

The question of awareness of troubles in Alzheimer s disease in low to moderate stage

P.Y. Malo, O. Michel, P. Jouanny Service de mÈdecine gÈriatrique CHU de Rennes 35000 Rennes France

Purpose Numerous authors focused on the frequent absence of awareness of the disease by Alzheimerís patients and depicted this as a part of the disease (anosognosia). We try to modelize this awareness/ recognition of their troubles by these patients. Methods Through a semi-structured questionnaire, we determined the status of 78 patients who were examined for cognitive decline and declared probable Alzheimerís in a low to moderate stage. We used five distinct categories: - group 1: patients aware of their troubles and expressing complaint - group 2: patients aware of their troubles, expressing them spontaneously but not in foreground - group 3: patients aware of their troubles, but not expressing them spontaneously (only after the question: what about your memory ?) - group 4: patients having a partial awareness of their troubles, but not expressing spontaneously and trying to minimize them - group 5: patients totally denying their troubles Results Repartition : Group 1: 32,05%; Group 2: 11,54%; group 3: 11,54%; Group 4: 21,79%; Group 5: 15,38%.NA: 7,69%.This shows that a large majority of patients, at these stages of the disease, have a definite awereness of their troubles and nearly the half expresses them spontaneously, without correlation to the MMS score. Conclusion The absence of correlation between awareness of the trouble and MMS score allows us to reconsider the cognitive substract of the lack of awareness of the trouble in Alzheimerís in a low to moderate stage, to the benefit of a psychological dimension based on mechanisms of defense of the Self, ranging from avoiding the evocation of the anxiogenous situation to denying it.

Working Memory and Balance in Older Adults and Patients with Dementia

Michael A. Rapp (Max Planck Institute for Human Development, Berlin, Germany)

PURPOSE: Recent research suggests a strong connection between sensorimotor and cognitive performance with aging. In the case of Alzheimer's disease, similar findings have been related to an impairment in executive control early in the course of the disease. We investigated the effect of divided attention between a working memory and a balance task under different complexity conditions in older adults and patients with Alzheimer's disease suffering from a specific deficit in executive functioning. METHOD: 10 young (aged 20-30) and 10 older (aged 65 to 75) adults, as well as 10 patients (aged 65 to 75) suffering from a dysexecutive syndrome in early stage probable Alzheimer's disease were tested for 5 sessions using a dual-task paradigm, combining two balance tasks (stable versus moving platform) with three levels of difficulty in a cognitive task (N-Back). RESULTS: When performing a monitoring task on a stable platform, sway is stable in older adults and in Alzheimer's disease. Sway increases differentially in older adults and in patients suffering from Alzheimer's disease when a working memory task involving visuospatial functioning is added, while younger adults seem to maintain their level of stability CONCULSION: The presented results speak to a possible role of working memory and executive control in the conncetion between sensorimotor performance and cognition in aging and Alzheimer's disease.

SESSION 352

Findings from the Canadian National Evaluation of the Cost-Effectiveness of Home Care

Neena L. Chappell (Centre on Aging, University of Victoria, Victoria, British Columbia, Canada) adn Marcus J. Hollander (Hollander Analytical Services Ltd, Victoria, British Columbia, Canada).

ISSUE: The international literature on the cost-effectiveness of home care services is mixed. There is a significant body of American literature which indicates that home care is NOT a cost-effective alternative to residential long term care. However, there have been a few Canadian studies which seem to indicate that home care may indeed be a cost-effective alternative to residential care, within the Canadian context of service delivery. In regard to the cost-effectiveness of home care compared to acute care hospitals the literature is more mixed. Given the existing literature, one could make the case that home care may be a cost-effective alternative to acute care under certain specific conditions. However, most of the literature is American and it is not clear if these findings would hold in the Canadian context. In order to provide decision makers with more information, the Canadian National Evaluation of the Cost-Effectiveness of Home Care conducted a series of 15 studies across Canada related to the cost- effectiveness of home care compared to residential care and acute care. STRUCTURE: The session will include five presentations. The first presentation will be 10 minutes, the second 20 minutes, the third 15 minutes, the fourth 20 minutes and the fifth 15 minutes. This will leave 10 minutes for questions. We expect that the Principal Investigators for all 15 studies will be present at the session to help answer questions at the session or after the session. CONTENT: The content of this session reflects the strategy deployed in selecting the 15 studies. The first presentation will present a rationale and overview for the program of research. The second presentation will summarize the results of five studies related to the cost-effectiveness of home care compared to residential care. The third presentation will provide an overview of the characteristics, service utilization and costs of short term home care clients. The fourth presentation will summarize the results of the cost-effectiveness of five hospital to home care initiatives such as day hospitals, home IV therapy, hospital based quick response teams, and early discharge for mothers with infants. The final presentation will deal with key issues and blockages related to implementing new, cost-effective home care programs. CONCLUSIONS/ANTICIPATED OUTCOMES: It is expected that Canadians and international members of the audience will have a better understanding of home care, and its relative cost-effectiveness, in the Canadian context.

Comparative Costs and Outcomes of Home Care and Residential Long Term Care

Marcus J. Hollander (Hollander Analytical Services Ltd, Victoria, British Columbia, Canada)

PURPOSE: To present findings from five studies related to the cost-effectiveness of home care compared to residential long term care. METHOD: A variety of qualitative and quantitative methods were used. RESULTS: Overall, it was found that home care services cost less than residential services for people with similar levels of need. However, there were a number of exceptions. For example, the costs for people in a transition state between levels of care or from home care to residential care were almost the same as those for similar clients in residential care. In addition, the costs were greater for home care clients who died than for residential clients who died. CONCLUSIONS: Many of the obvious savings from substituting home care for residential care may already have been achieved. Further savings may, however, still be obtained from specific, targeted programs.

Issues Related to Implementing Cost-Effective Home Care Services

Denise Alcock (Faculty of Health Sciences, University of Ottawa, Ottawa, Ontario)

PURPOSE: The National Evaluation of the Cost-Effectiveness of Home Care is a program of applied, policy-relevant research. The overall strategy of the program of research was to describe home care services because there is no national data base on home care and to determine which types of services are, or are not, cost-effective and under what conditions they may be cost-effective. It was also recognized early on that studies needed to be included in the program of research which would provide intelligence to decision makers about the kinds of issues or obstacles they may have to face in implementing new, cost-effective programs, and how to successfully address, or deal with, these issues and obstacles. Thus, two studies were commissioned to look at system of care related issues, one in the area of home care and residential care and one in the area of home care and acute care. METHODS: Qualitative methods such as interviews and focus groups were the main approaches to data collection. RESULTS: The presentation will present the results of a study of case managers and the issues they have to deal with in streaming new clients to home care or residential care. It will also present findings from a study designed to look at blockages in the hospital to home care interface. CONCLUSIONS: The results from these two studies will assist policy makers and planners to design, and implement, new, cost-effective home care initiatives.

Overview of the National Evaluation of the Cost-Effectiveness of Home Care

Neena L. Chappell (Centre on Aging, University of Victoria, Victoria, British Columbia, Canada)

PURPOSE: To provide an overview of the program of research, and the strategy for selecting studies, for the National Evaluation of the Cost-Effectiveness of Home Care. METHOD: A variety of qualitative and quantitative methods were used. RESULTS: The result was the successful completion of 15 studies in a $1.5 million integrated program of research on the cost-effectiveness of home care funded by the Health Transition Fund, Health Canada. CONCLUSIONS: It appears that there may be some situations in which home care can be a cost-effective alternative to residential care or acute care services.

The Cost-Effectiveness of Home Care Compared to Hospital Care

Peter C. Coyte (Department of Health Administration and Home Care Evaluation and Research Centre, University of Toronto, Toronto, Ontario)

PURPOSE: To provide an overview of the results of five Canadian studies on the cost-effectiveness of home care compared to acute care services. The topics for these five studies were selected based on a review of the international literature. This literature indicated that home and community care may be a cost-effective alternative to acute care for geriatric clients treated in a day hospital, clients receiving home based IV therapy, mothers with small infants with feeding difficulties who are discharged home early, and seniors receiving the services of a quick response team to route them from the hospital emergency department back to their homes rather than having them be admitted to the hospital. METHODS: Clinical trials and other quantitative methods. RESULTS: Research is still in progress on these studies but will be completed by the end of March 2001. CONCLUSIONS: The findings from these studies should highlight which of the above initiatives are cost-effective within the Canadian context. This will provide an opportunity for decision makers to act quickly on implementing new programs to increase the efficiency and effectiveness of health care in Canada.

SESSION 356

Physical Activities for Elderly People

L. Puggaard (University of Southern Denmark, Denmark) Maximal Oxygen Consumption and Coping with Everyday Tasks in Old Age. T.Rantanen (University of Jyväskylä, Finland) Muscle Strength, Physical Activity and Disablement in Old Age. J. Guralnik and S. Volpato (National Institute on Aging, Bethesda, USA) Exercise Potential in Non-Disabled but At-Risk Older Persons. W.J.Chodzko-Zajko (University of Illinois at Urbana-Champaign, USA) Physical Fitness and Cognitive Functioning in Old Age.

Issue: This symposium will examine the nature and strength of the relation between physical activity and physical and cognitive performance, as well as the role of physical activity in the disablement process in old age. Structure: Symposium will be introduced by E. Heikkinen followed by presentations of L. Puggaard, T. Rantanen, J. Guralnik & S. Volpato and W. J. Chodzko-Zajko. Fifteen minutes will be allocated for each presentation and the time remaining will be used for discussion. Content: Participants consider, from multiple perspectives, the evidence of the benefits of physical activity for older people. In the first paper in the session Puggaard describes age-related changes in maximal oxygen uptake and the association of maximal oxygen consumption and ability to carry out everyday activities. With advancing age, everyday tasks require a higher percentage of maximal oxygen capacity. The oldest women, aged 90-95 years, have to work on their maximal oxygen uptake level in most everyday tasks. The second paper by Rantanen, drawing from three epidemiological studies on ageing, will present analyses showing a powerful association of strength and disability in elderly people and discuss possible ways to explain this association. The third paper by Guralnik and Volpato is based on research carried out on persons age 75-85 who were not disabled but at risk for future disability. The findings suggested that this group of persons have a potential to begin an exercise program at a low level of intensity. Finally, Chodzko-Zajko examines the relation between physical fitness and cognitive performance in old age. He observes that there is some evidence to suggest that high-fit older adults process information in the central nervous system faster and more efficiently than less-fit individuals of the same chronological age. Conclusions: The current evidence suggests that benefits of exercise may be observed in cognitive performance but are particularly apparent in physical performance lowering the risk factors for future disability and maintaining the ability to carry out daily activities independently. Exercise interventions can be recommended for all older adults but the potential to begin an exercise program varies between the individuals and more research is required to further develop appropriate exercise counselling.

Exercise Potential in Non-Disabled but At-Risk Older Persons

J. Guralnik, S. Volpato (National Institute on Aging, Bethesda, USA), J. Cohen Mansfield (Research Institute, Hebrew Home of Greater Washington, Rockville, USA)

PURPOSE: It has been demonstrated in large, prospective epidemiologic studies that, in non-disabled older persons, physical performance measures are predictive of the onset of future disability. These non-disabled but at-risk persons represent an ideal target population that might benefit substantially from preventive interventions, including exercise. Although a great deal has been learned in epidemiologic studies about their characteristics, there is little information available about the potential for this group of persons to undertake an exercise program. METHOD: 447 persons age 75-85 were initially screened by telephone. Subsequent screening was done at home visits on 229 persons and 108 were found to be eligible (EPESE performance battery score of 4-9 (Guralnik et al. 1995) and MMSE score >24). Of these, 98 agreed to a comprehensive physical therapy evaluation of mobility, strength, balance, range of motion, and exercise limitations. RESULTS: Of 9 domains of impairment assessed, impaired physical endurance and pain had the greatest impact on the capacity to exercise. All persons were capable of beginning upper and lower extremity strengthening in a classroom setting. Over 85% were recommended for stretching and balance exercises in a class, with the remainder requiring individual attention. Walking intensity recommendations for this group consisted of walking at customary speed on level ground for 10-20 minutes (42.8%) and <10 minutes (42.9%), with a small minority able start with a more vigorous program. CONCLUSION: Non-disabled, but at-risk very old persons have the potential to begin an exercise program at a low level of intensity.

Maximal Oxygen Consumption and Coping with Everyday Tasks in Old Age

L. Puggaard (Institute of Sports Science and Clinical Biomechanics, University of Southern Denmark)

Aerobic capacity is usually measured by maximal oxygen uptake. A reduction in maximal oxygen uptake with increasing age has been reported to vary between 0-22% per decade. This reduction accelerates towards older age groups. Tasks requiring close to maximal oxygen consumption can only be performed for short periods, consequently older women, in particular, are at great risk of falling below the minimum aerobic threshold for independent living. There is not much previous research done on this topic; however, values from 13 to 15 ml oxygen/min/kg have been suggested as the criterion level for successfully coping with everyday tasks. PURPOSE: The aim of this study is to describe age-related changes in maximal oxygen consumption, and to analyse the association between maximal oxygen consumption and the ability to carry out everyday activities such as walking, dressing, cleaning and stair-climbing. METHODS: Four groups of healthy community-dwelling Danish women (age 30-35 (n=8), 50-55 (n=8), 75-80 (n=11) and 90-95 (n=4)) volunteered for the study. Direct measurements of maximal oxygen consumption were performed on a bicycle ergometer. The participants bicycled to exhaustion and the criterion for attainment of maximal oxygen uptake was Respiratory Exchange Ratio (RER) 1. A portable oxygen analyser (K2, Cosmed, Italy) was used to assess oxygen consumption in everyday tasks. Analysis of variance was used to evaluate between-group differences in oxygen consumption. Oxygen consumption in everyday tasks was estimated as a percentage of maximal oxygen consumption. RESULTS: The analysis shows that maximal oxygen consumption is 43 ml/min/kg for women aged 30-35 years and 35, 19 and 12 ml/min/kg for women aged 50-55, 75-80 and 90-95 years, respectively. With increasing age everyday tasks require a higher percentage of maximal oxygen capacity. Indeed, the oldest women performed on their maximal oxygen level in most tasks. CONCLUSION: Despite quite a low maximal oxygen capacity, the two oldest groups of women manage to cope with everyday tasks and live independently in their own homes. Different explanations are plausible, e.g. they may have many breaks in performing everyday tasks during the day. Another explanation may be their ability to modify the way they perform everyday tasks.

Muscle Strength, Physical Activity and Disablement in Old Age

T. Rantanen, (Department of Health Sciences and Finnish Center for Interdisciplinary Gerontology, University of Jyväskylä, Jyväskylä, Finland)

PURPOSE: The aim is to examine what is the role of muscle strength in the disablement process in old age. METHOD: Multiple analyses are presented. Data come from 1) Evergreen project, a 10-year prospective study on functional capacity among 679 initially 75-and 80-year-old people living in the City of Jyväskylä, Finland, 2) Honolulu Heart Program (HHP), a study on 8006 45-68-year-old men living on Oahu, HI, who have been followed-up since 1965, and 3) Womens' Health and Aging Study (WHAS), a study on causes and course of disability in 1002 women aged 65 years and older at baseline and living in Baltimore, MD. RESULTS: WHAS analyses showed that the association of knee extension strength and walking speed was positive but curved and included thresholds. A certain amount of strength is required to support and move body weight, which illustrates a biomechanical association. In prospective analyses over 25-30 years using HHP data after excluding from analyses all participants with diseases at baseline and adjusting for potential confounders, those in the lowest third of grip strength at baseline, were at increased risk of disability 25 years later, and mortality up to 30 years later. Greater muscle strength may be an indicator of constitutional robustness or vitality making people more resistant to disability and mortality. In the Evergreen study, after baseline strength tests, 82 people suffered a bone fracture and among them, 32 deaths occurred during the 10-year surveillance period. The adjusted RR of death after fracture was 4.17 greater in the lowest tertile of knee extension strength vs. the highest tertile (95% CI 1.32-13.1) measured before the fracture. In already aged and sick populations, muscle strength may be a good indicator of the burden of disease on an individual. CONCLUSION: Three ways to explain the powerful association of strength and disability were observed in these analyses. 1) In all populations, there is a biomechanical association between muscle strength and movement. 2) In healthy populations, strength may be an indicator of constitutional robustness. 3) In aged and sick populations, strength may be an indicator of frailty and burden of disease. Even though it has been established that muscle strength is modifiable, the effects of strength training interventions on functional mobility, risk of future disability and mortality, and vulnerability to external stress, need to be established.

Physical Fitness and Cognitive Functioning in Old Age

W.J. Chodzko-Zajko (University of Illinois at Urbana-Champaign, Urbana IL, USA)

PURPOSE: This paper will examine the nature and strength of the relation between physical fitness and cognitive performance in old age. METHOD: Both cross-sectional studies and training studies which have examined the effect of exercise training regimens on cognitive performance will be considered. RESULTS: In recent years extensive attention has focussed on the identification of various factors that may potentially alter the rate and extent of cognitive decline in aging. Of key interest to the present discussion is the notion that high levels of fitness may be associated with less pronounced cognitive decline in old age. There is now substantial evidence to support the hypothesis that physically fit older adults often process cognitive information more efficiently than less-fit individuals of the same chronological age. However, it is clear that the relationship between physical fitness and cognition is highly task dependent. Physical fitness effects are most likely to be observed in tasks that require a significant amount of executive control processing and are less likely to occur in more automated tasks. CONCLUSIONS: Despite the presence of an cross-sectional association between fitness and cognitive performance, no clear picture has emerged with respect to the effect of short term exercise training on cognitive performance. There is some evidence to suggest that high-fit adults process information in the central nervous system faster and more efficiently than less-fit individuals of the same chronological age. This increase in efficiency may be secondary to improvements in cerebral circulation, nerve cell regeneration, changes in neurotransmitter synthesis and degradation and/or reductions in cell damage due to free-radical oxidation.

SESSION 357

Assessment of Nursing Professionalization Following Geriatric Nursing Continuing Education

Ziva, Shapira (Director of Kaplan Academic Nursing School) Shlomit ,

Shick (Senior instructor at Nursing School)

Purpose : 1. To discuss how the training course on aging contribute to the quality of the work and the professional advancement of the institution and the individual . 2. To emphasize the need for such specialized course in light of the rapidity changing health care system as we enter the 21st century. Methods : Data on professional course graduates 1995-1999 was gathered through analyzing the researcher's own professional experience. Results : The course contribute to the professional capacity of the specializing nurses. Course goals were attained and maintained by the majority of the students for many years. Experienced graduates advanced in the profession ($p = 0.038$) while recent graduates were involved in instructing their patients. All the graduates - 100% ($p + 0.4$) expressed satisfaction . However there is a need to build in a dynamic process of updating and organizing professional training so as to best suit the changing needs of Israel's health care system , the profession , the students and the institution , while maintaining closest possible contact with all parties. Conclusions : Highly professional nurses improve the health and welfare of geriatric patients. It is extremely important to develop skills in this field : nursing directors should promote investment in such studies.

Course notes to courseware: computer-based education in health care of older people

Mira Vogel (St Bartholomew's and the Royal London School of Medicine and Dentistry, London, U.K.),Gerry Bennett (St Bartholomew's and the Royal London School of Medicine and Dentistry, London, U.K.)

The learning experience of students of geriatric medicine would be improved through the use of computer-based, needs-assessed, evaluated study guides in care of older people developed from paper-based core topics. The requirements of medical students using information technology to learn were identified through a survey. The available information technology infrastructure was investigated as a platform for distributing courseware. Expert authors of the original paper-based guide confirmed that the information was well structured, current and complete, and identified areas to enhance with multimedia or complementary material. Development tools were selected to fulfil the aforementioned requirements. Multimedia material was collected. An interface was designed to the specification of human-computer interaction guidelines, and the knowledge was inserted and extended. One study guide on gerontology was selected for evaluation. The students' knowledge was tested before and after using the computer-based guide. Academic progress was monitored and a comparison drawn with corresponding non-participating students. The sample completed a questionnaire on attitudes to aspects of the guide. Findings focus on effectiveness of communicating information, effects on student performance, pleasantness of use, and ease of use. Computer-based education has several well-established strengths. A relaxed, self-paced environment accommodates the heavy workload of medical students, while interaction and proactivity are promoted. Engaging communication of medical procedures and mechanisms can be achieved through judicious use of multimedia. Evolution, maintenance, and distribution of information is convenient and cheap, and so well suited for rapidly evolving medical knowledge. There is a healthy and growing infrastructure to support computer-based education.

Meeting the challenge of occupational therapy training in aging; clinical and academic collaboration.

Sylvia Davidson (Toronto General Hospital, Toronto, Canada), Debbie Rudman, Angela Colantonio (University of Toronto, Toronto, Canada).

Occupational therapists practicing within our current health care system are faced with numerous challenges due to an aging population. Many therapists feel unprepared for the realities of the demographics of their clinical caseload. Therapists must have an appreciation for complexities of aging, an understanding of theories of aging and their relevance for occupational therapy as well as an ability to explore various psychosocial and environmental issues pertinent to older adults. This has necessitated a thorough examination of the curriculum at one Canadian School of Occupational Therapy and some significant changes to how students learn about aging and health. As part of a revised curriculum, including an Older Adult block, students are involved in problem-based learning, with cases generated by clinicians. There are half-day fieldwork sessions to promote understanding of the experience of aging from the perspective of a community-dwelling older adult, lectures by clinicians and 'clinical experts' in aging, labs focusing on issues relevant to the older adult, such as cognitive assessment and home safety, and fieldwork placements with clinicians working in geriatrics. The students and clinicians have evaluated each component of this curriculum and changes to the program have been made based on these evaluations. This presentation will highlight components of the Older Adult block, emphasizing the link between academic theory and clinical practice. While challenges exist, collaboration and cooperation between academic institution and clinical community are facilitating better understanding of aging and the older adult, thereby producing occupational therapists who are highly qualified in the field of aging.

Nurses' formation on gerontology: From the curricular structure to basic concepts about aging

Maria Manuela Rino Mendes (University of São Paulo at Ribeirão Preto College Nursing, Ribeirão Preto, São Paulo, Brasil) Lisete Diniz Ribas Casagrande (University of São Paulo at Ribeirão Preto Faculty of Philosophy and Sciences, Ribeirão Preto, São Paulo, Brasil) Rosalina Aparecida Partezani Rodrigues (University of São Paulo at Ribeirão Preto College Nursing, Ribeirão Preto, São Paulo, Brasil)

Based on the presuppositions of the critical theory, one may establish relationships among education, work and societies. The guidelines of human education and professional formation ascribe to the universities the construction and dissemination of knowledge in favor of the humanization of a world in dynamic transformation. This research aims at analyzing the curricular structure of an undergraduate nursing program in order to identify the inclusion of the theme "aging" in professional formation, through contents, teaching-learning strategies as well as its determinant factors. The documental analysis included the pedagogical proposal of the program, courses, summary and teaching plans applied from August 1998 to July 1999; the above mentioned analysis was complemented by an inquiry with the coordinators of the courses about their program, the reasons for their inclusion in the curriculum, schedule and their theoretical or practical approach. Among the 43 regular courses, only 7 introduced the subject, such as: Psychology of Development, Nutrition, Women's Health, Public Health Nursing I, Epidemiology, Gynecological and Obstetric Nursing and Clinical Nursing, predominating brief contents of theoretical nature in a total of 88 hours. Only the Course on Gerontological and Geriatric Nursing (optional) approaches theoretical and practical aspects. The elderly's increasing demand regarding teaching was the determinant factor for the introduction of the theme in the curriculum. Nevertheless, nurses' gerontological formation will require an innovating interdisciplinary strategy, focussing on life cycle and aging as the fundamental axis of the pedagogical proposal.

Preparing for Practice: Current Trends in the Gerontological Curriculum in Canadian Health Sciences Programs

Jennifer Klein (University of Alberta, Edmonton, Canada), Jennifer Baumbusch (Simon Fraser Health Region, Burnaby, Canada)

PURPOSE: Two recent studies examined the present status of gerontological content in Canadian programs for nurses and occupational therapists preparing to enter clinical practice. Findings from each study will be presented and the common implications discussed. METHOD: Twenty-one Faculties and Schools of Nursing and ten Occupational Therapy programs participated. A retrospective survey design method was used to examine the quality and quantity of curriculum coursework and clinical placements of the 1999/2000 year. RESULTS: Findings reveal that there is great variation in the organization and content of gerontological requirements across programs. Some schools taught the gerontological content as a separate course and others had the gerontological content integrated throughout the programs. For clinical fieldwork, only 500f OT schools required students to take a placement specifically working with older adults while only 80f clinical hours for nursing students were in geriatric settings. Unfortunately, students are not choosing gerontology as their clinical specialty in numbers that reflect the needs of an aging population. Moreover, there is a limited number of faculty who are prepared to conduct research and teach gerontological content. CONCLUSIONS: The goal of including gerontological content in health sciences programs is to ensure students are prepared to provide excellent clinical care for older adults when they enter practice. Findings from these studies suggest that options to consider for increasing gerontological content include: interdisciplinary courses, greater focus on faculty development, and enhanced clinical practicums in geriatric settings with a broad range of older adults who represent the diversity of this population.

Retooling Gerontology Training for Community College Health Science Students and Practioners

C. Medlin (Tidewater Community College, Virginia Beach, VA, USA)

Allied health students and practitioners must strengthen gerontological competencies. Ten focus groups were undertaken in Virginia Beach, Virginia, USA to determine what these competencies should be. The focus of this session is on the development of a 28 credit, skills-based Certificate in Gerontology based upon data collected in local focus groups. Implications for faculty development and grant funding will also be addressed.

The Evolution of a Knowledge Transfer Centre at the Sherbrooke Geriatric University Institute.

Krystyna Kouri, Daniel Bergeron (Expertise Centre in Gerontology and Geriatrics, Sherbrooke Geriatric University Institute).

Formal and informal caregivers are confronted with the phenomenon of an accelerated rate of knowledge production in gerontology and geriatrics. A province-wide study in which five key sectors (N=258) in each of Québec's 18 administrative regions were surveyed, demonstrated the need for a single-point entry knowledge dissemination body for aging-related information. In response to these findings the Sherbrooke Geriatric University Institute (SGUI) created a bilingual knowledge transfer organism, the Expertise Centre in Geriatrics and Gerontology. Within a conceptual orientation which promotes self-care, and draws from teaching-learning principles of andragogy and geragogy, the Centre has developed, over the past five years, a variety of knowledge transfer modes; each targeting specific population groups. At the community level, and via an outreach orientation, dissemination strategies include interactive forums (lectures, workshops, etc.), a community information resource library, and affiliate partner links with the Internet-based Canadian Health Network. A consultancy service and a documentation centre provide province-wide access to a wide range of gerontological resources. Educational forums (colloquia, conferences, seminars, etc.) are organized regularly for caregivers, health professionals and researchers. The Institute's scientific publication, with a particular mandate to transform complex information, especially research outcomes, into an easier to understand format, is produced by the Centre. This publication is carried on the Institute's Web site along with more extensive information about the initiatives of the Expertise Centre. The new Development arm of the Centre serves as yet another knowledge transfer mechanism which facilitates the transformation of "innovations" (assessment tools, intervention instruments, etc.) produced by researchers and clinicians into marketable formats.

Web Delivery Modes for Gerontological Education

S. Hirst (Faculty of Nursing, University of Calgary, Calgary, Alberta, Canada). S. Raffin (Faculty of Nursing, University of Calgary, Calgary, Alberta, Canada).

Long before it was popular, health care professionals were caring for older adults. The knowledge and skills required to provide care to this population group were often acquired through trial and error. In the past several decades, the specialty of gerontological practice has experienced profound growth; and the growing complexity of and demand for such services while exciting is accompanied by the requirement for a strong knowledge base on which these services can be built. The importance of providing educational content and clinical opportunities related to older adults is of relatively recent recognition within academic institutions, and is heavily delivered by on-site courses and the use of nearby clinical experiences usually supervised by academic faculty members. Presented in this paper are specific World Wide Web based experiences with projects such as an theoretical aging and disability course, and an undergraduate nursing clinical experience. While some content will be presented as an overview of the design and issues, the focus of the paper is twofold: (1) the implementation of educational technologies for gerontological education within professional faculties, and (2) the use of computers as cognitive tools to facilitate learning in students. The opportunity to learn of the challenges and benefits associated with integrating educational technology into the gerontological teaching/learning process will be an integral aspect of this paper.

SESSION 358

Bioresonance Stimulation in Treatment of Elderly Patients with Knee Joint Osteoarthrosis

*V.V. Povoroznjuk, E.I. Bayandina, *A.B. Olekseyenko, *A.E. Kushnir (Institute of Gerontology, 04114 Kiev, Ukraine; *NIOKB NESSI, Dniepropetrovsk, Ukraine)*

Bioresonance stimulation (BS), a method which is based on activation and normalization of organism's biological rhythms at the expense of external source of acoustic energy, should be effective in the elderly with knee joint osteoarthroses. A study of BS was undertaken in a group of 15 patients with knee joint osteoarthroses (10 women and 5 men) aged 57-74 years. BS was performed for 10 min daily (modes 1 and 2), 10 sessions per one course. Methods used: orthopedic examination, x-ray of knee joints, visual analog scales and McGill questionnaire for measuring pain syndrome during different daily activities before and after treatment. According to data of a combined verbal-analog scale, the pain syndrome intensity reduced from (5.7+0.56)cm before to (4.0+ 1.1)cm after treatment); the volume of knee joint movements increased (from 103+5.5 before to 130+11.5 degrees after treatment) mainly at the expense of relieved painful contractures. After treatment the patients had reduced the starting pains, pains during a prolonged walk, and when walking down the stairs. The night pains showed a tendency to diminish. Thus, the bioresonance stimulation has proved to be effective in treating patients with knee joint osteoarthrosis.

Effect of One Yeaer DHEA Treatment on Bone Mineral Density and Bone-Turnover: The DHEage Study

JC. Souberbielle, F. Forette ** §, J. Raison &, C.Cormier***, C.Kindermans*, S Legrain****, V Faucounau §, EE. Baulieu §§. Physiologie, hôpital Necker (*), Broca Hospital, University Paris V (**), Endocrinologie-Nutrition, hôpital Hotel Dieu (&), Rhumatologie A, hôpital Cochin (***) AP-HP, Paris, Fondation National de Gerontologie (§) and INSERM U444 (§§), Le Kremlin-Bicêtre, France.*

The secretion of DHEA decreases with age, and the question is raised whether administration of DHEA counteracts defects associated with aging. Two hundred and eighty healthy individuals (70 women-70 men, 60-69 y old, and 70 women-70 men 70-79 y old) were given DHEA, 50 mg, or placebo (pl), orally, daily for one year in a double blind,placebo-controlled study. We measured hip and forearm BMD before and after 12 months (mo) of treatment, and markers of bone formation [serum osteocalcin (Oc) and bone alkaline phosphatase (bAP)] and resorption [serum Cross-laps (CTx)], before and after 6 and 12 mo of treatment. In men, no effect of DHEA was recorded, whether on BMD or biochemical markers, except an increase in bAP (+32%; $p<0.05$) at 12 mo in the older DHEA-treated men. However, differences in BMD change (expressed as median change in mg/cm2 [1st;3rd quartiles]) between pl- and DHEA-treated women were observed at the femoral neck (pl:-9 [-16;+18]; DHEA:+13 [+1;+13];$p<0.05$) and Ward's triangle (pl:-23 [-40;+6]; DHEA:+4 [-19;+25]; $p<0.05$) in the 60-69 y women and at the upper radius (pl:-10 [-19;+5]; DHEA:+4 [-8;+14]; $p<0.05$) and total radius (pl:-11 [-20;+5]; DHEA:+2 [-5;+10];$p<0.05$) in the 70-79 y women. CTx decreased by 11%

($p<0.05$) and 26%($p<0.01$) at 6 mo and 12 mo respectively, only in the 70-79 y DHEA-treated women, while Oc and bAP were unchanged. In the 70-79 y women with the sDHEA levels in the lowest quartile at baseline, the decrease of CTx was even larger (-43% at 6 mo and -35% at 12 mo; $p<0.01$) with a delayed decrease of serum Oc (-5% at 6 mo, NS, and -35% at 12 mo, $p<0.01$). These results suggest that daily oral treatment with 50 mg DHEA has favourable effects on bone in women, specially in those 70 y old and over, but not in men. Whether or not these effects are due to the formation of active estrogens and /or androgens deserves future studies.

Estriol (E3) replacement improves endothelial function and bone mineral density for two years in octogenarian women

Toshio Hayashi, Izumi Ito, Hatsuyo Kano, Akhisa Iguchi, (Department of Geriatrics, Nagoya University Graduate School of Medicine, Nagoya, JAPAN)

Background: Estriol (E3) is a weak estrogen and has little effect on genital organs. In hormone replacement therapy for postmenopausal women, administration of progestin is supposed not to be always necessary. However, its effects on elderly female are not available. PURPOSE: We investigated the long-term effects of estriol (E3) on endothelial function in octogenarian women. METHOD: Twenty-four octogenarian women (80+3.5 years old) were administered CaCl2 with or without estriol treatment (2 mg/day) for 104 weeks (HRT; hormone replacement group vs. control group). Plasma lipid and biochemical profile, endothelium-dependent flow-mediated dilatation (FMD), endothelium-independent dilatation by nitroglycerin in brachial artery, and bone mineral density (BMD) were assessed. RESULTS: 2 patients in HRT groups suffered of transient genital bleeding in the term. No other complications occurred such as venous thrombosis and body fluid retention. Plasma HDL-C and apo A1 concentration increased after 54 wks, however other lipids and apoproteins were not changed. Both plasma E3 and E2 were substantially increased by HRT during all over the experiment term (for example, E2, 4.6 to 31.3+ 8.1, E3, less than 5 to 45.3 + 7.9 pg/ml in 30 weeks). The FMD was also increased by HRT, as were the plasma nitrite/nitrate and cGMP values. The response to nitroglycerin was not changed. These changes of endothelial function continued from 30 weeks up to 104 weeks after prescription CONCLUSION: Endothelial function was improved in line with the anti-atherosclerotic effects. E3 might be effective drug for use in HRT in elderly patients.

Fosamax in Treatment of Involutional Osteoporosis and its Complications

V. V. Povoroznjuk

To study the efficacy of Fosamax in treatment of involutional osteoporosis and its complications (vertebrae fractures) 25 women aged 5675 years (mean age 63,61,2 years) were examined. To evaluate structural-functional state of bone tissue ultrasound densitometer "Achilles+" (Lunar Corp, Madison, WI) was used. Stiffness index of bone tissue (SI, %) was determined. Ultrasonometry, evaluation of pain syndrom's pronouncement were carried out in 3, 6, 12 months since the beginning of treatment: 17 patients (I group) were taking it for 6 months, 11 patients (II group) were taking it for 1 year. Patients ceased taking drug because of financial difficulties and not because of absent effect or side effects. 9 women taking Fosamax for 1 year were examined in 12 months after the end of treatment (they were included in the III group). Fosamax considerably reduced the pronouncement of pain syndrome and greatly improved structural-functional state of bone tissue: I group SI (before treatment 64,03,0%; in 6 months 68,72,9%; p=0,012); II group SI (before treatment 66,23,1%; in 12 months 71,22,7%; p=0,036); III group SI (before treatment 66,83,2%; in 12 months 73,12,6%; in a year after the end of treatment 69,64,3%). Results of our studies show Fosamax's efficacy in treatment of involutional osteoporosis and its complications. The drug increases bone mineral density, improves its solid characteristics, which is followed by a considerable decrease of pain syndrome's pronouncement and increase in functional abilities of patients

Intermittent intramuscular clodronate therapy in senile osteoporosis

M. Barbagallo, LJ Dominguez, GB Rini, MA Alessi Institute of Internal Medicine and Geriatrics, University of Palermo, Italy

PURPOSE: Bisphophonates are effective anti-resorptive treatments of osteoporosis in the elderly. Intramuscular clodronate is a potential alternative for osteoporotic patients who have contraindications or intolerance to the oral preparations. Aim of the present study was to verify the efficacy of an intermittent, intramuscular administration of clodronate (100 mg i.m. every 2 weeks) on vertebral and femoral bone mineral density (BMD) in elderly subjects. METHODS: 84 women older than 65 yrs, fulfilling the WHO criteria for osteoporosis (spine or hip T-score<-2.5) were recruited to a randomised, controlled study and followed for one year. Diet of all patients was adjusted to provide 1200-1300 mg/day of calcium, eventually by administration of supplements. Patients were then subdivided in two groups, group A including 42 patients which received 100 mg clodronate i.m. every two weeks and group B (42 pts) that did not receive additional therapies. BMD was measured at vertebral and femoral sites using dual energy X-ray absorptiometry (DEXA DPX-100 Lunar) at baseline and after 12 months. RESULTS: In the group given clodronate i.m. a significant increase in BMD was obtained at lumbar spine (+4.71%;$p<0.01$) and at all femoral sites (Wards: +4.00%, neck: +2.29%, trochanter: +1.18%; $p<0.01$ at all sites), while no significant differences were detected in pts receiving only calcium and vitamin D supplementation. CONCLUSIONS: Our present results demonstrate that an intermittent intramuscular clodronate administration twice a month is well tolerated and is effective in increasing bone mineral density at vertebral and femoral sites in elderly women with senile osteoporosis.

The use of Glucosamine products among older adults: Self treatment practices and perceived effectiveness

Violeta Ribeiro (School of Nursing, Memorial University of Newfoundland, St. John's, NF, A1B 3V6) Judith Blakeley (School of Nursing, Memorial University of Newfoundland, St. John's, NF, A1B 3V6)

Glucosamine products (GLS) are currently being used by many middle aged and older aults as a treatment for osteoarthritis. Produced by different companies, GLS are unregulated, sold under many different labels, in varying dosages and often in combination with other products. This raises several questions about the decision making and self treatment practices of older GLS users. The purpose of this research was to address some of these questions, namely: (1) what factors influence the consumers' decision to use GLS and their choice of GLS product?; (2) how do they manage and monitor their GLS therapy?; and what is their perception of the effectiveness, side effects and costs of GLS? The study used a descriptive/exploratory design and was based on a convenience sample of 65 adults aged 50 years and over. Data were obtained with a mail-out questionnaire. SPSS descriptors were used to provide an overview of the findings. Friedman's and Wilcoxon Signed-Ranks tests were conducted to compare the perceived effectiveness of GLS products with those of other treatments used for osteoarthritis. The results indicate that advice from friends was a major factor in the decision to take GLS. Cost was identified as major influence in the choice of type and brand name of GLS that was used. Almost all the subjects (92%) managed and monitored their own therapy. The vast majority (88%) took GLS regularly but only 33% took the recommended daily dose. Many (67%) perceived the product to be either very or moderately effective in relieving pain and stiffness and improving mobility. Reports of side effects were negligible. These findings support the need for public education and further research regarding the management and benefits of GLS.

SESSION 359

Comparison of Behavioral and Technological Approaches to Achieve A Useful Helping Technology for Elderly Consumers

M.H. Parker, [MKHP Associates, LLC, Alexandria, VA.]. D.M. Kutzik, Ph.D; A.P. Glascock, [Center for Applied Neurogerontology, Drexel University, Philadelphia, PA].

PURPOSE: To compare and discuss the outcome effectiveness of opposite approaches to achieving a passive computerized monitoring system. METHOD: Assistive technology targeted to older consumers is a growing area of research and business development. Questions arise about how to best develop new technology to meet the needs of an aging population. The presentation compares practical experience in developing analogous technologies to assist older adults with activities of daily living and safety issues. In one project, an existing signal processing method was adapted to detect certain behaviors of elderly and send an alarm. In the other project, behavioral research was used to identify measures for monitoring behavior of community resident elderly to detect change. Both projects used similar off-the-shelf technology of sensors and computer software, to perform non-obtrusive, continuous monitoring of activities of daily living. RESULTS: Analyses of these data showed that a normal activity profile can be developed and that variation from a person's normal routine or a fall can be detected. Contrasting design philosophies resulted in differences in the effectiveness of responding to problems and optimally implementing each system. CONCLUSION: The behavioral approach had greater flexibility in dealing with variation in performance among the older persons, an important factor in system efficiency and efficacy over time, while the technologically driven approach, which required consumers to adapt their behavior to the technological model, had a high error factor.

Design, Development and Testing of a Transport Chair System

G. R. Fernie, P. J. Holliday, M. Pacitto and P. Wilcox P (Sunnybrook & Women's College Health Sciences Centre, Toronto, Canada)

Many seniors are able to manage to function independently at home, but find the distances they encounter when visiting a hospital, airport or other large facility too great. In this presentation, we describe how a system was designed to meet these people's needs and report experience with the use of the system for two years. The system consists of corrals (similar to bus shelters) that are located by all entrances and at all levels in the car parks of our hospital. Transport chairs (known as StaxiTM) are nested together within these corrals in a manner similar to shopping carts. The Staxi was designed to be easy to push by a companion and to be safe for use without instruction. The ease of pushing was achieved by locating the centre of gravity of the user and the chair closer to the rear larger fixed wheels and applying very low loads on the front swiveling castors. An ergonomic pushbar enables a companion to manoeuver the chair easily. A major concern was the possibility that users might forget or be unaware of the need, to apply parking brakes before transferring on- and-off the chair. This was solved by incorporating an automatic brake.

The First Known Practical Multi-Directional Powered Wheelchair

G. R. Fernie, G. T. Griggs, P.J. Holliday, M. Pacitto and P. Wilcox (Sunnybrook & Women's College Health Sciences Centre, Toronto, Canada)

Powered wheelchairs and scooters are growing in popularity. The impact of these devices on quality of life and independent functioning of elderly people has been shown to be very high. Since approximately one-third of people over the age of 75 use some form of mobility aid, it will be increasingly important to design and adapt living, working and social environments to accommodate these products. Unfortunately, powered wheelchairs and, particularly scooters, require additional space for manoeuvering. In fact, there is even discussion of increasing the space requirements in barrier-free codes in Canada because of increased numbers of larger scooters. The economic cost of the need for extra space and the inconvenience of having to drive these vehicles using car-like manoeuvers, such as three-point turns and parallel parking, provided us with the motivation to develop a powered chair that is capable of spinning on-the-spot and moving sideways. In this presentation, we describe some of the rationale for design decisions that were made during the development of this multi- directional chair, which has been named the RocketTM. We also illustrate the functional advantages that this new design provides for the user. Some ongoing research into future enhancements is outlined. These include extending the use of powered mobility to seniors who are presently considered to be unsafe drivers for reasons of sensory and cognitive impairment.

Universal Design; An approach to designing for Seniors, addressing cultural, economic and gender disparities.

Pamela J. Cluff (Associated Planning Consultants Inc, Toronto, Canada.)

PURPOSE: The twenty first century provides us with an unprecedented opportunity to consider our social and physical world in relationship to the rapidly expanding numbers of seniors, surviving into old-old age. In community planning and design, the basic needs of all people, regardless of age, gender or ethnicity can be re-evaluated and past stereotypical solutions for accessible services and accommodation, put aside. The Universal Design approach is inclusive, not exclusive, allowing seniors and persons with disabilities to be dealt with, in the built-environment, as part of the complex matrix of humanity, as a whole. METHOD: Historical models and demographic data can be analyzed to demonstrate that both past and current solutions for shelter and care, have not always addressed the full spectrum of human needs, as defined by Maslow. RESULTS: A 'Universal Design' approach is flexible enough to accommodate the changing economic and health status of seniors, regardless of geography, culture, gender or historical norms. CONCLUSION: In certain countries the policy framework for Universal Design approach is already being systematically modified, as are design, construction and operational guidelines. In addition the rapid expansion of global communications networks will allow this information to be disseminated for the first time, to sponsors and designers, throughout the world.

Universal design for the ageing: simulation devices as tools of persuasion

Satoshi Kose (Building Research Institute, Tsukuba, Japan)

Purpose: The whole globe is ageing. From the viewpoint of professionals involved in providing the designed environment, whether products or dwellings and buildings, design concepts with due consideration of ageing users are the crucial issues to be tackled. How can we convey the ideas to designers who have never thought of the change and persuade them? Method: Lectures are the first steps to do to let them know the presence of the problems. The second step will be the simulated experience, both imaginary and real. Imaginary is to show them two contradicting examples, good and bad. If the examples are familiar to them, they will be fairly easily persuaded. If not, simulating experiences with quasi-ageing simulation devices such as goggles, earplugs and joint restraints might help. Unfortunately, existing devices do not allow easy comparison of getting much older. It was assumed to be the limitation. To break the ice, adjustable simulation devices were developed. The first attempt was to develop joint constraints with adjustable strength. Results: The effectiveness of the new devices are yet to be tested, but they are expected to tell people how they will deteriorate in their capability and experience further difficulties as they get older. It is what the previous devices failed to demonstrate. Further ideas for devices will be tried. Conclusion: To experience one's own ageing is an important step for the designers and decision makers to get involved in the practice of universal design. The new devices will serve the purpose.

Virtual Residential Care: Supporting Independent Living and Home Care Services by New (Geron-)Technologies

Richard Pieper (University of Bamberg, Bamberg, Germany)

Independent living at home - preference of the elderly and goal of social policy - has to be supported by new (geron-)technologies and technical, social, and health care services. But a systematic framework for the role of technologies and corresponding services is missing to understand the dynamics of non-/acceptance and to promote innovation in established care systems. The concept of virtual residential care is used in divers projects with new technologies and services. Three approaches are identified and discussed: 1. health care model - centering on ambulant health care/rehabilitation vs. hospitalization, 2. social care model - focussing on home care/ home help vs. residential care, 3. service housing model - centering on new housing projects with services and technical support vs. the risks of independent living. Three clusters of technologies and stakeholders are considered: telematics, smart home, and medical technology.In (1), telemedicine and new medical technologies promoted by innovative clinics are competing with ambulant health care networks having less developed technologies and fewer resources; in (2), home care is supported by social policy and client preferences, but residential care profits from lower costs with increasing client dependency both lacking resources and technological innovation; in (3), new models of residential living are developed introducing new technologies and services for safety and comfort, but insufficient concepts for social and health care. All models have an institutional bias expected to be influenced by proliferation of IT in private households and networks. The framework utilizes also experiences and results from three own projects.

SESSION 360

Demographic Patterns and Social Trends in Contemporary Grandparenthood: The Canadian Context

Candace L. Kemp (McMaster University, Hamilton, ON, Canada)

Although there exists a growing body of literature dedicated to understanding the complexities of grandparenting, few researchers have documented the demographic patterns and social trends that encompass contemporary grandparenthood. Concomitantly, in instances where researchers have described such patterns, data are largely derived from studies profiling American populations. In light of these observations, this paper examines social trends in grandparenthood and outlines the demographic context within which Canadians participate in grandparent-grandchild relationships. Drawing on nationally representative samples and data derived from both the 1990 and 1995 General Social Surveys of Canada, this study analyzes patterns influencing grandparenthood such as grandparents' rates of survival, the prevalence of grandparenthood, multi-generation families, step-grandparenthood and the availability of grandchildren. In addition, analysis considers the amount of contact adult grandchildren have with their grandparents, rates of intergenerational cohabitation and surrogate parenting as well as grandparents' participation in additional social roles. Results confirm that grandparenthood is a widespread occurrence for individuals aged 60 and over who have at least one child and further, that multi-generation families, adult grandchildren and grandparents with multiple roles are relatively common. A number of Canadian grandparents act as surrogate parents to their grandchildren or live in multi-generation households, yet as low percentages indicate, these family situations are not routinely encountered. Findings reveal significant variations in grandparenting patterns according to the age group and gender of both grandparents and grandchildren. Importantly, when compared to American studies, results vary slightly thereby demonstrating subtle national differences in grandparenthood trends.

Intergenerational family conflicts: Sources of disagreements between elderly mothers and adult daughters in Brazil

E.J. Barham, A.F. Alves (Universidade Federal de São Carlos, São Carlos, Brazil)

The difficulties that occur in the relationship between elderly parents and their adult children differ from one culture to the next. The purpose of this study was to determine the key difficulties in this relationship, in one region of Brazil. The objectives were: 1) verify whether conflicts occur, and if so, what they are about, 2) identify the consequences of these conflicts, and 3) investigate the strategies that are used to resolve them. Two versions of the data collection instrument were used, one as an interview protocol (with 21 elderly mothers) and the other as a questionnaire (with 13 adult daughters). The results indicate that: 1) mothers and daughters agree that there are misunderstandings in their relationship, primarily involving interpersonal factors, and both experience difficulty to express themselves when their opinions differ; 2) both perceive there to be positive and negative impacts of these conflicts; and 3) both believe that an improvement in their communication would help resolve these problems. It is important to note that the emotional exchanges (positive and negative) reported by the respondents occurred primarily in the family context, which reflects the emphasis placed on family ties, in Brazil. Given that interpersonal factors were those most strongly indicated as causing conflicts, interventions to improve the quality of this important relationship could include the strengthening of their interpersonal skills, thus improving the well-being of the elderly and their adult children.

Intergenerational Relationships and Old Age Security: A Case Study of India

1. Raj Dhruvarajan (Department of Economics, University of Manitoba, Canada) 2. Anitha Kumari (Department of Sociology, Heinrich-Heine University,Germany)

Abstract As a result of economic development and improved health care technology, India is currently witnessing rapid ageing of its population. At the same time, urbanisation, modernisation and globalisation have led to changes in economic structure, erosion of traditional societal values and the weakening of social institutions such as the joint family, in which older people occupied a position of prestige, respect and authority. As well, work related out- migration of children, especially from rural to urban areas, growing attitude of individualism' and increasing prevalence of dual career families have led to a decline in the traditional sense of duty and obligation of the younger generation towards the older generation. Thus, the increasing dependency of seniors for their care on family members and the simultaneous loosening of family ties place these seniors, especially those who are not financially independent, in a precarious position. The almost complete absence of an adequate social security system in the country further compounds the problem. The situation is particularly acute for women in general and widows in particular, who tend to be more dependent on their children. With declining support from families, there is clearly an urgent need for policies and programmes by governments for the security of senior citizens if a future crisis is to be averted. The more developed countries have tried to solve the problem through an old age social security system and a network of old age homes. This solution is expensive and currently beyond the capability of central and state governments in India. Also, old age homes may be appropriate for western countries, which emphasize individuality, nuclear families and a strong sense of independence, but not for India, where the tradition of filial obligation to parents still persists and where parents still prefer to stay with their children. In general, any solutions for the problem of aging in India should therefore take the country's social and cultural traditions into consideration. With this background, this paper tries to explore in detail the various issues of aging and old age security in India and to suggest some feasible policy options to overcome the problem.

Long Distance Contact and Care Between Adult Children and Their Aging Parents

M.W. Parker (School of Social Work, The University of Alabama, Alabama USA) V.R.A. Call (Department of Sociology, Brigham Young University, Utah USA) J.I. Kosberg (School of Social Work, The University of Alabama, Alabama USA)

Social and economic changes lead to increased geographic mobility among adult children (both within and between the countries of the world) thus challenging traditional assumptions regarding the existence of family caregivers for the elderly. Based upon a representative sample of 3352 American adult children, it has been found that geographic distance between elderly parent(s) (less than 50 miles, 50 to 90 miles, and greater than 90 miles) differentially affects the frequency of personal visits and telephone/mail contact. The health condition of the parent has almost no effect on the frequency of visits. The extent and type of contact and care were found to be associated with 1) adult child's perceived quality of relationship with the parent, 2) existence of siblings living in closer proximity to the parent, and 3) female gender of child and parent. Findings suggest that adult children and parents need to discuss plans for the time when their parents can no longer maintain independent living. This study has implications for both members of formal and informal care systems who are concerned about the possibility of unwanted geographic relocation of elderly parents closer to their adult children, or vice versa, in the face of parents' declining health condition and loss of independence

Meanings of Nonmarital Cohabitation for the Elderly in Korea

Seong Young Sohn (College of Liberal Arts, Dongduk Women's University, Seoul, Korea)

Nonmarital cohabitation is very rare and not welcomed in Korea. However, the elderly's case is somewhat different. The purpose of this paper is to study the meanings and situations of Korean elderly's nonmarital cohabitation. Using in-depth interview methods, I exlore the relationship of the nonmarital couples and their relationship with relatives including their own children. The findings indicate that adult children's recognition and emotional supports influence on the quality of the old nonmarried couple's relationship. Whether the cohabitation was initiated by the old couple or by their children also operates as a key factor in determining the old couple's status in the family.

Patterns of Intergenerational Financial Exchange

J. Ploeg (McMaster University, Hamilton, Canada) M. Denton (McMaster University, Hamilton, Canada) L. Campbell (McMaster University, Hamilton, Canada) A. Joshi (McMaster University, Hamilton, Canada) S. Webb (McMaster University, Hamilton, Canada)

The purpose of this study is to describe patterns of intergenerational financial exchange between older adults and their families, friends and neighbors. There is little data, particularly Canadian data, published on the patterns of financial exchange between generations. A self-administered survey questionnaire was developed to assess patterns of intergenerational financial exchange and was piloted with a small group of seniors. A convenience sample of persons aged 55 years and older from across Canada was obtained through advertisements in newsletters (e.g, Canadian Association for Retired Persons [CARP] News), newspapers, and other media (e.g, One Voice web site). This paper will present demographic characteristics of the sample and descriptive statistics of the types and amounts of financial assistance provided to and received from family members and friends (e.g, purchase of home, car, educational funds, etc). As well, participants' perceptions of the reasons for providing or receiving financial assistance will be summarized. This research makes a significant contribution to our understanding of intergenerational financial exchanges. This study is part of the Social and Economic Dimensions of an Aging Population (SEDAP) program of research funded by the Social Sciences and Humanities Research Council of Canada Major Collaborative Research Initiatives (SSHRCC).

Perceptions of selected familial supports for the Aged.

Sharada Akella (Smt V.H.D.Institute of Homescience,Bangalore,India) C.V.Geetha (Smt V.H.D.Institute of Homescience,Bangalore, India)

The present study was conducted to understand the developmental tasks and roles which give rise to the need for selected supports from family members to the Aged during these twilight years. The sample was seleted from North,South,East,and West zones of Bangalore Urban. the sample consists of '3067 Aged' called Group-I and '303 family members' called Group-II.Aged were of 60 and above years and Family members were between 15-59 years of age.The tool used in collecting data was an Interview Schedule.It was standardised after testing for its reliability. The selected familial supports studied were Economic,Sociological,Psychological,Biological conditions and Concept of Death against the variables Age and SES of the respondent.The data obtained was analysed statistically to arrive at significant results. Results show that there is a deficiency in the availability of Psychological and Sociological supports. Economic support is provided by the family members. the biological conditions of the sample was considerably favouravble. Death was a 'taboo' subject for conversation or discussion with no response. The conclusion is that adjustments and mutual respect between the two groups is to be encouraged. Also, activity in oldage instead of disengagement helps to attin an improved lifestyle in these years.

The relation between the elderly and their adult children after divorce

C.M. Fokkema, P.A. Dykstra (NIDI, The Hague, The Netherlands)

The present study addresses two research questions. The first is descriptive: Does divorce have a negative effect on the relationships between older parents and their adult children? This question will be answered by comparing the current contact frequency of (ever)-divorced parents with their adult children to that of parents in their first marriage. The second research question is explanatory: Which factors contribute to high-frequency interactions between older divorced parents and their adult children? To answer this question we will look at the kind of involvement of the parent with the children in the past, both during the marriage (division of caring and upbringing tasks between parents) and (soon) after the dissolution of the marriage (custody, visiting rights and remarriage). Other factors that will be considered, are the ages of the children at the time of the divorce, the life phase of the children, and the social economic status of the parents. The data are from the 1998-1999 survey 'Divorce in the Netherlands' (Scheiding in Nederland, SIN), which distinguishes three groups of men and women: first married, divorced and not remarried, and divorced and remarried.

SESSION 362

Health and Well-being: International Perspectives

Mary Luszcz (Flinders University, Adelaide, Australia). Generativity in the lives of adults; C.P.M. Knipscheer (Vrije Universiteit, Amsterdam, The Netherlands) Family cohesiveness and support received from children: their interdependence and its consequences for loneliness; Jacqui Smith (Max Planck Institute, Berlin, Germany). Health: An important predictor of decline in Well-being in Very Old Age; Linda S. Noelker (Benjamin Rose Institute, Cleveland, Ohio), Quality of life and subjective well-being in long term care. Discussant: James S. Jackson (University of Michigan, Ann Arbor, Michigan).

This symposium examines health and well being in later adulthood. The four papers each take a unique perspective to explore a range of issues which affect quality of life from middle age through late adulthood. In addition, the papers provide both theoretical insights as well as empirical evidence in the exploration of these issues. It is well know that people reach old age with diverse life experiences, having achieved various levels of well-being as well as having experienced different health problems. These papers consider how midlife concepts of generativity might apply to old age, how children affect the well-being of their parents as well as each other, the unique strategies used by older people to adapt to existent and emerging health problems, and offers a comprehensive theoretical perspective on maintaining well-being among long term care residents. The four papers also represent data from three continents, Europe, North America, and Australia. Luszcz, Boyd, Princi and Bennett expand the concept of generativity across adulthood as well as across several life domains. They view generativity not simply as a midlife concept but also as one which has important implications for late life. Their Australian data suggest that generativity improves self-esteem and well-being throughout adulthood. Knipscheer & van Tilburg examine the universal and unique contributions of specific children to the well-being of family elders. Very rarely do researchers investigate how different children contribute to their parents well-being and if they do so in unique or universal ways. Their Dutch data indicate that there can be important differences among children and that family cohesiveness is an important contributor to the well-being of older adults. J. Smith examines well-being and quality of life among the oldest old in Berlin. Her data indicate that self-regulatory processes help older people adapt to changing life conditions but only to a point. While older people, even the oldest old, are able to use multiple strategies to offset some health problems and maintain well-being, these techniques are not without limits. As health challenges accumulate, the ability of self-regulatory strategies to offset the negative impact on well-being is shown to diminish. And finally, Noelker considers quality of life in the unique housing setting of many people of advanced age, the long term residential care setting. She outlines a theoretical perspective which details four domains that influence quality of life. These are: safe and timely care, technically proficient care, individuation and respect. All of these factors are clearly important both for older people and the staff who cares for them. This broadened perspective both attends to the importance of well-being, despite health status, of older people and recognizes the multiple determinants, including self, staff and others, of well-being at this unique stage of life. These papers offer a broad array of issues, both theoretical and empirical, which are important to consider when attempting to achieve and maintain well-being in adulthood across a wide variety of health statuses.

Family cohesiveness and support received from children: their interdependence and its consequences for loneliness

C.P.M. Knipscheer, T. van Tilburg (Dept. of Sociology and Social Gerontology, Vrije Universiteit, Amsterdam, The Netherlands)

PURPOSE: It is very well documented that in general children provide much support to their old parents. However, most studies have focused on parent child dyads, in particular the relationship with the most supportive child. The current study adopts a family system approach. Research questions are: (1) Does instrumental and emotional support received vary across children? (2) Is there congruence of family cohesiveness among individual family members? (3) Does cohesiveness affect the support received from children? (4) What is the contribution of cohesiveness and support received from children in the explanation of differences in loneliness? METHOD: Data are available from 155 Dutch older adults, their spouse (if available; n= 111) and their children (n= 319). The mailed questionnaires included 12 questions on mutual supportive exchanges. Furthermore, both parents and children answered an item scale on family cohesiveness and on loneliness. RESULTS: Preliminary multilevel analyses showed that across children there was considerable variation in the intensity of the support provided to a parent. Furthermore, family members differed in their view on family cohesiveness. Parents viewed the family as more cohesive than children. The more cohesive the family, the more emotional support was provided by children. Differences in instrumental support were not observed. Finally, cohesiveness, the availability of a partner and number of children predicted differences in loneliness. Controlled for these effects, there was no contribution of support received from (multiple) children. CONCLUSION: The family of older adults should not be studied as a homogeneous system. Family cohesiveness is an important factor in wellbeing of older parents.

Generativity in the lives of adults

M.A. Luszcz, C.M. Boyd, R. Princi, K. Bennett (Flinders University, Adelaide, Australia)

We have been investigating links among generativity and variety of markers of psychological adaptation from young adulthood to later life in about 1000 adults. Our approach draws on the model originally proposed by Erikson, as well as more contemporary notions of generativity (e.g, McAdams), post-formal thought (e.g, Sinnott), psychosocial resources (e.g, M. Baltes; Thoits) and psychological well being (e.g, Diener; Lawton; Ryff). This paper will provide an integration and synthesis of some of our initial findings which indicate, for instance, that:(a) although generativity is a salient feature of mid-life, it is not restricted to that portion of the life span; (b) being generative is consequential for well being, although at midlife parental generativity may decrease with age and parenting experience, while post-formal relativistic thinking increases; (c) generative concerns feature in about half of the spontaneous responses from very old adults on what is important to them; (d) these concerns, which take the form of both producing and caring, are predicted by self-esteem, control expectancy, and social embeddedness. Emphasis will be placed on evidence for continuing generativity in older and very old adults and the central role it may occupy as a means whereby self-esteem leads to integrity or acceptance, at midlife and beyond. .

Health: An Important Predictor of Decline in Well-being in Very Old Age

Jacqui Smith (Max Planck Institute for Human Development, Berlin, Germany)

Assessments of well-being and quality of life are widely employed in the gerontological literature as indicators of the effectiveness of social policies and welfare programs, the success of medical and psychiatric treatments, and as global indicators of psychological adjustment and successful aging (P. B. Baltes & Baltes, 1990, 1992; Lawton, 1983, 1991; Patrick & Erickson, 1993; Rowe & Kahn, 1987; Ryff, 1989). In general, theories suggest that despite losses, subjective well-being and life satisfaction are maintained in old age. In this paper, we examine the idea that health is a central source of well-being in old age and that multimorbidity in very old age (>85 years) is realted to average decline in subjective well-being. Cross-sectional and longitudinal data from the Berlin Aging Study (BASE: Baltes & Mayer, 1999) is used to examine the extent to which objective and subjective indicators of different health statuses (e.g, specific illnesses, functional capacity) together with changes in health status predict overall individual well-being and changes in well-being. Results are multifaceted. At baseline assessment, the majority of participants reported satisfaction with their present life conditions (N = 516; M = 85 years). Over time, subjective well-being showed a linear decline. Older women, individuals aged 85 and over, and persons living in institutions where particularly at risk for decreased emotional well-being. Changing health status and multimorbidity was found to play a strong role in predicitn several dimensions of well-being (especially, satisfaction with one's own aging, and experience of positive affect). Our findings suggest that self-regulation processes that contribute to adaptation to changing life conditions operate effectively, at least up to the age of 80. However cumulative health challenges and losses appear to tap the limits of these adaptive processes, so that well-being declines for the majority of individuals after age 85.

Quality of Life and Subjective Well-being in Long Term Care

Linda S. Noelker (The Benjamin Rose Institute, Cleveland, OH)

Current research on well-being in long term residential care has shifted its emphasis from quality of care to quality of life as the focal outcome. This presentation details a conceptual model that incorporates four domains of quality of life essential to well-being in residential care: security, optimal health and functioning, autonomy, and affirmation of personhood. These domains are seen as key to maintenance of the self in environments where unwanted changes in living arrangements, life styles, social relationships, and interaction can occur and damage the integrity of the self. These four domains link to qualities of care that staff should demonstrate to enhance residents' sense of self. The qualities are: safe and timely care, technically proficient care, individuation, and respect. In order to enable staff, most of whom are paraprofessional workers, to display these qualities consistently, certain environmental, structural, organizational, and interpersonal characteristics must be in place. These characteristics, detailed in the model, provide the basis for interventions to enhance quality of life for residents. .

SESSION 363

A randomised controlled trial of vitamin D for physical capacity and fall risk in older patients

Craig Anderson (Clinical Trials Research Unit, University of Auckland, Auckland, New Zealand), Nancy Latham (Clinical Trials Research Unit, University of Auckland, Auckland, New Zealand), Arier Lee (Clinical Trials Research Unit, University of Auckland, Auckland, New Zealand), Anne Moseley (Rehabilitation Studies Unit, University of Sydney, Sydney, Australia), Ian Cameron (Rehabilitation Studies Unit, University of Sydney, Sydney, Australia), Caroline Stretton (Clinical Trials Research Unit, University of Auckland, Auckland, New Zealand)

PURPOSE: Frailty Interventions Trial in Elderly Subjects (FITNESS) was a randomised clinical trial that used a factorial design to assess the effectiveness of progressive resistance strength training (PRT) and vitamin D to improve physical capacity in frail elderly people. This abstract is for vitamin D. METHOD: FITNESS was conducted across five hospitals in Australia and New Zealand during 1999 and 2000. All older people who were admitted to acute geriatric wards, assessed as 'frail' by the attending clinician using broad criteria and able to participate were eligible. A central randomisation service was used. Patients were assigned either vitamin D (6x50,000 IU tablets) or matched placebo. Patients recorded any falls experienced in a calendar diary. Performance measures and self-report measures of health and activities were evaluated by assessors blind to treatment allocation at 3, 6 and 12 months post-randomisation. The primary efficacy endpoints were a 10 0ifference in the Physical Component Summary measure of the SF-36 at 3 months and a 30 0ifference in fall rate at 6 months. RESULTS: The study population (n=243) was 47% male, mean age 79 yrs (range 65-96). Baseline vitamin D levels were low (mean 18± 10 ug/L; 61% below 20 ug/L, 21% below 10 ug/L). CONCLUSION: The study results will be presented at the meeting. FITNESS will provide evidence of the effectiveness of vitamin D to improve physical function and reduce falls in frail older people.

Fall and injury prevention among older people in residential care - a randomised trial

J. Jensen, L. Lundin-Olsson, L. Nyberg, Y. Gustafson (Geriatric Medicine, Department of Community Medicine and Rehabilitation, Umeå University, Umeå, Sweden)

Falls and resulting injuries are particularly common among old people living in residential care but knowledge about the prevention of falls is limited. PURPOSE: The purpose of this trial was to investigate whether an intervention programme that targeted multiple risk factors for falls would reduce falls and fall-related injuries among old people living in residential care. METHOD: Nine residential facilities were distributed into two clusters. After assessments of 402 residents, all at least 65 years of age, the clusters of facilities were randomised into an intervention or a control group. The intervention programme included both general and individually tailored strategies. Strategies aimed at affecting all residents comprised measures such as staff education, medical review and environmental adjustment. Measures tailored to residents at high risk included physical training, supervision, adjustment of medication, aids and hip protectors (11 weeks). Falls and injuries were evaluated (34 weeks). RESULTS: The proportion of residents who fell was lower (44%) in the intervention than in the control group (56%), representing an adjusted odds ratio of 0.49 (95% CI: 0.31Δ0.78). The incidence rates of falling and of femoral fractures differed significantly between the intervention and the control groups (incidence rates ratio 0.80; 95% CI: 0.69Δ0.94, and 0.25; 95% CI: 0.08Δ0.82, respectively). The time to first fall also differed significantly between the groups (adjusted hazard ratio 0.66; 95% CI: 0.48Δ0.89). CONCLUSION: An interdisciplinary and multifactorial fall prevention programme directed to residents, staff and the environment has the potential to reduce falls and femoral fractures.

Falls and Fall-related Injury Long Term Residential Care Surveillance Project

Victoria J. Scott, (University of Victoria, Victoria, BC, Canada). Vikki Hay, (Director of Care, Oak Bay Lodge Society, Victoria, BC, Canada). Elain Gallagher (University of Victoria, Victoria, B.C.) Hansdeep Bhatia, Research Consultant, Victoria B.C. Andria Scanlan (B.C. Injury Research and Prevention Unit, Vancouver, B.C.)

Long term residential care administrators and clinicians have identified for some time a need to develop a standardized system of data collection for falls and injuries incurred by residents. The Falls and Fall-related Injury Surveillance System was initiated in September 2000 as a three-month pilot in the Capital Health Region of British Columbia. Its purpose was to trial a data collection tool as a provisional, standardized, falls prevention recording system. The findings include an analysis of the data collection tool in accordance with the following indicators: user (staff) friendliness; capacity to determine the incidence of falls, injuries and contributing factors; and efficacy in identifying appropriate prevention strategies. Data were collected on 60 falls on the 67-bed unit over the three-month trial, including details on potential contributing factors such as location and nature of the fall, resident activity and equipment condition at the time of the fall and resident condition, behaviour, mobility and medication use prior to the fall. Data on user friendliness of the recording system were collected through evaluation forms and a staff focus group session. An overview of the collaborative process used in the development of the tool is provided that reflects the multiple needs and uses of the data. Implications related to the generalizability and applicability of the tool at a provincial level are discussed, including the need for a central repository for data analysis, timely dissemination of findings directly to facilities, and identification of regional trends and differences to ensure best practices and benchmarking.

Falls and injury in residential care: rates and risk factors

N. Kerse, M. Butler (Division of General Pratice and Primary Health Care, University of Auckland, New Zealand), M. Todd, (Waitemata Health, Auckland, New Zealand) C. Coggan, (Injury Prevention Research Unit, University of Auckland, New Zealand)

Purpose To establish the rate of falls and injury in residential care settings and to prospectively identified risk factors for falls and injury. Methods Fourteen residential care facilities (93%), selected at random, were enrolled. Information including socio-demographic features, medication use, medical conditions, functional status and footwear was collected on 750 (86%) of residents. All institutions recorded falls and injury on standardised recording forms for 12 months (half of the homes participated in an intervention trial, commencing after 6 months). Falls and injury rates was calculated by number of falls or injury /1000 patient bed days. Risk factors were established using regression techniques controlling for the impact of clustering. Results Data from control group residents (n=275, followed for 12 months) and intervention group residents (n=304, followed for 5 months) is used in this analysis. 785 falls occurred in 222 residents (390f residents fell). 400f falls resulted in injury, (7 hip and 10 other fractures). Rates varied widely between homes, averaging 9 falls/1000 beddays (sd 25). Specialised dementia units had the lowest rate of falls. Being mobile, previously falling, restraint use and psychotropic drug use increased the likelihood of future falls. Having several cardiovascular diseases was protective as was wearing hard soled and shoes (compared with slippers). Conclusions Falls and injury are common in residential care, with up to 400f all residents falling in a year. Variability of fall rates between homes is high and risk factors differ from those predicting falls in community dwelling older people.

Follow-up data of a fracture prevention trial of nursing home residents

Th. Nikolaus, C. Becker, U. Lindemann

Purpose: we previously reported the results of a RCT to reduce fall and fractures. There was a major effect on falls, but no significant effect was seen for the incidence of hip or non-hip fractures. We hypothesised, that the fracture rate of the first and second year might differ considerably. This could be important to design studies but also to formulate realistic goals for fracture prevention programmes. Methods: observational study with pre-post design (first vs. second year). The intention of the study was a comparison of fracture rates over a 24 month period within a multifactorial intervention trial with waiting- list control design with 981 residents. The intervention consisted of a progressive training protocol, hip protectors, health education and environmental advice. Results: in the first year, there were 67 fractures in both groups. In the second year the total fracture number was 43 in all residents. The number of hip fracture declined from 32 to 22 (p=.09). Non-hip fractures were diagnosed in 35 residents in the first year and in 21 residents during the second year (p=0.03). Conclusions: the results show a notewothy trend with a remarkable decrease of hip and non-hip fractures rates in the second year. The overall fracture rate in the second year was similar to age-adjusted rates for home dwelling elderly. Successful fracture reduction are considerably harder to achieve than solely reduction of falls. This is presumably caused by learning and training effects of staff, residents and administrators.

Potentially amenable risk factors for falls

C. Becker, T. Nikolaus, U. Lindemann

Purpose: Many studies have looked for risk factors (RF) in different patient groups. However it is not clear whether which RF are potentially amenable. We compared RF in two groups that participated in a multifactorial intervention trial of exercise, health education and environmental adaptations that showed a major difference of fall rates (RR 0.56) between control (CG) and intervention group (IG). Objective: describe RF for falls of CG and IG of institutionalised elderly (total n=981) with a 12 month follow-up and daily fall diaries. Methods: observational study, univariate analysis of RI of fallers, assessment by study nurse administered MDS-RAI, daily injury diary Results: the following items were indicating an elevated fall risk in the CG (RR and 95%CI >1): independent walking and transfer, unstable gait, previous falls, impaired vision, motor agitation, wandering, depressive symptoms, incontinence, cognitive impairment and neuroleptic medication. In the IG impaired vision, incontinence and cognitive impairment were no longer independent RF for falls. The following items, even so often cited as RF for falls, where negative in indicating an elevated risk of falling in both groups: anxiolytic or hypnotic medication, multimedication, stroke, parkinsons' disease, bedrails, disruptive behaviour. Conclusions: RF in this high risk group include items that reflect activity and disease related RF. The diminishing of certain RF can indicate that subgroups might be easier to target. The persistence of depresssion is an example of a group that might be more difficult to include in succesful fall prevention programmes.

Prediction of falls among old people in residential care facilities by the Downton index

E. Rosendahl, L. Lundin-Olsson, K. Kallin, J. Jensen, Y. Gustafson, L. Nyberg (Dept. of Community Medicine and Rehabilitation, Geriatric Medicine, Umeå University, Umeå, Sweden)

PURPOSE: To investigate the prediction accuracy of the Downton fall risk index among old people living in residential care facilities at 3, 6 and 12 months, and with two different definitions of falls. METHOD: At baseline, Downton fall risk index was scored for each individual at a residential care facility. An index score of three or more was taken to indicate high risk of falls. The 78 participants, 56 women and 22 men, mean±SD age 81±6 years, were prospectively followed up regarding falls indoors for 12 months. RESULTS: At the three time-points of follow-up (3, 6 and 12 months), sensitivity ranged from 81% to 95% with highest value at 3 months, and the prognostic separation values ranged from 0.26 to 0.37. Within three months, the risk of falling was 36% in the high risk group (index score >=3) and 5% in the low risk group. The accuracy of the prediction did not improve using a fall definition where falls precipitated by acute illness, acute disease or drug side-effects were excluded. CONCLUSION: Downton fall risk index appears to be a useful tool for predicting falls among old people in residential care facilities. To enhance sensitivity, it may be recommendable to reassess regularly, for example every third month.

Preventing falls in residential care: a randomised controlled trial

N. Kerse, M. Butler (Division of General Pratice and Primary Health Care, University of Auckland, New Zealand), M. Todd, (Waitemata Health, Auckland, New Zealand) C. Coggan, (Injury Prevention Research Unit, University of Auckland, New Zealand)

Purpose A multidisciplinary fall prevention intervention (FIPPS Falls and Injury Prevention Pilot Study) was designed for residential care facilities and refined by a consultation process of multidisciplinary 'expert groups'. The intervention is a multidisciplinary risk factor management program. This study aimed to assess the 'acceptability' of the intervention for staff, and impact of the programme on falls care practices. Feasibility for a larger trial was evaluated. Method Fourteen randomly selected residential care facilities (93% response rate) were enrolled and personal risk factors collected on 541 (86% response rate) enrolled residents. All institutions recorded all falls on standardised fall recording forms for the duration of the study period (12 months). Seven institutions were randomly identified to receive the intervention. A 'care practices survey' established current falls prevention practices and was administered to all institutions before and after the intervention period. Focus groups with principal nurse managers, falls coordinators, and care givers determined the acceptability of the intervention. Fall and injury rates (falls or injuries / 1000 bed days) and changes in 'Care Practices' were compared between intervention and control groups. Results The intervention had a positive impact on vision and foot checks and medication use in intervention homes. The intervention was acceptable to staff and positive trends in falls and injury rates were observed. Conclusion Intervening with residential care staff is possible, acceptable and has an impact on care practices. Promising trends in falls rates were established. A larger trial, designed to test the efficacy of the intervention is feasible.

Risk Management of Falls Across the Continuum of Care

Erika Lavigne (SCO Health Service, Ottawa, Canada)

PURPOSE: The incidence of falls and the injuries that result has become an increasingly important focus of risk management in the health care of elderly clients. An integrated approach has been developed to address this concern within the Care of the Elderly and Rehabilitation program, which spans the continuum of care from inpatient rehabilitation to outpatient day hospitals to the community service of Helpline. METHOD: The approach will be reviewed by illustrating the role played by each of these three levels of patient/client care along the continuum outlining the processes of assessment, treatment / intervention/ education, and discharge planning (where relevant) with an emphasis on how integration is achieved. RESULTS: Outcome measures for the past two years will be presented for each level of the continuum in support of this approach. CONCLUSION: An integrated approach of thorough assessment, appropriate treatment / intervention / education, and support in the community serves to reduce and better manage the incidence of falls within the elderly population. Future plans for program enhancement will be reviewed

SESSION 364

Elderly Residents, making a film in an Old Age Home

M. BOCKER, D. SHALIF, A. VEBER (Occupational Therapy Dept, of UNITED AGED HOME JERUSALEM ISRAEL) R. FRIEDMANN (UNITED AGED HOME JERUSALEM, ISRAEL)

PURPOSE: Create a fictional film where the residents of the Old Age Home will be the main creators and also the actors. The intention is to improve the cognitive, emotional, and social skills. METHOD: Creating a fictional film within a group of older people; the majority are old, feeble and in nursing care status, eg. Using walkers or wheel chairs. The residents related stories from their daily life in the Home. Methods of drama therapy or dance therapy. The group gathered once a week for six months. The gatherings included relating stories and analyzing them. Then, the best stories were chosen for the script. Rehearsing, acting and filming followed. RESULTS: The group activity raised the older peoples self-esteem, improved the emotional awareness and enhanced the social atmosphere. A short fictional film was created which the families and the staff can have a better insight into the older persons life. The film is also on the agenda of the the community cable TV. CONCLUSIONS: Using the camera in a dynamic group of elderly, frail and nursing care residents can intensify their personal and social qualities; thus improving their quality of life. Using this method improves the technological gap between the generations. Such an experience can be a new frame of efficient view and treatment of the older population N.B. During the presentation part of the film will be shown.

Evaluation of cognitive and psychologic effects of a dog-based activities program in a nursing home

O. Michel, J-F. Sallard, J. Fauchoux, P. Jouanny (Geriatric Medicine Department, University Hospital, Rennes, France)

PURPOSE: Determination of the effects on cognition and mood of activities focused on a dog, initially educated for guiding blind people, in a nursing home population. METHODS: The whole population of a nursing home was evaluated with Mini Mental Status Examination (Folstein) and Geriatric Depression Scale (Yesavage) before being proposed the dog activities program. GDS scores over 15 were examined by a psychiatrist and, if verified depressive, treated and excluded from the study. The volunteers could attend the various activities twice a week. People who refused the program constituted the control. Any change in psychotropic treatment was a reason for exclusion. After six months, MMS and GDS were reperformed, and patients interviewed by a psychologist who analysed their reactions. RESULTS: among 25 patients in the study group (age: 76,9), 9 were excluded for prohibited treatment, 3 for insufficient participation, 3 died or were durably hospitalized. In the 19 control people (age: 73,1), 6 were excluded for prohibited treatment, 1 deceased. At baseline, no significative difference is found between the two groups, concerning disability (4,3 control vs 4 in AGGIR scale), MMSE (19,25 control vs 20,80) and GDS (9,58 control vs 11,50) After six months, MMS significantly increased in 1,5 point for test group, decreases in 0,65 point for control (p= 0,027). GDS scores improved in test group (1 point) and impaired in control (1,25 point).The subjective impression of the patients was positive. CONCLUSION: The introduction of a well educated dog in a nursing home can improve the wellbeing of the residents and has positive global cognitive effects.

Music Therapy and Occupational Therapy Applied to Speech Re-training in a Residential Care Setting

Brian B. Lam (Occupational Therapist, OT) and Brenda Lui (Music Therapist, MT) (Minoru Residence Extended Care, Richmond, British Columbia, Canada)

PURPOSE: To determine if a combined music therapy and occupational therapy speech re-training program is effective in improving communication and thus, quality of life in older adults in a residential care setting. METHOD: Residents were selected based on the following criteria: * have a speech impairment * have the ability to follow directions and cues * have the ability to concentrate 11 residents with this criteria were invited to participate in a weekly, 45 minute session for a 6 month period.The OT and MT lead residents through a series of neck, facial, mouth, and tongue exercises. To work on breathing and volume production, some exercises were sung. Residents chanted phrases and tapped out matching rhythm patterns on their laps. This combination of oral motor exercises, singing, and rhythm cueing allowed the residents to explore, experience, and practice certain skills required for verbal communication.Residents were videotaped monthly. Family and staff were consulted for their observations on any changes noted. RESULTS: Within the group, the following three changes were observed amongst the residents: * greater awareness of breathing * improved articulation of words and sounds * increased spontaneous responses through singing and rhythm cueing Independent of these weekly group sessions, family and staff identified improvements in the residents' desire to respond. Family and staff also commented on the increased clarity of the residents' responses. CONCLUSION: There is evidence which suggests that a combined music and oral-motor approach is effective in improving communication and thus, quality of life in older adults.

SESSION 365

Age correlations with brain atrophy and hyperintensities on MRI: the Sunnybrook Dementia Study

R.H. Swartz, S.E. Black (Department of Neurology, Sunnybrook & Women’s College Health Sciences Center, University of Toronto, Toronto, Canada)

PURPOSE: Evaluations of brain atrophy and white matter hyperintensities are usually performed blind to age on the assumption that individuals with cognitive impairment will differ on these measures from age-matched healthy controls across all ages. This study aimed to determine if the relationship between cognitive impairment and brain measures changes with age. METHOD: 205 individuals from a memory clinic underwent MRI and detailed cognitive testing. Segmentation techniques were used to determine the following volumes: ventricular (v-) and sulcal (s-) CSF, deep white, periventricular, basal ganglia, posterior and anterior thalamic hyperintesities, cortical strokes and medial temporal lobe thickness. RESULTS: All brain measures except cortical stroke were significantly correlated with age (R .26-.40). Cutoffs were determined based on the younger and older normal control sample distribution (n=15; n=19). 171 people with memory complaints were grouped into five categories by major imaging abnormalities: 20% were within normal limits on all measures; 29% had only atrophy; 6% had only small vessel disease; 25% had both and 19% had strategic infarcts. Those younger than 60 (63%) were within normal limits on imaging, while only 12over age 60 had normal appearing scans (p<0.0005), despite comparable neuropsychological impairments. CONCLUSION: Age was a major correlate of most brain volumes and must be taken into account in studies of atrophy or white matter. Younger individuals with memory complaints, often the most challenging to diagnose, were unlikely to have more atrophy or cerebrovascular disease than expected for their age. Functional imaging might be more useful for assessing these individuals.

Alzheimers disease, vascular and mixed dementia: a clinicopathological point of view.

D. Zekry, MD; C. Duyckaerts, R. Moulias, MD; J. Belmin, PhD; C. Geoffre, BA; F. Herrmann, MPH, J.-J. Hauw, MD. Laboratoire de Neuropathologie Raymond Escourolle (Drs. Zekry, Duyckaerts and Hauw), Hôpital de la Salpêtrière, INSERM U 106 and 360, Association Claude Bernard, Pierre et Marie Curie University, Paris, France; Hôpital Charles Foix (Moulias and Geoffre), Ivry-sur-Seine, France, Hôpital René Muret (Belmin), Sevran, France and Hôpitaux Universitaires de Genève (Herrmann), Thônex, Switzerland.

Purpose: To assess if patients with similar degrees of severity of dementia have fewer Aß plaques and neurofibrillary tangles if vascular lesions are present than those without vascular lesions, and to evaluate the validity of the mixed dementia concept. Background: The respective importance of degenerative and vascular lesions, their interaction in the genesis of dementia and the mere existence of mixed dementia are debated. Methods: We performed a prospective clinicopathological study in a long-stay care unit. The degrees of severity of clinical dementia were assessed by psychometry uniformly obtained at least 6 months before death. At autopsy, a volumetric study of cerebral structures and vascular lesions was performed. The density of neuritic plaques, Aß focal and diffuse deposits, and neurofibrillary tangles in the temporal and frontal isocortex was measured. Results: We studied 33 autopsies. According to the DSM III criteria, 28 patients had dementia. We excluded one Parkinson disease, one dementia with Lewy bodies, and two frontal lobe degenerations lacking distinctive histology. Among the 24 patients included for analysis, the degree of severity of clinical dementia was similar. The density of Aß focal deposits, neurofibrillary tangles and neuritic plaques in frontal and temporal isocortex was significantly lower when vascular lesions were present. Conclusion: This study shows that among elderly patients institutionalized in a long stay care unit who died with dementia and Alzheimer changes at post-mortem, those with any vascular lesions at autopsy had fewer Alzheimer pathological changes than those without vascular lesions.

Apolipoprotein E epsilon 4 allele and clinically defined vascular depression

AS Rigaud (Hopital Broca, 54-56 rue Pascal, 75013 Paris, France), L Traykov (Unite INSERM 324, 2 ter rue d'Alesia, 75014, Paris France), Remy Couderc (Hopital Armand Trousseau, 26 avenue du Arnold-Netter, 75012 Paris, France), Florence Moulin (Hopital Broca, 54-56 rue Pascal, 75013 Paris, France), Florence Latour (Hopital Broca, 54-56 rue Pascal, 75013 Paris, France), Francoise Forette (Hopital Broca, 54-56 rue Pascal, 75013 Paris, France)

The apolipoprotein E epsilon 4 allele was shown to be a risk factor for Alzheimer's disease. Its role in clinical cerebrovascular disease is controversial, while it is still unknown in vascular depression. Apolipoprotein phenotyping was performed in 50 patients with vascular depression and 122 controls. Inclusion criteria for vascular depression were fulfillment of the Diagnostic and Statistical Manual of Mental Disorders (DSM IV) criteria for a major depressive episode, brain computed tomography or magnetic resonance imaging findings of infarcts or lacunae, and a history of at least one of the following vascular factors: hypertension, heart disease, diabetes mellitus, hypercholesterolaemia, and peripheral vascular disease. The frequency of Apolipoprotein E epsilon 4 allele in patients with vascular depression did not differ significantly from control frequency (15% vs 12.3). Conclusions: The present study shows no association between the presence of Apolipoprotein E epsilon 4 allele and vascular depression and provides further evidence in support of the concept that Apolipoprotein E epsilon 4 allele is not associated with clinical cerebrovascular disease.

ApolipoproteinE epsilon4 allele and response to donepezil therapy in Alzheimer's disease

F. Latour (Hopital Broca, Paris, France), L. Traykov (Unite INSERM 324, Paris, France), F. Moulin (Hopital Broca Paris, France), M.L. Seux (Hopital Broca Paris, France), O. Hanon (Hopital Broca Paris, France) , F. Forette, (Hopital Broca Paris, France), A.S.Rigaud (Hopital Broca, Paris, France),

The objective was to evaluate the effects of the apolipoprotein E (ApoE) genotype and gender on the response to donepezil treatment in Alzheimer's disease (AD). ApoE genotyping was performed in 117 mild to moderate AD patients in a 36-week open label trial of donepezil therapy. Patients were treated blindly in relation to the ApoE genotype, with incremental dosages of donepezil. Of the 117 patients enrolled in the study (intent-to-treat population, ITT), 97 patients were treated with 5 mg of donepezil, but only 80 with 10 mg. The outcome measures were AD Assessment Scale-Cognitive Component (ADAS-Cog), Mini Mental State Examination (MMSE), Instrumental Activities of Daily Living (IADL), and the Caregiver-rated Clinical Global Impression of Change (CGIC). An ITT analysis did not reveal significant response differences between epsilon 4- carriers and epsilon4+ carriers on the outcomes (ADAS-Cog, $p = 0.28$; MMSE, $p = 0.1$; IADL, $p = 0.08$; CGIC, $p = 0.16$). When patients were stratified by gender, no differences were found between men and women (ADAS-Cog, $p = 0.81$; MMSE, $p = 0.47$; IADL, $p = 0.06$; CGIC, $p = 0.23$). There was also no significant interaction between genotype and gender (ADAS-Cog, $p = 0.09$; MMSE, $p = 0.44$; IADL, $p = 0.38$; CGIC, $p = 0.77$). Both doses of donepezil produced similar patterns of changes on outcome measures as those seen in the ITT population. These results do not support the hypothesis that the ApoE genotype and gender are predictors of the response to donepezil in AD patients.

Could Serum Paraoxonase1 Activity Be a Marker of Oxidative Stress in Dementia of the Elderly?

T. Dantoine (1), J. Debord (2), J-P. Charmes (1), L. Bernard-Bourzeix (1), L. Merle (2) (1: Gerontology, 2: Pharmacology departments, CHU, Limoges 87000, France)

HDL-linked paraoxonase1 (PON1) could be a factor of vascular ageing: PON1 decreases LDL peroxidation; serum PON1 activity (PON1a) decreases with ageing and chronic renal failure (CRF) and is a coronary risk marker in CRF patients who show accelerated atherosclerosis. Reactive oxygen species are PON1 substrates. Implication of vascular factors in Vascular Dementia (VD) and Alzheimer s type Dementia (ATD) is strongly suspected. METHODS: So we measured PON1a by spectrophotometry using paraoxon substrate in 180 healthy subjects (HS) [98 females (F), 82 males (M), mean age (A)= 75.3±8.9 years from 60 to 105 years] and 154 patients admitted for cognitive assessment. RESULTS: According to DSM IV/NINCDS/ADRDA/NINDS/AIREN criteria, 45 patients had Mild Cognitive Impairments (MCI) (28F, 17M, A=75.6 ± 9.3 yrs from 50 to 97 yrs), 60 had ATD (47 F, 13M, A=75.6 ± 8.3 yrs from 53 to 89 yrs) and 49 had VD (33F,16M, A=7.5 ± 7.2 yrs from 62 to 90 yrs). Age and creatinine clearance weren t different. PONa was lower in VD (0.25+/-0.1 U/ml) than in HS (0.41+/-0.2 U/ml)($p<0.01$). PONa in MCI (0.34+/-0.2 U/ml) and ATD (0.41+/-0.2 U/ml) weren t different. PONa in VD was lower than in ATD ($p<0.01$). Multiple linear regression showed PONa was correlated negatively with sex (M<F), age and VD but positively with ADT ($p<0.001$). CONCLUSIONS: This work confirms PONa is a marker of vascular disease (here decreased in vascular dementia). Its implication in oxidative stress and its variations in different types of dementia make us suggest PON1 plays an important role in dementias.

Oxidative stress, telomeres and replicative senescence

Violeta Serra, Thomas von Zglinicki (Dept of Gerontology, University of Newcastle, UK)

PURPOSE: Telomere shortening in human somatic cells leads eventually to replicative senescence. Telomere shortening is partially due to the inability of DNA polymerases to copy completely the very end of a linear DNA, but its major cause is stress-dependent telomere-specific accumulation of oxidative single-strand damage. We were interested in the role of individual differences in antioxidative defence capacity for telomere maintenance and replicative senescence in human fibroblasts. METHODS: Telomere length (Southern blotting), oxygen free radical generation (DCF fluorescence) and stress gene expression patterns (low density arrays) were measured in skin fibroblasts in vitro from different donors under normal and chronic mild stress conditions. RESULTS: We found significant correlations between donor age, replicative in-vitro life span of fibroblasts, and telomere length at explantation. However, none of these correlations was particularly strong ($0.03<p<0.05$). This is partly explained by the fact that fibroblasts from different donors senesce with different telomere length. Moreover, the rate of telomere shortening during in-vitro culture is largely dependent on the antioxidative capacity. Using expression array analysis, we identified EC-SOD (SOD 3) as the sole antioxidative enzyme which is strongly up-regulated in fibroblast strains with low telomere shortening rate and high antioxidative capacity, but is weakly expressed in strains which show fast telomere shortening and low antioxidative capacity. CONCLUSION: The pace of the "telomere clock" is set by free radical generation. It is not simply telomere length which triggers senescence.

Sex Differences in the Action of Cholinesterase Inhibitors

M. Weinstock, R-H Wang. (Department of Pharmacology, School of Pharmacy, Hebrew University Medical Centre, Ein Kerem, Jerusalem 91120, Israel)

PURPOSE: To investigate the possibility of a sex difference in rats in the pharmacological actions and cholinesterase (ChE) inhibitory activity of drugs used in the treatment of Alzheimer's disease (AD). METHOD: Tacrine, and rivastigmine (Exelon) were injected s.c. to male and female rats and their effects were measured on body temperature, spatial memory previously impaired by scopolamine, and ChE activity in several brain areas and heart in intact rats, after gonadectomy and hormone replacement. RESULTS: Significantly smaller doses of the drugs were needed to induce hypothermia and cause antagonism of scopolamine-induced memory impairment in females than in males This was due to greater dose-related ChE inhibition in the cortex, hypothalamus, hippocampus and striatum, but not in the heart of females. The sex difference was abolished by orchidectomy but not by ovariectomy. Testosterone reduced the responses to the ChE inhibitors in orchidectomized rats to those in intact rats. The concentration of tacrine reached in the brain after the same dose/body weight in females was double that in males. Orchidectomy increased brain concentration of tacrine in males to the level in females. CONCLUSIONS: There is a clear sex difference in rats in the effects of ChE inhibitors mediated by their actions in the brain. This results from a reduction by testosterone of the amount of drug reaching the male brain, thereby causing less ChE inhibition than in the female. It remains to be seen if women with AD are also more sensitive than men to the cognitive effects of these drugs.

SESSION 366

Adrenal secretion and aging

E.Ferrari, B. Pontiggia, R. Gornati, S.B. Solerte, M. Fioravanti, B. Vitali, M. Gandelli, F. Magri (Department of Internal Medicine and Medical Therapy, Chair of Geriatrics, University of Pavia, Italy)

We studied blood cortisol and dehydroepiandrosterone sulfate (DHEAS) in physiological and successful aging and in age-related pathological conditions. Serum cortisol and DHEAS were simultaneously evaluated in 23 old healthy subjects (76-96 y), 20 healthy centenarians (100-107 y), 23 old demented patients (68-91) including 12 patients with Alzheimer s disease (AD) and 11 patients with vascular dementia (VD), and 22 clinically healthy young controls (19-43 y). Only one blood sample in the morning was drawn in centenarians; in the other groups of subjects samples were collected every 4 h from 08:00 to 20:00 and every 2 h from 20:00 to 08:00, in order to study the hormonal circadian rhythms. A significant age-related decline of serum DHEAS occurred in elderly subjects, particularly if demented, by comparison to young controls. The morning DHEAS levels showed a further decline in centenarians. On the contrary, the morning levels of serum cortisol were not different in centenarians, young and old controls, and besides elderly subjects and especially AD patients exhibited a significant increase of the cortisol nocturnal levels. Therefore, the molar ratio between cortisol and DHEAS was significantly higher in elderly subjects and particularly in demented patients and it was significantly related to both subjects age and the degree of cognitive impairment (MMSE score). The cortisol/DHEAS molar ratio was very similar in centenarians and healthy old controls. The hormonal adrenal changes seem to be mainly related to the age, but the occurrence of senile dementia play an additive role. The evaluation of cortisol/DHEAS molar ratio represents an interesting marker of the neuroendocrine correlates of physiological and pathological brain aging.

Age Changes and Sex Differences in Serum DHEAS Concentration and its Related Factors

Chul-Young Bae, Seok-Kie Lee, Young-Gin Lee, MD (Department of Family Medicine & Geriatrics, Pochon CHA Medical University, Kyonggido, South Korea

There is no epidemiologic data of Dehydroepiandrosterone (DHEAS) in korea. We studied age changes and sex differences in serum DHEAS throughout adulthood and its related factors. Serum DHEAS and several biochemical markers (total cholesterol, triglycerides, HDL-cholesterol, glucose, etc.) were measured and structured questionnaires were administered to 1,710 healthy men (857) and women (853), aged 17-76 years. We also measured their height, weight, waist and hip circumferences and body fat contents with bioimpedance method. The DHEA concentrations showed a peak at age below 30 years in both sexes. The mean values of DHEAS declined steadily according to the ages in both men ($R=-0.38$, $p<.001$)and women ($R=-0.46$, $p<.001$). DHEAS concentrations were significantly higher in men than women at all age group except age group above 70 years. DHEAS levels in men were significantly higher with smoking, alcohol drinking, high BMI after adjusting age. On the other hand, DHEAS levels in women were higher with alcohol drinking and regular exercise after adjusting age. However, there were no significant association between DHEAS and lipid profile (total cholesterol, triglycerides, HDL-cholesterol), and fasting blood glucose level in both sexes. Our data suggest that serum DHEAS levels were influenced by several sociodemographic factors and body mass index, differently in men and women.

Biological screening of thyroid dysfunction in the Elderly patient

G. AIME, X. de PETIGNY, Y. HEMMENDINGER , M.C. SCHATZ (BISCHWILLER Gerontology Hospital France)

The aim of this study is to demonstrate the interest of biological screening of thyroid dysfunction in the older patient. This retrospective study is carried on two different populations; the first one is composed of 284 inpatients with acute diseases, the second one is composed of 132 patients of the Gérontology day hospital. This screening allowed us to discover that 8.8% of inpatients have abnormal TSH values, among them 4.6% are new cases. Among the day hospital patients we found only 2.3% of them with abnormal TSH values, but no new case at all. The biological screening of thyroid dysfunction in the elderly hospitalised because of acute disease is justified insofar as it permits us to discover an important percentage of patients with thyroid diseases often paucity-symptomatic or without symptoms. On the other hand, the screening of patients of the day hospital should be done only on a target population (dementia, past history of thyroid dysfunction,.......)

Dementia and primary hyperparathyroidism

O.CROIZIER, D.BESSEY*, C.LEPALLEC**,A.BIZIEN** *Centre hospitalier chateaubriant, 44110 Chateaubriant. France ** Hôpital Georges Clémenceau,AP-HP,91750 Champcueil.France*

Primary hyperparathyroidism is more and more often diagnosed in the elderly. This increase, related by several authors, is linked to the systematic computation of the corrected serum calcium, and to a best knowledge of clinical particularities. The most common signs are the psychiatric manifestations, until 65 0n some series. In old subjects, there is correlation between the intensity of psychiatric disorders and the level serum calcium. Sometimes, the serum calcium is normal. Chronic cognitive impairment linked to an hyperparathyroidism are not well-know. Our study of 31 olds patients shows a negative correlation between the score of the Mini Mental State Evaluation (Folstein) and the rate of parathormon ($r=0,21$). The physiopathology is complex. It would exist a direct effect of the parathormon on the cerebral cells by modifications of calcium and magnesium flows through membrane (the intravenous injection of parathormon increases the rate of cyclic AMP in the CSF). Precocious diagnosis and surgical processing allow a total disappearance of symptoms. A clinic study, some concrete cases and the review of the literature will be presented, and three questions will be discussed : 1° Is systematically parathormon assay necessary in the management of dementia ? 2° Is there a specific clinic form in the old subjects, whose symptomatology is essentially cognitive impairments ? 3° Is this only psychiatric symptomatology a surgical indication ?

Does Oral DHEA Supplementation Affect Bone Remodeling In Older Men?

B. Halloran (Divsion of Endocrinology, UCSF/VA Medical Center, San Francisco, CA USA), L. Brizendine (Department of Pyschiatry, UCSF Medical Center, San Francisco, CA USA), A.Kahn (Department of Growth and Development, UCSF Medical Center, San Francisco, CA USA)

Reductions in the circulating level of the steroid dehydroepiandrosterone (DHEA) in adults have been postulated to be responsible for many of the senescent changes seen in the elderly. This has led to efforts to slow or reverse these changes by providing DHEA supplementation. In the present, double blind study, we assessed the effect of oral supplementation on bone remodeling in older men. Ninety mg/day of DHEA or placebo was provided to 42 healthy subjects (56-80 years) for 6 months, followed by one month washout and a further 6 months with the opposite agent. Bone remodeling was assessed by measuring the biomarkers, serum osteocalcin (OC), procollagen peptide (PCP), bone specific alkaline phosphatase (BSAP) and urinary deoxypyridinoline (DPD). Our data show that serum DHEA and DHEAS levels increased about 2.5 to 4 fold respectively after 6 months treatment. There was also an ~20 0ncrease in estrogen. In contrast, levels of the remodeling biomarkers remained constant: PCP at ~9.0 ng/ml; BSAP at ~21.0 units/L; DPD at ~4.5 nM/L. The one exception was OC which showed a transient ~40% reduction in level (~10.2 ng/ml to ~6.2 ng/ml; p<.005 to p<.001) at three months but this occurred in both treated and placebo subjects. We conclude that DHEA supplementation does not affect bone remodeling in healthy older men when used for 6 months at doses targeted to restore circulating levels of the steroid to that of young adults. These findings suggest that DHEA, alone, is unlikely to be beneficial in limiting age-associated osteoporosis in older men.

Modulation of hepatic and renal glucocorticoid receptors during aging of mice

R. Sharma, H.S. Ranhotra (Department of Biochemistry, North Eastern Hill University, Shillong-793022, India

Glucocorticoids, acting through their specific intracellular receptors, influence variety of physiological processes. These receptors belong to a largest known family of eukaryotic transcription factors that modulate the cognate gene expression by changing the synthesis of mRNAs and related proteins, thus producing an appropriate cellular response. The regulation of hepatic and renal glucocorticoid receptors (GRs) in young (4-) and senescent (120-weeks) mice was studied. Significant changes in the level of GRs from liver and kidney were detected, whereas the affinity (Kd) for the hormone [3H]dexamethasone did not change in young and old mice. The concentration of GRs was markedly decreased in liver (25%) and kidney (33%) of old mice as compared to young ones. The magnitude of thermal activation of GR complexes was more pronounced in both the tissues at young age compared to old. In addition, we have found changes in the heat activation-inhibition studies of GRs, using polyunsaturated fatty acids (PUFAs) as measured by binding to DNA cellulose and purified nuclei. Linoleic acid (C18:2) exhibited significant decrease in heat activation of both hepatic and renal hormone-bound GR, with higher magnitude of inhibition (24%) in young as compared to old mice. Arachidonic acid (C20:4) was also found to be an inhibitor of activation causing significant decrease in hepatic GR activation, with greater inhibition in young liver with respect to old, however, without any such difference in the kidney of young and old mice. Furthermore, DNase I digestion and extraction of nuclear-bound GR-complexes from both the tissues reveal lesser extraction in old liver (26%) and kidney (24%)compared to young tissues, indicating chromatin condensation with aging,thereby controlling the accessibility to such transcription factors as GRs. These findings indicate that the changes in the GR concentration, activation-modulation by PUFAs and chromatin organization, that take place during aging, may contribute to functional changes in glucocorticoid action mechanisms in senescent animals.

Particular Aspects of Thyroid Status in Very Old Patients

C.R. Revnic (U.M.F."Carol Davila,Bucharest,Romania) G. Onose, T. Suloc, F. Revnic ("Ana Aslan"N.I.G.G,Bucharest,Romania)

Objective:The aim of our study was to investigate thyroid function in very old patients over 90 years by means of F.I.A. method.Design and methods:24 clinical euthyroid patients aged between 90-104 years old(20 females and 4 males),free of thyroid pathology in their hystory have been selected ,having the following medical and geriatric diagnosis at the admission in Geriatrics clinique :1)longevity associated with chronic degenerative rheumathoid diseases,B)longevity associated with systolic arterial hypertension,C)longevity associated with chronic painless cardiomyopathy with EKG modifications.The following parameters of thyroid function have been estimated in serum with DELFIA technology involving Eu+ labelled monochlonal antibodies:T3,T4,FT3,FT4,TBG and TSH.Statistical evaluation of data has been done with a Multical program. Results:Our data have pointed out a decrease in T3 levels both in men and women below normal values(1.3-2.5nmol/l).Extremely low values have been recorded in a 104 years old male patient(0.38nmol/l)A significant increse in TSH levels in female patients over 90 years old in comparison with age matched male patients have been recorded(p<0.001) TBG levels were very much increased both in male and female patientsIn 104 years old man the level of TBG exceeded 2 times the normal value.T4/TBG ratio in male was:7.7nmol/l above the average ratio(4.7 nmol/l),while in age matched female, the ratio was low. There is a correlation between FT3-T3 and FT4-T4 in relation with hTSH and autoimmunity.Conclussions:The dramatic change in T3 recorded in male patients over 100 years old can be attributed to a reduction in peripherial conversion of T4 to T3 reflecting nonthyroidal illness rather than a time effect of aging per se. Higher levels of hTSH are correlated with Tg levels accounting for the high incidence of autoimmunity in advanced age.

SESSION 367

Bloodstream infection in elderly :Differences between Young and Oldest Patients

G. GAVAZZI, [Department de medecine interne et gériatrie, Centre Hospitalier Universitaire,Grenoble, France M. R. MALLARET, [Unité d'hygiène hospitalière Centre Hospitalier Universitaire,Grenoble, France] N. P.COUTURIER, [Department de medecine interne et gériatrie, Centre Hospitalier Universitaire,Grenoble, France] O. A. IFFENERCKER, [Unité d'hygiène hospitalière Centre Hospitalier Universitaire,Grenoble, France] P. A. FRANCO. [Department de medecine interne et gériatrie, Centre Hospitalier Universitaire,Grenoble, France]

Purpose: In France, bloodstream infection (BI) are associated with the higher morbidity and mortality rate in elderly patients. To determine the epidemiology, microbiology and outcome of BI in elderly patients, we analyzed retrospectively data of 1740 episodes of BI occurred in patients over 65 years of age. Method: Study was conducted in 46 hospitals from southeast area in France. BI, polymicrobial, primary BI and contamination were defined according CDC data. Characteristics of patient, type of micro-organism, resistance to common antimicrobial therapy and source of infection were collected . BI was classified in Nosocomial (NBI) or Community-Acquired BI (CABI). All data were analyzed in 3 groups of age as follow: group A for patient 65 to 75 years of age, group B for patients 76 to 85 years of age and group C for patients over 85 years of age. Results: Of 1740 BI, 758 (43.6%) BI occur group A, 649 (37.3%) occur in group B and 333 (19.1%) in group C. Of 1740 BI, 898 (51.6%) are CABI and 842 (48.4%) are NBI. CABI are significantly more frequent in group C.

Concerning CABI, Source of BI and microorganism are not different ; resistance of Escherichia coli to ampicillin is significantly more frequent in group C . Concerning NBI, Urinary tract infection is significantly more frequent and indeterminate source less frequent in group C. Escherichia coli is more frequent and Staphylococcus epidermidis is less frequent in group C. Methicilline Resistance Staphylococcus Aureus (MRSA) is significantly more frequent in CABI whatever the group of age. Overall mortality rate was 14.2%. In multivariate analysis, presence of MRSA and bacteriological proven source of BI were significantly associated with death. Conclusion : epidemiological findings of BI are significantly differents between young and old elderly. The epidemiological data of Patients who are 75 years of age or younger is more closely related to that of young adult.

Endocarditis findings in eldelry people

Prieto A, Estrada A, Gómez L, Zamorano J.L., Almería C.*, Ribera J.M. (Geriatric and Cardiology* Services. Hospital Clínico San Carlos. Madrid. Spain).*

AIMS: To assess clinical characteristics, anatomic complications, and immediate evolution of infective endocarditis (IE) in elderly patients (A) compared with a younger group (B). PATIENTS AND METHODS: 103 patients (31 over 65 years), diagnosed according with Duke criteria between 1991-99. Retrospective study. Protocol includes clinical, anatomic and evolutive variables. Statistical analysis: Student t-test, chi-square test, p-value <0.05. RESULTS: Female patients were more common in A (45.1 vs 23.6%, p: ns). There were no significant differences regarding the localization of IE. Tricuspid valve were more frequently affected in B (26.0 vs 00<0.01), but this differences disappeared when IAVD patients were excluded. Heart failure was more frequent in A (41 vs 19%, p<0.05). Not other clinical (fever, leucocytoses, embolic complications, renal failure, vascular phenomena, murmurs, splenomegaly), microbiological, neither anatomical complications (abscess, rupture, perforation or fistule) differences were found. Surgery was equally performed in both groups (58 vs 46%, p: ns) and mortality was also similar (16.1 vs 12.5%, p: ns). CONCLUSION: Although it has been regarded that endocarditis in the elderly has a worse prognosis than young adults. In our group the IE in A and B have similar clinical, microbiological, anatomic and evolutive features (IAVD excluded). Its may be related to the use of more acute diagnostic methods and similar therapeutic options.

Flu vaccine is less efficient in elderly smokers

A. J. G. Bos, C. M. A. Bastos, M. R. Knorst (Institute of Geriatrics and Gerontology of Pontifical Catholic University of Rio Grande do Sul Δ PUCRS), M. F. Reis, A. P. Nogueira (Military Policlinic of Porto Alegre, RS Brazil)

In April 2000, almost 6,000 elderly (60 years old and over) were vaccinated for influenza at the Military Policlinic of Porto Alegre, as part of a national campaign. At the local set, subjects were randomly asked to fill-up a short questionnaire collecting data about prevalence of diseases, drugs in use, tobacco use, body weight and height. The volunteers consented in give a telephone number to get follow-up data collected 6 months latter. A total of 521 people could be contacted, 29% of those referred developed any cold or cold-like symptoms. Females were more likely to mention they had cold during the follow-up period. Age, body weight, height, body mass index, previous vaccination, suffering from asthma or bronchitis, diabetes, use of vitamins, aspirin were similar in average and distribution in both disease free and disease present groups. Twelve percent of the people who got cold smoked during the follow-up while this proportion in the disease free group was only 4 %. More than half of the smokers developed cold suggesting that the vaccination is less efficient in this group.

Lower respiratory tract infections in a geriatric long stay department

A. Chahwakilian, N. Schwald, S. Debray-Meignan

These one year study about lower respiratory tract infections concerns a geriatric long stay department which is divised in 3 floors, each floor corresponding to a 40 beds unit. One part of the staff is common to the 3 floors. The purpose of this prospective incidence study were to evaluate infectious risk factors and consequences in infected patients from january to december 1999. 145 infections concerned 89 patients (mean age : 86,3 years versus 85,5 years in whole of the department). The results differ between floors : 42 infections for 30 patients on the first floor, 63 for 39 in the second one, and 40 for 20 on the third one. The known risk factors were similar in each unit. The ratios of severe demented patients and of very dependent ones were lower among the infected subjects than in the whole of the department (respectively 70% and 65% versus 79% and 78%). In each unit, the ratio of infected patients was no correlated to the ratio of pneumococcal vaccinations. There was a summer epidemic on the second floor (18 infections in 2 monthes, versus 3 on the first and 9 on the third one). There was no significant epidemic observed on the third floor during the whole year. 12 patients on 89 died (13,5%). The results of this study suggest that small architecturally distinct units may contribute to prevent from spreading lower respiratory tract infections in a frail populations.

Lymphocyte profile in older patients with tuberculosis

A. B. Dey (All India Institute of Medical Sciences, New Delhi, India), Manav Wadhwan (All India Institute of Medical Sciences, New Delhi, India), H. Krishna Prasad (All India Institute of Medical Sciences, New Delhi, India), P.P. Chattopadhyay (All India Institute of Medical Sciences, New Delhi, India), V. Vohra (L.R.S. TB Hospital, New Delhi, India)

The prevalence of tuberculosis rises with age and it is ranked as the fourth major causes of death among older Indians. Cell mediated immunity declines with ageing, polypharmacy, malnutrition and active tuberculosis. CD4, CD8 and Natural Killer (NK) are important components of cell mediated immunity involved in cell lysis. The present study was carried out to assess the lymphocyte profile in older tuberculosis patients in order to measure the impact of active disease and its treatment on CD4, CD8 and NK (CD56) cells. Thirty older patients with microbiological or histological evidence of pulmonary or lymph node tuberculosis and 30 age and sex matched controls without systemic disease were recruited into the study. After confirmation of diagnosis and investigations to exclude secondary immunodeficiency states, peripheral blood mononuclear cells were collected by Hypaque gradient separation. These cell were counted by flowcytometer after staining by monoclonal antibody (Becton Dickinson CD4/CD8 Simultest and CD3/CD56 Simultest). The mean CD4, CD8 and CD56 cells were significantly lower in patients with tuberculosis compared to controls which showed significant improvement after 2 months of treatment. Lower CD4/CD8/CD56 cell counts were associated with extensive disease based on chest x-ray findings, multi-system involvement, lower nutritional status (BMI) and delayed treatment response. Two patients who died during treatment had very low counts. The effect of tuberculosis infection on NK cells have not been described earlier and is possibly due to decline in subsets of NK cells with T cell lineage.

Prospective study on the relationship between nosocomial infections and hypothyroidism in the aged

Lu Pei-Fang, Ma Yong-Xing, Yu Xiao-Feng (Department of Aging, Antiaging and Cognitive Function, Shanghai Institute of Gerontology and Geriatrics, Department of Geriatircs of Huadong Hospital,Shanghai,China)

Objective: Prospective study on the relationship between nosocomial infections and hypothyroidism in the aged. Methods: Prospective follow-up of elderly (>60 years) patients for nosocomial infections (N.I.) in geriatric ward from Jan. 1996 to Dec. 1997 after thyroid function tests (TT3, FT3, TT4, FT4, TSH) in 1995 in the healthy inspection of the aged in O.P.D. Results: The mean values of TT3, FT3, FT4 and TSH in 134 cases complicated with N.I. are significantly lower than that in 114 cases without N.I. The relative proportions of N.I. in various levels of TT3, FT3, FT4 and

TSH are significantly higher than that without N.I. Conclusions: Hypothyroidism is intimately correlated with N.I, and may be one of the important causes of N.I. in the aged. It is suggested that routine examination of thyroid function is very important for prophylaxis of N.I.

The burden of Chagas disease among Brazilian older adults: The Bambui Health and Ageing Study

MFF Lima e Costa 1,2,3, SM Barreto 1,2,3, HL Guerra 1,3 , JOA Firmo 1,3 , E Uchoa 1,2,3 and PG Vidigal 1,2,3 (1 Oswaldo Cruz Foundation Rene Rachou Research Institute, 2 Federal University of Minas Gerais Medical School, and 3 Research Group on the Epidemiology and Anthropology of Ageing - REGEA, Belo Horizonte, MG, Brazil).

Purpose: The prevalence of Chagas disease is decreasing in Brazil. Due to cohort effect, the disease might remain as a public health problem for some time among older individuals. The burden of T. cruzi infection in areas where the transmission has been interrupted is still unknown. This study aims at assessing the prevalence of this infection and its association with health status and health services use among elderly living in one of the oldest endemic areas in Brazil. Method: Seropositivity was determined by blood tests (IHA and ELISA) performed in 85.6% of all residents aged 60+ (1,496/1,742) and in 83.1% of sampled residents aged 5-59 years (1,212/1,458). Results: Seropositivity showed a cohort effect, with no cases below 20 years and high prevalence among those aged 60+ years (37.7%). After adjustments for confounders, seropositivity was associated with self-rated health reasonable (OR=1.43; 95%CI=1.03, 1.98) and bad/very bad (OR=1.89; 95%CI=1.30,2.75), staying in bed in past 2 weeks (OR=1.88; 95%CI=1.21, 2.92), hospitalization in past 12 months (OR=1.41; 1.05, 1.89) and use of 5+ prescribed medications in past 3 months (OR=1.75; 95%CI=1.15, 2.59). Conclusion: Our results are an example of how survival of individuals with past exposure to infectious disease may lead to a different picture of ageing in the developing world. Policy makers need to consider the overburden imposed by the increasing rates of non infectious diseases among the elderly (as observed in Brazil) with the consequences of T. cruzi infection in areas where the infection was widespread in the past.

SESSION 368

Metamorphosis of a Special Care Unit - Not your average LTC reno.

Laurie Gudmundsson-Egler, DT, Best Practice Specialist - Environment [The Good Samaritan Society, Edmonton, Alberta, Canada] Collaboration - to the benefit of all Edythe Andison, RN, BscN, GNC(C) [The Good Samaritan Society, Edmonton, Alberta, Canada] Old Building - Right Ideas Sherry Anne Chapman, Doctoral Student - Dept. of Human Ecology [Dept. of Human Ecology, University of Alberta, Edmonton, Alberta, Canada] Reminiscences of Home Pamela Otfinowski, Graduate Student - Family Studies [Dept. of Human Ecology, University of Alberta, Edmonton, Alberta, Canada] Partnering with Families

Metamorphosis of a Special Care Unit - Not your average LTC reno. This round table discussion will address the collaborative efforts of the Good Samaritan Society [a LTC provider in Edmonton, Alberta] and the Faculty of Human Ecology at the University of Alberta to turn a sterile institutional environment into a hospitable and meaningful one. The living space on this particular unit is typical of most older facilities built before the enlightenment of the 1990's. Design features such as concrete walls, long hallways with fire doors providing stairwell egress at the ends, one large common dining area and elevators situated close to the nursing station are just a few of the challenges. 73 residents with varying stages of Alzheimer=s type dementia live there. The initial desire was to dress up the freshly painted walls with new pictures since old ones had been relegated to the trash or other such storage areas. As discussion ensued, it became apparent that the exercise of hanging different pictures would create visual interest but would not facilitate tactile stimulation or bring real meaning to the lives of the residents. Contact was made with the Faculty of Human Ecology at the University of Alberta and a multifaceted research project was born. Evidence exists that individuals develop a self-identity through the meaning that is attached to and made from the home environment; when forced to leave one=s home, one=s self-esteem may diminish. This multi-disciplinary project considers older adults with dementia in continuing care and the sense of self experienced in relation to an aging facility. The team proposes to create murals, tactile wall hangings and reminiscence centres on the dementia care unit as a method of familiarizing and personalizing the space. Given the fact that the unit is, at present, a blank canvas, we have an opportunity to study the relationship between a sense of self and the environment in the context of people with dementia in a continuing care setting before, during and after completion. In the nature of client-centred care and the care-giving partnership, residents, formal care-givers and informal care-givers will be involved. The values, preferences and needs of residents will inform the project and determine elements that are comfortable, meaningful and stimulating. The four main components of this endeavour will be presented in this round table discussion. 1. Pre-data and expectations from family and staff focus groups. How can families potentially be involved with this project and to what effect? Will the results of the project have any effects on resident and/or family behaviour [ie. family visiting patterns, comfort and communication]? Will the results of the project have any effects on the interactions between residents and staff? 2. Pre-data and expectations from behaviour tracking and observations of residents. What changes might we see in behaviours? Will the changed behaviour activity have a positive effect on the quality of life for the resident community at large? 3. Findings from literature reviews re: effects of tactile/visual stimulation and reminiscence triggers for persons with Alzheimers type dementia. What kinds of visual and tactile triggers are most successful? Will the responses to the stimuli have direct/indirect effects for residents and/or families and staff? 4. Evaluation criteria and methodology. The last point we will stress is the importance of forging partnerships with other organizations. There has been an incredible synergy created by the union of minds within this group. One idea sparking another toward the achievement of a common goal. Individual Abstracts Reminiscences of Home Sherry Anne Chapman A reminiscence centre would create a place for residents to use as a meaningful living space. Domestic objects of living memory and rich texture donated by families and found in the community would assist in the creation of a centre. Residents values and preferences would inform the familiarization and personalization of this space. Sherry Anne Chapman is a doctoral student in the Department of Human Ecology seeking to develop relationships between health and museum professionals as they pool their resources towards supporting the quality of life of older adults. This project presents an opportunity to study a reminiscence centre as a museum in a continuing care environment. Partnering with Families Pamela Otfinowski Family members and staff are two key partners in this endeavour to recreate and enhance the environment for residents with Alzheimers type dementia. The special care unit is not only a place where people reside, it is also a place of work and a place for families to come together. Residents and their families will be involved in the research process to provide direction on making the space more hospitable and meaningful for themselves now and for others in the future. Pam Otfinowski is a graduate student in Family Studies/ Human Ecology, an RN. and someone who has experienced Alzheimers disease within her family circle. This project provides an opportunity to evaluate how and to what effect families and staff can be involved in an applied research study. Alzheimers - Finding the right environment Edythe Andison The structural design of the facility offers little for residents living with Alzheimers type dementia. A wandering path ends abruptly with a door that one cannot open, long hallways are devoid of interest but for a few pictures; not very inspiring or inviting to the 73 residents who call thishome. Edythe Andison, RN, BscN, GNC(C) is the Care Coordinator on this unit with a mission to create an environment that is not only aesthetically pleasing but also stimulating for some and relaxing for others. A place residents, families and staff alike can call home because, as stakeholders, they will participate in defining it. The presentation will elaborate on how everyone involved with the unit expects to reap the benefits of this research. Collaboration - of benefit to all Laurie Gudmundsson Egler The concept of this project was presented late one Friday afternoon and rather than checking watches and yawning, the participants sat forward and became excited. A collaboration of this magnitude had never existed between the Department of Human Ecology in the University of Alberta and The Good Samaritan Society before. The link is an important one for both parties and will likely survive this project. Laurie Gudmundsson Egler, DT. is the Best Practice Specialist - Environment for The Good Samaritan Society and is coordinating this joint venture. This portion of the discussion will focus on how we as a learning organization can apply our experiential data and extensive literature searches in a way that will have a lasting benefit to our clients.

Collaboration - To the benefit of all

Laurie Gudmundsson-Egler [The Good Samaritan Society, Edmonton, Alberta, Canada]

The concept of this project was presented late one Friday afternoon and rather than checking watches and yawning, the participants sat forward and became excited. A collaboration of this magnitude had never existed between the Department of Human Ecology in the University of Alberta and The Good Samaritan Society before. The link is an important one for both parties and will likely survive this project. Laurie Gudmundsson Egler, DT. is the Best Practice Specialist - Environment for The Good Samaritan Society and is coordinating this joint venture. This portion of the discussion will focus on how we as a learning organization can apply our experiential data and extensive literature searches in a way that will have a lasting benefit to our clients.

Old Building - Right Ideas

Edythe Andison [The Good Samaritan Society, Edmonton, Alberta, Canada]

The structural design of the facility offers little for residents living with Alzheimer's type dementia. A wandering path ends abruptly with a door that one cannot open, long hallways are devoid of interest but for a few pictures; not very inspiring or inviting to the 73 residents who call this 'home'. Edythe Andison, RN, BscN, GNC(C) is the Care Coordinator on this unit with a mission to create an environment that is not only aesthetically pleasing but also stimulating for some and relaxing for others. A place residents, families and staff alike can call 'home' because, as stakeholders, they will participate in defining it. The presentation will elaborate on how everyone involved with the unit expects to reap the benefits of this research.

Partnering with Families

Pamela Otfinowski [Dept. of Human Ecology, University of Alberta, Edmonton, Alberta, Canada

Family members and staff are two key partners in this endeavour to recreate and enhance the environment for residents with Alzheimer's type dementia. The special care unit is not only a place where people reside, it is also a place of work and a place for families to come together. Residents and their families will be involved in the research process to provide direction on making the space more hospitable and meaningful for themselves now and for others in the future. Pam Otfinowski is a graduate student in Family Studies/Human Ecology, an RN. and someone who has experienced Alzheimer's disease within her family circle. This project provides an opportunity to evaluate how and to what effect families and staff can be involved in an applied research study.

Reminiscences of Home

Sherry Anne Chapman [Dept. of Human Ecology, University of Alberta, Edmonton, Alberta, Canada]

A reminiscence centre would create a place for residents to use as a meaningful living space. Domestic objects of living memory and rich texture donated by families and found in the community would assist in the creation of a centre. Resident's values and preferences would inform the familiarization and personalization of this space. Sherry Anne Chapman is a doctoral student in the Department of Human Ecology seeking to develop relationships between health and museum professionals as they pool their resources towards supporting the quality of life of older adults. This project presents an opportunity to study a reminiscence centre as a 'museum' in a continuing care environment.

SESSION 369

Accidental hypothermia in the elderly

A.H. Ranhoff (Emergency Department, Ullevaal University Hospital, Oslo, Norway)

Accidental hypothermia is known to be a hazard to elderly people in temperate and cold climate. Purpose: To review the literature focusing on risc factors, epidemiology, clinical presentation and treatment of hypothermia in the elderly. To present and discuss three recent cases of severe accidental hypothemia in elderly patients, and from these give reccomendations on treatment. Method: Literature review and case reports from the Emergency Department. Results: The most important risk factors are connected to ageing itself and to the morbidity often found in elderly hypothermia victims. Knowledge about treatment of severe accidental hypothermia in elderly people is based on experience from few cases and some minor prospective studies mainly on rewarming of younger patients. Clinical treatment protocols seem to be based on experience from younger patients. In the winter of 1999 we treated three female patients aged 82, 90 and 102 years old, all with body core temperature < 30 (C. They were treated with external active rewarming using a warm air blanket (Bair Hugger), and they all survived. Conclusions: Based on review of the literature, general knowledge in geriatric medicine and experience from these three cases of hypothermia in the elderly, the use of careful, active external rewarming and a low stress strategy are recommended for elderly patients.

Acute functional impairment in elderly patients admitted to hospital

A.H. Ranhoff (Emergency Department, Ullevaal University Hospital, Oslo, Norway)

When elderly people are hit by diseases, they often present with diffuse and general symptoms. Symptoms of functional impairment are common. When caused by acute disease, these symptoms have a raoid appareance and prrogress as opposed to aging and chronical disease giving slowly progressing functional impairment. The following symptoms often cause referral of elderly people to hospital: Reduced mobility, falls, mental confusion, dehydration and malnutrition, and incontinence. Purpose: To find prevalence of acute functional impairment in elderly patients referred for urgent admittance in hospital for medical problems. Material and methods: Ullevaal University Hospital is a general hospital for a population of 200 000. All patients referred for medical problems and aged 75+ years were registered in the periode 01.11.98 to 01.03.99 (four months). Doctor on call in the Emergency department filled out a form after having taken history and examined the patient. Age, gender, first apparance or progress of functional impairment, presentation of reduced mobility, falls, mental confusion, dehydration or malnutrition, or incontinence within the last two weeks prior to admittance, were registered. Results: Of 537 patients, 294 (55%) had experienced a progress or first appearance of functional impairment within the last two weeks. 126 patients (23.5%) had a combination of impairments (>2). Conclusions: In patients 75+ years admitted for urgent medical problems 55 % had new or increased functional problems. In the care for these patients improvement of function and prevention of further functional decline are important tasks together with diagnostic and therapeutic efforts.

Body actimetry in frail elderly patients confined to bed

P. Couturier (LI2G, Université Joseph Fourier, Grenoble, France), A. Queroy (Unité de physiologie de la vigilance, Centre de recherche du service de santé des armées, Grenoble, France), A. Franco (LI2G, Université Joseph Fourier, Grenoble, France), Alain Buguet (Unité de physiologie de la vigilance, Centre de recherche du service de santé des armées, Grenoble, France).

The exploration of pathologies related to immobility in the frail elderly patient confined to bed requires a detailed analysis of the fragility factors and in particular by the study of motor behaviour. In this study an actimetric overmatress was used to measure the motor activity of patients confined to bed. We have schown that the use of this sensor was possible with a population who is frail and at risk of pressure sores. Specifically we investigated its biomechanical properties, patient's tolerance and unintrusiveness. The recording of movements in clinical settings also enabled us to judge the simplicity of its use.The actimetric data produced by the interface software has enabled us to characterize the motor behaviour of elderly patients confined to bed during rehabilitation or at risk of pressure sore. Specific indicators are proposed for characterising the individual psychomotor behaviour and the comfort in bed as well as the risk of developping pressures sores including the bed space occupancy, the relative rate of immobility of the sacral area and the pressure sore actimetric risk. Such parameters have been compared with a standard reference scale, the Norton scale. Thus, the monitoring of elderly patients during rehabilitation appears to be possible to prevent complications and to understand the mechanism of adaptation during prolonged immobilisation.

Discharge from hospital and elderly people: Data from medical GRDs, Spain

Guillén, F. (Hosp. Univ. Getafe, Getafe, Spain) Bravo G. (MediRuber, Madrid, Spain)

Purpose: Describe elderly people discharged from medical acute care hospitals in Spain through official data from the Diagnostic Related Groups (DRGs) from the National Institute of Health (INSALUD). Method: Retrospective analysis of data comprising all discharges from hospitals (INSALUD, approximately 34% of all in Spain) with a codified medical DRGs, excluding discharges of Major Diagnostic Categories (MDC) 14 and 15. 1998 is the analysed year. Results: A total of 864.829 discharges were recorded, of which 58.4% were medical, for people >64 years medical discharges represents 65.3% (73.2% for people >79 years). Major diagnostic criteria (MDC) with highest medical discharges for elderly people, in order, was MDC 5 (66.5%), 4 (68.0%), 6 (54.0%), 7 (53.0%), 1 (56.8%). (0f elderly people in the respective MDC). They explain 64.3% of total medical discharges, 76.2% for people 65-79 and 78.5% for >79 years. Using Diagnostic Related Groups (GRD), in those 65 to 79 years and those >79 gives the following order for the five more frequent medical GRD: 541, 88, 127, 14, 140, and 127, 541, 14, 88 and 544, respectively. Conclusions: 1. Medical GRDs represent nearly 60% of all discharges, but more than 70% for those aged >79 years. 2. Medical discharges classified under MDC 5, 4, 6, 7 and 1 represent 64.3%, but more than 78% in those over 79 years. 3. There is only a slight variation in GRD frequencies between age groups in the elderly.

Do-Not-Resuscitate Orders in Ontario Nursing Homes and Chronic Hospitals

Jeff Poss (Department of Health Studies and Gerontology, University of Waterloo, Waterloo, Ontario, Canada), John P. Hirdes (Department of Health Studies and Gerontology, University of Waterloo, Waterloo, Ontario, Canada and Canadian Collaborating Centre-interRAI, Providence Centre, Scarborough, Ontario, Canada)

Purpose: To investigate rates and factors associated with do-not-resuscitate (DNR) orders among Ontario nursing home and chronic hospital residents. Method: Data from a number of nursing homes in Ontario were collected using the Minimum Data Set (MDS) for long term care, a standardized multi-dimensional assessment. Data from Ontario chronic hospitals collected during the same time period were used to create a cross sectional sample. Analysis was done on those assessments with an indication (yes/no) of DNR. To control for a high proportion of terminal care residents in chronic hospitals, residents receiving hospice care were excluded. Results: DNR rates differed between nursing home (67%; N=921) and chronic hospital (44%; N=1379). In multivariate analysis, nursing home residents were found to have a DNR odds ratio of 1.8 compared to residents of chronic hospitals. Factors found to be predictive of higher DNR rates included having a substitute decision-maker, cognitive impairment, cancer, endstage disease, longer length of stay, bowel incontinence, functional impairment and older age, while lower DNR rates were associated with a primary language other than English or French. Conclusion: The MDS assessment allows residents in nursing homes and chronic hospitals to be compared. Advance directives such as DNR are an example of how standardized information may illuminate opportunities for improved care. Further study is suggested by the different rates of DNR by type of facility and by the influence of a substitute decision-maker in DNR likelihood.

Geriatric-based versus general wards for older acute medical patients: A randomized study

Asplund K, Gustafson Y, Jacobsson C, Bucht G*, Wahlin A, Peterson J, Blom JO, Angquist KA Department of Medicine, Geriatric medicine*, Advanced nursing, Administration and Surgery University Hospital, Umea, Sweden.*

The effects of residence in an acute geriatrics-based ward (AGW) with emphasis on early rehabilitation and discharge planning for older patients with acute medical illnesses were assessed. Outcome and use of resources were compared with those of patients treated in general medical wards (MWs). A per-protocol rather than intention-to-treat analysis was performed. METHODS: A randomized trial with 3-months follow-up. A total of 190 patients aged 70 years and older were randomized to an acute geriatrics-based ward, and 223 patients were randomized to general medical wards. RESULTS: The two groups were comparable at inclusion. However, after care in the AGW, 71% of patients could be discharged directly home compared with 64% of those treated in MWs (relative risk 1.17; 95% CI, 0.93-1.49). The length of stay was shorter in the AGW (mean 5.9 vs 7.3 days; P = .002). The proportion of patients in geriatric or other hospital wards or in nursing homes did not differ, but the proportion of AGW patients in sheltered living tended to be lower (P =.085). At the follow-up, case fatality, ADL function, psychological well-being, need for daily personal assistance, drug consumption, need for readmission to hospital, and total health care costs after discharge did not differ between the two groups. CONCLUSIONS: A geriatric approach with greater emphasis on early rehabilitation and discharge planning in the AGW shortened the length of hospital stay and may have reduced the need for long-term institutional living.

Short term readmission in elderly patients. Descriptive study and analysis of risk factors.

M.Rainfray (Centre de Gériatrie Henri Choussat - Université Bordeaux 2, France), K.Perez (U 330, Bordeaux, France), P.Barberger-Gateau (U 330, Bordeaux, France), I.Bourdel-Marchasson (Centre de Gériatrie Henri Choussat - Université Bordeaux 2, France), J-P.Emeriau (Centre de Gériatrie Henri Choussat - Université Bordeaux 2, France).

PURPOSE : The incidence of readmission is high (9-17%) in elderly patients. We present a descriptive study of short term readmissions in patients over 75 years hospitalized in a geriatric ward. METHODS : Three hundred and twenty-two consecutive patients (86+/-5 yrs) underwent a gerontological assessment and were followed during one month after discharge. A judgment on the usefulness of readmission was given by a multidisciplinary group, using the criteria of the Appropriateness Evaluation Protocol (AEP). RESULTS : Before entry, 56,60f the patients lived at home, 34,2 0n nursing homes. At discharge 42% were dependant for at least 1 ADL, 33eeded the assistance of a nurse, 13% a technical help for walking, 37,4% were incontinent. The most frequent medical conditions were dementia, heart failure, denutrition, stroke, diabetes.Mean length of stay was 15+/-9days. Seventy-four percent of the patients were satisfied of their life, 55,3 % had a feeling of empty life and 58,9 0.000000elt useless. Thirteen patients were lost of follow-up and 27 died. Fifty readmissions occurred in the month after discharge (16,%), 21 in the same ward, 29 in others. Five of the 21 readmissions were not appropriate according to the AEP criteria. In a multivariate analysis model, a short length of stay (less than 6 days), the absence of feeling of empty life and the need for assistance in walking were associated with an increased risk of readmission. CONCLUSION : Our work confirms the high incidence of readmission in frail elderly patients, and opens on potential preventive strategies.

The psychosocial risk factors for unplanned hospitalisation among community-dwelling elderly in Hong Kong

Liu CP, Leung AC, Tsui LL, Tang WY, Li SY (Aged Care Research & Development Unit, Haven of Hope Christian Service, Haven of Hope Hospital, 8 Haven of Hope Road, Tseung Kwan O, Hong Kong)

This is to identify the psychosocial risk factors of unplanned readmissions to hospitals among community-dwelling elderly in Hong Kong. 238 elderly persons were randomly recruited and assessed by using Minumum Data Set-Home Care in a half- yearly interval. Their hospitalisation patterns were recorded starting from July 2000. Clients¡≈ mean age was 74.1 (SD=7.2, range: 60-96), 54.4% of them were male, and in average have 2.3 types of chronic illness (SD=1.2, range: 0-7). The average number of bed-days in hospitals in 6 months before joining the study was 12.5 (SD=21.3, range: 0-126), and was 6.9 (SD=12.9, range: 0-87) in 5 months from July to November 2000. Logistic regression analysis shows that respondents¡≈ poor self-rated health (OR=2.8, 95%CI=1.5-5.1, P=0.001), and making negative statements frequently (OR=2.5, 95%CI=1.2-5.0, P=0.013) attributed to their hospitalization rate. In fact, for those whose perceived health was poor, their average number of bed-days in hospitals in 5 months was longer than those with better-perceived health (11.6 Vs 5.9, P=0.002). Those who made negative statements frequently also had a trend of staying longer in hospitals than those without depressed mood (9.9 Vs 6.4, P=n.s.). Results indicate that respondents¡≈ perceived health and psychological conditions have significantly influenced their hospitalisation patterns. Health education and promotional programs are useful in improving the self-care skills and confidence of the elderly and their informal carers. The elderly may internalize their depressed mood into physiological complaints and early detection of depression not only can eliminate their unnecessary hospitalization, but also provide appropriate preventive care in due time.

SESSION 370

The Need for Theory: Critical Approaches to Social Gerontology for the 21st Century.

Simon Biggs (Centre for Social Gerontology, Keele University, U.K.) Surface, Depth and Masquerade: An interrogation of the Personal and the Structural as factors influencing Age and Identity. Dr Ariela Lowenstein (Haifa University, Israel) Rethinking Family Development and Family Solidarity Carroll L Estes, PhD, (University of California, San Francisco)Theoretical Perspectives on Old Age Policy: A Critique and A Proposal World Congress of Sociology, Vancouver BC, Canada, July, 2001 Stephen Katz (Department of Sociology, Trent University, Peterborough, Ontario, Canada) Critical Configurations in Gerontological Theory: Multidisciplinarity or Nomadic Thinking? Ruth Ray (Department of English, Wayne State University, Detroit, USA) The Perils and Possibilities of Critical Theory: Lessons from feminist Criticism Jon Hendricks, (University Honors College, Oregon State University, Corvallis, OR 97331-221, USA) Structure and identity: Mind the Gap: Shaping the Self as we Age Hans-Joachim von Kondratowitz (Deutsches Zentrum für Altersfragen e.V. Berlin, FRG) The Double legacy of Constructivism for Gerontological Research Chris Phillipson, (Centre for Social Gerontology, Keele University) Globalisation and the Reconstruction of Old Age: Towards a New Political Economy of Ageing

Abstract ISSUE: This Double Symposium raises the question: what sort of theoretical issues will be key in developing a critical social gerontology for the new millenium? The focus of each session will be the conceptual frameworks, determining issues and critical positions that will contribute to a radical interrogation of contemporary ageing and our personal and societal responses to it. It is hoped that a possible geography for the study and experience of ageing may begin to emerge. STRUCTURE: Each session will consist of presentations by five leading speakers covering a key theoretical position or issue. Presentations will be followed by an opportunity for debate. CONTENT: In convening this double-symposium, we recognise the growth of dynamic and often challenging ideas that are emerging to develop a critical perspective on contemporary ageing. We also recognise the poverty of what could be thought of as the mainstream of gerontological thought. The scope of the issues to be addressed is formidable, including the place of feminist and political economic analysis, the role of identity formation and maintenance, the social construction of ageing, the effects of changing social institutions such as the family, critiques of power, marginalisation and globalisation, the relative merits of modern and post modern interpretations of contemporary ageing and beyond. An international grouping of speakers, who have been leading development in their particular fields, will expand upon key aspects of contemporary theory-building in social gerontology. Agreement is not expected. However, it is hoped that the symposia will work toward a more profound understanding of both the study and the experience of ageing as we move into a new millenium. OUTCOMES: A clearer understanding of the complex and contradictory nature of contemporary ageing. An exploration of the theoretical tools available to interrogate ageing as a field of study. The identification of core issues for a critical social gerontology in the 21st century.

Globalisation and the Reconstruction of Old Age: Towards a New Political Economy of Ageing

C.Phillipson, (Centre for Social Gerontology, Keele University)

This paper reviews the impact of globalisation on later life. The argument developed is that we are seeing a movement from, in the first place, a view of ageing populations as a challenge to be met within discrete geographical settings B part of a national project of social reform; to, in the second place, a paradigm focusing upon the emergence, following Beck, of the >risk society=, a setting in which managing ageing becomes just one of the many challenges of life, these framed increasingly as an individual as opposed to state responsibility. The paper examines three main areas: first, there is a summary of the key institutional changes associated with the post-war reconstruction of ageing, with a particular focus on the role of the welfare state, retirement and the intergenerational contract. Second, the paper reviews the new situation presented by the impact of globalisation, with an assessment of the role of transnational organisations. Third, these developments are considered in respect of the sociology of ageing, with an emphasis on some of the gains acquired from developing a global perspective.

Structure and identity: Mind the Gap

J. Hendricks, (University Honors College, Oregon State University, Corvallis, USA)

Shaping the Self as we Age The nature of human agency is grounded in ways of life. Regardless of personal attributes, individual actors do not arrive as self-consciousness alone. As Hegel pointed out so long ago, what we think and how we conceive reflect our social life space as it is defined through Anorms, entitlements and commitments. Certainly the relativity of one's self concept, as Mischel (1977) put it, is wrapped up in those shared experiences that accumulate in a lifetime=s experience. In turn, sense of self and perception by others is a key filtering lens for adapting to comes along. The two dimensions are not only reciprocal, they provide powerful pattern-maintenance mechanisms that help channel the experience of ageing though they are seldom analysed in a holistic fashion.Viewing self-concept and identity as outcomes of opportunity structures stemming from social engagements provides a valuable interpretative framework for understanding the role of social capital, to rely on Bourdieu=s term, in shaping who we are. Structural categories, those in which we reside, give shape to human experience. The recursive sweep of social roles, norms and expectations are the cradle not only of opportunity, but of knowledge, attitudes, and preferences that nurture personal initiative and shared experiences. It is from such groundings that habits of the mind derive. Of course the difficulty is in taking account of factors which are independent of actors. Such resources appear to be but are not really external to individuals. Furthermore, they are available to actors by virtue of their being grounded in social contexts.It is not an exaggeration to assert that contextual or structurally determined contingencies are the stuff from which sense of identity emerges. The resources that are accoutrements of structural location provide the frames of reference that are integral to identity: our own sense and others perceptions of us. To put the relationship in a nutshell: identity is a concomitant of economic, structural or social arrangements that provide the referential community for making sense of what goes on in life. In terms of specific affiliations-social class, age, occupation, organisational modes of production, vocational orders, ideologies, language, power and social processes characteristic of various structurally created niches constitute and social capital used by actors as they ply their way. From these forces come frameworks for the partitioning of valued attributes as well as the political and ideological trappings justifying the division. All such organisational arrangement spawn matrices of roles, values, norms, entire lifestyles that are embodied in the expression of identity. The goal of this discussion is to explore structural dimensions of social identity, to take discussions of identity out of the realm of human capital concerns falling within the purview of psychologists alone, and move them it an interactive framework so they can benefit from the insights of other social sciences and from critical analysis.

The Double legacy of Constructivism for Gerontological Research

Hans-Joachim von Kondratowitz (German Centre for Gerontology Deutsches Zentrum fur Altersfragen, Berlin, FRG)

During the last decades of gerontological research, it has been apparent that, as in other fields of social science research, the theoretical approach of social constructivism has gained considerably in importance and in impact for designing further research perspectives in gerontology. Several areas could be named in which this constructivistic line of reasoning has materialised: gender research, sociohistorical research, cultural studies in connection with migration and ethnicity research, professionalism and its impact on experts perceptions on ageing etc. All these research areas have favoured a more or less culturalistic approach to gerontology which has produced a double legacy while the advocates of constructivism have engaged in differentiating old age intensively, such an approach on the other hand has not been at all at ease with mainstream gerontology in its different academic representations. Insofar the orientation toward social constructivism implies a distinctive tension between different perspectives in social sciences which may also result in the necessity to practically negotiate the coexistence of these perspectives in certain areas of research activity. The paper will therefore first deal with a reconstruction of the constructivist legacy, will then proceed to antagonistically develop critical objections against this perspective and will finally try to develop a praxeology of negotiating areas of mutual interest and cooperation, but not without assessing the epistemological pitfalls of such a praxeology of research fields.

SESSION 371

Assessing the Well-Being of Midlife and Older Americans Via Chartbooks

Kristen Robinson [National Center for Health Statistics, Hyattsville, USA] ("Older Americans 2000: Behind the Scenes.") Victoria Velkoff [Aging Studies Branch, International Programs Center, Population Division, US Census Bureau, Washington Plaza II, Rm. 109, Washington DC 22309] ("65 Plus in America: The Making of a Chartbook.") Ellen Kramarow [National Center for Health Statistics, CDC, Hyattsville, USA] ("Health and Aging Chartbook, Health, United States, 1999.") John R. Gist [Public Policy Institute, AARP, Washington, DC, USA] ("Every Eight Seconds: Turning Age 50 and Above in America.")

ISSUE: Aging has often been associated with declines in economic security, health and wellness, functional ability, and connectedness with the rest of society. The aging of the population in the US and in other countries around the world has caused researchers to examine and challenge some of the traditional notions about aging by systematically assessing the well-being of older populations. A number of recent reports by both government and non-government organizations have assessed the relative well-being of older populations in the US. How is well-being best measured and how should we go about assessing the well-being of older persons? STRUCTURE: The session will consist of reports from (3 or 4) individuals who headed recent studies assessing the relative well-being of older Americans. Each person will present the purpose, structure, and audience of their respective reports, and discuss key findings and pitfalls in undertaking such projects. CONTENT: The panel members will discuss both the process of organizing a study assessing the well-being of older Americans and some of the substantive conclusions they derived from their data. With regard to substance, the panelists will discuss the motivation for the study they organized, the rationale for the indicators of well-being selected, issues and problems in decisions about the data to be presented, (e.g, what to include and what to exclude), the interpretation given to the various indicators, the central findings of the report, and any implications the report might have for government or voluntary action. In terms of process, the panelists will comment on the methodological and scientific as well as practical problems in assembling a databook assessing the well-being of the aging population using a team of experts. What problems were encountered in identifying content and issues, deciding on format and presentation, reaching consensus on objectives, and drawing conclusions, if any. CONCLUSIONS/ANTICIPATED OUTCOMES: The reports find general improvement in the well-being of the older population over time. There is some consensus on key measures of well-being, on the importance of diversity in the aging population in assessing overall well-being, and on issues of disparity in resources among older populations.

"Every Eight Seconds: Turning Age 50 and Above in America"

John R. Gist [Public Policy Institute, AARP, Washington, DC]

PURPOSE: "50-Plus America" is AARP's first annual report to the nation on the status of the population aged 50 and above. The purpose of this chartbook is to document for the first time in a single place the level of well-being of America's midlife and older population through a series of both objective indicators and attitudinal measures. It will also feature each year a substantive section on a different issue, starting with economic security in 2001. METHOD: Assembling extensive data from government surveys over a 20-year period in mostly graphical form to highlight the status of the population on 20-30 key measures of well being. The population is segmented somewhat unconventionally into ages 50-61, 62-74, and 75 and older to reflect the behavioral dynamics of retirement. The population is also segmented by income (top and bottom quartiles and middle half) to highlight distribution of well-being. RESULTS: The population aged 50 and older is in most respects noticeably better off than this age group was 20 years ago, although certain features show little change over time. Incomes did not grow significantly since 1980 in real terms until the past five years or so; net worth has increased much more in the top quartile than elsewhere. Other factors such as labor force participation, homeownership, living arrangements (alone), self-assessed health status, and disability status have not changed much, although they do vary significantly by age, income, or both. CONCLUSION: Overall, 50+ers are doing better in 2000 than they were in 1980, but the most striking outcome is the difference between the top and bottom quartiles, while the situation for middle-income earners remains precarious.

"Health and Aging Chartbook, Health, United States, 1999 "

Ellen Kramarow [National Center for Health Statistics, CDC, Hyattsville, MD]

PURPOSE: This special study on health and aging was part of the annual report on the nation's health submitted by the Secretary of the U.S. Department of Health and Human Services to the President and Congress. It summarizes the health of older people in the United States at the end of the twentieth century. METHOD: Nationally representative health surveys and vital statistics are used. Measures of health status, including mortality, the prevalence of chronic conditions, disability, oral health, hearing and visual impairments are presented. In addition, health care access and utilization measures such as hospital discharge rates, use of home health care services, and health insurance coverage are included. Special attention is paid to differences in health by age, sex, and race and ethnicity. RESULTS: There is much heterogeneity in the health of the older population. The largest differences are age-related. Persons 85 years of age and over, the majority of whom (71 percent) are women, have noticeably higher rates of illness, disability, and utilization of health care services than older persons who are less than 85 years of age.

Older Americans 2000: Behind the Scenes

Kristen Robinson [National Center for Health Statistics, Hyattsville, USA]

PURPOSE: In an effort to describe the overall status of the U.S. population age 65 and older, the Federal Interagency Forum on Aging-Related Statistics (Forum) has produced Older Americans 2000: Key Indicators of Well-Being (Older Americans 2000). The new report is divided into five subject areas (population, economics, health status, health risks and behaviors, and health care) and includes 31 key indicators carefully selected by the Forum to portray aspects of the lives of older Americans and their families. METHOD: While Older Americans2000 was a great success overall, the process of putting it together proved to be quite a challenge. Some of the difficulties the Forum encountered include 1) choosing a limited number of indicators to measure multiple aspects of older people's lives, 2) identifying reliable, nationally representative data to monitor these indicators over time, 3) finding the best ways to graphically present the data, 4) deciding what to say (and not say) about the data, and 5) coordinating and negotiating every step of this process with representatives from 12 Federal agencies. RESULTS: In general, the report found that older Americans are living longer and living better than ever before. However, not all older Americans are doing equally well. Many of those age 65 and older are still facing disability, chronic health conditions, and/or economic stress. CONCLUSION: Although the production of Older Americans 2000 was a difficult and sometimes frustrating process, the end result was well worth the effort. The report can be accessed via the Forum's Website - www.agingstats.gov.

"The Making of a Chartbook"

Victoria Velkoff [Aging Studies Branch, International Programs Center, Population Division, US Bureau of the Census]

The Census Bureau is currently producing two chartbooks on the older population. The first chartbook presents state-level data on the older population and the second gives information on the total US population aged 65 and older (65+ in the United States). The reason that chartbooks are often created is because we want to convey the information in an easy to understand way and we think that well-made charts do that. When planning a chartbook a lot of thought goes into the actual charts. For instance, what indicators will be included and how will these indicators be presented? In a true chartbook, the accompanying text is often limited so it is important that chart can stand on its own. Often we go through several versions of a chart trying to find one that presents the most interesting aspects of the data in a clear way. Another aspect to the planning of a chartbook and the ultimate usefulness of a chartbook is whether or not appendix tables are included with the background data for the different charts. Appendix tables can aid people using the chartbook who want to create a different chart with the data or use the data in another way. Census typically creates chartbooks with accompanying appendix tables.

SESSION 372

Healthy Aging in Developing Countries

M. Peláez (Pan American Health Organization/World Health Organization, Washington, D.C, USA) Health and Aging in Latin America and the Caribbean: Research, Policy and Practice, Adrian O Wilson (Department of Medicine, University of Cape Town, Cape, South Africa) Healthy Aging Δ the African Perspective and Potential, Peng Du (Institute of Population Research, People's University of China, Beijing, China) Healthy Aging-Chinese Perspective, Vinod Kumar (St.Stephen's Hospital, Delhi, India) Healthy Aging: South Asian Perspective, Hana M. Hermanova (Center on Aging, West Virginia University, Morgantown, WV, USA) Healthy Aging Strategies in Rural Aging and Joseph Troisi (Institute of Gerontology, University of Malta, Msida, Malta) Training for Healthy Aging.

ISSUE : Sixty percent of world's elderly population lives in developing countries and is rapidly growing. This will become seventy percent in next 25 years. Majority live in villages. Special issues include Resources are scarce and young age problems not yet solved. Urbanisation, nuclearisation of families and erosion of traditional values are rapidly taking place. Insanitation, unsafe drinking water, pollution, overcrowding and unhealthy housing are common. Double disease burden, poverty and lack of services are common. Appropriate cost effective and culture friendly healthy aging strategies are needed. STRUCTURE : The session based on paper presentations will Introduce concepts and practice of healthy aging in developing countries. Highlight aging and health perspective from Latin American, African, Chinese and South Asian viewpoint. Present minimal data sets on aging in developing countries. Address areas critical to healthy aging strategies. Emphasize on special aspects like rural aging and interdisciplinary training. Present a coherent healthy aging policy framework at different levels and its implementation. CONTENT : The symposium will present information on aging and an approach to healthy aging strategies from a developing countries' perspective. 1. It will highlight that (i) rapid population aging is happening in the face of serious inequalities of low per capita income, poverty, destitution, inadequate resources and low literacy where appropriate policies are frequently not in place, (ii) improvements in life expectancies are offset by lack of health promotion programmes and limited opportunities for life long individual development which act as impediments to quality of life in later years, (iii) rural environs where majority of elderly live are particularly vulnerable requiring special attention and (iv) strong informal support system and other traditional values though under threat, are still significantly operative in promoting healthy aging in developing countries. 2. Information to exemplify health related morbidity and socioeconomic status of elderly, changing family structures, living arrangements, intergenerational relationships and use of services by elderly in developing countries will be provided as a basis for policy formulations. 3. Regional examples will include : Survey data on health and aging in Latin America and the caribbean and its application to the development of health promotion and health education programme. African example to depict new responsibilities of elderly persons to care for multigeneration families in view of HIV/AIDS epidemic. Chinese example on concepts, targets and practice of healthy aging and various measures to promote healthy aging. Indian study, illustrating traditional factors known to promote healthy aging on one hand and multidimensional morbidity as impacted by socioeconomic status on the other. 4. Policy formulation and research needs will focus on local determinants and cost effective strategies of healthy aging and on education and training with different countries and settings in mind. Role of State, NGOs, communities, families and individuals for healthy aging will be outlined. CONCLUSIONS/ANTICIPATED OUTCOMES : are outlined below Dissemination of knowledge in healthy aging in developing countries. Identification of models of good practice. Identification of knowledge gaps. Recommendations on research needs and policy development for healthy aging.

Health and Aging in Latin America and the Caribbean: Research, Policy and Practice

M. Peláez (Aging and Health Programme, Pan American Health Organization/World Health Organization, 525 Twenty third Street, Washington, D.C, 20037, USA)

Most countries in Latin America and the Caribbean are developing countries with varying cultures and economies. In many countries, National Health Policies include focus on aging and health issues. However, there is general lack of health promotion and health education programmes in the region. This paper will present data from the Survey on Health and Aging in Latin America and the Caribbean and its application to the development of a health promotion and health education program. The programme was developed with different countries and settings in mind. The focus of the paper will be on the conceptual framework for the development of the program, a description of the contents of the program and the methodology used for its dissemination and evaluation. Health Promotion strategies appropriate to the requirements of older persons need participatory and constructional approach to community education. They also need to be implemented through community health centre or family centre. It is important for health professionals to possess knowledge of geriatric care in addition to analytical, communication and managerial skills.The described Health Promotion and Health Education Program was implemented with the collaboration of local health centers and the leadership of geriatric physicians. An important element of this program consists in the development of self-care groups focusing on promoting active aging and social participation in the community. In a broad sense, changing the public policies in response to needs and views of older persons in order to achieve active aging, also helps development and perfomance of such programmes.

Healthy Ageing : The African Perspective and Potential

Adrian O Wilson, (Director, African Foundation for Research and Interdisciplinary Training in Ageing (AFRITA), Institute of Ageing in Africa (IAA).)

Despite conventional dogma prevalent amongst world AIDS experts, many NGOs, and governments, Africa's aged are in the front line of exposure to the consequences of the HIV/AIDS epidemic. The risks they run are direct and indirect. These risks are compounded by recently described elder sexual abuse, particularly in some urban settings. Africa's older women will carry the responsibility of supporting their dying offspring, and their grandchildren, at a time when they could reasonably be expecting to be relieved of this burden. An almost complete lack of formal (institutional) support for older Africans, an HIV/AIDS induced loss of extended family (informal) support, and the reluctance of African governments to recognise the impact and consequences of HIV/AIDS will result inevitably in an unsustainable burden for older Africans, particularly the women folk. Multi-agency intervention is seen as the most practicable response. AFRITA/IAA have established a training programme which includes: Interdisciplinary training in healthy ageing for all health workers in rural and urban Africa Principles of HIV/AIDS management oriented to impact on older Africans Detection and management of elder abuse in HIV setting, Promoting inter-sectoral NGO collaboration through collaborative training, Constant communication with, and training participation from, target group, Target group awareness training, Pressure for policies and agendas to be driven by UNAIDS/ Commonwealth/WHO, Traditional healers trained alongside conventional medicine. The above interventions are discussed.

Healthy aging - A Chinese perspective

Peng Du (Institute of Population Research, People's University of China, Beijing, China)

China has the largest elderly population in the world, 130 million aged 60 and over and it is projected that the elderly population will increase to 450 million by 2050. At the same time China has one of the highest life expectancies in developing countries. Healthy aging is a relatively new concept for Chinese, but in the last few years it has been popularized and considered in policy making. This paper summarizes the concept, targets and practice of healthy aging from the Chinese perspective. China is facing rapid process of population aging, therefore the introduction of the concept of healthy aging is welcome and it helps the society to shift the focus from merely longevity to the quality of life - living longer and healthier. Healthy aging is regarded as one of the key strategies to meet the challenges of population aging in China. It is also regarded as an important precondition to eliminate the discrimination against the elderly both in the family and in society. The health of the elderly is affected by many socioeconomic factors and the promotion of healthy aging needs comprehensive policies. Three basic countermeasures have been put forward as follows: firstly, changing the administrative functions of the government to set up and improve the social security and social service system; secondly, set up a resource redistribution system to meet the needs of social development and multidimensional needs of the elderly population; thirdly, encourage and strengthen the existing cost effective preventive measures and traditional medicine, modern scientific knowledge as well as the healthy life style to promote life long health.

Healthy Aging: South Asian Perspective

Vinod Kumar, (St.Stephen's Hospital, Delhi, India)

South Asia having several mega-countries like India, Bangladesh and Pakistan represents big chunk of global population. It is one of fastest growing regions for population aging where 18% of world's elderly live. Countries in the region are largely agrarian with traditions of joint family system, active involvement with life, non-sedentarism and spirituality Δ factors known to promote healthy aging. However, increasing rate of youth migration in search of jobs, low literacy and grossly inadequate per capita income severely restrict opportunities for life long individual development and health related quality of life in later years. Indian data points to chronic diseases in over 50% of elderly persons and a relationship of low socioeconomic status with health problems, handicaps, widowhood and family headship. Double burden of noncommunicable (cardiovascular, respiratory, locomotor, visual, metabolic and neoplastic) and communicable (TB, infections, infestations) diseases is common amongst South Asian elderly persons. 38% of 70+ older Indians have chronic energy deficiency and geriatric anaemia is common. Pollution, insanitation, unhealthy housing, indifferent health attitudes and inaccessible and underutilized health services are special problems to developing countries. Policy formulations should focus on cost-effective strategies for achieving healthy aging. Culturally adjusted health promoting methods, preservation of traditional virtues and recognition of cheaper indigenous medical systems need special attention. Improving individual financial ability, imparting primary and adult education and strengething primary health care system also require emphasis. Identification and execution of roles of States, NGOs, communities, families and individuals for healthy aging need re-appraisal.

Healthy Aging Strategies in Rural Aging

Hana M. Hermanova, Director (Center on Aging, West Virginia University, Morgantown, WV, USA)

70% of populations in developing countries live in rural areas, and the elderly (60+) are over-represented. Rural areas continue to be disproportionately old. The topic of rural aging is therefore a key "aging" issue in developing countries. West Virginia University, in collaboration with international agencies, initiated a four year project in Rural Aging (1997 Δ 2000), which culminated in the first International Conference on Rural Aging in Charleston, WV, in June 2000. The conference track 2000 Forum-Policy Debate generated policy recommendations and consequently a Plan of Action in Rural Aging. The Plan of Action is designated to create a broad international collaborative network with strong participation of developing countries to address the major challenges in rural aging. Through the series of small scale consultations the collaborators will address issues of rural aging policy to be implemented at local level, generation of community based projects in active aging including persons with functional limitations, develop educational programs in rural aging for different categories of providers and the general public. In research, the group will rethink the current functional assessment to include social and physical environments and their interactions with functional capacities of an individual. A clearinghouse is being set at the West Virginia University to provide input into creating realistic policies on active aging in rural areas.

Training for Healthy Aging

Joseph Troisi (Institute of Gerontology, University of Malta, Msida, Malta)

The world is experiencing an extraordinary revolution in longevity. Since 1950, we have on average gained almost 25 years in our life expectancy. In spite of this, however, while the Western developed world has succeeded in adding years to life, it has not yet succeeded in adding life to years. Healthy aging is often confined to the absence of disease and infirmity. However, the health and happiness of older persons are dependent upon social, emotional, and psychological factors as well as the purely clinical aspects of physical and mental health. It is an undeniable fact that poverty and disease are the main opponents of a healthy longevity. Equally, if not more destructive, are the passivity and the feeling of oneself as a parasite. Older persons are becoming victims of professional models of care. They are often portrayed as slow, poor, weak and chronically sick. Consequently, we often tend to develop models of care to fit these images, little realising that the images are not the truth. To counteract this there is an urgent need for a radical change of perspective. Aging is a natural process. Often old age is the mirror of young age. Healthy and successful aging will only occur when an older person's personal dignity, sense of belonging and self-worth are maximised. Most people have, to a greater or lesser degree, the freedom to either flourish or to decay as they grow older. Our society can enhance this freedom and the opportunities for flourishing. Older persons themselves are fundamental partners in bringing about this cultural transformation. This is more easily achieved through education and training.

SESSION 373

Socio-cultural factors impacted on Japan's National Care-Services Insurance

Clayton Fong, Executive Director, National Asian Pacific Center On Aging, 1511 Third Ave. Suite #914, Seattle, Washington, 98101-1626 Teruhisa Mokuno, Chairman & CEO, Sun-Life Social & Welfare Organization(not for profit), 4-3-26, Sakae, Naka-ku, Nagoya, Japan Yusuke Kataoka, Acting Chairman & Executive Director, U.S.Foundation for International Economic Policy, 2-9-19, Hatsudai, Shibuya-ku,Tokyo, Japan

PURPOSE: Japan's Care-services Insurance System has been in place since April,2000. This system has advantages and disadvantages, which has divided the nation sharply in the process of implementation of this system as a law, designed to provide a comprehensive and uniform system for the delivery of care- services to all localities and to expand and enhance government policy. How the new plan can be implemented evenly throughout the nation is a question still surrounded by controversy and confusion. It is constantly faced with difficulties as to how duties should be performed to keep in compliance with health and welfare laws and regulations. The difficulty in meeting the guideline is primarily due to the absence of a unified, cohesive interpretation of the laws in question, and secondarily, to power struggles between the central government and regional bureaucracies maintain each respective areas as unique with different needs. The trial period of this system will reveal the roots of confusion, which will be of interest to the audiences. METHOD: A valuable interviews and in-depth researches are being conducted to see the pros and cons of this system. For comparative purposes, the same were conducted in several foreign countries, to see how historical, cultural and ethnic factors are impacted on the elderly of ethnic minority. RESULTS: The issue of Japan's National Policy on Social Welfare is sharply divided within the nation; and the issue of whether or not social welfare programs should be guaranteed by public funds or not, was debated not enough to bring about this system as a uniformly acceptable form. It was orchestrated as political approach rather than social approach. CONCLUSION: Japan is navigating in unchartered waters in the area of care-services for the elderly. This presentation will shed some light on the unknown territory in which Japan is traveling. Any system which deals with care-services for the elderly must be approached from socio-cultural view not political. December 20, 2000 The Secretarit The 17th Congress of the International Association of Gerontology Gerontology Reseach Center Simon Fraser University at Harbour Center 2800-515 West Hastings Street Vancouver, British Columbia, Canda V6B 5K3 Dear Sir, In accordance with the instruction given pertaining to transmission of Abstract, please find (4) copies of paper and a disk. I would appreciate it very much if you would be kind enough to forward to whoever in chage of presentation of subject as attached herein. Sincerely yours, Yusuke Kataoka Acting Chariman & Executive Director U.S.Foundation for International Economic Policy-Japan Office 2-9-19, Hatsudai, Shibuya-ku, Tokyo, Japan E-mail address: hoosiera@tke.att.ne.jp Fax: 81-03-3379-271

SESSION 374

Community Care for Seniors: Helping Family Caregivers of Seniors Overcome Barriers to Using Respite Services Project Overview

Taylor Alexander, President and CEO, Canadian Association for Community Care Norah Keating, Department of Human Ecology, University of Alberta Michael MacLean, Dean of Social Work, University of Regina Pat Corbett, Policy Analyst, Division of Aging and Seniors, Health Canada Linda Lysne, Respite Project Coordinator

The Canadian Association for Community Care (CACC), a national, non-profit voluntary organization, has received funding from the Population Health Fund to carry out a national respite study. For the purpose of the project, respite has been defined as "a break, time off or relief for the caregiver." Over a period of two years, a series of sequential consultations is taking place with service providers, family caregivers and community leaders to explore the barriers to respite for caregivers of seniors as well as identify strategies to address those barriers. During the same period, the project team is compiling the first-ever national inventory of programs and services that are models of best practice and will also produce a one-page "respite information sheet" for broad distribution across Canada. Five members of the project team will provide: · overview of this innovative project and its relationship to the findings of the first national respite study carried out by CACC (report published in 1998) · project goals/ objectives and their relationship to

Population Health Fund priorities · composition and role of the National Advisory Committee · sequential steps in the consultation process culminating in consultations with key provincial and territorial government representatives · research tools and evaluation framework · interim report and recommendations from regional focus groups held across Canada

Respite as Outcome for Caregivers: Stakeholders speak out

Linda Lysne (Canadian Association for Community Care, Ottawa, Canada)

Nearly one hundred service providers, community leaders and caregivers participated in focus group discussions in Halifax, MontrÈal, Halton, Winnipeg, Vancouver and Whitehorse during March, 2001. A local host organization was identified in each centre to assist with on-site arrangements. Some local host organizations worked in partnership with other community organizations to arrange space, recruit participants and offer respite care if needed.
Local host organizations recruited participants using tools developed by the project team: telephone screening guides, quota sheets and moderators' guides. The Project Coordinator moderated caregiver focus groups while moderators for service provider groups were locally recruited. Health Canada Program Consultants acted as moderators in Winnipeg, Halifax and MontrÈal. The Project Coordinator also facilitated a joint session for caregivers and service providers.
Participants brought considerable diversity to the discussions in terms of identifying barriers and proposing strategies. Some of the barriers identified: i) Lack of understanding of caregiver need for respite and the individual nature of caregivers' respite needs ii) Lack of recognition iii) Lack of information iv)Inadequate caregiver education, training, support and counselling v)Unmet service needs vi)Lack of workplace support for caregivers vii)Lack of service coordination vii) Staffing issues ix)Need for public awareness/advocacy) x)User fees xi)Inadequate transportation services xii) Challenges of navigating the system
A national survey was mailed out in May 2001 to 700 respondents across Canada for comment. It is based on fifty recommendations related to home care, long term care facilities, service providers, caregivers and the community at large.

Respite: Learning how to overcome the barriers

Michael J. MacLean (University of Regina, Regina SK Canada)

Respite is an important health and social service for seniors and their caregivers. It is well known, however, that formal programs described as respite services in Canada are not being adequately used by seniors and caregivers who could benefit significantly from them. This suggests that there are barriers to the use of respite services which are not fully understood. To date, there has been no systematic study of why these programs have not been used by those whose needs they are intended to meet.

The Canadian Association for Community Care is using a combined qualitative and quantitative methodology to better understand the barriers to the use of respite services by seniors and their caregivers in Canada and to identify strategies to address those barriers. A National Advisory Committee comprised of health and social service practitioners, researchers, educators and policy makers is guiding a sequential series of consultations, in which family caregivers, service providers and community leaders provide information about barriers to the use of respite care and recommendations to overcome these barriers. Their recommendations will be validated by a large number of family caregivers, service providers, health and social policy makers as well as representatives of organizations with a national perspective.
Consultations will also be held to inform provincial and territorial government officials with responsibility for respite services and to assess their receptiveness to implementation in their jurisdictions. The final recommendations will be incorporated into a fact sheet for broad dissemination to family caregivers, service providers and related organizations

Respite Revisited: Building on the first national respite study

Taylor Alexander (Canadian Association for Community Care, Ottawa, CANADA)

An innovative model of respite care is described in the Final Report of the first National Respite Care Project in which family caregivers, rather than care receivers are the primary focus. Traditional Canadian models of respite care for seniors have often focussed primarily on care receivers, overlooking many key needs of their family caregivers. If the latter's needs are not adequately met, there is danger of caregiver burnout and collapse of the care plan. Following an extensive initial phase of research and stakeholder consultation, many fundamental questions about respite care remained unanswered: i) What is respite care? ii)Who should be entitled to respite? iii)What are the barriers to developing or providing appropriate respite? iv)How do existing respite services fail to meet client i.e. caregiver need? v)How can existing respite care services be improved?Based on these challenging questions, the study team then developed, delivered and tested a caregiver-focussed respite program model in three community-based pilot sites in Canada for approximately one year. The purposes of the new model were to publicize respite services, assess caregivers and care receivers for their actual respite needs and develop strategies to meet those needs within and outside the formal care system. A wide range of data were gathered both on caregivers and care receivers. Numerous barriers to using respite services were identified and several successful innovations were developed to overcome those barriers. Innovations focussed on making existing respite services more flexible or introducing existing programs into new geographic areas.

Supporting Family Caregivers of Seniors: A Key Determinant of Health

Pat Corbett (Health Canada, Ottawa, Canada)

Respite is widely acknowledged as an essential support to family caregivers of seniors. Yet, despite the existence of formal respite programs, caregivers increasingly report stress and burden in their role. This has led to discussion among policy makers about the need to determine best practice models to assist caregivers of frail seniors in obtaining a break from their caregiving responsibilities.Health Canada has adopted a population approach to further its continuing mandate to improve the health of Canadians. This approach recognizes that in addition to the health care system, social, economic and environmental conditions have a strong influence on health.Research has shown the importance of supportive informal networks, enabling communities, and formal service systems that promote health and well-being. The challenge for action is to foster those personal support networks, caring communities, and appropriate health, social and other systems that support healthy aging. The goal of the Population Health Fund is to increase community capacity on or across the determinants of health including social support networks; education; personal health practices and coping skills; culture; health services and gender.The Population Health Fund seeks to achieve three objectives through project funding: (1) to develop, implement, evaluate and disseminate models for applying the population health approach; (2) to increase the knowledge base for future program and policy development and (3) to increase partnerships and intersectoral collaboration.
This initiative builds on an earlier national respite project funded by the J.W. McConnell Family Foundation and the Seniors Independence Program of Health Canada

Supporting Informal Caregivers: The place of respite

Norah Keating (University of Alberta, Edmonton, Canada)

Backed by perceived threats of population aging and the costs of providing support to frail seniors, Canadian policy makers increasingly have turned to family and friends as ideal caregivers to seniors. The informal care they provide is seen as better and cheaper than formal services provided by paid professionals. Yet there is growing evidence that caregivers and their families experience various economic and non-economic costs as a result of their caring responsibilities. Policy makers have begun to turn to the issue of how to provide support to this largely unpaid and unsupported workforce. Respite is seen as a key component of the strategy to support informal caregivers. However, attempts to provide services to lighten caregiver loads often have proven unsuccessful. One explanation for this poor fit between costs and support is that respite typically is conceptualized as a set of services provided from within health care portfolios. Yet recent research suggests that respite is a caregiver experience or outcome - of relief, a break or an opportunity to reconnect with others - - and that little public policy is focussed on needs of caregivers. The purpose of this presentation is twofold: to discuss conceptualizations of caregiver costs in order to determine in what areas caregivers might need a break; and to clarify conceptual definitions of respite to guide policy development and practice in support to caregivers. This discussion provides the backdrop for presentation of a national study on caregiver respite being conducted by the Canadian Association for Community Care.

SESSION 375

A Video Soundscape: Using Music and Nature Scenes to Facilitate Well-Being

C. LeNavenec & J. Parr Vijinski (University of Calgary, Alberta, Canada)

People experiencing a chronic illness are increasingly incorporating complementary treatment modalities (e.g. guided imagery, therapeutic touch, or the creative arts therapies) into their health care program as a means to promote health and well-being. This presentation will feature a video soundscape of two testimonials of older adults who have used music on their own accord for this purpose. It also includes two of the second author's original compositions set to beautiful nature scenes in Canada and the U.S. The video soundscape which is to be used in a world wide web-based University of Calgary nursing course on using music and guided imagery to promote health, affords insights about their responses to music combined withnature scenes such as what, why and how it helped to enhance well-being.

Feeling Arts as Material for Universal Healing

Y. Kitamura (Feeling Arts Committee, Osaka, Japan), T. Yoshioka (Department of Health and Behavioural Science, Kobe City College of Nursing, Kobe, Japan), Y. Ikawa (Department of Corporate Citizenship, Matsushita Electric Industrial Co Ltd, Osaka, Japan)

Artist Yoshihiro Kitamura uses original techniques and materials to perform an aesthetic experience he terms 'Feeling Arts'. He creates an abstract painting with soil, Indian ink and gold under such themes as the universe, life, heaven and earth before performing the 'Feeling Arts'. For his performance, he skillfully casts the light of three primary colors on the abstract painting and blends the image with selected music. The abstract painting shows subtle changes in shading, depth and color, almost as if it is an animated film. Individual viewers may feel, think and imagine something moving, peaceful or hopeful in their own world through this aesthetic experience. We think the 'Feeling Arts' is universally effective in healing, especially when a therapist asks a minimum question to his or her client without denial and force after appreciation of the 'Feeling Arts'. On this occasion, we introduce a video of the 'Feeling Arts' as a useful material for universal healing. Anyone can easily experience the 'Feeling Arts' with this material without distinction of religion, race or culture anywhere and anytime.

Springtime of Autumn: Creating Meaning in Times of Change

G. Marr Burdman (GeroWise (TM) International, Prescott, AZ, USA and University of Washington, Seattle, WA, USA)

SPRINGTIME OF AUTUMN: CREATING MEANING IN TIMES OF CHANGE focuses on practical applications of logotherapy and life review in the journey toward wholeness across the lifespan. Designed for health and social service providers and multidisciplinary students of gerontology, the video is designed to: highlight the holistic and developmental aspects of age related changes; explore the universal search for meaning in later years; emphasize timely life review and logotherapy techniques for creating meaning regardless of age or circumstance; present unique examples of living with dignity in the midst of major life challenges; and offer insights into a global web of connection and compassion that transcends cultural, gender and age differences.

SESSION 376

Community Capacity Development: Specialized Geriatric Services Beyond Canadian Academic Health Science Centres.

J. Puxty (Division of Geriatric Medicine, Southeastern Regional Geriatric Program, Queen's University, Kingston Ontario, Canada) Community Capacity Development within the Context of the Ontario Regional Geriatric Programs. D.P. Ryan (Regional Geriatric Program of Toronto, Faculty of Medicine University of Toronto, Toronto Ontario, Canada) Wrapping Multi-Media Around Remote Communities to Support Development in Aging and Health. W. Molloy (McMaster University, Hamilton Ontario, Canada) Geriatric Consultation and Education in Remote Northern Ontario Communities. W. B. Dalziel (Division of Geriatric Medicine, University of Ottawa Regional Geriatric Assessment Program of Ottawa-Carleton, Ottawa Ontario, Canada) Out and beyond: Developing Geriatric Capabilities in Rural Communities. J. Fitzgibbon (Southeastern Regional Geriatric Program, Queen's University Kingston Ontario, Canada) Community Development in Southeastern Ontario: Lessons from the Field. M. Borrie, J. Feightner (Division of Geriatric Medicine, Southwestern Ontario Regional Geriatric Program, University of Western Ontario, Lawson Health Research Institute, London Ontario, Canada) Rural Community Development of Geriatric/ Psychogeriatric Services in Southwestern Ontario.

Issue: Planning, implementing, and sustaining enhanced care of frail elderly persons in communities that are geographically remote from specialized geriatric services. Structure: A Canadian provincial program will present and discuss specific community development initiatives as they relate to planning, practice and research and evaluation. I. Community Development - Context of Community Development within Ontario Regional Geriatric Programs (15min.). II. Community Development Initiatives in Ontario's small urban, rural and remote northern communities (1.0hr.). III. Closing Comments (15 min.) Content: Community Development Initiatives in Ontario's small urban, rural and remote northern communities include: Presentation I: Geriatric Assessment, Consultation & Education in Remote Northern Ontario Communities (Ontario Regional Geriatric Programs of Toronto, Ottawa-Carleton, Central-West); Presentation II: Capacity Development Targeting Community Health Care Providers (Ontario Regional Geriatric Programs of Southwestern and Southeastern) Conclusions/Anticipated Outcomes: A roundtable discussion in which speakers will address progress and challenges in developing, implementing, and sustaining community-based health care services for the frail elderly in small urban, rural and northern geographic areas that are remote from larger health science centres. A Summary Report will be collated and mailed (hard copy or e-mail) to participants following the conference. This report will also be posted on the Ontario Regional Geriatric Program's Web-based Site.

Community Capacity Development within the Context of the Ontario Regional Geriatric Programs.

T.C. Knott, A. Jewell (Southeastern Regional Geriatric Program, Queen's University, Kingston Ontario, Canada) J. Puxty (Division of Geriatric Medicine, Southeastern Regional Geriatric Program, Queen's University, Kingston Ontario, Canada)

The planning and implementation of Five Regional Geriatric Programs (RGPs) commenced in 1986 as part of an Ontario Ministry of Health Provincial strategy for responding to seniors health care needs. Although the RGPs were established within urban academic health science institutions, their provincial mandate assured access to specialized geriatric services by up to 67% of Ontario's older population including those who lived in remote rural and small urban communities. In an attempt to ensure equitable access to specialized geriatric services and to enhance the capabilities of local healthcare providers, the RGPs have adopted a Community Development Approach integrating assessment, consultation, education, research and evaluation. A variety of models have been used to facilitate Community Development across the province, all of which incorporate local community partnerships and interdisciplinary teamwork. This roundtable discussion will focus on the successes and challenges in developing and sustaining enhanced community capacity development by presenting specific and illustrative examples.

Community Development in Southeastern Ontario: Lessons from the Field

J. Fitzgibbon, A. Jewell (Southeastern Regional Geriatric Program, Queen's University Kingston Ontario, Canada)

Sustainability of community development initiatives is predicated on building partnerships with local community stakeholders. A Core Team model comprised of Southeastern Regional Geriatric Program representatives and local health care system decision-makers within two small urban and rural counties was established in 1995. Using the collaborative Core Team model enhanced mutual learning and facilitated prioritization and implementation of community-specific initiatives related to health-care services for their frail, elderly populations. Examples of initiatives resulting from this model include a series of health-care provider workshops, a Seniors Steering Committee on Elder Abuse and A Community Health Centre Project.

Geriatric Consultation and Education in Remote Northern Ontario Communities

W. Molloy, I. Turpie (McMaster University, Hamilton Ontario, Canada)

Purpose: To describe models of specialized geriatric care provided in, Manitoulin Island and Sioux Lookout, Ontario, by the Central South Specialized Health Care for the Elderly Regional Program. Method/ Results: Outreach geriatric services have been provided on Manitoulin Island for over 10 years through special Ontario Ministry of Health and Long Term Care funding. Four visits are made annually by a geriatrician and another member of the specialized geriatric interdisciplinary team. During these site visits, consultation and educational sessions are provided to long term care facilities, geriatric medicine consultation is provided to the two hospitals, one in Mindemoya and one in Little Current and patients are assessed in their homes. Provider satisfaction is good and the ability of the facilities and area health professionals has improved. In addition, Geriatricians have provided specialized consultation to Sioux Lookout and neighbouring reserves. Conclusion: Successful models have been implemented to serve remote northern communities. Additional specialists and funding could expand these geriatric services to a larger number of these communities.

Out and beyond: Developing Geriatric Capabilities in Rural Communities.

W. B. Dalziel, (Division of Geriatric Medicine, University of Ottawa Regional Geriatric Assessment Program of Ottawa-Carleton, Ottawa Ontario Canada)

Models of service delivery in three small urban and northern communities initiated by the Ottawa Regional Geriatric Assessment Program will be described. A summary of the challenges and barriers to developing geriatric services in these communities, and an outline of the critical success factors for the development of geriatric capabilities in rural health systems will be discussed.

Rural Community Development of Geriatric / Psychogeriatric Services in Southwestern Ontario

M. Borrie (Division of Geriatric Medicine, South western Ontario Regional Geriatric Program, University of Western Ontario, Lawson Health Research Institute, London Ontario Canada) P. Stolee (South western Ontario Regional Geriatric Program, University of Western Ontario, Lawson Health Research Institute, London Ontario Canada) J. Feightner (Program Development and Coordination in Elderly Care, St. Joseph's Health Care, Department of Family Medicine, University of Western Ontario, London Ontario Canada) J. Devereux (Geriatric Assessment Unit, St. Joseph's Health Care, London Ontario Canada) D. Harvey (Southwest Region Health Care Programs, Ontario Ministry of Health and Long Term Care, MOH/MCSS, London Ontario Canada) M. Vickers (Geriatric Program, St. Joseph's Health Care, London Ontario Canada)

Purpose: This presentation will describe the evolution of community development within Specialized Geriatric Services in southwestern Ontario. Method and Results: Southwestern Ontario is a ten county, largely rural, area of 16,000 square miles with 200,000 people over 65 years. The Regional Geriatric Program (RGP), established in 1992 with a multidisciplinary outreach team of 10 clinicians supported by geriatricians, initiated the "Models Project" in 1995 to enhance capacity in two rural counties to provide local comprehensive geriatric assessment (CGA). Principles of community and organizational development guided these pilot projects. Two interdisciplinary "virtual teams", with members from community primary services agencies, were trained to serve as local resources in CGA. Lack of formal commitments to funding and infrastructure were two reasons the model was not sustained. A new initiative combines the resources of the RGP and emerging Regional Psychogeriatric Program (RPGP) and partners with the Ministry of Health and LongTerm Care (MOHLTC) Regional Office. The goal is to enhance CGA and Comprehensive Psychogeriatric Assessment (CPGA) capacity through organizing local resources into assessment teams, in each county, with formal links to regional specialized geriatric services. Four new provincial MOHLTC funding initiatives relevant to the frail elderly are being directed to identified regional needs. Consultation between county planning committees and regional resource people, and county-level human resource mapping of existing CGA/CPGA expertise, have resulted in plans to provide local services that network with each other and regional resources. Conclusions: Memoranda of understanding between the partner organizations will formalize clinical, educational, evaluation and funding responsibilities, as well as anticipated outcomes.

Wrapping Multi-Media Around Remote Communities to Support Development in Aging and Health.

D. P. Ryan, R. Fisher (Regional Geriatric Program of Toronto, Faculty of Medicine University of Toronto, Toronto Ontario, Canada)

As urban centres prepare for the boom in aging demographics in 2020, the future is already here in rural and remote regions of Canada. There is a dramatic shortage of health professionals knowledgeable in aging and health and significant obstacles to their recruitment. To provide clinical and educational services and overcome obstacles to recruitment a comfortable blanket of telehealth multi-media programming is wrapping itself around a remote community in Northern Ontario. The bundle of media include videoconferencing, webcasting, a web-based knowledge transfer center, online needs assessments and teaching case studies, email and chat, and POTS as well as bi-directional training visits. Participants include physicians, interdisciplinary teams, seniors and local community service groups. The framework reflects a model of changing practice behaviors through broad spectrum multi-mediated community development.

SESSION 377

Doppler Test for Predicting Stroke in the Elderly

G.I. Prada(Ana Aslan National Institute of Gerontology and Geriatrics, Bucharest, Romania)

The purpose of the investigation was to define a new test for early diagnosis of elderly at risk for developing stroke. A study has been carried out on 1093 consecutive patients referred for Doppler extracranial and peripheral investigations for various reasons (dizziness, occlusive peripheral arterial disease, sequelae of stroke). The age range was 60 to 105 years (mean 82.5 years). Prevalence of stroke among these patients was 17%, and gender distribution in stroke patients was: 43% women and 57% men. A so-called Doppler ischemic index was calculated as a ratio of ankle (posterior tibial artery) systolic velocity and wrist (radial artery) systolic velocity. Using both symmetrical parameter method and chi-square test we found that an index below 1.00 correlated strongly with the presence of stroke in a patients past medical history ($p<0.005$). The index correlated better if ankle (systolic velocity at posterior tibial artery) was also below or equal to 0.25 m/s ($p<0.001$). Sensitivity and specificity of this ;Doppler ischemic index were high enough (0.84 and 0.94, respectively) to warrant its use as a screening test that might define elderly patients at risk for stroke. The index correlated very well with the ischemic cerebral vascular accidents, but did not correlate with hemorrhagic cerebral vascular accidents. Consequently, it can be used in the elderly only for ischemic stroke.

Factors influencing hospital admission and radiological investigation in elderly Malaysian patients with acute stroke

Koh WK , Lee FS, Poi PJH, Srinivas P (Division of Geriatrics,Department of Medicine, University Hospital,Kuala Lumpur,MALAYSIA)

Purpose: Stroke is a leading cause of death and disability in older persons. To assess factors influencing the time to admission and investigation in acute stroke, we conducted a prospective study of all such patients admitted to the geriatric ward, University Hospital, Kuala Lumpur over a 4-month period. Methods: Structured interviews were used to investigate the timing of events preceding admission. Demographic and medical data, stroke knowledge and the timing of events were obtained from the patients and/or carers, and from the medical records. Results: Data from twenty nine patients were obtained during the study period. The median time from onset of symptoms to admission was 4 hours and 37 minutes. Sixteen patients (53.3%) were admitted within 6 hours. Factors associated with an earlier admission were age, 75 years and above ($p<0.013$), haemorrhagic stroke ($p<0.024$), knowledge of stroke symptoms ($p<0.025$), altered conscious level ($p<0.031$) and direct hospital presentation without prior GP consultation ($p<0.049$). Ethnicity, sex, education level, prior history of stroke or TIA, time of symptom onset, severity of motor weakness, admission Barthel index score, carer status and transportation used did not significantly influence the time of hospital admission. The conscious level of stroke patients was the main factor influencing time of CT brain scanning ($p<0.018$). Six (20%) patients had a CT brain scan performed within 6 hours of symptom onset. Conclusion: Public and medical personnel education could result in a significant reduction in the time taken to confirm the diagnosis of stroke.

Hemodynamic Study on Pathophysiology of Periventricular Lucency Using Second Derivative Plethysmography

T. Iwamoto, Y. Miyaji, A. Kiuchi, T. Umahara, K. Kanaya, H. Hanyu, M. Takasaki (Department of Geriatric Medicine, Tokyo Medical University, Japan)

To clarify the pathophysiology of periventricular lucency (PVL) on brain computerized tomography, we studied 307 elderly patients with a variety of diseases using newly-developed, second-derivative plethysmography (SD-PTG). The mean age was 77.7 years and 158 were men. PVL was graded into 4 scales according to the modified classification of van Swieten (grade 0 to 3). Grading of PVL was also assessed at 3 points: deep, anterior, and posterior PVLs. Hemodynamic parameters were calculated based on the b/a and d/a ratios with measurement made from the baseline to the top of each wave on the SD-PTG wave form. Grade 3 was seen in 16 of deep PVL, 21 of anterior PVL, and 22 of posterior PVL. In deep and anterior PVLs, significantly high b/a ratio and low d/a ratio of grade 3 cases were seen compared to those of the other grades. There was no difference of these parameters in posterior PVL. In patients with a more severe grade of deep/anterior PVL than posterior PVL, high b/a ratio and low d/a ratio were seen. The changes of b/a and d/a ratios, seen in severe PVL of deep frontal white matter, indicated that the pathophysiology of the PVL was associated hemodynamically with impaired recoil function of the aorta and accelerated circulatory resistance in the periphery. Furthermore, it is also suggested that a different pathophysiology might involved in other PVLs and the pathophysiology of PVL might differ according to area even in one brain.

Low well-being is a predictor for development of cerebrovascular disease in elderly diabetic patients

Yukari Murotani, Atsushi Araki, Toshiko Ohtake, Akinori Hattori, Hirohito Kazama, Toshiyuki Horiuti, Takayuki Hosoi, Hajime Orimo, Hideki Ito (Tokyo Metropolitan Geriatric Hospital and Tama Geriatric Hospital, Tokyo, Japan)

PURPOSE: To examine whether psychological factors are risk factors for the development of cerebrovascular disease in elderly diabetic patients in a 3-year longitudinal study. METHODS: One hundred ninety seven elderly diabetic patients free of cerebrovascular disease participated to receive a questionnaire about quality of life by an interviewer. They had a mean age of 75 ± 6 years (71 men, 126 women, treatment mode; 70 diet alone, 99 oral hypoglycemic drugs, 28 insulin therapy). The well-being in elderly patients was assessed by the PGC morale scale. Diabetes burden was assessed by the elderly diabetes burden scale, which consists of 6 sub-scales, symptom burden, life burden, diet burden, diabetic-specific worry, treatment dissatisfaction, drug therapy burden; 23 items). RESULTS: During 3 years follow-up period, fifteen patients (7.6 %) developed clinical cerebrovascular disease (CVD). The PGC morale scores in those who developed CVD were significantly lower than in those who did not develop (9.3 ± 4.8 vs. 12.0 ± 4.0, $P= 0.01$). There were no significant differences in elderly diabetic burden scores between the two groups. When multiple logistic regression analysis was performed using 8 variables (PGC morale scale, age, sex, HbA1c, total cholesterol, triglycerides, HDL-cholesterol, systolic blood pressure), both low morale scale and men were significant predictors for the development of cerebrovascular disease. CONCLUSION: In a 3 years longitudinal study, low well-being was a risk factor for cerebrovascular disease in elderly patients with diabetes mellitus.

Relationship Between Leuko-Araiosis and Blood Pressure Variability in the Elderly

F. Puisieux, P. Monaca , P. Dewailly (Service de Médecine Interne et Gériatrie, CHRU Lille, 59037 Lille Cedex, France), D. Deplanque (Service de Neurologie et de pathologie neurovasculaire , CHRU Lille, 59037 Lille Cedex, France), C. Delmaire (Service de Neuroradiologie, CHRU Lille, 59037 Lille Cedex, France), C. Di Pompeo (Département d'évaluation médicale, Faculté de Médecine de Lille, 59045 Lille Cedex).

Background: Although leuko-araiosis is a common finding on computed tomographic scan (CT) of the brain, its pathogenesis remains uncertain. Objective: To investigate the association between blood pressure (BP) disturbances and leuko-araiosis. Methods: We restrospectively reviewed CTs and 24-hour ambulatory blood pressure monitorings of 79 old patients (57 women and 22 men; mean age: 83*6). Among the 79 patients, 50 were demented (30 Alzheimer's disease and 18 vascular dementia) and 29 were non-demented. Leuko-araiosis score (LA score) was determined by using Rezek's scale. To evaluate short-term variations of BP, we determined (1) the variability of systolic and diastolic BPs (within-subject standard deviation (SD) of all readings over a 24-hour period (2) the coefficient of variability (variability of BP/mean BP), and (3) the maximal variation of BP (difference between the maximum and minimum 24-hour BPs). Results: Higher LA scores were associated with higher systolic BPs in 24-hour, diurnal and nocturnal periods, higher maximal variation of systolic BP, greater variability of systolic BP during 24-hour, diurnal and nocturnal periods, and greater coefficient of variability of SBP during sleep. Conclusions: Our study suggests that elevations of systolic BP and short-term variations in systolic BP may contribute to the pathogenesis of white matter lesions in old persons.

Significance Of MRI White Matter Abnormalities To Cognitive Ageing: Evidence From The Sydney Older Persons Study

O. Piguet, D.A. Grayson, (Centre for Education and Research on Ageing, University of Sydney, Sydney, Australia), L. Ridley, (Dept. of Radiology, Concord Repatriation General Hospital, Sydney, Australia), H.P. Bennett, W.S. Brooks, H. Creasey, T.C. Lye, (Centre for Education and Research on Ageing, University of Sydney, Sydney, Australia) & G.A. Broe, (Prince of Wales Medical Research Institute, Sydney, Australia)

Periventricular and deep white matter abnormalities identified on brain magnetic resonance imaging (MRI) are thought to represent evidence of vascular disease. These changes have been implicated as contributing to poor cognitive functioning, particularly affecting executive functions, although their respective and specific contribution remains unclear. Data from the most recent wave of the Sydney Older Persons Study (SOPS) are presented. SOPS is a longitudinal study following a cohort of 630 community dwellers living in the inner west of Sydney, Australia, aged 75 years and over at the time of recruitment in 1991. Brain MRIs were performed on 123 participants from this cohort (mean age: 86 years) and locations and size of periventricular and deep white matter lesions were recorded using a semiquantitative rating method. Presence of vascular risk factors was also investigated and nine tests of executive functions administered. Periventricular white matter abnormalities were found in all participants unlike deep white matter lesions. Statistical analyses revealed a lack of associations between white matter lesions and cognitive performance. In addition, evidence of white matter changes was not related to other vascular risk factors. These findings indicate that white matter changes are very common in elderly, non-demented participants. They also suggest that MRI abnormalities may not be evidence of a pathological process.

Tendency of mortality by cerebrovascular disease in the elderly population of Brazil - 1979 to 1995

N. E. Costa, S. Saldanha (Ministry of Health, Brazil), L. Vianna (University of Brasilia, Brazil)

PURPOSE: To analyze the tendency of the mortality by Cerebrovascular Disease (CVD) in the elderly Brazilian population, between 1979 and 1995, with stratification by sex and assortment by age groups above 60 years old. METHOD: Causes considered as CVD where contained in the CID 9, 4 digits (D 4), chapter VII, selection 430-438. The information where obtained from the Mortality System (SIM), Ministry of Health of Brazil. RESULTS: 1. The evolution of mortality by CVD between 1979 to 1995 in spite of the high coefficient (57/10000 in the year of 1979 and of 51,95/10000 in the year of 1995) has been showing a decrease tendency, through out of the years studied. 2. Considering gender, the speed of the fall of mortality is more accentuated in women, except in the 80 years-old age group and above, that were found the largest alterations in the mortality coefficients, making difficult the identification of tendencies, and the interpretation of the results. CONCLUSION: Given the dramatics of the acute CVD, its mortality and its sequels, the best treatment is its prevention, and knowledge of its risk factors is necessary, that subjected to control or suppression by preventive activities, adequate hospital assistance and prolonged health care, could contribute to reduce the mortality, the incapacity and to the improvement of live quality of the surviving elderly.

SESSION 378

Congruence in Perception of Problems of Community Living:Older Israeli's and Professionals Serving Older Persons

S.M. Neikrug (Tel-Hai, Upper Galilee, Israel)

PURPOSE: This paper evaluates the congruence between self-identified Problems of Community Living and related needs of older Israelis and perception of older persons' problems by professionals in various agencies serving the aged. METHOD: An instrument indicating 19 major problems of community living was developed by a panel of older persons was administered to a sample of older Israelis (60+) living in the community (n= 1164) and human service professionals (443) serving the aged. The panel concentrated on concrete problems as they felt that professionals dichotomize needs as 'concrete' or 'counseling' and accord higher status and preference to the latter. RESULTS: The results indicate major differences between older persons and professionals regarding the severity of the various problem of community living. The findings indicate that older persons often feel that there is no avenue to pursue redress for their complaints nor agency that has mandate to deal with common problems of community living. CONCLUSION: Quality of life in the community requires solution to clients' demands and self-identified problems. A commitment to quality of service together with a client centered approach and concern for client's quality of life is a basic recipe for successful service delivery. While many professionals are personally committed to a client centered approach, those who work in agencies sampled, are limited in terms of their knowledge of client problems (other than those they are mandated to serve) and are unable to provide solutions to problems not in their basket of services.

How Friendly Are We? Building an Evaluation for the Elder Friendly Hospital Initiative.

Belinda Parke (Capital Health Region, Victoria Canada) Doug Balson (Capital Health Region, Victoria Canada)

PURPOSE: To explain the evaluation process of the Elder Friendly Hospital initiative. The Capital Health Region, located in Victoria, Canada has endeavored to be responsive to the needs of older adults, the primary users of hospital services, with the establishment of the Elder Friendly Hospital initiative. This initiative has brought a developmental approach to acute intervention care. METHOD: A system wide, client/patient satisfaction program using qualitative and quantitative strategies in a phased-in approach to determine, from the older adults' perspective, what is important and how well does the health region meet what older adults' report as important. Included is translating the voice of older adults to the planning process to inform regional decision-making regarding health care processes. RESULTS: A model for measuring client/patient satisfaction in an integrated multi site health region that takes into account the lived experience of those who use health services. The model is sensitive to the varied needs and expectations of older adult populations as they change over time and as the location of service changes. CONCLUSIONS: Numerous challenges are inherent in building a program that cuts across time, context and is sensitive to individual differences. To evaluate and improve care delivery from the client/patient experience a long-range satisfaction measurement program is required that gathers information in an ongoing, systematic way across time and the care delivery context. Such a program integrates various approaches to gathering information and allows for client/patient profiles to be developed based experience of care rather than how care is delivered.

Seniors organizing in a city undergoing amalgamation: Lessons from a participatory research project

L. Letts (McMaster University, Hamilton, Canada), B. Berger, B. Berger, D. Dix, A. Knowles, B. McClelland, L. Wells (Toronto Seniors Council, Toronto, Canada)

PURPOSE: In 1998, Toronto faced municipal amalgamation of six former municipalities into one city. Older adults in the city were concerned that their voices would be lost in this new large municipality. A participatory research project was undertaken to identify if there was a need for a seniors' organization in the newly-amalgamated Toronto, and how such an organization could be formed. METHODS: The project involved three major phases: 1) reaching out to expand the planning group, link with other organizations, and seek funding; 2) bringing seniors together through a consensus conference, and 3) planning action following the conference which included modifying the organizational structure, evaluation, and beginning to address issues of importance to seniors in the city. RESULTS: A number of lessons were learned from the research. The importance of different roles in the work (including administrative tasks, leadership and facilitation) and the need for institutional and financial support were themes throughout the organizing process. Issues of power and trust within and between seniors' groups were important aspects of the process. Challenges associated with continually expanding membership were also identified. Although efforts were made to reach out to seniors representing the diversity of the city (including language, culture, socioeconomic status, and ability) further work in this area is needed. CONCLUSIONS: The Toronto Seniors Council was formed as a result of this initiative. The group continues its work to promote quality of life for older adults in Toronto.

The concept of expectations in relation to formal support for elderly

G. Samuelsson (Gerontology Reserach Center, Lund, Sweden)

The concept of client expectations has more and more come in focus for the planning process of the future social services and care. Also client expectations on service quality are in line with the strivings to "consumer adjustment". The concept of expectations is however complicated and multifaceted and it is influenced of many different factors as welfare system, family system and individual characteristics. A method to measure expectations is presented.

Using Focus Groups with Elderly for Developing a Local Strategic Plan for Service Development

Malka Korazim, Tali Goren - JDC-Brookdale Institue of Gerontology and Human Development, Jerusalem,Israel

In recent years there has been a growing interest in local strategic planning of services for the elderly. Focus groups with the elderly are becoming an important tool in the process of determining needs as well as involving elderly in the planning process. The purpose of this paper is to present the experience acquired using this method in developing strategic plans for the elderly in two big cities in Israel Tel Aviv and Jerusalem. In each city we conducted about 15 focus groups with different types of clients Jewish elderly, Arab elderly, elderly from low and high socio-economic levels, new immigrants, etc. The data collected through these groups revealed differences between the elderly and professionals with regard to determining needs and priorities. Main issues of concern to the elderly were the attitude to the elderly by service providers, the physical aspects of the environment and its safety, the need for upgrading recreational activities, and the cost of health services. The professionals were more often concerned with other issues: sheltered employment, services for the disabled elderly, and housing. The focus groups proved useful not only in raising new issues but also in providing concrete solutions for service development. At the same time, despite its advantages as an efficient resource on clients views and needs, there are still methodological and process-related questions that should be addressed, including how best to use focus groups as a tool for data collection and as a component and input resource in developing strategic plans for services for the elderly.

Working with older participants in a voluntary project to develop an evaluation tool for the project

Pat Chambers (Keele University, Staffordshire, UK) Jill Pickard (University College Northampton, UK)

The purpose of this study was to involve older participants from the Lifetime Project (which facilitates activities for older people over 50 in Northamptonshire, UK) in the design and pilot of an evaluation tool for the project. This tool was intended to reflect both the language and priorities of the participants and would be used as part of the ongoing evaluation and development of the project. A number of focus groups were held, comprising approximately one fifth of overall project membership. Firstly to ascertain the expectations and experience of project members to date and secondly to facilitate discussion on issues of quality. Key words and phrases were written down and agreed with participants and the resultant data collated and analysed using thematic analysis. Five themes were identified as indicators for evaluation: practicalities; social; education; health; challenging negative images of old age. These themes, in the words and phrases of the participants, were then incorporated into a questionnaire. The resultant questionnaire was piloted with some of the focus group participants, where it was favourably received and considered to reflect the flavour, content and language of the original focus group discussions. The project is now being evaluated using this tool. The project management team is committed to responding to these evaluations and both results and responses will be distributed to all project members via a newsletter. The study demonstrates the potential for older people to be active participants in the research process and thereby influence both practice and the delivery of services.

SESSION 379

A way to a qualitative policy on education: a bridge between elderly facilities and educational institutions

E. Messelis, H. Clincke & C. Geerts (Free University Brussels; Brussels; Belgium)

Elderly facilities often have to resort to external eductional institutions for organising a policy on education for their staff. To this day it is difficult to have a clear view on the ample amount of external educational organisations. The first part of the study examines by means of a written questionnaire, sent to the boards of 771 elderly facilities. They were asked which educational institutions they know, which they resort to and which experience they have with the latter. The second part examines, by means of a written questionnaire, 42 educational institutions, by assessing their view on their own internal quality. 67 boards have responded in the first part. The responding elderly facilities appear to know many educational institutions operating in eldery facilities (N=35). Half of the responding elderly facilities appear to resort to 24 of those educational institutions. Two thirds of the facilities which resort to external educational institutions claim to have a positive experience with the latter, as the supply of eductional institutions appears to meet the educational demands of them. Twelf educational institutions have responded in the second part of the study. All responding institutions appear to know quality systems (ISO 9000, CEDEO-EFQM,...). Only half of those institutions provide qualitative care according to a certain quality system. All responding institutions which resort to quality systems, are favourable to their use, as quality can be systematically examined. In conclusion, the study points out that the educational institutions can grow into a true partnership with the elderly facilities.

Creating a Bridge Across Cultural Divides: Ethnocultural Guide for Frontline Staff in Long Term Care

Saira Haq (Diversicare / Rockcliffe Long Term Care Facility, Toronto, Canada)

PURPOSE: In response to an increasingly diverse cultural population in our long term care facilities, the need to explore provision of culturally sensitive care became apparent. METHOD: Survey method was used to determine present understanding among staff of cultural differences and culturally sensitive care. Surveys were tabulated and trends were tracked. Based on survey results, a cultural assessment tool was designed to gather information from the resident, to guide the delivery of culturally sensitive care. Written information from the assessment was transferred to visual symbols at the bedside. Education for staff was done by the planning team, using case studies of residents within the facilities to enrich learning. RESULTS: Survey results suggest staff awareness of cultural differences, however a deficit in their ability to apply cultural knowledge to the provision of daily care. The three tiered model based on assessed needs, recognition of different learning styles and application of cultural knowledge to front line staff, has enhanced the delivery of culturally sensitive care to the residents. CONCLUSION: Post implementation survey results will show that the education guide and practical application to a long term care setting has enhanced transfer of knowledge to frontline staff, thus enhancing the provision of culturally sensitive care.

Cultivating Leaders for Today and Tomorrow: A Competitive Advantage

Helen Lantz (The CAPITAL CARE Group, Edmonton, CANADA)

The CAPITAL CARE Group, an innovative leader in continuing care, employs over 2400 staff. Following a staff survey that identified leadership as an area for improvement, The CAPITAL CARE Group developed a leadership profile defining critical and desirable leadership behaviors. This Profile was incorporated into recruitment processes, performance appraisals and education programs to enhance the quality of leadership. At the same time the organization identified recruitment and retention as a major cahleenge in the new millenium due to an increase in elderly clients and an aging workforce. Recently The CAPITAL CARE Group began looking for a systematic process of identifying, assessing and developing in-house high flyers to ensure qualified candidates for key clinical, research and managerial positions within the organization. A first step was to review and fine tune the Leadership Profile. Comsultants were hired to help develop a structured program to fit with the culture of the organizationand support other human resource practices. The consultants completed a benchmark study of comparable organizations' leadership programs and conducted research on various aspects of program development and implementation including coaching and mentoring models. This presentation will describe the journey to integrate strategic direction and business goals with career devlopment and personal learning plans, resulting in a Leadership Planning Model for The CAPITAL CARE Group. The goal of this Model is to create a culture and environment more favorable to undearthing the talent and skills of employees. Leadership Planning is a dynamic and continuous process of growing, cultivating and developing people and future leaders.

Intergenerational Service Learning: Effects on Attitudes Toward the Elderly

F. Butler (George Mason University, Fairfax, USA)

The purpose of this research was to determine attitude changes toward the elderly as a result of participation in a service-learning program over a three-month period. Intergenerational service learning components were incorporated into one undergraduate and one graduate gerontology course in a large university. The courses were modified to incorporate effective intergenerational exchanges and reciprocal learning. Nursing and health sciences students enrolled in either of these courses, partnered with older adults and provided practical health promotion and disease prevention information using email and the project’s web page and chat room. Seniors shared their life experiences with students and met with their partners face to face for socializing and joint computer classes. Students were encouraged to develop innovative teaching strategies to assist elders in maintaining function and independent living. The NIA Aging Knowledge test and The 14-Item Geriatrics Attitudes Scale were administered to 28 students prior to beginning the project and at the conclusion of the project. Results showed significant mean differences ($p<.001$) between pre and post attitudes tests for the entire group. Most of this is attributed to graduate students who had significantly ($p<.05$) higher aging test scores, and showed a significantly ($p<.001$) greater mean increase in positive attitudes toward the elderly on post attitude testing. This study suggests that ongoing exposure to the well elderly, meaningful exchanges, reciprocal learning and engaging in productive activities to enhance the well being of older adults are effective strategies for improving attitudes toward the elderly. Not surprisingly, knowledge of aging fosters more positive attitudes.

The Future of Long-term Care is at College

Peterborough, Ontario, Canada)

Two leading long-term care providers and a leading educational institution have partnered to build an exciting and dynamic vision of long-term care and education - St. Joseph's at Fleming. It will be built on the Sir Sandford Fleming College campus in Peterborough, Ontario. The college's innovative centre, the Institute for Healthy Aging will be situated in this facility. Residents will share their wisdom, knowledge and experience with students, staff and volunteers in this vibrant intergenerational community. People living at St. Joseph's at Fleming will have access to meaningful, challenging and satisfying activities. Both Fleming and St. Joseph's staff are developing a professional environment of discovery and learning that will attract researchers, teachers and learners from around the world. Training in geriatric care will be of such a high standard that it will become a sought-after specialty, meeting our community's needs and representing new models of care. The Institute for Healthy Aging will co-ordinate new courses, clinical practice and applied research for students, develop new College curriculum, promote healthy aging in the College and the community, pilot new technology initiatives with its partners, and provide development and educational opportunities for professionals. This is just a beginning. The College and long-term care partners see the potential for further relevant development that will benefit the region and the country.

SESSION 380

AD FitnessCare

P. Heyn (University of Central Florida, Human Services ad Wellness Department, Orlando, Florida, USA)

The purpose of this presentation is to demonstrate how to design an exercise therapy program for mentally impaired adults with Alzheimer's disease to improve their psychological and physical abilities. This program is designed to provide time for enjoyment through exercise. The exercises involved in this program are specifically designed for Alzheimer's Dementia type individuals and do not involve anything, which could be considered strenuous or dangerous. The physical assessments are noninvasive procedures. Objectives: Participants will: 1. Develop an awareness for the major components of wellness for dementia; 2. Identify the physiological and practical benefits of exercise; 3. Understand the therapeutic value of formal exercise program for the cognitive impair older adult; 4. Analyze the key assessment that we can use as markers to follow our risk factor progressions; 5. Identify the intervention strategies that will change lifestyle; 6. Experience the cultural support that will nurture adherence and compliance to an exercise program; 7. Develop exercises routines for the cognitive impair older adult; 8. Adapt and modify exercises for special conditions; 9. Decrease cognitive impairment through exercise application; 10. Develop proper, safe, and fun exercise to music; 11. Awareness of proper body posture, movement, and technique. Ultimately, participantswill be clear of how exercise can play an important role in maintaining independent and healthier living for Alzheimer's disease.

Cognitive decline and nutritional assessment

Gil P, Mesa C, López P, Silva L. (Geriatrics Service; Hospital Clínico San Carlos. Madrid. Spain.) and DEMENU Study (Nutricia).

AIMS: To know nutritional status on patients with Alzheimer's disease (AD) in moderate-severe stage living in nursing homes. METHODS: 99 AD patients according to NINCDS-ADRDA criteria moderate-severe stage (FAST 5-6) were included (DEMENU study). Terminal stage patients and/ or patients with enteral/parenteral nutrition were not included. The following data were collected: age, gender, timing of disease progression, Mini-Mental examination, nutritional assessment test (Mini Nutritional Assessment, MNA), behavioural disturbances (NPI), weight, height, skinford thickness and biochemical measurements: protein, albumin, cholesterol, calcium, iron, phosphor, zinc, magnesium, retinol, alta-tocopherol, vitamin B and flavonoides. Data base SPSS, statistical measurement of common tendency and dispersion and quantity comparative data t-Student (confidence interval 95%). RESULTS: Number of patients: 99 (mean age 88.5 +/- 6.1; women 79%; associated disorders 4.4 +/- 2). Cognitive Assessment, MMSE, 12.2 +/- 5.3. Blessed 13.8 +/- 4.2. NPI 10.8 +/- 5.7. Nutritional Assessment: MNA < or = 17: 17.5%; 17-23.5: 68.4%. BMI 24.3 +/- 2.8. Biochemical measurements: Zinc < 70 mcg/ dl: 80%; Fe < 68 mcg/dl: 47%; Albumin < 3.5 g/l: 30%; Total Protein < 6.5/ dl: 52.6%; Vitamin E < 5.8 mgr/dl: 23%. CONCLUSIONS: 1.- Alzheimer's disease patients living in nursing homes have a high frequency of protein-caloric malnutrition. 2.- Vitamin and mineral deficits must be carefully evaluated in these patients.

Coping patterns with eating for older adults suffering from dementia

Z. Guernina (Thames Valley University)

The purpose of this study is to show that problems with eating are increasing in prevalence among older adults, especially those suffering from dementia. The rationale is to identify coping patterns of eating among a sample of dementia sufferers in a hospital in Hull, UK. Observation and questionnaires filled in by carers were used. Different coping patterns are used by functional and organic patients. It is suggested that increasing awareness to the variety of patterns might reduce some of the problem beahviors, such as drooling, spitting or overfilling the mouth with food.

Influences on Mealtime Activities of Eating-Dependent People with Dementia Living in Long-Term Care

A.J. Gibbs, H.H. Keller, J.A. Tindale. (Department of Family Relations and Applied Nutrition, University of Guelph, Guelph, Canada)

Purpose: Promoting positive mealtime experiences for people with dementia contributes to quality of life. This study uses a Grounded Theory approach to address the current lack of Canadian research into eating dependency of people with dementia living in long-term care facilities (LTCFs). The aim is to develop a substantive theory about mealtimes in LTCFs that can guide multi-disciplinary clinical practice and research. Method: Initial data were collected through direct mealtime observations of residents with dementia living in Special Care Units (SCUs) at two publicly funded LTCFs in Ontario (n=20). Each resident was observed for nine meals, on three non-consecutive days. Early qualitative analysis suggested that interviews with key informants would contribute to the developing theory. Eight clinical dietitians, five registered nursing staff and eighteen health care aides working in LTCFs participated in personal, in-depth interviews. The Constant Comparison method of analysis was used to analyze and conceptualize the data. Results: A substantive theory entitled "Influences on Mealtime Activities of Eating-Dependent Residents with Dementia" emerged from the data. At the core of the theory are six categories of resident mealtime activities: arriving, eating, waiting, socializing, miscellaneous distracted activities and leaving. These activities appear to be influenced by internal factors (i.e. a resident's physical, clinical and social characteristics) and external influences (i.e. co-residents' activities, direct caregiving activities, indirect caregiving activities, organizational activities and governmental activities). Conclusion: Findings indicate that multi-disciplinary, multi-level mealtime interventions addressing all six categories of mealtime activities are needed to ensure optimal mealtime experiences for residents with dementia.

Psychocorrective methods in improving the activity of old age patients with vascular organic brain syndrome.

Kruglov L.S, M.D, (Saint Petersburg V.M.Bechterev psychoneurological institute, Saint Petersburg, Russia)

The Abstract. PURPOSE: To reveal the significance of psychocorrective influences for the clinical and social results of the therapy of patients suffering from the vascular organic brain syndrome. This condition is considerably spread in the old age and problems relating to its treatment are of significant importance. Today purely pharmacotherapeutic methods are insufficiently effective and there is a necessity to optimize the therapy of such patients, in particular by means of including the psychocorrective influences into the complex of care for them. METHODS. The test and control cohorts were selected. Each cohort included 48 patients. The cohorts were identical to each other in all main factors influencing the results of the therapy but differed in the volume of the psychocorrective influences used. For examination in the dynamics of treatment the SCAG scale, ten words memorizing test and Shulte's tables were used. The statistical processing of the obtained data was made using the Multiple Regression Analysis together with calculation of the average errors and chi-square. RESULTS. It was revealed that if the psychocorrective methods were used in the sufficient volume the patients' condition improved more considerably. Besides that, even in case of slight therapeutic reduction of the psychopathologic symptoms the above mentioned methods favour preserving a certain level of occupancy in the household and for some patients even improving it. CONCLUSIONS. The systematic use of psychocorrective methods is of considerable importance for the clinical results of the therapy of the vascular organic brain syndrome and for the social functioning of such patients. The positive influence on the level of the latter is connected not only with improvement of the clinical indices but also with direct optimizing the every day life occupancy level.

Reliability and validity testing of a feeding abilities assessment for persons with dementia

Wells, Donna L, RN, (University of Toronto, Toronto, Ontario, Canada) LeClerc, Chantale Marie, RN, (St. Michael's Hospital, Toronto, Ontario, Canada) Sidani, Souraya, RN, (University of Toronto, Toronto, Ontario, Canada) Dawson, Pam, RN, MSN (Baycrest Centre for Geriatric Care, Toronto, Ontario, Canada) Fay, Julie, MA (research assistant)

PURPOSE: The purpose of this study was to test the reliability and validity of a Feeding Abilities Assessment (FAA) developed for persons suffering from ideational apraxia as a result of dementia and living in long-term care facilities. The 32 item assessment determines the level of ability retained and suggests appropriate interventions to maximize a person's ability to self-feed. METHODS: A descriptive, comparative design was used to test the reliability (test-retest, inter-rater and internal consistency) and validity (content and construct) of the FAA. A sample of 259 residents (156 with dementia and a control group of 103 without dementia) was generated from four long-term care facilities within the greater Toronto Metropolitan area. The average age of those in the sample was 84 years. More than half were women (54%) and they had resided in the facilities an average of 2.4 years. Two research assistants were trained in the use of the FAA and administered the assessment. RESULTS: Data analysis showed that the FAA was both reliable and valid. Test-retest yielded a Pearson's r=.99. For inter-rater reliability, the Kappa coefficient=.98. The

FAA has internal consistency as evidenced by a Cronbach's alpha=.99. The content validity index (CVI) was equal to .80 and construct validity was determined by an independant sample t test, t=-10.10 [df=155, p<.01]. CONCLUSION: With a reliable and valid assessment of a person's feeding abilities, nurses and caregivers can determine the amount of assistance or intervention required by a resident during feeding. As a consequence, unnecessary dependence may be prevented.

SESSION 382

Assessing the risk of functional limitations among-low income elderly in Santiago, Chile

PP Marin, T Hoyl, H Gac, G Gonzalez, S Castro, E Valenzuela, R Kornfeld (Geriatric Program, Departament of Internal Medicine, School of Medicine, Pontificia Universidad catolica de Chile), SP Wallace (UCLA School of Public Health, Los Angeles, CA, USA)

PURPOSE: To determine the feasibility and utility of a short, simple screening tool for use in primary care clinics in low income communities in Chile and elsewhere in Latin America. METHOD: 1339 persons age 65 and over were screened in ambulatory clinics in two low income communities in Santiago, Chile between 1996 and 1999 as part of a larger program bringing geriatric services to those communities. The screening was completed using questions with yes/no responses that was completed rapidly by the primary physician or office nurse. RESULTS: The average of those screened was 72 years, and 74% were women. The most common health problems encountered were poor vision (77.8%), self reported depression (69.7%) and self reported memory problems (61.1%). Over one-third of the women reported falls and urinary incontinence. One or more of seven functional incapacities were reported by 10.6%. These disabled elders were older, more likely to have no living children, be underweight, depressed, incontinent, have poor hearing and be taking more than three medications. CONCLUSIONS: Urban low income elders in Chile exhibit alarmingly high rates of many risk factors for functional impairment. The instrument used (Ficha Valoracion Geriatrica Ambulatoria Universidad Catolica -FEGAUC) was found to be easy to administer and quickly identified risk factors for functional decline that could be modified in a primary care practice. Efforts to reduce these risk factors need to take a higher priority in the health care systems of Latin American countries such as Chile.

Elderly home care clients in three Swedish municipalities. Characteristics and health related problems.

C. Lindencrona (The National Board of Health and Welfare, Stock-holm Sweden) and B-G. Emtinger (The County Council, Linköping, Sweden)

PURPOSE: The purpose of the study was to explore and describe elderly homecare clients and their health related problems. METHOD: All elderly clients cared for in their own home were investigated in three municipalities (n=737). Data collection was carried out during one specific week through home visits. The data collector was known to the elderly and had experience of her/his care situation. In a conversational form, a structured questionnaire was completed. Also, patient records and official statistics were studied. RESULTS: The mean age of the home care client was 82 years. The majority women living alone (67%). The largest group managed with ADL-assistance from the social service agency (70%). Thirty percent received professional nursing by a district nurse and four percent advanced home care from the hospital. The most demanding group received care from both the social service agency and by the district nurse. This group represented the widest range of symptoms and care needs. Among them about 50 percent reported having pain; 40 percent that it daily interrupted their ADL-activities and 14 percent that medication did not give full relief. About one third suffered from urine incontinence (38%) and dizziness (35%). Home visits by a doctor was not documented. CONCLUSION: Separate groups of elderly home care clients emerged. The majority of elderly was cared for by a nurse aid. The most vulnerable and demanding group of elderly were those who in addition received care by a district nurse. For all home care clients, regular medical and professional nursing assessment need to be guaranteed.

Functional abilities and cognitive status of users of home care in Germany

V. Garms-Homolova (Institut fuer Gesundheitsanalysen und soziale Konzepte e.V, Berlin, Germany)

Purpose: At present 1.31 million Germans receive benefits in kind or money from the Social Insurance for Long Term Care. Little is known about the beneficiaries, since the Medical Service of the Insurance Institutions only collect data on applicants. A study in home care agencies - the empirical basis for this presentation - shed light on the status and disability profiles of population receiving benefits in kind. Method: MDS HC assessment of 477 clients (average age = 82 years) of home care agencies in Germany (service oriented sample). Results: Clients suffering from moderate to severe cognitive problems (worsening of memory, moderate to severe difficulties in everyday decision making) represent 39 per cent of the users of home care, i.e. the largest group. As frequent adjacent problems occur behavioural and mood difficulties as well as impaired communication. The portion of the clients with prevailing physical disabilities - those who serve as prototypes of beneficiaries when the long term care insurance was developed - amount "only" to 30 per cent. Nineteen per cent have serious psychological problems. Conclusion: The study shows a high prevalence of cognitive problems and prove, that the needs for care of the population actually served by the home care agencies differ considerably from the original intention of the Social Insurance for Long Term Care, which was designed mainly to cover the needs of the population with disabilities of elementary ADL.

Home visits - A means to prevent loss of function

Britt Mari Hellner (The National Board of Health and Welfare, Stockholm, Sweden)

This paper describes an experimental work where the aim is to develop knowledge about how to support health and well-being and prevent illness and need of care among the elderly. 21 municipalities received financial support from the Swedish government to develop home visiting programs. The municipalities had to fulfil certain demands to receive the governmental grant - that the preventive home visits were offered regularly during three years and carried out by professionals and that the project was monitored and evaluated. Within these frames the municipalities have designed their visiting programs according to local conditions. 3500 elderly persons participate in the project. The participants are citizens mostly over 75 years, living independently, i.e. in their own homes and without regular help from the municipality or health care system. Physical and mental health and functioning as well as social networks and well being are focused and evaluated during the visits. Most participants report that they are satisfied with their health, functional ability and well being. Although experiences from the first visit indicate that there are individuals as well as certain areas needing intervention. Frail elderly, caring for a demented spouse is one example of concealed problems revealed through home visits. Anxiety and depression are common problems among elderly emigrants and problems due to isolation and loneliness are common in the sparsely populated mountain districts. Until now the benefit of the home visits has been mainly individual. When the programs develop further hopefully results will be noticed in society as well.

The Home Independence Program.

Gill Lewin, Hilary O'Connell, Bev Wheeler and Brandi Acker (Silver Chain, Perth, Australia)

In recent years Silver Chain, like many other Home Care agencies, has found itself in a vicious cycle where demand forever outstrips supply. While one possible response would have been to continue to tighten eligibility criteria in an attempt to control demand, an alternative approach was to develop services which actively work to reduce the demand for ongoing home care. This was the approach adopted by Silver Chain. The result in service terms has been the development of the Home Independence Program (HIP) - a home based early intervention program directed at reversing or slowing down the disablement processes resulting from ageing and chronic diseases associated with ageing. Prior to embarking on a controlled intervention study, a pilot study of HIP was undertaken to trial and refine all aspects of the program. 49 individuals referred for home care have participated in the program. Preliminary results show that: 52% of participants demonstrated a measurable improvement in IADLs following the program whilst 81% reported experiencing less difficulty in their performance, and 82% required either a reduced level or no services following the intervention. The Home Independence program has been demonstrated to have the potential to reduce the demand for home care services. A controlled intervention study is required to determine the cost effectiveness of this program in both the short and longer term.

The Preventive Care Trial - A Three Year Randomised Controlled Trial of Home-based Health Assessments for the Over 70's

Julie E Byles (The University of Newcastle, NSW, Australia), Meredith Tavener (The University of Newcastle, NSW, Australia), Patrick Fitzgerald (The University of Newcastle, NSW, Australia), Balakrishnam R Nair (Division of Geriatric Medicine, John Hunter Hospital, Newcastle, NSW, Australia), Nick Higginbotham (The University of Newcastle, NSW, Australia) Claire Jackson (Centre for General Practice and Primary Health Care Integration, University of Queensland, Brisbane QLD, Australia), Richard F Heller (The University of Newcastle, NSW, Australia) Jonathan Newbury (Department of General Practice, University of Adelaide, South Australia, Australia)

PURPOSE: Health assessments for older people have potential to improve quality of life and reduce health care use. This study is an RCT of a series of home based preventive care health assessments with veterans/ war widows aged over 70 years. METHOD: The assessments were conducted over a three year period with 942 veterans randomly selected from 10 Australian regions. Veterans received an assessment in their home either annually or every 6 months, during which questions were asked from a specially developed checklist on topics such as nutrition, home safety, hearing, medications, vaccinations, and social support. A further 627 veterans acted as controls and took part in an annual telephone survey to collect outcome data on hospital and nursing home admissions, service utilisation and quality of life. RESULTS: Common health problems reported by veterans included no recent hearing check (63%), feet problems (45%), trouble sleeping (41%), and poor nutrition (37%). A total of 4304 medications were recorded during the first year of assessments with 53% of veterans taking 4 or more medications regularly. Interim results report no significant differences in hospital and nursing home admissions between control and intervention veterans, however significant differences existed in the emotional sub-scale and physical component score of the SF-36. CONCLUSION: The Preventive Care Checklist proved easy to administer, acceptable to participants and contained valid items for use with an older veteran population. The Trial demonstrated collaborative models for the conduct of assessments in the community, and the potential for non-medical health professionals to conduct visits in the home.

SESSION 384

Evaluation of transfer devices to reduce the risk of musculoskeletal injury to home care workers

Nancy Paris-Seeley (British Columbia Institute of Technology, Vancouver, Canada) Silvia Raschke, CO(C), (British Columbia Institute of Technology, Vancouver, Canada) James Watzke (British Columbia Institute of Technology, Vancouver, Canada) Yvette Jones (Simon Fraser University, Vancouver, Canada) Nigel Halsted (British Columbia Institute of Technology, Vancouver, Canada)

PURPOSE: The objectives of the study were to: (1) evaluate existing portable client transfer aids in terms of reducing the risk of MSI to home care workers in the bathroom setting, and (2) develop a detailed set of performance requirements for an optimal transfer device, or set of devices, for the bathroom setting. METHOD: A biomechanical evaluation and psychophysical assessment of a bathtub transfer board, portable bathtub side rail, raised toilet seat, walking transfer belt and baseline manual method for transferring clients into and out of the bathtub and on and off the toilet in the home bathroom setting were conducted. RESULTS: The results indicate that the devices tested did not reduce the moment on the home care workers L5/S1 joint under the tested condition. The bathtub transfer board and walking transfer belts demonstrated an increase in the moment. The study participants reported the perceived physical stress ratings to be low, even when the bio-mechanical data shows that they are at risk. Due to the perception of low risk, the worker's body bio-mechanics may not prepare them for a catastrophic failure of a transfer, such as a slip. CONCULSION: Opportunities for innovation exist in the development and commercialization of affordable transfer devices developed specifically for the home setting. One of the key performance requirements that must be met to substantially reduce risk of injury to a home care worker is to reduce loads on the L5/S1 joint to safe limits under the highest risk conditions.

Gateway to independence: assistive technology and older users

Claudine McCreadie,Anthea Tinker andJanet Askham (King's College London, Age Concern Institute of Gerontology. London. England); Alan Turner-Smith (King's College London, Centre of Rehabilitation Engineering. London. England)

Gerontologists and rehabilitation engineers have been working in partnership with older people to explore the feasibility of involving them in the early stages of engineering innovations. Two small projects have been funded under the U.K. government's EQUAL (Extending Quality of Life) initiative. One project focused on the development of a wayfinding device for use inside large complex buildings, the second on issues relating to indoor mobility. In both cases, a three stage methodology was employed. The first stage involved focus groups of older people in discussing their problems and solutions in relation to the two project topics. In the second stage, the engineers developed functional solutions based on the older users' views. In stage three, the older participants tried out the solutions. Older people, sometimes with substantial degrees of physical or sensory disability, were able to articulate clearly their views in a way that affected basic engineering design. They were enthusiastic about participating in the research. The engineers benefited, particularly by the involvement of the older users at two points in time. The approach enabled the ideas to be tested effectively without the large and costly investment of full prototype development. Finally, the research demonstrated the value of multi-disciplinary approaches, with social scientists and engineers collaborating in a way which opened the eyes of each to the input, knowledge and experience of the other.

Home for life: introducing assistive technology into the existing homes of older people

Claudine McCreadie,Anthea Tinker (King's College London, Age Concern Institute of Gerontology. London England.), Donna Cowan and Alan Turner-Smith (King's College London, Centre of Rehabiliation Engineering. London. England)Peter Lansley, Keith Bright and Susan Flanagan (University of Reading, Department of

Construction Management. London. England)

This multi-disciplinary project involving gerontologists, building surveyors and rehabilitation engineers begins from the recognition that much research on housing, technology and older people is based on NEW housing, whereas the vast majoirty of older people are living in older housing. The type and condition of the property may constrain the introduction of technology. This poses an important issue about how far technology can help older people remain in their own homes for life. The research has investigated with a range of social housing providers and with older occupants of their properties the feasibility, acceptability, costs and outcomes of technology that has been installed, using a combination of interviews, questionnaires and focus group discussions. The surveyors have audited the building types, and the engineers drawn up a package of assistive technology addressing three levels of hypothetical need. Assistive technology includes a full range of devices from stair rails and ramps to those based on electronics and computers. The paper will report on first year findings from the research which commenced in October 2000. These will cover: 1. the technology provision currently being made by our sample of social housing landlords; 2. the suitability of their housing stock for AT provision; and 3. the experience of older occupants of the provision and use of technology.

PROTOge : A Student Mentoring Program for Assistive Device Prototypes

James Watzke & Sara Frederking (Health Technology Research Group, British Columbia Institute of Technology, Burnaby, British Columbia, CANADA)

This paper presents a unique program designed to help post-secondary students explore the commercial potential of their assistive device prototypes, as well as raise students' awareness of the assistive device industry in British Columbia. Twelve individual inventors or teams and their assistive device prototypes are selected each year for the program, which is free for those accepted. Upon entering the program, a custom mentoring team and plan is created for each student/team, which exposes the inventors to a series of typical mentoring activities, e.g, 1) formal assessment of their prototype; 2) user testing (with carefully selected target consumers) with their prototype in a full-scale simulation laboratory or real-life setting, depending on which is most appropriate or practical; 3) design and engineering improvements to the prototype; and 4) guidance with the commercialization process, e.g, marketing research, patent searches, seminars on assorted commercialization topics by local industry experts. The program is in its second year, and has enjoyed significant success to date. The prototypes, experiences, and outcomes from Year 1 of the program will be highlighted, as well as information on how the program will be modified/improved for its forthcoming year.

Stimulating Mainstream Science and Engineering Research to Meet the Needs of an Ageing Society

P. R. Lansley (Research Group for Inclusive Environments, The University of Reading, United Kingdom)

The EPSRC EQUAL initiative encourages successful academics and researchers operating in the mainstream disciplines of architecture, building, surveying, industrial design, engineering and the physical sciences, to change the focus of their interests and to become committed to research into issues arising from the needs of older people and the ageing population as well as the needs of individuals with a range of physical and mental disabilities. Through a series of 22 large and small projects, engineering and physical scientists and social, medical and health scientists work with industry, government, voluntary agencies, other intermediaries and, particularly, users, on scientifically challenging user-defined problems concerned with achieving: a) inclusive environments and inclusive designs which are sympathetic to older people, and b) with the development of more effective approaches to rehabilitation. The initiative has successfully stimulated interest in ageing-related research and it has facilitated the initial development of a new inter-disciplinary community of researchers outside of conventional medical and health research communities. The main future challenges for the initiative are: a) maintaining momentum by establishing ageing-related research as a valued area within the mainstream of engineering and physical science, and b) sustaining the new research community with its vibrant links to users, industry, government and policy makers.

SESSION 386

A randomised trial of home-based strength training on physical health in frail elderly patients

Nancy Latham (Clinical Trials Research Unit, University of Auckland, Auckland, New Zealand), Craig Anderson (Clinical Trials Research Unit, University of Auckland, Auckland, New Zealand), Arier Lee (Clinical Trials Research Unit, University of Auckland, Auckland, New Zealand), Caroline Stretton (Clinical Trials Research Unit, University of Auckland, Auckland, New Zealand), Anne Moseley (Rehabilitation Studies Unit, University of Sydney, Sydney, Australia), Ian Cameron (Rehabilitation Studies Unit, University of Sydney, Sydney, Australia)

PURPOSE: Frailty Interventions Trial in Elderly Subjects (FITNESS) was a randomised clinical trial with a factorial design to assess the effectiveness of progressive resistance strength training (PRT) and vitamin D to improve physical capacity in frail elderly people. This abstract is for PRT. METHOD: FITNESS was conducted across five hospitals in Australia and New Zealand during 1999 - 2000. All older people admitted to acute geriatric wards, assessed as 'frail' by the attending clinician using broad criteria and able to participate were eligible. A central randomisation service was used. Patients assigned PRT used adjustable ankle weights to perform moderate-high intensity quadriceps training 3 times / week for 10 weeks at home under the supervision of a physiotherapist (weekly visits or phone calls). Control participants received frequency matched (social) visits. Performance and self-report measures of health and activities were evaluated by assessors blind to treatment allocation at 3, 6 and 12 months post-randomisation. The primary efficacy endpoint was a 10 0ifference in Physical Component Summary measure of the SF-36 between groups at 3 months. RESULTS: The study population (n=243) was 47% male, mean age 79yrs (range 65-96). Baseline Barthel Index scores (0-20) were 9-14 13%, 15-19 58%, and 20 290f participants (mean 17.8). Adherence to strength training was good, with a mean of 830f prescribed sessions completed. CONCLUSION: The study results will be presented at the meeting. FITNESS will provide evidence of the effectiveness of strength training to improve physical function in the frail elderly.

Coordination Exercise and Postural Stability in the Elderly People: Effect of Tai Chi Chuan

Alice M.K. Wong, Yin-Chou Lin, Shih-Wei Chou, Fuk-Tan Tang, Pong-Yeun Wong (Department of Physical Medicine and Rehabilitation, Chang Gung Memorial Hospital, Taiwan)

To evaluate the effects of coordination exercise on postural stability in older individuals by Chinese shadow boxing, Tai Chi Chuan (TCC). The TCC group, 25 subjects, had been practicing TCC regularly for 2 to 35 years. The control group included 14 healthy and active older subjects. They were tested by static and dynamic balance of Sensory Organization Testing (SOT) of the Smart Balance Master System. In static postural control, the results showed no differences between the TCC or control group in the more simple conditions, but in the more complicated SOT (eye close with sway surface and sway vision with sway surface), the TCC group had significantly better results than the control group. TCC group had significantly better results only in the rhythmic forward - backward weight-shifting test. Duration of practice seems not affect the stability of elder people. We proposed that the regular TCC practice could significantly improve postural stability in older individuals, especially in the more complicated conditions with visual and somatosensory conditions being disturbed. For the older persons, it seems never too late to begin an exercise regimen as TCC for coordination training.

Evaluation of Physical Training in Elderly Patients with Obesity

F.Revnic ("Ana Aslan" N.I.G.G, Bucharest, Romania) N.Teleki, M.Berteanu, C.Paraschiv (N.I.P.M.R, Bucharest, Romania), C.R. Revnic (U.M.F."Carol Davila", Bucharest, Romania)

Obesity is one of the most important health problem.Obese are perceived by others to have physical,metal,emotional and moral impairement.Inactivity may play a major role in body composition and metabolic status and could be related with GHRH-GHIGF1 axis.HGH is the locomotive that pulls all the hormones in the aging process.objective:The aim of this study was related with the effects of moderate levels of physical exercises upon endocrine(HGH,T3,T4,TBG,hTSH,Cortisol secretion),metabolical and physiological parameters in elderly female with obesity.Our study has been done on 24 patients aged between 45-75 years old) admited in Rehabilitation Clinique for osteoarticular and postraumatic pathologiesdivided into two groups:A:12 active patients and 12 from group B sedentary associated with obesity(10% with abnormal stereotyped pattern of food intake(night eatingsyndrome and 5% with bulimia). Standard physical training program(N.Teleki,F.Revnic,Geriatria VIII,5,1996) has been applied for 5 days consecutively.Cortisol,hTSH,hGH,T3,T4,TBG have been estimated in serum before and after training program with Delfia Research Spectrofluorimeter involving Eu+ labelled monoclonal antibodies with a FIA program and statistical evalualtion of data has been done using a Multicalc program.Serum cholesterol,Tg,Total lipids,Glucose,K+,Ca++,Mg++,TGP,TGO,CK,CKMB have been evaluated before and after training with Beckman ulrianalyser.Results: A decrease in hGH values has been recorded in sedentary obese patients associated with elevated levels of glucose and cholesterol.An increase in hTSH values in sedentary obese patients associated with an increase in T4/TBG ratio accaunts for a change in hypotalamo-hypophyiseal thyroid axis in After training,a decrease in cholesterol,Tg and total lipids has been recorded in group BMuscle adaptation to effort has been limited to a reduced efflux of CK in group A and elevated levels in group B accaunting for an impairement in sarcolemal integrity.Following training,there is an intimate modification in celular metabolism:the exit of K and Mg and entrance of Na,fixation of Pi by Pasteur effect,modifing cell membrane permeability.The relation between hGH levels and glucose before and after training is an inversely one.Following training an increase in hGH is conditioned by low levels of blood glucose.HGH and exercise may beneficialy sinergise in obese patients decreasing visceral adipose tissue.The improvement in performance of trained muscle is in part the result of intensified circulation in exercising muscle.Conclusion:Physical training in elderly obese patients leads to an increase in hGH secretion which in turn has a lipolitic activity,leading to a decrease in body fat and an increase in aerobic capacity with an improvement in emotional and mental health status.

Physical Activity Programme Evaluation in the Elderly

V. Diaz, I. Diaz, C. Villarroel, C. Acuna, A. Vives, A. Donoso, D. Nowogrodski. [HOSPITAL CLINICO UNIVERSIDAD DE CHILE, SANTIAGO, CHILE.]

Physical activity program evaluation in the elderly. Objective: To evaluate a physical activity program in low income elderly, changes in systolic and diastolic blood pressure,body hass index, depressive symptoms. Methods: Older adults who belonged to chronic diseases programs from 4 consulters (municipal) were included in a prospective, non randomized, interventional study. 2 techniques were used, first swimming twice a week during 3 months and second walking and breathing activities 3 times a week during 3 months. All participants were evaluated before and after activities. Statistical analysis included wilcoxon signed rank, t test and a probability of 0.05. Results: 134 elders participated, 116 women and 18 men. Age average was 66 years old, median 68 years old, 21 (15.67%) smoked, 73 (55.24%) had high blood pressure, 111 (82.84%) were receiving medicines, 32 (23.88%) drank alcohol, 2(1.5%) cardiac arrhythmia , and 7(5.22%) had diabetes mellitus. Average weight at the beginning was 68.27 kilograms (sd=10.30 and at the end was 67.73 kilograms (sd=13.37), t=2.47, (95% bmi: 0.1 to 0.9), wilcoxon for bmi, z:-3.35, p=0.001, t test for average systolic blood pressure at the beginning was 140.04 (sd= 14.7) and at the end was 132 (sd= 15.98), t test= 4.35, p=0.0001, (95% 2.8 to 7.5), average diastolic blood pressure at the beginning was 81.78 and at the end was 80.75, t test=1.4, p=1.16 not significant. Conclusions: Physical activity is highly beneficial for the elderly, getting better systolic blood pressure, body hass index, depressive symptoms, nocturia and joint symptoms.

SESSION 387

Dementia is predictive of poor outcome of hip fracture in elderly persons

A.S.Rigaud (Hopital Broca, Paris, France), L. Traykov (Unite INSERM 324, Paris, France), F Renaudin (Hopital Broca Paris, France), P Bouchacourt (Hopital Broca Paris, France), F Latour (Hopital Broca Paris, France), O. Hanon (Hopital Broca Paris, France), ML Seux (Hopital Broca Paris, France), H Barei (Hopital Broca Paris, France), F. Forette (Hopital Broca Paris, France).

This retrospective study was carried out to assess the relationship between hip fracture and dementia in the elderly. We included 154 elderly patients with a hip fracture (mean age 88±5 years) consecutively recruited in a geriatric hospital department. Patients were evaluated by detailed recording of medical history, physical examination, brain computed tomography and laboratory tests. Cognitive status was assessed by the Mini Mental State Examination and screening with a battery of neuropsychological tests. Dementia was diagnosed using the DSMIIIR criteria. The functional outcome of the rehabilitation and socio-economic consequences of the fracture were recorded. Our results showed that the percentage of demented patients was higher among hip fracture patients than in age-matched persons in the French population (54% vs 15% respectively). Sixty-two percent of the patients returned to their state of walking before the hip fracture, 27% had to use a frame and 11 0.000000ailed to regain the ability to walk. Poor functional outcome was more frequent in demented than non demented patients (p<0.001). Dementia and poor functional outcome of the rehabilitation were respectively associated with 3 and 4-fold increases in institutionalization rates. Dementia is frequent in elderly patients with a hip fracture and increases the risk of poor functional outcome and institutionalization for these patients. This suggests the need for multidimensional assessment and management of elderly persons with hip fracture.

Excess Mortality or Institutionalisation Following Hip Fracture: Men are at Greater Risk.

M.Fransen, M.Woodward, R.Norton (Institute for International Health, University of Sydney, Australia) E.Robinson, M.Butler (Clinical Trials Research Unit, University of Auckland, New Zealand) A.John Campbell (University of Otago, New Zealand)

Purpose: To assess the 2-year excess mortality or institutionalisation risk associated with hip fracture in people aged 60 years and over. Method: A cohort study of 565 community dwelling older people recently hospitalised with a hip fracture and 782 matched controls living in the same catchment area. At recruitment, information was gathered regarding marital status, cognition, vision, falls in the past year, comorbidity, medications, smoking, independence in activities of daily living, walking speed and general mobility. Mortality or institutionalisation was established 2 years later. Results: 2 years later, 52.1% of male hip fracture cases and 12.4% of male controls were dead or institutionalised compared with 39.2% of female hip fracture cases and 19.7% of female controls. Hip fracture patients were significantly more likely to be living alone, have a lower BMI, be cognitively impaired, have poorer vision, report more falls and have a poorer general health and physical function status prior to their hip fracture compared with controls. However, the (all) adjusted odds ratio for institutionalisation/mortality at 2 years was still 1.48 (95% CI 1.02, 2.19) for women and 6.89 (2.75, 17.27) for men. Conclusion: For both men and women who incur a hip fracture, the risks of death or institutionalisation within 2 years are increased compared with matched controls. The independent effect of hip fracture on this outcome was significantly greater for men than women. The marked influence of pre-fracture health status, physical limitations and gender on poor outcome have important implications for preventative strategies.

Hip Protectors: Experience in Residential Aged Care Facilities and the Community

Lockwood, K. (Hornsby Ku-ring-gai Hospital, Australia

Hip protectors have already been proven to be technically effective. However, a few hip fractures will occur despite correctly applied hip protectors being worn. This will occur in approximately one in 1500 falls. Adherence with hip protector use is variable and determines their overall effectiveness. There are many factors influencing compliance including where the older person is living.

In residential aged care facilities the staff will be the primary determinant of adherence. If the management of the facility is committed to hip protector use, high levels of compliance can be achieved, which may include the use of hip protectors at night. In these facilities it is likely to be beneficial if each resident has four or more pairs of hip protectors available for their use with the hip protector shields permanently sewn into the hip protector garment. The hip protectors should be easily laundered. Staff will require training in their use.

In community settings older people themselves will be primarily responsible for adherence to use. Encouragement from healthcare professionals, particularly a nurse or physiotherapist, will be beneficial as will the availability of a variety of sizes and styles of hip protector undergarments. Determining who should wear hip protectors is another area for consideration. Targeting on the basis of age and fall history is the simplest method. Other methods can be used including a more detailed falls risk assessment, or a bone mineral density measurement can be used. It may be beneficial to use hip protectors in conjunction with other fall or fracture prevention methods. This has not been studied in any detail but use of hip protectors in combination with exercise programs or medications to change bone quality may be effective.

Morbi-mortality in nonagenarians patients following hip fracture repair.

F.Formiga (CSU Bellvitge, L´Hospitalet de LL, Spain) , A.Lopez-Soto, R.Cristofol, E.Sacanella, F.Masanés, M.Crespo,H.Clinic, Barcelona, Spain), X.Valldeperas, D.Chivite J.Mascaró, R.Pujol.(CSU Bellvitge, L´Hospitalet de LL, Spain).

PURPOSE: To analize, prospectively, morbi-mortality following hip fracture surgery in nonagenarians patients. METHOD: Criteria for enrolment were: patients aged >89 years old admitted in two university hospitals because of traumatic hip fracture (n=117). Pathological fractures (n=2) and polifractures (n=3) were excluded. Barthel Index (BI) was measured in all patients at home, on admission, at discharge and at three moths of follow-up. Lower BI score (< 20) patients were excluded. Charlson comorbidity score (CS) and a validated mobility score, were also measured. All patients received comprehensive geriatric assessment. RESULTS: We included 106 patients (70% women); mean age was 92.4 years old; hospital stay was 16 ± 1 days. CS was 1.1 ± 0.2. BI previous to admission was 73 decreasing to 21 on admission (p<0.001). There was a persistent decline in BI at the moment of hospital discharge (24; p<0.001). BI three months later was 53; only 7 patients returned to base line ability. In-hospital mortality was 10 % and three-months accumulate mortality was 20%. Before injury 52% of patients were able to get about the house independently but only 6% at three months of folow-up. 88% returned to their prior dwelling. CONCLUSIONS: Nonagenarian patients have difficulties to recover their previous functional status after hip fracture repair. Nevertheless, the low mortality rate suggested that surgery followed by rehabilitation may be an effective therapy in this patients.

Sit-to-Stand test, a simple predictor of hip and other fractures in elderly women.

K.KAYAN, E.V.McCLOSKEY, R.U.ASHFORD, A.DEY, J.A.KANIS (UNIVERSITY OF SHEFFIELD, SHEFFIELD, U.K)

PURPOSE: We wished to assess whether a simple sit to stand assessment is associated with hip and other fragility fracture risk in elderly women. METHOD: 4346 women aged 75 years and above, at entry to a prospective, RCT study of the effect of a bisphosphonate on hip fracture risk were assessed for their ability to rise from a chair and classified into those who had difficulty to rise from a chair and those who had no difficulty. Median follow-up was 3.1 years and all incident fractures were verified radiologically. RESULTS: Women classified as having difficulty rising from a chair (31.8%) were significantly older (81.2±4.4 vs. 79.4 ±3.5 years, p<0.001), shorter (155.2±6.4 vs. 156.1± 6.0 cms, p<0.001), heavier (67.3±13.3 vs. 64.0±11.3 kg, p<0.001) and had a lower mean total hip BMD (0.74±0.15 vs. 0.76±0.13 g/cm2,<0.001) than those rising without difficulty. In women rising with difficulty, the incidence of hip fracture was increased two-fold compared to those rising without difficulty (3.3% vs.1.6%, p=<0.001; OR 2.18, 95% CI 1.45-3.30, p=0.0002). The risk of any non-hip fracture was also increased in women rising with difficulty (8.0 vs.6.1 %, p=0.015; OR 1.36, 95% CI 1.06-1.74, p=0.015). The increased risk persisted after adjustment for age, weight and hip BMD (OR 1.55, 95% CI 0.98-1.23, p=0.058 and OR 1.29, 95% CI 0.99-1.68, p=0.056 for hip and non-hip fractures respectively). CONCLUSION: We conclude that a simple test of the ability to rise from a chair to a standing position, is a good predictor of hip and other fragility fractures in elderly women.

SESSION 388

Assessing the Safety of the Cognitively Impaired Elderly Living in the Community

L. Poulin de Courval (CLSC Côte-des-Neiges, Montreal,Canada), D. Dastoor, S. Gauthier, I. Gélinas, M. Rossignol, J. Sampalis (McGill University, Montreal, Canada), L. Liu (University of Alberta, Edmonton, Alberta, Canada), David Gayton (Peace Arch Hospital, White Rock, B.C. Canada)

With the recent changes in Health care services, more seniors with cognitive impairments are cared for in their home. One major concern with this clientele is their safety as the nature of their condition puts them at risk for accidents. The purpose of this study is to develop a Safety Scale that could be used by community healthcare providers to: (1) evaluate the risk of accidents; (2) lower the risk of accidents; (3) assist with the evaluation of the need for institutionalization; (4) provide recommendations to family caregivers; and (5) enhance case management. The Safety Scale was validated in French and in English through a national study. It underwent content validation using experts in Montreal and Edmonton. The Scale was then administered at home to the caregivers of 175 community-residing patients with dementia in Quebec (92), Alberta (45) and British Columbia (38). Criterion validity was determined by correlating the Safety Scale scores with the patients' scores on the Modified Mini-Mental Status Examination (3MS) and the Neuropsychiatric Inventory (NPI). Construct validity was evaluated using 5 subjects in Edmonton, Alberta and 10 in White Rock, British Columbia who experienced a critical incident as a result of an accident. The test-retest and inter-rater reliability were also examined by administering the Safety Scale on three occasions, by 2 different interviewers.
Acknowledgement: This study is funded by Health Canada

Early psychosocial intervention in dementia through a memory clinic - a randomised controlled trial

E. Moniz-Cook , M.Wang, P. Campion (School of Medicine, University of Hull, UK) , E Gardiner (Department of Statistics, University of Hull, UK), I. Carr, G. Gibson, P. Duggan (Hull and East Riding Community NHS Trust, Hull, UK)

Memory clinics were established for the early diagnosis of dementia, but their value in psychosocial intervention remains uncertain. A randomised trial of psychosocial intervention in people over the age of 65 diagnosed with dementia in the Hull Memory Clinics, was undertaken. Subjects were stratified by MMSE score (>23; 17-23; < 17) and living situation (alone / with caregiver) and randomized to the experimental group(n=25) - 'memory clinic nurse intervention' or the control group (n=25) - 'usual intervention' by a community psychiatric nurse and a multidisciplinary EMI community team. The Clinic team offered all 50 families explanation of diagnosis and plans for follow-on support. The number of nurse-family contacts and the types interventions delivered were examined. These were: memory management, anxiety /depression management, delusion /hallucination management, family support/ monitoring and arranging practical services (e.g. benefits/ respite services) for caregivers. At six month follow-up there were: no significant differences in the number of nurse contacts with families; significant differences (p=0.05) in the day to day problems and burden reported by caregivers with the control group worsening; trends in lower depression in experimental dementia subjects (p=0.07); in both groups, where MMSE was low (<18) the number of nurse - family contacts were greater and the interventions used were practical services for caregivers; experimental subjects received more crisis preventive (memory / mood management) intervention. Early 'memory clinic' intervention may have potential in preventing family burden. These results are discussed in terms of community service provision (what works for whom when and where).

Evaluation of Three Generic Utility-based Quality of Life Measures in Alzheimer's Disease

G. Naglie, C. Tansey, M. Krahn, J. Irvine, P. Ritvo, G. Tomlinson, M. Silberfeld (University of Toronto, Toronto, Canada)

PURPOSE: To evaluate 3 generic utility-based quality of life (QOL) instruments to measure QOL in Alzheimers patients by self-report and by caregivers acting as proxy respondents. METHOD: Patients with mild or moderate Alzheimers disease (MMSE 10-27) and an informed caregiver were recruited from memory clinics and physician practices in Toronto. Patient-caregiver pairs were randomized to receive 1 of 3 utility-based instruments to be completed on 2 occasions (2 weeks ± 1 week apart): Quality of Well-Being Scale (QWB), Health Utilities Index (HUI), or European Quality of Life Instrument (EuroQol). RESULTS: We recruited 57 patient-caregiver pairs. The patients had a mean MMSE of 19.0. When patients self-rated their QOL, complete scores could be obtained on both occasions for 95.70sing the QWB, 81.20sing the EuroQol and 61.90sing the HUI. The test-retest reliability for patient self-ratings was 0.87 for the EuroQol, 0.80 for the QWB and 0.43 for the HUI. The test-retest reliability for caregiver proxy-ratings was 0.74 for the EuroQOL, 0.70 for the QWB and 0.77 for the HUI. For all 3 QOL instruments, caregiver proxy-ratings correlated poorly with patient self-ratings. Patients frequently rated their QOL higher than their caregivers. CONCLUSION: Alzheimers patients with mild to moderate disease could reliably rate their QOL using the QWB and the EuroQol, but not the HUI. Caregiver proxy-ratings correlated poorly with patient self-ratings.

THE COACH: A computerized cueing device to help people with dementia to be more independent

Alex Mihailidis (Centre for Studies in Aging, Sunnybrook & Women's College HSC, Toronto, Canada) Geoff R. Fernie (Centre for Studies in Aging, Sunnybrook & Women's College HSC, Toronto, Canada) Joseph C. Barbenel (Bioengineering Unit, Strathclyde University, Glasgow, Scotland)

Problem: Dementia often reduces independence because the affected person can not remember the sequence of steps needed to complete a task. The current solution is to have a caregiver assist using verbal reminders. This often leads to a loss of dignity and privacy. Method: We think that privacy can be restored by using a computerized device that provides reminders needed by the user and monitors progress. The COACH is a first prototype of a device that uses artificial intelligence to automatically adapt and to act intelligently when assisting a user. It was developed using a personal computer, and a video camera installed above the user's workspace that unobtrusively monitors his or her actions. When the user becomes confused, the device plays pre-recorded verbal prompts of varying levels of description to correct the user's actions. Currently, the device has been trained to assist a person during handwashing. Results: Preliminary testing with surrogate users, who simulated confused behaviour, showed that the device is operating with an efficacy of approximately 95 percent with respect to its ability to assist a person during handwashing. This efficacy will be improved with further refinements Conclusions: The preliminary trials have shown that the COACH has great potential in having a positive effect on the lives of people with dementia. These data support the decision to proceed to the next stage of this research, which is to begin testing with users with dementia.

The Social Networks of Demented Residents in Long-term Care

Hava Golander (Dept. of Nursing, Faculty of Medicine, Tel Aviv University, Tel Aviv, Israel) Perri Cohen (Dept. of Nursing, Faculty of Medicine, Tel Aviv University, Tel Aviv, Israel)

Dementia slowly and progressively erodes the cognitive, emotional, social and motor abilities of its sufferers causing great difficulties for the family and professional caregivers. Little is known about the remaining abilities preserved among the severely demented, therefore, the aim of this study was to learn about the remaining social skills of the demented resident living in long term care. This was done by examining the social networks that were formed among these residents and determining what factors influence the scope and nature of the interactions within the networks. The study focused on three principle questions: 1. To what extent do social networks exist among these residents? 2. What are the characteristics of the ties within the networks? 3. What factors influence the extent of involvement in the ties identified? The study included seven units for the mentally frail in three different long-term care institutions in Israel (n=212 residents). The instruments were specifically developed and modified for the present study based on existing literature concerning the morphological and qualitative aspects of social networks and included structured questionnaires, semi-structured interviews and non-participant observations. The nurses working with these residents were the main source of information. Preliminary analysis of the findings show that 420f the residents were involved in a social tie of some kind. Fifty-five social networks were identified and included a range of interactions, behavior patterns and types. The size of the networks varied from two to seven residents and included dyads, triads and clusters. Eleven different types of ties were identified among them close friendships, caring relationships and rivalries. We will discuss the factors that influence formation of these ties and the principle ramifications on a theoretical level and on the clinical level in caring for demented patients.

SESSION 389

Films and Videos on Art and Elderhood: Focus on InterArt, Life and Love

James Vanden Bosch (Terra Nova Films, Inc, Chicago, Illinois USA)

Young at Heart (28 minutes, released in 1988) - When a widow and widower, both artists, meet on a vacation tour, they start a tale that dreams are made of. Although their interest in art provides a strong bond, it is their differences which bring a fresh, lively element to their marriage and the film. Together they reaffirm that love and romance can happen at any age for the clear eyed and open hearted. // Shall We Dance? (24 minutes, released in 1995) - This documentary from Great Britain affectionately follows the preparations of a lively group of elderly women as they attend rehearsals for a dance performance at the famous Sadler's Wells ballet theater as part of a London cultural festival. The film touches on some of the deeper aspects of the women's lives as they experience the rewarding joys of self-expression. // Shared Visions (20 minutes, released in 1991) - A group of older artists share their work, their philosophy and their continued aspirations with a group of high school art students. The older artists and the students are filmed both in the artists' studios and in the art studio at the high school. A unique intergenerational exchange takes place as the artists and the students discuss each other's work philosophy and aspirations. // In This Very Room (12 minutes, released 1993) - This video clearly demonstrates that Alzheimer's residents can actively participate in many pleasurable and creative activities. It shows them engaged in music, dance, visual art and drama improvisations. These scenes are interspersed with statements by family members that confirm the value of these creative approaches for the Alzheimer's residents

SESSION 390

An Ethnography of Ban Bangkae: A Home for the Aged in Thailand.

S. Changmai (Faculty of Nursing, Christian College, Nakhon Pathom, Thailand)

The purpose of this ethnographic study was to explore, describe, and interpret the meaning of health, nursing and culture in Ban Bangkae: a home for the aged in Bangkok, Thailand. Data collection involved an observer-participation process with formal and informal interviews, field notes, and photographs. Fourteen residents, three nurses, and a warden joined in this study as 'informants'. The data were analyzed throughout the study, including staying close to the original data to depict the informants' words and their stories, identifying key factors and relationships among the information, and sorting the information, which described the culture of Ban Bangkae. Also, content analysis was utilized to inductively derive themes from the data. Residents indicated that the beginning of the old age was at 70 years because they related age to health. They agreed that health involved a strong and fit body and mind. Nursing services in Ban Bangkae were organized by four nurses and focused on health care and the residents' well-being. The culture of Ban Bangkae revolved around daily rituals. The residents mainly had similar rituals including waking up early, giving some food to the monks, exercising, doing some work in the Occupational room, joining some activities, enjoying recreation, and having meals. In conclusion, most of them were happy with the services provided for them and in spending their lives there. However, they identified some issues, including early dinner times, the taste of the food and its repeated menu. Moreover, some residents felt uncomfortable living with other people. Sometimes different opinions on issues culminated in arguments between residents.

Social Practices in Residential Care: A "Giddensian" Action Research Approach

J Jyrki (Department of Social Sciences and Philosophy, University of Jyv{skyl{, Finland)

The aim of this study is to develop and discuss a new theoretical frame of action research for use in institutional care. Some ideas of Anthony Giddens' structuration theory will be connected to the principles of traditional action research. Institutional care - for instance in residential homes - will be seen as a set of different social practices where both residents and members of staff participate in. These practices are in central focus of action research when trying to develop the quality of every day life in residential homes.Empirically the study is based on a ethnographical research work made in a Finnish old age home. The focus of the study, that was based on participant observation, was on how the daily routines and the social site of the home are worked into being in and through every day social practices. In my paper I will characterize some basic features of a "Giddensian" action research. Social practices will be conceptualized in the frame of his structuration theory. As a result, the idea of 'a social hologram' as an objective of action research in residential care is introduced. The study shows how concepts of structuration theory can be put to use when studying social practices in residential care using action research approach. It also shows the benefits of applying new theoretical approaches in gerontological research.

The constructivist approach in geriatric institution

M.P.Labernadie , B.Placines (Centre de Gérontologie de Pontacq-Nay , 64800 Nay , France), M.Wolf (Centre Hospitalier Général , 45300 Pithiviers, France)P.Duboe (Maison de retraite Saint-Joseph , 64800 Nay , France), J.P.Duviau(Maison de Retraite Saint-Joseph , 64800 Nay , France)

The different constructivist approaches admit the following hypothesis: the reality is the result of social interactions . She is a matter for a constructional dynamics , deconstruction , of an interpretation built through the communication processes. Going to an institution for the subject provokes a rupture with a previous reality and the subject becomes often a care object . The challenge of the institution is to fear the reality of the subject under two aspects: the temporality and the sense with the stake of the subject involvement to the production of his own reality . The micro-project of life generated of the organisational dynamic in struggle against the institutional conformism . He is necessary grants to consider a structural evolution , that it is possible to consider in term of quality indicator . A modelling of this constructivism gait in institution will be proposed then .

Vulnerability, Transcendence and Meaning in Life Amongst Elderly Nursing Home Residents.

E. B. MacKinlay (Centre for Ageing and Pastoral Studies, University of Canberra & St Mark's National Theological Centre, Canberra, Australia)

Transcending disabilities and finding meaning in life in the face of increasing frailty are major challenges for many nursing home residents. This study examined how a group of these people found meaning in life. A total of 20 in-depth interviews were conducted with residents, having a mean age of 78.7 years. Eighty percent of participants were widowed. Data were analysed based on grounded theory and the model of spiritual tasks of ageing (MacKinlay 1998). One component of this model is examined in this paper, self-sufficiency versus vulnerability: transcending losses and disabilities in ageing. All of these people lived with multiple chronic illnesses, yet 20% said they were in very good to excellent health, 15% claimed good health and 45% stated they were in fairly good health and the remainder in poor health. Analysis of interviews indicated that the ability to transcend disabilities was important in this self-perception of health. Those making this transition were moving from a 'doing' mode to a 'being' mode. They were still able to find meaning in their frailty. Fifty-five percent of the sample said they had no fears associated with growing older, contrasted with 100% of a sample of older independent living people expressing fears of future vulnerability in an earlier study. Awareness of the nature of spiritual tasks of ageing in the model provides essential information for spiritual interventions for frail older residents. Spiritual care is a multidisciplinary concern, being important in the practice of nurses, social workers, clergy and other health professionals.

SESSION 391

Cognitive function and mortality among nonagenarians. The Danish 1905-Cohort Survey.

Kjeld Andersen, Hanne Nybo, David Gaist, Hans Chr. Petersen, Bernard Jeune, James W. Vaupel, Kaare Christensen (Epidemiology, Institute of Public Health, University of Southern Denmark, Denmark)

PURPOSE: To examine whether cognitive impairment increases mortality among the very old. METHODS: In 1998, as part of a large nationwide epidemiological survey 1,794 nonagenarians underwent testing with the MMSE, verbal fluency, forward and backward digit span, and immediate and delayed recall of 12 words. The five latter tests were first standardized to a mean of 0 and a standard deviation of 1 and then a composite score was calculated as the sum of the standardized scores. According to the MMSE the participants were divided into three categories: no impairment (24-30 points) = reference group, mild impairment (18-23 points), and severe impairment (0-17 points). The composite score was divided into quartiles, the best performing quartile being the reference group. Based on Cox Proportional Hazards models we examined the association between cognitive impairment and mortality controlling for socio-demographic factors, sex, cardiovascular disease and stroke, self-rated health, depressive symptoms, smoking and alcohol use, and objective tests of physical performance (hand grip and walk speed). RESULTS: During the follow-up period from 1998 to 2000 (mean follow-up time: 1.6 years, SD: 0.5 years) 562 (31%) died. Compared to participants with no cognitive impairment the adjusted hazard ratio (95% CI) of death was 1.28 (1.03 - 1.60) for mildly impaired and 1.79 (1.41 - 2.28) for severely impaired. Using the composite score the adjusted hazard ratio was 1.39 (1.04 - 1.85) for the second quartile increasing to 1.88 (1.41 - 2.50) for the fourth quartile. CONCLUSION: Even very late in life, cognitive impairment independently predicts mortality.

Cognitive functioning of Finnish elderly people born in 1910: a follow-up from 80 to 90 years

I. Ruoppila, T. Suutama (Department of Psychology, University of Jyväskylä, Finland)

The purpose was to describe and analyze inter-individual and intra-individual changes in cognitive functioning among Finnish elderly people. As part of the Evergreen project, the data is based on the whole age-group born in 1910 and living in Jyväskylä in 1990 (N=283; 73.1% women). The participation rate was 72.4% at baseline, five years later it was 57.5% (n=96) from those eligible and 10 years later 48.8% (n=42). Those getting the lowest cognitive test scores at baseline or 5 years later were more often deceased or could not participate in the last phase than those getting higher test scores. The tests used were Digit Span, Digit Symbol, Word Fluency, and Mini-D, which is based on Luria's neuropsychological theory, covers major cognitive functions and is constructed for dementia screening purposes. Results: The findings showed a clear trend for cognitive functioning changing to a lower level from 80 to 85 years, but this decrease was not very significant. However, the decrease from 85 to 90 years was highly significant ($p<.01$, at least) in other tests except Mini-D. The deterioration of cognitive functioning from 80 to 90 years was found out in all tests. The retest correlations between baseline and the second assessment varied from 0.69 to 0.82, between the second and the third assessment from 0.55 to 0.84 and between baseline and the third assessment from 0.48 to 0.78. Digit Symbol and Word Fluency, which require speed and accuracy of performance, had the highest retest correlations. Some big intra-individual changes in cognitive performance occurred especially from 85 to 90 years. They were biggest in Mini-D. Conclusion: The stability of cognitive functioning seems to be quite high from 80 to 85 years. Some intra-individual changes occur from 85 to 90 years, but still the order of individuals remains mainly the same from phase to phase.

Cognitive Functioning of Finnish Older Persons: A Follow-Up from 75 to 85 Years of Age

T. Suutama, I. Ruoppila (Department of Psychology, University of Jyväskylä, Finland)

The purpose of the paper is to describe group level and individual changes in cognitive test performance among Finnish persons ageing from 75 to 85 years. 300 persons (66% women) aged 75 participated in a laboratory study of the Evergreen project in 1989, 190 of them took part in the 5-year follow-up, and 99 (70% women) in the 10-year follow-up (participation rates 78%, 72% and 59%, respectively). The subjects of this study were those persons who participated in cognitive testing at all three phases (n=76-91 by tests used). The psychometric tests used in about 30-minute test sessions were Digit Span, Logical Memory and Visual Reproduction from WMS, Digit Symbol from WAIS, a 5-minute version of Raven's Progressive Matrices, and an oral 3-minuteWord Fluency test. There was a trend in visuoconstructive tests, especially, that lower scores predicted drop-out because of death or other reasons. From 75 to 80 years of age, the decline in the test scores was more significant in visuoconstructive than in verbal tests, from 80 to 85 years also the latter tests usually showed highly significant decline. The test-retest correlations over the 5- and 10-year periods varied between 0.44 and 0.85, intelligence tests showing somewhat higher stability of the differences between the subjects than memory tests. In spite of the significant test score decline on group level, many kinds of individual changes were observed In all tests, a notable part of the subjects had a quite stable performance over the assessments, others showing more or less steep decline, and a small minority even improving their performance. On group level, test based cognitive functioning of older persons deteriorates significantly with increasing age. On individual level, however, various change patterns from steep decline to improvement of performance are possible.

SESSION 392

Canadian Health Network Senior's Affiliate Network

Linda O'Rourke, Joyce Springate, Susan Margles

Purpose: This presentation will provide a demonstration of the Canadian Health Network (CHN), an Internet-based source of health information. The mission of the CHN is "to enable Canadians to take action to improve their health and the health of their families and communities by disseminating knowledge and critical skills". CHN seeks to establish itself as the premier source for Canadians to access bilingual "health information you can trust" through its network of 22 affiliates from across the country. Method: One of those affiliates is the Senior's Affiliate, a consortium comprised of the Canadian Association on Gerontology (CAG), the Canadian Gerontological Nursing Association (CGNA) and Simon Fraser University Gerontology Research Centre (SFU-GRC). The consortium, now referred to as the Senior's Affiliate Network (SAN), have been working together, since August 2000, toward the goal of providing all Canadians with information which is "timely, credible, relevant and relates to health and well-being" of older adults. Results: The CHN provides several different ways to access the ever-growing collection of 6000+ Internet-based resources on the CHN site. Looking for and using the information is dependant on the interests and needs of the individual. As well, a rigorous quality assurance process ensures that the health information included on CHN is timely, relevant, current, and, and accessible. Conclusion: The Senior's Affiliate Network (SAN) encourages you to explore the CHN website at: www.canadian-health-network.c

Educational Need Assessment of Computer-Using Senior Citizens in Korea

Eunhee Jhoo (Hanyang Women's College, Seoul, Korea)

The purpose of this study was to assess the educational needs of computer-using Korean senior citizens in order to identify the factors consider for the instructional programme planning of the computer learning centres. The questionnaire were given to about 200 elderly attending several types of centres in Seoul and some focussed group were interviewed by the telephone, fax, or face-to-face to obtain more detailed information abut their motivation, difficulties and successful applications of computer-mediated communication skills. The questionnaire were comprised with factors related to learner, environment, instructional design and self-perceptions about the outcomes. For the overall view, the contents of computer learning networks, so called SilverNet and the programmes of other computer learning centres were surveyed and compared. The results show that Korean senior net lacks in organising social activities and inefficiently transits to on-line learning. Also, the findings from the data analysis reveal variations in the learner's motivation, preference for learning mode(on-line learning network vs off-line group activities), satisfaction of the programme and self-confidence in computer mediated communications. It is expected that the major factors varying their needs and satisfactions may be their educational background and instructional factors such as the interactions with instructors and teaching strategies. It is proposed that theses factors should be significantly taken into account for the effective instructional planning. *** It would be grateful that the platform presentation of this paper will be arranged on 4th or 5th of July because I am unable to arrive in Vancouver before 3rd of July.

Technology and Older Adults in Long term Care

S. Pratten (Social Service Worker Program, Sheridan College, Oakville, Canada

To determine the nature and extent of computer use by older adults, caregivers and service providers in long-term care facilities and day programs in the Halton and Peel Regions of Ontario. Completion of an informal questionnaire by Social Service Worker Gerontology students enrolled in a two-year diploma program at Sheridan College. The survey was based on the students' observations during their field practicum training at community based programs and facilities. These sites included nursing homes, retirement residences, supportive housing settings, and day programs for the frail and cognitively impaired elderly. The survey results were categorized into the types of computer use by the four user groups: active seniors, frail seniors, caregivers, and service providers. The applications for both active and frail seniors were mainly in the areas of 'Communication' and 'Research/Discovery'. Service providers used computers for 'Information Management' and to 'Produce/Present/Publish'. Caregivers used computers for all four applications. The survey results indicated that both active and frail older adults were enthusiastic computer users once they were provided with support and assistance. Quite a few settings had computer stations that had been donated but there were often not the resources to train the staff or volunteers to provide this support. Some of the staff admitted to not being computer literate themselves. There is a role for social service students to provide leadership in advancing the use of computers for the benefit of active seniors, caregivers and service providers in long-term care settings and day programs for older adults.

Web-Based Education: The 'E' Experience in Gerontology

Amy Finch Liane Connelly, Ron Fahey, | [Fort Hays State University, Hays. USA] |

Educators in gerontology must consider the use of distance | | education not only for providing initial courses for students | | in traditional university programs but also for providing | | continuing education for individuals who are currently | | employed. Distance education has become more convenient and | | accessible to all due to technological advances (Spodick, | | 1997). The purpose of this presentation is to provide | | participants the opportunity to learn about the development | | and use of long distance education courses in gerontology at | | a small rural university in the United States. Participants | | will learn about the issues involved in planning and | | developing long distance education courses using the World | | Wide Web, electronic tools and other electronic | | e-experiences. In addition, participants will be able to view | | three courses that have been developed using two different | | web course development tools. The three courses to be | | presented are Communication and Aging, Health Care Systems, | | and Learning in Older Adulthood. Education through this | | medium provides learners in a rural setting access to initial | | learning experiences or continuing professional development. | | Participants will evaluate two distinct web course | | development tools for use in the gerontology classroom.

SESSION 393

Clinical significance of soluble Interleukin-2 receptor and T-lymphocytes subsets in aging patients with pulmonary diseases

Zhang Yueli, Gu Zhengqi, Pang Zhonghua (Respiratory Department of Huadong Hospital, Shanghai 200040, P.R. China)

To examine the effect of T-lymphocyte subsets and soluble interleukin-2 receptor (sIL-2R) in the peripheral blood of subjects with pulmonary diseases. The levels of sIL-2R and the CD4, CD8 and CD4/CD8 of T-lymphocytes among patients with various pulmonary diseases were measured by sandwiched ELISH and alkaline phosphatase-antialkaline phosphatase (APAAP) methods. The level of sIL-2R was significantly elevated in patients with various pulmonary diseases when compared with healthy controls ($P<0.001$). Patients with lung cancer had the highest value of sIL-2R which was superior to that of control and patients with benign pulmonary diseases. The level of CD4 was lower in patients with pulmonary diseases than those in control ($P<0.05$). The level of sIL-2R and T-lymphocyte subpopulations may be useful in monitoring the abnormality of immunologic response in patients with pulmonary diseases, but can't be used as a referential indicator for various pulmonary diseases.

Diagnostic value and safeness of fiberoptic bronchoscopy for 70 year old patients suspected to have lung cancer

Sha Baokang, Ma Shoukang, Yan Dejun, (et al. Huadong Hospital , Shanghai 200040, P.R. China.)

Purpose: A retrospective analysis on the diagnostic value and safeness of fiberoptic bronchoscopy for 70 year old patients with suspected lung cancer. Method: Fiberoptic bronchoscopy was performed on 704 cases with lung cancer as shown by x-ray films. Before bronchoscopy examination, blood clotting time, electrocardiogram, arterial blood gas analysis were carried out regularly. To those abnormal cases, oxygen was given during examination and monitored with electrocardiogram. Modified Jackson spraying anesthesia and segmented spraying anesthesia was preferred. If the lesion was found, resected or brushed biopsy and douche solution were sent for check up. Results: 484 out of 704 cases were confirmed as lung cancer, among which squamous cell carcinoma occurred in 290 cases, adenocarcinoma in 123 cases, small cell carcinoma in 35 cases, adenosquamous carcinoma in 9 cases, and unidentified in 27 cases. During examination, there were 62 cases showed a change of ST-t wave on electrocardiogram, and 18 cases with oxygen partial pressure dropped to 50 mmHg but raised to 70 mmHg after inhaling oxygen. The examination continued on without anymore obvious harmful reaction. Conclusion: Fiberoptic bronchoscopy is safe for 70 year old patients, and is rather worthwhile for diagnosing suspected lung cancer.

Evaluation of CRP and bacteria culture, chest x-ray film in acute exacerbation of COPD

Zhang Yueli, Pang Zhonghua, Zhang Zhijie (Respiratory Department of Huadong Hospital, Shanghai 200040, P.R. China)

The aim of this study was to evaluation the relationship between C-reactive protein (CRP), chest X-ray and sputum cultures in acute exacerbation of elderly COPD. Forty seven elderly patients admitted to our hospital with an acute infective exacerbation of COPD were studied with the clinic data, chest X-ray film and sputum bacteria cultures. The patients were categorized according to the CRP level. CRP level was normal (<8 mg/L) in seven patients (group A), CRP was 9-39 mg/L in 11 patients (group B) and CRP >40mg/L in 29 patients. The sputum cultures were positive in 27 of 47 cases. The results of cultures in discovering microorganisms were about 57.5% (27/47). The positive rates of sputum culture were 14.3%, 54.6 % and 72.4% in groups A, B, and C, respectively, $P < 0.01$. The incidence of pneumonia in the group C was higher than that in the group B and group C, $P < 0.05$. The numbers of fever in the group C were the highest compared with that in the group B and group C, $P < 0.01$. There is a correlation between CRP and pneumonia, fever , the bacteria isolated from patients with acute infective exacerbation of COPD.

Interes of Fibreoptic Bronchoscopy in Lung Diseases of Olde People

M. Bégorre (Service de Médecine Interne et Gériatrie, Centre Hospitalier, OLORON, FRANCE), D. Bégorre-Bondroit (Service de Gériatrie, Centre Hospitalier, LOURDES, FRANCE)

Purpose : assess effectiveness and tolerance of fibreoptic bronchscopy to diagnose lung diseases in old peoples. Method : we collected during ten years in our two neighbourin hospitals indications and results of 450 lung examinations with fiberoptic bronchoscopy: airways obstruction, pulmonary infections, suspicious findings on chest xrays, benign ou malignant tumours. Results : In many cases we could diagnose ant treat lung diseases at the same time : inhalation of small particles (47 cases), or very plentiful mucous secretions without infection (32 cases). In case of pulmonary infections, microbial causal agent was indentified in 254 cases of 312, responsible primitive lung cancer was also identified in 39 of these 312 case. For all patients with primitive or secondary tumours, we made biopsies showing the histological type of tumour (59 cases). Conclusions : fibreoptic brochoscopy is a very easy method to complete clinical and xrays examination to diagnose pulmonary diseases. This method is also well tolerated especially in old patients if preparation and local anaesthesia is well done.

SESSION 394

Interdisciplinary Comprehensive Geriatric Assessment: Exploring Clients' and Caregivers' Perceptions of the Process and Outcomes

F. Aminzadeh, (Regional Geriatric Assessment Program of Ottawa Carleton, Canada)WB. Dalziel, FRCP (C) (RGAP of Ottawa-Carleton, Canada) A. Byszewski, FRCP (C)(RGAP of Ottawa-Carleton, Canada) S. Amos, (RGAP of Ottawa-Carleton,Canada)

PURPOSE: A growing recognition of the complexity of the health needs of older persons coupled with increasing evidence of the effectiveness of comprehensive geriatric assessment programs (CGA) have resulted in a more prominent role of these programs in the care of older persons. However, there is a paucity of research on clients' and caregivers' perceptions of the process and outcomes of these assessments. METHOD: This prospective study involved 3-month follow-up interviews with 116 clients/caregivers of a geriatric day hospital program in Ottawa, Canada. The participants had completed a Cognitive Change Care Map protocol. RESULTS: Quantitative analysis of participants responses to close ended evaluation questions revealed high levels of satisfaction with both the process and outcomes of the assessment, although, clients' evaluations were generally less positive compared to the caregivers. Qualitative analysis of participants' narrative comments provided additional insight into their experiences with, and expectations about, various aspects of the assessment, including: physical and social environment of care, affective quality of encounter, level of client/ caregiver involvement, educational needs, and the quality of life outcomes. CONCLUSION: This research provides valuable information regarding clients/caregivers' experiences with the CGA programs. This information guides protocol development and clinical interventions that enhance program sensitivity and effectiveness, particularly for clients with cognitive change.

Listening to Seniors: A qualitative study of seniors and acute care hospitalization

Peter Stephenson, (Department of Anthropology, University of Victoria, Victoria, Canada Belinda Parke, MSN (Capital Health Region, Victoria, Canada) Christina Holmes BA, MA (University of Victoria, Canada)

PURPOSE: The Capital Health Region in partnership with the University of Victoria Anthropology Department conducted a listening project to learn about the older adults' lived experience of hospitalization Older adults account for 62% of acute care medical and surgical hospital admissions in the Capital Health Region, Victora, British Columbia, Canada. Hospitals can unintentionally contribute to adverse clinical and social consequences for older adults. A cascade of events that results in poor outcomes and functional disabilites can flow from hopsitalization and seniors are especially vulnerable throughout this process. METHOD: A qualitative project, using semi structured face to face interviews with 25 older adults aged between 63 and 85, who experienced an acute care admission within the last two years. Older adults were recruited from senior's centers within the Capital Health Region. RESULTS: Themes that emerged from the stories captured the whole experience of arriving, being and leaving hospital. Being in and returning home from hospital commanded more attention. Of particular importance were issues related to staff identification, absence of care, feelings of being rushed and lack of communication between older patients, physicians and interdisciplinary team members. CONCLUSIONS: Within hospital practice can be an ageism that comes through in subtle ways that is often hidden and unknown.

Older adults' perceptions of blood pressure measurement and of health professional roles and activities

D. Bakker, G. Viverais-Dresler (Laurentian University, Sudbury, ON, Canada)

This descriptive study presents the findings from a group of older adults on their perceptions of: blood pressure measurement and its meaning to their health, and the health promotion roles of health care professionals. The convenience sample consisted of 51 community dwelling older adults recruited from either wellness clinics or senior citizens' clubs. Data were collected through indepth audiotaped interviews using both open and closed-ended questions. In regard to perceptions of blood pressure measurement the following three themes emerged: provision of reassurance, participation in self-care, and reliance on health care professionals. Health professionals were perceived most frequently as providing activities that were supportive and addressed primarily disease prevention. Less frequently, health professionals were perceived to partake in activities that focused on health promotion that included patient education. Findings give direction to the importance of taking into account the clients' perspective to better understand blood pressure management with the older adult.

SESSION 395

Adapting to Relocation: the effects of moving an elderly psychiatric population

W. Selzer (Gerontology Post Baccalaureate Diploma Program), J. Sun (Gerontology Post Baccalaureate Diploma Program), G. Gutman (Director, Gerontology Research Centre, Simon Fraser University, Vancouver, B.C, Canada), T. Unwin (SFU).

Purpose: Fifty-three residents aged 50 to 97 with a psychiatric illness were followed as they moved from a deteriorating institutional residence to a newly built intermediate care facility on the same site.

Method: Twenty six of the relocated residents completed both pre- and post- move interviews. Factors affecting adaptation to the move are examined specifically, characteristics of the residents, the environment, and the staff. Changes in weight and medications as well as mortality, morbidity, and hospitalizations rates were documented as indicators of relocation stress.
Results: At the end of three months there was only one death within the group of 53 transferred residents. There were two short hospitalizations and one temporary psychiatric admission amoung the 26 residents who participated in the interviews. Weight changes were recorded in 22 of the 26 interviewed residents. Generally, pre and post interviews showed consistency with regard to activity patterns, feelings about the new building, and feelings about the move (pre-move 65.4% were looking forward to the move and post- move 69.2% felt the move was good for them).
Conclusion: Residents appear to have adjusted well. Their degree of readiness and sense of choice and control about the move and the post-move environment, such as activities and private rooms, may have played a key role in positive adjustment. Other important factors included residents' familiarity with the site, pre-move preparations, and constancy of staff and activities. One point of interest was the post-move implementation of the Gentlecare model for facility care and residents' feelings of post- move improved care.

Institutional Relocation: Mortality and Emotional Aspects

Lars Bo Bülow (The Health Administration, City of Copenhagen, Denmark); Claus Holst (Institute of Preventive Medicine, Copenhagen, Denmark); Eva Bonde Nielsen (The Danish National Institute for Elderly Education, Denmark)

PURPOSE: To examine relocation effects on mortality and emotional aspects of nursing home residents living in the City of Copenhagen. Furthermore to examine relocation effects on emotional aspects of staff and family members. METHODS: The control material for this examination is a study of the mortality rate of the whole population of nursing home residents in the City of Copenhagen (n=17.095) since 1990. From 1998 and up to 2004 some of those (n= 850) were or will be relocated to new facilities. The mortality rate for those persons will be compared to the control material for the same period. Until now 176 persons have been relocated. Qualitative interview including residents (n=33), staff (n= 44) and family members (n= 16) are used before and after relocation to examine the effects on emotional aspects. RESULTS: For the persons already relocated (n=176) there were no increase in mortality after moving compared with the control group. Negative effects on emotional aspects were found in the first period after the information about the relocation was given. After relocation very few negative effects on emotional aspects were found and several positive outcomes were observed. CONCLUSION: The findings until now point out that relocation of nursing home residents do not influence mortality. Future findings might change this result. Negative effects on emotional aspects were found before relocation but very few afterwards.

Kiwanis Relocation Study: Implementation and Resident/ Family Perception of the Impact of Support Activities

Gloria Gutman (Simon Fraser University, Vancouver, Canada), Frances Hamm (Simon Fraser University, Vancouver, Canada) and Lenore Pickering (North Shore Health Region, Vancouver, Canada)

As part of a larger study, this analysis investigated the effectiveness of strategies developed and implemented to minimize the potentially stressful impact of a mass relocation of frail elderly residents. The study used a quasi experimental design to follow 149 residents (mean age = 87; 55.7% with moderate/severe dementia) during a move into a new multi level care facility from two closing intermediate care facilities. Qualitative and quantitative date were collected at 3 months pre-move and at 3 and 6 months post-move for the move facilities and for one non-move control facility (n=99 Mean age = 84; 67.4% with moderate/severe dementia). 31 of the planned 38 strategies were implemented, post-move interventions were the most difficult to conceptualize and implement. 77.8% of the residents interviewed were satisfied with the organization of the move, and 89.2% of families were motivated to help with the move. No statistically significant increase in physical dependence for ADLs, in falls, disturbed behaviour, or mortality rates was found. Well developed strategies can support relocating residents and their families. Future research should investigate support given to newly institutionalized residents, especially those with cognitive and sensory deficits

The Impact of Relocation on Adult Day Centre Clients with Dementia

S. Grant (Gerontology Programs & Gerontology Research Centre, Simon Fraser University, Vancouver, Canada)

Objective: To examine the psychosocial impact of a change in physical environment due to relocation on adult day centre (ADC) clients with dementia. Although extensive research has been conducted on relocation and seniors, very little work has been directed to the relocation of ADCs. In addition, limited research has been conducted on the subject of physical environments for ADCs, and it is anticipated that this study will make a contribution to bridging this gap in the literature. Method: The naturally occurring relocation of an ADC provides a rare and exciting opportunity for study. A pretest-posttest design was used and clients' behaviour and level of satisfaction with various design features was monitored approximately 1 month before and 1 month after they moved from a multipurpose environment to a purpose-built ADC. Data collection for the relocation group included the following: client, staff, and family interviews; Mini Mental Status Examination (MMSE); behaviour mapping; environmental assessment; and information from client records. The MMSE was administered at two points in time to an ADC with a similar proportion of clients with dementia to monitor the natural progression of dementia in an ADC not undergoing relocation. Results: Available at time of presentation. Implications: Determining the effect of various design features on clients in the context of ADCs is critical for the development of new ADCs. Ensuring that ADCs are well-designed from the outset will minimize the need for renovation or relocation. (Supported by a grant from the Alzheimer Society of B.C.)

Why do Arab-Israeli elderly leave the nursing home?

Khaled Suleiman, M.D. (Dabouriya Home for the Aged, Dabouriya, Israel); Noal Massalha (Dabouriya Home for the Aged, Dabouriya, Israel); Adrian Walter-Ginzburg, (Herczeg Institute on Aging, Tel Aviv University, Tel Aviv, Israel).

Purpose: Arab-Israeli society is undergoing economic and social changes which increase the propensity to make use of institutional settings for the elderly. However, the utilization patterns for these services are still affected by social norms. The goal of the study was to assess the reasons for the decision to leave the Dabouriya Home for the Aged, and especially to assess whether social norms affect the elderly and/or their families when taking this decision. Method: The study population included all of those who had voluntarily left the Dabouriya nursing home since it was founded in the early 1990s. The data were collected from the elderly and/or from their family by the nursing homes social worker. Results: During the eight years of the nursing homes operation, 297 residents had been admitted, and 69 (23%) had voluntarily left after an average length of stay of 2.9 months (s.d. 5.4); of these, the average age (76 years, s.d. 11) and gender (54% women) did not differ significantly from residents. Over the eight years, 180f those patients defined as nursingleft, compared to 340f the frail ($p<0.05$). Most of these reasons center on inability of the resident to adapt to the new environment (42%) , although the families are affect by social norms including the negative image of the nursing home and social pressure which defines nursing home placement as neglect. Other reasons include improvement in function and a large family support system. Conclusions: The Arab-Israeli nursing home provides a still-problematic solution to care of the disabled elderly Arab-Israeli.

SESSION 396

Effect of Melatonin on the Life Span and Biological Age Markers in CBA Mice

N. Yu. Zavarzina, I. G. Popovich, A. V. Shtylik, M. A. Zabezhinski, O. A. Zimina, V. N. Anisimov (N. N. Petrov Research Institute of Oncology, St. Petersburg, Russia)

PURPOSE: The goal of our study was to characterize the geroprotector potential of melatonin in mice. METHOD: 100 female CBA mice were randomly subdivided into 2 groups (50 mice per group) and starting at the age of the 6 months one of the group were exposed to melatonin with drinking water (20 mg/l) during night time 5 consecutive days monthly until the natural death. Body weight and temperature, food consumption, estrus function, locomotor activity, physical strenght, survival and tumor pathology have been monitored during all period of the observation. RESULTS: It was shown that the body weight gain and food consumption was similar in control and melatonin mice. As compared with the control, the body weight of mice treated with melatonin was increased at the age of 15, 18 and 21 months. Melatonin did not change the muscle strength evaluated in wire hang test. The rectal body temperature did not change with the age in control mice, whereas significantly decreased in the melatonin-treated mice. The treatment with melatonin was resulted in the decrease in the locomotor activity of animals as the age of 6 and 9 months as compared with the controls. The administration of melatonin slowed down the aging of the estrus function. The survival dynamics was similar in the control and melatonin mice from 6th to 23rd months of their life and than was reduced in melatonin-treated group. The maximum life span was increased by 2 months in animal treated with melatonin as compared with control. The treatment with melatonin was followed by increase in the incidence of lymphomas and lung adenocarcinomas. CONCLUSION: Our data suggest that melatonin should not be recommended as a potent geroprotector.

Factors Predicting Sexual Relationship Status in Older People

Victor Minichiello, Deborah Loxton, (School of Health, University of New England, Armidale, Australia)

PURPOSE: Recent studies are beginning to acknowledge that older people are sexual and that the expression of sexuality in later life is a basic human right. The aim of this paper is to determine the factors that predict sexual relationship status in older people. METHOD: A self-completed questionnaire was returned by 844 randomly selected older persons living in Melbourne, Australia. A model comprised of 11 predictors of sexual relationship status was tested. RESULTS: The results indicate that the model used in this study can reliably discriminate those in a sexual relationship from those not in a sexual relationship. Logistic regression analysis reveals that gender, general health, incontinence, attitude toward sexual issues, and changes in sexual activity and interest since mid-life were not significantly related to sexual relationship status. The following factors were found to predict an increased likelihood of being in a sexual relationship: those who were younger, married or living with a partner, satisfied with their health and physical condition, had a greater level of sexual knowledge, perceived sex as important to well being and who had one sexual partner in their lifetime. CONCLUSION: The implications of these results are discussed and suggestions to facilitate a more open and supportive environment for older people to maintain their sexual relationships are presented.

Identifying the sexual health needs of older people: findings from a programme of research

Merryn Gott, (Sheffield Institute for Studies on Ageing, Sheffield, UK). Sharron Hinchliffe, (Sheffield Institute for Studies on Ageing, Sheffield, UK). Ian Philp, (Sheffield Institute for Studies on Ageing), Sheffield, UK).

PURPOSE: The sexual health concerns of older people are rarely prioritised by academics, clinicians, policy-makers or society. This paper presents findings from research aiming to explore whether the sexual health needs of older people warrant further attention. METHOD: Research undertaken to date has involved: 1) an analysis of activity data from 3 UK Genitourinary Medicine (GUM) Clinics; 2) a questionnaire study of 224 older GUM clinic attenders; and 3) a general population questionnaire survey of 335 people >50 years. A study involving 60 people (30-49, 50-69, >70 years) from a GP setting is also in progress. This examines how sexual health is prioritised in relation to other aspects of health and overall quality of life (QoL) using depth interviewing and the WHOQoL-100. RESULTS: Findings from the first three phases of the research indicate that: 1) older people represent a consistent, distinctive minority of patients attending GUM clinics (approximately 5%) and present with a range of sexual health concerns; 2) within a community sample of older people, the majority were sexually active (80%) and one tenth reported concerns about their sexual health; and 3) older people with sexual health concerns experience significant barriers in presenting to health care professionals. Preliminary data from the study examining the prioritisation of sexual health in later life will also be presented. CONCLUSION: This research establishes that the sexual health needs of older people warrant further attention, especially given the context of an ageing population with changing sexual attitudes and behaviours.

Sexual Functioning in 55-80 Year Old Women

Simin Taavoni- (Iran University of Medical Sciences. Tehran. IRAN) Ramin Sarchami- (Qazvin University of Medical Sciences.Qazvin.IRAN)

It is important when considering the outcome of any health care intervention to measure how such intervention meets the patients needs and expectations. Sexual Functioning is an important aspect of health likely to influenced by medical conditions and health care interventions. Modern medicine has significantly increased the human life span, and today most women live one third of their lives after menopause. Although it is a natural phase of the life, but it bring along physical and mental problems for the women. PURPOSE: To determine sexual functioning in 55-80 years old women. MATERIALS AND METHODS: This is a qualitative and quantitative descriptive study. In this study 80 married healthy women with the age of 55-80 years, who were met in the public centers of North and East of Tehran City in autumn 2000 were interviewed. A valid and reliable questionnaire including the personal characteristics and sexual functioning were used. RESULTS: Some of the results were as followed: Only 5% of age 55-80 still had been working. l.25% of age 55-59 and 1.25% of age 70+ were post graduated and 8.75%of samples had finished high school. The average menopause age was 51.16 years old. 31.25% of the samples had been using HRT. There was significant finding in the women interest in sex, their sexual activity, sex life, sex feeling and ability to reach orgasm during the last months. Most of the samples had lower feeling in compare with pre menopause stage, and in the most groups who used HRT there were no differences. CONCLUSION: In the most of these women s believes sex was rather important and important (in HRT and none HRT groups)(52.5%). In comparison to previous years the importance of sex was decreased a lot (4.5%). Decreased somewhat (28.75%) and only for 26.25%of them it was not changed. Most of these groups have HRT and all of them were in the age less than 70 years old. Since the sexual relationship has a major role in reserving elder mental health and their life hopefulness it is essential that counseling with the clients and using HRT be recommended.

Supporting Sexuality - Management Roles and Responsibilities

S. Roach, R. Coates (Curtin University, Perth, Western Australia)

Presentation of part of the results of a doctorate investigating nursing home staff perceptions of residents' affectionate and sexual behaviour. A qualitative study was undertaken in Perth and Melbourne in Australia, and in Stockholm, Sweden. Interviews with nursing home staff were recorded, transcribed verbatim and then analysed using grounded theory methodology. Staff perceptions and responses to residents' sexual behaviour were found to be influenced by the level of support received from management. Negative consequences for residents result from unsupportive management practices, and this subsequently affects self esteem and health status. This paper outlines the role of nursing home management in either supporting or disregarding the sexuality of residents. Recommendations for change include education, staff recruitment, and selection and consensual policy development.

SESSION 397

Meet the Editors - Gerontology - Official Journal of the IAG

Mary Luszcz (Flinders University, Adelaide, Australia) Don Ingram (Gerontology Research Center, NIA, Baltimore, USA) Thomas Nold (Karger, Basel, Switzerland) A. Wister (Gerontology Research Center, Simon Fraser University, Vancouver, Canada)

PURPOSE: The purpose of the session is to introduce delegates to GERONTOLOGY, the official publication of the International Association of Gerontology. METHOD: Editors and Members of the Editorial Board will be present. Information will be disseminated on the range of areas encompassed by GERONTOLOGY, including experimental, clinical and behavioural gerontology. The audience will be encouraged to ask questions concerning the journal and publishing in it. RESULTS: Up to date information will be provided on the submission process, publication characteristics, e.g, where it is cited and the impact factor of GERONTOLOGY, style requirements, tips for prospective authors, etc. CONCLUSION: GERONTOLOGY provides a key means of communicating research results, theoretical reviews and debates across basic and behavioural sciences and clinical domains and supports the mission of the IAG.

SESSION 398

Clinical survey of 459 longevous persons

Zhu Yue, Ma Yong-Xing, Wang Zan-Shun (Department of Aging, Antiaging and Cognitive Function, Shanghai Institute of Gerontology and Geriatrics, Huadong Hospital, Shanghai, China)

The results of a clinical survey of 459 longevous persons were as follows: Age: 90-108yrs, M 116, F343. The age of death >70 yrs of their father, mother or parent were 13.4%, 31.3% and 16.0% respectively. There were only 15.6% and 12.6% of longevous with the habit of smoking and alcohol drinking. Self-dependence occurred in 73.5%. Cognitive function was apparently well or slightly impaired in 88.9%. Home care is emphasized for the life preservation of the longevous.

Consanguinity and Longevity

T.P.K. Reddy, A. Papa Rao, K.K. Reddy (Department of Anthropology, School of Biological & Earth Sciences, Sri Venkateswara University, Tirupati - 517 502. India)

Health and diseases are the expression of the degree of success or failure experienced by an organism it its effort to respond adaptively to an environmental challenge. Different health indicators reveal the structure and biological fitness of a population, resulting in the increase/decrease in (a) life expectancy and (b) the proportion of population aged 60+. The phenomenon of aging was done among Kurichians (who have high longevity), a tribal population of Kerala, by estimating fertility, mortality and morbidity. The consanguineous marriages percentage is high. The fertility is 1.01 times less in consanguineous than non-consanguineous. Among consanguineous, 1/3rd of the pregnancies proned to mortality and 1/4th in the case of non-consanguineous, which indicates high mortality among the offspring of consanguineous than non-consanguineous. Further, in total, it is to state that 1/6th of the offspring resulted to mortality. Due to consanguinity, the disease prevalence, prenatal and postnatal mortality is very high due to increase in homozygosity and enhanced risk of hereditary disease transmitted through recessive alleles. Further, among the ancestors of the consanguineous couples, the deleterious genes were eliminated through mortality, hence, observed a low mortality rates among consanguineous linearity when compared to the non-consanguineous. Thus, the effects of parental consanguinity of both the parents of the couples suggests that the practice of inbreeding had already reduced the burden of deleterious genes, thus leading to an increase in the fitness of an individual and hence, Kurichians having a maximum life expectancy.

Descriptive Epidemiology of Centenarians and Nonagenarians in a population based study, Kakegawa, Japan

Kanamori M. Suzuki M, (School of Medicine Hamamatsu University) Shiraki M. (University of Shizuoka, Hamamatsu College) Yamazaki S, Sato H, Ito S (Kakegawa Tokuiku Health Center) Kobashi G.(Department of Public Health, Hokkaido University School of Medicine) Yosimura K. (National Cancer Center), Uchida A.(Chiba University) Hirose N. (Department of Geriatric Medicine, Keio University School of Medicine)

Population based epidemiological study on centenarians and nonagenarians was conducted to examine whether centenarians are a special group genetically or not, to find a causal structure model emphasized body constitution, marital status, cognition and blood pressure as particularly important determinants for survival after 100 years. This paper is focused on the description of nonagenarians and centenarians in Kakegawa, Japan. The small town is famous for agriculture of green tea and orange, the one of the most longevous area in Japan. Methods: 1) Information of census data to obtain accurate frequency of the old living and survival rate from 90 years old to reach 100. Survival rate was calculated by the lifetime method. 2) Participants were free-living healthy volunteers; accept for interview, physical examination, blood sampling (12 volunteers of 12 centenarians,59 of 217 nonagenarians). Revised NEO Personality Inventory, life satisfaction index, activity of daily living were obtained using the questionnaire. Biochemical markers and peripheral blood count detected health and nutritional status. Results 1) Survival rate is 0.39 from 80 years old to reach 90, 0.05 from 90 years old to reach 100 2) Lp(a), a cholesterol-rich, low-density lipoprotein, is 21.6 (± 13.7) is low level. Liver function is almost all within normal, but Diabetes marker is slightly elevated. In factors of personality Neuroticism, Extraversion, and Openness are low scores, Agreeableness and Conscientiousness are increased. Conclusion: Survival rate is 0.05 from 90 years old to reach 100. The status without diseases such as liver, arteriosclerosis, mental activity, personalities are important to successful ageing.

The Emerging Face of Centenarians in Australia

John McCormack (LaTrobe University, Melbourne, Australia)

PURPOSE: This paper explores the changing prevalence and socio-health status of centenarians in Australia. The aims of the source study were (1) to identify and describe socio-demographic characteristics of Australian centenarians and compare them with centenarians from other countries; (2) to investigate whether there is social and health heterogeneity among Australian centenarians; and (3) to investigate whether there are social and health differences between centenarians and younger aged cohorts in Australia. METHOD: The study uses secondary sources of data to paint a preliminary picture of centenarians in Australia. Historical ABS census records and unpublished census data, as well as government departmental data were obtained to present a range of centenarian characteristics. Additionally, Aged Care Assessment Service (ACAS) data and acute hospital utilisation data for Victoria were obtained for centenarian health analysis. RESULTS: Centenarians appear to be a fast growing and heterogeneous group. As expected however, those presenting to ACAS are less independent in ADLs than younger cohorts. On the other hand, hospital data indicates they use less acute services than younger cohorts. Centenarians rate their own health as good, but there may be different groups within centenarians (ie the healthy & not so healthy). More research is needed. CONCLUSION: The author concludes by arguing for the establishment of a multidisciplinary Australian Centenarian Study.

Understanding Longevity: Beyond the conventional assessment in centenarians

D. Matallana, C. de Santacruz, C. Cano, C. Villaquirán, M. Benito (Aging Institute, Memory Clinic, Universidad JAveriana, Hospital San Ignacio, Bogotá, Colombia)

Though a hundred years humans used to be exceedingly rare, today we take notice of centenarians much more frequently since, probably, communication distances has been reduced and, on the other hand, populations in most countries are aging. Since our Memory Clinic, has seen, occasionally, centenarians, cognitive and functional outcome in nonagenarians and centenarians was, on the first place, the main purpose of the present research. Through a series of cases, 46 subjects had a comprehensive functional assessment (mean= 94 years, 8 were over 100 years, 63 0.000000emales and 37% Males). Results showed that at least 400f the sample had the expected associated diseases (high blood pressure; dementia and osteoarthritis = 37%). Limits on sensory functions were present in 400f patients. Instrumental activities (Lawton) were impaired in at least 900f cases, as well as their Basic activities (Barthell). Measurements based on execution were done to just 220f subjects. Cognitive functioning were accomplished to just 28 subjects through a complete neuropsychological evaluation. Descriptive analysis lead us to the conclusion that language, memory, visuoconstructional and executive functions were impaired in at least 2, or more, Standard Deviations bellow the expected levels. Since results were not sufficient, a qualitative approach -non clinical- were done. Forthcoming a comprehensive whole of the surrounding and relations through the subject and relatives narrative description of a day of his/her life (present and past), we pictured routines and did different analysis headed to understand the sense of longevity and vital circumstances of centenarians.

SESSION 399

Ethnic Diversity Issues Facing Elderly in the United States: Challenges, Opportunities and Social Policy Implications

Charlene H. James, MPH(City of Houston, Houston/Harris county Area Agency on Aging, Houston, TX USA) and Gerson David, ACSW(University of Houston Graduate School of Social Work, Houston, TX USA)

Purpose: This paper will address two important issues(1)the Area Agency on Aging's experience in advocating for and serving the growing number of ethnically diverse elderly and (2) policy modifications needed to insure access to health and social services, in light of restrictions on non-citizens' ability to receive public benefits. Method: The increasing number of ethnically diverse elderly in the greater Houston area has heightened the awareness of health and social service access issues. This is borne out where barriers to access are created by limited income, no health insurance coverage and the legal status of the elderly, since the enactment of The Personal Responsibility and Work Opportunity Reconciliation Act and the Illegal Immigration Reform and Immigrant Responsibility Act of 1996. The Agency mounted advocacy, education and constituent mobilization strategies to increase the awareness and availability of services and eligible public benefits. The Agency also formed partnerships by collaborating with organizations providing services and advocating on behalf of these individuals. Outreach efforts through the Agency's Benefits Counseling Program were accelerated. Results: Elderly persons were informed of available services for which they were eligible. Partnerships with organizations facilitated access to information in appropriate languages and access to needed services is occurring. Lastly,legislative advocacy is on-going at the local, state and national levels. Conclusion: Through the use of available service delivery network resources, elderly persons have been able to access services and improve their health status and quality of life.

Fears in Older Population in South Africa

Debo Akande (Potche University, Vanderbijlparke, South Africa)

The fear of elderly population may differ from one gender and cultural context to another. I explored this possibility in 430 male and female South African older adults between 67 and 77 years of age. Responses to a standard fear survey schedule revealed significant differences in the number, content, pattern, and level of fears. Female older adults endorsed fears at higher levels than older male adults who did not differ from one another. However, differences in the pattern and content of fears for men and women of different ages were noted across the races. Results were interpreted within a cultural context, which suggested that cultures which favour inhibition, compliance, and obedience serve to increase levels of fear. Possible generalisation of the findings in other collectivist cultures like Hong Kong and Asia are explored.

The elderly Arab population in Israel: Health and social support characteristics in context

Adrian Walter-Ginzburg, (Herczeg Institute on Aging, Tel Aviv University, Tel Aviv, Israel) Khalid Suleiman, M.D. (Dabouriya Home for the Aged, Kfar Dabouriya, Israel)

Purpose: Life expectancy in Israel is among the highest in the world, yet it varies among the subpopulations. This paper examines the health and functional differences and similarities in the Jewish and non-Jewish (Arab) elderly populations in Israel which may contribute to the observed patterns of life expectancy. Method: Analysis of a 1997 national survey of Israelis aged 60 and over, conducted by the Israeli Central Bureau of Statistics, as well as data available on the elderly in the Palestinian Authority, Jordan, and Egypt. We also use data gathered by the authors in the course of their work in the only public nursing home in the Arab sector in Israel. Results: The life expectancy of Jewish Israelis has increased over the past several decades for both Jewish and Arab residents, and although the Arab population in Israel has the highest average life expectancy of any Arab population in the region, yet it lags behind the Jewish population both in absolute years of life expectancy and in annual percentage increase in life expectancy over the past few decades, with a cross-over of mortality in the oldest age groups. The elderly Arab population has higher levels of disability and morbidity than the Jewish elderly population, as well as a high level of social support. We examine and describe the most salient socio-demographic and health differences between the two populations. Conclusion: In a system where there is universal health insurance and widely-available health care, there are still socio-economic differences in health and disability between the Jewish and Arab populations in Israel. These differences can be partly explained by health behaviors, access to health care, and social networks.

Understandings of successful aging in the context of migration: the case of Iranian immigrants to Sweden

Sandra Torres (Dept. of Sociology, Uppsala University, Uppsala, Sweden)

Inquiries into understandings of successful aging have been characterized by culture-specificity. This means that the understandings in question have only been studied in the specific cultural settings that have given them their meaning. Understandings that are simultaneously influenced by two cultures have yet to be studied. This study departs from a newly designed theoretical framework for the study of successful aging — a framework that aims to be culturally-relevant and that assumes that there is congruence between the manner in which sense is made out of the gerontological construct in question and the value orientations one upholds. Using this framework and the instrument designed to test it, this study focuses on the context of migration where culture of origin and host culture meet. Qualitative interviews using vignettes have been conducted with 30 Iranian immigrants to Sweden. The aim has been to study how prior and post migration understandings of successful aging differ from one another. The findings show that cultural contexts determine how the construct in question is understood and that migration to a culture that is different from one's culture of origin can challenge the manner in which successful aging is understood.

SESSION 400

Experience of a Lifetime

Terry Coles, (Maple Lake Releasing, Winnipeg, Manitoba, Canada)

EXPERIENCE OF A LIFETIME, is a documentary demonstrating the capacity of seniors to contribute to the growth of industry. Following 2 retired Canadian executives to their volunteer assignments in Asia and the Caribbean the documentary examines the two-way path of contribution and gain. What do a mattress manufacturer in Trinidad and a hospital in Thailand have in common? Morley and Tony, two enthusiastic retired businessmen who are volunteer mentors to companies and organizations in transition. Age is no barrier to making a difference for these men as they give and gain an experience of a lifetime

SESSION 410

Assessment and Management of Chronic Pain in Geriatrics

H. Eichbauer, I. Findl, K. Klaushofer, K. Koller (Hanusch-Hospital Vienna, Austria, Europe)

For lack of specialized pain centers, patients with chronic pain are referred to medical, neurological or geriatric departments. One third of patients are dissatisfied with pain management during stay in hospital (patient interviews 1998). To improve this situation, a pain management system was developed and tested under daily clinical conditions. If the history-taking resulted in chronic pain, we first found out the chronicity of pain by the Mainz Pain Staging System. In case of advanced chronic pain (stage II or III), a comprehensive history-taking of the patients pain including psychometric tests followed. For each patient we worked out an individual interdisciplinary therapy. To verify the results, patients were interviewed before dismissal. 27.8% of our patients during half a year (n = 381) suffered from chronic pain (N = 106; 38 men, mean age 64 years; 68 women, mean age 66 years), 68% of them suffered from non-malign pain, and 32% from cancer pain. By pain management activities we were able to raise significantly the satisfaction of the patients with pain therapy. Consequently, searching for chronic pain is necessary. Elderly people in particular do not mention their suffering, often believing that pain is an unavoidable sign of old age. Concentrating on medical reports alone is not adequate for chronic pain and can even aggravate the condition to a significant extent. Chronic pain can neither be explained nor treated without integrating psychological and social factors. A routine diagnostic and therapy practice facilitates an interdisciplinary pain therapy, raises the therapeutic capability of the staff and increases the therapeutic outcome.

Chronic Pain Conditions in Community Dwelling Elderly: Relationship with Physical Function and Disability.

A.K. Coppin, MD (University of Massachusetts, Boston, USA)

Purpose: The purpose of this research was to determine the association between chronic pain and disability among community-dwelling elderly individuals. Methods: Data from the first wave (1993) of the AHEAD survey were used. Separate measures of ADLs, IADLs and physical function were used as dependent variables. Multivariate regression analysis was utilized to estimate the impact of chronic pain. Results: The sample selection criteria included individuals of both sexes, 65 years and older, 7,136 subjects conformed the study sample. They were predominantly white (81%), and female (63 %), with a mean age of 77 (SD 6.5) years. Chronic pain was reported by 32% of the subjects; 14 % were overweight, 26% reported arthritis, and 13% reported diabetes mellitus. On average, the number of ADLs reported was just over one half (.54), IADLs was just over one third (.38), and the reported mobility limitations was almost one (.94). The results suggests that for ADLs and IADLs, the effect of chronic pain may be conditioned by older age, female gender, poor health, and overweight, or by the interaction with chronic conditions in which pain is a major component. The results showed a highly significant ($p<.001$) association between mobility limitations and chronic pain, which persisted even after the introduction of the interaction terms, suggesting a direct effect of chronic pain on the individual's ability to mobilize independently. Conclusion: This research highlighted the distinct impact of pain on mobility function and the multifactorial effect of pain on basic and instrumental activities of daily living.

Elderly Pain Caring Assessment (E.P.C.A.) : the first scale validated in noncommunicating elderly patients

R. Morello (Biostatistics, University Hospital, Caen, France), A. Jean (Geriatrics, La Rochefoucauld Hospital, Paris, France), J.C. Fermanian (Biostatistics, Necker University Hospital, Paris, France), J.F. Desson and M. Alix (Geriatrics, University Hospital, Caen, France).

Purpose Pain in noncommunicative elderly people is often misdiagnosed. Thus, appropriate management requires adequate assessment tools, like behavioural and multidimensional scales. It's a world-wide lack of this. E.P.C.A. is specifically presenting with chronic pain assessment in cognitively impaired older persons. Method Since 1992, E.P.C.A. has been elaborated in a collaborative, prospective and multicenter study (n=135 subjects). First words and signs reminding pain were listed by geriatric teams. Many reexaminations by experts created five successive patterns, refining the accuracy and exhaustivity of E.P.C.A.. Variability and reliability were explored, as well as face and content validities. Factorial analysis with varimax rotation was used to work out the construct validity. Result Intra-class correlation coefficients were higher than 0.80 and Cronbach's a coefficients greater than 0.70. Cross-validation and sensitivity to change studies were significant. Principal components have defined two different dimensions, before and during the nursing. Conclusion E.P.C.A. is the first validated behavioural pain scale for a reliable, easy and current use in geriatric practice.

Is Pain Under-recognized and Under-treated in Institutionalized Elderly Patients with Dementia?

P.A. O'Hara (SCO Health Service, Ottawa, Canada), C.I. Neutel (University of Ottawa Institute on Health of the Elderly, Ottawa, Canada), W. Walop (Laboratory Centre for Disease Control, Health Canada, Ottawa, Canada).

Although the literature indicates that the comorbidity of persons with dementia is similar to that of persons without dementia, evidence suggests that there may be differences in the way that their pain is acknowledged and treated. The purpose of this study is to determine whether or not such differences exist in the reporting of pain, and in the use of analgesics, among institutionalized elderly with and without dementia. As part of the National Population Health Survey (NPHS) conducted by Statistics Canada (1994-5), a randomly selected sample of long-term residents of health care institutions was surveyed. Data were collected for 1,727 residents who were 65 years of age or over, of whom 616 (36%) were classified as having dementia. While the proportion of residents having potentially painful conditions (e.g. arthritis, osteoporosis) was approximately the same, pain was identified less often in the dementia group (28%) than the non-dementia group (40%). The dementia group was also less likely to receive analgesics (38%) than the non-dementia group (55%). While residents receiving analgesics were 2.4 times more likely to be identified as having pain than residents not receiving analgesics, they were 0.6 times less likely to have dementia. In conclusion, although there are no definitive data to suggest that advanced age or dementia diminishes the experience of pain, the long-term residents of health care facilities in this study who were diagnosed with dementia were less likely to be identified as having pain, and less likely to be treated with analgesics.

The impact of chronic pain on elderly residents : a district-based cross-sectional study in Hong Kong

Yau Cheuk-ngok Daniel, Chiu Tak-yi, Chow Yuk-hing Ada, Wu Yee-ming, Liu Chi-pun, and Leung Chi-tat Antony (Aged Care Reseach & Development Unit, Haven of Hope Christian Service, Hong Kong, China)

PURPOSE: To understand the impact of non-malignant chronic pain experienced by elderly residents of residential care facilities in Tseung Kwan O (TKO) District, Hong Kong. METHOD: All six long-term care facilities in the local district were included in this study. The first part of the study included all the residents (n= 690) who were able to communicate if they were suffering from non-malignant chronic pain. Second part of the study consisted of 131 residents who were drawn from the identified pain sufferer's list. The Chinese version of the Brief Pain Inventory (BPI-C) was used to measure level of pain severity and interference of pain on the elderly residents. Open-ended questions were also included to gather qualitative data on the subjects' experience of pain. RESULTS: Mean age of subjects was 80.8 (SD 6.8). 80.20f the subjects were female. The overall prevalence of non-malignant chronic pain was 36.2%. Coefficient alphas for the four pain severity scales and the seven pain interference scales of the BPI-C were 0.82 and 0.87 respectively. While 80.70f the respondents reported that the average pain intensity in the past 24 hours was at mild to moderate level, 58.40f the respondents reported their perceived worst pain was at moderate to severe level. The common locations of pain were low-back region and lower-limbs. Mobility, daily living and mood were affected by the pain condition on 63.5%, 53.6% and 50.80f the respondents respectively. The most frequently mentioned activities being affected by pain were walking and transferring. CONCLUSION: Studies on non-malignant chronic pain in elderly populations in Hong Kong residential settings are scarce. Of concern is the high prevalence of pain being suffered by elderly residents in the care facilities. This study also provides evidence on how these older residents in Hong Kong are being affected by and coping with their chronic pain condition.

SESSION 411

Changes in self-reports and performance-based measures of mobility over 10 years among elderly people

Ritva Sakari-Rantala, Taina Rantanen and Pertti Era (Univ. of Jyväskylä, Jyväskylä, Finland)

PURPOSE: The purpose of this study was to describe the changes in self-reports and performance-based measures of mobility over 10 years, in two intervals of five years, among men and women who survived from 75 to 85 years. METHOD: The functional capacity of the 75-year-old citizens of Jyväskylä, Finland, was evaluated (n=355) and the measurements were repeated at age 80 and 85. In all three measurement occasions 146 men and women participated in interviews and 81 in laboratory tests. Difficulties in mobility were asked as perceived tiredness and slowness when moving about indoors, outdoors and climbing stairs. The maximal walking speed in a distance of 10 m and the stair-mounting ability were measured in a laboratory. RESULTS: Among men, there was no significant decline in self-perceived mobility over ten years. Among women, the decline in moving about indoors was significant between the age 80 and 85 (p=.040) and, in moving about outdoors, in both intervals of five years (p=.010 and p=.004). In the stair-mounting test, men improved their performance from 75 to 80 years (p=.039) but declined during the next five years (p=.002). Among women, a significant decline was seen in both five years' intervals (p=.001 and p<.001). Walking speed declined significantly from 75 to 80 years and from 80 to 85 years both in men and women (all p- values <.001). CONCLUSION: In this selected group of survivors, performance-based measures of mobility showed more linear decline over ten years than self- reports of mobility, except for the first follow-up period in the stair-mounting test among men. Perceived mobility declined differently among men and women and, among women, the patterns of decline varied according to different mobility tasks. The critical phase where faster mobility decline begins in old age is probably task and gender specific.

Development of training programs for health professionals in care of older people in India

A. B. Dey (All India Institute of Medical Sciences, New Delhi, India), S. Soneja (HelpAge India, New Delhi, India)

Several programs directed at the older population have been initiated in India following the declaration of the national policy, one of which is strengthening of the health services. Physicians are not trained enough to provide quality care as geriatrics is not a recognized specialty. Realizing the need for skilled professionals, a program for up-gradation of skills of health professional was initiated by the Government of India in 1998 with World Health Organization. The basis for this program was data derived from national sample surveys, research projects, authors data on morbidity profile of health seeking elderly and census of 1991. Pneumonia, IHD, stroke, carrier and tuberculosis were the most frequent causes of death; and hypertension, cataract, osteoarthritis, COPD, IHD, diabetes mellitus, prostatic hypertrophy, dyspepsia, irritable bowel syndrome and depression were most frequent morbidity in these reports. A group of experts prepared a comprehensive plan for training physicians in primary and secondary health care, undergraduate students, community health workers and non-formal carers. 80 consultants in medicine from 44 medical schools were sensitized in the discipline and were asked to prepare a training and practice manual for primary and secondary care physicians. As the follow up action 450 primary and secondary care physicians have been provided training in care of the older patient, which will continue for 2 more years. The current emphasis is on modification of the undergraduate curriculum and preparation of the postgraduate curriculum in order to produce trained doctors as well as specialists in health care of older patients.

From Early Diagnosis to End of Life Care: A Series of Online Teaching Case Studies in Dementia.

David Patrick Ryan, Rory Fisher, M.B. FRCP(C) (Regional Geriatric Program of Toronto & University of Toronto, Toronto, Canada)

An increasing number of physicians are using the internet for continuing education.To meet the needs of these physicians and especially physicians in rural or remote regions for whom access to continuing education in often logistically difficult, a series of online teaching case studies has been developed. The focus of the case studies is dementia because of demographic imperatives and dementia care is repeatedly identified in learning needs surveys. The learning materials were initially designed and continue to be available for small group learning but the process of transforming these materials for online learning has been challenging. This paper traces the transformation process through the stages of redefining educational objectives, instructional and multi-media design, progressive beta testing and the development of an evaluative framework. Data generated in these stages is reviewed while the case studies and associated online materials are demonstrated.

Involvement and participation of older clients in mental health care

C. Smits, W. de Vries and J. de Lange (Netherlands Institute of

Mental Health and Addiction)

The purpose of the present study was to develop a manual for mental health care staff to improve the involvement of older clients in their mental health care. The study took place in various mental health care settings in two regions in the Netherlands. In a survey 81 clients and their immediate caretakers were interviewed on their involvement and on factors facilitating and limiting client involvement. In-depth interviews with 13 client-staff combinations and observations of care situations provided information on latent factors. The survey results highlight the role of mastery and self-efficacy in clients. Furthermore, clients and staff estimates of client involvement do not always coincide. The observations and in-depth interviews showed a typology of clients varying in degree of autonomy and verbal assertiveness. A staff typology is being developed. A manual was written on the basis of the study results. Comments of an expert panel were used to improve the concept manual. The contents focus on relevant juridical and professional information, client and staff typology and strategies, client and staff matching, and helpful hints to facilitate older clients to verbalize or otherwise express their wishes in various stages of their care trajectory.

Involving the Whole Medical Team in Psycho-Geriatric Observation

M. Habrias (Centre Hospitalier de Bourganeuf, France)

The article gives an account of the basis of an original training scheme aimed at all members of the care team, in the 8 geriatric centers operated by a pension fund. It argued that neither nurses nor nursing aides are sufficiently familiar with the fundamental principles of psycho-geriatrics, whereas they do have a privileged view of behaviour troubles in institutions, which is different, complementary and helpful for diagnosis and subsequent therapeutic treatment. Four training days were set up for nurses and nursing aids, which aims were: to put in place a psycho-geriatric diagnostic tree diagram , accessible to these two categories, focusing on the distinction between : - cognition troubles - contact with reality troubles - anxiety troubles - mood troubles - relations with others troubles to list the main behavioural disorders and to state precisely their characteristics according to the chapters of the diagnostic diagram. to determine for each category of carers the appropriate level of observation. to research more particularly, according to work timetables : - problems of daily life activity (morning team). - instrumental and relational problems (afternoon team). - problems of actual instinctive-affective experience (evening/night team). The appropriation of this approach can put the members of the care team to advantage, enhance their understanding of behavioural disorders, contribute to diagnosis and result in greater support amongst the team for the different methods of care.

Physicians attitude towards prevention and ageing

Walter U (1), Schienkiewitz A (1), Bitzer E (2), Raum E (1), Schlaud M (1), Schwartz FW (1) (1) Medical School Hannover, Dept. of Epidemiology, Social Medicine and Health System Research, Germany (2) Institute of Social Medicine, Epidemiology and Health System Research, Hannover, Germany

Purpose: Prevention for the elderly has a high potential to reduce morbidity in old age. One important mediator are the physicians. The objective of our study is to examine the physicians attitudes of prevention and their images of ageing and in connection with their diagnostic strategies or therapeutic patterns of ambulatory medical care and patient age. Method: A representative sample of 574 office-based general practitioners was drawn out of 1.491 GP's in the north-west of Germany. End of October 2001 112 agreed to participate. The understanding of preventive medicine in ambulatory medical care for different target groups as well as physicians preventive provisions was studied. The questionnaire includes items for physicians attitudes towards prevention in general and its effectiveness, prevention for the elderly and patients view of prevention. The image of ageing was measured with a standardised instrument. Results: 76 % responded the questionnaire. The first analyse shows that nearly all physicians consult their patients individually about risk behaviour, 23 Offered preventive group programmes. 30 % are not informed about local preventive programmes. Traditional preventive programmes like nutrition counselling and smoking cessation are considered as less important for the elderly, whereas the importance of influenza vaccination, memory training and prevention of falls increase with age. In comparison to 65 + prevention has less priority for physicians to the oldest old. Important preventive programmes for 80 + are only a check up of the medication (91 %) and prevention of falls (75 %). Dental health is the most neglected issue for the elderly. Conclusion: Although physicians appreciate prevention as important for the younger old, future medical curricula has to improve the knowledge and skills about the potential and possibilities of prevention in old age.

Teaching Biology of Aging at Moscow State University

A. N. Khokhlov (Evolutionary Cytogerontology Sector, School of Biology, Moscow State University, Moscow, Russia)

Some years ago I initiated a course of lectures on biology of aging for the Schools of Biology and Basic Medicine at Moscow State University. The proposal maintained that, at the present time, quality biological and medical education cannot be provided without a good knowledge of consistent characteristics of aging and development. As a result, the appropriate changes were introduced in the curriculum of those schools. Today, the course contains, among other topics, the following: Definition of aging, mortality, maximum and average life span, life expectancy; Survival curves, life tables, Gompertz-Makeham law; Rate of aging, accelerated and premature aging; Age-related diseases; Longitudinal and cross-sectional studies; Aging and non-aging organisms; Longevity and long-livers; Biological age; Evolution and aging; Various theories of aging, requirements for new concepts; Cell cultures in gerontology - Hayflick's phenomenon, "stationary phase aging" model, cell kinetics model, and others; Telomeres and telomerase; "Gist" and "correlative" models in gerontology; Germ cells and aging, "immortality" of the germ line; Stem cells and aging; Aging of protozoa, bacteria, fungi, mycoplasmas, plants, etc.; Free radicals and aging; Experimental life span modifications, geroprotectors and geropromoters; Possible role in the aging process of membrane structure and function, as well as DNA, protein and lipid changes. The course content is incessantly updated on the basis of latest gerontological publications, with a special attention to any new findings in molecular gerontology. The lectures and the subsequent examinations proved the existence of a deficiency in students' perception of aging phenomenon, a deficiency that was redressed by the course. The author is grateful to Russian Foundation for Basic Research for support (grant 00-04-48049).

Using Gerontological Nursing Practice Standards to Develop Gerontological Nursing in Acute Care

K. Hunter McIlveen, D. Hendrick, P. Hennig (Royal Alexandra Hospital, Edmonton, Alberta, Canada)

Nursing practice standards are one component of the assessment of competency maintenance. The purpose of this presentation is to describe a process to support the nurses on an Acute Care of the Elderly Unit in reflecting on gerontological nursing practice standards, identifying learning needs and meeting those needs. This supports staff in fulfilling new professional licensing requirements as well as increasing knowledge in care of older adults in hospital. The framework is the Canadian Gerontological Nursing Association Standards of Practice. The process is a continuous loop in which practice standards, performance appraisal, and educational initiatives are linked. All nurses on the unit attended a one day education session at which the standards were reviewed and education specific to two standards provided. Feedback was sought from the staff regarding prioritization of further education relating to the standards. Staff feedback was the bases for inservice education planning. The orientation for new nursing staff was revised using the practice standards as a framework. A new performance appraisal approach in which the nurses use practice standards to complete a self appraisal is being introduced. Finally, monitoring of key indicators related to changes in patient care is being implemented. At this presentation, we will focus on the model used to develop the process, presentation of supporting material (e.g. orientation booklet, performance appraisal format), topic areas covered in education initiatives and feedback from the nursing staff on the standard based performance appraisal.

When the Patient Teaches the Doctor-A Revolutionary Approach to Geriatric Education

J. Tomkowiak, A. Gunderson (Southern Illinois University School of Medicine, Springfield, Il. USA)

The Geriatric Mentor Program at SIU School of Medicine is truly the touchstone of a new geriatric curriculum initiative. This session is designed to provide a description of this unique approach to geriatric education and to assist other health care professionals with the implementation of a similiar program in their setting. The Geriatric Mentor Program is an exciting idea that pairs medical students with a geriatric individual from the community. The program allows the patient to share their wisdom and life experiences with the student as they learn about the aging process. The student also develops a relationship with an older adult that allows them to see life changes through the eyes of that senior, and develop proactive, empathetic attitudes towards this population. Seventy seven students have been involved in the program and surveys of these students have revealed an increase in geriatric knowledge and improved attitudes toward caring for the geriatric patient. This program encourages students and health care professionals to proactively support the geriatric population in their successful aging through the enhancement of knowledge and attitudes.

SESSION 412

Participation of Elderly People in the Polish Society

B. Synak (Department of Sociology, University of Gdansk, Gdansk, Poland), P. Bledowski (Department of Social Policy, Warsaw School of Economics, Warsaw, Poland), M. Halicka (Department of Clinical and Social Gerontology, Medical Academy, Bialystok, Poland),

The purpose of the presented study is an examination of societal participation of the elderly in Poland in respect of their participation in working life, productive activities, political participation and leisure activities. This paper is based on the survey conducted in 2000, on a national random sample of 1821 people 65 +, and on 600 interviews. There is a very low rate of the elderly's participation in working life and a small part of retirees are interested in gainful employment. The new economic cicumstances produce ageism and social exclusion from working life. The elderly's participation in "productive activities" is relatively high but mostly it is limited to informal help for neighbors and friends. There is a very low rate of political participation . Elderly people are characterized by low engagement in local activities and little interest in social life of their settlements. Leisure activity is mostly of a solitary and passive type. Very few eldery people are involved in tourism and recreation. All kinds of social participation of the elderly are strongly differientiated by age, gender, social background and cultural environment. Elderly people in Poland live in a social niche, outside the mainstream of public life. This results from the exsisting social norms and lack of patterns of active participation. The political transformation has shaken the older generation's collective memory and does not favor to participation of the elderly in society.

Quality of life and frequency of going outside among the frail elderly living at home

Ayumi Kono, Department of community health nursing, Tokyo Medical and Dental University, Tokyo, Japan Ichiro Kai, Department of Social Gerontology, The University of Tokyo, Tokyo, Japan Shigeo Sasaki Senior Citizens of Welfare Section, Saku City Government Office, Nagano, Japan Chiyoko Sakato, RSenior Citizens of Welfare Section, Saku City Government Office, Nagano, Japan

Purpose: To investigate the relationship between quality of life and frequency of going outside among the frail elderly living at home. Methods: A total of 203 frail elderly residents were surveyed in Saku City, Japan. The data was collected by a questionnaire including the following items: frequency of going outside, ADL, instrumental ADL (developed by Tokyo Metropolitan Institute of Gerontology), fall-related self-efficacy (FES), self-efficacy for health promotion (SEHP), depression (measured by GDS), social support (measured by Social Support Scale developed by Noguchi), and daily activity. Results: The mean age of the respondents was 82.5 (SD 7.3) years, and 74.0% of them were females. They were classified into four groups according to the frequency of going outside: daily, once every 2-3 days, once a week and seldom. The scores of ADL, IADL and FES of the elderly seldom going outside were lower than the other three groups. Low SEHP and GDS as well as decreased social support from friends were associated with low frequency of going outside. Using ANOVA with ADL as a covariate, the elderly who seldom went outside received significantly less friend support than those who went outside daily. Conclusion: Results showed low frequency of going outside was associated with low physical and psychosocial function and decreased friend support. These findings suggest that the frequency of going out could be used as an index of quality of life among the frail elderly.

The role of leisure in enhancing physical and mental health in later life

Bryan J.A. Smale (University of Waterloo, Waterloo, Canada)

Considerable evidence has been generated in recent years that illustrates the critical role that participation in leisure activities plays in maintaining optimal physical health, improving one's sense of well-being, enhancing mental health, and reducing the effects of chronic stress. The purpose of this study was to examine the role that participation in active leisure pursuits plays in moderating physical and mental health in later life. Using data from the 1994 National Population Health Survey, adults aged 65 years and older were selected (N=5,093) and two key dependent variables were used in the analyses: a health utility index, which describes overall functional physical health, and a measure of mental health based on the mental distress scale devised by Kessler and Mroczek. Participation in active leisure pursuits was assessed according to a physical activity index that estimates the total amount of energy expenditure attributable to engagement in several different leisure activities. Other variables included in the study as control factors were an index of chronic stress, presence of a long term restriction to physical activity, level of social support received, and selected demographic factors including age, gender, income, and marital status. After controlling for the selected factors, the results indicated that active participation in leisure pursuits was associated with significantly higher levels of both physical and mental health. The results were consistent for both males and females, in all the older age groups, and especially for those with a long term limitation.

Walking and cycling among Finnish persons aged 55 and older; A follow- up study 1995-2000

Hirsiaho, Nina & Ruoppila, Isto (Department of Psychology, University of Jyväskylä, Jyväskylä, Finland)

The purpose of the MOBILATE follow-up study is to analyse and explain stability and changes in outdoor mobility among persons 55+ in Finland, Germany and Italy between 1995-2000. Methods: The sample in 1995 was stratified by age (55-74 and 75+ years), sex and the urban living area (centre, intermediate, outskirts). From the Finnish eligible sample (N= 1040) 618 persons were interviewed, the drop-out being 33.7%. For the 2000-study, from the eligible subjects (N= 438) of 95-study 294 persons were interviewed, the drop-out being 32.9%. The both data include standardised home interviews and trip-diaries. In 2000 psychological tests, physiological measurements and new questions on changes in mobility were included. Results: The 95-study revealed that "active bikers" (cycling 1-2 times/week, not driving a car) used public transportation more than the others. 92% of them were retired, and there were more people living alone than married among them. Of their accidents 77% happened during cycling whereas with the others 67% occured while walking. Health-satisfaction was higher among the active bikers. They informed less of illnesses preventing mobility and less mobility difficulties. They estimated their physical mobility being better, were more active in the outdoor mobility and had more physical hobbies than the others. From the 95-study subjects 88% were pursuing walking. Among the walkers 62% of their accidents happened while walking, 21% on cycling, and 12% when driving a car. Conclusions: In 2000 we expect the physically active subjects to differ from the others as in 1995.

SESSION 413

Cost-Effective Expansion of the Elderly Nutrition Program

E. A. Gollub, D. O. Weddle (National Policy and Resouce Center on Nutrition and Aging, Florida International University, FL, USA)

PURPOSE: The Elderly Nutrition Program (ENP), funded by the Older Americans Act, targets its home-delivered meals to a frail population at risk for malnutrition and poor quality of life. This study evaluates the cost-effectiveness of expanding the ENP to include breakfast as a second home-delivered meal. Program costs and effects on nutritional well-being and quality of life will be determined. METHOD: This cross-sectional field study is currently in progress. Clients receiving home-delivered breakfast in addition to noon meals are being compared to similar meal clients who are not receiving breakfast. Approximately 200 participants for each group have been recruited from 5 racially/ethnically and geographically diverse agencies currently administering traditional and expanded ENP home-delivered meal programs. Participant data is being collected through in-home interviews. A questionnaire that includes scales representing six distinct quality of life domains, malnutrition risk scores, and 24-hour food recalls is being used. Program costs are being collected from administrators. RESULTS: It is expected that breakfast clients will experience greater levels of quality of life and nutritional well-being. A cost of well-being ratio ($ meal service/quality of life score) will be developed. This will be the first time that the ENP breakfast service will be evaluated in terms of cost of influencing nutritional well-being and quality of life. CONCLUSION: This study will help determine whether the new program warrants promotion as a national model.

Dietary Quality and lifestyle habits of European and American elders

A. Haveman-Nies, C.P.G.M. de Groot, W.A. van Staveren (Wageningen University, Division of Human Nutrition & Epidemiology, Wageningen, the Netherlands), K.L. Tucker (Jean Mayer USDA Human Nutrition Research Center on Aging at Tufts University, Boston, USA)

BACKGROUND: Lifestyle habits play an important role in the onset of chronic diseases and disability. The prevalence of chronic diseases and functional limitations is rapidly increasing in the older population. Modifiable lifestyle factors can be important instruments in the postponement of morbidity and can have a major effect on the quality of life. PURPOSE: Lifestyle habits are changing over time and therefore this study describes dietary patterns and lifestyle factors, such as overweight, physical activity, and smoking habits of older Americans and Europeans. Further, the relationship between dietary patterns and lifestyle factors is investigated. METHODS: Two methods to make dietary patterns operational are cluster analysis and the calculation of diet scores. Both cluster analysis and diet scores can be used to classify persons into groups differing in nutritional status. In this study the Mediterranean Diet Score and the Healthy Diet Indicator are calculated for 2110 elders, aged 70-77 y, of the Europe-wide SENECA Study and the Framingham Heart Study. RESULTS AND CONCLUSION: Each dietary assessment method provided similar categorization of persons into groups of low and high dietary quality. In this older population, a high dietary quality was still related to other healthy lifestyle habits, implicating that a high quality diet is part of a healthy lifestyle and diet should be integrated in a multidisciplinary approach of health promotion.

Intermittent oro-esophagial tube feeding: Alternative alimentation for elderly with dysphasia or eating disorder

Akiko Kanemaru (Tokyo Metropolitan Geriatric Hospital, Tokyo, Japan), Ryutaro Takahashi (Tokyo Metropolitan Institute of Gerontology, Tokyo, Japan), Takayuki Kato,Junichiro Inoue, Sumiko Okada, Haruki Tobimatsu (Tokyo Metropolitan Geriatric Hospital, Tokyo,Japan)

PURPOSE: In dysphasic patients, social factors as well as medical indication affect the decision of feeding method. We examined the present status of alternative alimentation in our hospital. METHODS: We recruited subjects who received gastrostomy for tube feeding and those received rehabilitation for eating and swallowing disturbance from 1999 to 2000. Demographic, personal and medical records were collected. RESULTS: Information was collected form 52 subjects (mean age=75.8). Subjects were divided into 2 groups: those with a trial of intermittent oro-esophageal tube feeding (IOE) (IOE group; n=20) and those without challenge of IOE (ordinary care (OC) group; n=32). Mean ages were 69.6 and 79.8 years, respectively ($p<0.01$). Male:female ratios were 16:4 and 15:17 ($p<0.05$), incontinence was observed in 50% and 97% ($p<0.01$), respectively. OC group was more dependent at discharge ($p<0.01$), and more complicated suffering from degenerative disorder than IOE group (41%, 2%, $p<0.05$). At discharge, striking differences were found between the groups. In IOE group, 6 cases were eating orally, 7 were in combination of IOE and oral intake, 2 were on IOE and 3 were undergone gastrostomy and the last 2 were on other method. In OC group, 4 cases were eating orally, 24 were still on gastrostomy, 4 were in combination of continuous tube-feeding and oral intake ($p<0.01$). The percentage of discharge to home was 65% and 71% respectively (not significant). Conclusion: IOE seems to be a new choice when alternative alimentation is determined.

Older women and food: The influence of gender

Angela Dickinson (Oxford Brookes University, Oxford, UK)

PURPOSE Measures aimed at improving the nutritional status of older people require an understanding of their way of life and why and how they choose the food they eat, that is, the non-biological meanings and socio-cultural aspects of food. The aim of this study was to explore, in-depth, the food choices and eating habits of free-living people aged over 60. METHOD A qualitative, grounded theory study, where semi-structured interviews and food-diaries were used as data-collection tools. RESULTS The study provided an insight into the cultural complexity of the food choice decisions and eating habits of older people. Principally, this study found that food choice among older people was not determined so much by food preference or health consciousness as by the effect of income variations, restrictions imposed by gender, the social context of food and lay health beliefs. Gender can be seen to operate on several areas of this food-related work, which is done by older women. Empirical evidence will be presented to describe how gender influences the various components of the food-provisioning process, for example, food shopping, food preparation, clearing up and even the space within which these tasks are carried out. Much of this work is invisible, and the work requires investment of emotional energy. CONCLUSIONS Gender influences the food choices of women and has implications for the health of both women and men.

Successful Aging in Japans Longest-Lived People: The Role of the Traditional Okinawan Diet

B. J. Willcox (Division on Aging, Harvard Medical School, Boston, USA); D.C. Willcox (College of Nursing, Okinawa Prefectural University, Naha, Japan); D.J.A. Jenkins (Department of Nutritional Sciences, University of Toronto, Toronto, Canada); H. Todoriki and M. Suzuki (Divisions of Preventive and Community Medicine, University of the Ryukyus, Nishihara, Japan)

Introduction: The inhabitants of Okinawa, a Japanese prefecture (province) are among the worlds longest-lived people. Life expectancy is 77.2 years for men and 85.1 years for women (Japan Ministry of Health, 1995). Traditional dietary patterns may play a role in this phenomenon. Purpose: To assess the traditional diet of the Okinawans. Method: We recorded food intake for 3-7 days in 21 healthy community-dwelling Okinawan elderly (16 women and 5 men ranging in age from 72-88 years). Results: Vegetables and fruits, grains, and legumes were the most commonly consumed foods forming 40%, 32%, 120f the diet respectively. Fish and shellfish formed 11%, meat 3% and dairy products 20f the diet respectively. Caloric consumption averaged 1577.7 (SD 108.7) kcal per day, with 54%, 18% and 280f calories coming from carbohydrates, protein and fat respectively. Monounsaturated fat accounted for 40.7%, saturated 24.3% and polyunsaturated 17.80f total fat intake respectively. Flavonoid intake was 100.9 mg/day. Salt consumption averaged 7 grams per day. Conclusions: Most striking about the diet was the low caloric intake, the number and variety of plant foods, the high flavonoid content and the emphasis on monounsaturated fat as the principal fat. Healthy eating patterns may help to explain the successful aging of the Okinawans. Further study is needed to clarify the potential link between diet and longevity in Okinawa. We thank the Japan Ministry of Health and Welfare, the Medical Research Council of Canada, the Japan Foundation for Aging and Health (JAFAH) and Harvard Medical School for their support.

Undigested Discontent: The Gastrosemantic Senior

Sharon Koehn (Food For Life project, Vancouver, Canada)

'Gastrosemantics' denotes the "unusual powers of symbolization and communication" with which food is endowed (Khare). Here, this principle demonstrates how seniors communicate complex emotions as well as social relationships through the language of food. This presentation brings together the findings of Dr. Koehn's Ph.D. research and data collected for the Food For Life (FFL) project: a community-based study of seniors and nutritional changes triggered by life events. Both studies take a qualitative approach, relying primarily on in-depth interviews and utilizing Q.S.R. Nud.ist software for their analysis. Koehn's sample includes elderly Hindu women interviewed in India and Canada; the FFL data is derived from interviews and focus groups with seniors and care providers of various ethnic backgrounds. For Indian Hindus the medico-religious tradition of Ayurveda supplies a store of food prescriptions and taboos which are readily converted into metaphors of moral and social order. References to the digestive system in particular are symbolically loaded. 'Good digestion' may denote participation in social activities which promote some kind of 'mental digestion' of one's place in society. In parallel, the digestive problems of one woman in the FFL study were initiated by the departure of one friend, and resolved by the caring concern of another. Limiting one's food intake is another means by which relatively powerless women may send strong messages signaling their distress. Both sets of data yield examples. Caregivers who heed these messages may thus better serve their elderly clients through understanding the existential and social crises which underlie their nutritional shortfalls.

SESSION 414

Age-related changes of testosterone and estradiol fractions in men

Gorenoi Vitali Leifke Eckhard Brabant Georg (Department of Endocrinology, Hannover Medical School, Hannover, Germany)

The studies about changes in serum concentrations of testosterone and estradiol with ageing in men are inconsistent concerning study groups, age-intervals studied and reported parameters. Reported in this studies age-related changes are not readily comparable. Also only few data are presented about changes in bioavailable fractions of this hormones. Thus, we calculated age-trends/decade in serum concentrations of total, bioavailable and free testosterone (TT, BAT and FT), total and bioavailable estradiol (TE and BAE) and sex-hormone-binding-globulin (SHBG) in men from the data for the most representative studies (n>8000 for TT and TE and n>4000 for BAT, FT, BAE and SHBG) and for our own new study on n=514 20-70 years old healthy subjects, using the model of exponential regression. Whereas SHBG increases with age sex-hormone levels decreases with advancing ageing. The calculated age-trends/ decade were in the ranges of 8-15% (9%) for SHBG, -4-10% (-10%) for TT, -10-17% (-17%) for BAT and FT, -7-0% (-7%) for TE and -5-12% (-12%) for BAE for previously reported studies and for our study (in parenthesis). Results of our study based on information from a large study population qualitatively estimates (firstly to our knowledge) the range of age-related changes in serum concentrations of total and bioavailable testosterone and estradiol fractions. This results provide a broad data basis for therapeutic goals in the supplementation of sex-steroids in men.

Andropause: The Passage to the Second Half of Life

Jed Diamond [Director, Men Alive, Willits, California, USA]

Purpose: To demonstrate that andropause or male menopause is a real phenomenon, detail symptoms, treatment approaches, and show the importance of this critical transition period for a man's health and well-being. Method: Clinical evaluation and treatment of 300 men and their families ranging in age from 35 to 65 years of age. Results: Symptoms included reduced libido or potency in 800f the men, fatigue or loss of vitality in 80%, anger and irritability in 75%, depression in 65%, and nightsweats or hot flashes in 50%. Treatment approaches included hormone replacement therapy, exercise, dietary changes, stress reduction, couple counseling, career refocusing, and spiritual support. Improvement was demonstrated in 900f those treated. Conclusion: Andropause was shown to be a treatable change of life process and that a multi-modality approach was demonstrated to offer the best results.

Hyperplastical processes of the endometrium and the climacteric syndrome in premenopausal women

N.A. Omelchenko, V.A. Mityukov, M.A. Shemyakova

Individual means of the hormone replacement therapy (HRT) in women with hyperplasia of endometrium should be beneficial for the prevention of menopausal complications. 120 women aged 44 51 with neuro-vascular and psycho-emotional climacteric symptoms and hyperplasia of the endometrium were obtained during 6 months. All the patients were divided into two groups according to their hormonal status: group I included 76 women with absolute hyperestrogenemia and 44 patients with gestagen deficiency were included in group II. 66 women of group I were treated with Orgametril and Myrena, 36 patients of group II were used therapy with Climonorm. Other 18 women from groups I and II were treated with Livial. The women s state control was performed by ultrasonography of pelvic organs, biopsia of the endometrium, hormonal examination, determined of menopausal index by Kupperman (IK). The results obtained were: IK was found on 20% less in group I and 35% in group II then before the treatment. The regular menstrual function was restored and the volume of uterine bleeding was decreased in all the cases. Ultrasonography was found M-echo in 7 8 mm to the end of the menstrual cycle in 112 women (93.3 %). The data of control biopsia of the endometrium were shown the depression of the hyperplastical processes in the 34 cases (28.3%) and the absence in 86 patients (71.7%). Hyperplasia of the endometrium in premenopausal and perymenopausal women requires the individual methods of HRT according to age, pathohystological type, hormonal status.

Nutritional risk as a covariate in health related quality of life

of vulnerable, community-living seniors.
Heather H. Keller (University of Guelph, Guelph, Ontario, Canada)

PREVENTS is a pilot study exploring the association between nutritional risk and health outcomes in a convenience sample (n=367) of vulnerable community-living seniors. Baseline data from an extensive interview schedule were used to model health related quality of life. Standard multiple linear regression was used to specify final models that described the variance in two quality of life measures: number of days in past 30 where physical and mental health were good (Good Health Days); and, number of days in past 30 where activities were not limited by physical or mental health (No Bed Days). Conceptual models for full regression equations were based on the literature and included: demographics, psychosocial, mood, health, behavioural and nutritional risk variables. Nutritional risk was measured by SCREEN. The model describing Good Health Days was significant and explained 430f the variance in this dependent variable. 12 variables were included in the final model, although only five were significant at p<0.01 level. These variables included: satisfaction with amount of social contact with family or friends, having fallen inside during the past 6 months (negative association), income (negative association), lower nutritional risk, and not smoking. The regression for No Bed Days was also significant and explained 370f the variance in this dependent variable. This final model included 14 variables, of which three were significant; lower nutritional risk, falling inside in the past 6 months (negative association), and not smoking. Nutritional risk appears to be an important and modifiable covariate in health related quality of life.

SESSION 415

The International Consortium for Intergenerational Programs: An Approach to Global Aging Issues.

Alan Hatton-Yeo [The Beth Johnson Foundation, Stoke-on-Trent, England] ("Building Healthy Communities: An Intergenerational Approach") Ludger Veelken [University of Dortmund, Department of Sociology, Dortmund, Germany] ("Intergenerational Models of Learning in the University") Jumbo Klercq [Odyssee Project Office, Berg En Dal, The Netherlands] ("The Need for Intergenerational Cohesiveness in Dutch Society") Valerie Kuehne [University of Victoria, Office of the Vice President, Victoria BC, Canada] ("Intergenerational Program Research: Current Status and Future Directors".) Sally Newman [Generations Together, University of Pittsburgh, Pittsburgh, PA USA] ("The Impact of Intergenerational Programs on Young and Old in the USA".)

Issues - The symposium will describe how intergenerational programming as a global initiative can address issues of community regeneration, generational cohesiveness and quality of life of the old and young in many nations. It will also present information on the status and importance of international collaboration in addressing intergenerational issues. Structure and Content - The symposium will include five sections: (1) An opening statement made by the convener who will identify the goals of the symposium and present information on its unifying theme "The International Consortium for Intergenerational Programs (ICIP)". (2) Several panelists will address national or international issues and initiatives related to their country's intergenerational work. These will include: the learning dimension in intergenerational relationships, the necessity of training in intergenerational programming efforts, and how a critical review of national intergenerational problems can help solve social problems. The panelists will give examples of local, regional, or national intergenerational initiatives in their countries that impact on a community's young and old and benefit the community at large. Within each individual presentation, the panelists will reference how involvement in the International Consortium for Intergenerational Programs (ICIP) has been an asset to their countries' intergenerational initiatives. Finally, a panelist who has focused on research implications and outcomes in intergenerational work will review the current status and challenges of international research in intergenerational programs. (3) Two panelists, members of the initial management team of the "International Consortium for Intergenerational Programs" (ICIP), will present an overview of this newly formed NGO; its history, rationale, goals, structure, current membership, future plans, and role in addressing global intergenerational issues. (4) The audience will discuss with the presenters, intergenerational issues, such as networking, program development, evaluation, research and policy from a global perspective, and how their involvement in ICIP could support their countries intergenerational initiatives. (5) A closing statement by one of the panelists that will include outcomes of the symposium and some options for follow-up activities. Outcomes - Attendees will leave the symposium with a deeper understanding of the global social problems in aging that can be addressed through intergenerational initiatives, new information on the current status and impact of intergenerational programs internationally, answers to some questions related to intergenerational issues in their countries, and on the status of ICIP as an international organization dedicated to supporting intergenerational approaches to social issues. We also anticipate that some symposium participants will become members of ICIP as a vehicle to continue to connect with others interested in intergenerational issues.

Building Healthy Communities: An Intergenerational Approach

Alan Hatton-Yeo (The Beth Johnson Foundation, Stoke-on-Trent, United Kingdom)

Within the United Kingdom the current policy agenda is seeking to find effective ways to address Social Exclusion and the regeneration of disadvantaged communities. Fundamental to the success of this approach is the engagement of the young and old if effective, sustainable development is to take place. Informed by its contact with ICIP academics, policy makers and practitioners have begun to explore intergenerational programmes as a key potential agent of social change. The approach has achieved particular interest through its emphasis on seeing aging in terms of life course rather than chronology and recognizing the need to engage young and old if ageism is to be effectively countered. This paper will illustrate how this approach is currently effecting policy and practice in the United Kingdom. In particular it will illustrate how the newly launched United Kingdom Centre for Intergenerational Practice is drawing on the lessons from international collaborators, through the support of ICIP, to develop a conceptually sound approach to countering social fragmentation and building healthy connected communities.

Intergenerational Program Research: Current Status and Future Directions

Valerie S. Kuehne (University of Victoria, Victoria, Canada)

Purpose: The purpose of this presentation is to provide a survey of international research on intergenerational programs and describe the benefits and challenges of international collaboration in advancing the growing research program in this field. Method: Extensive literature review will be summarized and analyzed using themes. Areas in which researchers have generated more substantial knowledge will be contrasted with areas in which less is known. Results: A research agenda will be provided that is based on the state of current findings. Researchers and practitioners in this and allied fields will be encouraged to work from the strengths present in the current literature and their practice expertise to design and implement studies that will contribute to the growing knowledge base in this area. Conclusion: The potential value of international collaboration in designing and carrying out much needed intergenerational program research is substantial. The benefits and challenges inherent in such a collaborative approach will be discussed.

Intergenerational Programs in Germany and Models of the Intergenerational Learning in the University of Dortmund

Ludger Veelken, (University of Dortmund, Dortmund, Germany)

The conceptual level of Intergenerational Programs is still experimental with low professional standards. Intergenerational concepts are evident in demands for new ideas in educational work, consideration of assistance in living together, media expansion, internet cafes, and cultural activities. A special model in Germany is the intergenerational learning seminars integrated in the University of Dortmund where 20 years of experience has involved the learning together of College students and adults over 55 years of age. For the young and old students, the picture of the other generation has changed, the lectures have been higher quality and new models of cooperation result. The newly developed Intergenerational Consortium for Intergenerational Programs is important to this German co-learning experiment since it will help these students to disseminate to other countries information on how this model works and its successes.

The Impact of Intergenerational Programs on Young and Old in the USA

Sally Newman (Generations Together, University of Pittsburgh, Pittsburgh, PA USA)

This presentation will describe the impact of intergenerational exchange on children, youth, and older adults involved in a variety of intergenerational programs in the U.S. It will summarize data available from several types of intergenerational programs; those in which older adults serve children, those in which children serve older adults, and those in which the old and young team together to serve the community. The settings for these programs include schools, childcare centers, long-term care, personal care and adult day care settings, libraries, and community centers. The information presented will be drawn from a variety of data gathering instruments, such as questionnaires, surveys, interviews, standardized tests, and focus groups. These instruments completed by participants were used in evaluating programs or in applied research projects that examined specific aspects of intergenerational work. The material in this presentation will report on a diverse population of intergenerational participants including young children, school age children, and youth ages 3-20 (mainstream special needs and gifted) and older adults over 55, independent/high functioning and dependent/frail. The presentation will report representative quantitative and quality information available that gives some insight into the overall impact of intergenerational programs.

The Need for Intergenerational Cohesiveness in Dutch Society

Jumbo Klercq (Odyssee, Berg en Dal, The Netherlands)

With the increase in cultural diversity and generational separation within the Netherlands, there is a growing need for more cohesiveness in this country. This need is currently being addressed through a national intergenerational initiative that is creating a variety of intergenerational programs across the country. These programs which are being replicated in many communities recognize the necessity of training to help the participants and program specialists understand the intergenerational approach to program development. A characteristic shared by these programs is the learning dimension in the intergenerational relationships that are formed among the participants, old and young. A critical review of intergenerational programs as a solution for some social problems in our country translates to other countries and is fundamental to the mission of the newly formed Intergenerational Consortium for Intergenerational Programs (ICIP). ICIP an NGO based in the Netherlands has been formed in response to the growing need for a new intergenerational cohesiveness in countries across the globe.

SESSION 416

Analyses on the socioeconomic factors effect health care expenditures for the elderly in Japan

Manami Hori (Graduate School of Media&Governance, Keio University,Japan), Ichiro Innami (Faculty of Policy management, Keio University, Japan)

The purpose of this study is to explore the effect of socioeconomic factors on the regional gaps of the health care expenditures for the aged (HCEA) in Japan and evaluate the introduction of long term care insurance. Utilizing municipal health care demographic and socioeconomic data, this study develops a structural model on per capita HCEA determinants. The analysis reveals age structures, household structures, population density, municipal income, personal income of regions affect HCEA directly as well as indirectly through the availability of hospitals and long-term care facilities and services.

Change of cost for the care services by the long-term care insurance in Japan

Taishi Arimura (Faculty of Integrated Arts and Sciences, Hiroshima University, Hiroshima, Japan), Hiroshi Sumii (Hiroshima Prefectural College of Health and Welfare, Hiroshima, Japan), Takahisa Shimada (Keyaki Geriatric Nursing Home, Hyogo, Japan), Mika Kunisada (Fukuyama municipal Women$B!G)(Js Junior College, Hiroshima, Japan), Masami Hidaka (School of Medicine, Kobe University, Hyogo, Japan), Toshiya Oyamoto, Keiko Mori (Japan Kaigo Research)

Purpose: In Japan, the long-term care insurance started in April, 2000. We analyzed the change of cost in the special geriatric nursing home for the elderly in front and back of enforcement of the insurance. Method: With the economical data of elderly admitted in two special geriatric nursing home, we analyzed the cost to the provided services before and after April, 2000 by multivariate analysis of variance, and revealed the change of the cost by the insurance. Result: In the special geriatric nursing home, the cost to only four elderly out of 94 raised up. The other elderly paid the lesser cost after the long-term care insurance. In addition, in the two institutions, there is no relationship between the level of insurance benefit determined by long-term care insurance stage and the change of the cost. As more of the cost was paid before April, 2000 in the admission by welfare referral, as bigger the reduction of the cost after the insurance. Conclusion: The cost of the institutional services in the nursing home was significantly less after April, 2000 than before. The long-term care insurance reduced the cost in 2000 because the cost has been changed from pay-as-earn in welfare to pay-as-benefit in insurance. Decrease of the cost which had been paid more by pay-as-earn tends to be remarkable. However, when the cost had been considerably low by the case with low place profit, the cost tends to increase adversely by insurance. The cost is determined only by long-term care stage instead of income and family situation, and therefore there is a tendency to decrease in a case with much pay-as-earn with social insurance system.

Five years Long-Term Care Insurance in Germany: Has it stand the test financially?

Gerhard Naegele, Monika Reichert (University of Dortmund/ Institute of Gerontology at the University of Dortmund, Germany)

In 1995, the Long-Term Care Insurance (LTCI) was introduced in Germany. It follows the traditional Bismarck model of social insurance which is based on the pay-as-you-go-principle. It is a mandatory insurance scheme covering the whole population and all those who are (compulsory or voluntary) insured under the statutory health insurance scheme. The LTCI is administered by care funds and it is financed by contributions. These amount to 1.7 % of the qualifying income respectively the qualifying pension. But in sharp contrast to the tradition of the social insurance philosophy the contributions are limited to 1.7 %. This presentation will especially provide important information on the financial aspects of LTCI. For example, data show an increase in the costs which amounted to about 32 billion DM (approx. 14 billion US $) in 1999 and a further increase is predicted. Therefore, the aim of this paper is first, to analyse the reasons for this development (e.g, changing utilization patterns of the LTCI benefits) and second, present recently published proposals of different societal groups involved in order to protect the LTCI financially. The respective information basis is a public hearing of the German „Federal Parliamentary Study Commission on Demographic Change„ about the future of the LTCI which took place in September 2000. Third, the question whether resp. to what extent the LTCI has helped to lift the financial burden of care from care receivers and their families will be examined.

Geriatric Care in a Private Insurance Company: Sanitas Oro

Bravo, G. (Sanitas, Madrid, Spain) De la Fuente, C. (Sanitas, Madrid, Spain) Liaño, E. (Sanitas, Madrid, Spain) Ortiz-Mouliaá, J. (Sanitas, Madrid, Spain)

Purpose: Development of specific geriatric policies with a new medical policy directed to enroll only people aged 65 and over in the area of Madrid (Spain). Determine the impact of this population in the medical costs of a private insurance company. Methods: Retrospective administrative and economical analysis of Sanitas Oro and comparison with people of same aged with other insurance policy for all four years since its implementation in the insurance market (1996-1999). Results: In 1996 Sanitas Oro was launched to fill a gap in medical insurance policies in Madrid, it remains nearly the only choice for people of 60 years of age (yoa) and over, as most insurance companies limit their eligibility below this age (except for reimbursement policies, of much higher price). Compared to other products, Sanitas Oro has a smaller number of medical suppliers and the medical aspects are coordinated by geriatricians working with other specialties consulting teams. Since 1996 1,569 persons of over 60 yoa, have chosen this new product, while there are 105,204 older people in other policies in the same insurance company in Madrid. Mean age is 71.0 in Sanitas and 71.9 in Sanitas Oro. Sanitas Oro has a 17% reduction in medical costs, which represents mean savings of 52.67 Euros per person per year. This results have promoted Sanitas Oro to be offered in many other different places in Spain. Conclusions: A new medical policy for aged people has shown economical benefits through a reduction in medical costs. This results have led to a widespreading of the idea.

The Future of the German Long-term Care Insurance

J.Wilbers (Center for Psychological and Psychosomatic Reserach, University of Trier, Trier, Germany)

In 1995 an insurance to finance long-term care was introduced in Germany. Since then several amendments have been made but for financial reasons the benefits have not been increased. In the first decade of the 21st century a large number of elderly additionally will be entitled for the insurance. So at the same time the benefits of the insurance will devalue in real terms and the number of long-term patients will rise. Additionally more sophisticated concepts (e.g. for dementia patients), a higher quality of the care and better trained (and more expensive) staff are demanded by gerontological experts as well as the administration and the general public. Therefore the future of the long-term care insurance is at risk. The paper will present several projections for the forthcoming decades (life expectancy, need for care, financial conditions) and discuss the options for political decicions: increase of the insurance fees, cutting or abolishing some of the benefits, rising the requirements for application for the insurance, or replacing the insurance by another system. The German long-term care insurance thus may be an example that an innovative approach to help long-term care patients financially can run into serious difficulties only quite a short time after the start although the future demographic trends had been known at the time of introduction.

The German Long Term Care Insurance: Prospects after Six Years of its Existence

Hans-Joachim von Kondratowitz

In summer 2001 the German Long Term Care Insurance will exist six years which is the appropriate time for an evaluation of its effects and of the prospective developments of this nation-wide LTCI scheme. The contribution will therefore mainly concentrate on confronting the expectations and policy orientations with the real developments in the care sector within Germany. This means to concentrate on the following topics and discussing the effective developments and changes: the politically defined decision to design the LTCI essentially as granting benefits with a ceiling and a politically fixed contribution ratethe expectation to reduce the social welfare costs on the local level and use the saved money for reinvestments in the area of institutional care privileging home care (e.g. by giving the option between cash payments and benefits in kind for households in need of support) and putting pressure to selflegitimize and redefine itself on the side of institutional caredynamizing the care sector by opening up to privately organized care services and securing quality of care by introducing new quality assessment techniquesbeing more responsive to demographic and epidemiological changes and its effects on the care delivery process, but maintaining at the same time a balanced financial budget of the LTCI

SESSION 417

Peptide Regulation of Ageing

V. Khavinson (St. Petersburg Institute of Bioregulation and Gerontology, St. Petersburg, Russia) Peptide Regulation of Ageing. C. Franceschi, L. Piantanelli (Centre of Biochemistry, Italian National Research Centres on Ageing, Ancona, Italy), I. Kvetnoy (St. Petersburg Institute of Bioregulation and Gerontology, St. Petersburg, Russia), V. Anisimov (N. N. Petrov Research Institute of Oncology, St. Petersburg, Russia) Cell Biology of Gut Neuroendocrine Cells in Ageing. V. Morozov, V. Malinin (St. Petersburg Institute of Bioregulation and Gerontology, St. Petersburg, Russia) Geroprotective Properties of Dipeptides - Vilon and Thymogen. O. Korkushko, V. Shatilo (Institute of Gerontology of the Ukrainian Academy of Medical Sciences, Kiev, the Ukraine) Efficacy of Long-Term Application of Thymic and Pineal Peptide Preparations in the Treatment for Accelerated Ageing. A. Hipkiss (King's College London, the United Kingdom) Possible Mechanisms of Carnosine Anti-Senescence Effects. A. Boldyrev (M. V. Lomonosov Moscow State University, Moscow, Russia), T. Fedorova, G. Kramarenko, S. Stvolinsky, M. Yuneva (Institute of Neurology, Moscow, Russia), V. Lankin, E. Sorokina (Cardiological Research Centre, Moscow, Russia) Carnosine Compensates Deficient Anti-Oxidant System of Senescent Accelerated Mice. S. Gallant (Synthon International Ltd, Luton, Bedfordshire, the United Kingdom) Carnosine: the Prototype for a New Range of Anti-Ageing Molecules with Therapeutic Usefulness.

This symposium is arranged to highlight and discuss various aspects of peptide regulation of ageing processes - from cells to humans. The session is particularly focused on the anti-senescent effects of small peptide preparations (carnosine, Thymalin, Epithalamin, Vilon, Thymogen, Epitalon), whose geroprotective potentiality is supported by the results of cytological studies, animal experiments and clinical trials.

The symposium embraces six oral reports to the topic, each intended for about a quarter-hour talk, and one poster presentation at the Congress poster session. Questions are encouraged after every oral report and monitored by the symposium convenors. The preliminary speakers' order is adduced in Paragraph 2.

Dr. Khavinson will outline the symposium focus and share results of studying senescence-regulating peptide effects on animal and human organisms. Conducted research demonstrates peptide ability to accelerate tissue-specific protein synthesis and regulate expression of genes responsible for cellular differentiation and proliferation, thus providing preservation of the main physiological functions and inhibiting ageing. The report by Dr. Franceschi et al is dedicated to the effects of peptide hormones and biogenic amines upon the cellular homeostasis maintenance in ageing. The authors focus on the regulatory role of diffuse neuroendocrine cells in cell proliferation and apoptosis. Predominance of cell proliferation rate over the apoptotic one is supposed to be an ageing inhibition factor. In their poster presentation, Drs. Morozov and Malinin compare geroprotective properties of synthetic dipeptides Vilon and Thymogen on various animal models. Their prolonged administration is demonstrated to extend animal longevity by 20-30 % and significantly decrease spontaneous tumour incidence. Drs. Korkushko and Shatilo describe effects of prolonged application of peptide preparations Thymalin and Epithalamin in humans with accelerated ageing (cardiovascular system functional age decrease, physical working capacity and brain functioning enhancement, mineral saturation and bone tissue density rise), thus substantiating preventive and therapeutic potentiality of these preparations. Dr. Hipkiss will speak on the possible mechanisms of anti-ageing action of carnosine - a naturally occurring dipeptide delaying senescence and restoring juvenile phenotype in cultured human fibroblasts. The report by Dr. Boldyrev et al highlights the compensatory influence of carnosine upon the deficient antioxidant system in senescent accelerated mice. The obtained data demonstrate different roles of antioxidant enzymes in the compensation for increased reactive oxygen species production and highest efficacy herein of cytosolic Cu/Zn-SOD. Dr. Gallant's report is dedicated to the modulating potential of L-carnosine towards the ageing process in mammals. It considers effects of carnosine analogues, novel carnosine-containing compounds and usefulness of Drosophila screen for detecting carnosine-like agents or new anti-ageing molecules. Consequently, all the symposium participants declare the essential role of peptides in regulating the mechanisms of ageing at various levels of living material organisation.

The role of small peptides in the regulatory mechanisms of ageing has not been extensively investigated. The symposium is expected to reveal the fundamental problems in the present-day peptide science and share the knowledge of peptide-mediated mechanisms of senescence regulation. Such information exchange and discussion is highly expected to help potentiate research in this field.

Carnosine, Cell Senescence, Protein Carbonyls and Their Suppression

A.R. Hipkiss

Carnosine is a naturally-occurring dipeptide that can delay senescence and restore a juvenile phenotype in cultured human fibroblasts. This paper will discuss possible mechanisms by which carnosine might achieve its anti-ageing effects. Carnosine has long been thought to be an anti-oxidant and oxygen free-radical scavenger. However better anti-oxidants and free-radical scavengers than carnosine do not induce anti-ageing effects in cultured cells. Carnosine also appears to be an anti-glycating agent reacting readily with almost any deleterious aldehyde or ketone. Reaction of proteins with oxygen free-radicals and glycating agents results in the production of proteins carbonyl groups, typical of those known to accompany ageing. We have recently shown that carnosine can react with such "aged" proteins, most likely generating "carnosinylated" proteins i.e. protein-carbonyl-carnosine adducts. We suggest that formation of carnosinylated proteins couldoccur in cells cultured with carnosine. We propose that such carnosinylationof the carbonyls on glycoxidized proteins suppresses their reactivity andmay even promote their proteolytic destruction. Carnosine's potential tosuppress diabetic complications is consistent with this idea. The anti-ageingactivities of aminoguanidine and N-t-butylhydroxylamine, agents that are better anti-glycators than anti-oxidants, support our proposal. We propose that because ageing is multifactorial, effective anti-ageing agents should be pluripotent. Carnosine's ability to suppress protein carbonyl reactivity, as well as its previously described anti-oxidant, metal ion and free-radical-scavenging activities appears to fulfill this requirement.

Carnosine Compensates the Deficient Antioxidant System of Senescence-Accelerated Mice

A. Boldyrev (M.V. Lomonosov Moscow State University, Moscow, Russia), T. Fedorova, G. Kramarenko, S. Stvolinsky, M. Yuneva (Institute of neurology, Moscow, Russia), V.Z. Lankin, E. Sorokina (Cardiological Research Center, Moscow, Russia)

Senescence Accelerated Mice, SAM, is the model, in which Reactive Oxygen Species (ROS) play the major role in the process of aging. The mice are characterized with the normal development only till the age of 4 months and following accelerated aging accompanied by increased accumulation of age features as loss of hair, skin ulcers, periophthalmic lesions, and corneal opacity. This process of aging resulting in a shortening of a lifespan till 12-14 months instead of 3 years is considered to be caused by increased level of ROS as the result of dis-balance between ROS production and neutralization by the antioxidant system. We have found that while glutathione dependent enzymes (transferase, peroxidase and reductase) in liver, blood and heart, as well as brain glutathione level are values of the same order, the brain and blood Cu/Zn-superoxide dismutase and liver catalase activities are suppressed by 30-50% compared to control level. Moreover, SAM brain is characterized with higher NMDA binding and MAO activity as well as increased level of excitotoxic compounds like glutamate, aspartate and its amine. Hydrophilic antioxidant carnosine being used as dietary supplement in a daily dose of 150 mg/kg body weight significantly improved the antioxidant defense system with simultaneous supressing of NMDA binding and MAO B activity as well as decreased level of excitotoxic compounds. Animals treated with carnosine were characterized with better exterior and 20% longer average lifespan. The data obtained demonstrate different participation of antioxidant enzymes in compensation of increased ROS production with glutathione-dependent enzymes being the less important and cytosolic Cu/ZN-SOD being the most important. Efficiency of antioxidant therapy obtained in our experiments demonstrates that the disbalance in antioxidant system is one of the majo cause of accelerated aging in SAM animals.

Carnosine: The Prototype for a New Range of Anti-Ageing Molecules With Therapeutic Usefulness

Steven Gallant

We have shown that the naturally occuring dipeptide L-carnosine can modulate the aging process in mammals. I will briefly discuss the anti-aging effects of natural carnosine and then: 1) Describe the effects of carnosine analogues - herein including analogues involving alterations to the peptide bond but also modification of the histidine moiety 2) Describe the effects of novel compounds wherein carnosine is covalently attached to another molecule to create a third active compound 3) Describe the usefulness of the Drosophila screen as a means to detect carnosine like agents or indeed novel anti-aging molecules.

Cell Biology of Gut Neuroendocrine Cells in Ageing

C. Franceschi, L. Piantanelli (Centre of Biochemistry, Italian National Research Centres on Ageing, Ancona, Italy), I. M. Kvetnoy (St. Petersburg Institute of Bioregulation and Gerontology, St. Petersburg, Russia), V. N. Anisimov (N. N. Petrov Research Institute of Oncology, St. Petersburg, Russia)

Diffuse neuroendocrine system (DNES) cells regulate homeostasis via neurocrine, endocrine and paracrine mechanisms. Extensive effects of peptide hormones and biogenic amines necessitate studying of DNES cell biology and functional morphology in ageing.
Gut neuroendocrine cells (NEC) in 4-, 21- and 34-months old BALB/c-nu mice were identified and studied by argyrophilic Grimelius' method for total identification of DNES cell population in guts, argentaffine Masson's

method for serotonin-producing EC cells identification, Moser's method for identifying apoptotic cells, immunohistochemical methods, morphometry and image analysis.
Stomach: total number of NEC increased with age (604±42 - 4, 705±53 - 21, 753±53 - 34 months) though different NEC types behaved diversely. Serotonin/melatonin-producing EC cells equalled 325±52, 345±49, 389±46, respectively. Number of serotonin-producing D-like cells increased (95±12, 111±17, 126±24, respectively), while gastrin producing G-cells number diminished (400±27, 374±34, 327±55, correspondingly).
Duodenum: total NEC number also increased with age (196±14 - 4, 311±14 - 21, 303±11 - 34 months) Slight decrease by 34 months was not relevant. Serotonin/melatonin-producing EC cells increased, EC cell population grew 2.5-fold with age (186±7, 372±21, 431±22, respectively).
Total number of epitheliocyte nuclei did not vary significantly through life (6486±92, 6374±95, 6121±55, respectively) as well as mucous epitheliocyte proliferation activity (PCNA index equating 15.7±0.7 - 4, 15.7±0.8 - 21, 17.6±1.1 - 34 months). Conversely, apoptosis index rose with age (0.48, 0.47, 0.85, respectively).
Epitheliocyte proliferation activity was proven not to depend upon EC cells activity and remain unchanged while apoptosis index increased with age. Supposedly, cell proliferation level exceeded apoptotic elimination rate being a factor of ageing inhibition.

Efficacy of Long-Term Application of Thymic and Pineal Peptide Preparations in the Treatment for Accelerated Ageing

O. V. Korkushko, V. B. Shatilo (Institute of Gerontology of the Ukrainian Academy of Sciences, 04114 Kiev, the Ukraine)

Work was designed to study effects of long-term application of peptide preparations (PP) Thymalin and Epithalamin in humans with accelerated aging.
152 elderly subjects (aged 60-79) with biological age exceeding chronological one by over 5 years were observed. Among them, 58 persons received Thymalin, 46 - Epithalamin and 48 - placebo (saline solution). Patients received one of the PP in 6 courses during 3 years. Thymic and pineal PP efficacy was assessed by the patients' subjective indices characterising their general state, physical and mental working capacity, objective blood lipid spectrum indices, immune and bone tissue status, cardiovascular and central nervous systems functional age.
Effect duration and optimal intervals between single dose injections and consecutive treatment courses were assessed. Results confirmed both the efficacy of Thymalin and Epithalamin treatment and the long-term application thereof. Cardiovascular system functional age decreased, physical working capacity increased in 55 % and 72 % of subjects treated with Thymalin and Epithalamin, respectively. After 3 years of treatment, physical working capacity indices rose substantially comparing to the baseline. During PP treatment, blood cholesterol, beta-lipoprotein content and atherogenicity index decreased. Epithalamin significantly increased brain functional indices. Thymalin and Epithalamin raised mineral saturation and bone tissue density. Prolonged Thymalin administration normalised altered immune indices. It is noteworthy that PP effect was not stimulating but modifying. Thymalin and Epithalamin significantly improved life quality in the elderly inducing no essential clinical side effects.
PP thymic and pineal preparations (Thymalin and Epithalamin) may be applied in prevention and treatment for accelerated aging in humans.

Geroprotective Properties of Dipeptides - Vilon and Thymogen

V. G. Morozov, V. V. Malinin (St. Petersburg Institute of Bioregulation and Gerontology, St. Petersburg, Russia)

Role of small peptides in the regulatory mechanisms of ageing has not been extensively studied yet. We experimentally compared the effect of synthetic dipeptides - Vilon (Lys-Glu) and Thymogen (Glu-Trp) - on the cellular and humoral immunity, non-specific organism resistance, processes of antioxidation defence and tissue regeneration, carcinogenesis and longevity. Administration of Vilon and Thymogen to immunodepressed mice and rats increased their cellular and humoral immune response to thymus-dependent antigens. Besides, Vilon exerted a more pronounced effect upon the chemotaxis and phagocytic reactions of blood neutrophilic leukocytes. Prolonged administration of the studied dipeptides to mice extended the animals longevity on average by 20-30 % and significantly decreased spontaneous tumour incidence. Vilon and Thymogen raised the life span in Drosophila melanogaster and activated their antioxidation defence enzymes (catalase and superoxide dismutase). Still, Vilon influenced the regeneration processes in lymphoid and intestinal cells of X-rayed rats more prominently than Thymogen.
Comparative study on Vilon and Thymogen in the thymus and spleen tissue culture of rats of various ages displayed a difference in the drug action on the processes of lymphoid tissue growth and intralymphocytic synthesis of nucleic acids and protein. Biological properties of small peptides depend upon their structural and functional features, thus determining the further strategy of search for new regulatory peptides with the purpose to create effectual geroprotective agents.

Peptide Regulation of Ageing

V. Kh. Khavinson (St. Petersburg Institute of Bioregulation and Gerontology, St. Petersburg, Russia)

Study on the processes of age-related involution of the organism organs and tissues revealed a decrease in production of physiologically active peptide substances and intensity of protein synthesis. This prompted a conclusion on the essential role of peptides in the regulation of the mechanisms of ageing.
Indices of animal and human immune, endocrine, metabolic and antioxidation defence systems were investigated in dynamics.
Application of complex peptide preparations isolated from the thymus, epiphysis, prostate, cerebral cortex and retina was proven to restore the synthesis of tissue-specific proteins in these organs and tissues, to normalise their functional activity in various pathologic states and ageing, thus significantly extending animal longevity. Similar results were obtained in the research on the biological activity of peptides designed on the basis of amino acid analysis of the thymus, epiphysis, prostate, cerebral cortex and retina tissues.
Experimental and clinical results of studying peptide regulators demonstrate their geroprotective properties determined by the normalising impact of peptides on the main systems of the organism homeostasis maintenance and by the regulation of the tissue-specific mechanisms of ageing.
Peptides facilitate recovery of tissue-specific protein synthesis intensity and regulate the expression of genes responsible for cellular differentiation and proliferation. This secures preservation of the basic physiological functions and inhibits the processes of the organism ageing.

SESSION 418

A Comprehensive Geriatric-Palliative Approach in The Care of a Non-Cancer Incurable Young Patient

Shefer I, Berger S.I, Ben-Basat Z, Slizak G, Katav V, Gilis E, Garfinkel D. (Home Care Service - Dan District,Maccabi Healthcare Services, Israel).

A 29 years old male was admitted to our Home-Care Service presenting with a variety of symptoms and problems that are usually manifested by terminal cancer and/or elderly patients. Diagnosis of Localized Scleroderma Generalized Morphea was established six years earlier. Colchicine, methotrexate, cortico- steroids, extracorporal photopheresis and PUVA had been repeatedly tried with no beneficial effect on disease progression. Upon admission to our service, his thick, tough skin was already affected by ulcers with discharge and secondary infections, resembling pressure sores and quite resistant to therapy. Skin contraction resulted in joint disability, arthrosis and immobility. Prolonged steroid therapy had also induced diffuse osteoporosis that, in concert with the skin contractions, ulcers and arthrosis, set the stage for severe pain of various origins. Severe constipation resulting from the use of morphine, immobility or both, required frequent manual evacuations of fecal impactions. As external light induced skin itching and pain, it eventually resulted in photophobia that forced the patient to stay indoors in complete darkness. Eyelid thickening averted him from watching TV and reading. Physical disfiguration resulted in total disconnection from family and social activities. A chronic painful disease with physical disability, isolation, boredom and hopelessness, all resulted in reactive depression. This patient represents a complex of medical, nursing, nutritional, psychosocial and economic problems and we actually show, using a computerized video film, how achieving specific professional results by one team member may be in conflict with that of another. A comprehensive palliative approach with coordinated teamwork is needed, in order to alleviate some of the enormous physical and mental suffer of this non-elderly non-cancer incurable patient.

Defining the Role of Palliative Care in Residential Aged Care Facilities

Jill Pretty (Aged Services Association NSW & ACT. Sydney Australia)

This research sought to define the role of palliative care in nursing homes in relation to chronic diseases, to determine how staff perform this role and identify possible barriers to the provision of this care in aged care facilities. A literature review was undertaken followed by a small qualitative study involving the interviewing of two registered nurses providing specialised palliative care in nursing homes and one clinical nurse consultant working in an outreach program from a hospice. The literature review identified five key characteristics of palliative care. The results of the study supported these characteristics, but because of the difficulty in predicting the terminal stage of chronic illness, staff have defined palliative care into two levels: Level 1 - when a resident is assessed as totally depended on staff for all their care needs; Level 2 - when the resident showed significant changes in their care needs such as an inability to swallow, signs of agitation or increased levels of pain. Identified barriers to the provision of palliative care in aged care facilities included poor understanding of the role in of palliative care during the final stage of chronic disease by both medical practitioners and nursing staff. This study identified an expertise in the provision of palliative care, which has been adapted to meet the care needs of frail older people. Education of health professionals is an important factor in order to ensure quality palliative care for residents in these facilities.

Diagnostic Mix: Determinant of Nursing Home Admissions for Palliative Care Clients

Author: James Grealy [C&G Education and Research Pty. Limited]

Diagnostic mix is now used as the principal determinant for admission of palliative care residents to the nursing home. This admission protocol effected significant improvements in care and general services, whilst reducing intensely stressful periods for staff. Previously there was an expectation of continuously providing optimum quality care irrespective of resident needs and 'fixed' organisational resources. Thereby in 1999 the nursing home developed an approach of maintaining a 'palliative care' client group of particular diagnostic mix(es). Prior to instituting this protocol, the resident mix was such that quality care diminished because the facility services could not match resident need. METHOD: During the pilot program (1997; 2000) 70 residents were palliated with a mean admission period of 3 months. Diagnostic data was recorded under six categories according to complexity and length of stay. RESULTS: For example, residents with lung cancer had high complexity, high anxiety/ distress and the mean length of admission to death was 42 days. This contrasted with residents with gliomas having low complexity, low distress and a mean admission to death period of 112.8 days. Consequently, the nursing home could only provide optimum care to 3 residents with lung cancer at any time but up to 8 residents with gliomas. CONCLUSION: The admission protocol has assisted in determining the most appropriate admissions according to resident need and service capacity. Further, the data enabled mapping of clinical pathways, thereby assisting the health care team to plan for resources and care interventions in advance of symptom presentation and thereby also reducing staff stress.

Qualitative analysis of physicians' attitudes toward elderly terminally ill patients who refuse treatment

N. Poirier (Université de Moncton School of Nursing) & D. Poirier (Université de Moncton Law School)

PURPOSE : This study examined the reasons why physicians have difficulty respecting the wishes of their elderly terminally ill patients who refuse treatment. Consistent with the relevant literature, three alternative explanations were hypothesised in answering the question: fear of litigation, religious beliefs, and medical professional values. METHOD : Semistructured interviews were carried out with 24 emergency physicians from the southern part of the Canadian province of New Brunswick and submitted to both quantitative and qualitative content analysis. RESULTS : Four findings result from the analysis. First, the majority of interviewed physicians were not well aware of the administrative policies relating to refusal of treatment by their elderly patients. Most physicians believed that those policies are not useful. Second, in more that half of their statements, the respondent physicians expressed the opinion that it was the physician's decision to withdraw treatments, whereas in one third of those statements, respondent physicians identified the elderly patient as having the right to decide. Third, when there are conflicts between the law and medical professional values regarding the rights of elderly terminally ill patients, most physicians gave priority to their medical professional values. Finally, normative pluralism has revealed a valuable instrument capable of helping to understand why medical professional values are given priority over the wishes of terminally ill elderly patients. CONCLUSION : It is concluded from the study that any change affecting the professional medical values cannot simply be legislated but that legislators should embark on a process of discussion with the medical profession in order to bring the profession itself to recommend the adoption of particular rules and regulations.

Remaining at home to the end - quality of palliative care in Hospital-Based Home Care

B-G. Emtinger (County council, Linköping, Sweden), A. Milberg (Department of Geriatrics, University Hospital, Linköping, Sweden), P. Strang (Palliative Research Unit Linköping University, Sweden)

PURPOSE: The aim of this study was to investigate the quality of palliative care in advanced hospital-based home care (HBHC) through next-of-kins' satisfaction. METHOD: In the County of Östergötland about 400 patients are taken care of daily within HBHC in nine multiprofessional teams. The setting of this study was HBHC in three teams. Next-of-kins (N=99) whose spouses had died of cancer (N=73) and other diseases during the last 3 months completed a questionnaire about issues such as information, symptom control and quality of care. The questions were combined verbal and numerical, from 1-9, where 7-9 corresponded to I agree completely. RESULTS: The next-of-kin were very satisfied with the staff's care and attention (mean=8.3) and with the HBHC in total (m=8.3). Also the overall treatment was appreciated (m=7.8), whereas individual symptoms such as fatigue were problematic (m=4.3). In total, 71% of the next-of-kin were very satisfied with the overall symptom control (7 or more on the 9-point scale) and 94% had confidence with HBHC. The overall satisfaction was lower in cases where pain control had not been optimal. 97% would, without hesitation, choose HBHC again, in a similar situation. Four main categories were identified from the open-ended written comments reflecting satisfaction: feeling secure; being at home;being in the focus; and caring together. CONCLUSION: Next-of-kin who have chosen HBHC are very satisfied with the overall care and support, although certain symptoms still are problematic.

The role of the psychologis in a palliative care project

Zipora Charszan, CLSC Rene-Cassin, Quebec, Canada

Purpose: To provide families of terminally ill clients with psychological support and help duirng the dying process. Method: Observation of clinical practice and experience with clients and health care providers. Results: The role of the psychologist had a significant impact on the core team of health care providers in dealing with issues of burnout, frustration, anxiety, sadness, denial, and loss. Conclusion: The dual role played by the psychologist responded to the needs of the clients and the core team of health care providers. This enabled the initial core team to become an important resource and support for the entire HomeCare team of the CLSC Rene-Cassin working with this clientele.

SESSION 419

Reminiscence and Life Review: Clinical Applications

John Kunz (Center for Continuing Education/Extension, University of Wisconsin - Superior, Superior, WI, USA) Overview of clinical applications of reminiscence and life review across the continuum of care from prevention to intervention; Utilizing reminiscence matches and resource states Phyllis J. Meltzer (Gerontology Research Center, California State University, Fullerton, Fullerton, USA) Using life lines for health promotion and as therapeutic interventions Bob Woods (Dementia Services Development Centre, University of Wales Bangor, Bangor, UK) Randomized-controlled trial of life review with people with dementia on entry to residential care Florence Gray Soltys (School Of Social Work and Medicine - Univ. of North Carolina at Chapel Hill, USA) A theoretical framework for working with frail older adults at end of life Robert N. Butler (International Longevity Center USA, Ltd, New York, NY, USA) Discussant

ISSUE: This is the first of two symposia that address contemporary clinical applications and current research in the growing multidisciplinary field of reminiscence and life review. In this symposium, speakers from three different continents will present innovative strategic applications of their reminiscence and life review that affects mental and physical health as well as end-of-life issues for patients, clients, and community-dwelling older adults. STRUCTURE: Oral presentations including audiovisual examples will include speakers from the United Kingdom and the United States. The founder of the International Institute for Reminiscence and Life Review will convene the session. Key international leaders in clinical application will be featured as presenters. Robert N. Butler, who coined the term life review, will be the discussant. CONTENT: An overview of the clinical applications of reminiscence and life review the across the continuum of care from prevention to intervention will be provided. The clinical use of a reminiscence match and the resulting therapeutic resource states will be discussed in relation to mental health issues and problems with an emphasis on prevention and the treatment of clinical depression. A further discussion of the clinical uses of life review will include results of the application of the Self-Discovery Tapestry, a life review tool based upon research with older women. Clinical assessment, mental health counseling, and adaptive strategies utilizing this tool will be presented. The use of life review approaches with dementia patients in a residential setting will be discussed from both an anecdotal and controlled research perspective including a randomized controlled study. In this study, an intervention consisted of around ten individual sessions working chronologically through the person's life, and with the input of information and photographs from relatives, constructing with the person a life story book. The results indicated a significant decrease in depression as assessed by the Geriatric Depression Scale and an increase in autobiographical memory, compared with controls. Individual differences in response to life review were noted, and made the process of life review clinically demanding for the therapist. The session will conclude with a presentation of a theoretical framework for working with frail older adults facing the end of their lives. Photographs and video segments will illustrate the techniques that help terminally ill older adults reveal their life and address unresolved issues or past events in a way that enhances self-esteem and provide a sense of personal identity through recounting of personal achievements or experiences. CONCLUSIONS/ ANTICIPATED OUTCOMES: Participants in this symposium will be able to better understand the application of reminiscence and life-review approaches and instruments in clinical settings. By expanding their knowledge of these strategies for individuals coping with depression, dementia, end of life issues or those in need of self-affirmation and counseling the speakers will empower the participants to replicate these strategies with broader segments of their clinical populations.

SESSION 420

Combined albumin and cholesterol levels and decline of physical performance in the elderly.

B.W.M. Schalk,; M. Visser, ; D.J.H. Deeg, (EMGO Institute, Vrije Universiteit, Amsterdam, The Netherlands), B.W.J.H. Penninx, (Sticht Center on Aging, Wake Forest University, Winston-Salem, NC, USA), L.M. Bouter, (EMGO Institute, Vrije Universiteit, Amsterdam, The Netherlands)

PURPOSE: In recent years, blood markers are very often seen as a good predictor for health in the elderly. Serum albumin and cholesterol levels are associated with heart disease and mortality. However, evidence on the association of these blood markers with functional decline is rare. The aim of our study is to investigate the association between combined serum cholesterol and albumin levels with future decline in physical performance in the elderly. METHOD: We used data on 1042 men and women aged 55-84 years, participants of the Longitudinal Aging Study Amsterdam (LASA). Participants were classified into 3 categories, low, normal and high, for total cholesterol (< 5.20 / 5.20-6.20/  6.20 mMol/L) and albumin (44 / 45-46/ 47 g/L) using baseline (1991/92) blood samples. Physical performance (6-meter walk, putting on a cardigan, repeated chair stands) was assessed at baseline and 3-year follow up. Decline was defined as a difference < -5 %. RESULTS: In logistic regression models, adjusting for, age, performance score, body mass index, socio-economic status, exercise, smoking and chronic disease at baseline, we observed for the group with low albumin/ low cholesterol increased risk (OR=8.97; 95% CI 1.00-80.67) versus normal albumin/ low cholesterol. For participants with low albumin and high cholesterol levels versus normal albumin / high cholesterol, a decreased risk (OR=0.45; 95% CI: 0.22-0.91) was found. In all other groups no such relationship was found. CONCLUSION: Combined serum albumin and total cholesterol levels are usefull indicators for functional decline in the elderly.

Metabolic markers of Cobalamin deficiency in the elderly: Relation to cognition, hematological and clinica parameters.

Angela Garcia (Queen's University, Kingston, Canada) Alicia Paris-Pombo (Queen's University, Kingston, Canada)

We have investigated the relationship between metabolic markers of Cbl function, cognition, and clinical parameters of Cbl deficiency, in free-living, elderly, cognitively normal volunteers. Metabolic markers of Cbl deficiency included determinations of Methylcitric acid (MCTR) Homocysteine (HCYS) and Methylmalonic acid (MMA). Cognitive measures included the California Verbal Learning test (CVLT), Mattis Dementia Rating Scale (DRS) and Stroop. Clinical history, diet, vitamin intake, neurologic exam, standard hematological parameters, Cbl and Folate determinations were also performed. Data was collected in 248 subjects. Subjects with metabolic evidence of Cbl deficiency (elevated MCTR, HCYS or MMA, regardless of their Cbl levels) had significantly worse cognitive scores than subjects with normal metabolites. In particular, subjects with elevated MCTR used a deficient verbal learning pattern that has been associated with future development of dementia.

There was no difference in age, sex, years of education, or diet, between subjects with normal and abnormal metabolites. Subjects with metabolic evidence of Cbl deficiency did not show the classical haematological or clinical parameters associated with low Cbl levels. These results suggest that there is an association between the metabolic markers of tissue Cbl deficiency and cognitive impairment in the elderly. Cbl deficiency may have a pre-clinical phase during which cognitive changes leading to dementia may occur.

Nutritional indicators have association with the survival prediction in ambulatory Korean elderly

Eunju Lee, Young Soo Lee (Dept of Internal Medicine, Asan Medical Center, Univ. of Ulsan College of Medicine, Seoul, Korea), Dong Hoon Shin (University of Dankook College of Medicine, Cheonan, Korea)

Purpose: This study was performed to identify the normal distribution of the nutritional indices such as biochemical and anthropometric variables, showing the association between nutritional risk factor and mortality in ambulatory Korean elderly. Methods: Among 151,000 subjects over 40year olds in Jung-Up County, Korea, 1051 were selected for a random cluster sample. After the blood tests and anthropometric measurements were performed during Dec 1996 to Feb 1997, the mortality of the subjects, who had been over 65years at the enroll time, was followed up on Dec 2000. Results: (1) Of the 1051 subjects (M:F = 410:641), 340 were over 65years at the enroll time, while 711 were between 40 to 65 years. Triceps skin fold thickness (TSF), body mass index (BMI), serum protein and albumin showed a weak negative correlation with age, whereas not in the case of the waist-hip ratio (WHR), hemoglobin (Hb), hematocrit (Hct), leucocytes, serum cholesterol and creatinine. (2) Of the 340 elderly subjects, 34 (10%) died within 3 years. After the adjustment of age and sex, the decrease in Hb, Hct, serum protein and albumin and increase in serum creatinine seemed to associate with an increased risk of mortality among the variables ($p<0.05$). Especially in the case of serum albumin, it remained strong predictors of mortality after controlling for other significant variables (RR=0.15, 95% CI=0.03-0.63, $p=0.01$). Conclusion: We clearly showed the strong independent association of serum albumin with mortality among the ambulatory elderly Koreans in the rural community.

Optimal serum total cholesterol level in the Japanese elderly

S. Watanabe, S. Kumagai, S. Shinkai, H. Amano, T. Suzuki (Tokyo Metropolitan Institute of Gerontology, Japan), H. Shibata (Obirin University, Japan)

The association of serum total cholesterol concentration (TC) with all-cause mortality was investigated in the Japanese elderly from the Tokyo Metropolitan Institute of Gerontology Longitudinal Interdisciplinary Study on Aging (TMIG-LISA). In 454 men and 632 women aged 65 years and over at baseline who were ambulatory, TC was measured. Mortality risk during 6 years of follow-up was calculated using a proportional hazards model, adjusted for region, age, serum albumin, systolic blood pressure, body mass index, and smoking. Of 1086 subjects, 23 who took a medicine for hyperlipidemia, and 13 who died within a year were excluded from the analysis. During the 6-year follow-up, 22.4% of men and 12.1% of women died. TC for the young-old (65-74 years) elderly had a U-shaped relationship with mortality in both sexes. For the young-old, low TC (lowest quartile, <4.0 mmol/L for men (relative hazard (RH)=3.3), <4.7 mmol/L for women (RH=2.3)) was significant mortality risk, and high TC (highest quartile, >5.4 mmol/L for men (RH=3.3)) was also significant mortality risk for men. Lowest relative hazard in the young-old was at TC between 4.0 and 4.7 mmol/L for men, and between 4.7 and 5.3 mmol/L for women. While for the old-old (75 years and over) elderly, TC was not associated with mortality for men, furthermore, among women, a significant inverse association was found. Lowest relative hazard in the old-old women was at TC 6.0 mmol/L and over (highest quartile). The optimal TC for the old-old elderly appears to be different from that for the young-old elderly.

Prognostic Factors for Life Expectancy in Elderly Patients with PEG

Salles-Montaudon (Hôpital Xavier Arnozan, Pessac, France), I. Hamon (Hôpital Xavier Arnozan, Pessac, France), I. Bourdel-Marchasson (Hôpital Xavier Arnozan, Pessac, France), M. Rainfray (Hôpital Xavier Arnozan, Pessac, France), J.P. Emeriau (Hôpital Xavier Arnozan, Pessac, France).

Purpose : Percutaneaous endoscopic gastrostomy (PEG) is now a easily used tool for enteral nutrition, but the mortality rate remains high among frail elderly patients. The aim of our study was to define prognostic factors for life expectancy in elderly patients with PEG. Methods : We conducted a four years prospective study in all hospitalized patients in whom PEG was indicated for long term enteral feeding. Ansell Bioser kit was used for all the included patients and PEG was performed using antibioprophylaxy, antiseptic mouth wash and a sterile hydrocellular dressing around the cutaneous insertion site. Each patient was examined every three mounths in order to evaluate nutritional status (weight monitoring), and the rate of local or systemic complications. Results : We included 121 patients [47 men, 74 women, mean age : 83.5 +/- 7.6 years, indications for PEG : neurological dysphagia in 77 (63.6 %) patients and anorexia in 44 (36.4 %)]. Local complications were present in 25.6 0atients ; systemic complication in 23.1 %, and mortality rate in 57 %, including 30.4 0f early mortality (< 30 days). Mortality rate was correlated to swallowing difficulties and aspiration pneumonia ($p = 0.05$). No significant variation was found with age, gender, or PEG complication concerning the mean follow up duration (183.1 +/- 210 days). A lower life expectancy was found in demented patients with swallowing difficulties (277 versus 879 days). Conclusion : Neurological dysphagia increased the early mortality rate due to aspiration pneumonia especially when associated with dementia.

SESSION 421

Family Caregiving with Lifelong Disabilities: Research, Practice, and Policy Issues

T. Heller (Rehabilitation Research and Training Center on Aging with Developmental Disabilities, Department of Disabilities and Human Development, University of Chicago, Chicago, IL, USA) Family Support Interventions to Assist Family Caregivers of Adults with Intellectual Disabilities. E. F. Ansello, (Virginia Center on Aging, Medical College of Virginia Campus, Virginia Commonwealth University, Richmond, VA, USA) Building Intersystem Cooperation to Benefit Aging Adults with Lifelong Disabilities and Their Families. H. L. Sterns (Department of Psychology & Institute for Life-Span Development and Gerontology, The University of Akron, Akron, OH, USA) and E. A. Kennedy (Department of Social Science, Community and Technical College and Institute for Life-Span Development and Gerontology, The University of Akron, Akron, OH, USA) Person-Centered Planning for Later Life: Death and Dying Meeting Family and Staff Needs. A. Walker (Department of Sociological Studies, University of Sheffield, Sheffield, England), discussant.

Issue: Caregiving by family members is often at the heart of growing older with lifelong, developmental disabilities. This symposium addresses research, practice, and policy developments that strengthen the abilities of individuals with such disabilities and their family caregivers to continue living meaningfully in the community. Human service systems must pay particular attention to these family caregivers who need to be reinforced in maintaining care in this most natural of settings. Structure: After introductory overview by the convener of issues related to the unprecedented aging in developed nations of adults with lifelong disabilities, symposium members review their research on: interventions to strengthen families and individuals in caregiving, long-term planning, and dealing with death and dying; practice initiatives to improve coordination between human service agencies with little history of previous interaction; and comparative analyses of public policy to support family caregiving. Audience interaction is encouraged. Content: Heller discusses two interventions to support family caregivers of adults with intellectual disabilities (ID). The first involved 78 participant and 146 comparison families in a statewide cash-subsidy consumer-directed program over 4 years. Participant families had fewer unmet needs, experienced greater self-efficacy, and had greater increases in community involvement. In the second 37 families who received training and support (peer and professional) were more likely to develop plans with their relatives with ID for the permanency of that person's care. Ansello reviews research on the implementation of the Integrated Model to improve cooperation between aging and developmental disabilities service systems. Field-testing by 5 partnerships of aging and disabilities agencies in urban, rural, and suburban communities identified 3 core elements of intersystem cooperation and several universally effective strategies to realize these elements. Sterns and Kennedy report analyses of a death education and bereavement-counseling program for older adults with mild to severe ID. Focus groups of family caregivers and adults with ID helped identify major issues and content. The curriculum was shown to be effective in teaching issues related to death, dying, and loss. Walker, as discussant, provides an international perspective on these and other policies to strengthen caring by families. Conclusions: Human service systems have historically been somewhat narrowly categorical, e.g, serving elders or those with disabilities. Even systems with a presumed life-span approach, such as those in developmental disabilities, have understandably concentrated on early life and early intervention. The aging of people with lifelong disabilities has created a need to broaden such orientations. Attention must be given to the family caregivers of these aging adults. This research-based symposium demonstrates how human service agencies in the fields of aging and developmental disabilities can: initiate successful programs to improve the aging adult's and family's use of relevant services, engagement with the community, and planning for the future, including dealing with death and loss; improve intersystem cooperation to benefit aging adults, their families, and service providers; and develop effective policies related to meaningful aging with lifelong disabilities.

Building Intersystem Cooperation to Benefit Aging Adults with Lifelong Disabilities and Their Families

E. F. Ansello(Virginia Center on Aging, Virginia Commonwealth University, Richmond, VA, USA)

Purpose: In the United States the aging and the developmental disabilities systems have functioned along parallel tracks with little history of meaningful interaction until recently. With support from the U. S. Administration on Aging and other public sources the author directed a series of multi-year projects to improve intersystem cooperation in order to benefit aging adults with lifelong disabilities, family caregivers, and the staffs of human service agencies that serve them. Method: The most effective strategies for intersystem cooperation from previous projects were constituted "The Integrated Model" and were field-tested in Maryland and Virginia over 3 years. Through competitive applications five partnerships of aging and developmental disabilities agencies were selected to be trained in the Model and modestly funded to implement it in urban, rural, and suburban communities over an 18-month research period. Both initial training sessions and field implementation were pre-post-tested. Midterm and final plenary sessions provided qualitative data. Results: Core elements of intersystem cooperation proved to be structured collaboration, outreach (operationalized as both information dissemination and data gathering), and capacity-building of adults with lifelong disabilities, family caregivers, and community agency staffs. Several strategies to realize these elements proved to be universally effective. Initial training in the Model correlated with successful implementation. Local planning committees and statewide advocacy/ monitoring councils proved essential. Conclusion: The Integrated Model was demonstrated to be a cost-effective means of improving not only cooperation between the aging and developmental disabilities systems but also the individual's and family's capacities for continued community living.

Family Support Interventions to Assist Family Caregivers of Adults with intellectual Disabilities

T. Heller (Rehabilitation Research and Training Center on Aging with Developmental Disabilities, Department of Disabilities and Human Development, University of Illinois at Chicago, Chicago, IL, USA)

Purpose: This presentation describes research on support interventions for aging family caregivers of adults with intellectual disabilities (ID). It presents two studies, one examining a statewide cash subsidy consumer-directed program, and the other examining a family future planning training and support program. Method: The first study includes 78 participant and 146 comparison families. The family's unmet service needs, caregiving appraisal, need for out-of home placement and the community participation of the adults with ID were examined over four years. The second study assesses the Family Futures Planning Project in which 37 families received training and support in conducting long-term person-centered planning. This project uses ongoing peer (families and persons with ID) and professional support to help persons with ID and their families make plans, including residential, legal, and financial plans. Unique aspects of the program are the training and support provided to the persons with ID in future planning and the use of peer trainers with ID. Surveys regarding future planning were given to families (including 30 control families) before the intervention and 6 months later. Results: The first study's results indicated that, relative to the control group, participants had fewer unmet needs, used more services, were more satisfied with the services, experienced greater self-efficacy, were less likely to desire an out-of-home placement, and had higher increases in community participation. The second study found that families involved in the training were more likely than the other families to develop letters of intent and discuss future planning with the relative with ID.Conclusion: Both cash subsidy programs and ongoing peer and professional support were found to be effective interventions to help persons with ID and their families in continuing their community participation.

Person-Centered Planning for Later Life: Death and Dying Δ Meeting Family and Staff Needs

H. L. Sterns(Department of Psychology & Institute for Life-Span Development and Gerontology, The University of Akron, Akron, Ohio, USA)E. A. Kennedy(Department of Social Science, Community and Technical College and Institute for Life-Span Development and Gerontology, The University of Akron, Akron, Ohio, USA)

Purpose: Many have recognized the need for appropriate death education and responsive bereavement counseling for individuals with mental retardation and developmental disabilities (MR/DD), their families, and other care providers. Despite this, however, individuals with MR/DD may often be denied access to this important facet of the human experience. Method: Focus groups were conducted with care providers and families to determine major issues. In addition 41 participants were men and women aged 50 or older with mild to severe mental retardation, except for those with Down syndrome who were 35 or older. Participants were tested before (pre-test) and after the training (post-test) to find out if the training increased their understanding of death, dying, and loss. Results: Strong support for inclusion of death related issues was received from care providers and families. The pre- and post-tests Part I tested for key information and Part II was the Derry Death Concept Scale. Overall, both parts of the pre-test and post-test examined an individual's understanding of the 4 death concepts ? irreversibility, inevitability, finality, and causality. Results of the statistical analyses of these tests indicate that the training curriculum was effective in teaching issues related to death, dying, and loss. Conclusion: The post-test findings demonstrated that the curriculum was effective in increasing the understanding of death among adults with mild to severe levels of mental retardation. Staff concerns and family issues provided important information.

Who Cares? Supporting People With Intellectual Disabilities

and Their Family Carers in Older Age

Carol Walker (University of Lincoln and Humberside), Alan Walker, (University of Sheffield)

Despite the growth in independent living, most people with intellectual disabilities live in the family home. As their life expectancy increases, a growing proportion will continue to live with very elderly family members, usually parents, and an increasing number will survive them. Based on research undertaken in the UK, this paper will examine the main problems which such families face and the ways in which public services could better support them. The paper will then consider what, if any, steps are being taken both to support this much neglected group of lifelong carers to maintain, or disengage from, their role as primary carers, and to ensure that the transition to alternative forms of care which will inevitably occur when the family carer is unable to care because of ill-health or death, occurs in a sensitive and planned way. The paper will assess how far the British government's proposals to provide a national strategy for people with learning difficulties and another for carers acknowledge the special challenges presented by this group. The paper will also consider what lessons

SESSION 422

Family dynamics and chronic psychotropic drug use among home-care elderly women

Pérodeau,G,(UQAH, Hull, Québec),Collin,J. (U de Montréal, Montréal, Québec),Cohen,D,Florida (International University, Miami, USA) Ducharme,F. (U de Montréal, Montréal, Québec) Mishara,B. (UQAM, Montréal, Québec & Paradis, I (UQAH, Hull, Québec)

Prescribed psychotropic drug use among the elderly is widespread and often chronic. However, little is known of the effect of family pressure or attitudes toward drug use on actual consumption by seniors. The purpose of the present study is to examine psychotropic drug use by elders in relation with the family dynamics around medication use. We are interested in the social representations of psychotropic medication among chronic female psychotropic drug users. More specifically we examine family attitudes, beliefs, and health-related practices with regard to prescribed psychotropic medications. Forty face-to-face interviews were conducted at home with female chronic psychotropic drug users and, subsequently, their female caregivers, half of whom were drug users themselves. Respondents were recipients of a home care program. Input from caregivers represented the family viewpoint. The open-ended questions pertained to family traditions in terms of drug use, present habits, the symbolic role played by the medication in the family interaction and, finally the source of medical information on drug use. Results indicate both converging and diverging attitudes with regard to drug use between the elderly respondents and their caregivers. The role played by the drug in the family dynamics is presented. Maintenance of the drug habit can also be pinpointed to specific family patterns. Based on the results, recommendations are made geared toward integrating family members in prevention programs related to psychotropic drug use among elderly women.

Impact of a Medication Education Program Led by Trained Seniors

Patrick McGowan, (Institute of Health Promotion Research, UBC, Vancouver, BC, Canada); Neena Chappell, (Centre on Aging, U of Victoria, Victoria, BC, Canada); Heather Clarke, RN, (Research and Evaluation Consulting, Vancouver, BC, Canada); Lawrence Green, PH. (Centers for Disease Control, Atlanta, Georgia); Malcolm Maclure, S.D. (BC Pharmacare, Victoria, BC, Canada); Penny Miller, M.A. (Pharmaceutical Sciences, UBC, Vancouver, BC, Canada).

The objective of this research was to evaluate the impact of a lay-led medication education program for seniors. The one-hour program was led by trained seniors and focussed on ways to enhance safe and effective medication use. Subjects completed a questionnaire on medication knowledge and use before they received the program and again four-months later. During the project period 16 trained seniors led the program to 1600 seniors. Analysis was conducted using matched pre- and four-month post-program questionnaires completed by 550 seniors in the pilot community. To examine the effects of how medication information from the program is disseminated, random telephone interviews about medication knowledge and behavior were completed by nearly 1500 seniors in two comparison communities, at two points of time 12 months apart. At post-test, seniors in the pilot community were more knowledgeable and were practicing safer medication practices then they were at pre-test. Comparisons between the two time points in the comparison communities showed improvements in both communities, however, the benefits in one of the comparison communities can be attributed to an alternate intervention offered to seniors during the same project period. The results demonstrate benefits of a lay-led minimal intervention strategy aimed at improving seniors knowledge and medication-taking behavior.

Medication Practices in Community-Dwelling Chinese Elders

Lin Zhan, Jie Chen, An-li Jiang

Purpose. The purposes of this study were to: (a) explore the scope and methods of self medication practices among community-dwelling Chinese elders; (b) identify conditions and/or factors that influence older persons' decisions to use home remedies and/or a compliment to prescribed medications; and (c) develop culturally appropriate and ethnically sensitive intervention strategies to improve older persons' medication practices in the community. Background. Of the thirty-one million older persons today, more than 85% have one or more chronic conditions, such as arthritis, diabetes, hypertension, pulmonary disease, hearing and visual impairment, cancer, and mental illness (1). Multichronicity is often treated with multi-medications. Although people aged 65 or older comprise 12.6% of the nation's population, they account for one-third of all prescription drug use, and 40% of all the over-the-counter non-prescription drug purchases (2-3). On average, an older person receives between 12 and 17 prescriptions per year and consumes 4 to 5 prescription medications at one time (4). However, among Medicare beneficiaries who rate their health as poor, they report taking on average 31 prescriptions per year (5). In the institutional setting, one-third of the residents take between 8 to 16 medications at a time (6). Medication-related health problems account for 30% of the hospital admissions. Yet, data on medication practices in community-dwelling Chinese elders are lacking. Since more than 90% of older persons with chronic conditions live in communities, understanding their medication practices helps health providers intervene effectively. Method. Two phases of the study were designed. The first phase included focus group interviews with fifteen Chinese elders to explore the nature of medication practices in the sample. Major interview questions included: a) what self-initiated methods have older persons used in medication practices? B) Under what circumstances have older persons decided to take prescribed medications, to use home remedies, and/or over the counter drugs? C) What are factors or conditions that help or make difficult for older persons in adherence to the prescribed medication regimen? And d) how do older persons manage their medication use? In the second phase the researcher conducted a survey relating to medication practices in community-dwelling Chinese elders (N=210). Survey questionnaires included a) the Medication Practice Questionnaire, b) Health Status Questionnaire (SF-36), and c) Demographic Profile questionnaires. Comparative content analysis for interview data and statistical analyses for survey data were employed to identify the nature of medication practices and factors related to medication practices in community-dwelling Chinese elders. Findings. The results of the study revealed several medication practices behaviors in community-dwelling Chinese elders and barriers and facilitators relating to medication practices in the sample. It is suggested that culturally appropriate and ethnically sensitive intervention strategies need to be developed to enhance elders' capacity in medication management.

Predicting the probability of errors in a geriatric self-medication program

Sheri Laine Maddigan (The University of Iowa, Iowa City, Iowa, USA) Karen Bell Farris (The University of Iowa, Iowa City, Iowa, USA)

PURPOSE: Institutional self-medication programs allocate responsibility of medication administration to patients, within a controlled and monitored setting. The purpose of this project was to model direct and indirect relationships between demographic and clinical variables in predicting errors in a geriatric self-medication program. Independent variables were identified based upon the Theory of Self-Care Deficit and previous research. METHOD: A random sample of charts from 300 older adults in a self-medication program at a rehabilitation hospital between September 1, 1996 and December 31, 1999 were reviewed. Data were analyzed using path analysis for the probability of making an error during the first week and final week on the program, as these errors have been shown to vary. RESULTS: For initial and final weeks of self-medication, 6.7% and 29.70f variance in making an error was explained directly by visual impairment, hearing impairment, education, MMSE, medication complexity and the interaction between medication complexity and MMSE, respectively. For the initial week, MMSE showed a statistically significant direct path, and education was an indirect predictor through MMSE. For the final week, MMSE and education had statistically significant direct paths. Medication complexity was not significant in either model. A small significant correlation was found between managing money and making errors for the initial week. No statistically significant correlations were found between IADL's and making errors during the final week. CONCLUSION: Variance explained was not high. However, MMSE and education, not medication complexity, appeared to be important predictors of the probability of making errors during self-medication programs.

SESSION 423

Bacterial Sensitivity to Antibiotics, Over Time, in various Departments of a Long Term Care Center

R. Friedmann, H. Shulman, R. Hamburger. (Neve Horim Home for the Aged, Jerusalem, Israel), A. Yinnon, D. Raveh, (Shaare Zedek Medical Center, Jerusalem, Israel)

Purpose: To define the sensitivity of urine pathogens to antibiotics, in a comprehensive long-term-care center. Methods: The study was conducted over 30 months (1996-9), in Neve-Horim a long-term-care center, housing 286 residents in various departments. Unit A - 130 independent and frail residents - in which the antibiotic treatment is limited to oral medications only. Unit B - 120 nursing and demented patients. In this unit we also use first and second generation cephalosporins and gentamicin intravenously. Unit C - 36 complex nursing patients. In this unit ceftazidime, amikacin, timentin and imipenem, are also used. Urine cultures were taken according to clinical guidelines. Antibiotic therapy was administered as required. Results: 1401 positive urine cultures were obtained. There was a difference in frequency of pathogens between units; E. coli was found in 56 0n unit A, in 55 0n unit B and in 44 0n Unit C. Pseudomonas spp. were found in 1.6%, 5.0% and 11.0% respectively. There was no major difference in frequency of Klebsiella spp. 170r Proteus spp. 14%. Sensitivity to the various antibiotics was generally low across the study. Mean sensitivity to cotrimoxazole was 43%, to furadantin - 31%, ampicillin - 17%, cefuroxime - 42%, ciprofloxacin - 41%, gentamicin - 53%, and to imipenem - 93%. There was a difference of sensitivity to antibiotics across the three units; ceftazidime 71%, 73% and 44% respectively in units A, B and C, and amikacin 91%, 82% and 61%, respectively. There was also a reduction in sensitivity over time to the various antibiotics; e.g. - sensitivity to ceftazidime in unit C was 440ver the first three months and 180ver the last three. Sensitive to amikacin was 56% at the beginning, and 47% and at the end of the study. Conclusion: Choosing an antibiotic treatment for serious urinary tract infection for a resident of a comprehensive long-term-center should consider his specific microbial environment.

Chronic disease of gastrointestinal tract and microbiocenosis in elderly people

T.A.Chulok, K.G. Kaverina, S.L. Shumova, L.D Serova

The state of microbiocenosis in the intestine of 189 older (after 60) and 91 younger patients with chronic disease of gastrointestinal tract was determined. Dysbiotic disturbances of different severity were detected in 91,9 0f the examined persons. There are same principles of intestinal dysbacterious treatment: - Treatment of the main disease; - Selective decontamination of pathogenic; - Correction of autochthonous microflora; - Functional food. Two principles of intestinal dysbacteriosis treatment were compared: selective decontamination and autochthonous microflora correction. Application of antibiotics aggravated the state of dysbacteriosis, though it led to selective decontamination. The comparative study of the two preparations revealed that the use of probiotics containing Bifidobacterium bifidum was mainly substitutional, promoting the colonization of the intestine by Lactobacteria, which later determined the suppression opportunistic microflora. The effectiveness of Bifidobacterium forte, containing live B.Bifidum, immobilized on sorbent, provided to be the most pronounced. But only the application of probiotics did not lead to achievement the desired results during the period that patient stay at hospital. Unification of these two principles i.e. decontamination with further rehabilitation of microflora with probiotics may be considered optimum. The state of immune system and intestinal microflora of elderly man were studied. Dysbacteriosis and decrease in number of limphocutes in all subpopulations, especially of T-lymphosytes were detected in most cases. Application of immunotherapy of patients with increased level of conditionally pathogenic flora on the intestinal with help of cell-free vaccine from antigens of conditionally pathogenic with multiple and durable administration of the medicine results in patial restoration of microflora, allowed to correct secondary immunology insufficiency which accompanies dysbacterioriasis in elderly patients but did not exclude application of probiotics.

Computer Assisted Antibiotic Prescription in Pulmonary and Urinary Infections in Geriatrics

Drs W. Chatelier, M. C. Dellamonica, J. Falcot, C. Koubi, C. Obez (Clinique Les Sources,Nice,France) V. Mondain (Hop. de l'Archet I Service des maladies infectieuses, CHU,Nice,France)

PURPOSE To propose a reasoned, probability and consensus based antibiotherapy for elderly patients presenting pulmonary and urinary community-acquired infections, in order to improve therapeutic efficiency and molecule tolerance, and to prevent the already too frequent onset of antibiotic resistance. METHODS - analysis of the recommandations of the consensus conferences and guidelines in antibiotherapy; adaptation to the geriatric population. - taking into account of the clinical and paraclinical features of a given clinical situation requesting a determined antibiotherapy. - design of a database collecting all the clinical situations, with easy access to the different elements of the database. - typing on the PC keyboard by the prescriber of the specific patient data, the soft adapting the dosage to the renal function according to the Cockcroft formula. - before disposal of the soft, evaluation on a three month period of the infectious pathologies, the bacterial ecology and the treatement actually used in order to access the consequences of the use of the soft in the future. RESULTS - disposal on each medical PC of the antibiotic prescription guided by the soft, allowing to type on the PC keyboard the clinical and paraclinical data (biological and radiological), in order to get a well adapted and secure prescription. - printing and recording of prescriptions to have a permanent evaluation of the prescribed treatments. CONCLUSION Computer assisted antibiotic prescription according to the clinical, biological and radiological presentation, the general condition and the prognosis factors will allow to start an antibiotic therapy consistent with current recommandations, and well adapted to the ederly.

Lamivudine for chronic hepatitis B with cirrhosis in a 85 years old man

D Somme, J Ramanoelina**, E Pautas**, F Yvain*, O Saint Jean* * [Service de Gériatrie Hôpital Européen Georges Pompidou Paris France] ** [Service de Gériatrie Hôpital Charles Foix Ivry sur Seine France]*

PURPOSE : To evaluate if lamivudine is safe and effective for chronic hepatitis in a very old patient METHODS : An 8 months follow up RESULTS : A 85 years old patient was admitted for oedema and ascitis caused by cirrhosis. Chronic hepatitis B, with positive search for viral DNA, had been discovered five years before but no specific treatment had been proposed. Clinical status was poor. Biological findings associated both cytolysis and cholestatic disorders. Symptomatic treatment (rest, spironolactone, propanolol and salt-free diet) provides improvement. Lamivudine (60 mg/d) was started. Eight months later patient is asymptomatic, with lamivudine (60 mg/d) and propanolol (40 mg/d). Between the initial state and 8 months of treatment evolution of biological disorders were the following: ALAT (from 3 fold the Normal value (N) to N), 5'Nucleotidase (from 1.5N to N),Prothrombin rate (from 51% to N), Serum Albumine (from 24 g/l to 37 g/l), and DNA HBV (from >40 000 000 copies/ml to <400 copies/ml) CONCLUSION Lamivudine was well tolerated and effective in this patient, leading to the normalization of biological abnormalities and total suppression of viral replication. It is potentially useful in old patient with chronic hepatitis B and ongoing viral replication.

Susceptibility of Helicobacter pylori to Amoxicillin, Azithromycin, Clarithromycin and Metronidazole in Elderly Symptomatic Patients - A Central European Survey

S. Krcmery (Department of Geriatric Medicine, Comenius Univ. Faculty of Medicine, Bratislava), D. Ohlasova, N. Salyova (Department of Clinical Microbiology, Kosice), T. Jeger, I. Bunganic (Department of Internal Medicine), P. Jarcuska and I. Schreter (Department of Infectious Diseases, L. Pasteur University Hospital, Kosice, Slovak Republic)

The evidence for an etiologic link between Helicobacter pylori (H. pylori) infection and peptic ulcer disease is generally accepted. Among the most frequent antimicrobial agents used for treatment are amoxicillin (AMX), azithromycin (AZI), clarithromycin (CLA) and metronidazole (MET). Several strains of H. pylori have been previously described resistant to MET, also increasingly to macrolides (AZI and CLA) and more recently also to AMX. The objective of present study was to determine the susceptibility of H. pylori strains isolated from elderly (>65 years of age) symptomatic patients in Central European Region. Gastric biopsies were taken at routine endoscopy in 700 patients with peptic ulcer disease or chronic antral gastritis. 369 strains of H. pylori were isolated and identified by standard laboratory methods (gram stain microscopy, Urease test and culture). The plates were incubated at 35-37 degrees Centigrade under microaerophilic conditions for 3 days. Antibiogram was done by modified disk diffusion method (MDDM - Hachem 1996, Alarcon 1999). MET resistance rate in our group was 42%, higher than resistance rates found by Mégraud et al. in France (16%), Germany (19%) or Sweden (26%). The highest MET resistance rates are reported for South-east Asian countries (up to 95%). 12% of H. pylori strains were resistant to CLA and 10% to AZI, respectively. All isolates were found to be sensitive to AMX. In conclusion, newer macrolides (AZI or CLA) and amoxicillin should be used preferably in combination treatment with antisecretory agents to eradicate H. pylori infection in elderly patients.

The use of tele-medicine for determining infectious states among institutionalized elderly patients

T. Dwolatzky (Shaare Zedek Medical Center, Jerusalem, Israel), S Berliner (Sourasky Medical Center, Tel Aviv, Israel)

PURPOSE:The physician is often faced with a difficult decision when treating the elderly patient with a fever in a long-term care institution. Laboratory facilities are not always immediately available and in many cases the physician will try to avoid the transfer of a patient to an acute care facility. We have developed a simple blood test to determine the presence of infection. Our study examined the reliability of this test compared to other non-specific acute phase reactants. We also studied the possibility of adapting this test for widespread use via tele-medicine. METHOD: The inflammatory index test (IIT) determines the degree of leukocyte aggregation/adhesion on a slide prepared from citrated whole blood. The slide is scanned at the long-term care facility and transmitted via the internet to a central computer, where the picture is analysed. The result is returned within minutes to the treating physician. The IIT was correlated with the clinical diagnosis of the patient, as well as the total white blood cell count (WBC), the C-reactive protein (CRP), and the eryrthrocyte sedimentation rate (ESR). RESULTS: The sensitivity of the IIT was 84%, compared to 64 0.000000or WBC and the 44 0.000000or ESR. The correlation with the clinical diagnosis of infection was 87 0.000000or the IIT, compared to 82 0.000000or WBC and 64 0.000000or ESR. The IIT was as reliable as the CRP. CONCLUSION: The IIT is a reliable indicator of acute infections in elderly residents of long-term care facilities. The use of tele-medicine makes this test widely available.

SESSION 424

Dislypoproteinemia and the immune status in the elderly.

Speranta Babeanu Clinics of Natural Therapy Breaza, Romania, C.Balaceanu-Stolnici Ecology Faculty,Bucharest, Romania, C.Ursaciuc Institute of Genetics and Molecular Biology V.Babes, Bucharest,Romania, Laura Marinescu BA TouchTunes,Montreal,Canada.

Purpose: The study of the presence or absence of any disequilibrium of the immune status in the dislypoproteinemia in the elderly. Method: Sample of 320 patients aged from 47 to 107 years, 127 with dislypoproteinemis and other chronic diseases. Selection was done based upon Senieur Protocole requirements. The immune system was studied by: lymphocytes subpopulations with monoclonal antibodies: CD56,HLA-DR,CD3,CD4,CD6,CD19,CD45RO+,CD45RA+, seric IL:2, 6 and IL-2R, autoantibodies, lymphocytes blastic proliferation, delayed hypersensitivity tests(DHT). Multiple statistical analysis was used. Results: Immune tests showed: mild changes of the lymphocytes subpopulations, more important in the response to the anamnestic antigens, the significant decrease of the reactivity to IDR. The blastic changes of lymphocytes to PHA and PWM decrease with age. The Speraman correlations pointed out as the most important correlation is between age, total cholesterol, triglycerides, IL6, LTA, IDR tests (55% with negative responses). Conclusions: There are not any significant differences related to the immune status and dislypoproteinemia in the elderlies studied. The immunological data obtained mostly confirm the literature data but there are present the increase of BL and of Nkcells over the age of 80. DHT showed in 55% of cases a marked decrease especially to tuberculin as well as the lymphocyte proliferation to mitogens especially over the age of 8o. Concluding, the studied subjects proved to have a discreet immunodeficiency under the context of an associated chronic polipathology.

Immunity, autoimmunity and longevity or aging, and immunorestoration in the immunodeficiency arising from aging by traditional Chinese drugs and Germanium-132

Ma Yong-Xing, Wang Zan-Shun, Wang Chun-Fu (Department of Aging, Antiaging and Cognitive Function, Shanghai Institute of Gerontology and Geriatrics, Huadong Hospital, Shanghai, China)

1. The relationship between longevity or aging was studied by assay of nature killer (NK) cell activity in various age groups. NK cell activity was determined by 125IUDR method in 232 people including 72 youth,36 middle aged, 24 cases of 60-69, 30 cases of 70-79 yrs aged group and 70 longevous. The mean value of total (Male+Female) group were found to be 43.3±11.3, 44.8±15.1, 49.1±13, 43.0±19, and 49.3±14% respectively. NK activity tends to decline in 70-79 yrs group (this age period is coincided with the life span now in China), but to raise again in the longevous. The NK cell activity is surprisingly higher than that in the 70-79 yrs period and the young level (P<0.01), even though there was no significant difference of NK cell activity found between the longevous and 70-79 yrs group, probably because of rather small number in the 70-79 yrs group. We consider the higher NK cell activity of longevous group may be one for the mechanisms of long life span in >90 yrs group. That means better immune function, irrespective of its cause, may promote longevity by decreasing immunodeficiency related diseases, and probably by other possible mechanisms. Although the NK cell activity of the female is lower than that of the males in the preaged group, it tends to be higher than that of males in the aged group. This may be one of the factors related to the longer life span of the females. 2. No obvious correlation between NK cell activity and HLA-A, B, C phenotypes was observed. 3. RF(+), ANF(+) were observed only in 11.1 and 9.2% of 379 longevous. We consider the rather mild autoimmunity may be another one of the mechanisms of longevity because of the low positive rate of RF and ANF and no significant difference of SOD content of erythrocyte and NK cell activity between RF(+)+AnF(+) and RF(-)+AnF(-) groups. 4. We found Tribusponin, Ginseng and Vita-Rev (Vitality Revival; composed of six Chinese medicinal herbs, such as Polygonum multiform, Asrragalus membranaceus, Salvus miltiorrhiza, Lycium barbarum Polygonatum Kinglanum, Epimedium brevicornum) could exert bi-directional regulation of NK cell activity. Though the mechanism of this effect is not clear, it may be indicated that the immunostimulating agent including traditional Chinese drugs is not necessary for the preaged or aged if they have good immune functions, and it is beneficial for geroprotection in the immunodeficiency state arising from aging. 5. Long-Life SOD extracted from Cili Brain Gospel,composed of Rehmannia glutinosa (Gacrtn) Libosch+Cistanche Salsa (C.A. Mey.) G. Beck+Polyggonum Multiform Thumb, R. S.C. (Reinhart, Sea Snake Product), DHA+EPA and Ge-132 could increase NK cell activity, improve free radical metabolism, microcirculatory state and cognitive function. We consider these agents may have immunostimulating and some aging retarding effects.

Signal transduction changes in neutrophils and T lymphocytes with aging

T. Fulop Jr, N. Douziech, A.C. Goulet, G. Lacombe, D. Gagné, M. Arcand, G. Dupuis Inst. Univ. Gériatr, Lab. Biogérontol, *Dept. Biochim, Fac. Méd, Univ. Sherbrooke, Sherbrooke, Qc, Canada*

Purpose: We have demonstrated that we assist with aging to an alteration of the transmembrane signaling. We were interested at which level the alteration(s) could exist. Method: The granulocytes (PMNLs) and lymphocytes of healthy young (18-25 years) and elderly subjects (aged over 65 years) were studied, as a model. Results: The receptor number on cell surface (IL-2, FMLP, CD3) was investigated and was found not to change with aging. The subtype characterisation by anti-G protein antibodies demonstrated quantitative changes (mainly Gi and Gq) with aging. The study of PKC isozymes by Western blots demonstrated different resting and translocated patterns with aging in T lymphocytes compared to young subjects. The expression of tyrosine kinases in lymphocytes was not age-related. The exogenous and endogenous tyrosine kinase activities (ZAP70, p56lck) were decreased with aging under antiCD3 stimulation in lymphocytes. The p59fyn activity did not change, as well as the expression of CD45. The IL-2 signalling was also found to be altered with aging (Jak3 and STAT3 and 5). In PMNLs the GM-CSF signal transduction pathway was found to be altered by a diminished tyrosine phosphorylation of Jak2, STAT3 and 5. As it is known the cholesterol is increased in cell membranes resulting in an decreased membrane fluidity with aging. We tried to use the cyclodextrin (0.1mM to 20mM) to modulate the signal transduction and proliferation of lymphocyte through the TCR/CD3 receptor complex. The results indicate that with aging by extracting the cholesterol some degree of function (prolifeartion) could be obtained via the improvement of the decreased protein tyrosine phosphorylation. Conclusion: Thus, an alteration of signal transduction mechanism exists with aging and this might be caused by the alterations of cell membrane encountered with aging. These changes might contribute to the altered immune response observed with aging, but are subject to modulation.

The Effect of Long Life Superoxide Dismutase and Brain Gospel on Natural Killer Cell Activity

Ma Yong-Xing, Lu Pei-Fang, Zhu Yue (Department of Aging, Antiaging and Cognitive Function, Shanghai Institute of Gerontology and Geriatrics, Huadong Hospital, Shanghai, China)

1. Long Life Superoxide Dismutase (SOD) oral liquid, is composed of superoxide dismutase (SOD), polysaccharide, vitC, vitE and trace elements which were all extracted from a natural plant fruit Cili (Rosaroxburghii Tratt) in GuiZhou, China. A set of indices were evaluated after administration of SOD 10ml Bid for two months in 50~75 years old healthy people. The mean value of NK cell activity (22.4±10.8%, 27.5±12.9%, P<0.05), SOD (453.0±24.2, 468.6±21.3g/gHb, P<0.001), Catalase (15.5±1.7, 17.4±3.0U/mgHb, P<0.001) and GSH content (2.3±0.3, 2.6±0.5mg/gHb, P<0.001) in erythrocytes increased significantly, while the serum LPO level (4.20±0.78, 3.78±0.50 nmol/mL, P<0.001) decreased significantly. 2. Brain Gospel (B.G.) Capsule is composed of three Traditional Chinese Drugs (Rehmannia glutinosa (Gacrtn.), Libosh Cistanche Salsa (C.A.Mey.), G.Beck Polyggonum Multiflorum Thunb). A set of indices were evaluated after administration of B.G. 4 capsules tried for three months in 87 elderly, and 44 elderly as the control group of 50-85 years old. The nature killer cell activity (N.K.) increased significantly in the B.G. group (25.9±11.0, 33.5±13.4, t=2.71, P<0.01). There was no significant increase in the control group (24.2±14.1, 25.1±8.2, t=0.33, P<0.05). No significant effect on SOD and LPO were found in both B.G. and control group. 3. It is suggested that SOD and Brain Gospel can improve immunological function in the aged.

SESSION 425

Get me out of here!

Barbara Purdy, Reg. Physiotherapist/Occupational Therapist (Barbara Purdy Rehabilitation Consulting, Vancouver, Canada)

Get me out of here! video and manual teaches the latest techniques to effectively evacuate someone with a physical problem quickly and safely in the event of a fire, earthquake or an industrial accident. The primary focus is to prevent back injuries to the care giver while keeping the evacuee as safe as possible. Every year, people are needlessly injured as safety is often compromised by the need for speed in an emergency. Get me out of here! demonstrates procedures that incorporate ergonomically safe lifting and transfer methods that can be applied in hospitals, care facilities, businesses, industrial and hospitality settings as well as in private homes. The content includes techniques that quickly move a person who is walking, lying in bed or sitting in a wheelchair. Innovative ideas such as assisted standing, assisted speed walking and a controlled fall are used for a person who can walk. Safe maneuvers are shown for moving a person in bed to a wheelchair, from bed to the floor or down a flight of stairs. Techniques are demonstrated on how to move someone out of a wheelchair to the floor, or move the person and the wheelchair down the stairs. These maneuvers represent the most efficient combination of speed and safety, making the Get me out of here! video an invaluable tool for training to prevent injuries.

The Continuing Care Activity Measure (CCAM) Training Video

C. McCullough, M. Huijbregt (Baycrest Centre for Geriatric Care, Toronto, Canada)

Physiotherapy assessment and treatment for Long Term Care (LTC) clients addresses functional mobility activities such as bed mobility, transfers and locomotion. The expected outcome of intervention may be to improve function, to maintain the current level of function, or to offset expected deterioration. Evaluation is challenging as there are no standardised mobility outcome measures available for this diverse population. Traditional outcome measures are often diagnostic specific, target clients during active rehabilitation, and are not able to discriminate between different levels of functioning or to measure the subtle changes that occur in LTC clients. The Continuing Care Activity Measure (CCAM) was developed in reponse to the need for a mobility outcome measure that is sensitive enough to discriminate between clients at baseline assessment, to detect and evaluate change over time and to be applicable to a diverse diagnostic group. Preliminary reliability, validity, and responsiveness including the minimal clinically important difference have been determined. A multi-site validation study is currently in progress. To facilitate appropriate use of this tool, the CCAM Training Video has been developed. The video provides theoretical background on the CCAM and demonstrates three client assessments. Viewers are given the time to do their own scoring. Blank scoring sheets, criterion scoring and scoring rationale are provided. The CCAM is a promising LTC mobility outcome measure and the CCAM Training Video is a useful educational tool to assist in implementing and applying the measure in the clinical and research setting.

SESSION 427

[1] DRUG ABSORPTION MAY BE DELAYED AFTER STROKE

M. RIZEQ (1), S. GEORGE (2), R. A. BRAITHWAITE (1 and 2) AND P. CROME (3) (1)Combined Healthcare NHS Trust, (2)Regional Laboratory for Toxicology, City Hospital, Birmingham, (3)Department of Geriatric Medicine, Keele University, Keele, Staffordshire (UK).

Background Drugs absorption is delayed in acute migraine and a wide range of autonomic changes have been reported after acute stroke. It is possible, therefore, that gastric emptying may be impaired after acute stroke. We have investigated this using the paracetamol absorption test, a tool widely used to measure gastric emptying. Methods 12 patients with acute stroke were studied within 24 hours (T1) of the stroke and 7-10 (T2) days later. Patients with impaired swallow, oesophago-gastro-intestinal disease or receiving drugs affecting the autonomic or GI system were excluded. Oral paracetamol (1 g) was given with a glass of water. Blood samples for plasma paracetamol concentrations were taken for 240 minutes. Pharmacokinetic measurements Tmax, Cmax, AUC120 were measured from the plasma concentration time curve. The results were compared to age-sex matched controls (V). Results The patients were 8 women and 4 men aged 64-86 y (mean = 76). The volunteers were 64-84 y (mean = 73). Mean Tmax was 96.3, 58.3 and 46.2 min for T1, T2 and V respectively. Cmax was 16.1, 20.2 and 23.9mg/l and AUC120 was 1146, 1654 and 1510 mg/l.min for the same three groups. The difference in Tmax was statistically significant (ANOVA = 0.024) but the other measurements showed no significant difference. Conclusion These results suggest that pharmacological effect may be slowed in acute stroke because of delayed drug absorption. This may have proven detrimental when rapid a action is required and the iv route is not possible. Th relationship between stroke and drug absorption required further investigation which should include groups we excluded and the influence of pro-absorptive agents.

[2] Required dose of warfarin therapy in the elderly: a survey of 97 inpatients

E. Pautas (Hôpital Charles Foix, Ivry-sur-Seine, France), M. Debray, J.L. Bosson (Centre Hospitalier Universitaire, Grenoble, France), V. Siguret (Hôpital Charles Foix, Ivry-sur-Seine, France)

Purpose: We conduct a prospective study in elderly patients in order to evaluate: i/ the incidence of over-anticoagulation during the first month of treatment with warfarin ii/ the maintenance dose required to achieve an International Normalised Ratio (INR) between 2 and 3. Method: Over one year, elderly inpatients (age >70) requiring an oral anticoagulant treatment, with an INR range of 2-3, were prospectively recruited in our geriatric hospital. An initial low-dose warfarin regimen (4 mg daily) was recommended. Patients were followed up to one month after the first day of warfarin. Over-anticoagulation was defined as INR>4 and substantial over-anticoagulation as INR>6. Maintenance dose was defined as the warfarin dose required to obtain two consecutive INRs between 2 and 3 within 48 hours. Results: During the study period, a warfarin therapy was initiated in 97 patients, mean age 85.2 years (range 70-101). The mean follow-up was 26.1 +/- 12 days. Over-anticoagulation occurred in 33 patients (34%) and 7 (7.2%) had an INR>6. Minor and major haemorrhagic effects were collected. Fourty-five patients (46.3%) reached the maintenance dose. Mean maintenance dose was 3.3 +/- 1.36 mg. The mean delay to obtain it was 14.4 +/- 9.6 days. Conclusion: During the induction of warfarin therapy in the elderly, over-anticoagulation is common. It is confirmed that a low maintenance dose warfarin is required in the elderly, suggesting the use of low-dose warfarin induction regimen for elderly.

[3] Drug Disease and Age Peculiarities of Neuro-Hormonal Disorders

E. N. Soloshenko (Scientific Research Institute of Dermatology and Venerology ,Kharkov,Ukraine)

Purpose :Investigation of neuro-hormonal disturbances in organism of patients of different age with drug disease(Morbus medicamentosus). Method: Radioimmunological methods of hormone determination, methods of ECG and immunology Results:467 patients(348 women, 119 men of 20 and 60 years of age) suffering with drug disease had been examined. There were found evident disorders in diencephal-trunk area,endocrinous system and adreno-choline reactive structures of afferent organs. This is proved with low amplitude modulations of spindle-shaped nature on the background of the absence of registration for ECG of regional peculiarities; dissociation between too high ACTG content in plasma and relatively high cortisole level with very low tyrosine concentration; thyroid hormone level increase(aggregate thyroxin and 3-iod-thyronine);increase of noradrenalin content and adrenalin content in blood plasma and also of acethylcholine in blood serum and acethylcholinesterase activity, serotonin and histamine levels. Neuro-humoral regulation shifts result in changes in microcirculatory, acid-alcaline, water-electrolythic homeostasis, in content of some microelements-calcium, magnum, copper in drug disease patients. The disorders of normal lipids oxidation processes also occur. The secondary immunodeficiency was more pronounced in old patients. The correction of disorders found was accomplished with the help of piroxan adrenoblockers (butiroxan), antioxidants, cvaterone, corticosteroids, acupuncture and hypothermia, and more successfal of young age.

[4] Pharmacists' Perception of Geriatric Drug Therapy

William Simonson (President, American Society of Consultant Pharmacists) (Alexandria, Virginia, USA)

Purpose: Geriatrics has developed into a specialty within the practice of pharmacy. Dramatic scientific discoveries have lead to an increase in the number of new medications available for the treatment of diseases of aging. Increasing recognition of the significance of medication-related problems in the elderly has added to this geriatric focus. Since pharmacists play an important role in geriatric drug therapy, it is important to understand how they perceive the key issues in geriatric drug therapy. Method: This survey, which is currently being conducted, will report the perceptions of geriatric pharmacy specialists' on the most important issues in geriatric drug therapy. Responses will be assessed by category to determine their order of importance as reported by survey respondents. Results: The poster will report the responses of approximately six hundred certified geriatric pharmacists to determine their perceptions of the most important issues in geriatric drug therapy. Results will be compared to surveys conducted in the past to determine if recent developments in drug therapy have influenced their perceptions. Conclusion: This survey will explore the perceptions of pharmacists with special credentials in geriatric drug therapy to determine their perceptions of the important issues relating to the use and misuse of medications in the elderly.

[5] Autonomy and the Use of Drugs

Vicente Spinola Dias Neto; Giselle H. de P. Rodrigues; Juliana P. Magnatti (Pontifícia Universidade Católica de São Paulo Sorocaba Brazil).

PURPOSE: This study analyzed the influence of the quantity of medication used by a population more than 60 years old, their autonomy to do activities of daily living (ADL), instrumental activities of daily living (IADL) and the consequences in their quality of life. METHOD: Interviews, based on a standard questionnaire, have been done with all of the older people (n=409) from two city districts of Sorocaba, SP, Brazil. The software EPI-INFO 5.0 was used to compute the results. RESULTS: We observed that among those who had total autonomy in ADL, 52.3% were 60 to 69, and only 9.75%, 80 to 99. Among those who had difficulty to do four or more activities, 20% were 60 to 69 and 53.3% were 80 to 99. In IADL, those who presented total autonomy, 55.3% was 60 to 69 and only 4.56% was 80 to 99. Those who needed help to do four or more IADL, 31.34% was between 60 to 69 and 80 to 99. The ADL and IADL are influenced by the quantity of medication used by the patients too. Those who had total autonomy by ADL, 21% didn' t use any drug as 21.5% in IADL. Among those who used four or more drugs: 40% (ADL) and 34.32% (IADL) needed help to do four or more of these activities. Patients that didn' t use any drug: 45.6% were 60 to 69; 34.36%, 70 to 79; and 19.75%, 80 to 99. Among those who used four or more drugs, 52.5% were 60 to 69; 38.75%, 70 to 79; and 7.5%, 80 to 99. CONCLUSION: This study demonstrated that when lots of medication is used, the autonomy of the population decreases. This decrease of the autonomy is also seen with the increase of the age, mainly in the ADL. Furthermore, differently of what we expected, older patients are using fewer drugs than younger ones. So we conclude that the autonomy and consequently the quality of life of the patients are directly influenced by the quantity of medication used by them, and not only at their age.

[6] Prophylactic Ondansetron for postoperative nausea and vomiting in the aged

Guo Nailiang, Yang Lujun, Chen Peilian, Chen Xiongbin (Hua Dong Hospital, Shanghai Geriatrics Institute)

Objective: Postoperative nausea and vomiting is one of the most common complications. In recent years, Ondansetron was used to prevent postoperative nausea and vomiting in the aged in our hospital. Method: 138 selected aged patients (Male 66, Female, 72) 60-88 years old. 87 middle upper abdominal operations and 51 lower abdominal operations. ASA II-III. Laboratory studies showed that electrolyte, liver and kidney function were in the normal range. The patients were divided into two groups (70 cases in treatment group, 68 cases in control group) at random. Meperdine 0.5-1mg/kg+midazolam 0.05-0.08mg/kg were for premedication. No anti-emesis drugs were given before the operation. According to operation position, the puncture site at spinal segment was decided. The epidural catheter was inserted into the epidural space. Vital signs were monitored using the Detex AS3 Monitor. Then, the intravenous line was established. The local anesthesia was a mixture of 2% lidocaine 20ml and 1% decain, 5ml. When satisfactory anesthesia levels appeared, the operation began. In the treatment group, intravenous 8mg ondansetron was given to the patient about 30 minutes before the operation ended. Result: In the treatment group, nausea 11.4%, vomiting 7.1% was significantly lower than nausea 27.9%, vomiting 25% in the control group ($p<0.01$). There were no significant changes between these two groups in blood pressure, pulse rate, and oximeter ($p>0.05$). Conclusion: Ondansetron could reduce the incidence of postoperative nausea and vomiting.

[7] Evaluation of a prescriber guideline to improve oral anticoagulant induction in elderly inpatients

M. Debray (Centre Hospitalier Universitaire, Grenoble, France), E. Pautas (Hôpital Charles Foix, Ivry-sur-Seine, France), J.L. Bosson (Centre Hospitalier Universitaire, Grenoble, France), V. Siguret (Hôpital Charles Foix, Ivry-sur-Seine, France)

Purpose: We conducted a prospective study to determine the effectiveness of introducing a prescriber guideline to improve initiation of oral anticoagulant treatments in a 800-bed geriatric hospital. Method: Elderly in-patients (age>70) initiating an oral anticoagulant with a targeted INR between 2 and 3, were recruited prospectively. The first period (May-October1999) was a baseline-phase without intervention. For the second period (November 1999-April 2000), a pocket-sized guideline was distributed to all prescribers during a medical meeting. This guideline included a validated loading-dose warfarin protocol and essential information relating to the anticoagulant management. The number of over-anticoagulation (INR>4) during the first month of treatment and the time to achieve maintenance dose were compared between the 2 periods using Kaplan-Meier curves and a log rank test. Results: 99 patients, mean age 85.1 + 6.8 years, entered the study, 34 during the first period and 65 during the second. All except two patients during the first period were treated with warfarin. Prescribers correctly followed the induction protocol in only 21 patients among the 65 patients of the second period. There were no statistical differences between the 2 periods regarding the number of over-anticoagulation and the time to achieve the maintenance dose. Conclusion: The distribution of a prescriber guideline was not followed by an improvement of quality in oral anticoagulant induction. Low adherence to the prescriber guideline was noticed. Other training intervention should probably be coupled to the guideline to make it effective.

[8] Emergency Department Access to a Computerized Prescription Database: Its Impact on Hospitalized Geriatric Patients

J. Menezes, S. Shalansky (St. Paul's Hospital, Vancouver, BC, Canada), S Kulkarni, T Ellchuk (Faculty of Medicine, University of British Columbia, Canada)

PURPOSE: To investigate the impact of computer access to the British Columbia prescription database (PharmaNet) on geriatric patients admitted to hospital through the emergency room (ER). METHODS: Drug-related problems (DRPs) related to medications taken prior to admission were identified for all patients over age 65 admitted during two 4 week data collection periods. In phase 1 PharmaNet was available only to ward pharmacists, and in phase 2 PharmaNet was available to pharmacists and ER physicians. DRPs were defined according to previously published criteria. RESULTS: Study patients' (phase 1, N=115; phase 2, N=151) age (77.3 years versus 77.8 years) and number of medications prior to admission (4.5 versus 5.0) were similar between the two phases, however length of stay was longer in phase 1 (13.3 days versus 9.2 days). When PharmaNet was utilized in either phase, there were significantly more DRPs identified per patient (0.82 +/- 1.16 versus 0.27 +/- 0.56, $p<0.001$). However, implementing PharmaNet in the ER had little impact on the proportion of patients for whom PharmaNet was utilized (47.8% versus 50.3%). ER physicians accessing PharmaNet for only 2.6% of phase 2 patients. As a result, there was no significant difference in the number of DRPs identified per patient between phase 1 and phase 2 (0.59 +/- 1.0 versus 0.50 +/- 0.9, p=0.42). CONCLUSION: While use of PharmaNet resulted in identification of significantly more DRPs, ER physicians rarely utilized the database. Consistent use could result in improved patient care through more thorough detection and resolution of DRPs.

[9] Young-Old and Old-Old Adults Rate and Recall of Medication Instructions

L. McDonald-Miszczak, M. Cantrell, C. Funkhouser, A. Schneider (Dept. of Psychology, Western Washington University, Bellingham, WA, USA), & G. Gutman (Gerontology Research

Centre, Simon Fraser University, Vancouver, BC, Canada).

Proper adherence is dependent on remembering medication instructions (Morrow et al, 1988). Using specific guidelines to improve medication instructions (Morrow et al, 1991), we compared 71young-old (57-74 yrs.) and 62 old-old (75-89 yrs.) participants' (a) perceptions of memorability of instructions, and (b) cued recall. A MANOVA of cued recall indicated old-old adults recalled less information about when and how to take the medication than young-old adults. Zero-order correlations revealed that of the 14 analyses assessing participants' expectations of recall accuracy, only 3 were significant. Findings indicate (a) old-old adults' adherence may be impacted by poor recall of medication information, and (b) participants' expectations of recalling instructions do not closely map their actual recall. Findings suggest that health care professionals should emphasize the difficulty of instructions and they may even improve old-old adults' adherence by stressing how and when to take medication.

[10] 12-month trial demonstrating the safety and efficacy of transdermal fentanyl (Durogesic) in chronic non-cancer pain

Keith Milligan (Department of Anaesthesia, South Cleveland Hospital, Middlesbrough, UK)

A 12-month, open-label study of 532 patients with chronic non-malignant pain requiring continuous opioid therapy has evaluated the long-term efficacy and safety of transdermal fentanyl (TDF), patient preference (compared with previous analgesic) and the effect of pain control on quality of life. TDF was initiated at an equianalgesic dose to pre-trial opioids and titrated to maintain acceptable pain control and adverse events. Mean patient age was 51 years (range 22–88 years), with 94 subjects (18%) classified as elderly (at least 65 years of age). The 12 month drop-out rate was 32 0n the elderly compared to 22 0n the under 65 age group, but logistic regression of individual variables showed that age (unlike those <50 kg) was not a predictive factor for drop-out. There was no significant age-related effect on fentanyl clearance rate ($p=0.0745$) and, overall, the nature and incidence of adverse events was similar in the elderly and young sub-populations. However, headaches and increased sweating were more common in younger patients while somnolence, anemia, bronchitis and depression occurred more frequently among the elderly. The incidence of adverse events remained stable during the trial. Severe nausea was more common in the elderly than the younger subgroup (14% and 8%, respectively) while severe increased sweating occurred more frequently in the younger than the elderly subgroup (8% and 2%, respectively). This trial showed that TDF is well-tolerated and effective in both elderly and younger populations.

[11] Clinical benefits and NSAIDS´USE before and after an education program in osteoarthritis pationts.

A. Uribe, A. Rosete, M.L. Garduño, (Gerontology, Rheumatology and Rehabilitation Medicine Departments. Hospital Central Norte, Petróleos Mexicanos D.F. México)

PURPOSE: To determine whether exercise and education provide a better clinical outcome and decrease drugs use in osteoarthritis patients. METHOD: We trained 264 patients, in an open, 4 weeks educative and rehabilitation program, the intervention was measured with WOMAC (Western Ontario and Mac Master Universities Osteoarthitis Index), visual analogue scales for pain and wellbeing, and Calderon´s depression scale. Their NSAID´S use was evaluated with a specific cuestionary and the patient´s diary (pain + drugs use). The assessments were applied at week 0 and 4. Data analysis: Descriptive methods, T-paired and Wilcoxon rank tests. RESULTS: We studied 244 women (20 men), mean age 69.4 + 7 years, there were significant changes in health status perceived by patients in all scales and a decrease in NSAIDS'USE, it represented 30%. Our data found that 56% used antacids or another antipeptic protection, 30% had continuos NSAID intake and in 60% of patients it was just in case of symptoms. Obesity represented a risk factor in 24% of our patients. CONCLUSION: Our program helped patients to get clinical benefits, but we have to focus attention on risks factors as NSAIDS'USE in people after 60 and obesity.

[12] Telephone follow-up by a pharmacist improves medication therapy in geriatric medicine clinic patients.

Debora Kwan, Shabbir Alibhai, Tina Papastavros, Armi Armesto (Toronto Rehabilitation Institute, Toronto, Canada)

PURPOSE: Mismanagement of medications by the elderly can lead to significant morbidity and mortality. The objectives of this study were 1) to identify drug-related problems (DRPs) that require follow-up; 2) to find out if new DRPs arise at the time of follow-up; 3) to determine what interventions occur as a result of providing follow-up. METHOD: New patients referred to a geriatric medicine clinic were seen by a geriatrician, pharmacist and nurse. DRPs requiring follow-up were identified and categorized as one of the following: unclear indication, additional drug required, non-adherence, adverse reaction, drug interaction or, inappropriate dosing/administration. The pharmacist carried out follow-up by telephone. RESULTS: A total of 161 DRPs were identified in 33 patients (52 0.000000emale, mean age=79.6 years), over 12 months. The most frequent DRPs were adverse reactions (35.4%), non-adherence (29.1%) and inappropriate dosing/administration (21.7%). At the time of telephone follow-up, 103 additional DRPs were identified; most commonly non-adherence (27.2%), adverse reactions (22.3%) and one additional category: patient unclear about medication regimen (20.4%). There were 101 interventions, 2/3 of which were carried out by the pharmacist over the telephone and included medication education (40.0%) and dosing regimen modifications, e.g. timing, compliance aids (21.0%). New prescriptions constituted 130f interventions. Newly identified DRPs required further investigation or earlier clinic follow-up visits in 5 patients.CONCLUSION: Telephone follow-up is a convenient and feasible mechanism to detect and manage DRPs outside of scheduled patient visits. Provision of medication education to prevent non-adherence and manage adverse effects may contribute towards optimizing patient outcomes.

[13] Comparison of therapeutic effect between continuous and intermittent epidural injection in low back pain patients

Mi Jung Kim, Ki Seob Choi, Si bok Park, Sang Gun Lee(Dept. of rehabilitation Medicine, Hanyang University Hospital, Seoul, Korea)

Purpose: To compare the therapeutic effect between continuous epidural injection(EI) with catheter and intermittent EI without catheter in low back pain patients Method: 109 Patients with low back pain were randomly divided into two groups. First group(49 patients) were treated with 2 or 3 times of intermittent EI with steroid mixed with local anesthetics. Second group(60 patients) were treated with continuous EI with the same drug through catheter. The effect of EI was assessed by visual analogue scale(VAS) score at pre- and post-injection. Results: Pre-and Post-injection VAS scores of the first group were 6.5 ± 1.2 and 3.5 ± 1.5, respectively. Pre- and Post-injection VAS scores of the second group were 6.2 ± 1.6 and 2.3 ± 1.1, respectively. VAS score changes between pre- and post-injection were significant in both groups($p<0.01$). VAS score changes between two groups were greater in the second group($p<0.01$). The more severe the disc herniation(protrusion and extrusion) in MRI, the more marked VAS score changes in the second group. When morbidity period was less than one year, the VAS score changes in the second group were greater($p<0.05$). Conclusion: The therapeutic effect of catheter inserted continuous epidural injection is better than that of intermittent epidural injection in patients with low back pain.

[14] Prognostication of the needs in drugs for elderly people

V.V. Bezrukov, L.P. Kuprash, Yu.A. Grinenko, V.V. Chaikovska, L.P. Snigur (Institute of Gerontology, Kiev, Ukraine)

This work aimed to develop a methodology enabling to prognosticate the needs in drugs for treating deseases, which are commonly found in older people. Methods: sociological, pharmacological and mathematical. In developing such a methodology, we used the responses to a questionnaire, being provided by 7,500 patients in 14 geriatric units at the regional hospitals, to create a morbidity database. Having analyzed the data on morbidity and drug consumption among study subjects, we formed the clinico-statistical groups of patients. For each group, the drug standards and medicinal formulations were developed according to the geriatric pharmacology principles, with an account being taken of the efficacy and safety of drugs as well as the results of pharmaco-economical analysis. In conclusion, we've got a methodology enabling to prognosticate the needs in drugs for elderly in-hospital patients, thus ensuring efficacy of treatment and reducing costs of therapy.

[15] Ethnic Differences in Elders' Abilities to Obtain Prescription Medication

T.F. Borders (Department of Health Services Research and Management, Texas Tech University Health Sciences Center, Lubbock, Texas, USA)

PURPOSE: The health care needs Mexican-American elders have not been well studied. Of particular interest among health policy makers in the United States is whether elders have problems obtaining prescription medications. The purpose of this study was to determine 1) the percentage of elderly persons who report problems obtaining prescription drugs and 2) if Hispanic elders are more or less likely to have problems obtaining prescription medication than non-Hispanic whites. METHOD: The study is based on preliminary data from the Texas Tech 5000 (TT5000), a random telephone survey of 5,000 persons age 65 and older residing in Texas, an area with a relatively high percentage of Mexican-Americans. Andersen and Aday's behavioral model was used to determine the impact of health system, predisposing, enabling, and need factors. RESULTS: Only 17 percent of respondents reported having a problem obtaining prescription medication in the past 6 months. Hispanic elders, persons age 81 and over, employed persons, and individuals who had a lifetime incidence of myocardial infarction were less likely to have problems obtaining medication. Individuals with a lifetime incidence of coronary heart disease were more likely to have problems obtaining medication. CONCLUSION: In contrast to popular belief, the vast majority of elderly persons may not have problems getting medications when they need them. Population subgroups which are thought to be at the highest risk for not obtaining prescription medications, including the oldest old and Hispanics, may already have insurance coverage and other resources which enable them to obtain prescriptions drugs when they need them.

[16] Inappropriate Prescribing in Long Term Care Facilities: Prevalence and Associated Factors

M.J. Borrie (Division of Geriatric Medicine, South western Ontario Regional Geriatric Program, University of Western Ontario, Lawson Health Research Institute, London, Canada) C.D. Brymer (Division of Geriatric Medicine, University of Western Ontario, Lawson Health Research Institute, London, Canada) R.G. Crilly (Division of Geriatric Medicine, University of Western Ontario, Lawson Health Research Institute, London, Canada) D. Hindman (Shoppers Drug Mart, Toronto, Canada) R. Pavlakovic (Shoppers Drug Mart, Toronto, Canada) J. Esbaugh (Southwestern Ontario Regional Geriatric Program, London, Canada) P. Stolee (South western Ontario Regional Geriatric Program, University of Western Ontario, Lawson Health Research Institute, London Ontario Canada).

Purpose: The purpose of this study was to determine the prevalence of specific inappropriate prescribing (IP), using published Canadian criteria on prescribing long-acting benzodiazepines, anticholinergics, non-steroidal anti-inflammatories and tricyclic antidepressants in long term care (LTC) facilities in Ontario, Canada. A secondary aim was to determine physician-, pharmacist-, and facility-related factors associated with inappropriate prescribing. Methods: The Ontario Shoppers Drug Mart LTC facility database and additional characteristics, including physician and facility demographics, and consultant pharmacist time, were blinded and analyzed. Results: The analysis included 12,424 residents (age = 84.2 ± 7.6 years: 75.8% female) and 169 facilities. The total mean number of regular and PRN prescriptions was 9.0 ± 4.8 per resident. Of the residents, 13.6% were on at least one inappropriate medication studied; 2.7% were on a long-acting benzodiazepine, 2.0% on anticholinergics, 2.4% on non-steroidal anti-inflammatories without cytoprotection and 7.1% on tricyclic antidepressants. Regression analyses controlling for clustering effects suggest resident age, number of regular medications, and lack of physician CCFP certification are associated with IP ($p<.05$). Conclusions: Inappropriate prescribing in LTC facilities is relatively low. Clinical and resident characteristics not included in this analysis would likely increase explained variance in IP, but the results suggest potential for interventions aimed at physician and facility factors.

[17] Social marketing campaign to improve the quality of medication use among seniors

Karen Bell Farris (The University of Iowa, Iowa City, Iowa, USA Sheri Laine Maddigan (The University of Iowa, Iowa City, Iowa, USA) Sherry Dieleman (The University of Alberta, Edmonton, Alberta, Canada) Sarah Barber (The University of Alberta, Edmonton, Alberta, Canada) Cheryl Cox (The University of Alberta, Edmonton, Alberta, Canada) Jasneet Parmar (Northern Alberta Regional Geriatric Program, Edmonton, Alberta, Canada) Darryl Rolfson (The University of Alberta, Edmonton, Alberta, Canada)

Purpose: The purpose of this social marketing initiative was to (1) seniors and health professionals' awareness of the availability and need for structured medication reviews (SMR's) and (2) encourage action by target groups. Method: Non-equivalent control groups were used to assess the impact of the initiative in three study groups. Group 1 received the seniors' and health professionals' campaign; Group 2 received the health professionals' campaign only; Group 3 received no social marketing campaign. The seniors' campaign was comprised of self-screening forms, brochures, tabletop displays and presentations by seniors. The health professionals' campaign was focused on a toolkit for family physicians, community pharmacies and home care offices. A random sample of 900 seniors and 2600 health professionals were surveyed before and after the social marketing campaign. Results: The health professionals' response rate was 27%. Overall, 32.40f health professionals in Groups 1 and 2 reported that they received a toolkit and of those who received a toolkit, 54.4% reported that it helped to reduce the barriers to performing SMR's. At the post-intervention survey, health professionals who had received the social marketing campaign were more likely to have heard of an SMR; however, there was no difference in the likelihood of having performed an SMR or agreeing that it was feasible to incorporate SMR's into practice. Results from the seniors' survey will be available February 2001. Conclusion: While the social marketing campaign appeared to increase awareness of SMR's, it did not change the proportion of health professionals who performed SMR's.

[18] Medication Management Capacity and Adverse Drug Reactions in the Elderly with Cognitive Dysfunction

M. Akishita, K. Toba (Kyorin University, Tokyo, Japan), K. Nagano, N. Sudoh, Y. Ouchi (University of Tokyo, Tokyo, Japan)

We aimed at investigating whether the increased number of prescribed drugs and impaired medication management capacity would lead to the increase in adverse drug reactions (ADR) in the elderly. We conducted the database analysis of the patients (n=517) who were admitted to the acute geriatric ward of the University of Tokyo Hospital from 1995 through 1998. Of the patients, the information on ADR was obtained in 95% (n=490, 69±0.6 years old). The incidence of ADR was totally 12.7% and increased after 75 years of age. The incidence of ADR correlated with the number of prescribed drugs; ADR were found in <100f the patients who were taking <5 drugs, and in >150f the patients who were taking >5 drugs. Then, the relationship between medication management capacity and ADR was analyzed. Medication management capacity was assessed by instrumental ADL of Lawton & Brody; independent, assistance or dependent. As expected, impairment of medication management capacity was associated with the disturbance of ADL, as measured by Barthel Index, and with cognitive dysfunction, as measured by Hasegawa dementia scale-revised. The dependent group, however, showed a lower incidence of ADR with taking a smaller number of drugs than the assistance group. These results suggest that the increase in the number of prescribed drugs may lead to the increase in ADR, and that restriction of the number of drugs may prevent ADR in patients with cognitive dysfunction and thus with low medication management capacity.

[19] HIV Risk Behavior Profiles: Cohort Specific Differences Among Two Baby Boomer Cohorts of Substance Abusers

Marlies Schoeneberger, (University of Kentucky, Center on Drug & Alcohol Research, Lexington, Kentucky, U.S.A.)

While overall HIV infection rates have delcined consistently since the mid-1990s, they have increased steadily within the older adult population (CDC, 1999, NIH, 1994). The reported HIV and AIDS cases in the older populatin are considered very conservative and probably do not reflect a realistic picture of the extent of the HIV/AIDS epidemic in this population (Mack, & Bland, 1999; Stall, & Catania, 1994). It is being hypothesized that ageist stereotypes are to blame for the fact that older adults do not get tested routinely for HIV (Catania, et al, 1992; Stall, & Catania, 1994). PURPOSE: The purpose of this study was twofold: (1) to expose ageist stereotypes, and (2) to develop cohort specific HIV risk behavior profiles. METHOD: The study sample (N=20,987) was drawn from out-of-treatment substance abusers recruited into the NIDA Cooperative Agreement Project between 1990 and 1998 (N=27,882). The average age of subjects was 38 years, ranging from age 34 to age 52. More than two thirds were male (68%), African American (67%), and more than half had at least a high school education (62%). Two parallel analyses were conducted comparing two cohorts of male and female Baby Boomers. RESULTS: Results indicate that ageist stereotypes germane to substance abuse and sexual risk behaviors prevail and negatively impact drug use and related sexual behaviors in this population of older adult out-of-treatment drug users. Cohort specific HIV risk behavior profiles have been developed suggesting that certain demographic as well as behavioral characteristics either facilitate or deter HIV risk behaviors.

[20] Medication prescription in the elderly, on a survey in the North-East region of France

Durant R, Boulenger-Morel M, Blain H, Ferry JC, Jeandel C (Antonin Balmes Gerontology Center Montpellier, France)

PURPOSE: The study's aim is to evaluate polymedication frequency, to classify and quantify types of medication according to age, sex, and to appreciate seasonal factors on prescriptions for the elderly. METHOD: 4409 prescriptions in July 1998 (717 men, 1244 women) and 4400 prescriptions in January 1999 (772 men, 1335 women), chosen at random, amongst non hospitalised subjects over 60 years old affiliated to the French North-Eastern social security organism have been included in the study. Prescriptions have been analysed according to the international medication classification codes, and classified according to the anatomical therapeutical and chemical method. RESULT: number of prescription in July and January are comparable, but the number of lines is more important in the winter month (3,51 + 2,3 vs 3,43 + 2,3, p< 0,001). 630f the prescriptions are for women and their average number of lines is more important than men's (3,54 vs 3,24 in July, p<0,01 ; 3,59 vs 3,35 in January, p<0,01). Independently of age, sex and month, the most prescribed medications are in order: cardio-vascular system (35%), the central nervous system (15%), digestive and endocrine metabolism systems (14,5%). Prescriptions for the respiratory system are more important in January than in July (9,4 % vs 6,1%, p<0,01). CONCLUSION: Women consume more medication than men. The most prescribed medication is cardiovascular. The difference in prescription between the two months only exists for the respiratory system, January superior than July.

[21] Elderly Patients Attitude to the use of Loop Diuretics for the Treatment of Heart Failure

Rees, S, Thomas, P, Makinde, K, Olivan-Martinez, C, Baines, P. (Prince Philip Hospital, Llanelli, United Kingdom)

PURPOSE: To establish the views of elderly patients on information relating to their treatment with diuretics in heart failure. METHOD: Qualitative study, prospective semi-structured interviews of 70 elderly patients with heart failure recruited from Medical Wards, Day Care Unit and Outpatient clinics of a District Hospital. Main outcome measures were qualitative patient responses, patient knowledge base and self reported adherence. RESULTS: Male:Female 1:1 Median Age: 78 years Only 35% of patients knew they were taking diuretics for heart failure. 12% thought the diuretics were for urinary symptoms 33% thought they were for other reasons e.g. swollen ankles 36% were unsure or felt that the diuretic did not improve symptoms 53% were unsure or felt that stopping the diuretics would not be harmful Only 26% of patients felt they would like to receive more information Of the 70 patients interviewed :- 55% would go to their family physician for information 15% would approach their Pharmacist 12% would refer to the information leaflet 15% would ask the Hospital Physician and None would access the Internet. (some patients indicated more than one source) CONCLUSION: Elderly patients receiving diuretics for heart failure have an information deficit in relation to the indication for treatment. This is reinforced by the attitude to discontinuing treatment. There is a lack of interest in further information. However, the Family Physician has a key role in improving the knowledge base.

[22] Views of Elderly Patients Towards the Long Term use of Diuretic Therapy for Heart Failure

Rees, S, Thomas, P, Makinde, K, Olivan-Martinez, C, Baines, P. (Prince Philip Hospital, Llanelli, United Kingdom)

PURPOSE: To assess the relationship between patients views on loop diuretic therapy (for management of heart failure) and their adherence with their medication. METHOD: Qualitative study, prospective semi-structured interviews of 70 elderly patients with heart failure recruited from Medical Wards, Day Care Unit and Outpatient clinics of a District Hospital. Main outcome measures were qualitative patient responses, patient knowledge base and self reported adherence. RESULTS: 56% felt that stopping the medication would be harmful. Only 26% felt that knowing how the medication worked made them more likely to be compliant. 70% were indifferent. Only 2% felt that knowledge relating to mechanism of action made them less anxious. 90% were indifferent. Increased knowledge of the side effects made only: 3% more likely to be compliant. 65% were indifferent. Increased knowledge of the side effects made only: 3% more anxious. 60% were indifferent. 85% would not consider stopping the medication without consulting their Doctor but 9% would. 74% would not like to receive any more information regarding their medication. Conclusion: There appears to be a considerable degree of apathy amongst this group of patients regarding their medication. However, the patients appear to be highly compliant and very responsive to the advice of medical staff.

[23] Long term complications of anti-epileptics

Y.VASCHALDE, D.VASCHALDE** (*Service de Neurologie, ** Service de Gériatrie, Groupe Hospitalier du Havre, BP 24, 76083 LE HAVRE, FRANCE)*

Objectives and method : We report and discuss a clinical case of late complications of an anti-epileptic treatment in a sixty-nine years old man. Case description : A recently retired man suffering from a pharmaco-resistant cryptogenic epilepsia since childhood consults for a cerebellar syndrom and clinicaly confirmed cognitive impairment. The blood level of anti-epileptic drugs (phenytoin and phenobarbital) remained within the usual therapeutic margin. The patient's reluctance to change his treatment, wich has been the same since he entered his professional life, was difficult to fight. Five months after the replacement of phenytoin by carbamazepin, he realizes an improvement of his balance without worsening of his epilepsia. The persistance of a memory complain along with the worsening of former erection disorders make him accept the reduction of the dose of phenobarbital, and two years later interruption of the drug's prescription. Five years after the initial consultation he is put under a bi-therapy with gabapentin and carbamazepin. This treatment resoring his previous level of control of the epilepsia and the complete diseappearance of the cerebellar syndrom and memory disorder. Conclusion : We discuss the iatrogenic risks of antiepileptics in ages people and the insufficient diffusion of the knowledge aquired on aging of the epileptic in that particular population. Consequences are the risk of inappropriate treatment or a treatment difficult to accept. The pre-retirement period and the beginning of the third age appears to be the best moment to discuss those issues with the patients and anticipate, when possible, the potential complications.

[24] Use of inappropriate drugs in home dwelling elderly - a population-based survey

K.H. Pitkala, T.E. Strandberg, R.S. Tilvis, (Helsinki University Hospital, Department of Medicine, Geriatric Clinic)

Purpose was to investige the proportion of home-dwelling elderly using inappropriate medication according to explicit criteria developed by experts in United States through a modified Delphi consensus technique in 1997. In addition, drugs considered inappropriate related to certain medical conditions by same panel were analyzed in this population. A cross-sectional population based survey was made to a random sample of elderly living in Helsinki City area (N=3219, age groups 75-, 80-, 85-, 90- and 95-years of age retrieved from population register). Response rate of home-dwelling elderly was 78%. Altogether 11.3% of the home-dwelling elderly were using at least one innappropriate drug. 1.8% were on two innappropriate drugs and 0.2% were on three inappropriate drugs. The most commonly used contraindicated drugs were long-acting benzodiazepines (3.3%), dipyridamole (3.3%), amitriptyline (1.6%), ergot mesyloids (1.4%) and meprobamate (1.1%). Use of medications considered inappropriate related to certain medical conditions was high: 27.2% of COPD patients were on beta-blockers and additional 20.6% of them on sedatives. 25.4% of diabetics on oral hypoglycemics or on insulin had a concomitant beta-blocker. 37.9% of those with peripheral vascular disease had a beta-blocker. However, over 70% of all these patient groups had a comorbidity of coronary heart disease. Compared to previous surveys the usage of inappropriate medications in Finnish elderly population was considerably lower. Use of certain drugs considered inappropriate related to certain medical conditions was very high, though. However, contrary to the explicit criteria the use of some contraindicated medications may be justified when applying evidence to individual patients.

[25] Nutritional status among fifty elderly patients gone into a geriatric follow up and rehabilitation unit

F. Delahaye, Y. Grumbach (Gerontology Unit,University Hospital Center, Amiens, France)

Proteino-energetic malnutrition concerns more than thirty percents of hospitalized elderly. Sometimes very severe, her consequences worsen the prognosis, even if given a nutritional supplementation. We wanted to assess nutritional status among fifty elderly patients gone into a geriatric follow up and rehabilitation unit. Our tools have been the Mini Nutritional Assessment, the weight, the height, the body mass index and laboratory tests (albuminaemia, transthyrétin, C-reactive protein). 88% of our patients had a proteino-energetic malnutrition with hypoalbuminaemia. Our results confimed this fact under-estimated and seldom detected by non-geriatricians, and worsened by hospitalization.

[26] Orosomucoid : a mortality risk factor in elderly people living in the community?

A. Raynaud-Simon (Hôpital Charles Foix, Ivry sur Seine, France), S. Lafont (INSERM U 330, Bordeaux, France), J.F. Dartigues (INSERM U 330, Bordeaux, France), C. Berr (INSERM U 360, Paris, France), Y. Le Bouc (INSERM U 515, Paris, France).

PURPOSE We sought to explore the value of plasma orosomucoid, C-reactive protein (CRP), albumin and transthyretin concentrations and body mass index as prognostic factors for mortality in a general population of elderly subjects. SUBJECTS We studied 245 subjects aged 65 to 95 (mean age 75.9 ± 7.0 years) included in the PAQUID research program, a prospective cohort study of aging in elderly subjects residing in south-western France. METHODS BMI and albumin, transthyretin, CRP and orosomucoid plasma concentrations were determined at baseline. Mortality data were available for 6 years. Univariate and multivariate analysis of the risk of death was performed 2, 4, and 6 years after blood sampling using the Cox proportional hazards model. The most accurate threshold for prediction of death was determined by the Akaike criterion. RESULTS In multivariate analysis of nutritional and inflammatory parameters by quartiles, plasma orosomucoid concentrations in the highest quartile was the marker that was most strongly associated with mortality. An orosomucoid concentration of 1g/L was the most accurate threshold for prediction of mortality (RR = 12.8 after 2 years, 95% confidence interval 4.2 Δ 39.4 ; p< 0.001). CONCLUSION Orosomucoid concentrations above 1 g/L are strongly associated with the risk of death, independently from nutritional markers ; this may help identification of high-risk subjects for preventive interventions.

[27] Change in Circadian Eating Patterns in Nursing Home Residents with Alzheimer Disease

K.W.H. Young and C.E. Greenwood (Department of Nutritional Sciences, Faculty of Medicine, University of Toronto, Toronto, Canada and Kunin-Lunenfeld Applied Research Unit and Department of Food and Nutrition Services, Baycrest Centre for Geriatric Care, North York, Canada)

PURPOSE: Seniors with Alzheimer disease (AD) are susceptible to weight loss and malnutrition, which have not been associated with decreased food intake, to date. This study examined food intake patterns and how they change in relation to body mass index (BMI), behavioural function, and cognitive status in institutionalized seniors with AD. METHOD: 21 consecutive days of investigator-weighed food intake collections were conducted on 25 subjects (3 men, 22 women; age=85.9±7.6 yrs) with likely AD at a home for the aged, and the ability to self-feed. The Mini-Mental State Examination and London Psychogeriatric Rating Scale were administered to assess cognitive and behavioural function, respectively. RESULTS: Targeted energy needs were not met by 880f subjects, including an estimated 370revalence of protein inadequacy. Subjects with increased behavioural difficulties had reduced meal-related intakes that were associated with decreased energy intake at dinner. With increasing behavioural difficulties there was a shift in circadian eating patterns such that the greatest proportion of daily energy was consumed at breakfast. Individuals with low BMIs tended to be those with more behavioural difficulties, such that BMI also associated with the shift in overall eating patterns. CONCLUSION: These results suggest that increases in behavioural difficulties in seniors with AD result in a circadian shift in eating patterns, with peak energy consumption occurring at breakfast. This shift in eating patterns associates both with poor overall intake and poor BMI. (PFS & CIHR)

[28] Meal Delivery Practices Are Not Appropriate for Alzheimer Patients with Increased Cognitive and Behavioural Difficulties

C.E. Greenwood and K.W.H. Young (Department of Nutritional Sciences, Faculty of Medicine, University of Toronto, Toronto, Canada and Kunin-Lunenfeld Applied Research Unit and Department of Food and Nutrition Services, Baycrest Centre for Geriatric Care, North York, Canada)

PURPOSE: Shifts in circadian rhythms and increased behavioural difficulties alter meal consumption patterns in seniors with Alzheimer disease (AD). Despite these known changes, the profile of meals provided in long-term-care (LTC) parallel the needs of younger, free-living, healthy adults. This study examined the impact of food delivery patterns on achieved intake in LTC residents with AD and how this relationship changed depending on time of day, body mass index (BMI), behavioural function, and cognitive ability. METHOD: Food delivery and intake data (21 consecutive days; investigator-weighed) were collected on 25 seniors (3 men, 22 women; age=85.9±7.6 yrs) with likely AD. RESULTS: Overall, energy consumed was positively associated with energy delivered for the majority of subjects. However, energy delivered had the greatest impact on intake at breakfast and the least impact at dinner in those with the most behavioural difficulties and cognitive impairment. Although those with low BMIs were likely to be delivered more energy, the impact of delivery on intakes decreased as energy delivered increased. CONCLUSION: These data suggest that delivering excess food to those with poor BMIs likely does not result in increased consumption. Further, behavioural and cognitive deterioration lead to a shift in the time of day that energy delivered has an impact on energy consumption, with the most progressed individuals being most impacted by foods delivered in the morning, suggesting that traditional meal practices are inappropriate for institutionalized seniors with AD. (PFS & CIHR)

[29] Afternoon snacks are least beneficial to institutionalized seniors with Alzheimer disease at risk for under-nutrition

K.W.H. Young and C.E. Greenwood (Department of Nutritional Sciences, Faculty of Medicine, University of Toronto, Toronto, Canada and Kunin-Lunenfeld Applied Research Unit and Department of Food and Nutrition Services, Baycrest Centre for Geriatric Care, North York, Canada)

PURPOSE: Despite the lack of objective evidence, concerns are often expressed that afternoon snacks interfere with dinner intake in long-term care residents. This study explored the impact of eating an afternoon snack on dinner and total 24-hr intakes in seniors with likely Alzheimer disease and its relationship with body mass index (BMI), cognitive ability, and behavioural function. METHOD: Analyses were conducted on 21 consecutive days of investigator-weighed food intake in 19 women (age 86.4±7.7 yrs) who ate at least 7 snacks (1/3 of days) during the study period. RESULTS: Overall, dinner intakes were not lower ($p=0.56$) on days that snacks were consumed compared to days when no snacks were eaten, allowing for greater total 24-hr energy intakes ($p<0.01$). However, snack intake was least effective in boosting 24-hr intakes in subjects with greater cognitive impairment ($p=0.02$, $r2=0.27$) and behavioural difficulties ($p=0.04$, $r2=0.23$). Indeed, subjects with low BMIs were more likely to reduce dinner intake following snack consumption ($p=0.06$, $r2=0.19$), perhaps reflecting the fact that these individuals were given more calories at their afternoon snack. CONCLUSION: Since residents with greater cognitive impairment, behavioural difficulties and low BMIs are at greater risk for under-nutrition, these data suggest that the target group for intervention benefits the least from afternoon snack consumption and are consistent with the fact that these residents show shifts in their circadian eating patterns and are unresponsive to foods provided later in the day. (PFS & CIHR)

[30] Study on effect of medicated diet on chronic diseases in aged people

Zhang Dongshi Cao Yulin (Liaoning College of Traditional Chinese Medicine Shenyang City 110032 P.R. China)

The paper puts forth a new scientific conception of a "nutritiously medicated diet" for chronic diseases and difficulty in the recovery for the aged people. It is an important topic to delay aging process and keep healthy for the old people. The paper has studied the effect of the medicated diet on chronic diseases of the old patients by investigating some cases and basing on the theory of traditional medicated diet combined with modern nutriology, medicine and cooking technology. The nutritiously medicated diet is prepared through the combination of the method of traditional medicated diet with the technique of modern nutriology and medicine. The prescription is made up perfectly and it is processing carefully and scientifically. And the effects have been scientifically evaluated with a good reliability. The result has widened the category of researching further the nutritiously medicated diet in carrying on the essence of traditional medicated diet in China. It is also helpful to make the unique medicated diet spread worldwide serving for the health of the people all over the world.

[31] Prevalence and hematological effects of low serum vitamin B12 levels in geriatric out patients.

T. Vogel, C. Martin-Hunyadi, G. Kaltenbach, D. Heitz, M. Kiesmann, M. Berthel, Kuntzmann (Center of Gerontology, University Hospital of Strasbourg, France)

Prevalence of cobalamin deficiency is higher in old people. However the plasmatic threshold of the deficiency is badly defined and hematological disturbances usually associated are inconstant in this population. The purpose of this retrospective study realized in a geriatric day hospital is to appreciate the hematological repercussions of cobalamin deficiency according to 3 threshold of cobalamin plasmatic level. 460 patients without folate deficiency are involved and are divided into 4 groups: group1 ($n=44$): plasmatic cobalamin <150pg/ml; group 2 ($n=67$): plasmatic cobalamin between 150 and 250 pg/ml; group 3 ($n=62$) plasmatic cobalamin between 200 et 250 pg/ml; group 4 ($n=287$) is the reference group with a cobalamin plasmatic level over 250 pg/ml. Age, weight, sex and way of life don't differ in the 4 groups. Plasmatic folate level is increased and red cell folate concentration is lowered in the group 1 compared to group 4 ($p<0.05$) which illustrated the classic "folate trap". Count of platelets, leukocytes and lymphocytes and the hemoglobin rate don't differ in the 4 groups. The mean corpuscular volume is higher in the group 1 (92,5fl) than in group 4 (91,6 fl) ($p<0.05$) without any difference observed between groups 2, 3 and 4. In this study the amplitude of hematological anomalies is low and only observed if the choice of plasmatic cobalamin threshold deficiency is below 150 pg/ml. These findings are in contradiction with some other results which suggest that metabolical (hyperhomocysteinemia) and hematological (medullar megaloblastosis) repercussions could be observed with subnormal plasmatic level of cobalamin.

[32] The problem of age retarding diets optimisation

N.Potemkina, V. Kroutko, A.Dgigarev (National Gerontology Center, Moscow, Russia)

Modern gerontology considers a caloric-restricted but complete well balanced diet as being one of the most effective means of prolonging healthy and active life. The complexities of individual diet selection, and the difficulties of changing individual nutritional habits are the main problems here. We are now creating a method and computerized technology for the: 1 - development of nutritional rations, furthering maximum healthy active life spans, based on individual psychophysiological features and significant indices of personal health and ecological conditions; 2 - determination of the easiest and most rapid way for changing over to a new nutritional system, and providing psychological support during the person adaptation period. The technology is based on decision support system (DSS) "Geroprotecting Nutrition". This system includes some data and knowledge bases: "Chemical Composition of Foodstuffs", "Properties of Nutritional Components", "Food Pollution", "Food Components Consumption Norms", and "Recommendations for Healthy Diets". Diet is selected with the help of an optimization procedure. DSS "Geroprotecting Nutrition" was used for comparative analysis of nutrition for various groups of people: 1 - Swedish tourists from boarding houses on Koster Island; 2 - Moscovites with high incomes, who have some knowledge of healthy nutrition principles; 3 - Moscovites with low incomes, who do not think about healthy nutrition; 4 - Moscovites with low incomes , who follow healthy nutrition principles.

[33] Nutrition and Bone Tissue Functional State in Postmenopausal Women

V. V. Povoroznjuk, N. V. Grygoreva (Department of Clinical Physiology and Pathology of Locomotor Apparatus, Institute of Gerontology AMS Ukraine, Kiev, Ukraine).

There has been increasing evidence that balanced diet and maintained optimal status significantly reduce morbidity and mortality. High calcium intake prevents bone loss and osteoporotic fractures in postmenopausal women although the association is less obvious in the first years after menopause. Influence of diet on bone tissue functional state was investigated in 247 persons. Bone tissue functional state was determined by ultrasound densitometry (◊-osteoporosis, ◊◊-osteopenia, ◊◊◊-normal bone tissue). The diet of Ukrainian postmenopausal women is characterized by a reduced intake of proteins, especially animal; fats, especially vegetable; vitamins, main mineral macro- and microelements. The intake of main mineral element, necessary for bone turnover - calcium - is lower than reccomended. Results for main nutrients are presented in the table. Age Gr n Ca (mg/d) Mg (mg/d) P (mg/d) Vitamin D (mcg/d) 50-69 years ◊ 54 476,173,5 283,918,5 891,961,8 0.720,18 ◊◊ 40 471,337,01 287,618,8 863,961,77 0,440,07 ◊◊◊ 43 373,942,9 290,538,6 768,444,51 0,360,09 70 and more ◊ 63 486,236,77 264,010,1 865,738,78 0,380,07 ◊◊ 40 431,623,09 290,817,0 834,530,21 0,420,05 ◊◊◊ 47 439,384,83 273,925,8 876,478,41 0,360,08 It is evident that all elements essential for the bone are below the recommended values. It is advised that the diet must be rich in proteins, calcium and vitamin D

[34] Obesity in elderly people;its influence upon the nutritional status

Manuela Udrea (St.Luca Chronic Diseases and Geriatrics Hospital, Bucharest) Roman Speranta Babeanu (Centre of Diagnosis and Therapy Bucharest,Romania) Silvia Galaftion (Natl.Institute of Gerontology and Geriatrics Anna Aslan Bucharest,Romania)

Purpose:The nutritional assessment in a sample of people over 45 years old with obesity. Method: The study was performed on a sample of 340patients (89% women)dominating the age group of 70 to 79years old. The studied parameters comprised: BMI, mobility and physical activity, dietary inquiry, risk factors (dislypoproteinemia, BP, menopause age) social status, chronic diseases, immune status (peripheral lymphocytes, immunoglobulins, IDR to 4 anamnestic antigens). Statistic analysis included the symmetric paraeter. Results: Obesity dominated in the studied sample in the workers and less in intellectuals and among farmers. The sedentary life dominated among the obese persons As well as among those with unbalanced diets. As diseases prevailed the chronic degenerative rheumatism and atherosclerosis 37.5% of the subjects accumulating 6 concomittant diseases.. The analysis by symmetric parameter proves a significant correlation for the associations of obesity with one or two risk factors.The immunological indices studied did not show any differences compared with the rest of normoponderal people. Conclusion: The early diagnosis of the obesity and its association with any risk factors suggesting the necessity of its prevention sometimes very difficult to obtain in the elderly

[35] Vitamin C Deficiency In Hospitalized Old Patients : Prevalence And Signification

G. Sost, C. Jeanneau, C. Cattenoz, O. Petzaris, A. Le Treut, P. Jouanny (University Hospital Rennes, France)

PURPOSE: Recent data showed that scurvy occured in case of denutrition (cancer, restrictive regimen, chronic digestive trouble...). Denutrition is frequent in geriatric care. METHOD: We performed this deficiency survey in 72 old patients [67 to 101 years] consecutively hospitalized in an acute geriatric care unit. Vitamin C level in serum was measured in all patients and intraleucocyte level in half randomized patients. Clinical data, cognitive impairment, disability, nutritional status and various nutriments (vitamin D, folates, zinc, iron and calcium) were appreciated. RESULTS: 68 Of the patients were severily deficient in vitamin C (<3.5 mg/ml) et 22 % mildly deficient (3.5 to 6 mg/ml). 67 % had denutrition. No correlation between vitamin C and nutritional levels was observed. Serum vitamin C strongly correlated with zinc (p=0.0019), an other anti-oxydatant agent, suggesting that vitamin C could be rather an oxydation than a nutritional marker. No correlation was found between vitamin C level and degenerative pathologies (cardiovascular diseases, cataracte, cancers), disability, cognitive functions or clinical data, perhaps due to old age and bad general condition of population studied. Intraleucocyte vitamin C was correlated with folates (p=0.04), those two are given by fruit and vegetable. CONCLUSION: Vitamin C deficiency appears independant from denutrition but correlated with zinc and folates deficiency. One can ask if in case of exogen deficit, oxydative stress could facilitate the occurrence of deficiency secondary to increasing anti-oxydant needs. This study points out the frequency of vitamin C deficiency in hospitalized old patients, that is not observed in healthy old people. Nutritional therapy is necessary in acute care but also in prevention through varied regimen.

[36] Hypovitaminosis D is Common and More Severe in Winter in Institutionalized Older People in Sydney

Sitoh YY (Institute of Bone and Joint Research, University of Sydney, Sydney, Australia) Zochling J (Institute of Bone and Joint Research, University of Sydney, Sydney, Australia) Lau TC (Institute of Bone and Joint Research, University of Sydney, Sydney, Australia) Schwartz JM (Institute of Bone and Joint Research, University of Sydney, Sydney, Australia) Brnabic JM (Institute of International Health, University of Sydney, Sydney, Australia) March L (Institute of Bone and Joint Research, University of Sydney, Sydney, Australia) Cameron ID (Royal Rehabilitation Centre, University of Sydney, Sydney, Australia) Cumming RG (Health Services Research Dept, University of Sydney, Sydney, Australia) Lord S (School of Community Medicine, University of New South Wales, Sydney, Australia) Sambrook P (Institute of Bone and Joint Research, University of Sydney, Sydney, Australia)

Purpose: Hypovitaminosis D predisposes to increased bone loss and is important in the elderly, who are at increased risk of falling and sustaining fragility fractures. We studied the vitamin-D status, and associated determinants, in institutionalized older persons in Northern Sydney. Methods: Serum 25-hydroxyvitamin D (25OHD) levels were measured in a cross-sectional study of consenting adults aged 64 and older as part of an ongoing trial examining fracture risk and epidemiology in the elderly. Results: From May 1999 to May 2000, 252 women and 134 men (mean ages 86.7 and 84.8) from a random sample of 11 hostels and 18 nursing homes in Northern Sydney (latitude 33°55'S) were studied. Hypovitaminosis D (25OHD levels < 28 nmol/l) was seen in 87.7% of the women and 68.7% of the men. Mean levels of 25OHD differed significantly (p<0.001) between sexes (men 24.5± 18.0 nmol/l, women 17.2 ± 12.0 nmol/l). 25OHD levels did not vary significantly with age in both sexes. Only 8.0% of the women and 3.0% of the men took vitamin D supplements. Other factors significantly associated with 25OHD levels in women included season (summer levels significantly higher) (p=0.003), Short Mini-Mental State Examination (SMMSE) scores (p=0.032), and ease of access to sunlit areas (p=0.005). There was a trend for vitamin D supplementation to be associated with 25OHD levels (p=0.085). After multiple regression analysis, season and SMMSE remained as significant predictors. For men, only season was significantly associated with 25OHD levels. Conclusion: Hypovitaminosis D is common in institutionalized older persons in Northern Sydney and is currently under-treated.

[37] PEG (Percutaneous Endoscopic Gastrostomy) Patients in Nursing Homes: Carers' Perspective

U. K. SINHA, M. PARRISH, S. RAHA and W. E. WILKINS (Department of Integrated Medicine, Princess of Wales Hospital, Coity Road, Bridgend, U.K.)

Purpose To explore the views of nursing home staff regarding the patients on PEG feeds and the need for a formal training in this area. Method Structured interview with staff of 8 nursing homes in Mid Glamorgan (U.K.) area that were involved in caring for the patients on PEG feeding. The specific issues raised were training provided, problems encountered and their ability to manage these problems and availability of specialist advice. Results Thirty-two (52%) patients out of 62 discharged with PEG tube feeding over a period of two years were in 8 private nursing homes. Thirty-two registered nurses in these nursing homes were interviewed. Seven (21.9%) had formal training session on PEG arranged by the PEG clinic. Local infection (28%), leaking (12.5%), back flow (15.6%) and tube blockage (9.4%) were the problems frequently encountered. Twenty-eight (87.5%) felt they could deal with these problems and 29 (90.6%) had access to specialist advice in case of difficulties (from PEG clinic and/or dietician). Twenty-six (81.2%) felt the need for formal training and regular updating. Conclusion In spite of hospital and community based PEG clinic run by our hospital, staffs in local nursing homes feel the need for more formal training and regular updating of their knowledge. This study highlights the need for the local hospital performing PEG to run regular and structured teaching for the staff in private nursing homes along with dedicated follow up service.

[38] Age-related change in serum uric acid - 10-year longitudinal study in 80507 Japanese

H. Shimokata, F. Ando (Department of Epidemiology, National Institute for Longevity Sciences, Obu, Japan), M. Kuzuya (Department of Geriatrics, Nagoya University School of Medicine, Nagoya, Japan)

PURPOSE: To clarify 10-year longitudinal change in serum uric acid in Japanese men and women. METHOD: Subjects were 80507 Japanese (50157 men, mean age 44.5 years; 30349 women, 43.7 years), who had health examinations between 1989 to and 1998. Age-related change in uric acid was examined. The associations of uric acid with habit of drinking and body mass index (BMI) were also examined. RESULTS: Cross-sectional analysis: Serum uric acid decreased 0.086 mg/dl with 10 years of age in men, but increased 0.156 mg/dl in women ($p<0.001$). Alcohol and obesity significantly correlated with serum uric acid. Longitudinal analysis: Uric acid increased both in men and women (0.26 mg/dl and 0.14 mg/dl) between 1989 and 1998. The percentage of women who drink everyday increased from 5.9% to 10.3 during 10 years, but the percentage of men who drink everyday decreased from 55.6% to 52.5%. BMI in women was 21.8 both in 1989 and 1998, but BMI in men increased from 22.8 to 23.3 during 10 years. The birth cohort effects of longitudinal change in uric acid were examined by the mixed effect model. Uric acid generally increased with age in men and women, and uric acid was significantly higher in younger cohort in men. Serum uric acid also increased with age in the model controlled for BMI and drinking. CONCLUSION: Serum uric acid level significantly increased with age despite of changes in drinking and obesity in men and women, and there were significant birth cohort effects in men.

[39] Correlation of serum lipid peroxide level with antioxidant nutrients in the middle-aged and elderly Japanese

T. Imai, F. Ando, N. Niino, and H. Shimokata (Department of Epidemiology, National Institute for Longevity Sciences), S. Oka (Department of Nutrition, Tokushima University School of Medicine), K. Mori (Department of Living Science, Chukyo Junior College)

PURPOSE: Serum lipid peroxide level may be related to aging. The purpose of this study was to clarify the relationships between serum lipid peroxide level and antioxidant nutrient intakes. METHOD: The subjects were 1,021 males and 987 females who participated in the National Institute for Longevity Science-Longitudinal Study of Aging. They were random sampling from community living population. Antioxidant nutrient intakes were assessed by 3-day dietary record. Serum lipid peroxide level was measured by thiobarbituric acid reacting substances (TBARS). The correlations of antioxidant nutrient intakes with TBARS were analyzed in both genders ($p<0.05$). RESULTS: TBARS was 3.1 and 2.8 n mol/ml in male and female, respectively. There were significant differences in TBARS between genders. No significant differences were found between two age groups (middle; 40-59 yrs vs elder; 60-79 yrs). Carotenoid (middle male; $r=-0.12$, elder male; $r=-0.12$, middle female; $r=-0.13$, elder female; $r=-0.11$) and vitamin C (middle male; $r=-0.13$, elder male; $r=-0.13$, middle female; $r=-0.16$, elder female; $r=-0.13$) were significantly correlated with TBARS. But there were no significant differences in these correlation coefficients between age groups. As to isoflavonoid, genistein ($r=-0.12$) and daidzein ($r=-0.13$) were significantly correlated with TBARS only in elder male group. The correlation between TBARS and these antioxidant nutrient intakes were statistically significant even after controlling for covariates (energy intake, and smoking status). CONCLUSION: Carotenoid and vitamin C were inversely correlated with TBARS. Isoflavonoids were inversely correlated with TBARS only in elder male group.

[40] BMI and Waist Circumference Standards: a Critique in Younger and Older Caucasians and Japanese: Part-I

S. Iwao, N. Iwao, D.C. Muller, R. Andres (National Institute on Aging, Baltimore, USA), D. Elahi (Geriatric Research Laboratory, Boston, USA). M. Koda, H. Shimokata (National Institute for Longevity Sciences, Obu, Japan)

Purpose: To compare participants in similar longitudinal study populations in Nagoya and Baltimore with respect to anthropometric and plasma lipid characteristics as a preliminary step to testing the applicability of recently recommended standards for interpreting the Body Mass Index (BMI) and Waist Circumference (WC) in younger and older men and women (see Part II). Methods: 566 men and 329 women from the Baltimore Longitudinal Study of Aging and 868 men and 837 women from the National Institute for Longevity Sciences-Longitudinal Study of Aging (NILS-LSA) aged 39-64 and 65-80 years had anthropometric and plasma lipid determinations (Total-, HDL-, and LDL-cholesterol, and triglycerides). Results: BMI levels averaged 10-15 0gher in younger and older Caucasian men and women than in Japanese. Fat distribution pattern (WC) was also more favorable in Japanese (50wer in men and 140wer in women). Despite these characteristics, total-C and LDL-C were higher in Japanese, as were the triglycerides levels in older subjects. Counteracting these unfavorable characteristics, HDL-C values were considerably higher in the Japanese. As a result of these opposing characteristics the ∞gunfavorable: favorable∞h lipid ratios (LDL/HDL) were better in younger and older Japanese than Caucasian men; the ratios in women were, however, nearly the same in two populations. Conclusion: There are distinctive differences in anthropometric and metabolic characteristics in younger and older subjects of these two longitudinal populations, some distinctly more favorable in the Japanese, others not. Anthropometric standards recently promulgated need to be tested in population-specific studies. A test of these standards are presented in Part II (N. Iwao et al.).

[41] BMI and Waist Circumference Standards: a Critique in Younger and Older Caucasians and Japanese: Part-II

N. Iwao, S. Iwao, D.C. Muller, R. Andres (National Institute on Aging, Baltimore, USA), D. Elahi (Geriatric Research Laboratory, Boston, USA). M. Koda, H. Shimokata (National Institute for Longevity Sciences, Obu, Japan)

Purpose: To test whether guidelines recently proposed by NHLBI (NIH) and WHO for interpreting Body Mass Index (BMI) and Waist Circumference (WC) as indices of obesity and harmful distribution pattern of body fat are applicable in younger and older Caucasian and Japanese men and women. Methods: See Part 1 of this report describing the two longitudinal study populations in Nagoya and Baltimore. The anthropometric variables were dichotomized at BMI of 25 kg/m2 and WC of 80 cm (women) and 94 cm (men). Cut-points for abnormality of the plasma lipids were: total-C 240, HDL-C 35, LDL-C 160, and triglycerides 200mg/dl. Results: Correlation coefficients: r-values generally were higher for WC than for BMI, for woman than for men, for younger than for older subjects, but were very similar in the two population groups. The percentage of subjects exceeding the cut-points were much lower in the Japanese for BMI, WC and HDL-C and were slightly higher for total-C and LDL-C. Women had more abnormality in total-C and LDL-C, while men were more abnormal in TG and HDL-C. There were no consistent age differences. Striking differences occurred between the two populations in sensitivity and specificity of the BMI and WC cut-points for the four lipids; sensitivities were much higher for BLSA than for Japanese (60% vs. 24%), while specificities were lower (56% vs. 83%). Conclusion:

Clearly, BMI and WC are strongly related to the metabolic variables in both populations, but the striking differences in sensitivity and specificity suggest that NHLBI/WHO cut-points for abnormality of the anthropometric standards require racial/ethnic distinctions.

[42] Ultrasonographic Evaluation of Thyroid Gland in Elderly and Correlation with Thyroid Function and Malnutrition.

*Magnani L, Casarotti D, Cravello L, Agosteo E, Fontana I, Precerutti S, Rollone M, Ferrari E. (IRCCS, "S. Matteo" Polyclinic, Preside of Belgioioso, Pavia Italy*Department of Internal Medicine and Medical Therapy, Chair of Geriatrics, University of Pavia, Italy°II.AA.RR. ,"S. Margherita", Pavia , Italy)*

The aim of our study was to evaluate the morphological aspects of thyroid gland and its correlation with the parameters of thyroid function in elderly people. We studied a group of 267 old subjects 48 men (18%) and 219 (82%) women (mean 81 ± 7 ys, range 65-103 ys), admitted in Geriatric Hospital for different causes, excluding thyroid pathology. Thyroid gland was evaluated by ultrasonography; the parameters of thyroid function and of nutrition were measured. A thyroid volume increase was present in 105 patients (39,3%) and the goitre s prevalence was 37,7% in women and 48% in men. Solid nodules (diameter more of 0,5 cm) were observed in 149 patients (55,8 %). One nodule was found in 12,1%, two nodules in 36,2% and three or more nodules were present in 51,7% of patients. Solid nodules were prevalent in thyroid glands with increased volume (53%). The nodule s prevalence was statistically higher in women than in men (59,8 % vs 37,5%) without significant correlations with the subjects age. 94 patients (9,4 %) had a type III pattern of nodular vascularization, (namely an intra and perinodular vascularization). Liquid collections (more that 1 cm) were evident in 9 patients (3,4%). The thyroid retrosternal extension occurred in 3,2% of patients. Unhomogeneities of the echographic pattern were observed in 110 patients (41,2 %) and in 43,6% of the cases with increased volume thyroid gland. The presence of goitre was correlated either with higher T3 and FT4 levels ($p < 0,05$) and lower TSH levels ($p< 0,001$) or with lower cholesterol levels ($p < 0,05$). In this population we never found any correlation amoung the thyroid volume, the morphological pattern of the thyroid gland and the indexes of malnutrition.

[43] Factors implied in the feeding of the old persons

Haydée Morazzani (President Venezuelan Society of Geriatria-Gerontologia,at the Faculty of Medicine, Universidad Central de Venezuela, Caracas, Venezuela). Oara 3 Haydée Morazzani.

The purpose of this work is to identify the factors implied in the feeding of the old persons. The aging process runs parallel to a change in the style of life determined by diverse situations (health, personal level of income, necessities, changes in the time of leisure, among others). This implies adaptations of the economic resources and the nourishing factors. The objective of this work is to detect the factors implied in the feeding of olds to traves of the identification of physiological, psychological, educative indicators and the social-economics. Method: participant observation, design of field. Population and shows: 60 old persons. Instrument: questionnaire. Results: The age leads to changes in the nutritional ingestion - the health state is determining in the feeding of old - the diminution of the its self-esteem is responsible for the loss of interest by the food - habits, attitudes, - solitude situations are implied in the feeding of old - the technology leads to changes in the habits and nourishing patterns - the educative level and the cultural patterns are determining in the feeding of the old persons - the studied socioeconomic factors are implied in the nutritional diet of the old one. Conclusions: - the feeding of this group depends on its state of health, its cultural level, its social- economics conditions -the deficiency of resources for the necessities of feeding of the old persons goes in damage of their quality of life.

[44] Nutritional status and immunity: influence on 2 - year mortality in institutionalized elderly

M. Molaschi, C. Scarafiotti, M. Ponzetto, S. Raspo, P. Maina, M. Massaia, F. Fabris (Medical and Surgical Department, University of Torino, Torino, ITALY)

PURPOSE The study was conducted to evaluate the prognostic value on 2-year mortality of nutritional, immunological, mental and functional parameters in elderly institutionalized patients with steady clinical conditions. METHOD: The study population included 110 subjects aged 70-102 years, free from metabolic, haematologic and neoplastic diseases, not taking nutritional supplements and not showing signs of acute disease at time of enrolment. The study parameters included anamnestic data, use of drugs, mental status (MMSE), functional status (ADL), immunity (total lymphocyte count, lymphocyte subpopulations, immunoglobulins), nutritional patterns (MNA) and indicators (serum albumin, transferrin, prealbumin, Tcholesterol, triglycerides, haemoglobin, hematocrit). Independent parameters associated with 2-year mortality were identified using Cox proportional hazard models. RESULTS: On univariate analysis, patients who survived after 2 years showed significantly higher basal plasma values of albumin, Tcholesterol, transferrin, hemoglobin, hematocrit, B lymphocytes. MMSE, MNA total score and daily fluid intake were also higher in the surviving elderly, while age and number of lost ADL functions where higher for the elderly deceased in the 2-year observation period. The factors independently associated with 2-year survival were found to be serum albumin (OR 0.2295; IC 95% 0.0930 - 0.5660; $p < 0.01$), serum transferrin (OR 0.9930; IC 95% 0.9864 - 0.9996; $p< 0.05$), daily fluid intake (OR 0.3953; IC 95% 0.1760 - 0.8879; $p< 0.05$), total MNA score (OR 0.9002; IC 95% 0.8272 - 0.9795; $p< 0.05$). CONCLUSION: Our data confirm that nutritional status more than immunity is related to survival. MNA, fluid intake and some biochemical nutritional parameters can be considered in the multidimensional prognostic evaluation of the elderly patient.

[45] Acquired Factor VIII Inhibitor with Myelofibrosis

Edgar F. Hernandez, M.D. Shobhana Chaudhari, M.D. New York Medical College/Metropolitan Hospital Center, New York City, NY 10029

Case: An 81-year-old African American male patient with history of anemia presented to the emergency room complaining of generalized weakness, lightheadedness and weight loss. The physical examination revealed a patient in no acute distress BP 100/60, heart rate 90 /min, respiratory rate 15 /min, and afebrile. Pertinent findings were pallor, a soft systolic murmur at apex, and hepatomegaly. Stool occult blood was negative. WBC 9.14 K/cmm, Hb 6.3 g/dl, Hct 19%, Plt 59K/cmm, PT 14.3 sec, INR 1.3, PTT 54.4 sec. Peripheral blood smear revealed polychromatophilia, tear drop cells, blasts, and basophilia. Leucocyte alkaline phosphatase was normal. Bone marrow biopsy showed markedly hypocellular marrow, with marked decrease in hematopoietic elements and myelofibrosis. Mixing studies showed only partial correction of PTT (mixed PTT 40.3 sec). A factor VIII inhibitor assay was positive. The final diagnosis was idiopathic myelofibrosis, and acquired factor VIII inhibitor. The patient was initially transfused with packed red blood cells, and started on erythropoietin, after which he was discharged. Discussion: Factor VIII inhibitors are the most commonly encountered anticoagulant antibodies however; they are still rare, occurring in 1 in 5 million individuals per year. They are more common in patients over age over age 50. It is idiopathic in almost 500f cases, or in association with other diseases like hemophilia A, autoimmune diseases, dematological diseases malignancies(hematologic and nonhematologic), medications and pregnancy. To date, no cases of acquired factor VIII inhibitor have been reported in association with idiopathic myelofibrosis.

[47] Diagnosis and Nutrition Intervention of Protein-Energy Malnutrition in Institutionalized Elderly Chinese in Hong Kong

Cheung-Kei Lee, Bernard Kong, Sau-heung Li, Pauline Ku (Wong Chuk Hang Hospital, Hospital Authority, Hong Kong S.A.R.)

Protein-energy malnutrition (PEM) is associated with higher morbidity and mortality, and poor quality of life in elderly. A nutritional survey was conducted in a complex for the elderly to pick up the malnourished elders and identify the risk factors followed by nutrition intervention. 282 institutionalized elders were recruited into the study. 61 PEM cases were identified based on the defined criteria of PEM: anthropometric (Body mass index < 18.5kg/m2, or corrected-arm muscle area <16.1cm2 for male / <16.9cm2 for female) and biochemical indices (serum albumin <36g/L, prealbumin <180 mg/L, or Transferrin < 2.1g/L). Extremely dependent elders with poor cognition had higher prevalence of PEM. Dementia, feeding with gastric diet and chronic lung diseases were the significant risk factors for PEM. 2 stages of intervention (proprietary milk and high protein diet over 8 months) were given to the PEM cases. Body mass index, corrected-arm muscle area and serum albumin were significantly improved in medically stable elders. Serum albumin was the only prognostic indicator between the survived and deceased groups. Nutritional status should be monitored among the institutionalized elders particularly who are extremely demented and require modified diet and assistance in feeding. PEM in frail elders is a poor prognostic sign and low serum albumin predicts mortality. The majority of patients under stable medical conditions improved with some form of intervention. Moderate to severe PEM may be difficult to correct once it develops. The nutritional status of frail elderly should be properly assessed and a trial of intervention should be attempted.

[48] Descriptive Anthropometric Data of Community-Dwelling and Institutionalized Elderly Chinese in Hong Kong

Cheung-Kei Lee, Bernard Kong, Stella Yu, Sau-heung Li (Wong Chuk Hang Hospital, Hospital Authority, Hong Kong S.A.R.)

To accurately evaluate the nutritional status of older people, anthropometric reference data are required. A total of 1129 Chinese elders aged 60 years and older (347 from community and 782 institutionalized from 4 different types of long-term care facilities: 160 from an infirmary hospital, 341 from a Care & Attention Home, 167 from a Long Stay Care Home, and 114 from a Private Nursing Home, including 380 men and 749 women) were assessed by trained nurses from December of 1999 to November of 2000. Weight, height, skin-fold thickness, upper arm circumference were measured. Body mass index (BMI), arm muscle circumference, and corrected-arm muscle area were calculated. Data were categorized by types of living environments, sex, and 4 age groups (60 69, 70 79, 80 89, and 90 years and older). The extremely dependent group (Infirmary) had the lowest anthropometric indices. The indices decreased with increasing age. Men's indices were significantly different from women. Women had higher body mass index and fat storage but lower muscle reserves. The infirmary (18.8% and 6.9%) and private nursing (18.4% and 14.9%) groups had more grade III chronic protein-energy malnutrition (BMI < 16.0) and less grade I obesity (BMI 25.0 and 29.9), respectively. Screening to assess nutritional status should be considered an important component of regular health examinations of older adults. Anthropometry can be a reliable and specific indicator of malnutrition. For clinical and screening purposes, weight and BMI are most important anthropometric measures for both initial and follow-up assessment of nutritional status.

[49] Evaluation of diagnosis practices in elderly patients with iron deficiency

C. BUSSY, P. CHAIBI, A. LALHOU, Y. MARTIN, W. OURAD, F. PIETTE (hôpital Charles Foix, Ivry sur Seine, France).

Purpose: in a sample of hospitalised geriatric patients, to evaluate the management of iron deficiency, defined as serum ferritin less than 50 micrograms per liter. Method: we retrospectively studied the 260 last medical records in a general geriatric hospitalized population. Each patient underwent blood test at entry, with serum ferritin. When serum ferritin was less than 50 micrograms per liter without evident aetiology, care management was studied. Results : 12.3% (32) of our patients (mean age : 85.8 years, 81 0.000000emale) were classified as iron deficient, from the result of serum ferritin. For these 32 patients, 19 (59%) underwent a colonoscopy and an upper endoscopy. For 3 patients, only upper endoscopy was performed, without any explanation for the absence of colonoscopy in 1 case. For 10 patients, any endoscopic evaluation has not been performed, without any explanation in 5 cases. Thus, a logical explanation extracted from the medical file could be recognized for 7 patients, justifying the absence of a total endoscopic evaluation. Conclusion : in a geriatric hospital, optimal care management for iron deficiency occur for 81.20f the patients (26/32). Improvement of care management is a part of an accreditation step, which first needs an evaluation. Then, some propositions could be suggested, some modifications could be applied and evaluated.

[49] Underutilization of calcium and vitamin D supplementation in 3 Canadian long-term care facilities

L. T. Lee, W. M. Drake, D. L. Kendler (Osteoporosis Research Centre, St Vincent’s Hospital, Vancouver, BC, Canada)

PURPOSE: To assess the calcium and vitamin D intake of a sample of institutionalized elderly in 3 long-term care facilities in Canada. METHOD: Cross-sectional survey including a 3-day food record and pharmacotherapy records obtained through the pharmacy database. Dietitians at each of the 3 hospital sites randomly selected 53 patients in total; patients under age 65 were excluded. RESULTS: An inadequate intake for both calcium and vitamin D was evident: only 26% (n=14) of the 53 patients met the adequate intake (AI) for calcium and only 30% (n=16) met the AI for vitamin D. Twelve patients were diagnosed with osteoporosis, but only 42% (n=5) and 67% (n=8) of these patients achieved the AIs for calcium and vitamin D respectively. For the 24 patients with fracture(s) diagnoses (15 were hip fractures), 33% (n=8) met the AIs for each of calcium and vitamin D. Inadequate intakes of calcium or vitamin D were seen in 3 patients who were taking medications that interfered with bone metabolism. CONCLUSION: Ensuring adequate intake of calcium and vitamin may have been overlooked in the institutionalized elderly, who are at a high risk of osteoporosis and associated fractures. Dietary strategies for meeting the AIs for these 2 micronutrients include more appropriate supplemented foodstuffs, greater attention paid to feeding assistance and more awareness of dispensing medications that interfere with bone metabolism.

[50] Decreased Functionality and High BMI in Elder Mexican Americans: An Obese Model of Frailty.

EE Lazarou, TP Miles, DV Espino (University of Texas Health Science Center, San Antonio, TX USA)

PURPOSE: Examine whether high BMI is a risk factor for morbidity in community-dwelling Mexican American (MA) elders in the United States(US) METHODS: Physical function measures were obtained during a home interview with a probability sample of 2899 non-institutionalized MA's aged 65 and over living in the southwestern US. The physical performance score used to define frailty was based upon the assessment of the MA's ability to complete the task of walking 8 feet within 10 seconds. These subjects were followed in surveys 2 years apart(Fall 1993-Spring 1994; Fall 1995-Spring 1996). 258 subjects who took more than 10 seconds to complete the 8-foot walk, or were unable to perform this task were included in the analysis. The data results are based on those participants who were overweight defined as having a BMI >or = 27 (n=221) and who were determined to be frail based upon their ability or inability to perform the walking test. RESULTS: The Obese MA group were young-old (73.9 years) and female 69.7%. They were more likely than their thin counterparts to have arthritis (62.1 vs 56.8%), hypertension (56.4 vs. 31.4%), and diabetes (34.7 vs. 8.6%). They were also more functionally disabled; 42.90f obese MA's were unable to complete the 8 foot walk in less than 9 seconds after being able to 2 years prior. CONCLUSION: There appears to be an obese model of frailty in the Mexican American elder population. This concept deviates from the typical picture of frailty. Implications will be discussed

[51] Percutaneous endoscopic gastrostomy : A Chinese experience

T.Y. Lau, C.Y. Yung, T.C. Sim, K.Y. Sha, E.M.F. Leung (United

Christian Hospital, Hong Kong S.A.R, China)

In Hong Kong, percutaneous endoscopic gastrostomy (PEG) has become the preferred method to provide enteral feeding to older patients who have difficulties in eating, but the impact of PEG on patient outcomes is not well documented. This retrospective study reviewed a local experience with older patients in a regional hospital from January 1997 to October 2000. Working under a common care pathway, these patients were monitored closely by physicians, the Nurse Specialist (Geriatrics) and the community nurses. The sample consisted of 36 males and 35 females, mean age was 75.6 years, range from 35 to 96. The predominant indication for PEG placement was stroke (71.8%). At the time of review, 8 patients (11.2%) had had PEG removed and resume oral feeding, 22 (30.9%) had died with a functioning tube. Three patients (4.2%) died within a month of insertion, 16 (22.5%) died within 18 months. The mortality in days after PEG insertion was ranged from 4 days to 1,293 days with an average of 382 days. 24 patients (33.2%) reported tube dislodgment, 10 patients (14.1%) reported moderate amount of exit wound discharge and leakage of gastric fluid. Despite the fact that PEG can be accomplished safely, the implementation of PEG in a culture that is particularly fond of eating required much psychological preparation of the patient where nurses could contribute most.

[52] Changes in lipid levels with age - 10 year longitudinal study in a large Japanese population

Masafumi Kuzuya, Akihisa Iguchi (Department of Geriatrics, Nagoya University Graduate School of Medicine, Nagoya, Japan), Fujiko Ando, Hiroshi Shimokata (Department of Epidemiology, National Institute for Longevity Sciences, Obu, Japan)

PURPOSE: To determine the recent secular trends in serum lipids and characterize their influence on the aging process, we examined a large cohort of Japanese cross-sectionally and longitudinally. METHOD: The participants in this study were 80,331 Japanese men and women 20 to 79 years of age, who had received annual health examinations from 1989 to 1998. RESULTS: In cross-sectional analysis, an increase in total and LDL cholesterol as well as triglyceride levels was observed in the population during 1989-1998. Whereas HDL cholesterol level decreased in men and increased in women. The longitudinal changes in lipid levels, which were analyzed by the mixed effect model, showed that total and LDL cholesterol tended to increase with age in men between birth cohorts 1920s and 1960s. In women these cholesterol levels increased in 1930s and younger birth cohorts. HDL cholesterol tended to decrease in men of all birth cohorts. However, HDL cholesterol increased in women of 1940s and younger birth cohorts and tended to decline in 1930s and older birth cohorts. Triglyceride level increased in men of 1940s and younger cohorts but decreased 1930s and older cohorts. Triglyceride increased in women of 1930s and younger birth cohorts. Longitudinal analysis also suggested that there were birth cohort effects except for triglyceride level in women. CONCLUSION: These results suggested that Japanese serum lipid levels are still increasing and that there were birth cohort effects on serum lipid levels in the Japanese population.

[53] Motor performance and its relation to age, anthropometric characteristics and serum lipids in elderly women

Xinxin Guo, Michael Matousek, Valter Sundh, Bertil Steen Department of Geriatric Medicine, Göteborg University, Göteborg, Sweden.

Purpose: Motor performance and its relation to age, anthropometric characteristics and serum lipids were studied in a population-based sample of elderly women aged, 70, 74, 78 and 84 (n=488). Methods: Motor performance was measured by a precise laboratory test, Postural-Locomotion-Manual test, using an optoelectronic technique. Anthropometric measurements included body mass index and waist-hip ratio. Blood samples were drawn for the measurement of total cholesterol, high density lipoprotein (HDL) cholesterol, and triglyceride concentrations. Results: Motor performance was worse with advancing age in a curvilinear way. High body mass index, waist-hip ratio and serum triglycerides, and low HDL cholesterol, respectively, associated with poor mobility after adjustment by age, vascular disease, hypertension, diabetes, smoking, physical exercise and some chronic diseases. High waist-hip ratio, high triglyceride concentration and low physical exercise were independent predictors of poor mobility. Conclusions: Our results suggest that high waist-hip ratio and high serum triglycerides might serve as markers of motor impairment in elderly women. Monitoring these markers in clinical work may help to identify people with early motor impairment and prevent more severe mobility disability.

[54] Nutritional Status, Impaired Glucose Tolerance, and Hypertension in the Elderly

M.Georgescu,A.M.Georgescu(National Institute of Gerontology and Geriatrics,Bucharest, Romania)

Decreased synthesis of hepatic plasma protein (albumin)has been shown with diabetes. Similar,the concentration of albumin in serum has long been recognized as an indicator of the state of general health and nutrition of an individual. Modest to very low serum albumin concentrations are associated with morbidity and all cause mortality in older persons. Earlier studies often dealt with an association between hypertension and abnormalities of glucose metabolism.In an attempt to elucidate the correlations between the nutritional status , impaired glucose tolerance (IGT) and hypertension in Romanian elders we investigated a group of 126 (73 +/- 9 years) individuals with IGT together with a group of 111(74 +/- 10 years)normoglicemic control subjects. Serum albumin concentrations were (38 +/- 0,7) g/L among elderly with IGT and (42 +/- 0,9)g/L in normoglicemic control subjects,significantly higher (P<0.05)from the IGT group.Systolic blood pressure was (155 +/- 8)mm Hg, diastolic blood pressure was (96 +/- 5)mm Hg in IGT subjects. In normoglicemic control subjects systolic blood pressure was (151 +/- 6) mm Hg and diastolic blood pressure was (81 +/- 3) mm Hg. Our results show that higher (P<0.001)diastolic blood pressure was associated with IGT, probably as a feature of early stages of diabetic nephropathy. Interventions seeking to maximize nutritional status are needed and should be important in diabetic elderly.

[55] The relationship between age and visceral fat in middle-aged and elderly Japanese

Michiko Koda, Fujiko Ando, Naoakira Niino, Hiroshi Shimokata (Dept. Epidemiology, National Institute for Longevity for Sciences, Obu, Japan)

PURPOSE: The amount and distribution of body fat, which are related with many chronic diseases, are different by age and gender. The purpose of this study was to clarify the relationship among age, visceral fat, and body mass index (BMI: weight (kg) / height (m)2). METHOD: Subjects were 244 females and 260 males, aged 42 to 82 years, who were selected randomly from the neighborhood area of our institute. They were divided into four age groups: 42-49, 50-59, 60-69, and 70-82 years. Visceral fat area (VFA) was estimated using abdominal CT scans. Visceral fat obesity defined as VFA>=100cm2 following the Japan Society of Obesity. RESULTS: VFA was correlated with age in females (r=0.43, p<0.001). The mean VFA in females aged 70-82 years (98cm2) was twice of the mean VFA in females aged 42-49 years (50cm2). In males, there was no correlation between VFA and age. Those who had VFA>=100cm2 were 7 0n 42-49, 6 0n 50-59, 18 0n 60-69, and 43 0n 70-82 years among females, and 35%, 38%, 54%, and 46% among males, respectively. Females whose BMI<25kg/m2 but VFA>=100cm2 were 0 0n 42-49 and 50-59, 12 0n 60-69, and 26 0n 70-82 years. In males, they were 10%, 28%, 41%, and 39%, respectively. CONCLUSION: VFA increased with age in females. Those who were BMI<25kg/m2 but VFA>=100cm2 increased with age. BMI is used as indicators for obesity, but it is not sensitive to visceral fat obesity in elderly people.

[56] Diagnosis of denutrition in the elderly persons using dual

energy X-ray absorptiometry

C.JOCHUM and JL. NOVELLA and F. BLANCHARD (Departement of internal medecine and Gerontology , University Hospital, Rheims, France) and D. JOLLY and A. CLEMENT (Departement of Medical Information, University Hospital, Rheims, France)

Purpose : Denutrition in the elderly is frequently present with major consequences for the frailer ones. The classic investigation's tools had a poor level of reliability. The purpose of the study is to assess the validity of body composition by dual energy x-ray absorptiometry for a reliable diagnosis of denutrition. Method : One hundred one subjects aged over 70 were included in this prospective study. Biological and anthropometric variables were gathered as the Mini Nutritional Assessment (MNA) and the body composition by absorptiometry. A global index of denutrition was proposed combining anthropometric, biological criteria, and the MNA score. Two agreement analyses were made between classical diagnostic criteria of nutritional status and body fat and fat free mass assessed by anthropometry and absorptiometry. An association between nutritional status and body absorptiometric composition was studied with univariate analysis followed by a multivariate logistic regression model. This model allowed an elaboration of a Nutritional Absorptiometry Index (NAI). Results : Twenty-three of the 101 subjects were considered to be in a state of denutrition . Agreement was low between anthropometric and biological diagnostic criteria of denutrition. It was good between the different masses assess by anthropometry and absorptiometry. Subjects in a state of denutrition had significantly lower body fat and lower fat free mass. The NAI obtained by a logistic model (using fat free mass index and body fat mass) showed good diagnostic validity (sensibility :73.9% ; specificity : 95.2%) . Conclusion : In this study , the Nutritional Absorptiometry Index (NAI) appears to be a reliable diagnostic, a non-invasive tool for assessing denutrition in the elderly. Further studies should lead to a confirmation of this findings.

[57] Index of Malnutrition In Elderly People from Nursing Homes.

A.M.Garcia, (State University of Pernambuco, Recife, Brazil), P.C.Lira (Federal University of Pernambuco, Recife, Brazil)

The elderly population of the world is increasing. Ageing is a process that interferes in the nutritional state, therefore, the aim of this study was to evaluate of index of malnutrition in elderly people recruited in nursing homes. From June 1998 to January 1999, 308 individuals (men and women) between the ages of 60-99 were recruited from private, public and philanthropic nursing homes in the state of Pernambuco, Brazil. The anthropometric indicators of nutritional status used were BMI (Body Mass Index), arm-span and brachial circumference. Our results showed that 14.9% these individuals had malnutrition according to the traditional BMI method (using height and weight). Using weight and arm span as indicators, 23.1% had malnutrition, with a sensitivity of 93.5% and specificity of 82% (cut-off BMI= 18.5 24.9). Using the brachial circumference, 25% had the malnutrition diagnosis, with a sensitivity of 91.3% and specificity of 86.6% comparing to normal elderly. In conclusion the index of malnutrition observed in this work for the elderly people from Northeast of Brazil was elevated when compared to the rest of the country but was similar to poor countries of Africa and Malaysia. It can be due to the poorness of people from this region of Brazil leading to trouble in food access and food routine. A significant depression rate in this recruited population could have predisposed these individuals to malnutrition state.

[58] Validation of the Minimum Data Set 2.0 Section K in Residents of a Long-Term Care Facility

J. Bowman, H.H. Keller (Department of Family Relations and Applied Nutrition, University of Guelph, Guelph, Ontario, Canada), S.L. Kane (St. Joseph s Hospital and Home, Guelph, Ontario, Canada)

PURPOSE: The objectives of the study are to 1) determine if there is an association between nutritional risk, as assessed by a Registered Dietitian, and each of the variables in the MDS section K, 2) select the top three variables from MDS section K found to be associated with nutritional risk, and 3) determine if one or any combination of the top three variables has improved sensitivity and specificity for identification of residents at nutritional risk. METHODS: One hundred and twenty-eight participants residing in a long-term care facility underwent a comprehensive nutritional assessment performed by a dietitian. The dietitian s assessment of nutritional status was rated on a scale of 1-10. Nursing staff at the facility completed quarterly MDS reviews concurrently. Bivariate tests of association were used to determine the relationship between the dietitian s rating of degree of risk for malnutrition and each of the predictor variables in section K. The sensitivity (Se) and specificity (Sp) of specific variables, and combinations of variables was also determined. RESULTS: Prescription for enteral, parenteral, mechanical or syringe diet, supplement use, and swallowing problems were significantly associated with nutritional risk according to bivariate analysis. Body mass index (BMI), not currently an MDS trigger variable, was also significantly associated with nutritional risk. In general, Se and Sp analysis indicated that individual items and combinations of these items were only moderately useful as screening mechanisms. The highest Se and Sp was noted for BMI < 24 (0.83 and 0.57 respectively), a variable not currently used in Section K. The next best item was recent nutritional support (Se=0.60, Sp=0.70). CONCLUSION: Although individual items on MDS Section K appear to be associated with nutritional risk as identified by a Registered Dietitian, Se and Sp analysis suggests that these items and this section require further refinement and validation.

[59] Translation and Validation of a Spanish Version of the Mini-Nutritional Assessment

Flores-Castro M, Gutiérrez-Robledo LM, Romero-Velázquez KM, Llaca C (Instituto Nacional de Ciencias Médicas y Nutrición Salvador Zubirán, México City, México)

PURPOSE: The global nutrition evaluation (including anthropometric, biochemical and dietetic parameters) is the gold standard for nutritional diagnosis, but it's expensive, time-consuming and cumbersome. French researchers developed the simple and inexpensive Mini-Nutritional Assessment (MNA) to determine nutritional status in the elderly, with good results. We translated into spanish and validated this test in a cohort of elderly Mexicans. METHOD: From June 1993 to May 1995 we studied 217 elderly outpatients (75% women, mean age 79 ± 7.4) without physical or mental limitations from our institution's geriatric clinic, excluding patients hospitalized <4 weeks before testing, those with diabetic nephropathy, hypertension, history of radiotherapy or glucocorticoid use in the last 6 months. Was established the clinical nutritional status using the global nutrition evaluation and compared with the MNA score. RESULTS: The global nutrition evaluation showed subnutrition (low weight diagnosis + malnutrition diagnosis) in 23% and adequate nutritional status (normality diagnosis + overweight diagnosis) in 77%. Correlating these diagnoses with MNA results (<17 points = malnutrition, 17-23.5= risk of malnutrition, >23.5 = normal) was found that 1000f those with subnutrition were diagnosed either malnutrition (49%) or risk of malnutrition (51%). A significant difference in MNA scores between the patients with subnutrition and adequate nutritional status (p=0.001) was observed. CONCLUSIONS: The Spanish version of the MNA is a useful screening instrument for the detection of elderly patients with subnutritional status. MNA showed a diagnostic sensibility of 49% and a specificity of 89 0.000000or malnutriton. This instrument is simple, inexpensive and useful for detecting elderly Mexican individuals who would benefit from an early nutritional intervention.

[60] Nutritional status and basal metabolic rate of older persons in a Brazilian low-income community

E. Ferriolli, S. C. Miranda, R. Rigo, J. C. Moriguti, C. B. Nonino, A. Tannus, C. E. Paiva, J. S. Marchini (Division of General Internal and Geriatric Medicine and Division of Clinical Nutrition,

Department of Internal Medicine, School of Medicine of Ribeirao Preto, University of Sao Paulo, Ribeirao Preto, SP, Brazil)

Nutritional status is an important determinant of health condition and quality of life in the elderly population. Nutritional interventions to manage both undernutrition and obesity are central issues in public health and the assessment of nutritional status in older populations of developing countries is needed for strategies planning and implementation. This study was intended to assess the nutritional status and basal metabolic ratio of persons aged 60 years or over of a brazilian low-income community. Forty-four (26 female and 18 male, mean age 71.1 and 70.6 years, respectively) out of 104 older persons followed by a Family Medicine university program had their nutritional status assessed by clinical evaluation, anthropometry and blood biochemistry (serum albumin, transferrin, hemoglobin and iron concentration). Basal metabolic rate was determined by indirect calorimetry. Body mass index (BMI) varied from 16 to 41 Kg/m2 in the studied population. 34.10f the volunteers had BMI below 24 and 29.5% had BMI above 29. Overweight or obesity in various degrees were diagnosed in 23% of the women and 27% of the men and malnutrition in 38% and 27%, respectively. Tricipital and subscapular skinfold and arm circumference did not show a good correlation with the nutritional status in this population. Mean basal metabolic rate was 1663 Kcal and 1330 Kcal for male and female volunteers, respectively. This study shows that both obesity and malnutrition are very frequent among older persons of a low-income community in Brazil.

[61] Teaching Programme in Odontogeriatrics in a Brazilian Faculty of Dentistry

J.Baldisserotto, D.M.Padilha, L.Soll (Geriatric and Gerontology Institute - Pontificia Universidade Catolica and Faculty of Dentistryof the Federal University of R.G.S, Porto Alegre, Brazil)

The number of older people is increasing worldwide. This increase in the aged population is more rapid in developing countries, including Brazil. The growing need for oral health and tooth preservation among the aged has led to a increased interest in Geriatric Dentistry. Gerodontics is becoming an important topic in dental education and no time should be wasted to incorporate Geriatric Dentistry into undergraduate Dentistry curricula. In the present study we examine the demographic aspects and current concepts in Geriatric Dentistry, and we introduce new concepts and description of how Geriatric Dentistry has started to be taught as a discipline in the Dental school of the Federal University of Rio Grande do Sul.

[62] Development of systematic oral care in the elderly

Y. Sumi (Department of Dental Surgery, The National Chubu Hospital, Obu-city, Japan), Y. Nakamura (Second Department of Oral Surgery, School of Dentistry, Kagoshima University, Kagoshima-City, Japan), Y. Michiwaki (Department of Oral and Maxillofacial Surgery, School of Dentistry, Showa University, Tokyo, Japan)

PURPOSE: The purpose of this pilot study was to develop, implement and evaluate a systematic oral care procedure for community-dwelling dependent or institutionalized elderly and their caregivers Systematic oral care procedures: 1: Oral mucosa is swabbed completely with a foam-stick for one minute with 0.25 % of Povidone-Iodine solution. 2: Tongue is cleansed with a tongue brush for 30 seconds. 3: Teeth are cleaned with an electric toothbrush for 2.5 minutes with 0.4% stannous fluoride paste. 4: Mouthwash with 0.25% of Povidone-Iodine solution is used for one minute. MATERIALS AND METHODS: The subjects were 16 dependent elderly living in the community and their caregivers. After 8 weeks of systematic oral care, the plaque and gingival indices were scored and the subjects were asked a questionnaire which assessed the advantages, disadvantages and problems in providing systematic oral care. RESULTS: The results of this study demonstrated that the systematic oral care procedure reduced the plaque and gingival indices. In addition, the caregivers burden and fatigue was also reduced. CONCLUSION: A systematic oral care procedure was developed and implemented. The effectiveness of this procedure was evaluated. We hope the effective oral care system will spread in the caregiving field and the oral hygiene level of dependent or institutionalized elderly will improve.

[63] Attitudes to oral care among caregivers in Japanese nursing homes

Y. Sumi (Department of Dental Surgery, The National Chubu Hospital, Obu-city, Japan), Y. Nakamura (Second Department of Oral Surgery, School of Dentistry, Kagoshima University, Kagoshima-City, Japan), Y. Michiwaki (Department of Oral and Maxillofacial Surgery, School of Dentistry, Showa University, Tokyo, Japan)

PURPOSE: Aspiration pneumonia is a major problem for the elderly, leading to hospitalization, costly care, and at times, death. Recently, it was reported that oral care lowered the risk of pneumonia in the institutionalized elderly. This investigation of oral care practice and awareness among caregivers in Japanese nursing homes for the elderly seeks to provide a baseline reference for future research. METHODS: Subjects consisted of 410 individuals (mean age: 37.1 years; sex: 84 male, 326 female) employed as caregivers at 14 nursing homes for the elderly in Japan. Caregivers were surveyed by means of a self-administered questionnaire designed to elicit the following information: age, sex, occupation, awareness of oral care, importance of oral care, burden of oral care, and systemization of oral care. RESULTS: 77% of respondents had knowledge of the causal relationship between oral care and aspiration pneumonia and. Although 97% of respondents wanted training in oral care, only 39% had received it. Only 23% performed oral care systematically. 85% of respondents desired to use methods for cleansing the mouth in addition to those used in current oral care. CONCLUSION: Caregivers are adequately informed of the importance of oral care but inadequately educated on oral care and have little training in systematic oral care. The importance of providing appropriate and systematic oral care training to caregivers and of developing the equipment simplify and support oral care are stressed.

[64] A Study on Relation between Dependency and Oral Status of Elderly People

Honda E, Mutoh T, Maeda N, Morito M. (Tsurumi Univ. Sch. Dent. Med. Yokohama, Japan), Ishikawa M, Shibuya K. (LION Corp. Odawara, Japan)

Many researchers have reported the number of opportunistic candidiasis increases in the last decade. One of the most significant reasons of the fact is due to increase in the number of immunocompromised hosts including elderly people. It is well known that oral microbial flora might change not only with aging but also with denture wearing. The purpose of this study is to investigate relation among dependency, oral Candida carriage and halitosis of elderly people and to investigate affect of denture wearing on oral Candida carriage. We randomly chose dependent elderly people (n=47, mean age 73.1±4.6) in three institutions and independent subjects (n=56, mean age 74.7±5.4) living in their communities. The mean number of Candida of the dependent subjects was more than double times that of independent subjects. The amount of halitosis of dependent subjects was significantly higher than that of independent subjects (Mann-Whitney U test, p=0.001). In the independent subjects, the mean number of Candida and the level of halitosis were almost the same regardless of denture wearing. Whereas, in the dependent subjects, the mean number of Candida of denture wearers was 5 times higher than that of non-denture wearers and the level of halitosis of denture wearers was significantly lower than that of non-denture wearers (Mann-Whitney U test, p=0.013, 0.041, respectively). These results suggest that dependent elderly people wearing dentures harbour higher number of Candida and might be more susceptible to opportunistic candidiasis in oral cavity.

[65] Determining the factors associated with acceptance of oral rehabilitative therapy for elderly edentulous individuals.

Y. Kawai, A Savard, S Marcoux, J. S. Feine (Faculty of Dentistry, McGill University, Montreal, Canada)

Edentulism is considered to be a chronic condition, affecting function, appearance and quality of life. Once an individual has lost all teeth, therapeutic options are limited to prosthetic devices retained by bony ridges (conventional dentures) or by implants (implant prostheses). In determining prosthetic therapeutic success, there has been some discussion as to whether the primary outcome should be entrusted to ratings by the patients themselves or to ratings made by clinicians who provide these treatments. In addition, there is little solid evidence to assist the clinician in knowing what factors might predict a patient's acceptance of conventional therapy (dentures). In this pilot study (n=11; 6 male, 5 female; mean age =61), patients' ratings of satisfaction with their existing conventional dentures, measured with 100mm visual analogue scales (deGrandmont et al, 1994), were compared to clinicians' ratings of the dentures (Sato et al, 1998) (r=-0.55, Pearson's correlation). In addition, patients' satisfaction ratings were compared to the number of years the patient had been edentulous in the maxilla (r=0.61) and mandible (r=0.12), the number of dentures worn previously in the maxilla (r=-0.25) and mandible (r=-0.67) and the age of the existing dentures for the maxilla (r=0.51) and mandible (r=0.71). In this poster, we will present and discuss the results of these analyses using a larger sample of elderly edentulous subjects. This information will aid clinicians and their patients in determining whether conventional therapy would be satisfactory for individual patients.

[66] A Study on Microflora of Elderly Stroke Patients

Shuichiroh Nagaosa (Department of Dental Surgery,Tokyo Metropolis Rehabilitation Hospital,DDS,Japan),Yasunori Sumi (Department of Dental Surgery ,The National Chubu Hospital,DDS,Japan),Takashi Shinagawa (Department of Dentistry and Oral Surgery,Hitachi Totsuka Hospital),Yoshiroh, Sekine (Department of Dentistry and Oral Surgery,Taiseishinai Hospital,DDS), Minori Yoshida,and Terukazu Ueki (Department of Oral and Maxillofacial Surgery,Nihon University School of Medicine,DDS)

Importance of oral health care is emphasized since the care-requiring elders represented by stroke patients easily suffer from aspiration pneumonia because of dysphagia. It is very important to understand oral bacterial flora in order to maintain oral hygiene. In the present study, samples for cultivation were classified as follows; Group 1: Only Candida isolation from dorsal tongue of 28 healthy adults (18 men and 10 women, average age: 33.0±7.5 years) Group 2: Candida and aerobic bacterial detection from dorsal tongue of 30 elderly stroke patients (17 men and 13 women, average age: 70.1±6.9 years) Group 3: Candida and aerobic bacterial detection from both dorsal tongue and the pharynx of 32 healthy elders (7 men and 25 women, average age: 78.4±7.6 years). Its quantitative change and the change of normal microflora were evaluated from the viewpoint of oral hygiene. Candida isolation rate was 47 0n Group 2 and 59 0n Group 3 that showed no significance between the two groups. When compared among the subjects 1+ and higher (more than 10E+5CFU/mL) positive score at the dorsal tongue, however, it was 47 0n Group 2 and 12.5 0n Group 3. The number of 1+ and higher positive subjects in Group 2 was significantly higher (p<0.01) than that in Group 3. As a result of aerobic bacterial culture, P.aeruginosa was more frequently isolated from Group 2 and Group 3. It is suggested that in the elders, especially in elder stroke patients 1+ and higher positiveness of Candida and P.aeruginosa isolation from the dorsal tongue may indicate mal-oral hygiene.

[67] Understanding Nutritional Health in Older Adults: A Pilot Study

Bonnie Callen (University of Wisconsin-Madison, Madison, Wisconsin, USA)

PURPOSE: Assessment of nutritional risk among older adults can point the way to interventions based on specific risk factors or areas of need. However interventions are only effective when the individual recognizes himself or herself as at risk. A pilot study of adults over 65 admitted to an acute care setting was conducted. The purpose of this pilot was 1) to compare nutritional risk as measured by hospital dieticians on admission with two Nutrition Screening Initiative tools, the DETERMINE Your Nutritional Health Checklist and the Level I Screen, and 2) to elicit from patients their perceptions of their nutritional health. METHOD: A cross sectional convenience sample in an acute care setting was used for this descriptive study. RESULTS: Ten community living patients 65 and older (range 68-86) were interviewed during their hospital stay. While all ten were at nutritional risk as measured by both hospital assessment and nutritional risk screening tools, none of these patients believed themselves to be at risk and all perceived themselves as doing well nutritionally. All but one of these subjects had a BMI 27 putting them in the overweight category according to the Nutrition Screening Initiative categories. CONCLUSION: One conclusion of this pilot is that interventions and education need to include the perceptions of targeted individuals in order to be successful.

SESSION 428

Reaching Seniors with Government Information in the Electronic Age

David Foot (University of Toronto, Toronto, Ontario, Canada) ("Documenting the Growing Importance of the Senior Demographic in Society") Brian D. Ferguson (Assistant Deputy Minister Veterans Services Branch, Veterans Affairs Canada Charlottetown, Prince Edward Island, Canada) (Title of Presentation "Access Canada for Seniors - An Internet Portal Linking Government Information")

Issue The growing importance of the seniors' demographic in Canada and around the world will be documented and an Access Canada For Seniors Internet portal, which will provide single window access to and intelligent navigation of information relevant to seniors, their families and caregivers, will be demonstrated. Structure Dr. Foot will set the stage with the first 50 minutes documenting his work on shifting demographics and the growing importance of seniors in Canada and around the world. This will be followed by Brian Ferguson, who will take 40 minutes to describe a multi-jurisdictional initiative of the federal government to provide single window access to information relevant to seniors, their families and caregivers. Content Using global comparisons and demographic data from 100 different countries, Dr. Foot will document the growing importance of seniors as a market force and target audience for Governments as they work to provide quality service and information on government programs and services in health and finances. Mr. Ferguson will show how the Government of Canada is positioning to meet the challenge of engaging seniors in the information age. Conclusion/ Anticipated outcomes Participants will leave this Round Table with a growing understanding of the critical importance of positioning now to engage boomers and seniors in the knowledge society, ways to breakdown the silos of government so that citizens are able to access the information they need and want through one Internet portal. They will also get a glimpse of the payback on such an investment and envision what challenges the future will bring as we break down jurisdictional barriers in providing government information on health and finances.

SESSION 429

Social Theory and Gerontology: Making Connections Explicit

Merril Silverstein, Vern L. Bengtson and Eugene Litwak (Andrus

Gerontology Center, University of Southern California, Los Angeles, USA, School of Public Health, Columbia University, New York, USA), Theoretical and conceptual approaches to problems of families, aging, and social support. Chris Phillipson (Applied Social Studies and Social Gerontology, Keele University, Keele, UK). Social networks and social capital: Theorizing family support. Malcolm Johnson (International Institute on Health and Aging, University of Bristol, Bristol, UK), Theorising Long Term Care. Philippa J. Clarke (Institute for Human Development, Life Course and Aging, University of Toronto, Toronto, Canada) and Victor W. Marshall (Institute on Aging, University of North Carolina. Chapel Hill, USA). Social theory and the meaning of illness in later life.

ISSUE: The importance of theory in social gerontology is debated. This symposium seeks to make the links between theory and substantive research in gerontology explicit. STRUCTURE: The moderator will briefly introduce the session. Four papers address the explicit role of theory in different domains of social gerontology. The co-convener will conduct an open discussion first asking for panelist comments and then audience comments. CONTENT: Theoretical aspects of gerontology research addressed in four areas: families and social support, social networks and social capital, long term care, and the meaning of illness in later life. Discussion will focus on the nature and value of explicit theorizing in social gerontology. ANTICIPATED OUTCOME: A greater appreciation of the value of explicit theorizing in social gerontology. Thanks again, Diane Wurzinger UNC Institute on Aging 720 Airport Rd, Suite 100 Campus Box #1030 Chapel Hill, NC 27599-1030 Phone: 919-966-9444 Fax: 919-966-0510 email: diane_wurzinger@unc.edu

Social Theory and the Meaning of Illness in Later Life

Philippa J. Clarke (Institute for Human Development, Life Course and Aging, University of Toronto, Canada) and Victor W. Marshall (University of North Carolina Institute on Aging, University of North Carolina at Chapel Hill, USA).

Purpose: The experience of illness in later life is influenced by both micro level processes of adaptation, as well as social structural constraints and opportunities, including socio-economic position, social supports, and cultural beliefs surrounding aging, illness and chronic disability. However, there is often a failure to reconcile macro level determinants of well-being with micro level subjective processes. This paper investigates the impact of both micro and macro level factors on well-being following stroke. Methods: Data are drawn from a national survey of Canadian seniors, supplemented with qualitative interviews in a separate sample of community-dwelling stroke survivors. Results: Micro level characteristics, including poor health and functional disability, are associated with lower well-being following stroke, while macro level social supports and socio-economic position are related to higher well-being. However, greater explanatory value comes from empirical and theoretical interpretation incorporating interactionist and dialectical linking mechanisms between micro and macro levels of analysis. We find mediating and moderating effects between micro and macro level variables, whereby micro level experiences of disability are mediated and moderated by social supports and socio-economic resources. The qualitative interviews suggest a dynamic process of negotiation whereby survivors act back upon the constraints of macro level structures in an attempt to alter their impact on well-being. Conclusions: Both micro and macro level factors exist simultaneously and interactively in the lived experience of seniors following a stroke. Incorporating both perspectives within one integrated theoretical explanation can lead to a more comprehensive understanding of the processes influencing the experience of illness in later life.

The State and Social Capital: Theorising Family Relations and Family Support in Old Age.

Chris Phillipson (Keele University, Staffordshire, United Kingdom)

This paper reviews different theoretical perspectives for understanding the family life of older people. Two approaches are drawn upon: first, political economy arguments from critical gerontology; second, social capital and social network theory from political science. The paper explores some of the advantages to be gained from applying these perspectives to the study of family issues. The position taken is that these theories provide a corrective to existing models which have tended, in different ways, to segment analysis of family life from structural issues on the one side, and more generic social relations on the other. Studies of family life in gerontology were dominated, at least up to the 1980s, by functionalist, exchange and interpretivist perspectives, these focusing upon different issues relating to power relations within the family and the meaning of particular family ties. A common problem with these approaches, however, is their focus on family ties to the exclusion of other types of relationships, especially those relating to the state on the one side, and community ties more generally on the other. This paper will use ideas about the state, and about social capital, to examine different forces affecting family life. How the family links to public and private welfare states is one crucial queston; another concerns the role of wider friendship-based social networks. The paper will explore the theoretical basis of a move from family groups to personal communities, recognising the interplay of new structures and novel forms of social capital in the lives of older people.

Theoretical and Conceptual Approaches to Problems of Families, Aging, and Social Support

M. Silverstein and V.L. Bengtson (Andrus Gerontology Center, University of Southern California, Los Angeles, USA), Eugene Litwak (Columbia University, New York, USA)

PURPOSE: Demographic change is causing a rapid increase in the number of elderly members of society, at the same time that family structures and functions are changing as a consequence of reduced fertility, migration, divorce, and weakening norms of filial piety. Concern is especially acute in developing nations where systems of formal care remain limited. In more developed nations, the prospect of aging baby-boomers and the imperatives of a global economy have instigated a crisis of confidence in the ability of state systems to carry the burden of old age support. This paper examines how well several traditional orientations in social gerontology explain the shifting balance between informal family groups and formal government systems in the context of national and global change. METHOD: We systematically review three theoretical models concerning families, intergenerational mechanisms, and support to older generations: intergenerational solidarity and ambivalence, modernization theory, and primary group theories. Data on family and formal support are compared across nations in developed and developing regions of the world. RESULTS: Basic social theories in gerontology are shown to have sufficient explanatory power to incorporate modern contingencies related to aging, families, and social change. Trends in the developed and developing worlds appear to be converging in terms of the balance between family and formal care to the elderly. The empirical data suggest that attempts at macro-theorizing still have merit in social gerontology. CONCLUSION: We conclude by noting that intergenerational "strains" may have been exaggerated in late 20th Century conceptualizations about families, aging, and social support, and that 21st Century formulations must be based on greater attention to basic sociological theories and their integrative potential.

SESSION 430

Immigration and Aging: The Impact on Health and Community Care

F. Torres-Gil (Center for Policy Research on Aging, UCLA School of Public Policy and Social Research, Los Angeles, CA) The Policy and Politics of Aging along the United States and Mexico Border. I. Chi (Department of Social Work and Social Administration, The University of Hong Kong, Pokfulam Road, Hong Kong) Immigration and Aging: The Impact on LTC Services in Hong

Kong. Sara Carmel (Department of Sociology of Health and Gerontology, Ben-Gurion University of the Negev, Beer-Sheva, Israel) Health and Well-Being of Elderly New and Veteran Immigrants in Israel. J. Damron-Rodriguez (Department of Social Welfare, University of California, Los Angeles and Partners in Care Foundation, Los Angeles, California, USA) Worldwide Immigration: The Impact on the Demand and Supply of Eldercare.

Issue: The aging of the population and immigration are two of the major demographic dynamics. This session will examine the relationship of immigration to the health and long-term care of a country's older persons. National immigration policies vary greatly between countries, thus cross-cultural comparisons are important in understanding the relationship of immigration to the resources required to serve the increasing older population. Structure: The symposium will begin with a global overview of aging followed by the impact of immigration of population age. Presenters will describe immigrant older persons and their health, functional status, family supports and economic characteristics at the time of relocation. Content: Patterns of elder immigration and emigration will be distinguished. Immigration of younger persons and families, labor force participation and the impact on resources for the care of older persons will be discussed. Conclusions: Varying patterns of immigration impact a country's ability to build and enhance community care for growing older populations. Important factors to be considered in planning service delivery include major immigrant population, the pace of immigration and the level of development of national health and social services at the time of the immigrant influx. Panel Moderator: JoAnn Damron-Rodriguez, Ph.D, VA Geriatric Research, Education and Clinical Center and University of California at Los Angeles (UCLA), United States; Fernando Torres-Gil, Center for Aging Policy Research, Associate Dean, UCLA School of Public Policy and Social Research, United States; Sara Carmel, Ben Gurion University, Israel; Iris Chi, Ph.D, Chair, Department of Social Work and Social Administration, Hong Kong.

Health and Well-Being of Elderly New and Veteran Immigrants in Israel

S. Carmel (Head of the Department of Sociology of Health and Gerontology, Ben-Gurion University of the Negev, Beer-Sheva, Israel)

During the nineties about 750,000 immigrants arrived in Israel from the former Soviet Union. Among them the percent of elderly persons (65+) was significantly higher than that in Israel (16% versus 9.8%), significantly increasing the population of elderly and its socio- demographic composition. This study reports about two comparisons of elderly Israelis on indicators of health and well-being: one between the new immigrants and Israelis, and one between the new immigrants and veteran immigrants who immigrated to Israel at least two decades ago from Eastern European countries.Data were collected by structured home interviews from a sample of Israeli Jewish elderly aged 70 and over (n=1138). The results of both comparisons show that the new immigrants are relatively younger and have higher levels of education than the veterans, but their economic status is lower, and they have a lower percentage of men and married persons. The new immigrants also rank themselves lower than the veterans on a variety of measures of health and psycho-social indicators of well-being. It is suggested that the immigration experience and the stress caused by it, as well as factors related to the standard of living and health services in the countries of origin, outweigh the relative advantage that the new immigrants have, in terms of age and education, in influencing their health and well-being. Long-term effects of immigrating in old age, and implications of this situation on health and welfare services will be discussed.

Immigration and Aging: The Impact on LTC Services in Hong Kong

I. Chi (Department of Social Work and Social Administration, The University of Hong Kong, Pokfulam Road, Hong Kong)

The Long-term care services in Hong Kong have expanded rapidly in the past five years and this trend is very likely to continue in the coming two decades due to the fact that Hong Kong has a fast paced aging population. The government has adopted a mixed economy of care to involve more private sectors to provide long-term care services to the frail elders. Quite a number of residential care places are currently purchased from nursing homes operated by the private sector. At the same time, the new immigration policy allows 150 new immigrants each day to enter Hong Kong from Mainland China. The new immigration policy also allows private sectors to import workers from neighboring countries. Some of these new immigrants and most of the imported workers are working in the long-term care facilities. Because few of them have pre-service training in long-term care, the quality of care has been a major concern.

The Policy and Politics of Aging along the United States and Mexico Border

F. Torres-Gil (Associate Dean, Academic Affairs; Social Welfare and Policy Studies; Director, Center for Policy Research on Aging, UCLA School of Public Policy and Social Research, Los Angeles, CA)

This presentation examines immigration policy and politics as an essential element of population aging. The migration and immigration of individuals between and within nations has not been viewed as an important ingredient in understanding the advantages and disadvantages of world wide movements of people in a global economy. The United States in particular debates the benefits and problems associated with immigration from throughout the world including Mexico. Yet, immigrants can alter a nation's median age and bring a "youthfulness" and labor market advantage that it might not otherwise have. At the same time, immigrants can exacerbate social, cultural and political divisions and relationships. This presentation describes the case of the United States and Mexico in addressing immigration via population aging and draws on experiences of other nations to raise implications and suggest recommendations for incorporating immigrants into a more systematic public policy response to the aging of societies and the benefits of immigrants.

Worldwide Immigration: The Impact on the Demand and Supply of Eldercare

J.Damron-Rodriguez (Department of Social Welfare, School of Public Policy and Social Research, University of California, Los Angeles and Partners in Care Foundation, Los Angeles, CA, USA)

Issue: Immigration may impact a nation's demand for community and other long term services either through family caregiver's emigration or through older person's immigration. Also the supply of younger care providers formally and informally is influenced by immigration patterns. In some countries the demand for community and home care providers is dramatically increasing. Structure: This presentation will provide an overview of global aging and immigration patterns as a background to the papers presented in this symposium. Content: Age of immigration, country of origin, education and training of immigrants will all be discussed as influences on the demand and supply of care particularly non-institutional or community-based care. Both developing and developed countries will be presented in the overview. Implications: Policy implications will be framed which relate to the subsequent international studies.

SESSION 431

Cross-National Comparisons of Home Care with the MDS-HC: The InterRAI Experience

John N. Morris (Hebrew Rehabilitation Center for the Aged, Boston, USA) An Overview of the Development and Application of the MDS/RAI-Home Care; Roberto Bernabei (Catholic University of Rome, Rome Italy) Randomized Trials of the RAI-HC in Italy: A Prelude to the EU Study; Palmi V. Jsnsson (The Landspitali University Hospital, Reykjavik Iceland) A Pilot Test of the RAI-Home Care in Reykjavik; John P. Hirdes (University of Waterloo and Providence Centre, Toronto Canada) Quality Indicators for Home Care based on the RAI-Home Care; Naoki Ikegami (Keio University, Tokyo Japan)

ISSUE: Comprehensive geriatric assessment has been recognized as a fundamental tool that can be used to identify and respond to the needs of the frail elderly. However, until recently it has been difficult to engage in cross-national home care research because of the lack of comparable assessment systems in different countries. STRUCTURE: Various members of interRAI, a 20-country research network, will report on the results of research related to the RAI-Home Care (RAI-HC) in Canada, Iceland, Italy, Japan and USA. The RAI-HC is a comprehensive assessment instrument that directly supports the development of person-specific care plans through its Clinical Assesment Protocols (CAPs). The RAI-HC has also been designed to support case-mix based funding, outcome measurement, quality improvement and eligibility determination. CONTENT: The presentations will focus on various multinational research efforts to test, implement and develop new applications for the RAI-HC. These include validation studies, randomized clinical trials, pilot implementations and secondary analyses of MDS-HC data in jurisdictions where the instrument has been fully implemented. ANTICIPATED OUTCOMES: The symposium will demonstrate the RAI-HC's effectiveness as an assessment tool to support both clinical practice and research in home care internationally based on the interRAI experience.

A Pilot Test of the RAI-Home Care in Reykjavik

P.V. Jsnsson, H. Gupmundsdsttir, F. Fripbjvrnsdsttir, M. Haraldsdsttir, Slafsdsttir, A.B. Jensdsttir, H.Palsson, I. Hjaltadsttir, S. Harparson (The IceRAI study group - The Landspitali University Hospital, University of Iceland School of Medicine, Ministry of Health, Reykjavik, Iceland)

PURPOSE: Increasingly the frail elderly rely on home care. However, their needs are not well defined. We utilized the RAI-Home Care instrument to gather descriptive data on elderly people in home care in 4 community health centers in Reykjavik METHOD: Home care professionals assessed 257 individuals, 65 years of age and older who received home care in the autumn of 1997. The sample was comprised of 55 males and 202 women with a mean age of 82.7 years. RESULT: Short term memory deficits affected 36.7% of the individuals and depression was seen in 18%. Twenty one percent of clients were lonesome and 27% were always alone during the day. About 40 to 60% needed substantial help with IADL. Almost all were independent in ADL, but 53% needed assistance with bathing. Eighteen percent had not been out of doors for the last 30 days. Daily pain was seen in 47%, and the same proportion assessed their health as poor. Formal care was on average provided for 12.6 hours per 2 weeks. Medication intake was considerable: 34% took more than 9 medications. CONCLUSIONS: The RAI-HC provides a comprehensive, multidimensional view of the needs of the frail elderly receiving home care.

An Overview of the Development and Application of the MDS/RAI-Home Care

John N. Morris (Hebrew Rehabilitation Center for the Aged, Boston, USA);

PURPOSE: This presentation provides an overview of the on-going multinational efforts to develop and refine the MDS/RAI-Home Care (RAI-HC) and it discusses the applications of the RAI-HC including care-planning, resource allocation, outcome measurement and quality improvement. METHOD: The first version of the RAI-HC was developed by the interRAI group in 1997. Reliability was established through a 5-country study in which dual independent assessments were done on about 900 home care clients. Version 2 of the RAI-HC was released in 1999. Its Clinical Assessment Protocols (CAPs) were refined be evaluating their predictive validity for outcomes of interest (e.g, falls, institutionalization). Other research has established criterion validity against scales like the MMSE, Barthel and OARS IADL. Recently, a new 40-item screener has been developed for use in conjunction with the RAI-HC in order to identify persons in need of comprehensive geriatric assessment. RESULTS & CONCLUSIONS: The RAI-HC has been shown to be reliable and valid through extensive testing in North America, Europe and the Pacific Rim. The instrument can be used to create person-specific care-plans in a way that improves the likelihood of positive outcomes in a cost-effective manner.

Quality Indicators for Home Care based on the RAI-Home Care

John P. Hirdes (University of Waterloo and Providence Centre, Toronto Canada), Brant E. Fries (University of Michigan and Ann Arbor VA Medical Center, Ann Arbor USA), John N. Morris (Hebrew Rehabilitation Center for the Aged, Boston USA), Naoki Ikegami (Keio University, Tokyo Japan), David Zimmerman (Center for Health Services Research and Analysis, Madison USA), Dawn Dalby (University of Waterloo, Waterloo Canada), Suzanne Hammer (University of Michigan, Ann Arbor)

PURPOSE: The transition from institutional to community based care is a global trend. With the rapid expansion of home care services, there is a need to evaluate and monitor the quality of care to be sure that acceptable standards are met and quality improves on a continuous basis. METHOD: Researchers and clinicians from Canada, USA and Japan collaborated to develop and test a series of quality indicators for home care based on data available from the RAI-Home Care. These indicators included incidence and prevalence measures that deal with both the process and outcomes of care. Extensive consultation with home care professionals and researchers in Canada and the US provided one level of evaluation for the draft Home Care Quality Indicators (HCQIs). Michigan's MI CHOICE program (n~4,000) and a 14 city study of Community Care Access Centres in Ontario (n~2,000) provided data to test the distributional properties of the HCQIs. RESULT: HCQIs were developed for four main subgroups of home care clients: short stay/post-acute care, long term home care, palliative care and mental health. Not all HCQIs are used with every population, because of differences in the client populations and in the expected lengths of stay. Risk adjustments were developed whenever appropriate to ensure that comparisons across agencies are based on similar populations. CONCLUSIONS: The set of HCQIs developed by interRAI can be used by any home care agency employing the RAI-HC to benchmark the quality of home care on a regional, national or international basis.

Randomized Trials of the RAI-HC in Italy: A Prelude to the EU Study;

Roberto Bernabei (Catholic University of Rome, Rome Italy)

PURPOSE: This presentation deals with the standardisation of elderly care with a specific focus on home care. METHOD: The population characteristics and outcomes of more than 20 Italian Home Care Agencies that adopted a case management approach using the RAI-HC are examined. Moreover we collected data on structural/organisational characteristics of the Home Care Agencies to to understand their influence on the outcomes. In addition, a randomized clinical trial was conducted in which home care clients in Italy received either usual care or care based on the RAI-HC prior to its broad based implementation. RESULTS: Compared with home care clients in Canada and the United States, Italian home care clients are more cognitively impaired and have higher levels of ADL and IADL impairment based on the RAI-HC. Italian RCTs with the RAI-HC showed that it can significantly reduce health care costs (e.g, hospitalization) when used as a tool to support case management. Italian validation studies have shown that the RAI-HC is strongly correlated with industry gold standard scales for cognition and disability in home care clients. CONCLUSIONS: The promising findings related to the use of the RAI-HC in Italy have provided a basis for a new $1.5 US study of the instrument in 10 EU countries.

SESSION 432

Latest Data on the Efficacy and Treatment of Diabetes

Graydon S Meneilly (Professor and Head, Division of Geriatric Medicine University of British Columbia, Vancouver, BC Canada Title: Pathophysiology of Type II Diabetes in the Elderly) JaakkoTuomilehto (Professor and Head, Diabetes and Genetic Epidemiology Unit, Department of Epidemiology and Health Promotion Helsinki, Finland Title: Cardiovascular Risk Factors in Elderly Patients with Diabetes) Jeffrey Halter (Professor of Internal Medicine and Chief Division of Geriatric Medicine University of Michigan, Ann Arbor Michigan Title: Newer Therapies for Diabetes in the Elderly) Allan J Sinclair, Charles Hayward (Professor of Geriatric Medicine and Head of Department of Geriatric Medicine, University of Birmingham, Birmingham, England Title: Diabetes in Elderly Nursing Home Patients)

ISSUE: The symposium will address the pathophysiology and treatment of diabetes in the elderly. STRUCTURE: This session consists of four 20 minute talks which will outline important areas in the care of elderly patients with diabetes. CONTENT: Dr. Meneilly will discuss metabolic alterations which occur in elderly individuals with diabetes with particular reference to alterations in insulin release, insulin action and non insulin mediated glucose uptake. Professor Tuomilehto will discuss the effect of traditional cardiovascular risk factors such as hypertension and hyperlipidemia on the risk of cardiovascular disease in older people with diabetes as well as the benefits of interventions designed to reduce risk in these patients. Dr. Halter will discuss newer therapies for the treatment of diabetes in the elderly including the glitazones a new class of drugs which improve insulin resistance in patients with diabetes. Finally, Dr. Sinclair will discuss important aspects of diabetes in elderly nursing home patients including prevalence, clinical features and management issues. CONCLUSION: At the end of this session participants will have a greater understanding of the pathogenesis and treatment of diabetes in the elderly.

Cardiovascular Risk Factors in Elderly Patients with Diabetes

JaakkoTuomilehto, MpolSci, (Professor and Head, Diabetes and Genetic Epidemiology Unit, Department of Epidemiology and Health Promotion Helsinki, Finland)

PURPOSE: The purpose of this talk is to review the role of hyperglycemia and other cardiovascular risk factors on the risk of macrovascular events in older patients with diabetes. METHOD: Literature on the relationship between glucose levels, lipid levels and blood pressure on cardiovascular risk in the elderly was evaluated. RESULTS: Prospective epidemiologic studies suggest that improved glycemic control reduces the risk of macrovascular events in the elderly. In addition, recent data suggest that treatment of hypertension and hyperlipidemia may also reduce the risk of macrovascular events in the elderly. CONCLUSION: Physicians looking after elderly patients with diabetes should focus not only on blood sugar levels but also on modification of cardiovascular risk factors

Diabetes in Elderly Nursing Home Patients

Professor Allan J Sinclair (Charles Haywardof Geriatric Medicine and Head of Department of Geriatric Medicine, University of Birmingham, Birmingham, England)

PURPOSE: The purpose is to describe clinical features and treatment issues regarding elderly nursing home patients with diabetes. METHOD: The literature on elderly nursing home patients with diabetes will be reviewed in detail. RESULTS: This talk will address the incidence of diabetes in elderly nursing home patients; the clinical features of elderly nursing home patients with diabetes and contrast those to community dwelling elderly patients; and management issues in elderly nursing home patients with diabetes. CONCLUSION: There are many unique features in elderly nursing home patients with diabetes.

Newer Therapies for Diabetes in the Elderly

Jeffrey Halter FACP, (Professor of Internal Medicine and Chief Division of Geriatric Medicine University of Michigan, Ann Arbor Michigan)

PURPOSE: To review the role of newer therapies in the treatment of diabetes in the elderly. METHOD: The literature on newer therapies for diabetes in the elderly was reviewed. RESULTS: Recent data suggests that newer therapies such as alpha glucosadase inhibitors, insulin sensitizers such as the glitazones and newer drugs which stimulate insulin secretion have a role to play in the treatment of selected elderly individuals. CONCLUSION: Newer therapies will increasingly be used in the management of diabetes in the elderly.

t- Physiology of Type II Diabetes in the Elderly

Graydon S Meneilly, (Professor and Head, Division of Geriatric Medicine University of British Columbia, Vancouver, BC, Canada)

PURPOSE: To Review the Pathophysiology of Diabetes in the Elderly METHOD: Literature on Pathophysiology of Diabetes in the Elderly was reviewed RESULTS: In lean elderly patients there is minimal resistance insulin mediated glucose disposal. The principle defect is an impairment in glucose induced insulin secretion. In obese elderly patients glucose induced insulin secretion is relatively well preserved but there is marked resistance to insulin mediated glucose disposal. Both lean and obese elderly patients have impairments in non insulin mediated glucose disposal which may contribute to their elevated glucose levels. CONCLUSION: In lean elderly patients therapeutic intervention should focus on increasing endogenous insulin secretion or replacing the endogenous insulin deficit. In obese elderly patients with diabetes therapeutic efforts should focus should be on reversing the insulin resistance.

SESSION 433

Cultural Aspects of Quality of Life in Dementia Care

Atwood D. Gaines, MPH (Case Western Reserve U, Cleveland,OH, USA). Whose Quality, Whose Life?: Cultural Issues in Dementia Pharmacotherapy and Caregiving. Janice Graham, (UBC, Vancouver, BC, Canada)). If Meaning Counted: Measuring E/Affect in Antidementia Therapies. JoAnn Perry, (UBC, Vancouver, BC, Canada). The Care-Cure Tension in the Context of Quality of Life for Older Adults with Dementia. Peter Whitehouse, (Case Western Reserve U, Cleveland, OH, USA). Living and Measuring: Western Notions of Quality of Life and How to Measure It.

ABSTRACT Quality of life is an important concept in measuring the outcomes of health interventions. It has received more attention recently in the area of dementia care. Drug interventions are driving the process in part because of several cholinesterase inhibitors that have similar but subtle differences in mechanism of action. Associated clinical differences may be discovered by examining broad therapeutic outcomes such as quality of life. Concerns about interventions to slow progression of disease or even prevent Alzheimer Disease also raise issues about stage-specific quality of life. Pharmacoeconomic considerations are causing us to ask questions about the costs to society for improvements in quality of life. This symposium's interdisciplinary group consider quality of life as an important part of the social conversation about Alzheimer Disease, conversations that should include all participants from persons affected by these conditions to their families, communities, health care providers, and policy makers. Within the concept of quality of life panelists consider cultural, semantic (meaning), ethical and economic issues as well as important clinical and medical ones. Different societies see concepts related to quality of life through the eyes of their respective mythical and cultural traditions. Understanding the range of variation possible in different cultures and through different historical periods will enrich our opportunities to consider deeply the issues of quality of life and meaning of life that affect older people with dementia now and in the future and in different cultures.

SESSION 434

Comparative Analysis of the Prevalence of Depressive Symptoms in Japan, Sweden, and the United States

Kristen Suthers [University of Southern California, Los Angeles, USA] Yasuhiko Saito [Nihon University, Tokyo, Japan] Margaret Gatz [University of Southern California, Los Angeles, USA] Eileen Crimmins [University of Southern California, Los Angeles, USA]

PURPOSE: This paper provides a comparative analysis of depressive symptoms in adults aged 65 and over in Japan, Sweden, and the United States. Symptoms are compared by age group, as well as gender. METHOD: Items from the Center for Epidemiological Studies-Depression Scale (CES-D), were used to compare the prevalence of six depressive symptoms across Japan, Sweden and the United States. In Japan, data were analyzed from the Nihon University Japanese Longitudinal Study of Aging (NUJLSOA). In Sweden, data were analyzed from the Swedish Adoption Twin Study of Aging (SATSA). In the United States, data were analyzed from the Assets and Health Dynamics of the Oldest Old (AHEAD) longitudinal study. RESULTS: There is a strong similarity across countries in the type of depressive symptoms which are most frequent. Sleep disturbance is ranked high in all three countries, while reporting sadness or depressed mood is low. There is, however, some subtle variability between countries, whereas Japanese older adults were more likely to report loneliness, while greater numbers of Swedish older adults reported difficulty in getting oneself going. Cross-sectional results indicate that the frequency of depressive symptoms increases slightly across age groups in all three countries. Gender differences in depressive symptoms exist within all countries, however, this difference is greatest within the United States; the gender difference within Japan and Sweden is smaller and similar between these two countries. CONCLUSIONS: These international comparisons suggest that across these three countries there are more similarities than differences in depressive symptom profiles.

Deconstructing depression

Michael Stones (Lakehead University, Canada)

The psychiatric diagnosis of depression includes two main axes of anhedonia and dysphoria. The purpose of this paper is to explore differences in risk factors on each axis as they relate to age. The data are from English-speaking households in the Manulife Health Styles Survey. This survey is representative of Canadian households in 1999, with a response rate over 60 0.000000or the sample to be described. The findings indicate relative prevalence rates for depression, anhedonia, and dysphoria approximating a 1:2:4 ratio. Risk factors differentiating the axes include gender, which is associated more with dysphoria than anhedonia. Risk factors common to both axes include physical activity. The risk factors showed low interactions with age. The conclusions are that depression is not a homogenous contruct, but can be differentiated into two main types with different risk factors.

Depression in nursing homes

Gil P. Gregorio, Alonso P, Sánchez-Guevara A, Osuna C, Fariñas F. (Geriatrics Service; Hospital Clínico San Carlos. Madrid. Spain.) and ENERA Study (Pfizer).

AIMS: To analyze types, medical antecedents, precipitant factors and drug therapy of depression in nursing homes. METHODS: 1116 patients with depressive syndrome according to DSM-IV criteria were included in the study. DSM-IV classification of depression was used. The following data were collected: age, gender, period of disease progression, previous medical history, type of depression, Geriatric Depression Scale, related diseases, precipitant factors, functional assessment, treatment and drug response. Data base SPSS, statistical measurement of common tendency and dispersion and quantity comparative data t-student (confidence interval 95%). RESULTS: 1116 patients (mean age: 81.4 +/- 6.2; women: 72.4%). Type of depression: major depression 34.6%; dysthymia 32.2%; adjustment disorders 18.8%; mood disorders due to general conditions 16.2%. Most frequent precipitant factors were: mood disorder due to general conditions 48%, admittance in nursing home 22%, uncomplicated bereavement 16.5%. Therapy response was favourable in 70% of the patients. Major depression Dysthymia Adjustment disorders Men 31.9 20.3 20.6 Women 35.5 25 18 CONCLUSIONS: 1- The most frequent type of depression in nursing homes is major depression. 2- To suffer a disease and to be admitted in a nursing home are the more frequent immediate causes of depression. 3- Women suffer more frequently major depression and dysthymia.

High prevalence of Depression Among Estonian Older Population

K. Saks, H. Kolk (Department of Internal Medicine, University of Tartu, Tartu, Estonia), K. Jaanson (Mental Health Care Center, Tartu, Estonia), E. Tiit, E. Käärik (Institute of Mathematical Statistics, University of Tartu, Tartu, Estonia)

PURPOSE: Depression among elderly people could be high and undertreated in a society experiencing socio-economical transition. METHODS: A cross-sectional study was undertaken. A sample of persons 65+ (N=1000) was connected to the sample of general practitioners (GP;N=200) which was formed from the list of GP's through random numbers generator. Each GP interviewed five persons using an individual regulation for selection of subjects quaranteering the randomless of the sample. Questionnaires for GP's and older persons, Mini Mental State Examination (MMSE) and Geriatric Depression Scale (GDS, short version) were used. Data from 811 seniors were returned. Population estimates were calculated. RESULTS: GDS was above 5 points in 400f older persons (in 53% among persons 85+). Antidepressants were used by 50f elderly people. The best linear model for prognosing GDS score by questionnaire data contained the following variables: self-prognosis of the health status during next year, number of hobbies, number of functional complaints limiting everyday activity and the score of MMSE (all p's<0.0001), satisfaction with life (p=0.0017), self-assessment of the coping with everyday life (p=0.0091). The multiple R-square of the model was 42.7%. Such variables as the number of diagnosed illnesses, self-assessment of the health status, need for assistance in everyday life, number of regularly used medications but also employment status, self-assessment of the economic status, urban or rural location and sex were rather weakly correlated with GDS score and did not improve the model. CONCLUSIONS: Depression is a widespread, undertreated and multifactorial problem of Estonian elderly population.

Validating the SF-36 among older women with psychiatric diseases in Sweden - results from two population studies in Göteborg.

Silveira, E. (Department of Geriatric Medicine, Göteborg University, S-411 33, Göteborg, Sweden), Skoog, I. (Department of Psychiatry, Göteborg University) Sundh, V. (Department of

Geriatric Medicine, Göteborg University, Göteborg, Sweden), Taft, C. (Health Care Research Unit, Institute of Internal Medicine, Sahlgrenska University Hospital, Göteborg University), Palsson, S, Waern, M. (Department of Psychiatry, Göteborg University) Steen, B. (Department of Geriatric Medicine, Göteborg University, Göteborg, Sweden)

Introduction: Increases in population ageing world-wide lead to a higher demand for reliable cross-culturally validated health measures. The SF-36 has been shown to be a valid measure of general health in studies in Swedish older people. However, some of its components were found to be more related to mental health in Sweden than in U.S. studies, which is suggestive of cultural differences. There have been no detailed studies in Sweden on use of SF-36 mental health scores as a screening tool for psychiatric diseases (depression) in people aged 65 years and above. Purpose: To assess the validity and specificity of recommended SF-36 cut-offs i.e. mental health scale (MH-5) and mental component summary (MCS) scores against clinical diagnosis of depression in women from different age groups compared with "controls" in Göteborg, Sweden. Method: A total of 614 women (born in 1922, 1918, 1914 and 1908) interviewed in 1992 using a psychiatric interview schedule derived from the Montgomery-Åsberg Depression Rating Scale applied by psychiatrists as part of a large screening interview, the Comprehensive Psychopatological Rating Scale. Sixty-nine were diagnosed with depression (161 in total had any psychiatric disease). Additional data comprised SF-36 and other physical and social status measures. Results: The specificity of recommended cut-offs in the MH-5 and MCS (i.e. scores of 52 and 42) for diagnosis of depression (total sample) was 90.7% and 79.8%; sensitivity was 58% and 74.2%. No significant linear relationship was found between age and (low) scores either in MH-5 or MCS. Both the MH-5 and MCS were predictors of depression. However, variations in sensitivity and specificity were observed in the different samples despite similarities in prevalence of psychiatric disease. Conclusion: Overall, results seem to confirm the validity of SF-36 measures of mental health for diagnosis of depression in older women in Sweden despite variations in sensitivity and specificity.

Validating the SF-36 among older women with psychiatric diseases in Sweden - results from two population studies in Göteborg.

Silveira, E. (Department of Geriatric Medicine, Göteborg University, S-411 33, Göteborg, Sweden), Skoog, I. (Department of Psychiatry, Göteborg University) Sundh, V. (Department of Geriatric Medicine, Göteborg University, Göteborg, Sweden), Taft, C. (Health Care Research Unit, Institute of Internal Medicine, Sahlgrenska University Hospital, Göteborg University), Palsson, S, Waern, M. (Department of Psychiatry, Göteborg University) Steen, B. (Department of Geriatric Medicine, Göteborg University, Göteborg, Sweden)

Introduction: Increases in population ageing world-wide lead to a higher demand for reliable cross-culturally validated health measures. The SF-36 has been shown to be a valid measure of general health in studies in Swedish older people. However, some of its components were found to be more related to mental health in Sweden than in U.S. studies, which is suggestive of cultural differences. There have been no detailed studies in Sweden on use of SF-36 mental health scores as a screening tool for psychiatric diseases (depression) in people aged 65 years and above. Purpose: To assess the validity and specificity of recommended SF-36 cut-offs i.e. mental health scale (MH-5) and mental component summary (MCS) scores against clinical diagnosis of depression in women from different age groups compared with "controls" in Göteborg, Sweden. Method: A total of 614 women (born in 1922, 1918, 1914 and 1908) interviewed in 1992 using a psychiatric interview schedule derived from the Montgomery-Åsberg Depression Rating Scale applied by psychiatrists as part of a large screening interview, the Comprehensive Psychopatological Rating Scale. Sixty-nine were diagnosed with depression (161 in total had any psychiatric disease). Additional data comprised SF-36 and other physical and social status measures. Results: The specificity of recommended cut-offs in the MH-5 and MCS (i.e. scores of 52 and 42) for diagnosis of depression (total sample) was 90.7% and 79.8%; sensitivity was 58% and 74.2%. No significant linear relationship was found between age and (low) scores either in MH-5 or MCS. Both the MH-5 and MCS were predictors of depression. However, variations in sensitivity and specificity were observed in the different samples despite similarities in prevalence of psychiatric disease. Conclusion: Overall, results seem to confirm the validity of SF-36 measures of mental health for diagnosis of depression in older women in Sweden despite variations in sensitivity and specificity.

SESSION 435

Disability Prevention in Older Patients: The Pro-Age Study

Kharicha K, Iliffe S, (RFUCLMS, London, England) Swift C, (Kings College London, England) Meier-Baumgartner HP (Albertinenhaus Klinik, Hamburg, Germany), Stuck AE (University of Bern, Switzerland)

PURPOSE The population in all industrialized nations continues to grow older. Growing evidence indicates that the cost-effectiveness of timely therapeutic and preventive interventions in late life is at least as great as it is in younger people (or greater). This study compares the self-reported health behaviours, health care needs, and risk factors in older populations, in three European regions using the Health Risk Appraisal for Older persons (HRA-O) instrument. METHODS: A pilot study was carried out in three different health care systems in Europe (Switzerland, Germany and UK). Postal questionnaires were sent to all eligible patients, aged 65+, resulting in a sample of 213 in Switzerland, 149 in Hamburg and 235 in England. Questions derived from evidence based data covered health and disability risk factors which are known to be associated with a high yield for possible change. RESULTS: Differences in health behaviour and risk factors were found both between study populations and within study populations when stratified by age (65 - 74 and 75+). Key areas in which differences were found between areas include: nutrition, alcohol misuse, incontinence, depression, memory loss and uptake of preventive services. Associations were found between self-reported health behaviours and socio-economic factors. CONCLUSIONS: The HRA-O is a promising tool for identifying health and disability risk factors, cross-culturally in this age group. Findings from this pilot are used a basis for a newly started multi-centre randomised control study investigating whether risk factors for disability can be improved with an intervention based on HRA-O and health education in generalists' practices.

Fluctuating disability rather than progressive decline revealed by frequent re-assessment

I.P.Donald

A longitudinal study of disability (Study A) was conducted in the context of annual health checks for over 75 s in Primary Care. A subsequent intervention study (Study B) compared targeted nurse visiting with usual care. Disabled subjects in the intervention group received 4-monthly assessments over 1 year. Both studies used the Elderly At Risk Rating Scale (Donald IP, J Epidemiol Comm Hlth 1997;51:558-63) for the assessment of disability, defined as scoring >34. Functional change was defined as a move of at least 6 points (Donald IP, MD, Cambridge Univ, UK). In Study A, 1815 subjects were recruited, and 798 were seen in the final year. Study B included 4,865 subjects, and 442 with disability received repeated assessments. In Study A, 18% had functional decline, 2% functional gain, and 25% died over 3 years. However, each year 18.2% declined and 6.7% improved, while 8% died. In Study B, similar figures were seen at 1 year (17%,7%, and 9.4% respectively). For those with baseline disability, in Study A 17.8% further declined, 15.2% improved, and 18.7% died each year, while in Study B 12.5% declined, 12.1% improved, and 4.4% died every 4 months. Functional instability was constant during the course of each study, and associated with age, initial disability, and low energy. In conclusion, the magnitude of fluctuations in disability is related to the frequency of re-assessments, and is far larger than implied by studies over 2 or 3 years. Future work could understand factors that enhance functional stability.

Multiple Pathology and Tails of Disability

S. Matsushita (Shourakudo Social Welfare Hospital, Tokyo, Japan), M. Matsushita, H. Itou (Chuo University, Tokyo, Japan), R. Takahashi (Tokyo Metropolitan Institute of Gerontology, Tokyo, Japan), T. Ozawa, and K. Kuramoto (Tokyo Metropolitan Geriatric Hospital, Tokyo, Japan)

Disability is a serious issue in longevity. However its basic properties have not been identified besides increasing proportion and duration with advancing age. To unravel its fundamental nature and predict countermeasures we analyzed statistical properties of its duration and the effect of diseases obtained from the case records of the Tokyo Metropolitan Geriatric Hospital which is representative of the aged in the northwest of Tokyo. Duration of disability in transfer (mean 2.2 years) and voiding (mean 1.4 years) was assessed in 1017 cases (550 men, 467 women, mean age at death 79.3, range 41-104, average 3.7 diseases/ patient). Log number of patients (np) vs square of (age-mean) plots, log cumulative np vs log days plots, and multiple regression analysis were used for analysis. We found 1) duration of each disability showed log-normal distribution equivalent to the outcome of serial independent events and mimicked power distribution (npth degree of days, =1.4) or first passage time distribution of one-dimensional Brownian motion for 30-1000 days, 2) competing risk with multiple pathology diversely affected duration of disability, and 3) agewise np in disability showed a Gaussian distribution in accord with the central limit theorem since it is a summation of multiple pathology. While long tails like log-normal, power, or first passage time distribution identify disability as a step-wise stochastic process ubiquitous in nature, for example, phase transition, fragmentation of materials, and earthquakes, agewise bell-shaped distribution predicts a reduction in the amount of disability with postponing its onset and reducing premature rectangularization of disability-free survival curve.

Self-assessed energy provides a rapid predictor tool for survival and functional change

I.P.Donald, C.J.Bulpitt (Imperial College School of Medicine, London, UK)

Longitudinal studies of ageing have demonstrated the relation of self-rated health to outcomes. Expanding the assessment to a 5-point hierarchical scale could improve predictive power. A 3 year longitudinal study of disability on 1815 subjects was conducted in the context of annual health checks for over 75 s in Primary Care. The study used the 20 item Elderly At Risk Rating Scale (Donald IP, J Epidemiol Comm Hlth 1997;51:558-63) including one question on energy, for the assessment of disability. Functional change was defined as a move of at least 6 points (Donald IP, MD, Cambridge Univ, UK). Logistic regression was employed, adjusted by age and sex, with 95% confidence intervals. At baseline, 43% rated energy as average, 22% boundless, 22% limited, 9% very limited, and 4% none. All adverse outcomes showed a linear relation to the energy rating, and this item provided a greater range of relative risks than any other item. Using average energy as reference, boundless energy conferred reduced mortality (RR 0.7, CI 0.5-0.9), greatly reduced admission to care (RR 0.12, CI 0.02-0.9), and reduced functional decline (RR 0.62, CI 0.42-0.9) at 1 year. "No energy" conferred increased mortality (RR 9.9, CI 5.3-18.6), increased admission to care (RR 1.8, CI 0.5-6.7) and greater functional decline (RR 3.1, CI 1.1-8.3). In multiple regression, energy remained an independent predictor of all adverse outcomes. In conclusion, assessment of energy is strongly recommended in clinical practice, as its presence or absence provides strong predictive information, combined with an overall assessment of disability.

The determinants of locomotor disability

Shah Ebrahim (University of Bristol, Bristol, UK) Goya Wannamethee (University of London, London, UK) Olia Papacosta (University of London, UK)

Purpose. Reducing the prevalence of disability in old age requires an understanding of its causes. We examined the relationship between life-style and social factors measured at baseline in determining locomotor disability 12-14 years later. Method. Using data from the British Regional Heart Study, a cohort of 7735 men aged 40-59 at baseline in 1978-80, locomotor disability was assessed by postal questionnaire among 5717 men (880f survivors) based on ability to get outdoors, walk 400m, climb stairs, maintain balance, bend down, or straighten up. Results. At mean age 63 years, 250f the men reported locomotor disability. Lifestyle factors at screening (smoking, physical inactivity, obesity, heavy drinking) and manual social class were strongly and independently associated with increased odds of locomotor disability 12-14 years later. Surprisingly, blood cholesterol and blood pressure showed little relationship with locomotor disability. These findings appeared to be independent of diagnosed chronic diseases (ischaemic heart disease, stroke, chronic airways disease, arthritis). Conclusion. Lifestyle in middle-age is a strong predictor of disability later in life regardless of chronic disease. Leading a healthy lifestyle improves survival and reduces the incidence of disease. Healthy lifestyle also increases the odds of being-disability-free even in the event of developing major cardiovascular disease.

SESSION 436

Colorectal Cancer Screening

Davidovic Mladen, Bojic B, Milosevic D, Djurica S, Trailov D, Peric G, Stevic R, Mihajlovic G. (Clinical Institute of Geriatric Medicine, Beograd,Yugoslavia)

The reason for lack of improvement in survival is that in most cases of carcinoma coli ,the disease has already reached an advanced stage by the time of diagnosis. Therefore, the main goal of screening is to discover CC in early stage when successful radical treatment is possible. The aim of the study was the correlation between three groups of elderly individuals.One of 134 asymptomatic hospitalized persons(without symptoms of large intestines) , second of 405 old person in home for the aged(22 with symptoms of colon disorders) and third of 1512 rectosigmoidoscopy(53 polyps, 24 >65yr,6 agreement for endoscopy) . We have detected one cancer and 12 polyps in first group , 1 polyp in second group(with only nine agreement for the endoscopy) and none recidiv of polyp in the third group. We have selected three groups of elderly persons. The first one was the group of asymptomatic individuals(regarding digestive tract) hospitalised at our institute. The answer to the screening was optimal but it is really difficult to obtain such results in majority of the old population .The second trial was more selective. We have included in our endoscopy proposition only the persons with digestive disorders,after the assesment procedure in home for the aged. There was very low percentage of agreement to the endoscopy. And finally, we have reselected the elderly persons with previously diagnosed colon polyps to the control endoscopy. Only the 25% of the group was able for the control rectosigmoidoscopy.

Colorectal Cancer Screening

Davidovic Mladen, Bojic B, Milosevic D, Djurica S, Trailov D, Peric G, Stevic R, Mihajlovic G. (Clinical Institute of Geriatric Medicine, Beograd,Yugoslavia)

The reason for lack of improvement in survival is that in most cases of carcinoma coli ,the disease has already reached an advanced stage by the time of diagnosis. Therefore, the main goal of screening is to discover CC in early stage when successful radical treatment is possible. The aim of the study was the correlation between three groups of elderly individuals.One of 134 asymptomatic hospitalized persons(without symptoms of large intestines) , second of 405 old person in home for the aged(22 with symptoms of colon disorders) and third of 1512 rectosigmoidoscopy(53 polyps, 24 >65yr,6 agreement for endoscopy) . We have detected one cancer and 12 polyps in first group , 1 polyp in second group(with only nine agreement for the endoscopy) and none recidiv of polyp in the third group. We have selected three groups of elderly persons. The first one was the group of asymptomatic individuals(regarding digestive tract) hospitalised at our institute. The answer to the screening was optimal but it is really difficult to obtain such results in majority of the old population .The second trial was more selective. We have included in our endoscopy proposition only the persons with digestive disorders,after the assesment procedure in home for the aged. There was very low percentage of agreement to the endoscopy. And finally, we have reselected the elderly persons with previously diagnosed colon polyps to the control endoscopy. Only the 25% of the group was able for the control rectosigmoidoscopy.

Cost and Effectiveness of the Elderly Health Examination Program: Example of Hypertension Screening

H.C. Chiu B.H. Dang, L.W. Mau (Graduate Institute of Public Health, Kaohsiung Medical University, Taiwan), H.W. Liu (Department of Family Medicine, Kaohisung Medical University Chung-Ho Memorial Hospital, Taiwan)

The National Health Insurance (NHI) and social welfare agencies have implemented older adult health screening program for years. The purpose of this study was to explore the cost effectiveness of older adult health screening program by using the example of hypertension screening. Panel cohort study design was used for this study. Data sources were: 1) health screening information of older adults who had attended the 1995 and 1996 Health Examination Programs; 2) claim data of the National Health Insurance Program. Hypothetical models were developed to evaluate the cost and effectiveness of the screening program in different conditions. Sensitivity analysis also was used to evaluate the effect of each estimation indicator on the cost and effectiveness. There were 26,583 participants (26% of the eligible older adults) attending the health screening program in 1995. Among them, 15,531 participated the program in the next year (1996), had a retention rate of 58.24%. The incidence rate of hypertension was 6.6%. The ideal model implied that each early identified hypertension patient who had attended the health screening program not only saved medical expenses to US$104 but also prolonged the life for additional 128 days. The results indicated that health screening program was truly cost-effectiveness. More promotions for similar health examination programs are recommended. The implications of the findings are useful for health and social welfare policy planning for older adults. The budget for health care and social welfare of older adults should be relocated for preventive medicine.

Performance Rates of Mammograms among Elderly Women in Israel following Health Care Reform

Netta Bentur, and Revital Gross, (JDCΔBrookdale Institute of Gerontology and Human Development, Jerusalem, Israel)

Israel's National Health Insurance (NHI) Law, implemented in 1995, stipulates that women aged 50-75 are entitled to mammograms once every two years. Prior to the law's implementation, the health plans were entitled to determine whether or not to perform mammograms, in accordance with the basket of services they provided. Purposes: To monitor changes in performance rates of mammograms among elderly women in Israel since the law's enactment, to compare them to the patterns of younger women, and to identify the characteristics of those unlikely to undergo the tests. Methods: The survey is part of a comprehensive study examining the impact of the NHI Law on the Israeli population. For the purposes of the survey, three cross-sectional telephone surveys were conducted - at the end of 1995, at the end of 1997 and at the end of 1999 - among a random sample of adult residents of Israel. Results: The findings show that at the end of 1995, 28% of elderly women (65+) reported having had a mammogram during the past two years before the interview. In 1997, the percentage rose to 37% and in 1999, to 50%. While a small percentage of elderly women in the three surveys reported having had a mammogram more than two years ago, in 1999 almost half of the women had never had one. The proportion of younger women (aged 50-64) who had had mammograms was higher in all three surveys and was also found to be on the rise. Conclusion: While the performance rate of mammograms rose among older women, it is still low compared to younger women. Therefore, it is important to continue to promote the performance of screening tests among them and to continue monitoring them.

Prostate Cancer Screening for Older Men Among Primary Care Physicians

Jessica L. Harden, MPH (Houston Department of Health and Human Services, Houston/ City & Country Harris County Area Agency on Aging, Houston, Texas, USA)

PURPOSE: To identify the determinants of prostate-specific antigen (PSA) test and digital rectal examinations (DRE) used in prostate cancer screening by primary care physicians. METHODS: Sixty two articles were identified, meeting the following criteria: (1) published since 1987, (2) contain information on practices of primary care physicians in the United States, including age, gender and type of practice (not just their knowledge, attitudes or beliefs), (3) data related to the classification of preventive activities: early detection of disease (cancer screening). To create structure for this review, two different matrix of correlates to prostate cancer screening were developed. Data sources included physicians, and records of physicians? activities, such as charts, medical records and direct surveys of physician?s practices, questionnaires mailed in by physicians, articles reporting on the cumulative search of the subject. RESULTS: We found barriers to cancer prevention services were attitudes, beliefs and practices of patients and physicians.. Several studies tested patients on their knowledge and beliefs regarding prostate cancer and whether or not they would avail themselves to screening tests if offered, over 75% lacked correct knowledge about the disease. Payment for test was not a barrier, despite differences in socioeconomic status. Several factors were significantly related to physician?s use of PSA tests:conflicting cancer screening guidelines, lack of up-dated information through continuing education, inaccurate reports of actual screenings or referrals, time restraints and forgetfulness were barrier among single-practice physicians, however automated reminders systems significantly increased screenings. Patients relied more on primary care physician?s advice for screening(27% of studies) than self knowledge.

Uptake of Breast Cancer Screening Among Older People

Nia Edwards, Dee Jones

Current breast screening policy restricts routine invitation for mammography to women under 65 years-despite higher incidence and mortality of breast cancer amongst women aged over 65 years The aim of the study was to establish breast screening uptake history amongst older women and to ascertain their potential uptake of screening if invited . Method:A random sample of 1604 women,aged over 65 were interviewed at home regarding previous screening uptake and if they would attend if invited. Health and social characteristics were established using validated measures. Results: Response rate was 94%; 120 (8%) respondents had previously been screened - of these 63(16%) were aged 65 - 69 , 46 (6%) were aged 70 - 79 and 11(3%) were >80 . Married women (or widows) had a significantly higher acceptance rate compared with single women ($p<0.001$). More women in social class ! & II accepted screening than !!!& IV. Of previous non-attenders 853 (54%) would attend if offered and more younger than older women would attend ((287 (72%) aged 65-69years, 454 (56%), aged 70-79 years and 112(29%) aged >80)). Those who were prepared to accept were significantly less likely to be lonely or depressed but more likely to be anxious ($p<0.001$). Potential attenders were also less disabled($p<0.001$). Conclusion: Our study mirrors the results of ohers who report an annual uptake of 76% amongst women aged 65 - 69 years invited for breast screening . It would therefore appear unjustifiable to exclude women >65 from screening on the basis of low uptake rates. Categories of women need to be targeted in order to achieve maximum uptake rates - lower social classes and single women. Needs of disabled people will also have to be taken into account.

SESSION 437

Clinical Significance of Plasma Homocysteine and Cystatin C Levels for the Assessment of Renal Function in Very Old Subjects

Bonacasa R, Muzzoni B, Casarotti D, Cravello L, Albertelli N, Solerte S.B, Fioravanti M, Ferrari E. (Department of Internal Medicine and Medical Therapy, Chair of Geriatrics, University of Pavia, Italy)

The aim of this study was to evaluate the predictive role of plasma homocysteine and cystatin C concentrations in physiological aging and in healthy centenarians. We studied two groups of subjects: 29 healthy old subjects (aged 73-84 ys, mean 77,5 ± 0,65 SEM) and 45 healthy centenarians (aged 100-106 ys, mean 101 ± 0.2 SEM). Old subjects had been admitted in hospital for minor somatic diseases or for the rehabilitation after bone fracture; healthy centenarians lived at home or in nursing homes. Nobody had clinical relevant renal pathologies; indeed the values of serum creatinine, uric acid and blood urea nitrogen were within normal limits. The concentration of both plasma homocystein and cystatin C was higher in centenarians, where compared to old subjects (homocysteine 24,3 vs 18,9 mmol/L $p < 0.5$ and cystatin C 1,7 vs 1,3 mg/L $p < 0.5$). In the whole group both homocystein and cystatin C were significantly correlated with serum creatinine ($p < 0.01$, $p < 0.001$), uric acid ($p < 0.5$, $p < 0.001$) and blood urea nitrogen ($p < 0.5$, $p < 0.001$). Furthermore a positive correlation with age was found for homocysteine levels ($p < 0.5$). These findings may suggest that the age related increase of plasma homocystein concentration together with the increased levels of cystatin C may be considered as useful screening tests of the renal function even in the extreme segment of life.

Dementia In Aged Hemodialysis Patients.

JP Charmes (1), T Dantoine (1), L Bernard Bourzeix (1), D Benevent (2), C Leroux-Robert (2) (1: Gerontology, 2: Nephrology departments, CHU, Limoges 87000, France)

Poor data are available concerning the prevalence of dementia in aged chronic renal failure patients although dementia is known to be one of the first causes of dialysis withdrawal. Methods: We studied 120 dialysis patients (87 hemodialysis patients (HD) [mean age (A): 68.9 ± 1.4 years, 48 males (M), 39 females (F)] and 33 peritoneal dialysis patients (PD) [A :74.7 ± 1.8 yrs, 16M,17F]). Cognitive assessment used Instrumental Ability Daily Life scale (IADL) and Mini Mental Score (MMS) and diagnosis criteria of dementia reffered to DSMIV, NINCDS/ADRDA, NINCD/AIREN. RESULTS:MMS decreased with age (MMS=34.1 - 0.11.Age ; r=0.42 ; p<0.001). MMS was less than 24 in 32 patients [20 HD (10F,10M) and 12 PD (5F,7H)]. Mild cognitive impairments (MCI) concerned 3 HD and 3 PD. Diagnosis of dementia was confirmed in 7 HD and 9 PD: 3 HD and 3 PD died before the end of the assessment, 3 HD and 2 PD suffered from Alzheimer s type dementia, 1 HD and 2 PD suffered from vascular dementia. In 2 PD, dementia was related to drugs toxicity. CONCLUSIONS:This study emphasizes that dementia diagnosis in old chronic renal failure patients is under-assessed even if dementia is a contra-indication of the treatment by dialysis. It is important to correctly explore this population to find out patients suffering from dementia: this would improve understanding of patients cognitive dysfunctions and could improve their outcome by sooner treatments. This also underlines the importance of the global geriatric assessment in old chronically ill patients.

Influence of Enalapril on Progression of Chronic Renal Failure in Older Adults

Biljana Stojimirovic (Clinic of Nephrology, Clinical Center of Serbia) Jasna Trbojevic (Dept of Internal Medicine, Clinical Center "Dragisa Misovic") Dejan M. Nesic (Institute of Physiology, School of Medicine, University of Belgrade)

Hypertension, which is often associated with chronic renal failure (CRF), speeds up the progression of the disease, while adequate control of arterial pressure slows down the progression of the illness. Thanks to their specific influence on glomerular hemodynamics and permeability, as well as on mesangial proliferation, ACE inhibitors are especially efficient in controlling the development of CRF. The aim of this study was to assess the influence of ACE inhibitor enalapril on the progression of CRF in elderly patients. We examined 36 elderly patients at the Clinic of Nephrology, Clinical Center of Serbia. The first group of 22 pts (12 females and 10 males, mean age 72.67) with CRF and hypertension were treated with enalapril, and 14 hypertensive patients (8 females and 6 males, mean age 76) with CRF in the second group were treated with other antihypertensive drugs. All patients were followed for 4 years (1997-2000). Blood pressure, serum protein, urea, creatinine and calcium, as well as creatinine clearance were measured on monthly basis. Progression of CRF was represented by the slope of the regression line showing reciprocal serum creatinine values. No statistically significant differences were found between the two groups in neither of the examined variables. Also, the difference between the slopes of regression lines representing the progression of CRF were not statistically different (-0.04025 vs -0.025). Contrary to its effects in younger adults, enalapril didn't have significant influence in slowing down the progression of CRF in older patients.

Outcome of Acute Renal Failure in the Elderly: A Hospital Based Prospective Study

M. Uddin (Health Care of Older People Directorate, Kent and Canterbury Hospital, Kent, UK), I. Sturgess (Health Care of Older People Directorate, Kent and Canterbury Hospital, Kent, UK), I. John (Department of Renal Medicine, Kent and Canterbury Hospital, Kent, UK), and P. Stevens (Department of Renal Medicine, Kent and Canterbury Hospital, Kent, UK).

PURPOSE The purpose of this study is to compare the etiology, interventions and outcomes of acute renal failure (ARF) in under and over 75 years age group. METHOD Prospective data were collected on all patients with ARF in the East Kent Health Authority Area between March 1997 and February 1998. A total of 291 patients presented with ARF as defined by the Renal Association and were divided into 2 groups. Group 1= under 75 Years, n= 133, mean age 62. Group 2= over 75 years, n= 158, mean age 82.2. RESULTS The mean creatinine at referral, group 1 and group 2 was 519.6 and 527.7 umol/l respectively. Group 1 Group 2 p-value Causes Iatrogenic 44(33%) 55(34%) 0.26 Preventable 20(15%) 28(17%) 0.32 Interventions Critical Care 41(30%) 8(5%) <0.001 Central Line 59(44%) 34(21%) <0.001 Renal Replacement Therapy 38(28%) 8(5%) <0.001 Outcomes Survival to Discharge 83(62%) 93(58%) 0.26 Survival 3Months 68(51%) 60(38%) 0.01 Survival 1Year 57(42%) 38(24%) <0.001 Renal Outcome in Survivors 57(69%) 65(75%) 0.43 Chronic Renal Failure 21(25%) 26(28%) 0.34 Renal Replacement Therapy 5(6%) 2(2%) 0.09 CONCLUSIONS There is no significant difference between iatrogenic and preventable causes in both groups. Patients over 75 age group received significantly less investigations and interventions. Although there was an increased mortality at three and twelve months in the over 75 years age group as would be expected, there was no significant difference in the survival outcome and renal outcome of the two groups during the acute illness.

Quality of Life in Elderly Patients - Influence of Chronic Renal Failure

Biljana Stojimirovic (Clinic of Nephrology, Clinical Center of Serbia) Jasna Trbojevic (Dept of Internal Medicine, Clinical Center "Dragisa Misovic") Dejan M. Nesic (Institute of

Physiology, School of Medicine, University of Belgrade)

The aim of this study was to evaluate the impact of progression of chronic renal failure (CRF) on life style of elderly patients. Health related quality of life (QL) aspects were studied in 46 persons (26 males and 21 females) treated at the Clinic of Nephrology, Clinical Center of Serbia. The first group comprised 30 adult patients (16 male and 14 female) with mean age 46.25, while the second consisted of 14 older adults patients (8 male and 6 female), mean age 71.85. They were all in the final stage of CRF (creatinine clearance less then 20 ml/min), receiving the necessary conservative therapy. Using an original questionnaire sixteen QL variables were investigated: marital status, family relations, working ability, sleep, tiring, appetite, wound healing, hobby, sports, friendships, sexual activity, mood, traveling, self management and happiness. The results have shown that the progress of the disease has negative influence on all life functions in both groups. Only the marital status and relations with family members weren't influenced by the illness. Statistically significant differences were observed only in tiring (older patients tire more easily, $p<0.05$) and working ability (more diminished in older patients, $p<0.05$). Although we expected the results to be worse in the group of elderly patients lack of more statistically significant differences between groups suggests that CRF worsens the quality of life regardless of person's age.

SESSION 438

Designing the urban environment to improve the quality of life of older people with dementia

L. Mitchell, E. Burton, M. Jenks (Oxford Centre for Sustainable Development, School of Architecture, Oxford Brookes University, Oxford, UK), T. Blackman (School of Social Sciences, University of Teeside, Middlesborough, UK)

This paper will present early findings from a three-year research project, funded by the Engineering and Physcial Sciences Research Council, which began in March 2000. The project is investigating how people with dementia perceive, understand and utilise the external environment in order to develop guidelines listing criteria to be considered in the design of more inclusive urban environments. A study sample of 50 older people with mild to moderate dementia, and a control group of 25 older people without dementia, are being interviewed about their perceptions and experience of the local external built environment.The paper will present preliminary findings from interviews conducted over the next six months, under the following headings: i) Activities, including purpose, frequency, length and duration of trips around the local external environment ii) Personal experience, including sense of enjoyment, fear, confusion or disorientation iii) Wayfinding, including mental mapping abilities, understanding of the environment and coping techniques when lost iv) Influential environmental features, including how street layouts, pavements, road crossings, signs, public facilities, parks and so on help or hinder people with dementia in their engagement with the external environment The positive results of interior design guidelines indicate that certain design features, such as the configuration of buildings, the design, content and positioning of signs, and the use of colours, textures, lighting and familiar features can improve the wellbeing of people with dementia in institutions. The preliminary findings from our interviews will demonstrate the feasibility of translating these design considerations into the external urban environment.

Home Repairs and Adaptations to Assist Older People with Dementia in England

Terry McClatchey, Robin Means and Hazel Morbey

Home Repairs and Adaptation to Assist People with Dementia in England Purpose: The purpose of this project funded by the Nuffield Foundation is to investigate how Home Improvement Agencies (often known as "Care and Repair" or "Staying Put" projects) work with people with dementia. These agencies are well established in the UK and have considerable experience of assisting (mainly elderly) people with structural repairs and adaptations to assist mobility but little is known about how they assist (or do not assist) people with dementia. Method: The project involves a review of the literature, analysis of data that had been stored electronically on a national basis, a review of sample files at a number of fieldwork sites and detailed interviews with users, carers, HIA staff and related professionals in connection with specific cases. The fieldwork sites have been selected to represent a balance of demographic profiles in varying parts of England. Results: Findings include a clarification of the extent to which HIA's are used by other people with dementia who remain in the community and the ethical and financial issues they raise. They also illuminate some of the reasons why HIA's may be 'under used' by this group and how this might be tackled in the future. Findings also include firm recommendations on adaptations using both high and low technology solutions. Conclusions: Results have confirmed the potentially important role of HIA's in enabling other people with dementia to 'age in place' but suggest that this will only be realised through a greater understanding of their role by specialist dementia service providers.

Just Another Disability, Making Design Dementia Friendly, Concept Designs in Rural, Suburban, and Urban Contexts

Sandy Page and Sally Stewart(Mackintosh School of Architecture, Glasgow, Scotland)

Purpose Throughout 1999, as UK City of Architecture and Design, Glasgow carried out significant projects to demonstrate the City's understanding of the importance of design and architecture in our lives. Method One of these projects looked at making design dementia friendly by bringing together architects,designers and care professionals, people with dementia, their carers and families to create a comprehensive guide to that end. Results As members of the Architects Panel we would like to present a series of Concept Design Proposals based on private care provision with an emphasis being placed on rural, suburban and urban contexts. Conclusions Site specific proposals within the realms of the chosen contexts can be tested against the results. New care regimes need to be flexible to allow for contextual concerns.

The Gloucester Smart House Project

Jane Gilliard (Dementia Voice, Bristol, England) Roger Orpwood(Bath Institute of Medical Engineering, Bath, England) Teresa Parker (Housing 21, Taunton, England)

PURPOSE - The Gloucester Smart House is a unique collaboration between three organisations Dementia Voice, Housing 21 and the Bath Institute of Medical Engineering (BIME). Following a period of user consultation, the house has been equipped with assistive technology to help people with cognitive disability. METHOD - This paper will describe the method of consulting with people with dementia and their carers to identify those activities where they felt they had particular difficulty. This was followed by a period of development, in which the engineers designed devices that might help, or adapted existing technology to make it appropriate for people with dementia. People with dementia offered to try out these devices in their own homes, and the engineers conducted an iterative process of testing, refining and re-testing. RESULT - The Gloucester Smart House is now a demonstration unit, showing how new technology can facilitate independent living for people with dementia wherever they live. The house was a former resident manager s house in a sheltered housing complex. All the units of accommodation are single-bedded, so the Smart House had previously been used as guest accommodation for residents visitors. The partnership agreement honoured this arrangement. The Smart House therefore now has four key functions: - · A demonstration unit that is open to visitors interested professionals, people with dementia and their families · An on-going research and development project · Guest accommodation for residents visitors (during these times the house will not be open as a demonstration unit) · A facility where people with dementia and their carers can stay to try out the equipment

SESSION 439

Update on International Centenarian Research

L. Burrell and L.W. Poon (University of Georgia Gerontology Center, Athens, Georgia USA) Comparison Of Centenarians' Physical And Functional Health From The Georgia, Swedish, And Hungarian Studies. C. Franceschi (Universita di Bologna, Bologna, Itlay) Update On Genetic Research. P. A. Holtsberg and L.W. Poon (University of Georgia, USA) Patterns Of Longitudinal Change In Centenarians' Cognition. J.M. Robine (Equipe INSERM Dedmograhie et Sante, Montpellier, France) Update On Super-Centenarians. P. Martin (Iowa State University, USA), C. Rott (University of Heidelberg, Germany), B. Hagberg (University of Lund, Sweden) Personality and Coping Among the Oldest Old.

This symposium brings together international centenarian researchers to compare and contrast findings from different centenarian studies, and to provide updates on genetics, cognition, personality and coping styles of the oldest old as well as research and demography of the very old (super-centenarians). The goal of this symposium is to facilitate discussion and communication among researchers from different countries on the study of this unique and growing population.

Comparison of Centenarians'Physical and Functional Health from the Georgia, Swedish, and Hungarian Studies.

L. Burrell and L.W. Poon (University of Georgia Gerontology Center, Athens, Georgia USA)

This presentation highlights the similarities and differences in findings on the physical and functional health among centenarians from the Georgia, Swedish, and Hungarian centenarian studies. Although the methodologies and sampling methods are vastly different with the Georgia study sampling only cognitively intact and community dwelling centenarians, the Swedish study employing a population-based strategy, and the Hungarian study using a convenient sample, there are more similarities than differences along the abilities of the oldest old to function in the everyday environment.

Patterns Of Longitudinal Change In Centenarians' Cognition.

P. A. Holtsberg and L. W. Poon (Gerontology Center, The University of Georgia, GA, USA), A. S. Davey (Department of Child & Family Development, The University of Georgia, GA, USA)

In this paper, we examined patterns of longitudinal change in the cognitive functioning among a group of centenarians participating in the Georgia Centenarian Study. Particular attention was devoted to the impact and consequences of participant attrition and possible methodologies to ameliorate the impact of this confounding variable. Two basic patterns of change were discernable among centenarians retested at least 18 months after initial testing: stability and decline. An improvement pattern was not discerned among any of the cognitive functions assessed. Stability patterns were observed among the following cognitive measures: MMSE, total every-day problem-solving scores, free-recall memory for recent U.S. Presidents, WAIS-R arithmetic, and WAIS-R vocabulary. Patterns of decline were observed among the following cognitive measures: acquisition and retrieval of new information in paired-associates learning for pairs with or without mnemonic support, WAIS-R Block Design and Picture Arrangement. Results suggest that although some cognitive functions were stable for healthy centenarians, others showed marked decline.

Personality and Coping Among the Oldest Old

P. Martin (Iowa State University, USA), C. Rott (University of Heidelberg, Germany), B. Hagberg (University of Lund, Sweden)

Very old people face numerous physical, functional and psychosocial challenges. Personality and coping behaviors may serve as important resources to come to terms with late-life changes. This presentation provides an overview of recent research concerning personality and coping in centenarians. Overall findings suggest patterns of robust personality and specific coping behaviors, which are the basis for optimal adjustments in very old age. Important personality components include the personality traits of emotional stability, suspiciousness, conscientiousness, and optimism, as well as the personality states of extraversion and fatigue. Salient coping behaviors include cognitive coping, acceptance and religious coping. We conclude that centenarians draw from a number of unique personality traits and coping behaviors to buffer the effect of developmental challenges in their last years of their extreme long life.

Update On Genetic Research.

C. Franceschi (Universita di Bologna, Bologna, Itlay)

This presentation reviews research on genetic factors of longevity based on the findings from the Italian Centenarian Study.

Update on Supercentenarians

Jean-Marie Robine (INSERM, University of Montpellier, France)

The super-centenarians emerged in the middle of the 1960s. Their number has regularly increased since the middle of the 1970s. An International Database on Supercentenarians has been recently established. The current prevalence of known supercentenarians in the countries involved in the database is approximately 5 to 6 times more than in the middle of the 1970s. In roughly twenty years the maximum age observed has increased by about 10 years from 112 to 122 years. The annual probability of death at age 110 is as low as 0.50 when using only data from countries with exhaustive and validated data. The probabilities of death stagnate between 110 and 115 years and all the computed probabilities fall below the ceiling of 0.6. Our results are compatible with the last extrapolations of mortality trajectories using a logistic or a quadratic model. The last findings will be exposed.

SESSION 440

A profile of older informal caregivers in South Africa: prevalence, circumstances and lived experiences

J.D. Joubert, L. Khephe, C. Lombard, P. Reddy (Medical Research Council, Cape Town, South Africa)

Purpose: To investigate the prevalence of informal caregiving, and the environments and lived experiences of a sample of informal caregivers (ICs) in South Africa (SA). Only findings related to older ICs (55 years +) will be presented. Method: Both random and purposive methods were applied in different phases of the sampling process. Data were collected via a structured questionnaire during individual face-to-face interviews. Of 600 ICs interviewed, 160 were 55 years +. Results: The great majority of older ICs were female; over half were older than 65; 14% never attended school; and 31% held a primary school qualification only. The majority provided informal care to live-in family members. Analysed by relationship to the caree, the largest proportion of ICs (35 %) cared for their children and grandchildren; 31% for spouses, and 14% for parents. Amenities inside the place of care and the physical environment were less than ideal at times, e.g. 16% had no running water; 27% had no in-house toilet; and 8% lived in a squatter environment. Considerable proportions reported that their health, social life, and financial position had been adversely affected by their caring responsibilities. Although 76% were performing a caring role for >3 years, more than one fifth perceived themselves not to have the necessary skills, nor the appropriate knowledge to perform their caring tasks. Over half never received any professional information or advice about caring for someone. Conclusion: While developed nations appear to be saturated with research on informal caregivers, it is a severely neglected field in Africa. This first national empirical study of its kind in SA shows that older persons constitute a substantial portion of ICs in SA. Globally, many studies focus on the burden of ICs caring for older persons, but this study reinforces the need to acknowledge that older persons are not only care recipients, but indeed also caregivers—mostly without having a choice, and often amidst sombre circumstances and despairing poverty. SA's morbidity and mortality patterns show a triple burden of infectious disease, chronic ailments, and high levels of injury, assault and violence. Contributing to this burden, is the devastating HIV/AIDS epidemic with 1700 new infections per day. All these imply an enormous demand for care, exacerbated by the de-institutionalizing policies of health and welfare services. Older ICs are an indispensable asset in the current trend away from institutional care, and serious attention should be paid to their needs and concerns in order to sustain this essential community asset in SA.

Factors Influencing Perceived Level of Family Participation in Caregiving to the Impaired Elderly

Daisaku Maeda (Japan Lutheran College, Tokyo, Japan), Yutaka Shimizu (Sophia University, Tokyo, Japan), Koichi Hiraoka (National Ochanomizu Women's University), Torahiko Miura (Johchi School of Social Welfare, Tokyo, Japan)

PURPOSE: The purpose of this study is to find the variables that have statistically significant effects on the perceived level of family participation in caregiving to the elderly. METHOD: The respondents were the family members of impaired older persons who were randomly selected from among those who lived in N-ku of Tokyo. The sample size was 1,491, though the number of cases analyzed with ANOVA had shrunk significantly due to missing values. The perceived level of family participation was measured with 7-item 4-point Lickert scale. The analysis of variance and covariance was performed with the score of the level of perceived family participation as a dependent variable. RESULTS: Among eleven independent variables, the following seven variables were found to have statistically significant influence on the dependent variable. They are degree of physical impairment, degree of mental impairment, age of respondent, relationship of caregiver to the elderly, health status of main caregiver, whether an assistant caregiver is available or not, and the level of living of the household. On the other hand, age of the elderly, sex of the elderly, sex of respondent, and whether the main caregiver is working for income or not did not have statistically significant effect. The results were further analyzed carefully using MCA table, cross-tabulation, etc. CONCLUSION: The above analysis showed that the perceived level of family participation is one of the dependable tools to measure subjective as well as objective levels of well-being of the family-caregiver.

The Attitude of Middle-Aged Women towards Elderly Care in Korea

Ki Tae Kim, Ki Hyung Ryu, Byung Hyun Park (Department of Social Welfare, Pusan National University, Korea), Bong Kil Park (Department of Social Welfare, Choon Hae University, Korea)

The purpose of this study is to investigate the attitude of middle-aged women towards elderly care in Korea. We randomly selected a sample of 608 women aged between 40 and 59 from Pusan city, Korea. The method of face-to-face interview was used in this research. Interviewers visited and delivered a questionnaire to the selected women. The interviewer collected the questionnaire the following day. The survey was conducted in August 1999. The results of this research are as follow. 42 percent of the respondents reported that they have experienced living together with elderly parents. Of those, 23 percent of the women reported caring for their own parents, while 68 percent reported caring for their husband's parents. Our survey results showed that women with lower education are more likely to prefer to live with elderly parents than those women with higher education. Older women aged 50-59 are more likely to prefer to live with their elderly parents than younger women aged 40-49. Only 22 percent of the respondents reported that they wanted to live with the children when they become older. 47 percent of the respondents reported that they wished to live with their first son when they become older. This result confirms that the first son usually supports aging parents in Korea. Those women whose spouses are first sons expressed a strong sense of corporate responsibility towards family and society in the care for elderly parents. In conclusion, the consciousness of filial piety is gradually diminishing in contemporary Korea. However, the actual relationship between parents and children is still close. The Korean elderly are much more integrated into their families. At the same time, it is also true that the relationship between parents and children has been changing. Especially, those women who have higher academic background are not likely to prefer to live together with their elderly parents. Therefore, the government should prepare for the changing consciousness in the care of elderly parents.

SESSION 441

Music Therapy in Dementia Care across Various Cultural Settings

Susan Summers, MMT, BEd, MTA (St. Michael's Centre, Burnaby, British Columbia, Canada) The Voices of Dementia: Singing the cultural landscape. Nadine Cadesky, BMT, BA (Louis Brier Home and Hospital, Vancouver, British Columbia, Canada) Intuition, Improvisation and the Role of Heritage in Process-directed Music Therapy with Elderly Jewish Residents. Lennie Tan, BMT, MTA (Mount St. Joseph's Hospital, Vancouver, British Columbia, Canada). Music Therapy - Bridging Cultures: Meeting the needs of Chinese elderly through music.

The three presentations will demonstrate the effectiveness of music and music therapy techniques in addressing the cultural needs of persons with dementia who live in long-term care facilities. All three presenters work as music therapists within various cross-cultural milieu in long-term care facilities in the Vancouver area. They will share their unique experiences with persons with dementia in first, a "mixed" cultural milieu, secondly, a facility which is comprised primarily of older adults of Asian background, and thirdly, persons living in a Jewish multi-level facility. They will share their unique experiences with persons with dementia in first, a "mixed" cultural milieu, secondly, a Jewish multi-level facility and thirdly, in a facility which is comprised primarily of older adults of Asian background. For people of many cultures, placing an elder in a long-term care facility is a relatively new experience. The often difficult adjustment that needs to be made by the person with dementia, as well as by family members can often be softened by the introduction of well-chosen music. Music effectively addresses the cultural needs of those who live in institutional care through singing familiar songs of their culture, religion and homeland; by hearing familiar instrument sounds, melodies, genres and lyrics; by watching or listening to familiar recorded music and visual material and by joining together in a shared active experience of music making and vocalizing/singing. Each of the presenters have many years of experience working with older adults in care from a variety of cultural backgrounds. Their methods, philosophies, perspectives and models of practice will illuminate a variety of ways to bring integration and inclusion to those who may be isolated not only by dementia, but by their cultural or language differences as well. Presenters will share their experiences of working with persons with dementia from different cultural backgrounds. They will also offer delegates opportunities to participate in different music therapy and active music making experiences.

Intuition, Improvisation and the Role of Heritage in Process-directed Music Therapy with Elderly Jewish Residents

Nadine Cadesky, BMT, BA (Louis Brier Home and Hospital, Vancouver, British Columbia, Canada)

The presenter draws from five years working with the Frail Jewish Elderly to share her unique perspective on use of culturally appropriate music therapy in dementia care. Conference delegates will learn from her process-directed, intuitive and improvisational music therapy approach that respects and incorporates heritage and religion in relation to the materials and processes of therapy. Mention will also be made of how music can concurrently meet the needs of different cultures and religions. Methodology and examples will serve to emphasize the primary role voice plays in therapeutic interventions and provide a glimpse of how this powerful work can reach, engage and lead to meaningful response in residents with widely varied levels of functioning. Finally, delegates will learn how community expresses itself within this unique setting and how the therapist views and supports this community. The presenter has worked as Louis Brier Home and Hospital's Music Therapist since March of 1996. Louis Brier Home and Hospital is a multi-care-level facility built primarily to service British Columbia's Jewish Community.

Music Therapy - Bridging Cultures: Meeting the needs of Chinese elderly through music

Lennie Tan (Mount Saint Joseph Hospital, Vancouver, British Columbia, Canada)

In this presentation, the writer will talk about developing a music therapy program at an extended care facility where many of the residents come from an Asian background, i.e. Chinese from China, Hong Kong, Taiwan, Vietnam, Thailand as well as from the Philippines. Many of the Asian seniors did not receive much exposure to music in their younger years. For some, the music they heard was Chinese Opera. The writer started a percussion group using cymbals, gong and drums and wood blocks. These were sounds that were familiar, sounds that accompanied celebrations like Lion and Dragon Dances. To address self-esteem issues, a tone chime group was formed, where members learnt tunes to perform, first, for their peers, but later on for family and friends. In these groups music also brings together individuals from different cultures. Thus, even though it did not play an important part in their lives before, now in their twilight years, music serves to enrich and give new meaning to their lives as well as provide creative outlet for self-expression. There will be an experiential component to this presentation where the audience will be invited to participate in a music therapy experience.

The Voices of Dementia: Singing our cultural landscape

Susan Summers, MMT, BEd, MTA (St. Michael's Centre, Burnaby, British Columbia, Canada)

The diverse cultural composition of the Lower Mainland in British Columbia is reflected by a strong cultural presence in long-term care facilities. Older adults may experience cultural and language difficulties due to disabling conditions such as stroke or dementia. Together with feelings of being isolated due to multiple losses, their need for creative self-expression, for being listened to and understood, and for feeling a sense of belongingness and community becomes paramount. Music helps to address these needs. Music becomes a shared experience which dissolves borders, boundaries and limitations through vocalizing, through singing songs of their native lands and through playing music together. Based on findings from the presenter's qualitative research study and from her thirteen year experiences working with older adults in dementia care, this presentation will address the importance of active music-making and singing together within the multi-national culture of a long-term care facility in British Columbia. The presenter will share her qualitative findings as well as introduce interactive and experiential activities, including opportunities to sing and play instruments within a safe space. It will be demonstrated how active participation in music therapy programs, which emphasize music making and singing together, contributes positively to an older person's overall physical, emotional and spiritual health.

SESSION 442

Developments in bereavement theories and practice

Chris Powell (Age Concern England, Leeds UK / Westcliffe Medical Centre, Bradford, UK) Recent developments in bereavement theories and practice. Kate Davidson (University of Surrey, Guildford, UK) Gender Differences in Adaptation to Widowhood: A Qualitative Study. Terence A. Seedsman (Victoria University, Melbourne, Australia) Addressing Loss and Grief in Rural Communities Affected by Stock Diseases: An Australian Case Study. K. van den Hoonaard (Gerontology Programme, St. Thomas, University, Fredericton, Canada) Rediscovering Identity: Canadian Widows' Continuing Connections to their Husbands and the Rebuilding Their Identity.

This Round Table addresses recent developments in bereavement theories and models, and the relationship between these and current research and practice in bereavement and bereavement support. The presenters examine the implications of theories and research for policy makers and those responsible for providing support to bereaved people. The session will contain four presentations, each followed by brief discussion of the paper, and a final period of open discussion between presenters and audience. The opening paper provides the current context of thinking in bereavement and grief with a particular focus on recent debates generated by Walter's work on biography (1996), and other recent developments such as the Dual Process Model (Stroebe and Schut, 1995) and Continuing Bonds (Klass, Silverman and Nickman 1996). These theories are related to current practice in providing support to bereaved people. This concludes that Walters has not provided a genuine new model of grief but that his work is complementary to and integrative of older theories and others currently working in the field. Also that these developments are already reflected in practice by many providing support to bereaved people. The second paper presents a qualitative study which examines these issues in the context of gender difference and finds that while both widows and widowers travel along a 'chaos - coherence continuum' this journey varies by age, health status, social network involvement within the overarching variable of gender. There is consideration of the 'gaps' experienced following bereavement and strategies for filling them. The third paper reports on a recent government inquiry into the approaches taken to control a specific sheep disease in Victoria, Australia and looks at loss and grief in terms of social impact in rural communities. These impacts include the mental health impacts in communities where stock diseases are of major significance. Social impact is examined through the lens of grieving processes and recent models of loss and grief, and recommendations are given for the support of these communities. The final paper develops the theme of current thinking about continuing bonds in bereavement and their importance to identity. It presents an interview study of Canadian widows and the impact of the loss of a husband on the women's 'sense of self'. It demonstrates that many widows experience 'identity foreclosure' when their husbands die. Thus, bonds with the self as well as with the lost other must be examined in bereavement. It is anticipated that the session will underline the importance of using notions such as biography, continuing bonds, and the loss versus restoration orientation in current research into grief and bereavement, and in the practice of bereavement support. Many of these ideas are already being used in practice by researchers and bereavement support services, however, current theoretical debates are seeking to clarify the relationship of these ideas with older, more traditional theories of grief. It is hoped that the session will provide impetus for the closer examination of the relationship of theory and practice in bereavement research and support.

Recent developments in bereavement theories and practice

Chris Powell (Age Concern England, Leeds UK/Westcliffe Medical Centre, Bradford, UK)

This paper introduces a Round Table session on recent developments in bereavement theories and models and the relationship between these and current research and practice in bereavement and bereavement support. There is a review of the major models of grief followed by detailed examination of Tony Walter's contributions (1996 and 1999) and , along with the considerable discussion of this in the literature. There is also consideration of other recent developments including Klass, Silverman and Nickman (1996) and Stroebe and Schut (1995). Walter's paper (1997) in particular has sparked much debate with practitioners providing bereavement counselling or support taking exception to his description of professional support structures. This paper concludes by examining the relationship between theory and practice drawing on experience in the author's own practice and contributions by practitioners to the literature. I seek to show that Walters has made a significant contribution to our understanding of bereavement, particularly in his ideas about gender specificity, but that this is within the context of other significant changes in thinking about grief and bereavement which is already reflected in the practice of many who provide professional support to bereaved people. His model may be seen as complementary to and integrative of some other models, although presents more of a challenge to more traditional models than some are attempting to maintain (Parkes 1998).

SESSION 443

Caloric Restriction

Isao Shimokawa [Dept. of Pathology, Nagasaki Univ. School of Med, 1-12-4 Sakamoto, Nagasaki City 852-8523, Japan] ("A role for suppression of growth hormone in the antiaging action of caloric restriction") Richard Weindruch [Dept. of Med, Univ. of Wisconsin VA Hosp, 2500 Overlook Terrace, Madison, WI 53705, U.S.A.] ("Gene expression profile of aging and its retardation by caloric restriction") Yasuhiko Wada (Department of Hygiene, Hyogo College of Medicine. 1-1, Mukogawa-cho, Nishinomiya, HYOGO, 663-8501 JAPAN "Characterization of gene expression profile in heart after long-term energy restriction in mice") Mark A. Lane [Natl. Inst. on Aging, 5600 Nathan Shock , Baltimore, MD 21224, U.S.A.] ("The possible role of insulin signal transdcution in lifespan extension by caloric restriction")

ISSUE: Dietary caloric restriction (CR) is the only intervention conclusively shown to slow aging, extend lifespan, and maintain health and vitality in mammals. Despite 70 years of research using this model, its relevance to Although participants from the Natl. Inst. on Aging and Univ. of Wisconsin are currently addressing the former question with non-human primates, this symposium will focus primarily on the latter mechanistic area. Since identification and manipulation of specific genes is presently a major pardigm in biomedical research, this approach will be featured prominently. STRUCTURE AND CONTENT: One hypothesis for the biological efficacy of CR involves suppression of the growth hormone axis. Dr. Shimokawa is using minirats, with alterations in the genes of this endocrine pathway, to examine possible mechanisms of antiaging effects. Dr. Weindruch has achieved a broader characterization of changes in gene expression during aging and CR using muscle and brains of mice and monkeys. This approach has been extended to cardiac muscle by Dr. Koizumi, with a particular emphasis on the mechanisms of increased stress resistance in CR animals. Finally, Dr. Lane will explore the possible role of altered insulin action and changes in the expression of signal transduction components of this critical endocrine pathway in the beneficial action of CR. Mutations in genes for some homologs of the insulin signalling system lead to longer lifespan in nematodes, and reduced circulating insulin levels and greater insulin sensitivity are hallmarks of the CR state in rodents and monkeys. CONCLUSIONS/ ANTICIPATED OUTCOMES: Taken together, these findings provide a framework for a better understanding of the biological actions of CR, and the possible transcriptional regulatory mechanisms involved.

A role for suppression of growth hormone in the antiaging action of caloric restriction

Shimokawa, I. and Higami, Y. (Department of Pathology, Nagasaki University School of Medicine, Nagasaki, Japan)

Hereditary dwarf mice deficient in growth hormone (GH), prolactin, and TSH have been reported to live longer than their normal siblings. Caloric restriction (CR) also suppresses GH. Using a transgenic strain of rats, in which the synthesis of GH is selectively suppressed by overexpression of an antisense GH-RNA transgene, we have started a research project to explore a role for suppression of GH in the antiaging action of CR. Experimental groups of rats included control male Wistar rats, the transgenic rats (Mini), and their F1 hybrid rats. These rats were fed ad libitum (AL) or 30At 32 months of age, a survival analysis showed that the proportion of survival was greater in the following order; F1-AL, Wistar-AL, Mini-AL. CR also extended the lifespan in each group. These data suggest that moderate, but not severe, suppression of GH could extend lifespan in the rat; however, CR may prolong lifespan independently of suppression of GH.

Characterization of gene expression profile in heart after long-term energy restriction in mice

Akio KOIZUMI (Kyoto Univ. Schl of Pblc Hlth, Kyoto Japan), Yasuhiko WADA (Hyogo College of Medicine, Nishinomiya, Japan), Tsuyoshi KAYO (Akita Univ. Schl of Med, Akita, Japan)

Energy restriction (ER) is known to extend longevity but its mechanism remains enigmatic. ER is known to induce torpor in mice, which decreases core body temperature to a level as low as 25C. Cold temperature triggers fatal arrhythmia but life prolonging ER increases resistance to cold-induced arrhythmia. The aim of the present study is to characterize the gene expression profile associated with ER-induced cold resistance of heart. ER (200 kJ/week) and control (400 kJ/week) regimens were started on B6 male mice at 4 weeks of age and were continued until 11 months of age. mRNAs isolated from heart were pooled for three mice and were reverse transcribed to cDNA. The 32P labeled cDNA was applied to an expression array mounting 588 genes. Results were judged as positive when standardized hybridization signals were consistently higher by 1.5 times or lower by 1/1.5 times than controls in three independent hybridization experiments. We detected 88 genes expressed in heart. ER inhibited expression of several genes such as oxidative stress-induced protein, calcium-binding protein, and laminin receptor 1 gene. In contrast, ER increased expression of some genes including glutathione S-transferase Mu 1, transcription factor 1, and fetal myosin alkali light chain genes. Increased expression of glutathione Mu gene and decreased expression of oxidative stress-induced gene strongly indicate that ER induces protection against oxidative stress in heart. In terms of increased cold resistance, a change of myosin gene expression seems to be interesting. Obviously, further study is needed for better understanding of the molecular basis of cold resistance.

Gene Expression Profile of Aging and Its Retardation by Caloric Restriction

Cheol-Koo Lee, Tomas Prolla and Richard Weindruch, [University of Wisconsin, Madison, WI, USA]

PURPOSE: To provide the first global analysis of aging at the transcriptional level. METHOD: Oligonucleotide arrays representing 6347 genes were employed to determine the gene expression profile of aging and caloric restriction (CR) in the gastrocnemius muscle, neocortex and cerebellum in mice. RESULTS: In the gastrocnemius (Lee et al, 1999), aging resulted in gene expression profile indicative of a marked stress response and lower expression of metabolic and biosynthetic genes. Most alterations were either completely or partially prevented by CR, the only intervention known to retard aging in mammals (Weindruch and Sohal, 1997). Transcriptional patterns of calorie-restricted animals suggest that CR retards the aging process by causing a metabolic shift toward increased protein turnover and decreased macromolecular damage. In both regions of the brain, aging resulted in a gene expression profile suggestive of a marked inflammatory response, oxidative stress, and reduced neuronal plasticity and neurotrophic support (Lee et al, 2000). At the transcriptional level, brain aging in mice displays striking parallels with human neurodegenerative disorders. In the brain, CR selectively attenuated the age-associated induction of genes encoding inflammatory and stress responses. CONCLUSION: These observations are consistent with the idea that CR may slow aging, at least in part, by reducing molecular damage to tissues. References 1. Lee C-K, Klopp RG, Weindruch R, Prolla TA. Gene expression profile of aging and its retardation by caloric restriction. Science 1999;285:1390-1393. 2. Lee C-K, Weindruch R, Prolla TA. Gene expression profile of the ageing brain. Nat. Genet. 2000;25:294-297. 3. Weindruch R, Sohal RS. Caloric intake and aging. N. Eng. J. Med. 1997;337:986-94.

The Possible Role of Neuroendocrine Signaling in Lifespan Extension and Enhanced Stress Response by Caloric Restriction

Mark A. Lane, R. Michael Anson, and R. deCabo [Nutritional and Molecular Physiology Unit, Laboratory of Neurosciences, National Institute on Aging, NIH Baltimore, MD USA]

Caloric restriction (CR) is well known as the only nongenetic intervention that reproducibly extends lifespan and retards aging in mammals. In addition, rodents on CR exhibit an enhanced ability to deal with a variety of stressors including inflammatory agents, thermal and oxidative stress and neurotoxins. Although the biological mechanisms responsible for the effects of CR on aging, stress responsiveness and lifespan are not known, several lines of evidence suggest that neuroendocrine responses to reduced food are involved. For example, CR has robust effects on several important regulatory hormones including growth hormone/IGF-1, insulin and glucocorticoids. In addition, studies in several invertebrate models have implicated an insulin-like signaling pathway in lifespan regulation. Also, mice lacking p66Shc, an adapter protein in insulin signaling, lived longer and were more resistance to paraquat toxicity, compared to wild type animals. Our group and others have demonstrated that CR has several tissue specific effects on insulin and growth factor signaling. In addition, we have recently developed an in vitro model for investigation of altered stress response during CR. We have observed that rat hepatoma cell grown for only 48 hr. in serum isolated from rodents and monkeys on CR exhibit an enhanced response to serum withdrawal, heat shock, and hydrogen peroxide, compared to cells from the same line grown in serum from freely fed animals. Possible molecular mechanisms and implications for lifespan extension and retardation of aging will also be discussed.

SESSION 444

Negotiating Intergenerational Relations Across The Life Course: Interpersonal, Theoretical and Policy Considerations

Sara Arber and Khim Horton (University of Surrey, Guildford, UK), 'Doing gender': Risk and control in inter-generational relationships where older people have had falls; Karl Pillemer (Cornell University, Ithaca, N.Y, U.S.A.), Ambivalence In Parent-Child Relations In Later Life: Results Of An Exploratory Study; Ingrid Connidis and Julie Ann McMullin, (University of Western Ontario, London, Canada), Negotiating Family Ties Over Three Generations: The Impact of Divorce; Anne Martin-Matthews (University of British Columbia, Vancouver, Canada), Discussant.

As we begin the 21st century, the historical need for family members of different generations to work together and for public and social policy to respond to the needs of older persons and their families continues. Indeed, the drive to decrease public spending combined with population aging has escalated the need to both understand the private domains of family life and their connection to the public domains of social policy. The presentations in this session will address the negotiation of intergenerational relations at several levels and from different perspectives. Sara Arber and Khim Horton will discuss how gender shapes the negotiation of intergenerational relationships in situations where a parent has had repeated falls and a child serves as the primary caregiver. Karl Pillemer examines the ambivalent views of mothers regarding the quality of their relationships with children. Ingrid Connidis and Julie McMullin explore continuity and change in how family ties are negotiated across three generations, focusing on the impact of divorce.

Ambivalence In Parent-Child Relations In Later Life: Results Of An Exploratory Study

K. Pillemer (Dept. of Human Development, Cornell University,NY, USA)

This paper presents a study of 189 mothers aged 60 and over that examined ambivalence regarding the quality of their relationships with adult children. Both direct and indirect measures of ambivalence were used to address two research questions: 1. What is the prevalence of ambivalent assessments of the parent-adult child relationship? 2. What factors are correlated with such ambivalence? Ambivalence was uncovered in a number of domains of parent-child relationships. In addition, ambivalence in parent-child relations was strongly associated with several variables, including unequal exchange of assistance, value similarity, and educational attainment. Regression analyses found an association between a measure of ambivalence and both positive and negative affect.

'Doing gender': Risk and control in inter-generational relationships where older people have had falls

S. Arber, K. Horton (Centre for Research on Ageing and Gender(CRAG), Department of Sociology, University of Surrey, Guildford, UK)

The research examines the negotiation between older people who have had falls and their primary carers in relation to the meaning of risks and changes in behaviour consequent on repeated falling. The focus is how the gender of the older person and the gender of the primary carer influences the nature of this negotiated relationship in terms of control, autonomy and dependence. Forty in depth interviews were conducted with older people (20 men and 20 women) living in the community who had experienced two or more recent falls. In deph interviews were also conducted with their primary carer, 11 of whom were sons and 17 were daughters. In mother-son relationships, older women had less ability to negotiate in terms of control over what they should or could do to prevent falls, since their adult sons tended to assume the role of 'protectors' and instigated major changes to curtail the likelihood of falls but without negotiation or the consent of their mother. There was more subtle negotiation in father-daughter relationships where the older person was perceived as autonomous and in control of their subsequent actions. Daughters continued to perceive their older fathers as 'head of family' and in control, allowing them to maintain maximum independence. The paper shows how 'doing gender' shapes the experiences of older men and women, and the ways in which the gendered nature of inter-generational relationships are linked to differential perceived notions of dependency, power and control for older men and women.

Negotiating Family Ties Over Three Generations: The Impact of Divorce.

Ingrid Arnet Connidis, and Julie Ann McMullin, (University of Western Ontario, London, Canada).

This paper studies the impact of divorce on family ties in multi-generational families. Data are from interviews with three generations of ten families with number of participating members ranging from 4 to 13. For the oldest generation (generation one), one set of parent/s and all willing siblings were interviewed. For generation two, all children and their partners (current and former) of the generation one parent/s were contacted and those who agreed were interviewed. For generation three, consenting children of generation two who were aged 25 years or more and their partners, if any, were interviewed. Using a case study approach, we find substantial variations in the ways that family ties are negotiated following divorce in one generation, evident in patterns of relating between original and step kin, remarriage, divorce, and in views on marriage and relationships. These differences apply to both inter- and intra-generational relationships. Implications of these findings for research, theory, and policy are noted.

SESSION 445

Research and Development of the Canadian Centre for Activity and Aging's Leadership Training Initiatives.

G. Liz Cyarto (Canadian Centre for Activity and Aging, London, Canada) Research, development and delivery of the Seniors' Fitness Instructors Course (SFIC). Lynn Scholey (Canadian Centre for Activity and Aging, London, Canada) The Home Support Exercise Program (HSEP) for Frail Older Adults. Clara Fitzgerald (Canadian Centre for Activity and Aging, London, Canada) Restorative Care Education and Training in Long-Term Care Institutions (Nursing Homes).

Research in the area of physical activity and aging has demonstrated the importance of regular exercise for the older adult population. To implement physical activity programs, instructor training is critical. Instructors of physical activity programs for older adults require specific leadership training to ensure that they are providing safe and effective programs for their participants. This applies equally to community-based leaders and to individuals delivering programs to long-term care residents. Three education and training programs will be presented. These target older adults of different levels of functioning including the robust, community-dwelling older adults and those living in home-bound situations or institutional settings. In the early nineties, the Canadian Centre for Activity and Aging (CCAA) developed a peer leadership training program, the Seniors' Fitness Instructors Course (SFIC), to address the growing need for qualified instructors for community-based programs. More recently, the CCAA has initiated leadership training programs for individuals who work with frail older adults in long-term care settings and in the community (home support/care). These courses include the Functional Fitness in Long-Term Care Workshop, Restorative Care Education and Training (RCET), and the Home Support Exercise Program (HSEP). The Training for the Trainer course allows the CCAA to disseminate these training courses to other communities across the country. The transition from research to action, through the development and implementation of research-based education and training programs, is essential to ensure that older adults receive physical activity programs that are both safe and effective.

Restorative Care Education and Training in Long-Term Care Institutions (Nursing Homes)

Clara Fitzgerald (Canadian Centre for Activity and Aging, London, Canada), Nancy A. Ecclestone (Canadian Centre for Activity and Aging, London, Canada), Gareth Jones (Canadian Centre for Activity and Aging, London, Canada), JB Orange (Canadian Centre for Activity and Aging and The University of Western Ontario, London, Canada), Paul Stolee (Regional Geriatric Program, London, Canada), Darien Lazowski (Canadian Centre for Activity and Aging, London, Canada), Shanthi Jacob-Johnson (Canadian Centre for Activity and Aging, London, Ontario and Acadia University, Nova Scotia, Canada).

Physical activity programs in long-term care (LTC), regardless of the resident's ability, have typically focused on seated range of motion exercises. However, there is evidence to support the use of appropriate intervention strategies to improve the quality of life of frail older adults. The Restorative Care Education and Training (RCET) program was developed and implemented for restorative care staff in LTC facilities to improve physical and psychosocial functioning, and general quality of life for residents. This initiative assessed the impact of the RCET program on the physical and psychosocial functioning of 84 residents (mean age 83±8.5) from 12 facilities equally distributed across intervention and control groups. There was a significant improvement in measures of mobility, balance, functional independence of LTC residents following the program. The impact on staff (mean age 36±10) receiving the education was assessed using knowledge-based outcome measures for exercise, feeding, and communication. A significant improvement was also found in the knowledge level of LTC staff. This presentation will provide an overview of the 36-hour training program which includes components of communication, physical activity and aging, positioning and transferring, safe and effective eating, and assessment and evaluation. Older adults living in LTC can benefit from a challenging program. The adverse effects of frailty and deconditioning can be delayed, prevented or treated through restoration of function. Results of the present study emphasize the importance of RCET for staff and frail residents in LTC facilities.

The Seniors' Fitness Instructors Course (SFIC)

L. Cyarto, C. Fitzgerald, L. Scholey, G. Jones, D. H. Paterson and N. A. Ecclestone. (Canadian Centre for Activity and Aging, London, Ontario, Canada)

The Seniors' Fitness Instructors Course (SFIC) was developed in 1990 to address a need for training and information about appropriate physical activity programs for seniors. This course is available to those who have an interest in this area, regardless of educational background or previous experience. An emphasis is placed on training older adults and volunteers to become leaders of community-based programs. The theory portion of the course consists of 36 hours of in-class training, based on a comprehensive resource manual. Topics include an overview of aging and physical activity, exercise prescription and design, and programming for special conditions (osteoporosis, arthritis, diabetes, frailty, heart disease, and Alzheimer's Disease). The requirements for certification through the Canadian Centre for Activity and Aging are a minimum of 16 hours of practical teaching, CPR certification, and successful completion of a take-home assignment and practical evaluation. Over the past ten years, more than 1,000 individuals have been trained to lead safe and challenging physical activity programs in community centres, seniors' centres, churches, apartment buildings, and retirement homes. The SFIC is currently offered in two provinces in Canada (Ontario and British Columbia). This course has the potential to provide trained leaders in communities across the country.

SESSION 446

Reminiscence and Life Review: Current Research and Future Directions

Barbara K. Haight (College of Nursing Medical University of South Carolina Charleston, South Carolina, USA) Overview of current research; working with special populations Johannes J.F. Schroots (Faculty of Psychology and Education, Free University,Amsterdam, The Netherlands)The 'bump' effect in autobiographical memory: A new theoretical and empirical account Jeffrey Dean Webster (Psychology Department, Langara College, Vancouver, British Columbia, Canada) Measuring functions of reminiscence in adulthood: Psychometric, developmental, and cultural dimensions Toyoko Nomura (Faculty of Social Work, Iwate Prefectural University, Takizawa, Iwate, Japan) Evaluation research methods of reminiscence and life review group work with person with dementia

Issue: To examine the research in reminiscence and life review in the lastdecade, to summarize current understandings , and to propose future researchneeds to further clarify the phenomena of remembering.

Structure: There will be four presentations with Haight as convenor, followed by a discussion with all presenters and questions from the audience. Content: Overview of work in the field of reminiscence in the last decade with emphasis on working with special populations. Conclusions /Anticipated Outcomes: research presentations will present and discuss the most recent work in reminiscence and life review as interventions, as used for special andvarying populations, and as used by varying professional disciplines. Questions will beraised, discussed and answered as to the therapy of the life review and its use by varying age groups. The work will be summarized to provide a basis for future work and future needs will be delineated for the field in the area of research. Conclusions: An up to date understanding of the current work in the field with clear direction for future research

Evaluation research methods of reminiscence and life review group work with person with dementia

Toyoko Nomura (Faculty of Social Work, Iwate Prefectural University, Takizawa, Iwate, Japan)

Structure: (1) Brief review of Evaluation studies of reminiscence and life review group work with person with dementia (2) Discussion on two studies of reminiscence and life review group to identify problems of measuring the effect of this approach (3) Qualitative research methods on evaluating reminiscence and life review group work in conjunction with experience in Japan Content: Tentative qualitative evaluating methods of reminiscence and life review group will be proposed. Through two recent research on the effect of reminiscence and life review group work in Japan, we clarify problems of evaluating this approach. We will also discuss the differential effect on reminiscence and life review group work for person with dementia, with its focus on the person him/herself , care staff and family members. Conclusion: Along with quantitative methods, we need to develop more rigorous framework of qualitative methods in order to evaluate the effect of reminiscence and life review group work with person with dementia.

Measuring functions of reminiscence in adulthood: Psychometric, developmental, and cultural dimensions

Jeffrey Dean Webster (Psychology Department, Langara College, Vancouver,British Columbia, Canada)

The session will be organized in 3 parts: The introduction will highlight the need for adequate measuring tools and will briefly review prior measures. The second part will focus on the psychometric properties of the Reminiscence Functions Scale (RFS). The third part will use recent empirical research with the RFS to illustrate developmental and cultural variations in reminiscence in adulthood. Validity and reliability information will be provided and specific differences in reminiscence as a function of (1) age (e.g, younger adults score higher on Bitterness Revival) and (2) cultural (e.g, AfricanAmericans score higher than whites on Teach/Inform) will be presented. Conclusions state that psychometrically sound measures of reminiscence uses in adulthood are available and allow for a more precise delineation of individual differences which have heretofore been relatively neglected by reminiscence researchers

The 'bump' effect in autobiographical memory: A new theoretical and empirical account

Johannes J.F. Schroots (Faculty of Psychology and Education, Free University,Amsterdam, The Netherlands)

Review of the literature shows that the 'bump' effect is a universal phenomenon in autobiographical memory studies of older adults. The 'bump'effect refers to the observation that for older adults the period from 10 to 30 years of age produces recall of the most autobiographical memories (past events). Rubin et al. (1998) presents four theoretical accounts of the'bump',varying from a purely cognitive and cognitiveneural account to accountsbased on identity formation processes and/or genetic fitness. The issue isthat these accounts cannot explain the 'bump' in autobiographical memorydata in young, old and middleaged adults, as obtained with the Lifeline InterviewMethod (LIM) and Timeline (TL) . In search of a new theoretical account, the philosophical work of Whitehead(1929) provided the first clue for an autobiographical memory model that explains the 'bump' effect. Translated into psychological terms, the modelfeatures both retrospective and prospective memory and the unidirectionalflow of future events (expectations) into past events (experiences). . Schroots and Dijkema developed the Janus model, which is a dynamic model of autobiographical memory across the lifespan. The graphical reproduction ofthe Janus model by means of computer simulation will illustrate theautobiographical memory 'bump' and the close fit between model and empirical data for young, middleaged and older adults

SESSION 447

Best Practices in Elderly Mental Health Care - Outstanding Issues

M. Donnelly (Mount Pleasant Legionof Community Geriatrics, Department of Family Practice, University of British Columbia, Vancouver, Canada) Overview of Best Practices in Elderly Mental Health Care in BC; H. Tuokko, Associate Director, Centre on Aging, University of Victoria, Victoria, Canada) Issues in the Application of the Principles of Health Promotion, Prevention and Psychosocial Rehabilitation to the Psychogeriatric Population; P. MacCourt (President, BC Psychogeriatric Association, British Columbia, Canada) Barriers to Best Practices.

The Best Practices in Mental Health Care were developed in 1999, under the auspices of the Adult Mental Health Division, Ministry of Health and Ministry Responsible for Seniors in British Columbia. Although purported to be applicable to all adults, including elderly persons, they were generally not found to be appropriate or applicable to the elderly population, by those working in the psychogeriatric field. As a result, the British Columbia Psychogeriatric Association, with the support of the Mental Health Evaluation & Community Consultation Unit, UBC and the Adult Mental Health Division, spear-headed the development of Best Practices in Elderly Mental Health, using a consultative process that involved consumers and families, and relevant professionals and agencies. The principles of the BC Psychogeriatric Association were modified and adopted as fundamental guidelines in developing services for older adults with mental health problems and their families (ie: client-centred; goal oriented; accessible and flexible; comprehensive; specialized services, and accountable). Embedded in the document are certain assumptions that underlie best practices, the corner-stones of which are (1) mental health is defined as more than a lack of mental illness, and best practices must include health promotion and preventative strategies; (2) a collaborative team-based biopsychosocial-environmental approach to care that crosses sites and services is required; (3) the creation of an environmental milieu and culture of caring that utilizes principles of psychosocial rehabilitation, recognizes peoples' relational needs, and promotes quality of life and supportive/assistive environments, is imperative. In gathering information for our document from the scientific literature, we were struck by how relatively little is actually written about best practices in mental health for the elderly. In particular, deficits were noted in the literature in relation to psychosocial rehabilitation, health promotion and prevention, and the barriers that inhibit best practices. In this round-table session, an overview of the Best Practices in Elderly Mental Health document will be provided by Dr. Martha Donnelly. Dr. Holly Tuokko will talk about the application of health promotion and psychosocial rehabilitation principles to the psychogeriatric population. Penny MacCourt will talk about issues that create barriers to the development of best practices for care-receivers and their families, and for/by care-providers. Each presentation will be brief and serve as a spring-board for eliciting discussion with the audience about each area. This session will facilitate sharing of best practices in mental health for the elderly outside of BC, especially in relation to health promotion, preventative services, psychosocial rehabilitation, and identifying and over-coming barriers to best practices. It is hoped that the discussion will help to develop an international perspective and research agenda about best practices in elderly mental health care.

Barriers to Best Practices in Menta Health care of Elderly Persons

Penny MacCourt(President, BC Psychogeriatric Association, British Columbia, Canada)

In this presentation ideological and systemic barriers to developing and providing services for elderly persons with mental health problems that reflect the principles and assumptions underlying the Best Practices in Mental Health Care for the Elderly in BC, will be identified. It is hoped that participants will share ways that they attempt to overcome similar barriers in their geographic areas.

Issues in the Application of the Principles of Health Promotion, Prevention and Psychosocial Rehabilitation to the Psychogeriatric Population;

H. Tuokko, Associate Director, Centre on Aging, University of Victoria, Victoria, Canada)

In this presentation an over-view of literature and practices in the mental health care of elderly persons that utilize principles of health promotion, prevention and psychosocial rehabilitation will be presented. Suggestions will be made about how these principles could be applied to the psychogeriatric population. It is hoped that participants will share their practice experiences with these approaches and that the foundation for collaborative projects might be laid.

Overview of Best Practices in Elderly Mental Health Care in BC.

M. Donnelly (Mount Pleasant Legionof Community Geriatrics, Department of Family Practice, University of British Columbia, Vancouver, Canada)

The purpose of this presentation is to provide participants with an overview of the process by which Best Practices in Elderly Mental Health Care in BC were developed. The principles that underlie the guidelines for service development will be shared, as will be the underlying assumptions that we believe are corner- stones of best practices. The Best Practices is a living document and by presenting it at this round table , the input of participants may help us to incorporate an international perspective into its' continued development.

SESSION 448

The passive privatization of community long-term care and social welfare for seniors: Outcomes in Canada and UK.

Gillian Dalley (Centre for Policy on Ageing, London, UK) The passive privatisation of social welfare services for older people in the UK Ellen Gee (Simon Fraser University, Vancouver, Canada) The Canadian pension system-Travelling down the passive privatization path Diane Seddon (Centre for Social Policy Research and Development, Bangor, UK) Privatisation of community long term care in the UK Norah Keating (University of Alberta, Edmonton, Canada) Public policy and the costs of informal care Lillian Zimmerman (Canada), Vanessa Burholt (UK)

In the mid-twentieth century, many industrialized nations in the west developed social welfare states. In general, social policy and government programs were informed by an ethos of citizens' rights regarding health, pensions, unemployment etc. as a public good and thus by a value placed on universal access to services. In the past decade or so, an ideological backlash has put welfare states everywhere in some degree of disrepute. A parallel call for privatisation from the political/economic right, along with the 'rediscovery' of families as the main carers of seniors, means a shift from collective protection by the state to individual responsibility. This symposium examines the extent of this shift in Canada and the UK. Authors from both countries address the process and outcomes of this passive privatisation with the goal of comparing the winners and losers among public, private and seniors stakeholders. The session is chaired by Lillian Zimmerman (Canada) and Vanessa Burholt (UK). They will introduce the session by providing an overview of the issue of passive privatisation and will conclude with an analysis of similarities and differences in trends toward privatisation in the two countries. Four papers will be presented. Gillian Dalley discusses passive privatisation of social welfare services for older people in the UK. She describes the ideological and financial pressures that have resulted in the transfer of responsibility for care from the public to the private domain and reviews developments in social welfare services in the UK. Ellen Gee uses the Canadian pension system as evidence of passive privatisation in that country. She argues that fear of population aging is one reason for wide discrepancies in public sector involvement in meeting income needs in later life. In an examination of long term care for frail seniors, Diane Seddon considers the privatisation of community long-term care in the UK. She analyses the contradiction between public policy, which claims to be providing more care in the community and the movement towards a mixed economy of welfare and private parallel provision. Finally, Norah Keating presents an analysis of the impact of public policy in health, labour and income security in Canada on the costs experienced by informal caregivers. She describes a policy analysis framework developed to evaluate the direct and indirect impact of public policies on carers who are family members and friends. The first main outcome from this symposium is an analysis of the question of who benefits from the privatisation trend. The second is a consideration and of whether there should be interventions to reverse this trend.

Privatisation of community long term care in the UK

Diane Seddon (Centre for Social Policy Research and Development, Bangor, UK)

This paper presents an overview of community long-term care provision for older people in the United Kingdom and considers the passive privatisation of this provision over the past two decades. This paper draws upon the research, policy and practice literature, describing the mixed economy policies that emerged and are the legacy of 20 years of conservative government. It analyses the contradiction between public policy, which emphasises the importance of planning, organising and delivering care to older people in the community, whilst at the same time moving towards and mixed economy of welfare and a greater emphasis on payment and private provision in old age. The outcomes of passive privatisation for public and private sector organisations (for example their ability to respond to identified needs), older people (for example the impact on their quality of life and choices available to them) and their carers (for example their ability and willingness to continue caring) are considered. The paper concludes by exploring future options for community long-term care in the United Kingdom.

Public policy and the costs of informal care

Norah Keating, Janet Fast, Jacquie Eales (University of Alberta, Edmonton, Canada)

In Canada, a key justification of the shift toward privatisation of health and welfare has been that the best and least expensive care for frail seniors is informal care provided by families and friends. However, little is known about how individual policies actually influence the economic costs incurred by informal caregivers nor about the collective effect of policies and programs across policy domains and jurisdictions. In the project reported here, we undertook an analysis of the economic impact on informal caregivers of public programs in health, labour and income security. Methods included the determination of domains of economic costs; the development of profiles of caregivers from a Statistics Canada General Social Survey; and a scan of federal, provincial and regional policies across the domains of health, labour and income security. Findings are that the key factors that influence the economic impact of programs are gender, presence of young children, labour force status, geographic proximity, care receiver income and regional economy. There was a poor fit between program eligibility criteria and characteristics that predict negative economic consequences for caregivers, even among the few programs developed explicitly to reduce costs to caregivers. Informal caregivers least well served by existing policy instruments are women who are employed, who have concurrent child care responsibilities, and who live at a moderate distance from their care receiver. A policy analysis framework, developed from this project is presented as a template for tracking the impact of public policies on private costs.

The Canadian pension system-Travelling down the passive privatisation path

Ellen M. Gee (Simon Fraser University, Vancouver, Canada)

The purpose of this paper is to critically evaluate recent reform in and debate about public pensions in Canada. The paper begins with an overview of the Canadian pension system (and its three-tier composition which contains a built-in public-private mix) in comparison with other OECD countries. A brief overview of the current incomes of Canadian seniors is provided, focussing upon discrepancies based on gender and marital status. The main focus of the paper is the reforms and debates of the last decade. In the mid-90s, the federal government proposed a new pension system, called the Seniors Benefit. Before and after its defeat - largely at the hands of private sector purveyors of pension plans who feared it contained disincentives to save, i.e, to purchase their wares - the Canadian government has embarked on a series of acts and promoted a particular ideology that is creating a passive privatisation of pensions in Canada. The ideology is driven by what has been termed apocalyptic demography (fear of population aging and its demands on the welfare state). Acts taken involve the de-universalising of Old Age Security and an associated "social policy by stealth" mechanism regarding indexation of OAS limits; the tightening up of eligibility for disability benefits; the acceptance (due to costs) of marital status discrimination with regard to one benefit (the Spouse's Allowance); the privatisation of Canada Pension Plan investment funding; and an increased purported role for private pension plans and occupation pension plans. The paper concludes with an assessment of the consequences of such actions for the later-life income of future seniors in Canada.

The passive privatisation of social welfare services for older people in the UK

Gillian Dalley (Centre for Policy on Ageing, London, UK)

Two distinct trends in privatisation have been taking place in the UK over the past 20 years - one, the withdrawal of responsibility for the direct provision of services from public sector (state) authorities and the outsourcing of it to private companies and two, the transfer of responsibility for care from the public domain to the private domain as a result of both ideological and financial pressures. The first was prompted by the Thatcherite doctrine that 'private' was better (more efficient and morally superior) than 'public' (state). The second can be seen as the outcome of an ideological preference for private (family and individual) responsibility over collective responsibility for the care of dependent people along with the expression of a deep-seated though unarticulated prejudice against a generation of older people whose expectation of support from the welfare state - which they had established and contributed to since 1947 - has been dashed. The paper will review developments in social welfare services in the UK (including residential and domiciliary services and the interface of these with the National Health Service) within this explanatory framework.

SESSION 449

Problems of Dementia in Developing Countries (Indonesian View)

H. Samino &Tony Setiabudhi (Indonesian Association of Alzheimer's and Related Disease Jakarta/ Indonesia)

Since our Minister of Health inaugurated the existance of the 'Indonesian Association of Alzheimer's and Related Diseases' last July 2000; some activities were conducted. We realize that before this existing body was set up; we still do not have any data about the incidence of Dementia in our country. It is also related to the fact that our life expectancy is not so high in comparison to other developed countries.Nowadays the life expectancy was 63 for men and 65 for women. The AAzI (Asosiasi Alzheimer Indonesia) try to conduct a small survey which were coordinated by Prof K. Sidiarto (neurologist) and Prof. W. Sasanto (psychiatrist) from Jakarta during the celebration of the Alzheimer's day last October.There are 60 elderly clients were checked randomly (most of them are clients who stay at the home of the elderly in Jakarta Site) and some results is presented in this paper. We realize that there are still other developing countries which do not start with their activities in this field : We hope that our experience in clinical findings; campaigning the awareness program for laymen as well as for health/ social provider will perhaps can stimulate ideas to countries like Laos; Nepal or Ghana (because we got such a request via e-mail).

SESSION 450

Implementing an Internet-Based Functional Fitness Assessment and Health Promotion Plan for Older Adults

L. Stumpfhauser (Cramer Reed Center for Successful Aging, Wichita, Kansas, USA) Health and Lifestyle Review (HLR): An Internet-Based Standardized Assessment for Use in Placement and Health Promotion for Older Adults. M.E. Rogers (Center for Physical Activity and Aging, Wichita State University, Wichita, Kansas, USA) Assessing Functional Fitness with the HLR. B.S. Chaparro (Department of Psychology, Wichita State University, Wichita, Kansas, USA) Using the HLR to Compare Physical Performance Measures as Predictors of Mobility-Related Disabilty

ISSUE Much of the disability that occurs in later life may be reduced or prevented through early detection of physical deficits followed by appropriate physical activity intervention. This round table will demonstrate the use of the Health and Lifestyle Review (HLR) as an assessment tool, and as a basis for implementing health promotion programs for the young-old to the oldest-old populations. In addition, the use of the Guralnik and Fullerton physical performance measures to assess mobility-related disability will be presented. STRUCTURE This round table will consist of three brief presentations followed by discussion. CONTENT The Health and Lifestyle Review (HLR) is a standardized assessment and centralized database that includes such measures as vision, hearing, mental status, self-care, nutrition, mobility, chronicity, and social support. The HLR is user-friendly, requires minimal computer skills, provides instantaneous data transfer, and online technical support. Individual data from the HLR can be used to assess functional independence, need for support services, and provide basis for participation in health promotion/intervention programs and placement within the continuum of care. Group data are used to obtain a baseline for tracking the effectiveness of such programs, predict clients' probable future needs for intervention services, and provide reports for planning and risk management purposes. The HLR includes functional fitness measures for parameters including strength, mobility, balance, agility, flexibility, as well as activities of daily living (ADL), and instrumental ADL (IADL). The HLR was recently used to compare the efficacy of the Guralnik Test Battery (tandem balance, 5 chair stand, 8' walking speed) and components of the Fullerton Test Battery (30 s chair stand, 30 s arm curl, 8' timed up-&-go, 6 min walk) in identifying difficulties performing ADL and IADL in older adults living independently or in a continuing care retirement community (CCRC). General results of how well they predict mobility-related disability and their applicability to identifying those in need of specific health promotion programs will be discussed. CONCLUSIONS/ANTICIPATED OUTCOMES The HLR provides a viable means for assessing physical abilities in young-old to old-old adults and for measuring the effectiveness of health promotion programs. This round table will provide a means by which attendees can learn how to assess independently living seniors for potential mobility-related disabilities and how to counsel them into appropriate health promotion programs. Expanding the use of the HLR to other groups of older adults would enlarge the database for professionals to use to better understand the onset and progression of disability, and to evaluate the effectiveness of intervention programs that preserve function, enhance the quality of life, and potentially prolong active life expectancy.

An Internet-Based Standardized Assessment for Use in Placement and Health Promotion for Older Adults

Laszlo Stumpfhauser (The Cramer Reed Center for Successful Aging, Wichita, Kansas, USA), Michael E. Rogers (Center for Physical Activity and Aging, Department of Kinesiology and Sport Studies), and Barbara S. Chaparro (Department of Psychology, Wichita State University, Wichita, Kansas, USA)

The Cramer Reed Center for Successful Aging with faculty from Wichita State University and The University of Kansas School of Medicine-Wichita, Kansas, developed a standardized assessment for independently living older adults, called Health and Lifestyle Review (HLR). It consists of a functional assessment accessed by the World Wide Web and a centralized database. The HLR uses validated instruments to screen for hearing, incontinence, dementia, caregiver stress, nutrition, social support, medication interactions, mobility, strength, range of motion, ADL/IADL, fear of falling, healthy habits, and chronicity. Potential users of the HLR are (1) community and university based organizations that offer health promotion programs for older adults, (2) retirement communities, and (3) research entities. The HLR is user friendly: (1) requires minimal computer skills, (2) training is on line, (3) data transfer is instant and automatic (4) facilitates user networking, (5) technical support available online and by telephone. The database can be used to analyze demographic trends, establish functional fitness standards, develop and evaluate innovative health promotion/intervention programs, and to promote cooperative research. Retirement communities may use their own data also to gain objective information about potential residents' functional abilities to assure proper placement, make decisions regarding "life care", planning and risk management, and to identify trends in the market place. Medically prudent health promotion programs based on the HLR will also be discussed.

Assessing Functional Fitness with the HLR

Michael E. Rogers (Center for Physical Activity and Aging, Department of Kinesiology and Sport Studies) Barbara S. Chaparro (Department of Psychology, Wichita State University, Wichita, Kansas, USA), and Laszlo Stumpfhauser (Cramer Reed Center for Successful Aging, Wichita, Kansas, USA).

A number of studies have suggested that functional fitness may compromise both active life expectancy and the quality of life for older adults. However, effectively evaluating physical fitness in large groups of older adults is oftentimes difficult. The Health and Lifestyle Review (HLR) includes measures for many of the physical parameters that determine functional fitness including strength, cardiorespiratory capacity, balance, mobility, agility, and flexibility. These assessments can be grouped (HLRFF) and administered using a series of computer-networked stations. Each participant requires 5min to complete the tests at each station (total time35min). The data are immediately sent to the database and can be analyzed to recognize individual physical deficits, identify demographic trends, establish functional fitness standards, develop and evaluate the effectiveness of exercise intervention programs, and to promote cooperative research activities. Previous studies of young-old to old-old adults (aged 60-101 years) have indicated that the HLRFF is a viable tool for assessing functional fitness among older adults. Furthermore, the HLRFF has been used to assess older adults who participate in a variety of physical activity programs. This has allowed exercise specialists to substantiate the efficacy of programs designed to improve specific components of functional fitness (e.g, strength and balance) in older adults. Tracking functional fitness using the HLR provides valuable information that allows professionals to better understand the onset and progression of disability and to evaluate the effectiveness of intervention programs that preserve function, enhance the quality of life, and further prolong active life expectancy.

Comparing Physical Performance measures of the HLR as predictors of ADL/IADLs

Barbara S. Chaparro, Michael E. Rogers, and Laszlo Stumpfhauser

One characteristic of physical frailty is the inability to conduct activities of daily living (ADL) and independent activities of daily living (IADL). Within the HLR are physical performance measures including those of Fullerton and Guralnik. The HLR was recently used to assess the relationship between functional fitness and ADL/IADL capabilities. Seventy-three independently living older adults, age 66-101 years (85.96.3y; meanSD) from a retirement community were assessed over a span of two days. Relationships between the Guralnik Test Battery (tandem balance, 5 chair stand, 8' walking speed) and components of the Fullerton Test Battery (30 s chair stand, 30 s arm curl, 8' timed up-&-go, scratch test, chair sit-and-reach) and reported ADL/IADL scores were assessed. Results indicate that these measures of functional fitness are significantly related to the ability to perform both ADLs and IADLs. IADL was significantly correlated with tandem balance ($r=.535$; $p<0.001$), walking speed ($r=.408$; $p<0.001$), ability to stand from a chair ($r=.513$; $p<0.001$), 30 s chair stand ($r=.581$, $p<0.001$), 30 s arm curl ($r=.518$; $p<0.001$), 8' timed up-&-go ($r=-.707$; $p<0.001$), scratch test ($r=.285$, $p<0.05$), and chair sit-and-reach ($r=.354$; $p<0.01$). Similar relationships were found for ADLs. Results from regression analyses show the 8' timed up-&-go test to be best functional fitness predictor of daily functioning, accounting for 52% of the variance for ADL and 44% of the variance for IADL. Comparisons of young-old and old-old populations with respect to functional abilities will also be discussed.

SESSION 452

Altermatives: Prevention and Intervention for Alcohol and Drug Problems in Seniors

E. McKee (COPA, Toronto, Canada)

The demand for training on addiction treatment for older persons is greater than the resources available to respond with trainers. With the objective of disseminating information about addictions and older persons, Alternatives was designed. More than just a video, Alternatives is a complete presentation kit. In addition to the 29 minutes video containing two case scenarios and responses, Alternative also contains handout and overhead masters, background information on seniors and drug use, a step-by-step guide for organizing and delivering presentations, and two relevant information pamphlets. Alternatives presents an overview of the stresses facing seniors, the problems of decreased tolerance, the potential for prescriptions or over the counter drugs to be misused, and the problems of drug and alcohol interacting. Practical advice for either seniors or their caregivers, and healthy alternatives to alcohol and drug use are emphasized. Alternatives was a joint project of Addiction Research Foundation (now a division of Centre for Addictions and Mental Health), COPA and LESA (Both COPA and LESA are community-based addiction treatment programs for older persons.)

Haven in a heartless World - Abuse of elderly people in their homes.

Olaug Juklestad, National Centre for Information and Studies on Violence, Oslo University College

This video shows examples from Norway of abuse of elderly people. From research and also from working with elder abuse cases in Norway we know that women are the main victims of elder abuse. The perpetrators include daughters, grandchildren and sons-in-law, but consist mainly of husbands who mistreat their wives and sons abusing their parents or a single mother. One of the victims we met in our work, Anna, tells her story about a long-lasting marital conflict and what can often happen when an abuse victim doesn't receive necessary help even though many professions are involved. The video also includes a role play which illustrates reciprocal abuse between spouses, meaning that they alternate in taking the roles of victim and perpetrator. These cases typically include serious verbal and emotional/ psychological abuse, and some of these individuals (husbands) may resort to physical violence. The video also covers some aspects of elder abuse that we have uncovered through working in Elder Protective Service in Norway and insights in

SESSION 453

Sexuality and Health at the Menopause and Beyond

Fran E. Kaiser, M.D. [Merck & Co, Inc, Irving, Texas, USA]

This presentation will review the effects of estrogen deficiency on women and examine the interaction of aging and sexuality. Highlights will include the changing concept of the interaction of estrogen and cardiovascular disease and the role of estrogen and other agents in maintaining bone. The importance of the HERS study in altering estrogen utilization in older persons will be explored. Women maintain sexual function throughout life unless a medical disorder intervenes. The loss of estrogen can lead to dryness of the vagina. The role of testosterone decline at the time of the menopause in producing alterations in libido is controversial. Pain on intercourse (dyspareunia) is an important issue for some older women. Many patients are misinformed about sexuality. A sexual history should be a part of the general medical history. The effects of dementia on sexuality and the role of caregivers will be explored. One half of elderly women are widows and the health professional needs to be sensitive to their needs.

Potency in Older Men

Alvaro Morales, M.D. [Queens University, Kingston General Hospital, Kingston, Ontario, Canada]

Potency declines in many males with aging but is predominantly due to the aging process. Development of a penile erection requires the relaxation of cavernous smooth muscle. This involves the release of nitric oxide. the most common cause of erectile dysfunction (impotence) is vascular. Other causes include drugs (recreational such as tobacco and prescriptional such as beta-blockers), autonomic neuropathy, endocrinopathies and multiple sclerosis. Strength of erection is dependent on adequate levels of testosterone. testosterone is essential for the production of nitric oxide synthase. Diagnosis of erectile dysfunction involves a careful history and examination and then special tests as indicated. Males with vascular erectile dysfunction should be worked up for other atherosclerotic disease and risk factors for atherosclerosis treated. The management of erectile dysfunction now usually begins with the use of an oral phosphodiesterase-5 inhibitor such as sildenafil. A number of other phosphodiesterase-5 inhibitors are being developed. Slow release apomorphine (aprima) may be useful in some males. Other approaches include giving prostaglandin E1, either by urethral suppository or intracavernosal injection. Vacuum tumescent devices are useful in some older persons. In many men, penile prosthesis remains a major option. The details of a trial of oral testosterone therapy on sexuality in older men will be reviewed.

Sexuality and Aging

John E. Morley, M.B, B.Ch. [Saint Louis University Health Sciences Center and St. Louis VA Medical Center, St. Louis, Missouri, USA The Machopause] Fran E. Kaiser, M.D. [Merck & Co, Inc, Irving, Texas, USA, Sexuality and Health at the Menopause and Beyond] Alvaro Morales, M.D. [Queens University, Kingston General Hospital, Kingston, Ontario, Canada, Potency in Older Men

ISSUE: This symposium addresses the issues associated with aging and sexuality and also the broader effects of male and female hormone deficit on the aging process. STRUCTURE: John Morley will first address the effects of testosterone deficiency (machopause) in the aging male. Al Morales will discuss the causes and treatment of erectile dysfunction. Fran Kaiser will examine sexual issues facing the older woman and the effect of estrogen deficiency. CONTENT: 1. Testosterone decline in the older male plays a role not only in libido but also in sarcopenia, osteoporosis and altered cognition. A clinical diagnostic screening test is available and when positive bioavailable testosterone should be measured. 2. Vascular disease is the major cause of erectile dysfunction. The diagnostic approaches to erectile dysfunction will be discussed. The effects of testosterone on erectile dysfunction will be explored. Modern treatments of erectile dysfunction will be discussed. 3. Estrogen deficiency plays a role in osteoporosis in women. The changing view of estrogen in atherosclerosis prevention in view of the HERS study will be explored. The changes in female sexuality with aging will be reviewed. ANTICIPATED OUTCOMES: At the end of this symposium health professionals should be able to advise older persons the state of the art approaches to sexual problems that may occur with aging.

The Machopause

John E. Morley, M.B, B.Ch.[Saint Louis University Health Sciences Center and St. Louis VA Medical Center, St. Louis, Missouri, USA

The andropause or the symptomatic decline in testosterone in older males is now well accepted. Longitudinal studies have demonstrated that testosterone levels fall with aging and sex hormone binding levels increase. For this reason, bioavailable testosterone is a more appropriate measure of active testosterone in older persons. The majority of older males have secondary hypogonadism, i.e, a failure of the hypothalamic-pituitary unit. There are now a number of studies demonstrating that testosterone replacement improves libido, upper limb strength, bone mineral density, cognition and frailty. Testosterone may play an important role in the pathogenesis of sarcopenia. The major side effect of testosterone is an increased hematocrit. Effects of testosterone on the prostate are not clear at this stage. A clinical diagnostic questionnaire for andropause called the ADAM questionnaire has high sensitivity. ST. LOUIS UNIVERSITY ADAM: ANDROGEN DEFICIENCY IN AGING MALES QUESTIONNAIRE 1. Do you have a decrease in libido (sex drive)? 2. Do you have a lack of energy? 3. Do you have a decrease in strength and/or endurance? 4. Have you lost height? 5. Have you noticed a decreased enjoyment of life? 6. Are you sad and/or grumpy? 7. Are your erections less strong? 8. During sexual intercourse, has it been more difficult to maintain your erection to completion of intercourse? 9. Are you falling asleep after dinner? 10. Has there been a recent deterioration in your work performance? Yes responses to #1, #7 or any three other questions would be a positive questionnaire.

SESSION 455

Case management of pressure ulcers

Aviva Even Zahav, Geriatric Clinical Supperviser (Sheba Medical Center, Ramat-Gan, ISRAEL) Debora Muchnik, Nursing Standard and Procedures (Sheba Medical Center, Ramat-Gan, ISRAEL) Hana Kertzman, Reseach Unit(Sheba Medical Center, Ramat-Gan, ISRAEL)

Pressure ulcer is one of the main problems which delay the recovery process of patients, it also may detirurate patients clinical status along with pain and suffering. Universal hospitalisation data shows accurence of pressure ulcer in 3-110f all patient addmissions to general hospitals. Aditional data shows that 700f patients with pressure ulcer are at the age of 70 years and over. We found that the professional knowledge among medical staff in relation to the treatment of pressure ulcer is poor, and that there is an enourmus varaiety of methods of treatment and procedures among medical staff and wards. As a result, available resources were not used properlly and the effectiveness of clinical treatment was low. PURPOSE: To increase and improve knowledge among medical and nursing staff. METHOD: A multi proffesional team was formed. The team included senior nurses, physicians, a diatitian and a clinical pharmacist and it was leaded by the hospital geriatric suppervisor. The team performed a major audit of pressure ulcer among hospitalised patients, preventing means and treatment. RESULT: The outcomes of this audit were: poor documantation of treatment, lack of continuity and follow up of pressure ulcer condition, inconsistency of treatment and faliure of the preventing process. Following this process, we witnessed a major promotion in awareness of all medical and nursing staff. CONCLUSION: The team decided on designing a multidiciplinary protocol for prevention and treatment, professional workshops, structured audit system and consultation. Our presentation will emphassize the process stages and beneffits of it.

Determining When a Mattress Is Just Right - Prevention of and Intervention for Pressure Sores

Debra F. Elm (The Good Samaritan Society, Edmonton, Canada)

With the great variety of pressure relief and pressure reduction mattresses available determining which mattress is appropriate for specific resident/client needs is an ominous task. The Good Samaritan Society, a multi-site continuing care service provider set out to investigate the effectiveness of available mattresses for the prevention of and intervention for pressure sores. A literature search was done to determine the factors that cause pressure sores and the properties of a mattress that address these factors. A decision tree was developed which identified three categories of mattresses needed. The goal then was to determine which mattresses would be recommended for purchase for each category. Manufacture's information was obtained on mattresses available and was sorted into the three categories. Category one mattresses (the minimum standard for any resident) were reviewed first. The mattresses were short listed based on what the literature stated were acceptable properties. A vendor day was then held where staff and residents evaluated the mattresses. The evaluations were reviewed and four of the mattresses which scored the highest were brought in for trial for a two week period. Four residents were chosen to evaluate the mattresses for comfort and ease of movement, and the staff evaluated them of ease of resident transfers and manageability. A mattress was then chosen and recommended for purchase. Category two and three mattresses (increasing with pressure reduction need) are scheduled for evaluation in the same way, where an interface pressure sensor device will also be used. These results will be available for the presentation.

Epidemiology and characteristics of pressures ulcers in elderly in acute settings

Angela M. Botero, Fernando Gómez, Marta C. Bernal, Carmen Lucía Curcio, Arnoby Chacón [Geriatric and Gerontological Research Group, Caldas University, Manizales, Colombia]

Objective: to determine demographic, functional and epidemiological characteristics among elderly with pressure sores on admission to a referral teaching hospital for one year. Design: cross sectional and descriptive study. Setting and patients: nine hundred eighteen patients 60 years old and over admitted to Caldas Hospital in Manizales between September 1998 and September 1999. All patients were evaluated in initial 72 hours. Clinical data base were obtained from admission assessment. Demographic data and initial diagnosis were obtained. Skin was assessed systematically using the Fitzpatrick classification, ulcer were staged according to the National Pressure Ulcer Advisory Panel (1989). Area and localization of each ulcer was determined. Spanish version of Barthel scale for activities of daily living (ADL) was used with score ranged 0-100 points. Results: Eighty-seven of 918 (9.5%) subjects have pressure sores on admission. The age ranged between 65 and 95 years (mean 72.5 SD 8.1). The predominant age group of patients with pressure sores was 75-79 years (26.1%). Women were 53% and 90.8 Barthel scale scores ranged between 0 (54%) to 65 points. Most frequently occurring classifications of primary admitting diagnosis for the total sample were neurological diseases (28.7%) and Osteomuscular disease (23%). Two hundred nine pressure sores were found in 87 patients and one patient had 7 PS. The sacrocoxigea region was the most common site of PS (29.7%) followed by buttocks (21.5%), trochanter 16% and heel 11.2%. Less than 5% were found in other areas as dorsal column, omoplat, maleolo, knee, iliac spine, elbow and foot. Conclusion: The PS prevalence found is similar to literature reports in patients admitted to hospital settings and their characteristics are similar to other prevalence studies. It is necessary develop PS prevention programs in home for patients with neurological and osteomuscular diseases especially with stroke and hip fracture.

Platelet gel to improve wound healing and tissue regeneration in patients with pressure ulcers

Sacchi M.C.°, Perrero L, Bellora A., Levis A.°, Cornaglia E°, Sinaccio G. §, Laguzzi E.* *Division of Geriatric Medicine, SS Antonio e Biagio e C. Arrigo; Hospital, Alessandria, Italy; # School of Specialty of Geriatric Medicine, University School of Medicine, Turin, Italy; °Department of Hematology, SS Antonio e Biagio e C. Arrigo; Hospital, Alessandria, Italy; § Bioethical Service;National Institute Cancer Research (IST).*

INTRODUCTION. Pressure ulcers are associated with significant rates of morbidity and mortality in the geriatric population. Newer pharmacologically active therapies include the topical application of Growth Factors. By thinking about the importance to use a platelet gel as a source of multiple autologous GFs in the treatment of pressure ulcers, an easy, safe and economic technique has been recently set up to obtain quickly an autologous gel that can be used as routine in attempt to accelerate the healing of chronic wounds. The innovation of this technique consists in the substitution of the bovine thrombin, not biological safe and not saleable in Europe, with batroxobin. PATIENTS AND METHODS. Six elderly (>65) patients suffering from pressure ulcers, with the concomitant presence of more diseases (comorbidity: 4 ± 2 disease associated), have been selected. All patients were given informed consent before inclusion in the study. PC, prepared starting from a low quantity of whole blood (60 ml), is activated by a batroxabin-calcium gluconate blend to obtain a platelet gel. RESULTS. The results show, for all patients, an improvement in the cleaning and in the painful symptomatology, a reduction in ulcers’ sizes and, for five of the six treated patients, the recovery after 6 weeks from the first application. CONCLUSION. These excellent initial results demonstrate that the platelet gel stimulates repair of pressure ulcers resulting in accelerated granulation tissue formation and epithelization. ETHICAL ASPECTS. This study has been projected following the indications of Helsinki’s Declaration, Good Clinical Practice’s laws (GCP) and D.M. 18.3.1998.

Validity and reliability of the Spanish version of Braden scale for predicting pressure ulcers risk in elderly

Marta C. Bernal, Carmen Lucía Curcio, José Arnoby Chacón, José Fernando Gómez M, Angela María Botero [Geriatric and Gerontological Research Group, Caldas University, Manizales,

Colombia]

Objective: To determine the predictive validity and reliability of the Braden scale for predicting pressure ulcers in elderly people in a tertiary care hospital. Design: Cohort study. Methods: Eight hundred thirty one patients 60 years old and over without pressure ulcers admitted to Caldas Hospital in Manizales between September 1998 and September 1999 were included. Clinical data base were obtained from admission assessment. Demographic data and initial diagnosis were obtained. Skin was assessed systematically using the Fitzpatrick classification. Spanish version of Barthel scale for activities of daily living (ADL) was used with score ranged 0-100 points. A translated Spanish version of Braden scale was used. All patients were evaluated in initial 72 hours and observations were made every week for a minimun of 1 to a maximum of 3 weeks or until pressure sore was developed. Sensibility, specificity, predictive value of a positive test (PVP) and predictive value of a negative test (PVN) were calculated for different points over a range of Braden Scale scores. Main outcome measure: presence/absence of pressure ulcers according National Pressure Ulcer Advisory Panel classification. Results: The mean age was 71.9 (SD 8), 57% were men and 96.9%. The predominant age group of patients with pressure sores was 75-79 years (26.1%). Women were 53% and 90.8 The score in Braden scale ranging between 6 and 23 and interquartile range was 15, 21. A cutoff score of 16 was found to provide better predictive value with sensitivity 85.4% and specificity 63.2% and PVP was 12.5 and PVN 98.6. The Pearson correlation coefficents ranging between 0.70 and 0.81 Conclusions: These results suggest that Spanish version of Braden scale is valid and reliable scale to use in acute settings with a cutoff point of 16. However, several factors as age and functional status could be affected this cutoff point.

SESSION 456

How to build an Acute Care for Elders (ACE) program: a Canadian inter-disciplinary perspective

R.Y.M. Wong (University of British Columbia, Vancouver, Canada) Optimizing physician services in an Acute Care for Elders (ACE) unit. M. Shaw (Vancouver Hospital and Health Sciences Centre, Vancouver, Canada) Improving outcomes for the acutely ill elderly. M. McMillan (Vancouver Hospital and Health Sciences Centre, Vancouver, Canada) Physiotherapy service in an Acute Care for Elders (ACE) unit. E. Breurkens (Vancouver Hospital and Health Sciences Centre, Vancouver, Canada) Facilitating function - The role of Occupational Therapy in an Acute Care for Elders unit. S.M. Trautman (Vancouver Hospital and Health Sciences Centre, Vancouver, Canada) Systems Theory: A Social Work intervention when working with families/patients in an ACE unit

This Round Table session focuses on the planning and implementation of an Acute Care for Elders (ACE) program in a tertiary care hospital from an inter-disciplinary perspective. The session begins by discussing how proven effective strategies from research studies have been adapted and modified to address the unique local needs of a major Canadian health sciences centre, as well as some practicalities of developing and implementing an ACE program. This information will be provided via brief presentations from the perspectives of Medicine, Nursing, Physiotherapy, Occupational Therapy and Social Work, followed by ample opportunity for the audience to interact with presenters in a semi-formal way to address any pertinent issue. The target audience includes physicians, nurse practitioners, allied health professionals, administrators and other individuals who are interested in optimizing care for frail elders during their acute medical illnesses. The emphasis is on the practical aspects of building an ACE program. For instance, physician services within an ACE unit can be optimized by encouraging collaboration amongst different primary care providers (Family practitioners and Internists) and consultants (Geriatricians and Psychiatrists). Nursing practice is advancing in the care for older adults by focusing on their environmental, functional and cognitive requirements. Timely Physiotherapy assessment and intervention is important to prevent functional decline during hospitalization, especially when mobilization is a team effort with Occupational Therapy, Nursing, patients and families. To ensure "windows of opportunity" are not lost for older patients to return to the community at the time of discharge, Occupational Therapy can proactively intervene by early assessment, providing the relevant equipment and implementing preventative measures. Finally, effective discharge planning can be achieved by applying Systems Theory and the use of the Genogram as a Social Work intervention when dealing with families and/or patients in ACE unit. In summary, various health disciplines can contribute tremendously in the delivery of patient-centered care to acutely ill elders with an emphasis of preserving independence and function. At the end of this session, the audience will gain a deeper appreciation of how an ACE program can be constructed by pooling expertise and resources in an inter-disciplinary manner.

Facilitating function - The role of Occupational Therapy in an Acute Care for Elders unit

E. Breurkens (Vancouver Hospital and Health Sciences Centre, Vancouver, Canada), C. Sowden (Vancouver Hospital and Health Sciences Centre, Vancouver, Canada), C. Weihr (Vancouver Hospital and Health Sciences Centre, Vancouver, Canada)

Functional status or independence has been shown to be a cornerstone in determining length of stay and eventual discharge outcomes for elders admitted to acute care, regardless of the particular disease or symptom with which they present. The mandate of the Acute Care for Elders (ACE) unit is congruent with the current client-centered theories of Occupational Therapy (OT) practice. Thus the therapist is able to speak a common language with all team members and facilitate coordinated care with elderly clients. Through observation and interview, the OT begins identifying the Occupational Performance issues with the client. From these we are able to determine specific Performance Components and Environmental issues which are stumbling blocks for maintaining and/or improving function. Data from our assessments contribute to the individualized care plan on activities for daily living for each client. This ensures a consistent and congruent approach to care by all team members. Also, a baseline is established against which to measure effectiveness at time of discharge. Appropriate and timely interventions, provision of equipment and preventative measures ensure that "windows of opportunity" are not lost and discharge to the community remains a real option for our elderly clients. The occupational therapist has a multifaceted role on the ACE unit encompassing direct treatment of clients and developing the therapeutic milieu with other team members which makes this program successful.

Improving outcomes for the acutely ill elderly

M. Shaw (Vancouver Hospital and Health Sciences Centre, Vancouver, Canada), C. Acton (Vancouver Hospital and Health Sciences Centre, Vancouver, Canada)

Hospitalization is a critical juncture for acutely ill older adults and their families. For many frail elders, hospitalization marks the beginning of a downward trajectory characterized by declining physical strength and function, delirium, depression, adverse drug reactions, poor nutrition/hydration, cognitive deterioration, and loss of independent community living. While the downward trajectory is often attributed to an underlying disease process, considerable research suggests that hospitalization contributes to decline through iatrogenesis, polypharmacy, immobilization, and depersonalization. This presentation will describe the development of an ACE unit, an acute medical unit providing highly skilled health services and specialized geriatric interventions that aim to improve the outcomes of care for acutely ill older adults and their families. Specifically, we will address (a) redesigning interdisciplinary health care services during times of fiscal restraint, (b) lessons learned in the creation of a supportive environment for elder care, and (c) advancing nursing practice to address common issues in acute gerontological nursing such as medications of risk and immobility.

Optimizing physician services in an Acute Care for Elders (ACE) unit

R.Y.M. Wong (University of British Columbia, Vancouver, Canada), G.S. Meneilly (University of British Columbia, Vancouver, Canada), B. Stackhouse (Vancouver Hospital and Health Sciences Centre, Vancouver, Canada), R.N. Stanley (University of British Columbia, Vancouver, Canada)

To optimize patient-centered services in a 21-bed Acute Care for Elders (ACE) unit at a Canadian tertiary-care hospital, we have implemented a collaborative model of physician practice. Elderly patients with acute medical illnesses who require hospitalization are admitted through the Emergency Department to the ACE unit under the care of either family physicians or general internists based on medical complexity. For patients who present without an assigned family physician, hospitalists provide primary care during their hospital stay. To further enhance collaboration, the ACE unit is co-managed by a geriatrician and family physician. Guidelines are developed to define the physician roles and responsibilities in areas such as the frequency of patient rounds and response time when called by the unit. Consultations with Geriatric Medicine and Geriatric Psychiatry specialty services are readily available on a referral basis, with clear guidelines established in both cases. Constant medical review is possible during twice-weekly inter-disciplinary team rounds and morning reports 2 other days of the week. Continuing medical education on geriatric concepts is available to both attending physicians and their housestaff. Physician attitude towards providing care for elderly patients can also be assessed. In summary, encouraging collaboration among the various stakeholder groups involved and establishing the infrastructure to support physician activities, we can optimize physician services in an ACE unit.

Physiotherapy service in an Acute Care for Elders (ACE) unit

M. McMillan (Vancouver Hospital and Health Sciences Centre, Vancouver, Canada)

A goal of care for the elderly patient is to minimize muscle weakness, deconditioning and functional decline associated with acute illness and hospitalization. The ACE unit team identifies patients who are at risk. Physiotherapy (PT) assessment, recommendations and treatment plans are initiated within 24-48 hours. Particular attention is given to patients with repeat hospitalizations, especially if discharged recently. The physiotherapist (a) assesses functional ability and potential for improvement; (b) liaises closely with medical staff regarding functional status; (c) assists the patient and family to reach realistic functional short and long term goals; (d) provides a specific rehabilitation program which addresses the patient's problems. The PT Assistant assists with patients when two therapists are required, and supervises patients' daily exercise or ambulation programs as directed by the physiotherapist. Mobilization is a team effort with PT, Occupational Therapy and Nursing staff working collaboratively with patient and family. Family members are encouraged to be present during physiotherapy sessions and to assist as appropriate. A therapy room within the ACE Unit facilitates short treatment sessions, family participation and education. At twice weekly rounds, the team addresses medical, social issues and concerns regarding patient progress and discharge plans. Home-care PT follow-up is arranged as required. Patients who require further rehabilitation are transferred to the Sub Acute Medical unit that is in close proximity to the ACE unit. The expected outcomes are early mobilization, prevention of avoidable functional loss and successful discharge back to the community.

Systems Theory: A Social Work intervention when working with families/patients in an ACE unit

S. M. Trautman (Vancouver Hospital and Health Sciences Centre, Vancouver, Canada)

Systems Theory (ST) and the use of the Genogram is a useful Social Work (SW) intervention when dealing with families and/or patients from an Acute Care for Elders (ACE) unit. ST is a framework that views individuals, families, hospitals and other institutions as examples of systems. These systems are interdependent with other systems and each system is viewed to strive toward maintaining an overall equilibrium. When one system is stressed and no longer able to function, it has an effect on the other interconnecting systems. The entire system then struggles to maintain equilibrium. The role of SW is to identify which system is unbalanced and to intervene within that system to bring about greater change within the entire system. The use of a Genogram can identify which system requires SW intervention. A Genogram views the family as having a number of interconnecting systems (home support, hospital, extended family, physical, social and emotional) and demonstrates how these systems affect the family's overall level of functioning. The Genogram helps SW to think systematically about the systems in relationships to the family's life cycle and how they are related to patterns of health and illness. A Genogram is a tool for SW intervention that helps SW to keep in mind the complexity of a family's context, and identifies systems that need to be maximized for the overall functioning of the family.

SESSION 457

Community Based Elder Care in Asia: The Development of Home Help As a Critical Priority

Mary Ann Tsao (President/CEO, Tsao Foundation, Singapore) Susan Mende (RN, MPH, Aged Care Consultant, Sydney) Mala Manap (Vice President for Programme Development and International Affairs, Tsao Foundation, Singapore) Mark Gorman (Director of Programming, HelpAge International, London)

Ageing is one of the greatest challenges for 21st century Asia, as Asia will house almost two-thirds of the world's ageing population - the vast majority of whom will be in the developing countries of Asia.
With rapid ageing and a still infantile age care sector, Asia's growing population of the very old, frail, chronically ill or disabled older people are facing increasing difficulty as the gap widens between their needs and the care delivery capacity of the family and their country's health and social systems. For the many Asian countries still in development, the establishment of age care systems is further constrained by endemic poverty and other development priorities.
Other than family care, most countries still consider nursing homes the only other option for the frail and disabled older people for whom family care is not available. At the current accelerated rate of population ageing, institutional care as the only alternative is neither ideologically desirable, nor economically viable. This is especially true as the number of older people who need care will sharply increase, while the capacity for families to provide care decreases with smaller families, increasing female work force participation, immigration, changing family values and other factors.
Working with HelpAge International's Asian network of aged-care agencies, more than a dozen countries ranging from Sri Lanka to Cambodia - have identified home help as the most critically needed service for their country's frail older people. Relatively undeveloped, most Asian countries still lack home help and have varying levels of resource to establish such services at this time.This symposium will describe the status of home help in selected Asian countries and outline the challenges. The symposium will also address the role of care management, training, and a regional NGO to NGO home care initiative in the development of home help in the Asian region. Four speakers will address the following: i)Ageing demographics in Asia ii) An Asian multi-country survey study on home help iii) Singapore's experience with a socio-medical care management model iv) The role of training and a train-the-trainer model for home helpers/family carers v) The HelpAge International's regional home care initiative

"Ageing In My Own Place": A Sample of Home Help and Home Care Programmes in Fifteen Countries in the Asia-Pacific Region

Mende, Susan (RN, MPH, Aged Care Consultant, Sydney)

"When I am in good health, it is okay, but when I am sick I need to stay in bed. I am so lonely and I have no one to help me. I cannot clean my room and I cannot even wash my clothes because I am not in good health"
The fears of this older Korean woman are shared by millions of frail, vulnerable, older people across the Asia Pacific region.
Despite the continued prevalence of family care, family support is coming under strain at a time when the numbers of older people in the region are due to increase. This situation is even more critical for older people without families, who are reliant on community-based support for assistance with the all important activities of daily living. Home care services (health and support services provided to older people and their families in their own homes) can play a critical part in an overall system of care to meet the needs of frail older persons.
A number of service providers (mainly NGOs) in the Asia Pacific region have responded to the challenge of providing home-based care to this group of vulnerable elderly, and a sample of these programmes in selected countries are described in the report, "Ageing in My Own Place". Specifically, programmes in Australia, China, Fiji, Hong Kong, India, Indonesia, Korea, Macao, Malaysia, Mongolia, Philippines, Singapore, Sri Lanka, Thailand and Vietnam are described and analysed. The small and large Home Care and Home Help programmes across the region involve volunteers, paid staff, professionals and non-professionals, and a range of approaches to the provision of home-based health and support services. It is hoped that the experiences of these programmes will inform and support the development of home care services in the

Providing New Models of Care in Asia
Gorman, Mark

In the context of the changing demographic, economic and social situation in the Asia region, the need for researching and developing new forms of care for older people has become a priority. This presentation outlines the background of the HelpAge International home care initiative, a regional collaboration of HAI network members to provide best practice models with the aim of influencing policy and practice in home care.

The Role of Care Management in Community Based Care in Asia - The Singapore Experience
Tsao, Mary Ann (President/CEO, Tsao Foundation, Singapore)

As one of the fastest ageing countries in Asia and the world, Singapore has been challenged with the building of an effective age care system within a short time, and care management has emerged as a critical component of community-based elder care that serves to integrate the wide range of health and social needs of the frail, disabled and chronically ill older people throughout their life course. Two years ago, the Tsao Foundation's Hua Mei Care Management Service (HMCM) was established as a pilot.
A recent evaluation showed it to be effective in helping older people prolong their stay in the community and enhancing their quality of life. As in the West, care management helps older persons and their families manage the multitude of intertwining health and social services in order to ensure that the right service is delivered at the right time while containing cost.
Hua Mei Care Management, however, faced many challenges due to a weak primary health care system for older people, poor coordination between the various health care providers, insufficient and fragmented community services (such as home help and transport), absence of long term care financing for community care, low level of public understanding of geriatrics care and services, and decreasing family care capacities.
Because of these and other barriers to care, an effective care management service while difficult to run - is all the more valuable in supporting community living for frail older people.
This paper will describe the Hua Mei Care Management model and experience, its challenges and applicability in the Asian region. This paper will also discuss how care management together with home help is a priority and complementary service that can help maximize the impact and effectiveness of whatever limited resources that are available as Asia struggles to meet the health and social needs of its older people in the coming years.

Training in Home Care
Manap, Mala

Training for carers be they family caregivers, service providers or volunteers is critical for the effectiveness of any homecare programme. Training initiatives developed for homecare have to be strategic given the extensivness of the training needed, often nothing short of a national coverage. Strategies which have been developed in Singapore by the Tsao Foundation alongside partner organisations to achieve this maximum impact and coverage in homecare training will be discussed for possible adaptations in other parts of the Asian region.

SESSION 458

Tibor Janke: The Art of Survival
Pamela Brett-MacLean (The University of British Columbia, Vancouver, Canada)

This video celebrates Tibor Jankay, an impassioned artist, a lover, a survivor and a teacher. Born in a small Hungarian town in 1899 he began expressing himself through art at the age of six. As a victim of the holocaust, Tibor's artistic perspective and strong will helped him stay alive. He later immigrated to the United States with his beloved wife, and business partner, Irene. In this documentary film one experiences the sweep of passion, love, vision, colour and beauty that sustained and enervated him through to the end of his long life.

SESSION 461

[1] The clinical observation on the treatment of osteoporosis in males by dehydroepiandrosterone sulfate.
Sun Yiping, Mao Minwei, Sun lihua, Feng Yingying (Gerontology, The Shanghai Sixth People's Hospital, Shanghai China)

Purpose: To study the effect and security of dehydro-epiandrosterone sulfate (DHEAS) treatment of osteoporosis in males with TBMD 2.5sd . Method: 86 patients were divided randomly into two groups : the treatment group (n=44) and the control group (n=42), DHEAS (100 mg QD) was given to the treatment group for 6 months. The bone mineral density (BMD) biochemical markers of bone absorption and formation, and other serum biochemical markers were measured before and after DHEAS treatment. The drug side effects were also studied. Results: After oral administration DHEAS (100 mg QD) for 6 months, the serum concentrations of DHEAS and IGF-1 in the treatment group were respectively $93.75\pm16.1\%$ and $17.71\pm4.2\%$ higher than those in the control group ($P<0.01$). The BMD of L2, L3, L4, L2-4 and neck sections increased in the treatment group by $2.65\pm0.65\%$, $2.70\pm0.48\%$, $3.10\pm0.41\%$, $2.82\pm0.37\%$ and $2.32\pm0.31\%$, respectively, as compared with control group ($P<0.05$ or 0.01). No significant changes were observed in serum FT, E2 and PSA concentrations in the treatment group as compared with the control group. Conclusions: The treatment of osteoporosis in males with DHEAS is safe and effective.

[2] Distribution of osteoporosis risk factors among elderly women
Palma Reis, Helena (Algés Health Center, Lisbon ,Portugal)

Osteoporosis is an important Public Health problem owing to the risk of fracture. The factors implicated on bone mineral density are genetic, hormonal, ambiental and nutritional. Purpose: The aim of this study is to reveal the risk factors of osteoporosis among the elderly women living in the comunity, not in nursing homes and not dependent, followed by a general practitioner in a portuguese urban center. Methods and Results : A retrospective study was performed in 556 caucasian women aged 55 and over divided in groups: 193(55-64 years), 148(65-74 years), 215(<=75 years); medium age - 73.2 years The risk factors of osteoporosis were divided in the three age groups to compare them. Low BMI(17; 9; 4%); Family history of osteoporosis (29; 23; 25%); Early menopause(18; 17; 13%); Delayed menarch (10; 8; 10%); Nuliparity (10; 7; 5%); Menstrual problems (28; 15; 19%); Non breast feading (8; 10; 8%); Lack of physical activity (73; 81; 84%); Smoking habits (18; 10; 3%); Cofee intake (45; 27; 16%); Alcohol intake (18; 29; 12%); Inadequate calcium intake (72; 85; 88%); Lack of sun exposure (65; 80; 95%); Corticosteroids Therapy (12; 10; 8%); Anticonvulsivant therapy (2; 3; 3%); Hidroxid AL therapy (5; 3; 2%); Thyroid hormone (8; 5; 3%). Conclusions: There is no significant difference in the values of the three age groups. The high prevalence of the risk factors that can be changed (physical activity, smoking habits, calcium alcool and coffee intake, sun exposure) justify the efforts towards the preventive mesures, the earliest possible among all the population.

[3] Differential influence of physical activity on lumbar spine and femoral neck bone mineral density in elderly.

Vuillemin A 1,2, Guillemin F 2, Jouanny P 3, Denis G, Blain H 4, Durant R4, Jeandel C4 (1 Faculty of Sport, Nancy, France ; 2 School of Public Health, UPRES EA 1124, Faculty of Medecine, Nancy, France; 3 Department of Geriatrics, CHU Rennes, France; 4 Antonin Balmès Gerontology Center, Montpellier, France)

PURPOSE: This study investigates the relationship between lifetime physical activity and bone mineral density (BMD) at various sites in 129 healthy men and women aged 72.1±6.5 years. METHOD: BMD was measured by dual energy x-ray absorptiometry, and physical activity was assessed using the QUANTAP system (QUANTification de l'Activité Physique), a standardized and structured computer-assisted interview tool designed to assess lifetime physical activity. Linear regression models controlling for age, sex, height, body mass, lean mass and smoking habits were performed. RESULTS: Higher levels of Sporting activity during youth were associated with greater lumbar spine BMD ($p < 0.001$). Similarly, femoral neck BMD was greatest in subjects who reported regularly taking part in sport over the previous 20 years ($p < 0.05$) and during their whole lifetime ($p < 0.05$). Sporting activity at the time of bone mass development increases subsequent lumbar spine BMD, and more recent sport contributes to the preservation of femoral neck BMD. CONCLUSION: These results suggest that physical activity has a differential influence on BMD at different sites and at different ages, possibly related to the processes of bone construction and bone aging taking place at the time.

[4] Oropharyngeal Candidosis in elderly : Prevalence in a short-term hospital care

F. Retornaz, V. Seux, J. Soubeyrand (Hôpital Sainte Marguerite, Marseilles, France) A. Blancard (Hôpital Timone, Marseilles, France)

PURPOSE Prevalence of oral candidosis increases in elderly, specially in patients living in institution. METHOD We analyzed risk factors, symptoms and signs of oral candidosis in a cohort of 101 patients age * 65 years, mean age 72 (65 -96) and we compared the results of clinical suspicion of candidosis and microbiological results. When oral candidosis was suspected, empiric treatment was started before the results of yeast culture and then was modified if necessary according these results. RESULTS Yeast culture were positive in 51,5% (80% for Candida albicans, 10% for Candida glabrata and 4% for Candida tropicalis). Two different species of candida were isolated in 13%. 38% of patients were considered as infected. 12% were defined as carriers, 2% had symptoms without positive swabs. With the result of yeast culture, treatment was modified in 35 patients. 16 untreated patients received fluconazole (12) or amphotericin B (4). Treatment was stopped in 3 patients because of the negativity of the culture. Empiric treatment was modified in 16 patients (14 received fluconazole instead of sodium bicarbonate and 2 received amphotericin B instead of fluconazole). 57 patients remained untreated and only 9 patients continued the empiric treatment. CONCLUSION Prevalence of oral candidosis is very high in elderly subjects admitted on general hospitalization. An accurate diagnosis is assured if positive cultures are associated with signs and symptoms suggestive of candidosis. In hospitalized patients, management of oral candidosis requires yeast cultures because of the low specificity of clinical evaluation and the frequency of different species of Candida.

[5] Ultrahigh Frequency Electromagnetic Therapy in Treatment of Old Patients with Osteoarthrosis of Knee Joints

V. V. Povoroznjuk, E. I. Bayandina (Department of Clinical Physiology and Pathology of Locomotor Apparatus, Institute of Gerontology AMS Ukraine, Vyshgorodskaya St. 67, 04114 Kiev, Ukraine)

Ultrahigh frequency electromagnetic therapy (UFET, 10 mV/cm2) was used to accelerate metabolic processes in the knee joints, improve the joint's functional state and reduce the pronounced pain syndrome. The greatest effect of treatment was gained when action had been performed on the acupuncture points. Treatment was accomplished by means of an instrument "Elektronika-KVCh-101". This instrument is designed to carry on a microwave reflexotherapy by influencing reflexogenic zones with low intensity (10 mV/cm2) electromagnetic waves. The biologically active points were influenced during one seance of 30 min (15 min per each point). One course consisted of 1015 seances. The following points were involved: E35, E36 and R10. Twenty-eight patients aged 56 to 72 years, including 17 women, were examined. All of them had the diagnosis of knee joint osteoarthrosis of IIIII stage. The process was bilateral in 20 patients. The effectiveness of treatment was evaluated according to the dynamic of clinical and instrumental data obtained before and after treatment. As a result of treatment, the patients displayed a considerable increase (on the average by 1518 degrees) in volume of knee joint movements and reduced pain syndrome. The best results were seen in the patients having pronounced "night pains" caused by venous congestion in bone tissues. In 7885% of them night pains disappeared following a course of treatment. Thus, the UFET method can be recommended for treatment of patients with pronounced painful syndrome on the background of deforming knee joint osteoarthrosis.

[6] Anthropometric Data and Bone Tissue Functional State of Postmenopausal Women

V. V. Povoroznjuk, O. P. Dmitrenco (Department of Clinical Physiology and Pathology of Locomotor Apparatus, Institute of Gerontology AMS Ukraine, Vyshgorodskaya St. 67, 04114 Kiev, Ukraine)

There has been increasing evidence that anthropometric data are connected with bone state. In this study we've investigated anthropometric data and bone tissue functional state in 59 postmenopausal women. Bone tissue functional state was determined by ultrasound densitometry. Results are presented in the table. Bone density in postmenopausal women with osteoporosis was lower than in persons with normal or high weight ($p<0,05$). The women with normal bone mineral density have a higher body mass index, fold thickness on shoulder, back, stomach and shin than women with osteoporosis.

[7] Calcaneus Ultrasonometry in Pre and Post Menopausal Women: Comparison with Bone Densitometry

A. C. A. Souza, M Badalotti, R. H. Schneider, Y. Moriguchi (Laboratory of Osteoporosis and Bone Metabolism on Geriatric and Gerontology Institute PUCRS, Porto Alegre, Brazil)

Postmenopausal women have an increased risk of developing osteoporosis. Decreased bone mass is only one of a several factors known to bone fragility. We studied the calcaneus ultrasound profile in 114 premenopausal and 173 postmenopausal women (mean 55± 10 years). 100 women were selected for bone density comparison with DEXA. There was a negative correlation between ultrasound and age (r = -0.33, p<0.0001) and between ultrasound and menopausal time (r = -39, p<0.0001).There was a significant positive correlation between ultrasound and the density of spine and femoral neck (range 0.57 -0.62, p< 0.01). Linear regression showed that ultrasound is partially dependent of the bone density (R2 range 0.32- 0.34: p < 0.0001). Patients with osteoporosis showed a statistically significant decrease in BUA, SOS and QUI (p<0.002) when compared to normal women. In order to identify osteoporotic women, at the BUA cutoff point of 61.9 dB/MHz, at the SOS cutoff point of 1539.4 M/s and the QUI cutoff point of 85.4 the negative prediction value was 57%. In order to identify osteopenic and osteoporotic women, at the BUA cutoff point of 68.6 dB/MHz, at the SOS cutoff point of 1555.6 m/s and at the QUI cutoff point of 96, there was 87%, the specificity was 74%, the positive prediction value was 88% and the negative prediction value was 72%. These results suggest that postmenopausal bone alterations can be detected by ultrasound and this method can be considered a good population screening test for osteoporosis.

[8] Peripheral bone mineral density predicts fracture risk among women aged 65 and older

E. Siris (Columbia University, New York, NY), L. Wehren (University of Maryland, Baltimore, MD), E. Barrett-Connor (University of California, San Diego, La Jolla, CA), K. Faulkner (Portland, OR), P. Miller (Colorado Center for Bone Research, Lakewood, CO), T. Abbott (Merck & Co, Inc, West Point, PA), Y. Chen (Merck & Co, Inc, West Point, PA), M. Berger (Merck & Co, Inc, West Point, PA), A Santora (Merck & Co, Inc, Rahway, NJ), L. Sherwood (Merck & Co, Inc, West Point, PA)

Purpose. To determine whether peripheral bone mineral density (BMD) predicts fracture risk in women aged 65 and older, and to evaluate whether the relationship between BMD and fracture risk is the same for all ethnic groups. Methods. The National Osteoporosis Risk Assessment (NORA) program has enrolled over 200,000 postmenopausal women in the United States. Baseline questionnaire and peripheral BMD measurements (heel, forearm, or finger) and one-year follow-up fracture information were collected from 80,847 women. World Health Organization classification of BMD was used: normal (T-score >-1.0); osteopenic (-2.5 < T-score < -1.0); or osteoporotic (T-score < -2.5). Fracture rates were compared across BMD groups and for Caucasian vs non-Caucasian women. Results. Data were available for 73,485 Caucasian and 7,362 non-Caucasian women, of whom 3,614 women reported any new fracture and 1,903 reported fractures at typical osteoporosis sites (hip, wrist, forearm, rib, or spine)(shown in attached figure of fracture rates). BMD-adjusted fracture rates were much higher for women aged 80+ than for younger women. Conclusions. Low peripheral BMD predicted increased fracture risk in each group examined. BMD-adjusted incidence of fracture was relatively stable in women under the age of 80, and greatly increased in women 80+. The high incidence of fractures in women with low BMD emphasizes the need to identify and treat women with osteoporosis.

[9] Altered Hip Abductor Muscle Activation with Hip Osteoarthritis

KJ Sims, C Richardson, SG Brauer (Department of Physiotherapy, University of Queensland, St Lucia, Australia)

PURPOSE: Theoretical models suggest that hip abductor muscle activity may play an important role in controlling forces across the hip. Any alteration in muscle activity could influence the development or progression of hip OA. A recent gait study has suggested that there may be an alteration in the activity of the hip abductor muscles in some adults with hip osteoarthritis (OA). However, this study was descriptive only, lacking quantitative measures of muscle activity. The purpose of this study was to use quantitative measures to determine whether hip muscle activity was different in subjects with unilateral hip osteoarthritis in comparison to healthy older adults. METHOD: Thirty-eight older adults (19 healthy: 72±6 years; 19 unilateral hip OA: 69±7 years) performed a rapid, reaction-time step-up task. Surface electromyography was recorded from the stance-limb gluteus medius and tensor fascia latae. Onset and magnitude of activity were calculated. Components of the step, and centre of pressure were recorded with force platforms. Group, side and group x side effects were determined with repeated-measures ANOVA. RESULTS: Gluteus medius muscle activity of the affected side of hip OA subjects showed a delay in timing and a reduction in magnitude when compared to healthy subjects. Tensor fascia latae activity varied widely in OA subjects. CONCLUSION: Subjects with unilateral hip OA showed changes in hip abductor muscle activity when compared to healthy older subjects. Whether these changes occur prior to or as a result of joint disease is yet to be determined.

[10] An Interdisciplinary Approach to Osteoporosis Rehabilitation

E. Kilpatrick, J. Wilson, C. Young, P. Bond, D. DiCastri(Victoria Arthritis Outpatient Treatment Centre, Victoria, B.C, Canada)

PURPOSE: The Victoria Arthritis Centre's Osteoporosis Rehabilitation Program (OPRP) is a tertiary rehabilitation program for individuals with a diagnosis of arthritis and a secondary diagnosis of osteoporosis with moderate to severe impairment. The purpose of this interdisciplinary program is to test the efficacy of a clinically- based intervention on the functional ability and quality of life for individuals with osteoporosis. METHOD: The development of the OPRP followed from the identification of a treatment gap for individuals with significant impairment due to their osteoporosis. Provincial and international literature searches were conducted. From the information gathered, the OPRP was developed, consisting of combined group education and land/ water-based exercise sessions. Program instructors included Physical Therapists, Occupational Therapists, and the Nurse. The Social Work Counsellor was employed on a consultation basis. RESULTS: Groups of eight(8) participants met for seven(7), two(2) hour sessions. Health outcomes were measured at intake and discharge from the program using the McMaster Quality of Life Questionnaire (OQLQ) and the Modified Timed Up and Go(TUG) test. A six month follow-up assessment was conducted. Results indicate: 1) improved physical activity; 2) decreased pain related to postural deformity; 3) decreased risk of fracture; 4) increased use of fatigue management techniques; 5) improved nutrition and calcium supplement use. CONCLUSION: based on the early reasearch findings, the Victoria Arthritis Centre's OPRP has been successful in improving the functional ability and the quality of life of its participants.

[11] Compare Treatment Effect of Rocaltraol and Rocaltrol With Alendrenate on Senile Osteoporosis

Shen Ge, Gon Yun Xia, Peng Xiao Fen, Zhu Li Ming (Geriatric Department, Rui Jin Hospital Shanghai Second Medical University, China Shanghai)

Abstract: Purpose To compare the treatment effect of single Rocaltrol (Calcitriol) and Rocaltrol with Alendrenate (Bisphosphonates) on the senile osteoporosis. Methods 40 cases of osteoporosis patients (n=40, mean age=75 years) were randomly divided into 2 groups, 19 patients take the Rocaltro alone, 21 take Rocaltrol with Alendrenate. The duration of treatment was 6 month. The bone mineral densith (BMD) and symptoms were detected before and after treatment. Results In two groups, the BMD L2-4 increased significantly after treatment(p<0.01); the BMD L2-4 in single group increased 7.3%, the combination group increased 14.1%(p>0.05). The BMD of Hip also increased in the combination group , but the single not. Conclusions Both Rocaltrol and Rocaltrol with Alendronate were effective in treatment of O.P. The effect of Rocaltrol with Alendronate were superior to Rocaltrol alone

[12] Undiagnosed osteoporosis in women over age 65: the NORA experience

E. Siris (Columbia University, New York, NY), L. Wehren (University of Maryland, Baltimore, MD), E. Barrett-Connor (University of California, San Diego, La Jolla, CA), K. Faulkner (Portland, OR), P. Miller (Colorado Center for Bone Research, Lakewood, CO), T. Abbott (Merck & Co, Inc, West Point, PA), Y. Chen (Merck & Co, Inc, West Point, PA), M. Berger (Merck & Co, Inc, West Point, PA), A. Santora (Merck & Co, Inc, Rahway, NJ), L. Sherwood (Merck & Co, Inc, West Point, PA), S. Brenneman, (Merck & Co, Inc, West Point, PA)

Purpose: The National Osteoporosis Risk Assessment (NORA) has enrolled over 200,000 postmenopausal women, 95,156 of whom between 65 and 104 years of age. NORA participants had no prior diagnosis of osteoporosis and had not had bone mineral density (BMD) testing within the previous year. Methods: Questionnaire information and peripheral BMD measurements (at the heel, forearm, or finger) were collected on each woman. Results: Most participants (85,162) are Caucasian; however, African Americans (3440), Hispanics (3325), Native Americans (1095), and Asians (765) are included. The mean (SD) age was 72.8 (5.8) years; 6821(7.3%) currently smoke and 32683 (35.0%) previously smoked. Excellent or very good health was reported by 39.1%; 41.7% reported fair or poor health. 22.4% had previously used estrogen and 32.9riteria, 50.20f women had osteopenia and 13.0% had osteoporosis. The prevalence of osteoporosis increased with age (8.3% among women aged 65-74; 38.3% among women aged 85+), with decreasing body mass index (by quartile), and with lower self-reported health. By ethnicity, osteoporosis was most common among Asian and least common among African Americans. Over half (53.2%) met National Osteoporosis Foundation treatment guidelines. Conclusion: Women aged 65 and older should be routinely evaluated for osteoporosis.

[13] Evaluation of management of osteoporosis following an acute fracture

Anna Byszewski (Regional Geriatric Assessment Program, The Ottawa Hospital Civic Campus, Ottawa, Canada), Anne Cranney (Division of Rheumatology, The Ottawa Hospital Civic Campus, Ottawa, Canada), Malcolm Man-Son-Hing (Regional Geriatric Assessment Program, The Ottawa Hospital Civic Campus, Ottawa, Canada), Nahid Azad (Regional Geriatric Assessment Program, The Ottawa Hospital Civic Campus, Ottawa, Canada), Stephanie Amos (Regional Geriatric Assessment Program, The Ottawa Hospital Civic Campus, Ottawa Canada) Solange Dias

Osteoporosis is a leading health problem for the aging population. As new treatment options emerge, there is more evidence that these therapies are of benefit even for very old persons. Objective: To characterize the pattern of practice in the management of osteoporosis for patients admitted to an acute care hospital for acute hip/vertebral fractures. Method: Retrospective chart review (1 April 1999 Δ 31 March 2000): Data analyzed included standard demographics, assessment of risk factors, diagnosis and management of osteoporosis. Results: The average age of the 71 patients with hip fractures was 82.6 years. 30 returned to independent living. 89.50% underwent orthopedic surgery for the hip fracture. Cognitive difficulties were present in 54.9%. At discharge the majority were discharged from an orthopedic ward (55.5%) or geriatric assessment unit (34%). Average LOS 26 days. In the majority of cases, no risk factors for osteoporosis were recorded in the charts. 25% use sedatives and 27.80% of those on sedatives had previous falls. Only 4.2% had a DXA scan ordered, and 8.3% had a new diagnosis of osteoporosis. 33% had osteoporosis treatment ordered (mostly calcium and vitamin D). Lifestyle modifications such as fall intervention were addressed in 24.2%. No one received information about hip protectors. Conclusion: The management of osteoporosis continues to be a challenge in the older population. Interventions such as patient/physician information toolkits need to be developed in order to enhance the management of patients with osteoporosis.

[14] Vertiginous Syndrome in the Elderly

F. Halici, G.I. Prada, M. Mihalcioiu, S. Galaftion (Ana Aslan National Institute of Gerontology and Geriatrics, Bucharest, Romania)

We investigated the etiology of the vertiginous syndrome and its significance in the elderly. The study is based on 296 patients out of 1082 patients (27,4%), aged 70 years and over, admitted to Ana Aslan NIGG between January 2000-December 2000. We considered all patients presenting with dizziness or a vertiginous syndrome and established the diagnosis of them. The samplewas divided into three age groups: 70-79 years - 185 patients (62,5%), 80-89 years - 96 patients (32,4%), >90 years - 15 patients (5,1%). The age range was: 70-92 years (mean 81 years). Gender distribution was : women - 230 (77,7%), men - 66 (22,3%). The majority of the patients admitted to hospital with these symptoms, were women, especially in the age group 70-79 years. There were significant differences between patients belonging to different age groups. The oldest group had the least prevalence of all. There was also a significant difference, $p<0,05$, between women and men, in the age group of 80-89 years. The most frequent diagnosis of these patients was cervical osteoarthritis +/- dorsolumbar osteoarthrosis, 154 patients (52%), followed by orthostatic hypotension, 63 patients (21,3%) and depression, 35 patients (11,8%). The rest of them had sharp variation in hypertension, extrapyramidal syndrome, different forms of cardiac arrhythmia. We could observe the great impact of these symptoms on the elderly and the importance of a correct diagnosis, due to different ways of therapeutic approaches and various outcomes.

[15] A Systematic Literature Review and Best Practices in Falls Prevention for Older Adults

Victoria J. Scott (University of Victoria, Victoria, BC, Canada) Steven R. Dukeshire (Research Consultant, Truro, NS, Canada) Elaine M. Gallagher (University of Victoria, Victoria, BC, Canada) Andria M. Scanlan (BC Injury Research and Prevention Unit, Vancouver, BC, Canada) Safety and Security Working Group for Seniors (Federal/Provinical/Territorial Ministries Responsible for Seniors)

The multifaceted, interdependent complexity of fall risk factors makes it difficult to first identify and then change the constellation of factors that need to be targeted for an intervention to be effective in reducing falls and fall-related injuries that occur among older adults. The purpose of this project, funded by the Federal/Provincial/Territorial Ministers of Health and Responsible for Seniors, was to develop a Canadian guide for researchers, practitioners and educators in relation to preventing falls and fall-related injuries among community-dwelling seniors. This was accomplished under the direction of the F/P/T Safety and Security Working Group for Seniors through the following: 1) a systematic review of published and unpublished literature pertaining to interventions aimed at reducing falls and related injuries among seniors; 2) a comprehensive inventory of Canadian programs targeting the prevention of falls among seniors, and 3) a best practices guide to help practitioners develop, implement, and evaluate fall prevention programs among seniors. In addition to filling a void in the literature on falls prevention for the elderly, the project generated a unique, sophisticated framework for conducting comprehensive reviews of any sort, enabling the inclusion of both qualitative and quantitative research reports that meet with rigid criteria.

[16] Muscle and bone changes in hip fractures in the elderly over 75 years

P. Prokopova [Institute of pathology, 1-st medical faculty, Charles University, Prague, Czech Republic], Z. Kalvach [1-st medical faculty, Charles University, Prague, Czech Republic], M. Zeman [1-st department of surgery, Charles University, Prague, Czech Republic]

To assess muscle changes in hip fractures as well as correlation between involution of muscles and bones. Biopsies from muscular gluteus medius and bone tissue removed by surgery of hip fractures or serious osteoarthritis were investigated histologically in two groups of patients of the same age: patients with osteoarthritis [secondary muscular atrophy from inactivity] and patients with accidental injury without serious osteoarthritis [muscular involution]. The study is in progress and it is to be finished before the congress takes place. Preliminarily we suppose significance of muscle changes not only for instability and falls but also for bone resistance as well as parallel changes in muscle and bone tissue, probably in connection with worsening of neural regulation and influence on tissue nutrition.

[17] Fall related factors among a community-dwelling elderly cohort in Sao Paulo, Brazil

Monica Rodrigues Perracini (UNIFESP - Federal University of Sao Paulo - Sao Paulo - Brazil) Luis Roberto Ramos (UNIFESP - Federal University of Sao Paulo - Sao Paulo - Brazil)

This work represents a two-year prospective study, assessed in two waves of multidimensional household surveys (1991/92 and 1994/95), with a cohort of 1667 community-dwelling elderly citizens, aged 65 or older. The aim of this study is to identify factors relating to falls and recurrent falls, indicating the relative importance of each factor in terms of fall prediction and determining risk profiles. A stepwise logistic regression analysis was conducted with $p<0.005$ and 95% CI. The cross-sectional analysis revealed a model similar to that derived from the follow-up, with two fall related dependent variables: falls at any moment within the study and recurrent falls. The fall related factors at any moment within the study were: history of fractures (OR=4.6; 95% CI 2.23-9.69), female gender (OR= 2.3; 95% CI 1.70-3.06), poor or very poor sight (OR= 1.5; CI 1.12-1.97). Also, probabilities of a fall are amplified with the increased difficulty experienced in performing daily routine activities: around 1.5 times higher in elderly persons with 1-3 impaired activities (95% CI 1.14-2.03) and 2.5 times higher in elderly persons with upwards of 4 impaired activities (95% CI 1.47-4.05) in their daily routines. For recurrent falls, the predictive model is drawn up according to variables such as reading as a leisure activity and marital status, so that the recurrent falls related factors were: history of fractures (OR= 7.76; 95% CI 3.24-18.57), female gender (OR= 1.75; 95% CI 1.03-2.95), increase for elderly persons with no partner (OR= 1.59; 95% CI 1.00-2.52), and also increase for the group of elderly persons that do not read as a leisure activity (OR= 1.56; 95% CI 1.03-2.37), among the elderly whose sight is most impaired and finally, the chances of recurrent falls increase with the gradual reduction in functional capacity, so that for the elderly who are unable to perform 4 or more activities with little or no difficulty the odds are 3.3 times higher (95% CI 1.58-6.93). This study indicates the relevance of analyzing fall related factors in the elderly because it is possible to stress the chances of the occurrence of this type of event based on predictive models, estimating the individual risks and, above all, determining risk profiles to allow preventive intervention in elderly populations. The study also indicates the need to implement measures for prevention and rehabilitation in order to reduce the modifiable risk factors, such as in the case of functional capacity and sight, which exercise a fundamental role in influencing or determining a fall in the future.

[18] The Relationship between Physical Performance and Falls among the Japanese elderly Living in a Rural Community

S. Ueki, T. Kasai, J. Takato, Y. Sakamoto, H. Shimanuki, Y. Orii, H. Haga (Tohoku Bunka Gakuen University, Sendai, Japan), H. Imuta (Yamagata University, Yamagata, Japan), S. Yasumura (Fukushima Medical University, Fukushima, Japan), R. Kozakai, N. Niino (National Institute for Longevity Sciences, Ohbu, Japan)

The purpose of this study was to investigate the risk factors on falls among the elderly persons living in a Japanese rural community. We carried out the survey on falls and health among 507 elderly persons (189 males and 318 females) and the physical performance test among 287 elderly persons (100 males and 187 females), aged 75 years and over living in a rural community in Sanbongi town, Miyagi, Japan. We interviewed total health conditions, self-rated health, experience of falling, and measured grip strength, percentage of body fat, circumference of thigh and calf, flexibility of body bending in sitting style, one leg standing time with eyes open, total time during standing up a chair, walking for 6 meters, and sitting on a chair (Up & Go), and preferred and maximum speed walking for 10 meters. Annual incidence for falls for male and female subjects were 22.2% and 28.0%, respectively. On the relationship between the physical performance and experience of falling, the total point of motor fitness scale and preferred and maximum walking speeds of the subjects who fell was significantly lower than that of those who did not. In addition, one leg standing time and Up & Go time of the subjects who fell had a lower tendency than that of those who did not. These results suggest that motor fitness scale, one leg standing time and Up & Go time, in addition to walking speed, have discriminant and predictive validity for assessing the future occurrence of falls among the elderly aged 75 years and over.

[19] Maximal voluntary isometric knee extension strength in 64-74 years old female twins

K.Tiainen,M.Alen (Department of Health Sciences, University of Jyväskylä, Finland), J.Kaprio (Department of Public Health and General Practice, University of Oulu, Finland), E.Heikkinen, T.Rantanen (Department of Health Sciences, University of Jyväskylä, The Finnish Centre for Interdisciplinary Gerontology, University of Jyväskylä, Finland).

PURPOSE: Knee extension strength is important for functional independence in everyday life, yet little is known about the relative role of genetic and environmental influences on knee strength. The purpose of this study is to examine genetic influences on maximal isometric knee extension strength among older female monozygotic and dizygotic twins. METHOD: As part of the ongoing Finnish Twin Study on Aging (FITSA) 16 monozygotic (MZ) and 106 dizygotic (DZ) twin pairs have been investigated by December 2000.Participants were drawn from the Finnish Twin Cohort Study. The maximal voluntary isometric knee extension strength was measured in the dominant side using an adjustable dynamometer chair (Metitur LTD, Finland).The subject was in a seated position and the angle of the hip joint was 90 and the angle of the knee was 60 from the fully extended leg towards flexion. The ankle was fastened by a belt to a strain-gauge system. The best result of three measures was taken for the analysis. RESULTS: The mean maximal isometric knee extension strength in MZ twin individuals was 276 N (SD 97) and 287 N (SD 87, p= 0.535) in DZ twins. The mean height and weight in MZ twins was 158.0 cm (SD 6.1) and 72.4 kg (SD 11.1) The respective values in DZ twins were 158.5 cm (SD 6.0) and 70.2 kg (SD 11.9). In MZ twins, the within pair correlation for knee strength was 0.619, whereas in DZ twins it was 0.318, suggesting the influence of additive genetic effects and unshared (non- familial) environmental effects.Thus, the heritability of knee extension strength was estimated to be 60 %. CONCLUSION: The first analysis suggests substantial genetic effects on individual differences in knee extension strength among older women. Consequently, genetic influences may also play a role in disablement process. Results will be confirmed and examined in more detail after data collection in March 2001 is completed.

[20] Postural sway in 64-74 year-old female mono(MZ)- and dizygotic(DZ) twins

S.Pajala(Department of Health Sciences, University of Jyväskylä),P.Era(Department of Health Sciences,University of Jyväskylä),M.Koskenvuo(Department of Public Health, University of Turku), E.Heikkinen(Department of Health Sciences, Finnish Centre for Interdisciplinary Gerintology, University of Jyväskylä),T.Rantanen(Department of Health Sciences, Finnish Centre for Interdisclipinary Gerontology, University of Jyväskylä).

PURPOSE Recording postural sway is a widely used method in studying postural balance. The aim of this study is to investigate postural sway in MZ and DZ twin pairs to determine genetic effects on postural balance. METHOD As a part of Finnish Twin Study on Aging(FITSA) 14 MZ and 107

DZ female twin pairs aged 64-74 years recruited from Finnish Twin Cohort study participants, have been examined by December 2000. Postural sway was measured using force platform method. Data were collected in Good Balance NT system(METITUR LDT, Finland). Sway was recorded for 30 seconds in normal stance with eyes open and closed and for 20 seconds in semi-tandem stance with eyes open. Variables analyzed were: Total path of center of force movement in medio-lateral(mean X-speed,mm/s)and antero-posterio(mean Y-speed, mm/s)direction throughout the test and the mean moment of velocity(mm2/s).The within pair Pearson correlations were computed for MZ and DZ twins. RESULTS No differences in age, body height and mass and sway measures were observed berween MZ and DZ twins. The within pair correlations of sway in normal stance eyes open, in normal stance eyes closed and in semi-tandem stance in MZ pairs were 0.478, 0.272 and 0.086(X-speed), 0.484, 0.478 and 0.661(Y-speed)and 0.524, 0.376, 0.160(velocity moment). In DZ twins, the correlations were 0.133, 0.186, 0.261 and 0.180, 0.268, 0.205 and 0.200, 0.210, 0.130, respectively. CONCLUSIONS In this first analyse correlations varied among sway variables but slightly higher correlations in MZ twins suggests that there might be additive genetic component in balancing ability in older women. The recruitment of additional MZ twins is still in progress and the results will be confirmed and detailed after completion the data collection in March 2001.

[21] Frequencies and circumstances of falls among community-dwelling middle-aged and elderly people in Japan

H. Ogasawara, N. Niino, S. Tsuzuku, F. Ando, H. Shimokata (National Institute for Longevity Sciences, Aichi, Japan)

Purpose: The purpose of the present study was to report the result of fall surveys in NILS-LSA (National Institute for Longevity Sciences, Longitudinal Study of Aging). Method: Frequencies and circumstances of falls were assessed among 2255 middle-aged and elderly people who participated in the initial survey of NILS-LSA from November, 1997 to April, 2000 and responded to the questionnaires. The variables analyzed in the present study were demography and history of falls in the past one-year. Circumstances of falls, e.g. time, location, activities associated with falls, cause of falls and degree of injury due to falls were asked when the subjects experienced a fall. Fear of falling was also investigated in all subjects. Results: The prevalence of falls was 13.3 0n the middle-aged group (40-59yr.) and 18.7 0n the elderly group (60-79yr.). The distribution of time, location, activity associated with falls, cause and injury due to falls corresponded with previous falls studies among community-dwelling elderly people. The incidence of falls was extremely high during the daytime and outdoors. Falls occurred most frequently while walking. The majority of falls were due to extrinsic factors. About 40% of all falls caused no injury. As to the fear of falling, about 30% of the middle-aged subjects and about 60% of the elderly subjects reported that they were fearful. Conclusion: This paper revealed the frequencies and circumstances of falls among community-dwelling middle-aged and elderly people in Japan. The results suggested that fall accidents are not rare, even in middle-aged people.

[22] Effects of a four-week balance training intervention for elderly women

S. Sihvonen (Department of Health Sciences, University of Jyvaskyla, Jyvaskyla, Finland) P. Era (Metitur, Jyvaskyla, Finland and Department of Health Sciences, University of Jyvaskyla, Jyvaskyla, Finland)

PURPOSE: It is known that age-related degenerative changes in different sensory modalities effect the functioning of the postural control system in older adults. It has been suggested that despite of deterioration in many visual functions with aging their role in controlling balance become even more important than at younger ages. A randomized trial of four-week balance exercise intervention using visual feedback was carried out among women living in residential care facilities. METHODS: Subjects (N=16, mean age =81 years) were randomized to an exercise group (EG) (N=11) or to an control group (CG) (N=5). The EG attended 30 minute individualized balance exercise sessions on force platform balance measurement and training device (Good Balance, Metitur) three times a week for four weeks. Balance measurements for both groups were completed before the intervention, during intervention for EG and after intervention. Balance measurements included static and dynamic force platform balance tests and a functional balance test (Berg Balance Scale). RESULTS: This intervention differed from several other balance training studies among elderly by involving subjects to train with a device producing immediate feedback of their performances. The analysis of outcome variables including velocity of sway, sway amplitudes and velocity moment for static tests and total performance times and distances for dynamic tests are in preparation. CONCLUSION: Balance training using visual feedback may be an efficient way to enhance balance abilities of elderly adults.

[23] Evidence-based Guideline for the Secondary Prevention of Falls in Older Adults

J Moreland (St. Joseph's Hospital and McMaster University, Hamilton ON, Canada), J Richardson, D Chan (McMaster University, Hamilton, ON, Canada), J O'Neill, A Bellissimo (St. Joseph's Hospital, Hamilton, ON, Canada), Rosa Maria Grum, Lynne Shanks (Community Care Access Centre, Hamilton, ON, Canada)

PURPOSE: To develop an evidence-based practice guideline for the management of older adults who have sustained an accidental fall to prevent further episodes of falling. METHOD: An evidence model was developed. MEDLINE and CINAHL data bases were searched for studies of risk factors. We selected studies which were prospective and had greater than 80% follow-up. The estimate of the risk for each factor was abstracted and collated across studies. A method for rating the strength of evidence was developed and applied. The same data bases plus the Cochrane Library were searched for randomized controlled trials which evaluated interventions to prevent falls. Study quality was assessed and graded. Based on the evidence, recommendations for assessment and management were made. RESULTS: For community-dwelling older adults, the subjective assessment consists of 8 items. The objective examination includes 8 items and specific lab tests. Management addresses the findings and may include further investigation, medication adjustment, education, or referral to therapies. Institution-dwelling older adults should be assessed by a nurse on 13 items including environmental safety. Relevant findings are reported to the primary care physician. Eight lab tests are recommended. ECG and 24 hour Holter monitoring are also suggested. Medications should be reviewed. Identified medical problems are treated and referral to therapies, optometry, audiology or chiropody may be indicated. A user-friendly assessment and management checklist was developed to accompany the guideline. CONCLUSION: Evidence is present in the literature for the development of a comprehensive approach to the secondary prevention of falls in older adults.

[24] Nosocomial trauma of geriatric patients

Imre MOLNAR M.D. (Department of Internal Medicine and Geriatrics, Semmelweis Teaching Hospital, Miskolc, Hungary) Ildiko TORNAI M.D. (Department of Ophthalmology, Semmelweis Teaching Hospital, Miskolc, Hungary) Andrew EROS M.D. (National Institute of Primary Helath Care, Budapest, Hungary) Agnes KARPAT M.D. (Ophthalmologic Clinic, Health Sciences Faculty, Semmelweis University, Budapest, Hungary)

Purpose: To evaluate the effect of nosocomial traumas on qualitiy of life, length of stay and mortality of geriatric patients. The poster focuses mostly on accidents requirin surgery. Mthod: We collected data of noscűocomial traumas for four years in a general community hospital. teh patients were treated on our 96-bed geriatric department. We investigated the visual function too. Results: 3953 patients were studied. Among older adults, the presence of traumas is frequent. The traumas were found mainly on chest, upper arm, gluteal and sacral regions. The analyses showed, that predictor factor of hospital accidents was Barthel index on admission. The vision impairment is a risk factor to trauma in older adults. Conclusions: Limited activities of daily livind, dementia and geriatric problems on admission are the strongest predictor factors of traumas. Surgery influences the hospital mortality of geriatric patients.

[25] Risk Factors for Falls in Hospitalized Elderly

M. Molaschi, P. Maina, S. Speme, M. Ponzetto, M. Neirotti, S. Raspo, F. Fabris (Medical and Surgical Department, University of Torino, Torino, ITALY)

PURPOSE: Aim of the study was to evaluate risk factors for falls in a hospital setting. METHOD: The study was carried out on 301 patients (155 men and 146 women) consecutively admitted to University Geriatric Ward in Torino (Italy). Risk factors for falls were considered demographic variables (age, gender), functional status (IADL, ADL), presence of delirium, type of diagnosis and comorbidity, visual impairment, blood pressure, Body Mass Index, length of hospitalization, drugs, use of walking aids, impairment in balance or gait according to Performance-Oriented Assessment of Balance and Gait (M.E. Tinetti, 1986). RESULTS: Falls occurred in 33 patients (11%). Fallers were older (82.5 ± 7.1 yr.) than non-fallers (78.9 ± 8.2 yr.) The event was more frequent in subjects with impaired balance or gait. The prevalence of subjects using neuroleptics was higher among fallers than in the control group (24.2% versus 10.1%) ($p < 0.05$). Patients treated with narcotics were 9.1 0n the study group and 1.5 0n the control group ($p < 0.05$). Age (RR 1.06, IC 95% 1.01 - 1.13), length of hospitalization (RR 1.04, IC 95% 1.02 - 1.07), use of neuroleptics (RR 3.10, IC 95% 1.12 - 8.58) and narcotics (RR 4.14, IC 95% 1.01 - 16.9) were independent risk factors for falls. Walking without aid was a protective factor (RR 0.15, IC 95% 0.03 - 0.72). CONCLUSION: An assistential control should be planned when elderly patients need psychotropic drugs or are dependent in walking in order to prevent falls. The length of hospital stay of elderly subjects should be reduced by providing home care services.

[26] Validation of an instrument to measure fear of falling in nursing home residents.

Meyer G (University of Hamburg, Hamburg, Germany) Warnke A (University of Hamburg, Hamburg, Germany) Muehlhauser I (University of Hamburg, Hamburg, Germany)

PURPOSE: Assessment of fear of falling as part of a randomized-controlled-trial targeting prevention of hip fractures by external hip protectors.The hypothesis was that wearing the hip protector is instrumental to reduce fear of falling. METHOD: A new tool with 15 items in the 3 dimensions fear of falling, daily living and social life was developed. The Nottingham-Health-Profile (NHP) was used for validation. All 218 residents of 10 nursing homes who were recruited for the main study participated in a baseline assessment. A three months follow-up was pre-planned for 83 residents. Statistical analyses covered factor analysis, internal consistency of subscales, construct and discriminant validity. RESULTS: Of the 218 residents 61CONCLUSION: The new tool is a reliable and valid measure of fear of falling in nursing home residents. However, generalizability and applicabilty are limited by the small proportion of subjects able to complete the tests.

[27] 24 hour ECG Monitoring in Fracture neck of femur

Tayyab Haider, Jamal Karwan, Teshk Shawis (Care of Elderly Department Colchester General Hospital Colchester, UK)

Introduction. Fracture neck of femur (FNOF) causes high morbidity and mortality, hence its importance in health care economics. The main risk factors for (FNOF) include osteoporosis, the risk of falling one of the contributing factors for falls is cardiac dysrhythmia. Aims. To determine the prevalence of cardiac dysrhythmia in patients who had a fall resulting in (FNOF). Design. Case-controlled prospective series. Method. Consecutive cases that had falls resulting in (FNOF). Control was consecutive patients who underwent elective hip or knee replacement both groups had 24 hr ECG monitoring one week post operatively. Patients with dementia, history of syncope, dysrhythmia or who were terminally ill were excluded. Results. Fracture NOF Control Group n% n% Sex F 27 (84) 25 (78) M 5 (16) 7 (22) Age 71-79 72 - 94 mean 81.3 81.1 SVT 12 (38) 4 (13) VT 3 (9) 0 (0) Pauses >2000 ms 4 (12) 1 (3) Interventions 17 (53) 1 (3) Conclusions. Older patients with (FNOF) as a result of fall are likely to have cardiac dysrhythmia in their 24 hr ECG, which may be a contributory factor for the fall. 24 hr ECG monitoring is a non-invasive, non-expensive assessment. We suggest that 24-hr ECG monitoring should be part of orthogeriatric assessment in every fracture neck of femur resulting from a fall.

[28] A study of motion-stress effect on the body centroid, such as head-shaking and an alteration of the body position in old subjects.

Geun-Ho Lee, M.D.[Department of neurology, College of Medicine, Dankook university, Chonan, Korea]

It is well known that many patients with vertigo become vertiginous when an alteration of their body position occurs while either head-shaking or after standing up. Posturography conducted with those patients when standing still is thus not always successful in detecting abnormal symptoms. However, if the patients are subjected to motion-stress, such as head-shaking or alterations of the body position such abnormalities can be easily detected. To assess the effect of such motion-stress on the disturbance of the centroid in normal individuals, posturography was conducted on 40 normal subjects who were subjected to motion-stress in the manner mentioned above. And the results of this test were then compared with the findings of a conventional test. Through this comparison no increase in the imbalance, as a result of the applied motion-stress, was observed for the X distance (XD), Y distance(YD), and Length (LNG). However, a significant increase in the imbalance was found for the XD and LNG in old subjects. Therefore, motion-stress, such as head-shaking or alterations of the body position can be helpful in detecting vertiginous symptoms in vertigo patients. But in the elderly patients, the merit of above stimuli during the test should be yet clarified.

[29] Effects of Falling on the Quality of Life among the Elderly

H. Haga , S. Ueki, T. Kasai, H. Shimanuki (Tohoku Bunka Gakuen University, Miyagi, Japan), S. Yasumura (Fukushima Medical University, Fukushima, Japan), N. Niino (National Institute for Longevity Sciences, Aichi, Japan)

The present study was to examine the effects of falling on fear of falling, physical and emotional health, and social activity of elderly people. Method: Seven hundred and fifty four persons aged 65 and over living in Oiwake Town of Hokkaido, Japan participated in the baseline interview survey in 1998. Of all the subjects, 599 subjects who had never experienced a fall within one year preceding the baseline survey were followed-up for the present study in 1999, one year later. Five hundred and eighteen subjects (86.4%), 241 men and 277 women, responded to the follow-up interview survey. The questionnaire consisted of variables on age, gender, fall experience within the last year, fear of falling, self-rated health, history of diseases, life satisfaction, instrumental activities of daily living, social role, and social network. Results: Of the 518 subjects who did not experience falls at the baseline survey, 68 (13.1%) experienced falls, 452 (86.9%) did not experience falls within one year preceding follow-up survey. The rate of subjects with fear of falling at follow-up was likely to increase in the fallers, but not in the non-fallers. Although both scores of social role and life satisfaction and the number of neighbor with whom subjects associated significantly decreased at follow-up in the fallers, it was not found in the non-fallers. Conclusion: The results suggest that fall experience among elderly people not only increases anxiety about future falling but also causes a deterioration of subjective well-being as well as limitation in social activity.

[30] Fallers and non fallers in a geriatric gait and balance

clinic : a study of 1000 patients

C. Grosshans, MJ. Scheer, B. Peter Service de Gérontologie Clinique, Centre Hospitalier, Mulhouse, France

Methods: Between 1995 and 1999, 1000 elderly patients (mean age 83 years) were examined in a geriatric outpatient clinic specialized for gait and balance disturbances. We compared two groups: 1. Fallers n = 451 2. Non Fallers n = 549 Results: The two groups were comparable for age, sex, medicines (psychoactive drugs and diuretics) as well as cognitive capacities. Of interest are the following differences : group 1 group 2 Stat - more than 3 medicines 73% 68% $p = 0.05$. Spine abnormalities 41% 33% $p < 0.001$. Knee flexion 27% 17% $p < 0.001$. Hip limitations 33% 24% $p < 0.01$. Ankle limitations 41% 20% $p < 0.001$. Loss of proprioception 51% 46% $p = 0.08$. Previous great walker 37% 46% $p < 0.05$. Fallers walked less than non fallers during their active life. Conclusion - Slight limitations of ankle, knee and hip joint amplitudes are more frequent in fallers. Are these limitations likely to cause falls, or are they the consequence of reduced activity and poor gait ? This question needs further research. Careful examination can detect these slight limitations and may give way to the prevention of falls due to psychomotor de-adaptation.

[31] Hip Pads: Effective Hip Fracture Prevention

G Gross, T Chen, C Flaherty (Elder Service Plan, E. Boston, MA, USA)

Falls pose a serious health risk for the elderly. One of the most significant consequences of falls is hip fracture caused by the sudden transmission of a large mechanical load which damages tissues and cells. This review examines the results of a program which used hip pads in community dwelling, frail elders to dissipate the mechanical load over a larger area to prevent injury. This clinical trial compared the rate of hip fracture per fall in a study population wearing hip pads to the rate of hip fracture in a control population. Five hundred and sixty eight total falls were studied over twenty six months and the rates were compared using Fisher's Exact Test. The study population sustained no hip fractures over the twenty six month review for a very promising 0.0% rate compared to 4.3% in the control population. Fisher's Exact test yields a $P = 0.00089576$ and a highly significant difference suggesting that hip pads are an effective hip fracture prevention intervention in this population.

[32] Activity of Daily Living and Quality of Life in Patients with and without Hip Fracture

E.Kajita, N.Hirota (Dept. of Community Health and Gerontological Nursing, Toyama Medical and Pharmaceutical University, Toyama, Japan), Y.Moriguchi, M.Seki, Y.Kibayashi (The Nursing Dep. of SAINOU Hospital, Toyama, Japan)

Purpose: To establish an effective discharge guidance for patients with hip fracture to maintain activities of daily living (ADL) and quality of life (QOL). Methods: The subjects were 2 groups of 75 patients who admitted to a hospital for the treatment of hip fracture (Fx patients) or other chronic conditions (non-Fx patients). ADL and QOL were assessed using the instrumental ADL questionnaire (IADL) and the PGC morale scale, respectively. IADL before the admission and at follow-up and QOL at follow-up were evaluated by a mail survey followed by interviews or telephone calls by nurses for the confirmation of answers. Patients who developed mental illness or dementia, were institutionalized or died during the follow-up were excluded. Consequently 50 patients with hip fractures and 57 with other conditions were analyzed. Results The average age and days of hospital stay of Fx and non-Fx patients were 80.3 ± 7.2 vs 74.7 ± 6.4 years and 90.4 ± 45.4 vs 73.5 ± 115.0 days, respectively. The subjects with low ADL at follow-up were more frequent in Fx patients than in non-Fx patients ($p<0.01$). IADL score at follow-up was significantly lower in Fx patients ($p<0.05$). Having intimate friends was significantly less common in Fx patients than in non-Fx patients ($p<0.05$). However, custom of worship at a temple or shrine or participation to elections was maintained similarly regardless of the fracture. There was no difference in the PGC score between Fx and non-Fx patients. Conclusion The fracture patients QOL (IADL, social activities, PGC) for a discharge plan should be important in the guidance to patients.

[33] Compliance of Hip Protector Pads in severely demented, mobile elderly.

Angela Juby, Lorrie McAuley (Division of Geriatrics, University of Alberta, Edmonton, Canada)

Hip fracture has a mortality >20% and a significant morbidity in the elderly. Pharmacological agents take at least a year to provide measurable fracture reduction and improved bone density. Hip protector pads provide instant protection, but only if they are worn at the time of the fall. This study evaluates the compliance of hip protector pads in mobile, demented seniors residing in longterm care (LTC). A prospective study was undertaken at two LTC facilities admitting severely demented patients. Demographic data, MMSE score, Berg Balance Scale and timed "get up and go" were collected. Patient acceptance of hip pads, duration of wear and falls were recorded. 26 patients were entered into the study: 18 women; 8 men. The average MMSE score was 11.6 (0-25); Berg Balance scores from 3 to 54 with the average being 24.1 ; get up and go test average was 24.3 secs (8->40). 21 (81%) consented to wear hip pads, and wore them all day. There was no correlation between the MMSE score, the Berg Balance score or the get up and go test, and acceptance of hip protector pads. The refusers average MMSE was 17.4 (9-25). It is not possible to predict the acceptability of hip protector pads in severely demented patients using cognitive or mobility tools but in this study the majority (81%) consented to wearing them. Most hip fractures are secondary to falls. Fall risk education is not feasible in demented patients. Therefore, mobile patients should be offered this protection from hip fracture.

[34] Discontinuity of Care and Health Decline Associated with Hip Fracture

M. Cree (Department of Mathematical Sciences, University of Alberta), A. Sclater (Division of Geriatric Medicine, University of Alberta), Q. Yang (Alberta Health and Wellness, Alberta Government), D. Johnson (Director, Alberta Centre for Health Services Utilization), K.C. Carriere (Department of Mathematical Sciences, University of Alberta).

PURPOSE: This population-based prospective cohort study was undertaken to identify if discontinuity of care was associated with subsequent hip fracture and decline in health. METHOD: All Edmonton-area residents (n=607) aged 65+ years fracturing a hip between July 1996 - August 1997 were interviewed one week and three months post-fracture to collect data on pre and post fracture function, health perception, and social support. Alberta Health utilization data for two years pre and one year post fracture were linked to the cohort data and to an age-sex matched cohort of non-fracture (control) seniors to examine whether health utilization differed between the two groups. Annual number of physician visits and referral-adjusted continuity of care (0=low, 1=high) were measured for each patient. RESULTS: Hip fracture patients were more likely to be hospitalized pre-fracture [15%(yr. 1), 19% (yr. 2)] than controls [10% (yr. 1), 12% (yr. 2)]. Compared to the healthiest group of non-fracture seniors, fracture patients tended to have lower continuity of care over all four years ($p<0.006$ for each year) and a higher number of hospitalizations in the post-fracture year ($p=0.012$). Post-fracture health decline was more likely for patients with low continuity of care, a high number of co-morbidities and physician visits, low social support, and low in-hospital mental status. CONCLUSIONS: Seniors at high risk of a hip fracture tended to be: high users of health care, without a regular physician, burdened with three or more comorbidities, and physically dependent at the time of fracture. These patients may benefit from improved continuity of physician care to prevent further health deterioration.

[35] Falls and fear of falling: Which comes first? A longitudinal prediction model

S.M. Friedman (University of Rochester, New York, USA), B.

Munoz, S.K. West (Johns Hopkins University, Maryland, USA), G.S. Rubin (Institute of Ophthalmology, London, UK), L.P.Fried (Johns Hopkins University, Maryland, USA)

PURPOSE: Previous cross-sectional studies have shown a correlation between falls and fear of falling (FOF), but it is unclear which comes first, and whether the two outcomes have similar predictors. We hypothesized that each of these clinical outcomes might be a predictor for the other, and that the two syndromes might share risk factors. METHODS: We evaluated the 2212 participants in the Salisbury Eye Evaluation (SEE) project who had both a baseline and a 20 month follow-up clinic evaluation. At baseline, subjects were aged 65-84, community-dwelling, and had a mini-mental state exam score of 18 or greater. RESULTS: Falls at baseline were an independent predictor of developing fear of falling 20 months later (OR 1.69, $p<0.01$), and fear of falling at baseline was a predictor of becoming a faller at 20 months (OR 1.71, $p<0.005$). Age, white race, female gender, taking 4 medications, and a history of CVA were predictors for both falls and fear of falling at follow-up. In addition, poor balance and foot pain predicted falls, and mental health symptoms and knee strength predicted fear of falling. CONCLUSION: Individuals who develop one of these syndromes are at risk for developing the other. This may result in a spiraling risk for falls, fear of falling, and functional decline.

[36] Factors explaining falls in very old subjects leading to acute-care hospitalization

O. Beauchet,MD ; MA. Blanchon,MD; F. Eynard-Valhorgues,MD ; C.Terrat,MD; R. Gonthier,PhD. Hôpital de la Charité, Saint-Etienne, France

PURPOSE: Falls are a frequent reason for hospitalisation in short-Stay geriatric units. Paradoxically, the factors determining such hospitalisation remain unknown. The objective of this study was to identify the explanatory factors of falls leading to acute-care hospitalisation of very old subjects. METHOD : We prospectively compared 92 patients (means age 85,8 +/- 5,5 SD) hospitalised for falls and 163 (means age 85,1 +/- 5,5 SD) those hospitalised for another reason in short-stay geriatric unit. Data were collected over a 6-month period starting with a questionnaire and a physical examination. RESULTS: Patients admitted for falls were predominantly women (76,9%) living alone (76,9%). Falls depend mainly on intrinsic factors. The precipitating factor was a medical condition (84%) which was acute (96%). The pattern of multiple disease conditions was not specific for patients who fell. In the opposite, osteoarthritis and visual and auditory deficits with direct effects on motor functions were correlated with falls. The environment played a determining role, but was primarily a predisposing and not a precipitating factor as was directly the cause of falls in only 40f cases. The loss of self-sufficiency for daily activities was also significantly more frequent in patients who fell ($p<0,05$). CONCLUSIONS: The explanatory factors of falls as the reason for hospitalisation of very old subjects in short-stay geriatric unit are intrinsic factors. They are associated with a precipitating factor which is usually an acute medical condition and a chronic multiple disease state having an effect on postural balance leading to the fall. These factors are combined in a context of social and environmental isolation.

[37] Risk Factors for Falling Among Community-based Seniors Using the MDS-HC

Paula C.Fletcher, (Wilfrid Laurier University, Waterloo, Ontario, Canada) John P. Hirdes, (University of Waterloo, Waterloo, Ontario, Canada)

Falling has the potential to threaten the health and well-being of seniors. Each year approximately one third of individuals over the age of 65 experience a fall. Although the majority of falls do not lead to serious injury, hospitalization or death, seniors may acquire a myriad of other complications, such as impaired mobility, fear of falling, and restricted activity. Information to date would suggest that one-time and multiple fallers within the community represent two distinct groups; however, limited research has examined the specific characteristics that differentiate fall status among community- based seniors receiving home care. As such, this study investigated the factors associated with fall status using a sample of 2300 seniors receiving homecare services. Staff from ten home care agencies utilized the MDS-HC for assessment purposes during their regular visits to clients. The MDS-HC is a comprehensive and standardized assessment tool used to evaluate the needs and ability levels of older adults utilizing home care services. Logistic regression analysis revealed that the male gender, impaired gait and the presence of environmental hazards were significant predictors for fallers (1+ falls) and multiple fallers (2+ falls), although other risk factors indicative of frailty also remained significant within the final model for multiple fallers only. The full models and the implications for these findings will be discussed.

[38] Fear of Falling Among Seniors Receiving Home Care Services

Paula C. Fletcher, (Wilfrid Laurier University, Waterloo, Ontario, Canada) John P. Hirdes, (University of Waterloo, Waterloo, Ontario, Canada)

According to Tinetti & Powell (1993) fear of falling is a lasting concern about falling that leads to an individual avoiding activities that he/she remains capable of performing. This fear is not an inevitable consequence of aging, and more importantly may consist of risk factors that are amenable to intervention. Although there is some information about the covariates of fear of falling, detailed information about the risk factors for fear of falling, specifically among community-based seniors receiving home care services, is limited. The aim of this study was to examine the factors associated with fear of falling among 2300 seniors receiving homecare services. Home care staff from ten agencies assessed participants using the MDS-HC, a comprehensive and standardized assessment tool used to evaluate the needs and ability levels of older adults utilizing home care services. Logistic regression analysis revealed being female, having various impairments/limitations, lack of support and being a multiple faller significantly increased risk of fear of falling. Implications for these findings will be discussed.

[39] Accidental Deaths in Elderly Population in SO Paulo-Brazil: Retrospective Study

M..M.Amatuzzi; L.E. Garcez-Leme; C.R. Carelli. (Hospital das Clínicas da Faculdade de Medicina da Universidade de São Paulo, Brasil)

With the aim to study the rate of deaths by external causes in the elderly population of the city of São Paulo, the authors studied 29127 death declarations of the population over 65 years old of the city of São Paulo, in Brazil, in 1996, with attempting to identify the main cause of death. We could observe a decreased number of external causes as cause of death with the progress of age. The results show us the main causes of death in this population: Accident 40.4%; Fall 30.6%, Drowning 4.2%; Fire 1,2%; Poisoning 0.7%; Suicide 7.1%, Aggression 7.1%; Iatrogenic 8.3%. The external causes of death in the elderly population studied (2.3% of the total of deaths) were mainly related with accidents, mainly transit accidents and falls. The results show the need of ambient and preventive measures to prevent these fatal occurrences.

[40] Painful Vertebral Fracture in the Frail Elderly: A Commonly Overlooked and Underestimated Problem

W. E. DeCoteau, K. Dolgopol (Section of Geriatrics, Department of Medicine, University of Saskatchewan, Saskatoon, Sask, Canada)

A few years ago we had the opportunity to assess several elderly patients in our Geriatric Rehab program who had suffered extremely painful and disabling fractures of one or more vertebrae. We noted that the painful fractures had often gone undiagnosed for weeks or longer and often resulted in a prolonged hospital stay. Therfore, we decided to do a more systematic outcome study of this population. There were 26 subjects (mainly over 75 years and female); the majority had experienced prior falls. The severity of their pain and the liklihood of experiencing a fracture was often grossly underestimated by physicians, much to the chagrin of the patients and their families. The fracture was often masked by concomitant medical problems such as neurodegenerative or cardiovascular disease. Plain x-rays of the spine were not particularly helpful as the fractures were often obscured by degenerative arthritis or were interpreted as being "old". However, bone scanning was very useful in confirming the presence of a recent fracture. Some patients did well, but many were unable to return to their prior home setting; three have since died: another two have permanent paraparesis. At present the outcome of this study population is being compared to a similar age group of hip fracture patients. Our study suggests that physicians are not astute at recognizing severe vertebral fractures in frail elderly persons and further education is needed to understand the clinical picture in this group. We also urge less reliance on plain x-ray and more liberal use of bone scanning in the aforementioned setting.

[41] Rehabilitation of frail Chinese elderly with hip fractures in a community hospital in Singapore

David Yong (Ang Mo Kio Community Hospital Singapore)

PURPOSE: To study the outcomes of hip fracture patients in a geriatric rehabilitation facility of a community hospital METHOD: A prospective analytical study of 206 consecutively admitted patients with hip fractures in 1998-1999. RESULT: The patients were mostly women (2/3), more than 80yrs old (50%, mean age 79.5 yrs), had comminuted fractures (93.7%), had operations (87.1%) and were independent ambulators before the fracture (94.5%). During hospitalisation 84% were allowed weight-bearing, 16% had factors which precluded this. 16% had cognitive impairment, 28.6% sensory deficits and 31.6% neuromuscular deficits. 22.8% had post-operative complications with 32.5% still having an active co-morbid illness needing medical intervention. The incidence of wound infection was 5.4%. 48% regained prefracture ambulatory status, 38% were ADL independent; 78% were discharged home, 12% into residential care. Multivariate analysis showed that early weight bearing and absence of cognitive dysfunction predicted likelihood of regaining ambulatory status whilst being able to walk again and living with or having a carer predicted discharge home. CONCLUSION: The Chinese elderly admitted to a geriatric rehabilitative care unit were of advanced age, suffered comminuted fractures and postoperative complications and had multiple medical co-morbidities. These frail patients were likely to regain mobility status if treatments succeeded in optimising their physical function to permit early weight bearing and if they do not have cognitive impairment. Going home depended on walking again and presence of a caregiver in the Asian context.

[42] Acute diseases and drugs are important causes of falls among older people in residential care

Kristina Kallin, Jane Jenssen, RPT, Lillemor Lundin Olsson, RPT, Lars Nyberg, RPT, Yngve Gustafson, PhD. Department of Community Medicine and Rehabilitation, Geriatric Medicine, Umeå University, Umeå, Sweden.

PURPOSE: To study precipitating causes of falls among older people in residential care. METHOD: A cross-sectional design including 140 women and 59 men, mean age ± SD (range) 82.4±6.8 (65-97) living in four residential care facilities in Umea, Sweden. After base-line assessments the residents were prospectively followed up regarding falls during one year. With the purpose of preventing further falls a physician, a nurse and a physiotherapist followed up each fall and reached a consensus of the most probable cause of the fall. RESULTS: The most probable cause of the falls could be determined in 327 (68%), of the 481 registered falls. Acute illness or disease or symptoms of disease caused 153 (31.8%), of the falls. Forty-eight falls (10.0%) occurred due to delirium. Forty-one falls (7.9%) were caused by infections, most often urinary infections, and 11 (2.3 %) by acute stroke. Thirty-six falls (7.5%) were judged to be caused by drugs, of which 21 (4.4 %) were bensodiazepines. Drugs with anticholinergic properties were the cause of 14 (2.9%) of the falls. External conditions caused 39 (8.1%) of the falls, most often in form of obstacles or misuse of walking frames. CONCLUSION: Since acute illnesses and drug side effects are important precipitating factors, falls should be regarded as a possible symptom of disease or a drug side-effect until it is proven otherwise.

SESSION 462

Time for Life: Lifestyles of Seniors and Caregivers

J. Fast (Department of Human Ecology, University of Alberta, Edmonton Canada) and M. Bittmann (Social Policy Research Centre, University of New South Wales, Sydney, Australia) The Life and Time(s) of Informal Careers. T. Smeeding (Syracuse university, Syracuse, NY, USA) and A. Gauthier (University of Calgary, Calgary Alberta, Canada) Changing Patterns of Work and Leisure Among the Elderly: Some Cross-National Comparisons. L. Stone (Statistics Canada, Ottawa, Canada), A. Harvey (St. Mary's University, Halifax, Canada) and J. Légaré (Université de Montréal, Montréal, Canada) Relative Importance Of Factors Explaining Seniors' Activity Patterns In The Transitional Years To Total-Work Retirement, International Comparisons. Victor Ujimoto (University of Guelph, Guelph, Ontario, Canada) Discussant.

This symposium will address issues of time use and aging from an international perspective. The session will consist of three presentations followed by a discussant and general discussion. The issues to be addressed include the time use patterns of caregivers and the changing patterns of work and leisure among the elderly. The primary objective of the paper by Fast and Bittman is to enhance our understanding of careers' lives by: describing the time use patterns of informal careers; comparing the time use patterns of non-careers, co-residential and ex-residential careers; and to comparing the time use patterns of careers and non-careers in Canada and Australia. It is expected that the knowledge gained from the research will provide a better understanding of the specific challenges facing informal careers, uncover areas of unmet need for services, identify sub-populations of careers where extra supports are most urgently required, and assist in the more effective targeting of scarce resources. The paper by Smeeding and Gauthier uses time use surveys from six countries to examine the changes over time in patterns of time use of older adults: Canada, Finland, Germany, Netherlands, the United Kingdom, and the United States. Some of these countries have been collecting data since the 1960s, thus providing a window of nearly 30 years to examine changes over time in the work and leisure balance. The aim is to describe the country-level variations in patterns of time use, after controlling for individual-level factors such as age, gender, education, and health. Of particular interest is the extent to which there has been cross-national convergence in the way older adults spend their time. The paper by Stone, Harvey and Légaré will discuss the development of a classification of activity patterns from time-use diary data and its application to several countries' populations at different senior ages. Based on a general theory of activity-pattern occupancy, a multivariate analysis of these countries' time use data is used to rank pattern determinants on a scale of relative importance. Stability of the rankings across countries is examined. Implications of the results for prospects of increased active ageing by seniors are developed, with some commentary on related policy issues.

Changing patterns of work and leisure among the elderly: some cross-national comparisons

Anne H. Gauthier (University of Calgary, Calgary, Canada) and Timothy Smeeding (University of Syracuse, Syracuse NY, USA)

This paper examines trends over time in the patterns of time use of older adults, from the 1960s to the 1990s. Our aim is to describe the country-level variations in patterns of time use, after controlling for individual-level factors such as age, gender, education, and health. In particular, we investigate the extent to which there has been cross-national convergence in the way older adults spend their time. METHOD: We use time budget surveys from six countries to examine the changes over time in patterns of time use of older adults: Canada, Finland, Germany, Netherlands, the United Kingdom, and the United States. All these surveys relied on the diary method to collect data on daily activities. All surveys have been cross-nationally harmonized for the purpose of this analysis. RESULTS: Results reveal the well-known trend towards early retirement. But more interestingly, results suggest that although older adults retire earlier, they are not re-allocating time that used to be devoted to paid work to unpaid work and voluntary activities. The cross-national analysis furthermore suggests that the share of active and passive leisure activities has followed different trends in the different countries, with a trend towards active ageing being observed in only a few countries. CONCLUSION: While today's generation of older adults may expect to live more years after retirement than the previous cohorts, there is little evidence that the additional post-retirement years are spent doing more unpaid and volunteering work.

Relative Importance Of Factors Explaining Seniors' Activity Patterns In The Transitional Years To Total-Work Retirement, International Comparisons

Leroy O. Stone, Statistics Canada; Andrew Harvey, St. Mary's University and Jacques Légaré, University of Montreal

A classification of activity patterns derived from time-use diary data is developed, and applied to several countries' populations at different senior ages. Based on a general theory of activity-pattern occupancy, a multivariate analysis these countries' time use data is used to rank pattern determinants on a scale of relative importance. Stability of the rankings across countries is examined. Implications of the results for prospects of increased active ageing by seniors are developed, with some commentary on related policy issues.

The Life and Time(s) of Informal Carers

Janet E. Fast (Department of Human Ecology, University of Alberta, Edmonton, AB, Canada) Michael Bittman (Social Policy Research Centre, University of New South Wales, Sydney, Australia)

Policymakers, practitioners and researchers acknowledge the importance of informal care and the need to support carers in their work. Crafting supportive policies and programs requires thorough knowledge of caring work and how it affects caregivers' lives. Prior research tells us who carers are and what they do for others, and a little about the consequences of their efforts. But their lives still are poorly understood because much of what they do is hidden. In this study, national time use survey data were used to document the impact of caregiving on carers' ability to undertake paid work, their standard of living, and their quality of life. Comparative analysis of Canadian and Australian data reveal subtle differences in lifestyles, living standards, and quality of life under different social, economic and political conditions. Australians spent less time on caring work than Canadians (6 and 10 hr/week respectively). Both Canadian and Australian caregivers sacrificed paid work and leisure to meet care demands; co-residential carers also spent less time on social and community activities and engaged in more home-bound leisure pursuits. Caregivers also engaged in more activity episodes during a typical day, suggesting that their lives are more hectic. Co-residential caregivers also spent more time on unpaid domestic work than either non-carers or those caring for non-household adults, suggesting that much of their care work remains hidden. In sum, caregivers lead more hectic lives than others and are at greater risk of social isolation and economic hardship. This is especially true of co-residential caregivers

SESSION 463

Healthy Active Life Expectancy

(1) E. A. Kramarow (National Center for Health Statistics, Hyattsville, USA) New estimates of Active Life Expectancy of the Older U.S Population. (2) J. P. Michel and F. Hermann (Institutions Universitaires de Gériatrie) Survival rate of frail elders in Switzerland. (3) C. Jagger (University of Leicester, United Kingdom) and J.M. Robine (INSERM, Montpellier, France). Disability-free life expectancy at age 65 in the European countries: new results. (4) Y Saito (Nihon University, Tokyo, Japan) Health Expectancy in Asian Countries. (5) R. J. M. Perenboom (TNO, Prevention and Health, Leiden, The Netherlands) Health expectancies in the Netherlands. (6) E. Crimmins (Andrus Gerontology Center, University of Southern California, Los Angeles, CA, USA) A variety of approaches to measure healthy life expectancy.

As mortality rates decline and life expectancy increases among the elderly and the oldest-old, more and more questions arise about the quality of the years lived. The health expectancy indicators, namely disability-free life expectancy (DFLE), healthy life expectancy or active life expectancy (ALE), aim to provide new information on the functional states and the vitality of the ageing populations. They seem to be appropriate to the current demographic conditions. Six papers examining their use in the different parts of the world will be presented in this session. The first (Kramarow) presents new estimates of active life expectancy in the United States. The second (Michel et al) describes the increase in the survival rates of frail elders in Switzerland. The third (Jagger et al) compares the values of disability-free life expectancy in the European countries. The fourth paper (Saito) depicts health expectancies in Asian countries. The last two papers present different approaches to measure healthy life expectancy. The first (Peremboom) documents changes over time in health expectancy at age 65 in the Nertherlands. The last one (Crimmins) opposes a variety of approaches to assess healthy life expatancy in the United States. This session will provide an overview of the current use of health expectancy in the low mortality countries to assess the quality of the years lived by the elderly.

A variety of approaches to measure healthy life expectancy.

E. Crimmins, Andrus Gerontology Center, University of Southern California, Los Angeles, CA, USA]

Most research on active life expectancy has focused on life with and without disability. This paper moves further back in the process of disability to examine life with and without major diseases as well as functioning loss and disability. One reason for the focus on disease as well as disability is that most medical care is directed at the treatment of underlying diseases. Diseases examined include both mortal and morbid conditions. Health condition prevalence data are from the 1994 National Health Interview Survey for the United States. The Sullivan method is used to estimate life lived with and without disease for men and women at various ages.

Disability-free life expectancy at age 65 in the European countries: new results. Author's

C. Jagger, University of Leicester, United Kingdom and J.M. Robine, INSERM, Montpellier, France

To compare life expectancy and disability-free life expectancy at age 65 across the European Union, we used the cross-sectional data from the European Community Household Panel from fifteen European Union Member States participating in the third wave. Disability is assessed by a general question "Are you hampered in your daily activities by any chronic physical or mental health problem, illness or disability". Differences in disability-free life expectancy between Member States are greater than for life expectancy. A negative relationship between the proportion of life spent free of disability and life expectancy suggest a "longer life, worse health" scenario for Europe. To monitor health in the European Union, we must institute strictly comparable data collection across countries using measures that have direct relevance to public health policy.

Health Expectancy in Asian Countries.

Y. Saito, (Nihon University, Tokyo, Japan)

In Asia, the concept of health expectancy is not widely known yet, although it has been computed in several countries. In this paper, we review studies on health expectancy conducted in several Asian countries. Health expectancy was first calculated in 1974 in Japan by the Council of National Living among Asian countries. Since then several other studies have also been conducted and Japan has the largest number of studies in health expectancy. We begin by reviewing the Japanese studies, followed by those conducted in other Asian countries.

New estimates of Active Life Expectancy of the Older U.S Population.

E. A. Kramarow [National Center for Health Statistics, Hyattsville, USA]

Active life expectancy at older ages is calculated using the Medicare Current Beneficiary Survey (MCBS). The MCBS is a survey of the U.S. Medicare population (which includes almost all persons 65 and over) conducted continuously since 1991. The design of the survey includes rotating panels of respondents who are interviewed annually and remain in the survey up to 4 years. The MCBS should give better estimates of active life expectancy for two reasons. The survey includes the institutionalized population so that their prevalence and health status do not have to be imputed from other sources. Also, we can measure annual health transitions instead of the larger intervals (2 or more years) found in other studies. Active life expectancy by sex, age, race, ethnicity and educational attainment will be calculated and compared to previous work. Trends in active life expectancy will also be explored

Survival rate of frail elders in Switzerland

[J.P. Michel and F. Hermann, Institutions Universitaires de Gériatrie]

Abstract: The mortality rates among the oldest old decline in Switzerland with an unexpected pace. This paper will present the survival rate of different cohorts of frail elders in Switzerland and assess changes over time : survival after hospital discharge, survival of demented patients compared to non-demented elderly citizens living in Switzerland ; comparison between the 1986 and 1996 cohorts.

Trends in health expectancies for the elderly

Rom JM Perenboom (TNO Prevention and Health, Leiden, The Netherlands)

Is the increase of total life expectancy - even at the age of 65 years - accompanied by an increase in health or by an increase in ill health? The health expectancy indicator combines information on length of life with quality of life. Trends in activity restrictions-free life expectancy, disability free life expectancy, life expectancy in perceived good health and life expectancy in well-being will be presented for the elderly at the age of 65 years. For the calculation, Sullivans method is used. Data on activity restrictions, disabilities, perceived health and well-being is derived from the Netherlands Continuous Health Interview Surveys over the years 1983 to 1997. Results show that in terms of activity restrictions, disabilities and perceived health, that there is an increase in years in ill health and a decrease of healthy years. The increase in ill health is mainly caused by the number of years in mild ill health. Life expectancy in well being however is increasing and the number of years in distress is decreasing, both in absolute number of years as related to the increase in total life expectancy. It seems that in the Netherlands, severe ill health is well under control. Attention should now be focused more on mild health problems. The increase in well being can partly be explained by the this shift from severe ill health problems to mild ill health, but will also be related to the economic good situation in the Netherlands.

SESSION 464

Migration for Positive Later Life

Charles F. Longino, Jr (Wake Forest University, Winston Salem, NC, USA) 'Four-decade trends in retirement migration in the United States' Vicente Rodríguez (Institute of Economics and Geography, Madrid, Spain) 'The active retirement boom in southern Europe: a view from Spain' Rebecca Wong (Georgetown University, Washington DC, USA) 'Migration histories and health and wealth in old age among Mexican retirees' William Serow (Florida State University, Tallahassee, Florida, USA) and Klaus Friedrich (Institut für Geographie, Halle (Saale), Germany) Graeme Hugo (University of Adelaide, Adelaide, Australia) 'Migration in later life in Australia: recent trends and implications' Tony Warnes (Univ of Sheffield, Sheffield, UK) 'Summary: The diversity of positive migrations for and during later life'

A substantial minority of the population passing through the retirement transition change house and some their region of residence. After retirement there is a period of relatively low residential mobility but with increasing age from the mid-70s, a rising propensity to move is found, and among those who reach their 90s the rate is high. The motivations are diverse, and there are several types of moves which can in part be related to life course stage and age. Among young older people, positive and developmental motivations predominate. Some people move for family oriented reasons; others in search of improved amenities and life styles - these are often termed 'environmental preference' migrations. At older ages, however, 'defensive' reasons become more evident, as with 'down-sizing' moves to conserve income or energy, and moves to seek more support from relatives or from housing and social welfare providers as in congregate settings. A third category of moves are those for treatment and care which are made by those whose activities are restricted by ill-health and degenerative disorders. The symposium includes papers on the development and current state of migration in later life in Australia, Europe and north America and includes papers on specific features in Mexico and Spain. One of the best studied forms of later life mobility is 'Sunbelt' migration. Two papers will examine its development, in terms of both the favoured destinations and the economic impacts, in the United States. Another reports on the impacts of the concentration of northern European retiree migrants on the southern and eastern coasts of Spain; and a third will consider the relative importance of environmental preference relocations in Australia. Another important form of later life re-location is that associated with (skilled and unskilled) labour migrants, and has two sub-types. There are the relocations associated with the retirements of the labour migrants themselves, particularly those who return to their regions of nativity and childhood upon retirement. Secondly, there are moves of the parents of emigrants, to live near or with them in their adopted locations. These family oriented and 'return' migrations lead to lower concentrations of retired migrants and have been less studied, but will be examined carefully in two of the symposium papers. Migration in late life is often seen by policy makers and media commentators as problematic, but most decisions to relocate are made voluntarily and with good reasons; and the majority of participants report positive outcomes of their decision and related to their new lifestyles. The papers in the symposium will review trends in the development of later life migration and its impacts on the favoured destination areas and upon the demands for health and social services. The hypothesis of a common developmental model will be critically examined.

Aging, migration and well being: the case of Mexico

R. Wong (Department of Demography, Georgetown University, Washington, DC, USA)

This paper examines the patterns of past migration among Mexican older people, in particular international migration to the USA, and how these lifetime patterns are related to the individuals' well being in old age. This paper uses existing data sets from Mexico. However, its uniqueness resides in the fact that this presentation will be the first from an important new Mexican Health and Aging Study which is being produced in the Spring of 2001. Estimates of the prevalence of retirement migration to the United States have been difficult to make before this study.

Economic consequences of retirement migration: views from both sides of the Atlantic.

W. Serow (Population Center, Florida State University, Tallahassee, Florida, USA) and K. Friedrich (Martin Luther University, Halle (Saale), Germany)

This paper compares recent work evaluating the economic consequences of retirement migration in North American and European settings, particularly Germany. The paper argues that most economic research on retirement migration deals with short-term consequences for the migrant and the destination community. Short term effects predominantly stimulate housing construction and retail and housing services through the in-movement of housing capital and purchasing power. The long term effects tend to shift to the increasing demands for health and welfare services and therefore involve more public sector expenditure and impacts on local taxation. On the basis of existing research data from several countries, it will be argued that greater attention needs to be paid in future research to long-term, rather than short-term, outcomes.

Four-decade trends in retirement migration in the United States

C. Longino (Reynolda Gerontology Program, Wake Forest University, Winston-Salem, North Carolina, USA)

This paper provides an overview of retirement migration patterns in the USA over four census decades, 1955-60 through 1985-90, by analyzing public use samples from the four decennial censuses 1960-90. The proportion of retirement-aged persons making long-distance moves remained essentially stable over the four decades. The southward movement consolidated in the 1990s and spread to some new locations in the Sunbelt region. This growth is offset by very slight declines in the leading destination states of Florida, California, Arizona and Texas. Exceptions to these trends, such as the attraction of retirement destinations in New England, New Jersey and Pennsylvania, are presented. The active recruitment of retirees by economic development strategists in Sunbelt states seems to be having an influence on the trends. Such recruitment is a phenomenon primarily of the 1990s. Data from the 2000 census will be available in 2003 and findings from its study will be anticipated and predicted

Migration in Later Life in Australia: Recent Trends and Implications

G. Hugo (University of Adelaide, Adelaide, Australia)

The paper uses 1986, 1991 and 1996 census migration data to assess the changes occurring in the internal migration of the nation's older population. There is an analysis of the shifts which have occurred in the propensity to move at or near the time of retirement and in the oldest age categories. These are related to shifts in government policies concerning the aged but also to societal and cohort changes. Discernible shifts in the spatial patterning of movement are analysed with respect to moves between metropolitan and non-metropolitan areas, inter-regional migration and migration within large metropolitan areas. Changes in the characteristics of older internal migrants in Australia are assessed insofar as this is possible using census internal migration data. The final part attempts to draw out the implications of changes occurring in internal migration patterns for the well-being of the nation's older population.

The active retirement boom in southern Europe: a view from Spain

V. Rodríguez (Institute of Economics and Geography, Madrid, Spain)

Retirement migrations from northern European countries to the continent's southern coasts exemplify residential moves in search of improved amenities, environments and life styles. They are therefore modern expressions of a developmental and positive approach to later life. International European retirement migrations have many similarities with inter-regional net migration flows in other developed societies and regions, notably the United States and Australia. The eastern and southern coasts of Spain, and the Canary and Balearic archipelagos, have the largest concentrations of northern European retirees in the south. After reviewing the imperfections of the data sources and the origins, destinations and size of the flows, this paper draws on both official data and local surveys and projections to develop a detailed picture of current trends. The paper examines the increasing impacts of retirement migration from northern European countries to southern Europe on both the participants and the places involved. It also discusses the policy responses that are required to accommodate and manage the residential and service demands. The paper concludes, first, by evaluating the situation of the increasing number of elderly migrants in the most popular destination areas of Spain and, secondly, by evaluating the implications for the local environments and upon the activities and social relations and networks of the participants.

The diversity of positive migrations in and for later life

A. Warnes (Sheffield Institute for Studies on Ageing, Sheffield, UK)

This will be a summary and comparative review of the presentations. The objective is to identify the diverse types and motivations of migrations and changes of house at the onset of retirement and in later life. The relative importance of developmental, protective or defensive, and care-seeking motivations will be assessed, along with their relationships to age. Secondly, the relative prevalence of moves associated with family-oriented and self-actualising life styles will be examined. Consideration will then be given to whether a common international model of the development of later life migration applies, or whether the patterns described from north America, Europe and Australia are either place-specific or are on convergent paths. The summary will conclude with key points about the implications of later life moves both for the individuals concerned and for the areas which attract concentrations or retiree in-migrants, and with an assessment of the most likely developments in the patterns and impacts of later life migration.

SESSION 465

Comprehensive Geriatric Assessment: Clinical Use, Research and Education in Geriatric Medicine

M Nishinaga(Department of Geriatric Medicine, Kochi Medical School, Nangoku, Japan) Clinical use of CGA in Patients with Chronic Heart Failure. F Gómez (Geriatric and Gerontological Research Group, Caldas University. Manizales, Colombia, Canada) CGA in Latinoamerican Rural Elderly. K Matsubayashi(Center for The South Asian Studies, Kyoto University, Kyoto, Japan) Community-Based Comprehensive Geriatric Intervention for the Elderly. H Endo (Department of Geriatrics, National Chubu Hospital, Obu-city, Japan) Clinical Use of Comprehensive Geriatric Assessment in Japan. OFW James(Department of Geriatric Medicine, Newcastle, UK)

Education of CGA for Undergraduate Students.

This symposium is focused to clarify the problems underlying comprehensive geriatric assessment (CGA). In this session, CGA will be reviewed by several aspects including clinical application, research, spread and education. In clinical application, prognostic as well as medical cost saving effect of CGA is discussed. For research, CGA in Latinoamerican rural elderly and community-based comprehensive geriatric intervention for the elderly will be presented. CGA was first spread from UK to USA. Now CGA is well recognized in most advanced counties. However, nation-wide spread has not been surveyed. This topic is covered by the paper entitled clinical use of comprehensive geriatric assessment in Japan. Finally, we will compare education of CGA among UK, Canada and Japan.

CGA IN LATINOAMERICAN RURAL ELDERLY

Fernando Gómez [Geriatric and Gerontological Research Group, Caldas University, Manizales, Colombia]

The objective of this paper is to evaluate from Comprehensive Geriatric Assessment (CGA) conceptual model the particular and special characteristics in LatinoAmerican (LA) rural areas with emphasis in social, cultural and health care systems aspects. Rural elderly in LA is characterized for low economic incomes with annual income less than U$800 and low educational levels (820f the population have less than 5 years of education). There are a lot of risk groups as living alone (5%), dependence in physical ADL (10%), multipathology (osteoarticular problems, hypertension, heart failure, diabetes mellitus and COPD) and limited access to health services (less than 15% with social security). CGA is considered as a multidimensional interdisciplinary diagnostic process intended to determine a frail elderly persons medical, psychosocial and functional capabilities and problems in order to develop an overall plan for treatment and long-term follow-up. Interdisciplinary teams in LA rural areas include only physicians and nursing-technicians. The physician regularly attends patients for 2 or 3 hours twice or weekly, all age groups must be attended with 8 patients per hour. Other interdisciplinary team members as social worker or physiotherapist participate occasionally through university academic programs. There are difficulties with laboratory testing in older persons because the laboratories are rudimentary and imaging studies are scarce. Public transportation is less available than urban areas and due geographic distances there are difficulties to access quickly to hospitals during periods of crisis. Other problem is the health care costs must be assumed directly for relatives. In majority of rural LA areas no exist a whole integrated health system to attend elderly. The old people long-term follow-up is based in national health politics, with many changes and disruptions due that it is not a priority and there are other problems to solve, as childhood vaccination. Other difficulty is the rural urban migration in older groups especially women with catastrophic disabilities. However, the primary networks are strong and the home care of elderly is preserved. It is necessary to evaluate CGA major goals and purposes and adapt them to social, geographic and political LA characteristics. Improve diagnostic accuracy with a constant training and organize interdisciplinary team. Optimize medical treatment with a continuing health care system and improve medical outcomes with training in detect alarm signs and symptoms. Other mean goal in CGA in rural LA elderly is to arrange long-term case management permitting that elderly can access to health care systems.

Clinical use of CGA in patients with CHF

K. Nakahara, S. Matsushita, T. Ozawa (Tokyo Geriatric Metropolitan Hospital, Japan),

The treatment and management of elderly patients with congestive heart failure(CHF) have traditionally taken place in hospitals in Japan. These patients are prone to repeat exacerbation of their cardiac disease and therefore need recurrent and frequent hospitalization. The medical management of the elderly patients is associated with enormous socioeconomic burden. Then it becomes crucial to develop new strategies that are cost-effective to the patients with congestive heart failure. The purpose of this study was to examine the impact of the comprehensive geriatric assessment and the team-approach program in the hospital on readmission rates of elderly patients with CHF. Twenty-nine patients (mean age; 84 years old) who had CHF (New York Heart Association classes II through IV) received CGA and the team-approach program before their discharge. The year before the entry was compared to the first year of the program. The mean readmission rate was reduced from 2.4 times/year to 1.3 times/year ($p<0.05$) and duration from 103 days/year to 41 days/year ($p<0.05$). The functional status of them was markedly improved. The comprehensive assessment and the team-approach program were associated with a decrease in the need for hospitalization and improved the functional status of elderly patients with congestive heart failure.

Clinical Use of Comprehensive Geriatric Assessment in Japan

Hidetoshi Endo (Institute: National Chubu Hospital, Aichi, Japan)

Comprehensive geriatric assessment (CGA) in Japan started in 1990. Dr. Ozawa who was former professor of Kochi University was the first person that introduced the concept of CGA in Japan in early 1990. We surveyed 3 different types of medical institutions to make clear of clinical use of CGA in Japan, first, Hospitals approved by Japan Geriatric Society(JGS) as an educational institution (JGS-H). Second, long-term care hospital (LTC-H). is a hospital for chronic rehabilitation and extended care. Third, temporary care institution (TCI) which is called in Japanese Geriatric Health Facilities. This is primarily defined as an institution with temporary care less than 3 months. In summary, in spite of the fact that more than two-thirds of MDs know about CGA, less than half of institutions use CGA. The recognition and utilization of CGA was higher than expected. Many MDs appreciate CGA and are involved in the assessment. Except in JGS-H, assessment tools developed by Japan Ministry of Health and Welfare are well known and used. This is closely related to Long Term Care Insurance, because the record of these tools will become obligatory next spring. International tools for assessing basic ADL and cognitive function, such as Barthel Index and MMSE, are used in more than one-third of JGS-H. On the other hand, world standard tools for IADL or Mood are not common. We have to inform more the importance of these tools in Japan.

Community-Based Comprehensive Geriatric Intervention for the Elderly

Institute: Center for The South Asian Studies, Koto University , Japan

We reported the secular improvement in self-care independence of old people living in a Japanese rural community, Kahoku in which the annual community-based geriatric intervention was introduced since 1991. (Lancet,1996). The community-based geriatric intervention includes; 1) Geriatric examination of the elderly aged 75 years or older 2) Monthly report of the health condition of elderly subjects 3) Patrol visit by community nurses 4) Health lecture meetings 5) Exercise programs for the elderly 6) Daytime care services for the frail elderly. Our results as follows; (1) Independent rate of elderly in Kahoku improved from 71% to 87% during 8 years (Lancet, 1997). (2) Lower cholesterol group showed significantly faster decline in MMSE than higher cholesterol group during 3 years (JAGS, 1997). (3) Neurobehavioral functions were maintained in day-care participants, while those of non-participants significantly declined after 1 year and quantitative Zarit's scale of care burden was also significantly decreased during 1 year in day-care participant group. (4) Lower grade ADL, namely disability itself in the elderly is the risk of subsequent death independently from diseases themselves (Lancet, 1999). (5) Not only physical disabilities, but cognitive impairment measured by Mini-Mental State Examination was also a significant risk for subsequent death in older elderly subjects more than 75 years of age. (6) Community-based geriatric intervention may not only improve self-care independence in the elderly, but also may lower the increasing rate of medical expenses for community-dwelling older people in Japan (JAGS, 1998). In conclusion, community-based comprehensive geriatric intervention is useful for health promotion of the community-dwelling elderly population.

SESSION 466

Building bridges between scientific research, policy and practice

Longitudinal Aging Study Amsterdam (Vrije Universiteit, Faculty of Medicine, Amsterdam, the Netherlands), The Manitoba Centre for Health Policy and evaluation (University of Manitoba, Winnipeg, Canada) and the Canadian Health Services Research Foundation.

Building bridges between scientific research, policy and practice Policy, practice and research have their own dynamics, demands and pace. Policymakers generally need quick answers for political purposes and planning objectives; health and welfare institutions need practical information that can be applied as directly as possible in order to improve the quality of life of the elderly. Although (longitudinal) scientific research provides us with very important information on the processes of aging in the longer run, it develops rather slowly. At the risk that the results are not fully implemented and made use off especially when results are only or mainly presented in scientific publications without being disseminated further or translatedfor specific practical purposes and target groups. Therefore, researchers cannot expect nor benefit from comments coming from research-consumers In line of the 17th World Congress of Gerontology theme working together in a changing world we would like to stimulate a discussion between the participants in the Round Table on targeted (international) exchange between research, policymakers and (health)practice. Several examples of best practice will show how cooperation can be promoted and how fundamental or strategic scientific research is used to inspire and support policy making and quality practice. We will also point out how facts and experiences from policy and practice can be used for the development and the improvement of the research programme. · We will present a new initiative in the Netherlands, linked to the Interdisciplinary Longitudinal Aging Study Amsterdam (LASA, Faculty of Medicine, Vrije Universiteit), an intensive research project running now for ten years. The initiative is meant to get in close contact with the authorities and non governmental (health)institutions to inform, support and eventually train persons to apply the results and vice versa to learn from them. Co-presentation will be from ZON, the Netherlands Institute for the Implementation of Research. · We will present part of the work of the Manitoba Centre for Health Policy and Evaluation (MCHPE), a unit within the Department of Community Health Sciences, Faculty of Medicine at the University of Manitoba, that developed an on-going research agenda with the relevant provincial government departments (Health, Family Services and Education). They have done some excellent work relative to income levels and use of health services and to the delivery of health services in rural and remote areas, both policy and practice relevant. · The Canadian Health Services Research Foundation (CHSRF) is another excellent bridge builder. Grant applications are reviewed by peer review committees that include both researchers and policy makers and they explicitly acknowledge the necessity to communicate research findings to the scientific community and to policy makers and practitioners. It is acknowledged that these communications need to be especially tailored for policy makers and practice. We also will invite other organisations to contribute to building bridges between research, policy and practice to the benefit of all involved, especially the elderly.

SESSION 467

Aging, hyperglycemia, and asymptomatic cerebral infarction were associated with cognitive impairment in elderly diabetic patients

Atsushi Araki, Hideki Ito, Yukari Murotani, Hirohito Kazama, Junichirou Inoue, Toshiyuki Horiuchi, Akinori Hattori, Takayuki Hosoi, Hajime OrimoTokyo (Metropolitan Geriatric Hospital and Tama Metropolitan Geriatric Hospital, Tokyo, Japan)

PURPOSE: To examine the effects of hyperglycemia and brain MR-defined asymptomatic cerebral infarction on impaired cognitive function in elderly diabetes mellitus.METHODS: Two hundred thirteen elderly diabetic patients (59 men, 154 women) with a mean age of 75 years and 40 non-diabetic subjects participated in this study. Based on the brain MR findings and neurological deficits, the subjects were divided into 4 groups; symptomatic cerebral infarction (CI) group, asymptomatic CI group, diabetic control group without any CIs, and non-diabetic controls and the cognitive function was assessed using the WAIS-R, Stroop test, and Benton visual retention test. RESULTS: Some aspects of cognitive function (digit symbol substitution test, Stroop test, and Benton visual retention test) were more impaired in diabetic control group without any CIs than in non-diabetic control group. Among the whole diabetic subjects, age, HbA1c and serum AGE (carboxymethyllysine) were significantly associated with the cognitive impairment. The cognitive function as assessed by digit symbol substitution test and Stroop test in asymptomatic and symptomatic CI groups were declined as compared with non-diabetic and diabetic controls, while the similarity and picture arrangement in the WAIS-R were similar in the 4 groups after adjustment for age. CONCLUSION: Aging, hyperglycemia and the presence of asymptomatic cerebral infarction could explain for the impairment of some aspects of cognitive function, such as complex psychomotor skill and speed of mental processing in elderly diabetic patients.

Ambulatory blood pressure measurements in normotensive elderly type 2 diabetics with microalbuminuria - Indian profile

SK Agarwal, NP Singh, AK Kapoor, S Anuradha, Anupam Prakash (Maulana Azad Medical College & Lok Nayak Hospital, New Delhi, India)

Ambulatory blood pressure measurements in normotensive elderly type 2 diabetics with microalbuminuria - Indian profile SK Agarwal, NP Singh, AK Kapoor, S Anuradha, Anupam Prakash Maulana Azad Medical College & Lok Nayak Hospital, New Delhi, India Type 2 diabetics, normotensive on office blood pressure (BP) measurements, and having persistent microalbuminuria (urinary albumin excretion rate, UAER Δ 20-200 mg/l) form an interesting cohort for interventions to prevent morbidity and mortality in diabetics. However, scanty literature exists on this segment. Hence, we decided to study the 24-hour ambulatory blood pressure (AMBP) measurements in this cohort. Thirty type 2 diabetics with microalbuminuria (by Micral II Dipsticks), normotensive on office BP recordings were studied. Mean urinary albumin excretion rate was 37 ± 23.6 mg/l. 24-hour AMBP recordings were done at half-hourly intervals during day-time and hourly at night. Mean age of our cohort was- 57.93 ± 8.78 yrs, male to female ratio was 1.14:1. Average day time systolic and diastolic BP were 120.92 ± 9.48 and 71.53 ± 8.81 mm Hg. Average night time systolic and diastolic BP were 114.9 ± 10.11 and 66.05 ± 8.77 mm Hg. Only 4 (13.3%) were dippers, rest all had lost the normal dip in BP at night. Two patients (6.7%) had a significant BP load although they were normotensive on office BP recordings. There was no significant correlation of albuminuria with systolic or diastolic BP measurements. Hence, we infer that among normotensive microalbuminuric type 2 diabetics, there is loss of diurnal variation of blood pressure indicating it to be an early accompaniment of nephropathy, preceding onset of overt hypertension; and that AMBP has good correlation with office BP recordings in most of the cases.

Diabetes and dementia in elderly: lack of epidemiological association in the French PAQUID epidemiological study

I Bourdel-Marchasson, C Helmer. [Centre de Gériatrie Henri Choussat, 33604 Pessac Cedex, France INSERM U330-Université de Bordeaux 2 ; 33000 Bordeaux, France]

PURPOSE: The risk of dementia of Alzheimer type or vascular dementia could be increased in diabetic subjects due to some putative mechanisms: hyperglycemia or hypoglycemia toxicity, hyperinsulinism, hypertension, large cerebral vessels changes, oxidative stress, depression. Conversely, the risk could be hidden due to the increased death rate in elderly diabetic subjects. Thus, the risk of incident dementia during 8-year follow-up was studied in elderly diabetic subjects compared to others in PAQUID epidemiological cohort. METHODS: PAQUID epidemiological cohort consisted in 3777 subjects representative from subjects older than 65 years old in Gironde (South-West France). At baseline and every two years, subjects underwent a one hour-interview by a trained psychologist. Prevalent diabetic subjects were identified using the question: are you diabetic?, and the hypoglycemic treatment regimen record. Subjects who met the DSM-IIIR criteria for dementia diagnosis were further examined by a senior neurologist for possible dementia diagnosis. RESULTS 254 diabetic subjects (among them 201 with hypoglycemic treatment) were identified among 2721 who were visited (9.3%). 276 new cases of dementia were diagnosed, among them 186 from Alzheimer type. Diabetic subjects were not different from the others for the risk of dementia after adjustment on age and sex: relative risk (RR): 1.1, 95% Confidence Interval (CI): 0.7-1.8. Adjustment of analysis on other patients' characteristics (BMI, education level, cardiovascular antecedents) has no effect on the result. CONCLUSION This study did not evidence any epidemiological association between dementia and diabetes in French elderly subjects.

Factors that influence survival of diabetes inpatient elders: A case study in Taiwan

Cheng-Chieh Lin (Department of Family Medicine, Center of Community Medicine, China Medical College Hospital, Taichung, R.O.C.), Tsai-Chung Li (Department of Medical Research, China Medical College Hospital, Taichung, R.O.C.), Chiu-Shong Liu (Department of Family Medicine, Center of Community Medicine, China Medical College Hospital, Taichung, R.O.C.), Chia-Ing Li (Center of Community Medicine, China Medical College Hospital, China Medical College Hospital, Taichung, R.O.C.)

What factors predict survival among diabetic inpatients is rarely explored, so the objective of the current study is to examine the effects of sociodemographic factors, severity of diabetes, physical functioning, and supportive device use at admission to hospital on or survival among DM discharged inpatients. The study sample consisted of 110 consecutive diabetes inpatients admitted in China Medical College Hospital from July, 1998 to August, 1999. All diabetes inpatients were interviewed by a trained interviewer to collect variables such as sociodemographic factors, Barthel Index, Karnosky Scale, ADL, IADL, co-morbidity, diabetic control, complications, having one of catheter, naso-gastric tube, or Tracheotomy, etc. After a 6-month period, all diabetes inpatients were followed up to measure survival status. The statistical analyses were means, proportions, Student's t-test, Chi-square test, and Cox's proportional hazard model. Mean age of the study subjects is 66.8 years old and 62.7% of them are male. The survival rate in this sample is 80.0%. The significant factors that predict survival of diabetes outpatients are the duration of diabetes, Karnosky Scale, and kidney function. As the duration of diabetes increases by one year, the probability of survival for diabetes outpatients decreases by 0.93. As the Karnosky Scale increases by one, the probability of survival for diabetes outpatients decreases by 0.28. The probability of survival for those who had worse kidney function is 0.11 times less than the risk for those who had better function. The conclusion for our study is that the duration of diabetes, the Karnosky Scale, and kidney function influence survival of diabetes outpatients.

Self Care Factors Associated with Diabetic Foot Amputation in Adult and Old Patients.

E.D. Arias Merino, L.E. Navares Moreno (Gerontología, Universidad de Guadalajara) G. González Vasquez (OPD, Hospitales Civiles de Guadalajara)

PURPOSE: To quantify the risk of amputation associated with foot self care practice and co-morbidities conditions in diabetic patients through a case-control study. METHOD: We enrolled 144 patients (45 to 93 years old), age-gender matched. Cases: Thirty six patients with diabetic foot background and non-traumatic amputation (18 females and 18 males). Controls: 108 patients without diabetic foot and amputation (54 females and 54 males). All were evaluated for 53 factors associated with diabetic foot and amputation. RESULTS: The results showed that cases had significantly lower diabetic knowledge about exercise, medication and nutrition intake, and self-monitor blood glucose than controls patients. The risk of amputation was associated with peripheral neuropathy (OR 7.66, 95% CI 1.10-16.5) and peripheral vascular disease (OR 3.24, 95% CI 1.3-8.2). Foot care practices: trend analysis indicated that the risk on developing diabetic foot and amputation increase with errors in soaking, lubrication of their feet and between toes, foot wear, and inappropriate foot and shoes inspection. Cases and controls both not found differences in used unsafe methods when cutting their toenails, and callus care. CONCLUSION: There is not enough diabetic knowledge related to the illness and the foot care screening. The patients should receive education in these topics and physicians should made foot screening at the medical consultation.

THE COMPLEX URINE REFLECTION COEFFICIENT IN PATIENTS OF DIFFERENT AGE COHORTS WITH TYPE 2 DIABETES.

Nagibovich Oleg Alexandrovich, Russian Military medical academy, Saint-Petersburg, Russia. Zakharchenko Valentin Mikhailovich, Russian Military medical academy, Saint-Petersburg, Russia. Chernyakov Gennadiy Mikhailovich, Russian Military medical academy, Saint-Petersburg, Russia.

As type 2 of diabetes mellitus is a disease of people of the elder age cohorts and reserve possibilities of the elderly organism are much lower than those of the young one, consequently, the early diagnostics of complications caused by diabetes mellitus becomes more and more urgent in patients of the senior age cohorts. The object of this work was to assess the relationship between the age and the complex urine reflection coefficient (CRC) in patients suffering from type 2 diabetes. 27 patients at the age of 45-74 years suffering from type 2 diabetes with normal levels of albumins in the urine were selected. They were divided into three cohorts: 9 patients at the age of 45-54 years were included into the first cohort; the second cohort consisted of 9 patients at the age of 55-64 years; 9 patients at the age of 65-74 years were included into the third cohort. The cohorts under study did not differ in the main clinico-laboratorial indices. The CRC of the urine was measured using a special device. Condition of the urine was assessed according to the ratio of the amplitude signals reflected from the urine and the distilled water, respectively. The average values of CRC of the urine in patients of the first, second and third cohorts were 1,26±0,03; 1.25±0,02 and 1,22+0,03, respectively. The significant differences were not revealed. The CRC tended to decrease with growth of the age (r=-0.18). Definition of the complex urine reflection coefficient is perspective in diagnostics of diabetic nephropathy in patients suffering from type 2 diabetes mellitus.

The effect of aging and hyperglycemia on NO mediated action in rat aorta

Taku Tsunekawa, Toshio Hayashi, Navin Kumar Thakur, Hatsuyo Kano, Yuusuke Asakura, Daigo Sumi, Akihisa Iguchi, Department of Geriatrics, Nagoya University Graduate School of Mediicne, Nagoya, Japan

PURPOSE: We determined the effect of aging and hyperglycemia on endothelial and non-endothelial vascular responses, eNOS and soluble guanylate cyclase (sGC) using rats model. METHOD: Hyperglycemia was induced by intraperitoneal injection of streptozotocin in young (9wks), middle aged (54wks) and elderly (108 wks) male wister rats. After 1 to 12 weeks of hyperglycemia induction, rats were sacrificed and NO stimulated response by ACh and A23187 and tone related NO basal response were investigated in thoracic aortas. eNOS protein and sGC protein were quantified by western blot. Character of eNOS, iNOS, sGC and vessel component cells were studied by immunohistochemistry. RESULTS: The fasting blood glucose was increased 340 + 13 mg/dl in hyperglycemic induced rats. NO stimulated and basal responses were not significantly changed in younger (9wks.) rats when they were slightly decreased under hyperglycemia for more than 9 weeks. Endothelium independent response by NTG was diminished in elderly rats (108wks) as compared with those in younger and middle aged rats (54 wks.). Further, it was diminished in status of hyperglycemia for longer than 4 weeks. NO stimulated and basal responses were slightly decreased in aortas of elderly rats, and significantly decreased in hyperglycemia and depending on the duration of hyperglycemia. eNOS and soluble guanylate cyclase protein tended to decrease in aged diabetic rats. Further, O2- was increased by aging and hyperglycemia. CONCLUSION: NO and O2 play a role in changes of endothelial and smooth muscle function in aged diabetic rats.

The Glucose Tolerance Test (GTT) Controversy: Quantification of Delay in Diagnosis of Type 2 Diabetes

R. Andres, D.C. Muller, J.T. Carney, J.D. Sorkin (National Institute on Aging, Baltimore, USA)

Purpose: Two recent advisories differ in procedural recommendations for diagnosing diabetes. The American Diabetes Association (1997) advises against the use of the GTT; WHO (1998) strongly supports its use. There is clear evidence that the diabetic state is present for a number of years prior to onset of classical complications, and that glycemic control over a period of years delays development of complications. Early diagnosis of diabetes is therefore mandated. Methods: 984 male and 561 female participants in the Baltimore Longitudinal Study of Aging, aged 17 to 93 yr received glucose tolerance tests at approximately two year intervals. Fasting and two-hour plasma glucose levels were interpreted as Normal, Impaired, or Diabetic according to ADA/WHO standards. Age at development of first Impaired values (6.1-6.9 mmol/L fasting, 7.8-11.0 two-hour) and of first Diabetic values (7.0 fasting, 11.1 two-hour) were noted. Results: If only the fasting glucose levels had been obtained, the diagnosis of Impaired glucose metabolism would have been delayed in 770f the men and 880f the women. Similarly, delay in the diagnosis of Diabetes would have been delayed in 820f the men and 710f the women. The magnitude of the delay is remarkable: for the Impaired state, 11.1 yr in men and 8.4 yr in women, as well as long delays for the Diabetic state, 8.2 yr in men and 7.8 yr in women. Conclusion: Periodic glucose tolerance testing detects altered glucose metabolism at a significantly earlier stage than does testing for fasting glucose only. The ADA recommendation to discontinue the use of the GTT deserves serious reconsideration.

SESSION 468

A case of suicide in Elderly women

Nunez Lemus R.P. (Facultad de psicologia Universidad Autonoma de Queretaro, Mexico)

Show how psychotherapy can help elderly people with severe problems of depression, isolation and loneliness even living with family. The preventive alternative is weekly psichoanalitical therapy with some specific tasks to develop for the patient to change depressive attitudes. Three and a half years attended a female old patient who intended suicide. By now she is taking care of herself in different daily life activities. The suicide will be prevent with adequate psychotherapy.

A short-term schedule for withdrawal from benzodiazepines in geriatric inpatients: experience and suggestions for guidelines

M. Petrovic, D. Pevernagie, A. Mariman, G. Van Maele, M. Afschrift (Departments of Internal Medicine and Psychiatry, Ghent University Hospital, Ghent, Belgium)

Purpose: We tested the hypothesis that an immediate withdrawal from benzodiazepines (BZD) is feasible in hospitalised geriatric patients. Methods: Geriatric patients taking BZD for at least 3 months were eligible to participate in the study upon admission to the inpatient ward. Patients with dementia or other severe psychiatric disorders were excluded. Forty patients agreed to stop BZD. A withdrawal programme including initial substitution therapy combined with psychological consulting was offered. The daily BZD medication was substituted by either lormetazepam 1 mg or placebo, double blind, administered at bedtime. After one week the replacement therapy was stopped. The Pittsburgh Sleep Quality Index was used to register subjective estimations of sleep quality. It was evaluated 5 times during a period of four weeks (upon intake and 4 times at preset intervals: 3, 8, 15 and 30 days after the start of the study). A one-year follow-up of benzodiazepine use was also conducted by contacting the treating general practitioners. Results: Seven patients (17.5%) relapsed while in the hospital and another 7 patients (17.5%) restarted BZD use after discharge. The overall success rate was 65%. Major withdrawal symptoms were documented in only 2 patients (5%). The subjective quality of sleep was significantly better in the Lormetazepam substitution group. The success rate was also significantly higher in the Lormetazepam substitution group (80% vs. 50% in the placebo group). One year after discontinuance, 42.5 % of the discontinuers remained off their benzodiazepines. Conclusions: Therefore, short-term withdrawal from BZD was achieved in two thirds of elderly hospitalised patients without dangerous side effects. Nevertheless, a short-term substitution therapy, using short to intermediate acting benzodiazepine should be considered since subjective sleep quality may deteriorate following an immediate withdrawal and because a higher success rate is obtained.

Actualization of potential and depression during post-stroke rehabilitation

M. Couture, J. Desrosiers, G. Leclerc (Centre de recherche en gériatrie et gérontologie, Institut universitaire de gériatrie de Sherbrooke et Université de Sherbrooke, Canada)

PURPOSE : Many studies have tried to determine which factors are associated with depression after a stroke. However, most of them were only interested in biological or clinical variables, thus leaving out psychological variables. The purpose of this study was to verify whether the degree to which a person who had a stroke actualizes his/her potential is related to the development of post-stroke depression during or after the rehabilitation period. The actualization of potential is a psychological process aimed at developing a person's resources and abilities while taking into account individual and environmental characteristics. METHOD : Participants (n = 32, mean age = 71 years) were assessed at the beginning and at the end of their intensive functional rehabilitation program with the Beck Depression Inventory and the Measure of Actualization of Potential. RESULTS : Near 160f the participants were treated for depression during their rehabilitation and 500f the participants showed signs of depression at the end of their rehabilitation program. The results demonstrated that the actualization of potential is negatively correlated with depressive symptoms (p = 0,008). CONCLUSION : Since the degree to which a person actualizes his/her potential is a relatively fixed personal attribute, it can be hypothesised that it is the actualization of potential that influences the likelihood of not developing depressive symptoms rather than the depression affecting the actualization of potential. Measuring the actualization of potential at the beginning of a rehabilitation program might be useful for detecting individuals most at risk for developing post-stroke depression.

Back To Nature : The Use of Herbs/ Phytopharmaca Against Depression and Anxiety

Tony Setiabudhi PhD. (Trisakti Medical School/ Indonesian Society of Gerontology Jakarta/ Indonesia)

During his presentation at the European Association of Geriatric Psychiatry Symposium last September 2000 in Romania; the author mentioned that : Kraepelin was visiting our country in early 20th century. At that time he disclosed that in the Netherlands Indies (the name of our Archipelago during Dutch Occupation) there were no "Melancholia/ Depressive Disorder's Patient" was found. At that time several new opinions cropped up and developed, that the Indonesia community who live in a tropical country always able to enjoy SUNSHINE. That's why; since that time some theory and approach was introduced to treat and prevent the recurrence of depressive patients through both Natural or Artificial light. To day when we have to face the globalization; we notice that anxiety as well as depressive mental disorders are found everywhere in this world; and most of them are treated by using psychopharmaca (anxiolytics/ anti depressants or both). While we still trying to study the effect and psychopharmacological action of the medications we are also get a lot of data relating to the latest discovery of neuritransmitters and its reliances that we can understand that between ANXIETY and DEPRESSION there are so many correlations. On the other hand; some herbs (and its alkaloid/ ingredients) are also explored and proved that it has affinity to GABA or other neuro-transmitters.. When Germany/ United Kingdom confess the efficacy of hypericum for treating Anciety and Depression, and is now used by millions of their patients why don't we try to carrying out some herbs in this eastern region which perhaps has a better future ? Some recent findings on hypericum in developed countries are also presented in this psper.

Depressed Mood in Elderly Medical Inpatients: Promoting, Enhancing Or Confounding Factor Of Adverse 6-Month Outcome?

V.Wietlisbach, B.Burnand (Institute of Social and Preventive Medicine, University of Lausanne, Switzerland), B.Yersin (Emergency Service, University Hospital, Lausanne, Switzerland) and C.J.Bula (Geriatric Service, University Hospital, Lausanne, Switzerland).

Purpose: To determine whether hospitalized elderly persons with depressed mood are more likely to experiment adverse outcomes (rehospitalization, nursing home admission or death) in the next 6 months, independently of or in interaction with their comorbidity, functional and cognitive status. Population: Every other non-institutionalized patient aged 75+ admitted to the internal medicine service of an academic hospital in Western Switzerland (n=401). Method: Data on patient characteristics and health status were collected upon admission. Patients scoring >5 on the 15-item Geriatric Depression Scale were considered as having depressed mood. In this analysis, high comorbidity, functional limitation and cognitive impairment were defined as a Charlson index >2, an IADL score <4 and a MMS score <24 respectively. Results: In bivariate Cox regression models, depressed mood was associated with rehospitalization (Hazard Ratio: 1.56; p=0.017), nursing home admission (HR: 2.10; p=0.033) and death (HR: 1.57; p=0.059). In multivariate Cox regression models including the other health indicators, independent predictors were depressed mood (adjusted HR: 1.47; p=0.050) for rehospitalization, cognitive impairment (HR: 3.63; P=0.001) for nursing home admission and functional limitation (HR: 2.58; p<0.001), along with high comorbidity (HR:2.95; p<0.001), for death. When interaction terms between depressed mood and the other factors were added to the multivariate models, a nearly significant interaction with cognitive impairment (HR: 2.09; p=0.078) was found for the prediction of nursing home admission. Conclusion: In this population, depressed mood came out as an independent predictor only for rehospitalization and tended to be associated with a higher likelihood of nursing home admission in patients with cognitive impairment.

Identification and treatment of late life depression in residential care: changes between 1990 and 1997.

Arthur A, Matthews R, Lindesay J, Jagger C. (University of Leicester, Leicester, UK).

PURPOSE: To report the proportion of residents in care homes identified as depressed by care staff, and the level of, and predictors for, use of antidepressants in 1990 and 1997. METHOD: Censuses of those aged 65 years and over in any type of residential care at midnight on 27 November 1990 and 30 November 1997, in Leicestershire, UK. Care staff were asked to complete an assessment form for each resident which included a rating of depression and use of antidepressants. RESULTS: In 1990 10.5% (465/4410) of residents were considered almost always depressed by care staff compared to 8.0% (329/4123) in 1997. Among depressed residents, the use of antidepressants increased over this period from 25.1% (114/454) to 44.8% (143/319). Treatment with antidepressant medication was associated with younger age in both 1990 (p=0.011) and 1997 (p=0.038) and better physical functioning in 1990 (p=0.012). CONCLUSION: Increased use of antidepressant treatment appears to be due to the wider range of antidepressant drugs available since 1990. However there is a need for better methods for care staff to detect depression in residents and for appropriate action to be taken by those responsible for their medical management.

Psychotherapy for Depression in Australia: Are Older Clients as Accepted as Younger Ones?

E. Helmes (Edith Cowan University, Perth, Australia), S. Gee (Victoria University of Wellington, Wellington, New Zealand)

Current cohorts of older adults are often reluctant to seek psychological treatment and therapists often parallel attitudes with a reluctance to treat older adults. Such reluctance to treat older people can reflect ageist attitudes or limited professional education on working with older adults. We surveyed psychologists and counselors in Australia to determine practice patterns and aspects of treatment practices for depression in older adults. A vignette based upon one used by James and Haley (1995) depicted either a 43- or 72-year old depressed woman. A total of 1682 surveys were mailed to practicing psychologists and counselors in all states and territories of Australia. The return rate was 42%. Here we report on the responses of 414 psychologists and 293 counselors to five questions that asked therapists' ratings on a 7-point scale as to their ability to form a therapeutic relationship with the woman, the likely prognosis, their competence to treat the woman, her appropriateness as a client, and their willingness to accept her as a client. These five variables were used as dependent variables in a 2x2 MANOVA. The interaction and main effect for professional group were not significant. The main effect for client age was significant for the MANOVA and for the univariate effects for all five dependent variables. Results are discussed in terms of Australian society's attitudes towards older people and training standards for psychologists in Australia with regards to older clients.

SESSION 469

Age-related changes in the state of chromatin in human buccal epithelium cells

Yury G. Shckorbatov (Institute of Biology, Kharkov National University, Ukraine)

The main nuclear component, chromatin, may be divided into two parts: euchromatin and heterochromatin. The increase of the facultative heterochromatin quantity may be an evidence of decrease in nuclear activity. The hetrochromatin granule quantity (HGQ) after orcein staining was investigated in buccal epithelium cells of different age donors (non-smokers). It was shown that the HGQ increases after 50 years but the process of HGQ changes with donor's age was not monotonous. The mean HGQ level in a group of donors of 20-29 years age was 15.4±1.0, and in a group of donors of 30-49 years it was the same -15.4±1.6. In groups of donors aged 50-59 and 60-79 years old HGQ was significantly higher: 23.9±1.8, and 23.2±1.1, respectively. The process of age-related HGQ changes is well approximated by the equation y=44.2 - 2.43x + 0.608x2 - 0.431x3 (y - HGQ, x - age, years). The correlation between HGQ and donors age is r=0.734 (p>0.99). Thereafter we observed the age-related increase of chromatin condensation. The stabilization of the heterochromatinization in the group of donors of age 60-79 years may be related to different processes. This may be connected to advanced mortality among persons with a high HGQ level or to process of decondensation of chromatin in cells of persons of age after 70. For elucidation of the problem the longitudinal investigations are necessary.

Apolipoprotein E and aging among Han Chinese population

Ma Yong-Xing, Lu Pei-Fang, Zhu Yue (Department of Aging, Antiaging and Cognitive Function, Shanghai Institute of Gerontology and Geriatrics, Department of Geriatrics of Huadong Hospital, Shanghai, China)

Objective: To observe the correlation between APOE alleles and aging in Han Chinese population. Methods: APOE Alleles were determined in 1800 Han Chinese (Male 1532, Female 268) of various age groups: Youth (20-39 years old) 137, Middle (40-59) 232, Old (60-84) 1360, Very Old (~85) 71. APOE was amplified by one-stage PCR using the forward primer: 5'-GGC ACG GCT GTC CAA GGA GCT-3' and reverse primer: 5'-GAT GGC GCT GAG GCC GCG CT-3'. The PCR product was digested directly with 5U of Cfol and separated by a 20% polyacrylamide (acrylamide:bisacrylamide=29:1) nondenaturing gel. Results: APOE4 frequency of the very old age group (2.8%) were significantly lower than old (7.6%, p=0.03), Middle (8.4%, P=0.02) and youth (8.4%,P=0.03) respectively. Conclusion APOE4 is significantly correlated with aging.

Influence of the seasonal factors in early ontogenesis and programming of human longevity

A. Vaiserman, N. Koshel, I. Belaja, V. Voitenko (Institute of Gerontology, Kiev, Ukraine)

PURPOSE: The probability of occurrence of many adult diseases depends on developmental conditions during fetal and postnatal stages (Barker's hypothesis). A logic consequence of a Barker's hypothesis is the assumption that human longevity can also depend on the features of early development. Since the human development is greatly influenced by factors of a seasonal nature in conditions of a moderate climate (temperature, insolation and, first of all, qualitative and quantitative structure of nutrition), the dependence of longevity upon month of birth is investigated. METHOD: The archival records of Kiev area (Ukraine), involving a sample of people who died during 1990-2000 years (44307 men and∫ 45117 women), were used in the study. RESULTS: It has been shown that relation of longevity to month of birth has, both in men and in women, an U-shaped character: longevity of people, who were born in the middle of the year, had lowest values, and longevity of∫ people, who were born at the end of the year had highest values. Thus, the longevity of women, who were born in May, makes 69.70±0.36 years, and of those born in December - 73.67±0.30 years; the longevity of men, who were born in May, was 59.30±0.46 years, and of those born in December - 63.04±0.39 years (the distinction between minimum and maximum longevity values was significant, $p < 0.001$). CONCLUSION: The obtained results confirm our assumption, that not only adult diseases, but also human longevity can be programmed by the environmental factors in early ontogenesis.

Parental Age Effects on Human Longevity

L. A. Gavrilov, N. S. Gavrilova, (Center on Aging, NORC/ University of Chicago, Chicago, IL, USA), G. N. Evdokushkina, V. G. Semyonova (Institute of Public Health, Moscow, Russia)

This study is focused on the following scientific problem: does the parental age at child conception affect progeny lifespan? Our previous studies found that daughters conceived to older fathers (above age 45) live shorter lives (Gavrilov, Gavrilova, 1997, Science, 277: 17), and more research is required for understanding the mechanisms of parental age effects. These studies are also of practical importance, because persons conceived to older fathers are at higher risk of prostate cancer (Zhang et al, 1999) and Alzheimer's disease (Bertram et al, 1998). In this study we used high-quality genealogical data for European aristocratic families where the exact lifespan and parental ages at conception are known for each person. The methodology of historical prospective study of extinct birth cohorts (born in 1800-80) was applied to individual lifespan (more than 6,000 cases per each sex) as a dependent variable in multivariate regression analysis with nominal variables. The following additional predictor variables are also taken into consideration: parental and spousal lifespan, year and month of person's birth, ethnicity and birth order. We found that daughters conceived to older fathers live shorter lives, while sons are not affected. Maternal age effects on lifespan of adult progeny are negligible compared to effects of paternal age. Conception to old father is not dangerous when father lives more than 80 years. Surprisingly, children conceived to particularly young fathers also live shorter lives, especially in the case of long-lived fathers. This study was supported in part by grants from the National Institute on Aging.

Study of the Inheritance of Human Longevity

N. S. Gavrilova, L. A. Gavrilov (Center on Aging, NORC/University of Chicago, Chicago, IL, USA), V. G. Semyonova, G. N. Evdokushkina (Institute of Public Health, Moscow, Russia)

Understanding the mechanisms of familial transmission of human longevity is an important, still unresolved scientific problem. Our preliminary studies found very unusual non-linear (accelerating) pattern for the dependence of offspring lifespan on parental lifespan in humans, suggesting increased genetic heterogeneity among longer-lived parents (Gavrilova et al, 1998, Human Biology, 70: 799). The purpose of this study is to validate these findings on a larger dataset (more than 12,000 cases) and to consider possible alternative explanations by controlling for the effects of other important predictors of human longevity. In this study we collected, computerized and analyzed particularly accurate and reliable genealogical data for European aristocratic families (taken from professional data sources), where the destiny (lifespan) of each person (born in 1800-80) was traced in history. The methodology of historical prospective study of extinct birth cohorts was applied to individual lifespan as a dependent variable in multivariate regression analysis with nominal variables. To control for possible confounding effects of socio-cultural differences between families, the spousal lifespan was included into analysis as an additional predictor variable. We found strong non-linear, accelerating pattern for the dependence of progeny lifespan on parental lifespan, even after adjusting for the effects of other predictor variables: spousal lifespan, parental ages at person's conception, year and month of person's birth, ethnicity and birth order. Daughters demonstrated particularly sharp, non-linear pattern of lifespan inheritance. Our findings support genetic explanation for exceptional human longevity. This study was supported in part by grants from the National Institute on Aging.

The Principal Mechanism of Ontogenic Aging and Rejuvenation

Valery G. Shakhbazov (Department of Genetics and Cytology, Kharkov State University, Ukraine)

The process of aging is as complex as life itself and the general theory of aging is not elaborated yet. The author previously reported about his studies of the role of different causes of aging: decrease of bioelectric properties of cell nuclei, processes of cohesion of macromolecular structures of chromatin and establishing of the electric equilibration in these structures. We revealed the dependence of the bioelectric properties of cell nuclei upon ontogenesis, used as a method of biologic age determination. The data obtained prove the connection between the process of aging and nucleus and chromatin potential decrease. Thereafter, the process of ontogenetic aging is accompanied with the process of phylogenetic rejuvenation. The main cause of rejuvenation is the sexual process and meiosis. This process takes place in the period of intensive accumulation of the electric charge in the nucleus and results in division of homologous chromosomes. In the later steps of ontogeny, during amphimixis, in the new organism are transferred the nuclear structures with restored electric unequlibration and potential possibility of a new energetic wave. The great significance of nuclear structures in the process of aging in the process of aging is connected with the meiosis process dividing the homologous chromosomes. The additional proof of presented theoretic considerations is the observed by many authors increase of longevity in heterotic organisms that are characterized by advanced degree of unequlibration in homologous chromosomes.

The risk of mortality in carriers of the hereditary hemochromatosis gene (HFE).

M.O. van Aken, A.J.M. de Craen, D.L. Knook, B.T. Heijmans, P.E. Slagboom, J. Gussekloo, R.G.J. Westendorp (Gerontology and Geriatrics, Leiden University Medical Center, Leiden, the Netherlands).

Purpose: Hemochromatosis is associated with homozygosity for the mutation Cys282Tyr in the hereditary hemochromatosis gene (HFE). The estimated population frequency for HFE heterozygosity is 10 to 15 percent and for HFE homozygosity it is 0.5%. Some, but not all HFE carriers have lifelong increased levels of serum ferritin and serum iron. Because iron is thought of as a determinant of atherosclerosis by promoting oxygen radical formation and lipid peroxidation, HFE homozygous and heterozygous subjects may be at risk for atherosclerotic events and mortality. Methods: Within the Leiden 85-plus Study, a longitudinal population-based study of inhabitants of Leiden aged 85 and over, HFE-genotypes and serum ferritin levels were determined for 661 participants (187 men/474 women). After the baseline measurements (1986-1988) all participants were followed for mortality and primary causes of death during a 10-years follow-up period. As a control group, the HFE-genotype was also determined in 248 young subjects, aged 18-40 years. Results: The prevalence of HFE heterozygosity was similar in old and young subjects (82/661 (12.4%) versus 30/248 (12.1%), p=0.9). The prevalence of HFE homozygosity among the oldest old was 0.2% (1/661), instead of 0.5 0.000000e+00xpected. During the10-years follow-up period, the risk of mortality of all cause (Relative Risk 1.1, 95 Conclusion: HFE homozygous subjects suffer an increased mortality risk, although some survive until very old age. HFE heterozygous subjects do not suffer an increased mortality risk.

SESSION 470

Attitudes of families of Arab-Israeli residents of a nursing home towards the institution.

Khaled Suleiman, M.D. (Dabouriya Home for the Aged, Dabouriya, Israel); Assad Azaiza, (The Dabouriya Association for the Aged, Dabouriya, Israel); Adrian Walter-Ginzburg, (Herczeg Institute on Aging, Tel Aviv University, Tel Aviv, Israel).

Purpose: Although provision of formal service sector services to the Arab-Israeli elderly is contrary to existing norms and traditions in Arab society, social and needs-based changes have made them necessary. The goal of the study is to assess the attitudes of the families of Arab-Israeli elderly towards the nursing home in which their relatives live. Method: A 65-question anonymous instrument was administered to families of nursing home residents that ranked both the opinion of the family member, and of the elderly resident him/herself (as the family understood it). The questionnaire was distributed to 60 families, of which 41 (68%) answered all the questions (470f all 87 nursing home residents at the time of the study). Respondents were: child, 49%; spouse, 5%; sibling, 5%; grandchild, 5%; more distant relative, 36%. Results: The families of Arab-Israeli nursing home residents think of the home primarily as a place for treatment and rehabilitation (90%). After their relative entered the home, they accept the situation despite contrary cultural norms (83%) and despite the fact that the elderly resident him/herself does not always accept the move (66%). The relatives visit very frequently, and are primarily concerned that their relative be treated with dignity and that they maintain a presentable appearance. The families wish to be active partners in the nursing home treatment and activities. Conclusions: The nursing home provides a necessary solution to care of needy elderly in traditional Arab society, with families maintaining an active role.

Decision Making in Institutionalization & Intergenerational Relationship—A Study of Four Major Chinese Cities

KWAN Yui-huen, Alex & CHONG Ming-lin, Alice (City University of Hong Kong, Kowloon, HONG KONG)

As a Chinese society, it is only natural for the Chinese culture to exert an influence on how elderly people are being treated regarding institutionalization. In traditional China, taking care of the elderly is an obligation in filial piety, and most of the frail older adults are being taken care of in their own home by their children or other family members. Yet in face of the challenge of population aging, and changing social values, more and more families find it difficult to take care of the frail elderly members at home. This paper intends to report a comparative study of four major cities (Hong Kong, Guangzhou, Beijing, and Shanghai) in China on decision making in institutionalization and intergenerational relationship between the elderly residents and carers. A total of 1,680 respondents (280 carers and 280 residents in each city) were successfully interviewed using questionnaire. Among them, 280 matched pairs of residents and their family carers were from Hong Kong, Shanghai, and Beijing, but only 197 matched pairs of residents and carers from Guangzhou. Findings suggest that poor health and inability of family to take care of the elderly were the two main reasons leading to institutionalization. It was mostly the older adults themselves or their son that initiated the idea of institutionalization. Before institutionalization, the residents' relationship with their carers was the worst in Hong Kong. After institutionalization, this relationship tended to level off in all four cities. In conclusion, this study sensitizes policy-makers, researchers, and home administrators about important issues in institutionalization. It provides rich empirical data about ways to improve service quality; gives direction for formulation of long term care policy, and for training and staff development.

Development and Testing of the Relatives' of Aged Care Residents Assessment of Staff Support Tool

Toye, C. (Edith Cowan University, Perth, Western Australia) Kristjanson, L. J. (Edith Cowan University, Perth, Western Australia) Helmes, E. (Edith Cowan University, Perth, Western Australia)

The researchers purpose was to develop and test a questionnaire for use in aged care facilities (ACFs) to measure residents' family members' perceptions of support from the staff. Items for the questionnaire, the Relatives' of Aged Care Residents Assessment of Staff Support Tool (RACRASST) were developed from data obtained at interviews with family members of Western Australian ACF residents and with staff, and from a literature review. Response options added ranged from strongly agree to strongly disagree, with a not applicable option. Testing has been as follows: Firstly, a panel of experts assessed the clarity, content validity, and internal consistency of the scale and its hypothesised sub-scales. Secondly, the instrument was pre-tested with a small sample of ACF residents' family members and findings of reliability/validity analyses were used to select items to retain. Thirdly, data collected from a large sample using the resultant, 32-item questionnaire were subjected to a factor analysis and three items were deleted because of a high rate of missing/ not applicable responses. Fourthly, the test-retest reliability coefficient for the scale was determined. Finally, the RACRASST was used to measure family members' perceptions of staff support in a study, and its properties were reassessed after two more items were deleted because of missing/ not applicable responses. The 27-item RACRASST is a unidimensional scale. The test-retest reliability coefficient for the scale was found to be 0.99 over 23 days and Cronbach's alpha coefficient was 0.96 in recent testing. The RACRASST is a promising but immature instrument, requiring further assessment.

Family Caregiver's Preference and Its Determinants for the Long-Term Care Service Use for the Impaired Elderly

Heung Bong Cha (Graduate School of Social Welfare, Hallym University, Kangwondo, Korea)

This study is aimed to examine the relative weight of four determining factors for the family caregiver's attitude toward long-term care service use for the impaired elderly: (1) the predisposing factors (age, sex), (2) need factors (types and levels of disability and illness), (3) enabling factors (home ownership and family income), and (4) family care factors (the relationship of a family caregiver to the elderly and the extent of family care burden). Of four factors, this study focuese, especially, on the rold of family care factors: how and to what extent it directly influences on the caregiver's attitude toward long-term care service use, and also indirectly mediates effects of the other factors on this attitude. The data for this analysis is taken from the 1997 Survey for the Impaired Elderly conducted by Seoul Metropolitan City. With regard to the preference for each type of long-term care services, the results of this study indicate that amont of burden demanded from the family caregiver plays the primary rold in determining his/her preference for long-term care services. When need and enabling factors are controlled, families overburdenended by caring for the impaired elderly are significantly more likely than those less overburdended to prefer institutional care and community care services. In addition to its direct effect, family caregiver's burden also mediates the effect of home ownership on the preference for long-term care services. In terms of the relative preference between family care and social care, more than half of surveyed families prefer the complementary use of community care services to alleviate family care. This study shows that the importance of the family care context in shaping the caregiver's preference of long-term care services. When family caregivers feel overburdened by caring for the elderly, he/she is likely to seek the alternative resources of social care services. Still, family caregivers prefer to use social care services as a supplementary resource rather than the substitutional one for long-term care services. These results produce a useful suggestion for the future orientation of family policies which aim to alleviate many imposing types of family care burdens and, instead, to enhance access to community care services

Family involvement in the homes for the aged

Paivi Voutilainen, Seija Muurinen, Marja Vaarama (National Research and Development Centre for Welfare and Health / Policy and Services for Ageing People) & Arja Isola (University of Oulu, Dpt of Nursing Science and Health Care Administration)

Close collaboration between residents, their family members and nursing staff in homes for the aged is considered as an important indicator of high quality nursing care. However, little is known of the process of families with nursing staff to become actively involved. The aim of this study was to describe the family members' views on their possibilities to participate in planning and decision making and find out the most common ways of participating in nursing care. The study was guided by the framework of need theories. The data was collected using structured questionnaire developed for this study. 474 family members from 4 institutions (36 wards) returned the questionnaire, response rate being 81,9 %. The mean age of the respondents was 59,5 years. The respondents were spouses (10 %), children (66 %) and other relatives/ friends (23 %). The results imply that family members involved in nursing care by responding residents' social and emotional needs. The main activities were to maintain residents' social contacts (59 %) and to mentally support residents by discussions (68 %). Responding residents' physical needs was insignificant. The respondents expressed their willingness to participate in planning and make decisions on nursing care but only 41 % of them had been offered an opportunity to do so. The information received from nursing staff was considered inadequate and didn't support family members' involvement. It was concluded that the role of family members has to be discussed and the ways to be involved created. Modes of family centered nursing care are to be implemented and staff trained to allow more family involvement.

Negotiating Professional and Family Caregiving Boundaries in Long-term Care

C. Ward-Griffin (University of Western Ontario, London, Canada), N. Bol (Regional Psychogeriatric Program), K. Hay (Parkwood Hospital)

PURPOSE: Previous research suggests that positive relationships between professionals and family caregivers are a critical dimension of ensuring quality, continuous, client-centred care. However, little is known about the process of negotiation between nursing staff and families in long-term care facilities (LTCF). The major purpose of this qualitative study was to critically analyze the relationship between registered nurses and family members caring for a veteran diagnosed with Alzheimers Disease and Related Disorders (ADRD). Specifically, we were interested in knowing how formal and informal caregivers negotiate the caregiving situation in a LTCF. METHOD: Guided by a critical ethnographic method, purposive sampling was used to obtain 20 nurse-family caregiver dyads. Separate in-depth interviews, direct observations of the nurse-family caregiver interaction and field notes provided data for analysis. RESULTS: Findings revealed four different types of relationships between nurses and family members: conventional, conflictual, collaborative and carative. Each typology conceptualizes the roles of the nurse and family member differently, and each uses different negotiation strategies resulting in different outcomes. The conflictual relationship was the most stressful of all the typologies for both nurses and family caregivers. Findings also suggest specific factors that facilitate mutual collaboration between families and staff caring for people with ADRD in LTCF. CONCLUSION: Relationships between staff and families in LTC are dynamic and multifaceted. This study found that the development of certain types of nurse-family relationships depend on a number of influencing factors, suggesting a need for changes in practice and long-term care policy.

The effect of a relationship enhancing program of care on residents, family members and careproviders.

Katherine Simone McGilton (University of Toronto, Toronto, Canada) Linda O'Brien-Pallas (Univeristy of Toronto, Toronto, Canada) Dorothy Pringle (University of Toronto, Toronto, Canada)

Quality of life for residents in long-term care institutions has been linked with meaningful and genuine relationships with their careproviders, who are mainly health care aides (HCAs). Despite this evidence, there remains an absence of controlled studies concerning the benefits of restructuring caregiving in order to enhance relationships. A 7 month intervention with 3 distinct components (continuity of careprovider, relationship enhancing skills, and support from supervisors) was developed with the objective of enhancing the quality of relationships between the careprovider and the resident. A quasi-experimental comparison design was used to evaluate the intervention on 40 residents, 42 family members and 19 careproviders on 2 long term care units (1 intervention and 1 comparison). Data was collected at baseline and at 4 months post intervention. Results indicated that, over time, residents perceived changes in their relationship with careproviders ($t = 2.88$, $p = .008$) as did family members ($t = -3.84$, $p = .001$). Finally, the quality of the careproviders' interactions improved ($t=3.25$, $p=.003$) as did the continuity of careprovider assignment ($t=-11.6$, $p=.001$). No statistically significant changes were found for the comparison unit on any variable. The intervention did lead to a change in the way careproviders related to residents which indicates that relationships can be enhanced for residents living in long-term care environments.

The Roles of Adult Sons in Institution-Based Elder Care

Sherry L. Dupuis (Brock University, St. Catharines, Ontario, Canada)

Although our understanding of the roles of community-based family caregivers has been expanding rapidly over the past decade, our understanding of the roles of family members in long-term care settings remains limited. Our understanding of the roles of male caregivers in long-term care facilities is even less developed. Guided by symbolic interactionism and the conceptual framework of the caregiving career, the purpose of this study was to examine men's involvement in institution-based elder care by focusing on adult sons caring for a parent living in a long-term care facility. Data for this study came from in depth, active interviews with 50 adult sons caring for parents in one of four long-term care facilities in Southern Ontario. In a previous study focussed on the roles of adult daughters in long-term care facilities, five caregiving role manifestations were developed from the data. Although some of the adult sons felt that they approached their caregiving roles differently than their sisters, the stories told by the adult sons in this study suggest that adult sons think about their institution-based elder care roles in similar ways as adult daughters, with four of the five caregiving role manifestations emerging in the adult sons' stories. In conclusion, the adult sons in this study expressed a strong sense of family responsibility and placed importance on monitoring care and in maintaining normalcy in their parents' lives, primarily by providing emotional and social support to their parents.

SESSION 471

A SURVEY ABOUT AGED LIFE STRESSORS IN TEHRAN CITY

Ramin Sarchami- (Qazvin University of Medical Sciences. Qazvin. IRAN) Simin Taavoni- (Iran University of Medical Sciences. Tehran. IRAN)

BACKGROUND: Nowadays the most concerning consideration in human life is not only the length of life but also the quality of life, and it should be emphasized that people live healthier in the end stage of life in all aspects such as physical, emotional, psychosocial, etc. Researches have demonstrated that there are a lot of stressors in the life of aged people and these stressors vary from a society to another. PURPOSE: This study is performed to determine the aged life stressors in Tehran city in autumn 2000. METHODS AND MATERIALS: In this study 100 aged people of Tehran city have been involved by a simple random sampling from four main part of Tehran (North, South, East, West). A questionnaire consisted of 25 questions was used. 9 questions were about demographic characteristics and the next 16 questions were about the factors that may cause a stressful life. Findings: Results were as followed: %66 were married and lived with their legal partner, %55had above 5 children, %54 were retired and %69 lived in their personal house. %60 of them have an income about 500-700 thousands Rails monthly, and %36 had 2-3 children to support, %88 of them lived independently of their children. %73 of these aged were concerned about the future of their children, and only %6 were concerned about changes in appearance due to aging. Also %83had a gastrointestinal problem and were obliged to follow a food regimen. CONCLUSION: Quality assurance of aged life is partly related to their life style during youth, and partly a social responsibility to provide necessary supports in different stages of life and specially in elderly, and finally it is partly due to chance. Any way since the society has a lot of potentiality to help aged people there should be special considerations to support aged people. It should be noticed that the more we prepare an assured social support for aged people now the less we will have stress about our coming future.

Challenges in assessing quality of life for older people

Lynne Corner (Centre for Health Services Research, University of Newcastle, Newcastle upon Tyne, UK) John Bond (Centre for Health Services Research, University of Newcastle, Newcastle upon Tyne, UK)

The abstract must not exceed 1,600 characters (250 words) and should be organized as follows: PURPOSE: Statement of the purpose of the study or program being presented. METHOD: Description of the method used. RESULTS: Summary of findings in sufficient detail to support conclusions. Vague statements such as "will be presented and discussed" should be avoided. CONCULSION: Statement of the conclusion based on the findings of the study. PURPOSE: The theoretical, methodological and practical challenges in assessing quality of life are considerable. It is important to involve direct expression of views by consumers and it is also recognised that traditionally defined outcomes need to be complemented by approaches that focus on the person's concerns in order to evaluate interventions and identify more relevant and appropriate forms of service provision. Positivist approaches to method dominate and there is now an array of questionnaires and interview schedules that have been developed. However, an understanding of what meaning the outcomes have for individuals or groups is lacking in traditional outcome methods. Approaches which focus on the individual alone ignore the wider, social, political and economic context in which individuals are situated. Appreciating the dynamics of interactions and relationships is crucial in assessing quality of life. METHOD & RESULTS: A study exploring person-centred outcomes from the perspective of older people using qualitative methods, identified public and private accounts. CONCLUSION: This has implications for the future development in methods of assessing outcome in health and social care research.

Catherine Brennand Centre for Health Services Research 21 Claremont Place University of Newcastle upon Tyne NE2 4AA UK Tel: +44 (0)191 222 7046 Fax: +44 (0)191 222 6043 Email: C.M.Brennand@ncl.ac.uk

Concern Themes as Correlates of Subjective Well-being: A study with elderly residents of Beijing

Lena Fung (Department of Physical Education, Hong Kong Baptist University, Hong Kong)

PURPOSE: Recent growth in literature concerning subjective well-being (SWB) reflects its place as a valued outcome in and of itself. However, despite the stream of information generated, a crystallized body of knowledge is still lacking, especially knowledge about the determinants of high and low levels of SWB in different cultures. With the view of making a contribution towards understanding SWB, the present investigator undertook a study on the SWB of elderly residents of Beijing and investigated the relationship between Concern Themes (CTs) and SWB. METHOD: Volunteered participants were recruited from Beijing community centers. With the help of research assistants, 312 male and 305 female elderly persons aged between 60 and 89 completed three sets of questionniares: 1) The Satisfaction with Life Scale, 2) The Positive Affect and Negative Affect Scale, and 3) The Concern Themes Questionnaire. To identify the relative contribution of different CTs to SWB, a hypothesized model was developed for fitting with obtained data. Furthermore, differences in perceptions of CTs between male and female elderly persons were examined by means of One-way MANOVA. RESULTS: Result from the Structural Equation Modelling showed that among the CTs of Social and Family Support, Health and Mobility, Food, Shelter and Income, and Safety, concerns about Social and Family Support was significantly linked to feelings of SWB. This was followed by concerns about Health and Mobility. With respect to differences in perceptions of concerns, males were significantly less concerned about Social and Family Support and significantly more concerned about Food and Income than females. CONCLUSIONS: Concerns of elderly persons are varied. As concerns are related to SWB, one approach to assist elderly persons advance their level of SWB would be to provide means to minimize their feeling of anxiety from such concerns either through counselling or actual improvement of conditions which cause concerns.

Interest and limits of a quality of life questionnaire Euroqol in dementia

J Ankri (Université de Paris V, Paris, France). B. Beaufils (Université Paris VIII,Saint-Denis, France). J-L Novella (hôpital Sébastopol Reims, France). I Morrone (hôpital Sébastopol Reims, France). F Guillemin: Ecole de Santé Publique EA 1124, BP 184 54505 Vandoeuvre les Nancy. D Jolly (DIM, hôpital Maison Blanche Reims, France). L Ploton (Université Lumières, Bron, France). F Blanchard (hôpital Sébastopol, Reims, France)

Purpose: To study the feasibility and validity of a generic quality of life instrument, the EuroQol (1), in a sample of dementia patients. Method: The French version of the EuroQol questionnaire was administered to a sample of 142 subjects with dementia according to the DSM III-R criteria. Feasibility of administration and acceptability of the questionnaire were determined by the refusal rate, type of administration, time of administration, and number and distribution of missing data. Test-retest reliability and inter-rater concordance (patient, family proxy, care-provider proxy) were analyzed Results: Administration time varied considerably around a mean of 15 minutes. The response rate of 83.2% to the five items on the questionnaire was satisfactory, and the non-response rate rose as a function of dementia severity. The instrument's sensitivity was good and discriminated well among the subjects. Test-retest reliability was average for the dimensions taken as a while but weak for pain evaluation. The external validity as indicated by inter-rater concordance was poor, except for the mobility dimension; other criteria produced better results. An overall score appeared justified, with good reproducibility, good discriminating power, and satisfactory validity. Conclusion: A generic health-related quality of life questionnaire such as the EuroQol can be administered to dementia patients. The instrument is reliable for this population in dimensions that are stable over time. Assuming that dementia patients are capable of expressing their quality of life, at least up to a certain level of deterioration, the EuroQol is a fairly valid instrument for use with this population.

QUALITY OF THE LIFE A FUNDAMENTAL VISION

M. Dumitru, H. Thadepalli (UCLA Drew University, USA), E. Telford (Center of Biogerontology, Canada).

The paper presents a holistic vision regarding the main gerontological issue, how to age and to maintain Quality of the Life (QOL). We believe that our 10 years studies conceptualizes QOL as an ontogenetic process that is produced by a complex of individual, social and environmental factors. Study design: cross sectional survey. Participants: 370 people aged between 65 and 89. Methods: .health related, social, economical, nutritional variables. .Physical complains and diseases. .Measurement of QOL: well being scale life satisfaction. In our vision the individual is a landmark influenced by subjective, objective, negative and positive factors. Without a right attitude we aren't able to implement this concept no matter how much we know, because we are immobilized by a number of myths about aging. The most significant roadblock is that of identifying the many misconceptions we have conscious or unconscious. The search for criteria of QOL is a complex endeavor and is not possible to solve it without a fundamental vision. The only way to think is in terms of multicriteria approach, and a dynamic vision has to be used to clarify the complex relationship between multiple indicators in order to construct a positive image of the old age and aging. We forcefully promote the QOL as a guiding theme in gerontological research and as a challenge for the design of social policy.

Spiritual Practice and Well-being of Indian elderly

Kumari, V (VHD Homescience College, Bangalore, India)
Prakash, I.J. (Bangalore University, Bangalore 560056, India)

People who are following spiritual practice are expected to cope with aging better. A purposive sample of men and women in three age groups - young, middle aged and old- all belonging to a religious mission were interviewed and assessed for Psychological and spiritual well-being, purpose in life and death anxiety. There were 60 subjects, 30 male and 30 female in each group. Older people who had longer years of practice were found to have less stress, better sense of well-being and higher purpose in life. Usually Indian studies find women to be lower on well-being. In this study, gender differences were surprisingly absent. The role of spiritual practice in successful aging is examined in detail.

The subjective well-being of the older people in the sparsely populated areas of Lapland

Simo Koskinen, University of Lapland, Department of social work. ELVI-project. Rovaniemi. Finland

Purpose: To analyse the experiences of olde age, aging and well-being among the older people who are living at their own homes in the villages of Lappish sparsely populated areas. Method: The study is the part of the multidisciplinary ELVI-project (The Aiding the Lives of of the Aging) at the university of Lapland, where 158 persons more than sixty-five years of age were interviewed in nine villages of Lapland. The questionnaire included mainly structured questions but also open questions. The data was analysed using quantitative and qualitative research methods. Results: The own home was experienced as a life's resource. At home you can realize autonomy, self-determination and freedom. There are the own paths to walk. When the functional capacity is decreasing many risks can emergence also at home. The experiences of work and war are central elements in older people's life. The physical health was estimated good by more than 33% and the mental health by 72%. 44%of the respondents estimated their own age lower than it was in fact. The economic situation was estimated good by 33% and 89% was satisfied with their dwelling. 22% of the older people felt lonely almost sometimes. Different services were lacked by 40%. Conclusion: The experiences of well-being are in connection with the cultural background of the villages and with the past life of the older persons. The subjective well-being has an important meaning to developing living at own home.

The Well-being of the Aged People in the Rural Areas of Lapland

Katri Ylikulppi (University of Lapland, Department of Social Sciences, Rovaniemi, Finland)

Purpose: The purpose of this study is to describe how the aged people living in the rural areas of Lapland manage to live at home. The typology of the elderly (N=158) in the basis of well-being and managing at home were constructed. Method: The study is part of a Elvi- research and development project, which research and develop the means and aids to help people to manage at home. The study included a large survey. The well-being was examined through income, housing conditions, mood, social relationships, health and functional ability. Quantitative analysis were made by factor analysis and cluster analysis. Results: Four groups were founded in the basis of analysis. Half of the aged (53 %) formulated the first group which was managing very well in their daily living. The second group (19 %) were having good external circumstances (health, income, dwelling), but weak internal circumstances (sosial relationships). Third group (17 %) was opposited to previous group. It had the weakest external circumstances especially in income and housing conditions, but fine internal elements especially in social relationaships. The fourth group (11 %) was having the most vulnerable situation in managing at home. They had the lowest functional capasity and also self-rated health. The social relationships and self-rated mood were also weak. Conclusion: The majority of the aged were managing well in living at homes. Also the income and housing conditions were quite good or average in all presented groups. The most differentiated factors that separated the groups were related to health and functional capasity, self-rated mood and social relationships.

SESSION 472

New Models of Continuing Care in Alberta, Canada

Vivien Lai (Alberta Health and Wellness, Edmonton, Canada), Future trends and rationale for new models of continuing care in Alberta, Canada. Phil Gaudet (The Good Samaritan Society, Edmonton, Canada), Assisted Living in Alberta. Helen Lantz (The Capital Care Group, Edmonton, Canada), Laurier House, an example of innovative supportive living in Edmonton, Alberta, Canada. Phil Gaudet (The Good Samaritan Society, Edmonton, Canada), Wedman Village, Dementia Duplex. Helen Lantz (The Capital Care Group, Edmonton, Canada), McConnell Place, an example of dementia care in Edmonton, Alberta, Canada. Corinne Schalm (The Capital Care Group, Edmonton, Alberta, Canada), Research and Evaluation Findings on New Models of Continuing Care in Alberta, Canada

This symposium discusses new models of continuing care. The symposium will first address future trends and the need for developing new models of continuing care to provide services to clients traditionally served in nursing homes. New models piloted in Alberta for supportive living (Wedman House Assisted Living and Laurier House) and dementia care (McConnell Place and Wedman Village) will be presented. Evaluation findings showing results and benefits of the new models of care in comparison with traditional nursing homes will be presented. The expected outcome of the symposium is to demonstrate that innovative residential models piloted in Alberta provide better quality services at a lower cost than those provided by traditional nursing homes.

Assisted Living, The Good Samaritan Society: A Unique Alternative To Traditional Continuing Care in Edmonton, Alberta, CANADA

Phil Gaudet (THE GOOD SAMARITAN SOCIETY, Edmonton, CANADA

In the early 90's there was little choice for individuals whose services were beyond those of Home Care, but did not want, nor necessarily require institutional care. The Good Samaritan Society set about to fill that gap. With this in mind, residential options were investigated, and Oregon's Assisted Living model was adopted. As a result, the first Assisted Living facility, Wedman House, officially opened in April of 1994. The success of this program has lead to the opening of several more Assisted Living facilities in Alberta by The Society. As a social model of care, Assisted Living offers a home-like, residential experience for people who desire privacy and maximum involvement in decision making. The facility features individual suites, with kitchenettes and private bathrooms included. Several communal areas, including a large dining room allows for the choice of private time versus group involvement. Thus, the concern of social isolation is alleviated. Our services reflect the value that residents place on independence, choice, dignity, individuality, privacy and a home-like environment. These essential elements, along with the operational concepts of shared responsibility, bounded choice, and managed risk, are the keys to attaining the goals of the Assisted Living concept. The philosophy is to support individual life-style choices. The presentation will describe these principles and concepts. In addition, the difference between The Good Samaritan Society's Assisted Living model and those of other supportive housing models will be clarified.

Future trends and rationale for new models of continuing care in Alberta, Canada

Vivien Lai (Alberta Health and Wellness, Edmonton, Canada)

The presentation will discuss future trends of the aging population, as well as rationale for the need of new models of continuing care. It will outline common features of the new models that address the needs of the new aging population. It will compare these features with those of the traditional nursing homes. The conclusion is that the features of these new models of care address the needs of the new aging population more successful than those of the traditional nursing homes

Laurier House, an example of innovative supportive living in Edmonton, Alberta, CANADA

Helen Lantz (The CAPITAL CARE Group, Edmonton, CANADA)

Laurier House is a unique accommodation alternative that offers continuing care services with life lease care housing. The CAPITAL CARE Group designed Laurier House with independent living suites that retain the privacy, space and quality of a home for residents who require personal and medical care and may wish to have a spouse or partner living with them. Residents, who are assessed as needing facility based care, are admitted to Laurier House through Alberta's single point of entry system. Residents invest their housing dollars in the accommodation and pay monthly upkeep fees, similar to condominium charges. As with other continuing care facilities in the province, Alberta Health pays the full cost of required health services. When the residents leave Laurier House, the life lease payment minus a small percentage for a reserve fund, is returned to the resident or estate. The presentation will explain what differentiates Laurier House from conventional continuing care facilities and describe the building, the multi-skilled staff, the health and medical services and the life lease agreement. The CAPITAL CARE Group is the largest public continuing care organization in Canada. In operation since 1964, the organization provides services to more than 1400 residents in nine facilities, offers a variety of community based programs and employs over 2400 staff from diverse health care disciplines.

McConnell Place, an example of dementia care in Edmonton, Alberta, CANADA

Helen Lantz (The CAPITAL CARE Group, Edmonton, CANADA)

Caring for residents with a dementia has been a challenge to caregivers for many years. Often residents were confined to an institution such as a mental home or a long-term care facility. The CAPITAL CARE Group has taken a new approach to care for residents in the mid-stage of a dementia by building two free standing residential Alzheimer Care Centres with a third Centre close to completion. McConnell Place North, built in 1995, was the first residential Alzheimer Care Centre in Canada and McConnell Place West, built in 1998, was the second such facility in Canada. The Centres are replicas of the successful Woodside Place in Oakmount, Pennsylvania and incorporate some modifications based on formal evaluations and consultations with staff. Each home consists of three houses to accommodate twelve residents in private rooms with an ensuite bathroom. The philosophy is "to make every day a good day for the residents" and emphasis is on maintaining independence and dignity in a home-like environment. Residents are encouraged to participate in everyday activities with staff providing support that enables residents to do as much as possible on their own. This model of care is believed to reduce disruptive behavior, improve the quality of life and retain functional skills for a longer period of time. The presentation will describe how environment can have a beneficial effect on behavior and include information on multi-skilled staffing, family involvement, community linking programs and the Research Program.

Research and Evaluation Findings on New Models of Continuing Care in Alberta, CANADA

C. Schalm (The CAPITAL CARE Group, Edmonton, Alberta, CANADA), L. Gardner (Leslie Gardner Consulting, Edmonton), N. Keating (The University of Alberta, Edmonton), D. Milke (The CAPITAL CARE Group), J. Ross Kerr (The University of Alberta), S. Warren (The University of Alberta)

Each of the four models of continuing care presented in this symposium was the first of its kind in Canada. They were developed as alternatives for clients who otherwise would have been admitted to a traditional nursing home type setting. As new models, they have been evaluated by a number of research studies. This presentation integrates the findings of those studies which demonstrated these models as cost effective options that clients and families prefer to more traditional long term care facilities. Study findings include: residents are comparable in care requirements to those in traditional long term care facilities in Alberta but target groups are more specific; all of these sites have multi-skilled staff rather than traditional staffing patterns; costs are lower; families participate extensively in supporting the quality of life of their relative; families and residents are more satisfied with these residential environments and there is more emphasis on independence and choice.

Wedman Village Homes, a Residential Model of Care for Alzheimer Residents in Edmonton, Alberta, CANADA

Phil Gaudet (THE GOOD SAMARITAN SOCIETY, Edmonton, CANADA

The Good Samaritan Society has demonstrated a strong commitment to special programs which focus on the care of people with Alzheimer's Disease. Wedman Village Homes consists of three, 10 - bedroom duplex homes (30 beds) for the care of elderly persons with Alzheimer and related dementia. It is designed to meet the personal needs and support requirements of individuals in the early to mid stages of dementia. The program is based upon The Good Samaritan Society's Shared Living model. It is a residential model that is well rooted in the values of privacy, dignity, choice independence and a home-like environment as espoused by The Society's Assisted Living program. The homes provide alternatives for people with dementia who can no longer benefit from other community-based services such as home care or day care programs. As with Assisted Living, the care component of the "Village" is based more on a social rather than a medical model of care. Personal autonomy and competencies are emphasized. This is an interactive program. One purpose is to assist the residents in maintaining their functional skills for as long as possible. With this in mind, residents are encouraged to participate in daily activities associated with a homelike environment such as laundry, housekeeping, food preparation and social activities. The presentation will describe staffing patterns, environmental features and programming concepts that contribute to the resident's safety, self-esteem and over-all well-being.

SESSION 473

The UK Growing Older programme on Extending Quality Life

A. Walker (Department of Sociological Studies, University of Sheffield, Sheffield, UK) The Growing Older Research Programme. K. Davidson (Centre for Research on Ageing and Gender, Department of Sociology, University of Surrey, UK) Older Men: Their Social World and Healthy Lifestyles. M. Evandrou (Age Concern Institute of Gerontology, King's College London, London, UK) Family, Work and Quality of Life. T. Maltby (Department of Social Policy and Social Work, University of Birmingham, Birmingham, UK) Older Women's Lives and Voices. K. McKee (Sheffield Institute for Studies on Ageing, University of Sheffield, Sheffield, UK) The Impact of Reminiscence on Quality of Life. T. Scharf (Centre for Social Gerontology, School of Social Relations, Keele University, Keele, UK) Older People in Deprived Neighbourhoods: Social Exclusion and Quality of Life. A. Withnall (Department of Social Policy and Social Work, University of Warwick, Coventry, UK) Older People and Lifelong Learning. Christina Victor (Department of Public Health Sciences, St George's Hospital Medical School, London, UK) Loneliness, Social Isolation and Living Alone.

This round table introduces the UK national research programme on extending quality life: Growing Older. It comprises 24 projects examining different dimensions of quality of life in old age and how it can be extended. This session will provide an overview of the Programme and brief introductions to seven of the projects. The discussion will focus on early findings and methodological issues in quality of life research. The round table aims to introduce this major programme to conference participants and to exchange information with researchers involved in similar work in other countries and practitioners working with older people.

Family, Work and Quality of Life: Changing economic and social roles

Maria Evandrou, Karen Glaser and Ursula Henz (Age Concern Institute of Gerontology, King's College London, London, Great Britain)

Individuals undertake a variety of roles within work and family life. Balancing various responsibilities among those in middle and later adulthood is of particular interest given socio-economic and demographic changes, such as rising female labour force participation, increases in longevity, and rises in the age which children leave home, which are likely to create additional roles. This paper investigates the complex inter-relationships between the multiple roles of mid-life individuals, focussing on work and family commitments. The extent to which men and women in mid-life undertake a multiplicity of roles is explored using a series of typologies. The degree of variation in patterns of multiple role occupancy by socio-economic group, ethnic origin, education, health and material resources is also examined. The project also investigates the likely effects of multiple work and family responsibilities in mid-life on measures of quality of life and well-being in later life (health, financial resources and social activities). The research is based upon secondary analysis of longitudinal data containing paid work and caring histories (Family and Working Lives Survey, and the Retirement and Retirement Plans Survey). Initial results indicate that although the proportion of mid-lifers occupying multiple roles at one point in time is low, this proportion rises to 24% when we examine occupancy over the lifecourse. There is an association between paid work and caring which has implications for the accumulation of future pension entitlements and health status. The findings will inform debate on how policy can best aid those endeavouring to balance paid work, family life and caring responsibilities.

Investigating quality of life among older women in Sheffield using participatory research: preliminary findings.

Tony Maltby, University of Birmingham, UK; Lorna Warren and Joe Cook, both University of Sheffield, UK

PURPOSE: To investigate and explore 'life-story' and autobiographical methods within a participatory framework to provide an understanding of the complexity of older women's quality of life and attempt to provide a platform for their 'quiet voices'. METHOD: This paper presents the preliminary findings of the first phase of this project and in particular the methodological challenges of using a 'participatory' approach. Eleven small pre-established discussion groups of older women (50+) were drawn to reflect the ethnic mix of Sheffield, UK. These discussions (all tape recorded) have allowed the development of a range of themes to be used as a basis of individual interviews to be conducted by volunteers from within the discussion groups during the second phase (now in progress). RESULTS: These can be grouped under three headings. 1. Working with the community; 2. Usefulness of a 'discussion group' format; the challenges and successes; 3. Participatory methods and their role in quality of life research. Preliminary findings indicate that the locally based participatory research method can elicit a complex yet rich source of data that can elevate the importance of quality of life issues often assumed as unimportant by service providers and local policy makers. However, part of this problem maybe the imprecision of the term 'quality of life' since it had little meaning to the 'discussion group' women. CONCLUSION: When given an appropriate platform older women can make valuable contributions to the local policy making process. This has wide implications for the planning and implementation of services to local communities.

Marital Status and the Social Worlds and Health Behaviours of Older Men

K. Davidson (University of Surrey, Guildford, UK) T. Daly (University of Surrey, Guildford,UK)

Our research examines the lives of older men in order to understand what influences their social relationships, lifestyles and well-being. Most men are married when they die, however, older men who live alone represent a small but significantly increasing population which has hitherto been largely ignored in research on gender and later life. In this phase of the project, we have conducted 50 in-depth interviews with married, widowed, divorced and never married men over the age of 65. We analyse firstly, how older men's involvement with family and friends of both sexes, and their participation in the wider community (formal organisations, leisure and social activities), are influenced by their marital status and living arrangements. Secondly, we investigate to what extent older men's informal support networks and participation in formal organisations influence their health-related behaviour (diet, physical activity, drinking and smoking) and their subjective well-being. Preliminary findings suggest that quality of life is mediated by a complex intersection of marital status, life course history and access to social capital. Whilst widowhood and divorce indeed present severe challenges to the older man, the response to these events varies considerably. A better understanding of the gendered experiences of later life can contribute to the promotion of supportive social relationships within the community, more appropriate social organisations and strategies for encouraging healthier lifestyles in older, non-married men.

Older People and Lifelong Learning

A. Withnall (University of Warwick, UK)

Recent UK and European educational policy documents on lifelong learning tend to focus on vocational education and largely exclude the post-work population. This research aims to understand the contribution which learning in later life in both formal and informal contexts might make towards improving the quality of older people's lives. Adopting a life course approach, 10 focus groups with older learners have been conducted and a conceptual model of the pathways towards learning in later life constructed. This is being tested with 50 older people learning formally and with 50 not so involved with the aim of exploring whether they may be involved in other kinds of learning. It is intended to follow this up with 25 in-depth interviews and a series of learning diaries; a fieldwork team of specially trained older people themselves will carry out the interviews. Participants are invited to comment on findings at every stage and results are being systematically disseminated to user groups. It is expected that results will be used to inform both educational policy and practice and to provide information about the possible value of later life learning to older people themselves.

Older people in deprived neighbourhoods: social exclusion and quality of life

Thomas Scharf, Chris Phillipson, Paul Kingston, Allison Smith (Centre for Social Gerontology, School of Social Relations, Keele University, UK)

This paper derives from a research project, supported by the UK's Growing Older Programme that seeks to generate new insights into the experience of inequality in later life. The project aims to explore relationships between older people's quality of life and aspects of their residential environment. In particular, ideas relating to current social policy concerns about social exclusion are to be examined in relation to older people. The focus for the research is a detailed examination of the quality of life of older people living in socially disadvantaged neighbourhoods in three English cities. The paper outlines the aims of the study and discusses key methodological issues that arise from the study of potentially marginalised older populations. Specific issues addressed include research ethics, sampling strategies, survey design and fieldwork experiences. It is argued that these issues may be of relevance to gerontology researchers engaged in studies of older people living in different residential environments.

The Impact of Reminiscence on Quality of Life

Kevin J McKee, Helen Elford, Fiona Wilson, Sharron Hinchliffe (University of Sheffield, Sheffield, UK), Fiona Goudie (Community Health Sheffield, Sheffield, UK) Man C. Chung (University of Plymouth, Plymouth, UK), Gillie Bolton (University of Sheffield, Sheffield, UK).

PURPOSE: Claims have been made that reminiscence activity in older people produces benefits for psychological well being and Quality of Life (QoL). Key issues to be answered include: (1) Whether disclosure, reminiscence or life review have different impacts on QoL; (2) The importance of context (one to one, group, alone) and activity form (writing, verbal); (3) How cognitive impairment moderates the influence of these activities on QoL; (4) The potential role of, and benefits for, informal carers and care staff in facilitating reminiscence-type activities. As part of the ESRC Growing Older Programme designed to generate new knowledge on extending the quality of life of older people, this study will aim to address the above issues. METHOD: 200 older people from residential and community care settings will be invited to take part in a comprehensive evaluation of reminiscence-type activities. Older people will participate in four reminiscence activity sessions, over a period of one month. QOL assessments will take place one week before activities begin, during and after each session, and at one month follow up. In addition older people, their carers, and care staff will be invited to take part in qualitative interviews and focus groups. CONCLUSIONS: This approach enables contextualisation of the meanings of reminiscence, and exploration of the perceived benefits and barriers to reminiscence-type activity for both carers and older people themselves. The findings will have considerable implications for policy, and will advance current therapeutic activity with older people closer to the goal of evidence based practice.

SESSION 474

Differences in sources and impacts of social supports between older and younger caregivers

Hyeji Choi-Ko & Letha Chadiha (George Warren Brown School of Social Work, Washington University, St. Louis, MO, USA)

PURPOSE Sources of social supports for elderly caregivers (EC) and their impacts on EC's physical, mental, and social health should be differentiated from those of young caregivers (YC). METHOD The preliminary data set of the Black Caregiver Project was analyzed for this paper. In the project, caregivers of frail elders in St. Louis and southern Missouri were interviewed. Subjects (N=80, mean age= 54) were categorized as EC (N= 40, 18< age<55) or YC (N=40, age<55). RESULTS Significantly less EC (17.5%) received supports from their friends or neighbors than YC (50%) (c2= 9.45, p= .002). Also, EC were significantly less likely than YC to get help out with money (c2= 4.2, p= .04) and advice on dealing with life's problems (c2= 7.72, p= .005) from church members. Consistently, EC was significantly less likely to be satisfied with the supports from church members than YC (t= 2.44, p= .02) although there was no significant difference in satisfaction between EC and YC with supports from family (t=1.84, p= .07) and friends (t= -.13, p= .90). An examination of the impact of the supports received shows that for the EC getting supports from friends was associated with a significantly lower level of stress (t= -2.06, p= .04) and getting supports from church members was significantly related to a lower level of depression (t= 2.24, p= .03). However, this is not true for the YC, there was no significant association between getting supports and levels of stress or depression. CONCLUSION In sum, EC were less likely to receive intensive supports, less likely to be satisfied with supports received, but more likely to be influenced by receiving supports. This suggests necessity of developing social service programs for EC to develop and extend their support systems.

Elderly people acting as caregivers

Y. M. Garcia, V. C. Aranha, E. L. Klein, Y. C. M. C. Fernandes, C. K. Sznaider, E. M. S. Gonçalves, A. C. B Oliveira, E. Marangoni, F. M. Ajjar, C. Farneda, R. Barone (Disciplina de Geriatria Δ Medical School of São Paulo University, São Paulo, Brazil)

PURPOSE: To determine the presence of elderly people acting as caregivers in a specialized geriatric out-patient unit from a University Hospital. METHOD: from the patients attending to routine medical consultation, 103 were randomly assigned to undergo an interview, reviewing patterns of caregiving they received or offered, and also the patients' feelings about it. RESULTS: 95 patients were interviewed and 8 refused. Their mean age was 76.5 years. 75.3% were females. Their number of clinical diagnoses varied from 1 to 7, with a mean of 4.0 diagnosis. 28 patients (30.4%) were caregivers, 6 of spouses, 6 of siblings, 4 of their children, 3 of friends, 2 of grandchildren or nephews, 3 of more than one person. 29 (31.5%) patients received care, 18 from their children, 8 from spouses, 2 from siblings or grandchildren. From those receiving care, 6 (20.7%) also offered care to others and 22 (75.9%) took part on housekeeping, while in the whole group 76 (82.6%) did it. 20 (21.7%) worked, 77 (91.7%) took part of house expenses. 24.2% offered financial support to others. During psychologic interview, only 5. CONCLUSIONS: despite high morbidity, there was a large number of caregivers among those elderly, even when they received care themselves; most of them participated on housekeeping and expenses and an expressive number offered financial support; in their subjective point of view, they tend to underestimate their role as caregivers, although having a positive opinion about this activity.

Groups of patients and their families in the Geriatric System

Aviva Even-Zhav, Clinic Supervisor of Geriatrics, The Chaim Sheba Medical Center Monica Gun-Usishkin, Clinical Supervisor of Psychiatric, The Chaim Sheba Medical Center. Tel Hashomer 52621, ISRAEL

In old age, when loss of health is accompanied by other significant losses in life and there is a rise of chronic diseases, nurses play an important role in diagnosing, treating, preservation, advancing and amelioration life quality of the elderly and their families. For the purpose to help patients and their families was decided on a project of groups for patient and families in all the geriatric system. Senior nurses which are clinic specialist in geriatrics and psychiatric managed this project. The groups meet once a week for one hour. In several words the nurses led the groups and in other wards the social worker led the group together with the nurse. Groups purposes: 1. Guiding patients and families, providing information on relevant subjects. Offerings help in the process of hospitalization and release. 2. Coping with losses and physical inability. 3. Creating a supporting and encouraging environment, and Strengthening relations and contact with the system. Main conclusions of this initiative are: 1. In the wards in which this project took pace was positive response of patients, families and staff. They expressed satisfaction and learned about ways of copping with the condition. 2. The groups gave responses to the problems discussed. It is recommended to enlarge and continued this project.

Older Persons Caring for Disabled Adult Sons/Daughters

Gordon Flowerdew, Kathleen MacPherson, Steve Adams (Dalhousie University, Halifax, Canada)

PURPOSE: This study examines the prevalence, and the distribution of scenarios, of older persons caring for adult sons or daughters with long-term disabilities. This caregiving situation is particularly vulnerable to changes in the health and functional status of the parent(s). However, even basic prevalence estimates are not available. METHOD: The data are from the population-based 1996 Canadian General Social Survey (GSS). All 12,756 respondents aged 15 or over provided demographic and health information about themselves and were asked to identify and describe persons with long-term health or physical limitations whom they helped, or persons from whom they received help because of their own long-term health or physical limitations. They also described the types of assistance or care provided, adequacy of help from others, and some of the impacts of caregiving. RESULTS: Seventy-seven respondents (21 male, 56 female) reported giving help to a son or daughter with a long-term health or physical problem requiring specific types of support. Of these, 46 (15 male, 31 female) were aged 65+. Using the weighting variable provided for the GSS, the estimated number of elderly Canadians providing such care to their adult sons or daughters is 20,000. The specific types of care provided include child care (11.50f the estimated 20,000), meal preparation and housework (52.5%), assistance with shopping, transportation or banking (56.5%), and personal care (20.0%). CONCLUSION: Older persons caring for disabled adult sons or daughters represents a demanding, complex, and not uncommon situation. Yet there has been little investigation of the related health and social service/policy implications.

Sons and daughters as primary caregivers - a Norwegian experience based on longitudinal population data

T. I. Romoren (Norwegian Social Research, Oslo, Norway)

The purpose of this study is to compare types and duration of informal care given to an elderly person when a son or a daughter is the primary caregiver. Data are from the Larvik study, which has an event oriented panel design. All residents 80+ who lived in the coastal town of Larvik, Norway as of January 1, 1981 (N=434) were followed until death (mean age 89) registering long-term disabilities, informal and formal care use both prospectively and retrospectively. 36 % of the primary caregivers were daughters, 19 % sons. Mean age was 60 for both groups. The proportion married, in full-time work, with good health and getting support from other family members was higher among sons, while the proportion living together with the elderly was higher among daughters. Differences in type of care (emotional support, practical help (with IADL-functions) and personal care (ADL-functions) were small and insignificant between daughters and sons. Total duration of informal care was 7.3 years for daughters and 3.9 for sons. This difference, however, was due to a small minority of daughters (n=14) with extreme lengths of caregiving episodes (14-33 years). The mean duration of long-term institutional care was the same for the elderly in both groups (3.9 years). These results suggests that gender differences in children's caregiving activities may be smaller than expected in some cultures and that the differences in the duration of caregiving may be due to differences in the threshold for transition into the caregiving role and not in the threshold for leaving it.

SESSION 475

The Gesher Project: Healing Holocaust Trauma Through Art

Linda Frimer, (Co-founder, Artist, and Facilitator of the "Gesher Holocaust Project", Vancouver, British Columbia, Canada)

The purpose of this presentation is to share the experience of the creative bridging of cultural trauma between the generations of the Holocaust through art. The "Gesher Holocaust Project" has provided an opportunity for elders from disparate cultures to visually express their stories, and to enable appreciation, understanding and respect between generations and nations. Over a six-month period, Gesher intergenerational participants met and through the creative processes of writing, painting and talking, and began to bridge the protective silence between the generations. The Gesher Project has had a tremendous impact upon both survivors and second generation participants. It has greatly expanded their understanding of the Holocaust experience, the effects upon their lives and its effect on their intergenerational relations. Roberta S. Kremer, Executive Director, Vancouver Holocaust Education Centre, has described the quality of the creative work, both in terms of content and artistic expression as "outstanding". As artist/facilitator and co- founder of our project, I created a series of art exercises to move form silence to expression. Participants worked on themes such as "darkness and names". They worked with cultural colour associations and personal symbols, with emphasis always on what the art evoked rather than on how it appeared. Together they created a collective "Bridge" mural and a commemorative "hands" painting. Their final project was the creation of individual, large format, mixed media works of art. Using enlarged family photos and personal symbols these powerful paintings created visual "memory banks". The results of the Gesher Project have been life changing for its participants and brought to a public forum, its exhibit elicits healing, compassion and education.

Youth, Elders, and Art Experiences: Best practice in intergenerational learning

Bill Zuk (University of Victoria, Victoria, British Columbia, Canada); Robert Dalton (University of Victoria, Victoria, British Columbia, Canada)

In many homes and communities across North America today, young people have little contact with the elderly. In our highly specialized and mobile society we find it efficient to organize ourselves by age, interests, and needs. Where elders once lived with their children and grandchildren, seniors today often live independently, in retirement communities, or extended care facilities. Schools, hospitals, businesses, churches, recreation centers, and other institutions often contribute to the separation of youth from elders. But separation comes at a cost. Elders may feel detached from life and from opportunities to share their knowledge and wisdom. Youth may lack the perspective that comes from experience and can feel rootless, knowing little about local and family history and cultural heritage.This presentation examines initiatives by public school and post-secondary teachers to use art as a means of bringing youth and elders together in learning experiences that enable them to benefit from what each has to offer. Harmful stereotypes are set aside and relationships are built through these kinds of initiatives. The ideas expressed in the artwork, and the words and actions of participants bear witness to the mutual trust and appreciation that develops through such experiences. The encouraging results suggest further possibilities for intergenerational art activities should be explored, ones that provide unique and relevant educational opportunities for youth and elders while fostering understanding that benefits individual participants and entire communities

SESSION 476

Age-dependent effects of mitochondrial factors on nuclear apoptosis

T G.Mozzhukhina, A.I.Bazhinova, À.Ya. Litoshenko (Institute of Gerontology, AMS of Ukraine, Kyiv, Ukraine)

Apoptosis is important for normal development and tissue homeostasis. But the role of apoptosis in aging still completely understood. The experimental data show that (1) mitochondria exert a decisive role in apoptosis control; (2) mitochondrial damage and proportion of effete mitochondria in cells increase with age; (3) the accumulation of injured nuclei and disturbed chromatin, and nuclear DNA is function of age. These three notions determined the aim of this investigation: to study age-dependent effects of mitochondrial factors on nuclear apoptosis. The adult (6-8 mo) and old (26-28 mo) Wistar rats were used. Subcellular fractions were isolated from liver homogenate by differential centrifugation. Cell-free systems contained nuclei, and intact mitochondria or extracts of intermembrane proteins from mitochondria subjected to hypotonic shock. Apoptosis was estimated by ethidium bromide agarose gel electrophoresis followed by densitometry. It was found that the intact mitochondria as well as extracted mitochondrial proteins added in vitro to purified nuclei induced DNA degradation by apoptotic mechanism (nucleosomal-size ladder). The mitochondrial proteins denaturated by heating also caused DNA degradation, but to a lesser degree. It may be signify that mitochondria contain certain nonprotein components which can serve as apoptosis inductors. It was shown that mitochondria and their components isolated from liver cells of old animals had more expressed effects as compared with ones from adult rats. Interestingly, DNA in the old animal nuclei was more susceptible to mitochondrial apoptotic stimuli as compared with DNA in the adult nuclei. Thus, the probability of apoptotic cell death rises with aging as result from age-associated increase in apoptosis stimulating activity of mitochondria and vulnerability of chromatin.

Aging and Working Capacity: Methodology of Biological Age and Age Changes Tendencies

L.M.Belozerova. Ontogenesis laboratory. Perm State Medical Academy

The aim of the research is the methodological treatment of biological age methods creation according to working capacity and estimation of different factors influence on aging tempi. Mental working capacity on the basis of short-time memory, psychic productivity, thinking and attention registration has been studied in 442 persons; bioelectric activity of the brain has been estimated in 138 examinees, physical working capacity has been measured in 732 people of child's, young, maturity, elderly and old age by means of stepergometry. On the data bases we have elaborated four methods of biological age determination: 1) according to mental working capacity; 2) according to physical working capacity; 3) according to mental and physical working capacity; 4) according to the brain biolectric activity. The creation of biological age determination method includes the following stages: 1) the task determination; 2) the treatment of indices complexes (markers) 3) different age groups examination; 4) computer data treatment (correlation and multiple regression); 5) preliminary decision adoption); 6) determination of biological age and proper biological age of the group and individual; 7) control of method objectivity. We have found the following age changes: 1) mental and physical working capacity decrease begins in the maturity period and goes on in the old; 2) the decrease of lability, receptive ability, ability to take and transform information (data on reduction of the brain biolectric activity of the main rhythms); 3) the aging tempo according to mental working capacity is higher in the women but in the men - according to the both kinds of working capacity; 4) the tempo of aging in people of physical labour in all models is higher than in ones of mental labour; 5) sportsmen-veterans who continue to go in for sports grow old slower than people with routine motion regimen.

Circadian Rhythm of Body Temperature Induced by Age and Gerovital H3 Treatment in Rats.

Ileana Turcu ("Ana Aslan" National Institute of Gerontology and Geriatrics, Bucharest, Romania), Amalia Gabriela Diaconeasa ("Ana Aslan" National Institute of Gerontology and Geriatrics, Bucharest, Romania), Lucia Dutu ("Ana Aslan" National Institute of Gerontology and Geriatrics, Bucharest, Romania)

Purpose: the aim of our present study was to assess the changes induced by aging, the chronic treatment with Gerovital H3 or both, on the fundamental periodicity of animal body, in order to figurate these changes as markers of aging and chronopharmacology. Method: the circadian rhythm of body (rectal) temperature was investigated in Wistar rats of both sexes, 4 as well as 27 months of age, in chronically, 20 mg/kg b.w. i.p. administered Gerovital H3, by comparison with controls (saline). Inner (rectal) temperature was automatically recorded using an "Ellab" thermometer with thermistors. Cosinor analysis was applied. Results: the age as well as Gerovital treatment proved able to induce detectable and reproducible changes of the pattern of body temperature circadian bioperiodicity parameters (amplitude, phase, mesor, period). Conclusions: the detected changes proved able to be taken into account as possible markers for biological age and treatment efficiency. They also support the quality of circadian rhythm as methodological instrument useful in gerontological research.

Correlative links between the rate of gaseous exchange and antioxidant enzymes in the heart of young and old mice

N. Utko, Kh. Muradian (Institute of Gerontology AMS Ukraine, Kiev, Ukraine)

Purpose: There is a strong rationale in clarifying the interrelationship between subsystems from both "sides" of the oxidative stress in the aging heart by focusing on coordinated alterations within the subsystems rather than on comparison of parameters mean values. Materials and methods: The rates of oxygen consumption and carbon dioxide exhalation, as well as the heart superoxidedismutase (SOD), catalase (CAT), and glutathione-peroxidase (GP) activities were determined in young (3-5 mo.) and old (22-26 mo.) intact and moderately stressed (by bringing from the vivarium and handling) female CBA mice. The number of mice was increased up to 15 animals in each group, to enable the analyses by routine and multivariable regression, correlation, three-dimensional plotting, etc. Results: Positive pair, partial, and multiple correlations were found between the gaseous exchange and SOD activity in the heart of intact or stressed mice of the both age-groups. These functionally logical positive correlations, nevertheless, were not supported by the expected positive correlations with CAT and GP. Moreover, CAT and GP tended to be negatively correlating with SOD, probably promoting accumulation of H_2O_2 and related free-radical products. Three-dimensional plotting and multivariable analyses revealed several interesting relationships. For instance, "cup"-like response surfaces were found for both young and old heart SOD, CAT and GP, showing that SOD activity was minimal with CAT and GP close to the mean values. At the CAT or GP activities lower or higher these obviously optimal (tracing?) levels, SOD activity was increased. Conclusions: The results highlight possible disharmony in antioxidant defense, obviously contributing to failures of the aging heart. The seemingly bizarre interrelationships between the regulatory and executive subsystems of free-radical generation and scavenging are too multivariable for their analysis by one- or two-dimensional descriptive or statistical methods, rather favoring three- and higher-dimensional analytical methods.

IGF-I mediated activation of MAP and PI 3-kinase pathways in young and old mouse skeletal muscle following exercise

M. Li, C. Li , W. S. Parkhouse (School of Kinesiology, Simon Fraser University, Vancouver, Canada)

The purpose of this study was to examine the effect of aging on the ability of IGF-I to activate MAP and PI 3-kinase pathways following an acute exercise bout. Mice were sacrificed 12 hours after a low intensity treadmill run following an IP injection of des-IGF-I. Control mice were similarly treated. Mice were sacrificed and blood and skeletal muscle were collected. MAP kinase and PI 3-kinase proteins and their phosphorylation state were determined by immunoblotting. Injection of des IGF-I decreased blood glucose concentration in both young ($p<0.01$) and old animals ($p<0.01$). Basal phosphorylation of protein kinase B (PKB) in skeletal muscle decreased with aging ($p<0.01$) while basal phosphorylation of transcription factor FKHR increased with aging ($P<0.01$). In both young ($p<0.01$) and old ($p<0.01$) animals, IGF-I significantly increased the phosphorylation of PKB. In young mice following exercise, p70 S6K phosphorylation was increased ($p<0.01$) by des IGF-I administration while this was not seen in old mice. IGF-I and exercise together significantly increased phospho-ERK2 per ERK2 ($p<0.05$) in young but not old mice. It is concluded that aging dampens some of the responses of PI 3-kinase and MAP kinase signalling pathways to IGF-I following exercise in mice skeletal muscle.

Lipoprotein Metabolism in Japanese Centenarians

Y. Arai, N. Hirose, S. Nakazawa, K. Yamamura, K. Shimizu, M. Takayama, Y. Ebihara, Y. Osono (Deptartment of Geriatric Medicine, Keio University School of Medicine)

PURPOSE: To assess the complex interaction of apolipoprotein E (apo E) polymorphism and nutritional status, inflammatory parameters, physical and cognitive function in explaining lipid profiles in centenarians. METHOD: Seventy-five centenarians (54 female and 21 male, mean age 100.7±1.2 years, range 100-105 years) and 73 healthy elderly volunteers (37 female and 36 male, mean age 63.1±10.0 years, range 50-79 years) were studied. Plasma lipids and lipoproteins, apo E phenotype, nutritional indices, inflammation markers (C-reactive protein (CRP), Interleukin-6 (IL-6)) were determined by a standard procedure. Cognitive function of centenarians was assessed according to the clinical dementia rating (CDR). RESULTS: In comparison with the elderly, the centenarians had low concentrations of total and low-density lipoprotein (LDL-C) cholesterol and a relative predominance of high-density lipoprotein 2-cholesterol (HDL2-C). The number of apo ƒÃ2 allele was the only significant determinant of LDL-C and apolipoprotein B (apo B), suggesting that the low apoB-containing lipoprotein in centenarians may be attributable to a genetic nature. Centenarians had elevated level of Lp(a) and decreased HDL-C which seem to be unfavorable lipoprotein profiles. Lower levels of HDL-C in the centenarians were associated decreased serum albumin, elevated CRP and IL-6 levels, cognitive impairment, suggesting that HDL-C could be a sensitive marker for frailty in the oldest old. CONCLUSIONS: Apo E polymorphism, nutritional status and inflammation process were principal for regulating lipoprotein metabolism in centenarians. To measure these factors is of great use for evaluating dyslipidemia in the oldest old.

Mitochondria and Peroxisomes Alterations in Rat Liver of Different Ages Chronic Intoxicated with Potassium Cyanide

E.Lupeanu ("Ana Aslan" National Institute of Gerontology and Geriatrics, Bucharest, Romania)

The aim of this study is to demonstrate that the mitochondrial dysfunction and the limitation of oxygen supply at cells could lead to the age-related progressive decline of energy metabolism and purine catabolism rise. Experiments were carried out on 48 females Wistar rats, aged 8 and 24 months, grouped in four different lots according to age and treatment procedure. Potassium cyanide was administrated by i.m. injections, a sublethal dose of 4mg/kg b.w, once at 48 hours for 4 months. Mitochondrial NADH oxidation was reduced ($p<0,01$) in adult and old cyanide intoxicated rats. NADH cytochrome c reductase, succinate dehydrogenase and succinate cytochrome c reductase activities decreased ($p<0,05$), but NADH dehydrogenase and NADH-NBT reductase activities significantly increased ($p<0,01$) in adult intoxicated rats. Cytochrome c capacity to stimulate mitochondrial NADH oxidation declined in adult and in old rats treated with KCN. On the contrary, Fe(III)-EDTA complex capacity to stimulate mitochondrial NADH oxidation was greater in adult and old rats intoxicated with KCN than in untreated rats of similar ages. Xanthine oxidase activity significantly rose (0,01) only in adult rats intoxicated with KCN, not in old ones. Urate oxidase activity increased (p0,01), while catalase capacity to protect cells against H_2O_2 toxicity declined ($p<0,01$) in adult and old cyanide treated rats. Results sustain our supposition relared to purine catabolism stimulation by functional alteration of mitochondria and limitation of oxygen supply at cells, characteristic feature of aging.

Positive Correlation betwenn Leptin and Fat Mass in Hospitalized Elderly

O.BOUILLANNE (CH Emile Roux, Assistance Publique-Hôpitaux de Paris, Limeil Brévannes, France), V.NIVET-ANTOINE (CH Charles-Foix, Assistance Publique-Hôpitaux de Paris, Ivry/Seine, France), C.COUSIEU (CH Hôtel-Dieu, Assistance Publique-Hôpitaux de Paris, Paris, France), J.PELLERIN, A.LAHLOU, D.DURAND, F.PIETTE (CH Charles-Foix, Assistance Publique-Hôpitaux de Paris, Ivry/Seine, France)

Purpose : Leptin released from adipocytes is thought to play a key role in the regulation of energy intake and body weight. Studies in middle-aged groups have found a strong positive correlation between leptin concentrations and fat mass. The ageing process is associated with a progressive gain of fat mass and loss of muscle mass. However it has been found that elderly people have lower leptin concentrations than the young and that the relationship between circulating leptin and total body fat mass was disrupted. Other studies have showed that subcutaneous fat tissue has a higher secretion rate of leptin than visceral fat tissue. Then we study the relationships between leptin and subcutaneous fat mass measured by the skinfold thickness. Method : Leptin, insulin-like growth factor (IGF-1) ; IGF-binding proteins 1 and 3 (IGFBP-1 and IGFBP-3) cortisol, testosterone, estradiol, albumin, glycemia, transthyretin, C-reactive protein, creatinine, body mass index, triceps, biceps, subscapular, supraliac skinfold thickness, midarm circumference and calf circumference were assessed on the day 0 and on day 45 in hospitalized elderly. We studied 117 patients (92 women and 25 men). Mean age was 86 years. Results : leptin levels (10.2±11.3µg/L in women and 4.8 ± 6.6µg/L in men) and skinfold thickness were higher for women than for men ($p < 0.05$). The first explanatory variables for leptin levels in both sex was the skinfold thickness (model R◊ = 0.8 for men and model R◊ = 0.4 for women). Leptin levels and skinfold thickness were not different between Day 0 and Day 45. Conclusion : In elderly subcutaneous fat mass is a significant derterminant of leptin levels.

Protective effect of L-carnitine against DNA damage caused by aging

P.Juliet Arockia Rani, C.Panneerselvam(AL Mudaliar Post Graduate Institute of Basic Medical Sciences, University of Madras, India)

Oxidative damage to DNA is shown to be extensive and could be a major cause of physiological changes associated with normal aging. Previous studies in our laboratory have shown that L-carnitine promotes antioxidant status in aged rats. The present study was aimed to find out the neuroprotective role of L-carnitine during. Male albino rats of Wistar strain were administered L-carnitine for 7,14 and 21 days. Comet assay was used to measure DNA damage in cortex, straitum, cerebellum, hippocampus, and hypothalamus of young and aged rats. Results show that there is a considerable DNA damage caused in aged rat brain regions we have examined. L-carnitine is capable of reducing DNA damage in a duration dependent manner. The alkaline comet assay proves to be a sensitive and simple method to detect DNA damage and estimate the neuroprotective effect on antioxidant like L-carnitine.

SESSION 477

Learning About Aging from the study of Rare Diseases: The Molecular Biology of Werner Syndrome.

George M. Martin [Univ. Washington, Seattle, USA] Yasuhiro Furuichi[AGENE, Kamakura Kanagawa, Japan] Lawrence A. Loeb [Univ. Washington, Seattle, USA] Junko Oshima [Univ. Washington, Seattle, USA]

We shall address the issue of how research on rare diseases can provide information on the mechanisms of aging and the genesis of major geriatric disorders in human subjects. The focus will be upon the prototypic human segmental progeroid syndrome, the Werner syndrome. We shall begin with an overview of the nature of gene action in the modulation of aging and geriatric disorders by George M. Martin, followed by a systematic review of the discovery of the family of helicase enzymes of which Werner syndrome is a member, by Yasuhiro Furuichi. Lawrence A. Loeb will focus upon biochemical aspects of the Werner helicase itself, with special emphasis upon the nature of the rather special exonuclease domain of that protein. Finally, Junko Oshima will present an interesting theory of the mechanism whereby severe deficiencies of the Werner helicase can result in the abnormalities seen in that disorder. We can conclude, from the several presentations, that genes that control the integrity of our genome are likely to be of great importance in protecting us from major geriatric disorders, but that not all of our geriatric diseases are mainly the result of genomic instability. A major challenge for the future is to discover if more subtle variations in the expressions of genes such as the Werner helicase can make a difference in patterns of aging and the timing of the unfolding of major geriatric disorders in human subjects.

Biochemistry of the Werner Helicase

Michael Fry [Technion - Institute of Technology, Haifa, Israel], Ashwini Kamath-Loeb, James Shen, Ann Blank and Lawrence A. Loeb [University of WAshington,Seattle, WA USA]

The Werner syndrome gene encodes a protein (WRN) of 1432 amino acids that belongs to the RecQ family of DNA helicases. WRN is unique among known RecQ helicases in that it is also a 3'->5' exonuclease. WRN helicase unwinds a variety of DNAs containing alternative structure, including tetraplex structures, three-way junctions and Holliday junctions, and other structures that mimic replication forks. The 3'->5' exonuclease activity of WRN is stimulated by neighboring alternative structures, including extrahelical loops, that may be present at the replication fork. WRN exonuclease also preferentially excises mismatched nucleotides from the 3'-terminus of DNA, suggesting a role in proofreading of replication errors; however, WRN differs from known proofreading exonucleases in that it does not cleave single-stranded DNA. Alternative secondary structures in DNA have been shown to impede progression of DNA synthesis by DNA polymerases. Unwinding of these structures by WRN helicase, and excision by the exonuclease of 3'-terminal nucleotides downstream of alternate secondary structure, suggest that WRN may function in rescuing replication at forks stalled or collapsed by unusual secondary structures. Such secondary structures may accumulate during cellular aging, either as a result of DNA damage, or processes involved in repairing damaged DNA, or processes that occur during DNA replication.

Functional Assays for Werner Helicase Mutations

Junko Oshima (Department of Pathology, University of Washington, Seattle, WA, USA)

WRN gene encodes a nuclear protein which has both exonuclease and helicase functions. Homozygous null mutations of the WRN locus causes Werner syndrome (WS), a disorder similar to accelerated aging. It is not clear whether the loss of either exonuclease or helicase activity alone would cause this conditions. Biochemical and cell biological line of evidence suggest that WRN may be involved in multiple DNA metabolisms, including replication, repair, recombination and transcription. In human cells, absence of WRN protein facilitates extensive deletion of endogenous and exogenous DNA. It is conceivable that, in normal cells, WRN protein and other exonucleases and/or helicases are working in concert during the process of DNA repair or recombination. In WS cells, overcompensation by more efficient enzymes may be responsible for the extensive deletions or hyperrecombination.

Lessons from Human Progeroid Syndromes

George M. Martin [University of Washington, Seattle, USA]

The goal of this introduction will be to put the study of the molecular biology of the Werner syndrome (WS) into the broader context of our current understanding of molecular processes of aging. This will be done by interpretations of a broader array of the world literature. Like all phenotypes, senescence is a result of interactions between genes and interactions between genes and environment. The genetic part of the equation accounts for about one third of the variance of life span in humans, but there are potentially thousands of genes, mutation or polymorphism at which can modulate rates of development of geriatric disorders; severe deficiency of the Werner helicase impacts upon a large number (cataracts, arteriosclerosis, cancer, diabetes, osteoporosis, hypogonadism). There are three major types of gene action that modulate aging: good alleles with bad effects late in the life span; good alleles that may be down-regulated for good reasons; bad alleles or slightly bad alleles that do not show their true colors until late in life. WS perhaps fit best with the third of these, although given the fact that there is pathology before maturation is complete, WS does not fit a evolutionary biological definition of aging, which invokes gene action that escapes the force of natural selection. It is thus important to determine if more subtle variations in gene action at that locus (WS heterozygotes and polymorphisms) can modulate geriatric disorders. There is some evidence in favor of that postulate, but the results are still inconclusive.

The biochemistry of WRN helicase

Yasuhiro Furuichi (AGENE Research Institute Kamakura, Japan)

To date, five DNA helicases that belong to the RecQ family exist in humans. The list of human RecQ helicase comprises RecQ1, BLM (Bloom syndrome), WRN (Werner syndrome), RTS (Rothmund-Thomson syndrome) and RecQ5b1-2. Of these, the defective BLM, WRN and RTS helicases are responsible for distinct but overlapping clinical features suggesting premature aging and an enhanced risk of cancer, which apparently stems from chromosomal instability in the cells of tissues and organs where expressions of these helicase genes are specified. Our biochemical studies on WRN helicase showed that (1) it unwinds not only

DNA, but also DNA-RNA heteroduplexses, and contains an exonuclease activity, (2) it exists mainly in the nucleoplasm, but can exist also in the nucleolus of growing cells but disappear from the condensed chromatin at the M-phase, (3) it forms nuclear foci when cells are treated with genotoxic agents that result in double-strand breaks, suggesting the involvement in DNA repair and transcription, (4) the protein level of WRN helicase is upregulated in growing cells or tumor cells, while it is down-regulated by p53 tumor suppressor protein. We conclude that WRN helicase controls the genomic stability tissue specifically, and that the diverged clinical symptoms of Werner syndrome stem from the defective gene expression in relevant tissues. The biological significance of WRN helicase as a guardian angel of genomes, will be discussed in relation to the natural aging and the diseases associated with human aging.

SESSION 478

Intergenerational Bonds and the Life Course

G.O. Hagestad (Agder University College, Kristiansand, Norway & Northwestern University, Evanston, IL, USA) Interdependent Lives across Generations: Bridging Micro- and Macro-perspectives; L.M. Burton (Center for Human Development and Family Research in Diverse Contexts, The Pennsylvania State University, PA, USA) Intergenerational Family Support in the Context of Welfare Reform: Ethnographic Insights from the Three-City Study; A. Biddlecom (Survey Research Center, University of Michigan, Ann Arbor, USA) Patterns of Informal Support among Older Asians: A Comparative Analysis; C. Holland (Open University, Milton Keynes, UK) Older People Living with Family Change; P.A. Dykstra (Netherlands Interdisciplinary Demographic Institute, Den Haag, The Netherlands) Late Life Family Constellations: A Cohort Analysis.

The contributors to this symposium focus on the links between older adults' lives and those of their family members, within the context of social change. The aim is to gain insight into the implications of demographic changes (such as increasing longevity, the declining birthrate, and the rise in divorce), cultural changes (such as increased individualism), and economic changes (such as increasing income differentials) for exchanges within families. Both 'upward' (i.e. support provided to the older generation) and 'downward' transfers (i.e. support provided to the younger generation) will be considered. Findings from both developed and developing countries will be presented. The papers in the symposium represent a mix of large-scale quantitative and in-depth qualitative research. The prevailing view, particularly in policy circles and in the media, is that the recent demographic, cultural and economic developments serve to put older adults at risk of being without the family supports they require. How correct is this view? Through an analysis of the assumptions underlying this view and by presenting empirical findings on the lives of older and younger family members, this symposium will help providing a basis for separating myth from reality.

Interdependent lives across generations: Bridging micro- and macro-perspectives

Gunhild O. Hagestad (Agder University College, Kristiansand, NORWAY; and Northwestern University, Evanston, IL, USA)

Interdependent lives across generations: Bridging micro-and macro-perspectives. The life course perspective has emphasized the importance of studying interdependencies among lives in the family. In this presentation, I use a variety of data sources to illustrate the importance of considering such interconnections on different levels of social reality. First, I examine patterns of interdependence on the micro-level of family groups and provide research illustrations of shared constraints, support and resources, interlocked transitions, constellations of developmental tasks, reciprocal socialization and what I have called indirect relationships. Secondly, I explore chains of interdependence created by the wider societal context through the family as a social institution. Using examples from the United States and countries in Western Europe, I discuss how social policy structures intergenerational interdependence. Thirdly, I ask how structural conditions on a macro-level may bolster or weaken micro-level interdependencies. In addition to discussing relevant laws and policies, I explore possible consequences of age- segregated institutions for patterns of family transfers, socialization and support. Finally, I raise some unanswered questions about how demographical, social and cultural change may forge new forms of interdependencies.

Intergenerational Family Support in the Context of Welfare Reform: Ethnographic Insights from the Three-City Study

L.M. Burton, T.R. Hurt (Center for Human Development and Family Research in Diverse Contexts, The Pennsylvania State University, PA, USA), D. Skinner (Frank Porter Graham Child Development Center, University of North Carolina, Chapel Hill, NC, USA)

The 1996 United States federal welfare reform law, known as the Personal Responsibility and Work Opportunity Reconciliation Act [PRWORA] constitutes the most significant change in public policy for low-income families since passage of the Social Security Act of 1935. Using longitudinal, ethnographic data on 215 African-American, Latino, and Non-Hispanic White families who participated in the federally-funded research project, Welfare Reform, Children, and Families: A Three-City Study, this presentation will describe the structural and exchange features of the intergenerational support networks families experience as they make welfare reform-related life course transitions (e.g. parent moving from welfare to work). Findings suggest that families construct a range of intergenerational support networks that vary notably in composition and patterns of resource exchange over relatively short periods of time. This variability appears to be a function of families= consistent attempts to simultaneously meet the needs of elderly and child family members in the context of tenuous resources related to long-standing personal circumstances (e.g, health problems) and family and household economic transitions related to welfare reform

Late Life Family Constellations: A Cohort Analysis

P.A. Dykstra and A.C. Liefbroer (Netherlands Interdisciplinary Demographic Institute, Den Haag, The Netherlands)

Patterns of changes in life expectancy, childbearing, home-leaving, marriage, divorce and remarriage tend to be analyzed at the macro level. Little is known about how these patterns come together at the level of individuals. This paper traces changes in the life courses of successive birth cohorts as they shape conditions for the exchanges of support in late life families. Piecing together data from eight Dutch surveys with retrospective life history information on the 1900-1970 birth cohorts, findings are presented on developments in (a) the likelihood of living with a partner in old age, (b) having children in the household in old age, (c) having siblings in middle age with whom to share parent-caring tasks, and (d) being sandwiched in middle age between caring for elderly parents and having dependent children. Compared to the cohorts that preceded them and those that will follow, current cohorts of Dutch older adults are well embedded in extensive and intact family networks.

Older People Living with Family Change

J. Bornat, B. Dimmock, S. Peace, C.A. Holland (Open University, Milton Keynes, UK)

Increasing rates of divorce and separation are sources of change and reconstitution within families. How do these factors affect the lives and family relationships of the oldest generation and how in turn do older people respond to such changes? What implications do these changes and responses to them have for the ways in which older people are supported within families and the wider community? Evidence from 60 in-depth interviews, some of which are forming part of a longitudinal study, in the town of Luton, England, will be used to explore implications for social policy of shifting meanings for care, independence, interdependence and intergenerational exchanges in step-families. The data, drawn from genograms and from interviews, with older people or their family members, suggests a need to pay attention to the plurality of family forms, the possible exclusion of older men and the importance of parenting roles in later life. All imply a life course and lifelong family policy perspective which tends to be absent from social policy debates.

Patterns of Informal Support among Older Asians: A Comparative Analysis

A. Biddlecom (Survey Research Center, University of Michigan, Ann Arbor, USA)

Throughout Asia the family has had a long-standing role as the primary provider of support for elderly persons. In recent decades, however, rapid population aging and dramatic social and economic changes have led to growing concern that the traditional system of familial support for the elderly will erode and, thereby, engender greater difficulty or uncertainty for the elderly in securing physical and material support in old age. Despite strong economic gains, many countries are not yet at a stage to develop broad social security and health care programs, and there is often a strong desire on the part of government planners and individuals to preserve the long-standing cultural and family arrangements. This paper presents recent empirical evidence of informal support in four Asian countries to evaluate whether there is indeed cause for concern. Analyses are based on representative samples of persons age 60 years and over from a recent round of national surveys in the Philippines, Singapore, Taiwan and Thailand. The types of support examined include social support in the form of visits, and monetary and material transfers. Results confirm the continued centrality of the family as a support provider in all countries under study, yet reveal key differences in the levels and providers of support across the countries

SESSION 479

Analysis of the factors affecting out-of-pocket health expenditures among Korean elderly with chronic illness

Mee-Hye Kim and So Hee Kim (Department of Social Welfare, Ewha Womans University, Seoul, Korea)

The major purposes of this study are 1) to estimate the ratio of out-of-pocket health care expenditures of Korean elderly with chronic illness to their total household income; 2) to analyze the factors affecting health care expenditures; 3) to identify the characteristics of Korean elderly suffering from the overburden of health care expenditures; 4) to suggest social policy buffering against overburden of health care expenditures among Korean elderly. This study employs the secondary analysis of data from the 1998 National Survey of Health and Nutrition collected by the Korean Institute for Health and Social Affairs. The variables used for this study are out-of-pocket health care expenditures, demographic characteristics (gender, age, education, living arrangement), health status (ADL, IADL, subjective health), economic status (family income, subjective economic status). Statistical methods employed are correlation, multiple regression, frequency and percentage. This study shows that Korean elderly with chronic illness paid 25.0% of total income as health care expenditures on the average. The more aged, unhealthy, and poor they are, the more they pay on health care. In the case of Medicaid beneficiaries, households composed of elder persons pay more on health care. The variables of sex and education do not affect health care expenditures. Korean elderly are overburdened by health care expenditures because of low income, characteristics of developmental stage such as age, number of chronic illnesses, and inappropriate coverage of national health insurance. National health insurance needs to be modified to lessen the burden of out-of-pocket health care expenditure through expanding medical coverage and decreasing personal expense.

Costing and Evaluation of Diabetes Care for Seniors: The Ontario Diabetes Status Index

A. Sclater (Division of Geriatric Medicine, University of Alberta, Edmonton, Canada), J. Canavan (Ministry of Health and Long-Term Care, Toronto, Canada).

The Diabetes Advisory Committee created a costing and evaluation committee to develop a framework for assessing the impact of diabetes on the people of Ontario. Ten indicators were identified and developed to measure the effect of diabetes on health and health care services during the period 1990-2000. The four weighted indicators chosen to monitor service utilisation were (1) separations from acute care hospitals (2) total inpatient days (3) physician office services and (4) admissions to home care. The six weighted indicators selected to monitor complications included (1) photocoagulation procedures, (2) severe visual impairment, (3) vitrectomies on in-patients, (4) dialysis (new cases), (5) kidney transplants, and (6) amputations. Taken together these indicators form the Ontario Diabetes Status Index. Although seniors comprise only 11% of the Ontario population as a whole, they account for 50% of the hospital expenditures with diabetes as the most responsible diagnosis, and 44% of all expenditures paid for physician services related to diabetes care. Representative data indicates certain trends emerging related to both services and complications. From 1989-1990 to 1992-1993, both services and complications increased, with complications rising at a faster rate. Services began to decline in 1993-1994. Concern has been expressed by health care professionals regarding the rising rate of diabetes complications in the context of decreasing services. Further work needs to be done to link the negative impact of decreasing services to identified health outcomes. These data will help in planning and evaluating services and in deciding whether changes in services improve health outcomes.

Efficacy of a psycho-educative group program for informal caregivers of patients with dementia

R. Hébert (Sherbrooke Geriatric University Institute, Sherbrooke, Qc, Canada), L. Lévesque (Montreal Geriatric University Institute, Montreal, Qc, Canada), J.P. Lavoie (Directory of Public Health, Montreal, Qc, Canada), J. Vézina (Laval University, Québec, Qc, Canada), C. Gendron (Douglas Hospital, Montréal, Qc, Canada), F. Ducharme (Montréal Geriatric University Institute, Montréal, Qc, Canada), M. Préville and L. Voyer (Sherbrooke Geriatric University Institute, Sherbrooke, Qc, Canada)

PURPOSE: To test the efficacy of a psycho-educative group program for informal caregivers of patients with dementia. METHOD: The study was a multicenter randomised controlled trial. Eligible subjects (primary caregivers of community-dwelling patients with dementia) were blindly assessed before the randomisation and after 16 weeks, that is at the end of the 15 weekly sessions of the program for the study group. Randomisation were stratified according to sex, center and kinship. Subjects randomised to the control group were referred to the traditional support groups of the local Alzheimer's Society. Outcome measures were: the reaction to behavioural problems (primary), burden, psychological distress, anxiety, perceived social support, and personal efficacy. RESULTS: A total of 158 subjects were randomised to the study (n=79) and control (n=79) groups in 12 successive waves. Preliminary results shows that study subjects present a significant ($p<0.05$) decrease in psychological distress and in their reactions to the behavioural problems of the care-receivers. There was no significant effect on the other outcome variables. CONCLUSIONS: This is one of the first study showing a significant effect of such a support group program for the caregivers of subjects with dementia. Long-term effect (after 6 months) and impact of the program on institutionalisation will have to be demonstrated.

ISO-SMAF Profiles: A Classification System Based on the Functional Autonomy Profile for Continuing Care services in Québec

N. Dubuc R. Hébert, J. Desrosiers, (Faculty of medecine,

University of Sherbrooke, Canada) M. Buteau. (Faculty of Administration, University of Sherbrooke, Canada) L. Trottier (Gerontology and Geriatrics Research Centre, Sherbrooke Geriatric University Institute, Canada).

Purpose : To develop a Resources Utilization Classification System based on the Functional Autonomy Measurement System (SMAF) scale. Method : The ISO-SMAF Profiles were generated by using a systematic process of cluster analysis together with validation procedures. The data came from a provincial study with a multistage probabilistic sampling of 1977 elderly people with disabilities who lived in different living environments (home to institutions). The study included a clinical evaluation and a cost estimation of the required services (health care, lodging, administrative support) and yielded the determination of the number of carehours required and received, and the costs incurred (public, private, and volunteer). Results : The 29 items of the SMAF generated 14 ISO-SMAF Profiles. From the first to the last group, an increasing loss of autonomy from a score of 9.1 to 73.8 (out of 87) can be observed. The first three groups show disabilities mainly on the domestics activities, whereas the group 14 shows an important loss of autonomy on all dimensions of the SMAF. Between these extreme groups, we observe a progression of disabilities on domestics activities and on activities of daily living within two separate patterns of profiles: those with disabilities appearing first in mobility and those with predominant disabilities in mental functioning. Conclusion : This system allows for allocating care and services in an efficient way to the frail elderly and monitoring the services delivered to this population.

Resources and costs associated with disabilities of elderly people at home and in institutions.

R. Hébert, MD MPhil1,2; N. Dubuc, PhD(c)1,2; M. Buteau, DSc1,3; J. Desrosiers, PhD1,2; G. Bravo, PhD1,2; L. Trottier,1; C. St-Hilaire, PhD(c)1; C. Roy, DSc3 (1 Gerontology and Geriatrics Research Centre, Sherbrooke Geriatric University Institute; 2 Faculty of Medicine, University of Sherbrooke; 3 Faculty of Administration, University of Sherbrooke)

PURPOSE: This study was carried out in order to: 1) to determine the level of disabilities and resources involved in the care of elderly people living at home or in institutional settings; 2) to estimate the costs (public, private, voluntary) of these resources; 3) to compare the costs according to the level of disability; and 4) to predict the costs associated with disabilities. METHOD: A representative sample of elderly subjects living at home (n=300), in intermediate facilities (n=271) and nursing homes (n=774) from metropolitan, urban and rural areas in the Province of Quebec (Canada) were assessed. Measurements included a disability scale (SMAF), a cognitive test, a scale to calculate the received and needed nursing care time, and an estimation of the cost. RESULTS: There were significant differences but large overlap in the disability level, cognitive status and nursing care needed and received between subjects from the three settings. The disability score explained 850f the variance in nursing care time and 55% (home), 15% (intermediate facilities) and 68% (nursing homes) of the variance in the cost. Nursing care was responsible for most of the cost in all settings. Regression equations were generated to estimate the cost associated with disability scores at home, in intermediate facilities and in nursing homes. CONCLUSION: These data can help in the planning and management of services for frail elderly people and can be used in cost-benefit analysis to estimate the benefit of an intervention.

Social Security Policies for Ageing With Disabilities and Disabled Aged : Indian Experiences

M N Usha (INSTITUTE for Social and Economic Change NAGARBHAVI BANGALORE 560072. INDIA)

Ageing with disabilities in Indian context is a difficult process.The multiple deprivations faced by disabled aged are more pronounced among illiterates,disadvantaged and women living in rural ,Tribal and hilly areas. The paper highlights the Social Security policies (such as Home for the Aged,Free medical assistance, Pensions, Free Aids and Appliances ,Travel concessions and Sheter workshops and so on) thatare available in India to enable disabled persons lead a smooth and happy life. Community Based Rehabilitation Programmes have been implented in a big way by NGOs. The paper presents a few Case studies that have both success stories as well as episodes that need greater attention by policy makers. However, the adequacy and quality of and delivery of services are partially satisfying those who avail of services offered by state governments and Non government Organizations. The paper is an out come of a study conducted in Karnataka in South India. Some of the recommendations made are : To Carry out need assesments of the disabled aged and identify the priority areas of Action. To expand the facities given to Aged persons , especially Vocational Rehabilitation and Skill development programmes coupled with Continuing education and Life Long Education programmes. To supplement the support systems that are made available to disabled aged with Well being programmes such as health care, income generating activities and enhanced Pension schemes. Finally the paper presents a few action plans for future.

SESSION 480

Feeling of Pride, Occupational History, and Retirement Transition

J. Seitsamo (Finnish Institute of Occupational Health, Helsinki, Finland)

The purpose of this study is to find out, which associations there are between occupational history, retirement transition, and personal feelings of pride, and further, how pride is related to the level of self-reported functional capacity. The study material is based on a follow-up study of Finnish Elderly Workers (n=6257) which started in 1981 and reached it's endpoint in 1997. At the baseline, the subjects were aged 44-58 years, and they were all occupationally active. In 1997, the mean age was 65 years and all the respondents had retired. The measure of pride was based on the question: "Do You have any particular skills, talents, or know-how which you are proud of?" (0=no special, 1=yes). Occupational status had a far-reaching effect on pride even beyond retirement transition. The proportion of those who reported to have some groud for pride in 1997 was 29% if their occupational history consisted of physically demanding work. However, in those whose occupational history was mainly mentally demanding by nature the proportion was 46%, respectively. If a person did have some causes to be proud of, his or her functional abilities were significantly better than in those who didn't have any causes at all. This was true in all occupational groups. The results indicate, that person's feeling of pride may have an important role in contributing person's well-being, and sustaining self-assessed functional capacity as well.

Labour market, employment and unemployment of the elder workers

M.J.Oddone, L.B.Chernobilsky (University of Buenos Aires/ CONICET,Argentina)

Purpose: This project concerns with labour conditions of the elder workers (45 and older), taking into consideration the process related to the worker separation from the labour market, the unemployment and the time of being unemployed, and also the different surviving strategies developed by these unemployed workers. Method: This study is focused on the data provided by the National Survey (May 1998) in the metropolitan area of Buenos Aires. Also focused on is the typology created from the surviving strategies to solve the every day life of this group of unemployed people based on the life cases study methodology. The software SPSS for quantitative data and Atlas/ti for qualitative data were used to analyse secondary data. Results: In the labour market remains 11.05% of retired people distributed equally between men and women. One third of the unemployed are 45 years old and older.

Considering the variable "time of being unemployed", when greater than one year's time, this percentage is increased up to 45.2%. 41% of under-employed and 45.2% of informal workers are 45 years and older. Being self employed is the only activity that allows one to get a minimal income due to the discrimination factors against these elder workers.
Conclusions: The economically working population shows an ageing pattern according to the demographic structure of the country. Once the workers become retired, they do not continue in the labour market. The elder workers are unemployed longer than the younger workers and the only solution is to work in the informal market as self employed.
Considering the labour conversion, the life case study indicated that education should be the result of an integrated planning between supply and demand. Myths and stereotypes based on an organisational ideology about "development of the worker career", increase the social isolation suffered by them in the labour market.

Older farmers and retirement in Australia

Roslyn Foskey (Institute for Rural Futures, University of New England, Armidale, Australia)

In Australia few people remain in the workforce beyond 65 years and there has been a trend towards retirement between the age of 55 and 65 years. In contrast, a high proportion of owner / managers in Australian farming are aged 65 years and over. This project, supported by the Australian Rural Industries Research and Development Corporation explores farmers' expectations about, and experience of, retirement. The research is being undertaken against a background of significant structural change in Australian farming.
Four areas of northern New South Wales, two coastal and two inland, were selected for the fieldwork that used both focus groups and interviews to explore the issues. The project involved a sample of 58 active, semi-reitred and retired farmers aged 55 years and over, and 11 professional advisers to farmers. Participants in the research were recruited through a combination of media publicity, community and government agencies. The next stage of the project is piloting a retirement education program to meet the specific needs of the farm sector.
The study findings are consistent with a number of factors identified in the International literature as influencing the decision to remain in, move into, or retire from, farming in later life. These include physical capacity and health status, attachment to place and farm succession issues. In addition the study revealed that economic change, market forces, polulation movement, environmental and land use issues all impact on the later life choices of farmers in Australia.

The Age Segregation Hypothesis and the New Retirement in Canada

Lynn McDonald (Faculty of Social Work, University of Toronto, Toronto, Canada) Peter Donahue (Faculty of Social Work, University of Calgary, Calgary, Canada) Joanne Daciuk (Centre for Applied Social Research, University of Toronto, Toronto, Canada) Malcolm Stewart (Toronto, Canada)

PURPOSE: The debate surrounding the shifts in the life course have spilled over into a new debate about the nature of retirement or what some call the new retirement. One of the dimensions of the new retirement is the return to work after retirement, which throws the age-segregation hypothesis of education, work and retirement into question. This paper examines the socioeconomic characteristics of men and women age 45+ who have returned to work after retirement. METHOD: Data from the General Social Survey, (1994) are used to compare men and women who remain retired with those who have returned to work (N=2880). Using logistic regression, three labour force re-entry models are estimated for men and women separately: a general model for re-entry, a model assessing full-time re-entry and a model for part-time re-entry to work. RESULTS: The findings indicate that, for men, reasons proximate to retirement influence the return to full-time work, namely mandatory retirement provisions and forced retirement due to unemployment, while part-time work is a function of previous professional occupation. For women, part-time returnees are those who have wealth, who worked in a skilled or professional occupation and who wanted to stop work full-time, while full-time returnees have a strong work history and little wealth. In brief, full-time re-entry is related to involuntary retirement for men and financial need for women.
CONCLUSION: The policy implications of these findings highlight the serious mismatch between peoples' lives and Canadian pension policy which is based on the age segregation hypothesis and which is insensitive to gender differences.

The Solution to the Costs of Population Aging: "Put the Old Folks Back to Work"?

J. Schulz (Brandeis University, Massachusetts, USA), A. Taqi (International Labour Office, Geneva, Switzerland)

The paper addresses the fear that rising "dependency ratios" threaten to raise public pension costs to unprecedented levels. It focuses on one commonly proposed solution: encouraging or requiring older people to work longer. Case study research was carried out in four industrialized countries looking at the many obstacles that determine whether this solution is viable (discrimination, inadequate training programs, pension disincentives, and possible age differences in productivity, efficiency, health, adaptability, etc.). The study found little evidence that the labor force participation of older workers is likely to rise in various countries. Particular attention was given to the United States, where older worker participation is relatively high and pension costs relatively low (compared to most countries in Europe). Even in this more favorable environment, the study found that significant problems remain and that little progress has been made.

What retirement does to health

Lars Andersson (Stockholm Gerontology Research Center, Box 6401, S-113 82 Stockholm, Sweden)

The deterioration of health with age has several determinants. In addition to aging effects, one important determinant is work life. Data from the Swedish Annual Surveys of Living Conditions ULF conducted by Statistics Sweden, clearly shows a retirement levelling or even a retirement dip (i.e. a long-lasting improvement in health) with regard to several indicators of subjective health. The data set is based on interviews with 40,829 individuals aged 55-84, during the period 1980-1998. Keeping in mind that mortality is higher in the blue-collar group, it is also evident how surviving blue-collar workers health-wise to some extent catch up with white-collar workers after retirement. A challenging question is how the ambitions of the government in many countries to raise the retirement age in order to secure the pensions for future retirees can correspond with the sharp improvement in health in connection with retirement.

WORK AFTER 62?

P. E. Solem (NOVA - Norwegian Social Research, Oslo, Norway) R.J.Mykletun (Norwegian School of Hotel Management, Stavanger, Norway), and A. Mykletun (Institute for Research Methods, Bergen, Norway)

PURPOSE: To identify factors contributing to intention of continuing in paid work after age 62. METHOD: Survey of a representative sample of Norwegian municipality workers (N=903), having an optional pensionable age of 62. Multiple logistic regression analyses. RESULTS: Only 14 % of the sample had decided to continue after 62, while 32% would consider it. The rest was uncertain (30%) or would most probably not (14%) or definitely not (9%) continue. Workers who intended to continue, esteemed the development gained through the work itself as well as the social recognition earned from it. They did not bother too much about wages and working hours, and they did not report exposure to recent organisational relocations. Especially, they reported recent participation in longer training programs, and they were quite optimistic about the future of their own work. They reported a career history of varied work content, and had also better health and working ability. The same main pattern of predictors applied for both the total sample and the subgroup of workers aged 45+. The youngest and the oldest workers most frequently reported the intention to work after 62, while the middle aged most frequently reported the intention to quit. CONCLUSION: Workers intending to continue beyond 62 seem more internally motivated by work itself and less by wages. Possibilities of learning, and receiving support and recognition from the employer, are strong motivating factors. A majority of about 2/3 were indecisive about work after 62, which indicates a potential for effects of interventions.

SESSION 481

Comprehensive Assessment for the diagnosis of the Nutritional State in 60 year-old and over

Y. Aravena (Instituto Nacional de Geriatría. Santiago. Chile) J. Silva (Instituto Nacional de Geriatria. Santiago. Chile) J. Espinola (Instituto Nacional de Geriatria. Santiago. Chile)

OBJECTIVE: To validate anthropometric measurements and biochemical exams applied to people of 60 years-old and over in the diagnosis of the nutritional state. METHOD: The study was carried out as a retrospective traversal cut of the nutritional state of 200 people over 60 year-old functionally healthy of an area of Santiago from Chile. Anthropometric Parameters were measured: weight, height, circumference: brachial, calf, waist, pleats: triceps, bicipital, subscapular, suprailiac; biochemical parameters: albumin, protein and lipid levels. RESULTS: The sample was constituted by 96 women and 104 men, between 60 and 92 years old. The diagnosis of the nutritional state according to Body mass Index (BMI): Nutritional state Men% Women% Undernourished 1.9% versus 1.2%; Normal: 32.7% versus 19.7%; Overweight: 48.1% versus 32.6%; Obese: 26.3% versus 46.5%; Corporal composition: 98.8% of the women and 68.3% of the men have more than 30% of body fat, the muscular mass is diminished 58.1% in the women and 61.5% in the men. Calf circumference: it is diminished in 16.3% of the women and in 18.3% of the men. Biochemical analysis: normal proteinemia levels were found in all people, and only 1.2% of the women had low albuminemia level. Total cholesterol presents high levels in 50% of the women and in 26.9% of the men, the triglycerides values were high in 75% and 79% in men and women respectively. CONCLUSIONS: 1. Both women and men had high levels of triglyceride, but only the women's group present more obesity, higher percentage of body fat, and higher levels of total cholesterol than men. So we think that women have more risk factors of losing their autonomy than men. 2. In the integral diagnosis of the nutritional state of those 60 years and over, it is necessary to use the studied indicators assessment.

Correlates of anthropometric measures in older Quebecers

Bryna Shatenstein, P.Dt. (Centre de recherche, Institut universitaire de gériatrie de Montréal and Département de nutrition, Université de Montréal. Montréal, Canada) Sylvie Nadon, Dt.p, (Centre de recherche, Institut universitaire de gériatrie de Montréal. Montréal, Canada) Guylaine Ferland, (Centre de recherche, Institut universitaire de gériatrie de Montréal and Département de nutrition, Université de Montréal. Montréal, Canada)

PURPOSE: Information is needed on seniors' anthropometric characteristics and their correlates. METHODS: Weight, height, waist and hip circumference, measured by a nurse in clinic, were examined in Quebecers aged 55-74 (weighted n=448) from the 1990 Enquête québécoise sur la santé cardiovasculaire (EQSC) and Enquête québécoise sur la nutrition (EQN) datasets. Body mass index (BMI) and waist-hip ratio were calculated. Diet quality was scored from a 24-hour diet recall. Relationships were examined between anthropometric measurements and sociodemographic and lifestyle characteristics and dietary issues. Significant independent variables and diet quality indices were retained in multiple regression analyses. RESULTS: BMI distributions and proportions at a 'healthy weight' (BMI<27) were similar in men and women (median=26). Relatively more women had an acceptable waist-hip ratio based on Canadian standards (41% vs 24%, p<.001). In men, regular physical activity and weight concerns were correlates of higher weights and BMI. Weight was higher in those who chose foods to avoid weight gain, and in ex-smokers than current or non-smokers. These models explained 16.8% (weight) and 12.9% (BMI) of variance. Among women, negative correlates of weight and BMI included dietary supplement use, a dietary recall having 2 or fewer meals, and the contradictory beliefs that having a nice body requires effort, but overweight is preferred to food intake control. Better diet quality was a correlate of higher weight, and weight concerns were associated with higher weight and BMI. These models explained 24.7% (weight) and 28.5% (BMI) of variance. CONCLUSIONS: Older Quebecers have gender-based lifestyle attributes, dietary beliefs and eating habits which influence anthropometric characteristics. Targeted initiatives should focus on healthy weights in aging people.

Estimating geriatric patient's body weight using the knee height caliper in Hong Kong

Jung, M.Y, Chan, M.S, Chow, S.F, Chan, Y.T, (United Christian Hospital, Dietetic Department, Kwun Tong, Hong Kong SAR, PRC) Lau, T.Y, Leung, M.F, Man, C.W. (United Christian Hospital, Medical & Geriatric Department, Kwun Tong, Hong Kong SAR, PRC)

PURPOSE: The use of the knee height caliper is a convenient way to estimate a patient's body weight since it is lightweight, portable, and only requires one person to use. However, the equation devised to estimate an individual's body weight (using the knee height caliper) was specifically designed for Caucasians and Blacks. Therefore, this study is to assess the suitability of the knee height caliper among Chinese geriatric patients or old aged home residents residing in Hong Kong. METHOD: Over a six month period, all geriatric patients in an acute care hospital and old aged home residents in Kwun Tong area were included into the study. Only patients/residents that were considered unstable with ascites; low blood pressure; on cardiac monitors or had respiratory difficulties were excluded. The four examiners compared techniques with trial measurements of five subjects to minimize inter-rater variability. The actual body weights measured with a bed scale or chair scale (which were calibrated) were compared with the calculated body weights from the knee height caliper measurements. A total of over 200 subjects will be recruited into the study RESULTS: A total of over 200 subjects will be recruited into the study and the result of actual body weight compared against the body weight as estimated by the formula of the knee height caliper CONCLUSION: The present study serves to validate the utility of knee height caliper in the estimation of body weight in Chinese elderly.

Estimation of calorie and protein intake in aged patients: validation of meal-portions method.

G. Berrut, A.M. Favreau, E. Dizo, B. Tharreau, C. Poupin, Ph. Fressinaud, P. Ritz (Centre hospitalier Universitaire, Angers, France)

Purpose : Malnutrition is highly prevalent in hospital, mainly in geriatric wards. Estimates of calorie consumption by patients are not performed routinely owing to technical difficulties. Method: The meal-portion (MP) method has been designed to estimate calorie and protein consumption from the portion of the food items actually eaten by the patient, which is evaluated at the time plates and dishes are cleared away. Results: Comparison of estimates and true values (obtained by weighing) show a mean difference of Δ 2 kcal/ - 0.8 g protein from evaluations of portions (n=50 meals) and Δ 7 kcal/ - 1.0 g from fl portion, only being significant for protein and fl portions (P=0.03). When evaluations are performed by observers of different professional categories (nursing staff, medical doctors, dieteticians) on actual meals consumed by 30 diseased elderly people, no statistical differences are evidenced. This inter-observer agreement remains regardless of the cognitive or physical status of the patient. A third study performed after one year of no retraining showed that the method is robust enough but prone to clerical errors. Conclusion: valid estimates of calorie and protein consumption can be obtained with the MP method, quoting in portions. Quality controls are required both at the food production site (in order to avoid propagation of errors arising from food composition) and in data collection (to eliminate clerical mistakes). These results suggest that the MP method could be a tool for estimating calorie and protein intakes in many clinical situations.

Malnutrition in Geriatric Longstay Units: A Painful Established Fact

L. COCHART , Y. HEMMENDINGER , R. ILTIS, M.C SCHATZ (BISCHWILLER Gerontology Hospital)

A recent study about malnutrition conducted in geriatric long stay units in northern Alsace (East of France) pointed that about 66 % patients were undernourished. The study indicate the problem seems mostly due to exogenous reasons such as dependency on feeding linked to physical and psychological dependency, thymic troubles, neuronal pathologies and dental status. We have to add to these impairments an hyper catabolism generally associated to a deep state of malnutrition . Today it happens the evaluation tools we are using are not sufficient to express a definitive view on this particular problem. Furthermore , there is no consensus about tools and limit values to estimate malnutrition especially in long stay units. We are witnessing in the increase of under nourishment in elderly patients and our inability to give practical as well as theorical answers. We should try to prevent and correct malnutrition throughout a pluridisciplinary approach. Geriatricians an caretakers must be further awared of this problem. We have to improve quality of food in a better environment an quality of the relationship between caretakers an elderly patients. The results of the study will be presented and we could talk about the question of caring and 'miss-caring' in a short discussion.

Mechanisms of Hyperhomocysteinemia in Hospitalized Elderly Patients

N. Salles-Montaudon (Hôpital Xavier Arnozan, Pessac, France), F. Parrot (Hôpital Pellegrin, Bordeaux, France), D. Balas (Laboratoire d'Histologie, Nice, France), E. Bouzigon (Hôpital Pellegrin, Bordeaux, France), M. Rainfray (Hôpital Xavier Arnozan, Pessac, France), J.P. Emeriau (Hôpital Xavier Arnozan, Pessac, France).

Purpose : Total homocysteine level is a sensitive marker of vitamin B12 deficiency especially in the elderly. The aim of the study was to examine the association between hyperhomocysteinemia and chronic atrophic gastritis or poor nutritional status in hospitalized old patients. Methods : During a 12-month period, all the consecutive hospitalized patients who underwent gastric endoscopy were recruited in this observational prospective study. Clinical, histological and biological data concerning nutritional status (using the Mini Nutritional Assessment (MNA), albumin level), histological gastric analysis (Sydney system, Helicobacter pylori), homocysteine, plasma folate and vitamin B12 concentrations were collected for each included patient. Results : 196 patients (132 women, 64 men ; mean age : 85.3 ± 5.7 years) were included. Thirty three percent had plasma vitamin B12 £ 150 pmol/l and 45.4 % had increase homocysteine concentrations (>18 mmol/l). After adjustment for age and sex, the strongest predictors of the total homocysteine level were serum vitamin B12 level [relative risk (RR) 0.997, p = 0.007] ; creatinine clearance [RR 0.94, p = 0.001] ; serum albumin level [RR 0.92, p = 0.04] and MNA score [RR 0.92, p = 0.03]. No correlation was found between homocysteine concentration and chronic atrophic gastritis or Helicobacter pylori infection. Conclusion : Plasma homocysteine concentration is a sensitive marker of cobalamin deficiency in the elderly. Atrophic gastritis seems to be a relatively rare cause of hyperhomocysteinemia, whereas poor nutritional status plays an important role in old hospitalized patients.

Nutritional Assessment adapted to evaluate a geriatric population in sub-acute care

F. Bloch, G. Abitbol, S. Haulon, J.-M. Odinot and N. Charasz (Department of Geriatrics, Hopital Broca, Paris, France.), L. Maudieu (Department of Dietetics, Hopital Broca, Paris, France.)

PURPOSE: Malnutrition is known to be a cause of increased mortality and morbidity in the elderly hospitalized population. Presently there are no generally accepted methods for assessing malnutrition in a geriatric population hospitalized in a sub-acute care unit; the goal of this study was to define a method that could be used for evaluating malnutrition in this group of people. METHOD: One hundred patients hospitalized in a geriatric sub acute care unit of the Broca hospital (Paris-France) were studied between June and November 2000. Each patient was studied at the time of admission and one and two months later. In addition to biological indexes and Body-Mass-Index (B.M.I.) three other parameters were used: Mini-Nutritional-Assessment (M.N.A.), Nutritional-Risk-Index (N.R.I.) and Prognostic Inflammatory and Nutritional Index (P.I.N.I.). RESULTS: N.R.I. was the least expensive, easiest, and fastest to perform. It was directly correlated with M.N.A. (r=0.557; p<0.0005), with B.M.I. (r=0.503; p<0.0005) and serum albumin level (r=0.559; p<0.0005). CONCLUSION: We found that the N.R.I. can be successfully used to evaluate the risk of malnutrition in a hospitalized geriatric population. In addition, it was easier to perform and was less expensive than the other commonly employed methods.

The Mini Nutritional Assessment (MNA) in elderly hospitalised subjects; Comparison between Otago and Belfast.

I.M.Rea, McClean A, McGarry M,(Department of Geriatric Medicine, Queens University, Belfast, UK), Busby L (Otago General Hospital, New Zealand).

PURPOSE: The Mini Nutritional Assessment (MNA) tool was used to compare nutrition between acute and rehabilitation elderly hospitalised patients in Otago, New Zealand and Belfast, Northern Ireland. METHOD: The MNA, previously used as a quick screening tool of nutrition in adults, includes anthropometric, functional, dietary, global and general assessment questions and categorises subjects as well nourished (>24), at risk of malnutrition (17-23.5) and malnourished (<17) out of a total score of 30. MNA assessment was used in 60 subjects in Belfast and 60 subjects in Otago with 30 in acute and rehabilitation categories, with no age or sex difference between countries. RESULTS: MNA score for all subjects was 19.5 with no difference MNA between male (19.7) and female (19.4) patients. Subjects categorised as acute (less than 14 days post admission) had MNA score of 19.1 compared with a value of 20.1 for subjects categorised as rehabilitation (greater than 14 days in hospital) with no significant difference between groups (p=0.5). There was a significant difference in mean MNA scores between the two countries with MNA score of 20.4 in Otago and 18.7 in Belfast (p=0.05) with significant differences for female rehabilitation patients in Otago compared to Beflast (22.3 v 17.3) CONCLUSION: These results suggest that in similarly categorised hospitalised elderly subject groups in Otago and Belfast there were differences in nutrition, as assessed by MNA, between country and between rehabilitation subject groups, which deserve further investigation.

SESSION 482

Family network, well-being and elderly's perception of formal and informal home care

Eric Olsson and Bengt Ingvad (School of Social Work, Lund University, Lund, Sweden)

PURPOSE: In this study we explore how the family with the old person and the public home help services contribute to the care of the frail elderly and how they interact. The study focuses on the significance of extended family network and the elderlys' health and well-being on experiences of the received care. METHOD: Thematic deep interviews with the elderly are used. Forty elderly 80+ with formal home help twice a week or more are interviewed. RESULTS: The formal care was in all cases more extensive than the informal care. The majority of the elderly had limited contact and care from their families and 25 percent had no contact at all. In cases with contact they were often disappointed with the intensity and the frequency of contact and help. Only a few of them had everyday care from a relative. For a majority the formal care was very important both practically and emotionally. Those who had no contact with relatives had developed strong emotional bonds to the home helper. The well-being and the subjective health were not clearly related to the experience of informal and formal care. CONCLUSION: The elderly in this study mainly depends on formal home help services for their daily living. It fulfils needs of social contact for a majority. The results imply the significance of a public welfare system for securing the practical and social needs for frail elderly.

Managing Exclusion and Resisting Diminished Identities: Home Care Users 'Living On The Edge.'

Jane Aronson (School of Social Work, McMaster University, Hamilton, Canada)

Home-based care is, typically, provided for frail elderly people with the intention of enabling them to live independently in their own homes. However, in a political and discursive context that prizes active or 'successful' aging and material self-sufficiency, the very fact of needing help to manage at home represents a threat to care recipients' identities and reputations. This paper explores how elderly home care users strive to maintain and construct viable identities for themselves in these contradictory conditions. A longitudinal, qualitative study of women receiving tightly-rationed, long-term home care in Ontario illuminates service users' isolation and exclusion. In successive interviews, study participants speak of both taking on and resisting the constraints on identity that this social exclusion generates. They describe efforts to conform to dominant depictions of successful aging by being uncomplaining and undemanding, as well as strategies to expand their possibilities, maintain lifelong expressions of themselves and engage in valued exchanges with others. Theoretically, the study offers insight into the tensions of managing identity in the face of bodily decline and social marginalization, and into the complexities - especially heightened for women - of home care's intrusion into the self-defining and private arena of the home. Practically, the study suggests some directions for social care policies and practices that seek to foster and buttress the identities and engagements of elderly citizens.

Perceived Needs for Home Help Services Among Frail Israeli Elderly

Esther Iecovich (Department of Social Work, Bengurion University, Beer Sheva, Israel)

This study examines perceived ability to perform IADL tasks and perceived needs for home help services among frail Jewish and Arab elderly people, and investigates the determinants that best predict perceived needs for assistance in IADL. Data are based on a national survey conducted in 1997 by the Central Bureau of Statistics in Israel and included 5055 respondents, aging 60 and over of which 601 (523 Jews and 78 Arabs) were frail and handicapped. Data collection was conducted by face to face interviews. The findings show that the majority of the respondents had difficulties in performing IADL activities, specifically, cleaning, laundry and shopping. More Arabs than Jews reported they did not need help in either of the IADL tasks due to their living arrangements, i.e. many of them lived alone, however, more need for help was reported as compared to their Jewish counterparts. Regression analyses reveal that ethnicity variables are significant predictors of perceived need for help in IADL. Among Jewish elderly measures of perceived health, functional status, and income were strongly correlated with perceived need for help in IADL. For the Arab respondents, perceived ability to perform ADL was significatnly correlated with perceived need for help in IADL. The results imply that when assessing needs for home help services and preparing care plans, not only objective criteria of functional status and living arrangements have to be taken into account but rather ethnic and cultural variables should be considered as well

Personal Care Workers: Perceptions of their Role

Malka Korazim, Tali Goren, JDC-Brookdale Institute of Gerontology and Human Development, Jerusalem, Israel

Personal care services for the elderly are provided in Israel to over 80,000 people under the long-term care insurance law. The service includes 10-15 hours of care per week provided by a worker employed by a public, voluntary or private agency. The estimate is that in Israel there are about 35,000 personal care workers enrolled in the provision of this service. A nationwide study was initiated by the National Insurance Institute in order to provide some basic information on the characteristics of the personal care workers, the nature of their job and their role perception. The study is based on a sample of 400 workers currently providing services under the law. The purpose of this paper is to present some of the major findings related to the unique features of this role. The findings confirm that the job of a personal care worker is a low-status female occupation. However, the findings also indicate that the occupation is gradually undergoing some type of professional upgrading. It was found that about half of the workers had undergone training and that a more skilled type of care is being provided by an increasing percentage of workers. A large percentage of the workers (75%) perceive themselves as a formal, professional service provider and rely less on their relationship with their clients as a basis for role definition. Formal training was found to have an impact on job performance and its perception. These findings raise clear implications for the future development of this occupation.

The Discoursive Formulation of Mental Health Issues in the Context of Home Care

M. Saarenheimo (The School of Public Health, University of Tampere, Finland)

Mental health problems of the elderly have become one of the central concerns of the home care professionals. In the context of everyday care mental health questions are addressed with a diversity of concepts ranging from the discourses of professional psychiatry to the everyday vocabulary of the care professionals and their clients. The choice of a discourse has, in its turn, important consequences for the care practices. This paper deals with the different patterns used in the home care interactions to formulate mental health issues. A qualitative group interview was conducted with 6 groups of home care professionals. Each group was interviewed twice. In addition, 4 home care managers were interviewed individually. The data was analysed using a discoursive and dialogical framework. The purpose of the analysis was to detect regular patterns of formulating mental health problems and interventions in the interview conversations. The recognition of the patterns was based on analysing the different vocabularies and discourses, negotiations of moral codes and expressions of personal attitudes and emotions. The conceptions concerning the mental health of the elderly clients appeared to be constructed in a variety of ways depending on the specific context of care as well as the context of conversation. When describing their clients and reflecting care episodes the home care professionals collectively used explanations, theories and everyday beliefs that offered the most satisfactory explanation for action in a specific situation. Recognition of the professionals' construction of conceptual patterns can be of help when planning new educational and supervisory models for mental health work in home care organizations.

Views of older people on the desirable qualities of home care services

Professor Norma V Raynes (University of Salford, Salford, ENGLAND)

Delivery of client centred home care services requires views of older service users to be accessed. A 10% random sample of all service users aged 60 plus stratified by age was undertaken.(N=300). Focus groups and home interviews were used to access people's views of a quality service and round table meetings with politicians, senior managers and older service users. Older people's views of quality differ from those of providers, there are differences as well as overlap in the views of those over and under 80. They do not differentiate between the what and how of service quality. Detailed planning as well as resources are essential to access views. Older people's views on quality are clear and realistic. Clients can be taught ranking techniques and a number of practical low cost means of putting their ideas into practice to influence quality standards and monitor these have been identified.

Working Toward More Empowering Care: An Exploratory Study of the Experience of In-Home Service Delivery.

Carol McWilliam (University of Western Ontario, London, Canada) Catherine Ward-Griffin (University of Western Ontario, London, Canada)

Abstract: PURPOSE: The purpose of this study was to explore the shared experience of in-home service delivery in a Community Care Access Centre in Ontario. To inform the development of client-driven service delivery, researchers aimed to discover how empowerment (the equitable balancing of knowledge, status, and authority) was enacted in care management relationships. METHODS: Interpretive phenomenology with in-depth interviewing from a purpose- ful sample of 3 clients, 6 informal caregivers, and 9 providers (homemakers, nurses and therapists) was used to elicit an understanding of the processes and content of shared service delivery experience. Applying immersion and crystallization techniques, the researchers conducted individual and team analyses to inductively derive a hermeneutic interpretation of the shared experience. RESULTS: Clients, caregivers and providers experienced varying degrees of empowerment in their shared enactment of in-home care management. Two dimensions illuminated the structure of their experience: empowerment as a process of sharing power in the relationship, and empowerment as an outcome of predominant focus on limitations, or on strengths. The nature of the shared experience of empowerment in in-home care predominantly reflected the traditional expert model of service delivery, with limited awareness of empowerment as an equitable sharing of knowledge, status and authority in the care management relationship. CONCLUSION: Education related to the philosophy and techniques of an empowerment model of service delivery and facilitative changes in the organizational context are required if in-home care is to reflect a more client-driven approach to service delivery.

SESSION 483

National Policies on Aging: Why have them?

David R Phillips and Alfred Chan Cheung-ming (Asia Pacific Institute of Aging Studies, Lingnan University, Hong Kong) (National policies on aging in the Asia-Pacific region: the examples of Hong Kong and Singapore) Anna Howe (Australian Association of Gerontology, Melbourne, Australia) (The National Strategy for an Aging Australia: Old Politics or New Policy?) Mark Rosenberg (Queen s University, Kingston and Canada) (Assessingthe Outcomes of Two Federal Elections: Policy Concerns of Seniors - the Forgotten Issues) Ryoji Kobayashi (Tokyo Metropolitan University, Tokyo, Japan) (Long term care insurance in Japan: the first step in major reforms in national policies for the aged)

The International Year of Older Persons in 1999 was expected to see increased attention to the development of national policies on aging, yet such integrated policies remain the exception rather than the rule. This symposium examines the circumstances giving rise to national policies on aging in some countries and why they have not developed in others. As well as reviewing the conceptualization of aging as a field warranting integration across different policy areas, the goals and content of such national policies, particular attention will be given to the role of older people s representative organizations relative to other participants in the policy development process, and the influence of international agencies. In countries that do not have national policies on aging, the balance between age-based policies vis-à-vis inclusion of older people in generic policies will be canvassed. These issues will be examined in: ·Singapore and Hong Kong, which have high level coordinating bodies charged with developing national policies on aging; ·Australia, where several states have attempted "whole of government" approaches to aging and where a national strategy on aging has been developed; ·A comparison of Canada and the US, focusing on aging policy in recent national elections; and ·Japan, which is seeing significant reforms in major elements of a national policy on aging, but which are not yet integrated.

Assessing the outcomes of federal elections in the US and Canada: Policy concerns of seniors - the forgotten issues

Mark Rosenberg, (Queen s University, Kingston and Canada)

Federal elections were held in November 2000 in both Canada and the United States. As among the most committed voters and recognizing that demographically seniors will be a growing force in both countries over the next thirty years, seniors might have expected their policy concerns to be addressed by the main party leaders during the elections campaigns. Focussing mainly on social security, health care and drug policies, this paper assesses the positions of the major parties in both countries, seeks to explain the differences in policy between the parties and the countries, and suggest the likely directions of Canadian and United States policy in the near future. I will argue that seniors in both countries should be pessimistic that major improvements in social security, health care and drug policies are likely to occur in the near future. Seniors groups tend to over-estimate the extent to which they are a force in shaping policy directions. Although they have major lobbying organizations to try to influence policy (e.g, the Association of American Retired Persons), seniors in these organizations and in general reflect the diversity of political interests which exist in both countries, placing their party loyalties before their loyalties to seniors causes. As a result, no significant policy changes are likely to occur in the United States, while the changes likely to occur particularly in Canada will move policies closer to those which exist in the United States in the coming years.

Long term care insurance in Japan: the first step in major reforms in national policies for the aged

Ryoji Kobayashi, Tokyo Metropolitan University, Tokyo, Japan

Japan is facing the fastest population aging of any country in the world, with heavy demands of support for the elderly. The government has increased expenditures on pension, health care, long-term care and welfare services in the last three decades. However, the growing elderly population and its changing needs have prompted the government to review the whole structure of policies for the aged as well as the financial arrangements. The introduction of long-term care insurance in April 2000 is supposed to be an initial step towards changing the whole structure of policy for the aged. This paper tries to examine some basic principles underlying the present policies for the elderly and the recent development of debates on policy approaches in the future, mainly through major policy documents issued by the central government

National policies on aging in the Asia-Pacific region: the examples of Hong Kong and Singapore

David R Phillips and Alfred Chan Cheung-ming (Asia Pacific Institute of Ageing Studies, Lingnan University, Hong Kong)

This paper reviews the emergence of nascent national policies on aging in two areas of the Asia-Pacific region, Hong Kong and Singapore. Whilst it is important to recognize that both are in many respects special cases in the region, as a Special Administrative Region of China and a city-state respectively, they do illustrate rapid demographic aging with concomitant public policy responses emerging. The two territories have adopted somewhat different approaches. Hong Kong s policy has evolved rather piecemeal over the past 30 years, reflecting the utilitarian, residual nature of social welfare in the colony and SAR. The policy has been somewhat fragmented, based on specific departments, agencies and programs. There have been a number of White Papers on the needs of older persons, with particular focus on social welfare and financial support. Housing has become a more recent focus. Arguably, only since 1997 has a more coherent territory-wide strategy begun to be developed under the auspices of the Elderly Commission and with the aim of promoting "healthy aging". Singapore by contrast has developed programs and policies rather more recently than Hong Kong, mainly over the past decade or so, in the wake of a number of reports and reviews. It has adopted a more top-down approach, based on an Inter-Ministerial Committee s recommendations and the reviews of some specific areas such as health and financial provision. The paper considers whether these attempts in both Hong Kong and Singapore might be considered as the development of national policies on aging. In addition, the cultural context, which heavily emphasis family responsibility for older people, is evident in both societies, as in many other countries of the region. The paper also considers the extent to which such philosophies can assist, or undermine, the development of national policies on aging in the region.

The National Strategy for an Aging Australia: Old Politics or New Policy?

Anna Howe, Australian Association of Gerontology, Melbourne, Australia

The timing of the announcement of the initiative to develop a National Strategy for an Aging in late 1997 and the subsequent course of development raises a number of issues concerning its purpose and likely outcomes. This paper reviews these issues against the background of earlier initiatives at state level aimed at developing integrated policies on aging. The aim of the National Strategy was stated as "to take a longer term, whole of government approach to identifying, and develop proactive policies to meet the challenges and opportunities arising in the course of population aging in Australia". The four key themes of Strategy are (1) healthy aging, (2) independence and self provision, primarily for retirement income, (3) world class care and (4) attitude, lifestyle and community support. Discussion papers on these themes were released through 1999-2000 and the final strategy is expected to be released by mid 2001. This paper examines four aspects of the strategy: (1) the changing political context in which it was initiated, developed and released; (2) the scope of the elements of the Strategy compared to the range of policy instruments available to government; (3) the reception by older persons representative groups, aged care organizations and the community more widely; and (4) the symbolic goals and outcomes of the strategy in terms of changing thinking about aging vis-à-vis attention to differentials in well-being among the present and future older populations.

SESSION 484

Population Ageing and Socioeconomic Development

I. Hermalin and Mary Beth Ofstedal (Population Studies Center, University of Michigan, USA) (How are the Elderly in Asia Faring under Rapid Demographic and Socioeconomic Change.) Kevin Kinsella (International Programs Center, Census Bureau, Washington, D.C, USA) (Recommendations for Research on Population Aging and Development.) Alfred Chan Cheung-ming and David Phillips (Asia Pacific Institute of Ageing Studies, Lingnan University, Hong Kong) (Healthy Ageing: The Best Way to Combat Problems of an Ageing Society.) Alberto Palloni and Martha Pelaez (University of Wisconsin-Madison and Pan American Health Organization) (Population Ageing in Latin America and the Caribbean.)

This Symposium critically assesses the intricate relationship between population ageing and socioeconomic development. As most countries in the world would experience a rapid increase in the number and proportion of older persons in the next two decades, it is useful for us to understand the impact of this critical process on socioeconomic development, especially among the developing countries. In turn, it is also important for us to appreciate the impact of development (or the lack of it) on the well-being of the older persons. The Symposium contains five papers by well-known researchers and policy makers. The first two deal with broader issues that cut across national boundaries. The first paper by Hermalin and Ofstedal will assess the key indicators of well-being among older persons in Asia and their policy implications. Kinsella will present the second paper drawing from the findings of a special panel convened by the National Academy of Sciences. The paper will describe an international research agenda and data gaps as recommended by the panel that would help enhance deeper understanding of the interrelationship between aging and development. The third paper will shift focus to national experiences in dealing with the ageing process. Kawasaki from Japan's Cabinet Office will examine Japan's policy on ageing and its future directions. The fourth and fifth papers deal with the issue of health and well-being of the older persons. Chan and Phillips will examine the Hong Kong experience in the context of a community strategy to promote healthy ageing. Pelaez and Palloni will present the experiences in Latin America and the Caribbean and the determinants of well-being among older persons in that region. We anticipate interesting discussions on both policy and research issues.

Healthy Ageing: The Best Way to Combat Problems of an Ageing Society

Alfred Chan Cheung-ming and David Phillips (Asia Pacific Institute of Ageing Studies, Lingnan University, Hong Kong)

Abstract: Parallel with technological advancements and improvements in most health and social care systems, many people,s lives have been prolonged and even deaths averted from conditions previously deemed incurable. The bad news that counters this is that people may spend their later years in illness and disability — some of which conditions were not recognized until longevity set in, such as Alzheimer,s disease and osteoporosis. The result of this, however, is a rapid increase in the number of the older people who will meet with disabilities and degenerative diseases. The healthcare system is much less capable of preventing or curing such conditions. For a simple answer, additional funding to improve medical interventions including adoption of a dvanced technologies for old age ailments appears to be the solution. Years of experience in North America and other countries whose population have aged earlier than those in Asia have shown that medical interventions for old age illnesses are expensive yet the outcomes are only mediocre. Money spent on advanced care and technologies alone cannot solve the challenges. The present paper, addressing the above challenges that appear to accompany population ageing, proposes that healthy ageing, as a medium long term community strategy, should be adopted in the hope to prolong quality life years and to compress morbidity in later years. The paper focuses on the strategy being evolved in Hong Kong as a particular example of healthy ageing being promulgated as a national theme.

How are the Elderly in Asia Faring under Rapid Demographic and Socioeconomic Change

Albert I. Hermalin and Mary Beth Ofstedal (Population Studies Center, University of Michigan, Ann Arbor, USA)

Abstract: The history of Western industrialized countries and theory on the consequences of rapid socioeconomic change have led to concerns that rapid changes underway in much of Southeast and East Asia will have adverse consequences on the well-being of the elderly on several dimensions, but there has been little systematic assessment of the evidence to-date. This paper reviews data from Asia and particularly from a detailed comparative study of four countries to look at key indicators of well-being, including living arrangements and intergenerational support, work and retirement trends, economic well-being and health status. Findings indicate that while there has been change on several dimensions, there is also considerable persistence of traditional arrangements, and accommodations within families to changing conditions. The program and policy implications of these changes are also discussed.

Population Ageing in Latin America and the Caribbean

Author,s name and in brackets institution, city and country: Alberto Palloni (University of Wisconsin-Madison, USA) and Martha Pelaez (Pan American Health Organization, World Health Organization, Washington, D.C, USA)

This paper evaluates the nature of the aging process in Latin America and the Caribbean through an examination of the demographic profile of the 60+ population, its health and disability status, its composition by social and demographic characteristics, and the prevailing patterns of living arrangements. The data presented is from a multicenter study on the Health and Wellbeing of Older Persons in seven urban centers in Latin America and the Caribbean. In the study we highlight a number of features that will inevitably play a role in the design and implementation of public policies. These include the following: accelerated pace of aging, massive socioeconomic differentials, sharp gender inequalities, unfavorable composition by health and disability status, erosion of traditional family-based support system, and insufficient development of institutional transfers. The prospects that emerge are not optimistic, all the more so because rapid aging will occur within institutional contexts that until recently have been characterized by untamed inflationary pressures, frequent recessionary set backs, high levels of unemployment, increasing absolute poverty, expansion of social and economic inequalities, and continued growth of the informal sector.

Recommendations for Research on Population Aging and Development

Author,s name and in brackets institution, city and country: Kevin Kinsella (International Programs Center, Census Bureau, Washington, D.C, USA)

To provide the scientific basis for policies designed to deal with the opportunities and problems associated with major shifts in population age structures, the U.S. National Academy of Sciences recently convened a panel of U.S. and non-U.S. experts to explore the scientific opportunities for conducting policy-relevant comparative research on aging. The focus was on behavioral, socioeconomic, and health aspects of human population aging. The panel was asked to provide suggestions for an international research agenda and recommendations for the kinds of data needed to carry out that agenda in the context of rapid demographic aging. Through regular meetings and cross-country interaction with colleagues, the panel examined the advantages of multidisciplinary involvement in data development; identified areas in which cross-country analysis is critical; considered the process by which the scientific community could develop and implement a data-driven research agenda; examined the advantages that would ensue from combinations of survey and administrative record data; and considered privacy and confidentiality issues relating to the dissemination and use of basic data. This presentation will highlight the overarching and topic-specific recommendations of this study, including the arguments for comparative cross-national research, harmonization of data, and linkage among data sets. The most important recommendation relates to the necessity of developing multidisciplinary longitudinal data collection instruments that allow researchers and policymakers to understand interactions among various life domains (e.g. health, work, family), and how these interactions change as soc ial policies and conditions change. Particular emphasis will be given to those topics that affect the process of socioeconomic development.

SESSION 485

Aging in Asia: Social and Cultural Perspectives

Hyunsook Yoon (Graduate School of Social Welfare, Hallym University, Kangwondo, Korea) H. Kendig (Faculty of Health Sciences, University of Sydney) and S. Quine (Department of Public Health and Community Medicine, University of Sydney) The Development of Community Care Services in Australia Sung Jae Choi (Department of Social Welfare, Seoul National University, Seoul, Korea) Economic Status, Work, and Retirement of Elderly Koreans. Koichi Hiraoka (Department of Sociology, Ochanomizu University, Tokyo, Japan) Long-Term Care Insurance System in Japan Peng Du (Institute of Population Research, People's University of China, Beijing, China) Economic Status, Work and Retirement in China Shengming Yan (Department of Sociology, Peking University, Peking, China) Living Arrangement and Parent-Child Interactions in Urban China Iris Chi (Department of Social Work and Social Administration, University of Hong Kong, Hong Kong, China) Social Support and Depression among Elderly Chinese People in Hong Kong.

Among the facotrs thought to affect and alter the experience of growing older in Asian countries, culture, politicis, demographics, and social economic change have been acknowledged as highly influential. Existing family structures, as an outgrowth of each of the above are alos importan. The relatvie importance and shifting alighment of these factors emerges from a cross-national comparison of aging in Asia and the goal of this symposium is to explore the permutations as they are found in five selected Asian countries where aging issues have emerged as increasingly important. Shifts in cultural preferences are brought about as the population itself grows older and as productive and economic pursuits come to reflect the global marketplace. Certainly, there are generalizations to be made, yet the experience of diverse Asian countries may suggest alternatives and options for each other while recognizing that universal remedies applicable to all nations do not exist. Gerontologists need an adequate base of concrete knowledge of the particular circumstances and changes affecting the lives of older people and their families in individual Asian countries. Korea, Japan, China, Hong Kong, and Australia each face unique circumstances but at the same time reflect the influence of global economic linkages.

Economic status, work and retirement in China

Peng Du (Institute of Population Research, People's University of China, Beijing, China)

In China, retirement system and social security system mainly exist in urban areas, but the proportion of urban population is only a quarter in the total population. For the majority of the elderly, especially those living in rural areas, children are still the best investment for old-age security. Even in large cities today, many elderly people still believe that the son is their most reliable security for later life. Among all older persons aged 60 and over in China, 57.1% depend dominantly on the financial support from their children and other relatives; in rural areas this proportion is 64.2%. Research findings also reveal that the elderly who are depending mainly on their children's support usually live with their children together. The relative poverty of the older persons affects their economic status. Beyond retirement age, 25.0% of the elderly are still working and regard their income as the main economic resources. These elderly workers are mainly engaged in agricultural industry and other traditional work. In general, female elderly have poorer economic status than their male counterparts, due to the high illiteracy rate and low economic participant rate. Therefore the gender difference exists among the elderly as for the economic status and labor force participation, and a key factor for such a situation in cities is the different retirement age. Although there is some debate focusing on the postponement of retirement, in the background of labour surplus nationwide, it seems impossible to change the existing regulations in the near future.

Economic Status, Work and Retirement of Elderly Koreans

Sung-Jae Choi (Department of Social Welfare, Seoul National University, Seoul, Korea)

The modernization, that has seen rapid acceleration for the past 40 years has changed Korean society from an agricultural one to an industrial one. In the process of rapid modernization current generation of elderly Koreans has sacrificed themselves for their families' immediate daily living and education of their children with little consideration of their old age. A system of mandatory retirement at the age of 55, which has been prevailing in Korean society and is contrary to the unprecedentedly rapid lengthening of life expectancy of Koreans, has kicked out the non-elderly workder from the labour market and made them premature elderly persons without adequate income maintenance programs. This paper will first review the employment status, retirement system and the economic status of elderly Koreans. Then, this will cirtically examine current income maintenance and reemployment policies for the elderly and their problems. In relation to these problems this paper will deal some issues associated with ths income maintenance and reemployment policies: for example, filial responsibility, supports through informal network, level of minimum guarantee by the state, pensionable age, contribution and benefits of pensions, productive welfare, etc, and finally will suggest some policy recommendations for income maintenance and reemployment for the elderly.

Living Arrangement and Parent-Child Interactions in Urban China

Shengming Yan (Department of Sociology, Peking University, Beijing, & Department of Social Work and Social Administration, University of Hong Kong, Hong Kong, People's Republic of China)

With dramatic sociodemographic changes since 1949, what are the patterns of the elders' living arrangement and their interactions with adult children in mainland China, where coresidence with son and daughter-in-law and reciprocity between generations are stressed by the traditional norms, is of particular interests. Using probability survey data in a Chinese city, this paper examines the patterns of living arrangment of older parents, their interactions with adult children, as well as the related factors. Results indicated that coresidence with adult children is still the predominant pattern of the living arrangements. Nevertheless, there is some variability. More than one third of the parents live either alone or only with spouse, and among those who have conresident children in their homes, about 15 percent actually lives with daughters. Age and employment status are the main factors that predict parents' living arrangement. On the other hand, for adult children, gender, age, educational level, and marital status are the major factors that predict coresidence with older parents. With respect to the interactions, the non-coresident children maintain frequent contacts with parents. The majority of them visit their parents at least at weekly level. In addition, about one third of them uses other means, such as writing letter or making call to contact their parents. There are intensive exchange of services and help between parents and children. The patterns of living arrangement are closely associated with children's support for the parents, with coresidence significantly promoting children's financial and emotional support after they got married and their help with household chores. The implications of changing patterns of living arrangement for the parent-child interactions are discussed.

Long-Term Care Insurance System in Japan

Koichi Hiraoka (Department of Sociology, Ochanomizu University, Tokyo, Japan)

The Long-Term Care Insurance Law that created a universal long-term care insurance system came into force in April 2000 in Japan. This paper aims to analyze the significance of the establishment of this system for the development of long-term care services for the elderly in Japan. The first part of this paper focuses on the development of long-term care services since the 1970s and analyzes socio-economic and political factors that led to the introduction of the long-term care insurance system. The second part of this paper describes the institutional design of this program. A comparison is made between the Japanese and the German system of the financing of long-term care, and special attention is drawn to the limited role played by the public assistance program in Japan. The third part of this paper, based on the survey and the care studies of local government that I conducted in 2000-2001, analyzes the changes in the provision and utilization of long-term care services that have been taking place since the beginning of this program.

Social Support and Depression among Elderly Chinese People in Hong Kong

Iris Chi (Department of Social Work and Social Administration, University of Hong Kong, Hong Kong, China)

This study examines the association between social support and depressive symptomatology in a representative community sample of 1106 Chinese people in Hong Kong aged sixty years or older. Significant relationships were found between depression and all dimensions of social support including social network size, network composition, social contact frequency, satisfaction of social support, instrumental/emotional support, and helping others. The authors found that social support from family is important for elderly Chinese people in Hong Kong, and satisfaction with support is a more imprtant predictor of depression levels than other objective measures of network relationships. Lastly, it was found that material aid and instrumental support is more important in preventing depression for elderly individuals in Hong Kong than emotional support. Although Hong Kong is mainly a Chines society with 980f its residents are ethnic Chinese, the urbanization and morenization in the past two decades has reduced the family support fuctions in care for its older members. While majority of elders are still living with children, more elders tend to live with spouse only or live alone. More elderly persons in Hong Kong are relying on friends, neighbors and formal social service providers to provide the needed social support in their daily lives. How would this transition of social support patterns affect the psychological well being of the elderly persons in Hong Kong is an interesting research question, which needs to be explored.

The Development of Community Care Services in Australia

H. Kendig (Faculty of Health Sciences, University of Sydney) and S. Quine (Department of Public Health Community Medicine, University of Sydney)

PURPOSE: The paper provides a review of the policies, programs, and practices of community care services in Australia as developed over the past 20 years and assesses their effectiveness as well as issues for further developments. The influence of applied research is considered. METHOD: The paper draws on a review of policy papers and inquiries and related academic literature; service and program evaluations; national data on service needs and use patterns; and interviews with key policy makers and service providers. RESULTS: Australian community care services were initially developed by the voluntary sector and government involvement at the time was limited to modest supplementary grants. During the 1980s the case for more government direction and support was strengthened when policy makers became concerned about the escalating public costs of residential care services and the stresses experienced by informal carers of frail older people. The Home and Community Care Act of 1985 provided national and state funding for community services that aimed to prevent inappropriate entry to residential care and to maintain the quality of life of vulnerable older and younger people. Subsequent service innovations and evaluations have shown the increasing capacities of community services and practitioners to provide flexible and appropriate client-centred care. CONCLUSION: Major issues remain in terms of fragmentation between services; continuity with the acute and residential sectors of care; and financial disincentives between levels of government. Applied research has been important in identifying individual and community needs, and also in promoting service innovation and more effective program management.

SESSION 486

Muscle function and Everyday Activities among Elderly People

Jacob-Steen Madsen and Lis Puggaard (Institute of Sports Science and Clinical Biomechanics,University of Southern Denmark, Odense University, Odense, Denmark)

In the time of information technology, the ways of spreading knowlegde are changing. In the future computer- and internet- based learning will be very important. The new medias of computertechnology offers several advantages. The student can educate him/her-self independent of time and place. Compared to books the new medias are easy to update and it is possible to mix a variety of inputs. For instance video, audio, animations, pictures and text. This is the background for making a CD-ROM. The CD-ROM describe: How musclefuntion deteriorates with increasing age, the effects of poor musclefunction on independent living and the importance of regular exercise on musclefuntion. In this context musclefunction is elucidated by musclestrength, -power, -endurance and Δflexibility. The interaction of these parameters in everyday movements is described and the importance of exercise is elucidated. This CD-ROM aims to: - educate health-care staff (Doctors, therapists, nurses, healtcare-workers and sports instructors) in the importance of preservation of musclefuntion and independent living. - inspire health-care staff on how to develop trainingprograms. - promote exercise as an efficient mean to independent living and wellbeing among elderly people. The CD-ROM sends the message that: - training of musclefunction is beneficial among elderly people. - it is never to late to start training. - training can postpone the time of dependence. - muclefunction is one of the cornerstones in an independent lifestyle.

Restorative Care: The Best You Can Be.

Clara Fitzgerald (Canadian Centre for Activity and Aging, London, ON, Canada) Nancy A. Ecclestone (Canadian Centre for Activity and Aging, London, ON, Canada)

Restorative Care: The Best You Can Be, was produced by the Canadian Centre for Activity and Aging as a resource for the Restorative Care Education and Training (RCET) program. Restorative Care helps residents achieve the best quality of life by maximizing their abilities. This video is for clients/residents who live in long-term care (LTC), their caregivers, and all staff/health care providers and administrators who work in LTC. The RCET trains staff in long-term care institutions/nursing homes to implement a restorative care program in their facility. The five main components of the 36-hour training program include: Communication, Physical Activity and Aging, Positioning and Transferring, Safe and Effective Eating and Assessment and Evaluation. Also, it includes information on creating a restorative environment, team building, the impact of learned helplessness and the importance of maintaining physical function for the clients/residents. This video was produced from results of a randomized control trial investigation in 12 LTC facilities in Ontario, Canada.

Seniors - fit for life

Bjarne andersen (University of Southern Denmark, Odense, Denmark) Kirstine Langagergaard (Municipality of Aalborg, Aalborg, Denmark)

This video presents a project containing physical-, cultural- and social activities for elderly people. The video illustrates the character of exercise in a group of rather unfit elderly participants Δ several of them totally unfamiliar with exercise or sports. Through interviews of a few participants and their relatives the video gives an impression of the significance of participation for these people: Physically, mentally and socially. The video sends througt its content a message that: Δ it is never to late to start Δ you always benefit from exercise Δ exercise gives energy to handle the physical challenges of everyday life Δ daily routines become easier to cope with Δ being independent gives a higher quality of life.

Who Wants to Be Healthy

Yosefa Ben - Moshe (ESHEL, The Association for the Planning and Development of Services for the Aged in Israel, Jerusalem, Israel)

This film was created with the objective of informing the broad population of the elderly about principles of proper nutrition in old age. The main topics are: The importance of diversity in food consumption, familiarity with nutritional risk factors related to daily living problems and life - style, misinformation on over the counter products, the relationship between drug use and nutrition, skills in purchasing and choosing food products' the interrelation with physical activity and food consumption. The film presents a plot based on the T.V. popular game " Who Wants to Be a Millionner ".

SESSION 487

A cross-cultural approach to intervention in cases of senior mistreatment

Maxine Lithwick (CLSC René-Cassin/Institute of Social Gerontology of Quebec, Montreal, Quebec, Canada); Iryna Dulka (The Centre for Applied Family Studies, McGill University School of Social Work, Montreal, Quebec, Canada)

Detecting and intervening in cases of senior mistreatment is complex. Case managers find it even more difficult when they are confronted with situations of mistreatment where non-mainstream cultural factors must be considered in order to detect and intervene. An educational program was developed to educate case managers on risk factors associated with senior mistreatment in non-mainstream populations and the development of an intervention plan using a cross-cultural approach. This program was developed from a study that examined how abuse is defined is 8 different cultural communities, where older persons seek help and what are their obstacles to seeking help from government-sponsored organizations. Representatives from different cultural communities helped finalize the curriculum. The program was tested in 6 different sites where social workers provide services. The main content of the program will be presented as well as the impact that this program has had on providing a framework for working with older victims from various non-mainstream cultural groups.

Developments in Education on Elder Abuse in UK

Author: Bridget Penhale (University of Hull, UK)

Developments in Education on Elder Abuse in the UK Purpose: This paper will provide an overview of developments in education concerning elder abuse in the UK as they have been developing over the last decade. Method: There are a number of issues and developments in relation to education on abuse that have been taking place in the UK. Consideration of some of these necessitates an examination of structural aspects such as institutionalised ageism. The results of an earlier survey of schools of medicine, nursing and social work will be drawn on in relation to this. There will be a particular focus on elder abuse, but some consideration will also be given to other adults who may be vulnerable and at risk of abuse by way of comparison. Specific attention will be given to the recent development of a Comparative European module concerning the protection of vulnerable older people. This is a programme, funded by the European Commission that has been developed in partnership with colleagues from Germany, Austria and France. The module has been designed to elicit maximum participation from students, and to introduce and develop comparative perspectives, in this case from Europe. The development, content and assessment of the module will be discussed. Results: The findings of the evaluation of the module, and possible future developments will be examined. Conclusion: The potential for this type of student-centred learning to be utilised within gerontology will be emphasised.

Domestic Elder abuse

Jyothirmayee Kidambi[ARYARAMA A COMMUNE FOR SENIOR CITIZENS, HYDERABAD, ANDHRA PRADESH, INDIA]

PURPOSE: understand the factors that lead to elder abuse in different family settings Δ rural, tribal, slum and urban. METHOD: A personal Interview Schedule [inventory] of Elder abuse developed and revised by the author is used along with observational notes. The aim of the study was to procure information on nature, severity, causes, gender & economic differences and abuse reporting patterns of elder abuse in four different settings - slum, urban, tribal and rural areas.RESULTS: the study in addition to the information on patterns of elder abuse, highlighted gaps and total absence of social support system for victims.CONCLUSION: based on the findings of the study a model for abuse prevention is suggested.

Domestic Violence and Elder Protective Police Stations in Brazil

G. G. Debert (Department of Anthropology, UNICAMP, Sao Paulo, Brazil)

In the last decade violence against the elderly and elder abuse were transformed into a Brazilian political concern and Special Police Stations for the Protection of the Elderly were created in 1992. The aim of this paper is to describe Δ through an ethnographic account - the practice carried out in these institutions. The analysis of the documentation they produced reveals a disparity between the number of people who seek out the police stations and the number of reports filed, and the fact that a small number of reports result in police official inquiries. The idea of "domestic violence" is used to explain this disparity: the complaints involve relatives and the complainant does not want her or his aggressor to be prosecuted or punished. I argue that the way the Police Stations are structured privileges the complaints that older person makes against his or her own children, transforming this institution almost exclusively into an agency for the protection of individuals from their families. Police Station staff, especially when they are sensitive to elderly problems, are caught between the real world and the legal sphere, and in practice they translate one domain to the other. To offer instruments of pressure and negotiation for the complainants, they are forced to give up some of the legal norms and procedures. From their point of view traditional juridical procedures are characterized as inefficient and slow and the conciliatory practices they adopt expresses a moral agenda that requires families and communities to fulfill new duties and obligations.

ELDER ABUSE AND RESTORATIVE JUSTICE: AN INTERVENTION OPTION?

Arlene Groh (Community Care Access Centre of Waterloo Region, Waterloo, Canada) Michael Stones (Lakehead University, Thunder Bay, Canada)

Four main types of abuse are identified in the literature: physical, emotional, financial and neglect (Podnieks, 1990, Dow, et al. 1995, Wolf, 1998). In the national study, Services for Abused Older Canadians (Pittaway, et al. 1995) patterns of service utilization were identified along with client barriers. The interventions most commonly used in cases of elder abuse that were examined included adult protection, domestic violence, advocacy, family systems, and multi-disciplinary models. A three-year project in Waterloo, Ontario, Canada, funded by the Trillium Foundation, focuses on the use of Restorative Justice as one intervention model. The challenges of different theoretical perspectives and intervention models will be outlined. The Restorative Justice Model focuses on a) healing following an incident, b) restoration of relationships more than on retribution, and c) values democracy by hearing all participant’s voices. A community development process was utilized in bringing together the Community Care Access Centre of the Waterloo Region along with Community Justice Initiatives, Kitchener-Waterloo Multicultural Centre, The Network for Conflict Resolution, the Waterloo Region Committee on Elder Abuse, the Waterloo Region Police Services and White Owl, an aboriginal resource in the region. The successes and challenges of the process to-date will be outlined. Some of the project evaluation outcome measures are partially based on adherence of principles and values. Preliminary results of the evaluation will be presented and discussed.

Elderly at Risk. Developing Elder Protective Services in Norway.

Olaug Juklestad, (National Centre for Information and Studies on Violence, Oslo University College, Oslo, Norway)

Experience from Norway about the progress in the work of highlighting the issue of elder abuse from its start until today. Awareness of the problem of elder abuse was awakened in Norway in the early 80's . The first survey amongst a small sample of home nurses in Oslo, showed that some of their patients were known to suffer abuse by a family member. Following presentation of these results, the Ministry of Health and Social Affairs started the task of accumulating knowledge and implementing measures. Since 1986 the Ministry has funded several projects with the aim of gathering information about and evolve measures directed at elderly people prone to abuse in the home. Research made it clear that, in spite of welfare, it did not follow that elderly victims received the necessary help. Violence to the elderly will not have priority unless there is, at least, one key-person who has some knowledge of the subject and has a key role to play in the local assistance agencies. The Ministry therefore funded a new project, Elder Protective Services" project, (1991-94) in one community in Oslo. The project was able to demonstrate significant practical results. As the government funding came to an end, the local authorities incorporated Elder Protective Services as part of their organisation. Last year Oslo City Council decided that all of Oslo's urban administrations shall have Elder Protective Services. Two municipalities outside Oslo have also opened a service.

How Bankers View Elderly Customers: Issues of Protection vs. Privacy in Financial Transactions

Karen F. Stein (University of Delaware, Newark, Delaware, USA)

Purpose: An individual's right to privacy has become an increasingly important issue. Adult Protective Services, for example, generally respects the autonomy of the individual even when decisions arising from that autonomy may place or keep an elderly person in an abusive or exploitive situation. Banks have been recruited as "frontliners" to prevent financial exploitation of the elderly.A concern for both banks and the banking public, is the tension between the right to privacy in financial transactions vs. protection against possible financial exploitation (even at the risk of violating the right to privacy). This research explores bank branch managers' attitudes towards the relative importance of privacy vs. protection for their elderly clients who withdraw large sums. Method: 120 bank branch managers were personally interviewed about their practices and attitudes regarding privacy concerns. Banks were located in rural, suburban and urban areas of Delaware, USA. Results: 34% of the banks had prevented a potential scam or financial exploitation by questioning a large withdrawal. In 85% of these cases, the victim was elderly. Regardless of whether the bank had ever prevented financial exploitation, 66% of managers believed that privacy is less important than protection against victimization for elderly customers, and would question a withdrawal even at the risk of violating privacy concerns. Conclusion: The right to privacy is seen as less important than the right to protection. Much of this seems to be due to stereotypical attitudes about the capacities of older persons to conduct their own financial affairs, than to any experience with actual prevention of financial exploitation.

Preventing and Treating Elder Abuse - an Educational Program for Professionals in Israel.

Sarah Alon (ESHEL, Tel Hashomer, Israel); Tali Tzuk (ESHEL, Jerusalem, Israel).

The purpose of this presentation is to describe the content, process and outcome of a course on elder abuse provided to Israeli practitioners in two cycles in 1999-2000. As professional awareness has been named to be the most important variable to the identification, prevention and treatment of elder abuse, a special course was based on the following instructional objectives: 1. To develop skills for individual casework (i.e. detection assessment and intervention strategies). 2. Acquiring orientation to community cooperation (i.e. raising awareness, pooling resources, establishing multi-disciplinary teams.) The participants represented all the settings of elder care consisting of nurses and social workers. Methods of instruction included: lectures, case presentations, interactive discussions, videotapes. The course yielded several products: 1. Shifting attitudes among participants. 2. Gaining skills in detection, assessment and intervention 3. Identifying and clarifying ethical dilemmas. 4. preparing an organizational plan for dealing with elder abuse.

The End of Elder Guardianship?

Israel Doron (D. Jur. Candidate, Graduate Programme in Law, Osgoode Hall Law School, York University, Toronto, Canada)

The purpose of this study was to examine the ability to abolish the legal regime of elder guardianship. The method used by this research was based on multi-level examination of Ontario's elder guardianship law reform. The different levels of research included historical, political, comparative and empirical dimensions of Ontario's elder guardianship laws. All the different levels of examination suggest that a total abolishment of elder guardianship will not benefit the elderly and will probably harm the most vulnerable portions of the elderly, i.e. the poor, lonely, institutionalized elderly women. However, elder guardianship law reform can significantly limit and narrow the need to resort to formal legal guardianship, reaching de-facto to a similar result. While legal abolishment of elder guardianship is not recommended, changing the current structure and content of the law could significantly reduce formal legal guardianship over the elderly and preserve their fundamental rights.

SESSION 488

Ageing in Place in Ageing Communities: Elderly Women s Accounts of Growing Older in Rural Saskatchewan

Patricia A. MacKenzie (School of Social Work and Center on Aging, University of Victoria, Victoria, B.C.)

Purpose - Only a handful of studies have examined the lives of older rural women (Cape, 1987; Shenk and McTavish, 1988; Shenk, 1991; Keating, 1997, McCullough and Kivett, 1998). No previous studies have been completed in Saskatchewan, a province in the central agricultural core of Canada and the consummate rural location. The purpose of this 1998 study was to explore what it is like for older women to experience ageing in place in ageing, rural prairie communities. Method - Interviews were conducted with 18 elderly women living alone in six non-urban proximate villages within the Central Plains Health District of Saskatchewan, Canada. Using the constant comparative method of Grounded Theory, the analysis of the narrative text produced several categories that were used to describe and interpret the data. These categories include: the relationship of health to living alone, personal attitudes, receiving help, kinship networks, peer networks, non-peer/family supports, the importance of spirituality, attachment to place, and worries over rural sustainability. Results - Two major themes tie the categories together and describe how the women managed their lives and coped with ageing in place. These themes, CONNECTEDNESS and RESILIENCE, describe both the resiliency noted to be present in individuals and communities and the sense of connectedness to both people and place which was found to exist in most cases. Conclusions Three factors were found to essential to allow older women to grow older in an ageing, rural community. These factors are health status, access to social support and having the right attitude. Several recommendations for programs and service delivery systems to benefit older rural residents emerged from the study.

Challenges in utilizing national secondary databases to explore the health of rural seniors

Fran Racher (School of Health Studies, Brandon University, Brandon, Canada), Barbara M. Gfellner (Department of Psychology, Brandon University, Brandon, Canada) & Betty Havens (Department of Community Health Sciences, University of Manitoba, Winnipeg, Canada)

In the first phase of a three-year project funded by SSHRC, a research team assembled by the Rural Development Institute of Brandon University is exploring the health of the rural population of Canada. As senior citizens comprise a substantive proportion of the rural population, attention to their health status and health care needs is paramount. Researchers are analyzing data from the 1996/97 National Population Health Survey and the General Social Survey Δ Cycle 11 to depict the health status, well being and social support as well as health care access and utilization of rural populations in general and rural seniors in particular. This presentation will emphasize the challenges we experienced in defining and operationalizing the concept of "rural" for use in the analysis of large secondary databases and how these insights may be applied to evaluating differences between the provinces and regions in Canada. The findings of our work focus on issues related to health status, social supports and health care utilization of rural seniors and how the results from the analysis of these secondary databases may be utilized to the benefit of specific rural populations.

COMPARISON OF HEALTH INDICATORS AMONG URBAN AND RURAL OLDER COLOMBIAN POPULATION.

Carmen Lucía Curcio, Carolina Alzate, Fernando Gómez. [Geriatric and Gerontological Research Group, Caldas University, Manizales, Colombia]

Objective: To compare 60 years and older urban and rural people with respect to demographic characteristics and health indicators: self-perceived health, self-reported symptoms, medications use and social networks in elderly Colombian population. Design: Descriptive epidemiology and cross-sectional study. Setting: Two rural coffee grower areas and urban area in a 400.000 inhabitant city in Colombian Andes Mountains. Subjects: A randomized sample of rural area of 113 persons and 370 randomized urban inhabitants Measurements: A precoded questionnaire applied by personal interview adapted from a World Health Organization original version. Results: The mean age for the urban sample was 71.2 years (SD 8.12) and for the rural 70.2 years (SD 7.9) with similar gender distribution (65% women and 45% men). A higher percentage in urban single people than rural group was observed (9.7% vs. 4.4%, $p < 0.05$). The low scholarity in rural group was notorious compared with urban sample: 94.7 vs. 52.7% ($p < 0.01$) with less than 5 years of education. Concerning self-perceived health rural elderly referred it as fair or bad compared to urban elderly (74% vs. 48%) with significative differences between rural and urban women. The prevalence of symptoms during the last two weeks -very often or near continuously- were pain in the joints or back trouble (39.1% vs. 44.20rban-rural), difficulties in falling asleep (27% vs. 250rban-rural) and worsening of memory (20% vs. 270rban-rural). The consumption of at least one prescribed medicine during the last week was 52.2 0n rural elderly and 58 0n urban elderly. Concerning hypnotics use no differences in urban and rural were found (7.2% vs. 6.2%). The mean of person living with in both samples was 4.2 persons and 750rban and rural elderly people living with their children. CONCLUSIONS: There are important differences among urban and rural older Colombian population concerning self-perceived health, self-reported symptoms and medication use. The social network was preserved in rural and urban areas. The rural elderly is a group with higher risk factors to develop disability.

Establishing a Senior Center: An Innovative Project in a Rural Philippine Setting

Gregoria Go Beltran (Retired Principal, Hope Christian High School, Manila, Philippines)

The establishment of senior centers to meet the needs of the elderly is rather common in Western industrialized countries. Such an attempt, however, is rare and innovative in developing countries. PURPOSES: This paper focuses on the discussion of the establishment of a senior center in l997 in a rural community in the Philippines. Its purposes are: to trace the background factors that led to its establishment; to discuss its objectives, development, and growth; to evaluate its contributions in enhancing the well-being of seniors; to identify its problems and how these are overcome; and to provide suggestions for similar projects in developing countires. METHOD: The method used is an in-depth case study of a senior center based primarily on participant observation. RESULTS: Although there are positive contributions made to promote the welfare of the seniors, there are also shortcomings that have to be identified early on and rectified accordingly. Activities and programs have to be introduced through trial and error attempts with imputs from the seniors themselves. As a non-government project, financial support from private sources external to the community has remained a strong force since its founding. CONCLUSION: The stability of the center depends upon the combination of a strong leadership sustained by a strong faith, a positive and supportive attitude shown by the seniors themselves and an on-going support from the larger com munity.

Interventionist Strategies for Empowering Rural Aged Women In Himalayan Area.

Aabha Chaudhary (Anugraha, New Delhi, India)

India remains predominantly an agrarian society with 80.8% of total elderly population living in rural areas. The proportion of elderly to the total population has been rising from 6.7% in 1991 to an estimated 7.3% in 2000. In India, majority of rural women are illiterate, financially insecure and socially dependent. Due to early marriage they commonly suffer from widowhood in old age. Inhospitable conditions and unfriendly terrain in remote rural Himalayan regions further marginalize women due to social and economic constraints and health related morbidity. The Intervention Plan, an outcome of the need assessment study conducted in over fifty villages, covering one thousand aged women, aims at their socio-economic empowerment. This paper highlights the intervention strategies for promoting productive ageing and in gaining a sense of self worth, social respectability, economic security and holistic well being. The nodal agency for implementation at the village level is the Community based Elders' Organisation. The interventions suggested in the social sector include networking and advocacy to liaison between older women and public authorities, communication and publicity of gerontological issues, counselling and guidance on old age pension scheme. Preventive and promotive aspects of health are emphasized along with home remedies and herbal cures for improved health status. By instilling entrepreneurial skills and developing livelihood options which are multigenerational and remunerative would give the aged women much needed economic security. These measures one hopes would go a long way in initiating the process of empowerment for the "Productive aged" womenfolk in the rural Himalayas.

The Meaning of Health and Well-being for the Rural Older Widowed Woman: An Australian Perspective

Beth de la Rue [University of Southern Queensland, Toowoomba, Queensland, Australia]

PURPOSE: This presentation, a PhD thesis, focuses upon the meaning of health and well-being for the elderly widowed woman who lives on the land in Australia. In addition it explores the influence geographic location and gender relations have on the lives of these women. METHOD: Qualitative life history narratives, social constructionism and Gubrium's socio-environmental theory were used to provide the theoretical directions for this study. 5 older women, with no major illness or disability, living on the land away from any major provincial centre and widowed for at least 2 years, voluntarily participated in the study. Data collection was collected from each informant by in-depth interviews, photo-analysis and autobiographies. Data analysis was by life history narrative analysis. RESULTS: Thematic analysis using a life history approach revealed that geographic location had a profound influence on the lives of these women from pre-widowhood to post-widowhood in their journey through the process of widowhood. Spirituality, reminiscing, and past role models all had a role to play in surviving their widowhood journey. Widowhood also had consequences which were new challenges and threats to their security and safety net. CONCLUSIONS: Geographic location plays an active intimate role in an older widowed rural woman's management of life, health and well-being. This has profound implications for health promotion and relocation to another place of living in the face of inevitable advancing age.

SESSION 489

A utility-based measure of social care outcome for older people

Ann Netten (Personal Social Services Research Unit, University of Kent) Mandy Ryan (Health Economics Research Unit, University of Aberdeen, UK) Diane Skatun (Health Economics Research Unit, University of Aberdeen, UK) and Paul Smith (Institute of Psychiatry).

Purpose:. In the field of health services research there is increasing use of measures that aim to reflect utility gains from health related quality of life (Qalys). The objective of this UK government funded study was to develop a similar measure that reflects the objectives of social care services for elderly people. Method: After an extensive consultation exercise outcome of social care was defined as meeting needs in five key domains: food and nutrition, personal care, social participation and involvement, safety, and control over daily life. Discrete choice conjoint analysis was used on a sample of 350 people over the age of 60 to derive utility weights. Respondents were also asked to rate the vignettes used for discrete choices using a visual analogue scale. Sub-samples were re-interviewed to test re-test reliability and to investigate incorporating a monetary domain. Results: A series of analyses revealed a broadly consistent pattern with personal care weighted as most important, with a sense of safety lowest, and insignificant in some analyses. Significant variations in preferences were associated with living circumstances and experience of services. There was evidence of good reliability (Kappa=.64) and validity when predicted scores were compared with average ratings (R2=.81). Conclusions: If we are to reflect the impact of services designed to meet the needs of older people in evaluations of the efficiency and effectiveness of services policy options we need measures that reflect the benefit gain. The results suggest that conjoint analysis provides a valid and reliable way to derive such a measure.

Health status of the elderly people and their provision with medical services in Ukraine

V.Chaikovska, N. Verzhikovska, V. Bezrukov (Institute of Gerontology, Kiev, Ukraine)

Present research aimed at the development of geriatric care system according to health status and medical care needs of the elderly residing in various regions of Ukraine. In the course of study we used complex health assessment method and recently elaborated computer-based system for quantitative evaluation of older person s dependance on medico-social care. 8574 elderly residents of various regions of Ukraine were examined. Findings revealed that morbidity levels for urban and rural population of retirement age were, respectively, 4412.4 0 and 4115.3 0. However, low accessibility of services was reported. Elderly population needs in outpatient care were met by 53.0 %, in rehabilitative outpatient treatment by 19.0 %, in home-based care by 28.9 %, in urgent medical services by 67.5 %, in institutional care by 73.8 %, and in social care for the elderly who were living alone by 79.5 %. Necessity for restructuring medical and social care sector and ways of setting up more adequate system of geriatric services in Ukraine are substantiated. Findings mentioned above also allow to suggest that such innovations as changing focuses from institutional care use to intensive use of outpatient and home-based care may be economically advisable for Ukraine. It would have allowed to reduce annual state costs by 40 % in addition to significant clinical benefits.

Quality of Health Care Services among the Elderly in Israel following Health Care Reform

Netta Bentur, and Revital Gross, (JDCΔBrookdale Institute of Gerontology and Human Development, Jerusalem, Israel)

One of the main objectives of the National Health Insurance (NHI) Law, implemented in Israel in January 1995, was to increase equity among different population groups and improve services for vulnerable populations. Since 1998, there has been a significant modification of the NHI Law due to budgetary restraints and increased co-payments, which have influenced the provision of health services. Purpose: To follow the changes in the public's perception of the quality of health care services. Methods: Two cross-sectional telephone surveys were conducted at the end of 1997 and at the end of 1999, among a random sample of adult residents of Israel. Results: The findings show that in both surveys, a larger proportion of elderly reported an improvement in health services compared to the proportion reporting deterioration. However, the percentage reporting an improvement declined (from 28% to 18%) while the percentage reporting deterioration rose (from 7% to 16%). Nevertheless, the percentage of elderly reporting an improvement in services exceeded the comparable percentage of younger adults (aged 22-64) in both surveys. Most of the elderly in both surveys reported that the office hours of the family physician, specialists, administrative services and laboratories were convenient. A smaller proportion of younger adults reported this way. Conclusions: The findings indicate that the elderly's situation is on a par with that of younger adults, and even better in some areas. At the same time, it is important to continue monitoring the impact of the law on the need for health services of vulnerable groups such as the elderly, especially the chronically ill and disabled elderly.

Regionalization and health service utilization among older adults: Rural-urban differences

Allan DE, Penning, MJ (Centre on Aging, University of Victoria, BC, Canada)

Purpose: In 1997, British Columbia joined the majority of Canadian provinces in introducing regionalization as a means of moving toward a population health model of health care delivery. Among other objectives, the transfer of decision-making authority from a provincial to regional level was designed to make health services more appropriate to the needs of the local community, thereby enhancing regional equity. This paper assesses the extent to which this occurred by focusing on regional similarities and differences in older adults' use of health services over time. In particular, it examines the impact of regionalization on the utilization patterns of older adults residing in comparatively urban (Regional Health Boards) and rural (Community Health Service Societies) areas of the province. Method: Data for the analyses are drawn from administrative health data collected by the provincial government and available through the British Columbia Linked Heath Data resource. Rates of physician, hospital and community-care service utilization among older adults are examined across a nine-year period (1990-1999), and presented for RHBs, CHSSs and the province as a whole. Results and Conclusion: Findings point to the increasing similarity of the older populations of RHBs and CHSSs with regard to visits to general practitioners and outpatient hospital separations over time. Differences in visits to specialists and inpatient hospital separations have remained constant over time. These trends appear to be a continuation of trends established earlier rather than since the introduction of regionalization

Service productivities, efficiencies and the analysis of alternative policies for community care

Bleddyn Davies (PSSRU, London School of Economics and University of Kent, Canterbury, England) and José Fernandez (PSSRU, London School of Economics, England)

PURPOSE. Policy-making requires estimates and methodologies to predict what service combinations would most efficiently achieve alternative outcome priorities given different scenarios about service supply. The paper illustrates the use of estimated impacts of service inputs on outcomes ('service productivities') to consider whether less costly community care packages should be allocated to the more highly dependent to free resources for the less dependent, many arguing that British success in supporting more persons for longer in the community rather than in homes has been at the cost of preventing deterioration among those of lower dependency.) METHODS. Econometric production function techniques were used to estimate the impacts of varying levels of community nursing and social care services on seventeen outcomes of value in their own right to stakeholders. These are used to simulate the scenario in which all producers combined services around user and caregiver circumstances as efficiently as the most efficient. Evidence is from the ECCEP project for a cohort of 419 triads comprising new users of home and community services, their principal informal caregivers (if present), and their care managers, recruited from 12 areas in England and Wales. RESULTS. What input mix is most efficient depends on user circumstances and outcome prioritised. Optimally efficient mixes would create gains for many outcomes for most user types, and allow reprioritisation between user types without losses to others, but only if service supply is flexible without great price changes. CONCLUSIONS. The new approach could usefully complement others in contributing to more evidence-based policy-making.

The Chronic Care Paradox

R.L. Kane (University of Minnesota School of Public Health, Minneapolis, USA)

Despite the demographic reality of a preponderance of chronic disease, the medical system is still organized for acute illness. This presentation will describe the necessary changes in our conceptualization and organization or health care including prevention, monitoring, patient roles, definition of successful outcomes, and the use of information technology. It will review the evidence of successful approaches and discuss the reasons why they have not been more widely adopted.

The Impact of Continuing Care Reforms to Home Support Services on Senior Clients: A Regional Assessment

Georgia Livadiotakis (Simon Fraser University, Vancouver, Canada)

In 1994, the British Columbia Ministry of Health capped community health care funding across the province. In order to respond to the growing demand for service delivery within their budget, in March 1999, approximately 1300 personal care and intermediate care level 1 clients, (the two highest functional care levels) in the Simon Fraser Health Region (SFHR) were discharged from the Continuing Care Program.
This study examined quantitatively and qualitatively the impact of this discharge on 141 senior clients level of care and current support network. Of the 141 study participants, 77.3% were female. Participants mean age at the time of their discharge was 79.87 years (SD= 7.06 years, range= 61-

100). Approximately 66.0% were assessed at the personal care level and 34.0% were at the intermediate care 1 level. In comparison to seniors who made a successful appeal to continue their service, discharged clients were more likely to be male, were married and had an adequate income. Additionally, discharged clients were more likely to be assessed at the personal care level and self rated their health as good/excellent. Discharged clients were also more likely to be assessed as being independent with instrumental activities of daily living and activities of daily living.
Findings reveal that at follow-up approximately 60.9% of participants were assessed at the same level of care, while 10.9% improved from the intermediate care 1 level to the personal care level and 28.3% were reassessed to a higher care level (intermediate care 1 or 2 level). Changing to a higher or less functional care level was significantly associated with a decline in ADL and IADL performance, while experiencing a negative health change when service was not delivered had an indirect relationship. Substitution for government service was greatest for seniors who remained at the same care level or improved. Payment for formal service delivery was associated with older age and having no proximate children.
Qualitative reports revealed that approximately 34.3% of participants reported experiencing physical and/or emotional hardship as a result of performing their own housekeeping tasks. Approximately 29.2% of participants reported the involuntary shift of responsibility to themselves or to their family and/or friends, while 28.5% reported being more independent. Remaining participants reported mixed feelings about their discharge from service. Overall, the study's findings suggest that the preventive and maintenance functions of home care may have been compromised with this discharge policy.

Third Age Ontario: An Electronic Seniors' Sensitivity Kit for Ontario Government Policymakers and Planners

Wendy Hulko (Ontario Seniors' Secretariat, Toronto, Canada)

PURPOSE: To assist Ontario government policymakers and planners in developing and reviewing policies and programs that have the potential to impact the quality of life of seniors. METHOD: A seniors' sensitivity kit delivered electronically to policy makers and planners within the Ontario government, developed in partnership with the Ontario Gerontology Association. RESULTS: Third Age Ontario, an Ontario government Intranet site, was developed and promoted amongst policymakers and planners across the Ontario government. Some of the features of the site are an aging quiz, statistical and demographic information (tables and graphs) on seniors and resources and links related to aging and seniors. The development of the site, feedback from users on the impact on their policy and plannning work and the current status will be detailed. CONCLUSION: Ontario is home to over 1.47 million people aged 65 years and older and this number is expected to grow to 1.86 million by 2011. Third Age Ontario addresses the urgent need for policymakers and planners across government to become sensitized to the implications of an aging population and the unique needs and characteristics of seniors in Ontario to inform their policy and planning work.

SESSION 490

Goal setting for rehabilitative care to the elderly disabled in a special geriatric nursing home

Masami Hidaka, Seiichi Takemasa, Tomoaki Shimada, (Kobe University School of Medicine) Mika Kunisada, (Fukuyama municipal Women's Junior College) Sachiko Kasahara, (International Buddhist College) Hiroshi Sumii, (Hiroshima Prefectural College of Health and Welfare)

Purpose: The purposes of this study are to reveal the characteristics of the functional grouping among the elderly disabled at the special geriatric nursing home(SGNH), and to plan the appropriate rehabilitation goals. Method: Subjects were 100 persons (29 males, 71 females, average ages 79.6 years old) in two SGNHs. Their level of the bedridden and the burden score of the dementia were evaluated with the criteria determined by Japanese Ministry of Health and Welfare scores, which were divided into six groups according to their stage between the level of bedridden or the burden score of dementia, as well as MOSES. Results: Those in group I or II are almost able to look after themselves in SGNH, and the rehabilitation goals are to maintain their living function. Those in group III or IV are major purposes in the improvement of the mobility and the activation of life. For those in group V with poor independence on ADL complicated by the emotional problem with dementia, acquirement of the sufficient communication means and the support of safety should be considered. As those in group VI are completely bedridden, and cannot perform roll over the bed by themselves, it is more important to activate the mobility and activities from bed to the wheelchair, and the need of care is highest.
Conclusion: The rehabilitation goal must be making up to be optimal and successful for the elderly disabled in SGNH, according to their need of care. The more serious their disabilities are, the more important the cooperation of medical treatment with careworks becomes.

Independent living rehabilitation; an ergonomic approach to gerontology by physical therapists.

Klari Varallyai, Campbell River Physiotherapy Clinic, Campbell River, BC, Canada

To develop independent living rehabilitation. To focus on the development of a structure and a process of rehabilitation and physical therapy that is sensitive to the unique physiology, psychology, and sociology of the aging. Combining the above with the science of ergonomics, independent living rehabilitation will become a realistic goal for seniors. Definition of Ergonomics the word ergonomics is derived from the Greek words ergos "work" and nomos "laws or study". The science of ergonomics and information about human abilities, limitations and other characteristics to the design of tools, jobs, environments for safe effective use, and to optimize the functioning of a system by adapting it to human capacities and needs. Ergonomic interventions are more commonly utilized in the work place to prevent workplace injuries as well as to promote safe and efficient productivity. However, benefits of ergonomics, extends far beyond the workplace. The knowledge of ergonomics adds to independence in our homes as well as the recreational and educational environment. The practical application of ergonomics for the retiring and aging population offers: · a greater ability to utilize all aspects of self care. · a wide range of environmental control leading to greater independence. Physiotherapists, with their background in anatomy, physiology, psychology, and biomechanics, are in the front throes of assisting the aging population, helping to identify the limiting activities and analyze how to lessen or modify the physical and environmental demands of the aging population so they are able to "remain independent" and to exert some influence over their environment, to maintain physical mobility, and to help to alleviate the problems associated with micturition. Independent Living The value of independence also carries in itself, an appreciation of the need to remain inter-dependent. Independent Living Rehabilitation is a realistic and achievable attainment for the majority of seniors 65 105.

Job Satisfaction in the Era of Efficiency

M. Blondin, F. Knoefel (SCO Hospital, Ottawa, ON, Canada)

There has been much focus on Quality Improvement and improving efficiency in the Health Care sector over the last few years. The Geriatric Rehabilittion Program of the SCO Health Service successfully implemented changes that reduced length of stay and improved patient outcome with a near tripling of rehabilitation efficiency. There were no direct costs associated wtih these changes, so that cost efficiency improved as well. But what has not been well described is the cost on employee's job satisfaction. We used a modified Job Satisfaction Questionnaire to retrospectively measure the indirect cost of significant job change.

Planning a Specialized Geriatric Rehabilitation Service for Hemodialysis Patients

Adler, L, R(Toronto Rehabilitation Institute, Toronto, Canada) Holmes, C, R(Toronto Rehabilitation Institute, Toronto, Canada) Spevakow, D, (Toronto Rehabilitation Institute, Toronto, Canada)

Title: Planning a Specialized Geriatric Rehabilitation Service for Hemodialysis Patients Purpose: This presentation will describe the planning process for elderly hemodialysis patients who will be receiving care on an inpatient geriatric rehabilitation service in a large metropolitan center in Canada. Description: The current system of service rarely offers the opportunity to provide focussed rehabilitation to the frail elderly receiving hemodialysis in our area. The vast majority of new patients started on dialysis are over the age of 65 years and future trends predict considerable growth in this population. This presentation will focus on specific aspects of developing an inpatient rehabilitation service for this special geriatric population. One aspect of the planning process involved identifying the educational needs of interprofessional staff from both the rehabilitation and dialysis settings. Another consideration included identifying the implications of integrating dialysis patients into an established geriatric rehabilitation service and planning for this to occur. Decision-making concerning advanced directives is one ethical issue related to caring for this population that was identified through the planning process. Finally the opportunity to identify and plan for a variety of research initiatives to evaluate the new service were identified. Conclusion: This presentation will be helpful for caregivers, interprofessional staff and administrators eager to learn about the planning process of this important care initiative for geriatric patients.

Using a Real-Time Database to track outcomes in Geriatric Rehabilitation part II: Demonstration

F. Knoefel, D. Dalle (SCO Hospital, Ottawa, ON, Canada)

The trend to increasingly measure outcomes in health care has been facilitated by the wide-spread use of computers. In geriatric rehabilitation the use of tools, such as the Functional Independence Measure (FIM), allow for outcome measurement of both indivudual patients as well as groups of patients or programs. Because of treatment group variability though, various other measures are needed to describe the patient population for research, including cognition measures, depression rating scales, and medical co-morbidity scales. With limited health care resources, it is difficult to balance the requirements of staff for clinical time, team rounds, and otcome measurement. This presentation will demonstrate the data base developed in our institution using Microsoft Access software, which integrates the data requirements for research with goal setting and patient follow-up at team rounds. Simulating team rounds, a particular patient's evolution in the progtram will be tracked. Some examples of the reporting capabilities of the software will also be shown.

Using a Real-Time Database to track outcomes in Geriatric Rehabilitation part I: The process

F.Knoefel, D. Dalle (SCO Hospital, Ottawa, ON, Canada)

The trend to increasingly measure outcomes in health care has been facilitated by the wide-spread use of computers. In geriatric rehabilitation the use of tools, such as the Functional Independence Measure (FIM), allow for outcome measurement of both individual patients as well as groups of patients or programs. Because of treatment group variability though, various other measures are needed to describe the patient population for research, including cognition measures, depression rating scales, and medical co-morbidity scales. Wtih limited health care resources, it is difficult to balance the requirements of staff for clinical time, team rounds, and outcome measurement. This presentation will describe the process of developing a database which would satisfy research needs and allow data inut in a real-time basis. Issues include: data coompleteness, software limitations and staff buy-in.

SESSION 492

End-of-Life Care for Seniors: Canadian Initiatives

Honourable Sharon Carstairs (Senate of Canada, Ottawa, Canada) Quality End of Life Care: The Right of Every Canadian Jane McNiven (Canadian Pensioners Concerned Inc, Halifax, Canada) My Plans for Me: Educational Information Packages and Training Workshops on Advance Health Care Directives D. W. Molloy (McMaster University, Hamilton, Canada) "Let Me Decide" An Advance Health Care Directive Rory Fisher (University of Toronto, Toronto, Canada) A Guide to End of Life Care for Seniors

Canada's population is aging dramatically and as a result the care of seniors at the end of life becomes a national priority. This symposium highlights recent Canadian initiatives addressing concerns surrounding end of life care for seniors. Presentations will be made by a legislator, a representative of a seniors group and health care professionals. These will be discussed from an international perspective. A Senator will discuss the recommendations of a sub-committee of the Senate of Canada regarding "Quality End of Life Care: The Right of Every Canadian". This recommends the development of a national strategy on end of life care, coordinated by the federal government in full partnership with the provinces and the volunteer sector. The report also recommends the establishment of a national pharmacare program for the dying, and the implementation of income security and job protection for those who care for dying family members at home. The National Canadian Pensioners Concerned Incorporated (CPC) have undertaken a national project to develop practical, easy to read, accessible information on advance health care directives. Entitled "My Plans for Me: Educational Information Packages and Training Workshops", this will be presented as a seniors initiative in this area. This is followed by a perspective on Advance Directives by a geriatric physician with discussion of the use of one particular directive "Let Me Decide" which has been implemented in the community, retirement home, nursing homes and hospitals using systemic implementation processes. Results and current and future projects in this area will be given. The last presentation will discuss "A Guide to End-of-Life Care for Seniors", developed with a broad interdisciplinary input from both geriatrics/gerontology and palliative care to reflect a consensus of best practice in this area. This guide has been widely distributed and is available in both French and English at www.rgp.toronto.on.ca/iddg Finally, the international discussant from Switzerland will comment on these initiatives and provide an international perspective. The symposium will provide the perspectives and efforts of several policy-makers, seniors' organizations, and health and social care professionals concerned with improving the quality of end of life care for seniors.

A Guide to End of Life Care for Seniors

Rory Fisher (University of Toronto, Toronto, Canada) Margaret Ross (University of Ottawa, Ottawa, Canada) Michael MacLean (University of Regina, Regina, Canada)

Presentation and discussion of a Guide to End of Life Care for Seniors. The purpose was to develop a guide, reflecting the consensus of best practices in health care and social service delivery. The guide was funded by Health Canada. The concept was to bring together the fields of geriatrics/gerontology and palliative care to focus on seniors' issues specifically. A national advisory committee was formed and it brought together lead expert authors from various disciplines and organizations around the country. The first draft was reviewed by the National Advisory Committee and revised with input from Canadian and international expert reviewers. The main audience is for health care and social service providers but the Guide has been of interest to the public at large. Aspects of optimal care covered include living and dying well, maintaining comfort, service delivery and care for caregivers. Also, included are ethical, spiritual, cultural and Aboriginal issues. Key points in the various chapters of the Guide will be addressed with regard to their value to providers. Twenty three thousand copies have been distributed and the full Guide is available in French and English on the website www.rgp.toronto.on.ca/iddg The response has been very favourable and the demand has exceeded the supply. Future initiatives will be addressed.

"Let Me Decide" An Advance Health Care Directive

D. W. Molloy (McMaster, University Hamilton, Ontario L8V 1C3 Canada)

Advance directives are documents that people fill out when they are capable to tell others what health and personal care they want should they become incapable in the future. They allow individuals to maintain control over their health and personal care and maintain autonomy in spite of incapacity. They promote autonomy, take the burden of decision making off family, friends and health care workers, and reduce health care costs. Although the majority of people support the use of directives, few have completed them. We have performed a variety of studies on one particular directive, the "Let Me Decide" over the last fifteen years and published over thirty peer reviewed papers on them. We have a wide range of educational tools to teach the public and health care wonders about directives. We have developed instruments to measure barriers to their use, capacity to understand them, satisfaction with communication around health care needs, attitudinal questionnaires and applied them in these studies. We have implemented them in the community, retirement homes, nursing home and hospitals using systematic implementation processes. Patients, families and staff enthusiastically support them. Yet directives have never "caught on" because they have not been promoted widely or the general public have not been educated about them. Some are afraid advance directives will lead to euthanasia, others believe they will reduce the rights of the disabled. Yet they likely will reduce the "demand" for euthanasia and promote patients' rights. This published research, current projects and future directions are described and discussed.

My Plans for Me: Educational Information Packages and Training Workshops on Advance Health Care Directives

Jane McNiven (Canadian Pensioners Concerned Inc, Halifax, Canada)

In 1997, National Canadian Pensioners Concerned Incorporated (CPC) undertook a national project to develop practical, easy to read, accessible information on advance health care directives. Seniors and professionals participated in workshops held across Canada to assist in the preparation of the educational information package, 'My Plans For Me' which includes: 1) an overview of advance directives and its various forms, information on provincial legislation, answers to commonly asked questions, and a resource directory; 2) a manual for professionals or volunteers to use in educating or informing others, either in group or individual sessions; 3) a booklet designed to be used by seniors, their families and friends in discussing and preparing advance directives; and 4) a provincial information kit on advance directives in each province. Many issues concerning the use of advance directives were identified during the course of the project and after dissemination. These include: 1) potential conflict between the rights of the individual to determine medical treatment and the rights of the institution; 2) inability of directives to take into account cultural diversity and limited literacy skills; 3) provision of clear instruction regarding the control of pain at the end of life. "My Plans for Me" has provided a valuable tool to guide seniors, their families and health care providers in preparing advance health directives. It has also underscored many limitations of written advance directives that need to be addressed to ensure that all seniors are able to determine the care they receive at the end of life.

Quality End of Life Care: The Right of Every Canadian

Subcommitte to Update "Of Life and Death" of Standing Senate Committee on Social Affairs, Science and Technology (Senate of Canada, Ottawa, Canada)

Canada needs a national strategy on end-of-life care, coordinated by the federal government in full partnership with the provinces and the volunteer sector. This was the first of fourteen recommendations in Quality End of Life Care: The Right of Every Canadian, the final report of a Subcommittee of the Senate of Canada which was tabled in June 2000. This Subcommittee of the Senate was given a mandate to review the progress of the implementation of the unanimous recommendations of an earlier report on end of life issues, titled Of Life and Death. The Subcommittee received input from 50 witnesses, including medical doctors, national health organizations, ethicists, lawyers, the Minister of Health and government departments on the issues of palliative care, withholding and withdrawal of life-sustaining treatment, research and training, advance directives and pain control. The Subcommittee found that in the past 5 years we have made little progress in the area of quality end of life care. Canadians are still dying in needless pain. Only an estimated 5% of dying Canadians receive integrated and interdisciplinary palliative care. There is a patchwork of care available. Access to palliative care depends on geography and most of the costs of home care are assumed by the family, and more often women. Along with a national strategy, the report also recommended the establishment of a national pharmacare program for the dying and the implementation of income security and job protection for those who care for dying family members at home.

SESSION 493

Same Patients, Different Systems: Clinical Implications for the Care of the Frail Elderly Population

A. Mark Clarfield (Sarah Herzog Memorial Hospital, Jerusalem, Israel) Same Patients, Different Systems: Clinical Implications for the Care of the Frail Elderly Population. David B. Hogan (University of Calgary Medical Clinic, Calgary, Canada) Same Patients, Different Systems: Clinical Implications for the Care of the Frail Elderly Population. Jean-Pierre Michel (Département de gériatrie, Hôpitaux Universitaires de Genève, Thônex-Genève) Same patients, different systems: Clinical implications for the care of the frail elderly population. Carlos Alberto Cano Gutierrez (Hospital San Ignacio, Bogotá, Colombia) Same Patients, Different Systems: Clinical Implications for the Care of the Frail Elderly Population.

Influenced by history, demography, availability of resources, etc, countries have developed systems of care for the frail elderly population. These systems vary in the public/private mix, the strength of the hospital or community model, the link between continuing care and acute care, the relationship between medical care and social care and the level of accessibility and equity. This symposium will examine systems of care in countries from four different regions of the world with very different healthcare systems (Canada, Colombia, Israel, Switzerland). The approach will not be based on a description and analysis of each of these systems of care or on an attempt to develop indicators which can be used to judge and rank their performance. Rather, the focus will be on a case study approach. A case scenario combining acute and chronic medical problems in a frail elderly person will be presented. Following the presentation of the case, members of the panel from each of the four countries will describe concretely the itinerary and management of the elderly person in the country's health care system. The presentation will focus not on the ideal but on the real situation. The objective is to develop a concrete understanding of each of the systems of care and an awareness and comparison of the strengths and weaknesses. Following the presentations, the panel will then engage in a discussion with the audience. This will be followed by the presentation by the Chair of a summary bringing together the key points.

Same Patients, Different Systems: Clinical Implications for the Care of the Frail Elderly Population - Israel

A. Mark Clarfield, MD

Israel offers its citizens a universal, publicly funded and administered healthcare system. Taxes are collected by the National Insurance Institute and distributed via a capitation system to one of four non-profit sick funds. All primary, acute, rehabilitation and complex long-term nursing care in both out and in-patient facilities as well as medications (small co-payment) are provided according to a defined basket of services according to the National Health Insurance Law (1995). With respect to institutional long-term care, the Israeli system is more like American Medicaid with patients, spouses and children formally required to fund this service. If the family cannot afford such care (expensive in comparison with the average income), like Medicaid they must approach a government ministry in order to receive subsidy, which is offered on a sliding scale. Poor families pay almost nothing up to the need to pay for 950f the service. Long-term care patients are defined as regular (900f cases) and complex nursing (10%). The former is funded under the subsidy mechanism alluded to just above, while the latter care is included in the same basket of services as acute and rehabilitation care under the National Health Law. This illogical division of fiscal responsibility leads to confusion on the part of the patient, the family as well among the formal care-giving network. Under the National Health Insurance Law, by 1998 regular long-term care was meant to be absorbed into the basket of services. Unfortunately, to date this vital transfer has not yet taken place.

Same Patients, Different Systems: Clinical Implications for the Care of the Frail Elderly Population - Colombia

Carlos Alberto Cano Gutierrez, MD

Colombia is a developing country with a population of more than 42 millions and about 3 millions (7%) are older than 60. Life expectancy has been modified and is actually 70.6 years (67.3 for male and 74 for women). Our Health System is poor in comparison with developed countries but doing efforts to grow better in coverage and quality. Law 100 for Social Security System was signed in 1993 and by its means has been possible the coverage in health care to grow up. At the beginning of this law less than 200f people older than 60 years was covered. Actually, 63% has either contributive (66%) or subsidized (34%) way of social security system. However, 370f older people has no any system of social security. Health Promote Entities (EPS in Spanish) have the duty of include at least 60f people older than 60 years. Care for older people in Acute Units is good but with big troubles in mean and long term because its coverage is extremely low and achieved for just a few of these so called entities. Community based care for frail elderly is limited to realize a medical and nurse control. The System allows frail elderly to obtain assistance services but the law is very vulnerable in its practice.

Same Patients, Different Systems: Clinical Implications for the Care of the Frail Elderly Population - Canada

David B Hogan, MD

Under our federal system, the ten Canadian provinces have ultimate responsibility for the regulation and delivery of health care within their boundaries. The central or federal government influences this by linking tranfers of money to pay for these services with adherence to certain principles (i.e, universality, comprehensiveness, public administration, portability, accessibility). The Canadian health care system provides universal, publically-funded coverage for medically necessary hospitalizations and physician services. Continuing care is a complex array of services built on the principles of universality and selectivity (certain payments are made by the consumer on the basis of their income). The private sector has a large role in continuing care. Each province has defined, organized, and funded continuing care in its own fashion. It incorporates both community-based (e.g, home care) and facility-based (e.g, nursing homes) services. Publically-funded drug-benefit programs for seniors are also available though they vary markedly from province to province. Compared to many other countries, Canadian families are smaller, separated by longer distances, and are arguably both less able and willing to provide family-based care to functionally dependent members. Challenges exist for frail seniors, their families, and their practitioners in navigating this potentially complex, fragmented system.

Same patients, different systems: Clinical implications for the care of the frail elderly population - Genève

Professor Jean-Pierre Michel

The alliance treaty signed in 1291 by the representatives of three cantons still presides over the federal cohesion of Switzerland. This federalist will is clearly reflected in the sharing out of responsibilities in health matters. Each of the 26 cantons constituting the Swiss confederation profits from a legislative and executive autonomy, which means that each canton, establishes its own health policies and budget. In fact there is no health ministry at the country level: the government of each canton has a health department responsible for the implementation of the programs elaborated by the canton authorities. The co-ordination between cantonal activities and the international liaisons are in the hands of the Federal Office of Public Hygiene. The smooth and harmonious functioning of Swiss institutions is noteworthy, although the cantonal diversity of health services and the powerful private insurance companies. Their activities are nationally co-ordinated by a very new law. · confirming the obligation for everybody to undertake an insurance policy · obliging the insurance companies to welcome everyone whatever his health status and · establishing new competitive rules of funding insurance and refunding care. Questions concerning the role and place of the aged vary from canton to canton and depend upon the particular character of the canton: whether it is industrial or agricultural, whether it is or not university. There are five medical universities in Switzerland and only two of them have a chair of geriatrics.

SESSION 494

Couples, Careers and Retirement

Maximiliane E. Szinovacz [Eastern Virginia Medical School and European Centre for Social Welfare Policy and Research (Vienna, Austria), Norfolk, Virginia, USA]; "Couples' Joint Retirement Patterns: An International Comparison" Phyllis Moen [Cornell University, Ithaca, New York USA]; and Stephen Sweet [Cornell University, Ithaca, New York USA]; "Planning for Retirement: American Workers and The Setting of Career Clocks" Keiko Katagiri [University of Tokyo, Tokyo, Japan]; "Transition into Retirement: Challenge for Middle-aged Japanese Couples" Sonja Drobnic [Universitat Bremen, Bremen, Germany]; "Retirement Timing in Germany: Does the Spouse Matter?"

Retirement as a structural aspect of the life course is a relatively recent phenomenon, institutionalized in industrialized societies only in the 20th century. "Retirement" is typically defined as later life withdrawal from the workforce, often in conjunction with public and/or employer-provided pension benefits. But growing numbers of workers retire from their career jobs and then take on employment in another job and/or unpaid community service. Retirementin terms of eligibility for a pensioncan no longer be equated with a one-way, one-time individual (rather than couple) exit from the workforce or with the cessation of all productive activity. Neither is retirement occurring at one set age (such as 62 or 65). The proliferation of public and private retirement income programs have encouraged a world-wide trend toward progressively earlier retirement from career jobs and greater heterogeneity in the age and nature of retirement. The papers in this symposium look at retirement as a couple-level process, involving the planning and transitions of two-spouses, in a world with outmoded templates of the retirement status passage.

Couples' Joint Retirement Patterns: An International Comparison

Maximiliane E. Szinovacz [Eastern Virginia Medical School and European Centre for Social Welfare Policy and Research (Vienna, Austria), Norfolk, Virginia , USA]

Past research indicates that spouses tend toward joint retirement. However, the extent of this pattern and national variations in it are not known. Further investigation of such patterns is particularly important in view of planned retirement reforms (changes in retirement age, elimination of gender-based differences in eligibility in some European countries). This paper addresses this issue, using panel data from the European Household Surveys as well as from the U.S. Health and Retirement Survey. Specifically, we will show for the U.S. and each of the European Community countries: a. timing patterns of spouses' exit from the labor force and receipt of pensions; b. to what extent selected timing patterns of spouses' retirement in relation to each other are associated with "early" and regular retirement of either spouse; and c. to what extent selected timing patterns evolve from health problems of and/or caregiving for a spouse.

Planning for Retirement: American Workers and The Setting of Career Clocks

Phyllis Moen [Cornell University, Ithaca, New York USA] Stephen Sweet [Cornell University, Ithaca, New York USA]

American workers are experiencing conflicting trends regarding later life career planning and possibilities. Retirement transitions remain embedded in established social and organizational policies and practices which, by the second half of the 20th century, came to be normatively defined in terms of timing and legitimacy. These normative expectations, in conjunction with the institutionalization of income supports (in the form of Social Security benefits and private pensions) set retirement apart from unemployment as a later life work exit that can be planned for, anticipated, and positively defined (Costa 1998; Graebner 1980). Unlike previous generations of workers, the transition to retirement can be planned and timed according to personally customized career clocks. How workers are preparing for these transitions, though, is not fully understood. In this presentation, we focus on couples surveyed in the Cornell Couples and Careers Study (1998-99, N=2216) and couples in the Cornell Midcareer Paths and Passages Study (1999-2000, N=887). These data sets comprise hour long telephone interviews with couples who have at least one partner working in one of eleven companies located in upstate New York. These data indicate that women were less likely to have begun retirement planning, and older workers were more likely to have reported engaging in any retirement planning. A sense of efficacy also has significant effects, as referents reporting greater perceived constraints begin retirement planning later. Resources, biographic pacing, and life stage influence the levels of financial and lifestyle planning for retirement. One of the strongest predictors of the anticipated transition into retirement, aside from the predicted impact of planning, are the anticipated transitions of coworkers, reaffirming the normative influence of anticipated life stage transitions.

"Retirement Timing in Germany: Does the Spouse Matter?"

Sonja Drobnic [Universitat Bremen, Bremen, Germany]

Using longitudinal data on employment and family careers, this paper examines the timing of retirement in a household context. It investigates retirement decisions of non-married and married elderly men and women. Since in (West) Germany, patterns of investment in alternative family and market roles over the life course are highly gendered, a separate analysis is also performed on working married couples where both spouses were employed at age 50. The determinants of retirement decisions considered in the models are: early life course employment patterns, employment characteristics in later life, health situation, and household circumstances, including the income level. Data come from the German Socioeconomic Panel Study. An event history analysis is conducted using a piece-wise constant hazard model with time-varying covariates. The analysis indicates that there are indeed important differences in retirement behavior between men and women as well as between non-married and married individuals. Thus, the spouse does matter in retirement decisions but the study discloses gender asymmetry in response to marital status, and displays differences between those spouses where both are employed in late life and those with a traditional division of paid/unpaid labor.

Transition into Retirement: Challenge for Middle-aged Japanese Couples

Keiko. Katagiri [University of Tokyo, Tokyo, Japan] and H. Akiyama [University of Tokyo, Tokyo, Japan]

Successful transition into retirement is a widely held concern in Japan. Long life expectancy requires exploring the marital relationship of retired couples. Both of the middle-aged couple is afraid of their life after retirement. Wives worry how to manage the life with their retired husbands all day long. Husbands also don't want to be treated as a nuisance. Given little empirical research in the literature, this study explored the marital relationship of Japanese middle-aged and retired couples. There were three objectives: 1) to examine the marital relationship of retired couples in Japan; 2) to explore the difference of marital quality between the dual career couples and traditional couples, that is, working husband and full-time housewife; and 3) to explore the change of marital quality between the middle-aged couples and the retired couples. Focus groups were conducted with married persons: Japanese male and female retirees, and middle-aged working men and women. A systematic content analysis was conducted with the tape-recorded statements. First, dual career couples whether working or retired, hold better marital relationship than traditional couples. They are characterized by good communication, sharing housework, independence that leads to have established good relationship. Conversely, traditional couples reveal their discrepancy in their perception of marital relationship. While husbands assume their marriage is going well, poor communication and workaholic life prevents them from constructing good relationship with wives. Retirement had a serious effect on their life. Husbands lose almost all resources, such as social status, work role, financial status and work-related networks at that time. When they face their wives, expecting to get support, they notice their relationships are about to break up. Second, most of the working women and some of the working men in their fifties mentioned the importance of equal partnership, which is a new idea for Japanese marital relationship. This study does not necessarily indicate that dual career couples are always happier than others. Participants can be seen as happy survivors of a long striving marriage life. Many of the wives, either having part-time jobs or full-time housewives, are not included in this study. Discrepancy between couples suggests the necessity that marital relationship should be explored from both the wives' and the husbands' side.

SESSION 495

Cross-European Longitudinal Study of Aging (EXCELSA): Preliminary Results

("European Survey on Aging Protocol (ESAP): Translation and adaptation to six European languages") Fernández-Ballesteros, R. (Autónoma University of Madrid, Spain), Hambleton, R.K. (Massachusetts Univ, USA), Schroots, J.J.H. (Free Univ. of Amsterdam, The Netherlands), Rudinger, G. (Bonn Univ, Germany), Drusini, A. (Padova Univ, Italy), Heikkinen, E. (Jyvaskyla Univ, Finland), Paul, C. (Porto Univ. Portugal), Charezewska, J. (Polish National Inst. Nutrition, Poland), Rosenmayr, L. (Vienna Univ, Austria); ("Aging Protocol (ESAP): Reliability and Validity") Rudinger, G. (Bonn Univ, Germany), Kleinemans, U. (Bonn Univ, Germany), Fernández-Ballesteros, R. (Autónoma Univ. of Madrid, Spain), Schroots, J.J.H. (Free Univ. of Amsterdam, The*

Netherlands), Drusini, A. (Padova Univ, Italy), Heikkinen, E. (Jyvaskyla Univ, Finland), Paul, C. (Porto Univ, Portugal), Charezewska, J. (Polish National Inst. Nutrition, Poland), and Rosenmayr, L. (Vienna Univ, Austria) ("Measuring Competence: The European Survey on Aging Protocol (ESAP)") Fernández-Ballesteros, R. (Autónoma Univ. of Madrid, Spain), Zamarron, M.D. (Autónoma Univ. of Madrid, Spain), Schroots, J.J.H. (Free Univ. of Amsterdam, The Netherlands), Rudinger, G. (Bonn Univ, Germany), Drusini, A. (Padova Univ, Italy), Heikkinen, E. (Jyvaskyla Univ, Finland), Paul, C. (Porto Univ, Portugal), Charezewska, J. (Polish National Inst. Nutrition, Poland), Rosenmayr, L. (Vienna Univ, AustriA) (*"Self-rated health and health behaviors among 30 to 85-year-old people living in seven European countries") Heikkinen, E, Suutama, T, Hietanen, A. (The Finnish Center for Interdisciplinary Gerontology, University of Jyvaskyla, Finland), Fernández-Ballesteros, R. (Autónoma University of Madrid, Spain), Schroots, J.J.H. (Free Univ. of Amsterdam, The Netherlands), Rudinger, G. (Bonn Univ, Germany), Drusini, A. (Padova Univ, Italy), Paul, C. (Porto Univ, Portugal), Charezewska, J. (Polish National Inst. Nutrition, Poland), Rosenmayr, L. (Vienna Univ, Austria)*

In terms of population, Europe is the oldest continent in the world. This demographic situation is giving rise to the implementation of social and health programs, as well as other policies, by the European Union. Since 1993, the European Commission has supported two Concerted Actions on Gerontology in order to proceed to a European longitudinal study on ageing. After the drawing up of a general plan for EXCELSA, as a pre-requisite, a pilot study was conducted. The main purpose of EXCELSA-Pilot was to adapt and validate the European Survey on Ageing Protocol (ESAP) in several European Countries (Austria, Finland, Germany, Italy, Poland, Portugal, and Spain). The ESAP was administered to a sample of 96 people aged 30 to 85 per country (one third of participants were re-tested). Our total sample was 672 people. Structure and Content: a general overview of EXCELSA-Pilot, and the main results of the ESAP will be presented and discussed. The ESAP contains ten general areas (Social relationships, Intelligence, Self, Life satisfaction and Well-being, Personality, Self-reported health, Life styles, Mastery and perceived control, Bio-behavioural measures, and Anthropometric measures and Sociodemographics). Guidelines for the ESAP translation/adaptation, problematic issues during the ESAP translation to six European languages, and statistical analysis conducted for testing score generalizability will be presented, and recommendations with regard to the ESAP discussed. Moreover, all measurement procedures and instrument should demonstrate scientific guarantees. In order to assess test-retest reliability a third of each sample was re-tested after two months; reliability analysis follows the classical test-retest-approach that incorporates the relative invariance of interindividual differences (test-retest-correlation) and differences in central tendencies (mean or median). The validation strategy focuses primarily on the cross-national equality of the instruments used, and attempts to answer the questions arising. However, the ten dimensions assessed through the ESAP are selected because of their relevance to the study of ageing, and specifically to the study of competent ageing. Therefore, the research will deal with results regarding differences in ageing, as well as in other socio-demographic variables. Furthermore, since the definition of competence is an empirical issue, exploratory and explanatory factorial analysis will be presented in an attempt to identify the most sensitive measures of competence, as well as psychosocial factors related to competence. Finally, EXCELSA is devoted to subjective health and life style. Conclusions and Outcomes: The procedure followed for adaptation to several European languages yielded quite satisfactory results. Test-retest analyses show moderate reliability. Cross-European reliability can be assumed for 7 Scales. However, the validity of the postulated theoretical (factorial) models underlying the instruments could not be proved. Cross-European validity was demonstrated only for the instruments related to Mental Abilities. The consequences of the empirical results are discussed with respect to changes and improvements of the instrument set to be used within the planned EXCELSA main study. The majority of our variables and measures discriminate across age group. The ESAP sections fit quite well into our exploratory analysis. The equation model yielded a complex modeling of competence. With regard to the health and life styles analysis, pilot studies in seven European countries on different aspects of self-reported health, physical capacity and health behaviours among 30 to 85-year-old men and women showed both similarities and differences between countries related to gender and age group.

SESSION 497

An Innovative and Successful Facility - Home Care Services

K R Gangadharan, (Reddy's Heritage Foundation, Hyderabad, India)

Purpose An Innovative Community Model of Home Care Services developed for the first time in India where in trained Bed Side assistants provide care at homes of the elderly. This model if replicated elsewhere would benefit several millions of the elderly in the Globe. Method The hospital that offer in house facility realised that over a long period of hospitalisation, older patients feel exhausted and prefer returning home. Therefore, this new programme was developed. Results Heritage Hospital, India's premier hospital for the elderly was established in 1994. The facility thereafter widened its scope of activities to include many programmes for the elderly, one amongst them being Home Care Services. In India majority people pay their health care costs, as health insurance is not popular. Though a lot is deliberated about fragmentation of joint family system, plenty of people care for their older adults. As in any other part of the World, Older sick patients prefer staying and dying at home. To meet this expectation, Heritage Home Care Services was started. In a short period since its evolution, the programme has attracted hundreds of members within a year. The Bedside Assistants render yeoman services at homes thereby reducing the burden of the families while facilitate employment of young girls who would have otherwise wasted their time. Results The programme found to be a successful model is being replicated in other parts of India. The Government has enlisted Heritage to offer this programme in South India and the first batch of Training of Trainers was completed in September 2000.

Care satisfaction: Advanced hospital-based home care - or Geriatric care in Hospital?

A. Ekdahl (Geriatric Department, University Hospital in Linköping, Sweden), B-G. Emtinger (County council, Linköping, Sweden)

PURPOSE: To answer the questions: What are the differences/similarities in patient groups? What are the differences/similarities in care quality viewed by the patients and their next-of-kin? METHOD: Interviews of randomly chosen patients in advanced hospital-based home care (HBHC)(N=46) and Geriatric care in Hospital (N=57) in the same population and at the same clinic in Sweden. Questionnaires were sent to the next-of-kin by letter and a collection of background data such as age, diagnosis, ability to perform daily activities were made in the beginning and end of the time of care. RESULTS: The mean age (=82 y) and the main groups of diagnoses were the same, although the diagnoses were more concentrated in HBHC versus care in a Geriatric Clinic. The patients were more independent in their functions of daily living in HBHC. More patients in hospital were living alone and there were prominently females dominant. There were no significant differences in how the patients perceived their healthy life situation based on a simple question. When it came to level of information (who are responsible, information about routines, information about their illnesses) HBHC was prior to hospital in all parts. That goes too for the patients and next-of-kins´ judgement of the positive effect of the care time on the illness. CONCLUSION: Both HBHC and care in Hospital are needed in fore geriatric patients. The patients in HBHC were more satisfied with their care than the patients in hospital. The feeling of security in the staff and the home itself were the dominant themes in the verbal comments. The staff is guest in the patients home not the other way around. It is important to develop the care in Hospital in a way that makes it more homelike.

Factors influencing utilization of hospital-based home care service among CVA and DM discharged inpatient elders

Cheng-Chieh Lin (Department of Family Medicine, Center of Community Medicine, China Medical College Hospital, Taichung, R.O.C.), Roger L. Amidon (Department of Health Administration School of Public Health University of South Carolina; USA), Tsai-Chung Li (Department of Medical Research, China Medical College Hospital, Taichung, R.O.C.), Chia-Ing Li (Center of Community Medicine, China Medical College Hospital, China Medical College Hospital, Taichung, R.O.C.)

Home health care has served as a hospital bed and nursing home bed replacement program. To provide home health care for dependent elderly has become one increasing important hospital trend as well as one main mode of long-term care in Taiwan. The aim of this study is to examine what factors influence utilization of hospital-based home care service among CVA and DM discharged inpatient elders. The study sample consisted of 87 consecutive CVA or DM discharged inpatient elders who were eligible for home health care criteria, Barthel Index below 60 with one of catheter, naso-gastric tube, and tracheotomy in China Medical College Hospital from July, 1998 to August, 1999. All eligible discharged inpatient elders were interviewed by a trained interviewer to collect variables about patients such as sociodemographic factors, Barthel Index, ADL, IADL, number of chronic illnesses, home care use, etc. and variables about caregivers such as life satisfaction, care conflict, etc. The statistical analyses were Chi-square test and odds ratios. Mean age of the study subjects is 69.2 years old and 45.8% of them are male. Among patient variables, both number of chronic illness conditions and status after hospitalization reach statistical significance at 0.05. As chronic illness condition increases by one, the odds of utilizing home care service increase by 1.56. The odds of utilizing home care service for those who institutionize is 0.21 times less than the odds for those who stay at home. Among caregiver variables, only caregivers' life satisfaction reaches statistical significance at 0.05. As life satisfaction increases by one, the odds of utilizing home care service decrease by 0.74. The conclusion for our study is that we identified number of chronic disease, residential status after hospitalization, and caregiver's life satisfaction significantly influenced utilization of hospital-based home care service.

Hospital and Home Care for the Elderly Client

M.S. Sheppard (Saskatoon District Health, Saskatoon, Canada), J.M. Franko (Saskatoon District Health, Saskatoon, Canada), M. Rathgeber (Saskatoon District Health, Saskatoon, Canada), D. Treppel (Saskatoon District Health, Saskatoon, Canada), C. Neudorf (Saskatoon District Health, Saskatoon, Canada), S.E. Card (Saskatoon District Health, Saskatoon, Canada), A. Hergott (Saskatoon District Health, Saskatoon, Canada), J. Mann (Saskatoon District Health, Saskatoon, Canada), S. McNeil (Saskatoon District Health, Saskatoon, Canada)

Purpose: To determine the outcomes, care needs and costs of services for elderly patients (age >75 years) following an acute care hospitalization. Method: Patients (N=972) were enrolled upon admission to medical and surgical hospital units. Non-acute hospital days were determined by InterQual(r) ISD-A 2000 criteria. Outcome measures, including self-reported physical and mental health (SF-12), and restrictions in activities of daily living (Stanford Health Assessment Questionnaire), were collected by telephone 2, 4 and 13 weeks post-discharge. Caregiver burden was collected 2 weeks post-discharge. Outcomes and costs for patients provided with home care were compared to those for patients who received non-acute convalescent care days in hospital using logistic regression. Adjustments were made for previous health status and other patient, caregiver and health system characteristics. Results: Preliminary analyses show disposition on discharge was 51.50me, 31.10me with home care, 7.40ng-term care/private care home and 4.7 0eceased. The average length of stay was 11.66 days (s.d.= 11.88, median=8, mode=5). Approximately 200f hospital days reviewed were used to provide non-acute care. The alternate level of care for non-acute days was 330ng-term care and 270me-based care. Analyses in progress will evaluate the outcome status of all patients and caregivers in the study and make comparisons among those who received post-acute home care, post-acute days in hospital, and no post-acute care. Conclusion: This study will have implications for the most appropriate type of post-acute care for elderly patients and the costs associated with each.

Similarities and Differences Between Users of Home Health Services and Home Support Services and Non-Users of Home Care Over Time

Dorothy FORBES, R(University of Saskatchewan, Saskatoon, Canada) Norma STEWART, (University of Saskatchewan, Saskatoon, Canada) Malcolm ANDERSON, (Queen's University, Kingston, Canada) Debra MORGAN, (University of Saskatchewan, Canada) Karen PARENT, (Queen's University, Kingston, Canada)

Funding has not kept pace with the increased demands placed on Canadian Home Care programs. The response has been to attempt to meet the more pressing needs of short-term, post-acute clients and reduce or eliminate home support services. The purposes of the research are to determine the similarities and differences over time between 1) those who use formal, publicly funded home care services and those who do not, and 2) those who use home health services (e.g, nursing and other health care services) and those who use home support services (e.g, housework, personal care, and meal preparation). Analyses of three waves of the National Population Health Surveys (Statistics Canada) will be conducted: 1994/95 n= 17,626; 1996/97 n= 81,804; 1998/99 to be released Dec. 2000. The independent variables include age, gender, living arrangement, education, income levels, availability of informal support, sense of coherence, restriction of activities, perceived health, number of overnight hospitalizations, and number and type of chronic conditions. The dependent variable, use of home care services, is measured in terms of frequency of use and types of services. The analyses consist of data description, bivariate, and multivariate analyses using SPSS 10.0 for WindowsTM. Multiple logistic regression analyses examine the associations of the independent variables with type of home care use. Preliminary findings reveal an increase in the numbers of old-old Canadians who use home care (primarily assistance with personal care, meal preparation, and housework). However, there is a trend towards home care programs offering more professional home health services and less home support services. Identifying the predictors of use of home health care and home support services will assist decision-makers in targeting funding and services to those who will most benefit from these services over the short- and long-term.

Telemedicine and elderly people : application in hospital home

L. Nicolas, A. Franco, L. Amico, S. Paliard-Franco (Hospitalisation à Domicile, Département de Médecine Communautaire, CHU, Grenoble, France), P. Couturier, M. Frossard (Laboratoire Interuniversitaire de Gérontologie, LI2G, CHU, Grenoble, France), H. Provost, A. Chemarin (France Telecom R&D, Meylan, France)

The Grenoble hospital home network takes part in a research, called ViSaDom, in partnership with France Telecom R&D and LI2G. In this research, a telecare system is installed at patient's home. Continuous and coordinate care, are provided for these patients. The device of visiophony is equiped with a video camera, driven from the hospital home offices, and allows to communicate orally and visually, with the patient at home, from the hospital : to see oneself, to pass on documents, to show pressure ulcers, to take photos. The patient has the call's initiative and is free to answer or not, when he's called. Thirty patients have been selected, sixteen have the visiophony's device and fourteen are witness, after drawing lots. The functional dependence (ADL), the state of health (KARNOFSKY), the depression and anxiety (Hospital Anxiety and Depression Scale) and interviews were conducted. The first results, find 370 communications for sixteen patients (on average, twenty-three calls per patient and six minutes per call). Four categories of communications are identified : patient's or family's education, forwarding of medical data, forwarding of logistic information, cooperative work between general practitioner, nurse, patient at home and hospital practitioner in the hospital home offices. A large number of communications is an help to medical decision, at distance, in real time. The anxiety score is significantly lower for the patients with visiophony than for the witness patients ($p<0.05$). The tele-assistance allows new professional behaviours, a better coordination, in real time instead of delayed time, and increases, for the patient the feeling of safety.

SESSION 498

Active Ageing: Changing the Paradigm

Alexandre Kalache, Irene Hoskins, and Peggy Edwards (World Health Organization)

ISSUE: Population ageing raises worrisome questions for policy-makers. Will a proportionately smaller number of working adults be able to provide the support that older people need? Will larger numbers of older people bankrupt our health care and social security systems? How do we ensure that older people remain independent, healthy and active for as long as possible? What are the supportive environments and healthy lifestyles that prevent disease and ensure the highest capacity and autonomy possible? How do we best balance the role of the family and the state when older people do need assistance? How can we best make use of older people's wisdom, experience and talents? How can we improve the quality of life in old age? STRUCTURE: Chair: Alexandre Kalache Speaker: Irene Hoskins, Peggy Edwards and two other speakers from developing countries. Active interaction with audience will be sought. CONTENT One useful way to shift the paradigm from population ageing as a burden on society to older people being a resource is to think about enablement instead of disablement. Disabling processes increase the needs of older people and lead to isolation and dependence. Enabling processes restore function and expand the participation of older people in all aspects of society. If ageing is to be a positive experience, longer life must be accompanied by continuing opportunities for independence, health, productivity, security and enhancement of the quality of life. While the likelihood of experiencing disabilities increases as people age, many disabilities can be prevented or delayed. The World Health Organization and other international organizations (OECD, European Commission, ILO, UNESCO, and others) have adopted the term "active ageing" to express this vision. CONCLUSION The World Health Organization believes that we can afford to grow old if countries enact active ageing policies that enhance the health, independence and productivity of their older citizens. But the time to plan and to act is now. In all countries, measures to help older people remain healthy and active are a necessity, not a luxury. The proposed session will provide the opportunity to explain the concept, review the evidence in favour of active ageing policies, and discuss the actions necessary to ensure an active and healthy old age for people in both developed and developing countries.
Peggy Edwards will provide further clarification regarding the development of WHO's policy framework. Based on her extensive work in the area of health promotion in Canada, she will discuss the conceptual approach behind the development of the policy framework and how the framework could be adapted to fit a large variety of cultural, economic, health and social circumstances in different countries and at various stages of development. More specifically, she will discuss the concept from the perspective of current health policy and health promotion approaches in Canada.
Irene Hoskins will provide a brief overview of the intersectoral origins of the term "active ageing" and how the concept is linked with healthy ageing. She will explore some of the dimensions of social, economic and cultural determinants of health and speak about selected policy responses, particularly in the area of creating a more age-friendly environment. She will also explore the gender perspectives of active ageing in both developed and developing countries. The discussion will include an overview of how new concepts are applied in the current activities of WHO's Ageing and Life Course Team in the areas of preventing disability, creating age-friendly standards, and contributing to the policy debate leading to the Second World Assembly on Ageing.
Alex Kalache will provide the introduction on behalf of WHO. He will discuss the new paradigm on active ageing which affirms the roles of older people as resources and contributors to their communities, societies and the global economy. He will look in particular at health as a central issue in development planning and how health can be maintained both at older ages and throughout the entire life course. Health and barrier-free environments are essential for older people to be part of social and economic development and to ensure a productive old age with a good quality of life. He will link the discussion to the current preparations for the Second World Assembly on Ageing (Madrid 2002).
Alex Kalache will also serve as the moderator for the Round Table.

SESSION 499

Overcoming the Challenge of Attrition in Geriatric Longitudinal Research: Issues and Strategies

C.C. Hogue and W. Somboontanont (University of North Carolina at Chapel Hill, NC, USA)

Attrition threatens validity of longitudinal studies of older adults. Attrition often exceeds 20 0n longitudinal studies that test interventions. Five classes of factors influence attrition: subjects, sites, treatment or intervention, other aspects of design, and implementation. Overcoming potentially biasing losses of subjects requires understanding those factors. Using a single-masked study of integrated resistance training for sedentary, rural community-residing older adults with arthritis as a model, this paper will describe why attrition is a problem, what the likely causes are, and what strategies and techniques were used to limit attrition. In this study, 128 eligible subjects were screened, 106 were enrolled, and 97 completed the study. The attrition rate was 8.5%. The study investigated whether a 16-week training program designed to increase muscle strength, flexibility, aerobic capacity, and speed of task completion, as well as knowledge about, acceptability of, and support for exercise would lead to improved health status and physical activity among the subjects. All subjects (mean age = 72 years) had arthritis of the hip or knee and nearly all had additional chronic conditions Experimental intervention required subjects attendance three mornings a week for 4 hours each time The training was demanding, though individualized and progressive. The control intervention required subjects attendance once a week. Control subjects were very disappointed to have been randomized to the control group. The measurements at 3 times over an 11-month period were challenging because of the nature of the tests, and sometimes because of the frailty of the subject.

Usability of Handheld Technology for Self-Report Survey-Based Instruments in the Elderly

Patrick Boissy [Sargent College of Health and Rehabilitation Sciences, Department of Physical Therapy, Boston University, Boston, USA] Karen Jacobs [Sargent College of Health and Rehabilitation Sciences, Department of Occupational Therapy, Boston University, Boston, USA] Serge Roy [Sargent College of Health and Rehabilitation Sciences, Department of Physical Therapy, Boston University, Boston, USA]

Background Paper and pencil have prevailed as the de facto method of data collection by clinicians and researchers using outcome assessment based on standardized questionnaires and survey instruments. Traditionally, data is transformed into a digital format suitable for computerized quantitative data analysis either by manual data entry or scanner technology. Purpose This pilot study evaluates the usability of a novel approach to collect data digitally from self-report survey-based instruments in the elderly. Elderly subjects (n=25) completed a 48 questions survey instrument on participation and activity (PDI) under development by the Roybal Research Center in Applied Gerontology at Boston University. A data collection program running on a Palm OS handheld device (TRG Pro) connected to a bar code wand scanner (Socket Bar Code Wand CF Card) was used to collect digitally data from the PDI. The instrument paper interface was adapted for self-report use by the elderly. An optimized layout to ensure readability was designed and answer fields to questions from the PDI were coded using bar codes. Method After completing a 5-minute tutorial subjects scanned their answers for each questions from the paper interface using the bar code reader. Participants were filmed while completed the survey to document and identify potential problems. User satisfaction with this new approach was evaluated with a questionnaire and a filmed interview after they completed the survey. Conclusion Preliminary results suggest that data entry on a paper interface using a bar code reader is suitable for elderly subjects and that it doesn't compromise the integrity of the data.

Use of Modern Databases for Analysis of Trends in the Gerontology Development: Possibilities and Perspectives

Yu.K. Duplenko, S.G. Burchinsky (Institute of Gerontology, Kiev, Ukraine)

At the present stage of the science and science-of-science, a great significance is attached to a quantitative evaluation of the main trends in developing a certain research area or research problem and to the assessment of priorities of this development. It is thought that among the most accessible and informative approaches to solving these tasks is analysis of the dynamics of the number of publications or a bibliometric method. To identify the currently developing trends and priorities in gerontology research (1990es), we carried out a bibliometrical analysis of publication massive by the key aspects of aging problem, being reflected in Medline database (internet). The search in the base was conducted in conformity with the occurrence of concrete key words and their combinations, characteristic of the given massive with an interval of 3 years (1991, 1994, 1997, 2000). The most significant result of this search has been the finding of an absolute increase in the total number of publications in gerontology during 1990es. There is an increase in the relative share of works dealing with functional shifts during aging and age-dependent pathology. Of special note is a significant rise of the share of the publications, which consider different aspects of life span prolongation. In the biology of aging, a characteristic phenomenon is an increased proportion of works devoted to the mechanisms of cellular aging. Thus, the analysis that has been made permits to identify research priorities at the turn of the two centuries and opens up possibilities for optimization of future planning.

SESSION 500

Correlates of Subjective Health in Older Adults: A Meta-Analysis

M. Pinquart (Department of Developmental Psychology, Friedrich Schiller University, Jena, Germany)

The paper addresses age-associated changes of subjective health and associations of subjective health with physical health, functional health, and mental health. 180 empirical studies on subjective health in older adults (60+ years) were analyzed using the meta-analytic approach by Rosenthal (N = 177,721). Using longitudinal data-sets, we found an age-associated decline of subjective health (r = -.13), which was stronger in old-old samples (r=-.26) than in young-old samples (r = -.11). Subjective health was correlated with physical health (e.g, symptom checklists; r = .34), functional health (ADL/IADL; r = .32) and mental health (depression; r = .33). However, the size of correlation varied by respondents' age: Correlations of subjective health with physical health and functional health were lower in the old-old than in the young-old. Furthermore, the size of the association between subjective and objective health varied by the method of assessment of objective health, showing highest associations with symptom-checklists and results of medical examinations due to strict protocols. Because of the age-associated decrease of the relationship of subjective health with objective health, we conclude that older adults have higher abilities to adapt their criteria of perceived health to deteriorating objective health so that the age-associated growing number of objective health problems has only limited influence on health perception. However, these coping processes appeared to be insufficient to protect one's health perception totally against deterioration in the old-old, given the stronger age-associated decline in the ratings of absolute health in this group.

Explanatory Factors in Functioning Differences at Elderly- A cross disciplinary perspective -

Tatiana Olteanu, Doina Roditis, Gh. Ghenciu, Liliana Susman, Oana Cuzino

The aim of the study was to understand the extent to which the psychosocial, behavioral, socio - economical risk factors and lifestyle aspects constitute explicit factors of differences in daily functional ability of elderly people. A study sample of 417 elderly subjects, over 65 years, was evaluated (mean age = 73,2 years, SD =+5,6). Socio - medical investigations were carried out for a complex gerontology assessment. We applied the medical and social interviews and we used the assessment methods for the mental and physical functional ability, the functional ability assessment scale ADL/IADL; the Linn's dependency scale, Mini Mental Test - Folstein, the MOS - SF 20 General Health Scale. For statistical processing, we performed comparative, correlational and multiple regression analysis. An increased prevalence of chronic degenerative pathology, with great influence on the functional ability for the entire sample and significant differences in functional ability between men ! and women, were pointed out. Among the explicative variables of functional differences in elder dependency degree found out, those relevant were the pathological configuration and the following variables: perceived health condition, social support interactions, social functioning - social roles and socioeconomic status. These study grounds the need for global evaluating the elder health condition and for optimizing the social and medical support pointed strictly to the aged population necessities.

Functional capacity and self-rated health among elderly people in St. Petersburg

Ilkka Pietila (Kuntokallio Centre for Gerontological Training and Research, Helsinki, Finland) Pertti Pohjolainen (Kuntokallio Centre for Gerontological Training and Research, Helsinki, Finland)

A demographically comprehensive interview study about the living conditions, health status, functional capacity and service needs of 60-89-year-old people in St. Petersburg was carried out in April 2000 as part of a project financed by the European Commission. The research data consisted of 1216 structured interviews (412 men, 804 women). Since there were no up-to-date registers available in St. Petersburg, the sample was made by searching for appropriate people for the sample from door to door. The original sampling frame included regional lists of interviewable groups which represented the age and sex distribution of the regions. Based on the number of interviews (1216) and refusals (176), response rate (87%) could be measured after the sample was completed. Self-rated health was measured with a five-step scale (1=very good, 5=poor). Of the men, 17% felt their health was very good or good, 53% felt it was average, and 30% felt it was rather poor or poor. Among women the corresponding percentages were 7, 46, and 47. On average, older respondents reported poorer health than younger respondents both among men and women. Self-rated health was related to education: people with more than eight years of education reported better health than people with less education. Functional capacity was measured with several questions concerning everyday activities, classified in PADL and IADL activities. For independent living, the most important PADL activities included walking between rooms, use of bathroom, washing, dressing, getting up from bed, and eating. In the youngest age group (60-69), 23% had at least some problems with daily activities. In the age groups 70-79 and 80-89, the respective figures were 41% and 70%.

Health-related quality of life in English & Japanese elderly subjects

M H Shamssain (The Institute of Pharmacy, Chemistry and Biomedical Sciences, School of Sciences, University of Sunderland, Sunderland, United Kingdom) I Ohtsu, A Naito, M Inoue, T Homma (The Institute of Respiratory Medicine, Tsukuba University, Tsukuba, Japan)

PURPOSE: To compare the health-related quality of life between English and Japanese elderly subjects. METHOD: We studied 119 English and 101 Japanese elderly subjects who were randomly selected from the north east of England and Tsukuba in Japan. Health-related quality of life was assessed by SF-36 questionnaire. RESULTS: Mean (SD) age and body mass index (BMI) in English subjects were 76.7 (6.4)y, and 26.7 (5.4) kg/m2 while in Japanese subjects, they were 73.0 (5.9) y and 22.2 (3.60 kg/m2), respectively. Mean subscores of physical functioning (PF), role physical (RF), bodily pain, vitality (V) and social functioning (SF) in Japanese subjects were significantly higher than English subjects (p<0.001). There was negative correlation between age and PF sub-score in English while there was positive correlation between age and general health (GH) sub-score in Japanese subjects. There was negative correlation between BMI and SF in English subjects. There was significant correlation between PF and SF and also between PR and RE in both groups. CONCLUSION; The present study illustrates that, compares to Japanese elderly subjects, English elderly generally have limitations in physical activities or daily activities due to physical health problems and / or emotional problems.

Self-Rated Health and Functioning Among Older People in the Far East: Japan and Korea

Y. Lee (Ajou University School of Medicine, Suwon, Korea), S. Shinkai (Tokyo Metropolitan Institute of Gerontology, Tokyo, Japan)

PURPOSE: To compare and identify factors associated with self-rated health and functional limitations among Japanese and Korean community-dwelling elderly people METHOD: Data from the 1987 National Survey of the Japanese Elderly and the 1994 Survey on the Living Status of the Korean Elderly were used. A nationally representative sample of non-institutionalized persons aged 60 and over was obtained from the two surveys, with 2,200 and 2,058 completed in-person interviews. Multiple regression analysis was conducted to identify significant factors associated with self-rated health and functioning. RESULTS: The percentage of older persons who assessed their health to be “excellent,” “very good,” or “good” was 56.3 0n the Korean sample, compared to 82.6 0n the Japanese sample. In activities of daily living (ADLs), instrumental ADLs, and mobility, the Korean elderly also showed higher levels of functional impairment compared to their Japanese counterpart. Factors associated with these two measures, however, were found to be similar between the two populations, with older age, female, lower socioeconomic status and higher levels of comorbidity and depression being significantly associated with poor self-rated health and functioning. CONCLUSION: A significant gap in the health and functional status between the Japanese and Korean elderly was observed, which may be partially explained by differences in socioeconomic status and chronic disease prevalence. Findings of common factors associated with health and functioning among elderly people in the two countries suggest that health policy for the aged targeting vulnerable segments of the population would be mutually beneficial.

Self-Ratings' Stability or Lability? A Twenty-Year Journey of Self-Rated Health in Germany

Sunkyo Kwon [Technical University Berlin, Institute for Health Sciences, Berlin, Germany]

PURPOSE: During the last two decades, self-rated health (SRH) has been demonstrated in numerous studies to be a valid predictor of mortality and functional capacity even though the underlying (causal) mechanisms of the construct have not been yet unveiled. To understand the meaning of SRH better, it is necessary to grasp its characteristics across different cultures and time frames. In this study we explored whether there were SRH differences across a 20-year period in the Federal Republic of Germany. METHOD: Nationally representative data from the German Federal Center of Health Education (BZGA) were scrutinized for the measurement points 1975, 1980, 1984, 1990, and 1995 (N=10,570, 45.2% male, age range 14-95, mean age 45 years). These included a 6-point Likert-type item on global assessment of one's one health. RESULTS: Former East Germans for whom data were available in 1995 revealed slightly less positive estimates of SRH compared to the West German counterparts (T[3540]=4.56, p=.000). This subsample was excluded in the main analyses. A 5 (measurement points) x 3 (age groups) x 2 (gender) analysis of covariance (with the covariate "no. of symptoms reported which correlated r=.4 with SRH) revealed main effects for measurement points, age groups, and the time by age interaction, but not for the often-cited gender factor. CONCLUSION: SRH in this study showed age differentials and an inverted U-shaped SRH level across the 20 years covered. Self-appraisals of health should be assessed regarding possible age and cohort effects; particularly the latter is subject to the discussion whether it merely reveals differences in level or even in meaning conveyed within a particular time frame.

The Impact of Population and Social Characteristics on Perceived Health and Happiness of the elderly in China

Xiaochun Qiao and Chirayath Suchindran (Carolina Population Center and Department of Biostatistics, The University of North Carolina at Chapel Hill)

Purpose: to analyze the differential impacts among rural and urban areas, sex, age, race, education, and marital status on perceived health and perceived happiness of Chinese elderly. Data and Method: A sample survey on the Support Systems for Elderly was conducted in 12 provinces, autonomous regions and municipalities in mainland China in January 1, 1992. According to the sample coverage this survey can generally represent the status of the elderly in China to a greater and lesser extent. There were 20083 respondents aged 60 and over enumerated in this survey. Perceived health and perceived happiness were asked. This paper examines differences in the perceived health and happiness among regions, sex, age, race, education, marital status and some socioeconomic variables. Logistic regression models with perceived health and happiness coded as binary variables are used for this purpose. Results: Older people in rural areas report higher levels of perceived health than the elderly in urban areas, even though the health expectancy in rural areas is less than that in urban areas in China. Health for females is not as good as for males. The influence of age on health is also highly significant. In general, the higher the age of the elderly, the less healthy the people possess. The minority elderly people are less healthy than the Han, majority people, with an odds ratio of 0.67. The level of education clearly has a positive impact on health, that is the higher education the healthier the elderly have. The marital status is not significant on health influences. Comparing with the elderly who is living with their spouses, the only variable of the elderly whose spouse has already passed away is significant, with an odd ratio of 1.1. Considering the happiness perceived, the elderly living in rural areas are less happy than that living in urban areas. The female elderly feel happier than males. Almost all the dummy variables for age are not significant, but the race, education and the marital status are all highly significant. The minority elderly are less happy than the elderly living in the urban areas. The educated elderly feel happier than illiterate one. And married elderly who have still lived with their spouse feel much happier than the elderly who have no or not lived with their spouses. Some socioeconomic variables are also taking a positive role on health and happiness. Conclusion: Self-perceived health and happiness depend upon not only the physical and mental health status but also their expectation on health. Age is an important variable to health but not to happiness and variables of marital status and education are all-important to health and happiness to the elderly.

SESSION 501

Associations Between Panoramic Radiographic Findings and Self-Reported Medical Conditions in Older Subjects

R.E. Persson L.G. Hollender, Hujoel, P.P, G.R. Persson, Powell, L.V, H.A. Kiyak (University of Washington), M.I. MacEntee, C.Wyatt (University of British Columbia).

Abstract: Older people are at greater risk for systemic and oral diseases. Specifically, periodontitis has been associated with several systemic conditions. It is important to assess risks before the disease advances. Purpose: To analyze patient-based health information (PHI) and findings from panoramic radiographs PMXs. Older subjects included 485 men and 579 women (mean age 67.2, SD +4.7) enrolled in a clinical trial in Seattle or Vancouver. PMXs identified carotid calcification (CC), osteoporosis (OP), and horizontal alveolar bone loss (HBL). Number of vertical defects >3mm and molars with furcation invasion were identified. Results: Mean teeth remaining was 21.8 (SD +8.1). Self-reports (PHI) of OP revealed an 8.2% prevalence overall, 12.9% in Caucasian women. The Klemetti PMX Index identified 11% with signs of OP, and high correlations between PHI and PMX. Odds ratio for PMX findings of OP and HBL was 1.8 (95% CI 1.0-3.0) in Caucasian women. Intraclass correlation was not significant between PHI of heart disease and CC on the PMX, but was for a positive PHI of a stroke and CC on the PMX (ICC=0.21, 95% CI=0.06-0.33, $p<.01$). Elders with HBL had significantly fewer teeth ($p<.001$). Conclusions: Radiographic signs of osteoporosis are correlated with patient-reports of this condition, as are signs of carotid calcification with stroke. There is less association between self-reports of heart disease and PMX-detected carotid calcification. Risks for periodontitis (positive HBL score), osteoporosis, and stroke are significant in older persons. Panoramic radiographs can be very helpful in detecting early signs of these conditions. This clinical trial is monitored by an independent Data & Safety Monitoring Board, and is supported by NIH/NIDCR Grant No. RO1 DE12215.

Ethnic Differences in Preventive Health Behaviors and Oral Health Status

H.A. Kiyak, P.P. Hujoel, R.E. Persson, G.R. Persson, L.V. Powell (Univ. of Washington), M.I.Macentee, C. Wyatt (Univ. of British Columbia).

Abstract: "TEETH" (Trials to Enhance Elders' Teeth and Oral Health) is a randomized clinical trial to prevent tooth loss in older adults. Purpose: This presentation describes ethnic differences at baseline in oral health status and preventive health of elders in one research site(Seattle). Criteria for participation included: no preventive dental visits in >1 year, >4 teeth, age >60. The sample included 700 elders in Seattle and 400 in Vancouver, B.C, but only the 270 Caucasians and 230 Chinese in Seattle were compared. Oral exams were conducted using NIDCR criteria. Interviews were completed in English or Chinese on demographics, diseases, medications, and preventive behaviors. Results: Ethnic differences emerged on oral health status and health behaviors. Caucasians had fewer sound coronal and root surfaces ($p<.0001$ each), resulting in 21.7 teeth vs. 22.7 for Chinese elders ($p<.05$), and higher DMFS scores ($p<.0001$). Chinese elders displayed worse periodontal health, with deeper pockets, more exposed root surfaces, and greater attachment loss (AL), including more sites with AL >5 mm (all at $p<.0001$). Caucasian elders practiced prevention more than Chinese elders, including limiting red meat, sugar and salt in their diet, using vitamins, and consuming more foods with fiber, flossing and performing self-exams (all at $p<.001$). Both groups were irregular dental service users, but Caucasians had had more recent check-ups for general health ($p<.04$), blood pressure ($p<.0002$), vision and foot health ($p<.001$ each). Conclusion: Although all participants in this clinical trial are low income and irregular dental care users, cultural factors influence health behaviors and oral health outcomes. This clinical trial is monitored by an independent Data and Safety Monitoring Board, and is supported by NIH/NIDCR Grant No. RO1 DE12215.

Health-related behaviours reported by three ethnic groups of older adults in British Columbia.

M.I.Macentee, C. Wyatt (Univ. of British Columbia, Vancouver, BC, Canada); H.A. Kiyak, P.P. Hujoel, R.E. Persson, G.R. Persson, L.V. Powell (Univ. of Washington, Seattle WA. USA).

Abstract: Purpose: Ethnic diversity in western societies produces a need for sensitivity to health-related beliefs and practices of ethnic minorities. Subjects aged 60-75 years in Vancouver, BC who participate in a multi-centre (Seattle and Vancouver) clinical trial to enhance elders' tooth and oral health (TEETH) were recruited from ethnic groups in community centres and through newspaper announcements. They were interviewed in their own language to identify preventive health-related behaviours. This investigation focuses on nutritional, hygienic and self-examination behaviours reported at baseline by subjects from Caucasian, Chinese or Indian backgrounds who live in the Lower Mainland of BC. Information was recorded from at least 213 subjects, about two-thirds of whom were Caucasian, one-fifth were from India, and the remainder from China. We analysed dichotomous responses relating to behaviours to quantify ($p<0.01$) relationships between variables using contingency tables with chi-squared statistics. Results: Subjects from India, compared to the others, were less likely to have smoked tobacco, but they were more likely to limit consumption of red meat, salt and sugar, and to conduct physical self-examinations. Caucasians, in contrast, were more likely to consume fibrous foods and vitamins. There were no significant differences in the oral hygiene behaviours of the three groups - nearly everyone brushed their teeth but few used dental floss. Conclusions: concerns for nutrition and hygiene were more prevalent among elders from India than among Caucasian or Chinese elders. The trial is monitored by an independent Data and Safety Monitoring Board, and is supported by the NIH (USA) RO1 DE12215. a

Oral Health Beliefs and Attitudes of Greek and Italian Older Adults

Rodrigo Mariño (University of New England, Armidale, NSW, Australia) Victor Minichiello (University of New England, Armidale, NSW, Australia) Clive Wright (Dental Health Services Victoria, Australia) Margot Schofield (University of New England, Armidale, NSW, Australia)

INTRODUCTION: Oral health status of immigrant groups, particularly older immigrants, is a major public health challenge in Australia. However, oral health is a less studied area of older immigrants' health and quality of life. Little is known about their oral health needs, what they think about their oral health needs and their knowledge of and attitudes to oral health. AIMS: This paper describes a qualitative approach to obtaining information needed for designing and evaluating a culturally appropriate oral health intervention for Greek and Italian older persons living in Melbourne. The study was particularly concerned with understanding the oral health meanings and experiences of older migrants. METHODS: 17 focus group discussions were conducted between June and July 2000. 172 participants were recruited from Italian/Greek elderly clubs in Melbourne. Transcripts were analyzed for themes and key concepts. RESULTS: Participants were highly aware of the major oral disease and the treatments available. They were also aware of dental caries preventive measures. Findings indicate that, although they received the message of periodic dental check-ups, barriers interfering with seeking check-ups included past experiences with treatments, cost, the waiting period for treatment and the location of public services. It was also found that participants held a number of false beliefs and myths, and strong negative attitudes towards dentistry, in particular towards public oral health services. CONCLUSION: These results were important precursors in the design of an oral health intervention program for migrant groups. The data suggest that to increase use of oral health services, as well as reducing costs and waiting periods, specific myths, misconceptions and negative attitudes must be addressed.

Oral Health Status and Dental Care in a Hospitalized Elderly Group

J.Baldisserotto, D.M.Padilha (Geriatrics and Gerontology Institute of Pontifícia Universidade Católica and Faculty of Dentistry of Federal University of Rio Grande do Sul, Porto Alegre, Brazil.

The aim of this work was to identify the oral health status of a group of hospitalized elderly patients and to provide them with basic dental care. This is a pioneer programme involving dental students as a part of their learning in Odontogeriatrics Discipline. All patients were examined by dental students using W.H.O. methods.Dental care was also provided by the students. The programme was carried out on a weekly basis and lasted for an academic year. The majority of the elderly were edentulous and needing dentures mainly for the lower jaw.Root caries was a serious problem related to the remaining teeth.The hygiene of the phrotesis were bad. It was also identified that the caregivers did not peform any activities related to patient's oral hygiene, independently of their impairment. It was concluded that the hospitalized elderly patients need dental care and the health caregivers should be prepared to develop preventive actions. This experience was also very important for the improvements in the teaching programme in Odontogeriatrics at the Dental Faculty of the Federal University of Rio Grande do Sul.

Relationship Between Systemic Diseases and Periodontal Disease in Three Mexican Elderly Community's

R. Merchant, R. Reyes, L.M. Gutierrez, C. Yaca, (Institute of Medical Sciences and Nutrition Salvador Zubiran department of geriatric medicine), A. Borges, (Universidad Nacional Autonoma de Mexico, facultad de odontología) Mexico City, Mexico.

Purpose: The aim of this study is to clarify the relationship between systemic diseases and periodontal disease, we wanted to know if periodontal disease could be consider as a risk factor which modifies the course of many systemic diseases: Diabetes Mellitus, Pneumonia, Infectious endocarditic, Hypertension, and osteoporosis. Methods: Three communities of at least 600 individuals were selected. All people who had lived for at least 5 years in the community and who were able to answer the questionnaire by their selves were included in the study. Sociodemografic conditions were divided into urban (Urban Center president Aleman CUPA), periurban (Isidro Fabela) and rural (Solís valley) populations. The sample was selected by aleatory and systematic system. The information was collected by two forms: clinical examination which included the extension and severity index to periodontal disease, dental prosthesis examination and interview to answer the questionnaire. Information was captured in SPSS program using numerical codes, and the statistical analysis was made with OTTS ratio, Xi square for establishing associations between demographic topics and clinics, and multivariate analysis. Results: in a preliminary analysis was observed relationship between periodontal disease, total dental prosthesis with several systemic diseases and periodontal disease with glucemia control. Conclusions: the principal characteristic in all patients show changes in the bolus consistence, maybe this change is the principal reason to start the frailly in the older people, and its possible if would describe the oral status in patients whit frailly.

Secondary Dentin Formation is Associated with Age and may be Linked to Heart Disease

S. Woo, H. Goodis (UCSF School of Dentistry, San Francisco, CA USA), R. Garcia (Boston University School of Dental Medicine, Boston, MA USA), A. Kahn (UCSF School of Dentistry, San Francisco, CA USA)

Secondary dentin formation (SDF) occurs throughout adult life leading to the complete occlusion of the tooth root canal (pulp) space in some individuals. Here we examined whether SDF (canal occlusion) occurs steadily with age or is influenced by select local and systemic factors. Dental x-rays of healthy mandibular first bicuspids (premolars) were scanned and the images analyzed from a cohort of 72 middle-aged to elderly men. These x-rays had been taken at 3-year intervals in a long-term study that also included a dental exam and a medical questionnaire. Periodontal disease (PD), cervical wear, occlusal wear, smoking and heart disease were recorded for each tooth/patient. The extent of SDF-induced canal occlusion was determined by calculating root canal height to tooth height, and canal width to root width at the cervico-enamel junction (CEJ) and at increments down the root surface. At 1/4 and 3/4 distances from the CEJ, the root canal was scored as being occluded or open. The degree of SDF (canal occlusion) was significantly associated with subject age by all criteria ($p<.0001$ to $p<.0003$). An association was also observed between heart disease and SDF using measurements of CEJ ratio and 3/4 distance ratio ($p<.014$ and $p<.05$). No relationship was observed between SDF and smoking, periodontal disease (PD), tooth occlusal or cervical wear. These results confirm age as a (the?) major risk factor for the rate/ degree of SDF (occlusion) and suggest a possible association between SDF and heart disease, a new finding reminiscent of reports linking PD to heart disease.

SESSION 502

A Cooperative Continence Program that Works

M. Foley (Carewest, Calgary, Canada), C. Richardson (SCA Hygiene, Calgary, Canada)

The purpose of this paper is to outline the development of a continence program (bladder and bowel) and the benefits to Carewest, its residents and staff. Continence is a key component of caring for elderly clients in the community and continuing care centres affecting resident comfort and dignity. It can also be costly in terms of nursing time and budget. Carewest is a public provider of Continuing Care in Calgary, Alberta, Canada. In partnership with SCA Hygiene (an international manufacturer of incontinence products), Carewest has developed an interdisciplinary program, meeting resident needs by thorough assessment, appropriate product usage, education and ongoing cost analysis. This ongoing comprehensive managed care approach has resulted in cost effective, quality continence care for a population of over 1,000 residents.

A Piddly Problem? Designing an Intervention to Improve Continence Care in a Primary Care Context.

Farida Tilbury and Sally Roach (Royal Australian College of General Practitioners Research Unit, Perth, Australia)

Incontinence is a potentially 'socially terminal' condition which is sometimes inadequately treated. GPs often share the commonly held, but incorrect, assumption that it is a normal part of aging. Older patients frequently receive inadequate or inappropriate care because of low levels of GP knowledge about effective treatments and the services provided by allied health professionals. The paper describes the development of an intervention designed to raise public awareness; decrease the taboo nature of the subject; train GPs to treat the condition; and enhance integrated care from a number of health professionals. The ultimate goal of the intervention is to enable continued community dwelling among the older population. Findings of the research, which included surveys, interviews and focus groups with patients and health care providers, indicate that improved care results from better communication between health providers themselves and between health providers and patients. A specific mode of training for GPs which includes academic detailing and integrated provider workshops is described. Examples of posters, pamphlets and clinical practice guidelines developed for the intervention are used as illustrations.

Development and application of urinary incontinence self care program for community elderly women

M. Song (College of Nursing, Seoul National University, Seoul,

Korea)

The Purpose of this study were to develop urinary incontinence self care program for the community older women and to evaluate the effect of the program. The program was developed based on literature review and author's experience from the previous study. the program consisted with 4 weeks of group education which includes anatomy physiology of urinary and reproductive system, health promoting life style for continence and pelvic floor muscle exercise training. In order to evaluate the effect of the program, 8 weeks of research was carried out. Eighteen elderly mildly incontinent women was recruited from the two senior citizen's center in the community. For the first 4 weeks of base line data collection period (period I) , only general health promotion education was given. For the next 4 weeks (Period II), incontinence self care program was applied to the subjects. Subjective report of degree of incontinence was compared between the period I and Period II and there was significant reduction in degree of incontinence from period 1 to period II (p=.014). There was no significant difference in self esteem between the two period. In conclusion, the program showed effectiveness and feasibility to be utilized for mildly incontinent community elderly women.

Enhancing Sleep for Nursing Home Residents and Reducing Costs: Changing Night Practice and Introducing a New Incontinence Product

Susan Slaughter, Bev Neault, Connie Haseldon, Wendy Ryan (Bethany Care Society, Calgary, Canada)

Purpose: To facilitate an undisturbed night sleep for nursing home residents, night nursing practice was reviewed and adjusted. Method: On a trial basis for 7 days, nursing staff were instructed not to awaken any residents to turn or change them. Changing and turning occurred only at the request of the resident. Resident characteristics were monitored on all shifts. Observations included any signs of skin breakdown, wetness of the bed linen, and unit cost of incontinence products. The few residents who were wet in the morning were provided with a more expensive and extra absorbent incontinence product. Resident characteristics and costs were monitored following this change in practice for 7 days. Staff also reported on the impact the practice change had on the quality of their work. Results: Residents slept through the night. Call bells were less frequently used. Staff had time to respond promptly to the special needs of the few residents who were unable to sleep. Bed linen was less often soiled. Unit cost of incontinence products was reduced. Conclusion: The routine of turning and changing residents several times through the night was adjusted according to the individual needs of residents. Shifting from routine to individualized care at night has resulted in enhanced sleep for residents, increased job satisfaction for nursing staff, and reduced costs for administrators.

The Prevalence Of Faecal Incontinence Amongst Community Residing Older People

Nia Edwards, Dee Jones (University of Wales College of Medicine, Cardiff, UK)

Purpose: Faecal incontinence (FI) has significant impact not only upon quality of life but upon provision of care amongst older people in the community. FI may ultimately lead to a breakdown in coping strategies of informal carers and subsequent preventable institutionalisation. A reluctance to report symptoms due to embarrassment , perceived lack of effective treatment and management has led to a recognised underestimation of the problem. Our aim was to ascertain the prevalence of FI and identify the health and sociodemographic characteristics of those afflicted. Method; A sample of 3000 older people was selected randomly from Family Health Services Authorities. 2818 men and women aged 65 years and over were interviewed in their own homes: a response rate of 96%. Validated quetsionnaires were used to measure health and social characteristics. Results: 78(3%) of respondents admitted FI. No significanct association was found between increasing age and FI; 38 (2%) aged 65-74 years and 40 (3%) >75 years (p=0.1). A significant association between FI and gender was found ((15 (1%) of men v 63(4%) of women (p,0.0005)). Similarly there was a significant association between FI and anxiety (p,0.00001), FI and depression.(p<0.0001), FI and disability (,p,0.000. Of those with FI 69% had coexistent urinary incontinence. When contact with professionals was explored over 50% stated they had not discussed their FI problem with a health care profesisonal. Conclusion: Appropriate therapeutic intervention and treatment of FI can improve symptoms and quality of life. This together with patients' reluctance to report symptoms leads us to suggest that older people should be specifically and proact ively assessed for continence problems. The associated health characteristics can not be assumed to be caused by FI due to the cross-sectional nature of this study but the findings indicate that these people have a great deal of morbidity that requires thorough assessment and management.

Urinary incontinence and subsequent mortality among the elderly living in the Canary Islands (Spain).

B.J. Anía (Hospital Doctor Negrín and Universidad de Las Palmas de Gran Canaria, Spain), A.J. Santana, J.L. Suárez, C.D. Acosta, S. Rodríguez, L. Guerra (Sociedad Canaria de Geriatría y Gerontología, Spain).

Purpose: To ascertain the prevalence of urinary incontinence in the population of elderly people living in the Canary Islands and its effect on subsequent mortality. Method: A random sample was drawn that was representative of the people aged 65 and over living in the Canary Islands. Sampled subjects were asked to participate in a survey about functional status done in their homes by physicians. Survival was ascertained more than three years later. RESULTS: We studied 285 elderly subjects, of whom 278 (109 males and 169 females) provided data on incontinence. Sixty-eight (62.4%) of the males and 86 (50.9%) of the females had never experienced any trouble with continence. Occasional incontinence was reported by 34 (31.2%) of the men and 53 (31.4%) of the women. Incontinence was deemed frequent by 7 (6.4%) of the males and 30 (17.8%) of the females. Undergarment pads were worn by 5 (4.6%) males and 24 (14.2%) females. Only 1 man and 1 woman had a permanent urinary catheter. Mortality of subjects with frequent incontinence was 42.4%, whereas only 15.6% of those with occasional incontinence and 10.0% without incontinence died during follow-up. Frequent incontinence was found significant as a risk factor for mortality independent from age. Conclusion: Frequent incontinence is found about three times more often among elderly females than males, and is a risk factor for subsequent mortality. Percentage of use of undergarment pads approximates the prevalence of frequent incontinence.

Urinary retention in the elderly.

de PETIGNY , G. AIME, S. BAMBIS, R. ILTIS, M.C SCHATZ (BISCHWILLER Gerontology Hospital)

This prospective study includes the aged patients (75 years and more) who are admitted in the Clinical Gerontology Ward of BISCHWILLER Hospital, to estimate the prevalence of urinary retention and to analyse the predictive factors. An ultrasonic examination is done for all the patients included , in the first 48 hours of the admission, to evaluate the quantity of urine retained after miction. The criterion to consider the urine residue as pathologic is a residue volume more then 250 cc or more then 20 % of miction volume. Among the 141 patients included in the study 22,7 % have a urinary retention. This anomaly should be sought after, even if there are no urinary incontinence (31 % of the studied population) or other clinical sign. Urinary retention, even without symptoms may give rise to complications ; there is more urinary infection 47 % of the studied population (p < 0, 001). The better management of these patients may reduce the prevalence of urinary retention by acting on the factors which initiate this disorder : bladder irritation (constipation), drugs and ecological factors (the motor impairment is very strongly related to urinary retention).

SESSION 503

A Comparison of Life Satisfaction and Mood in Community Dwelling Elders and Nursing Home Residents

S. Gueldner, S. Loeb, J. Penrod {School of Nursing, The Pennsylvania State University, University Park, PA, USA}

The purpose of this study was to compare life satisfaction and mood in a sample of 70 nursing home residents and 68 dwelling elders of comparable age and health status. A two-group comparative design was used. Instruments used included Pfeiffer's Short Portable Mental Status Questionnaire, the Profile of Mood States, and Life Satisfaction Index A. The questionnaires were administered in a one-to-one interview format. The sample was provided by six nursing homes and community facilities where seniors are likely to gather. Even after controlling for the effects of gender and age, respondents living in the community had higher life satisfaction scores than nursing home residents ($p<.001$). Likewise, nursing home residents scored higher on the Tension-Anxiety ($p<.01$), Depression Dejection ($p<.001$) and Confusion-Bewilderment ($p<.05$) sub-scales of the Profile of Mood States, and lower on the Vigor-Activity subscale. As age increased, elders scored lower on the Anger-Hostility and Vigor-Activity indexes. These findings confirm the sensitivity of these instruments for eliciting differences in life satisfaction and mood between groups of elders with different characteristics or life circumstances. These findings serve as compelling evidence that the nursing home environment gives rise to unhealthy feelings among the residents. Focus groups could be conducted to provide mentally alert residents the opportunity to tell us, in their own words, what it is about their environmental experience that makes them feel less satisfied, more depressed, and less vigorous than those who live in the community.

CONSTITUENTS OF HEALTHY AGEING IN THE INDIAN ELDERLY

D. Jamuna & K. Lalitha, Centre for Research on Ageing, Dept. of Psychology,S.V. University, Tirupati Δ 517 502, INDIA.

Promoting "healthy ageing" is one of the major concerns of Gerontological research. Healthy ageing has been defined in many ways in Gerontological studies. In the present study healthy ageing was measured in terms of different facets of Quality of life in a sample of 640 community dwelling elderly (60-89). The subjects with no marked disabilities and cognitively intact were included. The subjects who have reported good quality of life were screened and included to investigate the psycho-social constituents of healthy ageing among them. Healthy agieng constitutes physical, psychological, level of independence, social, environmental and spiritual domains. Results indicate that age, economic condition, type of living arrangement, flexibility of behaviour, satisfaction with familial contacts, acceptance of personal ageing changes, physical and mental activity and certain life values were the significant constituents of healthy ageing. The implications of the findings and significance of interventions to promote healthy ageing are discussed.

Quality of Life among Indian Elderly with specific reference to Urban-rural Differences.

M.Easwaramoorthy (Personality Division, Defence Institute of Psychological Research, Delhi, India

Quality of Life was studied among elderly with reference to urban rural differences. Sample (N=380,236 from Urban and 144 from rural areas ,Aged 60+) was drawn using multi-stage stratified random sampling procedure from the state of Tamil Nadu, India. Quality of life was studied using various Standardized measures relating to Economic, Physical, Psychological and social well-being. The data was analysed using Descriptive and inferential statistics the results indicated that elderly living in urban areas have significantly higher mean scores than the elderly living in rural areas on personal income, perception of financial status, health awareness, mental status, leisure activities and self rated quality of life. The rural aged in comparison to urban aged has significantly higher mean scores on self-rated health. The results suggest that urban elderly have a better quality of life than the rural elderly

Reminicing and Sentiments as a Strategy for Social Welfare

D. Garcia-Puebla (Casa Club del Jubilado y Pensionado del ISSSTESON, Hermosillo, Sonora, México)

PURPOSE: To Provide an economical resource where reminiscing and sentiments are used as a strategy for a successful aging process. Stimulating the principles of aging given by the United Nations: independence, participation, care, fulfillment and dignity. METHOD: The memories written by 25 subjects (range 60-85 years) during a literature workshop, where the basic material is their reminiscences written following a pattern offered them. And the application of an instrument to know if there are personal and social improvement. RESULTS: Enhance the quality of life of the participants. Improvement their personal care and appearance. Their relationships and share with relatives and social acquaintances become more fulfilling. They learn and develop their potentialities. They find more meaning to their lives. They feel again able to give and that satisfy them. CONCLUSION. This is a strategy recommended in countries where low budgets are assigned for elderly programs also in wealthy to preserve their traditions. This activity improve on their relationships and give the elderly the opportunity to approaching the new generations.As far as they leave their work written also they satisfy the need of transcend. By the way they leave a legacy of history, folklore and culture for new generations to look back on.

Successful Aging from the perspective of elderly people.

M.von Faber (Leiden University Medical Center, Leiden, The Netherlands)

PURPOSE: Although Successful Aging is an often used phrase, it is not clear which indicators characterize elderly people as 'successful'. In the Leiden 85-plus Study, we combined quantitative research and qualitative research about the concept of Successful Aging. METHODS: We screened a population based sample of citizens of Leiden (n=705) aged 85 years for optimal physical, psycho-cognitive and social functioning and feelings of well-being. If Successful Aging is considered as optimal functioning and well-being, 100f the participants could be classified as such in the first cross-sectional analysis. In addition, we performed in-dept interviews with 27 participants about the concept of Successful Aging. RESULTS: It appeared that most elderly people viewed 'success' as a process of adaptation rather than an optimal state of being. They valued well-being and social functioning more than optimal physical and psycho-cognitive functioning. Well-being is linked to Successful Aging and means maintaining a feeling of continuity of the self-identity. Remarkable is the different view on physical functioning in old age.This might be explained by the ambiguity in perceptions on 'normal' aging from elderly persons and their social environment. Furthermore, adaptation related to decreased functioning, the social context and well-being plays a role. CONCLUSION: Both quantitative and qualitative research showed that a feeling of well-being was not directly related to optimal physical functioning. The in-dept interviews showed that maintaining a satisfactory balance between adaptation and identity contribute to a feeling of successfulness in old age despite physical limitations. From this perspective, many persons can be considered to be successfully aged.

The Myth of "Successful Aging" in Western Cultures

Helga Reimann, rer.pol.habil, phil. (retir.of Sociology, University of Augsburg, Germany)

The concept of "successful aging" is to be analyzed as to its meaning and realization in developed countries as well as to its relation to the overall cultures. It is also examined whether it is transferable to other, less modernized cultures. Several methods from cultural sociology are used: the "Verstehen" of Max Weber, the "Relationieren" of Karl Mannheim etc.. Visual material from advertisement is used to exemplify. The ideal of "successful aging" proves to be mostly unatainable, and is still widely influential, especially for the beliefs and practices of the "new elderly" (a category in German gerontological studies). It is deeply imbeded in the protestant ethic of an active, rational and self-disciplined life-style promising "rewards" in a blessed long life. "Problematic aging" is often denied and seen as an individual failure rather than as the course of nature, the result of adverse living conditions, and as a collective responsability. On the other hand the few "successfully aging persons" could help to dissolve the negative image of the aged. The Western myth of "successful aging" does not seem to be a promising item for globalization, except for the elites of those regions that are already strongly "westernized". The cultures and especially the religions in traditional societies or settings provide them with other ideals of well-being in old age and adequate rituals to reach them (like meditation) that are in turn "imported" by discontent "Westerners" - an example of the interchange characterizing cultural globalization.

SESSION 504

Elder care and work-family problems in Brazil

Karsch, Ursula (Catholic University, São Paulo, Brazil)

This paper address issues related to work and elder care in Brazil, focusing the work-family problem in the country, particularly with respect to the care of elders family members. The data were derived from various sources, including own research, publications, government documents, and personal communications. The family in Brazil is undergoing a transformation as a result of social and demographic changes. Brazil's older population is rapidly growing, but neither the society nor the government have given much attention to issues concerning the aging of its population. The increase in elderly women so that they outnumber elderly men, unemployment and the informal labour market, the labour force participation rate of women age 40 to 60 (25% in 1980 to 43% in 1995) and patterns of marriage and divorce contribute to changes in family structure and new roles in family support. A continuous internal migration from rural to urban areas, predominantly by young people in search of opportunities in city labour markets are changing Brazilian household composition. The proportion of elderly living alone is also increasing, especially for women, and the percentage of older women living alone grew from 9.4% in 1970 to 14.5% in 1989. A study in the city of São Paulo (1989) revealed that 90% of elders lived with at least one other person (31% with persons of the same generation). A mutual support system can be observed whereby the younger help the older in their personal and physical needs and the other help the younger with housing and monetary support.

Eldercare in an Aging Society: Analysis of Health Professionals' Work and Family Lives

C. Ward-Griffin, J.B. Brown, A. Vandervoort, S. McNair (University of Western Ontario, London, Canada)

PURPOSE: Although a number of studies have examined the effects of combining work and eldercare family responsibilities, little is known about a unique group of employed family caregivers- those who provide care simultaneously to patients/clients and to elderly relatives. The purpose of this qualitative study was to examine the ways in which women representing four different health professions (nursing, medicine, physiotherapy, social work) experience their dual roles both as health providers and as family caregivers. METHOD: Purposive sampling was used to obtain 10 “double duty” caregivers from each profession, who provided at least one hour of care per week to an elderly relative. During in-depth individual and focus group interviews, participants were asked about the conditions, processes, and consequences of combining professional and family caregiving roles. RESULTS: Study findings revealed that health professionals who assume family caregiving responsibilities are located at the juncture of public and private domains of caregiving where they must constantly negotiate and redefine the boundaries between their professional and personal caregiving roles. Due to competing work and family demands and contradictory expectations, participants reported difficulty in assuming these dual caregiving roles, especially within the current climate of health care restraint CONCLUSION: Boundaries between professional and personal caregiving are continuously negotiated by health professionals who also assume elder caregiving responsibilities within the family. Changes in both practice and policy are needed to address the difficulties encountered by double duty caregivers.

Ever-Single, Older Women's Caregiving Dilemma

Jennifer Baumbusch (Simon Fraser Health Region, Burnaby, Canada)

PURPOSE: A larger study on ever-single, older women's relationships with the health care system uncovered the dilemma of access to informal care that confronts this population as they age. METHOD: A critical, feminist theoretical framework was used to guide this qualitative study. The sample consisted of 8 ever-single women between the ages of 65 and 77 living in a mid-sized, Southwestern Ontario city. Data were generated using semi-structured interviews. RESULTS: Most of the women were experienced informal caregivers, having cared for aging parents, siblings, and friends. For themselves, potential sources of informal care were siblings and friends, and occasionally nieces and nephews, however, most of the women were unable to identify an individual who would be available to provide informal care on an ongoing basis. They demonstrated great reluctance to burden anyone with taking on this role for themselves. Overall, the women were willing to use their financial and material resources or relocate to a residential care facility rather than have family or friends provide long-term informal care in the community. CONCLUSIONS: There is growing pressure on older Canadians and their informal support networks to manage health care needs in the absence of formal services. For often-invisible populations, such as ever-single, older women, this may put greater demand on their material resources or put them at risk for premature institutionalization. Greater recognition of the needs of subgroups of older adults is required to meet the diverse health care needs of an aging population.

Nonsupport and Conflict in the Relationships of Women Caregivers

Anne Neufeld, RN, (Faculty of Nursing, University of Alberta, Edmonton, CANADA) Margaret J. Harrison, RN, (Faculty of Nursing, University of Alberta, Edmonton, CANADA)

PURPOSE: The purpose of this qualitative study was to examine women caregivers' descriptions of nonsupport and conflict. Nonsupport and conflict in caregivers' relationships with family and friends may have a greater impact on functioning and health outcomes than support, but have received limited attention in research. METHOD: From a larger study of social support and caregiving with 20 women caring for a relative with dementia we identified 8 women who reported both support and nonsupport. Each woman was interviewed at least 3 times over a period of 2 years. The interviews were tape recorded, transcribed verbatim and subjected to thematic content analysis. RESULTS: In relationships with family members women caregivers described dissonance between their appraisal of the care recipient's needs and the views of other family members. They also reported that family members criticized their caregiving decisions. Offers of aid were often absent or unfulfilled in relationships with both family members and friends. In relationships with friends, the women described exclusion from social activities and subsequent isolation. CONCLUSION: The findings of this study indicate that nonsupport as well as support exists in caregivers' relationships and varies with the type of relationship. This information extends theoretical perspectives on social support and can assist professionals to develop interventions that are specific to the type of relationship and the form of nonsupport that caregivers experience.

Relation Between Perceived Role of Family and Behavior of the Person with Dementia

G. deGeest (Centre on Aging, University of Victoria, Victoria, BC, Canada)

The relation between perceived role of family and the behavior of the person with dementia was examined in a population of older adults. The researcher utilized two instruments in data collection: The Family Perceptions of Caregiving Role (FPCR), and The Cohen-Mansfield Agitation Inventory (CMAI). A total of 40 persons with dementia each had a family respondent and a nurse respondent. Results from the analysis used to examine the predictive difference between the behavior for the person with dementia and the frequency of family visits revealed little or no significant difference. Correlational analysis provided little evidence of a strong link between the family's perceived role in partnering, and the behavior of the person with dementia, specifically the agitation levels. Interventions by family and staff may have a profound effect on behavior, but there may be additional influences responsible for the agitation levels observed in this study.

The Impact of Cultural Changes on the Traditional Roles of Elderly Men and Women

J.G. Garcia (Department of Gerontology, University of South Florida, Florida, USA), J.I. Kosberg (School of Social Work, University of Alabama, Alabama, USA)

Worldwide, women have been the major family caregivers; men have been in positions of economic and social power. Traditional gender role distinctions have continued into old age. As a result of changing values in many countries, females are increasingly pursuing careers and education, and are less-likely to be economically, socially, and psychologically dependent upon male relatives. Aging males, influenced by pressures for gender equity, are becoming less domineering and more caring. There is evidence that older males are becoming caregivers and experiencing caregiving adversities, as do females. Also, older wives, caring for impaired husbands and witnessing the freedom of younger women, can become dissatisfied with their marriages. The possibility of anger, marital conflict, and abuse can result. It is suspected that such problems are likely to occur in developing nations and in rural areas where traditional norms are more likely to be maintained. To be discussed are the experiences and research findings in the U.S. with regard to individual, family, marital, and intergenerational conflicts resulting from cultural changes that affect and challenge traditional male and female roles of elderly populations. Aging men will need new skills, education, and sensitivity for taking on different roles and older married couples will need awareness of tensions that result from changes in their relationships. Those responsible for formal resources in countries of the world will need to ensure that programs and services for the elderly (often female-oriented) reach and serve older males as well as females, in both rural and urban settings.

SESSION 505

"The Raging Grannies": Live theatre as a tool for exploring political passion

Kathleen Weiss (Western Gold Theatre, and The University of British Columbia; Vancouver, British Columbia, Canada), and Joanna Nagle (Organizer) and Members of "The Raging Grannies", (Vancouver, British Columbia, Canada)

The Raging Grannies is an ad-hoc group of older women who use street theatre to make their views known about the political and social issues that matter to them. The purpose of this session is to acquaint participants with "The Raging Grannies" approach to street theatre. The Grannies will share stories of their experiences, and sing a number of original song parodies they have developed for different political demonstrations. The session will also include information on the basics of "forum theatre", an approach to addressing social issues through theatre which empowers spectators and actors alike. Many older adults feel strongly about political and social issues, but lack a mode for expression of their views. This workshop will demonstrate how this kind of theatre can empower the older adult to speak out and give them a means of expression. Practical exercises to beginning this kind of work will be introduced to participants.

SESSION 506

AGEING and SPEED of BEHAVIOR in the ELDERLY SUBJECTS

Alexander A. Polyakov (Institute of Gerontology Academy of Medical Sciences, Kiev, Ukraine)

The purpose of this study was to evaluate a role of slowing down of a psychomotor speed with age as factor of mental performance. METHOD: Study was made of 80 men aged 30-74 yrs. Volunteers (engineers) were recruited at a local plant. The psychomotor speed and mental capa- city was measured with a battery of computerized reaction time tests in different regimes (free, imposed and on-line). A computer using applied programs has processed the results obtained. RESULTS: This study suggested that reaction time of men beginning to increase significantly after 50 years. It was established that dynamics of speed of behavior has rhythmic nature. Thus with age increases deviation of speed behavior. In experiment the age differences in dynamics of mental work capacity; namely low speed, low reliability and high fatigability of elderly subjects are detected. It was found that in a condition of the expressed lack of time for test solution 15 % of people could work in experiment only. Test condition at which the time for the answer four times exceeded individual time was optimal even for the elderly people. The reliability of their operation in this condition reaches level for the young people. In this condition there were no "blocks" of activity. CONCLUSION: The schedule, which is taking into account age slowing down of information processing, can play a role "of the exterior modulator ", boosting performance and reliability of mental activity of elderly people.

Generativity in Midlife and Older Adults: Its Structure and Relationship to Well-being

BOYD, Lyn (Flinders University, Adelaide, Australia). LUSZCZ, Mary (Flinders University, Adelaide, Australia).

PURPOSE: Generativity, Erikson's notion of a preoccupation with establishing and guiding the next generation, and with leaving a lasting legacy of the self, is thought to reach a peak in midlife and decline in older age. Drawing from two recent models (McAdams & de St. Aubin, 1992; Stewart & Vandewater, 1998), this study investigated whether three hypothetical components of generativity, namely concern (valuing generativity), current engagement (perceptions of present generativity), and lifelong accomplishment (generativity over the life span), might display different patterns of age differences, and whether the relationship between generativity and well-being might be moderated by age. METHOD: Young, midlife and older adults (N = 300; mean age = 48.22 + 21.54), were administered an expanded version of the Loyola Generativity Scale (McAdams & de St. Aubin, 1992). RESULTS: Confirmatory factor analyses identified three factors corresponding to those hypothesized, together with a fourth, generative commitment (effort toward generativity). Midlife adults' ratings of current engagement exceeded those of older adults, but contrary to predictions, older adults did not report higher levels of lifelong generativity. The two groups did not differ on concern or commitment to generativity. Lifelong and current generativity, but not concern, were related to well-being, particularly at midlife. At midlife, self-appraisals of generative engagement and accomplishment were both directly and indirectly related to well-being, while for the older adults they were only indirectly related through their effect on integrity or self-acceptance. CONCLUSION: Findings suggest that perceiving oneself to be generative may be more central to the well-being of midlife adults than of older adults.

Goal Attainment Scaling and Rehabilitation Outcomes

Lindsay Gething, Judith Fethney & Cate Carey (Research Centre for Adaptation in Health and Illness),University of Sydney, Sydney, Australia

The ageing of the Australian population has led to policy makers calling for implementation of strategies which provide improved health outcomes and "consumer focus" while enhancing cost effectiveness of care. This project aimed to evaluate the applicability of Goal Attainment Scaling (GAS) as a method that facilitates consumer input. Two Sydney, Australia based hospitals participated in a longitudinal study that explored success at achieving rehabilitation goals jointly set by therapist and client. Participants were drawn from Concord Repatriation General Hospital (n = 43, mean age 71.5 years, SD 10.1, all admitted for orthopaedic surgery) and the War Memorial Hospital, Waverley (n = 27, mean age 77.9 years, SD 8.1, admitted for strokes and hip fractures). For the Concord group, outcomes were very promising, with 75% of participants achieving rehabilitation goals. For the older War Memorial Hospital clients, however, only 33% achieved rehabilitation goals, even though significant improvements in mobility and confidence in avoiding falls were made by this group over the interview period. Results indicate that while GAS does show promise for enhancing client/therapist collaboration in achieving positive health outcomes, clients who are frail aged still present many challenges to health professionals.

Goal-Setting Effects on Memory Across the Life Span

R. L. West (Institute on Aging and Department of Psychology, University of Florida, Gainesville, FL, USA)

Goal-setting as a self-regulatory process has rarely been examined in memory and aging research. This study evaluated goal theory and tested the impact of goal-setting on performance and self-efficacy. Participants were assigned randomly to an easy condition or difficult condition with difficulty varying as a function of goal challenge. In baseline assessments, 127 adults completed self-efficacy measures. A shopping list of 15 items was then presented for the baseline recall trial, followed by three other recall trials. In the easy condition, a categorizable list for each subsequent trial included words recalled on the first trial plus five additional words. In the difficult condition, the list was not categorizable and the list for each subsequent trial consisted of the recalled words plus 15 additional words. All participants received feedback on memory gains over trials. After the four recall trials, self-efficacy measures were repeated. With difficulty levels set in relation to individual baselines, older and younger adults responded to goal-setting conditions, showing increased self-efficacy, especially in the easy condition, and improved performance across trials, with greater gains for the most challenging goals. The expected crisscross pattern of self-efficacy and performance in relation to goal challenge was found only for the younger adults, with lower self-efficacy and higher performance for the difficult goal condition, and higher self-efficacy and lower performance for the easy goal condition. These empirical results verified that self-regulatory processes related to goal-setting apply to the memory domain, but more strongly for younger than for older adults.

Inhibition, naming and aging

Sarah M. Harrington & Catriona M. Morrison (Cardiff University, Cardiff, Wales U.K.)

PURPOSE. In order to examine the different accounts of cognitive aging, normal, healthy, ageing individuals (ages 64-80) were compared to young adults (ages 18-26) on three confrontation naming tasks-word naming, picture naming, and naming from a definition. These tasks were chosen as, collectively, they help isolate different levels of lexical processing. METHOD. Participants were presented with single words, photographs or definitions (short sentences) and were instructed to name the object represented as quickly and accurately as possible. RESULTS. The young adults were faster and more accurate than the old adults at picture naming. They were also faster at word naming. There was no difference in accuracy between young and old in word naming or definition naming and there was no difference between young and old in reaction time on definition naming. CONCLUSION. We suggest that these results best support inhibitory deficit accounts of cognitive aging, and the implications of the results are discussed.

Life Span Perspective: The analysis of aging within the Colombian context

Elisa Dulcey-Ruiz, M.A. Psychologist (CEPSIGER - Center of Gerontological Psychology- Bogota, Colombia. Raul Perez-Varon, Gerontologist, researcher (CEPSIGER - Center of Gerontological Psychology - Bogota, Colombia.

Life Span Perspective: The analysis of aging within the Colombian context Purpose: To present a critical analysis of the process of aging and the possibility to build a peace culture in Colombia, taking into account the Life Span Perspective and the historical, socio-cultural Colombian context. Method: Descriptive In the context of a country experiencing both demographic transition and social instability, this document aims to present the Life Span Perspective as a principle concept. >From this Life Span Perspective (which talks about the influence of the historical, socio-cultural context and the permanent change in the building of the life cycle) it is possible to analyse the process of aging and the condition of old age in Colombia. The document takes into account the actual Colombian context analysed from the view point of building social stability. Conclusion: Clonclusions reached were of the significant rola and influence the historical, socio-cultural context ahd upon building the process of aging and peace culture.

Prospective memory abilities in later adulthood

Claudia Jacova, Peter Graf & Beat Meier (University of British Columbia, Vancouver, Canada)

Prospective memory (ProM) is the ability to remember at some future moment that something needs to be done. ProM is affected by normal ageing. However, reports differ with regard to the onset and the size of the age-related decline. The purpose of the study is to 1) determine at what age ProM begins to decline; 2) examine the contribution of processing resources to the decline in ProM; and 3) compare performance on two ProM tasks, one cued by activity-initiation, one by activity-completion. 140 adults between 45 and 85 years of age are given two naturalistic ProM tasks, embedded in a 4-hour testing session. The first task requires participants to remember to write the date on a sheet of paper before they start a designated task (activity-initiation). The second task requires participants to remind the experimenter of an additional test at the end of a designated task (activity-completion). Several measures of cognitive and attentional functioning are also assessed in the session. The results show a decline in ProM performance from the youngest (45-49 years) to the oldest participants (80+ years). Age-related changes in processing resources contribute to the decline in ProM. Age effects are larger on the task cued by activity-initiation than on that cued by activity-completion. It is concluded that ProM is not preserved until the 7th decade of life, as reported in previous studies, but begins to decline much earlier. Additionally, decline in ProM performance is influenced by specific task attributes such as the position within the ongoing activities.

Variation in Inhibitory Deficits in Relation to Depth of Processing

Tannis Y. Arbuckle, Kirsten Fabi, Michaela Georgescu, & Lucie Bonneville, (Concordia University, Montreal,Canada)

The inhibitory deficit hypothesis has been challenged by negative priming studies that have shown equivalent inhibitory control for young and old adults. In the present study the negative priming effect (NPE) was used as an index of inhibitory control to test the hypothesis that whether or not older adults will show an inhibitory deficit depends on the depth of processing of the stimulus information. The target stimulus for the negative priming task was always the larger of a pair of pictured animals. In the perceptual judgment condition (shallow processing), the animal that was larger in reality was pictured as larger; in the semantic judgment condition (deep processing) the two animals were pictured as the same size. Results showed that both young (n = 26) and older participants (n =24) had large NPEs in the semantic judgment condition whereas young adults had a small NPE and older adults no NPE in the perceptual judgment condition. A replication experiment, currently ongoing, includes a third condition, interference, where the larger animal in reality is pictured as being the smaller one. The discussion and conclusions will focus on whether inhibitory deficits are better understood as one possible manifestation of an age-associated decline in attentional control, with the precise behavioural effects of that decline varying depending on how deeply the stimulus information is processed.

SESSION 507

Chromosomes and Aging

T. Lezhava (Department of Genetics , Tbilisi State University)(Chavchavadze 1,Tbilisi, 380028, GEORGIA) T.Jokhadze (Department of Genetics, Tbilisi State University) (Heavy metal induced chromosome changes in vitro and in vitro aging) N.Dvalishvili (Department of Genetics, Tbilisi State University) (Long-term cultures of human lymphocytes as a model of in vitro aging) T. Kadotani (The Kadotanin Medical Research Foundations)(Chromosomal study in ageing)

Aging is one of the most complex issues in biology.The aging process is a graduel deterioration of body functions.The deterioration becomes recognizable at the end of the reproductive span, as it merges into the aging period.The functional decline in humans is a linear process with insidious manifestations beginning at the age of 20 +/- 10. Most of normal homeostatic changes, especially age-related loss of cell functions occur in the chromatin domens functional units of hereditary structures (formation of "active genes" is not enough for transcription, existence of "active chromatin" is nessesery as well). Gerontochromosomology is a complex science applying biological, physical and chemical methods for the studies of numerous issues related to agespecific changes of functional characteristics of nucleoprotein structures chromosomes. Importent clues to chromosome function at late developmental phases and to senile diseases may be obtained by cytogenetic evaluation of chromosome structure and function. At the Symposium chromosome functional and stractural charasteristics will be discussed. The following issues are planned to be considered: cyclical properties, eu- and heterochromatin, heterochromatinization, nucleolar organizing ragions, sister chromatid exchanges, reparation, spontaneous (including telomeres) and induced (by heavy metal salts, radiation) chromosome aberrations, premature aging and in vivo and in vitro aging. Long term culture of lymphosytes on the basis of chromosome caracteristics will be presented as a model system of aging. The submitted reports will present new data concerning chromosome functional and structural changes related to in vivo, in vitro and the premature aging.

Chromosomal study in ageing

Tetsuji Kadotani (The Kadotani Medical Research Foundation, Higashi-Hiroshima, Japan), Tomiko Kadotani

Chromosomal study was carried out to investigate the influence on the chromosomes in ageing. Satellite associations in chromosomes and chromosome fragile sites were studied in the newborns, middle-aged women and the aged women over 60 years old. The lymphocytes were cultured for 72 hours in the minimal essential medium without folic acid (MEM-FA) supplemented with 5% calf serum. The slides were made by means of the flame-drying technique. The chromosome observation was made with the frequency of the break and/or gap and also the satellite associations were calculated for each one with 50 well-delineated metaphases. The locations of the break points were identified by conventional Giemsa staining and by G-banding technique after decolorizing them. The satellite association in the newborn group was statistically higher than both the 40-45 and 60-76 years old groups. In the newborns, 6 fragile sites were observed. In the aged women over 60 years old, 8 fragile sites were observed. The statistical difference was not recognized between in the newborns and in the aged women. Now, we are investigating fragile sites on people over 90 years old.

Chromosome functional changes in aging

T.A.Lezhava (Department of Genetics, Tbilisi State University) (Chavchavadze 1,Tbilisi, 380028, GEORGIA)

Chromosome is known to be a heterogenous structure withgenetic activity, replication time and degree of condensation varying over its length. Structural condensation in chromosomes closely correlates with functional heterogeneity: tightly condensed (heterochromatin or heterochromatinized) regions are genetically inactivated (characterized by late replication, lack of transcription), while decondensed (euchromatin) regions display active function and contain the RNA and DNA capable of rapid incorporating labels. The purposes of the present work were: 1.To define the level of chromosome modification - heterochromatinization (condensation of eu- and heterochromatin regions) in aging ; 2.To study the correlation between chromosome mutation, repair capacity and heterochromatinization in order to define which of them is primary in aging 3.To propose the conception concerning the mechanisms of senile pathologies. The MUTATION level (chromosome aberrations, including telomere regions); MODIFICATIONS of CHROMOSOME STRUCTURE level of condensed chromatin identified by the techniques of differential scanning microcalorimetry and electron microscopy; level of transcriptional activity of DNA-dependent RNA polymerase; Ag-positive NORs and associations of acrocentric chromosomes; REPARATION intensity of unscheduled DNA synthesis and the frequency of sister chromatid exchanges have been studied in lymphocyte cultures from individuals at the age of 72-114 to reveal the chromosome functional organization at late stages of ontogenesis and to find explanations of some senile pathologies. The analysis of obtained results showed: 1.Chromosome progressive heterochromatinization (condensation of eu- and heterochromatin regions) occurs at aging; 2.Decrease of repair processes and increase in frequency of chromosome aberrations in aging are secondary to the progressive heterochromatinization. 3. Chromosome heterochromatinization may be the reason for some senille pathologies; 4.Chromosome heterochromatinization is an area where one should seek the ways for prolonging the lifespan. 5. Chromosome heterochromatinization is a key factor of aging.

Heavy metal induced chromosome changes in vitro and in vitro aging

T. Jokhadze (Department of Genetics, Tbilisi State University) (Chavchavadze 1,Tbilisi, 380028, GEORGIA)

Three metal salts ($CuSO_4$,$CdSO_4$,$NiCl_2$) have been used in our experiment for studyng sensitivity of human chromosomes to metal ions at aging in vivo and in vitro.The studied metals are known as chromatin modifiers.PHA stimulated cultures of peripheral blood lymphocytes from virtually healthy donors of two age groups from 18 to 25 and from 75 to 93 yrs were used as objects.Cultivation and harvesting of materials were performed by standart methods.In addition to the short term (50hrs) cultures prolonged 144 hrs (in vitro aging) cultures were studied for the first age group. 0.5×10^{-4} M concentration for copper and cadmium and 10^{-5} M concentration for nickel ions were tested. The results of the analysis proved that chromosome sensitivity to the damaging activity of the agents was unlike at different stages of ontogenesis. All three metals caused increase of mutation level in short term cultures of middle aged individuals, while they expressed different activities in cultured cell of aged individuals and at in vitro aging. In particular,the effect was significantly noticeable in aging as compared with midll aged individuals.Copper and nickel, known to couse chromatin condensation, reveald higher activity. Cadmium salt, the chromatin decondensating agent, did not induce chromosome aberrations in both in vivo and in vitro aged cells.

Long-term cultures of human lymphocytes as a model of in vitro aging

N.Dvalishvili (Department of Genetics, Tbilisi State University) (Chavchavadze 1,Tbilisi, 380028, GEORGIA)

Various chromosome characteristics of human lymphocytes have been studied at different times of cell cultivation in order to represent a longterm culture of lymphocytes as the model system of cell aging.Long-term cultures of peripheral blood lymphocytes were harvested at 144 hrs of incubation(4th and later mitosis) and the studied values were compared with those obtained from 51 hrs and 72 hrs cultures (1 st and 2 nd mitosis) of the same individuals.Cells in long - term cultures were regularly supplied with fresh media .Increased frequercies of spontaneous and mutagen induced chromosome aberrations,aneuploidy,polyploidy (endoreduplication mainly) and sister chromatid exchanges have been observed at 144 hrs of culturing. .The ribosomal gene activity was significantly reduced at in vitro aging expressed in decreases of the counts of Ag-NOR positive acrocentric chromosomes,lack of of association incidence and the level of endogenous DNA dependent RNA polymerase activity. Centromeric heterochromatin (C-band) variants were evaluted for chromosomes 1,9and 16 and a dimensional variability of C-heterochromatin was observed enlarged patterns of C bands in chromosomes 1 and 9 were registered for 144 hrs of culturing. Our results are in correspondence with the published date concerning the cytogenetic characteristics of aged individuals that allows us to represent the prolonged cultures of human lymphocytes as a model of in vitro aging.

SESSION 508

Cultural Constructions of Alzheimer's Disease

Anne Basting (University of Wisconsin, Oshkosh, USA) ("God is a Talking Horse" and Other Lessons From Stories by People with Dementia) Lawrence Cohen (University of California, Berkeley, USA) (A theory of senility and culture) Annette Leibing (Universidade Federal do Rio de Janiero, Rio de Janiero, Brazil) (The Ôglocal culture of Alzheimers disease in Brazil) John Traphagan (California State University, Fullerton, USA) Margaret Lock (McGill University, Canada) (Discussant)

ISSUE: This invited symposium examines the relevance of the cultural and structural practices, in local and comparative contexts, through which the dementias are understood and treated and through which demented persons are framed. STRUCTURE: The session begins with a discussion of epistemological and pragmatic issues raised in efforts to link knowledge production in molecular and neurobiologies, clinical neurology, neuropsychology, and geriatrics, anthropology and sociology, political economy, and phenonomenological and narrative analysis. It turns to critical anthropological case studies from Brazil and Japan, and then to a North American study of how narrative and personhood are related in a storytelling intervention. A critical discussion concludes the session. CONTENT: Cohen proposes three axes for a critical cultural analysis of what he as an ideal type terms senility: (1) phenomenological, (2) discursive, and (3) materialist. He uses ethnography from India and the United States and Canada. Leibing examines how dementia is covered in both popular and scientific discourse in Brazil to unravel how both "local" and "global" forces come together in the articulation of specific clinical and social local worlds. Traphagan looks closely at several axes of social and institutional settings in Japan to demonstrate how local worlds in which senility takes shape and is medicalized are themselves politically constituted. Basting examines Time Slips, a creative storytelling project she directed with people with AlzheimerÕs disease. The project demonstrates that the social identity of persons with AlzheimerÕs can be strengthened to improve their quality of life, and raises questions about phenomenology. CONCLUSIONS/ANTICIPATED OUTCOMES: The session seeks to move beyond the use of "cultural difference" and "social construction" in much social science dementia literature. By bringing together scholars working on senility and dementia in cosmopolitan but non Euro-American settings (Cohen, Leibing, Traphagan), on narrative and voice in the intersubjective construction of the person with dementia (Basting), and on the current genomics of AlzheimerÕs (Lock), a critical new articulation of biology, society, phenomenology, and political economy is attempted.

A theory of senility and culture

Lawrence Cohen (University of California, Berkeley, USA)

PURPOSE: To propose three axes for a critical cultural analysis of what will be broadly termed senility: (1) phenomenological, (2) discursive, (3) materialist. METHOD: Utilizing field materials from India and the United States to demonstrate the utility of each and the necessity of linking them. RESULTS: A phemonology of senility locates the narrativity of selfhood within the contested politics of a voice: how are demented persons heard, or not heard, and what are the grounds for interpretation? How do different and changing social and juridical spaces of kinship and care articulate dependent bodies as variably coherent subject positions? Attention to discourse locates senility within a relationship to modernity and its biopolitics and raises the question of whether, after Agamben, senility comes to stand as mere "animal" or "bare" life, not life within the space of sovereignty and law. It pushes us to think about postcoloniality, globalization, and other processes of articulation. If kinship and care are central to the phenomenology of senility, these must be engaged as contingent biopolitical processes. Attention to materiality is twofold: technique and political economy. Shifting techniques in the biomedicine of late life disorders simultaneously operate as powerful clinical breakthroughs and as products of massive transnational and sovereign industries. CONCLUSION: The impact of these material, discursive, and phenomenological processes and structures of senility need be located within a political economy of the life course (who survives, and how?), one attentive to contestations over voice and the withholding of the status of "living" from the demented.

"God is a Talking Horse" and Other Lessons From Stories by People with Dementia

Anne Basting (University of Wisconsin, Oshkosh, USA)

PURPOSE: Scholars and activists within fields of disability and age studies have fought to have people of all ages recognized as people with disabilities. These broad categories are peopled with individuals with opinions not just needs to be attended. But how can the voices of people with dementia be heard? In what form can and do their voices have meaning? METHOD: My presentation follows Time Slips, a creative storytelling project with people with Alzheimers disease. As Project Director, I organized 18 weeks of storytelling workshops in two cities and trained students and staff of two adult day centers to facilitate the group workshops. RESULTS: The founding assumption of the project is that the self is relational. When ones personal control of their environment is challenged in dementia, literature suggests that their self is lost. But Time Slips assumes that ones social identity can be strengthened to improve ones quality of life. Interviews with students, staff and family caregivers reveal that the experience was effective in shifting perspectives of people without dementia. CONCLUSION: Creative storytelling offered the people with Alzheimers an avenue for self-expression and a social role. The Time Slips stories are composites of the voices of all participants, facilitators and storytellers. They help us hear the experience of dementia without mistakenly falling back on a pure sense of the individual. For asserting the voice of the disabled can mistakenly reify a mythic sense of independence that drives cultural biases against the disabled in the first place.

Senility and the Politics of the Disintegrated Self in Japan

John Traphagan (California State University, Fullerton, USA)

PURPOSE: To consider the politics of senility in Japan, with a focus on how a discourse of non-use has emerged in relation to the recently promulgated national Long-Term Care Insurance (LTCI) program. METHOD: Analysis of various government publications and field work among government employees and users of programs and facilities for older people. RESULTS: Local governments in Japan construct and disseminate a public discourse on aging which situates senility within a conceptual frame that ties individual well-being to collective well-being. A variety of facilities and programs have been developed as contexts in which older people can engage in care of self and through that, it is hoped, avoid or delay senility. This is not only seen as being individually beneficial, but also as a social responsibility of older people. Well-being is achieved through self-discipline and self-cultivation, which are viewed as central in maintaining an integrated self. The collapse of this integrated self, evident through the onset of senility, is not only a problem for the well-being of the individual and his or her family, but is problematized as challenging the integration, and thus the well-being, of the social whole. Older people are encouraged to engage in self-discipline and self-cultivation through government (and other) organized facilities and activities in order to avoid using LTCI. CONCLUSION: Care of self can be understood as a central features of a political economy of growing old in Japan in which the onset of senility is, in part, constructed in terms of burdening limited care resources

The global culture of Alzheimers disease in Brazil

Annette Leibing (Universidade Federal do Rio de Janiero, Rio de Janiero, Brazil)

PURPOSE: To show the inter-relatedness of local and global clinical realities by looking at the popular and scientific production of knowledge regarding Alzheimers disease. As a local example urban Brazil (Rio de Janeiro) and its geronto-geriatric styles of reasoning have been chosen. METHOD: Analysis of popular and scientific publications and technologies in Brazil and abroad RESULTS: Two main threads can be observed within the local history of AD, one linked mainly to biomedicine, another to alternative or more person-centered approaches and a third one emerging now with the genetic explanation. By looking at global and local practices, different aspects appear which show that local practices can neither be seen as passive receivers of hegemonic theories and ideologies, nor that they are free of wider influences, interests and worldviews. CONCLUSION: The term "local Alzheimers" makes sense when considering the variety of incorporations of biomedical realities into Brazilian cultures of aging and its memory practices

SESSION 509

Retirement and Pension Reform in the New Millennium

Yung-Ping (Bing) Chen (Gerontology Institute, University of Massachusetts Boston, MA, USA) 'Social Security Reform: Individual Accounts as an Experiment' Bert Jonker (Cap Gemini Ernst & Young, Utrecht, The Netherlands) 'The Dutch pension system reconsidered in the perspective of an ageing population' Tony Mallier & David Morris (Coventry Business School, Coventry University, Coventry, United Kingdom) 'Pension Reform in Britain: a return to basic principles' Gerhard Naegele (Institute of Gerontology, Dortmund University, Germany) 'The Retirement and Pension Reform in Germany: some aspects of the current discussion' Eskil Wadensjo (Swedish Institute for Social Research, Stockholm University, Stockholm, Sweden) 'The Swedish Old Age Pension Reform: A New Model'

Issue: There is evidence in the older industrial nations to indicate pension schemes, both public and private, face unanticipated escalating costs relative to the available resources pension funds hold. The aim of the symposium is to consider the evolving policy responses of governments to the challenge of pension provision.Structure: The symposium contributors recognising the influence of the differing approaches in the past to pension provision will examine the contrasting strategies now being developed in six nations in response to the anticipated changing demographic, economic and social environment of the twenty-first century.Content: In the course of the twentieth century governments became increasingly involved in facilitating the provision of retirement pensions by encouraging the introduction of mechanisms, both public and private, to provide income security for older citizens. In the development of their strategies for pension provision governments have, until recently, made three basic assumptions:* adult males would normally spend their lives in full-time employment but in the latter part of the 20th century new work patterns have been developing;* that the number of young people entering the labour force would always exceed the number of older people retiring and thus the relative size of the inter-generational financial transfers required for pensions would remain relatively stable;* continuing economic growth would enable the employed and retired to continue to experience higher living standards.The phenomenon of demographic ageing, characterised by a growing proportion of the retired to the active working population, and the slowing down of the rate of economic growth in the older industrial nations have resulted in these assumptions being questioned. Conclusions: The symposium will provide the opportunity to compare the differing policy options now being developed by governments as they seek to evolve programmes which will be economically viable while ensuring older citizens have an appropriate standard of living.

Dutch pension system reconsidered in the perspective of an ageing population

B. B. (Bert) Jonker (Cap Gemini Ernst & Young, Utrecht, The Netherlands)

There are three levels to the Dutch pension system mirroring the World Bank recommendations for a three-pillar system.* Level one: the national insurance scheme (AOW) financed on a pay-as-you-go basis, guarantees all residents a basic minimum income pension, independent of former earnings, from the age of 65 years.* Level two: capital funded occupational or supplementary pensions, practically all employers offer a supplementary pension scheme although this is not a legal requirement. These schemes provide the major part of an individual's pension income and are usually earnings based.* Level three: voluntary pension provision provided by private insurance contracts individuals enter into on their own initiative and account. The Dutch tax system allows income devoted to pension provision to be tax exempt and individuals have exploited this facility to minimise their income tax.A number of factors have given impetus to the current reforms. The anticipated increase in the percentage of the Dutch population aged over 65 years. The increase in the number of older people since the 1980's taking early retirement, this being financed on a pay-as-you-go basis. Finally shifts in career patterns (extended education and earlier retirement) have reduced the financial base for pension provision.Entering the new millennium the Dutch government together with employers' and employees national organizations are developing pro-active strategies in relation to the system and funding of collective old age provision (AOW); a business oriented approach to early retirement and private pension provision; and encouraging continued labour market participation of ageing employees. These strategies are designed to sustain the social security and pension systems while ensuring the Dutch economy remains prosperous and retains its competitive edge.

Pension Reform in Britain: a return to basic principles

Tony Mallier & David Morris (Coventry Business School, Coventry University, Coventry, United Kingdom)

The absolute and relative number of older people in Britain is increasing and this demographic change has lead to a renewed debate relating to the provision and financing of pensions in Britain. Recent legislation will continue and extend the existing practice whereby the responsibility of the State is restricted to the provision of a welfare floor by providing a means-tested minimum income guarantee (MIG) for all pensioners. The MIG will be higher than the Basic Pension which, for the majority of pensioners, will become increasingly irrelevant.All employees with incomes above £ 10,000 will be required to save for their retirement through either a Private Pension Plan, an employer sponsored Occupational Pension or the new Stakeholder Pension Schemes. The former State Earnings Related Pension is being phased out and it is anticipated all Second Pillar pension provision in future will be the result of personal saving in one of the above alternatives. Reflecting changes in the labour market and new tax measures employers are shifting from providing defined benefit to defined contribution schemes. Similarly the low cost Stakeholder Pensions, which employers must provide in the absence of alternative provision, while allowing flexibility in contribution levels are based on the defined contribution principle. Upon retirement contributors will have to purchase an annuity which provides the actual pension.The paper will outline the changes arising from the recent legislation and evaluate the potential consequences for pension provision in Britain.

Social Security Reform: Individual Accounts as an Experiment

Yung-Ping (Bing) Chen (Gerontology Institute, University of Massachusetts Boston, MA, USA)

During the Presidential Election both Democratic and Republican candidates advocated differing "individual accounts" models to enhance retirement income. However, as far as Social Security was an issue in the election, voters were ambivalent. This ambivalence reflected the hypothetical and ideological nature of the issues involved. This paper will examine an alternative "individual account" model and its potential.The starting point is that US payroll tax is higher than required for existing Social Security commitments: consequently the revenue 'surplus' could be diverted to create mandatory "individual accounts". By utilizing the payroll tax 'surplus' individual pension supplements could be provided for retirement, resulting in a better balance between Social Security and private pension provision. The "individual account" funds could be invested in a way similar to the existing Thrift Savings Plan where the funds are held and managed by a central authority with constrained investment options. However the objective of supplementing private pension coverage would be achieved by investing solely in government bonds.After an experimental period, the transfer of payroll tax funds to "individual accounts" would cease. Individuals would then have the opportunity either to continue voluntary contributions or, should the initial experience of the accounts prove unsatisfactory, the right to discontinue contributing. Mandatory now but voluntary later would be a unique feature of this model. These suggested "individual accounts" are akin to the pilot programme of medical savings accounts and the authorised demonstration programme of individual development accounts. A demonstration programme of "individual accounts" to supplement existing Social Security provision would provide all workers with benefits upon retirement especially the 50% who rely heavily upon Social Security payments.

The Retirement and Pension Reform in Germany: some aspects of the current discussion

Gerhard Naegele (Institute of Gerontology at the Dortmund University, Dortmund, Germany)

Primarily due to labour market reasons and to demographic changes the income security systems in Germany are under economic pressure. After a description of these reasons and changes, the current reform debate will be illustrated with regard to the Statutory Pension System for the employees in the private sector (Gesetzliche Rentenversicherung, GRV). The GRV is the most important pension system covering about 80% of German workers. It follows the traditional Bismarck model of social insurance and is based on the pay-as-you-go principle. In Germany, efforts to reform the GRV have already began in 1992. Out of the proposals that have been discussed and partly introduced since then, the following ones can be mentioned: raising the legal retirement ages, making early retirement more difficult, introducing partial retirement schemes, raising public grants from tax money, lowering the level of pension payments and introducing a complementary capitalized based second (private) old age income security system. This paper will present and evaluate the final proposals to reform the GRV which presumably will pass Parliament in the spring of 2001.

The Swedish Old Age Pension Reform: A New Model

Eskil Wadensjo (Swedish Institute for Social Research, Stockholm University, Stockholm, Sweden)

The old age pension system in Sweden of the last decades was established in 1960. It was a pay-as-you-go system with some funding, and with earnings-related pensions. Financing problems induced a new pension reform. A preliminary decision was taken by the parliament in 1994 and the final decision was taken in 1998. The new pension system has gradually started and all parts of it are now being enforced. The main idea behind the new pension system is to increase work incentives by making the pension system actuarially fair and thereby make the pension system viable. The system should be more an insurance system and less a system of income redistribution. A second aim of the reform is that the pension system should guarantee a basic income for everyone at old age. This means that some redistribution should take place but it should be more visible than in the present system. The major change is the change from a defined benefit system to a defined contribution system. This new defined contribution pension system is partly a pay-as-you-go system and partly a premium reserve system with the pay-as-you-go system as the main part. The construction of the defined contribution pay-as-you-go system is an interesting innovation.

SESSION 510

Differences in quality of life perceptions among COPD patients and their non-COPD spouses

G. Low and G. Gutman (Gerontology Research Center and Program, Simon Fraser University, Vancouver, Canada)

Purpose: The purpose of the study was to determine whether there are significant and specific differences in patient quality of life perceptions among COPD patients and their non-COPD spouses. Method: 67 community-dwelling COPD patients and their non-COPD spouses participated. Subjects were recruited from physicians offices, out-patient hospital programs, Continuing Care, and newspaper advertisements. Patients and spouses completed the Sickness Impact Profile (SIP) and the St. George's Respiratory Questionnaire (SGRQ). Results: For both questionnaires, the higher the score, the lower the perceived life quality. Overall, spouses' scores of patient life quality were higher than those of COPD patients. At the bivariate level, statistically significant differences were found on the SIP for the physical domain and on the SGRQ for the psychosocial domain. At the multivariate level, only the SGRQ findings were replicated. Age and gender of both the patient and spouse accounted for 39.9% of score differences. Conclusions: Spouses perceived patient life quality to be significantly lower than patients did. Discordance was greatest among the oldest couples with a female non-COPD spouse. Discordant beliefs may generate friction among couples as a result of differing expectations of coping with COPD. Differences may also lead to difficulties with nursing care planning when a spouse is a primary caregiver. Alternately, perceptual differences may reflect a COPD patient's efforts to buffer his/her spouse's quality of life through minimizing disease impact. Domain specific differences provide direction for supportive nursing interventions.

Gender, Age and Spiritually Oriented Copin in Sweden

F. Ahmadi Lewin (Department of Sociology, Uppsala University, Uppsala, Sweden)

There has not been much systematic research in Sweden examining the existential and spiritual aspects of coping with different serious illnesses.

Taking one step towards redirecting the attentions towards this research area, this article discusses some findings and barriers being important when investigating the religious and spiritually oriented coping strategies among ill persons in the context of Swedish culture. The paper concludes that a new alternative scale of the measuring spirituality among ill persons and new models of meaning and importance of religious and spiritual coping with serious illness should be developed from perspectives which consider the cultural context of the societies like Sweden where people practice their religion in a spiritual, subjective and/ or nonorganizational way rather than an organizational way and therefore practicing organizational religiousness is not an important health-related measure. In this relation Religious Orientation Scale (ROS) and The Spiritual Assessment Inventory (SAI) are seemed to be appropriate methods which the new models can be based on.

Grief, Faith and Healing: The Chaplain's Role in a Supportive Housing Complex

Debby Vigoda (Ontario Gerontology Association, Toronto, Canada)

It is widely accepted that almost everyone is in need of some kind of healing, regardless of age. There is a need for healing of physical and mental health, for the individual, loved ones and friends. Current research shows that there is a significant growth in the number of people, health care professionals and patients, who believe that religious belief has the capacity to assist in healing, through spirituality and reflection. The Director of Pastoral Care at Toronto's Baycrest Centre for Geriatric Care developed an intensive screening and training program for volunteer chaplains. Through these chaplains, the residents in the supportive housing complex of Baycrest are provided with spiritual support and avenues for religious expression. An added challenge for the Department of Pastoral Care is the significant proportion of residents (almost fifty per cent) who are Holocaust survivors. The role and responsibilities of the chaplains will be described as well as the involvement of the residents.

Groupwork for Elderly in Singapore

Helen Ko (Singapore Action Group of Elders Counseling Centre, Singapore) Chiang Hai Ding (National University of Singapore Society Senior Circle), Singapore

This is a pilot programme of Support and Guided Autobiography groups. The purpose is to investigate the efficacy of groupwork as a modality for working with the elderly in Singapore. With the help of a facilitator, group norms, topics and the number of sessions are determined by the group in the initial phase of the programme. These groups met regularly for two-hour sessions to discuss issues and topics pertinent to them in the context of ageing in Singapore. Guided Autobiography groups met to share their life-stories in a safe group environment. Evaluation of the programme was done through feedback forms administered to participants and in a group setting with the facilitator. Initial feedback suggests that the group experience had been therapeutic, reduced social isolation and enhanced psychological well-being. Existing friendships were strengthened and new friends were found. The results of this project is significant in that prior to it, it was often assumed that the elderly in Singapore will not self-disclose in a group environment. The reason cited is that most of the current cohort of elderly in Singapore, being of Asian origin, subscribe to the belief that family and personal problems should be kept private. As such, it was thought that a groupwork modality as utilised in this pilot project will not be effective for such a client group. The initial findings indicate otherwise.

Self-Care and Illness Self-Management in UK and USA: Consumer Acceptance and Policy Significance

GH DeFriese (University of North Carolina at Chapel Hill, NC, USA), A Rogers (University of Manchester, UK)

PURPOSE: To describe the way and the extent to which the concepts of self-care and disease self-management have been incorporated into the fabric of national health care systems serving older adults in the UK and the USA. METHOD: Four aspects of self-care and illness self-management serve as the framework for this analysis: (1) the general culture of health care consumerism in each country; (2) the overall supply and accessibility of personal (especially primary) health care services; (3) the way in which information about health is seen as empowering individuals as consumers/users of health care and in enabling laypersons to interact with professionals more effectively; and (4) the way in which the terminology of self-care and self-help is used in the two countries. RESULTS: Very different histories of the two national health care systems, differences in the size and composition of these national populations, and differences in the levels of demand on formal and informal care providers have allowed these ideas to be expressed differently in the two countries. CONCLUSIONS: Consumerist values, far stronger in the USA than in the UK, encourages UK consumers to internalize strong medicalized norms, take more frequent self-action in response to illness symptoms, and express a strong desire to not waste the doctors time. This self-rationing of the use of formal health services in the UK is very different from the situation in the US, where active promotion of greater self-reliance has become a central feature of recent health plan approaches to demand reduction.

Social Predictors of Recovery in Older Persons after Injury to the Extremities. A Prospective Study

G.I.J.M. Kempen, W. Scaf-Klomp, A.V. Ranchor, R. Sanderman, J. Ormel (Department of Health Care Studies, Section of Medical Sociology, Maastricht University, The Netherlands)

PURPOSE: to study the impact of educational level and social support on short-term and long-term recovery of (instrumental) activities of daily living after injuries to the extremities in late middle-aged and older persons. METHOD: 171 patients who had sustained fall-related injuries (hip fractures, other fractures or contortions and dislocations) participated in the study. Data were collected at baseline before the injury and 8 weeks, 5 months and 12 months after the injury. Analysis of variance was used to assess possible differences between three levels of education and social support with respect to changes in disability scores from baseline to the three follow-up measurements. RESULTS: pre-injury assessed educational level or social support did not play a role in short-term changes. In the long-term (5 and 12 months after the injury), recovery was significantly associated with social support: those with higher levels of support had a better recovery. Long-term recovery (12 months after the injury) was only borderline associated with level of education. Short-term changes in disability appeared to be determined by the severity of the injury; level of education and social support only began to influence recovery when the impact of severity expired. CONCLUSION: patients recovering from fall-related injuries who had reported high levels of education and social support before their injury had recovered better at 12 months. Encouragement and special attention given by health professionals to low and medium educated patients to maintain social support may be beneficial for rehabilitation after fall-related injuries in older persons.

The Chronic Disease Self-Management Program - What Happens After a Pilot?

Faye White, BSW (Vancouver Richmond Health Board), Patrick McGowan, (Institute of Health Promotion Research, University of British Columbia, Vancouver, BC, Canada)

The Chronic Disease Self-Management Program (CDSMP), a lay-led education initiative, gives people the knowledge, skills, and motivation they need to manage their chronic health problem(s). It is led by pairs of trained leaders to groups of 10 persons once a week for six consecutive weeks. The CDSMP was introduced into Vancouver and Richmond as a pilot program funded by the Vancouver/Richmond Health Board through the Community Health Initiative Fund. During the one-year trial, 90 leaders were trained to deliver the program. The evaluation involved pre- and six-month post-program questionnaires that examined attitudes, behaviours, health status, and impact of illness. The qualitative evaluation involved 30 program participants and leaders. Subjects provided opinions and perspectives on topics such as program impacts, best and worst parts of the program, and what it was like taking a health education program as part of a group. With the pilot phase completed new decisions about the future of the CDSMP needed to be made. This presentation will use the CDSMP as a case study to illustrate the planning decisions that need to be made when programs successfully complete their pilot stage. Topics that will be discussed include: determining the ongoing size and scope ot the program; selecting a home for the program; developing administrative guidelines and relationships with existing programs; and determining monitoring and quality assurance mechanisms to ensure program integrity.

SESSION 511

A Cross-national Qualitative Assessment of Elderly Goals and Health Care Needs in Two Rural Communities

G. Gairola (University of Kentucky, Kentucky, USA); I. Greaves (Gnosall Surgery, Staffordshire, England); and S. Thornett (Gnosall Surgery, Staffordshire, England)

The development of home and community based care (HCBC) is important in any national effort to address the growing need for health care among the elderly. This is especially true when HCBC is viewed as a cost-effective alternative to institutionalization. Traditionally, planning and evaluation for HCBC have relied on lists of medical problems and functional deficits generated from standardized medical and functional protocols. However, there is growing interest in including a more client-centered approach. A client-centered approach takes into account individual and family personal goals and perceptions of needs. This approach helps empower elderly to design their own care services and assists communities in designing programs specific to the needs of their area. This paper describes a cross-national collaborative study in which two rural communities, one in England and one in the United States served as sites for a qualitative study of the goals and needs of the elderly as they relate to the provision of health services. Focus group interviews were conducted in each country, including elderly persons in both community and institutionalized settings. Institutionalized elderly were interviewed to retrospectively assess whether or not they could identify HCBC services that would have been critical in preventing their institutionalization. Findings from this study suggest that the elderly failed to plan for debilitating life events. They most commonly feared a loss of independence, a loss of their right to choose care during a time of crises, and social and family isolation. HCBC is an additional burden to the stressful self-reliant.

An International Comparison of Payment Incentives and Rehabilitation Therapy for Elderly Institutional Residents.

Walter P. Wodchis (University of Michigan, Ann Arbor, USA)

PURPOSE: To examine the effect of resident factors and health system payment incentives on the delivery of ancillary rehabilitation therapy to elderly institutional long term care residents. METHODS: Data are based on Minimum Data Set resident assessments from Ontario residents between 1996 and 1998 (n=24,880) and Michigan residents in 1998 and 1999 (n=32,870). Multivariate analyses were used to determine the effect of resident factors and payment methods on the provision of ancillary rehabilitation therapy. Payment methods used by public payers in this study were cost-based, case-mix, and global budget payment. RESULTS: Fifty-nine percent of Ontario residents received either physical or occupational therapy, while 20 percent of Michigan Medicaid, 88 percent of Medicare and 37 percent of private-pay residents received therapy. Recent falls and fractures were positively associated with receipt of therapy, while cognitive disorders and lower physical functioning were negatively associated with receipt of therapy. After controlling for resident diagnoses and functioning, Ontario residents were more likely to receive some rehabilitation therapy but received less total therapy time. A program change for Medicare residents from cost-based to case-mix payment led to less rehabilitation time and no difference in the likelihood of receiving therapy. CONCLUSIONS: This study finds that Michigan Medicare and Ontario residents have similar characteristics and that differences in payment incentives play an important role in the provision of ancillary rehabilitation therapy to residents.

Case Study Cost Analysis of Community-Based Services Initiated From A Quick Reponse (QRP) Program

J. Franko, D. Treppel, C. Neudorf (Strategic Health Information & Planning Services, Saskatoon District Health, Saskatoon, Canada)

PURPOSE: To examine the system costs associated with providing community-based services initiated by a Quick Response Program (QRP) in 3 emergency rooms (ER) in Saskatoon. METHOD: This study was a retrospective review of all ER records of potential QRP clients over a 12 week period. We collected community services utilization data 30 days before and after the date of the ER visit. RESULTS: 145 people who met the study criteria, were studied further. Community services data were available on 129 people. There was an increase in utilization of community physical therapy, occupational therapy, social work, nursing, and home health aid service after people visited the ER. This was reflected both in total time spent providing service and in the number of people who received services. Individually, some saw an increase, some saw a decrease, and some saw no change in service. The total amount of time spent providing community services/person after ER visit ranged from 40 to 6350 minutes, with a median of 320 minutes. The total cost of community services was ~$30,500 or $407/person prior to the ER visit and ~$47,600 or $369/person after the ER visit. CONCLUSION: Overall, there was an increase in community services provided to people who presented at an ER and were seen by QRP. Some changes in service utilization may reflect increased reliance on private services, stabilization of medical condition, or an opportunity for re-assessment of services actually needed. System costs vary, depending on the community service provided and the needs of the clients.

Effectiveness of Anticipatory Care Interventions with Community Dwelling Elderly: Meta-analysis

J. Ploeg (McMaster University, Hamilton, Canada) J. Feightner (University of Western Ontario, London, Canada) B. Hutchison (McMaster University, Hamilton, Canada) C. Patterson (McMaster University, Hamilton, Canada) C. Sigouin (McMaster University, Hamilton, Canada) M. Gauld (McMaster University, Hamilton, Canada)

The purpose of this project was to assess the impact of anticipatory care interventions with community dwelling elderly on mortality, admissions to long-term care, admissions to acute care hospital, use of homemaking and Meals on Wheels, and falls. Anticipatory care was defined as proactive, provider initiated primary care that is above and beyond demand-led usual care, provided in a community setting, and linked to the usual care system. A meta-analysis of randomized trials comparing anticipatory care interventions with usual care in community dwelling elderly was conducted. Published research studies were identified by searching Medline (1966-1999) and CINAHL (1982-1999) and by reviewing reference lists of retrieved articles. Eighteen randomized trials with 14,028 patients were reviewed. Anticipatory care interventions were associated with a reduction in mortality (Common Odds Ratio [OR] 0.81, 95and fewer admissions to long-term care (Common OR 0.83, 95% CI 0.70 to 0.98). We found no evidence that anticipatory care results in reduced admissions to acute care hospital, increased use of homemaking or Meals on Wheels, or reduced falls. Anticipatory care interventions can be expected to reduce the odds of death by 19% and admission to long-term care by 17%. Such interventions can prolong life and reduce dependency among the elderly. Study findings are significant as they represent the first known meta-analysis of such interventions in the primary care setting.

Evaluation of an enhanced service delivery model for frail

seniors.

D. Papineau, F. Hamm (North Shore Health Region, North Vancouver, Canada), J. Hirdes, (University of Waterloo, Canada).

New ways of providing community health services to frail seniors with complex multidimensional health needs are being explored collaboratively by stakeholders who offer or receive services. The goal is to provide cost-effective community-based services that enable clients to remain at home. The present study used a quasi-experimental design to examine the cost-effectiveness of a new integrated service model for geriatric clients with complex needs. This new model was compared with the care model currently in place. Key aspects of the new model included a case manager with a caseload of 25 clients providing care coordination and home nursing care, and recreation therapy for isolated clients. The new model was found to be more cost-effective, clients in that group (n=30) remained significantly longer at home (p<.01) than those in the service-as-usual group (n=27). The total cost of services for the new model of care group during the six-month study period was $208,735 compared with $304,538 for the usual care group. The lower costs were attributable to lower hospitalization and care facility costs. There were no significant between-group differences in health outcomes. Clients receiving the new model of care improved significantly over time on three RAI-HC outcome scales. Information from client RAI-HC assessments was used in developing an algorithm to serve as a reliable adjunct to current criteria for selecting appropriate clients for this new treatment model. Suggestions for further research include replicating this exploratory study using an experimental design with a larger number of clients selected using the RAI-HC algorithm.

Quality indicators across ten Community Care Access Centres in Ontario

Dawn M. Dalby (Department of Health Studies and Gerontology, University of Waterloo, Waterloo, Ontario, Canada), John P. Hirdes (Department of Health Studies and Gerontology, University of Waterloo, Waterloo, Ontario, Canada and Canadian Collaborating Centre-interRAI, Providence Centre, Scarborough, Ontario, Canada)

Purpose: To develop and utilize a set of Quality indicators (QIs) for home care to compare Community Care Access Centres (CCACs) across Ontario. Method: Ten CCACs completed a minimum of 100 assessments using the Minimum Data Set-Home Care (MDS-HC), which represents a standardized multi-dimensional assessment instrument with good validity and reliability. Each CCAC completed one assessment per client. Representatives from six Canadian provinces, the United States and Japan developed the preliminary list of approximately 30 QIs, each representing a prevalence rate. This project is ongoing and the final list of QIs is expected in early 2001. Results: The sample included a total of 1952 clients. Most clients were female (71.4%) with a mean age of 76.3 years. Prevalence rates varied by CCAC and by age group on several QIs. For example, the rate of inadequate pain control varied by CCAC from a low of 17.7% to a high of 45.0%. In the youngest age group (18-64) the rate was 42.9 Conclusion: The implementation of the MDS-HC allows CCACs to assess their performance relative to their peers. The QIs can be used as performance indicators to evaluate quality at both the local and provincial level. Ongoing efforts will refine these QIs and continue to explore client characteristics important in explaining agency-wide variation.

Quality services in a diversified environment: Accrediting elderly service assessors and providers

Lam, Zarina (Accreditation Consultant, Centre on Aging, The University of Hong Kong)

The paper describes the recent experience of elderly service reform in Hong Kong. The training and accreditation of assessors and providers was newly adopted as an essential step to the reform. 1000 health assessors were required for the implementation of new care standard in elderly service delivery within a diversified service community. A structured training program was provided. This study intended to understand the implementation process a comparative study of health assessors (N=300) recruited from different organizations and having experience varied from 3 months to 20years. A 10 cm visual analog scale was used to measure the self-reported pre-and-post training scores. Implications on these new roles of assessors in the implementation of new standard of care requirement for elderly persons on providers and service standardization will be discussed.

The Victoria Geriatric CARE Program - Measuring Outcomes

Ted Rosenberg MD, Vicki McNulty and David Brook MD Dept of Geriatric Services, Victoria, Canada

Purpose The Victoria Geriatric Community Assessment Rehabilitation and Education (CARE) is an integrated regional geriatric program for frail elderly people living in the community. It combines specialized individual geriatric assessment and management with targeted 3 hour group interventions (for Falls/Immobility, Dementia Caregiver Education and Bladder Health) and long-tern follow up. This integrated model of care has replaced our previous model, which included a geriatric medical clinic and day hospital. Our challenge has been to measure health outcomes and develop meaningful evaluation indicators with scarce resources. Methods In the year prior to the development and implementation of the CARE program we evaluated our entire regional geriatric program (inpatient and out-patient) in the Victoria Geriatric Outcomes Evaluation Study (Victoria GOES).Outcome measures included the SF-36, GDS, MMSE, ALSAR,TUG, BERG and CRA. We met with the team to determine a way to integrate these scales from a research setting into our regular interventions. Results Results form the Victoria GOES showed that the scales used were valid, reliable and responsive improved health outcomes (eg SF-36, GDS, Berg Balance Scale, ALSAR) for patients and good rationalization of the overall service. We will discuss which outcome measures were included into our usual care and their impact on resources. Conclusions It is possible to include valid, reliable and responsive outcome measures into routine geriatric clinical practice. These tools better define patient needs and outcomes of care.

SESSION 512

Intergenerational Relations in Asian and South Asian-Origin Families in North America

T. Shibusawa (Columbia University of Social Work, New York, USA) and J. Lubben (Departments of Social Welfare and Urban Planning, University of California, Los Angeles, USA) Intergenerational Support and Psychological Well-Being Among Older Chinese and Japanese Americans Living in Los Angeles. K. Kobayashi (School of Social Work and Family Studies, University of British Columbia, Vancouver, Canada) The Impact of Family Composition on Intergenerational Exchanges in Later-Life Japanese Canadian Families. B. Mitchell (Department of Sociology and Anthropology, and Gerontology Programs, Simon Fraser University, Vancouver, Canada) Ethno-Cultural Diversity in Intergenerational Support Systems: A Comparative Analysis of Asian and British-Canadian Midlife Families). P. Dave (Department of Human Development and Family Studies, M.S. University of Baroda, Vadodara, India) Older Asian Indian Women in the US and Canada: Implications for Social Policies.

In both Canada and the United States, the numbers and percentages of elders of Asian and South Asian-origins is increasing. This is partly due to the aging of the North American-born (especially among the Japanese), but more a result of recent changes in the ethno-cultural composition of immigrants, who either age in the North American context or are relatively recent immigrants. This roundtable provides a relatively informal venue in which scholars from Canada, the US, and India discuss the latest research on the generally neglected topic of social support within families of Asian and South-Asians origins in North America.Two major dimensions of social support are explored Δ the support provided by children to aging parents (Shibuzawa and Lubben, and Dave), and the degree and nature of reciprocal support across generations (Kobayashi, and Mitchell). Two papers are comparative (Mitchell, and Shibuzawa and Lubben) and two are focussed on one ethno-cultural group (Japanese Canadians -Kobayashi, and Indo-Canadians/Americans - Dave). One of the important themes to emerge is the wide diversity, both within and across ethno-cultural groups. Within groups, differences are related to gender and marital status, illustrating the gendered nature of intergenerational relations in intersection with "race." Across groups, significant differences relate to timing of immigration, living arrangements, and traditional cultural orientations. Some categories of these populations are in more vulnerable situations than others. Special attention is paid to the extent and characteristics of multi-generational living arrangements, and their role in social support and social exchange across generations.Outcomes of this roundtable include an analysis of the degree of diversity in family social support and exchanges, an identification of sub-groups most at risk, and social policy implications for the provision of social services to an increasingly heterogeneous aging population.

Ethno-Cultural Diversity in Intergenerational Support Systems: A Comparative Analysis of Asian- and British-Canadian Midlife Families

B. Mitchell (Dept of Sociology and Gerontology Programs, Simon Fraser University, Burnaby, Canada)

This presentation addresses ethno-cultural diversity in intergenerational support systems between Canadian young adults (aged 19-35) and their midlife parents. Specifically, relationship quality and patterns of affective and instrumental support are compared and contrasted among Chinese- ,Indo- and British-Canadian families. The data used are a sub-set of the Culture and Coresidence Study (Gee, Mitchell, Wister & Lai, 1999-2000), which is comprised of a sample of 1,907 young adults living in the Greater Vancouver Regional District of British Columbia. These data are unique in that they entail detailed information on the family life of young adults for selected ethno-cultural groups with large enough sub-samples to allow comparative analyses. The three ethno-cultural groups in this research are analyzed according to a number of dimensions of intergenerational support, including: relationships closeness, bi-directional provisions of emotional support, and a number of other helping behaviours (e.g, instrumental and financial assistance). These associations are also examined by gender and living arrangements of the young adults. Results show that Indo-Canadians display the strongest patterns of intergenerational support between young adults and their parents. For example, 73.4% of Indo- Canadian young adults describe their relationship with their mothers as "excellent," compared to only 24.9% of Chinese-Canadians and 33.3% of British-Canadian young people. Furthermore, 79.6% of Indo-Canadians are "very likely" to ask parents for child care, if ever needed, compared to only 54.8% of British- and 49.8% of Chinese-Canadian young adults. However, while the Chinese and British generally exhibit lower levels of affective intergenerational closeness and various other types of parent-child support, these patterns are less uniform. Findings are discussed in terms of their implications for intergenerational relations and solidarity in ethnically diverse contexts.

Intergenerational Support and Psychological Well-Being among Older Chinese and Japanese Americans Living in Los Angeles

T. Shibusawa (Columbia University of Social Work, New York, USA), J. Lubben (Departments of Social Welfare and Urban Planning, University of California, Los Angeles USA)

This paper examines the relationship between intergenerational support and psychological well- being among Chinese and Japanese elderly persons residing in Los Angeles. The purpose is to examine the nature of familial social exchanges and their possible impact on mental health. Methods: Data are from the Cross-National Study of Chinese and Japanese American Elderly, funded by the University of California, Center for Pacific Rim Studies. Randomly selected Chinese American (n=204) and Japanese American (n=137) adults aged 60 years and over were interviewed regarding social support networks, physical health status, stressful life events, attitudes toward aging, and psychological well-being. Results: Whereas 92% of Japanese American elders were born in the US, a large majority of (95%) of the Chinese American elders were foreign-born. There were more intergenerational social support exchanges among Chinese American elders and their adult children than among their Japanese American counterparts. Intergenerational support was shown to be a significant predictor of psychological well-being among Chinese American elders whereas it was not as strong a predictor among the sampled Japanese American elderly. Conclusions: Japanese Americans tended to receive less support from their children, and their well-being was less dependent on intergenerational support than Chinese American elders. These differences in intergenerational support are discussed in the context of relative acculturation and socio-economic status among the two groups of Asian Americans.

Older Asian Indian Women in the US and Canada: Implications for Social Policy

P. Dave (Department of Human Development and Family Studies, M.S. University of Baroda, Vadodara, India)

Increasingly, younger people from a number of Asian countries are immigrating to other places, including North America. The current situation in India exemplifies this trend. In the Indian case, older parents, especially mothers, are expected to immigrate along with their adult children. Their contributions to household/family work - including cooking, cleaning, and child care - are noteworthy. In return, what do their families and/or the state have to offer them? Are social policies friendly to these immigrant elderly women? To what extent are these women able to use social services? This paper offers a critical analysis of these issues, focussing on the social policy implications of increased numbers of Asian Indian elderly women in North America.

The Impact of Family Composition on Intergenerational Exchanges in Later-Life Japanese Canadian Families

K. M. Kobayashi (School of Social Work and Family Studies, The University of British Columbia, Vancouver, Canada)

This paper uses a life course perspective to explore the effect of family composition on intergenerational exchanges in older nisei (second generation) - adult sansei (third generation) dyads in Japanese Canadian families. An examination of the nature of family relationships in later-life, this research focuses on the impact of composition variables (i.e, family size, gender, and marital status) on social and emotional support exchanges in older parent-adult child dyads. Methods: This study uses data gathered in semi-structured, face-to-face interviews with a random sample of 100 parent-child dyads in British Columbia collected in 1995-1998. The age range for parents is 55-86 years, and for children, 31-50 years. Results: Both qualitative and quantitative analyses indicate a high level of support exchange between older parents and adult children. Further, family size, marital status of parent, and gender of child and parent are significant predictors of intergenerational exchanges in Japanese Canadian families. Conclusions: The results suggest that that there is a two-way flow of support in Japanese Canadian families as older parents and adult children both provide and receive support. With regard to the exchange of support within the family, a gendered pattern emerges. In line with other literature on intergenerational exchanges in later-life, mothers and daughters both provide and receive more support, particularly in the areas of service and emotional assistance, than do fathers/sons. Findings are discussed in the context of acculturation and ethnic identification in post-immigrant Japanese Canadian families.

SESSION 513

Co-ordinating Health and Social Care: Historical and Contemporary Critiques of UK and Australian Experiences

Robin Means (Faculty of Health and Social Care, University of West of England, Bristol, UK) Shifting Boundaries: Historical Reflections on the Changing Nature of the Health and Social Care Divide in the UK; Caroline Glendinning (National Primary Care Research and Development Centre, University of Manchester, Manchester, UK) The New Collaborators - Bringing Primary Care into Health and Social Services Collaboration for Older People; Michael Fine (Department of Sociology, Macquarie University, NSW, Australia) From Alternative Provisions to Coordinated Care: Changing Links Between Hospitals, Residential Facilities and Care at Home for Older People; Diane Gibson (Australian Institute of Health and Welfare, Canberra, Australia) Exploring the Boundary: the Health-Social Care Interface in Australia; Helen Bartlett (Oxford Centre for Health Care Research and Development, Oxford Brookes University, Oxford, UK) Discussant.

Issue: This symposium combines cross-national with historical perspectives on the development of services for older people; the shifting boundaries between acute and community, health and social services; and endeavours to improve co-ordination between the various service sectors. Structure: Four papers will be presented, one each on historical and contemporary developments in each of the UK and Australia and one examining statistical and evidence of changes in the linkages between services. They will be drawn together by a discussant familiar with historical and contemporary developments in both countries. Content: The papers in this symposium will: trace the fragmentation of services for older people into distinctive 'health' and 'social' care elements, and the institutional and professional factors behind this fragmentation; review the pressures to renegotiate the boundaries between the various service domains; and evaluate the histories of strategies to reduce fragmentation through various co-ordinating mechanisms. Conclusions/outcomes: By combining both comparative and historical analyses of policies designed to improve service co-ordination across the 'health'/'social' services divide, this symposium will identify both the common trends and continuities within and between countries, and the differences which may impact differentially on the success of service co-ordination policies. It will therefore enhance understanding of the problems, barriers and 'success factors' affecting this intractable policy area.

Exploring the Boundary: the Health-Social Care Interface in Australia

Diane Gibson (The Australian Institute of Health and Welfare, Canberra, Australia)

Purpose: To explore the interface between residential and acute hospital care. Methods: Records from two national databases containing information on episodes of care in long term institutional care and hospitals were linked using probabilistic statistical linkage. Results: The findings describe the changing patterns of length of stay and episode type in acute care hospitals for older people during a period of progressive reduction in the availability of long term institutional care in Australia. Geographical differences are also presented. The interface between acute and long term care is thus explored in empirical terms in the context of the changing policy context. Conclusions: It is argued that monitoring of the acute care-long term care interface is a critical activity informing policy development in the health and social care fields. Too often planning and policy development in one field proceeds in the absence of information on trends in the other, and the actual interface is all too rarely the subject of large scale national empirical investigation.

From 'Alternative Provision' to 'Coordinated Care': Changing Relationships Between Hospitals, Residential and Domiciliary Care.

Michael Fine (Department of Sociology, Macquarie University, Sydney, Australia)

Purpose: In Australia and Britain, as in most comparable developed societies, aged care has long held a rather ambivalent position alongside, yet also as part of, the health care system. This relationship is under pressure at the present time as there is a search for new constellations of care which link hospitals, ongoing residential care, and care provided at home. From being an alternative form of provision, it is becoming increasingly popular to regard aged care as a form of complementary service for whichever closer linkages with more expensive, institutionally based, and professionalised medical services are sought in order to produce what is described as continuity of care. In this paper attention will be given to some of the numerous initiatives in this field and to the historical circumstances that shaped them. However, evidence suggests that such policies have typically fallen short in practice. Methods: Primary research undertaken by the author, as well as on other Australian and international research, this paper examines ideological, economic and social structural barriers to the achievement of better coordinated systems of care. Results and Conclusions: It will be argued that there is a need to acknowledge the conflicting nature of power and interests involved in the provision of aged care.

Shifting Boundaries: Historical Reflections on the Changing Health and Social Care Divide in the UK

Robin Means (Faculty of Health and Social Care, University of West of England, Bristol, UK)

Purpose:Any study of the development of welfare services for elderly people in the UK needs to consider the ever-changing interface between social services and health. This paper examines this interface, and the development of debates about it, from the creation of social services departments in 1971 through to the implementation of major community care reforms in 1993, in four contrasting local authorities. Methods: Analysis of policy documents and empirical findings from research in four contrasting localities Results and Conclusions: The data will illustrate the constant nature of the debate about 'what is health care?' and 'what is social care?' ; this will be linked to the impact upon social services of the withdrawal of the NHS from much of its continuing care provision.

The New Collaborators: bringing Primary Care into Health and Social Services Collaboration for Older People

Caroline Glendinning MPhil (National Primary Care Research and Development Centre, University of Manchester, Manchester, UK)

Purpose: The paper will describe and critically evaluate current policies to give primary care a key role in the planning, commissioning and delivery of co-ordinated services for older people. Method: The paper will use policy analysis, national survey data and qualitative data from local case studies. Results and Conclusions: The history of collaboration between health and social services in the UK has had limited success. Moreover, GP and other primary care services were largely excluded from the planning and commissioning of those joint or integrated services which did develop. However, since the early 1990s, and particularly since 1997, primary care has been given a lead role in health services development and in the development of partnerships with other services. The paper will review the progress made towards closer collaboration between health and social services and critically evaluate the prospects for future success.

SESSION 514

Activities, Preparation and Retirement Adaptation

Marlene M. Rosenkoetter, RN, FAAN John M. Garris, [University of North Carolina at Wilmington Wilmington, NC USA]

Purpose: As employees leave the workforce and entire retirement, they experience the freedom from the responsibilities of employment, but they also enter a new time in their lives. Planning for retirement in the United States (US) generally focuses on the financial aspects, with little emphasis placed on preparation for the many other aspects of life after retirement. The purpose of this study was to examine the preparation of employees for retirement, and their activities and adaptation following retirement. Method: A population of 1565 retirees from an international company residing in seven southeastern states in the US were surveyed using a 72-item questionnaire designed by the researchers. Results: Of the 764 respondents (48.82%), what they did to prepare for retirement was vastly different from what they believe others should do in preparation. No significant differences were found between men and women. Sedentary activities, such as watching television and reading, increased significantly while exercise and social activities remained constant. Slightly over 48% reported no volunteer activities, and of these, 44% reported less than one hour or no regular physical exercise; yet the vast majority were in good or better health. Numerous psychosocial changes were found following retirement and these were influenced by retirement preparation. Conclusions: Retirement preparation had impacted psychosocial adaptation for these subjects, and problems were noted in activity patterns. The findings have ramifications for pre-retirement planning, human resource personnel and health care providers working with retirees and those about to retire.

Making Economic Decisions at Retirement: Choices in Situations of Uncertainty

Diana Olsberg, Director, University of New South Wales Research Centre on Ageing & Retirement (RCAR), Sydney, Australia

Responding to demographic changes and ageing populations, governments in many countries are cutting back on government-provided pensions and other welfare benefits. Policies are being introduced which require increasing levels of personal individual responsibility for retirement needs, and rhetorics of choice have moved to the forefront of the policy agenda. However, the efficacy of people's choices, their capacity to make informed choices and the processes of personal individual decision-making - particularly in the areas of economic decision-making - are largely under-researched. This paper presents a report of a national study in Australia amongst recent retirees who have received a lump sum retirement benefit, and examines their economic decision-making at retirement. A number of questions direct the analysis. How does gender affect economic decision-making? Does social connectedness affect processes of economic decision-making? Is the amount of money correlated with patterns of economic decision-making? How does occupational background affect economic decision-making? The research findings offer important insights for people interested in planning and policy-making which concern the devolution of government services. The paper presents illuminating insights into the social context and predictors of peoples' economic decision-making in situations of uncertainty at retirement, and thereby is also of interest to anyone interested in aspects of social action.

Productive activity in later life: from work to work

Donna Dosman (Department of Human Ecology, University of Alberta), Janet Fast (Department of Human Ecology, University of Alberta), Norah Keating (Department of Human Ecology, University of Alberta)

ABSTRACT It is commonly believed that, as people age and leave the paid work force, they disengage from "productive" activity and become unproductive and dependent. This may be consistent with the conventional economic view of what constitutes productive activity, but is inconsistent with a contemporary view of unpaid work (domestic, volunteer and caring work) as equally economically valuable (i.e. productive) activity. It also is believed that participation in productive activity contributes to healthy aging and quality of life. The purposes of this study are: to investigate differences in how people allocate their time among productive and other activities pre- and post-retirement; and to examine the effect that different time use patterns have on perceptions of health and quality of life. Data from a subset of 4,890 respondents aged 45 and over from Statistics Canada's 1998 General Social Survey on time use were analyzed using a range of descriptive, bivariate and multivariate techniques. Results indicate that people remain engaged in productive activity even as they move out of the paid work force, substituting unpaid for paid work. Only respondents who have exceeded their normal life expectancy greatly reduce their productive activity. Somewhat different patterns of substitutions are apparent for men and women. Further, engagement in productive activity is positively related to respondents' perception of their health and quality of life. That is, previous assumptions about the connection between engagement in productive activity and well-being of seniors are supported, but those about seniors' withdrawal from productive activity on retirement are not.

The Attitudes of Professional Baby Boom Women Toward Retirement: A Cohort Comparison

Kari A. Brozowski, (Nipissing University, North Bay, Ontario, Canada)

Baby boom women in Canada will begin to flood into retirement within the next decade. Given that women have traditionally had problems with financial well being in retirement, it's important to determine if there are any problems for this large group of women in preparing for the transition. Pinpointing what problems exist enables us to offer solutions. This study investigated the differences that exist between professional baby boom women and an older and younger cohort, born between the years 1931-1945 (pre-baby boom), 1946-1955 (early baby boom), 1956-1965 (later baby boom), 1966-1973 (post-baby boom), in their attitudes toward retirement, presence of children, intermittence in employment history, retirement income security, and retirement planning knowledge. A sample of 320 was drawn from four cities in Ontario including Windsor, London, Toronto and North Bay. Respondents were asked to complete a 65-item questionnaire, which included questions about whether or not they were financially prepared for retirement, and how much they liked the idea of retirement. Differences between baby boom women and the older and younger cohorts were examined. By means of Multivariate Analysis of Variance, it was found that significant differences only existed for Cohort Groups in Intermittence in Employment History. For Women With and Without Changes in Marital Status, differences were displayed in Retirement Attitudes, Retirement Income Security, and Retirement Planning Knowledge. Overall, results suggested that early professional baby boom women could have financial problems in retirement if they experienced a divorce or separation

The Impact of Divorce on Women's Preparations for Later Life

Sharon Webb and Margaret Denton (McMaster University, Hamilton, Ontario Canada)

The purpose of this paper is to examine the impact of divorce on the preparations that women make for later life. Using the reflexive planning for later life conceptual model developed by Denton et al. (2000) we consider both collective and individual financial and non-financial preparations for later life. We draw on data from 20 life history interviews with married, separated and divorced women ages 45 and older. Comparisons are drawn between married and separated and divorced women. Overall, results show the significant impact of divorce on preparations for later life. Divorce impacts lifestyles, financial plans, residential mobility, family and social life. This study suggests public policy changes could minimize negative financial impacts of divorce on later life.

THE INCREASE OF PENSIONS PAYMENT - THE WAY TO SOFT CONTRADICTION BETWEEN GENERATIONS IN

ALBANIA
ILIA TELO (Director of Labour Institute, Tirana- ALBANIA).

The economic situation of pensioners during the period of transition remain unsatisfactory. The average real payment of pensions in year 2000 was only 2/3of the level of 1990. While the level of average pensions payment in comparison with average wages actually is 45 percent towards 70 percent ten years ago. This is why there are created disproportions and contradictions between generations. The analysis of situation and proposals for the softening of this problem are the purpose of this study. For this are using statistical data prepared by INSTAT (The Albanian Institut of Statistics) as well as SII (The Albanian Social Insurance Institut). In addition we have accomplished a survey by 1000 questionaries on family budgets of pensioners in five districts of the country. For the data analyzing in using the comparative method between districts , with the period of pre-transition, as well as with CEESs. Results of the study are showing that the edlery are within boundaries of living or surving. The main reasons for this situation are the low level of employment rate, the high rate of unemployment, as well as the enlargement of informal work. In conclusion, to raise pension payment, and the well-being on the whole, firstly it is necessary to increase the employment rate, decrease unemployment, reduce "black" and "grey" work as well as raise contributions for the budget of social Insurance Institut. These factors will impact to improve the ratio between contributors and benefits of the social insurance budget, which till now is only 1 with 1, towards 3 with 1 ten years ago. In the period, the government budget must contribute much more than actually, in absolute and, especially in relative ciphres toward GDP .

Well-Being in Retirement: Is it Money or is it People?

Peter Donahue (Faculty of Social Work, University of Calgary, Calgary, Canada) Elsa Marziali (Faculty of Social Work, University of Toronto, Toronto, Canada)

PURPOSE: Well-being, or the lack of, in retirement has been attributed to a number of factors including: finances, health, self-efficacy, and social support. This study compares and contrasts various criteria used to determine whether individuals make successful or unsuccessful transitions into retirement. METHODS: Sixteen cases were selected from a qualitative study of 100 men and women that had experienced involuntary retirement. Of the 16 cases, 8 were selected as examples of a successful retirement transition and 8 were selected as examples of an unsuccessful retirement transition. The initial grouping of the cases was based on two criteria developed by one of the investigators: whether the individuals discussed their retirement transitions in positive or negative terms, and the financial status of the individuals. The second investigator was given the same cases blind to previous group assignment and rated cases independently on quality of interpersonal relationships and social support. RESULTS: The investigators matched on poor versus good outcomes on 65 percent of the cases. On seven of the cases, the raters disagreed; one rated all seven as successful and the other rated them all as unsuccessful. Upon reviewing these seven cases, all subjects were aware of their financial constraints, but were not overly concerned nor upset by them. Rather, they stressed the importance of their social lives, connections with family and friends and overall well-being. CONCLUSION: Financial Status post-retirement is an important factor for quality of life and well-being, but social contact and important interpersonal relationships provide an important buffer for maintaining well-being.

SESSION 515

A cardiovascular life history: the Framingham Heart Study

Peeters A (Erasmus University, Rotterdam, The Netherlands), Mamun AA (Gronigen University, Gronigen, The Netherlands) Willekens F (Gronigen University, Gronigen, The Netherlands) Bonneux L (Erasmus University, Rotterdam, The Netherlands)

PURPOSE: In low mortality countries cardiovascular disease is the leading causes of death in adults, causing up to 500f deaths at the oldest ages. Although it is known that risk doubles approximately every decade at middle ages, the consequent impact on healthy aging has not been extensively analysed. Here we transform epidemiological occurrence rates into time-based measures of years spent with and lost to cardiovascular disease. METHOD: Using the age-schedule of cardiovascular disease observed during forty years of follow-up in the Framingham Heart Study we constructed multi-state life tables describing the human life course with cardiovascular disease. RESULTS: Within this cohort 40 year old men (women) live 35 (41) years; 28 (36) free of cardiovascular disease, 5.1 (3.7) with coronary heart disease, 3.2 (1.2) with myocardial infarction, 1.0 (1.2) with stroke, and 0.74 (0.88) with congestive heart failure. From the age of 40, 33% men (17% women) will ever suffer a myocardial infarction; 16% (21%) a stroke; and 18% (19%) congestive heart failure. Once an event has occurred, 60 year old men (women) with a myocardial infarction will lose on average 9 (13) years of life compared to individuals without cardiovascular disease. Those with stroke will lose on average 12 (14) years of life. CONCLUSION: We illustrate the power of transforming occurrence rates into time-based measures of saved and lost health. From age 70, a striking 320f remaining life expectancy is lived with cardiovascular disease. To ensure healthy aging, changes in population trends of cardiovascular disease, its risk factors and its treatment strategies need to be similarly analysed for their impact on the prevalence of cardiovascular disease at the oldest ages.

Social Factors as Predictors of Death in Canadians Aged 55 or Older

K. Wilkins (Health Statistics Division, Statistics Canada, Ottawa, Ontario, Canada)

The goal of this analysis was to examine selected social and demographic characteristics measured in 1994 in people aged 55 or older in relation to death at any time within the following four years. Longitudinal data from Statistics Canada's National Population Health Survey were used; multiple logistic regression was used in order to control for the effects of age, major chronic diseases and smoking. In the sample of 3,907 people aged 55 or older who were followed longitudinally, 482 deaths (255 men, 227 women) occurred from 1994 to 1998. For men, but not for women, being unmarried was independently predictive of death (odds ratio=1.9; 95% confidence interval 1.2, 2.9) after controlling for other relevant influences. For women, but not men, dependency on other people to carry out activities of daily living (ADL) was strongly predictive of dying (odds ratio=2.6; 95% confidence interval 1.2, 5.8). This finding may in part reflect the much higher likelihood of men than women who were ADL-dependent in 1994 to be married (66% and 35%, respectively) and thus perhaps to be cared for by their spouse. Other social factors, including perceived social support, frequency of social contacts and level of income, were not significantly associated with death for either sex. The results of this analysis illustrate the importance of sex-specific analysis in examining social factors as predictors of death.

Stability and change in self-rated health as a predictor of mortality: A 10-year follow-up study among older people

Raija Leinonen (The Finnish Centre for the Interdisciplinary Gerontology, Department of Health Sciences, University of Jyvaskylä, Finland), Eino Heikkinen (The Finnish Centre for the Interdisciplinary Gerontology, Department of Health Sciences, University of Jyvaskylä, Finland), Marja Jylhä (School of Public Health, University of Tampere, Finland)

Purpose: To examine how change or stability in self-rated health evaluated over a 5-year period predicts mortality. Methods: The study is a part of the Evergreen project with the subjects comprising all the inhabitants of Jyväskylä, central Finland born in 1914 (N=382). At baseline, in 1989, 91.6 % and in the second wave measurements, 5 years later 87.3% of those who were eligible participated in the interview; 77.2%

participated in the study centre examinations at baseline. Sixty-nine persons died over the five years after the second wave measurements between 1994 and 1999. The data were collected by interviews, questionnaires and examinations in the study centre, focusing on different domains of health and functional capacity. Dates of death were obtained from the population register. Four groups were constituted for the analysis according to self-rated health in 1989-1994: 'good-good' (n=81), 'good-bad' (n=37), 'bad-good' (n=35) and 'bad-bad' (n=64). Cox proportional hazard models adjusted for the number of chronic diseases, maximal walking speed over 10 meters and cognitive capacity (sum score of three tests) was used to compare mortality between the groups. Results: The relative risk of death in the 'bad-bad' group was 2.2 (1.09-4.45) compared with the 'good-good' group and 2.9 (1.18-6.96) compared with the 'bad-good' group. In men only the death rate in the 'good-bad' group was 3.9 (1.32-11.4) compared with the 'good-good' group and 6.0 (1.24-28.68) compared with the 'bad-good' group. Conclusions: Both stability and change in self-rated health over the 5-year period seem to be more important predictors of subsequent mortality than the baseline self-rated health in itself among older people.

The Pattern of Survival Improvement Changed during Last Century: What Does It Tell Us about Aging

A.I.Yashin (Max Planck Institute for Demographic Research, Rostock, Germany), S.V. Ukraintseva (Research Center for Medical Genetics, Russian Academy of Medical Sciences), S.I. Boiko (Max Planck Institute for Demographic Research, Rostock, Germany), A.S. Begun (Max Planck Institute for Demographic Research, Rostock, Germany), James W. Vaupel (Max Planck Institute for Demographic Research, Rostock, Germany)

The goal of this study is to evaluate the patterns of improvement in human survival during last century, analyze causes of such an improvement and discuss possible future changes in survival patterns. Despite the fact that the decline of mortality during last century was the subject of numerous discussions in demographic literature the consensus about the pattern of this decline has not been reached. We analyze time series of last century mortality data in developed countries of Europe, USA and Japan. We find that the pattern of correlation between the slope and intercept of the Gompertz part of the mortality curve (the Strehler and Mildvan correlation) experienced several changes during last century. We calculate respective changes in survival curves corresponding to period mortality data. We find that the improvement in survival, observed during last century followed two different patterns. The major change in the pattern took place in the middle of the century for countries of Western Europe and USA. During the first half the clear trend to rectangularization of survival curve was observed. The second half was characterized by almost parallel shift of the survival curves to the right. In Japan similar changes in the pattern of survival improvement happened in 1968. We show that the model of changing heterogeneity may explain observed trends and predict future survival patterns. This explanation suggests the presence of groups of individuals, which experience different rate of aging. We present the evidence about existence of such individuals in human population.

SESSION 517

Education, Challenges, and Dreams for Students and Elders

Polly McMahon, {Spokane Falls Community College; Spokane Falls, WA USA} *CD ROM Presentation and Discussion on Educational Opportunities for Entry Level Students from Welfare-Work Programs*

Issue: In the USA welfare cutbacks have focused on work oriented educational benefits known in WA state as WorkFirst or in some cases as Worker Retraining. There is high demand for training competent skill based individuals in the aging field. This roundtable would focus on the integration of student needs with those of the elderly population especially in rural areas. Structure: The presentation would provide six two minute CDROM interactive video segments describing the student experiences from this training and feedback from the elders with whom they worked. Following this presentation time would be permitted for discussion regarding challenges, next steps, and questions. Content: This is an interactive presentation in which the participants could gain immediate contact with non-traditional students who had previously been welfare recipients, disabled, or unable to secure employment and who are now successful in providing direct care and service to elders in rural areas of WA state. Feedback from the elders would also be integrated into this presentation. Conclusion/Anticipated Outcomes: The final product of this session would be encouragement for other health care providers and educators who are confronted with a lack of skilled labor in the rapidly expanding aging community. Different types of educational programs and training models would be discussed.

Multidisciplinary geriatric evaluation and intervention in a Geriatric Day Hospital: seven-year experience.

G. Sergio, L. Bartorelli (UOC Geriatria, Dipartimento Tutela della Salute dell'Anziano, ASL Roma C, Roma, Italia

The Authors show the organization of the Geriatric Day Hospital (DH), focusing on the multidisciplinary approach used to the elderly both in evaluation and intervention. At this moment the team consists of 28 multidisciplinary professionals.. On average 24 patients (mean age 74) a day are admitted at 8 AM and remain until 3 PM (for those patients living in the same district of the Hospital a minibus service is provided). About 55% of the patients are admitted for diagnostic assessment and all technological services of this general hospital are provided. The other 45% receive rehabilitation and/or medical treatment (venous infusions, medication, O2 therapy, etc.). Physical rehabilitation for neurological, osteoarticular, respiratory and cardiovascular problems consists of special exercise programs performed individually and/or in small groups (according to the method "body/conscience") during an 8-16 day cicle (on average 12). The neuropsychological rehabilitation for Alzheimer or vascular demented patients consists of 1) "formal" Reality Orientation Therapy (ROT) for small groups of 5 patients (MMSE=14-24) for a 45 min session, 4 days a week, for 4 consecutive weeks, twice a year; 2) individual cognitive rehabilitation (MMSE=10-24)with computer memory training using programs with various levels of difficulty (duration 30 min, 2-3 days a week, for 4 weeks, cycle can be repeated twice a year or see ROT frequency); 3) occupational therapy (MMSE=10-24) for 2 hrs a time (see above) in group and individually, in our garden too.

Third Age Care Service

Dra. Diana Scharovsky (Hospital Privado de Comunidad, Mar del Plata, Argentina), Julia Bidonde

The Third Age Care Service arises from the definition of health provided by the WHO which describes it not only as the absence of an illness but as the physical, social, spiritual and psychological well being. It is then possible to elaborate programs which interact with all the factors mentioned above, and which can contribute to humankind culture and environment. In order to understand the relationship between a person, his/her group and the community, it essential to comprehend these interrelationships. According to this approach, health promotion constitutes the basic axis of the activities addressed to our patients and which have as their main goal to modify behaviors, change surroundings in a positive way oriented towards the increase of health level starting from a multidimensional paradigm. It lays the foundations of its actions on three prevention levels, primary, secondary and tertiary prevention. Interventions are carried out according to four axis: patient, family, community and teaching Programs for: Patient: therapeutic exercise, falls, cognitive stimulation, strokes, back pain, risk factors, obesity, back pain. Family: self-help groups for families with patients suffering from dementia, stroke and falls. Community: creation of the following non-governmental organism: GAMA (Alzheimer s Support Group), CERAM (Meeting and Rehabilitation Center for the Elderly), Physical Activities

Center Teaching: Health Education, School for Hypertension, Dyslipidemia Workshop, Adult Primary School, Gerontology Oriented Course for Physical Education Teachers.

SESSION 518

Elder Abuse Femicides

Patricia Brownell, (Fordham University Graduate School of Social Service, New York City, USA); Jacquelin Berman, (New York City Department for the Aging); Susan Wilt (Office of Health Promotion and Prevention and Research, New York City Department of Health)

Purpose of Study: to examine elder abuse femicides with the goal of identifying factors that can lead to more effective safety planning for at risk victims. Data were obtained from 315 cases of homicides involving women victims age 50 years and older from the New York City Medical Examiner's records over a ten year period. Data elements include age, race, nativity of victims, relationship to alleged perpetrator, time and place of death, method and type of crime, living arrangements and other people in victims' households at time of death, substance abuse status of victim and perpetrator (if applicable). Secondary data are supplemented with archival research using newspaper accounts of elder abuse femicides occurring during the time period covered by the study as reported by local journalists. Findings include husbands were most likely to be known perpetrators followed by adult children, and victims were most likely to die from stabbings, followed by death from gunshot wounds. Protective strategies for older women at risk of homicide are discussed, as well as implications for future research.

Financial literacy in later life

Joanna Walker (University of Surrey and Pre-Retirement Association, Guildford, UK)

Purpose: was to discover and address the financial education needs of people in the pre-retirement phase (45-60 years) as part of a larger UK Government funded project on financial literacy in later life. Methods: involved focus group discussions with mid-lifers whose existing skills and understandings about money management, together with their perceptions of previous or current learning needs, were elicited using guided and open questioning. Learning materials were developed and presented to the original group, and to a further one, for their comment and further reflection. A chairperson and a participant observer ran the group sessions, yielding field notes and records of discussion. Results: Focus group data showed high concern about financial issues in the short and the longer term, but this sense of responsibility was hampered by being overwhelmed with information and by feelings of inadequacy when faced with facts and figures. Basic skills in financial management had been mastered mostly through experience, and coping strategies had arisen. Learning was perceived as possible, especially where it built on previous experience, however haphazard. Personal styles with money were significant insofar as they affected people's financial goals and strategies. Conclusions: Learning about financial management could be progressed at this stage in life by helping people review their existing skills and ways of managing, assessing their current and future challenges, and providing a 'safe' learning opportunity. Whereas the plethora of 'experts' in this field tended to disempower, learning should aim to put people more in control by developing confidence to apply basic principles.

Is it Elder Abuse or Violence Against Women? Hearing the Voices of Abused Older Women

Jill Hightower M.A.(B.C. Coalition for The Prevention of Abuse of Seniors, New Westminster, B.C. Canada) M.J. (Greta) Smith (BC// Yukon Society of Transition Houses, Vancouver, B.C.Canada) Henry C. Hightower, (University of British Columbia, Emeritus, Halfmoon Bay, Canada)

This work investigates a gap in the academic literatures, and in field practice. There are growing literatures on both elder abuse and violence against women, but neither gives much attention to issues of partner violence among older people. Even in qualitative work on violence against women, the voices of older women are virtually absent. Empirically, our earlier study showed that women aged 50 and older were greatly under-represented among those served by women's shelters. This is inconsistent with prevalence survey findings on domestic abuse of older women. Using a guided focus group approach, including providers of health and social services for older persons, community advocates for the prevention of elder abuse, and women's shelter staff, participants identified services to older victims of domestic violence, and gaps among these services. Focus group results highlight service gaps, incompatible service strategies, and provide illustrations of perverse results in practice. In multi-cultural communities such as British Columbia the added complications of foreign languages and diverse cultures make it both more difficult and more important to elicit the concerns and perceptions of victims. Development of sound and effective strategies to end abuse within the family and promote safety for the older victim must be based in the realities of the lives of older victims. Conclusions highlight the need for an interdisciplinary approach based in qualitative research using victims' insights, and interdisciplinary cooperation between those who work with older adults and those who work primarily in the field of violence against women.

Older Abuse and Neglect: An Enigmatic Dilemma to Ethonocultural Minorities and Faith Leaders.

Salim S. Bheriani (Hamilton Urban Core Community Health Center

Abuse and Neglect of Older Adults is prevalent throughout the world. Lack of appropriate support and resources, inadequate training with lack of sensitivity amongst service providers, and definitive studies and inadequate definition creating further potential risk, re-victimization, and compromising health of older adults, families, and entire community. These issues are not only challenging the developing countries, but also for the developed nations like United States, and Canada. The Canadian research in the area has been rudimentary; hence insufficient data exist to provide meaningful studies and prevalence rates. Furthermore, older abuse and neglect in general perceived from dominant culture with secular social service; yield convergent views and enigmatic dilemmas. More so, lack of understanding of several barriers add further to the complexity in ethonocultural minorities and making respective faith leaders vulnerable to their spiritual roles. My presentation paper and brief interviews with ethnic seniors and their faith leaders will challenge the professionals to gain better understanding to this new social problem and defining and solving it in ways that are sensitive to each individual cultural beliefs. The brief study results indicated that the seniors and particularly faith leaders are more comfortable taking holistic and spiritual healing approach rather than operating in a context of medical model and professional service providers in dealing with older abuse and neglect.

The Significance of Quality Relationships: older women's understandings of elder abuse

Hazel Morbey (University of the West of England, Bristol, UK)

Specifically feminist perspectives are largely absent from the developing discourse of elder abuse in the United Kingdom. This is also the case for research that focuses on older people as primary informants about the issue. Focus groups were used as a participative research method, to gather older women's understandings and experiences of elder abuse. Eight scenarios of abusive situations were developed as a research tool to explore the significance of gender, age and social relationships to understanding abuse in later life. Quality of relationships emerged as a central feature of the older women's discussions around the stresses of familial caregiving. For the participants in this research quality of relationship and quality of caregiving are inextricably linked, to the point that the older women questioned whether a stressed and unsupported informal caregiver could provide quality care. A scenario depicting a marriage with a history of violence is used to illustrate the significance of quality of relationships to caregiving. Familial relationships, which develop into active caregiving relationships, are likely to have been in existence for many years. A number of research participants believed that the nature of such relationships through their life-course should be of concern to practitioners. If previous significant conflict and abuse have existed or are identified then it is important that practitioners are aware of these, in order to feed such information into formal assessments of risk and vulnerability.

Violence and Abuse Against Older Women in Australia

Jane Mears (University of Western Sydney, Sydney, Australia)

Purpose: To examine the issue of violence and abuse directed against older women, by talking in focus groups and seminars to older women about their experiences of violence and abuse. These seminars also provide the opportunity for women to share experiences and talk through ways of dealing with violence and abuse. Method: For a 2-year period leading into the study, the researchers ran seminars with groups of older women. With the permission and informed consent of the women involved, these group discussions were recorded. In addition, older women who wished to tell individual stories were invited to do so. A booklet that put together all these stories was produced and used as the basis of a pilot study. Forty older women were invited to read the booklet and fill in a questionnaire recording their responses, ideas and reactions to the book. Results: The results of this pilot study are essentially that violence is a problem of major concern to older women in Australia. A large proportion of the women who participated in the study had experienced violence towards them at some time in their lives and were still dealing with the effects and consequences of this violence. The second stage of the study, the distribution of 10,000 booklets and questionnaires is well underway. Conclusion: It is clear that the problem of violence against older women needs to be taken seriously at all levels of policy making and service delivery. The paper proposes some strategies that will support and assist older women to deal with this problem.

Why Is It so Difficult to Combat Elder Financial Exploitation of the Elderly?

D. Poirier (Université de Moncton Law School) & N. Poirier (Université de Moncton School of Nursing)

PURPOSE: The scientific community and the general population are now fully aware that economic abuse is the most frequent form of elder abuse. However, no satisfactory answer has been given to why it is so difficult to fight elder economic abuse. Three hypotheses have been advanced to explain that phenomenon: the inadequacy of existing law, the inefficacy of existing law, and family values conflicting with the application of the law. METHOD: The authors have undertaken a three stage analysis of the empirical data available on the subject of elder financial abuse. Firstly, the authors have analysed the adequacy of the different components of Canadian law (criminal, civil, guardianship). Secondly, they have analysed the efficacy of the various components of the Canadian law in combating elder financial abuse. Finally the authors have constructed a conceptual model to answer their initial question. RESULTS: Three main finding are reported by the authors. Firstly, they found that the Canadian law currently in effect is adequate to combat the various forms of elder abuse, including financial abuse. Secondly, they found however that the relevant components of the Canadian law were ineffective mainly with regard to financial exploitation. Thirdly, normative pluralism is presented as a theoretical model for the better understanding of the different normative orders which may conflict in the complex issue of elder economic abuse. The domestic normative order (family values) may in fact conflict with the professional normative orders of protection officers (social workers, police officers, and others) and with the territorial normative order (the law of the land). CONCLUSION: The theoretical modal may help decide which solutions and interventions have more chances of success in combating elder financial abuse

SESSION 519

Trends in the Care of Dependent Elders in Four Countries: Family and Formal Services

Y. Arai and M. Sugiura (National Institute for Longevity Sciences—NILS, Aichi, Japan), New Japanese Insurance for Elderly: A Welcome but Difficult Break with Tradition. L. Trahan, (Ministry of Health and Social Services, Québec (Québec) Canada), Organization of Services for Frail and Dependent Elders in Québec. G. Sundström (Institute of Gerontology, University College of Health Sciences, Jönköping, Sweden and L. Johansson (National Board of Health and Welfare, Stockholm, Sweden, Long-term Care in Sweden: A Fifty Years Perspective on Change. S. H. Zarit (Gerontology Center, Penn State University, University Park, PA USA) and D. Shea (Department of Health Policy and Administration, Penn State University, University Park, PA), Sources of Help to Dependent Elders: A Comparison of the US and Sweden. M. Downs (University of Bradford, Bradford, UK), Discussant.

ISSUE: The social and cultural traditions of countries influence the extent to which families or the state assume responsibility for care of dependent elders. Systems that emphasize family responsibility may place excessive burden on families to provide care. Conversely, extensive public systems are under increasing pressure to cut costs and provide services in cost-efficient ways. A comparison of how different societies meet these challenges can illuminate strengths and limitations of their approaches, and identify optimal strategies for maximizing social and family resources for providing care. STRUCTURE: This symposium will examine the role of family and public services in four countries with very different traditions and procedures for organizing care. The countries are: Japan, Québec province in Canada, Sweden and the USA. These countries range in their traditions from a strong family orientation in Japan to an emphasis on communal responsibility in Sweden. Examining care in these different contexts will bring new perspectives to the challenges faced by families and society in caring for disabled elders. CONTENT: In Japan, the Confucian tradition of family responsibility for its elders remains strong, but the pressure of an expanding older population as well as women's increased involvement in the workplace has reduced the ability of the traditional family caregiver, the daughter-in-law, to provide care for her parents-in-law. The implications of a new public long term care insurance provide the potential for increased access to formal services, but the cultural stigma about using services has contributed to low rates of service use. In Québec, a well-developed care system is being reorganized to meet the dual challenge of increased need among a growing population of disabled elders and pressures for efficiency in service delivery. New models of integrated community services offer the possibility of providing high quality care to this population. In Sweden, recent emphasis has been to control the costs of public old age care in a system that proportion of elders receives help today compared to 25 years ago. This broad coverage has been achieved by substituting less expensive kinds of support for more expensive services. Family help and private services are playing an increasing role in filling gaps in services. Finally, in the USA, responsibility for providing and paying for help lies mainly with families. The implications of this approach were examined by comparing elders in the USA with Sweden, where formal help is more accessible. The results showed that families provide as much help in showed that families provide as much help in both systems, but that formal help is higher in Sweden. The effect of higher levels of formal help in Sweden was to reduce unmet needs among elders to a negligible amount compared to the US. CONCLUSIONS: Despite the differences in history and tradition in these four countries, common themes of social change in the roles of families and the need for cost efficient strategies have emerged, which provide the context for developing new approaches to care.

Long-term Care in Sweden: A Fifty Years Perspective on Change

G. Sundström (Institute of Gerontology, University College of Health Sciences, Jönköping, Sweden and L. Johansson (National Board of Health and Welfare, Stockholm, Sweden)

In the first half of the 20th century in Sweden, pensions for the aged expanded to cover everyone and by 1948 provided a level that (barely) sufficed to live on. In 1950, old-age care meant institutional care, covering 20% of the oldest (80+). Half of the residents were single, many were childless, and most were poor. After public scandals involving the old age homes, national guidelines that emphasized community care for the elderly were established in the 1950s. This was and is mainly public Home Help (help with shopping, cooking, cleaning, toileting, bathing, getting out of bed, etc.). Home Help targeted 38% of the elderly 80+ in 1975 and used an estimated third of the budget for old-age care. Yet, at the same time, institutional care had expanded to cover 30% of the same age group. By that time, services were quite "egalitarian" as they were used equally by all social classes, if one adjusted for class differences in morbidity. Institutional care also had developed in the same direction. After this crescendo, these forms of public old age care levelled off and diminished gradually to current levels of 22% of the 80+ population in institutional care and 20% with Home Help. In many localities, community care now consumes an estimated fifth of the budgets; locally even lower figures are reported. (Local variations in old age care are sizable indeed.) Yet, other types of support for the elderly have expanded in the last decades, to 'cover up' for ever more heavily rationed Home Help. Therefore the same proportion of the elderly is targeted by some kind of public support today (1999) as in 1975: they may not use Home Help but seem to make do with transportation services and/or alarm systems and/or meals-on-wheels. A further ingredient of this mixed picture is the fact that an increasing fraction of needy elders receive support from their children and other informal helpers and fewer use public Home Help. Also, more elderly purchase private out-of-the-pocket paid help, in all social classes but especially among the most affluent. Private retirement housing also expands, and though basic patterns remain, these developments imply inherent change of old-age care in the welfare state.

New Japanese Insurance for Elderly: A Welcome but Difficult Break with Tradition

Y. Arai and M. Sugiura (National Institute for Longevity Sciences—NILS, Aichi, Japan)

The new public Long-Term Care insurance scheme ("Kaigo Hoken"), in place since April, 2000, radically departs from the traditional Japanese idea that the family is the prime resource of long-term care. Home care availability is no longer the benchmark. There has long been tremendous social pressure for families to provide care, particularly by female kin, partly due to the Confucian stress on filial piety. Caregiving used to be a legal obligation for the eldest son, something the government "took advantage of" even after World War II. However, the recent huge numbers of impaired elderly and concomitant decrease in informal care capacity have made "caregivers' burden" a social issue. Overemphasis on family values and self-help now serve to stigmatize social services in Japan. The new insurance covers institutional and home care not only for those aged 65 or more, but also for people over 40 with "age-related" diseases such as dementia. Municipal governments are the insurer, and the level of services is decided by patient impairment. Monthly premiums cover half the cost for people over 40, with 10% copayment at the service point. Rates are adjusted for low income, and taxes pay the balance. Unexpectedly, there has been no rush to use the new services, largely because some families feel a cultural stigma attached, and premiums can be high. These obstacles must be quickly overcome for clients and caregivers to benefit from this inevitable departure from traditional Japanese care for the impaired elderly.

Organization of Services for Frail and Dependent Elders in Québec

L. Trahan (Research and Evaluation, Ministry of Health and Social Services, Québec, Québec G1S 2M1 Canada

The growing elderly population represents a challenge to public services but it is not the only factor to take into account while restructuring services for the frail and disabled elderly. Technological advances which led to major reforms in several countries have resulted in fewer acute care beds in hospitals, decreasing the length of stay and increasing pressure on home care. Furthermore, it is important to pay attention to the emergence of new models of organizing care like integrated community-based services. How to adjust the amount and the types of services such as home care, residential care, geriatrics, etc. to respond adequately to the needs of the frail elderly is the real challenge of any policies for the future. The new policy of the Ministry of Health and Social Services then focus on the organization of health and social services for the elderly and their delivery and financing.

Sources of Help to Dependent Elders: A Comparison of the US and Sweden

S. H. Zarit (Gerontology Center, Penn State University, University Park, PA USA) and D. Shea (Department of Health Policy and Administration, Penn State University, University Park, PA).

PURPOSE: The growth of the older population has placed increasing burdens on families and society to provide care. Different approaches to organizing and funding care may have different implications for the amount of family involvement and the care that elders receive. In this study, we compare two countries with very different systems of financing and access to care: Sweden, which has an extensive system of publicly funded, community- based long term care services, and the USA, where services are largely privately financed. METHOD: Data were drawn from national surveys in Sweden and the USA which had comparable questions. The Swedish survey was the 1994 Aging in the Community Study, which had a representative sample of 1,378 community-dwelling people aged 75 and older. The US survey was the 1992 Medicare Current Beneficiary Study, which included 4.583 community-dwelling people aged 75 and older. RESULTS: Rates of disability were comparable in the two countries. Among elders who needed assistance, families provided similar amounts of help in the two countries. Elders in Sweden were more likely to receive formal services. Unmet need, defined as an ADL for which the person needed, but did not receive, assistance, was much higher in the US than Sweden (29% compared to 1%), and was concentrated most among people living alone. CONCLUSION: This comparison shows that families remain involved in care of elders in countries that have extensive public care systems, and that services in that context can fill gaps where family help is not available.

SESSION 520

Calf muscle metabolic and functional changes during recovery in malnourished elderly subjects

I Bourdel-Marchasson, E Thiaudière, P-A Joseph, P Dehail, M Biran, P Faux, M Rainfray, J-P Emeriau, P Canioni. [Centre de Gériatrie Henri Choussat, 33604 Pessac Cedex, France RMSB, UMR 5536-Université de Bordeaux 2 ; 33000 Bordeaux, France]

PURPOSE: The loss of muscle strength and mass is one of the consequences of malnutrition, and therefor the possible reversibility of these changes is a major concern in elderly subjects. METHODS: 24 hospitalized clinically stable elderly patients were explored by isokinetic plantar flexor torque measurements and NMR imaging for medial gastrocnemius mass assessment and 31P and 13C NMR spectroscopy for inorganic phosphate (Pi), phosphocreatine (PCr), and glycogen quantitation. Eleven patients from 24 were considered as malnourished and nine were explored twice within a one-month interval. RESULTS The malnourished subjects had lower muscle mass (P<0.02), and tended to have lower strength than control-hospitalized subjects. Muscle strength increased after refeeding in the malnourished (P<0.01), whereas muscle mass was unchanged. Pi/ATP ratio was decreased in the malnourished as compared to controls (P<0.001) and increased during refeeding (P<0.01). Mean PCr/ATP ratio was decreased in malnourished patients (P<0.01) and reached the control values after nutritional repletion. Mean glycogen muscle content was not different in both groups, although with very scattered distribution for malnourished patients, becoming not different to that of controls after refeeding. CONCLUSION The decrease in PCr/ ATP ratio could result either from the decrease in total muscle creatine or reduced oxidative capacities. High or normal values of glycogen associated with low Pi/ATP ratios in the malnourished was interpreted as a preferential use of lipid than carbohydrate oxidation for energy supply, which is known to result in lower muscle performance. All the data suggest that normalization of muscle metabolite content following refeeding resulted in muscle strength improvement in malnourished subjects.

Correlates of body composition assessed by multiple-frequency bioelectrical impedance with bioclinical markers of the nutritional status in elderly inpatients.

C. Oasi, J. Sibony-Prat, A. Bruhat, J. Belmin (Service de Gériatrie, Hôpital R. Muret et Université Paris Nord, Sevran, France).

PURPOSE : To investigate correlates of body composition assessed by multi-frequency bioelectrical impedance (MFBI) with bioclinical markers of nutritional status in commonly used in geriatric medicine.. METHODS : We assessed the nutritional status of 100 consecutive patients (29 men and 71 women, 81.8 + 8.1 years) admitted in an acute care geriatric hospital ward, by measuring body mass index (BMI), arm muscle circumference (AMC), sum of 4 skinfold thickness (SST), Mini Nutritional Assessment (MNA) score, albumine (Alb) and prealbumine (PA) plasma levels. Moreover, body composition was determined by MFBI analysis (Analycor, Spengler, France). RESULTS : Lean body mass was positively correlated with BMI, AMC, SST (r : 0.55, 0.40, 0.27 respectively p<0.01) and negatively with age (r :0.38, p<0.01). Body fat was positively correlated with BMI, AMC, SST and MNA score (r : 0.78, 0.40, 0.71, 0.33 respectively, p<0.01). Body cell mass was positively correlated with BMI, AMC and SST (r : 0.56, 0.41, 0.27 respectively, p<0.01) and negatively with age (r : 0.40, p<0.01). None of body composition parameters was significantly correlated with Alb or PA values. CONCLUSION : Body composition parameters determined by MFBI were hignly correlated with anthropometric markers of the nutritional status, but not with Alb and PA. Since MFBI is highly reproducible, this method is promising to assess longitudinal changes in body composition in elderly patients with an impaired nutritional status.

Effects of Age on Energy Expenditure and Respiratory Quotient During Experimental Underfeeding in Healthy subjects

J. C. Moriguti (Faculty of Medicine of Ribeirão Preto of São Paulo University, Brazil and Human Nutrition Research Center on Aging at Tufts University, Boston, USA), S. K. Das (Human Nutrition Research Center on Aging at Tufts University, Boston, USA), M. A. McCrory (Human Nutrition Research Center on Aging at Tufts University, Boston, USA), E. Saltzman (Human Nutrition Research Center on Aging at Tufts University, Boston, USA), A. S. Greenberg (Human Nutrition Research Center on Aging at Tufts University, Boston, USA) and S.B. Roberts (Human Nutrition Research Center on Aging at Tufts University, Boston, USA)

PURPOSE: The effect of aging on energy regulation remains controversial. We compared the effects of underfeeding on changes in energy expenditure and respiratory quotient in young normal weight men and women {YNW, age 25.7 ([3.2][SD]) years}, young overweight men and women {YOW, age 26.1 ([3.5][SD] years}, and older (OLD) men and women {age 68.4 ([3.3][SD])}. METHOD: The thermic effect of feeding (TEF) during weight maintenance, and changes in resting energy expenditure (REE) and respiratory quotient were determined in response to undereating by an average 896 kcal/d for 6 weeks. In addition, body composition was measured. RESULTS: No significant differences among the groups were observed in TEF, fasting and postprandial respiratory quotient, or the change in fasting respiratory quotient with underfeeding. However, REE adjusted for fat free mass and fat mass was significantly lower in old subjects compared to YNW and YOW subjects (P lower than 0.05). In addition, the REE response to weight change was significantly attenuated in the OLD subjects in models controlling for weight change (P=0.026). CONCLUSION: These data suggest that the responsiveness of energy expenditure to negative energy balance is attenuated in old age, and provide further support for the hypothesis that mechanisms of energy regulation are broadly disregulated in old age.

Malnutrition and obesity among elderly in a Brazilian community. The Bambui Health and Ageing Study.

S. M. Barreto1,2,3, V. M. A. Passos1,2,3, E. Uchôa1,2,3 , H. L. Guerra2,3, J. O. A. Firmo2,3, P. G. Vidigal1,2,3, M. F. F. Lima e Costa1,2,3 (1Federal University of Minas Gerais Medical School, 2Oswaldo Cruz Foundation René Rachou Research Centre, and 3Research Group on the Epidemiology and Anthropology of Ageing (REGEA), Belo Horizonte, Brazil)

PURPOSE: Very little is known on the anthropometry and associated functional status among elderly in developing countries. This study describes the distribution of body mass index (BMI) among elderly in a formerly endemic area for Trypanosoma cruzi infection in Brazil and investigate factors associated with obesity and malnutrition. METHODS: All residents of Bambui town, aged 60+ years were invited for this study (n=1742) and 1451 (85,8%) participated. Obesity was defined as BMI>30kg/m2 and malnutrition as BMI<20kg/m2. Associated factors were investigated using multinomial logistic regression, taking individuals with 20>BMI<30 kg/m2 as the reference group. RESULTS: The mean BMI was 25.1 ± 4.9kg/m2, being 23.9 ± 4.1kg/m2 for males and 25.8 ± 5.2kg/ m2 for females. BMI significantly decreased with ageing (25.5 ± 5.0kg/m2, 24.7 ± 4.9kg/m2 and 23.3 ± 4.5kg/m2 for age 60-69, 70-79 and 80+ years, respectively). Obesity was prevalent among 12.8% of participants, being directly associated with female sex, higher family income, hypertension and hyperglycemia, and inversely related to walking >3 times/week. Malnutrition affected 14.8% of participants, increased with age and was lower among women and higher income families. It was negatively associated with hypertension and hyperglycemia and directly related with T. cruzi infection and >2 hospitalisations in past 12 months. DISCUSSION: Population ageing is the most striking demographic change occurring in Brazil. The metabolic alterations associated with obesity are consistent with results found elsewhere. Malnutrition is highly prevalent in this community. The association of malnutrition with T.cruzi infection, increased hospital admissions and low income may reflect illness-related weight-loss and social deprivation of elderly in this community.

Nutritional assessment in an elderly sample.

Speranta Babeanu (Clinic of Natural Therapy Breaza, Romania Manuela Udrea St.Luca Chronic Diseases and geriatrics Hospital, Bucharest) Romania Laura Marinescu BA TouchTunes,Montreal, Canada)

Purpose:The discrepancies in the literature regarding the nutritional assessment in the elderly, usually referred to the adult values and which are not taking into consideration the concomitant pathology, made us to assess the nutritional status in a representative sample of elderly subjects. Method:200 subjects from 50 to 107 years old mostly included into the age group of 70 to 79. The pathology consisted of chronic rheumatism and cardiovascular diseases. The subjects were evaluated clinically, socially, nutriti onally and paraclinically(various protein indices, minerals, immune data). The nutritional data comprised: analysis of caloric, nutrients and liquid intake as well as anthropometric data). Various nutritional assessment indices were used. All the data were analyzed by various statistical methods. Results:Decrease of BMI over the age of 80, decrease of lean body mass over 80 and of muscular mass over 7o, increase of procentual adipose mass until the age of 75 especially in women. As biological markers: a slight decrease of serum albumin but significant of transferrin: the positive correlation between the age and some lipidic parameters until the age of 80. As immune data: the relative decrease of total TL and increase of ICC and of BL. The nutritional assessment indices show the important decrease over the age of 90. Conclusions: drawn from the study: - unbalanced food intake with the prevalence of hydrocarbonates, and diminished liquid intake; - lack of a close relationship between BMI and the caloric intake; - influence of age upon some components of protein and lipid metabolism; direct relationship between some instruments of nutritional assessment and the global health status.

Plasma levels of DHEA sulfate and nutritional status of elderly women in a geriatric hospital ward

C. Oasi, J. Sibony-Prat, A. Bruhat, J. Belmin (Service de Gériatrie, Hôpital R. Muret et Université Paris Nord, Sevran, France).

PURPOSE : To investigate plasma levels of DHEA sulfate (DHEAs) and nutritional status in elderly women.

METHODS: Nutritional status of 71 elderly women (85 + 7 years) consecutively admitted in a acute care geriatric ward was assessed by body mass index (BMI), arm muscle circumference (AMC), sum of 4 skinfold thickness (SST), Mini Nutritional Assessment (MNA) score, body cell mass determined by multifrequency bioimpedance analysis (Analycor, Spengler, France), albumine (Alb) and prealbumine (PA) plasma levels. In all patients, plasma levels of DHEAs (umol/l) were determined at entry by radioimmunoassay.

RESULTS: We found positive correlations between DHEAs values and plasma Alb ($p<0.01$), PA ($p<0.03$), MNA score ($p=0.07$) and a negative correlation between DHEAs and age ($p<0.02$). The other parameters were not significantly correlated with DHEAs levels. Multivariate analysis showed that age, MNA and Alb were independent factors correlated with DHEAs. Plasma levels of DHEAs of women with Alb under 35 g/l were significantly lower than those with Alb above 35 g/l (1.03 ± 0.81 mmol/l and 1.63 ± 1.69 mmol/l , $p=0.04$). Plasma levels of DHEAs were significantly lower in women with undernutrition defined by MNA score under 24 than in those without undernutrition (1.09 ± 0.82 mmol/l and 1.93 ± 0.70 mmol/l, $p=0.04$). Plasma levels of DHEAs were 0.84 + 0.71 mmol/l in patients whose body mass cell was under mean of age-ajusted reference value minus 2sd, and 1.32 + 0.93 mmol/l in those whose body mass celle was above this value ($p=0.07$).

CONCLUSION: In these elderly women, plasma levels of DHEAs are correlated to several indicators or the nutritional status, independently from age, and were significantly decreased in women with an impaired nutritional status. These results support the view that DHEAs deficiency may be involved in causes or consequences of undernutrition in elderly women.

The diagnosis of malnutrition in elderly inpatients : comparison of diagnosis criteria

C. Oasi, J. Sibony-Prat, A. Bruhat, J. Belmin (Service de Gériatrie, Hôpital R. Muret et Université Paris Nord, Sevran, France).

PURPOSE : To compare the diagnosis of malnutrition in elderly patients using different diagnosis criteriae commonly used. METHODS : We assessed the nutritional status of 100 consecutive patients (29 men and 71 women, 81.8 + 8.1 years) admitted in an acute care geriatric hospital ward, by measuring body mass index (BMI), arm muscle circumference (AMC), sum of 4 skinfold thickness (SST), Mini Nutritional Assessment (MNA) score, albumine (Alb) and prealbumine (PA) plasma levels. Nine different diagnosis criteriae of malnutrition (I to IX) were considered : BMI (I), AMC (II), SST (III) values below the mean of age-ajusted reference values minus 2 sd, MNA score below 24 (IV) or 17 (V), Alb below 35 g/l (VI) or 30 g/l (VII), PA below 0.20 g/l (VIII) or 0.15 g/l (IX). RESULTS : Mean values were : BMI : 24.9 + 4.3 kg/m2, AMC : 20.3 + 4.7 cm, SST 36.7 + 15.4 mm, MNA : 19.3 + 4.2, Alb : 34.7 + 5.4 g/l, PA : 0.22 + 0.06 g/l. The percentages of patients considered as malnourished according each criteria were : 4% with I, 84% with II, 40% with III, 87% with IV, 26% with V, 56% with VI, 16% with VII, 38% with VIII, and 10% with IX. The concordance between the diagnosis of malnutrition according these different methods was poor (kappa values below 0.20), except for those related to Alb and PA (kappa 0.47 between VII and IX, kappa 0.38 between VI and VIII). CONCLUSION : There are large differences between the criteria used to diagnose malnutrition in elderly inpatients. This might have important issues in clinical practice to diagnose malnutrition and to implement nutritional assistance.

SESSION 521

Decapation hypothesis of the chromosome stability and aging

Kh. Muradian (Institute of Gerontology AMS Ukraine, Kiev, Ukraine)

The ends of eukaryotic linear chromosomes (LC) are highly vulnerable and have to be protected by the nucleoprotein caps. Due to the non-canonical G:G paring, the cap DNA forms unusually stable two-, three- and four-stranded DNA constructs. According to our model, a LC contains two relatively massive and stable elements the body and caps at 3'ends of the body DNA. However, these well protected parts are linked by a flimsy single stranded-DNA "neck" which could be easily broken. The resulting decapped chromosome can swiftly undergo dysfunctional modifications, ultimately leading to LC aberration or loss, followed by cellular senescence and death. The cap breakage and related DNA loss should be frequent events at incoherent fluctuations of LC body and cap, inevitable in situations associated with LC condensation or movement, e.g. at the mitotic LC "horsetail" dragging. In fact, there are two alternative strategies, differing around 10 times in a human cell DNA loss: i) parsimonious - associated with untangling the cap DNA and replication from the very beginning of the matrix (lesser 15-20 nucleotides loss per replication); ii) exhaustive - cutting off the cap and copying only the body DNA (wasting up to 150-200 nucleotides per replication). It is obvious that in the first case the DNA loss is lesser but it needs a rather difficult target the end of the cap DNA. The second alternative seems easier to realize but it is associated with higher DNA wasting. Depending on the age and other variables, a cell probably uses any of these alternatives. The assumption is supported by existing data and could explain why DNA losses (40-200 nucleotides per cell division) vary in different cells and culture conditions and are much higher than it could be expected from the "DNA-end replication" problem. Switching from the exhaustive to parsimonious strategy seems a promising mode of the cell replicative life-span extension, applicable for both medicine and biotechnology.

Gene Promoters and Aging

M.S. Kanungo, Rashmi Upadhyay, K. Shanti, S. Gupta Molecular Biology Laboratory, Department of Zoology Banaras Hindu University, Varanasi - 221005, India

Transcription factors and RNA polymerase that bind to transcription start sites of genes carry out basal transcription. However, stimulation or repression of genes is brought about by nuclear trans-acting factors (TAF) that bind to specific sequences (cis-acting elements) of the promoter located upstream of the transcription start site. Our objective was to find out if the levels of the trans-acting factors change after adulthood, which would alter the expression of genes and lead to deterioration of functions in old age. Fibronectin (FNT) is responsible for wound healing. Its gene is expressed in the liver of mammals, and it is stimulated by cAMP that binds to an 8-base pair DNA sequence (CRE) located in its promoter. Electrophoretic mobility shift assay (EMSA) using the CRE and nuclear extract (NE) of the liver of rat showed that three TAFs bind to the CRE in the young in which wound healing is fast, whereas only one TAF is present in the old in which wound healing is slow. Creatine phosphokinase (CPK) is essential for ATP production from phosphocreatine. Several cis-acting elements, MEF, E-box, and (A)22 and (GTTT)8 repeats located in its promoter bind to specific TAFs present in the NE of the heart of mice. Their levels are far lower in the old. Vitellogenin (VTG) and ovalbumin genes of the bird, Japanese quail, code for the egg yolk and egg white proteins and are expressed in the liver and oviduct, respectively. Their expression declines after adulthood, but is enhanced by 17 B-estradiol that binds to tissue specific TAFs which then bind to cis-acting elements in their promoters. The levels of the TAFs decrease after adulthood, when egg laying declines. Administration of the hormone raises the levels of these TAFs. Thus, the promoters of genes play an important role in the regulatory changes in the expression of genes that occur during aging and alter the levels of corresponding proteins/enzymes. This leads to deterioration of functions after adulthood and leads to aging. However, it is possible to delay or prevent at least some of the changes by administration of hormones and effectors, and thereby prolong the adulthood period.

Hyperhomocysteinemia and methylenetetrahydrofolate reductase gene polymorphism in Japanese centenarians

S.Nakazawa, N.Hirose, Y.Arai, K.Yamamura, Y.Ebihara, M.Takayama, K.Shimizu, S.Homma (Department of Geriatric Medicine, Keio University, School of Medicine, Tokyo, Japan) Y.Gondo, H.Inagaki, K. Kitagawa, Y.Masui (Tokyo Metropolitan Institute of Gerontology, Tokyo, Japan)

PURPOSE: The prevalence of hyperhomocysteinemia is relatively high among the elderly. The aim of this study was to evaluate clinical relevance of hyperhomocysteinemia and methylenetetrahydrofolate reductase (MTHFR) gene polymorphism in centenarians. METHOD: We investigated 92 centenarians (66 female, 26 male). Total homocysteine (tHcy) level was measured by HPLC. As possible determinant of tHcy, the serum levels of folic acid, nutritional indices, creatinine were measured. Frequencies of A223T-missense mutation in the MTHFR gene were analysed by PCR method. Cognitive function of centenarians was assessed by using clinical dementia raring (CDR). RESULT: Mean level of tHcy of centenarians was 14.5±5.2 nmol/mL, which was relatively high as compared with reference data. The frequencies of A223T mutation in MTHFR gene among centenarians were as follows; AA 34%, AV 48%, VV 18%), which were not significantly different from those among 120 healthy volunteers (female 58, male 62, mean age 50±7 years). In centenarians, the level of tHcy tended to be higher in VV group as compared to AV and AA group ($p=0.058$). There was no significant association of tHcy with the levels of folic acid or any nutritional indices. Centenarians with elevated tHcy levels (tHcy>15nmol/mL) had significantly lower body mass index, higher serum creatinine, and relatively lower cognitive function than those with lower tHcy levels. CONCLUSION: A223T mutation in MTHFR gene had no impact on longevity. Hyperhomocysteinemia in centenarian was associated with renal insufficiency but not with low levels of folic acid or poor nutritional status.

Oxidative stress, telomeres and vascular dementia

Thomas von Zglinicki, Violeta Serra, Gabriele Saretzki (Dept of Gerontology, University of Newcastle, UK), Elisabeth Steinhagen-Thiessen (Evangelisches Geriatriezentrum Berlin, Germany)

PURPOSE: Specific risk factors with prognostic relevance for Vascular Dementia (VaD) are not known, and known genetic risk factors for Alzheimer´s Dementia (AD) have generally low penetrance. Oxygen free radical mediated brain damage has been suggested as a major cause of dementias. Telomeres shorten with each cell division in human somatic cells due to the telomere-specific accumulation of oxidative single-strand damage We hypothesized that telomere length might be useful as cumulative indicator for antioxidative defence capacity in vivo. METHODS: Telomere length and shortening rate (Southern blotting), and oxygen free radical generation (DCF fluorescence) were measured in skin fibroblasts in vitro. Peripheral blood mononuclear cell (PBMC) telomere length was measured from 190 donors: patients with either AD or VaD or cognitively normal patients with severe cerebro/cardiovascular disease (CVD) or healthy control donors. RESULTS: There is a significant correlation between telomere shortening rate and antioxidative capacity in fibroblast strains derived from donors from all four groups. In vivo we found a very strong correlation between the incidence of VaD (but not AD) and short telomere length (adjusted for age) in PBMC, while there was no significant correlation to APOE or GST genotypes. Short telomeres in VaD patient PBMC are not the results of faster proliferation of hematopoetic stem and/or progenitor cells, because lengths of telomeres in PBMC and fibroblasts from these patients are closely correlated. CONCLUSION: Telomere length might become a prognostic risk indicator for VaD.

Paraxonase gene polymorphisms PON 55 and 192 and longevity in Belfast Elderly Longitudinal Free-living Aging STudy (BELFAST)

I.M.Rea, C. Belton, D.McMaster, I.S.Young, P.P. McKeown (Departments of Geriatric Medicine, Clinical Chemistry and Medicine, Queens University Belfast, UK)

PURPOSE: PON1, known to hydrolyse substrates including organophosphates, is also associated with high density lipoprotein (HDL), and reported to protect low density lipoprotein (LDL) against oxidative modification 'in vitro'. Since very elderly people seem protected from early mortality from vascular disease, it was of interest to carry out genotyping of the PON55 and PON192 polymorphism in elderly survivors. METHOD: 296 subjects (80-103 years), enlisted as part of a study of aging (BELFAST), were well, free-living, independently mobile and cognitively intact. Control subjects were sex -matched subjects (12-23years) from Young Hearts Study. PON155 and 192 polymorphisms were studied using standard PCR-RFLP approach. RESULTS: PON1 genotypes were in Hardy-Weinberg equilibrium. PON55 frequencies for LL, LM and MM in elderly subjects were 0.41, 0.46 and 0.13 and not significantly different from the control population. PON192 frequencies for QQ, QR and RR genotypes in the elderly group were 0.47, 0.44 and 0.09 respectively with no significant change compared to controls but Q and R alleles were significantly different (0.69 and 0.31) in elderly compared to young subject groups (0.73 and 0.27) ($p<0.01$). CONCLUSION: This data suggests that carriage of the PON192 polymorphism allele may be associated with longevity in the BELFAST longitudinal group. This is of interest because of its association with a lower ability of HDL to protect LDL against oxidative modification which is converse to the original proposed hypothesis. On the other hand, the 192R allele has increased enzymatic activity which could potentially accentuate a protective role in detoxification and a role in healthy ageing.

Selfish-transposon "exiling and sloughing" hypothesis of aging and gene circulation

Kh. Muradian (Institute of Gerontology AMS Ukraine, Kiev, Ukraine)

A significant part of the genome consists of selfish transposons (ST), known also as egoistic or parasite-like jumping genes. Unlike the workaholic "bee" genes, ST uppermost concern is their own propagation, with all destructive consequences for the genome. Since ST often encompass several bee genes, their relocation could be aggravated by impairment of these and other "innocent" by-standing genes. It is plausible, though unproved, that the ratio ST/bee gene could be critical for a cell survival and should have a tolerance range, close to the upper limit in modern species. Furthermore, constant balancing between the "bees and STings" could be a real "headache" for the evolution, necessitating development of mechanisms for active removal of ever-growing number of ST. Two features of telomeric and subtelomeric regions (TSR) make it tempting to speculate that the ends of linear chromosomes are used for ST muting and removal. Firstly, TSR exhibit strong "silencing" effect, i.e. even genes with hyperactive promoters stop expressing when inserted into these regions. Secondly, TSR hastily replicate at the very end of the S-phase, with occasional incomplete replication at emergencies. Therefore, TSR can be regarded as potential "exiling" sites or convenient "reservations" where ST are muted, due to the silencing effect, and periodically sloughed off, due to the incomplete replication. It seems important that the incomplete replication could be caused by excessive ST number, thus forming a negative loop. The self-propagation and negative-loop could create a circulation cycle, necessary for ST and the encompassed genes regulation in phylo- and ontogenesis. It is noteworthy that TSR are enriched by transposons, obviously highlighting the active "exiling" into the peripheral mute regions, for to keep ST off from the events in the central parts of the genome. In the generally disregulated aging genome, ST "exiling and sloughing" and the resulting ST/bee ratio could be impaired.

SESSION 522

comparison of specific knowledge (physical activity and hypertension) of groups- IMMA Project

Elizabeth Carvalho Lugão (MAster degree student, universidade do Estado do Rio de Janeiro, Uerj; Ufrj teacher, Rio de Janeiro ,Brazil

Trying to follow P.Freir steps: education as a practice of freedom, we try to clear up people. Our purpose is to evaluate knowledge about quality of life of groups in RJ (IMMA Project participants). Knowing about physical activity and hypertension, looking for better quality of life, it implies participation in health maintenance by using the knowledge of injuries provoked by hypertension, and the benefits of adopting a healthy lifestyle. Method: open questions for 167 people (60-90 years old), 56 of Caxias, 1st group (52 women, medu=ium age=65, modal age=63); 44 Andaraí, 2nd group (39 women, me=69,mo=68); 40 S.Gonçalo, 3rd group(36 women, me=65,mo=68); 27 Niterói, 4thgroup(26 women, me=69, mo=58;68;73). The illiterate (5%) people were helped. About hypertension, 1st group: 21% knew (48% hypertensive); 2nd group: 43% knew (41% hypertensive); 3rd group: 42,5% knew (50 % hypertensive); 4th group 45% knew (30 5 hypertensive). About physical activity: 1st group didn't know; 2nd group 20,5% knew; 3rd group 7,5% knew; 4th group didn't know. Conclusion: knowledge about hypertension was low, but about physical activity is lower. We found out that in every group people ignored the hypertension meaning, worst about physical activity meaning; they confound physical activity effects and modalities with its concept.

Health Promotion Education Programs to Address Inequalities in Old Age

Pamela Elfenbein (Southeast Florida Center on Aging, Florida International University, Miami, Florida, USA) Gema Quintero (Southeast Florida Center on Aging, Florida International University, Miami, Florida, USA)

PURPOSE: Development and implementation of a health education and wellness program to address inequalities in old age. Program goals: increase health literacy, promote positive health behaviors and attitudes, improve overall health status and quality of life of program participants. METHOD: A program was established to provide health education programming at 11 Miami-Dade County senior public housing developments. In cooperation with the schools of social work and nursing and the departments of occupational therapy, physical therapy, and dietetics and nutrition, multidisciplinary teams of students where created. A programming assessment was designed to identify knowledge deficiencies and health topics that interested the program participants. The multidisciplinary teams developed and implemented site specific programming. A brief participant satisfaction survey was developed. Students were surveyed on their knowledge and attitudes on aging and older adults. RESULTS: Participants described their time as 'very well spent' and desired to have health promotion activities repeated. Changes in life styles were observed when non-disabled program participants took the initiative and independently organized health promotion activities in the absence of program staff. Students and faculty displayed significant ($p<.05$) shifts in preference for working with older adults, and an expansion of scientific and practical horizons. CONCLUSION: Health education and promotion programming resulted in positive lifestyle change and sense of well being for program participants. Students and faculty provided the opportunity to work with older adults in community health promotion settings demonstrated a significant change in population preference favoring older adults.

Promoting the elderly's health - educational and interactional strategies

Rosalina Aparecida Partezani Rodrigues (University of São Paulo at Ribeirão Preto College of Nursing, Ribeirão Preto, São Paulo, Brazil) Maria Manuela Rino Mendes (University of São Paulo at Ribeirão Preto College of Nursing, Ribeirão Preto, São Paulo, Brazil) Sueli Marques (University of São Paulo at Ribeirão Preto College of Nursing, Ribeirão Preto, São Paulo, Brazil) Luciana Kusumota (University of São Paulo at Ribeirão Preto College of Nursing, Ribeirão Preto, São Paulo, Brazil) Suzele Cristina Coelho Fabrício (University of São Paulo at Ribeirão Preto College of Nursing, Ribeirão Preto, São Paulo, Brazil) José Gustavo Camargo (University of São Paulo, Ribeirão Preto, São Paulo, Brazil)

This investigation aims at characterizing the participants in a group of elderly people who develop health-promotion activities. It also aims at developing educational proposals for health promotion and protection within the studied group. Thirty subjects who lived in the City of Ribeirão Preto and whose ages ranged from 52 to 84 years, mostly females (93.4%), participated in this study. The theoretical framework of the Pedagogy of Liberation proposed by PAULO FREIRE and the research-action methodology were used. Data collection was carried out by means of participant observation, semi-structured interviews and observation of the educational group activities. Data analysis was conducted according to the presuppositions of data analysis preconized by FREIRE, that is, the analysis of the generating topics was divided into four phases: assessment of generating topics, choice of generating topics, creation of typical existential situations with the elderly and the elaboration of guiding forms to record the topics. The main health-related topics concerned health promotion and illness prevention, that is, medication, memory, diet, physical activity, culture, leisure, among others. Thus, the elderly verbalized their learning of methods that changed their habits, attitudes and behaviors in order to experience their old age with health and life quality.

Randomized Controlled Trial of a Health Promotion Program offered to Seniors in Subsidized Apartments

J. C. Ross-Kerr, M. J. Wood, S. Warren, L. Hayduk, S. O'Brien-Cousins, K. Ferris, K. Raine-Travers, M.D, Godkin, M. Woolley (University of Alberta, Edmonton, AB, Canada)

The purpose of the Seniors ALIVE project was to study the effect of a health promotion program on health outcomes measured as physical, functional and psychosocial well-being. The study involved a repeated measures, quasi-experimental 2-group design with outcomes measured at the outset, 4 and 8 month intervals. The target population was seniors living in subsidized housing in metropolitan Edmonton. The housing units for the intervention and control groups were randomly selected on the basis of building size from listings in a seniors accommodation guide for the area. Buildings selected were randomly assigned to the experimental or control group. The intervention group received the health promotion program, while the control subjects did not. Initially 131seniors enrolled in the intervention group and 111 in the control group. At the second data collection point numbers were just under 100 for each of the two groups and at the final data collection point there were 96 in the experimental group and 88 in the control group. Reasons for subjects leaving the groups included moving from the building, illness and hospitalization, loss of interest in the project, and death. An expected substantial dropout from initial to final data collection points was accounted for in initial calculations. Background variables included age, gender, marital status and education, while outcome variables were: health status; functional status; cognitive status; quality of life; group participation; and health care utilization. The health promotion program consisted of three key activities exercise sessions, health corners and a health promotion newsletter. Results indicated gains in several areas of health and well-being.

SESSION 526

Aging, the web and you: Online information, education and training

M. Haug (Novartis Foundation for Gerontology, Basel, Switzerland) ('Untangling the Web: Trends and Opportunities in Senior e-Health'.) R. Roush (Texas Consortium of Geriatric Education Centers, Houston, Texas, USA) ('Older People on the Web: What they Want, What They Need'.) C. L Russell, M. J. Mahony, T. Shaw, A. Sefton, G. Ryan, and S. Barnet (University of Sydney, Sydney, Australia) ('Planning for Gerontology Online'.) G. Andrews and J.Lawrence (Centre for Ageing Studies, Flinders University, Adelaide, Australia) ('Going Virtual - Some Early Reflections'.)

Advances in Web-related technologies have created many new opportunities for educating and informing older persons themselves and those providing services to them. World wide a broad spectrum of older people and aged care professionals are 'getting online' and discovering the advantages of this new medium. New websites have provided increasing opportunities for sourcing information on all aspects of aging. In addition educational institutions are increasingly offering on-line training options using a variety of web-based delivery platforms. This symposium will highlight issues associated with using the web for information and education of older persons and those providing services to them including development of on-line graduate courses; identify recent growth trends and future prospects for advances in this area; demonstrate some examples of current practice; and explore the challenges posed by on-line delivery and possible strategies for dealing with these. Future directions for further development of on-line information, education and training resources will be explored and debated. Issues such a quality control of information and educational offerings will be canvassed; multidisciplinary and multidimensional elements of on-line materials will be discussed; cultural issues and the scope for both formal and informal learning will be examined. Participants will be invited to contribute to an interactive debate and discussion of the issues highlighted by presenters.

Going Virtual? Some Early Reflections

G R. Andrews and J. Lawrence (Centre for Ageing Studies, Flinders University, Adelaide, Australia)

Launching a Gerontology program online for a global market has highlighted a range of complex issues for the Centre for Ageing Studies. These key underlying issues for our online course developers include: defining, achieving and sustaining quality online learning criteria, action, and continuous improvement; maintaining leading edge currency expert networks, content reviews and upgrades; meeting both formal and informal learning agendas' content, design and delivery for differing markets and needs; representing multidisciplinary online effective models of interdisciplinary exchange and shared care; cultural inclusiveness and language barriers respecting cultural and linguistic diversity; content vs. problem-structured processes (ie how is knowledge to be organised?); teacher vs. learner-centred learning (ie how are learners' individual learning needs to be met); maximising access for students' technical and financial tradeoffs. This presentation will address each of these issues and the strategies we are evolving within the Applied Gerontology Education Program to address them. While such issues are not unique to an online environment, we believe that resolving them will prove a significant factor in the success and growth of our online program.

Older People on the Web: What they Want, What They Need

R. Roush (Texas Consortium of Geriatric Education Centers, Houston, Texas, USA)

That older adults want health information from the Web is evident in reviewing the findings contained in the recent report, ?Pew Internet & American Life Project: Online Life Report,? (November 2000). Highlights of the Pew report revealed: · 52 million American adults (550f those with Internet access) have used the Web to get health or medical information. Dubbed ?health seekers,? these mostly middle-aged, Web-savvy persons (63 0.000000emale) go online at least once monthly for health information, with 92aying the health information found was useful; · Of the 21 million health seekers who say they were affected by what they found on their Internet searches, 70aid the information influenced their decision how to treat an illness or condition; and · 860f health seekers are concerned about getting health information from an unreliable source online, with the overwhelming majority finding these information sources from searches rather than having been directed by a knowledgeable person. While these results constitute good news, too few older people and their doctors have the tools with which to ferret out the good from the bad information, nor are they aware of the features of well designed Web sites. What older adults need from the WWW is valid, reliable health information on user-friendly sites adjudged by content experts and human factors researchers. This presentation will address issues associated with meeting those needs.

Planning for Gerontology Online

C. L. Russell, M. J. Mahony, T. Shaw, A. Sefton, G. Ryan, and S. Barnet (University of Sydney, Sydney, Australia)

The University of Sydney's College of Health Sciences is designing an online flexible learning system to meet the needs of health professionals concerned with best practice in serving the ageing. This presentation will highlight the possible and practical, with online demonstrations. Practitioner relevance, modularisation and learner support are key elements. Sophisticated educational (not just technological) design is fundamental. Included in the design is the use of both on-line cases and application in the learners' own contexts. This is a program designed for a wide range of health professionals by a multi-professional team. The challenges emerging in designing for the online environment and widely distributed learners will be discussed.

Untangling the Web: Trends and Opportunities in Senior eHealth

M. Haug (Novartis Foundation for Gerontology, Basel, Switzerland)

It's a reality?the Internet is here to stay. And with every day new trends and opportunities emerge, stretching the boundaries of communications and technology. Originally billed as a novelty for the young and computer savvy, the Internet already has a reach that took television over 20 years to achieve. The fastest growing segment? - Seniors. And one of their top interests? - Health. With a focus on Internet content, Melanie Haug will present an overview on the current offerings for both consumers and professionals in senior eHealth. Using the HealthandAge.com (the Number #1 website focussing on healthy aging, and the Number #4 Health website overall) experience as an example, she will discuss the benefits provided to a cross-section of those interested in senior health

— from the worried well to the chronically ill, from researchers to clinical practitioners — and the important role these sites can play in both education and the patient-provider relationship.

SESSION 527

Integrating traditional and modern medicine in the care of elderly

Sylvester Yong - (Dotolo Research - Asia Singapore. Traditional Medicine vs Modern Medicine - recognizing the relevance of both practices. · Invited presenter from China. Traditional Medicine in China co-existing alongside modern medicine to offer better care options · Invited presenter from UK. Modern Medicine - advancement in care option with a price tag · Invited presenter Issues of significance in the integration of traditional with conventional medicine)

The symposium will discuss the reason underlying the growing interest towards traditional medicine and its impact on care of the elderly. The invited presenters will touch on specific issues relating to traditional medicine, modern medicine, and issues relating to its integration. Discussions will center on how an integrated system is likely to benefit the elderly more in terms of care options available. The need to address chronic degenerative problems and disease state that lead to disability and demand for long term care and services in old age remain a major concern for all communities. These demands for services by the elderly makes it critical for governments and policies planners to explore care options that are not only practical but also affordable. Modern medicine must continue to offer the best solution in acute and life threatening situations such as infection, trauma and disease state that demand the best in conventional therapy. Evidence based findings from scientific research must continue to determine the best approaches and modalities available. Is there a part for traditional medicine to offer? If so, how can it be integrated into modern medicine? These are some of the issues which will be highlighted during the presentation. Many traditional medical practices are ingrained in the culture and customs of various societies. Some have existed for several thousand years. Many of them have withstood the test of time. In spite of the lack of scientific basis for their use and recommendation, their health potentials are based on careful observation, documentation and evaluation of outcome over time. Many individuals have also sought out traditional medical practices and have benefited from these approaches. n various culture, such as China and India, Traditional Chinese medicine (China) and Ayuverdic medicine (India) have co-existed alongside conventional practices from time immemorial. They fulfill a complementary roles to conventional practices and expand the therapeutic options available. Even though some of these practices may not be appreciated by other cultures and less so by the medical fraternity, they should not be ignored and disregarded. Modern medicine must recognize the relevance of some of the more establish practices and explore means of defining those that are likely to be useful. Major academic and research institutions around the world are already embarking on key research projects to determine the effectiveness of various traditional recommendations, especially the use of local herbal preparations available in different settings. New research findings are confirming the benefits of various traditional medical approaches such as acupuncture, homeopathy, qigong, meditation, massage therapy etc. In the next few years, new research findings are likely to offer new options that not only effective, but also safe, less costly and probably less traumatic. It is timely to examine closely the management options presented by traditional medicine and determine who best it can be integrated into the modern medical care system. The challenge lies in maintaining an open mind to the possibilities and capturing the best outcome that will be brought about by the integration of tradition with convention.

Integrating Traditional and Modern Medicine in the Elderly.

The UK experience and its Academic Implications.

M.Impallomeni

Several surveys carried out in the United Kingdom (UK) during the last decade have confirmed the trend towards increased consumption of Complementary and Alternative Medicine (CAM) also seen in other industrialised Countries. It has been estimated that 20% of the UK population used at least a form of CAM during the year 1999. Most of these therapies are practised in the private sector, but some are becoming patchily available within the National Health Service (NHS). Most are delivered in Primary Care, but some are also provided in Secondary care, especially acupuncture, chiropractice and aromatherapy. Successful models of integration with Western Medicine have been described in Geriatrics Departments, as well as in Oncology and Palliative Care Units. Regulation, both statutory and voluntary, has not yet been established for the majority of CAMs in the UK, but is expected by her Majesty's Government to become "an essential element in the delivery of quality patients services", as specified in a recent Government paper. This will be necessary both for the patients' protection and for clear professional accountability. Modern Western Medicine is generally backed by solid scientific research regarding its efficacy and safety. Although not all CAMs have been subjected to equally rigorous studies some have already been the object of serious research. Acupuncture, osteopathy, chiropractice and, to a lesser degree, herbal medicine have been subjected to scientific scrutiny. There are potent reasons to explain this dearth of solid clinical evidence for CAMs, such as the difficulty of standardising therapies which are essentially personalised in order to assess them through the yardstick of randomised controlled (blind when possible) trials. Such difficulties however are being gradually overcome. There have recently been remarkable success stories of integration of Traditional and Western Medicine, such as all-trans-retinoic acid (ATRA) and artemisin. Both originated from Traditional Chinese Medicine: the first has been so successful in the treatment of some forms of Leukaemia that its introduction has been considered a revolution in their treatment. The second is on the brink of large scale studies as it is thought to be particularly effective in drug resistant malaria. An open trial of Marma Therapy, a form of Auyrvedic Medicine massage therapy which has been in use in India for 3000 years, was performed in my Geriatric Medicine Department at the Hammersmith Hospital. The patients were bed-bound as a result of strokes which had occurred more than a year prior to the commencement of the study. This was made possible by a grant from the Foundation for Integrated Medicine (FFIM) and was carried out in collaboration with the Hale Clinic of London. After six months, one quarter of all patients had become capable of walking with only the support of a walking aid. Despite this apparent success, applications to research founding bodies were unsuccessful, largely because some anonymous referees could not support research in what they considered to be unorthodox therapies. This prejudice should not be allowed to occur in future. I am convinced that it will be deemed unethical not to research treatments which appear to be effective especially where no other form of successful therapies exists. The future of Medicine Worldwide will in my opinion see an inexorable integration of Modern and Traditional Medicine. This will follow the use of rigorous scientific research to establish evidence which will be equally expected of both forms of therapies. The many prejudices against this integration will have to be acknowledged before being overcome. Ring fencing of research funds for CAM therapies will probably be necessary for this to happen. The elderly will be the section of the population which is most likely to benefit from such integration and therapeutic progress.

SESSION 528

Issues in the Study of Well-being and Health in Later life

Dorly Deeg (Faculty of Medicine/Longitudinal Aging Study Amsterdam, Free University of Amsterdam, Van der Boechorststraat 7, 1081 BT Amsterdam, The Netherlands). The social identity of older persons: beneficial to quality of life? Paul

Higgs (Department of Psychiatry and Behavioural Sciences, University College London, Wolfson Building, Riding House St, London W1N 8AA. England). The theoretical grounding of quality of life research: towards a needs satisfaction model. Christoph Rott (German Centre for Research on Ageing, Department of Adult Development, Bergheimer Str. 20, 69115 Heidelberg, Germany) The nature of subjective wellbeing and mental health in the oldest old. Kevin Morgan (Gerontology Research Unit, Department of Human Sciences, Loughborough University, LE11 3TU, England). Sleep as a critical health correlate of subjective wellbeing. Mary Gilhooly (Centre of Gerontology and Health Studies, University of Paisley, PA1 2BE, Scotland): Discussant.

An essential component of health outcome measurement, and an enduring element of psychological and sociological research for over 40 years, the construct of wellbeing continues to attract critical attention. While much has been learned, questions concerning the nature, origins, structure, correlates, measurement and value of quality of life continue to be raised. Drawing on work in progress from major projects in Europe and the United States this symposium examines current issues in the use and interpretation of health-related wellbeing and quality of life data. Taking a pragmatic approach to wellbeing assessment, the symposium papers focus specifically on three issues: the theoretical underpinnings of subjective wellbeing; the use of wellbeing measurement to assess psychosocial and health dynamics in later life; and the use of health 'proxies' as indicants of wellbeing and quality of life. Using data from the Longitudinal Aging Study Amsterdam, paper 1 (Deeg) will examine relationships between quality of life (SF-36) assessments, self-rated health, and the construct of social identity. Extending the issue of the theoretical basis for quality of life measurement, paper 2 (Higgs) describes the development of a new instrument grounded in a model of human needs. Moving the focus away from assessment onto the assessed, Paper 3 (Rott) addresses the phenomenology of wellbeing among society's oldest citizens, and explores the mediating role of fatigue in changing levels of depressive symptomatology among sexagenarians, octogenarians and centenarians from the Georgia Centenarian Study. Finally, the use of health proxies for general wellbeing is critically examined in paper 4 (Morgan) in relation to insomnia, a symptom widely included in quality of life assessments. Overall, the presenters will introduce areas of current debate, provide authoritative updates of research findings, and describe agendas for future research.

Quality of life in Early Old Age[QoLEOA]: Development of a Needs Satisfaction model

Paul Higgs (Department of Psychiatry and Behavioural Sciences, University College London, Wolfson Building, Riding House St, London W1N 8AA UK), David Blane (Department of Social Science and Medicine, Imperial College of Science, Technology and Medicine, St Dunstan's Rd, London W6), Dick Wiggins (Department of Sociology, City University, Northampton Square, London EC1), Martin Hyde (Department of Social Science and Medicine, Imperial College of Science, Technology and Medicine, St Dunstan's Rd, London W6)

Despite becoming established as a medical outcome measure and the subject of much and varied research, Quality of Life [QoL] remains poorly defined and lacks an agreed upon theoretical basis. This is especially so in QoL studies with older populations where (ill) health has for too long been used as a proxy measure. Using a postal questionnaire, sent to stratified sample of 286 people aged between 65 and 75 years, who have been previously sampled in the 1930's as participants in the Boyd-Orr study (Gunnell et al; 1996) and subsequently interviewed (Blane; 1999; Holland et al 2000; Berney et al, 2000) , we tested a 'needs satisfaction' model of QoL in Early Old Age. The 22 item, 4 dimension, scale is theoretically derived and ontologically grounded in a model of human needs. The scale was developed in two stages. Firstly it was tested with focus groups. Following amendments suggested in the focus groups it was subject to self completion pilot and cognitive interview testing. Concurrent validity was measured using the Life Satisfaction Index - Well Being (James et al; 1986). Reliability analysis suggests only slight modifications to our model. The modified domains have alpha's between .59 and 0.77. A second order factor analysis reveals that the modified versions of the dimensions tap a single latent QoL factor. Associations between each of the dimensions and between the overall scale and the LSI-W were statistically significant.

Sleep as a critical health correlate of subjective wellbeing in later life

K Morgan (Gerontology Research Unit, Department of Human Sciences, Loughborough University, Leicestershire LE11 3TU, UK)

As a correlate of psychological wellbeing, sleep disturbance continues to be regarded as a critical indicant of both psychological wellbeing and quality of life at all ages, appearing as a prominent diagnostic feature in both DSM-IV and ICD-10 (particularly in relation to depression and anxiety states) and included in many of the most commonly used health outcome measures, including the Nottingham Health Profile and the SF-36. The symptom of disturbed sleep is also included in many schedules for assessing the mental health and wellbeing of elderly people, including the GMS, CAMDEX, and the CARE. In all cases the assumption is made that sleep disturbances are associated with, and consequently predict, lowered morale, compromised subjective wellbeing and reduced quality of life. This presentation investigates the strength and nature of relationships between quality of sleep and quality of later life. In 1985 detailed profiles of lifestyle, health and subjective wellbeing were collected in face-to-face interviews from a community-dwelling random sample of 1042 people aged 65+. Follow-up interviews with survivors were conducted in 1989 and 1993 (n = 690 and 410 respectively), with complete mortality data collected to February 2000. The baseline prevalence of insomnia was 21.2%, while 4 and 8-year follow-up analyses showed a stable incidence of 3.1% per person year at risk. Prevalent and incident cases of insomnia showed significantly differing trajectories for psychological wellbeing, health and mortality. Sleep problems comprise heterogeneous elements in later life, and can show a low specificity for mood and wellbeing outcomes.

The Nature of Subjective Well-being and Mental Health in the Oldest Old

C. Rott (German Centre for Research on Ageing, University of Heidelberg, Germany), P. Martin (Iowa State University, USA), L.W. Poon, M.A. Johnson, (University of Georgia, USA)

In spite of the low prevalence of diagnosed depression in old age some studies with very old participants suggest elevated levels of depressive symptoms in the oldest old. Traditionally, these mental health problems are related to increased functional limitations, illnesses, and losses. An alternative explanation emphasizes the role of fatigue as a mediator of this relation. This study investigates age differences in depressive symptoms, compares longitudinal changes, and examines whether fatigue predicts levels of and change in depressive symptoms. Two hundred and eighty four sexagenarians, octogenarians, and centenarians were assessed with measures of subjective well-being, depressive symptoms, and fatigue. After 5;0 (60s and 80s) and 1;9 (100s) years, 152 subjects were reexamined. Both, significant age differences and age changes were obtained. Overall findings revealed that centenarians had the most unfavorable levels of depressive symptoms. Octogenarians showed the most negative development. Change in fatigue was related to changes in depressive symptoms especially for people in their 80s and to a decline in positive affect within centenarians. The oldest old demonstrated substantial interindividual differences in intraindividual change. Some of these survivors into extreme old age seem to be fairly resistant to depressive symptoms, but most of them are characterized by a dramatic lack of and decrease in subjective well-being.

The social identity of older persons: beneficial to quality of life?

DJH Deeg PG Klandermans, CPM Knipscheer (Faculty of Medicine/Longitudinal Aging Study Amsterdam, Vrije Universiteit, Amsterdam, Van der Boechorststraat 7, 1081 BT Amsterdam, The Netherlands).

Elder-identity is the extent to which older persons identify with their age peers. Its association with quality of life is studied in the Longitudinal Aging Study Amsterdam (LASA). LASA is based on a nation-wide cohort, initial ages 55-85 years, with oversampling of men and older-old. During baseline (1992-93), 3107 subjects were interviewed. In the third cycle (1998-99) a questionnaire on social identity with respect to the older age group was included (n=1465). Three dimensions of social identity could be distinguished: cognitive, evaluative, and emotional, indicating the awareness of being part of the older age group, the value attached to belonging to the older age group, and the involvement experienced with the older age group. As expected, the association of social identity with age was positive. The associations of the three components with quality of life (measured by SF-12) and self-rated health (measured by single question), however, showed different directions. The evaluative component showed positive associations, but the opposite was true for the two other components. Thus, a positive value attached to belonging to the older age group increased quality of life; awareness of being older and involvement with the older age group, however, was associated with lower quality of life. Since social identity may be expected to differ cross-culturally, it is a likely candidate for explaining differences in older persons' quality of life levels between countries.

SESSION 529

Falls and Injury Prevention in Later Life

David Buchner (United States Center for Disease Control, Atlanta, Georgia, USA), Elaine Gallagher (School of Nursing, University of Victoria, BC, Canada), Jes Bruun Lauritzen (Orthopedics Dept, Hvidovre, Denmark), Jake Pauls (Consulting Services in Building Use and Safety, Silver Spring, Maryland, USA), Laurence Rubenstein (UCLA School of Medicine and Sepulveda VA Geriatrics Center, Los Angeles, California, USA)

Falls and related injuries are common and devastating among older adults. State-of-the-art approaches for preventing these problems will be discussed in this session by researchers and policymakers. Dr. Buchner will discuss the FICSIT trials of multi-component exercise interventions and new initiatives from the US Centers for Disease Control. Dr. Gallagher will discuss interventions targeted toward community-based falls prevention using participatory action research and collaborative inquiry methods. Dr. Lauritzen will present an overview of one the most promising fracture-preventive interventions yet to come along-hip protectors. Dr. Pauls will present a pictorial overview of environmental hazards in the community and what can be done about them. Dr. Rubenstein will provide an overview of the epidemiology of falls and injuries and discuss the new evidence-based fall prevention guidelines recently completed by the American Geriatrics Society and the evidence-based quality of care indicators for falls and instability recently completed by the RAND corporation as part of the ACOVE project.

Are Environmental Factors in Falls Adequately Evaluated?

Jake Pauls (Consulting Services in Building Use and Safety, Silver Spring, Maryland, USA)

PURPOSE: Falls often occur as a result of environmental defects; however such environmental defects are often not adequately identified and evaluated in research. Common environmental factors, chiefly those pertaining to elevation changes, are described along with methods for their evaluation, especially those methods used in post-injury litigation. METHOD: A fairly thorough list of environmental factors was developed based on literature and experience in the field. Techniques for field documentation and evaluation are presented. Comparisons are made with evaluations described in papers typically published in medical journals. RESULTS: Important environmental factors are sometimes given short shrift in research papers and conference presentations because of limited resources available for documenting and evaluating such factors. Litigation-spurred investigations can be much more extensive and intensive and are often more critically evaluated. CONCLUSION: Given their importance in fall prevention strategies, environmental factors warrant more careful identification and evaluation. A balance must be found between detail in and number of cases of individual falls investigated to form the basis for insights into causes and prevention.

Community-based falls prevention using participatory action research and collaborative inquiry methods

Elaine Gallagher (School of Nursing, University of Victoria, BC, Canada)

Most injury prevention research is aimed at the level of individuals - either in terms of improving their personal health or balance, increasing their awareness or fitness, or improving the safety of their homes. According to Labonte's theory of health promotion, prevention can also be targeted towards small groups, whole communities, and society as a whole. This paper will describe programs of research aimed at community and societal levels of change, utilizing participatory action research and collaborative inquiry methods. Advantages and disadvantages of these approaches will be examined in light of the fall prevention outcomes achieved.

Effect of Hip Protectors Against Hip Fractures

Jes Bruun Lauritzen, (Department of Orthopedic Surgery, Hvidovre Hospital, University of Copenhagen, Denmark)

Increased research and understanding of the biomechanics of hip fracture has made hip protection a recommended strategy by The European Commission in the "Report on Osteoporosis in the EC - action for Prevention 1998", and a Cochrane review (1999) concludes, that hip protectors seem to reduce the occurrence of hip fractures in selected populations with high risk. The effect of external hip protectors has been studied in five randomized trials in nursing homes. No of hfx/subjects Hip fractures avoided Study Follow-up(mths) Intervention Control RR 95%CL No Lauritzen 1993 11 8/247, 31/418, 0.44, 0.20-0.95 10; Ekman 1997 11 4/302, 17/442, 0.34, 0.12-1.0 7; Heikinheimo 1997 12 1/36, 5/36, 0.20 4; Harada 1998 19 0/30, 4/24, 0.0 5; Kannus et al 2000 18 13/653, 67/1148, 0.4, 0.2-0.8 15; RR; relative risk. CL; confidence limits. Hfx; hip fractures. Data are sparse among home-dwellers. One controlled case cohort study among elderly orthopedic in-patients indicate a comparable effect among those with risk factors for hip fracture (Hindsø & Lauritzen, 2001). Follow-up 1 to 1 year; n 1590. Primary acceptance was 57%. Users reported 143 falls with impact on the hip protector, and no hip fractures occurred. Two hip fractures occurred while the patients used their hip protectors, but no impact on the hip was reported. Long-term adherence at two years was 40%. Preliminarily, the hip protectors seem cost-saving. Conclusion: Hip protectors are an important supplement in the prevention of hip fractures.

Physical Activity and Fall Prevention: More than Just Exercise Classes

David Buchner (Division of Nutrition and Physical Activity, Centers for Disease Control and Prevention, Atlanta, GA, USA)

Physical activity is commonly recommended as a component of fall prevention programs. This paper will review the evidence from the FICSIT studies and other exercise studies as to the role of physical activity in fall prevention. Despite longstanding public health recommendations that older adults adopt an active lifestyle, older adults are the least active age group and national surveillance data show no change in physical activity levels over the past decade. The paper will also discuss strategies and next steps for increasing physical activity in older adults and the relationship of these efforts to fall prevention. In particular, the presentation will identify environmental determinants of physical activity and the potential of promoting activity and preventing falls by environmental changes not usually considered as related to fall prevention.

Preventing falls in clinical practice: Evidence-based fall prevention guidelines and quality of care indicators.

Laurence Rubenstein (UCLA School of Medicine and Sepulveda VA Geriatrics Center, Los Angeles, California, USA)

The catastrophic problem of falls in older persons results from multiple, diverse and interacting underlying risk factors and situational causes, many of which are correctable. Frequently older people do not appreciate or report these problems to their physician and, even if reported, physicians often do not respond with appropriate assessment and intervention-which allows occurrence of considerable preventable injury and disabilities. Recent evidence-based work by the RAND Corporation and an international task force led by the American Geriatrics Society and British Geriatrics Society have produced a set of clinical practice guidelines for approaching and preventing falls in clinical practice and a set of quality of care indicators for assessing quality of medical care for vulnerable elders at risk of falling. Both are intended to lead to improved clinical practice, and ultimately better outcomes, for older persons who fall or who are at risk of falling. The background and substance of these two projects will be presented in detail.

SESSION 530

Geriatric Rehabilitation: Best Practices and Best Outcomes

M. Borrie (Division of Geriatric Medicine, South western Ontario Regional Geriatric Program, University of Western Ontario, Lawson Health Research Institute, London Ontario Canada) Geriatric Rehabilitation: Best Practices and Emerging Trends M. A. Acanfora (Regional IAG Latin American Committee, Buenos Aires, Argentina) Geriatric Rehabilitation: The Latin American Practice P. Stolee (Southwestern Ontario Regional Geriatric Program, University of Western Ontario, Lawson Health Research Institute, London Ontario Canada) Goals and Outcomes of Geriatric Rehabilitation F. Knoefel (Sisters of Charity Ottawa Health Service, St. Vincent Hospital, Dept. of Family Medicine, University of Ottawa, Ottawa, Ontario, Canada) Co-morbidity and Rehabilitation Outcome

Issue: This round table forum will review and discuss current Canadian and international practices and outcomes in geriatric rehabilitation. The presentations will focus on published and unpublished best practices from Canada and the world, and on the identification and measurement of outcomes that are relevant to the geriatric population. The impact of demographics, comorbid illnesses, and different approaches to rehabilitation resources in Canada and other parts of the world will be discussed. Structure: Summary presentations will set the stage for wide ranging discussion during the second half of the round table session. Content: (Presentations) A summary of the published and emerging best practices in geriatric rehabilitation from Canada and the published best practices in the international literature will be presented. This is based on the published abstracts and papers from members of the Canadian Geriatrics Society 1981-2000, a systematic literature search of the literature using specific criteria for best practices and levels of evidence, and surveys to each of the 16 Canadian academic centres in Geriatric Medicine. The demographic trends over the last 10 years from the Canadian Institute for Health Information (CIHI) influencing the need for, as well as the availability of inpatient and outpatient resources in Ontario will be discussed. Goals and outcomes of geriatric rehabilitation vary widely among rail older persons undergoing rehabilitation. Goal Attainment Scaling (GAS) is an individualized, client-centred, objective outcome measurement approach that has properties that make it particularly suitable for use in geriatric care. Use of GAS has yielded insights into the goals and outcomes of geriatric rehabilitation. GAS data from two Canadian centres will be used to describe the goals of geriatric rehabilitation and the merits of an individualized approach to outcome measurement for these programs. Comorbid illnesses in the older population increase the complexity of care and influence the realistic approaches, goals and outcomes in the elderly. Different measures, such as the Functional Independence Measure (FIM) and Minimum Data Set - Post acute care (MDS-PAC), are instruments increasingly used in rehabilitation. Multiple comorbid illness in the frail elderly may make the instruments less clinically relevant in this population. Comorbid illnesses also have a significant impact on the choice of rehabilitation venue(s) and resources. Data from chart review of two Canadian centres will be used to illustrate these points. The current practices and future directions of Geriatric Rehabilitation in Latin America will be addressed and compared to the Canadian situation. The barriers to developing an adequate rehabilitation system will be discussed. Conclusions / Anticipated Outcomes: The roundtable will consider the relative merits of examples from different international settings for geriatric rehabilitation approaches and outcome measures. There will be opportunities to discuss the priorities in different countries to meet the anticipated demand for effective geriatric rehabilitation resources for the frail elderly and their caregivers. We wish to acknowledge the Ministry of Health and Long-Term Care for their financial support of Dr. Borrie's, Dr. Stolee's, and Dr. Knoefel's contributions to this roundtable. The views presented in the abstracts and by the members of the roundtable have not been endorsed by the Ministry of Health and Long-Term Care and do not necessarily reflect their views.

Co-morbidity and Rehabilitation Outcome

F. Knoefel (SCO Health Service, St-Vincent Hospital, Department of Family Medicine, Ottawa. Ontario, Canada)

PURPOSE: A) To review the literature regarding medical co-morbidities and geriatric rehabilitation outcomes, and B) to present the findings of a study comparing co-morbidities in two Ontario Geriatric Rehabilitation and Physical Medicine and Rehabilitation populations. METHOD: A) Literature review. B) Retrospective chart review of 100 patients each (geriatric and physical medicine) at two rehabilitation centres in Ontario, Canada. Co-morbidity will be measured using the Cumulative Illness Rating Scale and outcomes will be measured using the Functional Independence Measure. RESULTS: The analysis has not been completed. CONCLUSION: Will depend on the Results, but the hypothesis is that one of the primary differences in populations between the two types of rehab programs is co-morbidity. ROUND TABLE DISCUSSION: The role of co-morbidity in geriatric rehabilitation outcome measurement will be discussed. Participants will be invited to discuss other tools for measuring co-morbidity.

Geriatric Rehabilitation: Best Practices, Ontario Resources, and Demographic Trends

J. Wells (Division of Geriatric Medicine, South western Ontario Regional Geriatric Program, University of Western Ontario, Lawson Health Research Institute, London Ontario Canada) M. Borrie (Division of Geriatric Medicine, South western Ontario Regional Geriatric Program, University of Western Ontario, Lawson Health Research Institute, London Ontario Canada) F. Knoefel (Sisters of Charity Ottawa Health Service, St. Vincent Hospital, Dept. of Family Medicine, University of Ottawa, Ottawa, Ontario, Canada) P. Stolee (South western Ontario Regional Geriatric Program, University of Western Ontario, Lawson Health Research Institute, London Ontario Canada)

Purpose: To present an overview of published Canadian, international, and current unpublished Canadian best practices. Ontario acute care hospital demographic trends in rehabilitation and geriatric services will be reviewed with designated inpatient and outpatient resources in Ontario. Method and Results: A computerized search of the published literature on Geriatric Rehabilitation for the last 5 years have revealed over 700 publications. The search of the Canadian Geriatric Society database for the last 20 years has revealed 30 publications and abstracts on rehabilitation. In evaluating Best Practice, we have used established frame works and standards for Clinical bench-marking and best practice and standardized levels of evidence to assess strength of evidence. The resources available in Ontario for rehabilitation vary from inpatient geriatric rehabilitation units, outpatient geriatric Day hospitals in the 5 academic centres with active Divisions of Geriatrics, to very limited accessibility to rehabilitation for frail elderly in rural and remote areas. In the academic centres the average inpatient length of stay was 47 days, mean age 81, with 70% of patients returning home. However, there was large variability in a number of important parameters including staffing, waiting lists, and primary diagnoses (Knoefel et al). Demographic and service utilization data analysis of the 10 year trend (in 2-year increments 1989-1999) of rehabilitation and geriatric service utilization from acute care hospitals will gathered from the Canadian Institute for Health Information and be presented showing the influence of increasing comorbid diagnoses on rehabilitation services. Conclusions: The implications and results will be discussed in the roundtable discussion.

Geriatric Rehabilitation: The Latin American Practice

*Miguel Angel Acanfora, Carmen Luz Catalan, Susana Hierrezuelo (*Regional IAG Latin American Committee, ** Hogar Frances, Buenos Aires, Argentina, *** Centro Ibero Latinoamericano para la Tercera Edad, La Havana, Cuba)*

Purpose: To present an overview of the Practice of Geriatric Rehabilitation in several centres of different countries in Latin America. Methods and results: We shall present the method of admission and outcome measurement in different Latin American centres offering Geriatric Rehabilitation as well as show the current trends and a prediction of the future of geriatric rehabilitation. The different resources available in most of the countries in Latin America make the practice of geriatric rehabilitation a challenge, and this area often remains unknown to other members of the medical field. A demographic view and the utilisation of geriatric services in acute hospital and long term institutions will be discussed. The outcomes of these approaches will be compared with others. Conclusions: The reality and benefits of the Rehabilitation Practice will be discussed in the round table discussion.

Goals and Outcomes of Geriatric Rehabilitation

P. Stolee (Southwestern Ontario Regional Geriatric Program, London, Canada; University of Western Ontario, London, Canada)

Goals and outcomes of geriatric rehabilitation vary widely among frail older persons undergoing rehabilitation. Goal Attainment Scaling (GAS) is an individualized, client-centred, objective outcome measurement approach that has properties that make it particularly suitable for use in geriatric care. GAS data from two Canadian centres [(Halifax (N=170) and London (N=128)] will be used to describe the goals of geriatric rehabilitation and the merits of an individualized approach to outcome measurement for these programs. Interdisciplinary teams typically identified four to six individualized goals in consultation with each patient. In both centres, the most common goal areas included mobility, discharge planning arrangements, and activities of daily living. Other common goal areas included: bowel and bladder problems, skin problems, pain, nutrition, and medical problems. GAS was found to be more responsive to change than commonly used standardized measures such as the Barthel Index, Functional Independence Measure and Spitzer Quality of Life Index [Standardized Response Mean (SRM) for GAS >1.7; SRM < 1.0 for other measures]. Content analysis of individualized GAS goals provides information on the level of patient improvement that is considered clinically important. Goal attainment can also be equated to standardized outcomes using receiver operating characteristic curves. GAS is a clinically meaningful and responsive approach for the measurement of outcomes in complex patients of geriatric rehabilitation programs. Use of GAS has yielded insights into the goals and outcomes of geriatric rehabilitation.

SESSION 531

A do-it-yourself programme of mental health promotion among seniors in Singapore.

CHIANG Hai Ding (National University of Singapore Society Senior Circle) and Helen KO (Singapore Action Group of Elders Counselling Centre).

PURPOSE. What can they do: some educated seniors in Singapore who are concerned that they may lose their cognitive abilities, family and friends, and become isolated and lonely. METHOD. Find a convenor and a facilitator to organize these programmes. Three groups of about a dozen each met regularly for two-hour "Discussion Group" sessions on the meaning of "Being old in Singapore". The first three topics, based on "Seniors and ..", were "ageism", "losses", and "engagement". They were chosen by the convenor. However, participants went on to discuss "health", "housing", "finances" and "relationships". A smaller group of half a dozen met to share their "Guided Autobiographies" (as taught by American psychologist Professor James Birren). They chose the themes of "family", "life work" and "friendships and loves". RESULTS. All the Discussants declared that they were intellectually stimulated. They also appreciated hearing views other than their own. They found support from among their peers. They continued to meet socially after the sessions ended. The Autobiographers declared that they were stimulated, relieved and inspired by remembrances. Through sharing lives they validated each other's life experiences. They became more confident. These seniors bonded with each other. Most proposed introducing similar programmes for other seniors, and a few undertook to create a body to promote activities for seniors in Singapore. CONCLUSION. Activities for seniors in Singapore have tended to be organized for seniors by Government or other agencies. However, pro-active educated seniors can themselves organize and benefit from such programmes which promote mental health, and which draw on their education, life experiences and memories.

Elderly volunteers in a decreasing welfare society

F. Kolland (L. Boltzmann Institute of Social Gerontology and Life Course Research, Vienna, Austria)

The sobering frustration of high expectations arising from a central state's freedom of implementing social welfare has brought back an increased interest in the decentralization as well as self-regulatory production of welfare. The objective here is to build the skills and acceptance necessary for living a self-responsible life during all its stages with a stronger than usual commitment to civil duties. Thus, the elderly may be regarded as a challenging social potential. This paper discusses extent, motivation, and effects of volunteer work on the background of a random sample (n=1.000) of older adults (60+) living in the urban area (Vienna). Statistical data for Austria show a decrease in the social commitment within organisations and societies in the past 25 years. On this basis the hypothesis has been derived that volunteer work in organized or formalized communities is dwindling away. Still, does this mean interest in social engagements within organisations demanding duty and responsibility is slackening off? The results of this study show that the total volume of volunteer work has not decreased, but even continued to soar. 30% of the elderly are engaged in voluntary work. However, the ways of participation have changed as well as the motives of volunteers. The majority prefers not just to act exclusively on behalf of others, or altruistically, but also on their own behalf (self care). Inherent in individualisation, a tendency towards meaningful activities reflecting upon the self is not contradictory to the inclination to do voluntary work. From these results, further insights into the activity theory of the process of aging can be obtained.

Manual for Senior Peer Counselling of B.C. Trainers' Training

Truda Loewen (B.C. Senior Peer Counselling, B.C. Coalition for the Elimination of Elder Abuse, Abbotsford, B.C. Canada.)

People who teach elder volunteers can be of any age. They do not all understand the best way to teach elders using the students' vast store of knowledge accumulated during their long lives. This presentation is based on two volumes. The first one is the actual Masters' Project of the presenter which explains in detail the necessity for a Trainers' Training Manual, and includes history, the research and conclusions drawn therefrom, as well as the impact the research has on the Manual itself. An inventory of the sessions is included. The second volume is the actual Manual itself with detailed lesson plans, pre-reading on Teaching the Elderly, overheads and handouts. With little adaptation this Manual can be used for teaching any group of senior volunteers. The results of the research were that the present course being taught peer counsellors is adequate and well received, but there are areas which were found to be especially useful which need to be augmented. There were also some other areas which could be added to the course. The conclusions drawn from this study and compilation of the Manual are that it is necessary to ensure that the trainers' of peer counsellors are well trained themselves. This can be validated by their experience in training peer counsellors and completion of this course. which has been adopted by Senior Peer Counselling of B.C. as necessary for certification as a Senior Peer Counsellor Trainer.

The Evolution of Rehabilitative Peer Groups in CNIB Manitoba Division - Response to the Needs of Blind and Visually Impaired Older Persons 1984-2001

Joan Weselak and Dorothy Orebanjo (Client Services Department, Canadian National Institute for the Blind, Manitoba Division, Winnipeg, MB, Canada)

The peer group program purpose is the rehabilitation of isolated, blind and visually impaired older persons through sharing the experience of vision loss. Participation in groups facilitates independence, self-esteem and acceptance. These program goals are achieved by establishing a senior advisory board, exploring needs through senior forums, and assessing individual clients. In response to expressed needs group support programs are then tailored, involving an activity base, grief counselling or caregiver support. Peer leaders are empowered while staff provide facilitation and counselling, using speakers and demonstrations as required. Evaluation is a key tool. A successful outcome of this group work includes the moving of the individual through the grief process. Participants are better prepared to complete rehabilitation training. Groups are empowered to advocate within their communities for equal access. Individuals are enabled to develop their potential and expand their horizons. As a result confident, healthy older persons require fewer community and family resources. Participation in group settings for blind and visually impaired older persons promotes the rehabilitation process. This develops ongoing social contacts and strengthens the individual, family and the community.

Understanding Seniors' Peer Counselling Experiences in Service Delivery to Mistreated Older Adults.

J. Harbison (Maritime School of Social Work, Dalhousie University, Nova Scotia, Canada)

PURPOSE: Mistreated seniors are frequently unwilling to confide in professional helpers. Older volunteer counsellors may therefore have an important role to play in addressing mistreatment in their peers. However research addressing this question is limited. An exploratory study examined senior peer counselling contributions to service delivery for abused older adults in five Canadian provinces. METHOD: To gain an understanding of the infrastructure and agency missions within which the seniors provided counselling program (n=6) documents were examined and interviews held with administrators (n=8) responsible for program delivery. To understand seniors' experiences focus groups (n=6) were held with senior counsellors (n= 30). Analysis includes content analysis of documents, selective coding procedures for interpreting interview transcripts, and feedback from participants. RESULTS: There are diverse ways in which peer counselling is incorporated into service delivery. These range from situations where seniors' contact is by telephone "help line" to those where seniors engage in face-to-face ongoing assistance. Some counsellors questioned the legitimization of their roles by professionals. Whatever the degree of support and training from agency personnel seniors tended to see their involvement in peer counselling as both rewarding and stressful. While some had direct and/or personal experience of mistreatment others did not. Most had other volunteer roles and many saw their work with the senior abuse program as time-limited. CONCLUSION: In partnership with seniors further research is needed to understand what contributions seniors can best make in the `elder abuse' counselling field and what training and supports are required.

SESSION 532

Old Age and Autonomy: The Role of Service Systems and Intergenerational Family Solidarity - Oasis

Ariela Lowenstein and Ruth Katz (Center for Research and Study of Aging, Faculty of Welfare and Health Studies, The University of Haifa, Haifa, Israel) Clemens Tesch-Roemer, Hans Joachim von Kondratowitz and Andreas Motel-Klingebiel (German Center for Gerontology, Berlin, Germany). Quality of life and intergenerational relations - A comparative approach Paul Kingston, Judith Phillips and Mo Ray (Applied Social Studies and Social Gerontology, Keele University, Keele, UK). The experience of conflict and ambivalence in intergenerational exchange Svein Olav Daatland and Katharina Herlofson (Norwegian Social Research, Oslo, Norway). Families and services in elder care - substitution or complementarity in a comparative perspective. Ruth Katz, Ariela Lowenstein, Dana Prilutzky and David Mehlhausen-Hassoen (Center for Research and Study of Aging, Faculty of Welfare and Health Studies, The University of Haifa, Haifa, Israel). Intergenerational family solidarity and its relation to autonomy and life satisfaction in old age

ISSUE: The importance of intergenerational family solidarity, ambivalence and conflict, service systems and family care as related to quality of life is presented within an international perspective and debated. This symposium seeks to make the links between theory and empirical research in the above areas regarding different age cohorts. Special attention will be devoted to the old-old (75+). STRUCTURE: The moderator will briefly introduce the session. Five papers address the explicit role of intergenerational family solidarity, ambivalence and conflict, within an international perspective, and their impact on family care and quality of life in different cultural contexts and different welfare regimes. The co-convener will conduct an open discussion first asking for panelist comments and then audience comments. CONTENT: Theoretical aspects and empirical data of intergenerational family solidarity, ambivalence and conflict are presented and addressed in five areas: family care and social support, quality of life, autonomy and life satisfaction and the role of service systems as substituting or complementing. Discussion will focus on the nature and value of explicit theorizing in intergenerational family relationships. ANTICIPATED OUTCOME: A deeper understanding of the meaning of different cultural contexts and different welfare regimes to explicit theorizing in intergenerational family solidarity, conflict and ambivalence.

Families and Services in Elder Care - Substitution or Complementarity in a Comparative Perspective

S.O Daatland and K. Herlofson (Norwegian Social Research, Oslo, Norway)

All welfare states are concerned about how they may build supportive relationships between families and services in elder care. In so doing they will inevitably be dealing with questions like: what is the actual and preferred balance between families and service systems? Are families and services substituting or complementing each other? In its simplest form, the substitution thesis states that there is an inverse relationship between services and family care. When service levels are low, family care is high, and vice versa. Substitution theory also assumes that services and family care will most probably appear as alternative sources of help and not as both sources. Do families and services tend to substitute or complement each other, and do these patterns tend to vary between countries with different welfare regimes? These questions are addresses in the Oasis project based on a survey among the urban population aged 25+ (N=1200) in each of five participating countries (Israel, Spain, Norway, Germany, UK). The present paper focuses on the balance of help to persons aged 75 and older, living at home.

Quality of Life and Intergenerational Relations: A comparative approach

Clemens Tesch-Römer, Andreas Motel-Klingebiel, Hans-Joachim von Kondratowitz

Purpose: Quality of life is a main indicator for wellbeing in modern welfare states and a measure for the effectiveness of socio-political interventions. With respect to old age it can be shown that quality of life is conceptually strongly connected to the family as an institution delivering help and assistance to their frail members. The dimensions of quality of life will be discussed theoretically and empirically. Method: The results are part of the cross-national comparative project OASIS. A random sample of n=6,000 (age 25 to 95) from five countries (United Kingdom, Israel, Spain, Norway and Germany, n=1,200 per country) was interviewed with an standardised survey instrument (ti=60 min). Comparative descriptive analyses and multivariate models will be presented. Results: Since the study is still in the field at the time of the abstract submission expected results are described as hypotheses (at the conference data will be presented). We expect a strong relation between family support and the indicators of quality of life. The strength of this connection probably varies between different welfare state regimes and strongly depends on the support available in the formal service system but it should be of significant relevance under all welfare regimes. Conclusion: We expect that the availability of support from any source belongs to the most important predictors of quality of life in old age. Independent from the societal support systems the family acts as an Δ to a large extent independent Δ institution in providing support and maintaining quality of life of the elderly.

Intergenerational Solidarity and its relation to Autonomy and Life Satisfaction in Old Age

R. Katz, A. Lowenstein, D. Prilutzky and D. Mehlhausen-Hassoen (Faculty of Welfare and Health Studies, The University of Haifa, Israel).

Purpose: The model of intergenerational family solidarity of Bengtson and others was developed based on classical theories of social organization, exchange theory, group dynamics and the developmental family theory. According to the model, intergenerational family solidarity includes six dimensions: structural, functional, affective, consensual, associational and normative. The goal of this study is to test the links between the different dimensions and autonomy and life satisfaction of elderly population. Method: The results are part of the cross-national comparative project OASIS. A random sample of n=6,000 (age 25 and older) from five countries (United Kingdom, Israel, Spain, Norway and Germany, n=1,200 per country) was interviewed with a standardised survey instrument. Comparative descriptive analyses and multivariate models will be presented. Results: It is expected that the various solidarity dimensions will be differentially related to indicators of autonomy and life satisfaction. For example structural solidarity will be inversely related to the degree of autonomy while normative solidarity will be positively associated with the degree of autonomy. Conclusion: It is expected that the strength and the direction of the different solidarity dimensions to autonomy and life satisfaction of the elderly will vary between different family cultures within and between the five participating countries.

SESSION 533

Interactive Discussion of Leadership Training Courses for Physical Activity Programming

L. Scholey, L. Cyarto, C. Fitzgerald (Canadian Centre for Activity and Aging, London, Ontario, Canada) ("Leadership Training for Physical Activity Leaders in Long-Term Care Institutions")

More older adults are recognizing the importance of physical activity to maintain their independence and quality of life. Instructors require specialized training to design and implement appropriate programs for this diverse population. The Canadian Centre for Activity and Aging (CCAA) has developed training courses to prepare individuals to lead programs for older adults. The courses offered by the CCAA are the Seniors' Fitness Instructors Course, Functional Fitness in Long-Term Care Workshop, Home Support Exercise Program, Restorative Care Education and Training, and Training for the Trainer. Trained leaders provide programs to older adults in their community, their home, and within long-term care facilities (nursing homes). Conference delegates are invited to attend this round table discussion to share their interest or expertise in the area of leadership training for physical activity programs for the older adult.

Leadership Training for Physical Activity Leaders in Long-Term Care Institutions (Nursing Homes)

Lynn Scholey, Liz Cyarto, Clara Fitzgerald (Canadian Centre for Activity and Aging, London, Ontario, Canada)

Traditionally, long-term care (LTC) facilities (nursing homes) have not placed value in the maintenance or improvement of the abilities of their residents. Physical activity programs have typically consisted of seated range of motion exercises, regardless of ability. This component of the roundtable will focus on training developed by the Canadian Centre for Activity and Aging for staff in LTC facilities. Functional Fitness for Long-Term Care is a 24-hour workshop that prepares individuals to design and implement exercise programs for frail older adults. These programs include exercises to improve or maintain residents' balance, strength, and mobility. The Restorative Care Education and Training program prepares staff to work with residents in achieving their highest level of function possible. The 36 hours of training includes modules on communication, physical activity, mobility, feeding/eating programs, and assessment.

SESSION 534

Community-Based Care: A Changing Research, Education, and Practice Environment

H.M. Young (ERA Care Communities and University of Washington, Seattle, WA, USA), S.K. Sikma (University of Washington, Bothell, WA, USA), B. Belza (University of Washington, Seattle, WA, USA), C. J. Leppa (University of Washington, Bothell, Bothell, Washington, USA), B.J. Bowers (University of Wisconsin, Madison, WI, USA)Discussant

Abstract ISSUE: Community based gerontological care is a growing area of practice due to the change in demographics and increased desire of consumers to reside in the least restrictive environment possible. Philosophical polarities exist around approaches to treatment, choices and decision making, professional role, and societal expectations. The regulatory and policy environment for long-term care is compelling, and has far reaching implications for practice. The purpose of this symposium is to highlight contemporary issues and opportunities in community-based long-term care drawing from data, theoretical frameworks, policy, and practice exemplars. STRUCTURE: Following an introduction by the convener, four related papers will be presented, highlighting scholarship, research, and educational initiatives in community based long term care settings, followed by an integrative response led by a discussant. Audience members will be invited to participate in a discussion of the issues. CONTENT: The first paper focuses on a theoretical model for community based long term care practice. Traditional gerontologic nursing education curricula have often reflected deficit models focusing on disabilities, diseases and losses of chronological age. This paper proposes an alternative framework focusing on wellness, healthy aging, and developmental and environmental aspects of this practice arena for educating providers to work with older adults living in community-based,residential long term care settings. The second paper provides exemplars of the community health nursing model and highlights a systematic and programmatic approach to integrating theory in a retirement community through nursing practice and student experiences. The third paper discusses challenges in adopting a palliative care philosophy in long tern care, gives an overview of the regulatory context, and outlines potential barriers to assessment and delivery of quality end of life care in the nursing home environment. The final paper provides a theoretical model of polarities in policy development derived from an evaluation study of nurse delegation in Washington State. Implications of a change in community-based long term care policy for the system, professional, and consumers are discussed. The discussant is Dr. Barbara Bowers, Professor at University of Wisconsin, Madison. Dr. Bowers will reflect on themes across the papers, will respond to critical issues raised, and will suggest directions for the future. CONCLUSIONS: This symposium will serve as an opportunity for consideration and dialogue about the philosophical, policy, and practice dilemmas in the delivery of community based long term care for older adults and strategies for influencing educational, regulatory, and practice systems to promote healthy aging.

Community Based Long-Term Care: Building Links Between Education and Practice

B. Belza (University of Washington, Seattle, WA, USA), H.M. Young (ERA Care Communities and University of Washington, Seattle, WA, USA), S.K. Sikma (University of Washington, Bothell, WA, USA)

Abstract PURPOSE: To highlight systematic and programmatic approaches to integrating theory in a retirement community through practice and student experiences. CONTENT: The community health nursing framework and theories of person-environment fit and transitions provide a basis for person-centered community programs that promote healthy aging and optimal functioning throughout late life transitions. The presentation will emphasize program development through an academic-clinical partnership, with integration into clinical experiences for undergraduate and graduate nursing students, as well as student-led health education projects in the communities. A successful educational opportunity that paired residents (informants) with graduate nurse practitioner students will be highlighted. The experience provided a new perspective on aging issues from the point of view of older adults, helped students confront myths of aging, and reinforced the importance of resilience, social engagement and regular physical activity for older adults. CONCLUSION: Theoretical models of aging (e.g, person-environment fit, transitions) can provide a context for learning and a structure for student experiences in a long-term care setting.

Community-Based Long-term Care: A Framework

S.K. Sikma [University of Washington, Bothell, Bothell, Washington, USA] and H.M. Young [ERA Care Communities and University of Washington, Seattle, WA, USA]

Abstract PURPOSE: Traditional gerontological nursing education curricula have often reflected deficit models focusing on disabilities, diseases and losses of chronological age. Older adults have been characterized as frail or vulnerable rather than possessing relatively high levels of wellness, health and functioning and wanting to have a strong voice in defining what wellness is, where care occurs, and who delivers it. This paper proposes an alternative framework for educating providers to work with older adults living in community-based, residential long term care settings. CONTENT: Based in multidisciplinary theories relevant to aging, the framework synthesizes an understanding of aging in all of its bio-psycho-social aspects and the strengths of adults as they age. Appropriate for gerontologic practice, education and research, the framework reflects several conceptual models: Lawton's ecological model of aging; Bridges'and Meleis's life transitions models; and Prochaska's stage of personal change model. The framework reflects a respect for client autonomy, an ethical principle of paramount importance to health care consumers in US society. It addresses the conflict inherent in the demand by consumers for professionals to respect the dignity of risk and the right to failure, rooted in the ethical principles of autonomy and self-determination and the long held professional ethical principle of beneficence, often expressed as parentalism. CONCLUSION: This framework provides a useful structure for emphasizing the consumer values of self-direction and control, while applying sound principles to promote health and optimal person-environment fit across a continuum of older adults with widely ranging competencies.

Nurse Delegation: Practice Implications for Community Based Long Term Care

H.M. Young (ERA Care Communities and University of Washington, Seattle, WA, USA) and S.K. Sikma (University of Washington, Bothell, WA, USA)

Abstract PURPOSE: Community-based long-term care balances consumer preferences, option availability, and cost. An approach to managing costs is assigning professional nursing tasks to assistive personnel. This study evaluated implementation of nurse delegation in community based long-term care settings in Washington State. METHODS: Qualitative data were collected and analyzed using grounded theory methodology. Seventy-eight in-depth focused interviews were conducted with consumers, RNs, Nursing Assistants, providers, and case managers, followed by expanded participation and public forums where preliminary research results were presented to individuals engaged in nurse delegation (n = 248). RESULTS: The overarching social process identified in this study was balancing freedom with risk creating tension at the intersections, evident from three main perspectives: consumers, professionals, and the health care system. Consumers balance personal freedom with taking risks. The health care system balances the constraints of costs and reimbursement structures with client choice, with protecting public safety, and fear of policy "creep". Professionals balance new opportunities for redefining the nature and scope of nursing practice in community based settings with concerns about safety and choice. CONCLUSION: Implications for: 1) professional expectations for RN practice; 2) tension around overlapping roles, responsibilities, and reimbursement; 3) consumer expectations for expect greater control over their daily lives and more power in their partnerships with health care providers; 4) tension and competing demands inherent in a delivery system with strong vested interests and philosophical underpinnings; and 5) opportunities to partner with consumers to expand nursing's scope of influence in the community, enhancing quality of life and care.

Palliative Care in Long-Term Care Nursing: Taking Care of the "Dwindles"

C. J. Leppa [University of Washington, Bothell, Bothell, Washington, USA]

Abstract PURPOSE: This paper will explore a palliative care approach to end of life care for those nursing home patients in progressive decline from chronic illness - those who "dwindle to death." CONTENT: While long term care nurses are working to provide good end of life care with expected and supported decline and death, they work in an environment that is heavily regulated based on a philosophy of patient/resident improvement and discharge (Shield, 1995). The Omnibus Budget Reconciliation Act of 1987 created the Minimum Data Set (MDS) in the U.S. - a patient assessment requirement intended to identify and/or prevent LTC resident abuse or neglect. While LTC staff deal with the expected decline and death of some of their patients, "state surveyors view the facility's role as one of restoring health or providing rehabilitation" (Gage et al, 2000). For example, a resident's unwillingness to eat can be seen as either a dying patient's right to refuse food or as evidence of a malnourished and dehydrated resident that results in a citation for substandard care (Gage et al, 2000). A new palliative care assessment section to the MDS is currently in development in the U.S. that begins to address these issues but implementation will take time and it is not clear how the new material will integrate with the current MDS assessment. CONCLUSION: This paper discusses the challenges in adopting a palliative care philosophy in long-term care nursing and outlines potential barriers to assessment and delivery of quality end-of-life care in the nursing home environment.

SESSION 535

Effects of life events on the dietary habits of seniors

B. Grice (Vancouver/Richmond Health Board & Food For Life project, Vancouver, Canada); S. Koehn (Food For Life project, Vancouver, Canada); S. Crawford (Gerontology Research Centre, SFU, Canada).

The eating habits and food intake of seniors are thought to be influenced by their experience of a life event. Our research strategy was primarily qualitative such that our current findings are based on case studies of ten seniors plus data collected from twenty focus groups. Each was analyzed using Q.S.R. Nud.ist software. Adopting a 'participatory action research' (PAR) model, we have ensured that seniors were involved in meaningful decision-making roles and that our research findings were validated with the research participants. The life events most commonly identified as associated with a nutritional change were the death of a loved one, illness of a spouse, a move, a familial break-up, and financial hardship. Isolation and substance abuse additionally affected nutritional intake. Of the 15 different dietary changes identified, the most frequently reported were insufficient caloric intake (often associated with a loss of motivation), eating out more often, nutritional improvement, replacement of meals with tea and toast, etc, difficulty shopping or preparing foods, and increased consumption of "convenience" foods. Valuable coping resources and strategies included social supports (especially family), health/community and church-based programs (although there were reported barriers to access) and personal resources (e.g. notions of independence). Our findings confirm the premise that health and community service providers should consider the psycho-social dimensions of seniors' lives in order to support their nutritional requirements. Dietary crises triggered by social losses require solutions that give priority to addressing those losses; socialization may be as important to good eating as the food itself.

Lifestyle in Middle Aged Men and Cardiovascular Health in Older Age: A 15-Year Follow-Up

*Z. Mikes, M. Kornitzer, J. Simková, M. Dramaix, A. Dukát, J. Kolesár, V. Strelková (Department of Geriatric Medicine, Comenius Univ. Faculty of Medicine, Bratislava, Slovak Republic, * Universite Libre de Bruxelles, Belgium)*

The aim of the study was to assess the impact of physical activity and some risk factors in middle aged men on cardiovascular mortality during long-term follow-up. The authors performed a long-term follow-up in 2000 40-55-year old men without any signs of cardiovascular disease. A thorough physical examination was performed, blood pressure and serum lipid values were set. Aside of the personal questionnaire, the probands filled-in their job and leisure time activity questionnaires. Physical working capacity was assessed by the exercise test. Physical activity at the baseline examination was lower in smokers (129.4 W vs. 125.5 W, $p < 0.005$) and was decreasing with the number of the cigarettes smoked. 5 years after the baseline examination, the cardiovascular mortality was higher in smokers and was rising in due proportion with the value of systolic blood pressure and total serum cholesterol level, but not the BMI value and intensity of the physical activity. The results of the 15-year follow-up proved the risk character of smoking and systolic blood pressure. Furthermore, cardiovascular mortality was increasing with the BMI value and age, and it was decreasing with rising values of heavy leisure time physical activity. The results show that risk character of obesity and protective influence of the heavy leisure time activity in the middle aged men can rebound in older age. Healthy lifestyle in middle age decreases the risk of cardiovascular mortality in older age.

Prevalence and factors associated with intermittent claudication among elderly. The Bambui Health and Ageing Study.

V. M. A. Passos1,2,3, S. M. Barreto1,2,3, H. L. Guerra2,3, J. O. A. Firmo2,3, P. G. Vidigal1,2,3, M. F. F. Lima e Costa1,2,3 (1Federal University of Minas Gerais Medical School, 2Oswaldo Cruz Foundation René Rachou Research Centre, and 3Research Group on the Epidemiology and Anthropology of Ageing (REGEA), Belo Horizonte, Brazil)

PURPOSE: Intermittent claudication (IC) is the clinical manifestation of the chronic atherosclerotic occlusive disease of lower extremities, being an important cause of morbidity in the elderly. This is the first study in Brazil to determine the prevalence and factors associated with IC in the elderly (60+ years). METHOD: A cross-sectional population-based study was conducted in Bambuí, Southeast Brazil. After a written informed consent, prevalent cases were defined by the London School of Hygiene Cardiovascular Disease Questionnaire Information included: 1) a self-report of social-demographics, activity, smoking, drinking and other cardiovascular diseases, 2) a physical examination for height, weight and blood pressure and 3) laboratory tests for glucose, total cholesterol and triglycerides. Multiple logistic regression was used to investigate the relationship among the variables and IC. RESULTS: 1485/1742 (85.2%) elderly residents of Bambuí participated in this study: 37 (2.5%) were identified as having IC; 28 (4.8%) were male, 9 (1.0%) were female, 16 (1.8%) aged 60-69 years, 17 (3.7%) aged 70-79 years, and 4 (2.7%) aged 80 years or more. IC prevalence were significantly higher for male (OR=5.1; 95%CI:2.4-11.0), current smokers (OR=3.1; 95%CI:1.2-8.5), ex-smokers (OR=3.4; 95%CI:1.3-8.7) and those who reported more than two hospital admissions in the last 12 months (OR=2.8; 95%CI:1.1-7.2). CONCLUSION: The total and sex-specific prevalences observed are comparable to those found elsewhere. The association with smoking reinforces the importance of this risk factor for peripheral artery disease, and the association with an increased number of hospital admissions may express the higher morbidity of affected individuals.

Prevalence of risk factors and of preventive healthcare use: The Bambuí Health and Ageing Study

MFF Lima e Costa 1,2,3, SM Barreto 1,2,3, E Uchôa 1,2,3, JOA Firmo 1,3, PG Vidigal 1,2,3, HL Guerra 1,3 (1 Oswaldo Cruz Foundation Rene Rachou Research Institute, 2 Federal University of Minas Gerais Medical School, and 3 Research Group on the Epidemiology and Anthropology of Ageing - REGEA, Belo Horizonte, MG, Brazil).

Purpose: This study describes for the first time in Brazil the prevalence of risk factors and preventive healthcare use among older adults. Method:

All residents of Bambuí aged >60 (n=1742) and a sample of those aged 18-59 years (n=1020) were selected, for comparison. Results: Response rates were: 92.2 and 89.1%, respectively. Prevalence of the following risk factors were higher among older than younger adults: physical inactivity (47.7 vs. 28.0%); blood pressure >140-159/>90-99 mmHg (25.8 vs. 8.7%) and >160/>100 mmHg (19.1 vs. 4.1); total cholesterol >240 mg/dl (40.6 vs. 9.8%); blood glucose >126 mg/dl (12.4 vs. 2.2%). Daily consumption of fruits/vegetables (51.9 and 51.7%) and body mass index >25 kg/m2 (51.6 and 56.2%) were similar between the two groups. Smoking was lower among older (18.7%) than younger adults (31.1%). The proportion of participants with blood pressure checked in past year was high (86.6% and 61.2%), suggesting that the high prevalence of uncontrolled hypertension among older adults was not due to low access to healthcare. Conclusion: For a long time, it was believed that these risk factors were public health problems in large Brazilian cities. The high prevalence of most risk factors indicates a great demand for prevention and health promotion in this small town. There are no reasons to suppose that this is an isolated finding. Further investigations are needed to verify whether this reflects the reality of other towns in Brazil and other developing countries.

Smoking and alcohol consumption in relation to cognitive performance at middle age

Kalmijn S, Tijhuis MAR, Verschuren WMM (National Institute of Public Health and the Environment, Bilthoven, the Netherlands), Launer LJ (NIA, NIH, Bethesda, USA)

Purpose: In the elderly, smoking and alcohol consumption is related to cognition. We examined these associations at middle age. Method: Data are from the population-based Doetinchem cohort study, which started in 1987. In the second follow-up (5 years later) cognitive function was assessed in 1,928 subjects, aged 45-65 years. We constructed compound scores for three cognitive domains (memory, psychomotor speed, and cognitive flexibility) and one overall cognitive index. Multiple linear regression analyses were performed, with alcohol consumption (glasses/day) and cigarette smoking (current, former, never) at baseline as independent variables, adjusting for each other, and for age, sex, education, and cardiovascular risk factors. Results: Average alcohol consumption among drinkers (68%) was 1.6 glasses/day (SD=1.4) and 29.7Conclusion: Even at middle age, current smoking was inversely and alcohol consumption positively related with psychomotor speed and cognitive flexibility, although the effects were small. This suggests that in order to postpone or prevent cognitive decline, preventive actions can already be taken at middle age.

SESSION 537

Coping With Chronic Illness: A Study of Time Use Patterns Among Seniors in Canada 1998

C. C. Victorino (University of Calgary, Calgary, Alberta, Canada)

PURPOSE: This paper uses data from the 1998 Canadian time use survey to examine variations in the patterns of time use of seniors affected by chronic health conditions. It aims at describing the level of activity limitations experienced by seniors as captured by the variation, type, and duration of daily activities. The paper aims also at exploring the extent to which socio-economic characteristics such as education and income can mitigate the impact of chronic conditions on patterns of time use of seniors. METHOD: The study uses multivariate tobit regression to examine the impact of chronic conditions and various individual-level socio-economic characteristics on the patterns of time use of seniors. The study considers the following chronic conditions: heart, respiratory and musculoskeletal diseases, arthritis, diabetes, and cancer. The dependent variables are time spent on specific activities such as sport, personal care, and passive leisure. RESULTS: The results are expected to show that, compared to their non-chronically ill counterparts, chronically ill seniors have less variation in the activities they are engaged in, spend more time at home, and spend more time on passive activities. These findings are expected to vary by type of chronic condition, age, gender, education, income, marital status, and religion. CONCLUSION: Although time use surveys have a long history, they usually do not collect information on the health of respondents. The 1998 Canadian time use survey is unique in this respect and is expected to provide national-level estimates of the impact of chronic illness on the patterns of time use of seniors.

Disability Among Older Women and Men in Fiji: Concerns for the Future

Sela V. Panapasa (Institute for Social Research, Population Studies Program, University of Michigan, 311 Maynard Street, Ann Arbor, MI 48104 USA)

The purpose of this paper is to present differences in the disability status of older individuals in Fiji based upon gender, marital status and family socioeconomic structure. Using aggregate data from the 1966, 1986, and 1996 censuses of Fiji, this paper presents life table estimates of life expectancy across time for older people in Fiji and projects future longevity trends. Using survival analysis on individual level census data for the same time periods this paper also estimates the determinants of disability and how disability relates to productive years of life lost as well as overall life expectancy. The analysis resulting from this study shows that, while life expectancy in Fiji is on the rise, disability is a central determinant in the quality of years gained across time. Specifically, chronic disabilities related to both life style and diet such as diabetes, hypertension and emphysema are central to longevity and the quality of life among the elderly. Survival analysis also reflects the importance of family structure, and socioeconomic status in moderating the impacts of disability on longevity and quality of life. The results also show, however, that the ability of the elderly respondent to contribute to the family of residence plays a key role in determining the level and quality of support they received from their family. The paper concludes from a planning perspective, describing the policy implications of the findings. While focusing on the elderly in Fiji, it generalizes the implications of the findings for elderly throughout the Pacific Islands.

Gender Specific Changes in Health-Related Quality of Life Following Cardiovascular Disease: A Prospective Study

C.H.M. van Jaarsveld, R. Sanderman (Northern Centre for Healthcare Research, University of Groningen, The Netherlands), G.I.J.M. Kempen (Dept. of Health Care studies, Section Medical Sociology, Maastricht University, The Netherlands).

PURPOSE: The objective was to study gender specific changes in Health-Related Quality of Life (HR-QL) following cardiovascular disease in elderly people (>57 yr). METHOD: HR-QL was conceptualized and measured by physical, psychological (depressive symptoms/anxiety), and social (and role) functioning. Pre-morbid data (T0) were available from a community-based survey in 1993. Incident cases with Acute Myocardial Infarction (n=89) or Congestive Heart Failure (n=119), developed after 1993, are prospectively followed. Assessments were done at 6 weeks (T1), 6 (T2) and 12 months (T3) after diagnosis. RESULTS: Analysis includes 108 male and 100 female patients. At the pre-morbid assessment, gender differences on covariates were found: female patients were on average significantly older, lower educated, lived more often without a partner, had more co-morbidity and more severe disease compared to males. Moreover, females had significantly worse pre-morbid HR-QL compared to males. Unadjusted follow-up results showed worse HR-QL at all 3 post-morbid assessments in females. However, multivariate analyses on the changes from baseline in HR-QL including adjustment for the just mentioned covariates, showed no significant gender differences for physical and psychological adaptation to disease. Large individual differences in both gender groups were observed. Disease specific analyses revealed similar results. CONCLUSION: Gender differences in HR-QL following cardiovascular disease are mainly the result of pre-morbid differences in HR-QL and possibly not the result of gender specific adaptation processes.

Health status of elderly people living in a low-income community in Brazil

Cleusa Ernestina dos Santos (Instituto de Geriatria e Gerontologia - PUCRS, Porto Alegre, Brazil) Elisabete Michelon (Instituto de Geriatria e Gerontologia - PUCRS, Porto Alegre, Brazil), José Bergamaschi (Pontifícia Universidade Católica do Rio Grande do Sul, Porto Alegre, Brazil)

PURPOSE: Study the prevalence of chronic health conditions and functional status of elderly people living in a low-income community. METHODS: A random sample of 106 among approximately 350 individuals aged 60 years and older living in a low-income community were interviewed. The presence of chronic health conditions was assessed questioning the individual whether her/she has ever been told by a physician to have the following diagnosis: arterial hypertension, diabetes mellitus, dyslipidemia, heart disease, cerebrovascular disease, pulmonary disease, arthritis and cancer. Functional status was evaluated using the Katz Activities of Daily Living (ADL) scale and the Lawton Instrumental Activities of Daily Living (IADL) scale. Self-perceived urinary incontinence, gait disorders, falls, hearing and visual impairment were assessed. RESULTS: Mean age of the individuals was 68 years, 65% were women. and 80% had an income lower than US$150. Prevalence of chronic conditions were the following: arterial hypertension (60%), diabetes mellitus (16%), dyslipidemia (24%), heart disease (39%), cerebrovascular accident (11%), pulmonary disease (28%), arthritis (60%), cancer (6%). The majority (95%) were independent for all ADL and 69% were independent for all IADL. Urinary incontinence was referred by 30%, gait disorders by 53% and falls by 28%. CONCLUSION: The most frequent chronic conditions in this low-income elderly group were arterial hypertension, arthritis and gait disorders. There was a low rate of dependence for ADL and IADL.

Longitudinal changes in higher-level functional capacity in Japanese urban and rural community older populations

Y. Fujiwara, S. Shinkai, S. Watanabe, S. Kumagai, H. Yukawa, H. Yoshida, T. Ishizaki, T. Suzuki, H. Amano (Tokyo Metropolitan Institute of Gerontology, Tokyo, Japan), H. Haga (Tohoku Bunka Gakuen University, Sendai, Japan), H. Shibata (Ohbirin University,Tokyo, Japan)

Purpose: to examine the longitudinal changes in higher-level functional capacity in Japanese urban and rural community older populations. Method: population-based cross-sectional and prospective cohort studies on 793 subjects in urban Koganei and 725 subjects in rural Nangai, both 65 to 84 years of age. Main outcome measures were disability in instrumental activities of daily living (IADL), intellectual activity or social role, as measured by the Tokyo Metropolitan Institute of Gerontology Index of Competence. Results: At baseline, older persons in rural Nangai had a higher prevalence of disability in intellectual activity compared with their respective counterparts in urban Koganei. By contrast, disability in social role was more prevalent in Koganei than in Nangai. In both areas older persons had lowest prevalence of disability in IADL among three subscales. The six-year longitudinal survey on older persons who had no initial disability in all three subscales demonstrated that in Koganei older persons were most likely to be disabled in social role with advancing age, followed in turn by intellectual activity and IADL. By contrast, older people in Nangai were most likely to be disabled in intellectual activity, followed by social role and instrumental ADL. The Cox-proportional hazard model analysis revealed that the baseline level of intellectual activity or social role significantly predicted future onset of IADL disability in both areas even after controlling for sex, age, and chronic medical conditions. Conclusions: In both urban and rural community older populations, disability in social role and intellectual activity preceded IADL disability, and predicted significantly the future onset of IADL disability.

Public health priorities in rapidly ageing populations: The value of a disability survey

S. Jitapunkul (Faculty of Medicine, Chulalongkorn University, Bangkok, Thailand), C. Kunanusont, W. Phoolcharoen (AIDS Division, Department of Communicable Disease Control, Ministry of Public Health, Nonthaburi, Thailand), P. Suriyawongpaisal (Thailand Health Research Institute, National Health Foundation, Bangkok, Thailand), S. Ebrahim (Department of Social Medicine, University of Bristol, UK)

Purpose: To determine which diseases and health problems are most strongly associated with long-term disability among the Thai elderly and to determine their public health priority. Design: A cross-sectional mulitistage random sampling survey Setting: Nationally representative communities throughout Thailand Subjects: 4,048 participants aged 60 years and over Results: Overall, 769 (19%) people reported with long-term disability. Participants with long-term disability (LD) reported having between one and 21 long-term diseases or health problems. Eighteen of these problems were independently associated with LD in logistic regression analysis. Nearly half of the cases with LD (46.4%) suffered from two or more health problems. The odds of LD increased with the number of problems suffered. The problems contributing most to the population burden of disease as assessed by population attributable risk fractions were hemiparesis, arthritis, accidents (unintentional injuries), blindness and other eye diseases, kyphosis, weakness of limbs, deafness, and hypertension. This ranking of public health priority differs from conventional approaches using mortality statistics and disabililty adjusted life years (DALYs). Conclusion: National disability surveys provide an valuable means of assessing the population burden of disability and determining the underlying causes of disability. These methods provide a direct assessment of disability prevalence and disease priorities for rapidly ageing transitional countries where death certification may be incomplete or inaccurate.

The impact of chronic condition on functional disability in an older population in Taiwan

H.C. Chiu, L.W. Mau,. W.L. Tasi (Graduate Institute of Public Health, Kaohsiung Medical University, Taiwan), Y.H. Hsieh (Department of Social Welfare, National Chung Cheng University, Taiwan)

This study evaluated the impact of chronic condition on incident functional disability, while controlling for demographic characteristics and cognitive function. A prospective cohort of 1,286 community-dwelling elders was studied over a four-year period (1994-1998), which was a representative sample of urban elderly population in southern Taiwan. Only the sample who reported no functional limitations at baseline was included into analyses (i.e, 865 subjects free of physical ADL disability and 713 subjects of IADL disability). The measurement instrument was the Chinese-version Multidimensional Functional Assessment Questionnaire. Two logistic regression models were established for identifying predictors of ADL disability. The results indicated that the subjects with specific chronic conditions at baseline significantly had a higher risk of incident ADL disability at follow-up. With the adjustment of control variables, arthritis, diabetes, and hypertension were significantly predictive of physical ADL disability, while diabetes was the only chronic condition associated with incident IADL disability. The present findings cross-nationally confirm the impact of chronic conditions on future functional disability. For health promotion and disease prevention, the community-dwelling elders at risk should not be only those who are disabled, but also include those who have initial chronic condition, especially for older persons with diabetes.

SESSION 538

Co-operation in home care: - Home nurses' point of view

P.Pöyry,M-L.Perälä,T.Hammar,A.Noro, P.Rissanen,J.Teperi (National Research and Development Centre for Welfare and

Health, STAKES,Helsinki,Finland)

PURPOSE: In Finland as in many other countries home care of elderly people is highly emphasised while institutional care is reduced. Advances in the treatments and technology for independent living have allowed an increasing number of elderly people to maintain their independence in their home setting, thus increasing the need for home care services. Broaden range of home health and social care services are rising the need for the integration of the services. Responsive co-operation and communication of the home care personnel is therefore an important research topic at the moment. One aim of our survey about discharge and home care practices in Finland was to study co-operation of the personnel in home nursing and home services: (1) How much does the personnel in home nursing and home services have administrative co-operation and client-specific co-operation, (2) how sufficient is the co-operation and (3) how it relates to organisational solutions. METHOD: The study data was collected in 320 municipalities. A questionnaire was sent to one public health nurse in charge of home nursing (n=320). Response rate was 91%. The data was analysed quantitatively (frequencies, percentages, cross-tabulations). RESULTS: Most often arranged administrative co-operation practices were meetings of permanent multidisciplinary teams. Client-specific information was most often delivered by written. Most of the respondents considered co-operation sufficient. Certain organisational solutions were related to the intenseness of co-operation.

Home Care Training A Beginning in the Ageing World

S.Soneja, S.S.Sandhu (HelpAge India, New Delhi, India)

India is growing old! Decrease in mortality rates due to fall in infections, has resulted in increase in life expectancy of the Indian population. Life expectancy has increased from 40 years in 1951 to 64 years today. So, effectively, a person today has 20 years more to live than he would have 50 years back. However this in not without problems. In this kind of an ageing scenario where increase in life span also results in chronic functional disabilities make us realise the need for assistance to manage activities of daily living of the older persons. This assistance comes by way of family member, a volunteer or a paid worker who can be trained to provide safe, competent care and help to maintain dignity and very high quality of life in the older person. A home care worker provides companionship, emotional support, and looks after personal care of the older person like bathing, dressing etc. Apart from that the home carer also provides critical support as an information provider on certain health matters as well as helps in handling other aspects of social care like cash management. It is therefore essential to train family members of the society and equip them with theoretical and practical knowledge, skills and attitude, necessary to provide care to the aged elderly. This development of home care in the region can help the older persons as well as provide an employment opportunity to active and needy younger generation who are sensitive to the issue.

Nurses' Experience of Empowerment in their Provider-client Relationship in In-Home Care

Barbara Godfrey, RN,N (cand) (University of Western Ontario, London, ON Canada); Carol McWilliam, RN, EdD (University of Western Ontario, London, ON Canada); Mary-Anne Andrusyszyn, RN, EdD (University of Western Ontario, London, ON Canada)

PURPOSE: The purpose of this research was to gain and understanding of the nurses' experience of knowledge, status and authority (empowerment) in the nurse-client relationship in in-home care. METHOD: Using phenomenological research methodology, the researcher purposefully selected eight community nurses varying in age, years of experience, nursing agency and visiting versus shift nursing. Narrative data were collected through in-depth interviews averaging 55 minutes in length, using a semi-structured interview guide. Hermeneutic analysis was used to elicit interpretive findings illuminating themes and patterns of the balancing of power as experienced by nurse providers of in-home care. RESULTS: Themes and patterns contained in the findings illuminate the nurse participants' stage of evolution in integrating the theory of empowerment into their everyday practice in providing in-home care. CONCLUSION: The results of this study increase understanding of the balance of knowledge, status and authority within the nurse-client relationship as experienced by community nurses today. These understandings have an impact on the implementation of client-driven care in the community setting, as well as on nursing practice and nursing's knowledge base related to empowerment.

The construction of caring relationships in home help services

Bengt Ingvad (School of Social Work, Lund university, Lund, Sweden)

PURPOSE: The aim is to study social interaction in care-giving work. The focus is the relationship between the elderly and the home helper. how it develops an changes during the care-giving work. METHOD: Interviews, questionnaires and case studies with observations have been used. 70 home helpers and 500 home help recipients are included. 20 case studies were performed. RESULTS: The two parties exercise a strong emotional influence on each other. Often their relationship is characterised by a well functioning interaction. The parties adapt to each other´s expectations of emotional exchange. In some cases conflicts concerning these expectations may arise. In such critical situations, psychological constructions, like attributing personal traits and stereotypes, are created. The basis for these constructions is different for the parties. For the recipient this is a way to satisfy emotional needs and retain self-image. For the home helper this is a way to endure emotional strain and cope with acts in conflict with the norms and ethics of care-giving. CONCLUSION: The elderly´s and the home helpers´ psychological constructions play an important role in care-giving work. The constructions influcence the two parties´ experience of the care-giving work and the content of the work.

The Relationship between Dementia Family Caregivers and Home Care Workers

Margaret A. Perkinson, (Washington University School of Medicine, St. Louis, USA)

There is surprisingly little research on the relationship between family caregivers of persons with dementia and their home care workers, and how that relationship impacts the quality of care provided. Little is known about the ways home care workers are incorporated into family households and how families and home care workers view this process. In an attempt to understand home care from both perspectives, ten focus groups and twenty key informant interviews were conducted with home health aides currently working with persons with dementia and with family caregivers of persons with dementia who receive home care. The aides discussed their views of their work, their interactions with family members, their greatest concerns working in homes and with persons with dementia, and their thoughts on ways that families can contribute to the effectiveness of home care workers. Families discussed their greatest problems and concerns with home care and described instances of good and unsatisfactory home care workers. Respondents provided suggestions for developing good relationships between families and home care workers, and identified the kinds of information families can share with aides (e.g, the relative's preferences and routines) that can help the home care worker provide better quality care. Based on this data, educational materials for both family caregivers and home care workers were developed. (Funded by the AARP Andrus Foundation.)

Whose Responsibility is It? Formal Service Practitioners' Views of Family Caregivers' Responsibilities and Difficulties.

J.P. Lavoie (Direction de la santé publique de Montréal-Centre and CLSC René-Cassin, Montreal, Canada), Jacinthe Pepin (Université de Montréal, Montreal, Canada), Nancy Guberman (Université du Québec à Montréal, Montreal, Canada), Sylvie Lauzon (Université de Montréal, Montreal, Canada), Maria-Elisa Montejo (CLSC René-Cassin, Montreal, Canada)

A small number of studies have examined relations between home care practitioners and their clients, but very few have explored the relationship between the former and informal caregivers. However, the main services asked for and used by informal caregivers are home care services. This lack of interest is probably due to the ambiguous status of caregivers in home care policies and services. The research presented here, which draws on both Schön's concept of the reflexive practitioner and Callon and Latour's notion of social translation, examines the views of home care practitioners (workers, professionals and administrators) with regards to caregivers' responsibilities, difficulties and need for support. Semi-structured interviews were conducted with 70 practitioners from 10 governmental home care agencies located in rural, urban and metropolitan areas of Quebec (Canada). The majority saw compensation for disabilities as being primarily the responsibility of disabled individuals and their families. The role of home care agencies was seen as being to provide the latter with support when their task became too difficult. However, almost all respondents considered the support offered to caregivers to be insufficient and proposed a few additions to current services. Perceptions of the problems experienced by caregivers and the services that should be provided to them varied depending on the professional group. Only a few practitioners considered compensation for disabilities to be a social responsibility as well. They commented on the half-heartedness of home care policies and services and their lack of coherence, calling for more political measures and greater community action.

Working in Clients' Homes: the Impact On the Health and Well-being of Visiting Home Care Workers

Margaret Denton, Isik Zeytinoglu and Sharon Webb (McMaster University, Hamilton, Ontario Canada)

The purpose of this paper is to examine the effects of working in clients' homes on the health and well-being of visiting home care workers. This paper reports the results of a survey of 674 visiting staff from three non-profit home care agencies in a medium sized city in Ontario, Canada. Survey results are also complimented by data from 9 focus groups with 50 employees. For purposes of this study, home care workers include visiting therapists, nurses, and home support workers. Health and well-being is measured by three dependent variables: stress; job stress; and intrinsic job satisfaction. Multiple least squared regression analyses show several structural, emotional, physical, and organizational working conditions associated with the health and well-being of visiting home care workers. Overall, results show that workload, difficult clients, clients who take advantage of workers, sexual harassment, safety hazards, a repetitious job, and work-related injuries are associated with poorer health. Being fairly paid, having good benefits, emotional labour, organizational support, control over work, and peer support are associated with better health. Results suggest that policy change is needed to encourage healthier work environments for employees who work in clients homes.

SESSION 539

The Art of Life: Interart, collage, reflection ... and transitioning

Pamela Brett-MacLean (The University of British Columbia, Vancouver, British Columbia, Canada); Joy Coghill (Western Gold Theatre Company, Vancouver, British Columbia, Canada), Marilyn Magid (George Derby Centre, Burnaby, British Columbia, Canada); Susan Summers (St. Michael's Centre, Burnaby, British Columbia, Canada); Kathleen Weiss (Western Gold Theatre, and The University of British Columbia, Vancouver, British Columbia, Canada)

This transitional session will provide an opportunity for participants to reflect on the proceedings of the conference and their experience of the "Creative Aging through the Arts" conference programme, and discuss the importance of creativity through the life course. Participants will be able to share information and resources, and identify needs and opportunities. All participants will be invited to engage in individual and collaborative art making, and celebrate "creative aging through the arts" through music and song, collage and sculptural play. The session will end with a simple closing ritual that will acknowledge the connections between us, as we live and love, and work to remake the world through compassionate caring, through our relationships with one another, ...as we live our lives of, and through, art. The session will be informed by an improvisational approach to engaging with all the might arise, and be revealed within the moment as we renew our engagement with, and wonder of, the possibilities of life, ... living lives of art. Within the space of "presence", an art-based, aesthetic visioning of hoped-for futures will be used to close the session.

SESSION 540

Effects of Senior Center Types on Patterns and Levels of Utilization among Elderly Korean-Americans

W. Kim (Graduate School of Social Service, Fordham University, New York, USA)

This study was undertaken to address the effects of type of senior center (Korean-specific and mainstream) on the patterns and levels of utilization (frequency of use, duration of use, activity participation, and service use) among elderly Korean- Americans. Data were collected through face-to-face interviews with 120 senior center users (60 from a Korean-specific center and 60 from 10 mainstream centers in New York City) using a non-probability sampling procedure. The study findings include: 1) Senior center type was significantly related to four dimensions of senior center use on the bivariate level; 2) Hierarchical regression analyses — with each dimension of center use as the criterion and several selected variables as covariates — indicate that type of senior center was a significant independent contributor to all dimensions of senior center use; and 3)Determinants of center use levels were convincingly different between elderly Korean-Americans attending the Korean-specific center and those attending mainstream centers. This study highlights the usefulness of type of senior center (ethnic-specific and mainstream) as an explanatory variable in understanding senior center utilization by elderly Korean-Americans. Policy makers and service providers must be sensitive to specific sub-group differences when planning and delivering senior center programs and services to minority elders who experience cultural and language barriers in utilizing services.

Social Integration, Social Support and Medical Utilization of the Elderly in Taiwan

Peter S.K. Chi [Cornell University, Ithaca, NY, USA] Ping-Lung Hsin [Chung-Hwa Institution for Economic Research, Taipei, Taiwan]

PURPOSE: This study,based on data from the 2000 Taiwan Elderly Survey attempts to test an integrated model, linking Andersen and Newman's behavioral systems approach with two key sociological concepts: social integraiton (as measured by an index of multiple roles) and social support (as measured by financial support and instremental support). it is hypothesized that social integration may reduce the elderly's need for care, which will in turn change their medical utilization patterns; it is also hypothesized that among the elderly who have used formal health care, social support may reduce their out-of-pocket expenditures. METHOD: We use logit regression to analyze the determinants of physician visits and hospitalization, while variation in health expenditures among the elderly is examined using the Tobit model with sample section. RESULTS: Findings show that elderly with good or poor health conditions are less likely to use medical services than the frail elderly and that married elders are less than the non-married to use medical care. The higher the educational level, the lower the probability of using medical services. The elderly who live with their children are less likely to use formal medical services than those who do not live with their children. CONCLUSION:

Finally, social integration and social support are found to be effective mechanisms for minimizing the moral hazard problems in Taiwan's newly established national health insurance program.

The help-seeking behavior of community dwelling Chinese older adults in Hong Kong

Esther Chow, Agnes Yeung (City University of Hong Kong, Kowloon, Hong Kong SAR, CHINA)

PURPOSE: Instances that happened during the year between 1995 to 1997 alarmed the community's concern towards the Seniors' vulnerable situation in Hong Kong. The winter monsoon death toll took more than 60 older adults at the 1996 Chinese Lunar New Year, the suicidal death rate increased 126%, and the use of destructive means in settling problems increased. Studies revealed that single elderly living alone have a small network for social and emotional support, and living in the community does not guarantee the presence of care and the natural development of informal helping networks. This paper aims to understand the help-seeking behavior of the community dwelling Chinese Older Adult and to explore its various correlates, after the implementation of "Community Care" Policy for 20 years. METHOD: A cross-sectional survey is used. A total of 393 elderly aged 60 and above single living alone and those living with family were selected through random sampling within a designated public housing estate for interview. RESULTS: Findings reveal strong correlation among various factors with help-seeking behavior. They are: gender, age, the number of relatives living together, living arrangement, health conditions, activities of daily livings, the social networks of the elderly, involvement in family activities, free from problems, attitude of help-seeking, locus of control, and self-esteem scores. CONCLUSION: Findings provide relevant and substantial information, and guidelines on planning and delivery of Seniors social services, and are collected as part of the study on the impact of Networking Strategies Initiative (NSI) on changes the help-seeking behaviors and patterns of support networks of the elderly in the community. Meaningful conclusion and recommendations can be drawn concerning the future policy directions and services delivery models.

The Need, Use, Effectiveness and Target Efficiency of Formal Elderly Care at Home

M.Vaarama, A.Hakkarainen (Stakes, National Research and Development Centre for Welfare and Health, Helsinki, Finland)

Purpose: to explain the use/non-use of formal care by people 75+ living at home/shelter in 1998, and to evaluate the target efficiency of the given service Methods: we examined: (1)interaction between individual, environmental and social resources, self-perceived need and actual use of formal care; (2) self-perceived effectiveness of formal care (3) targeting of formal care across the client groups. From randomly sampled 21 municipalities, a random sample of 6530 persons 75+ was taken. 3183 self-completed questionnaires (61,4 %) and 386 interviews (42,1 %) were obtained. Official statistics served as secondary data. The primary factors studied covered socio-economics, living environments, health, functional ability (IADL/PADL) and sense of coherence, social networks and informal care, need and actual use of formal care, targeting of care, client-satisfaction and need of additional help. Statistical analyses were linear and log-linear regression analyses. Results: Living alone, poor housing environments, low sense of coherence, loneliness, ADL-difficulties and problems with indoor and outdoor mobility cause the need of external help. Support from social networks and informal care decrease the use of formal care. The more intensive the formal care, that higher the self perceived effectiveness. Unmet need exists both by the users and non-users. The needs of most deprived clients are under-covered, while the objectively not-needy persons receive formal care. Conclusions: The demand of formal care is connected to livability of the environment and living-ability of an older person. The target efficiency of formal care could be improved by re-distribution of current resources, but also new resources are necessary.

SESSION 541

Longevity and Anti-Aging Interventions

1. Vladimir Anisimov [N.N. Petrov Research Institute of Oncology, St. Petersburg, Russia] 2. Etienne-E. Baulieu [Professor of Endocrinology, Collège de France, Le Kremlin Bicetre, FRANCE] 3. Kenichi Kitani [Director General National Institute for Longevity Sciences(NILS, Obu, Aichi, JAPAN] 4. George S. Roth [National Institute on Aging, Baltimore, MD USA]

With the graying of the world population, gerontologists are increasingly addressing the issue of whether interventions can be identified that slow the rate of aging and increase lifespan as well as healthspan. Although various anti-aging interventions have been investigated in this regard, little consensus has emerged to identify leading candidates for further study. This symposium will review a variety of dietary, pharmacological, and hormonal interventions to assess their potential for slowing the rate of aging and increasing longevity. Dr. V. Anisimov will review a range of pharmacological and dietary interventions that purport to alter the rate of aging. He will offer a classification system by which various geroprotectors can be assessed and will emphasize their impact on cancer risk. Dr. E. Baulieu will discuss the research that has been conducted on the adrenal steroid, dehydroepiandrosterone (DHEA), that shows marked age-related decline in serum levels in humans and other animals. As a dietary supplement, DHEA is currently being consumed by thousands of persons expecting beneficial effects on aging and promoting longevity. Dr. K. Kitani will present an overview of studies on the drug, L-deprenyl, and particular derivatives, which have shown potential for increasing lifespan in laboratory rodents. These drugs act in a complex manner to enhance antioxidant defense mechanisms. Dr. G. Roth will discuss a novel strategy for developing caloric restriction mimetics. Such nutraceutical and pharmacological interventions are being evaluated for their potential of increasing lifespan and healthspan by mimicking the metabolic effects of a low calorie diet without actually reducing caloric intake. Thus, the objective of the symposium is to expose weak areas of research in anti-aging interventions but then to discern the most promising areas for future efforts. If such interventions were realized, then enormous potential exists for increasing lifespan and healthspan and reducing the economic burden in aging populations.

Effect of "anti-aging" interventions on cancer risk

V.N. Anisimov (N.N. Petrov Research Institute of Oncology, St.Petersburg, Russia)

A significant increase of the elderly in populations of developed countries has been associated with increased morbidity and mortality from the major age-related diseases - cardiovascular, cancer, neurodegenerative, diabetes mellitus, decreased in resistance to infections. Obviously the development of means to prevent premature aging in humans is crucial to offset this trend. However, data on such treatments are scarce, contradictory and often unreliable from the points of view of the adequacy of the experiments to current scientific requirements as well as the interpretation of the results and safety. Available data on life span extension and adverse effects of the following geroprotectors will be critically reviewed: antioxidants, chelate agents and lathyrogens, succinate, adaptogens and herbs, neurotropic drugs, inhibitors of monoamine oxidase, glucocorticoids, DHEA, sex and growth hormones, melatonin, pineal peptide preparations, protein inhibitors, antidiabetic biguanides, thymic hormones and peptides, immunomodulators, enteroadsorbents, lypofuscin inhibitors, as well as calorie intake restriction and special diets. Most of the available results are insufficient and cannot provide convincing evidence of life span extension and safety of the putative geroprotectors. Effects of genetic manipulations (mutant, knockout and transgenic animals) on longevity and cancer will be evaluated as well. Drugs and means for prolonging life span can be subdivided into 3 categories: a) geroprotectors equally prolonging the life span in all the members of the population: these postponed the beginning of the population's ageing; b) geroprotectors decreasing the mortality rate in a long-lived subpopulation, which raised their maximal life span: these slowed down the population's aging rate; c) geroprotectors increasing the survival rate in a short-lived subpopulation without changes in the maximal life span: in this case the ageing rate rose. There was a high positive correlation between the type of geroprotector-induced aging delay and the pattern of tumour development in the same population of animals. Type A geroprotectors did not influence the incidence of tumours but increased a tumour latency. Type B geroprotectors were effective both in the inhibition of spontaneous carcinogenesis and in tumour latency increase. Certain drugs of the Type C category raised tumour incidence in the exposed populations. According to the multistage model proposed, geroprotectors either inhibit or accelerate the passage of carcinogen-exposed cells from one stage to another. Thus, the efficacy of geroprotectors as preventive means of cancer development will decrease with respect to the age of exposure onset. Recommendations regarding the available drugs and means of life span extension should be carefully reconsidered under international scientific control.

How does (-)deprenyl affect animals, their survivals in particular?

K. Kitani, C. Minami, K. Isobe, K. Maehara (National Inst. Longevity Sci, Obu, Japan) S. Kanai (Tokyo Metropolitan Inst. Gerontology, Japan) G.O.Ivy (Univ. Toronto, Scarborough, Canada), M.C.Carrillo (National Univ Rosario, Rosario, Argentina)

PURPOSE : We and others have shown that chronic treatment with (-)deprenyl can significantly prolong survivals of animals. Antioxidant enzyme activities such as superoxide dismutase (SOD) and catalase (CAT) can also be significantly increased by (-)deprenyl in brain dopaminergic regions and we suggested a causal relationship may exist between these two effects of the drug. The aim of this study is to further clarify how the drug actually affects animal bodies and their survivals. METHOD & RESULTS : We have further confirmed the effect of the drug on survivals of Fischer rats of both sexes at a dose of 0.25 mg/kg/inj (3Å~a week), which is one half that of the dose successfully used in our previous study (0.5 mg/kg), while a two fold higher dose (1.0 mg/kg/inj) shortened the survival of rats. Furthermore, a 13-month treatment at this higher dose lost its effect on enzyme activities, showing comparable values for control and treated rats. These observations are consistent with our previous notion that animals can survive longer while antioxidant enzymes are maintained at levels higher than their natural levels. We have also found that the drug increases SOD and CAT activities in selective tissues outside of the brain (e.g. the heart, kidneys, adrenal glands and the spleen) as well. Accordingly, (-)deprenyl is not a mere neurotropic drug but is a more systemic one, which may be related to anti-tumorigenic and immunomodulatory effects reported for the drug, releasing many humoral factors such as various cytokines, TNFÉø, etc. CONCLUSION : Collectively, the drug may generally affect the neuro-immuno-endocrine axis regulating homeostasis during aging as an anti-aging drug.

Intermediary Steroids: A New Class of Molecules for Biomedical Interventions in Aging

Etienne-Emile Baulieu, (Collège de France and INSERM, Paris, France)

DHEA(S) [dehydroepiandrosterone(sulfate)] and PREG(S)[pregnenolone(sulfate)] are known as intermediary steroids in the biosynthesis of classical hormones in glandular cells, testosterone and estradiol for DHEA, PROG[progesterone] and corticosteroids for PREG. However, besides identical metabolic transformation obtainable after administration in vivo, DHEA and PREG have activities of their own, as indicated by the following examples related to possible biomedical intervention in aging, particularly at the nervous systems where their synthesis has been demonstrated ("neurosteroids"). 1/ DHEA(S) is inhibitor of GABAA-R function, and neuroprotective against glutamate neurotoxicity was observed in vitro 2/ PREG(S) also inhibitor of GABAA-R and stimulatory of NMDA-R, and the physiological implication of its decrease in hippocampus in aged-related memory deficit has been demonstrated, with repair by administration (PNAS, 1997, 94, 14865) 3/ The formation of PROG from PREG in the peripheral nervous system is involved in myelin repair (Science, 1995, 268, 1500) 4/ PREG binds with high affinity a Microtubule Associated Protein MAP2 and consequently stimulates tubulin polymerization to form Microtubules (PNAS, 2000, 97, 3579). There is potential role for PREG and synthetic analogues to treat/ prevent brain alterations associated to aging. Oral, double-blind, one year administration of 50mg/d of DHEA ("DHEAge") was performed in 280 60-80 y old men and women (PNAS, 2000, 97, 4279). Physical and mental effects will be reported, and the currently studied PREG administration protocol "PREG-MEM" will be described.

SESSION 542

The Masters Degree in Gerontology: Is it necessary?

JoAnn Damron-Rodriguez (UCLA, and Partners in Care Foundation,Los Angeles, California, USA - Gerontology in the United States: the Disciplinary Dialogue) G. Gutman (Is The Master's Degree in Gerontology Necessary? The Canadian Experience) Martha Meyer (Bremen University, HB, Bremen, Germany - Postgraduate education in Gerontology in Western Europe: Current state and future developments) Graham D. Rowles (University of Kentucky, Lexington, Kentucky,USA - Doctoral Education in Gerontology: Do we need it?)

Abstract ISSU: Over the past three decades, Gerontology education has expanded considerably in many countries around the world. Students in higher education can now participate in courses at all levels, through from undergraduate work to taught doctoral programs. Courses differ in content and orientation, from the highly theoretical to the very practical, and there is now a very wide variety of programs on offer under the rubric of 'gerontology'. In this symposium, we focus on postgraduate education in gerontology as it is currently delivered in a number of countries and institutions. Contributors to the symposium will present details of their programs but crucially, and based upon evidence from program evaluations, will be asking the critical question about whether, in the 21st century, we really need such courses. Between them, the symposium contributors have a wide range of both academic and practical experience in this field and will be able to draw out key issues regarding how such programs have developed over the years, and what the future might hold. STRUCTURE: Chair : Professor Sara Carmel Discussant: Professor Miriam Bernard - Introduction and opening remarks - Prof. Sara Carmel (10 minutes) - Gerontology in the United States: the Disciplinary Dialogue - Prof. JoAnn Damron-Rodriguez (15 minutes) - Is The Master's Degree in Gerontology Necessary? The Canadian Experience Dr. Gloria Gutman (15 minutes) - Postgraduate education in Gerontology in Western Europe: Current state and future developments - Dr. Martha Meyer (15 minutes) Doctoral Education in Gerontology: Do we need it? - Prof. Graham Rowles (15 minutes) DISCUSSION: LEARNING THE LESSONS - Prof. Miriam Bernard (10 minutes) Questions/comments from the audience (10 minutes). CONTENT: Professor Sara Carmel will introduce the symposium, and as part of her opening remarks, will make reference to the first two Israeli MA programs, which were opened in 1999. Professor JoAnn Damron-Rodriguez will reflect on the American experience, by focusing on the benefits and limitations of gerontology graduate programs in comparison to geriatric professional programs. Professor Gloria Gutman will present the Canadian experience with academic gerontology programs. Dr. Martha Meyer will describe the current state of academic gerontological education at a Europe-wide level, and the foreseen developments in designing a curriculum that is multidisciplinary and valid throughout the European Union. Professor Graham Rowles' will discuss experience with taught Ph.D programs in the USA. He will present a number of central questions and dilemmas that have to be addressed by such programs in the future. CONCLUSIONS: Professor Miriam Bernard will summarize the contributions by addressing three issues: a) How gerontology programs have been developed, in terms of their orientation/rationale, and methods of instruction; b) What are the expected developments in these programs, and c) To what extent, are such programs really necessary.

Gerontology in the United States: the Disciplinary Dialogue

JoAnn Damron-Rodriguez (Department of Social Welfare, University of California, Los Angeles, and Partners in Care Foundation, Los Angeles, California, USA)

PURPOSE: Gerontological education in the United States has been in a state of uneven development for the last 50 years. A key issue is the designation of the study of aging as a specific discipline or as an interdisciplinary field versus a content arena within a discipline. Focusing on graduate education, this presentation will compare and contrast gerontology degrees to geriatric professional degrees in the health professions. METHOD: The presentation will use data from California Geriatric Education Center funded by the US Bureau of Health Professions, the California Council on Gerontology and Geriatrics with comparison USA data from the Association of Gerontology in Higher Education. Specific disciplinary references will be made to social work from evaluation data from the Geriatric Social Work Consortium funded by the John F. Hartford and Archstone foundations. RESULTS: Though progress has been made in the preparation of well-qualified professional to serve the growing number older Americans the challenge is growing. The varying benefits of gerontological vs. professional preparation are compared for both benefits and limitations. CONCLUSION: A continuum of gerontological and geriatric educational options is presented including specializations within disciplines and dual degrees in gerontology and a health profession.

Is The Master's Degree in Gerontology Necessary? The Canadian Experience

G. Gutman (Director, Gerontology Program, Simon Fraser University, Vancouver, Canada)

While many universities offer some courses or subspecialties within traditional departments, currently in Canada, there are only three universities which offer Masters degrees in Gerontology: The University of Sherbrooke in Quebec, The University of Waterloo in Ontario and Simon Fraser University in British Columbia. The Sherbrooke program, the first to be established, is linguistically distinct (courses are offered in French while at the other two universities English is the language of instruction), but like Simon Fraser University the degree offered is a Master of Arts in Gerontology. The University of Waterloo, in contrast, offers a MSc in Health Studies and Gerontology. All three programs are interdisciplinary but differ in their areas of specialization. At SFU students choose between two streams: 1) aging and the built environment and 2) health promotion/population health. At Waterloo there is more emphasis on the biological perspective and on epidemiologic methodology. At Sherbrooke the emphasis has moved from philosophic/humanistic to professional education. Strong research training is an underlying theme of all three programs .

In terms of evaluation, since all are "regular" senate-approved graduate programs, they are subject to the same type of periodic review as other departments within the university. Using the Ontario Council of Graduate Studies guidelines as an example, rating criteria include evidence of student demand, ratio of degree completions to admissions, time to graduation, and post-graduate employment of students in a cognate area. As well, faculty productivity (grants, publications, peer recognition, service) is considered. All three programs have successfully passed external academic review. All three have also pass "community" and "alumni" tests - i.e. their graduates are valued locally and nationally by community groups and agencies and they have strong alumni support. All three offer a depth of instruction in Gerontology that is not possible in a subspecialty situation.

Postgraduate education in Gerontology in Western Europe: Current state and future developments

M. Meyer, (Bremen University, HB, Germany)

Highly qualified gerontologists are of fundamental importance to meet the challenges of ageing societies. No significant efforts have been made at a Europe-wide level to develop standards and to introduce comprehensive academic training in gerontology. An inventory carried out involved 18 European countries. The document analysis elaborated the current state of academic gerontological education, structures of higher education as well as different conceptual frameworks, contents and degrees. Out of a total of 60 programmes, 49 lead to an academic degree: 42 of these are postgraduate degrees to Master' s level or equivalent, 7 programmes out of 49 are undergraduate programmes leading to a BSc or equivalent. The evaluation of the current state of higher education in Gerontology shows a heterogeneous picture with a great structural diversity of programmes, the lack of guidelines for entry requirements and course contents. The distribution of programmes across Europe is uneven and the regional and national density varies considerably: More or less „blank spots"- especially in Southern Europe- are contrasted with a wide variety of programmes in terms of quantity and quality in Western and Middle European countries. From 1998 to June 2000 the European Commission DG-V- funded a working group in order to develop an European Master programme in Gerontology. The overall aim of this projekt was the development of a model curriculum that is both multidisciplinary and „European" and valid throughout the European Union. It aims to optimize the use of existing Masters programmes in Europe and to develop new programmes in European countries which currently have no such provision.

Doctoral Education in Gerontology: Do we need it?

Graham D. Rowles (Sanders-Brown Center on Aging, University of Kentucky, Lexington, Kentucky, USA)

Rapid growth of graduate education in gerontology in the United States culminated in 1989 with creation of the first Ph.D. Program in Gerontology at the University of Southern California. There are now six doctoral programs and several others in various stages of development. Against the backdrop of the experience of the Ph.D. Program in Gerontology at the University of Kentucky, with its explicit focus on aging and health, the purpose of this contribution is to address critical questions in the development of such programs. These include: the viability of gerontology as an emergent research discipline with its own theory; the issue of a multidisciplinary versus interdisciplinary focus; the relative balance of theoretical and applied themes in the curriculum; and the need for truly groundbreaking educational innovation. The rich potential for advanced gerontology education is tempered by pragmatic concerns such as: placing doctoral gerontology education within the predominantly disciplinary structure of the contemporary academe; developing appropriate curricula for persons with widely divergent intellectual backgrounds, experience and professional training; program evaluation and accreditation; the placement of graduates; and the receptivity of society and its institutions to a new field. It is concluded that global demographic trends are making training opportunities in gerontology at the doctoral level both necessary and inevitable and that we are in the midst of an era of educational experimentation and innovation that is likely to have profound implications for the quality of life of elders in the twenty-first century.

SESSION 543

Unique Challenges of Geriatric Rehabilitation

Ruth Berekoff (Rehabilitation Program, Holy Family Hospital, Vancouver, Canada) Overcoming Feelings of Hopelessness in the Geriatric Rehabilitation Setting. Maureen Desborough (Rehabilitation Program, Holy Family Hospital, Vancouver,

Canada) Patients Tell Us Where to Go. Abdollah Rezazadeh (Rehabilitation Program, Holy Family Hospital, Vancouver, Canada) Easy Street: Enabling success in Daily Occupation for Geriatric Population. Barb Lang (Rehabilitation Program, Holy Family Hospital, Vancouver, Canada) Designing, Implementing and Evaluating an Interdisciplinary Dysphagia Management Program for Geriatric Rehabilitation. Sandra Whytock (Rehabilitation Program, Holy Family Hospital, Vancouver, Canada). Planning Education Programs for Elderly Learners.

This symposium addresses the challenges of providing rehabilitation programs for the elderly. The symposium begins with a description of geriatric rehabilitation programs at Providence Health Care, Holy Family Hospital site. Holy Family Hospital provides rehabilitation for elderly patients who are living with the experience of arthritis, joint replacement, fracture, amputation and stroke. Five presentations will illustrate selected management strategies designed specifically to accommodate the challenges of aging. "Overcoming Feelings of Hopelessness in the Geriatric Rehabilitation Setting" presents a bio-psycho-social assessment tool used by the interdisciplinary team to assist elderly patient to come to terms with loss. "Our Patients Tell Us Where to Go" outlines a team process designed to guide elderly patients to set and work towards their goals in a manner which is respectful of their hopes and autonomy. "Easy Street: Enabling Success in Daily living tasks" describes a functional approach to rehabilitation for the elderly which encorporates the use of "Easy Street", a simulation of challenges the patient will experience in their own community. "Designing, Implementing and Evaluating an Interdisciplinary Dysphagia Management Program for Geriatric Rehabilitation" describes a team strategy to assist patients and their families to manage dysphagia, a common and significant problem for the elderly. "Planning Education Programs for Elderly Patients" focuses on challenges encountered by elderly learners, and the use of curriculum principles to design flexible education programs to meet their needs. At the conclusion of these presentations participants will be able to use the principles described to design strategies to manage the unique challenges of providing geriatric rehabilitation

Designing, Implementing, and Evaluating an Interdisciplinary Dysphagia Management Program for Geriatric Rehabilitation

M. Desborough, J. Gjessing, B. Lang, C. Ong, S. Whytock (Providence Health Care, Holy Family Hospital, Vancouver, Canada)

Up to 47% of patients at 2-3 weeks post-stroke reportedly present with dysphagia. Earlier discharge from acute care has in turn caused dysphagia management to become integral to a geriatric rehabilitation program. The identification and management of swallowing disorders has traditionally been considered the realm of the S-LP and/or OT. The current trend in the literature, however, appears to be towards a coordinated interdisciplinary approach to dysphagia management. The Interdisciplinary Dysphagia Committee at Holy Family Hospital has worked to design a protocol to formalize the roles that several core disciplines play in early identification of a swallowing problem and in providing a comprehensive management program. The protocol begins with a swallow screening conducted by nursing on admission to the rehab program, and links the interventions of the S-LP, RDN, OT, PT and RN in developing and discussing the dysphagia management plan along with the patient and family from admission through to discharge. The program is individualized and includes team plans for supporting the patient/ family who decides to live at risk. An implementation plan will be presented which was devised to meet the challenge of ensuring consistency of practice among all rehab staff. The committee has outlined clear outcomes for the project. Preliminary results will be presented. At the conclusion of this presentation participants will be familiar with the scope of the interdisciplinary dysphagia protocol and appreciate how effective implementation allows team members to provide early, consistent, and comprehensive care to the patient with a swallowing disorder.

Easy Street: Enabling success with daily living tasks for the geriatric population.

Abdollah Rezazadeh (Occupational Therapy Department, Holy Family Hospital, Vancouver, Canada)

LCD projector The challenge of Geriatric Rehabilitation is to help patients return to the community safely and for the long term. Holy Family Hospital's Easy Street offers patients a safe environment in which to practice daily living tasks prior to leaving the hospital. Holy Family is the only Rehabilitation site in British Columbia and one of a few in Canada that provides geriatric rehabilitation patients with a transitional environment in which to practice daily living skills. Easy Street is a strong assessment tool and guides the patient's treatment plan by providing the therapist and patient with information on the skills and resources the patient will need to live a full and active life. A large number of Holy Family Hospital's patients have found the Easy Street environment to be instrumental to their return to the community. Case studies will be presented to illustrate the successful use of Easy Street with geriatric patients.

Overcoming feelings of hopelessness in the geriatric rehabilitation setting.

Ruth Berekoff, Amy Freeman, Social Work Department Holy Family Hospital, Vancouver, Canada

Adjustment support is a critical component of a geriatric patient's treatment plan and successful discharge from hospital into the community. Geriatric patients presenting for rehabilitation at Holy Family Hospital are coping with loss of independence and increasing dependency. How can the multidisciplinary team work together to help their clients manage this life challenge? What information is important for the team to know to help the client with this process? The multidisciplinary team at Holy Family has developed a bio-psycho-social assessment tool to guide their interventions with this population. This tool considers the developmental stage of the geriatric patient, the socio-economic status, the individual's uniqueness, the psycho-social situation, and the barriers the aged face in society. Using case studies the presenters will detail how a geriatric patients' adjustment to a disability affects their discharge into the community. The presenters will demonstrate the impact of the assessment tool on discharge outcomes.

Patients Tell Us Where To Go

Maureen Desborough (Providence Health Care, Holy Family site, Vancouver, British Columbia Canada

The presenter will outline an approach to patient goal setting which begins with the patient articulating her/his desired goals in his/her own words, without influence. These goals form the foundation of the interdisciplinary team's work with the patient. The team collaborates with the patient to develop short term, achievable goals while assisting the patient toward the gradual identification and acceptance of realistic long-term goals. Patients at Holy Family are active participants in the goal setting process. Their involvement helps the team identify patient priorities, focus resources on those priorities and design an appropriate care plan. At the conclusion of this presentation participants will be familiar with the goals setting process at Holy Family Hospital. Participants will be provided with a copy of the format used to develop patient goals.

Planning Education Programs for the Elderly

Sandra Whytock (Holy Family Hospital, Vancouver, Canada)

Education is a key component of rehabilitation for any age group. However, providing education for an elderly population in rehabilitation brings unique challenges that accompany aging. Memory loss, sensory impairment, fluctuating energy and concentration and highly individualized learning needs are just some of the effects of aging that impact learning. Delivery of educational programing is further challenged by the need to accommodate therapy and medical appointments, by changes in staff and by changes in patient participants due to open access. At Holy Family Hospital individual instruction is provided as needed to all patients and their families, and group educational programs are offered to the major client populations that we serve. The group educational programs are provided for clients with arthritis and for those who experience stroke or amputation. This presentation will focus on the use of principles of curriculum development to plan an educational program and to develop instructional approaches that respond to the unique challenges of aging in this population. Included will be: how to identify essential concepts, how to identify content areas, how to plan evaluation, how to develop a lesson plan, and lessons learned about implementation. Each of these steps will be illustrated by examples taken from planning, implementation and evaluation of the group education programs offered. At the conclusion of this presentation, participants should be able to use the principles described to plan an educational program for elderly clients and their families.

SESSION 544

Inequal mobility? The effect of residential area, age, socio-economical status and gender on the mobility of persons 65+.

Anu Siren (University of Helsinki, Helsinki, Finland) Liisa Hakamies-Blomqvist (1. University of Helsinki, Helsinki, Finland; 2. VTI, Linköping, Sweden)

PURPOSE: The purpose of the study was to examine how certain social background factors, such as place of residence, age, socio-economical status, and gender, affect the mobility of older citizens. METHOD: Data were collected by mail survey. The survey questionnaire was sent to a random sample of Finnish persons aged 65 and over (N=2500). The survey questionnaire consisted of questions about e.g. travel patterns, trip lengths, and experienced problems. A total of 1516 persons participated to survey and the overall response rate was 61%. RESULTS: The results showed that the place of residence, age, and gender were significant predictors on older persons' mobility. Rural residents, persons aged 75+, and women made fewer trips and they also experienced their mobility being limited. The socio-economical status was a predictor of travel frequency, but not a significant predictor of self-experienced mobility. The most often named factors restricting free mobility were poor health, lack of public transport, and high cost of private car driving. CONCLUSION: Certain sub-groups of older persons are more vulnerable to lack of adequate mobility. These groups also often experience their travel as being limited and would like to do more trips if traveling was easier. Thus, actions promoting independent mobility of older persons should be directed especially towards those sub-groups whom we now know to be in the poorest situation in terms of independent mobility.

LIVING ARRANGEMENTS AND LEVEL OF WORRY AMONG THE KOREAN ELDERLY

Jibum Kim [Center on Aging, The University of Chicago and NORC, Chicago, USA] Yun-Suk Lee [The University of Chicago, Chicago, USA] Eung-Ryul Kim [Korea University, Seoul, Korea]

Traditionally, Korean elderly have coresided with their children. From 1981 to 1996, the percent living alone increased from 4.3% to 13.7%. This change has not been accompanied by increased government’s support for formal care. The resulting lack of support may have caused those living independently of their children to worry more about health and finances. Thus, we examine the relationship between elderly living arrangements and multiple measures of worry. Using cross-sectional data from 1996 International Study on Living and Consciousness of Senior Citizens, we first describe living arrangements and their association with four measures of worry (health, being alone, finances, and children caring). Then, we adjust for age, sex, home ownership, number of children, and contact with children living separately. Most elderly have high levels of worry in all domains. Elderly living alone show the highest levels of worry, after adjusting social and demographic factors. Further there is no differential worry level among single with children, couple only, and couple with children households. The findings support that elderly living alone are not well adapted to the rapidly changed social conditions in Korea. Future studies on subjective well-being of Korean elderly should pay attention to worry and the function and meaning of living arrangements. Increased government attention and support for the elderly living alone is needed.

Living Arrangements of the Elderly in Ghana

Ishmael Okraku (Department of Sociology, Saint Mary's University, Halifax NS Canada)

Data on Ghanaian households were analysed to provide some indication of the living arrangements of the elderly and the potential for social support. The data for the study were collected by the World Bank and Ghana Statistical Services as part of the 1993 Ghana Living Standards Survey (GLSS). The survey used a national sample of 4552 households with 20,403 individual respondents, including 1229 aged 60+ (male 618, female 611). The results show that most elderly Ghanaians live in fairly large households surrounded by family members and other relatives. Most of the men were married (82%; 11% had two or more wives) and lived with spouse(s), children and/or grandchildren, and other relatives (62%); nine per cent lived with spouse only. About 11 0ved with children and grandchildren but no spouse, while 14 0ved alone. Whether living with or without spouse, elderly males usually were heads of their households (93%). For elderly females, only 21 0ved with a spouse. Most were widowed (56%) and tended to live in households with an adult child and grandchildren, often headed by the child (39%) or lived alone (18%). However, a sizable portion (15%) headed households with grandchildren only. The above patterns of living arrangements were evident in both urban and rural areas and would seem to suggest a fairly strong base for family support for most of Ghana's growing numbers of elderly people.

Mid-Life Patterns and the Residentail Mobility of Elderly Men

L. M. Hayward (Centre for Gerontological Studies, McMaster University, Hamilton, Canada)

There are numerous ways to better integrate the elderly into communities, many of which are contingent upon whether older people will remain in their pre-retirement homes or make a move. The objective of this paper is to establish that mid-life patterns can be related to residential mobility in later life. Using a life course theoretical perspective, it is argued that life course trajectories, in particular residential history, social and family relations, socio-economic status, and health, are associated with moves in later life, either directly or indirectly through their effect on earlier residential trajectories. These relationships are examined with multi-variate Cox proportional hazards and Poisson regression models, using data from a sample of 1063 men studied over a period of 30 years - the Ontario Longitudinal Study of Aging. The findings indicate that mid-life measures of these trajectories, specifically the number of mid-life moves, housing tenure, children, contact with family, continuity of social activity, overall social relations, occupation, retirement age, education, health rating, and years with declining health, are associated with the likelihood of moving in later life. Moreover, length of residence prior to mid-life, housing tenure, marital status change, period of empty nest, family contact, occupation and education, are associated with the number of moves made during mid-life, and hence are indirectly related to the likelihood of moving in later life. With the "baby boomers" just entering mid-life, these findings suggest a number of directions for future research with associated implications for the development of public policy for Canada's aging population.

Supplemental Transportation for Seniors

Helen K. Kerschner & Rhonda Aizenberg [Beverly Foundation, 44 So. Mentor Avenue, Pasadena, CA 91106 USA]

This paper presents results of two US initiatives. The first involves an opinion-gathering study on the transportation concerns and needs of seniors. The second, an outgrowth of the first, involves an effort to identify and promote community-based supplemental transportation programs for seniors. The opinion study used focus groups and written surveys to collect qualitative and quantitative data from seniors and lay caregivers. The follow-up project used an interactive inquiry to identify existing programs and a mail survey to collect detailed data on their structural and operational components. Over 370 programs were identified, and 236 returned completed surveys. Project staff and an expert panel reviewed responses and selected program "models of excellence." Profiles were developed for all programs, and case studies and program reviews were prepared for "models." Project materials were distributed to encourage adaptation and innovation. Results demonstrate the significance that supplemental transportation programs have for seniors. When seniors can no longer drive, they usually are too impaired to use traditional forms of public and paratransit. Often, supplemental transportation programs make the difference in whether a senior is isolated, continues to drive unsafely, or needs institutionalization. Results also show how organizational and administrative variables affect service delivery. However, in spite of significant differences in program characteristics, there is at least one thing in common: The belief that these programs are critical to the quality of life of seniors. Project conclusions highlight the increased significance these programs will have as the population ages. Guidelines for establishing programs will be presented.

SESSION 545

A RCT of low dose recombinant human growth hormone in the treatment of malnourished elderly medical patients

Leung-Wing Chu (Division of Geriatric Medicine, University Department of Medicine, Queen Mary Hospital, the University of Hong Kong, Hong Kong SAR), Karen SL Lam (Division of Endocrinology & Metabolism, University Department of Medicine, Queen Mary Hospital, the University of Hong Kong, Hong Kong SAR), Sidney CF Tam (Division of Clinical Biochemistry, Queen Mary Hospital, Hong Kong SAR), Wayne JHC Hu (Division of Geriatric Medicine, University Department of Medicine, Queen Mary Hospital, the University of Hong Kong, Hong Kong SAR), Sau-Lan Hui (Division of Geriatric Medicine, University Department of Medicine, Queen Mary Hospital, the University of Hong Kong, Hong Kong SAR), Anna Chiu (Department of Dietetics, Queen Mary Hospital, Hong Kong SAR), Ka-Chun Chiu(Division of Geriatric Medicine, University Department of Medicine, Queen Mary Hospital, the University of Hong Kong, Hong Kong SAR), Pauline Ng (Department of Dietetics, Queen Mary Hospital, Hong Kong SAR)

Background: High dose recombinant human growth hormone (rhGH) has been shown to improve the nutritional status of malnourished older adults. It is uncertain whether low dose rhGH is effective and whether its effect on nutritional status will lead to any improvement in physical function. There is also no data on the outcome after a short course of rhGH treatment. Objectives: To determine the efficacy of low dose rhGH treatment for 4 weeks in malnourished elderly patients, its effect on physical functions and the intermediate term outcome after a 4-week rhGH treatment. Design: Randomized, placebo-controlled, double-blind trial. Setting: An university teaching hospital. Patients: 19 medically stable malnourished elderly subjects Interventions: Low dose rhGH or placebo: in the rhGH group, rhGH (SaizenR) 0.09 iu per kg BW 3 times weekly were given together with appropriate dietary intervention as prescribed by the dietitian. In the placebo group, equal volumes of normal saline per kg. BW three times weekly were given together with the dietary intervention. Results: The baseline demographic, anthropometric, nutritional, hematological variables, measures of physical function and IGF-1 levels in both groups were comparable. Compared to the placebo group, the GH treated group showed a more rapid gain in body weight (after 3 weeks, +1.27 ¡Ó 0.36 vs. -0.28 ¡Ó 0.37 kg; p=0.008), total lean body mass (change after 3 weeks by bio-impedance analysis: +1.45¡Ó0.36 vs. -0.37 ¡Ó0.48 kg, p=0.009) and a faster improvement in 5-meter walking time (decrease after 4 weeks: 23.79¡Ó9.41 vs. 0.45¡Ó4.62 sec.; p=0.047). The haemoglobin level rose more in the rhGH than the placebo groups (change at 8 weeks: +0.84¡Ó0.34 vs. -0.42¡Ó0.29 g/dL; p=0.012). Serum albumin level also showed a greater delayed increase in the rhGH group than in the placebo group (change at 8 weeks: +5.1¡Ó0.8 vs. 1.6¡Ó1.2 g/dL; p=0.023). There was no statistically significant difference for other nutritional variables. There was a greater rise in the mean serum IGF-1 level at 4 weeks in the GH than in the placebo groups (47.2¡Ó14.0 vs. 13.0¡Ó6.3 ng/mL; p=0.034). The improvement in the rhGH group gradually diminished on follow up, and became statistically insignificant 8 weeks after stopping rhGH treatment. There were no GH-related adverse effects. Conclusions: Low dose rhGH was an effective and safe adjuvant to dietary augmentation for stable malnourished elderly subjects. It led to a faster gain in total lean body mass, which was associated with greater improvement in walking speed when compared with dietary intervention alone. There were no apparent side effects.

Carotenoids and vitamin A plasma levels in a geriatric ambulatory population

Y. M. Garcia (Disciplina de Geriatria Δ Medical School of São Paulo University, São Paulo, Brazil) M. J. Roncada (Department of Nutrition Δ Public Health School of São Paulo University, São Paulo, Brazil) D Wilson (Department of Nutrition Δ Public Health School of São Paulo University, São Paulo, Brazil) E. T. Carvalho Fo (Disciplina de Geriatria Δ Medical School of São Paulo University, São Paulo, Brazil)

PURPOSE: Determine in elders of an out-patient geriatric unit plasma levels of carotenoids and vitamin A, and compare them to the consumption of vitamin supplements. METHOD: elderly patients randomly taken had a blood sample collected for determining their carotenoids and vitamin A plasma levels by Neeld and Pearson method. They were also interviewed for investigating their vitamin supplements usage. They were divided according to gender, age (group1=60-79 years, group2=80 and more), and usage of supplements containing vitamin A. Plasma level considered critical for vitamin A is below 20mg/dL. RESULTS: 828 elderly persons (586 females) were evaluated. Their ages varied from 60 to 101, mean=74.2. Mean level of carotenoids was 152.1+79.2mg/dL, 162.3+80.9mg/dL for females and 134.0+71.6mg/dL for males (difference statistically significant by ANOVA, p=0.0000). Mean level of group1 was 159.9+83.3mg/dL, and of group2 was 133.2+59.9mg/dL (difference statistically significant, p=0.0000). Mean level of vitamin A was 39.4+17.5mg/dL, 38.2+12.0mg/dL for females and 42.2+26.2mg/dL for males (difference statistically significant, p=0.0027). Mean level of group1 was 39.9+18.6mg/dL, and of group2 was 37.6+12.4mg/dL (difference not significant). 3.4% of patients were below critical level. Users of vitamin A supplements had a mean plasma level of 42.8+13.8mg/dL, and non users of 39.1+12.7mg/dL (difference not statistically significant). CONCLUSIONS: most patients had normal levels of carotenoids and vitamin A; carotenoids levels were higher in females and younger patients; vitamin A levels were higher in males; vitamin A supplementation did not alter significantly plasma levels.

Effects of exercice and nutritional supplements on muscle mass and function in frail elderly

M.Bonnefoy (Gériatrie - Hôpital Lyon Sud - Hospices Civils de Lyon - France ; INSERM U449 ; Faculté de Médecine Lyon-Sud ; Centre de Recherche en Nutrition Humaine de Lyon) ; S.Normand and C.Pachiaudi (Centre de Recherche en Nutrition Humaine de Lyon) ; M.Laville (INSERM U449 ; Centre de Recherche en Nutrition Humaine de Lyon) ; C.Cornu (Service de Pharmacologie Clinique ; Lyon).

Purpose : Both physical inactivity and inadequate nutritional intake are main factors contributing to sarcopenia and reduction in muscle function in frail elderly. The potential reversibility of both sarcopenia and undernutrition is of utmost importance .Until now only few studies have examined the effects of dietary supplements combined with exercise training. Methods Aproximately 2000 residents of 16 homes for the elderly in the city of Lyon-France received an information during 16 introductory meetings. 57 subjects met the inclusion criteria and volunteered to participate .The study was a 9 months randomized controled trial with a factorial design comparing exercise training, nutritional supplementation, both interventions, and neither in 57 frail elderly. Primary outcomes measures were fat free mass (FFM) measured by labelled water and quadriceps muscle power measured by leg extensor machine. Results Mean age was 83 years. Muscle power increased in supplemented group(p=0.055) (+69.73%+/-27.72). 5 times chair rise improved in exercise group (p=0.014).There was a tendency toward an increase in FFM (p=0.09) in supplemented group ; the greatest improvement on body composition was observed with combined intervention (+2.46%+/-1.08) versus -1.48%+/-1.59 in exercise alone. BMI was increased in supplemented group (p=0.01). A tendency toward increase in resting metabolic rate (RMR) was observed in exercise group (p=0.08). Conclusion The nutritional supplement was effective on muscle function and nearly effective on body composition. Exercise improved function. The best results on FFM, BMI, RMR were observed in exercise plus supplement group.The interest of a combined intervention can be emphasized to counteract sarcopenia and muscle weakness in frail elderly.

Results of a one year nutritional supplementation and resistance training program in free living elders

Daniel Bunout (INTA and Faculty of Medicine, University of Chile, Santiago, Chile), Gladys Barrera (INTA, University of Chile, Santiago, Chile), Sandra Hirsch (INTA, University of Chile, Santiago, Chile), María Pía de la Maza (INTA, University of Chile, Santiago, Chile), Mercelo Avendaño (INTA, University of Chile, Santiago, Chile), Vivien Gattas (INTA, University of Chile, Santiago, Chile), Margarita Petermann (INTA, University of Chile, Santiago, Chile).

Purpose: To assess the effects of a one year nutritional supplementation and resistance training program on nutritional status and muscle strength in free living elders. Method: Healthy elders aged 70 years or more, participated in the study. Half were receiving a nutritional supplement given by the Chilean government that provided 400 Kcal, 15 g/protein and 50% of vitamin DRVs per day. Half of the subjects were randomly assigned to a resistance exercise training program. Every six months, a full assessment was performed. Results: One hundred forty nine subjects were considered eligible for the study, and 108 (31 supplemented and trained, 28 supplemented, 16 trained and 33 without supplementation nor training) completed the year of follow up. Overall compliance with the supplement was 48 ± 22 % and trained subjects assisted to 56 ± 21% of programmed sessions. By DEXA, no changes in lean body mass were observed, but fat mass increased from 22.2 ± 7.3 to 22.9 ± 7.21 kg in all groups. Bone mineral density and content remained constant in both supplemented groups and decreased significantly in the non supplemented groups (ANOVA $p < 0.01$). Serum cholesterol and triglycerides remained constant in both supplemented and in the trained groups, but increased significantly in non supplemented non trained individuals (ANOVA $p < 0.05$). Upper and lower limb strength and walking capacity increased significantly in trained subjects. Conclusion: Nutritional supplementation and resistance training avoided a derangement in bone mineral density and serum lipid levels and improved muscle strength.

Weight loss in dementia; can it be prevented?

Heather H. Keller (University of Guelph, Guelph, Ontario, Canada)

Weight loss is common in dementia. This quasi-experimental study compared the weight patterns over a nine-month period in an intervention facility and control facility (not randomly selected). Residents in special care units at the intervention site received clinical nutrition services at approximately 1 hour/resident/month. This individualized intervention included more frequent follow-up and responsive care to the changing needs of these dementia residents. The control site continued to receive minimal clinical nutrition services as mandated by the Ontario government. Although there were institutional differences, weight change during the nine months was significantly different by site and associated with the amount of time and number of visits provided by the dietitian. 56.8 0f the control group residents maintained their weight, although 36.40st on average 50f their baseline weight, and only 6.8 0ained weight. Two-thirds of the intervention residents maintained their weight, 27.3 0ained at least 50f their baseline weight during the nine-months, and only 6.10f these residents lost weight. Weight gainers, whether at the control or intervention site, received significantly more dietitian time and visits (mean 421 minutes and 8.6 visits vs. weight loss group mean of 74.3 minutes and 1.9 visits). Average weight change per month was - 0.46 +/- 0.91 kg for the control site and 0.32 +/- 0.05 kg for the intervention site ($p<0.01$). Individualized care from a clinical dietitian promotes weight maintenance or gain in dementia clients. Weight loss can be prevented in these residents of long term care facilities.

SESSION 546

The Journey to Excellence: Dementia Care Programs in Two Canadian Cities

Helen Lantz (The CAPITAL CARE Group, Edmonton, AB, CA, THE JOURNEY TO EXCELLENCE: DEMENTIA CARE PROGRAMS IN TWO CANADIAN CITIES) Connie F. Wark (The CAPITAL CARE Group, Edmonton, AB, CA, TWELVE HOUR DEMENTIA CARE EDUCATION PROGRAM: CONTENT AND EVALUATION) Marlene Foley (Carewest, Calgary, AB, CA, DEMENTIA CARE EDUCATION IN A CONTINUING CARE ORGANIZATION; FROM THE CLASSROOM TO THE BEDSIDE) Iris Neumann (The CAPITAL CARE Group, Edmonton, AB, CA, DEVELOPMENT AND IMPLEMENTATION OF A LEAST RESTRAINT POLICY) Connid F. Wark (The CAPITAL CARE Goup, Edmonton, AB, CA, MANAGIN CHANGE: IMPLEMENTATION AND EVALUATION OF A DAILY LIVING PROGRAM FOR RESIDENTS WITH DEMENTIA) Marlene Collins (Carewest, Calgary, AB, CA, COMPETENCY PROFILE FOR THE DEMENTIA CARE SUPPORT WORKER)

Moving from a medical model to a social model of care that focuses on the individual is a widely accepted goal for programs that provide care to residents with dementia. The CAPITAL CARE Group (TCCG) in Edmonton, and Carewest in Calgary, are both multi site, public sector organizations operating 1400 and 942 beds, respectively. Both provide continuing care, respite, outreach, and other innovative services. All long-term car2e centres operated by these organizations have a mandate to ensure that residents receive the highest possible quality of life during their stay. Leaders in both organizations needed innovative and evidence based care giving practices to move away from the medical model. The purpose of the symposium is to share the steps these two organizations have taken to move to a social model of care. A descriptive overview of the current status of dementia care in the organizations' long term care centres will be presented, followed by a review of two staff education programs. The Carewest staff competencies document will be shared as well as TCCG's restraint reduction program. Presentations will discuss the strengths and weakness of the educational methods, as well as, organizational strategies, change process steps, the dynamics of change management, managing teams, and confronting resistance to change. Both organizations have independently initiated a number of strategies for managing large-scale system changes in dementia care. Education programs for staff have been an essential organizational strategy, but unit-based assessments and mechanisms to address deficiencies have also been employed. In effecting change, the Calgary Regional Health Authority initiated a program called Dementia Care Network and developed staff competencies, which were considered vital to improved care for residents with dementia. Staff competencies are achieved through staff development and evaluation. The content of staff competencies will be reviewed and how these factors contribute to an improved care will be discussed. TCCG began to effect change through a Restraint Reduction Task Force that reviewed the current status of restraint use, wrote new policies, developed an education program, and then rolled out the education program to each of it’s centres. The outcomes of the Restraint Reduction program will be presented. The two organizations’ educational programs for staff on dementia care units will be reviewed and contrasted. Carewest’s educational program, entitled Supportive Pathways, provides 18 hours of staff training and focuses on building empathy for the resident, whereas TCCG educational program is 12 hours long and focuses on interactive learning of skills and knowledge. For TCCG, training has preceded the implementation of a Daily Living Program which is a unit based assessment and the subsequent action plan to deal with deficiencies that provides a method for on-going staff development. Although their routes are different, both organizations expect to have a similar outcome, that is, they will move away from a medical model to a social model of care which focuses on the individual resident.

Competency Profile For The Dementia Care Support Worker

Calgary Regional Health Authority, Dementia Care Network, Calgary, Alberta, Canada

The Competency Profile for the Dementia Care Support Worker was developed by the Calgary Regional Health Aughority Dementia Care Network. The Steering Committee formed a working group comprised of personal care workers, educators and managers working in the field of dementia care, teh Alzheimer Society and family representatives. The Competency Profile describes the knowledge and skills that are required by support workers to provide quality care to individuals and families experiencing dementia. The support worker may be employed in a variety of settings, including home, facility and community settings such as personal care homes or assisted living complexes. The Profile also addresses the attitudes of the worker that contribute to a therapeutic relationship with the client/family.

Dementia Care Education in a Continuing Care Organization: From The Classroom To The Bedside

M. Foley (Carewest, Calgary Regional Health Authority, Calgary, Alberta, Canada)

Carewest embarked on a process of reinvention in the early 1990's. The vision was to be the Provider of Choice, committed to value in Continuing Care. After extensive research and consultation with stakeholders, it was determined that customer service would be enhanced in a program-based model. A Dementia Care (Supportive Pathways) Program was developed, with education being a key component. This paper addresses the education program developed and how the transfer of learning is reinforced on a day-to-day basis on the units.

Development and Implementation of a Least Restraint Policy

Iris Neumann (The CAPITAL CARE Group, Edmonton, Alberta, Canada)

In the past, caregivers in continuing care have viewed restraints as a safety measure: a way to prevent residents from climbing out of bed or a wheelchair and sustaining a serious fall. Staff decided when a resident was at risk and when to use a restraint. Current research indicates that restraints may actually cause physical and emotional harm. With the knowledge of what best practice should be, The CAPITAL CARE Group began a review of the organization's restraint policy. The policy and procedure for restraint use was revised and included practice change. For this practice change ot be successful the organization formulated, implemented and evaluated an intervention and education strategy. The intent was to improve knowledge, attitudes and behaviors of staff, families and physicians in an effort to reduce restraint use. The education consists of a three hour workshop describing the history of restraint use, potential effects of restraints, alternatives to restraints, an assessment form as well as family education. Following the workshop, an implementation committee was formed to assist staff with the changes in practice. For a resident at risk, a decision must be reached about what is best for that person - application of a restraint or restraing free living. Both the benefits and risks are explained and all options explored with the resident, family, and interdisciplinary team in an effort to secure a balance of quality of life and safety.

MANAGING CHANGE: IMPLEMENTATION AND EVALUATION OF A DAILY LIVING PROGRAM FOR RESIDENTS WITH DEMENTIA

Connie F. Wark (The CAPITAL CARE Group, Edmonton, AB, Canada)

To improve the quality of life for residents on dementia care units, The CAPITAL CARE Group implemented a Daily Living Program (DLP), which involves a unit-based assessment and evaluation following a 12-hour staff education program. A multi-disciplinary team, and a family representative, assessed unit care practices (flexibility, dignity, individuality, choice) related to resident care, families, staff and environment. They developed an action plan noting areas of success and concern. The DLP evaluation assesses improvement in residents' Quality of Life by measuring staff behavior, knowledge of residents, and changes in envrionment. The tools include Self-Monitorting and Therapeutic Environment Screening Scale (TESS-2+). The evaluation appears to be a sound method for promoting continual self-monitoring and improvement.

Twelve Hour Dementia Care Education Program: Content And Evaluation

Connie F. Wark (The CAPITAL CARE Group, Edmonton, AB, Canada)

This presentation will review the implementation and evaluation of a multi-disciplinary dementia care education program for continuing care staff that instills individualized, client-centred care, focusing on transfer of learning and content. Preparatory reading introduces 12 hours of training for long-term care staff. During each 3-hour session staff participate in group activites and commit to making a change the next day at work. Training is evaluated using a pre and post questionnaire. Tools taught for managing change include: Self-monitoring Checklists (modified from Burgio, n.d.), ABC (problem solving) meetings, Visual Care Plans, and the Personal Care Book (Alzheimer Society of Canada). A consistent educator supported by Unit Managers at each session implements the program. Evaluation results are communicated directly to the centre involved. Staff need to be involved in their learning and encouraged to make changes as soon as possible.

SESSION 547

Telehomecare: The Intelligent Future of Long Term Care

C. Miller & V. Riley (Honeywell Laboratorys, Minneapolis, USA) Independent LifeStyle Assistant. M. Groves (Gerontology Research Centre, Simon Fraser University, Vancouver, Canada) Action Sequencing: The Intelligent Home as an Assistive Device. S. Kose (Housing, Urban Planning & Building Design Research Group, Building Research Institute, Tatehara, Tsukuba, Japan) Housing Performance for Long Term Care. S Robinovitch (Kinesiology, Faculty of Applied Science, Simon Fraser University,

Vancouver, Canada) The relations between risk for falls in the elderly and characteristics of the home environment. J. Barlow (SPRU - Science and Technology Policy Research, University of Sussex, Brighton, UK) Smart Housing Technologies and the Delivery of Care and Support Services to People at Home.

Technology has expanded the capability for patient care beyond direct person-to-person contact within traditional organisational confines of space and time. E-health initiatives have improved access to specialized knowledge, skills and information, reduced hospital admissions, advanced hospital discharges, and enhanced service delivery in urban, rural and remote communities. Increasingly, the home has become central to care, health care professionals are working as consultants, patients are becoming more self-sufficient and there is greater reliance on community-based staff and volunteers. This symposium looks at the role of smart housing in long-term care and includes presentations on smart housing to support independence; the potential of smart housing as an assistive device for persons with cognitive impairment; the longevity of dwellings and legislative initiatives to improve housing performance in Japan; the risk of falls for home based care; and pilot projects in healthcare technologies that have demonstrated the potential of information and communication technology for home based care. This symposium will provide an introduction to the intelligent future of long term care.

Independent LifeStyle Assistant

C. Miller & V. Riley (Honeywell Laboratorys, Minneapolis, USA)

The goal of the Independent Lifestyle Assistant research program is to develop an intelligent home automation system with situation awareness and decision-making capabilities that can be easily integrated with a diverse set of sensors, medical devices and "smart" appliances to enable elderly and infirm users to live and function safely at home.

Action Sequencing: The Intelligent Home as an Assistive Device

M. Groves (Gerontology Research Centre, Simon Fraser University, Vancouver, Canada)

Impaired memory (e.g, procedural, visual recognition, spatial, verbal) limits performance on individual actions or series of actions for which physical capacities and/or suitable non-personal assistance exists (e.g, assistive devices, technical aids, adaptations, prostheses, wheelchair, cane and other material help). Performance of goal directed activities of daily living can be enhanced by segmented the activities into a series of actions with the intelligent home cueing the action sequences, enabling persons with impaired memory to complete activities. Through Action Sequencing, the intelligent home becomes an assistive device that replaces the supervision and/or cueing components of personal assistance provided by caregivers, enables persons' with cognitive impairment to live independent lives in their own homes for longer, makes the residence a safer place to live, and reduces expenditures associated with the home care.

Housing Performance for Long-Term-Care

S. Kose (Building Research Institute, Tatehara, Tsukuba, Japan)

Telehomecare cannot occur without dwellings that have been designed to support the longevity of inhabitants. Like most countries, Japan has a Building Standard Law that sets minimum requirements with which any building must comply. However, the requirements are for safety and sanitation, and do not address people's needs regarding usability, comfort and longevity. To respond to the issue, the government introduced legislation (Autumn 2000) that will assist in improving the quality of Japanese dwellings through performance indicators. The "Housing Quality Assurance Law" relates to basic building design, excluding most of the building hardware and appliances. The performance indicators allow building quality standards to be set, this way dwellings are somewhat treated like products in terms of encouraging quality assurance. This paper reports the recent introduction of housing performance indicators, with particular emphasis on housing performance for aging.

The relations between risk for falls in the elderly and characteristics of the home environment

S Robinovitch (Kinesiology, Faculty of Applied Science, Simon Fraser University, Vancouver, Canada)

Falls are the number one cause of unintentional injury in the elderly, and it is commonly believed that elimination of environmental hazards can reduce falls. However, several studies have shown that there is little or no association between risk for falls in the elderly and the presence of environmental hazards, or attempts to eliminate environmental hazards. There are several possible reasons for this, related either to study design or the multi-factorial nature of falls. This paper provides a critical overview of the relations between risk for falls in the elderly and characteristics of the home environment, including evidence for the benefit of specific environmental modifications and the value of home monitoring or "fall alert" devices.

Smart Housing and the Delivery of Care and Support Services to People

J. Barlow (SPRU - Science and Technology Policy Research, University of Sussex, Brighton, UK)

The introduction of telecare on a mass basis will be critical if governments are to cope with the demands of a growing elderly population on the care services over the next 2-3 decades. While the technologies for delivering health and social care to individuals whenever and wherever they need them are developing rapidly, less attention is being paid to fundamental question of who will pay for them and what impact they will have on existing health and social care systems. In the UK, government and major players in the ICT industries are beginning to consider how care will be provided in the future and what role telecare will play. The Telecare Planning and Implementation (TCPI) project is addressing this question. The project is exploring the business and care models by which telecare can be delivered to individuals within their homes, and elsewhere. The TCPI vision involves bundling services to the home, including a range of care services customised according to individual needs. The project is (1) developing four telecare scenarios for 2020, (2) trialling various telecare models in individual homes and (3) developing a simulation model to evaluate the effects of different approaches to telecare.

SESSION 548

Aged Interest Groups in Developed and Rapidly Developing Countries

Elizabeth Ozanne (The University of Melbourne, Victoria, Australia) A Sociopolitical Analysis of the Australian Council on the Ageing AssociateJean-Philippe Viriot Durandal (Franche Comte University, IUT Belford, France) Senior Lobbies in France: Two Directions for an Institutional IntegrationNana Apt (The University of Ghana, Legon, Ghana) The Role of Organized Aged Interest Groups in Situations of Rapid Development AssociatePing-kwong Kam, (City University of Hong Kong, Hong Kong) A Political Economy Analysis of the Role of Older Person's Interest Groups in Hong Kong

ISSUE: The shifting roles and organization of aged interest groups in developed and developing countries have been the subject of recent research and interest in both the U.S. and Europe and in rapidly changing regions like Ghana in Africa and Hong Kong in China. While some researchers have questioned the impact of age-based interest groups on the policy making process, others see renewed activity in both defense of existing aged based policies and utilization of both more participatory strategies as well as more sophisticated technologies of mass marketing to engage an ever broadening aged constituency. STRUCTURE: This symposium will seek to explore both the phenomena of aged interest group organization in the five different countries/regions of France, Australia, United States, Ghana and Hong Kong, as well as examine the variety of strategies being utilized by groups in these countries to impact on the policy making process. CONTENT: The key peak body representing aged interest groups in Australia is the Council of the Ageing, originally formed in the 1950's by the National Council of Women and Rotary and built on the model of the Old Peoples Welfare Council in Britain. Along with other modern-day peak councils however, both the structure and strategies adopted by COTA to impact the policy making process have shifted radically over time as the contingencies in the environment have changed. This paper will explore the development of the organization over three time periods from the early 50's, through the 70's & 80's to the late 90's using a political economy and resource mobilization framework. With budgetary restrictions on public expenditure on the aged in France in the 90's, a new coalition of independent senior lobbies has been observed to emerge in opposition to both state agencies and traditional political parties and trade union intermediaries. Frustrated by existing insider players, these new groups have adopted both radical strategies outside the existing institutional structure to get their point across, as well as seeking to increase their technical expertise to directly impact the policy making process. The success of these various strategies are explored. In Ghana, the role of organized aged interest groups has been strategic in a situation of rapid development. This paper will explore the nature of emergent groups in urban and rural townships and their role in the AIDS crisis and the social development of the country. The limited power of older people's pressure groups in Hong Kong is explored by the fourth paper which examines the way in which the broader political context and the constrained socioeconomic circumstances of the majority of older people compounds their powerlessness. The roles and impact of three key organized interest groups are examined. The final paper explores the response of aged advocacy groups in the U.S. to the changed political environment that has emerged in the 90's by utilizing interviews with interest group leaders and congressional staff members to examine emergent patterns of organizational maintenance, contemporary political strategies, and new patterns of coalition and competition. CONCLUSIONS/OUTCOMES: The above papers explore continuity and diversity in aged interest group politics in both developed and rapidly developing countries. The picture is one of dynamic and continuing change in relation to shifting local circumstance and history and provides a rich comparative tapestry against which to reflect on the individual national pictures.

A Sociopolitical analysis of the Australian Council on the Ageing

Elizabeth Ozanne, Brenda Keogh (The University of Melbourne, Victoria, Australia)

PURPOSE: Council on the Ageing Australia was formed in the early 1950's as a joint initiative of the National Council of Older Women and Rotary building on the model of the U.K. National Old Peoples Welfare Council. It is the key aged peak council recognized by government and has continually evolved in its structures and strategies with changing social and political circumstances. The paper examines the evolution of the organization over three major time periods from the early 50's through the 70's and 80's, into the contemporary period, utilizing a political economy and resource mobilization framework. METHOD: Analysis of archival data, interviews with key stakeholders and review of the Australian and international literature on aged interest groups was undertaken as part of this Australian Research Council funded study which constitutes one of a number of sociopolitical histories of key Australian aged interest groups. RESULTS: This study is a work in progress but the preliminary results of the evolving organizational form and strategies of COTA over three distinctive time periods will be presented. CONCLUSION: There has been only limited exploration of the range, nature and impact of aged interest groups in Australia and few historical or sociopolitical histories have been completed on the more significant players. This grounded historical analysis of COTA is the first in a series of individual organizational studies aimed to provide a broader picture of aged interest group politics in Australia.

Political Economy Analysis of the Role of Older Persons Interest Groups in Hong Kong

AssociatePing-kwong Kam, (City University of Hong Kong, Hong Kong)

This paper explores the relatively limited power of older persons in Hong Kong, determined both by the constrained social and economic circumstances of the majority of older people, the residual nature of old age policy and the few organized interest groups. Though there are three relatively large older persons pressure groups or coalitions in Hong Kong their representation is narrow and influence limited. The first one is the Association of Rights of the Elderly which is regarded as a professional advocacy group, rather than a pressure group with full participation from older people. The second is the League for the Rights of the Elderly which, because of its radical image and the adoption of more militant strategies, has difficulty in involving a broad constituency and is therefore marginalized to represent a small disadvantaged sector of older persons. The third group, the Coalition of Senior Citizens serves primarily as a co-ordinating body for several older peoples user groups and is not involved in progressive or radical action. The lack of a territory wide age concern group in Hong Kong is seen as a major handicap in profiling the interests of older persons with key decision makers.

Senior Lobbies in France: Two Directions for an Institutional Integration

Jean-Philippe VIRIOT DURANDAL (Franche Comte University, IUT Belfort France),

In France, like in most western European countries, public policy shifted >from a large and generous coverage of social risks to budget restrictions >in the beginning of the 90's. Within this context, a coalition of >'independent' senior lobbies emerged in France opposed to the public >decision makers (government, SSA) as well as to the traditional political >and social intermediaries (such as political parties, or trade >unions). They were primarily motivated by the desire to maintain pension >levels and to keep the purchasing power of senior citizens. These >organizations tried to gain institutional integration within decision >making bodies in the field of aging. The responses of the 'insiders' of >the institutional game did not meet their expectations. The limited range >of political opportunity paper deals with the main two responses of >seniors organizations in France to the question How can senior citizen >groups find a place in the public arena? The strategy of integration >followed by the main 3 'independent' French senior citizen groups was >twofold (both of them based on resource mobilization and competition or >opposition to the traditional players (state and trade unions): 1. They >switched from a passive mode (memo, consultation,...) to a more radical >mode, in which the strategies of resources mobilization and collective >actions are designed to apply sanctions or strong pressure on public >decision-makers (demonstrations in the street, law suites, appeals to >political sanctions against candidates,...) This repertoire takes place >outside of institutional confines (streets, courts, media,....). 2. At the >same time the senior groups converted the expertise of their 'young >retirees' to gain more weight in the public arena. The emergence of this >new social movement in the 90's mainly composed of former executives gave >senior groups considerable resources to develop technical knowledge and to >promote a real pool of expertise on public policy on aging. It is argued >in this paper that this second aspect of the strategy of resource >mobilization, can be considered as an instance of both radicality and >legitimacy within the public decision process. >

The Role of Organized Aged Interest Groups in Situations of

Rapid Development

N. Apt (The University of Ghana, Legon, Ghana)

This paper explores the role of organized older persons (largely women's) organizations in social development in Ghana in both urban and rural settings. The origins and development of two major urban organizations are examined and the pattern of older person's associations in rural townships explored. The contribution of older persons to the national fight against aids is also examined. The paper is based on a series of studies conducted out of the University of Ghana Centre of Social Policy Studies looking at self help and social support provided by and for older persons in urban and rural townships.

SESSION 549

Ethical Implications of Models of Mediation for the Vulnerable Old and Their Adult Children

Brian W. W. Aitken (Huntington College, Laurentian University, Sudbury, Ontario, Canada, P3E 2C6 Ethics and Mediation in a Post Modern World) John Della Bosca (Huntington College, Laurentian University, Sudbury, Ontario, Canada, P3E 2C6 A National Report: Mediation with Frail Seniors) Peggy English (Vancouver Based Family Mediations, A Family Mediation Checklist for the Elderly" Douglas Joblin, Laurentian University, Gerontology Department, The Problem of Mediation with Older Men)

This round table will attempt to demonstrate the lack of a fitting model of mediation for dealing with various conflicts that emerge between the frail elderly and their adult children. Current models of family mediation tend to be judgemental or paternalistic and do not explicitly recognize the vulnerability of the frail elderly nor do they protect their autonomy and dignity. This presentation will first present the findings of a national survey sponsored by Family Mediation Canada of patterns in mediation between the frail elderly and their adult children. Next an outline of the evolution of family mediation through three distinct models will be given; these models reflect ethical values and conventions of communication implicit in what historical/cultural analysis has termed the pre-modern/ modern and postmodern age. Case studies will be used to illicit from the attendees a discussion of the ethical appropriateness of each model of mediation for seniors in a postmodern age. Thirdly, an attempt will be made to build a model of mediation for a postmodern age based on the ethical insights of feministic ethics which emphasize connectedness rather then rightness, the contractual thought of John Rawls which sees fairness as creating a level playing field in all relationships and the Aristotilean notion that friendship is the end of all relating so it is the process that counts in mediation not a predetermined, desirable outcome. Finally, some insights from the field of gerontology will be presented which give a holistic understanding of the vulnerability many frail seniors experience as well as supporting the contention that on-going significant relationship with younger family members is critical for happiness and quality of life in later life. The presentations, therefore, will be fourfold: 1) "A National Report: Mediation with Frail Seniors" (Della Bosca) 2) '"The Evolution of Family Mediation in Canada: A Stage Approach."(Della Bosca) 3) "Ethics and Family Mediation in a Post Modern World." (Aitken) 4) "Gerontological Reflections on the Vulnerability of Frail Seniors and Their Need for Relationship." (Aitken) Anticipated Outcomes or Conclusions might be as follows: (1) The field of family mediation is unprepared for the onset of family crises between the frail elderly and their adult children, (2) practitioners in the field of family mediation have no background in gerontology, and (3) their is widespread acceptance among practioners in the field of family mediation for a new a model of mediation based ethical values that strength the inclusivesness of seniors in the lives of their families.

A Checklist for Family Mediation with Seniors

Brian WW Aitken (Huntington College),Douglas Joblin (Huntington College), Peggy English, John Della Bosca

This presentation will outline the Family Mediation Canada Checklist for family mediation skills. Although this tool is used primarily for divorce and family breakdown mediation, the presentation will show how it might be utilized by mediators dealing with the frail elderly and their adult children in conflictual situations such as institutionalization, naming power of attorney, control of finances, making wills, etc.

A National Report: Mediation with Frail Seniors

Brian WW Aitken (Huntington College),Douglas Joblin (Huntington College), Peggy English, John Della Bosca

The findings of a national survey sponsored by Family Mediation Canada will be outlined. The questionnaire attempted to find any patterns in mediation between the frail elderly and their adult children when a crisis occurs. The findings show that there is no model for mediating this sort of conflict, that mediation trainers do not have any background in gerontology and that there is a universal interest in applying relevant gerontological knowledge to this sort of mediation.

Ethics and Mediation in a Post Modern World

Brian WW Aitken (Huntington College),Douglas Joblin (Huntington College), Peggy English, John Della Bosca

This presentation starts with the premise that current models of family mediation tend to be judgemental and paternalistic and do not explicitly recognize the vulnerability of the frail elderly nor do they protect their autonomy and dignity. An attempt will be made to construct a model of mediation for a post-modern age based on the ethical insights of feminist ethics which emphasize connectedness rather than rightness, the contractual thought of John Rawls which sees fairness as creating a level playing field in relationships and then on the Aristotilean notion that friendship is the end of all relating,so it is a process that counts in mediation not a predetermined, desirable outcome.

The Problem of Mediation with Older Men

Brian WW Aitken (Huntington College),Douglas Joblin (Huntington College), Peggy English, John Della Bosca

All acts of successful mediation require excellent interpersonal skills. Men, particularly senior men, have not been nurtured well in these ways. The negative and tyrannical characteristic of men's four archetypes, which have shaped and directed men through the last four thousand years of patriarchalism, have blocked such development. They have nurtured more violent than peaceful warriors, more possessive than nurturing lovers, more rigid than compassionate kings, and more seductive than healing magicians. This presentation will examine these archetypal patterns so as to help mediators and men themselves better understand the reasons for their weal interpersonal communications skills, especially when dealing with conflict. It will also examine ways in which the positive characteristics of these four male archetypes might help mediators and men embrace a new post-patriarchal and dialogical mediating power in their own lives, in the lives of others around them and in the systems that contain them.

INDEX

Gerontology 2001; 47(suppl 1):1-718